CLARKE'S
ISOLATION AND IDENTIFICATION
OF DRUGS

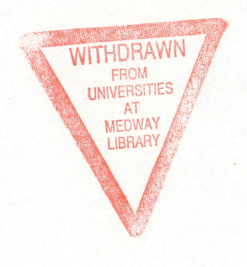

CLARKE'S
ISOLATION AND
IDENTIFICATION
OF DRUGS

in pharmaceuticals, body fluids, and
post-mortem material

Second Edition

Senior Consulting Editor
A. C. Moffat

Consulting Editors
J. V. Jackson   M. S. Moss   B. Widdop

Assisted by E. S. Greenfield

Prepared in the Department of Pharmaceutical Sciences of
The Pharmaceutical Society of Great Britain

London
THE PHARMACEUTICAL PRESS
1986

Copies of this book may be obtained through any good bookseller or, in any case of difficulty, direct from the publisher or the publisher's agents:

The Pharmaceutical Press
(publications division of The Pharmaceutical Society of Great Britain)
1 Lambeth High Street, London SE1 7JN, England

Australia
The Australian Pharmaceutical Publishing Co. Ltd
35 Walsh Street, West Melbourne 3003

Canada
McAinsh & Co. Ltd
2760 Old Leslie Street, Willowdale, Ontario M2K 2X5

Japan
Maruzen Co. Ltd
3–10 Nihonbashi 2-chome, Chuo-ku, Tokyo 103

New Zealand
The Pharmaceutical Society of New Zealand
124 Dixon Street, PO Box 11–640, Wellington

U.S.A.
Rittenhouse Book Distributors, Inc.,
511 Feheley Drive, King of Prussia, Pennsylvania 19406

Senior Consulting Editor

A. C. Moffat, BPharm, PhD, DSc, FPS, CChem, FRSC
Assistant Director, Home Office Forensic Science Laboratory, Huntingdon, Cambridgeshire, England, formerly Head of Drugs and Toxicology Division, Central Research Establishment, Home Office Forensic Science Service, Aldermaston, Berkshire

Consulting Editors

J. V. Jackson
Late of the Metropolitan Police Forensic Science Laboratory, London

M. S. Moss, MSc, PhD, MIBiol, CChem, FRSC
Director, Racecourse Security Services Laboratory, Newmarket, Suffolk

B. Widdop, PhD
Consultant Biochemist, Poisons Unit, Guy's Hospital, London

THE PHARMACEUTICAL SOCIETY OF GREAT BRITAIN

Department of Pharmaceutical Sciences

Director: W. G. Thomas

General Editor: A. Wade

Clarke's Isolation and Identification of Drugs

Editorial Staff

E. S. Greenfield

Janet Batson
Christine Maule
D. K. Mehta
P. Gotecha

Contents

*Deceased June 1984

†Deceased December 1982

Preface

Isolation and Identification of Drugs was first published in 1969 from an idea developed by Professor E. G. C. Clarke, who edited that first edition. Regrettably, Professor Clarke did not live to see the inception of a new edition. It seemed fitting, therefore, to call this new edition *Clarke's Isolation and Identification of Drugs*, especially as the book is affectionately known as 'Clarke'.

The first edition became a standard reference text for those concerned with the identification of drugs, gaining its reputation by providing a dependable source of analytical data for drugs and allied substances. The dog-eared, stained copies on laboratory benches are a testament to its usefulness.

Accidental or suicidal poisoning, the abuse of narcotics and other drugs, the dangerous habit of glue-sniffing, and drug abuse in sport have increased enormously during recent years. The information in this book has been planned to provide the means for detecting, identifying, and quantifying most drugs and other toxic substances which are likely to be encountered in these situations, and to assist in interpreting the analytical results.

The book was planned for use not only in hospital and toxicological laboratories, but also in numerous other analytical establishments—including hospital and industrial quality control laboratories, and clinical laboratories engaged in drug investigations for purposes such as therapeutic drug monitoring or research into pharmacokinetics and patterns of drug metabolism. Also, there is much information which will be of use in certain areas of environmental toxicology, particularly the analysis of toxic metals and pesticides. Finally, the needs of students who are studying drug analysis and its applications have been kept in mind during the writing of the book.

There have been many developments in analytical techniques since the first edition was published, and this has necessitated rewriting the whole of the text and the inclusion of new data throughout. Nevertheless, the style and presentation used in the first edition have been retained.

The amount of text in the book has been increased by about 60% which has been made possible by increasing the page size and using a double column format throughout. Whenever possible, the data have been verified from at least one independent source.

The book is divided into four parts.

Part 1: Analytical Techniques

This part contains 18 chapters on analytical techniques and allied subjects. New chapters in this edition include descriptions of hospital toxicology and drug abuse screening, forensic toxicology, drug abuse in sport, therapeutic drug monitoring, the analysis of metals and anions, and the analysis of pesticides, together with information on sampling procedures and on the use of quality control in clinical analysis.

The information on analytical techniques has been extended and brought up to date, particularly with the inclusion of high pressure liquid chromatography, fluorescence spectrophotometry, and nuclear magnetic resonance spectroscopy. Each chapter provides a description of the technique, practical hints on its use, and information on the application of the technique to problems.

The chromatographic systems have been completely revised and made more comprehensive and systematic. The general screening system using thin-layer chromatography has been extended and, for the first time, general screening systems employing gas chromatography and high pressure liquid chromatography are described.

The information on colour tests has been completely revised and extended. The older methods of paper chromatography and microcrystalline tests have been omitted from this edition.

A final chapter brings together the knowledge of pharmacokinetics and drug metabolism which is needed for the interpretation of the qualitative and quantitative results obtained from the analyses.

Part 2: Analytical and Toxicological Data

This part contains monographs for over 1300 drugs and related substances. About 160 substances which were included in the first edition, but which are now of little interest, have been deleted (see p. xvii). However, about 300 substances not described previously have been added.

A new feature of this edition is the inclusion of ultraviolet spectra. These, together with infra-red spectra, now appear within the monographs for ease of reference.

The ultraviolet and infra-red data have been completely revised, as have the chromatographic data which now include high pressure liquid chromatography. Analytical information on many major metabolites is presented for the first time, and many monographs include the eight major mass spectral peaks for the substance and its major metabolites.

References to published methods for quantifying drugs in various biological fluids are given in the monographs, where available.

Many of the drug monographs contain a new section entitled 'Disposition in the Body'. This section details the absorption, distribution, and excretion of the drug, notes the major metabolites and therapeutic and toxic plasma concentrations, and gives values for pharmacokinetic parameters such as half-life, volume of distribution, clearance, and protein binding. In addition, abstracts from published clinical studies and case histories are included.

The presentation of literature references has been changed in this edition so that they now appear within the text rather than being collected together in an appendix.

Part 3: Indexes to Analytical Data

This part contains 64 indexes of analytical data, tabulated in numerical order, and includes all the data for chromatography, spectrophotometry, and mass spectrometry, together with indexes of molecular weight and melting point.

Part 4: Appendix of Reagents and Proprietary Test Materials

This part contains descriptions of reagents referred to in analytical procedures in Parts 1 and 2.

It has taken nearly 6 years to produce this second edition and during the whole of that time it has been very much a team effort with many collaborators. In particular, I give my warmest thanks to Eric Greenfield and Janet Batson who throughout the whole period have worked unstintingly to bring the book to fruition. Although the work was detailed and exacting, they always managed to keep both their patience and their sense of humour. They have been ably assisted in the later stages by Christine Maule, Rosalind McLarney, Dinesh Mehta, and Prakash Gotecha at the Department of Pharmaceutical Sciences of The Pharmaceutical Society of Great Britain, and I thank them all for their stalwart work.

Three consulting editors have also made invaluable contributions to the book and I am greatly indebted to John Jackson, Michael Moss, and Brian Widdop who not only provided advice, enthusiasm, and data, but also contributed chapters on their own specialist subjects.

Thanks are due in particular to the Central Research Establishment, Home Office Forensic Science Service, Aldermaston, for permission to use their analytical data and spectra, and to Mrs Myra Clarke FRCVS, for permission to use the name 'Clarke' in the new title of the book.

My former colleagues Howard Stead, Richard Gill, and Robert Ardrey at the Central Research Establishment, Home Office Forensic Science Service, have similarly given their time and enthusiasm and I owe a special debt of thanks to them for providing so much of the information included in the monographs as well as for their own chapters.

I also gratefully acknowledge the co-operation of the other authors of chapters in providing up-to-date accounts of their respective topics. There has also been a whole host of friends and colleagues who have helped one way or another to put this book together. Many who gave specific assistance are acknowledged on p. xviii, but I take this opportunity to give my most grateful thanks to all those who have helped in the production of the book.

I must also record here the deaths of John Jackson and Donald Chapman during the preparation of this second edition. Their contribution will be used by others for years to come, and I deeply regret that John and Donald will not see the success of their work.

A. C. Moffat

July 1985

General Notices

The following explanatory notes are provided so that the reader can interpret and use the information given in the book. They should be studied before using the data given in the monographs in Part 2.

Health and Safety

This work is intended to be used by appropriately qualified and experienced scientists. Processes and tests described should be performed in suitable premises by personnel with adequate training and equipment. Care should be taken to ensure the safe handling of all chemical or biological materials, and particular attention should be given to the possible occurrence of allergy, infection, fire, explosion, or poisoning (including inhalation of toxic vapours). Cautionary notes have been included in a number of monograph entries, but the possibility of danger should always be kept in mind when handling biological samples, and medicinal or other chemical substances.

Classification

At the head of each monograph an indication is given of the classification of the compound according to its therapeutic or commercial use or its pharmacological action. The substance may, of course, have other uses or actions in addition to that stated.

Nomenclature

MONOGRAPH TITLES. The main titles of the monographs in Part 2 are usually British Approved Names, United States Adopted Names, or International Non-Proprietary Names, where these exist. For pesticides the nomenclature generally follows the British Approved Names, the British Standard Recommended Common Names, or the names issued by the International Organisation for Standardisation (ISO). In some approved names it is now general policy to use 'f' for 'ph' in sulpha, 't' for 'th', and 'i' for 'y'; for this reason entries in alphabetical lists and indexes should be sought in alternative spellings if the expected spellings are not found.

The main title of a monograph is generally that of the free acid or base as this is the form in which the compound will usually be isolated in an analysis; details of the commonly available salts are included in subsidiary paragraphs within the monograph.

The following abbreviated names for radicals and groups are used in the titles.

Recommended name	Chemical name
acetonide	isopropylidene ether of a dihydric alcohol
aceturate	N-acetylglycinate
besylate	benzenesulphonate
camsylate	camphor-10-sulphonate
caproate	hexanoate
closylate	4-chlorobenzenesulphonate
cypionate	3-cyclopentylpropionate
edetate	ethylenediamine-NNN'N'-tetra-acetate
edisylate	ethane-1,2-disulphonate
eglumine	N-ethylglucamine
embonate	4,4'-methylenebis (3-hydroxy-2-naphthoate) (=pamoate)
enanthate	heptanoate
estolate	propionate dodecyl sulphate
esylate	ethanesulphonate
gluceptate	glucoheptonate
hybenzate	2-(4-hydroxybenzoyl)benzoate
isethionate	2-hydroxyethanesulphonate
lauryl sulphate	dodecyl sulphate
meglumine	N-methylglucamine
mesylate	methanesulphonate
napadisylate	naphthalene-1,5-disulphonate
napsylate	naphthalene-2-sulphonate
pivalate	trimethylacetate
steaglate	stearoyloxyacetate
tebutate	tert-butylacetate
theoclate	8-chlorotheophyllinate
tosylate	toluene-4-sulphonate

CHEMICAL NAMES. The nomenclature generally follows the definitive rules issued by IUPAC, 1979.

PROPRIETARY NAMES AND SYNONYMS. A selection of proprietary names have been included in the monographs in Part 2. In general, they apply to the United Kingdom, United States of America, Canada, and certain European countries. Comprehensive lists of proprietary names, world-wide, can be found in *Martindale, The Extra Pharmacopoeia*, 28th Edn, London, The Pharmaceutical Press, 1982. Only single-substance preparations have been included except in the case of certain major classes of drugs for which the names of some compound preparations have been added. Some proprietary names which are not in current use have been retained.

Names under the heading 'Synonyms' include alternative names, common titles, and abbreviations.

CAS REGISTRY NUMBERS. Chemical Abstracts

Service (CAS) registry numbers are provided, where available, in the monographs to assist readers to refer to other information systems.

Molecular Weights

Molecular weights have been calculated using the table of Atomic Weights as revised in 1977 by the Commission on Atomic Weights, XXIX IUPAC General Assembly, and based on the ^{12}C scale. Molecular weights have been corrected to four significant figures and are listed in ascending order in the index of Molecular Weights (p. 1073).

Physical Characteristics

DISSOCIATION CONSTANTS. Numerous methods can be used for the determination of dissociation constants, and there are often differences in the various values reported in the scientific literature. The pK_a values given in the monographs have been taken from published data and should be regarded only as approximate. The temperature at which the determination was made is given where known.

Information on the theory, measurement, and evaluation of dissociation constants is given in *The Pharmaceutical Codex*, 11th Edn, London, The Pharmaceutical Press, 1979.

MELTING POINTS. The melting points recorded in the individual monographs in Part 2 are listed in ascending order in the index of Melting Points (p. 1085).

PARTITION COEFFICIENTS. Values for log P are given in a number of monographs. Where the pH of the aqueous phase is stated, the values given are apparent coefficients at that pH (not ion-corrected). Where no pH is stated for the aqueous phase, it can be assumed that log P is for the neutral form of the substance even though it is potentially ionisable.

The values given are approximate only but they serve to indicate the characteristics of the substance when it is submitted to an extraction process.

For a comprehensive collection of partition coefficients for drugs see C. Hansch and A. J. Leo, *Substituent Constants for Correlation Analysis in Chemistry and Biology*, Chichester, John Wiley, 1979. Information on the theory, determination, and use of partition coefficients is given in *The Pharmaceutical Codex*, 11th Edn, London, The Pharmaceutical Press, 1979.

SOLUBILITY. The solubilities given in the monographs in Part 2, unless otherwise stated, apply at ordinary room temperature. They have been obtained from various sources and should not be regarded as precise because of variations depending on the method and conditions of determination. In general, approximate values are given when a substance is soluble in less than 1000 parts of solvent. Where no figure is given, the usual solubility terms have been adopted:

very soluble	1 in less than 1
freely soluble	1 in 1 to 1 in 10
soluble	1 in 10 to 1 in 30
sparingly soluble	1 in 30 to 1 in 100
slightly soluble	1 in 100 to 1 in 1000
very slightly soluble	1 in 1000 to 1 in 10 000
practically insoluble	1 in more than 10 000

In the solubility statements, the word 'water' refers to purified water, the word 'ether' refers to diethyl ether, and the word 'ethanol', without qualification, refers to ethanol (95%).

TEMPERATURE. Temperatures are expressed throughout the text in degrees Celsius (Centigrade).

Analytical Data

All analytical data in the monographs in Part 2 apply to the form of the substance described in the main title of the monograph, unless otherwise specified.

In all lists or indexes of chromatographic data, a dash indicates that the value is not known, not that the substance does not elute.

EXTRACTION. It has not been possible to give direct information on the best method for extracting individual substances from various biological samples. However, useful information can be gained from the data on solubility, dissociation constant, and partition coefficient. The best solvent can be chosen by reference to the solubility, the pH for extraction is indicated by the pK_a value, and the partition coefficient gives a quantitative measure of the phase volume ratios needed for a successful extraction.

COLOUR TESTS. Where colour tests are given in the monographs in Part 2, the names of the tests are printed with initial capitals. These names refer to the tests described under Colour Tests (pp. 128 to 147) where complete tables of colours are provided. Reference should be made to this chapter for an explanation of the system used for describing the colours.

Colour tests applicable to biological fluids are described under Hospital Toxicology and Drug Abuse Screening (pp. 3 to 34).

THIN-LAYER CHROMATOGRAPHY. The thin-layer chromatographic systems referred to in the monographs in Part 2 are described on pp. 167 to 177, together with lists of data for drugs in important chemical and pharmacological classifications. General screening systems (Systems TA to TF), which include over 700 drugs, are provided. System TA is the same as System T1 which appeared in the first edition but the data have been completely revised and extended. In order to clarify the presentation of values, the data are expressed in terms of Rf × 100. Complete lists of data, in ascending order, are given in the indexes of Thin-layer Chromatographic Data (p. 1094).

GAS CHROMATOGRAPHY. The gas chromatographic systems referred to in the monographs in Part 2 are described on pp. 192 to 200, together with lists of retention data for drugs in important chemical and pharmacological classifications. A general screening system (System GA), which includes over 700 drugs, is provided. For most of the systems, the data are given in terms of Retention Index (see p. 190). Retention times or relative retention times are used in a few systems. Complete lists of retention data, in ascending order, are given in the indexes of Gas Chromatographic Data (p. 1112).

HIGH PRESSURE LIQUID CHROMATOGRAPHY. The high pressure liquid chromatographic systems referred to in the monographs in Part 2 are described on pp. 213 to 220, together with lists of retention data for drugs in important chemical and pharmacological classifications. A general screening system (System HA), which includes over 400 drugs, is provided. For the majority of the systems, the data are given in terms of column capacity ratio, k' (see p. 204). Complete lists of retention data, in ascending order, are given in the indexes of High Pressure Liquid Chromatographic Data (p. 1121).

ULTRAVIOLET ABSORPTION. The wavelengths of principal and subsidiary peaks, in the range 230 to 360 nm, are recorded in each monograph for acid, alkaline, and neutral solution, where available. Values in neutral solution are given for compounds for which values in acid or alkaline solution are not available or when the values in neutral solution differ significantly from those in acid or alkaline solution.

In many monographs, the ultraviolet spectrum is reproduced. In these spectra the following notation is used:

——————— acid solution

·········· alkaline solution

– – – – – – – neutral solution

Where more than one curve is shown, they do not necessarily relate to the same concentration and, consequently, points where the curves cross cannot be taken as true isosbestic points. The wavelengths

of peaks in a few of the spectra may differ very slightly from those stated in the text. Where there is doubt, the values given in the text should be used. In monographs where the spectrum is reproduced, the A_1^1 value for the major peak only is given; if no spectrum is reproduced, the A_1^1 value for each peak is stated, if available. The A_1^1 values apply to the form of the substance described in the main title of the monograph, unless otherwise stated.

The A_1^1 values are divided into three categories in order to provide an indication of reliability:

The letter 'a' after a figure indicates that the value is a mean value based on several reported figures all of which lie within a range of $\pm 10\%$ of the mean.

The letter 'b' after a figure indicates that the value is a single reported value of unknown reliability.

The letter 'c' after a figure indicates that the value is a mean value based on several reported figures some of which lie outside $\pm 10\%$ of the mean.

The phrase 'no significant absorption' indicates that no peaks are found at the concentrations normally used.

The A_1^1 values quoted in the monographs may be useful in identification, and may help in determining the strength of a solution which is required to obtain a curve within the instrumental range of absorption. They may also be useful to give an approximate indication of the amount of drug present in a solution. However, because of instrumental differences and the possible effect of solvent and pH, A_1^1 values are subject to considerable variation and the values quoted should not be used when an accurate assay is required. In this case, a reference specimen should be examined at the same time as the sample.

The wavelengths of main peaks are listed for acid, alkaline, and neutral solution in the index of Ultraviolet Absorption Maxima (p. 1128).

INFRA-RED ABSORPTION. The wavenumbers of the six major peaks in the range 2000 to 650 cm^{-1} (5 to 15 µm), in descending order of amplitude, are recorded in the monographs in Part 2. In many cases the infra-red spectrum is also reproduced. When selecting the six principal peaks, those which are in the region where Nujol absorbs (1490 to 1320 cm^{-1}, 6.7 to 7.6 µm) have been omitted. Corrections for calibration errors have been applied where these are known.

The six principal peaks, in ascending order of the main peak, are listed in the index of Infra-red Peaks (p. 1141).

MASS SPECTRUM. The m/z values of the eight most abundant ions, in descending order of intensity, are included in many monographs in Part 2. Where dashes occur in the listing this indicates that less than eight ions have been observed.

The eight principal peaks, in ascending order of the main peak, are listed in the index of Mass Spectral Data of Drugs (p. 1152). A separate index for pesticides is on p. 1161. The full mass spectra for the majority of the listed compounds are displayed in *Pharmaceutical Mass Spectra*, London, The Pharmaceutical Press, 1985.

QUANTIFICATION. The methods referred to in the references quoted under the heading 'Quantification' in the monographs in Part 2 are not intended to be recommended methods. These references are intended to be used as a guide to the literature on the particular subject.

REAGENTS. Reagents required for specific tests or methods are generally described fully in the appropriate place in the text. However, certain common reagents which are used throughout the book are italicised in the text and are described in Part 4: Appendix of Reagents and Proprietary Test Materials (p. 1169). Reagent solutions are made in purified water unless otherwise specified. When ethanol, without qualification, is stated to be used, this refers to ethanol (95%).

Unless otherwise stated, solutions of solids in liquids are expressed as percentage w/v, and solutions of liquids in liquids as percentage v/v. When acids of various strengths are specified, e.g. 50% sulphuric acid, this implies the appropriate dilution by volume of the strong acid in water.

Disposition in the Body

Many of the monographs in Part 2 contain a section with the heading 'Disposition in the Body'. The information in these statements has been obtained from a detailed survey of published papers and other reference sources. Certain monographs have a single reference at the end of the statement and this indicates that all the disposition information has been obtained from that source. Wherever possible, information is included on absorption, distribution, metabolism, excretion, therapeutic concentration, toxicity, and pharmacokinetic parameters.

Entry to the literature is provided by the inclusion of abstracts of published papers on clinical studies or case histories. These abstracts include details of drug concentrations in plasma or other body fluids or tissues; in these data a dash means that the particular value was not determined, and ND or 0 means that the substance was not detected. Concentrations in body fluids or tissues are expressed in μg/ml or μg/g.

In some monographs the information is incomplete, the amount of detail being dependent upon that available in the literature searched. It should not be assumed that the statements presented reflect the only significant factors in the disposition of the drug concerned.

THERAPEUTIC CONCENTRATION. This is the concentration range usually observed after therapeutic doses, as reported in clinical studies and other research projects. It should not be interpreted as the concentration range required for optimum therapeutic effect.

TOXICITY. This statement may include drug concentrations in blood or other body fluids or tissues, which have been reported to be associated with toxic or lethal effects. Because of intersubject variations or other variable factors, the reported toxic or lethal concentrations may occasionally lie close to or within the therapeutic range.

In some monographs, the toxic or lethal blood concentrations are stated in the form 60 to **89** to 150 μg/ml. These figures have been obtained from a survey of a number of reported cases and represent the maximum concentrations found in 10%, 50%, and 90% of the subjects, respectively.

Maximum permitted concentrations in air (8-hour exposure limit) are those recommended by the Health and Safety Executive in *Occupational Exposure Limits 1985*, Guidance Note EH 40/85, London, HMSO.

VOLUME OF DISTRIBUTION. This relates to plasma concentrations after intravenous administration, unless otherwise stated. Values are based on a body-weight of 70 kg.

CLEARANCE. This usually refers to the total plasma clearance (or total whole blood clearance) after intravenous administration. In some instances the total clearance after an oral dose has been included if the drug is known to be well absorbed and is not subject to significant first-pass metabolism.

Numerous factors and intersubject variations may affect the absorption, distribution, metabolism, and excretion of drugs. These include age, sex, and disease states such as renal impairment. In addition, results of analyses may be subject to unavoidable analytical inaccuracies. Consequently, there may be considerable variations in the observed drug concentrations and in values for pharmacokinetic parameters in individual cases. Hence, the values given in the monographs should be used only as a guide and should not be taken as absolute values.

Dose

The dose recorded under this heading in the monographs in Part 2 indicates the usual daily dose (oral unless otherwise stated) that may be administered for therapeutic purposes. It is intended solely as a guide in deciding whether the amount taken by an individual falls within the normal dosage range and should not be taken as a recommendation for treatment.

More detailed information on doses in different conditions and age groups may be found in *Martindale, The Extra Pharmacopoeia*, 28th Edn, London, The Pharmaceutical Press, 1982, or in the manufacturers' data sheets for the products.

This second edition of Clarke could not have been completed without the comments on the first edition and the contribution of analytical data from many scientists involved in the analysis of drugs. In order to assist in the preparation of a third edition, the reader is invited to send any constructive comments and relevant new data concerning the analysis of drugs in biological materials to the Editor, Clarke's Isolation and Identification of Drugs, Department of Pharmaceutical Sciences, The Pharmaceutical Society of Great Britain, 1 Lambeth High Street, London SE1 7JN, England. In this way, future editions of the book will be improved to the benefit of all those who use it.

Deletions

The following substances which were included in Volumes 1 and 2* of the 1st Edition are not included in this edition.

Acetyldihydrocodeine
Adrenalone
Allantoin
Allylprodine
Alphameprodine
Alphamethadol
Aminometradine
Aminopentamide
Amisometradine
Amolanone
Amopyroquine
*Amotriphene
Amprotropine
Amydricaine
Amylocaine
Apoatropine
Azacosterol

Azamethonium Bromide
Benzalkonium Bromide
Benzamine
Benzathine Penicillin
Benzethidine
Betameprodine
Betaprodine
*Brocresine
Butallylonal
Butethamine
Butoxamine
Cetoxime
Chlorisondamine Chloride
Citronella Oil
Clamoxyquin
Clonitazene
*Cloponone

Codeine N-Oxide
Cyclamic Acid
Cyprenorphine
Demecolcine
Demeton-O
Desomorphine
Diampromide
Dibutoline Sulphate
*Diethylaminoethyl Diphenylpropionate
Dimenoxadole
*Dimethocaine
Dimethylthiambutene
*Dimophebumine
Dioxaphetyl Butyrate
Dioxathion
*Dioxyamidopyrine
*Diphenazoline
Dithiazanine Iodide
Embramine
Erythrityl Tetranitrate
*Ethylisobutrazine
Ethylmethylthiambutene
*Ethylpiperidyl Benzilate
Etonitazene
Etoxeridine
Etymide
Fenimide
*Fenmetramide
Furethidine
Hydromorphinol
Hydroxypethidine
*Imidocarb
*Iminodimethylphenylthiazolidine
*Iopydol
*Iopydone
Isobutyl Aminobenzoate
*Isometamidium
Isomethadone
Laudexium Methylsulphate
Leucinocaine
Levomethorphan
Levomoramide
Levophenacylmorphan
Lucanthone
Metabutethamine
Metabutoxycaine
Metazocine
*Methadone Intermediate
Methaphenilene
Methoxypromazine
Methylaminoheptane
Methyldesorphine
Methyldihydromorphine
Methylhexaneamine
Methyridine
Metofoline
Metopon
*Moramide Intermediate
Morpheridine
Morphine N-Oxide
Mustine
Myrophine
Naepaine

*Naftazone
Narcobarbital
Nicocodine
Nicomorphine
*Nifuroxime
Noracymethadol
Norbutrine
*Nordefrin
*Norgestrel
Norlevorphanol
*Octacaine
Octaverine
Orthocaine
Pamaquin
*Panidazole
*Paromomycin
Pentaquin
*Pethidine Intermediate A
Phenadoxone
Phenamidine
Phenampromide
*Phenatine
Phenisonone
Phenomorphan
Phenoxypropazine
Phenylpropylmethylamine
*Phthivazid
*Picloxydine
Pipamazine
Piperoxan
Pipethanate
Plasmocide
*Proadifen
Probarbital
Proheptazine
Properidine
Pulegium Oil
*Pyrrocaine
Quinapyramine Chloride
Racemethorphan
Racemoramide
*Resorantel
*Rifamide
*Rolicypram
Stilbamidine
Sulphasomizole
Sulphonal
*Taurolin
Teclothiazide
*Terodiline
*Tetracosactrin
*Tetraethylammonium Bromide
*Thozalinone
Thurfyl Nicotinate
*Tiletamine
Tolonium Chloride
Tolycaine
Triclobisonium Chloride
Tropacocaine
Tropine
Tymazoline
Viomycin
Xenysalate

Acknowledgements

Special acknowledgement is made to the Controller, Her Majesty's Stationery Office for permission to publish analytical data and spectra provided by the Central Research Establishment, Home Office Forensic Science Service, Aldermaston.

Acknowledgements are gratefully made to the following establishments, individuals, and manufacturers for the provision of analytical data, spectra, advice, or samples.

Can-Test Inc., Vancouver; Lynn & Johnston Laboratories Ltd, Montreal; Mann Testing Inc., Toronto; Metropolitan Police Forensic Science Laboratory, London; Poisons Unit, Guy's Hospital, London; Racecourse Security Services Laboratory, Newmarket; The Laboratory of the Government Chemist, London; The Medicines Testing Laboratory, PSGB, Edinburgh.

R. Bain, H. J. Battista, T. M. Callaghan, D. Carson, P. G. W. Cobb, A. S. Curry, T. Daldrup, M. Donike, B. S. Finkle, R. S. Frank, G. V. Fraser, D. Harvey, L. Kazyak, S. S. Kind, G. Machata, G. A. March, R. J. Mesley, M. R. Moller, R. K. Müller, J. Oliver, R. Osland, D. A. Patterson, H. W. Peel, R. Permisohn, B. Perrigo, H. Schütz, S. Shouten, R. Spragg, C. Sutton, C. B. Teer, E. Tomlinson, D. Uges, V. Westenberger, R. A. de Zeeuw.

A/S GEA Pharmaceutical Manufacturing Co., Astra Pharmaceuticals Ltd, Bayer AG, Boehringer Ingelheim Ltd, The Boots Co. plc, Bristol-Myers Co. Ltd, A. Christiaens, Delagrange International, Delandale Laboratories Ltd, Du Pont Pharmaceuticals, Farmitalia Carlo Erba Ltd, Glaxo Laboratories Ltd, Grünenthal GmbH, Hoechst UK Ltd, Imperial Chemical Industries plc, Janssen Pharmaceutica, Laboratoires Anphar-Rolland, Eli Lilly and Co. Ltd, May & Baker Ltd, MCP Pharmaceuticals Ltd, Norwich Eaton Ltd, Riker Laboratories Ltd, Roche Products Ltd, Roussel Laboratories Ltd, Sandoz Products Ltd, Schering Pharmaceuticals Ltd, E. R. Squibb & Sons Ltd, Upjohn Ltd, Winthrop Laboratories, Wyeth Laboratories.

Abbreviations

A number of units, terms, and symbols are not included in this list as they are defined in the place in the text where they are used. Very common abbreviations (gram, centimetre, etc.) have been omitted. The titles of journals are abbreviated according to the general style of *World List of Scientific Periodicals* (London, Butterworths, 1963–80).

A_1^1—specific absorbance (abbreviation of $A_{1\,cm}^{1\,\%}$)

AFID—alkali flame ionisation detector

agg.—aggregate (in botanical names), including 2 or more species which resemble each other closely

AUC—area under the curve

B.P.—British Pharmacopoeia

b.p.—boiling point

CAS—Chemical Abstracts Service

CI—Colour Index (*Colour Index*, 3rd Edn, 1971 and supplements)

Cl—clearance

ECD—electron capture detector

Ed.—editor(s) *or* edited by

Edn—edition

et al.—*et alii*, 'and others': for three or more co-authors or co-workers

eV—electron volt(s)

fg—femtogram(s)

FID—flame ionisation detector

f.p.—freezing point

FPD—flame photometric detector

ft—foot (feet)

GC—gas chromatography

GC–MS—gas chromatography–mass spectrometry

GCDP—gas chromatographic decomposition product

GSC—gas-solid chromatography

h—hour(s)

HPLC—high pressure liquid chromatography

HPLC–MS—high pressure liquid chromatography–mass spectrometry

ibid.—*ibidem*, 'in the same place' (journal or book)

idem—'the same': used for the same authors and titles

in—inch(es)

IR—infra-red

k'—column capacity ratio

λ—wavelength (nm)

log—logarithm to the base 10

ln—logarithm to the base e (natural logarithm)

μg—microgram(s)

μm—micrometre(s)

M—molar, i.e. the strength of a solution in moles per litre

mEq—milliequivalent(s)

MID—multiple ion detector

min—minute

mol—mole

m.p.—melting point

MS—mass spectrometry

m/z—mass to charge ratio

v—frequency (Hz)

$\bar{v}$—wavenumber (cm^{-1})

ng—nanogram(s)

nm—nanometre(s)

NMR—nuclear magnetic resonance

P—apparent partition coefficient

pg—picogram(s)

PID—photoionisation detector

pK_a—the negative logarithm of the dissociation constant

PMR—proton magnetic resonance

ppm—part(s) per million

PTFE—polytetrafluoroethylene

RI—retention index

RIA—radioimmunoassay

RRT—relative retention time

RT—retention time

s—second(s)

s—standard deviation

sp.gr.—specific gravity

sp.—species (plural spp.)

$t_{\frac{1}{2}}$—half-life

TCD—thermal conductivity detector

TIC—total ion current

TLC—thin-layer chromatography

UV—ultraviolet

V—volt(s)

V_d—volume of distribution

var.—variety

Vet.—veterinary

vol.—volume(s)

v/v—volume in volume

w/v—weight in volume

w/w—weight in weight

PART 1 : Analytical Techniques

Hospital Toxicology and Drug Abuse Screening

B. Widdop

When tablets or capsules are found in the immediate vicinity of, or in the possession of, an unconscious patient, it is reasonable to assume that a drug overdose has been taken. If the patient responds to supportive treatment and no active measures are contemplated, toxicological analyses are of historical interest only. Conversely, when circumstantial evidence is lacking, a diagnosis of poisoning may be difficult to sustain simply on the basis of clinical examination, since coma induced by drugs is not readily differentiated from that caused by disease processes. The role of the laboratory is important in several types of poisoning cases.

In the diagnosis of brain death, the presence of depressant drugs with prolonged duration of action should be excluded. Episodes of cardiac arrest, hypoxia, or severe circulatory insufficiency occur frequently in severely-overdosed patients, and can lead to cerebral anoxia and brain death. Measurement of the plasma concentration of the drug(s) to establish the presence or absence of toxic concentrations is invaluable in this context.

Poisoning in children is mainly accidental but deliberate poisoning by parents or guardians may go unrecognised. Suspicions are aroused when a child shows bizarre symptoms and signs for which there is no obvious pathological explanation. The detection of drugs in samples from these cases does not prove that the child has been wilfully poisoned, but sufficient concern may be generated to ensure future supervision by the social services.

In the diagnosis and monitoring of drug abuse, clinicians rely heavily on laboratory tests. The analyses guard against the issuing of drugs to patients who may not be dependent on them, and help to assess the progress (or otherwise) in treating genuine addicts.

Signs of endogenous mental illness are often hard to differentiate from those induced by psychoto-mimetic agents (e.g. amphetamine, cannabis, lysergide), and laboratory analyses can be an invaluable diagnostic aid.

In certain poisoning cases a specific antidote may be available, e.g. for carbon monoxide, cholinesterase inhibitors, cyanide, heavy metals, iron, methanol, ethylene glycol, opiates, paracetamol, and some halogenated hydrocarbons. If the circumstantial and clinical evidence is clear, the clinician may administer the antidote without waiting for confirmatory laboratory tests. However, subsequent analyses may be a useful guide to the need to continue therapy. For example, parenteral therapy of iron poisoning with desferrioxamine is indicated if the clinical state of the patient deteriorates and the serum-iron concentration is extremely high; information about cholinesterase activity in serum or erythrocytes is useful when massive doses of atropine are being infused into patients suffering from organophosphate poisoning; intravenous infusions of acetylcysteine can be discontinued if the plasma-paracetamol concentration demonstrates that a patient is unlikely to sustain liver damage.

The abuse of solvents ('glue-sniffing') is increasing, and patients who reach hospital have a variety of neurological signs. The detection of the responsible agents in blood proves the diagnosis.

Covert ingestion of laxative drugs is a lesser known facet of drug misuse. These patients, convinced that daily evacuation of the bowel is essential for survival, take laxatives in quantities which lead to persistent gastro-intestinal and systemic disorders. Other patients self-administer diuretic agents, usually to lose weight, and again systemic disturbances are induced. Analytical tests to detect all these drugs can avoid months of fruitless clinical, biochemical, and haematological investigations.

COLLECTION OF SAMPLES

Urine

A urine specimen should be obtained from the patient on admission to hospital, preferably before any drugs (e.g. diuretics, tranquillisers) which may interfere with the tests have been administered.

Unconscious patients are usually catheterised and, in this case, the sample may be contaminated with the catheter lubricant which frequently contains lignocaine as a local anaesthetic. Urine is ideal for qualitative screening as it is available in large volumes, and usually contains higher concentrations of drugs or poisons than blood. The presence of drug metabolites can be used to assist identification if chromatographic techniques which can separate them are used. A 50-ml sample is sufficient for a comprehensive series of tests, and no preservative should be added.

Stomach Contents

This sample includes vomit, gastric aspirate, or stomach washings. It is important to obtain the first sample of washings rather than a later sample which will be considerably diluted. This is the most useful sample on which to carry out qualitative analyses; if it is obtained soon after the overdose was taken it may be possible to recognise the presence of undegraded tablets or capsules. An immediate clue may be obtained by detecting the characteristic odour of certain compounds. However, the main virtue of this sample is that the drugs are present in high concentrations. The sample is also devoid of metabolites which complicate some assays. At least 50 ml of sample is required to carry out a wide range of tests, and no preservative should be added.

Blood

Samples which should be taken on admission of the patient are 10 ml of heparinised blood, 2 ml of fluoridated blood, and 10 ml of blood without preservative or anticoagulant. The use of disinfectant swabs containing alcohols, and of heparin containing phenolic preservatives, should be avoided. The sample should be dispensed with care; for example, the vigorous discharge of blood through a syringe needle can cause sufficient haemolysis to invalidate a serum-iron assay. Any drugs administered to the patient for treatment of the poisoning must be reported to the laboratory.

Rapid Detection of Drugs Commonly Taken in Overdosage

Two analytical schemes are presented, both of which have been devised to give a simple method for indicating the identity of the drug or drug-type which may be present in a sample of blood, urine, or stomach contents.

Scheme 1 is designed to produce the maximum amount of useful information in the minimum time. It includes preliminary direct tests followed by solvent extraction and thin-layer chromatography, and a test for benzodiazepines in urine. If evidence exists which suggests a specific drug, the appropriate test should be carried out first. However, it must be remembered that patients frequently ingest more than one drug, and it is unwise to discontinue the analysis at the first sign of a positive result. When a drug has been detected, it can be identified and quantified using tests described later in this chapter.

Scheme 2 can be used when more time is available for the analyses. It involves a more elaborate extraction procedure, with separation into strong acid, weak acid, neutral, and basic fractions.

SCHEME 1

Direct Tests on Urine, Stomach Contents, and Blood

DIRECT TESTS ON URINE

1. *Glucose, ketones, and pH—'Labstix' test*. Dip a 'Labstix' strip briefly into the urine and read after 10 to 15 seconds. For glucose, the result should be correlated with a blood-glucose determination. A positive result for ketones may indicate intoxication by acetone or isopropyl alcohol. This test may also be positive in starvation or in diabetic ketosis.

2. *Salicylates—Trinder's test*. To 1 ml of urine add 5 drops of *Trinder's reagent*. A violet colour indicates the presence of salicylate or salicylamide. A positive result is obtained after therapeutic doses of aspirin or aminosalicylic acid.

3. *Volatile reducing substances (including alcohols and aldehydes)—dichromate test*. Place 1 ml of urine in a test-tube; apply 1 drop of 2.5% potassium dichromate in 50% sulphuric acid to a strip of glass-fibre filter paper, insert the paper in the neck of the test-tube, lightly cork the tube, and place in a boiling water-bath for 2 minutes. A colour change to green indicates a positive result. Ethanol, the most commonly found member of this group, gives a positive reaction if present above 400 µg/ml and the blood-ethanol concentration should then be measured (p. 19).

4. *Phenothiazines—FPN reagent*. To 1 ml of urine add 1 ml of *FPN reagent*. A variety of colours ranging through pink, red, orange, violet, and

blue indicates the presence of a phenothiazine derivative. The colours are transient and should be observed immediately. Positive results can be obtained after therapeutic doses.

5. *Imipramine, desipramine, and trimipramine—Forrest reagent*. To 0.5 ml of urine add 1 ml of *Forrest reagent*. A green-yellow colour darkening through dark green to blue, depending on the amount of drug present, immediately appears. Phenothiazines may also give a positive result, but the test is more sensitive than FPN reagent to imipramine.

6. *Trichloro-compounds—Fujiwara test*. To 1 ml of urine add 1 ml of *sodium hydroxide solution* and 1 ml of pyridine, and heat in a boiling water-bath for 2 minutes. The development of a red colour in the pyridine layer indicates ingestion of a trichloro-compound. A blank urine sample and an authentic solution of trichloroacetic acid should be tested at the same time, both blank and control solutions being treated in similar fashion to the sample, because contamination of the atmosphere with laboratory reagents may give positive results.

Metabolites of carbon tetrachloride may also give a positive result with this test, but carbon tetrachloride is only partially metabolised to trichloromethyl compounds and the test may fail to detect this agent. If carbon tetrachloride poisoning is suspected, evidence of hepato-toxicity should be sought by carrying out appropriate serum-enzyme assays.

7. *Paracetamol—Cresol–ammonia test*. To 0.5 ml of urine add 0.5 ml of *hydrochloric acid* and heat for 10 minutes at 100°; to 2 drops of the mixture add 10 ml of water, 1 ml of 1% o-cresol in water, and 4 ml of 2M ammonium hydroxide. A blue colour appears if paracetamol is present. The test is very sensitive and can detect therapeutic concentrations. The presence of the parent drug and its conjugated metabolites can be detected for several days after overdose. If a positive result is obtained, a plasma-paracetamol determination should be carried out immediately (p. 23).

8. *Ethchlorvynol—diphenylamine test*. Sprinkle a few mg of diphenylamine sulphate on to the surface of 2 ml of urine in a test-tube, incline the tube, and carefully trickle in 1 ml of *sulphuric acid*. A red colour forms on the surface of the crystals if ethchlorvynol is present.

The test is specific, and is sufficiently sensitive to detect therapeutic concentrations.

9. *Paraquat and diquat—dithionite test*. To 1 ml of urine add 1 ml of a freshly-prepared 0.1% solution of sodium dithionite in M sodium hydroxide. A blue colour indicates the presence of paraquat. A green colour is given by diquat, but paraquat may also be present.

A strong blue colour obtained with a urine sample taken more than 4 hours after ingestion suggests a poor prognosis. Confirmation of the severity of the poisoning is obtained by measuring the plasma-paraquat concentration (p. 25).

DIRECT TESTS ON STOMACH CONTENTS

1. *Odour, colour, and pH*. Characteristic smells may indicate the presence of substances such as camphor, cresol, cyanide, ethanol and other organic solvents, ethchlorvynol, methyl salicylate, paraldehyde, and phenelzine. A high pH may indicate ingestion of alkali. Undegraded tablets or capsules should be retrieved and examined separately. A green or blue colour suggests the presence of iron salts.

2. *Salicylates—Trinder's test*. To 2 ml of the sample add 2 ml of 0.1M hydrochloric acid, boil for 10 minutes, filter if necessary, neutralise the filtrate with 0.1M sodium hydroxide, and add 3 drops of *Trinder's reagent*. A violet colour indicates the presence of salicylate.

Aspirin itself will not react with the reagent as preliminary hydrolysis is required.

3. *Oxidising agents—diphenylamine test*. Filter a portion of the sample and add 2 drops of the filtrate to 1 ml of a 1% solution of diphenylamine in *sulphuric acid*. A deep blue colour, appearing immediately, indicates the presence of an oxidising agent. The test will detect hypochlorite (from domestic bleach), bromates, chlorates, iodates, nitrates, and nitrites. Tests to distinguish between certain anions will be found under Metals and Anions (p. 64).

A light blue colour, caused by organic matter, should be ignored. Note that nitrate and nitrite from meat products will give a positive reaction.

4. *Ferrous and ferric iron—ferricyanide and ferrocyanide tests*. To 2 drops of sample add 3 drops of 2M hydrochloric acid and 1 drop of 1% potassium ferricyanide solution. A deep blue precipitate indicates ferrous iron. Repeat the test but adding 1 drop of 1% potassium ferrocyanide solution. A deep blue precipitate indicates ferric iron.

5. *Phenothiazines—FPN reagent.* Carry out the test as described for urine (above) using a suitable volume of the filtered sample.
6. *Imipramine, desipramine, and trimipramine—Forrest reagent.* Carry out the test as described for urine (above) using a suitable volume of the filtered sample.
7. *Trichloro-compounds—Fujiwara test.* Carry out the test as described for urine (above) using a suitable volume of the filtered sample.
8. *Ethchlorvynol—diphenylamine test.* Carry out the test as described for urine (above) using a suitable volume of the filtered sample.
9. *Paraquat and diquat—dithionite test.* Carry out the test as described for urine (above) using a suitable volume of the filtered sample.
10. *Organophosphorus compounds—inhibition of cholinesterase.* To each of two tubes add 3 ml of *dithiobisnitrobenzoic acid solution*, 0.1 ml of 5% acetylthiocholine iodide solution, and 20 μl of normal serum; to the first tube add 0.2 ml of water and to the second tube add 0.2 ml of the filtered sample and allow to stand for 2 minutes. Any significant difference in colour between the tubes is suggestive of the presence of an organophosphorus compound or other cholinesterase inhibitor.

The method given for the quantification of cholinesterase activity in serum (p. 23) may also be applied to stomach contents.

DIRECT TESTS ON BLOOD
1. *Glucose.* Measure the blood glucose by a standard method or, approximately, by the 'Dextrostix' or similar method. Hypoglycaemia is a feature of overdosage with insulin, hypoglycaemic agents, and ethanol. It can also occur in the early stages of liver damage following severe poisoning with paracetamol.
2. *Urea.* Measure the blood urea by a standard method or, approximately, by the 'Urastrat' method (see Reagent Appendix), to exclude uraemia.
3. *Carbon monoxide—carboxyhaemoglobin test.* Dilute a sample of the blood 1 in 20 with 0.01 M ammonia and compare the colour with a sample of normal blood treated similarly. A pinkish tint suggests the presence of carboxyhaemoglobin.
4. *Salicylates—Trinder's test.* To 0.5 ml of plasma add 4.5 ml of *Trinder's reagent*, shake well, and centrifuge. A violet colour in the supernatant liquid indicates the presence of salicylate or salicylamide. A quantitative method for salicylate in plasma is given on p. 26.
5. *Volatile reducing substances (including alcohols and aldehydes)—dichromate test.* Carry out the method described for urine, above.
6. *Organophosphorus compounds—inhibition of cholinesterase.* To each of two tubes add 3 ml of *dithiobisnitrobenzoic acid solution* and 0.1 ml of 5% acetylthiocholine iodide solution; to the first tube add 20 μl of normal serum and to the second tube add 20 μl of the sample serum and allow to stand for 2 minutes. Any significant difference in colour between the tubes is suggestive of the presence of an organophosphorus compound or other cholinesterase inhibitor.

A method for the quantification of cholinesterase activity in serum is given on p. 23.

Extraction of Urine and Stomach Contents
This procedure gives an extract which can be analysed by thin-layer chromatography. If both types of sample are available, they should both be examined. If necessary, particulate material in stomach contents should be removed by filtration or centrifugation, and the clarified filtrate or supernatant liquid extracted. Direct extracts of stomach contents, when evaporated to small bulk, are difficult to apply to thin-layer chromatographic plates because of the presence of fats and other dietary material. For this sample, therefore, a back-extraction step is included in the procedure.

Half-fill each of two 20-ml screw-capped glass bottles (McCartney bottles) with sample, and make one acidic by the addition of 1 to 2 ml of M sulphuric acid, and the other alkaline by the addition of 1 to 2 ml of M sodium hydroxide (check the pH with an indicator paper). Label the bottles A and B (acids and bases) respectively, fill them with chloroform, screw on the plastic caps, shake gently for about 5 minutes, and centrifuge for 5 to 10 minutes. Remove the top aqueous layer using a Pasteur pipette connected to a water-operated vacuum pump.

For samples of stomach contents, carry out the following back-extraction procedure. Add 3 ml of 0.5M sodium hydroxide to the acid chloroform extract (A), and 3 ml of 0.25M sulphuric acid to the alkaline chloroform extract (B). Shake the bottles again, centrifuge, and discard the organic solvent layers. Make bottle A acid by the addition of 0.5 ml of 3M sulphuric acid, and make bottle B alkaline by the addition of 0.5 ml of 6M sodium hydroxide.

Add 10 ml of chloroform to each bottle, shake, centrifuge, and remove the aqueous layers as above. Remove residual moisture from the two extracts from either urine or stomach contents by filtering through phase-separating paper, and collect the filtrates in 10-ml conical test-tubes. Add a little tartaric acid to the basic extract to prevent the loss of volatile bases, and evaporate to dryness under a stream of air or nitrogen. Dissolve each residue in 0.1 ml of chloroform.

Thin-layer Chromatography of Extracts

ACIDIC AND NEUTRAL EXTRACT

Reference Solutions. Prepare solutions in chloroform of authentic samples of drugs as indicated in Table 1, each drug being at a concentration of 1 mg/ml.

Method. Divide a TLC plate (silica gel G, 250 μm) into 8 equal columns by scoring lines with a spatula, and draw a horizontal line 10 cm from the origin. Apply 10-μl aliquots of the reference solutions and 25-μl aliquots of the sample extract to the columns on the plate in the sequence shown in Table 1. Evaporation of the spots can be hastened by the use of a cold air blower.

Table 1. Sequence of application of acidic extract to TLC plate

Column number	Solution
1	amylobarbitone and phenobarbitone
2	sample extract
3	phenobarbitone and phenytoin
4	sample extract
5	glutethimide
6	sample extract
7	meprobamate
8	sample extract

Develop the plate in a tank containing 100 ml of a 4:1 mixture of chloroform:acetone (System TD, p. 168). Alternatively, System TE (p. 168), or System TF (p. 168) may be used. After development, remove the plate from the tank and dry under a stream of cold air.

NOTE. Chloroform and acetone can form an explosive mixture in the presence of alkali and should be disposed of immediately after use.

Location Reagents. Examine the plate under ultra-violet light.

Cover columns 3 to 8 with a glass plate and spray columns 1 and 2 with *mercuric chloride–diphenylcarbazone reagent*. White spots on a violet background indicate the presence of barbiturates or related compounds (e.g. glutethimide).

Cover columns 1 and 2 and 5 to 8 with glass plates, and spray columns 3 and 4 with *mercurous nitrate spray*. Black spots are given by barbiturates and related compounds (e.g. glutethimide).

Cover columns 1 to 4 and 7 and 8 with glass plates, and spray columns 5 and 6 with *Dragendorff spray*. An orange spot is given by methaqualone and by glutethimide (weak reaction).

Cover columns 1 to 6, and spray columns 7 and 8 with *furfuraldehyde reagent*. A violet spot is given by meprobamate.

The chromatographic system distinguishes between certain types of barbiturates, and for most clinical situations this is sufficient. If doubt exists, or if it is crucial to know which barbiturate is present, the sample should be examined by gas chromatography. Certain antibiotics give white spots with *mercurous nitrate spray*, but do not react with *mercuric chloride–diphenylcarbazone reagent*.

Table 2. TLC data for some acidic and neutral drugs

Compound	Rf Values Systems			Mercuric chloride–diphenyl-carbazone reagent	Mercurous nitrate spray
	TD	TE	TF		
Primidone	08	39	26	+	+
Meprobamate*	09	60	34	–	–
Paracetamol	15	45	34		
Phenytoin	33	36	53	+	+
Salicylamide	38	46	55		
Barbitone	41	31	61	+	+
Phenobarbitone	47	28	65	+	+
Cyclobarbitone	50	35	64	+	+
Butobarbitone	50	38	65	+	+
Heptabarbitone	50	30	65	+	+
Amylobarbitone	52	36	65	+	+
Pentobarbitone	55	45	66	+	+
Quinalbarbitone	55	44	68	+	+
Glutethimide†	63	78	62	+	+
Methaqualone‡	63	—	—	–	–
Phenylbutazone	78	66	68		+

*Violet with *furfuraldehyde reagent*
†Weak reaction with *Dragendorff spray*
‡Positive reaction with *Dragendorff spray*

An alternative sequence of spray reagents, and alternative reference compounds, are given for Systems TD, TE, and TF on p. 168, and a comprehensive list of Rf values in these systems will be found in the indexes to Thin-layer Chromatographic Data in Part 3.

BASIC EXTRACT

Reference Solutions. Prepare solutions in chloroform of authentic samples of drugs as indicated in Table 3, each drug being at a concentration of 1 mg/ml.

Method. Divide a TLC plate (silica gel G, 250 μm)

into 8 equal columns by scoring lines with a spatula, and draw a horizontal line 10 cm from the origin. Apply 10-μl aliquots of the authentic solutions and 25-μl aliquots of the sample extract to the columns on the plate in the sequence shown in Table 3. Evaporation of the spots can be hastened by the use of a cold air blower.

Table 3. Sequence of application of basic extract to TLC plate

Column number	Solution
1	codeine
2	sample extract
3	amitriptyline and nortriptyline
4	sample extract
5	chlorpromazine
6	sample extract
7	*suspected drug
8	sample extract

*Column 7 is reserved for an authentic solution of any basic drug which may be suspected on clinical or circumstantial evidence.

Develop the plate in a tank containing a 100:1.5 mixture of methanol:*strong ammonia solution* (System TA, p. 167). After development, remove the plate from the tank and dry under a stream of cold air until the plate no longer smells of ammonia. (Avoid using hot air to dry the plate as this can volatilise certain drugs.)
Alternatively, System TB (p. 167) or System TC (p. 167) may be used. For these systems, plates impregnated with potassium hydroxide are used.
Location Reagents. Examine the plate under ultraviolet light.
Cover columns 3 to 8 with a glass plate and spray columns 1 and 2 with *acidified iodoplatinate solution.*

Violet or blue colours are given by most basic drugs.
Cover columns 1 and 2 and 5 to 8 with glass plates, and spray columns 3 and 4 lightly with *Mandelin's reagent.* Various colours are given by many basic drugs (p. 137).
Cover columns 1 to 4 and 7 and 8, and spray columns 5 and 6 lightly with 9M sulphuric acid. Most phenothiazines are extensively metabolised, and urine extracts yield a number of spots on the chromatogram with colours ranging from pink to blue.
If a pure solution of a suspected drug has been applied to column 7, spray this and column 8 with a reagent with which it is known to react. Alternatively, if the Rf values and spray reagent reactions derived from columns 1 to 6 suggest the presence of a drug for which a further detection reagent exists, use this reagent on column 8 to obtain additional evidence.
Details of Rf values and spot colours are given in Table 4.
Acidified iodoplatinate solution reacts with many basic drugs to give violet or blue colours. False positive reactions can occur with endogenous urine components; urine extracts from heavy smokers contain nicotine, the metabolites of which coalesce to give a brown spot. Mandelin's reagent reacts with fewer compounds, but gives more distinct colours, and some spots exhibit characteristic fluorescence under ultraviolet light. The presence of drug metabolites in urine extracts can result in a characteristic pattern of spots on the chromatogram.

Table 4. TLC data for some common basic drugs

| Compound | Rf Values in Systems | | | Acidified iodoplatinate solution | Mandelin's reagent | | Metabolites in System TA |
	TA	TB	TC		visible	UV (350 nm)	
Maprotiline	15	17	05	—	—	—	
Protriptyline	19	17	07	violet	pink	green	
Desipramine	26	20	11	violet	blue	—	
Dihydrocodeine	26	08	13	blue	white	—	One at Rf 16; drug and metabolite have elongated spots
Codeine	33	06	18	blue	—	—	
Nortriptyline	34	27	16	violet	violet	yellow (violet centre)	
Morphine	37	00	09	blue	—	—	
Promazine	44	41	30	green	—	—	Many, which give pink or blue spots with 9M sulphuric acid
Brompheniramine	45	33	16	blue	—	—	One, below the parent drug
Chlorpheniramine	45	33	18	violet	—	—	One, below the parent drug

Table 4. TLC data for some common basic drugs (*continued*)

Compound	Rf Values in Systems			Acidified iodoplatinate solution	Mandelin's reagent		Metabolites in System TA
	TA	TB	TC		visible	UV (350 nm)	
Imipramine	48	49	23	violet	blue	quenches	Desipramine; a second metabolite sometimes occurs between imipramine and desipramine
Methadone	48	61	20	pink (grey rim)	—	—	Methadone degradation product at Rf 15
Procyclidine	48	63	31	violet	—	—	
Thioridazine	48	43	30	brown (blue rim)	blue (violet rim)	quenches	Pair of blue spots, with pink spots above and below with *Mandelin's reagent*
Chlorpromazine	49	49	35	violet (blue rim)	pink	yellow (weak)	Many, which give pink or blue spots with 9M sulphuric acid
Promethazine	50	37	35	violet (blue rim)	pink	—	One, below the parent drug
Quinine	50	02	11	violet	—	blue (strong)	One immediately below and one immediately above the parent drug; both strongly fluoresce
Amitriptyline	51	55	32	violet	violet	yellow (violet centre)	Nortriptyline; a second metabolite sometimes occurs between amitriptyline and nortriptyline
Clomipramine	51	54	34	violet	blue	quenches	One or two, both below the parent drug
Dothiepin	51	50	42	red (blue rim)	white	blue (weak)	One or two, both below the parent drug
Doxepin	51	52	37	violet	grey	blue (orange rim)	One or two, both below the parent drug
Pethidine	52	37	34	violet	—	—	One, below the parent drug
Dibenzepin	54	20	35	violet	blue	quenches	Two, both just below the parent drug
Nicotine	54	39	35	brown	—	—	Metabolites coalesce to give spot at Rf 60
Opipramol	54	06	22	blue	yellow	green	
Diphenhydramine	55	45	33	violet	—	—	One or two, both just below the parent drug
Orphenadrine	55	48	33	violet	yellow	blue	One, below the parent drug and with the same reactions to *Mandelin's reagent*
Chlorprothixene	56	51	51	violet	pink	orange	
Cyclizine	57	49	41	violet (blue rim)	—	—	One, below the parent drug
Mianserin	58	39	58	blue	violet	quenches	Two, below the parent drug
Butriptyline	59	61	48	pink	grey	green	One or two, both below the parent drug
Trimipramine	59	62	54	violet	blue	quenches	One or two, both below the parent drug
Carbamazepine	60	04	56	—	yellow (blue rim)	green (strong)	
Pentazocine	61	15	12	violet	grey	white	
Dextropropoxyphene	68	59	55	violet	grey	—	Several; one at Rf 40 which gives a blue streak with *acidified iodoplatinate solution*; the parent drug is rarely seen in urine extracts
Lignocaine*	70	35	73	blue	—	—	
Buclizine	75	61	83	red	—	—	

*Lignocaine is present as a local anaesthetic in various catheter lubricants; urine samples are frequently contaminated with it.

An alternative sequence of spray reagents, and alternative reference compounds, are given for Systems TA, TB, and TC on p. 167, and a comprehensive list of Rf values in these systems will be found in the indexes to Thin-layer Chromatographic Data in Part 3.

Detection of Benzodiazepines in Urine

This test relies on the hydrolysis of benzodiazepines or their metabolites to the corresponding amino-benzophenones. The product is extracted, chromatographed, and detected by the formation of an azo-dye (Bratton Marshall reaction).

Reference Solution. Prepare a solution containing 10 mg of oxazepam and 10 mg of nitrazepam in 100 ml of M hydrochloric acid.

Method. Take two 20-ml screw-capped glass bottles (McCartney bottles) and to the first add 10 ml of the urine and 3 ml of *hydrochloric acid*, and to the second add 9 ml of 'blank' urine, 1 ml of the reference solution, and 3 ml of *hydrochloric acid*. Screw on the caps and heat the bottles in a boiling water-bath for 15 minutes. Cool the solutions, add to each bottle 10 ml of petroleum spirit (b.p. 40°–60°), shake for 5 minutes, and centrifuge. Transfer the solvent layers to 10-ml conical test-tubes, evaporate to dryness under a stream of air or nitrogen, and dissolve the residues in 0.1 ml of methanol.

Divide a TLC plate (silica gel G, 250 μm) into two equal columns and apply 50 μl of each extract to the plate. Develop the plate in a tank containing a 4:1 mixture of chloroform:acetone (System TD, p. 168). After development, dry the plate in a stream of cold air.

Location Reagents. Spray the plate with the following reagents in the sequence shown, drying the plate under warm air after each application.
1. 9M sulphuric acid (spray lightly)
2. A freshly prepared 1% solution of sodium nitrite
3. A 5% solution of ammonium sulphamate
4. N-*(1-naphthyl)ethylenediamine solution*

Chlordiazepoxide, oxazepam, and the metabolites of diazepam and medazepam are hydrolysed to 2-amino-5-chlorobenzophenone, which forms a violet dye with the reagents. The test does not distinguish, therefore, between these drugs.

The test will detect benzodiazepines in urine at therapeutic concentrations but it is not specific. Any compound that yields an aryl amino group on hydrolysis, e.g. phenylbutazone, will respond to the test.

SCHEME 2

Direct Tests on Urine, Stomach Contents, and Blood

Carry out the direct tests described under Scheme 1 (p. 4).

Extraction of Urine

To 10 ml of urine add sufficient *phosphoric acid* or tartaric acid to adjust the pH to 3, extract with two 30-ml portions of ether, combine the ether extracts, wash with 5 ml of water, add the washing to the sample, and retain the aqueous solution for later extraction. Extract the combined ether extracts with 5 ml of saturated sodium bicarbonate solution and retain the aqueous solution for possible examination for the presence of salicylate (Strong Acid Fraction A).

Extract the ethereal solution with 5 ml of 0.5M sodium hydroxide and retain the extract for examination for the presence of barbiturates and other weakly acid substances (Weak Acid Fraction B)—see Table 5.

Wash the ethereal solution with water, discard the washing, dry the solution with anhydrous sodium sulphate, and evaporate to dryness. The residue may contain neutral drugs (Neutral Fraction C)—see Table 5.

To the aqueous solution retained after the first extraction add sufficient *dilute ammonia solution* to adjust the pH to 8, extract with two 10-ml portions of chloroform, wash the combined extracts with water, filter, add a little tartaric acid to prevent the loss of volatile bases, and evaporate to dryness. The residue may contain basic drugs (Basic Fraction D)—see Table 5.

Adjust the aqueous solution obtained after extraction of Fraction D to pH 3 by the addition of *hydrochloric acid*, heat at 100° for 30 minutes, cool, and extract with two 10-ml portions of ether. Reserve the aqueous solution. Wash the combined ether extracts with 5 ml of M sodium hydroxide, and evaporate the ether to dryness. The residue may contain benzophenones (Fraction E)—see Table 5.

Adjust the reserved aqueous solution to pH 9, cool, extract with a mixture of ethyl acetate and isopropyl alcohol (9:1), and evaporate the solvent layer to dryness. The residue may contain opiates (Fraction F)—see Table 5.

Extraction of Stomach Contents

Any fragments of capsules or tablets or any powdery

Scheme for the extraction of drugs from urine and stomach contents

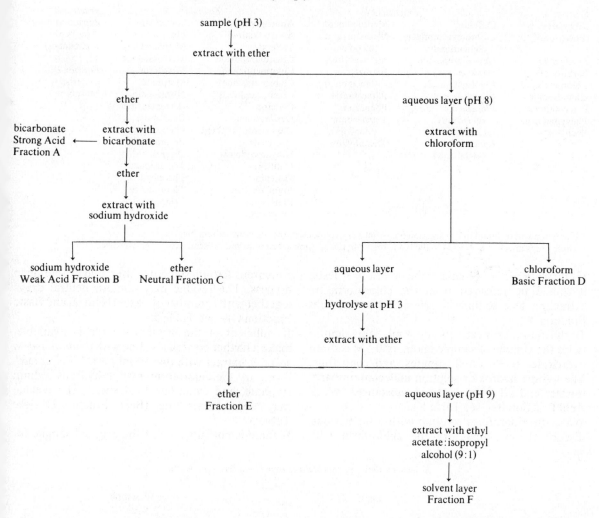

material should be removed and suspended in water for extraction. If the sample contains much food residue or mucus, stable emulsions will be produced during the extraction procedure and the following pre-treatment is necessary.

Add an excess of solid ammonium sulphate together with a few drops of 10% phosphoric acid, heat and stir well, and filter. The filtrate is then extracted by the method described for urine, above.

Extraction of Blood

Because blood, plasma, or serum samples are small and only a limited number of drugs may be easily detected and identified in them, this extraction procedure differs slightly from that for urine and stomach contents.

The initial extraction is carried out at pH 7.4 as many basic drugs are recovered by chloroform extraction at this pH. As a result, the substance looked for is most likely to be found in either fraction B or C, and preparation of fraction D is only necessary either to ensure that nothing has been missed or where no drug has been found in fractions B and C.

To 4 ml of the sample add 2 ml of *phosphate buffer (pH 7.4)* and 40 ml of chloroform, shake vigorously, add about 2 g of anhydrous sodium sulphate, and shake again to produce a solid cake. Decant the chloroform through a filter, extract the cake again with a further 20 ml of chloroform, and combine the chloroform extracts. Retain the sodium sulphate cake.

Table 5. Drugs commonly taken in overdosage, which may be found in the various fractions obtained in the extraction process

Fraction A	*Fraction C*		*Fraction D*		*Fraction E*
Salicylates	Caffeine	Meprobamate	Amitriptyline	Lorazepam	Benzodiazepines
(Phenytoin)*	Carbromal (stomach	Methaqualone	Amphetamine†	Maprotiline	(as benzo-
	contents only)	(blood only)	Caffeine	Methadone	phenones)
Fraction B	Chlordiazepoxide	Methyprylone	Chlordiazepoxide	Methaqualone	
Barbiturates	(blood only)	Nitrazepam	Chlormethiazole	Mianserin	*Fraction F*
Chlorpropamide	Chlormethiazole	(blood only)	Chlorpromazine†	Morphine	Codeine
Glutethimide	Ethchlorvynol	Paracetamol	Clomipramine	Nitrazepam	Morphine
Paracetamol	Flurazepam	Phenazone	Codeine	Orphenadrine	
Phenylbutazone	(blood only)	Temazepam	Desipramine	Oxprenolol	
Phenytoin	Glutethimide	(blood only)	Dextropropoxyphene	Phenelzine†	
	Lorazepam	Theophylline	Diazepam	Propranolol	
	(blood only)		Dihydrocodeine	Quinine	
			Dothiepin	Temazepam	
			Doxepin	Theophylline	
			Ergot alkaloids	Thioridazine†	
			Flurazepam	Trimipramine	
			Imipramine		

* Phenytoin will be found in this fraction only after very vigorous extraction with sodium bicarbonate.
† These drugs may be undetected in the blood owing to the very low concentrations present, even after overdose.

If salicylate has been found in the preliminary tests, it should be removed from the chloroform by extraction with sodium bicarbonate (Strong Acid Fraction A).

To the chloroform extracts add 8 ml, equivalent to twice the volume of sample taken, of 0.5M sodium hydroxide, shake for 2 minutes, and centrifuge. The sodium hydroxide solution may contain barbiturates and other weakly acid substances (Weak Acid Fraction B)—see Table 5.

Wash the chloroform solution with a little water, discard the washing, dry the chloroform with anhydrous sodium sulphate, filter, and evaporate to dryness. The residue may contain neutral drugs together with a number of bases (Neutral and Basic Fraction C)—see Table 5.

If sufficient of the original sample is available, make a further portion alkaline with *dilute ammonia solution*, extract with two 10-ml portions of chloroform, dry the chloroform with anhydrous sodium sulphate, and evaporate to dryness. The residue may contain basic drugs (Basic Fraction D)—see Table 5.

If there is not sufficient of the original sample for

Scheme for the extraction of drugs from blood, serum, or plasma

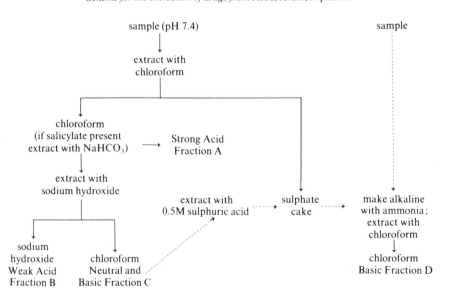

this extraction, the following procedure may be carried out. After fraction C has been examined by the methods described below, dissolve any remaining residue in chloroform and extract with 0.5M sulphuric acid. Add this extract to the sodium sulphate cake retained after the first extraction, make alkaline with *dilute ammonia solution*, and extract with two 10-ml portions of chloroform. Dry the chloroform with anhydrous sodium sulphate and evaporate to dryness. The residue may contain basic drugs (Basic Fraction D)—see Table 5.

Ultraviolet Spectrophotometry of Fractions

The analyst should familiarise himself with the ultraviolet absorption of normal samples of urine, stomach contents, and blood; endogenous substances may interfere with the spectra of any drugs that may be present.

EXAMINATION OF FRACTION B

Barbiturates are a frequent cause of serious poisoning and should be sought first in samples from unconscious patients. The ultraviolet method given below will give a clinically acceptable quantitative result for the blood-barbiturate concentration; the method also permits the detection of other compounds in fraction B.

The method does not distinguish between the common 5,5-substituted barbiturates. If the physician proposes to institute a forced alkaline diuresis or haemodialysis, it is essential to confirm the presence of a long-acting barbiturate (e.g. barbitone, phenobarbitone) by thin-layer chromatography or gas chromatography.

Scan the fraction B extract from 220 to 400 nm against 0.5M sodium hydroxide as the blank. Particularly note the absorbance reading at 255 nm at this pH of 13.

Add 1 ml of a 16% solution of ammonium chloride to the sample and blank solutions and re-scan at this lower pH of 10. Particularly note the absorbance at 240 and 255 nm.

Add a few drops of 10M sulphuric acid to both cells to give pH 2 or less, and re-scan, particularly noting the absorbance at 240 nm. When spectrophotometry is complete, add the pH 2 solution to the remainder of fraction B, acidify the solution, extract with ether, pour the extract through a Whatman No. 90 filter paper, and evaporate to dryness. The residue is retained for chromatographic examination.

Table 6. Ultraviolet spectrophotometry of fraction B

Compound	Absorbance maximum		
	pH 13 nm	pH 10 nm	pH < 2 nm
Chlorpropamide	232	—	232
Barbiturates, N-methyl-substituted	246	246	end absorbance
5,5-substituted	254	239	end absorbance
Paracetamol	257	—	245
Phenylbutazone	264	264	237
Barbiturates, S-substituted	303	—	285

Quantification of Barbiturates

If a 5,5-substituted barbiturate is present, the approximate concentration (μg/ml) in the original sample can be calculated in two ways:

1. (absorption at 255 nm of pH 13 solution) − (absorption at 255 nm of pH 10 solution) × 160
2. (absorption at 240 nm of pH 10 solution) − (absorption at 240 nm of pH 2 solution) × 88

If only a barbiturate is present, good agreement should be obtained from the two calculations. A marked difference between the two suggests the presence of some other substance. The factors given are a compromise; if greater accuracy is required, the modified procedure described by P. M. G. Broughton (*J. Biochem.*, 1956, *63*, 207–213) can be used.

EXAMINATION OF FRACTION C

Dissolve the dry residue in 3 ml of dry methanol and scan the solution between 220 nm and about 320 nm, using methanol as the blank. If no absorbance peaks are detected, it is still possible that a substance with a weak ultraviolet absorbance is present and so the solution is then retained for chromatographic examination. If any absorbance peaks are detected, the solution is acidified by the addition of 2 drops of *hydrochloric acid* and the scan repeated. The ultraviolet spectra of basic compounds extracted from blood at pH 7.4 may differ

Table 7. Ultraviolet spectrophotometry of fraction C

Compound	Absorbance maximum	
	Neutral nm	Acid nm
Lorazepam	230	230 (316)
Methaqualone	265 (306)	234 (269)
Temazepam	230 (314)	237 (284)
Flurazepam	—	240 (284)
Phenacetin	244	244
Chlordiazepoxide	247 (266)	246 (308)
Chlormethiazole	250	258
Caffeine	273	273
Nitrazepam	—	280

considerably from those of the pure compound because of the presence of lipid material and possibly of metabolites.

If the methanol solution has been acidified, dilute it with about ten volumes of water, make alkaline with *dilute ammonia solution*, extract with two 5-ml portions of chloroform, and evaporate the combined chloroform solutions to dryness. The residue is retained for chromatographic examination.

EXAMINATION OF FRACTION D

Dissolve the residue in 4 ml of 0.05M sulphuric acid and scan the solution between 220 and 360 nm. Make the solution alkaline with *dilute sodium hydroxide solution* and again scan the solution. Extract the alkaline solution with chloroform, evaporate the extract to dryness, dissolve the residue in methanol, and scan this neutral solution. The solution is retained for chromatographic examination.

Table 8. Ultraviolet spectrophotometry of fraction D

| | Absorbance maximum | | |
| | Acid | Neutral | Alkaline |
Compound	nm	nm	nm
Dothiepin	230	—	—
Lorazepam	230	230 (316)	—
Methaqualone	234 (269)	265 (306)	—
Temazepam	237 (284)	230 (314)	231 (313)
Amitriptyline	239	239	—
Nortriptyline	239	239	239
Flurazepam	240	—	231
Diazepam	242 (284)	—	—
Chlordiazepoxide	246 (308)	—	262
Desipramine	250	—	250
Trimipramine	250	—	—
Clomipramine	251	—	—
Imipramine	251	—	252
Chlormethiazole	258	—	250
Orphenadrine	264 (258)	—	264 (258)
Maprotiline	272	—	—
Caffeine	273	273	273
Oxprenolol	273	—	—
Mianserin	279	—	—
Nitrazepam	280	—	—
Dihydrocodeine	283	—	283
Codeine	285	286	—
Morphine	285	287	298
Propranolol	288 (305, 319)	290 (306, 319)	—
Doxepin	292	—	—

For data on other compounds see the index of Ultraviolet Absorption Maxima in Part 3.

Chromatography of Fractions

Evaporate to dryness the extracts for fractions B, C, and D, dissolve each in 100 µl of chloroform, and examine by thin-layer chromatography as described for Scheme 1 (p. 7). For fraction B and fraction C use Systems TD, TE, or TF (p. 168), and for fraction D use Systems TA, TB, or TC (p. 167). Fraction E may be examined by gas chromatography using System GA (p. 192); retention indices for benzophenones are given on p. 196.

Fraction F may be examined by thin-layer chromatography using Systems TA, TB, or TC (p. 167), or by gas chromatography using System GA (p. 192). Rf values and retention indices for opiates are given on p. 174 and p. 198, respectively.

GAS CHROMATOGRAPHY FOR DRUG SCREENING

Gas chromatography is a useful adjunct to the schemes previously described. The fractions remaining from Scheme 2 can be examined directly by gas chromatography or, alternatively, the micro-extraction method, described below, can be used.

The most generally useful system for screening is one using a dimethylsilicone stationary phase such as SE-30, OV-1, or OV-101. Volatile amines elute with a better peak shape on alkaline columns such as Apiezon L coated with potassium hydroxide.

Micro-extraction Method

Rapid gas chromatographic screening can be carried out using direct solvent extraction of small volumes of samples. Extractions are performed in small disposable test-tubes, and no transfer or evaporation of solvent is involved, so that drugs are not lost in the procedure. Accurate micro-pipetting and the use of internal standards enables quantification of drugs detected in serum or plasma samples.

Disposable test-tubes approximately 6 cm long with an internal diameter of 5 mm (Dreyer tubes or their equivalent) are used. Samples and aqueous reagents are dispensed using high-precision pipettes (Eppendorf or their equivalent); organic solvents are dispensed using a Hamilton gas-tight, Luer-fitting, glass syringe fitted with a Hamilton repeating mechanism and a stainless steel needle. A standard bench centrifuge (3000 rpm) is adequate for these procedures, but separations are achieved more quickly by using a high-speed (10 000 rpm) centrifuge, although the test-tube adaptors supplied may have to be drilled out to accept Dreyer tubes. The technique is simple, but the analyst should pay careful attention to detail, especially when withdrawing solvent extracts for chromatography.

Method. Dispense appropriate volumes of sample and reagents (e.g. 200 µl of plasma and 50 µl of chloroform) into duplicate test-tubes, and mix for 30 seconds, gently at first and then more vigorously. Centrifuge the tubes for 5 to 10 minutes at 3000 rpm (or 2 to 3 minutes at 10 000 rpm); if emulsions persist after centrifuging, these are readily dispersed by vigorously mixing for 10 seconds and then centrifuging again.

To withdraw an aliquot of the chloroform extract, draw 5 µl of air into the syringe, pass the needle through the aqueous/solvent interface and into the chloroform phase, expel the air gently to dislodge any debris from the needle and draw up the required volume of chloroform, wipe the needle with a tissue, and inject the extract into the chromatograph.

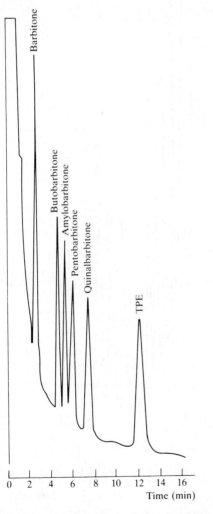

Fig. 1. Chromatogram of a standard solution of barbiturates on System GF, together with tetraphenylethylene (TPE).

Barbiturates and Other Acidic and Neutral Drugs

The plasma or serum extract is examined on two independent columns using 2.5% SE-30 on Chromosorb G (System GA, p. 192), and 3% Poly A103 on Chromosorb W HP (System GF, p. 195). Compounds are identified by reference to retention data derived by chromatographing a solution of the pure drugs in chloroform.

Reference Solutions. Prepare a chloroform solution containing 10 µg/ml of each of barbitone, butobarbitone, amylobarbitone, pentobarbitone, quinalbarbitone, and tetraphenylethylene (internal standard), and inject 3 µl on to both columns to obtain standard chromatograms (e.g. Fig. 1).

Method. To 100 µl of the serum sample add 10 µl of *phosphate buffer (pH 5.6)*, and extract with 100 µl of chloroform containing 10 µg/ml of tetraphenylethylene using the micro-extraction method, above; inject 3 to 5 µl of the chloroform extract on to both columns.

Identify any peaks which appear on the chromatograms by reference to the standard chromatogram and to the retention data listed in Table 9; the index of Gas Chromatographic Data in Part 3 may also be consulted. Corroborative evidence must be obtained from both systems.

For quantification, prepare standard solutions of the identified drug containing 0, 10, 20, 50, and 100 µg/ml in plasma. Examine at least three standards by the same method as used for the sample. Duplicate analyses of samples and standards are essential.

Table 9. Retention indices of some acidic and neutral drugs

Compound	System GA	System GF
Barbitone	1497	2230
Allobarbitone	1606	2340
Butobarbitone	1665	2390
Butalbital	1668	2395
Amylobarbitone	1718	2430
Pentobarbitone	1740	2465
Vinbarbitone	1740	2495
Quinalbarbitone	1791	2510
Meprobamate	1796	2460
Glutethimide	1836	2315
Phenazone	1848	2445
Hexobarbitone	1857	2380
Phenobarbitone	1957	2960
Cyclobarbitone	1963	2825
Heptabarbitone	2058	2940
Methaqualone	2125	2580
Phenylbutazone	2365	2860

Extracts from plasma samples derived from patients intoxicated with glutethimide give rise to several peaks due to the presence of metabolites (see monograph for Glutethimide).
Retention indices for other drugs in these two systems will be found in the index to Gas Chromatographic Data in Part 3.

The standard solutions of various drugs in plasma may be dispensed into aliquots of 0.5 ml, and stored frozen until required for use.

Measure the peak-height ratio of the drug to the internal standard for each extract, and construct a calibration curve by plotting the mean peak-height ratio against the known concentration of the drug. Read off the concentration of drug in the sample directly from the graph. Alternatively, calculate the mean calibration gradient from the standards and divide this into the mean peak-height ratio of the sample duplicates.

Standard solutions of drugs can also be prepared in chloroform and these can be injected directly on to the chromatograph. The solutions should contain 10, 20, 50, and 100 µg/ml of the drug together with 10 µg/ml of tetraphenylethylene; they can be stored at 4° in the dark when not in use. If these standards are used, account must be taken of the incomplete recovery of the individual drugs from plasma. Thus, having derived the apparent drug concentration in the sample by measurement of the peak-height ratio, this value should be multiplied by the appropriate recovery correction factor (Table 10).

Table 10. Correction factors for the recovery of acidic and neutral drugs from plasma

Allobarbitone	1.32	Hexobarbitone	1.10
Amylobarbitone	1.10	Meprobamate	1.56
Barbitone	2.33	Methaqualone	1.14
Butalbital	1.00	Pentobarbitone	1.10
Butobarbitone	1.20	Phenobarbitone	1.28
Cyclobarbitone	1.12	Phenylbutazone	1.25
Glutethimide	1.00	Quinalbarbitone	1.18
Heptabarbitone	1.15	Vinbarbitone	1.00

Basic and Neutral Drugs

The preferred sample for this analysis is stomach contents, since the quantities of drug present are normally higher than in a urine sample. Urine can be used, but a concomitant analysis by thin-layer chromatography is advisable. The extract from stomach contents or urine is examined on two independent columns using 2.5% SE-30 on Chromosorb G (System GA, p. 192), and 3% Poly A103 on Chromosorb W HP (System GF, p. 195). Compounds are identified by reference to retention data derived by chromatographing a solution of pure drugs in chloroform.

Reference Solutions. Prepare chloroform solutions containing standard mixtures of drugs, all at concentrations of 10 µg/ml, and inject 3 µl on to both columns. The composition of these solutions

and the appearance of the chromatogram are shown in Fig. 2.

Method. To 100 µl of stomach contents or urine add 50 µl of M sodium hydroxide and extract with 100 µl of chloroform containing 10 µg/ml of tetraphenylethylene by the micro-extraction method, above; inject 3 to 5 µl of the chloroform extract on to both columns.

Identify any peaks which appear on the chromatograms by reference to the standard chromatogram and to the retention data listed in Table 11; the indexes of Gas Chromatographic Data in Part 3

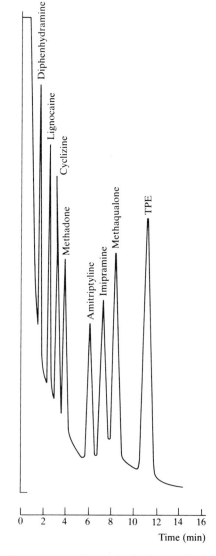

Fig. 2. Chromatogram of a standard solution of basic drugs on System GF, together with tetraphenylethylene (TPE).

may also be consulted. Corroborative evidence must be obtained from both systems.

Note that when urine samples are analysed, two or more peaks may appear on the chromatogram due to characteristic metabolite patterns.

Table 11. Retention indices of basic and neutral drugs and some metabolites and degradation products

Compound	System GA	GF
Methyprylone	1529	2090
Norpethidine	1745	—
Pethidine	1751	1995
Meprobamate	1796	2460
Pheniramine	1804	2100
Caffeine	1810	2340
Glutethimide	1836	2315
Phenazone	1848	2445
Ethoheptazine	1857	2110
Lignocaine	1870	2240
Diphenhydramine	1873	2105
Doxylamine	1906	2170
N-Monodesmethylorphenadrine	1920	—
Imipramine N-oxide (degradation product)	1920	2280
Amitriptyline N-oxide (degradation product)	1930	2320
Iminostilbene	1930	2620
Orphenadrine	1936	2185
2-Ethyl-5-methyl-3,3-diphenyl-1-pyrroline (methadone metabolite)	1950	2190
Atropine degradation product	1970	2240
Nefopam	2000	2380
Chlorpheniramine	2002	2335
Cyclizine	2020	2320
Carbamazepine-10,11-epoxide	2030	2560
2-Ethylidene-1,5-dimethyl-3,3-diphenylpyrrolidine (methadone metabolite)	2030	2280
Atropine degradation product	2040	2340
Norcyclizine	2050	—
Benzoctamine	2082	2445
Hyoscine degradation product	2085	2440
Brompheniramine	2096	2470
Dicyclomine	2097	2265
Diphenylpyraline	2099	2405
Methaqualone	2125	2580
Methadone	2148	2370
Hyoscine degradation product	2150	2520
Procyclidine	2156	2485
Butriptyline	2181	2465
Dextropropoxyphene	2188	2370
Amitriptyline	2196	2510
Atropine	2199	2660
Trimipramine	2201	2505
Nortriptyline	2210	—
Mianserin	2211	2595
Doxepin	2217	2570
Mepyramine	2220	2560
Imipramine	2223	2540
Chlorcyclizine	2225	2560
Monodesmethyldoxepin	2235	—

Table 11 (*continued*)

Compound	System GA	GF
Desipramine	2242	—
N-Monodesmethyltrimipramine	2250	—
Promethazine	2259	2675
Protriptyline	2261	2590
Pentazocine	2275	3030
Carbamazepine	2290	2610
Hyoscine	2303	2885
Promazine	2316	2745
Maprotiline	2356	—
10-Hydroxyamitriptyline (stereoisomers)	2360	2830 or 2880
Dihydrocodeine	2363	2840
Codeine	2376	2860
Dothiepin	2380	2770
10-Hydroxynortriptyline	2385	—
Monodesmethyldothiepin	2390	—
Clomipramine	2406	2795
Diazepam	2425	3045
Dibenzepin	2443	2885
Dothiepin sulphoxide	2450	2820
Dipipanone	2474	2710
Chlorpromazine	2486	2940
Disopyramide	2495	2910
Metoclopramide	2630	—
Trimethoprim	2638	—
Trifluoperazine	2683	3050
Flurazepam	2785	3210
Prochlorperazine	2954	—

Amphetamines and Other Volatile Bases

The extract from stomach contents or urine is examined on two independent columns using 2.5% SE-30 on Chromosorb G (System GA, p. 192), and 10% Apiezon L with 2% potassium hydroxide on Chromosorb W HP (System GB, p. 193). Compounds are identified by reference to retention data derived by chromatographing a solution of pure drugs in chloroform.

Reference Solutions. Prepare chloroform solutions containing standard mixtures of drugs, all at concentrations of 5 µg/ml, and inject 3 to 5 µl on to both columns to obtain the standard chromatogram.

Method. To 100 µl of stomach contents or 500 µl of urine add 100 µl of M sodium hydroxide, and extract with 100 µl of chloroform by the microextraction method (above); inject 3 to 5 µl of the chloroform extract on to both columns. Identify any peaks which appear on the chromatograms by reference to the standard chromatogram and to the retention data given on p. 193. Corroborative evidence must be obtained from both systems.

Volatile Hypnotics

This procedure uses gas chromatography to identify and quantify chlormethiazole, ethchlorvynol, and trichloroethanol in plasma. System GA (p. 192) may be used as an alternative to the system described below.

Reference Solution. Prepare a solution in chloroform containing 30 μg/ml of ethchlorvynol, 50 μg/ml of each of chlormethiazole and trichloroethanol, and 25 μg/ml of 2-methylnaphthalene (internal standard). Inject 3 μl of this solution on to the gas chromatographic column to obtain the standard chromatogram.

Method. Extract 100 μl of plasma with 100 μl of chloroform by the micro-extraction method (described above), and inject 3 to 5 μl of the chloroform extract on to the column, using the following system.

COLUMN. 2% w/w Carbowax 20M and 5% w/w potassium hydroxide on 80 to 100 mesh Chromosorb W HP.

COLUMN TEMPERATURE. 140°

CARRIER GAS. Nitrogen at 60 ml/min.

Identify any peaks which appear on the chromatogram by reference to the standard chromatogram and to the retention data listed in Table 12.

Table 12. Retention data for some volatile hypnotic drugs

Compound	Carbowax RRT	System GA RI
Trichloroethanol	0.52	857
Ethchlorvynol	0.69	1030
2-Methylnaphthalene	1.00	—
Chlormethiazole	1.28	1230

For quantification, prepare standard solutions of the identified drug in chloroform using the concentrations shown in Table 13. Add to each solution 20 μg/ml of 2-methylnaphthalene as internal standard. The standard solutions can be stored at 4° protected from light.

Table 13. Standard solutions of volatile hypnotic drugs

Compound	Concentration (μg/ml)			
Chlormethiazole	10	20	30	40
Ethchlorvynol	20	50	100	150
Trichloroethanol	50	100	150	200

Inject 3 to 5 μl of at least three of the standard solutions on to the column. Duplicate analyses of samples and standards are essential. Measure the peak-height ratio of the drug to the internal standard for each solution, and construct a calibration curve by plotting the mean peak-height ratios against the known concentrations of the drugs. Read off the apparent concentration of drug in the sample directly from the graph. The values for each

duplicate sample extract should agree to within 10%; if the difference is greater, further duplicates should be extracted.

Alternatively, calculate the mean calibration gradient from the standard solutions and divide this into the mean peak-height ratio of the sample.

The mean apparent drug concentration should be multiplied by the appropriate recovery correction factor in order to take account of the incomplete recovery of the individual drugs from plasma. These correction factors are, for chlormethiazole 1.04, for ethchlorvynol 1.05, and for trichloroethanol 1.33.

Tests for Specific Compounds and Groups of Compounds

ALCOHOLS

Ethanol is frequently taken at the same time as other drugs and can intensify the action of depressant drugs. A blood-ethanol determination assists in distinguishing this from normal alcoholic intoxication; it is also useful in the clinical assessment of unconscious patients admitted with head injuries and smelling of drink. Children are particularly at risk from hypoglycaemia which may follow ingestion of alcohol.

Methanol is available in a variety of commercial products (antifreeze preparations, windscreen-washer additives, duplicating fluids). Poisoning is often associated with a delayed onset of coma, marked metabolic acidosis, electrolyte imbalance, and hyperglycaemia, with a raised serum amylase. Therapy with ethanol infusions must be instituted without delay.

A qualitative test for alcohols in urine or blood is given on p. 4. Alcohols are preferably detected and measured in blood by gas chromatography, see below.

An enzymatic assay kit for ethanol in blood is available (see Reagent Appendix).

CONFIRMATION OF METHANOL

To 1 ml of urine add 1 drop of 2.5% potassium dichromate in 50% sulphuric acid and allow to stand at room temperature for 5 minutes. Add 1 drop of ethanol and a few milligrams of chromotropic acid and then add *sulphuric acid* so that it forms a layer in the bottom of the tube. A violet colour at the interface indicates methanol. Note that formaldehyde will also give a positive reaction in this test.

Gas Chromatography of Alcohols

This procedure will identify and quantify the common alcohols in blood and urine. The column used is 0.3% Carbowax 20M on Carbopak C. The system is the same as System GI for Solvents and Other Volatile Compounds (p. 199) except that for this purpose it is operated isothermally at 120°.

IDENTIFICATION OF ALCOHOLS

Reference Solution. Prepare an aqueous solution containing 0.2 mg/ml of each of ethanol, methanol, isopropyl alcohol, and propanol, and inject 1 µl on to the column. The retention data for these compounds are listed in Table 14.

Method. Add 50 µl of whole blood or urine to 0.5 ml of distilled water in a stoppered test-tube, mix in a vortex mixer, and inject 1 µl on to the column. Identify any peaks which appear by reference to the standard chromatogram.

Table 14. Retention times of alcohols relative to propanol

Water	0.30	Isopropyl alcohol	0.79
Methanol	0.36	Propanol	1.00
Ethanol	0.50		

QUANTIFICATION OF ETHANOL OR METHANOL IN BLOOD OR URINE

Standard solutions should be prepared at least once a week and stored at 4°. Hamilton dispensers should be used to deliver accurate small volumes of the solutions, and great care should be taken to avoid cross-contamination of solutions if the same dispenser is used for different solutions.

Internal Standard Solution. Add 100 µl of propanol to 500 ml of distilled water. This gives a solution containing 0.16 g/litre.

Standard Alcohol Solutions. Add 100 µl of dehydrated alcohol or of methanol to 100 ml of distilled water. Add 50 µl to 250 µl of this solution, in increments of 50 µl, to 1.0-ml aliquots of the internal standard solution in stoppered test-tubes. This gives standard alcohol solutions equivalent to 0.04, 0.08, 1.20, 1.60, and 2.0 g/litre.

Method. Add 50 µl of the blood or urine sample to 0.5 ml of the internal standard solution in a micro test-tube (Dreyer tube), mix for a few seconds, and inject 1 µl on to the column. The test samples should be analysed in duplicate.

Inject 1-µl aliquots of at least two of the standard alcohol solutions.

Measure the peak-height ratio of ethanol (or methanol) to that of the internal standard for each sample extract and each standard solution. Plot the peak-height ratio value against the designated alcohol concentration for each standard, and use the mean peak-height ratio for the sample duplicates to read off the alcohol concentration in the sample.

Alternatively, divide the peak-height ratio for each standard by the designated alcohol concentration to obtain calibration gradient values. Take the mean of these, and divide this figure into the mean peak-height ratio value for the test sample, to give the alcohol concentration directly.

AMITRIPTYLINE AND OTHER TRICYCLIC ANTIDEPRESSANTS

In overdose, these drugs have a cardio-respiratory depressant action leading to hypoxia and either respiratory or metabolic acidosis. Deep coma and convulsions can occur.

Alkaline extracts of samples of urine or stomach contents may be examined by thin-layer chromatography using Systems TA, TB, or TC (p. 167). Alternatively, the samples may be examined by gas chromatography using Systems GA or GF (p. 192) together with the micro-extraction method (p. 14). High pressure liquid chromatography systems for antidepressants (Systems HA and HF) are described on p. 214.

Note that amitriptyline, imipramine, and other tertiary amines give rise to the corresponding demethylated metabolites in urine samples. Measurement of plasma concentrations of these drugs is rarely necessary and should only be carried out by specific gas chromatographic procedures.

AMPHETAMINES, OTHER STIMULANTS, AND ANORECTICS

These drugs can be analysed by thin-layer chromatography using Systems TA, TB, or TC (p. 167). However, samples of urine or stomach contents are best analysed by gas chromatography (p. 17).

BARBITURATES

Barbituric acid derivatives account for a high proportion of poisonings, the severity being related to the amount and type of barbiturate ingested. For example, blood concentrations of phenobarbitone or barbitone which do not cause unconsciousness would cause deep coma in the case of pentobarbitone or quinalbarbitone.

Gas chromatography applied to plasma or urine samples is the method of choice (p. 15), as this simultaneously identifies and quantifies the drugs. Alternatively, extract a urine sample with chloroform at acid pH, identify the barbiturate by thin-layer chromatography (p. 7), and determine the concentration by ultraviolet spectrophotometry (p. 13). Chromatographic systems for barbiturates are described on p. 171 (thin-layer chromatography), p. 196 (gas chromatography), and p. 216 (high pressure liquid chromatography).

If more than 2 hours have elapsed since the overdose, barbiturates may have passed from the stomach to the small intestine; in these circumstances, stomach aspirate or washings may give negative analytical results.

BENZODIAZEPINES

Benzodiazepine tranquillisers are widely prescribed and therefore occur more frequently than any other type of drug in overdose cases. Fortunately, the effects of these drugs in overdose are usually mild, although they may have a synergistic effect when taken with alcohol or other drugs. They are extensively metabolised prior to excretion in the urine.

A thin-layer chromatographic method for their detection in urine is described on p. 10; the method cannot distinguish between the various benzodiazepines (other than nitrazepam), but this is rarely important in the acute clinical situation. Concentrations in plasma can be measured by gas chromatography with electron capture detection, but the technique is difficult due to the instability of some of the drugs and their metabolites. Chromatographic systems for benzodiazepines are given on p. 196 (gas chromatography), and p. 216 (high pressure liquid chromatography).

CARBON MONOXIDE

Common sources of carbon monoxide are automobile exhaust fumes, improperly maintained and ventilated heating systems, smoke from fires, and household gas (other than natural gas). The affinity of carbon monoxide for haemoglobin is about 240 times that of oxygen, so that poisoning can occur when only small quantities of the gas are present in the atmosphere. When patients are removed from the contaminated atmosphere, the carboxyhaemoglobin disappears rapidly, particularly if oxygen is administered. Only traces may remain by the time the patient reaches hospital and, therefore, carboxyhaemoglobin measurements are rarely justified in clinical toxicology.

A qualitative test for carbon monoxide in blood is given on p. 6.

Quantification of Carbon Monoxide in Blood

The following method is based on that of E. J. van Kampen and H. Klouwen, *Ned. Tidschr. Geneeskd*, 1954, *98*, 161–164, and *Rec. Trav. Chim. des Pays Bas*, 1954, *73*, 119–128.

The method depends on the fact that normal blood contains several forms of haemoglobin, e.g. the reduced form, the oxygenated form, and a small amount of methaemoglobin. If a reducing agent such as sodium dithionite is added to the blood, both the oxygenated form and the methaemoglobin are quantitatively converted to the reduced form, which has the visible spectrum B shown in Fig. 3. Carbon monoxide has a much greater affinity for haemoglobin than has oxygen, and carboxyhaemoglobin is not reduced by sodium dithionite. Thus, even when treated with sodium dithionite, carboxyhaemoglobin retains its normal twin-peaked spectrum, marked A in Fig. 3. The wavelength of

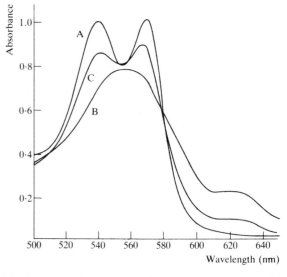

Fig. 3. Ultraviolet spectra of (A) carboxyhaemoglobin, (B) reduced haemoglobin, and (C) a blood sample from a patient poisoned with carbon monoxide.

maximum absorbance difference for spectra A and B is at 540 nm, whilst at 579 nm the spectra have the same absorbance (isosbestic point). The percentage carbon monoxide-saturation of a blood sample can be calculated from measurements of the absorbance at these wavelengths of the carbon monoxide-saturated sample (A), the carbon monoxide-free sample (B), and the untreated sample

(C), after reduction of each with sodium dithionite. *Method.* Dilute 0.2 ml of the blood sample (mixed well) with 25 ml of a 0.1% solution of ammonia and divide the resulting solution into three approximately equal parts labelled A, B, and C. Saturate solution A with carbon monoxide by bubbling the gas through it in a wide container and at a rate which minimises frothing. A few minutes bubbling should suffice. Saturate solution B with pure oxygen for 10 minutes to displace all the strongly bound carbon monoxide.

Add a small amount of sodium dithionite to each of the solutions A, B, and C, and also to 10 ml of 0.1% ammonia solution, and mix well. Place matched 1-cm cells containing the ammonia solution into the sample and reference beams of a spectrophotometer which has been set to record between the wavelengths 500 and 650 nm, in the superimposed, repeat-scan mode on a range of 0 to 2 absorbance units. Record the baseline for the determination. Then record the absorbance spectra for solutions A, B, and C. Wash out the sample cell thoroughly between the recordings and wash the cell with a little of the solution whose absorbance is about to be recorded.

If the blood sample was from a person who died from inhalation of carbon monoxide, a set of spectra as shown in Fig. 3 should be obtained.

Measure the absorbances of each solution at 540 nm and 579 nm, and calculate the ratio of absorbance at 540 to that at 579 nm for each of the solutions A, B, and C.

The percentage carboxyhaemoglobin-saturation is calculated as follows:

$$\% \text{ saturation} = \frac{\text{ratio for C} - \text{ratio for B}}{\text{ratio for A} - \text{ratio for B}} \times 100$$

Approximate normal values for the ratios of absorbance are: saturated carboxyhaemoglobin 1.5, and reduced haemoglobin 1.1.

Note that the haemoglobin content of blood can vary, and therefore the volume of diluent may also need to be varied. A dilution giving a maximum absorbance of about 1 is ideal.

Carbon monoxide in blood may also be quantified using an automated visible spectrophotometer (IL 282 Co-oximeter, see Reagent Appendix), which utilises four wavelengths to measure haemoglobin, oxyhaemoglobin, carboxyhaemoglobin, and methaemoglobin in small blood samples. Reference standards are commercially available (see Reagent Appendix).

CARBROMAL

This bromureide derivative is considered obsolete but may still occur in cases of poisoning. The symptoms following overdose are similar to those of barbiturate poisoning.

Test for Carbromal and Other Organic Bromine Compounds
Acidify a portion of stomach contents with 2M hydrochloric acid, and extract with four times its volume of chloroform; evaporate the extract to dryness, dissolve the residue in 0.5 ml of ethanol, transfer the solution to a white porcelain dish, add 2 drops of 2M sodium hydroxide, and dry with gentle heat. Cool, add 2 drops of a 1% solution of fluorescein, 4 drops of *acetic acid*, and 4 drops of *strong hydrogen peroxide solution*, and evaporate to dryness on a boiling water-bath. A red colour, due to eosin, indicates the presence of carbromal, bromvaletone, or other organic bromine compounds.

CHLORMETHIAZOLE

Chlormethiazole is widely used as a sedative in the treatment of alcoholism but tolerance develops rapidly. However patients often stop taking the drug. If, following a bout of heavy drinking, a large dose of chlormethiazole is taken, the patient collapses into deep coma accompanied by respiratory depression, hypotension, and hypothermia.

Test for Chlormethiazole
To 2 ml of plasma add 0.5 ml of M sodium hydroxide, extract with 5 ml of chloroform, centrifuge, discard the aqueous phase, and filter the chloroform. Extract the filtrate with 2 ml of 0.1M sulphuric acid, and scan the ultraviolet absorption of the acid solution between 200 and 300 nm. Chlormethiazole gives a well-defined absorbance maximum at 258 nm.

The above procedure may be used as the basis of a quantitative determination. Alternatively, gas chromatography may be used (p. 17).

CHLORATES AND OTHER OXIDISING AGENTS

Sodium and potassium chlorates are popular weedkillers which are highly toxic after oral ingestion. Cyanosis and methaemoglobinaemia are common features of poisoning with these substances. A test for oxidising agents in stomach contents is given on p. 5.

ETHCHLORVYNOL

The clinical features of overdose with ethchlorvynol resemble those due to poisoning with other hypnotics, but coma is often prolonged and accompanied by severe respiratory depression. Ethchlorvynol has a pungent odour which is often detected in the stomach contents. A qualitative test for ethchlorvynol in stomach contents is given on p. 6. A gas chromatographic method for the quantification of ethchlorvynol in plasma is given on p. 17.

GLUTETHIMIDE

Glutethimide intoxication resembles that of barbiturates in many respects, but is characterised by a fluctuating state of consciousness which may be due to the production of the active derivative, 4-hydroxyglutethimide.

Test for Glutethimide

To 1 ml of blood or stomach contents add 10 ml of chloroform, shake gently for 5 minutes, centrifuge, and filter the chloroform layer through a Whatman No. 1 filter paper. To the filtrate add 2 ml of 0.5M sodium hydroxide, shake for 2 to 3 minutes, centrifuge, separate the chloroform layer, filter it into a dry tube, and evaporate to dryness. Dissolve the residue in 2 ml of methanol and scan the ultraviolet absorption of the solution from 220 to 270 nm. Glutethimide has a maximum at 235 nm.

Add 2 drops of 10M sodium hydroxide and immediately scan the solution again. If glutethimide is present, the peak at 235 nm diminishes rapidly due to hydrolysis of the piperidine ring.

Glutethimide can also be detected by thin-layer chromatography (p. 7). For quantification, gas chromatography is the method of choice (p. 15).

IRON

Poisoning with iron salts is extremely dangerous, particularly in young children. Rapid necrosis of the gastro-intestinal mucosa occurs, with haemorrhage and fluid and electrolyte loss. The absorbed iron rapidly exceeds the binding capacity of transferrin, and free iron accumulates in the serum. The determination of the serum-iron concentration is required when intravenous infusions of the chelating antidote (desferrioxamine) are given.

A green or blue colour in the vomit or stomach aspirate suggests the presence of iron salts.

A qualitative test for the presence of iron salts in stomach contents is given on p. 5, and a quantitative method to determine serum-iron concentration is given on p. 60.

Commercial serum-iron assay kits are available (see Reagent Appendix).

MEPROBAMATE AND OTHER CARBAMATES

Meprobamate causes coma, respiratory depression, and hypotension when taken in overdose.

Test for Carbamates in Stomach Contents

Acidify a portion of the sample with 2M hydrochloric acid, extract with four times its volume of chloroform, separate the chloroform layer, and evaporate to dryness. Dissolve the residue in 0.5 ml of ethanol and spot a 0.1-ml portion on to a filter paper; stain the spot with 0.01 ml of *furfuraldehyde solution*, allow to dry, and expose the paper to the fumes of hydrochloric acid for 2 to 3 minutes. A black spot indicates the presence of a carbamate.

Meprobamate can be detected and quantified by gas chromatography (p. 15).

ORGANOPHOSPHORUS PESTICIDES

There are no simple direct chemical tests for organophosphorus compounds. The toxic effects are usually associated with depression of the cholinesterase activity of the body, and measurement of the plasma or serum cholinesterase can be used, therefore, as an indication of organophosphorus poisoning.

Plasma or serum cholinesterase (pseudocholinesterase) is inhibited by a number of compounds and can also be decreased in the presence of liver impairment. Erythrocyte cholinesterase (true cholinesterase) reflects more accurately the cholinesterase status of the central nervous system. However, pseudocholinesterase activity responds more quickly to an inhibitor and returns to normal more rapidly than erythrocyte-cholinesterase activity. Thus, measurement of pseudocholinesterase activity is quite adequate as a means of diagnosing acute exposure to organophosphorus compounds, but cases of illness which may be due to chronic exposure to these compounds should also be investigated by determining the erythrocyte-cholinesterase activity. A colorimetric method for this purpose has been reported (K.-B. Augustinsson *et al.*, *Clinica chim. Acta*, 1978, *89*, 239–252).

A test for cholinesterase inhibitors in serum is given on p. 6.

Quantification of Cholinesterase Activity in Serum
Adjust the temperature of 3 ml of *dithiobisnitrobenzoic acid solution* to 25°, add 20 μl of the serum sample and 0.1 ml of a 5% solution of acetylthiocholine iodide, mix well, and record the absorbance of a 1-cm layer at 405 nm at 30-second intervals over a period of 2 minutes. If the change in absorbance exceeds 0.2 in 30 seconds, dilute the sample 1 in 10 with normal saline and repeat the measurements (the readings must then be multiplied by 10). The concentration of cholinesterase is calculated as follows:

Cholinesterase (milliunits/ml)
= change in absorbance in 30 seconds × 23 400

Normal values for cholinesterase in serum are 1900 to 4000 milliunits/ml. Commercial kits for the determination of cholinesterase activity are available (see Reagent Appendix).

Alkyl phosphorus compounds can be detected in serum by performing the cholinesterase determination on (a) a sample of normal serum, (b) the test serum, and (c) 10 μl of normal serum + 20 μl of test serum. If a low value is obtained from (b), this could be due to a low cholinesterase from liver disease or other causes. A value for (c) which is lower than the sum of the results from (a) and (b) indicates the presence of an inhibitor. Usually, in organophosphorus poisoning, the result from (c) is lower than that from (a).

PARACETAMOL

Overdose of paracetamol can cause severe and sometimes fatal liver damage. Few symptoms appear on the first day after ingestion, although nausea and vomiting can occur. Liver-function tests become abnormal 12 to 36 hours after overdose, with raised concentrations of serum aminotransferase and bilirubin, and prolongation of the prothrombin time. Antidotes are available (oral methionine, intravenous acetylcysteine), but these are effective only when given within 12 hours of the overdose. The plasma-paracetamol concentration is a reliable indicator of the likelihood of liver damage (see monograph for Paracetamol).

A sensitive direct test on urine is described on p. 5.

Quantification of Paracetamol in Plasma by Colorimetry

After J. P. Glynn and S. E. Kendal, *Lancet*, 1975, *1*, 1147–1148.

Standard Solutions. Dissolve 1 g of paracetamol in the minimum volume of dehydrated alcohol, and dilute to 100 ml with water to give a stock solution containing 10 mg/ml. This solution should be stored frozen. To 20-ml aliquots of normal plasma add 100, 200, 400, 600, and 800 μl of the stock solution to give standard solutions containing 50, 100, 200, 300, and 400 μg/ml of paracetamol. Note that paracetamol is unstable in plasma; fresh plasma standards should be prepared each week and stored at 4° when not in use.

Method. Prepare seven 10-ml centrifuge tubes each containing 2 ml of a 10% solution of trichloroacetic acid. To five of the tubes add 1 ml each of the five standard solutions, and to the other two tubes add 1 ml of normal plasma and 1 ml of the plasma sample respectively. Agitate each tube for a few seconds, and then centrifuge at 3000 rpm for 5 minutes to deposit the protein precipitate.

Prepare seven 30-ml tubes containing 1 ml of 6M hydrochloric acid and 2 ml of a 10% solution of sodium nitrite (freshly prepared); this procedure should be carried out in a fume cupboard.

Carefully remove 2 ml of the supernatant liquid from each of the centrifuge tubes, add to the appropriate 30-ml tube, and allow to stand for 2 to 3 minutes. To each of the tubes add, dropwise, 2 ml of a 15% solution of ammonium sulphamate to remove excess nitrous acid (vigorous frothing occurs), followed by 2 ml of 6M sodium hydroxide; mix for a few seconds to remove any gas bubbles, and measure the intensity of the yellow solutions at 450 nm against the plasma blank. Calculate the concentration of paracetamol in the sample by reference to a calibration curve prepared from the values for the standard solutions. Duplicate analyses of samples and standards should be carried out.

Paracetamol concentrations below 50 μg/ml cannot be measured accurately by this method; for such samples a chromatographic method should be used (see below).

Salicylic acid undergoes a similar reaction, but plasma containing 1000 μg/ml of salicylate yields a colour intensity equivalent to only 20 μg/ml of paracetamol. Samples contaminated with heparin which contains cresol as a preservative can give spurious results as high as 200 μg/ml.

Quantification of Paracetamol in Plasma by an Enzymatic Method

P. M. Hammond *et al.*, *Lancet*, 1981, *1*, 391–392.
This method is based on the enzymatic degradation

of paracetamol by an aryl acylamidase, to yield 4-aminophenol which then reacts with o-cresol in the presence of ammonia and copper ions to give a blue indophenol dye. This method is highly specific; common metabolites of paracetamol (glucuronide, sulphate, mercapturate) do not react. The limit of accurate measurement is approximately 10 µg/ml. The method is available in kit form (see Reagent Appendix).

Quantification of Paracetamol by High Pressure Liquid Chromatography

Standard Solutions. Prepare standard solutions of paracetamol as described in the colorimetric method, above.

Internal Standard Solution. A solution containing 125 µg/ml of N-propyl-4-aminophenol in methanol.

Method. To 50 µl of plasma, serum, or whole blood in a 1-ml polypropylene centrifuge tube add 100 µl of the internal standard solution, mix, and centrifuge for 2 minutes in a microcentrifuge. Examine 5 µl of the supernatant liquid by high pressure liquid chromatography, using the system described below, with ultraviolet detection at 240 nm.

COLUMN. ODS-silica (ODS-Hypersil, 5 µm, 15 cm × 4.6 mm internal diameter).

ELUENT. Methanol:water:*acetic acid*:sodium acetate (200:800:5:5).

Examine the standard solutions by the same procedure.

Paracetamol metabolites, salicylic acid, and salicylic acid metabolites also elute from this system. Retention times relative to paracetamol for these substances in this system are:

Paracetamol glucuronide	0.30
Paracetamol sulphate	0.48
Gentisic acid	0.50
Paracetamol	1.00
Salicylic acid	1.22
Salicyluric acid	1.37
N-propyl-4-aminophenol	1.85

Quantification of Paracetamol by Gas Chromatography

A. Huggett *et al.*, *J. Chromat.*, 1981, *209*, 67–76.

Standard Solutions. Prepare standard solutions of paracetamol in plasma as described for the colorimetric method, above.

Internal Standard Solution. A solution containing 200 µg/ml of N-butyryl-4-aminophenol in chloroform; it should be stored in the dark at 4°.

Acetylating Reagent. A freshly prepared mixture of acetic anhydride:N-methylimidazole:chloroform (5:1:30).

Method. To 100 µl of plasma or serum in a small test-tube add 50 µl of the internal standard solution, 50 µl of *phosphate buffer (pH 7.4)*, and 20 µl of the acetylating agent. Mix for 30 seconds, and centrifuge at 7500 rpm for 3 minutes. Withdraw 3 to 5 µl of the chloroform extract and examine by gas chromatography using the system described below, and a flame ionisation detector.

Examine the standard solutions by the same procedure.

COLUMN. 3% Apolane-87 on 100–120 mesh Chromosorb W HP, 1.5 m × 4 mm internal diameter glass column.

COLUMN TEMPERATURE. 235°

CARRIER GAS. Nitrogen at 40 ml/min.

Paracetamol and N-butyryl-4-aminophenol elute with retention times of approximately 2 minutes and 3 minutes, respectively.

PARAQUAT AND DIQUAT

Granular preparations usually contain 2.5% of paraquat and 2.5% of diquat; liquid preparations may contain 20% w/v of paraquat only. Treatment consists of reducing paraquat absorption by administering copious amounts of the adsorbents Fuller's Earth or bentonite, with cathartics. Active elimination techniques (forced diuresis, haemodialysis, charcoal haemoperfusion) may also be applied.

A plasma-paraquat assay is a reliable indicator of whether a dangerous amount of the herbicide has been ingested. Patients whose plasma concentrations do not exceed 2.0, 0.6, 0.3, 0.16, and 0.1 µg/ml at 4, 6, 10, 16, and 24 hours, respectively, after ingestion are likely to survive. The main use of an assay is in the prevention of overtreatment of patients who are not at risk.

Test for Paraquat and Diquat in Urine or in Stomach Contents

Paraquat and diquat are readily detected in urine or stomach contents by the test given on p. 5.

This test may also be carried out by an alternative procedure in which the reducing reagent is prepared in encapsulated form. Mix together thoroughly 10 g of sodium dithionite, 6 g of disodium tetraborate and 25 g of sodium bicarbonate; pack the mixture into gelatine capsules (gauge 0) to produce about 40 capsules. To carry out the test, tip the contents of 1 capsule into 10 ml of urine or stomach contents, and shake to dissolve. A blue colour, due to the reduction of paraquat to its free radical, indicates the presence of paraquat. A reference solution of paraquat (5 µg/ml) should be tested at the same time. The contents of the capsules are stable for at least 6 months at room temperature.

Quantification of Paraquat in Plasma by Colorimetry

After D. R. Jarvie and M. J. Stewart, *Clinica chim. Acta*, 1979, *94*, 241–251.

Standard Solutions. Prepare standard solutions of paraquat in plasma containing 0, 0.1, 0.2, 0.5, 1.0, and 2.0 µg of paraquat ion per ml; store frozen until required.

Extraction Solvent. Mix 50 ml of water-saturated isobutyl methyl ketone with 50 ml of water-saturated isobutanol, and add 0.5 g of sodium dodecyl sulphate.

Method. To 2 ml of plasma in a 15-ml glass-stoppered centrifuge tube add 2 ml of water and 10 ml of the extraction solvent, mix gently for 5 minutes on a roller mixer, and centrifuge for 5 minutes at 3000 rpm. Carefully remove 8 ml of the solvent phase, transfer it to a second tube containing 0.8 ml of 2.5M sodium chloride, stopper the tube, shake vigorously for 5 minutes, and centrifuge for 2 minutes at 3000 rpm. Carefully remove the solvent phase, transfer 0.7 ml of the aqueous phase to a 4-ml glass tube, add 100 µl of a freshly-prepared 3% solution of sodium dithionite in 0.3M sodium hydroxide, shake the mixture briefly, transfer to a semi-micro quartz cuvette, and immediately scan the solution between 384 nm and 460 nm against a blank containing 0.7 ml of 2.5M sodium chloride and 100 µl of the sodium dithionite solution.

The absorbance due to paraquat is obtained by subtracting the reading at 460 nm from that at 397 nm. Results for standard solutions treated in the same way are plotted and the concentration in the sample is deduced from the calibration curve.

The method is capable of measuring plasma-paraquat concentrations down to 0.05 µg/ml.

If diquat is also present, this will be extracted and gives rise to additional small peaks between 430 and 460 nm. Corrections can be made for this, but the increase in paraquat concentration is small (10 to 15%) and is usually insignificant in clinical situations.

Quantification of Paraquat in Plasma by Radioimmunoassay

This is the most sensitive and specific method, and can measure plasma-paraquat concentrations as low as 6 ng/ml. No interference with other bipyridyl herbicides occurs. For information see T. Levitt, *Proc. Analyt. Div. Chem. Soc.*, 1979, *16*, 72–76, and D. Fatori and W. M. Hunter, *Clinica chim. Acta*, 1980 *100*, 81–90.

PHENOTHIAZINES

Tests on Urine
1. To 1 ml of urine add 1 ml of *FPN reagent*. A pink, red, orange, violet, or blue colour indicates the presence of a phenothiazine derivative. The colours are transient and should be observed immediately. Positive results can be obtained on urine samples from patients receiving therapeutic doses.
2. Mix together 98 ml of 30% sulphuric acid and 2 ml of *ferric chloride solution*, and add 1 ml of this reagent to 1 ml of urine. A pale pink colour deepening to blue indicates ingestion of thioridazine. Other phenothiazines can give colours, but the test is more sensitive than FPN reagent towards thioridazine.

Phenothiazines may be determined in urine by the thin-layer chromatographic method described on p. 7. Thin-layer chromatographic systems for phenothiazines are described on p. 174, gas chromatographic systems on p. 198, and high pressure liquid chromatographic systems on p. 219.

PHENYTOIN, PRIMIDONE, AND PHENOBARBITONE

These drugs are commonly prescribed in combination in the treatment of epilepsy. Symptoms of acute overdose simulate those of barbiturate poisoning. Laboratories which offer a routine therapeutic drug monitoring service for these drugs will have little difficulty in adapting their normal procedures to the occasional overdose case. These drugs can be measured simultaneously in plasma samples by gas chromatography using the method described for Barbiturates and other Acidic and Neutral Drugs (p. 15), except that the column used is 2% SP-2110 and 1% SP-2510-DA on Supelcoport (System GE, p. 194).

Two standard plasma solutions are used, the first containing 50 µg/ml of phenobarbitone and 20 µg/ml each of primidone and phenytoin, and the second containing 100 µg/ml of phenobarbitone and 50 µg/ml each of primidone and phenytoin. The internal standard used is either 5-methyl-5-phenylhydantoin or 5-*p*-methylphenyl-5-phenyl-hydantoin.

A high pressure liquid chromatographic system for anticonvulsants is described on p. 215.

QUINIDINE AND QUININE

These stereoisomers have similar toxic properties, severe overdose resulting in cardiac arrhythmias and visual disturbances which sometimes lead to permanent blindness.

Test on Urine for Large Amounts
Make 20 ml of urine alkaline with *dilute ammonia solution*, extract with an equal volume of chloroform, shake the chloroform extract with 3 ml of 10% sulphuric acid, and centrifuge. A blue fluorescence in the acid phase, more noticeable under ultraviolet light, suggests the presence of quinidine or quinine.

Quantification of Quinine and Quinidine by Fluorescence Spectrophotometry

Standard Solutions. Prepare solutions in plasma containing 5, 10, and 20 μg/ml.
Method. To 200 μl of the plasma sample in a 10-ml conical test-tube add 40 μl of 2M tris(hydroxymethyl)methylamine and 4 ml of a mixture of chloroform and isopropyl alcohol (3:1); mix for 30 seconds, and centrifuge for 5 minutes. Carefully transfer the solvent layer to a second test-tube containing 4 ml of 0.05M sulphuric acid, mix, centrifuge for 5 minutes, and carefully transfer about 2 ml of the acid layer to a 1-cm quartz fluorescence cuvette. Excite the extract at 350 nm and measure the intensity of emission at 450 nm. The standard plasma solutions are processed similarly at the same time.

SALICYLIC ACID

Salicylic acid is often found as the hydrolysis product of aspirin or other salicylic acid derivatives. Aspirin is one of the most commonly used analgesics and accounts for a high proportion of serious accidental or deliberate poisonings. Ingestion of more than fifty 300-mg tablets can cause serious toxicity in adults.
The ingestion of methyl salicylate is less common but is particularly dangerous due to rapid absorption; one 5-ml spoonful of methyl salicylate is equivalent to 12 aspirin tablets. Plasma-salicylate measurements are a reliable guide to the severity of poisoning (see the monograph for Salicylic Acid).
Respiratory alkalosis and metabolic acidosis are characteristic features of salicylate poisoning, and blood-gas analyses (oxygen and carbon dioxide) are mandatory. Loss of consciousness is rare except in cases of very severe poisoning with acidaemia. Forced alkaline diuresis is considered if plasma-salicylate concentrations exceed 500 μg/ml, and if marked clinical features or acidosis are present.

Tests on Urine and Stomach Contents
Tests for the presence of salicylates in urine or stomach contents are given on p. 4 and p. 5, respectively.

Quantification of Salicylic Acid in Plasma by Colorimetry

Standard Solutions. Prepare aqueous solutions containing 0, 200, 500, and 800 μg/ml of salicylic acid; they should be stored frozen when not in use.
Method. Place 1 ml of the plasma sample in a 15-ml centrifuge tube, add 5 ml of *Trinder's reagent*, mix for 30 seconds, centrifuge for 5 minutes at 2400 rpm, and measure the colour intensity of the supernatant liquid at 540 nm. Determine the concentration by comparison with the standard solutions.

Quantification of Salicylic Acid in Plasma by High Pressure Liquid Chromatography

Salicylic acid may be determined by the method described for paracetamol, p. 24, using standard solutions in plasma or whole blood containing 0, 100, 200, 400, and 800 μg/ml of salicylic acid.

THEOPHYLLINE

Serious overdose with this xanthine bronchodilator can provoke serious hypotension, cardiac arrhythmias, and convulsions. These symptoms indicate a poor prognosis, particularly in elderly patients. Symptoms of poisoning after a high dose of a slow-release preparation can be delayed for several hours as the drug gradually accumulates to toxic concentrations. Patients with plasma concentrations greater than 60 μg/ml may require charcoal haemoperfusion.
Commercial immunoassay kits are available for the determination of theophylline in serum or plasma.

Quantification of Theophylline in Plasma by High Pressure Liquid Chromatography

Internal Standard Solution. A solution containing 5 μg/ml of 8-chlorotheophylline in M sodium acetate.
Method. To 50 μl of plasma (or serum) in a 10-ml

centrifuge tube add 100 µl of internal standard solution, and 2 ml of a mixture of chloroform and isopropyl alcohol (9:1); mix, and centrifuge at 3000 rpm for 5 minutes. Transfer the solvent phase to a second tube, and evaporate to dryness under a stream of air or nitrogen at 50°. Examine the residue by high pressure liquid chromatography, using the system described below, by dissolving the residue in 20 µl of the eluent and injecting 10 µl on to the column.

COLUMN. ODS-silica (ODS-Hypersil, 5 µm).

ELUENT. Mix together 100 ml of methanol, 30 ml of tetrahydrofuran, and 900 ml of water, add 1 ml of *acetic acid*, and adjust the pH to 5.6 by the addition of *sodium hydroxide solution*.

The adjustment of the pH is critical for the separation of 8-chlorotheophylline. UV detection is at 280 nm.

Other xanthines and xanthine metabolites also elute from this system. Retention times relative to theophylline are: 3-methylxanthine, 0.49; theobromine, 0.63; paraxanthine, 0.88; caffeine, 1.36; 8-chlorotheophylline, 1.46.

TRICHLORO-COMPOUNDS

Chloral hydrate and dichloralphenazone are metabolised to trichloroethanol, which is the major active product of these drugs. Trichloroethanol can be determined in plasma or serum by gas chromatography (p. 17).

A test for the presence of trichloro-compounds in urine is given on p. 5.

Screening for Drugs of Abuse

Analytical methods for use in the investigation of drug dependence are given below, together with techniques for the detection of other substances which may be abused. These include volatile solvents (p. 31), diuretics (p. 32), and laxatives (p. 32).

EXTRACTION OF URINE FOR DEPENDENCE-PRODUCING DRUGS

Patients attending a clinic for the treatment of drug dependence are routinely asked for a sample of urine for analysis. Thereafter, periodic tests are carried out as a check on whether the patient is complying with prescribed medication or is also taking drugs obtained illicitly. Laboratories which offer a routine service to treatment clinics may have to cope with batches of 50 or more samples at a time. The scheme described below has been designed with this in mind, although single samples can be dealt with in the same way.

Two methods are described, one using direct solvent extraction, and the other a solid-liquid elution system which is quicker and more amenable to processing a large number of samples. In both methods, a pH of 9 is selected to ensure good extraction of morphine. In strongly alkaline conditions, morphine forms a phenolic ion which has poor solubility in the solvent used.

Solvent Extraction

Place 10 ml of urine in each of two 20-ml glass bottles fitted with plastic screw-caps (McCartney bottles), and to one bottle add 1 to 2 ml of M sulphuric acid and to the other add sufficient sodium bicarbonate to saturate the solution. Label the bottles A and B (acids and bases) respectively. Fill each bottle with a mixture of chloroform and isopropyl alcohol (9:1), screw on the caps, shake for 5 minutes, and centrifuge for 5 to 10 minutes. Aspirate the top aqueous phase using a Pasteur pipette connected to a water-operated vacuum pump, filter the chloroform extracts through phase-separating paper to remove residual water, and collect the filtrates in 10-ml conical test-tubes; evaporate to dryness under a stream of air or nitrogen, reconstitute the residues in 100 µl of chloroform, and analyse by thin-layer chromatography.

Solid-liquid Extraction

This method uses commercially-prepared columns containing granules of diatomaceous earth with a large pore volume (e.g. Tox Elut, Extrelut, see Reagent Appendix). The urine sample is poured on to the column followed by organic solvent which percolates rapidly through the granules and extracts lipid-soluble drugs and metabolites. Particulate material, pigments, and polar metabolites are retained in the diatomaceous earth. Further purification of the organic extract takes place as it passes through the dry region of the column.

Add 20 ml of urine to the column (use a ready-buffered column at pH 9), and allow the sample to soak into the packing material for 2 minutes. Place a 50-ml test-tube under the column outlet, and pour 15 ml of a mixture of chloroform and isopropyl alcohol (9:1) on to the column. When the first elution is complete, add a further 15 ml of the solvent and collect the eluate in the same test-tube.

Insert into the top of the column a hollow rubber stopper connected by a rubber tube to a pressure bulb, and apply gentle pressure to discharge residual solvent. Place the tube containing the eluates in a beaker of hot water and evaporate the extract to dryness under a stream of air. Dissolve the residue in 50 μl of the solvent mixture and analyse by thin-layer chromatography.

In this system, weakly acidic drugs (barbiturates), as well as neutral and basic drugs, are extracted together at pH 9. Phenobarbitone extraction is poor (recovery approximately 20%), but is still sufficient to allow detection of the drug in dependent patients.

THIN-LAYER CHROMATOGRAPHY OF DEPENDENCE-PRODUCING DRUGS

Use plastic sheets or glass plates (20 × 20 cm), coated with silica gel (250 μm thick). Score vertical lines on the plates in order to bring about an even movement of the developing-solvent front; if large batches of samples are being processed, each plate can be scored to produce 12 columns to accommodate the reference mixture and 11 sample extracts. Score a horizontal line about 10 cm from the bottom of the plate to mark the distance to be travelled by the solvent front. Four plates are required.

Acidic Drugs

Reference Solution. Prepare an ethanolic solution containing 1 mg/ml of each of amylobarbitone and phenobarbitone.

Method. Apply 25 μl of the reference solution to the first column of the plate, and apply 25 μl of the acidic extract from the solvent extraction method, or of the column extract, to the next column on the plate. Use a 100-μl gas-chromatography syringe for the application, taking great care to wash the syringe several times with chloroform between the application of each extract. Develop the plate in a tank containing chloroform:acetone (4:1) (System TD, p. 168). After development, remove the plate and dry under a hot-air blower.

Location Reagents. Spray the plate with *mercurous nitrate spray*. Barbiturates give black spots initially which turn chalky-white as spraying is continued. This reagent is quite sensitive, 1 μg of a barbiturate being easily discerned. Glutethimide and phenytoin (sometimes used to control withdrawal symptoms) also react with this spray.

Rf values for some common acidic drugs of abuse are given in Table 15. System TE (p. 168) can also be used.

Table 15. TLC data for some common acidic drugs of abuse

Compound	System TD	System TE
Phenytoin	33	36
Phenobarbitone	47	28
Amylobarbitone	52	36
Quinalbarbitone	55	44
Glutethimide	63	78

Basic Drugs

Reference Solution. Prepare an ethanolic solution containing 1 mg/ml of each of morphine, codeine, methadone, and cocaine.

Method. Apply 25 μl of the reference solution to the first column of each of three plates. Divide the basic extract from the solvent extraction method, or the remainder of the column extract, equally between the three plates. Develop one plate in a tank containing 100 ml of methanol:*strong ammonia solution* (100:1.5) (System TA, p. 167). Develop the other two plates in a tank containing ethyl acetate:methanol:*strong ammonia solution* (85:10:5) (System TE, p. 168). After development, remove the plates from the tanks and dry under a stream of cold air until they no longer smell of ammonia. Avoid using a hot-air blower as methadone may volatilise.

Location Reagents. Spray the plate developed in System TA, and one of the plates developed in System TE, with *acidified iodoplatinate solution*. Lightly spray the remaining plate developed in System TE with 9M sulphuric acid; phenothiazine drugs and their metabolites give pink, red, or blue spots. Overspray with *acidified iodoplatinate solution*; the presence of the acid deepens the blue colour produced when morphine reacts with iodoplatinate solution, and this increases the sensitivity of detection of this compound.

The three plates should be examined side by side immediately after spraying. A list of Rf values in the two systems for the major narcotic drugs and their metabolites is given in Table 16. However, many other basic drugs will react with acidified iodoplatinate solution. Rf values for many substances in these two systems will be found in the index to Thin-layer Chromatographic Data in Part 3. Thin-layer chromatographic data for narcotic analgesics in other systems is given on p. 174.

Interfering Substances

Heavy smoking is very prevalent amongst the drug-dependent community, and the presence of nicotine and its metabolites in the basic extract can confuse the interpretation of the TLC plates. In System TA, nicotine and its metabolites coalesce with an Rf

Table 16. TLC data for some common narcotic drugs and metabolites

Compound	System TA	TE
Norcodeine	13	—
Methadone metabolites	15	98
Nordihydrocodeine	16	25
Dihydrocodeine	26	36
Codeine	33	40
Morphine	37	20
Methadone	48	98
Quinine	51	36
Pethidine	52	80
Nicotine	54	70
Cotinine	60	40
Hydroxycotinine	60	20
Norcotinine	60	20
Cocaine	65	98
Dextropropoxyphene metabolites (streaking)	70	40

value of about 60. However, in System TE, three spots can be distinguished due to nicotine, cotinine, and norcotinine with hydroxycotinine. The spots give grey-brown colours with acidified iodoplatinate solution, but in urine samples from heavy smokers, the colours are darker and can easily be mistaken for codeine (Rf 40) or morphine (Rf 20). The situation is resolved by the simultaneous viewing of both plates. To gain experience, urine samples from volunteers who smoke should be processed.

Phenothiazines are sometimes administered by clinicians as part of the treatment of drug abuse. These produce so many urinary metabolites which react with acidified iodoplatinate solution that the detection of other drugs on the plate is made difficult, if not impossible. Detection of morphine in such samples is particularly difficult.

Cocaine

Cocaine gives a bright blue colour with acidified iodoplatinate solution, and has the same Rf value as methadone in System TE; the two are well separated in System TA. In practice, cocaine is rarely detected in urine samples by this technique. The drug is rapidly metabolised to benzoylecgonine, a polar substance which extracts poorly into organic solvents.

Immunoassay kits which are highly specific for benzoylecgonine are available, and this method should be used if it is essential to detect cocaine abuse.

Codeine

It is essential to distinguish between codeine, a common constituent of cough medicines, and morphine. A small amount of codeine is thought to be O-demethylated to morphine in man, but morphine is not detected by the above procedure, even when very large doses of codeine have been taken. A high intake of codeine can give rise to the detection of the N-demethylated metabolite, norcodeine. This appears on both thin-layer systems, and is likely to be confused with nordihydrocodeine.

Dextropropoxyphene

Dextropropoxyphene is extensively metabolised in the liver, and the parent drug is not detected in urine samples. The appearance of the metabolites is quite characteristic. In System TA they give a tailing blue spot at an Rf of about 70. In System TE they appear as a blue streak running from an Rf of about 40 down to the base-line.

Diamorphine

Diamorphine is rapidly de-acetylated to morphine in the body, and is not excreted in the urine. The detection of diamorphine is based, therefore, on the identification of morphine in urine (see below). If diamorphine is detected in an extract, this may indicate an attempt by the patient to deceive the analyst by the direct addition of the drug to the urine sample.

Dihydrocodeine

This drug gives two spots which have a distinctive appearance on the TLC plate. These spots are due to the drug itself and its metabolite, nordihydrocodeine, both of which react with acidified iodoplatinate solution to give deep brown-violet spots.

Methadone

Methadone is N-demethylated in the body to give a product which undergoes spontaneous cyclisation to yield two metabolites in the urine. In System TE, methadone and the metabolites run almost coincidentally on the solvent front, whereas in System TA, methadone runs just above morphine and is separated from the metabolites which run at about Rf 15. Both methadone and the metabolites give characteristic red-violet colours with acidified iodoplatinate solution. Methadone and the metabolites are usually found in most samples, but occasionally only the metabolites are detected.

Morphine

Morphine and codeine run together in System TA, but are well-separated in System TE; they appear as blue spots.

Morphine is excreted in the urine mainly as morphine-3-glucuronide, a water-soluble metabolite which is not extracted into organic solvents. Less than 10% of the drug is excreted as unchanged morphine. Thus, the sensitivity of the test for morphine can be considerably increased by hydrolysing the conjugated metabolites to yield free morphine. This can be achieved either by acid hydrolysis at a high temperature, or by incubating the urine sample with β-glucuronidase. The latter method is a more gentle procedure than acid hydrolysis which can destroy other drugs present in the sample. For routine work, all samples can be spiked with the enzyme solution when received, incubated overnight, and analysed on the following day.

The solutions produced after hydrolysis are examined by the methods for dependence-producing drugs described above under Extraction of Urine, and Thin-layer Chromatography.

ACID HYDROLYSIS

To 10 ml of urine in a screw-capped bottle (McCartney bottle) add 2 ml of *hydrochloric acid*, screw the cap on to the bottle and allow to stand in a boiling water-bath for 15 minutes. Cool the bottle, transfer the contents to a 250-ml beaker, add solid sodium bicarbonate to adjust the pH to 8.5 and, when the frothing has subsided, transfer the solution back into the McCartney bottle.

ENZYME HYDROLYSIS

Dissolve 5000 Fishman units of mixed glucuronidase/sulphatase (from *Helix pomatia*) in 1 ml of *acetate buffer (pH 5)*. Adjust 10 ml of the urine to pH 5 with 0.1M hydrochloric acid, add 1 ml of the enzyme solution, and incubate at 37° for about 12 hours.

GAS CHROMATOGRAPHY OF DEPENDENCE-PRODUCING DRUGS

Spots of doubtful identity on the thin-layer chromatographic plates can sometimes be characterised by gas chromatography on two independent columns using 2.5% SE-30 on Chromosorb G (System GA, p. 192), and 3% Poly A103 on Chromosorb W HP (System GF, p. 195).

Reference Solution. Prepare a solution in chloroform containing 10 μg/ml of each of codeine, cyclizine, diphenhydramine, dipipanone, methadone, and pethidine.

Method. Inject 5 μl of the reference solution on to both columns to ensure that the instruments are functioning properly. The retention indices of these substances are listed in Table 17, together with those of other abused drugs.

To 0.5 ml of urine in a micro test-tube add 100 μl of 2M sodium hydroxide, and 100 μl of chloroform, mix for 30 seconds, centrifuge in a high-speed centrifuge for 2 minutes, and inject 3 to 5 μl of the chloroform extract on to both columns.

Identify any peaks which appear by reference to the retention data listed in Table 17. Further systems and data for the gas chromatography of narcotic analgesics are given on p. 198.

Table 17. Retention indices for some commonly abused drugs and their metabolites

Compound	System GA	GF
Norpethidine	1745	—
Pethidine	1751	1995
Glutethimide	1836	2315
Diphenhydramine	1873	2105
2-Ethyl-5-methyl-3,3-diphenyl-1-pyrroline (methadone metabolite)	1950	2190
Cyclizine	2020	2320
2-Ethylidene-1,5-dimethyl-3,3-diphenylpyrrolidine (methadone metabolite)	2030	2280
Norcyclizine	2050	—
Methadone	2148	2370
Dextropropoxyphene	2188	2370
Pentazocine	2275	3030
Dihydrocodeine	2363	2840
Codeine	2376	2860
Dipipanone	2474	2710

Amphetamine and methylamphetamine are also frequently abused. Because of their volatility and the lack of specific detecting agents, gas chromatography is the method of choice (see p. 17).

CANNABIS

The abuse of cannabis cannot be detected by thin-layer chromatography or by conventional gas chromatography because the concentrations of cannabinoids in urine are too low. Immunoassay, applied to either blood or urine, is the best method (see B. Law *et al., J. analyt. Toxicol.*, 1984, 8, 14–18).

Cannabis and cannabis resin can be presumptively identified using the Duquenois Reagent (p. 133). Individual cannabinoids can be separated by thin-layer chromatography (p. 172), gas chromatography (p. 197), or high pressure liquid chromatography (p. 217).

SCREENING FOR ABUSE OF SOLVENTS

The term 'glue-sniffing' derives from the abuse of adhesives which often contain solvents such as toluene, ethyl acetate, acetone, or ethyl methyl ketone. These, and similar compounds, also occur in a diverse range of other commercial products which may be abused, e.g. shoe-cleaners, nail varnish, dry-cleaning fluids, bottled fuel gases (butane and propane), aerosol propellants, and fire extinguishers (bromochlorodifluoromethane).

The gas chromatographic method given below uses head-space sampling and split flame ionisation:electron capture (9:1) detection. This increases the sensitivity towards halogenated solvents without unduly decreasing the flame ionisation detector response of non-electron-capturing species.

Collection and Storage of Samples. Blood samples should be taken as soon as solvent abuse is suspected because some inhaled compounds are excreted rapidly. Solvents can be identified in samples collected into plastic tubes which have been transported at ambient temperature and stored at 4°. However, for quantitative work, samples should be collected in stoppered glass bottles with a metal-faced wad (with 1% sodium fluoride added to inhibit esterase activity), refrigerated whilst being transported, and analysed immediately, especially when very volatile agents may be involved. Qualitative assay of volatile substances such as dichloro-difluoromethane, propane, butane, and isobutane is still possible in blood specimens stored at −20° for 3 months.

Blood specimens should be packaged separately from any material thought to have been abused in order to avoid contamination. Pressure-sensitive adhesive tapes which contain solvents such as toluene should not be used to seal the sample containers.

Gas Chromatography of Solvents

The column used is 0.3% Carbowax 20M on Carbopak C. This is System GI (p. 199), and reference should be made to this system for full details of operating conditions and retention data.

Reference Mixture. This is prepared in three stages.
1. Prepare a mixture of the substances listed below. This mixture should be stored in a glass-stoppered bottle at −20°.

Acetone	20 ml	Isopropyl alcohol	20 ml
Carbon tetrachloride	200 µl	Isopropyl nitrate	1 ml
Chlorbutol	10 mg	Methanol	15 ml
Chloroform	1.5 ml	Tetrachloroethylene	100 µl
Ethanol	20 ml	Toluene	50 ml
Ethyl acetate	20 ml	1,1,1-Trichloroethane	1 ml
Ethyl methyl ketone	20 ml	1,1,2-Trichloroethane	2 ml
Ethylbenzene	10 ml	Trichloroethanol	50 µl
Hexane	40 ml	Trichloroethylene	1 ml
Isobutyl methyl ketone	5 ml		

2. Introduce the following volumes of the three gaseous compounds into an evacuated gas-sampling bulb: bromochlorodifluoromethane 20 µl, dichlorodifluoromethane 750 µl, and trichlorofluoromethane 20 µl.
3. Admit air to the gas-sampling bulb to atmospheric pressure and introduce 25 µl of the liquid mixture prepared above.

Inject aliquots from 0.01 to 1.0 µl of this reference mixture on to the column to produce the standard chromatogram.

Internal Standard Solution. Prepare two stock solutions containing, respectively, 50 mg of 1,1,2-trichloroethane and 50 mg of ethylbenzene, each in 50 ml of whole blood. The purity of these substances should be checked by gas chromatography, particularly for the presence of 1,1,1-trichloroethane and toluene.

Dilute 1 ml of the trichloroethane solution and 2.5 ml of the ethylbenzene solution to 100 ml with glass-distilled water containing 100 mg of sodium azide. This working internal standard solution can be stored in 1-ml portions at −20°.

Method. Using a 1-ml disposable plastic syringe, transfer 100 µl of the internal standard solution to a 7-ml nitrogen-filled vial sealed with a crimped-on PTFE-silicone disk, and maintain the vial at 65° in a heating block for 15 minutes. Remove 400 µl of the head-space in the vial with a warmed (40°) gas-tight glass syringe, and inject on to the chromatographic column to check for any extraneous peaks contributed by the vial, cap, syringe, or laboratory environment.

Add to the vial 200 µl of the sample (whole blood, plasma, or serum), using a disposable syringe, heat at 65° for a further 15 minutes, and inject 400 µl of the head-space on to the column.

Disks faced with PTFE should be used in the head-space vials as some solvents may be absorbed by butyl-rubber caps. Contamination of samples with chloroform, usually from the laboratory environment, is common. An artefact eluting with a retention time of 33.2 minutes derives from the gas-chromatograph septa.

After sample injection, the gas-tight syringe should be purged by removing the plunger and drawing ambient air through the barrel and needle using a vacuum pump.

SCREENING FOR ABUSE OF DIURETICS

Benzothiadiazine diuretics (thiazides) may be abused by patients who are obsessed with losing weight; prolonged use can cause severe hypokalaemia and hypomagnesaemia.

Diuretics can be detected by high pressure liquid chromatography using System HN (p. 217).

Detection of Diuretics in Urine by Thin-layer Chromatography

Reference Solutions. Prepare reference solutions containing 1 mg/ml of each of the substances listed in Table 18, using ethyl acetate as solvent.

Table 18. TLC data for some common diuretics

Compound	System TF Rf	Colour after diazotisation
Frusemide	12	red
Chlorothiazide	16	pink
Hydrochlorothiazide	39	pink
Hydroflumethiazide	47	orange
Cyclopenthiazide	62	pink
Bendrofluazide	71	orange

Method. To 10 ml of urine add 1 ml of M hydrochloric acid and 10 ml of ethyl acetate, mix on a rotary mixer for 10 minutes, and centrifuge. Transfer the ethyl acetate layer to a second tube, add 10 ml of a 5% solution of lead acetate, stopper the tube, and mix gently for 1 to 2 minutes (washing with lead acetate solution removes urinary pigments from the extract). Centrifuge, transfer the solvent extract to a 15-ml conical test-tube, and evaporate to dryness under a stream of air or nitrogen.

The extract is examined using silica gel G plates and ethyl acetate as the mobile phase (System TF, p. 168). Score the plates vertically to bring about an even movement of the mobile phase, and score a horizontal line 10 cm from the bottom of the plate to mark the distance travelled by the solvent front. Dissolve the residue from the extract in 100 μl of acetone and immediately apply 30 μl to the plate; at the same time apply 10-μl portions of each reference solution. After development, dry the plate with a hot-air blower.

Location Reagents. Spray the plate with *hydrochloric acid* and heat in an oven at 100° for 10 minutes in order to hydrolyse any thiazide present to the corresponding sulphonamide derivative. Then spray the plate with the following reagents in the sequence shown, drying the plate under warm air after each application.

1. 9M sulphuric acid (spray lightly)
2. A freshly-prepared 1% solution of sodium nitrite
3. A 5% solution of ammonium sulphamate
4. N-(*1-naphthyl*)ethylenediamine solution

Further data on the thin-layer chromatography of diuretics is given on p. 172.

INTERFERING SUBSTANCES

Interference may arise from the presence of benzodiazepines; these are hydrolysed to aminobenzophenones which also undergo diazotisation. Sulphonamides are also detected by this procedure, and can be distinguished by either of two methods. The unhydrolysed plate may be sprayed with *Van Urk reagent*, then heated at 100° for 5 minutes. This gives yellow colours with sulphonamides but not with thiazides. Alternatively, hydrolysed extracts of urine and of reference solutions can be chromatographed by the following procedure.

Reference Solution. Prepare a solution containing 10 μg/ml of bendrofluazide, chlorothiazide, and frusemide in normal urine.

Method. Extract 10 ml of the reference solution and 10 ml of the urine sample by the method given above. To each dried extract add 1 ml of 10M sodium hydroxide, heat in an autoclave for 15 minutes at 121°, cool, acidify the solutions, extract each with 10 ml of ethyl acetate, and evaporate the extracts to dryness. Dissolve the residues in 100 μl of acetone and chromatograph 30 μl of each as described above.

Table 19. TLC data for the hydrolysis products of some common diuretics

Parent drug	Hydrolysis product	System TF Rf	Colour after diazotisation
Frusemide	2-amino-4-chlorobenzoic acid-5-sulphonamide	17	red
Chlorothiazide Cyclopenthiazide Hydrochlorothiazide	4-amino-6-chlorobenzene-1,3-disulphonamide	48	pink
Bendrofluazide Hydroflumethiazide	4-amino-6-trifluoromethylbenzene-1,3-disulphonamide	61	orange

SCREENING FOR ABUSE OF LAXATIVES

Colonic stimulants are the most commonly misused laxative preparations. These include bisacodyl, danthron, oxyphenisatin, and phenolphthalein. Some vegetable laxatives, for example aloes, cascara and senna, give rise to the anthraquinone derivative rhein (1,8-dihydroxyanthraquinone-3-carboxylic acid).

A 50-ml sample of urine should be collected on three successive days in order to improve the chances of catching a laxative abuser. The colour of the urine should be noted; heavy use of danthron colours the urine pink or blue. If the urine turns red when made alkaline, this may indicate the presence of phenolphthalein or a vegetable laxative.

Detection of Laxatives in Urine by Thin-layer Chromatography

F. A. de Wolff *et al.*, *Clin. Chem.*, 1981, *27*, 914–917.

Laxatives can be detected in urine by this method for at least 18 hours after ingestion.

Reference Solutions. 1. Dissolve 2 mg of phenolphthalein in 1 ml of ethanol and dilute to 10 ml with chloroform.

2. Dissolve 2 mg of danthron in 10 ml of chloroform.

3. Dissolve 2 mg of rhein in 10 ml of chloroform. (A method for preparing rhein from sennoside A or B has been described by J. Lemli, *J. Pharm. Pharmac.*, 1965, *17*, 227–232.)

4. Bisacodyl and oxyphenisatin are substantially metabolised in the liver by a hydrolytic process, and far more of the hydrolysis product is excreted in the urine than unchanged drug. Hence, the reference solutions contain both the parent drug and the hydrolysis product, and are prepared in the following manner. Dissolve 2 mg of each substance in 2 ml of ethanol, add 20 µl of 6M sodium hydroxide, heat for 30 minutes at 70°, cool, neutralise with 20 µl of 6M hydrochloric acid, and add 8 ml of chloroform and 2 mg of the parent substance to each corresponding solution. (The precipitate of sodium chloride which forms on neutralisation does not interfere with the chromatography.)

Method. Enzymatic hydrolysis of the glucuronide metabolites is essential before extraction.

Adjust 20 ml of urine to pH 5 with 0.1M hydrochloric acid, add 2 ml of *acetate buffer (pH 5)*, and 10 000 Fishman units of mixed glucuronidase/sulphatase (from *Helix pomatia*), and heat in a water-bath at 60° for 2 hours. Pour the urine on to an unbuffered Tox Elut column (see Reagent Appendix) and leave for 2 to 3 minutes to allow the sample to soak into the column. Place a 50-ml test-tube under the column outlet and pour on to the column 20 ml of a mixture of chloroform:isopropyl alcohol (9:1). When the elution is complete, insert

into the top of the column a hollow rubber stopper connected by a rubber tube to a pressure bulb, and apply gentle pressure to discharge residual solvent. Place the tube containing the eluate in a beaker of hot water and evaporate the extract to dryness under a stream of nitrogen. Dissolve the residue in 100 µl of chloroform just prior to examination by the following thin-layer chromatography systems.

System 1

PLATES. High performance silica gel (10 × 20 cm) with fluorescent indicator and concentration zone (see Reagent Appendix).

MOBILE PHASE. *m*-Xylene:isobutyl methyl ketone:methanol (10:10:1).

System 2

PLATES. As used for System 1.

MOBILE PHASE. Hexane:toluene:*acetic acid* (3:1:1).

Score two plates vertically to divide them into two (10 × 10 cm) zones, and score a horizontal line parallel to the concentration zone at a distance of 5 cm.

To one plate apply 5-µl aliquots of the reference solutions of bisacodyl, danthron, oxyphenisatin, and phenolphthalein to each zone, together with a 3-µl and a 10-µl aliquot of the urine extract, also to each zone. Develop the plate using System 1.

To the second plate apply 5-µl aliquots of the reference solutions of danthron, phenolphthalein, and rhein to each zone, together with a 3-µl and a 10-µl aliquot of the urine extract. Develop this plate using System 2.

Remove the plates and dry under a hot-air blower. *Location Reagents*. Danthron is visible as a yellow spot on the first plate, or as an orange spot on the second plate. Examine the plates under ultraviolet light at 254 nm and 366 nm. All the substances absorb at 254 nm; danthron and rhein give an orange fluoresence at 366 nm.

Spray the left-hand side of each plate with 6M sodium hydroxide. Bisacodyl and its hydrolysis products give violet spots; oxyphenisatin appears as three faint pink spots; phenolphthalein and rhein give a violet and a red spot, respectively.

Spray the left-hand side of the first plate with a freshly prepared 1% solution of potassium ferricyanide.

Heat both plates to 100° and spray the right-hand side immediately with *Mandelin's reagent*.

The Rf values and colour reactions of these compounds and their hydrolysis products are listed in Table 20.

Table 20. TLC data for some common laxatives and their hydrolysis products

Compound	System 1 Rf relative to phenolphthalein	System 2 Rf relative to rhein	Visible colour	Colour after spraying with sodium hydroxide	Colour after spraying with Mandelin's reagent
Bisacodyl	98	—	—	violet	violet
hydrolysis product	71	—	—	violet	violet
Danthron	138	138	orange	red	brown
Oxyphenisatin	98	—	—	pink*	pink
hydrolysis product 1	80	—	—	pink*	pink
hydrolysis product 2	63	—	—	pink*	pink
Phenolphthalein	100	08	—	violet	brown
Rhein	—	100	yellow	red	green-yellow

* Violet after spraying with potassium ferricyanide

Bibliography

Analytical Methods in Human Toxicology, Vol. 1, A. S. Curry (Ed.), London, Macmillan, 1985.

R. C. Baselt, *Analytical Procedures for Therapeutic Drug Monitoring and Emergency Toxicology*, Davis, California, Biomedical Publications, 1980.

R. C. Baselt, *Disposition of Toxic Drugs and Chemicals in Man*, 2nd Edn, Davis, California, Biomedical Publications, 1982.

A. S. Curry, *Advances in Forensic and Clinical Toxicology*, Cleveland, Ohio, CRC Press, 1972.

A. S. Curry, *Poison Detection in Human Organs*, 3rd Edn, Springfield, Illinois, Charles C. Thomas, 1976.

R. H. Dreisbach, *Handbook of Poisoning: Prevention, Diagnosis and Treatment*, 11th Edn, Los Altos, California, Lange Medical Publications, 1983.

S. Kaye, *Handbook of Emergency Toxicology*, 4th Edn, Springfield, Illinois, Charles C. Thomas, 1980.

Poisoning: Diagnosis and Treatment, J. A. Vale and T. J. Meredith (Ed.), London, Update Books, 1981.

The Poisoned Patient: The Role of the Laboratory, R. Porter and M. O'Connor (Ed.), Amsterdam, Elsevier North-Holland, 1974.

Topics in Forensic and Analytical Toxicology, R. A. A. Maes (Ed.), New York, Elsevier, 1984.

Forensic Toxicology

J. V. Jackson

The first complete work of international importance on the subject of forensic toxicology was written by Orfila in 1813 ('Traité des poisons tirés des regnes minéral végétal et animal, ou toxicologie générale, considerée sous les rapports de la pathologie et de médecine légale'). It was an immediate success and won him the title of 'Father of Toxicology'. "The chemist", said Orfila, "horrified by the crime of homicidal poisoning, must aim to perfect the process necessary for establishing the case of poisoning in order to reveal the crime and to assist the magistrate punish the guilty". It is interesting to note that he realised the necessity of adequate proof of identification, emphasised the importance of what we now call quality assurance (purity of standards etc.), and anticipated the need for pharmaceutical, clinical, industrial, and environmental toxicology.

The term 'forensic toxicology' covers any application of the science and study of poisons to the elucidation of questions that occur in judicial proceedings. The subject is usually associated with work for the police, the coroner, and the criminal law courts. However, the analysis and identification of controlled drugs and the maintenance of agricultural, industrial, and public health legislation (to ensure clean air, pure water, and safe food supplies) are all aspects of forensic toxicology. Like the forensic toxicologist, analysts employed in these areas may at times find their work the subject of severe public scrutiny in a law court, and both groups should be aware of the strengths and limitations of each other's methodology.

Accidental self-poisoning and attempted suicide cases are generally the responsibility of the clinical toxicologist or the hospital biochemist, working in conjunction with a poison control centre. A small proportion of these cases is referred to the forensic toxicologist, either because of an allegation of malicious poisoning, or because the patient dies and a coroner's inquest is ordered. The preliminary analysis may already have been carried out, and close co-operation between the forensic and hospital laboratories is obviously desirable. What follows is an attempt to provide an account of the principles, methodology, and special problems encountered in forensic toxicology for all workers in these related fields, and for chemists and pharmacists in more remote areas of the world who may be faced with the request 'test for poisons'.

PRINCIPLES OF FORENSIC TOXICOLOGY

The forensic toxicologist is expected to detect and identify poisons, but if we define 'poison' as a chemical substance harmful to living organisms, it is obvious that 'harmfulness' is not a property that can be measured by any chemical method of analysis. Toxicity is a biological concept, usually determined by some form of bioassay. Although a bioassay may be used to detect the presence of a poison it does not provide the specific identification which is a prime requirement for forensic work. Prosecutions based almost entirely on animal experiments have succeeded in the past (for instance the trial of Dr Pommerais, Paris, 1862, was the first successful detection of digitalis poisoning), but this method alone would not be considered adequate in a modern trial. However, bioassays are probably the most rapid way of detecting poisoned food. For example, contaminated flour was implicated as the cause of a large outbreak of poisoning in the Middle East by feeding pigeons with samples of the food eaten by the victims. Subsequent chemical analysis of the flour identified the contaminant as endrin. Chemical analysis of all the various food samples would have taken weeks.

If official regulations permit this method to be used, it can be useful provided that the analyst is aware of the problem of species differences which can lead to erroneous conclusions. If the animal is more sensitive to the toxin than man (e.g. benzoic acid in the cat), a false positive result would be obtained. Alternatively, a false negative result would be obtained if the animal were more resistant (e.g. *Amanita phalloides* and the rabbit). This aspect is illustrated by TCDD (2,3,7,8-tetrachlorodibenzo-*p*-dioxin), the extremely persistent impurity, present in the systemic herbicide trichlorophenoxy-acetic acid, which was released in the Seveso disaster in 1976. Species differences for the LD50 (mg/kg) of this substance have been reported to be: guinea pig 0.0006, mouse 0.001, rat 0.04, and dog 0.1.

This apparently simple and logical method of testing for the presence of a poison has its limitations as far as the forensic toxicologist is concerned, and the bulk of all forensic analyses must be submitted to the chemist. However, all the techniques of analytical chemistry, from colour tests to mass spectrometry, are based on the molecular structure of the compounds involved, whereas toxicity is related to the dose. Anything can become a poison if it exceeds the threshold limit of the organism's ability to deal with it. Without a living organism as a test reagent, the word 'poison' is an abstract concept.

If the poison is not specified by name, the request to 'test for poisons' is a major problem for the chemist, because there is no single chemical method of analysis capable of detecting all the various poisons. At least seven different analytical schemes are required to exclude even the most commonly encountered poisons (Fig. 1). Compared with toxicologists in academic research or industry, the task of the forensic toxicologist is made more difficult because the analytical material, the available time, and the resources are all severely limited. He has scarcely any control over the sampling time or the selection of material for analysis, and no certain knowledge that a poison is present.

Forensic toxicology demands an overall analytical system designed to exclude or indicate the presence of any poison in each of the chemical groups shown in Fig. 1. Most of the numerous screening procedures reported in the literature are too limited to permit a confident negative report. All too often they are drug oriented, despite the fact that two-thirds of all discovered criminal poisonings are due to compounds other than drugs.

Apart from these analytical problems, the legal aspect of the work demands a scrupulous attention to details which are of little or no importance in other types of toxicology. Failure to make full descriptive notes on the items received, a simple error in the date the analysis was performed, or neglecting to check reagent purity, can become evidence of careless work in the hands of an astute lawyer. He may, with justification, explore the extent of the toxicologist's experience and knowledge, demand a detailed account of the analytical methods, and challenge the integrity of any opinion. The crucial evidence of identification and quantifi-

cation of the poison may be faultless and the conclusions correct but, if the court's confidence in the forensic toxicologist as an unbiased scientific expert is destroyed, the case may be lost.

Orfila was well acquainted with this aspect of forensic toxicology, and the guiding principles he established over 100 years ago are still applicable. These may be summarised as follows:

All chemists undertaking this work must have toxicological experience.

The analyst must be given a complete case history containing all the information available.

All the evidential material, suitably labelled and sealed in clean containers, must be submitted and examined.

All the known identification tests should be applied, and adequate notes made at the time.

All the necessary reagents used for these tests should be pure, and blank tests should be performed to establish this fact.

All tests should be repeated, and compared with control samples to which the indicated poison has been added.

Strict adherence to these principles makes forensic toxicology one of the slowest and most expensive forms of analysis. However, this must be accepted not only to ensure justice for the poisoned victim and for the accused, but also to protect the integrity and reputation of the analyst and the laboratory he represents.

RANGE OF CASES SUBMITTED

The ultimate objective of any forensic scientist is to attempt to provide answers to questions that may arise during criminal investigations or in subsequent court proceedings. The traditional question which must be answered is 'Has this person been poisoned?', together with the supplementary queries that follow if the result is positive such as 'What was the nature of the poison?', 'How was it administered?', and 'Was it a dangerous or lethal amount?'.

Laws governing the possession and use of narcotic and stimulant drugs, and legislation concerned with the influence of drink or drugs on driving skills, have increased the work-load of many forensic laboratories; these cases can account for over 70% of the total submitted.

Modern analytical methods can give the forensic toxicologist the ability to answer questions which previously were considered either hopeless or not worth considering because the results were so often negative. For example, in the 1960's over 90% of all allegedly poisoned food and drink samples submitted for analysis to the Metropolitan Police Forensic Science Laboratory were negative. Today, over 60% are positive. Methods which are sensitive to 1 μg or less of an increasing number of drugs and poisons make it worthwhile to undertake an analysis, even when the plate, cup, or container has apparently no food or drink left in it.

Drugs may be detected in blood at therapeutic concentrations, and it is possible, therefore, to obtain clues to the clinical history of the deceased, the victim, or the accused, even when they are unable or unwilling to provide this information for themselves. Thus, the discovery of drugs used in the treatment of epilepsy, diabetes, etc., in a blood sample taken from an unidentified body, may start a new train of inquiries leading to successful identification of the body. Similarly, allegations of doping prior to rape or robbery may be refuted or confirmed.

The final example of what might be termed the 'new forensic toxicology' concerns the analytical checking of statements made by witnesses during the course of a police inquiry. Provided that a blood or urine sample is taken within about 12 hours of an event, there is a good chance of checking the truth of statements such as 'I don't remember what happened because I was high on drugs at the time', 'I used to be an addict, but I haven't taken anything for over a year', or 'I killed him in self-defence because after taking LSD he went berserk and attacked me with a knife'.

Stains can also be examined for drugs and poisons. For example, if the victim notices a nasty taste and spits out the drink, the allegation that someone tried to poison him can be investigated if the stained garment is submitted for analysis. Certain drugs can be detected in blood stains, and this has proved to be useful evidence additional to examination for the blood group, especially when the blood group is common. The request 'test for drugs' is almost as much a routine request by the detective investigating a murder as the request for serology.

In most cases, the results obtained in the various types of cases mentioned above can be proved conclusively, i.e. the identity of the poison can be confirmed by more than one method, and it can be quantified. Even when specific identification is not feasible, an opinion as to whether the suspect is most probably telling the truth or is lying, can be of value to the investigator.

ANALYTICAL REQUIREMENTS

It is impossible to design a single analytical scheme which is both capable of detecting all the drugs and poisons now available and suitable for all the various purposes mentioned above. The forensic toxicologist needs a repertoire of standard methods which he can modify according to the nature of the investigation, the type and amount of material for analysis, and the time and resources he has available. This collection of standard methods should include about a dozen general screening methods and as many special methods as he can acquire and practise.

General screening methods are designed to detect, or exclude, the majority of poisons in a particular group in a single series of operations. Because the main objective is detection rather than quantification, general screening methods are usually more flexible than special methods and can therefore be applied to a wide variety of materials. They are essential for the investigation of unknown poisonings, and have some advantages even when the toxic agent is known or suspected. A good general method will provide a provisional identification which can then be confirmed by the application of a quantitative special method.

Special methods will only detect, or exclude, a limited number of related chemical compounds. Because of their more limited purpose they can be made more efficient, rapid, and selective than general methods but in certain circumstances they waste both time and material. The temptation to screen for poisons by employing a whole series of special methods should be resisted. Some of the specialised methods designed to detect a particular poison or a chemically-related group of drugs (e.g. barbiturates, phenothiazines) are not as selective as they purport to be. This is because the extraction procedures have been simplified for rapid processing, because they utilise a non-specific identification technique, or, more frequently, because they are designed to quantify the drug rather than identify it. For example, many methods based on a colour reaction only require the preparation of a protein-free filtrate; consequently, the drug or poison is never really separated from most of the endogenous material and the only evidence of identification involves the dangerous assumption that the positive response is due to the compound sought. If possible, non-selective special methods should be avoided in forensic toxicology. Unfortunately they are often the only type the manufacturer of the compound can supply.

Classification of Poisons

Drugs and poisons can be classified alphabetically, pharmacologically (antidiabetic, anticonvulsant, etc.), or by chemical structure (barbiturates, phenothiazines, etc.). However, for analytical purposes it is more useful to classify poisons according to the method used for extraction. Five major groups are usually considered:

(a) gaseous and volatile substances isolated by diffusion or distillation;
(b) organic non-volatile substances isolated by solvent extraction;
(c) metallic poisons isolated by ashing or by wet oxidation of the organic matter;
(d) toxic anions isolated by dialysis; and
(e) miscellaneous poisons which require special extraction techniques such as ion-exchange columns, formation of derivatives or ion-pairs, freeze-drying and continuous extraction with a polar solvent.

Some of these groups have been sub-divided because they are too large or because alternative methods of extraction are available. The seven groups so formed are illustrated in Fig. 1.

which can be applied to the sample directly without the need for any isolation or purification processes are indispensable in the initial stages of an analysis. Immunoassay techniques also eliminate the need for many separate operations and, like colour tests, can provide a tentative identification and approximate quantification of the poison. However, a disadvantage of both these methods is that a negative result eliminates only a few of the possible toxic substances. Consequently, additional colour tests or immunoassays are required before that particular group of poisons can be excluded. This type of sequential testing can waste much time.

A broad-spectrum screen, capable of detecting or eliminating most of the poisons in a group, usually requires a combination of three or more of the available techniques. For the drug and pesticide groups, the only combination potentially capable of encompassing all the required steps is mass spectrometry coupled with either gas chromatography or high pressure liquid chromatography. However, a simple, direct solvent extraction scheme is generally employed to eliminate endogenous substances which might otherwise reduce the efficiency of the system.

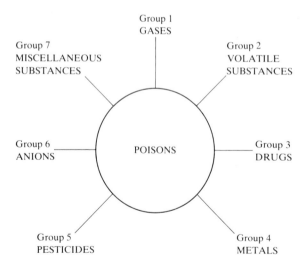

Fig. 1. The seven major groups of poisons.

Most analyses require several unit operations, namely separation of the poison from the biological material, isolation and purification of the toxic substance and its metabolites, identification, confirmation of identity, and quantification. The most useful methods are those which combine two or more of these unit operations. Thus, colour tests

Case Investigation

Analyses may be required to answer specific questions concerning, for instance, the amount of alcohol in blood. Alternatively, the enquiry may be more general, such as 'Was this food poisoned?'. This latter type of case is termed a 'general unknown' (that is, those cases where the analyst knows nothing about the nature of the poison, if any). All 7 groups of poisons shown in Fig. 1 should be excluded before a negative report can be given. Fortunately, group tests are available for four of these groups, i.e. volatile compounds, drugs, metals, and pesticides. Specific tests must be used to detect gases, anions, and miscellaneous compounds. Obviously, the choice of which group should be eliminated first is critical if a rapid answer is expected.

Intuitive considerations or 'guesswork' nearly always predominate in a 'general unknown' case. It is common to commence with a drug screen, and this is usually confined to those drugs which are soluble. If the case is a suicide attempt or a suspect doping, the choice is justified but, if all the circumstances have not been reported to the analyst, it may not be right to make the assumption that a drug is present.

Most poisoning cases involve alcohol, carbon monoxide, hypnotics, narcotics, sedatives, or tranquillisers. However, it may be that these are the most common poisons because they are sought more often than other toxic substances, and because they are almost the only poisons for which comprehensive screening systems have been published. There are inherent dangers in this pragmatic approach because there is no differentiation between self-poisonings and criminal poisonings. On the other hand, a completely systematic and comprehensive analytical scheme covering all the poison groups is extremely costly.

The first essential task of the analyst must be to ensure that the so-called 'general unknown' case is an authentic unknown poisoning. Only about 10% of submitted cases do not have any guiding features, and these cases consist mainly of unidentified drowned, burnt, or decomposed bodies, or of the submission of some untasted, but allegedly poisoned, food sample. In most cases there are nearly always some facts available which can provide clues to the most likely group of poisons to be excluded as a first action. Thus, if the time of onset of the symptoms was less than 1 hour, and there is no evidence of injected material, then the sample should be examined for gases and volatile poisons before other groups. Severe vomiting and diarrhoea provide an indication of possible metal poisoning.

The age and occupation of the victim or the site of the incident may guide the choice of the first group screen to be employed. For instance, few elderly people indulge in solvent sniffing, farm workers have easier access to the more toxic pesticides, and a death in an electroplating factory would certainly require cyanide to be eliminated. These facts are not freely given but must be sought.

If no circumstantial details are provided the most useful preliminary analytical instrument is the telephone!

The prerequisite for a case to be accepted into a forensic toxicology department is suspicion. Details of the circumstances leading to the conclusion that a criminal action has taken place must be supplied to the analyst in order for him to plan his analysis.

Every case submitted must be accompanied by a form similar to that shown below and every effort must be made to obtain the information requested on the form. If possible, a personal consultation with the investigating officer should also be arranged.

Information to be submitted with the exhibits in all cases where there is suspicion of poisoning or doping

Name of victim   Sex
Age   Weight or height
Nationality   Recent foreign travel?
Occupation (give details of end-product of factory or firm).

Medical History

Did victim suffer from viral hepatitis or any other infectious disease?

Any recent illness or chronic disease? What drugs were prescribed?

Was victim an alcoholic, drug addict, smoker?

What poison is suspected? How much?
(Tablet bottles, syringes etc., found near body should be submitted.)

Give names of any drugs or poisons to which victim or associates had access (apart from any mentioned above).

Times

Date and time victim last seen to have been in normal health.

Date and time of illness or death, and where found, e.g. at work, in bed, outdoors etc.

If these times are not known, when was the victim found?

Time and details of last meal.

Treatment

Any medical attention given after the suspected poisoning or doping?

Time of hospital admission. Date and time discharged.

Details of any treatment given (volume of stomach wash, time when blood/urine samples taken).

Hospital analysis: supplied/not done/not available

Tick any of the following symptoms that apply:
Diarrhoea, vomiting, thirst, blindness, constipation, cyanosis (blue tinge to skin), jaundice, loss of weight, shivering, convulsions, eye pupils dilated, eye pupils constricted, delirium, coma, sweating, renal failure.

Name of pathologist or doctor. Autopsy report sent Yes/No

Date of autopsy and possible cause of death.

Any further information which could be useful to the laboratory, e.g. victim pregnant, details of suspect (especially occupation and end-product of factory or firm, comments made by victim, witnesses or suspect).

Samples Required

If victim alive: vomit, stomach aspirate or wash, blood and urine.

If victim dead:

Stomach contents	All available (no preservative); enquire if stomach wash or vomit is available. If no contents, submit stomach.
Blood	
Femoral vein	30 ml unpreserved and 5 ml preserved (for alcohol analysis). Identify source. Do not mix.
Heart	All available from intact heart chambers. Avoid body cavity samples. Enquire if antemortem samples are available.
Urine	All available, however small a volume (preserved). Enquire if antemortem samples are available. If no urine, submit kidney and bile.
Liver	250 g. Gall bladder should not be included with this sample.

If the suspected poison is a volatile substance, brain and lungs will be required. Bone and hair are needed if metal poisoning is suspected. Brain should always be submitted if the body is decomposed. If in doubt, consult the laboratory.

Glass jars should be used whenever possible. Samples should be properly labelled and sealed. The label should include the name of the victim, signature of pathologist, and the date.
Antemortem samples should also specify time of sampling.

Although investigation should always precede analysis, there is no need to wait for full completion of the questionnaire because some poisons are so common that they should always be eliminated. These include ethanol, aspirin, paracetamol, barbiturates, and carbon monoxide. Many of these can be checked by rapid analytical probing tests before a full group screen is applied. Completion of the following analytical probing tests will, in many cases, provide clues to the nature of the poison.

Analytical Probing

MEDICAMENTS NEAR THE BODY

It is a common mistake to spend too much time identifying every tablet or capsule found at the scene (in many cases they have nothing to do with the event). However, it is equally foolish not to have a quick attempt at identification before analysing body fluids (see p. 50).

FOOD OR DRINK RESIDUES NEAR THE BODY

The priority given to this aspect will depend on the case history, but a rapid initial examination at an early stage is often useful (see p. 48).

BODY FLUIDS

A number of preliminary tests should be carried out in order to confirm or exclude the most common toxic agents.

Urine

The following tests, details of which are given on p. 4, should be performed: Trinder's test for salicylates, cresol–ammonia test for paracetamol, FPN reagent for phenothiazines, Fujiwara test for trichloro-compounds, and the dithionite test for paraquat and diquat. In addition, the content of alcohol should be determined by gas chromatography (p. 19).

Stomach Contents

This sample should be examined visually for colour and the presence of tablet residues or excipients (often maize starch). The odour should be noted as this may indicate the presence of alcohols, aldehydes, ketones, phenols, cyanide, ethchlorvynol, nicotine, etc. The following tests, details of which are given on p. 5, should be performed: Trinder's test for salicylates, cresol–ammonia test for paracetamol, FPN reagent for phenothiazines, Fujiwara test for trichloro-compounds, and the diphenylamine test for oxidising agents. In addition, the Reinsch Test for heavy metals (p. 57) should be carried out, and a diluted, filtered extract examined by direct ultraviolet spectrophotometry for drugs with high A_1^1 values.

Blood

Tests on this sample should include a quantification of alcohol by gas chromatography (p. 19), and detection and quantification of carbon monoxide by spectrophotometry (p. 20).

The precise order in which these tests are carried out will depend on the information available, but most of them will need to be done at some time, unless the evidence overwhelmingly indicates a specific poison (e.g. cyanide). Even in these cases, ancillary questions may arise in court, for instance, was the victim doped or drunk prior to the administration of the fatal poison? A careful toxicologist should, therefore, carry out most of the above plus a routine drug screen in every case. For example, not all carbon monoxide cases are suicidal or accidental, even if the circumstantial evidence seems to indicate a non-criminal cause of death.
The flow chart (Fig. 2) shows how the information obtained from the questionnaire and the suggested analytical probing are combined to obtain a probable identity, or at least the type of poison involved.
If the analytical probing suggested above is compared with the poison group classification shown in Fig. 1, it can be seen that every group has been

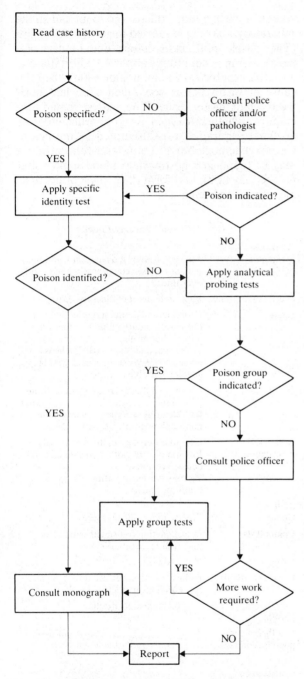

Fig. 2. Analytical probing flow chart.

digoxin, and insulin. If the laboratory has facilities for immunoassay, tests for this most difficult group can be started. Radioimmunoassays are essential for traffic-offence cases (drug-driving cases), and can assist greatly in the probing phase of an investigation. Immunoassays are not specific, and advantage can be taken of this cross-reactivity to provide general tests for barbiturates, benzodiazepines, tricyclic antidepressants, and opiates.

A simple drug screen of the urine and stomach contents, such as Scheme 1 (p. 4), may be undertaken as part of this probing phase, but it is better to carry out a more traditional multi-fractional screen (Scheme 2, p. 10) rather than risk the need to repeat this part of the analysis when nothing has been detected by the simple screen. Both approaches are valid depending on the type of case predominating in the laboratory. If most of the work is undertaken for the coroner and pathologist and concerns mainly the investigation of suspected suicidal overdoses, then the simple drug screen is probably better. However, if there is a large number of antemortem investigations (i.e. non-fatal doping, poisoning, traffic and drug offences), then the traditional multi-fraction screen is more economical of both sample and time, in the long-term. Moreover, there is an increasing demand for the forensic laboratory to investigate the possibility of drug involvement in murder and manslaughter cases. In these cases, proof is required of drug ingestion rather than of the consumption of an overdose, so that a simple drug screen might not suffice.

Only a small number of qualitative tests utilise the blood sample. This is because it is generally the most limited sample, and is also the most valuable for the confirmation and quantification phases of a toxicological analysis.

The analysis of tissue samples was formerly a prerequisite of any toxicological examination, but it is less important now provided that the laboratory has sensitive, instrumental methods in routine use. However, analysis of the liver is essential when a full range of body fluids cannot be obtained, or if the detailed analysis of these fluids fails to provide an answer. For these reasons, liver should still be requested as a routine specimen in every post-mortem case. It is doubtful if the supply and analysis of a full set of body organs, advocated by many classical toxicology textbooks, can now be justified for there is little evidence that such routines have uncovered homicidal poisonings that would otherwise have been overlooked. In general, the

checked by at least one test designed to confirm or exclude one or more of the most common toxic agents within that classification, with the exception of Group 7, Miscellaneous Poisons. The most common poisons in Group 7 are cannabinoids,

analysis of liver specimens need only be considered in those cases where the circumstantial evidence conflicts strongly with the analytical results.

Toxic blood concentrations of some drugs (e.g. thioridazine) are not significantly higher than therapeutic concentrations. This is not generally true of liver concentrations which, in postmortem specimens, may be over ten times higher than those obtained from patients on therapeutic dose regimens. Liver analysis in these cases will provide a more certain indication of a fatal overdose.

Tissue analysis is obviously a necessity for exhumed or decomposed bodies or when the victim has survived for several days following ingestion of the poison. In all these cases the routine samples (stomach contents, blood, and urine) may not be available or if available may not produce meaningful results.

GROUP TESTS

In the following pages, each classified group of poisons is discussed in turn. The group tables summarise the type of circumstantial evidence usually characteristic for the majority of poisons, list possible spot or probing tests to confirm or refute the circumstantial indications, and indicate analytical methods required for the group. A general method is suggested where this is available. The figure given under 'number of compounds reported' is the number of compounds in the group that has been reported to the International Association of Forensic Toxicologists as being involved in poisoning cases over a fifteen-year period. The figure given under 'number of compounds to be excluded' is a very rough estimate of the total number of poisons within that particular group.

Group 1 Poisons: Gases

The presence of this group of poisons is usually indicated by the circumstances of the incident (providing they have been reported in full to the analyst). Furthermore, the identity of the actual gas involved is often indicated by the circumstantial evidence. This is fortunate since no single-stage group test or analytical method is available for this group (Table 1). However, a few points need careful investigation. For instance, a portable heater may have been removed from the room where the death occurred. In one case, a devoted mother warmed her son's cold bedroom before he was awake using a defective paraffin heater, which was subsequently transferred to warm the bathroom before he took a bath. He was found dead in bed with no visible

source of carbon monoxide in the room and so the laboratory was only requested to analyse for drugs. (The classic pink skin colour due to carboxyhaemoglobin is not always apparent!) Fortunately, a routine test for carbon monoxide established the cause of death before too much time had been wasted looking for drugs. The analyst should also enquire whether oxygen was administered or artificial respiration was attempted before death. Carboxyhaemoglobin at a non-fatal concentration may be found in a postmortem blood sample, but no one may think to inform the analyst of the first-aid which has been given.

Table 1. Group 1 Poisons: Gases

Indications	
Symptoms	Apnoea, asphyxia, dyspnoea, vomiting; pink or red skin colour (carbon monoxide or cyanide)
Onset of symptoms	Very rapid onset of illness or death
Scene	Hospitals and dental surgeries (anaesthetic gases), industrial sites, laboratories, mines. Victims found in bathrooms, boats, caravans, cars, fires, kitchens Presence of fire extinguishers, gas fires, geysers, portable heaters
Occupation	Chemical industry, electroplating, fumigation, furnaces, glue factories, industrial tank cleaning, jewellery, metal treatment, mines, photography, sewers, tanneries
Additional investigations	Examination of equipment or vehicle Examination of clothing if stained or if odours are noted Postmortem examination of lung and brain specimens
Analysis	
Odour	Carbon monoxide, cyanide
Colour tests	Direct reading colorimetric indicator tubes (Draeger tubes)
Group tests	Not available
General methods	Diffusion in Conway cell (cyanide), headspace gas chromatography
Commonest poisons	Carbon monoxide, cyanide
Number of compounds reported	5
Number of compounds to be excluded	30

Some compounds which are gases at normal temperature and pressure can be detected by headspace gas chromatography (p. 187), using Systems GA or GI (p. 199). System GI will detect butane, ethane, methane, nitrous oxide, and propane, and also several of the low boiling-point fluorocarbons in blood samples.

Only two poisons in this group require routine exclusion. These are cyanide and carbon monoxide. The main exceptions to this general recommendation are cases arising from an incident on industrial premises, or the use and abuse of compressed solvent fuels and aerosols. In the former case, a list of the industrial gases used or available on site should be requested; in the latter case, most of the relevant compounds are covered by head-space gas chromatography as mentioned above.

CARBON MONOXIDE

The detection and measurement of carbon monoxide in blood samples is frequently required in forensic toxicology for the investigation of deaths in fires, cars, caravans, etc. and it is essential for all routine screening schemes. A preliminary colour test may be used (p. 6), but the most rapid and convenient method of detecting and quantifying carbon monoxide as a primary or secondary cause of poisoning is by using a spectrophotometric method (p. 20).

CYANIDE

In most cases this poison is self-indicating by its odour of bitter almonds. However, there is a very variable ability amongst the population to detect cyanide by its odour, so a colour test is useful (p. 65). For blood and tissue specimens it is preferable to use the quantitative method using Conway micro-diffusion cells (p. 65).

Group 2 Poisons: Volatile Compounds

Rapid onset of symptoms, followed by serious illness or death is the most valuable clue to the presence of this group. The probable identity of the particular poison may be indicated by the nature of the symptoms (Table 2). Physical evidence at the scene (e.g. bottles, residues in cups, etc., tubes of adhesives, and plastic bags with characteristic odours) frequently leaves little doubt of the nature of the intoxicant, if the material is submitted within 48 hours. If death has been delayed for several days by hospital treatment, it is imperative to obtain for analysis any antemortem samples taken on admission to hospital, no matter how small.

If several days have elapsed before the body is discovered, there is a tendency to think that analysis for volatile poisons would be futile. In fact it should be one of the first groups to be checked. The presence of alcohols, toluene, and halogenated hydrocarbons has been shown in many such

Table 2. Group 2 Poisons: Volatile Compounds

Indications	
Symptoms	Abdominal pain (especially with phenols), convulsions (especially with glycols), delirium, drunken behaviour (drowsiness, ataxia, speech and vision disturbance), jaundice (aniline, nitrobenzene), tremors, vomiting
Onset of symptoms	Rapid onset of illness or death when inhaled, slower if taken orally
Clinical history	Alcoholism; 'glue-sniffing' habit (more common in children and teenagers)
Scene	Domestic locations; hospitals and research laboratories; industrial locations. Presence of liquor, methylated spirit or surgical spirit; glues or polishes associated with plastic bags; unusual siting of anti-freeze or other domestic products
Occupation	Degreasing plants, dry cleaners, printing; manufacturer of adhesives, dyes, paints, petroleum products, plastics, polishes, perfumes, rubber
Additional investigations	Bottles or containers found near victim, even if empty. Examination of clothing if stained or if odours are noted. Antemortem examination of blood or urine samples. Postmortem examination of lung and brain specimens; also vitreous humour, especially if the body is decomposed
Analysis	
Odour	
Colour tests	Dichromate test for ethanol, aldehydes, and ketones; colorimetric indicator tube (e.g. Alcotest); Fujiwara test for trichloro-compounds
Group tests	Head-space gas chromatography
General methods	Gas chromatography
Commonest poisons	Chloral hydrate, ethanol, methanol, toluene
Number of compounds reported	25
Number of compounds to be excluded	60

samples, although the interpretation of the detected concentrations may present problems.

Special care is needed if the samples have been frozen; volatile poisons may be missed if the analytical material is not allowed to thaw, preferably at room temperature, before examination.

The frequent abuse of toluene, acetone, and other solvents associated with the 'glue-sniffing' habit should be remembered in all poisoning cases. Because the addict is now turning his attention to a wide variety of industrial solvents, a good general screening method backed up with a large data base is required. Gas chromatography is the only way of achieving this coverage since all other methods require the application of separate colour tests or chemical reactions for each volatile substance.

Head-space gas chromatography (p. 187) is probably the most widely used method for general screening of volatile poisons, Systems GA or GI (p. 199) may be used. Steam distillation of the sample prior to analysis by gas chromatography can be helpful with the less volatile materials.

Group 3 Poisons: Drugs (Solvent Soluble)

In general, postmortem stomach contents, blood, and urine samples may be analysed by immuno-assay (see under Immunoassays, p. 148), and by the same methods as those detailed for patients' samples (see under Hospital Toxicology and Drug Abuse Screening, p. 3), provided that the objective is identical, i.e. to obtain evidence of a drug overdose (Table 3). However, in some suspicious deaths or criminal cases, stomach contents, blood, and urine samples cannot be obtained and tissue samples have to be examined. Most screening systems for biological fluids are easily modified by the introduction of a few additional clean-up procedures to permit the utilisation of homogenates of liver or other tissues. There is much to be said for having a few routine extraction methods of general applicability rather than a large number of detailed methods each designed for a specific purpose. The inherent defects of a few routine systems are soon discovered through constant use, but this is preferable to the unknown defects of a multiplicity of systems which are rarely used. Enzymatic digestion allows the extension of stomach content, blood, and urine extraction routines to samples of solid tissue.

Table 3. Group 3 Poisons: Drugs (Solvent Soluble)

Indications

Symptoms	Effects are variable but the following information may be used as a guide:
Analgesics	Gastric irritation, haematuria, tinnitus, sweating, coma, convulsions
Opiates and synthetic narcotics	Contracted pupils, muscle twitching, slow respiration, hypotension, coma
Sedatives and hypnotics	Ataxia, slurred speech, drowsiness, stupor, coma
Stimulants and antidepressants	Dilated pupils, dry mouth, headache, tachycardia, tremors, convulsions
Onset of symptoms	Relatively slow unless injected (i.e. 2 to 48 hours)

Indications

Age	Illicit drugs more common in 16 to 30 age group. The elderly use their own prescribed drugs
Scene	Illegal lodgings, colleges, discos, clubs, mental homes
Additional investigations	Antemortem samples if the victim is admitted to hospital. Postmortem examination of nasal swabs, injection marks and a control area of skin

Analysis

Colour tests	No general tests, only selective tests for salicylates, phenothiazines, sulphonamides, etc.
Group tests	Direct solvent extraction and examination by TLC and immunoassay. Confirmation and quantification by UV, GC, HPLC, MS
Commonest poisons	Amitriptyline, amylobarbitone, butobarbitone, diazepam, imipramine, morphine, orphenadrine, paracetamol, pentobarbitone, quinalbarbitone, salicylates
Number of compounds reported	200
Number of compounds to be excluded	>1000

TISSUE ANALYSIS

Direct solvent extraction before or after acid or enzymatic digestion has almost superseded the classic protein precipitation methods. Due to the more sensitive detection methods of gas chromatography and mass spectrometry, much smaller amounts of tissue can be processed. Consequently, any emulsion problems that arise are more easily resolved than in the past when several hundred grams of liver and large volumes of solvent were required.

Enzymatic Digestion. This method is usually the best choice for general screening. It is simple, readily adaptable, and gives a protein-free filtrate from which any drugs present may be extracted. It also gives enhanced extraction of many drugs compared with the tungstate, ammonium sulphate, or Stas-Otto methods.

A suitable procedure is as follows: macerate 10 g of liver or other tissue with 40 ml of M tris(hydroxymethyl)methylamine; add 10 mg of Subtilisin A (see Reagent Appendix) and incubate in a water-bath at 50° to 60° for about one hour, with agitation. Filter the digest through a small plug of glass wool to remove undissolved connective tissue.

Aliquots of this digest may be substituted for the specified biological fluid in most routine screening procedures. The filtered digest has a pH of 8.0 to 9.5.

This method is very useful for the analysis of sectioned injection marks. The superficial fatty skin layer is removed and the remaining muscle layer analysed as above. If the injection was intramuscular and of recent origin, the drug concentrations should be greater than in a similar tissue sample not showing an injection mark. If the injection was intravenous, such a distinction cannot be expected.

The method's superb ability to 'liquidise' solid tissue can be used for many purposes apart from drug analysis. The recovery of shot-gun pellets and small bomb fragments in body tissues is one such application. The preparation of solutions for direct aspiration into atomic absorption instruments for the detection of some metals has been studied. Its use for the detection of toxic anions and some pesticides also seems feasible.

GENERAL DRUG SCREENS

A multipurpose drug screen such as Scheme 2 (p. 10) may be applied to samples of body fluids, especially when there is a limited amount of sample.

DRUG SCREENING IN NON-FATAL CRIMINAL CASES AND TRAFFIC OFFENCES

Many forensic enquiries entail analytical investigations which require detection of therapeutic drug concentrations rather than toxic concentrations. For example, in driving offences a screen is required for drugs which can impair judgement and psychomotor activities (e.g. sedatives, tranquillisers, stimulants, and narcotics). This type of analysis may also be needed to check allegations that the victim or accused is a drug addict or was under the influence of drugs at the time of the crime. The amount of blood and urine available for analysis in these cases is usually very limited and irreplaceable; additional samples taken several days after the event are useless.

Background information is of paramount importance, and the following information should be requested as a matter of routine. Were there any drugs in the possession of the victim or the defendant? What was the subject's condition (e.g. drowsy, asleep, confused, agitated, etc.)? Did the police doctor certify impairment of driving ability? Is the subject prescribed any drugs by his own doctor and, if so, when was the last dose taken? Is the subject a known drug addict?

When the identity of the suspect drug is not known before analysis, the successful detection of thera-

peutic concentrations of many of the basic drugs in blood alone is extremely difficult. Blood and urine samples should be obtained whenever possible in this type of investigation; when the blood sample is small, the chance of detecting and confirming residual traces of some antidepressant or stimulant drug is almost zero. If there is no urine sample, prescreening by radioimmunoassay methods is essential to provide an analytical guide to the nature of any drug present in the blood sample.

For forensic purposes, at least two uncorrelated methods of identification are required (e.g. TLC and GC, or GC and MS). Immunoassay methods provide good exclusion evidence, but poor confirmation of identity, although they are vital for the detection of insulin, lysergide, and the cannabinoids.

When drug concentrations are liable to be low, the extraction of separate aliquots of urine or stomach contents is recommended (Scheme 1, p. 46).

Group 4 Poisons: Metals

Historically, poisons in this group (Table 4) have been used frequently, probably because in general they are potent, tasteless, readily available, and produce symptoms similar to many common diseases. Consequently, suspicion is rarely aroused until it is too late.

For example, the substitution of arsenious oxide for the contents of one or two prescribed capsules can have fatal results with all the appearance of a straightforward drug overdose suicide. A drug-screen analysis in these circumstances will result in a very perplexed analyst and a lot of wasted time and case material. This is not a theoretical possibility, it has happened on more than one occasion!

Table 4. Group 4 Poisons: Metals

Indications	
Symptoms	Anaemia, cramps, diarrhoea, gastric pain, hair loss (thallium and selenium), jaundice, metallic taste, paralysis, peripheral neuritis, salivation, urine retention, vomiting, weight loss
Onset of symptoms	Usually after several hours; death may occur within 24 hours but more commonly after several days
Scene	Industrial locations, laboratories
Occupation	Electroplating, smelting; manufacture of agricultural chemicals, alloys, batteries, ceramics, glass, paint, petroleum products
Additional investigations	Antemortem examination of blood and urine. Postmortem examination of kidney, intestinal contents, bone, hair, nails

Table 4 (*continued*)

Analysis	
Colour test	Reinsch Test
Group test	Atomic emission spectroscopy
Commonest poisons	Arsenic, antimony, lead, lithium, mercury, thallium
Number of compounds reported	9
Number of compounds to be excluded	20

Group 4 poisons should be checked as a matter of routine if vomiting and diarrhoea are noted as symptoms, no matter what other poisons may be suggested by medical opinion or circumstantial evidence. Although the Reinsch Test (p. 57) will detect only seven of the twenty potentially toxic metals, it can be applied to almost any material (body fluids, slurried tissue, food and drinks) without any elaborate preparation, and it is sensitive enough to detect toxic concentrations of the most common poisonous metals in a few minutes. However, it misses too many metals for it to be considered as a complete group exclusion test.

If the suspect metal is specified, a laboratory equipped with atomic absorption spectrophotometry should have little difficulty in confirming the medical or police suspicions. Details of the identification and quantification of the most common metal poisons are given under Metals and Anions (p. 56).

However, the clinical symptoms are often not specific for the diagnosis of the actual metal involved and circumstantial evidence may be unavailable. In many forensic toxicological investigations there is, therefore, a requirement for a general screening method for metals.

A satisfactory routine metal screening method must be capable of analysing any biological material, without drastic modifications and with detection limits which provide reliable exclusion of minimum quoted toxic concentrations. Fortunately for most metals the lower threshold of toxicity is at least an order of magnitude higher than the normal level. A semi-quantitative rapid screening method for metals in biological samples using atomic emission spectroscopy is described on p. 56.

Group 5 Poisons: Pesticides (Solvent Soluble)

Most of the published work on the analysis of pesticides (insecticides, herbicides, rodenticides, etc.) makes the assumption that the analyst knows the identity of the actual compound or that he has some knowledge of the particular type of pesticide present in his analytical sample. This is rarely true in forensic work and until this information has been obtained, many excellent published methods are not suitable. This group is illustrated in Table 5.

Table 5. Group 5 Poisons: Pesticides (Solvent Soluble)

Indications	
Symptoms	Principal features are vomiting and convulsions. The following additional symptoms may be used as a guide:
Chlorinated hydrocarbons	Dizziness, headache, muscular weakness, tremors
Chlorinated phenoxyacetic acids	Burning sensation, low blood pressure (convulsions are not a main feature for these substances)
Organophosphates	Contracted pupils, salivation, sweating, dyspnoea, anoxia, cyanosis
Phenols and cresols	Fever (main symptom), thirst, sweating, anoxia, haematuria, jaundice
Onset of symptoms	Rapid (within 30 minutes) if product contains a petroleum solvent or is inhaled. Otherwise, slow (1 to 6 hours)
Scene	Farms and horticultural nurseries, food processing factories, domestic premises
Occupation	Manufacture of agricultural chemicals, farm workers, gardeners, pesticide officers
Additional investigations	Stained clothing, vomit, drink, stomach contents
Analysis	
Visual appearance	Abnormal colours in food, drink, or stomach contents (pesticides often contain dyes)
Odour	Hydrocarbon solvents or odours which are fishy, sulphide, or urine-like
Colour tests	Fujiwara test for trichloro-compounds Sulphuric Acid–Fuming Sulphuric Acid Test for aldrin, dieldrin, and endrin Cholinesterase inhibition test for organophosphates Dithionite test for paraquat and diquat
Group tests	Ultraviolet spectrophotometry, gas chromatography (see chapter on Pesticides)
General methods	Solvent extraction; most pesticides extract into acid and neutral groups
Commonest poisons	Chlordane, dichlorophenoxyacetic acid, lindane, mevinphos, nicotine, paraquat, parathion, trichlorophenoxyacetic acid
Number of compounds reported	20
Number of compounds to be excluded	> 500

With the exception of the world's poor peasant populations who have little access to modern synthetic drugs, few people with suicidal intentions choose to use pesticides for this purpose. This is not true of poisoners; in fact many of the chemicals used for homicidal poisoning have been pesticides. Arsenic, thallium, phosphorus, and strychnine preparations have been used as rodenticides, and nicotine and mercury salts as insecticides and fungicides. The criminal use of the herbicides sodium chlorate and paraquat is fairly common, and only a few years after its commercial introduction as an insecticide, parathion was used to commit a murder. Contrary to popular opinion, many malicious poisonings are not premeditated. The necessary warning labels present by law on most pesticide containers seem to provide an irresistible temptation to the neighbour seeking revenge, or to the jealous lover. The solvent soluble pesticides must therefore be considered in the forensic investigation of a malicious food poisoning, sudden illness, or suspicious death. An exclusion screening method, rather than a series of individual tests, is of vital importance. In view of the criminal use of pesticides in the past, the discrepancy between the number of pesticides available and the number actually detected in criminal cases is perhaps an alarming indication of how few forensic science laboratories have an adequate routine method.

The analysis of pesticides is described under Pesticides (p. 71).

Group 6 Poisons: Anions

The medicinal use of bromides and other toxic anions has declined, but most of the substances in this group are still readily available, and poisoning cases do still occur. However, detailed information on actual cases (blood and tissue concentrations etc.) is scarce. This may be because most of these poisonous salts are taken in such large amounts that their presence is usually indicated by the circumstantial evidence, and so analytical confirmation is not sought. Conventional inorganic tests applied to a filtered sample of the contents of the gastro-intestinal tract will often suffice to confirm a diagnosis. Nevertheless, an attempt at isolation, identification, and quantification in blood and tissues should be made to assist in the interpretation of an atypical case where symptoms and circumstances do not provide the usual clues. The forensic toxicologist in particular should remember Orfila's maxim—"The presence of a poison must be proved

in the blood and organs before it can be considered as a cause of death."

The toxic dose of most of the chemicals in this group is relatively large, about one or two teaspoonfuls. This may explain why, with the exception of chlorates and fluorides, they have not featured in many homicidal poisonings. However, toxic anions occur quite commonly in malicious poisoning cases, so food, drink, vomit, stomach washings, gastric aspirates, and urine should always be examined for their presence. In non-fatal cases, blood samples are usually inadequate, and should be reserved until the results of the work on other samples is known. Table 6 summarises the common features of this group.

The diphenylamine test for oxidising agents (p. 5) has a sensitivity of about 1 ppm and, if negative, excludes most of the toxic anions in this group.

Table 6. Group 6 Poisons: Anions

Indications	
Symptoms	Violent vomiting, diarrhoea, abdominal pain, cyanosis (methaemoglobin formed with oxidising agents), stained skin and mucosa (permanganate, oxalate, iodide, and bleaching agents) Exceptions to these symptoms are fluoride and bromide
Onset of symptoms	Usually within one hour, death may occur within several hours (note that the toxic dose of this group is relatively large, > 10 g)
Scene	Agricultural sites (nitrate, chlorate, fluoride, and fluoroacetate) Industrial sites (nitrite, oxalate, and sulphite) Domestic sites, drain and lavatory cleaners (hypochlorite and persulphate), weed killers (chlorate), insect powders (fluoride) Laboratories
Occupation	Sewer workers, rat catchers (fluoroacetate), factory workers
Additional investigations	Vomit, stained clothing, cups, etc. found near victim, stomach contents or washings, antemortem blood
Analysis	
Visual evidence	Chocolate-coloured blood, blood-stained vomit or urine, crystalline residues in food and drink
Colour test	Diphenylamine test for oxidising agents which covers about 50% of the group
Group tests	Not available
Number of compounds reported	7
Number of compounds to be excluded	15

A method for the isolation of toxic anions by dialysis, and procedures for identification and quantification are given under Metals and Anions (p. 55).

In non-fatal poisoning cases, the sample of food, vomit, etc. may be very limited. If this is the case, the sequential method described under Examination of Food and Drink, below, should be used.

EXAMINATION OF FOOD AND DRINK

Most malicious poisoning cases involve the addition of toxic substances to food or drink. The analysis of suspected poisoned food or drink presents different problems from the detection of drugs and poisons in body fluids. The concentration of the toxic agent is usually higher than that found in blood, urine, or postmortem tissue samples, but the available material for analysis is often more limited, and of much greater variety. The routine analysis of blood and urine samples soon ensures recognition of endogenous substances (urea, tryptamine, cholesterol, etc.) and of common exogenous chemicals such as caffeine and nicotine when they occur in extracts, spectra, and chromatograms. But one scarcely knows what to expect from the analysis of chicken curry or chocolate gateau. Packet labels demonstrate that even simple foodstuffs may contain several unfamiliar chemical additives. The parallel analysis of a purchased sample of the same food may be necessary to check that inexplicable reactions or unfamiliar spectra are normal or abnormal for that type of material.

Before starting the analysis every effort should be made to obtain details of the circumstances leading to the complaint or suspicion of doping or poisoning. Every case must be accompanied by an enquiry form similar to that shown on p. 39, and this should be supported, when possible, by an interview with the police officer. Was the suspect material tasted? If not, what aroused suspicion? Is the victim ill? What are the symptoms? Without clues to guide the selection of tests and screening systems, the sample is a 'general unknown'.

Depending on the case history, it is sometimes useful to request a urine and a blood sample from the victim; they may have been poisoned, but not by the food or drink submitted for analysis! Alternatively, the food may contain a poison, but there may not be any evidence of the poison in their blood or urine. Fake poisonings are not uncommon, especially in marital cases. Another type of fake poisoning is the misguided joke of putting some obnoxious material (e.g. urine, aloes, soap, mustard, etc.) into a person's food or drink.

About 10 g of food or 10 ml of drink (which may be all that is available) is adequate, providing that there is some guide to the nature of the poison. However, this would not be sufficient for twenty or thirty individual colour tests. A drug screen alone is not sufficient, unless the circumstantial evidence indicates that the intention was to dope rather than to poison the victim. The method must utilise techniques which are non-destructive and eliminate large numbers of compounds.

The method described below is designed to obtain the maximum amount of analytical data from the minimum quantity of material. It is very flexible and can be applied to tea, coffee, milk, alcoholic drinks, sandwiches, cakes, pies, sausages, and numerous other types of food. Vomit and food stains may also be examined.

Analytical Procedure

Make a full description of the exhibit, noting type of container, labels, seals, stains or identification marks on the outer surface, and total volume and/ or weight. Note the colour, odour, presence or absence of suspended solids or sediment, pH, and whether material has a tendency to form a stable froth on shaking.

COLOUR

The presence of abnormal colours may indicate the presence of inorganic pigments (e.g. copper, nickel, or cobalt salts), dyestuffs from tablets, capsules, medicines, pesticides, and rodent baits, especially those containing warfarin, reserpine, chloralose, or diphenadione. Common rat-bait colours are blue, green, or red and are usually associated with oatmeal or cereal grain.

ODOUR

Material taken straight from the refrigerator should be warmed gently prior to examination for odour. If possible, the opinions of several colleagues should be obtained on any abnormal odour. Many poisons can be detected in this way, but the test is very subjective, and some people have a poor sense of smell (e.g. cyanide detection by odour is an inherited ability). In favourable circumstances it is a very sensitive test; for instance, cyanide, chloroform, and toluene can be detected at about 1 ppm.

Apart from the usual characteristic odours of sulphides, aldehydes, ketones, and esters, etc., the analyst should be familiar with the smell of chloral hydrate, ethchlorvynol, methylpentynol, phenelzine, thiamine, penicillamine, penicillins and other common antibiotics. The latter compounds are typical of substances found in joke or fake poisonings.

These cases can be most frustrating to the analyst for a negative report cannot be given when there is a most obvious detectable abnormal odour whose source has not been identified. If the material has a distinct odour, a comparative head-space gas chromatographic screen is indicated.

SEDIMENTS AND SUSPENSIONS
Sediments may be due to insoluble or sparingly soluble tablet or capsule excipients such as talc, starch, or calcium phosphate, certain poisons such as arsenious oxide, or sometimes to an interaction of the added contaminant with the beverage or drink (e.g. battery acid producing a coagulation of protein material). Microscopic examination of the sediment or filtered suspension may give a clue to the nature of the material.

The presence of insoluble inorganic crystalline sediments is often due to the addition of cleaning powders (especially when accompanied by a faint odour of bleach or ammonia). Nevertheless, a spectrographic analysis for metals should be undertaken at some stage (p. 53). When crystalline material can be isolated from the material under examination, X-ray diffraction and infra-red spectrophotometry are valuable non-destructive techniques if they are readily available and are backed up by good spectral libraries.

FROTHING
The presence of stable froth when the sample is shaken (with water if necessary) may indicate contamination with soap or detergents. Acidify the sample, shake again, and if froth still forms, a detergent rather than soap is present. Although of low toxicity, soap, detergents, and cleaning powders are frequently the cause of complaints of poisoning.

DIRECT ULTRAVIOLET SPECTROPHOTOMETRY
In poisoned food or drink samples, concentrations of 0.1 to 10% are not uncommon so that direct ultraviolet spectrophotometry may often be used. This is in contrast to biological samples for which prior solvent extraction is required because of the very low concentrations (less than 0.01%).

If a sample of food contains a foreign substance with an $A_1^1 > 200$, and it is present at a concentration of 0.1%, the material may be diluted 50 times and still show the characteristic spectrum for that substance when examined by direct ultraviolet spectrophotometry. This is a very useful, rapid and non-destructive exclusion method for the large number of drugs, disinfectants, and pesticides with high specific absorbances.

Direct ultraviolet spectrophotometry is invaluable as an initial screening technique for all alcoholic drinks, and for beverages such as tea, coffee, milk, and soup. It may also be applied to solid foods (cakes, sweets, bread, etc.), and to complete meals (meat, stews, vegetables) either by application to a diluted homogenate or by examination of a copious water-wash of the food material. The latter method is preferable as most poisoners tend to sprinkle the poison on the surface of the food rather than adding it during the cooking process. A note of the weight of the material used and the volume of added water should be made to facilitate calculation of the approximate quantity of poison present.

If possible, a control sample of the particular food or drink should be examined at the same time. If the spectra obtained with the control sample are similar to those obtained with the sample, a large number of substances are excluded (Table 7) without loss or destruction of what may be an extremely limited amount of original material.

Table 7. Some compounds detectable in food and drink by direct ultraviolet spectrophotometry

Analgesics: acetanilide, aspirin, benorylate, cinchophen, etenzamide, ethoxazene, flufenamic acid, mefenamic acid, paracetamol, phenacetin, phenazone, phenylbutazone, propyphenazone, salicylamide, salicylic acid
Antidepressants: amitriptyline, butriptyline, clomipramine, desipramine, dibenzepin, dothiepin, doxepin, imipramine, iprindole, isocarboxazid, maprotiline, nortriptyline, opipramol, protriptyline, trimipramine
Antidiabetics: acetohexamide, chlorpropamide, metformin, tolbutamide
Antihistamines: antazoline, carbinoxamine, chloropyrilene, chlorpheniramine, cyproheptadine, dimethothiazine, diphenhydramine, doxylamine, isothipendyl, mepyramine, methapyrilene, promethazine, trimeprazine, tripelennamine, triprolidine
Antimalarials: amodiaquine, chloroquine, chlorproguanil, cinchonidine, cinchonine, primaquine, proguanil, pyrimethamine, quinine
Barbiturates: all
Benzodiazepines: all
Disinfectants: acriflavine, aminacrine, chlorhexidine, chloroxylenol, cresol, dofamium chloride, domiphen bromide, hexachlorophane, parachlorophenol, phenol, proflavine
Diuretics: amiloride, bendrofluazide, benzthiazide, chlorothiazide, clopamide, cyclopenthiazide, cyclothiazide, ethacrynic acid, frusemide, hydrochlorothiazide, polythiazide, quinethazone, spironolactone, triamterene
Local anaesthetics: benzocaine, butacaine, chloroprocaine, cinchocaine, cocaine, cyclomethycaine, dimethisoquin, diperodon, dyclonine, lignocaine

Table 7 (*continued*)

Pesticides and herbicides: ametryne, atrazine, benzyl benzoate, carbaryl, demeton-S, desmetryne, dinitro-orthocresol, diquat, methoprotryne, nicotine, paraquat, pentachlorophenol, rotenone, simazine, terbutryne
Purgatives: aloin, bisacodyl, danthron, oxyphenisatin, phenolphthalein
Rodenticides: coumatetralyl, diphenadione, warfarin
Sulphonamides: all
Tranquillisers: benperidol, captodiame, clopenthixol, flupenthixol, haloperidol, phenothiazines, prothipendyl, trifluperidol
Vitamins: acetomenaphthone, ascorbic acid, ergocalciferol, nicotinamide, pyridoxine, riboflavine, thiamine
Xanthines: acepifylline, bamifylline, bufylline, caffeine, diprophylline, etamiphylline, theobromine, theophylline
Miscellaneous substances: aminosalicylic acid, benzoic acid, betanaphthol, carbamazepine, chlorphenesin, dibromopropamidine, diethylpropion, halquinol, isoniazid, methaqualone, metronidazole

COLOUR TESTS

After ultraviolet spectrophotometry, the diluted liquid or washings is available for further preliminary tests, using a small aliquot for each test.
1. Apply the Fujiwara Test for trichloro-compounds (p. 135). The aqueous layer in this test can be used to test for the presence of oxalate (p. 67).
2. Apply the Diphenylamine Test for oxidising agents (p. 132).
3. Test for the presence of halides with silver nitrate (p. 64).

Warm the main bulk of the sample on a waterbath, note any odour, and test the sample with appropriate test papers (pH, lead acetate, silver nitrate, starch). Apply the Reinsch Test for metals (p. 57).
After the application of the Reinsch Test, filter the sample and retain the solids and the filter paper.
Use small aliquots of the filtrate to test for borate (p. 64), and phosphate.

EXTRACTION SCHEME

The preliminary observations often allow the tentative identification of a poison so that specific tests can then be made. If this is not so, the extraction procedure outlined below should be applied to the filtrate obtained above.

ANALYSIS OF TABLETS AND CAPSULES

Excipients. Most tablets and capsules are complex mixtures containing a small amount of one or more drugs together with a larger amount of excipients. The following substances are frequently used as excipients.

Adhesives/binders: acacia, ethylcellulose, gelatin, liquid glucose, methylcellulose, polyethylene gly-

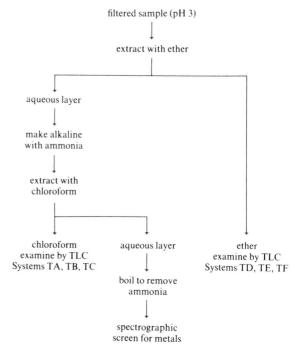

Scheme for the extraction of toxic substances in food and drink

Details of the thin-layer systems are given on pp. 167 to 169, and information on a spectrographic screen for metals on p. 56.

cols, polyvinyl pyrrolidone, sodium alginate, sodium carboxymethylcellulose, starch, and starch derivatives.

Diluents: calcium phosphate, calcium hydrogen phosphate, calcium sulphate, glucose, kaolin, lactose, mannitol, colloidal silica, sodium chloride, sodium sulphate, sorbitol.

Disintegrating and wetting agents: agar, alginic acid, bentonite, microcrystalline cellulose, gelatin, magnesium aluminium silicate, methylcellulose, sodium lauryl sulphate, starch, and starch derivatives.

Glidants and lubricants: boric acid, colloidal silica, hydrogenated vegetable oils, magnesium stearate, polyethylene glycols, stearic acid, talc.

Flavouring agents: cocoa, glucose, liquorice powder, sodium citrate, sucrose.

A combination of visual and microscopic examination, colour tests, chromatography, and ultraviolet and infra-red spectrophotometry is employed in the analysis. If the preparation is fairly common and does not contain a complex mixture of drugs, two or three of these techniques will usually succeed in establishing the identity of the tablet or indicating the nature of the drug or drugs it contains. The first step is to make careful notes about the container and its contents.

Container. This may be a tube, envelope, folded paper packet, box, or bottle. Note any seals and labels. Make full notes of the information given on the label.

Contents. Note the total number of tablets or other preparation in the container, together with an estimate of the total number which the container could hold if filled. Note the shape (flat, bevelled, biconvex, etc.), whether compression-coated, film-coated, enteric-coated, or sugar-coated, markings (numbers, letters, symbols, or score marks), exterior and interior colour, layered and core tablets, and mean weight, diameter, and thickness.

Visual Recognition

This can only be regarded as a useful clue; even tablets with well-known brand names may be faked, and placebo tablets are sometimes made. Every laboratory should maintain a reference collection of authentic tablets and capsules and reference can be made to published collections of tablet identification data. If the container bears the name of the pharmaceutical manufacturer a telephone call giving the details of the tablets (even if they are unmarked white ones) may enable the firm to suggest a limited number of their products sold in that form. Especial care is required with capsules because their contents may readily be changed. (Arsenic, cyanide, and lysergide have been substituted in the past.)

The analyst should be aware of certain less common preparations which may be encountered.

Homoeopathic Preparations. These are usually round, flat/flat tablets with rough surfaces, 5 to 6 mm in diameter, and contain mainly lactose.

Injection Tablets. Small, totally soluble tablets used for making solutions for injection. The most commonly encountered until recently were diamorphine tablets. These were round, flat/flat tablets, 4 mm in diameter and 2 mm thick, weighing 30 mg. They have been discontinued but they may still be seen, having been burgled from pharmacies. These tablets should not be confused with LSD microdots which are usually highly coloured.

Health Food Preparations. These usually contain vitamins, minerals, herbal extracts, yeast, etc. There are too many different brands to incorporate in any collection.

Sex-shop Preparations. These usually contain substances reputed to be aphrodisiacs such as vitamin E and ginseng.

Non-medicinal Preparations. These include a variety of preparations such as sweetener tablets, fertiliser tablets, stink bombs, indoor fireworks, and slug pellets.

Analytical Procedure

MICROSCOPIC EXAMINATION

Place a small amount of a crushed tablet or capsule contents on a slide, mix with a drop of water, and cover carefully with a cover-slip avoiding trapped air bubbles. Observe under low-power magnification. Effervescence will be obvious. If crystalline material is visible, note if it is water-soluble. Check the pH of the solution. An alkaline reaction may indicate the presence of a sodium salt of an acidic drug. Introduce a small drop of *silver nitrate solution* along one edge of the cover-slip; a visible precipitate indicates the possible presence of a hydrochloride salt of a basic drug.

Note the presence of any organised plant material. In most cases this will be corn (maize) or wheat starch which can be confirmed by the blue colour obtained with iodine solution or by examination under polarised light (starch grains exhibit a distorted cross). The ability to recognise the various commercial starches is a useful skill. The presence of a large amount of uncooked starch grains in a sample of stomach contents often provides a useful clue to the ingestion of an unsuspected overdose of tablets or capsules, even when the deceased survived for several hours after their ingestion.

The presence of other types of plant material indicates the tablet is probably a herbal remedy. These are frequently very complex mixtures and are unlikely to be identified by the simple methods proposed in this chapter. However, the examination of an alcohol extract by ultraviolet spectrophotometry and thin-layer chromatography is worth attempting.

ODOUR

A few drugs have distinctive odours and this can provide a clue to the compound or at least to the type of preparation. A yeast-like or meaty smell may indicate a harmless vitamin preparation, an odour of peppermint may indicate a non-toxic indigestion remedy. Antibiotics, especially of the penicillin group, sometimes have a rather unpleasant sulphide-type smell. Other drugs with characteristic odours are chlormethiazole, phenelzine, amitriptyline, ethchlorvynol, chloral hydrate, and methylpentynol.

SIZE

The size of the tablet, which should be measured with callipers having a vernier reading to 0.1 mm, can provide a rough guide to the general class of preparation. Large diameter tablets (i.e. > 10 mm) are unlikely to contain potent alkaloids (except codeine) and conversely, tablets with diameters less than 5 mm could not contain drugs with medicinal doses of 200 mg or more.

There is an approximate correlation between tablet diameter and the amount of drug contained in the tablet (Table 8), and this may be used as a rough guide.

Table 8. Relationship between tablet diameter and probable drug content

Tablet diameter mm	Probable drug content mg
less than 6	less than 5
,, ,, 7	,, ,, 15
,, ,, 8	15 to 100
,, ,, 9	30 to 200
,, ,, 10	200 to 300
greater than 11	250 to 500

A useful table of tablet diameters and related drug content is given in *The Pharmaceutical Codex*, 11th Edn, London, The Pharmaceutical Press, 1979, pp. 909–912.

COLOUR TESTS

These should be tried only if an adequate number of tablets or capsules is available, as they are destructive tests. They may provide a clue to the identity of the unknown but they are rarely specific. However, they are useful when the appearance or markings suggest an identity.

1. Heat some of the powdered material on a metal spatula. Little or no charring is indicative of an inorganic preparation.
2. Marquis Test (p. 139). Many basic drugs produce colours with this reagent. It is a good test for opiates, stimulants, antihistamines, and phenothiazines.
3. Koppanyi–Zwikker Test (p. 135) for barbiturates and sulphonamides.
4. Mercurous Nitrate (p. 140) and Nitrous Acid (p. 143) for sulphonamides.
5. Ferric Chloride (p. 133) for phenols.
6. Forrest Reagent (p. 134) or FPN Reagent (p. 134) for phenothiazines.
7. Iodoplatinate Test (p. 135). This is a valuable test if the test material does not contain starch. If a colour is not obtained, most of the basic narcotic, antidepressant, antihistamine, and tranquilliser drugs can be eliminated.

EXTRACTION OF TABLETS AND CAPSULES

Elaborate solvent fractionation schemes are not usually necessary for solid dosage preparations. Most drugs are soluble in methanol and most of the excipients are not; therefore the preparation of a simple methanol extract is all that is required. However, if the methanol extract is too concentrated, the spot on the TLC plate will be overloaded and the resultant chromatogram will be useless. Any subsequent ultraviolet spectrophotometric examination of the extract may give spectra which are not on scale. This cannot always be avoided, but the following guide-lines have been found useful.

If a possible identity is suggested by the case notes or by visual examination of the sample, check the published content of medicament and adjust the amount of methanol to produce an approximate concentration of 1 to 20 mg/ml.

If there are no clues to the identity (e.g. a plain white tablet), measure the diameter. For a diameter of 5 to 6 mm, use 1 or 2 ml of methanol per tablet; for diameters of 8 to 9 mm, use about half a tablet in 5 to 10 ml of methanol; for diameters greater than 9 mm, use about one quarter of a tablet in 20 ml of methanol.

THIN-LAYER CHROMATOGRAPHY

The great majority of drugs present in pharmaceutical products are nitrogenous bases. The extract should be examined, therefore, by Systems TA, TB, or TC (p. 167). If these fail to reveal any positive reacting spots with the suggested location reagents, the possible identity of the unknown substance is reduced from a large number of basic drugs to a few hundred acidic and neutral drugs. The extract should then be examined by Systems TD, TE, or TF (p. 168).

ULTRAVIOLET SPECTROPHOTOMETRY

A portion of the methanol extract is diluted with water and examined at both acid and alkaline pH by ultraviolet spectrophotometry. The features of any resultant spectrum should be checked in the index to Ultraviolet Absorption Data in Part 3. If the identity is suspected, the spectrum may be compared with that given in the monograph in Part 2.

INFRA-RED SPECTROPHOTOMETRY

Extract a small portion of the crushed tablet or capsule contents with chloroform; to a portion of the chloroform extract add solid potassium bromide, dry under an infra-red lamp, prepare a compressed disk, and examine by infra-red spectrophotometry. The features of any resultant spectrum should be checked in the index of Infra-red Peaks in Part 3. If the identity is suspected, the spectrum may be compared with that given in the monograph in Part 2.

Many theoretical reasons can be put forward to suggest why such a procedure would be useless (e.g. the product may contain more than one drug, or the contents may be insoluble in chloroform). However, in practice it is often a rapid, nondestructive method of identification. Even when the product does contain more than one drug, infrared spectrophotometers often have spectral subtraction routines which enable a pure spectrum to be obtained from a mixture.

For the majority of compounds, a mixture of 1 mg of drug with 150 mg of dry potassium bromide will produce a good spectrum. It is not too difficult to obtain a rough estimate of the amount of sample needed to achieve this concentration if the product has been partially identified by other means. However, when the identity is completely unknown, it may require several attempts to obtain a disk with the correct concentration. Table 8 may be used as a rough guide.

LOW DOSE PREPARATIONS

When the results of all the above analytical methods are negative, this information still may provide a useful clue to the possible identity of the sample. Homoeopathic and other low dose preparations should be considered.

If the unknown preparation contains less than 1 mg of active drug, the amount of substance extracted for each test may be too small to react under the test conditions. This is especially true if only one tablet has been analysed and the particular compound has few reactive functional groups. Tablets and capsules of modern high potency drugs usually have distinctive shapes, colours, or markings. If the tablet is small, white, and unmarked, it may be one of the established drugs with very low effective doses. A list of tablets and capsules which may contain 1 mg or less of active ingredient is given below.

Antihypertensives and drugs used in cardiac disorders: clonidine, deserpidine, digitoxin, digoxin, glyceryl trinitrate, lanatoside C, reserpine, warfarin.

Diuretics: cyclopenthiazide, polythiazide.

Ergot alkaloids and related drugs: dihydroergotamine, ergometrine, ergotamine, lysergide, methysergide.

Hypnotics, sedatives, and tranquillisers: benperidol, clonazepam, flunitrazepam, flupenthixol, haloperidol, lorazepam, lormetazepam, triazolam, trifluoperazine.

Steroids, hormones, and related compounds: betamethasone, dexamethasone, dienoestrol, ethinyloestradiol, ethynodiol diacetate, fludrocortisone, liothyronine, lynoestrenol, mestranol, norethisterone, stilboestrol, thyroxine.

Miscellaneous drugs: atropine, colchicine, folic acid, hyoscine.

EXAMINATION OF SYRINGES

A syringe found at the scene of an incident or in the possession of the victim or suspect should always be examined by the toxicologist, even if it has been stated that it is clean or empty.

If the syringe contains a few drops of an aqueous solution, remove a portion with a small TLC-spotting pipette, and examine by the usual routine TLC systems. There is a high probability that a narcotic drug will be present, but barbiturates, amphetamine, or methylphenidate may also be abused using a syringe. Wash the syringe with 1 ml of water and use this solution for ultraviolet spectrophotometry in acid and at pH 10. If a drug is indicated, a pure sample of the substance should be examined in conjunction with the original undiluted aqueous solution.

If the syringe is dry, introduce one or two drops of methanol into the syringe, and proceed as described above.

The volumes of water used and any dilutions necessary for the ultraviolet examination must be noted in order to give a quantitative estimate of any drug present. Apart from the small amount used for TLC, the bulk of the extract is still available should analysis by gas chromatography or mass spectrometry be required. Direct solvent extraction can be applied to the extracts, and dilutions used for ultraviolet spectrophotometric analysis. This may also be necessary if the syringe is heavily blood-stained. It is important to remember that some of the drugs encountered in syringes are susceptible to alkaline hydrolysis (e.g. diamorphine, methylphenidate, and barbiturates). Thus the addition of strong sodium hydroxide solution to the syringe should be avoided.

Bibliography

Advances in Analytical Toxicology, Vol. 1, R. C. Baselt (Ed.), Davis, California, Biomedical Publications, 1984.

Assay of Drugs and Other Trace Compounds in Biological Fluids, E. Reid (Ed.), Oxford, North Holland Publishing Co., 1976.

Blood, Drugs and Other Analytical Challenges, E. Reid (Ed.), Chichester, Ellis Horwood, 1978.

Chemist and Druggist Directory and Tablet Identification Guide, London, Benn Business Information Services, 1985.

W. A. L. Collier, *IMPREX: Index of Imprints used on Tablets and Capsules*, 10th Edn, Cambridge, IMPREX, 1984.

A. S. Curry, *Advances in Forensic and Clinical Toxicology*, Cleveland, Ohio, CRC Press, 1972.

A. S. Curry, *Poison Detection in Human Organs*, 3rd Edn, Springfield, Illinois, Charles C. Thomas, 1976.

Forensic Toxicology, J. S. Oliver (Ed.), London, Croom Helm, 1980.

Forensic Toxicology: Proceedings of a Symposium held at the Chemical Defence Establishment, Porton Down, 29–30 June 1972, B. Ballantyne (Ed.), Bristol, John Wright, 1974.

Handbook of Pharmaceutical Excipients, Washington, American Pharmaceutical Association and London, Pharmaceutical Press, 1985.

Introduction to Forensic Toxicology, R. H. Cravey and R. C. Baselt (Ed.), Davis, California, Biomedical Publications, 1981.

The Poisoned Patient: The Role of the Laboratory, R. Porter and M. O'Connor (Ed.), Amsterdam, Elsevier North-Holland, 1974.

S. Thomas, Tablident: A New Method of Solid Dose Form Identification, *Pharm. J.*, 1983, *231*, 261–263.

Topics in Forensic and Analytical Toxicology, R. A. A. Maes (Ed.), New York, Elsevier, 1984.

Toxicology Annual, Vols 1 and 2, C. L. Winek (Ed.), New York, Marcel Dekker, 1974 and 1978.

Metals and Anions

W. B. Yeoman

Samples

The samples usually available in suspected cases of non-fatal poisoning include stomach washings or vomit, blood, and urine. In postmortem cases, samples of stomach contents, blood, and urine should be obtained.

It is good practice to store all samples at $-20°$ if analyses cannot be made immediately, and to retain all residues similarly, after reporting of results. It often becomes necessary to carry out further analyses on the samples or to submit them for validation of the findings by another laboratory. However, the samples must be allowed to return to room temperature gradually as the application of direct heat or even placing them in a low-temperature water-bath may result in the loss of unstable or volatile components.

Stomach Contents

Vomit or stomach contents aspirated before any wash-out procedures are the most suitable samples for analysis. Any unusual odours, the presence of food residues, or of 'altered' blood ('coffee grounds'), and the presence of any other foreign material should be noted. Both stomach contents and vomit are mucoid and frequently viscid and require filtration before further examination. Normal filtration of the sample may be difficult; a more satisfactory method is to force the sample through a 2-cm layer of cotton wool held in the barrel of a syringe. Stomach contents obtained at autopsy can be treated similarly.

Alternatively, prepare a filterable slurry by adding water, mixing thoroughly, and filtering through a coarse grade filter paper. If the filtrate is too turbid or the slurry will not filter, add a suitable volume of a 10% solution of sodium carbonate, heat with continual stirring, and filter.

Although stomach contents are usually concentrated enough to allow direct analysis, stomach washings may be too dilute to yield meaningful results. Such a sample may be concentrated by distillation or by dialysis procedures, but this often leads to the loss of certain anions, such as hypochlorite, sulphide, and sulphite.

Isolation of Toxic Anions by Dialysis. Dialysis in cellophane bags or Visking tubing frequently succeeds where filtration procedures fail. However, it is more time consuming and may give low yields for borate, chlorate, and oxalate even after dialysis for 16 hours. It is rarely necessary for samples of food or drink. The dialyser should be as flat as possible. The thinner the layer in the inner container, and the larger the volume of water in the outer vessel, the more rapid the diffusion. Prepare a slurry of about 25 g of the gastric or intestinal contents, place it in the inner container, add 250 ml of water in the outer vessel, and dialyse for at least 2 hours. Carefully evaporate the dialysate (the contents of the outer vessel) to dryness in a platinum dish and dissolve the residue in a little water.

Isolation of Toxic Anions by Protein Precipitation. Prepare a slurry of the sample, coagulate the proteins with ammonium sulphate, filter, precipitate ammonium sulphate remaining in the filtrate with methanol, and evaporate the supernatant liquid (F. Rieders and F. J. Frere, *J. forens. Sci.*, 1963, *8*, 46–53).

Blood

Venous blood (30 ml) should be obtained in all cases of suspected poisoning; a 5-ml portion of the sample should have an anticoagulant added to it. Heparinised sample containers should be avoided as the heparin may contain trace elements related to its animal source. If such a container is used, then a duplicate blank container should also be subjected to the assay to take account of possible contamination. In assays for lead and cadmium, either disodium or dipotassium edetate is the preferred anticoagulant.

Blood obtained at autopsy may be grossly contaminated by other fluids released during the autopsy procedure. A blood sample should therefore be obtained from a major artery or vein, e.g. the femoral artery. However, even these samples are likely to be highly haemolysed and give a poor yield of serum. It is therefore useful to perform some simple digestion procedure, such as the enzyme digestion method for tissues (see p. 44), before analysis. If this approach is used, then the subsequent analysis performed on the sample must be repeated on a reagent blank. It is not unknown for a reagent blank to yield high concentrations of the analyte.

Low temperature ashing techniques for the assay of cations, using mixed reactive gases at low pressure (1 Torr) have been reported (F. G. Carter and W. B. Yeoman, *Analyst, Lond.*, 1980, *105*, 295–297; H. T. Delves, *Prog. analyt. Atom. Spectros.*, 1981, *4*, 1–48).

Urine

The largest possible volume of urine should be submitted to the laboratory soon after the incident. To avoid the possibility of contamination, preservatives should not be added to the sample. The total volume should be measured immediately after receipt. A 20-ml portion of the sample should be stored at $-20°$ for future reference.

Metals

The analysis of trace metals in biological fluids has been carried out for many years. An increased interest in environmental pollution, together with health-monitoring of individual workers has resulted in the rapid development of both sensitive instruments and sensitive techniques.

Atomic absorption spectrophotometry (AAS) is one of the most widely used methods. Either flame atomisation or electrothermal atomisation (ETA) using the graphite furnace is employed. Some useful references are given in the Bibliography.

The control systems in each atomic absorption instrument will have individual settings, and in all cases the manufacturer's instructions should be followed. Whichever instrument is used, a facility for background correction is mandatory in order to compensate for interference from the complex biological medium. However, background correction does have limitations when wavelengths below 300 nm are used.

Another approach to trace metal analysis has been the development of anodic stripping voltammetry (ASV), a derivative of classical polarography. An advantage of the method is that it requires relatively small volumes of blood. The need to subject samples to digestion procedures prior to ASV poses some difficulty, although digestants are available commercially. The advent of inductively coupled plasma/atomic emission spectroscopy (ICP/AES) which uses an argon plasma as a heat source enables temperatures of up to 10 000° to be attained and is potentially capable of enhanced sensitivity. Present practice, however, suggests that for many elements the ICP/AES may not offer superior sensitivity over conventional atomic absorption spectrophotometry.

Interference from endogenous biological materials in the sample poses problems with all these techniques and many workers routinely use preliminary digestion procedures. However, such an approach is not expedient in an emergency situation and generally, the simplest preparative steps yield the best results.

In the analytical methods which follow, the water used for making solutions should be double-distilled, and high-purity grade acids which are low in trace metals should be used. It is advisable to carry out all assays in duplicate. Dilute standard solutions should be freshly prepared.

Screening for Metals by Atomic Emission Spectroscopy

E. C. Blacklock and P. A. Sadler, *Clinica chim. Acta*, 1981, *113*, 87–94.

A method which can be used as a screen for all heavy metals has not yet been devised. However, the following method will detect antimony, arsenic, bismuth, cadmium, lead, mercury, and thallium. Certain metals do not form complexes, e.g. barium and chromium, and these may be detected in trace amounts by direct application to the Lithium Fluoride–Graphite Mixture.

Reagents. Complexing Agent. Dissolve 10 g of ammonium pyrrolidine dithiocarbamate, 10 g of sodium diethyldithiocarbamate, and 10 g of potassium sodium tartrate in sufficient water to produce 1000 ml.

Lithium Fluoride–Graphite Mixture. Dry lithium fluoride at 250° for 1 hour, cool, and grind 1 part with 9 parts of non-pelletable graphite powder for 5 minutes.

Method. Liquid samples such as urine, spirits, beer, and lemonade can by assayed without prior extraction. Samples of food, stomach contents, or blood must be extracted as described below.

To 1 g of food or stomach contents or 1 ml of blood in a screw-capped test-tube add 1 ml of *nitric acid* and allow to stand overnight. Centrifuge at 3000 rpm for 15 minutes and to 1 ml of the supernatant liquid from the sample tube add sufficient water to produce 10 ml. Adjust the aqueous solution to pH 4, transfer to a glass separating funnel, add 1 ml of the Complexing Agent and 4 ml of chloroform, and shake vigorously for 2 minutes; allow to separate and collect the chloroform layer in a glass vial. Repeat the extraction with a further 2 ml of chloroform and combine the chloroform extracts. Repeat the procedure using 1 ml of water (blank).

Add the combined chloroform extracts (or 2 ml of a liquid sample) to 50 mg of the Lithium Fluoride–Graphite Mixture and evaporate by means of an infra-red lamp. Cool the mixture and tamp it into an anode cup for emission spectroscopy. Burn in a DC arc at 15 A, using a 3 mm rod as the counter electrode, using the following (or similar) conditions: Spectrograph—Hilger and Watt 3 metre grating; plate mask—2 mm; slit width—0.015 mm; analytical gap—6 mm; electrode mask gap—6 mm; exposure time—20 s; current—15 A; top electrode (negative)—Ringsdorff 3 mm graphite rod; bottom electrode (positive)—Ringsdorff RW0078 anode cup; charge weight—20 mg $\pm$ 1 mg; photographic plate—Kodak Spectrum Analysis No. 1 (SA1); wavelength range—200 to 350 nm.

The method may be used in a semi-quantitative manner by visually comparing the sample plate against plates prepared with known concentrations of metals.

The identity of any metal found in abnormal amounts should be confirmed by specific methods described later.

Reinsch Test

To 15 ml of the sample of body fluid or homogenised tissue extract, add 3 ml of *hydrochloric acid*, and immerse in the liquid a 5 mm × 10 mm copper strip or a spiral of copper wire formed by winding the wire around a glass rod ten times; heat gently for 2 hours. Remove the metal, wash gently with water and examine the surface.

A silver deposit indicates the presence of mercury; a shiny black deposit which is insoluble in *potassium cyanide solution* is given by bismuth; a dull black deposit which is soluble in *potassium cyanide solution* indicates the presence of arsenic; a purple deposit which is insoluble in *potassium cyanide solution* is given by antimony. Dark deposits may indicate selenium or tellurium, whereas a speckled discoloration is given by high concentrations of sulphur.

The test is sensitive to approximately 0.5 μg/ml of arsenic, 1.0 μg/ml of antimony and bismuth, and 2.5 μg/ml of mercury.

Arsenic

Two methods are described below. A colorimetric method which is applicable to blood, and an atomic absorption spectrophotometric method which is applicable to urine. Both methods employ an arsine generating vessel. A large volume of blood (up to 50 ml) or urine (25 ml or more) may be required because concentrations of arsenic in the body may be near the detection limits of the assays.

COLORIMETRIC ASSAY FOR ARSENIC IN BLOOD

Standard Arsenic Solutions. Dissolve 2.4196 g of arsenic trichloride in sufficient M hydrochloric acid to produce 1000 ml. This solution contains 1 mg of As in 1 ml. Serially dilute the solution with water to produce solutions containing 0.5, 2.0, 5.0, and 10.0 μg of As in 1 ml.

Reagents. Silver DDC Solution. A 0.5% solution of silver diethyldithiocarbamate in pyridine. This reagent should be stored in amber bottles.

Stannous Chloride Reagent (40%). Dissolve 40 g of stannous chloride dihydrate in sufficient *hydrochloric acid* to produce 100 ml.

Digestion Mixture. To 3 volumes of *nitric acid* add 1 volume of *sulphuric acid* and 1 volume of *perchloric acid*.

Method. In cases of suspected arsenic poisoning, 5 ml of blood should be used; a larger volume may be required from unexposed subjects.

Place 5 ml of the blood sample in a 125-ml flask, add 5 ml of the Digestion Mixture, heat, gently at first, then at about 150°. When the solution boils and begins to char, add 2 ml of *nitric acid*; continue to add 1-ml quantities of *nitric acid* and a few drops of *perchloric acid* until a clear straw-coloured solution is obtained. Maintain the temperature until white fumes of sulphur trioxide are evolved and the solution is free from nitric acid. Cool, transfer quantitatively to a 10-ml volumetric flask, and dilute to volume with water.

Transfer 3 ml of the digested sample to the arsine generating vessel, add sufficient water to produce 35 ml, and then add 5 ml of *hydrochloric acid*, 2 ml of a 15% solution of potassium iodide, and 0.5 ml of Stannous Chloride Reagent (40%); swirl the solution, and allow to stand for 15 minutes. Insert a pad of glass wool moistened with *lead acetate solution* into the lower tube of the generating vessel. Introduce 3 ml of the Silver DDC Solution into the absorber tube, and 3 g of granulated zinc into the flask, and immediately assemble the two parts of the apparatus. Allow the evolution of arsine to continue for 1 hour. Transfer the Silver DDC

Solution from the absorber tube to a 1-cm cell, and record the absorbance at 540 nm, using in the reference cell a blank prepared by treating 5 ml of water in the same manner.

Repeat the procedure using 5 ml of each of the diluted standard solutions.

Plot the absorbance of each standard solution against the concentration of arsenic, and read off the concentration in the sample.

ATOMIC ABSORPTION ASSAY FOR ARSENIC IN URINE
In this method, the arsine generator is suitably connected to the atomic absorption spectrophotometer.

Standard Arsenic Solutions. Prepare diluted standard solutions as described in the colorimetric assay, above.

Reagent. Stannous Chloride Reagent (20%). Dissolve 20 g of stannous chloride dihydrate in sufficient *hydrochloric acid* to produce 100 ml.

Method. To 25 ml of the urine sample, add 1 ml of a 20% solution of potassium iodide and 0.5 ml of Stannous Chloride Reagent (20%), mix, and allow to stand for 10 minutes. Isolate the arsine generator from the spectrophotometer, and introduce into the vessel 10 ml of the sample solution; add 0.5 g of granulated zinc and 1 ml of *hydrochloric acid*, immediately assemble the two parts of the generator, and stir with a magnetic stirrer for 2 minutes. Connect the arsine generator to the spectrophotometer and record the absorbance at 193.7 nm.

Repeat the procedure using 25 ml of each of the diluted standard solutions and 25 ml of water (blank).

Plot the absorbance of each standard solution against the concentration of arsenic, and read off the concentration in the sample. The calibration curve is non-linear.

INTERPRETATION
Arsenic is distributed into all human tissues and fluids.

The concentration of arsenic in urine from unexposed subjects is less than 0.05 µg/ml. In cases of chronic poisoning, values between 0.05 and 5 µg/ml may be found. Acute poisoning is usually associated with values in excess of 1 µg/ml and may reach 20 µg/ml.

Arsenic is metabolised to monomethylarsonic acid and dimethylarsinic acid. Individuals exposed to arsenic, such as glass workers, may have a total arsenic concentration in the urine of up to 0.07 µg/ml, more than 50% of it appearing as dimethyl-

arsinic acid. High excretion of arsenic is also seen in consumers of seafood such as crab meat.

Blood concentrations in unexposed subjects are usually in the range 0.001 to 0.025 µg/ml. Smokers may have slightly higher concentrations.

Cadmium

H. T. Delves and J. Woodward, *Atomic Spectroscopy*, 1981, *2*, 65–67.

The following atomic absorption spectrophotometric technique is applicable to blood, and involves atomisation in a graphite furnace assembly. Blood samples should be anticoagulated with dipotassium edetate. If heparin is used, a blank containing heparin of the same batch should be carried through the preparative and assay procedures.

Standard Cadmium Solutions. Dissolve 2.7442 g of cadmium nitrate [$Cd(NO_3)_2,4H_2O$] in sufficient M nitric acid to produce 1000 ml. This solution contains 1 mg of Cd in 1 ml. Serially dilute the solution with a 0.05% solution of *nitric acid* to produce solutions containing 0.0005, 0.001, 0.002, 0.004, 0.006, 0.008, and 0.01 µg/ml.

Method. To 100 µl of the sample of whole blood add 100 µl of a 0.05% solution of *nitric acid* and 100 µl of a 1% solution of ammonium dihydrogen phosphate, and mix thoroughly. Introduce 20 µl of the mixture into the graphite furnace, dry, ash, atomise, and record the absorbance at 228.8 nm.

Repeat the procedure using, in place of the sample, solutions prepared by adding 100 µl of each of the diluted standard solutions to 100 µl quantities of pooled normal blood.

Plot the absorbance of each standard solution against the concentration of cadmium, reduce the intercept to zero by drawing a parallel line through the origin, and read off the concentration in the sample. The calibration curve should be linear in the range 0 to 0.01 µg/ml.

INTERPRETATION
Blood-cadmium concentrations in non-smokers are less than 0.0025 µg/ml whereas smokers may exhibit concentrations of up to 0.0065 µg/ml; 50 to 70% of the cadmium is present in erythrocytes. Symptoms of cadmium toxicity appear at blood concentrations of 0.015 µg/ml or more. Concentrations in the urine, although variable, may be of a similar order to those found in blood.

Chromium

The following atomic absorption spectrophotometric technique is applicable to urine, and involves atomisation in a graphite furnace assembly. The method of standard additions is used. Contamination from stainless steel needles should be avoided. The use of polystyrene test-tubes is recommended. This method may be modified to determine chromium in blood, but the assay conditions are much more critical.

Note. In an emergency, the sample of urine may be aspirated directly into a conventional air–acetylene flame and its absorbance at 357.9 nm compared with urine from an unexposed subject.

Standard Chromium Solutions. Dissolve 7.6958 g of chromic nitrate $[Cr(NO_3)_3,9H_2O]$ in sufficient M nitric acid to produce 1000 ml. This solution contains 1 mg of Cr in 1 ml. Serially dilute the solution with 0.01M nitric acid to produce solutions containing 0.01, 0.02, 0.03, 0.04, and 0.05 µg of Cr in 1 ml.

Method. To 10 ml of the urine sample add 0.1 ml of *nitric acid* and allow to stand for 1 hour. Transfer three 1-ml portions of the solution to separate test-tubes and to two of them add, respectively, 1 ml of standard solutions containing 0.02 and 0.05 µg/ml of Cr; to the third tube add 1 ml of 0.01 M nitric acid. Introduce 5 µl of each solution into the graphite furnace, dry, ash, atomise, and record the absorbance at 357.9 nm.

Record the absorbance of each of the diluted standard solutions in a similar manner.

Plot the absorbance of each standard solution against the concentration of chromium, read off the concentration in the three sample tubes, and calculate the concentration in the sample. The calibration curve should be linear at least in the range 0 to 0.03 µg/ml.

INTERPRETATION

The concentration of chromium in urine samples from unexposed subjects is usually in the range 0.002 to 0.04 µg/ml. Whole blood concentrations of chromium are generally between 0.001 and 0.005 µg/ml.

Copper

The following colorimetric and atomic absorption spectrophotometric methods are applicable to serum. The atomic absorption method uses a conventional air–acetylene flame atomiser.

COLORIMETRIC ASSAY FOR COPPER IN SERUM

Standard Copper Solutions. Dissolve 1.000 g of copper foil in the minimum volume of a 50% solution of *nitric acid*, and add sufficient of a 1% solution of *nitric acid* to produce 1000 ml. This solution contains 1 mg of Cu in 1 ml. Serially dilute the solution with water to produce solutions containing 0.5, 1.0, 1.5, and 2.0 µg of Cu in 1 ml.

Reagent. Oxalyl Dihydrazide Reagent. To 12 ml of *strong ammonia solution* add 8 ml of a saturated solution of oxalyl dihydrazide, 20 ml of a 40% solution of acetaldehyde, and 20 ml of water.

Method. To 1 ml of the serum sample in a plastic centrifuge tube add 0.7 ml of 2M hydrochloric acid, mix, and allow to stand for 15 minutes; add 1 ml of a 20% solution of trichloroacetic acid, mix thoroughly, allow to stand for a further 15 minutes, and centrifuge. Transfer 2 ml of the supernatant liquid to a test-tube, add 3 ml of Oxalyl Dihydrazide Reagent, mix, and allow to stand for 20 minutes.

Record the absorbance of the solution at 542 nm, using in the reference cell a blank prepared by treating 1 ml of water in the same manner.

Repeat the procedure using the diluted standard solutions.

Plot the absorbance of each standard solution against the concentration of copper, and read off the concentration in the sample. The calibration curve should be linear for concentrations in the range 0 to 2 µg/ml.

ATOMIC ABSORPTION ASSAY FOR COPPER IN SERUM

Standard Copper Solutions. Prepare a solution of copper containing 1 mg in 1 ml as described in the colorimetric method, above. Serially dilute the solution with *sodium chloride–potassium chloride solution* to produce solutions containing 0.5, 1.0, 1.5, 2.0, and 2.5 µg of Cu in 1 ml.

Method. Dilute 1 ml of the serum sample with sufficient of a 6% solution of butan-1-ol to produce 10 ml, mix, aspirate into an oxidising (blue) flame, and record the absorbance at 324.7 nm.

Repeat the procedure with 1 ml of each of the diluted standard solutions, and with 1 ml of *sodium chloride–potassium chloride solution* (blank).

Plot the absorbance of each standard solution against the concentration of copper, and read off the concentration in the sample. The calibration curve may be non-linear.

INTERPRETATION

The concentration of copper in normal serum samples is in the range 0.7 to 1.6 µg/ml. Hormone levels may affect the concentration of copper, and women using oestrogenic oral contraceptives may show concentrations as high as 3 µg/ml. Significantly lower serum concentrations are found in Wilson's disease (below 0.7 µg/ml). In cases of copper poisoning, concentrations in excess of 3 µg/ml have been reported.

Gold

The following atomic absorption spectrophotometric technique is applicable to serum, and uses a conventional air–acetylene flame atomiser.

Standard Gold Solutions. Prepare a solution containing 1 mg of Au in 1 ml. Serially dilute this solution with *sodium chloride–potassium chloride solution* to produce solutions containing 0.5, 1.0, 1.5, 2.0, and 2.5 µg of Au in 1 ml.

Method. Dilute 1 ml of the serum with sufficient of a 6% solution of butan-1-ol to produce 4 ml, mix, aspirate into an oxidising (blue) flame, and record the absorbance at 242.8 nm.

Repeat the procedure with 1 ml of each of the diluted standard solutions, and with 1 ml of *sodium chloride–potassium chloride solution* (blank).

Plot the absorbance of each standard solution against the concentration of gold, and read off the concentration in the sample. The calibration curve should be linear in the range 0.5 to 2.5 µg/ml.

INTERPRETATION

Trace amounts of gold present in serum from unexposed subjects may not be detected by this method. There appears to be little agreement regarding the interpretation of serum-gold concentrations, and it is difficult to correlate serum concentrations with dose. Following a dose of 50 mg of sodium aurothiomalate, serum-gold concentrations of 1.5 to 2 µg/ml have been obtained, whereas values of up to 15 µg/ml following an overdose of 500 mg have been reported. Gold appears to cross the placental barrier and has been detected in foetal kidney and liver. Excretion in the urine is extremely slow and the presence of gold in tissues has been demonstrated 1 year after a single dose.

Iron

The following atomic absorption spectrophotometric method is applicable to serum and uses a conventional air–acetylene flame atomiser.

Note. In emergencies, especially involving young children, the serum sample may be aspirated directly into the flame to give an indication of intoxication. A screening test for ferrous and ferric iron is given on p. 5. Commercial kits for the assay of iron in serum are available (see Reagent Appendix).

The assay of a urine sample in the presence of a chelating agent such as desferrioxamine involves elaborate sample preparation to hydrolyse the chelate, and electrothermal atomisation.

Standard Iron Solutions. Dissolve 0.484 g of ferric chloride hexahydrate in sufficient M hydrochloric acid to produce 100 ml. This solution contains 1 mg of Fe in 1 ml. Serially dilute the solution with *sodium chloride–potassium chloride solution* to produce solutions containing 0.5, 1.0, 1.5, 2.0, and 2.5 µg of Fe in 1 ml.

Reagent. Trichloroacetic Acid–Mercaptoacetic Acid Reagent. Dissolve 100 g of trichloroacetic acid in 500 ml of water, add 30 ml of mercaptoacetic acid and 166 ml of *hydrochloric acid*, allow the mixture to cool to room temperature and dilute to 1000 ml with water. The reagent should be stored in an amber bottle.

Method. To 2 ml of the serum sample add 2 ml of Trichloroacetic Acid–Mercaptoacetic Acid Reagent, mix thoroughly, allow to stand for 5 minutes, and centrifuge at 1700 rpm for at least 10 minutes. Aspirate the supernatant liquid into an oxidising (blue) flame, and record the absorbance at 248.3 nm.

Mix 25 ml of each of the diluted standard solutions and 25 ml of *sodium chloride–potassium chloride solution* with 25 ml of Trichloroacetic Acid–Mercaptoacetic Acid Reagent. Aspirate these solutions into the flame as for the sample.

Plot the absorbance of each standard solution against the concentration of iron, and read off the concentration in the sample.

INTERPRETATION

The concentration of iron in the serum of normal subjects is in the range 0.8 to 1.6 µg/ml. Iron is concentrated in the erythrocytes and whole blood concentrations in healthy subjects are in the range 380 to 560 µg/ml for females, and 450 to 625 µg/ml for males. The accidental poisoning of children with iron preparations is common and serum concentrations greater than about 3 µg/ml indicate the need for immediate therapy. Serum concentrations of up to about 25 µg/ml have been reported in intoxicated children, and up to about 50 µg/ml in cases of fatal poisoning.

Lead

Numerous procedures for the determination of lead in blood by atomic absorption spectrophotometry have been reported. The first method described here uses a nickel cup to contain the sample, a conventional air–acetylene flame atomiser, and a nickel absorption tube. The second method uses a graphite furnace assembly. Both methods are applicable to whole blood.

FLAME ATOMISATION ASSAY FOR LEAD IN BLOOD
H. T. Delves, *Analyst, Lond.*, 1970, *95*, 431–438.
Standard Lead Solutions. Dissolve 0.16 g of lead nitrate [$Pb(NO_3)_2$] in sufficient 0.1M nitric acid to produce 100 ml. This solution contains 1 mg of Pb in 1 ml. Serially dilute the solution with water to produce solutions containing 0.1, 0.2, 0.4, 0.6, 0.8, and 1.0 µg of Pb in 1 ml.
Method. The blood sample, and a quantity of pooled normal blood to be used for preparing the standards, should be agitated for at least 30 minutes immediately before transferring to the vessel for atomisation.
Transfer 10 µl of the blood sample to a 10×5 mm nickel crucible (Delves cup), add 10 µl of water, and heat at 150° for 1 minute or until sputtering occurs. Add 20 µl of *strong hydrogen peroxide solution*, and evaporate to dryness at 150°. Place the cup in the air–acetylene flame and under the nickel absorption tube, and record the absorbance at 217 nm. The correct positioning of the cup is crucial.
Repeat the procedure using a series of nickel crucibles containing, individually, 10 µl of the pooled normal blood and 10 µl of each diluted standard solution.
Plot the absorbance of each standard solution against the concentration of lead, reduce the intercept to zero by drawing a parallel line through the origin, and read off the concentration in the sample.

GRAPHITE FURNACE ASSAY FOR LEAD IN BLOOD
M. Stoeppler *et al.*, *Analyst, Lond.*, 1978, *103*, 714–722.
Standard Lead Solutions. Prepare diluted solutions of lead as described in the flame atomisation method, above.
Method. The blood sample, and a quantity of pooled normal blood to be used for preparing the standards, should be agitated for at least 30 minutes immediately before transferring to the vessel for atomisation.
Transfer 100 µl of the blood sample to a polystyrene test-tube, add 150 µl of water and 150 µl of 2M nitric acid, mix vigorously for 30 seconds, centrifuge, and transfer the supernatant liquid into a 1-ml polyolefin cup. Introduce 10 µl of this solution into the graphite furnace, dry, ash, atomise, and record the absorbance at 217 nm.

Repeat the procedure using a series of polystyrene test-tubes containing, individually, 100 µl of the pooled normal blood and 150 µl of each of the diluted standard solutions.
Plot the absorbance of each standard solution against the concentration of lead, reduce the intercept to zero by drawing a parallel line through the origin, and read off the concentration in the sample.

INTERPRETATION
About 95% of the lead content of blood is in erythrocytes. The distribution of blood-lead within the normal population is skewed. The usual range of blood concentrations is between 0.06 and 0.35 µg/ml with a median value of 0.13 µg/ml. Lead concentrations in adult females are between 0.02 and 0.03 µg/ml lower than those in males of the same age groups. Concentrations in excess of 0.3 µg/ml in children should be investigated further. Exposed subjects may have concentrations between 0.36 and 0.8 µg/ml but be free from symptoms of intoxication. Values of 0.8 to 1.2 µg/ml are associated with mild symptoms and such concentrations in children may cause 'lead encephalopathy'. Concentrations above 1.2 µg/ml are usually associated with severe symptoms.

Lithium

The following method employs atomic emission spectrophotometry (flame photometry), and is applicable to serum.
Standard Lithium Solutions. Dissolve 4.3516 g of lithium chloride monohydrate in sufficient 0.1M hydrochloric acid to produce 100 ml. This solution contains 5 mg of Li in 1 ml. Serially dilute the solution with *sodium chloride–potassium chloride solution* to produce solutions containing 5.0, 10.0, 15.0, 20.0, and 25.0 µg of Li in 1 ml.
Method. Dilute 1 ml of the serum sample to 50 ml with water, aspirate into an air–acetylene flame in a flame photometer, and record the emission intensity at 670.8 nm.
Repeat the procedure with 1-ml portions of the diluted standard solutions, and with 1 ml of *sodium chloride–potassium chloride solution* (blank).
Plot the emission intensity of each standard solution against the concentration of lithium, and read off the concentration in the sample.

INTERPRETATION
Concentrations of lithium in normal serum are less than 0.5 µg/ml. For details of therapeutic and toxic

concentrations of lithium, see the monograph on Lithium Carbonate.

Mercury

K. C. Thompson and G. D. Reynolds, *Analyst, Lond.*, 1971, *96*, 771–775.

Flame atomisation is not necessary for the atomic absorption spectrophotometry of mercury. The cold vapour technique described here employs a reduction vessel (which may be purchased) to produce mercury vapour; the vapour is led to a quartz absorption cell within the atomic absorption instrument. The method is applicable to inorganic and organic mercurial compounds in urine.

Standard Mercury Solutions. Dissolve 0.1353 g of mercuric chloride in sufficient 0.1M hydrochloric acid to produce 100 ml. This solution contains 1 mg of Hg in 1 ml. Serially dilute the solution with water to produce solutions containing 0.05, 0.10, and 0.15 µg of Hg in 1 ml.

Reagents. Stannous Chloride Solution. A 5% solution of stannous chloride dihydrate in a 25% solution of *hydrochloric acid*.

Hydrogen Peroxide Solution (50 volume). *Strong hydrogen peroxide solution* diluted with an equal volume of water.

Method. Transfer 5 ml of the urine sample into a 35-ml stoppered tube, add 1 ml of *hydrochloric acid*, mix, and allow to cool; add 10 ml of a 5% solution of potassium permanganate, mix, stopper loosely, and allow to stand overnight. Remove the excess potassium permanganate by adding, dropwise, Hydrogen Peroxide Solution (50 volume). Transfer 0.5 ml of the Stannous Chloride Solution to the reduction vessel, turn on the magnetic stirrer and the argon gas flow, and record the baseline absorbance at 253.7 nm. Add 3 ml of the prepared sample, immediately close the reduction vessel, stir for exactly 2 minutes, and record the absorbance at 253.7 nm.

Repeat the procedure using 5 ml of each of the diluted standard solutions and 5 ml of water (blank). Plot the absorbance of each standard solution against the concentration of mercury, and read off the concentration in the sample. The calibration curve should be linear for concentrations in the range 0 to 0.15 µg/ml.

INTERPRETATION

Urinary concentrations of mercury found in normal subjects are usually less than 0.05 µg/ml, although concentrations up to 0.1 µg/ml may be occasionally found. However, values up to 0.3 µg/ml are not considered to be clinically significant. Excessive consumption of fish may produce urinary concentrations between 0.2 and 0.35 µg/ml without symptoms of intoxication. Children suffering from acrodynia (Pink disease) display urinary concentrations up to 4 µg/ml. In general, concentrations greater than 0.3 µg/ml are considered to be indicative of exposure to mercury. Elemental mercury is poorly absorbed from the gastro-intestinal tract and is not considered toxic by this route. Mercury vapour is absorbed through the skin and lungs and may produce toxicity; personnel engaged in the manufacture of mercury thermometers may excrete up to 3 mg/day. High urinary excretion of mercury may also be observed occasionally in subjects who have persistently used mercurial ointments for psoriasis.

Mercuric chloride is highly toxic, and ingestion of 1 g may prove fatal. A postmortem urine sample with a mercury concentration greater than 0.1 µg/ml is highly indicative of mercury poisoning.

Thallium

The following atomic absorption spectrophotometric method is applicable to blood and urine, and uses a conventional air–acetylene flame atomiser.

Standard Thallium Solutions. Dissolve 1.3034 g of thallous nitrate ($TlNO_3$) in sufficient water to produce 1000 ml. This solution contains 1 mg of Tl in 1 ml. Serially dilute the solution with water to produce solutions containing 0.2, 0.5, 1.0, 2.0, and 4.0 µg of Tl in 1 ml.

Reagent. Sodium DDC Solution. A 1% solution of sodium diethyldithiocarbamate.

Method for Blood. Transfer 5 ml of the anticoagulated blood sample to a screw-capped centrifuge tube, add 1 ml of the Sodium DDC Solution, and 1 ml of a non-ionic surfactant (such as a 5% solution of Triton X-100), mix thoroughly, and allow to stand for 10 minutes. Add 3 ml of isobutyl methyl ketone, shake thoroughly, and centrifuge. Aspirate the organic layer into an oxidising (blue) flame, and record the absorbance at 276.7 nm.

Repeat the procedure with 5 ml of each of the diluted standard solutions, and with 5 ml of water (blank).

Plot the absorbance of each standard solution against the concentration of thallium, and read off the concentration in the sample. The calibration curve should be linear in the range 0 to 4 µg/ml.

Method for Urine. The method is the same as that given for blood, above, except that the pH of the sample and of the standard solutions should be adjusted to 7 to 7.5 before addition of Sodium DDC Solution, and the non-ionic surfactant is omitted.

INTERPRETATION
Concentrations of thallium in the blood or urine of unexposed subjects are usually less than 0.01 µg/ml. Clinical symptoms of intoxication are associated with blood concentrations of about 0.1 µg/ml; values of 8 to 10 µg/ml have been reported. Urinary concentrations of up to 20 µg/ml may be seen in exposed subjects. Thallium salts are highly toxic and doses of about 12 mg/kg of a soluble salt may be fatal.

Zinc

The following atomic absorption spectrophotometric method is applicable to serum, and uses a conventional air–acetylene flame atomiser. Zinc is present in erythrocytes and assays of whole blood are difficult to calibrate.
Note. Laboratory reagents, glassware, and other apparatus are likely to be contaminated with zinc. The use of zinc-free polypropylene test-tubes is recommended.
Standard Zinc Solutions. Dissolve 2.0846 g of zinc chloride in sufficient M hydrochloric acid to produce 1000 ml. This solution contains 1 mg of Zn in 1 ml. Serially dilute the solution with *sodium chloride–potassium chloride solution* to produce solutions containing 0.5, 1.0, 1.5, 2.0, and 2.5 µg of Zn in 1 ml.
Method. Dilute 1 ml of the serum sample to 10 ml with a 6% solution of butan-1-ol and mix. Aspirate into an oxidising (blue) flame, and record the absorbance at 213.8 nm.
Repeat the procedure with 1 ml of each standard solution, and 1 ml of *sodium chloride–potassium chloride solution* (blank).
Plot the absorbance of each standard solution against the concentration of zinc, and read off the concentration in the sample.

INTERPRETATION
Normal serum concentrations of zinc are in the range 0.7 to 1.7 µg/ml. Zinc salts are considered to be poisonous, but there appears to be no consensus of opinion on the minimum lethal dose. However, fatalities have been recorded following a dose of as little as 10 g of zinc sulphate. A number of suicides have been attempted with eye lotions containing zinc salts. Zinc derived from galvanised pipes occurs as a contaminant of drinking water.

Anions

Most commonly-encountered anions may be found in biological fluids, albeit at low concentrations. Possible sources for excessive concentrations of some anions of toxicological significance are listed below. The list is by no means exhaustive.

Anion	Possible source
Borate	Eye-drops, eye lotions, depilatory agents, topical preparations such as boric acid ointments and powders, and water softeners
Bromide	Sedative medicines, photographic chemicals, and industrial fumigants
Chlorate	Throat gargles, toothpastes, fireworks, matches, and weed killers
Cyanide	Amygdalin, metal polishes, insecticides, and metallurgical processing (plating)
Fluoride	Dentifrices, toothpastes, insecticides, and rodenticides
Hypochlorite	Bleaching agents and disinfectants
Iodine/Iodide	Antiseptics
Nitrate	Anti-anginal vasodilators, antiseptics, fertilisers, preservatives, and explosives
Nitrite	Preserved meats, from nitrate metabolism, and explosives
Oxalate	Rhubarb leaves, bleaching agents, cleaning agents, ink erasers, metal polishes, and anti-rust agents
Phosphate	Laxatives, matches, anti-rust agents, and water softeners
Sulphate	Electrical storage batteries and in industrial processes (as sulphuric acid)
Sulphide	Depilatory agents, paints, and hydrogen sulphide gas
Thiocyanate	Sodium nitroprusside, amygdalin, and insecticides

Qualitative tests for anions may be performed on stomach washings, gastric contents, or vomit. Anions may be extracted from the sample by the methods described on p. 55, although extraction by dialysis may result in the loss of borate, chlorate, and oxalate ions. In an emergency, the quantitative tests described below may be modified to identify anions present in serum, plasma, or urine samples. Where a sample of the suspected poison is available, tests should be carried out on it alongside those on the biological sample. Where the manufacturer of the suspected product can be identified, either the company or a Poisons Information Centre should be contacted for details of the formulation of the product. A useful source for information on the ingredients of medicinal products and some products of toxicological significance is *Martindale, The Extra Pharmacopoeia*, 28th Edn, J. E. F. Reynolds (Ed.), London, The Pharmaceutical Press, 1982.

Screening for Anions

A good deal of information is obtainable by acidifying the samples with dilute mineral acids and observing the reaction, first at room temperature and then after gentle application of heat. Bicarbonates, carbonates, cyanides, hypochlorites, nitrates, and nitrites yield characteristic gases following such treatment. Care must be exercised when cyanide intoxication is suspected as hydrogen cyanide may be evolved.

Transfer to 2 test-tubes either 1-ml portions of filtered or clarified gastric contents, or 5-ml portions of stomach washings. To one tube add an equal volume of *silver nitrate solution*, observe the reaction and then add a 30% v/v solution of *nitric acid*. To the second tube add an equal volume of *barium chloride solution*, observe the reaction and then add a 30% solution of *nitric acid*.

INTERPRETATION

Result	Indication
A precipitate with silver nitrate solution which is insoluble in nitric acid; no reaction with barium chloride solution	Presence of bromide, chloride, cyanide, hypochlorite, iodide, or thiocyanate
A precipitate with silver nitrate solution which is soluble in nitric acid; no reaction with barium chloride solution	Presence of cyanates, sulphites, or boric, carbonic, iodic, oxalic, and nitrous acids
A precipitate with silver nitrate solution, and with barium chloride solution, soluble in nitric acid	Presence of silicates, thiosulphates, or arsenic, arsenious, chromic, or phosphoric acids
No precipitate with silver nitrate solution or with barium chloride solution	Presence of hydrochloric, nitric, or perchloric acids
No reaction with silver nitrate solution; precipitate with barium chloride solution which is insoluble in nitric acid	Presence of fluoride or sulphate. High concentrations of sulphates give a precipitate with silver nitrate

Tests for Specific Anions

The presence of a particular anion may be confirmed by qualitative tests performed on 5 ml of filtered gastric contents or 10 ml of stomach washings. Quantitative assays may then be performed if necessary.

Borate

COLOUR TESTS

1. Acidify a portion of the sample with *dilute hydrochloric acid*, and apply the solution to turmeric paper. A brown-red colour, which intensifies when the paper is dried indicates the presence of borate.

Moisten the paper with *dilute ammonia solution*; a green-black colour is produced. The test is sensitive to 20 µg/ml of borate.

2. Transfer a portion of the sample to an evaporating basin, add 1 ml of *sulphuric acid* and 3 ml of ethanol, and ignite. A green border around the flame indicates the presence of borate.

COLORIMETRIC ASSAY FOR BORATE IN SERUM

Standard Borate Solutions. Dissolve 0.210 g of boric acid in sufficient water to produce 100 ml. This solution contains 2 mg of BO_3^{3-} in 1 ml. Serially dilute this solution with pooled normal serum to produce solutions containing 20, 50, 100, and 200 µg of BO_3^{3-} in 1 ml.

Reagent. Carminic Acid Reagent. Dissolve 0.02 g of carminic acid in sufficient *sulphuric acid* to produce 100 ml.

Method. Transfer 1 ml of the serum sample, and 1 ml of pooled normal serum (blank) to separate 15-ml centrifuge tubes and carry out the following procedure on each tube. Add 5 ml of a 4% solution of ammonium sulphate, mix thoroughly, and heat in a boiling water-bath for 15 minutes. Centrifuge at 3500 rpm for 10 minutes, and transfer the supernatant liquid to a 10-ml volumetric flask. Wash the precipitate in the centrifuge tube by shaking with 2 ml of water, centrifuge, and add the supernatant liquid to the volumetric flask. Add sufficient water to the flask to produce 10 ml and mix. To 1 ml of this solution add 5 ml of *sulphuric acid*, mix thoroughly, add 5 ml of the Carminic Acid Reagent, mix thoroughly, and allow the colour to develop for 10 minutes. Record the absorbance of the solution obtained from the sample at 600 nm, using the solution obtained from the pooled normal serum in the reference cell.

Repeat the procedure with the diluted standard solutions.

Plot the absorbance of each of the standard solutions against the concentration of borate ion, and read off the concentration in the sample.

INTERPRETATION

The concentration of borate ion in normal serum is up to about 7 µg/ml; concentrations between 20 and 150 µg/ml are associated with toxicity. Concentrations from 200 to 1500 µg/ml have been reported in fatalities.

Bromide

COLOUR TESTS

1. To a portion of the sample add an equal volume of *silver nitrate solution*. A yellow precipitate which

is insoluble in a 30% v/v solution of *nitric acid* and slightly soluble in *dilute ammonia solution*, indicates the presence of bromides.

2. To a portion of the sample add 5 ml of *chlorine solution* and 3 ml of chloroform. A yellow colour which is extracted into the chloroform layer indicates the presence of bromide; iodides give a violet colour and chlorides do not react.

COLORIMETRIC ASSAY FOR BROMIDE IN SERUM

Standard Bromide Solutions. Dissolve 1.2877 g of sodium bromide in sufficient water to produce 500 ml. This solution contains 2 mg of Br^- in 1 ml. Serially dilute this solution with water to produce solutions containing 200, 400, 600, 800, 1200, and 1600 μg of Br^- in 1 ml.

Reagent. Chloroauric Acid Solution. Dissolve 0.5 g of chloroauric acid (gold chloride, $HAuCl_4, xH_2O$) in sufficient water to produce 100 ml.

Method. Transfer 2 ml of the serum sample, and 2 ml of water (blank) to separate centrifuge tubes and carry out the following procedure on each tube. Add 4 ml of a 20% solution of trichloroacetic acid, mix thoroughly, allow to stand for 15 minutes, and then centrifuge at 2000 rpm for 5 minutes. Transfer 4 ml of the supernatant liquid to another tube, add 1 ml of the Chloroauric Acid Solution, and record the absorbance of the solution obtained from the sample at 440 nm, using the blank solution in the reference cell.

Repeat the procedure with the diluted standard solutions.

Plot the absorbance of each of the standard solutions against the concentration of bromide ion, and read off the concentration in the sample.

INTERPRETATION

Bromide concentrations in normal serum are usually less than 10 μg/ml. Following therapeutic administration of bromides, concentrations of up to 80 μg/ml are attained. Toxicity is usually associated with concentrations above 500 μg/ml, although some individuals may show signs of intoxication at values as low as 300 μg/ml. Bromide has a plasma half-life of about 15 days.

Chlorate

COLOUR TESTS

1. Acidify a portion of the sample with *dilute sulphuric acid*, and add 1 ml of a 1% solution of indigo carmine. A deep blue colour is given by chlorates.

2. To 5 ml of vomit add 5 ml of a 20% solution of trichloroacetic acid and filter. Divide the filtrate into two equal portions; to the first portion add 2 ml of aniline and 1 ml of M hydrochloric acid. A blue-green colour is given by chlorates. To the second portion, add 2 ml of a 1% solution of diphenylamine in *sulphuric acid*. A blue colour is given by chlorates.

Ingestion of chlorate renders the blood brown due to the formation of methaemoglobin. To 1 ml of blood, add 2 drops of *potassium cyanide solution*. An immediate red colour confirms the presence of methaemoglobin; sulphaemoglobin does not give this colour.

INTERPRETATION

Serious and sometimes fatal poisoning occurs after the ingestion of 15 g or more of sodium or potassium chlorate.

Cyanide

COLOUR TESTS

Distil the sample into a 10% solution of sodium hydroxide, and carry out the following tests on the alkaline distillate.

1. Add a freshly prepared 10% solution of ferrous sulphate in freshly boiled and cooled water; a precipitate of ferrous hydroxide is formed. Add sufficient *dilute hydrochloric acid* to dissolve the precipitate; a blue colour (Prussian Blue) indicates the presence of cyanide.

This test is specific for cyanides and in an emergency can be performed directly on gastric contents without prior distillation.

2. Add *ammonium polysulphide solution* and evaporate to dryness on a water-bath. To the residue add a few drops of *dilute hydrochloric acid*, filter, and to the filtrate add a few drops of *ferric chloride solution*. A deep red colour due to ferric thiocyanate indicates the presence of cyanide.

COLORIMETRIC ASSAY FOR CYANIDE IN SERUM OR WHOLE BLOOD

Cyanide may be lost or produced during storage of whole blood; samples should be stored at 4° and analysed as soon as possible. Cyanide concentrations may decrease significantly after death.

Standard Cyanide Solutions. Dissolve 0.025 g of potassium cyanide in sufficient water to produce 10 ml. This solution contains 1 mg of CN^- in 1 ml. Serially dilute this solution with normal blood or serum, as appropriate, taken from non-smokers, to produce solutions containing 0.5, 1.0, 2.0, and 5.0 μg of CN^- in 1 ml. The diluted solutions should be freshly prepared.

Reagents. Barbituric Acid and Pyridine Reagent. Dissolve 3 g of barbituric acid in 15 ml of pyridine in a 25-ml volumetric flask, slowly add 3 ml of *hydrochloric acid*, and dilute with sufficient water to produce 25 ml. The mixture may be warmed to effect solution.

Phosphate Solution. Dissolve 15.6 g of sodium dihydrogen phosphate dihydrate in sufficient water to produce 100 ml.

Method. To the outer compartments of two Conway microdiffusion cells add 0.5 ml of *dilute sulphuric acid*, and to the inner compartments add 0.5 ml of 0.1M sodium hydroxide. To the outer compartments add 0.5 ml of the serum or blood sample, and 0.5 ml of normal serum or whole blood (blank) respectively; immediately close the cells and carry out the following procedure on each cell. Gently agitate the cells, ensuring that the contents of the two compartments do not mix, and allow to stand for at least 2 hours. Transfer 0.1 ml of the solution from the inner compartment to a tube containing 1 ml of the Phosphate Solution, add 0.5 ml of a 0.25% solution of Chloramine-T, mix, allow to stand for 3 minutes, add 1.5 ml of the Barbituric Acid and Pyridine Reagent, mix, and allow to stand for 10 minutes. Record the absorbance of the solution obtained from the sample at 580 nm, using the blank solution in the reference cell.

Repeat the procedure with the diluted standard solutions.

Plot the absorbance of each of the standard solutions against the concentration of cyanide ion, and read off the concentration in the sample.

INTERPRETATION

Blood-cyanide concentrations of up to $0.02 \mu g/ml$ may be found in normal individuals who do not smoke; smokers may have concentrations of up to about $0.05 \mu g/ml$. Acute toxicity is associated with blood concentrations of $0.5 \mu g/ml$ or more; such concentrations may be encountered during sodium nitroprusside therapy for hypertension. Concentrations above $1 \mu g/ml$ have been reported in fatalities. Cyanide is concentrated in the erythrocytes.

Fluoride

QUALITATIVE TESTS

1. To a portion of the sample add a 25% solution of calcium chloride. Fluorides give a white gelatinous precipitate which is insoluble in a 30% v/v solution of *acetic acid*, and slightly soluble in *dilute hydrochloric acid*.

2. Dry a portion of urine or vomit, and fuse with calcium hydroxide. Add 0.2 g of purified sand and transfer to a lead dish. Smear a film of soft paraffin on the reverse of a glass cover plate, and expose part of the glass by making an identifiable sign on the paraffin film. Add 5 ml of *sulphuric acid* to the dish, place the cover plate on it with the paraffin layer on the inside, and heat gently for 20 minutes. Remove the paraffin film from the cover plate. An etched mark on the plate, corresponding to the mark made, indicates the presence of fluoride.

ASSAY FOR FLUORIDE IN PLASMA OR URINE BY ION-SPECIFIC POTENTIOMETRY

Standard Fluoride Solutions. Dissolve 0.221 g of sodium fluoride, previously dried at 300° for 12 hours, in sufficient water to produce 1000 ml. This solution contains $100 \mu g$ of F^- in 1 ml. Serially dilute this solution with the Buffered Sodium Chloride Solution to produce solutions containing 0.01, 0.05, 0.10, and $0.20 \mu g$ of F^- in 1 ml. All standard fluoride solutions should be stored in polyethylene containers.

Reagent. Buffered Sodium Chloride Solution. Dissolve 6.4 g of sodium chloride, 13.6 g of sodium acetate, and 6 ml of *acetic acid* in sufficient water to produce 1000 ml. The solution should be stored in a polyethylene container.

Method. For plasma samples, dilute 1 volume with 1 volume of the Buffered Sodium Chloride Solution. For urine samples, dilute 1 volume with 9 volumes of the reagent. Insert the electrode of an ion-specific fluoride meter into the diluted sample and allow to equilibrate for 30 minutes. Record the ion potential of the solution.

Dilute 1 volume of each of the diluted standard solutions with 1 volume of the Buffered Sodium Chloride Solution, and record the ion potential of each solution.

Plot the ion potential of each standard solution against the concentration of fluoride ion, and derive the concentration in the sample.

INTERPRETATION

Plasma concentrations of fluoride are normally less than $0.2 \mu g/ml$; urine concentrations are usually less than $1 \mu g/ml$ but up to $4 \mu g/ml$ is not considered harmful. Blood concentrations greater than 2.6 $\mu g/ml$ have been reported in fatalities.

Young children may ingest up to 0.5 g of fluoride by swallowing fluoride toothpaste. Stannous fluoride is a common ingredient so that a test for excess tin may aid interpretation.

Hypochlorite

COLOUR TESTS

1. Acidify a portion of the sample with *dilute hydrochloric acid*. Evolution of chlorine indicates the presence of hypochlorite; the solution may be yellow.

2. To a portion of the sample add *silver nitrate solution*. A white precipitate is given by hypochlorite.

3. Moisten *starch-iodide paper* with the sample. A blue colour is given by hypochlorite.

4. Filter a portion of the sample and add 2 drops of the filtrate to 1 ml of a 1% solution of diphenylamine in *sulphuric acid*. An immediate blue colour is given by hypochlorite.

Iodide

COLOUR TESTS

1. To a portion of the sample add 5 ml of *chlorine solution* and 3 ml of chloroform. A violet colour in the chloroform layer indicates the presence of iodide.

2. To a portion of the sample add *silver nitrate solution* and an equal volume of a 30% v/v solution of *nitric acid*. A curdy yellow precipitate which is insoluble in *dilute ammonia solution* is given by iodides.

Nitrite

COLOUR TESTS

1. To 10 ml of gastric contents, stomach washings, or vomit, add 10 mg of diphenylamine sulphate and then carefully add 5 ml of *sulphuric acid* to form a separate layer. A blue ring at the interface is indicative of nitrites.

2. To 10 ml of the sample add 10 mg of brucine sulphate and carefully add 5 ml of *sulphuric acid* to form a separate layer. A red ring at the interface is given by nitrites.

3. To a portion of the sample, add 0.5 ml of a 10% solution of potassium iodide and 0.5 ml of *dilute hydrochloric acid*. Liberation of iodine which turns *starch mucilage* blue is indicative of nitrites.

The presence of nitrites in blood renders it brown due to the formation of methaemoglobin. To 1 ml of blood add 2 drops of *potassium cyanide solution*. An immediate red colour confirms the presence of methaemoglobin.

COLORIMETRIC ASSAY FOR NITRITES IN URINE

The nitrite ion is rapidly eliminated from blood and it is best to assay urine in cases of suspected overdose.

Standard Nitrite Solutions. Dissolve 1.5 g of sodium nitrite in sufficient water to produce 1000 ml. This solution contains 1 mg of NO_2^- in 1 ml. Serially dilute this solution with water to produce solutions containing 10, 20, 50, and 100 µg of NO_2^- in 1 ml.

Reagents. Naphthylamine Solution. Dissolve 0.48 g of 1-naphthylamine in sufficient of a 20% v/v solution of *hydrochloric acid* to produce 100 ml.

Sulphanilic Acid Solution. Dissolve 0.6 g of sulphanilic acid in sufficient of a 20% v/v solution of *hydrochloric acid* to produce 100 ml.

Method. Add 1 ml of the urine sample and 1 ml of water (blank) to two separate 50-ml volumetric flasks, and carry out the following procedure on each flask. Add 1 ml of the Sulphanilic Acid Solution, mix, and allow to stand for 10 minutes. Add 1 ml of the Naphthylamine Solution and 1 ml of a 16.4% solution of sodium acetate, dilute to 50 ml with water, mix, and allow to stand for 10 minutes. Record the absorbance of the solution obtained from the sample at 510 nm, using the blank solution in the reference cell.

Repeat the procedure with each of the diluted standard solutions.

Plot the absorbance of the standard solutions against the concentration of nitrite ion, and read off the concentration in the sample. The calibration curve should be linear in the range 0 to 50 µg/ml.

INTERPRETATION

In reported cases of overdose, the blood and urine concentrations have been extremely variable. High concentrations may be found after heavy consumption of preserved meats. The concentration of methaemoglobin in the blood is an indication of the degree of toxicity.

Oxalate

COLOUR TESTS

Acidify the sample with *dilute hydrochloric acid*, add 3 ml of ethanol, and heat to precipitate the proteins. Extract the sample with 3 quantities of ether; combine the organic layers and evaporate to dryness. Dissolve the residue in 3 ml of water and carry out the following tests:

1. To 1 ml of the solution, add 2 drops of *dilute sulphuric acid* and 3 drops of a 1% solution of potassium permanganate. Disappearance of the violet colour is indicative of the presence of oxalate.

2. To 1 ml of the solution add 1 ml of *silver nitrate solution*. A white precipitate which is soluble in a 30% v/v solution of *nitric acid* is given by oxalates.

3. To 1 ml of the solution add 1 ml of a 25% solution

of calcium chloride. A precipitate which is soluble in a 30% v/v solution of *acetic acid* but insoluble in *dilute hydrochloric acid* is given by oxalates.

A method for the determination of oxalate in serum by gas chromatography has been described by P. Nuret and M. Offner, *Clinica chim. Acta*, 1978, *82*, 9–12.

INTERPRETATION

Trace amounts of oxalate in urine are not usually significant as oxalates are present in many plant foods; approximately 2 to 10 mg is excreted daily in the urine. Oxalate may also occur in urine as a result of poisoning with ethylene glycol.

Sulphide

COLOUR TEST

To a portion of the sample add 3 ml of *dilute sulphuric acid* and heat the solution. Hydrogen sulphide fumes which turn *lead acetate paper* black are given by sulphides.

COLORIMETRIC ASSAY FOR SULPHIDE IN BLOOD

Standard Sulphide Solutions. Prepare a solution of sodium sulphide to contain 1 mg of sulphide ion in 1 ml. Serially dilute this solution with pooled normal blood to produce solutions containing 0.5, 1.0, and 2.0 µg of sulphide ion in 1 ml.

Reagents. Acidic Ferric Chloride Solution. Dissolve 0.2 g of ferric chloride in sufficient *dilute hydrochloric acid* to produce 100 ml.

Dimethylphenylenediamine Solution. Dissolve 0.1 g of *NN*-dimethyl-*p*-phenylenediamine in sufficient of a 50% v/v solution of *hydrochloric acid* to produce 100 ml.

Method. To the outer compartments of two Conway microdiffusion cells add 4 ml of 0.5M sulphuric acid, and to the inner compartments add 3 ml of 0.1M sodium hydroxide. To the outer compartments add 4 ml of the blood sample and 4 ml of normal blood (blank), respectively; immediately close the cells and carry out the following procedure on each cell. Gently agitate the cells, ensuring that the contents of the two compartments do not mix, and allow to stand for at least 2 hours at 37°, or for 4 hours at room temperature. Transfer 2 ml of the solution from the inner compartment to a 15-ml centrifuge tube, add 2 ml of a mixture containing equal volumes of the Acidic Ferric Chloride Solution and the Dimethylphenylenediamine Solution, mix thoroughly, and allow to stand for 10 minutes. Record the absorbance of the solution obtained from the sample at 670 nm, using the

solution obtained from the blank in the reference cell.

Repeat the procedure with the diluted standard solutions.

Plot the absorbance of each of the standard solutions against the concentration of sulphide ion, and read off the concentration in the sample.

INTERPRETATION

Sulphide concentrations in the blood of unexposed subjects are usually less than 0.05 µg/ml. Fatalities have been associated with concentrations between 1 and 5 µg/ml which indicate ingestion of about 10 g of a soluble sulphide.

Sulphite

COLORIMETRIC ASSAY FOR SULPHITE IN URINE

Urine is the preferred sample but the method may also be used for stomach washings.

Standard Sulphite Solutions. Dissolve 1.5746 g of anhydrous sodium sulphite in sufficient water to produce 1000 ml. This solution contains 1 mg of SO_3^{2-} in 1 ml. Serially dilute this solution with water to produce solutions containing 0.5, 1.5, 3.0, 6.0, and 10.0 µg of SO_3^{2-} in 1 ml.

Reagents. Magenta Solution. Dissolve 0.02 g of basic magenta (fuchsin, CI 42510) in sufficient M hydrochloric acid to produce 100 ml. This reagent should be protected from light.

Formaldehyde Reagent. Dilute 1 ml of methanol-free *formaldehyde solution* to 1000 ml with water.

Method. To 50 µl of the sample add 1 ml of the Magenta Solution and 3 ml of Formaldehyde Reagent, and allow to stand for 5 minutes. At the same time, prepare a blank solution by adding 1 ml of Magenta Solution and 3 ml of water to 50 µl of the sample. Record the absorbance of the first solution at 570 nm, using the second solution in the reference cell.

Repeat the procedure for the diluted standard solutions.

Plot the absorbance of the standard solutions against the concentration of sulphite ion, and read off the concentration in the sample.

INTERPRETATION

The normal urinary concentration of sulphite ion is less than 6 µg/ml. The estimated lethal dose of sulphurous acid is 10 g.

Thiocyanate

COLOUR TEST

To a portion of the sample add 1 ml of *ferric chloride solution*. A deep red colour is given by thiocyanates.

This test may also be performed on serum or plasma after precipitation of the proteins.

COLORIMETRIC ASSAY FOR THIOCYANATE IN SERUM AND PLASMA

Standard Thiocyanate Solution. Dissolve 9.718 g of potassium thiocyanate in 100 ml of water and dilute with sufficient water to produce 1000 ml. This solution contains 0.1 mmol of CNS^- in 1 ml. Its exact strength should be ascertained by titration with silver nitrate. Dilute 0.5 ml of this solution to 100 ml with water.

Reagent. Acidic Ferric Nitrate Solution. Dissolve 80 g of ferric nitrate nonahydrate in 250 ml of 2M nitric acid, dilute with sufficient water to produce 500 ml, and filter.

Method. To 0.5 ml of the sample add 4.5 ml of a 5% solution of trichloroacetic acid, allow to stand for 15 minutes, and centrifuge. Transfer 2 ml of the supernatant liquid, 2 ml of the diluted standard solution, and 2 ml of water (blank) to 3 separate tubes. Whilst excluding light, add 4 ml of the Acidic Ferric Nitrate Solution to each tube, mix, and record the absorbance of the sample and standard solutions at 460 nm, using the blank solution in the reference cell.

Calculate the concentration in the sample by comparison with the standard solution.

INTERPRETATION

Thiocyanate is a metabolite of cyanide and in addition to its toxicological significance, measurement of blood-thiocyanate concentrations aids in the verification of an individual's compliance with an anti-smoking programme.

Plasma concentrations in non-smokers range from 0.1 to 4 µg/ml, whereas in smokers concentrations range from about 5 µg/ml up to 20 µg/ml. Serum concentrations of up to about 200 µg/ml have been recorded in fatalities.

Bibliography

E. Berman, *Toxic Metals and their Analysis*, Chichester, Heyden, 1980.

Chemical Toxicology and Clinical Chemistry of Metals, S. S. Brown and J. Savoy (Ed.), London, Academic Press, 1983.

G. D. Christian and F. J. Feldman, *Atomic Absorption Spectroscopy: Applications in Agriculture, Biology & Medicines*, Florida, Krieger, 1979.

Clinical Chemistry and Chemical Toxicology of Metals, S. S. Brown (Ed.), Amsterdam, Elsevier North-Holland, 1977.

A. S. Curry, *Poison Detection in Human Organs*, 3rd Edn, Springfield, Illinois, Charles C. Thomas, 1976.

Ion Chromatographic Analysis of Environmental Pollutants, Vol. 2, J. D. Mulik and E. Sawicki (Ed.), Manhattan, Ann Arbor Science, 1979.

J. Michal, *Inorganic Chromatographic Analysis*, New York, Van Nostrand Reinhold, 1973.

Pesticides

R. R. Fysh and M. J. Whitehouse

Several hundred compounds are available for use as pesticides and there is a need for systematic screening methods for use in forensic or clinical toxicology laboratories. The methods should be sensitive, specific, and applicable to the examination of proprietary formulations, food and drink, or biological fluids. A number of such methods are described here, ranging from simple tests to a comprehensive scheme based on gas chromatography and combined gas chromatography–mass spectrometry (GC/GC–MS). The simple methods are particularly useful when a specific pesticide, or one of a group of pesticides, is implicated by the case history because of exhibits found at the 'scene' or from signs and symptoms shown by the victim. However, the GC/GC–MS method is likely to be the most successful approach when little or nothing is known about the suspect material and only limited quantities are available.

CLASSIFICATION OF INSECTICIDES AND HERBICIDES

The terms 'pesticide' and 'insecticide' are often confused or used interchangeably. This is incorrect since the word 'pesticide' is a general one which covers a wide variety of substances and may be applied to any substance which is used to destroy undesirable life forms. Pesticides therefore include insecticides, fungicides, herbicides, rodenticides, nematocides, molluscicides, and acaricides. Only insecticides and herbicides are dealt with here since the other pesticides are encountered only rarely in toxicology.

In the following classification, insecticides and herbicides are distinguished by chemical type. However, this classification is not unique since some may be used for both purposes. Combinations of herbicides or insecticides may be found in some commercial formulations.

The common names approved by the British Standards Institution (BSI) and the International Organization for Standardization (ISO) have been used throughout for convenience and brevity. The preferred names of the International Union of Pure and Applied Chemistry (IUPAC) can be obtained from the Pesticide Manual (see Bibliography).

Insecticides

These may be classified into four chemical groups:

Chlorinated hydrocarbons which include dicophane (DDT) and its analogues (e.g. dicofol and methoxychlor), hexachlorocyclohexane isomers (e.g. lindane), and bridged polycyclic chlorinated compounds (e.g. chlordane);

Organophosphorus insecticides which include phosphorodithioates (e.g. malathion), phosphorothionates (e.g. parathion), phosphorothiolates (e.g. omethoate), and phosphates (e.g. mevinphos);

Carbamates which are essentially *N*-methylcarbamates (e.g. carbaryl);

Alkaloidal insecticides which include natural and synthetic pyrethrins, rotenone, and nicotine.

Herbicides

These may be classified into at least eleven groups but the five most important groups are:

Chlorinated phenoxy acids, e.g. 2,4-dichlorophenoxyacetic acid (2,4-D) and dichlorprop;

Substituted ureas, e.g. linuron and chlorbromuron;

Triazine herbicides, e.g. simazine;

Uracil herbicides, e.g. bromacil;

Quaternary ammonium compounds, e.g. paraquat and diquat.

Table 1 (p. 81) gives an alphabetical list of over 200 compounds together with their uses and chemical classification.

Toxicity

Pesticides include such a diversity of chemical types that it is not surprising that their toxicity covers a very wide range. For example, as little as 100 mg of mevinphos or of nicotine may cause death, whereas 1.5 kg of the herbicide aminotriazole is unlikely to endanger human life. Even within a particular class of pesticide the lethal dose may vary considerably.

In Table 1 the pesticides have been classified arbitrarily into six groups according to their toxicity rating and these ratings are related to the estimated lethal dose. The majority of the ratings have been derived from determinations of median lethal doses (LD50) in small laboratory animals. They are intended to be a guide to their relative toxicities and should only be used in this manner.

Although certain pesticides may be considered to be only moderately or slightly toxic, the vehicle in which they are formulated (e.g. kerosene or toluene) may be more toxic and can be, in some cases, the main causative agent for the symptoms observed.

For a more detailed discussion of the toxicities of pesticides, see the references in the Bibliography.

TECHNIQUES OF ANALYSIS

Available methods range from simple chemical tests to those which utilise instrumental techniques of varying degrees of sophistication. The ideal method should be specific, sensitive, of wide applicability, simple, and rapid, with results which can be easily interpreted. Unfortunately, no technique combines all these attributes and the analyst is advised to be aware of the limitations of a particular method.

Colour Tests

Although lacking in specificity and, in some cases sensitivity, these tests can be extremely valuable in indicating the class of compound. They may also be used as a quick confirmation of the constituents of a proprietary formulation. In order to ensure that false positives are not obtained and to check the reagents, a reference compound together with a blank solution should be carried through the same procedure as the sample.

Some colour tests for pesticides are described under Colour Tests, including Nitric–Sulphuric Acid (p. 143) for dicophane, Phosphorus Test (p. 144) for organophosphorus compounds, Sodium Dithionite (p. 144) for diquat and paraquat, and Sulphuric Acid–Fuming Sulphuric Acid (p. 146) for dieldrin, aldrin, and endrin.

In addition, many other tests described on pp. 129–147 may be used for pesticides, especially Aromaticity (Method 2), Diphenylamine Test, Fujiwara Test, Koppanyi–Zwikker Test, Liebermann's Test, Marquis Test, Methanolic Potassium Hydroxide, Palladium Chloride, Sodium Nitroprusside (Method 2), and Sulphuric Acid. Certain pesticides are included in the Tables of colours, where appropriate.

A test for the presence of cholinesterase inhibitors in blood is given on p. 6, and a method for the quantification of cholinesterase activity in serum is given on p. 23.

Spectroscopic Methods

Ultraviolet, infra-red, nuclear magnetic resonance, and mass spectrometry all find a role in the analysis of pesticides, but only ultraviolet and mass spectrometry are suitable for screening purposes. Infra-red and nuclear magnetic resonance require extensive clean-up procedures before they can be used and the sample requirement is not consistent with the concentrations usually available in toxicology cases. However, both these techniques are valuable in the differentiation of isomers.

ULTRAVIOLET SPECTROPHOTOMETRY

Pesticides in food, drink, and biological fluids may be detected by ultraviolet spectrophotometry, usually after a simple extraction procedure. However, care must be taken to ensure that there are no ultraviolet-absorbing co-extracted compounds which could interfere. The main drawback of the method is a lack of specificity, because the UV spectrum usually only indicates the group to which a particular pesticide belongs. In addition, those pesticides which lack a chromophore, e.g. chlorinated hydrocarbons, cannot be screened by this method. Nevertheless, UV data can be useful when used in conjunction with data derived from chromatographic methods. Table 2 (p. 85) gives data for those pesticides which show significant UV absorption.

MASS SPECTROMETRY

This technique, when combined with gas chromatography, provides the most comprehensive screening method available, with high specificity and sensitivity, and wide applicability. It can be used for identification and quantification down to very low concentrations, using the technique of selected ion monitoring whereby the mass spectrometer acts as a sensitive and specific detector for the gas chromatograph. Further information on this technique may be found under Mass Spectrometry (p. 259).

Chromatographic Methods

THIN-LAYER CHROMATOGRAPHY

This technique represents a cheap, simple, and quick method for screening pesticides, but it suffers from the disadvantage that there is no single system and location method to cover all the compounds of interest. Nevertheless, when combined with ultra-violet spectrophotometry, it can provide a useful first approach to screening for pesticides. Alternative methods can then be used for confirmation. Further information on the technique can be found under Thin-layer Chromatography (p. 160). A thin-layer system for the separation of organophosphorus pesticides (System TW) is described on p. 177.

HIGH PRESSURE LIQUID CHROMATOGRAPHY

This method is of value for dealing with compounds which are thermally labile and therefore are not suitable for gas chromatography. However, reported methods have usually described the analysis of specific pesticides, or groups of pesticides, and screening methods are not yet available, partly because pesticides which do not absorb in the ultraviolet cannot be detected with the commonly-used UV detector.

GAS CHROMATOGRAPHY

This is the most useful technique for screening pesticides since it has wide applicability and sensitivity, and utilises equipment which is readily available in most laboratories. Over 95% of all pesticides may be chromatographed intact or as a simple derivative; in some cases there is a clearly defined decomposition product although quantification may be difficult if the extent of decomposition is not reproducible. The sensitivity of the method is high using a flame ionisation detector; when specific detectors are used, e.g. electron capture, alkali flame ionisation, or flame photometric detectors, even lower concentrations in body fluids may be detected.

COMPREHENSIVE SCREENING PROCEDURE

This procedure employs an initial gas chromatographic screen followed by gas chromatography–mass spectrometry to provide the final confirmation. The details suggested here will cover most compounds and situations which are likely to be encountered by the toxicologist, but they may be varied to suit a particular analysis.

Extraction

Samples which are encountered may be proprietary formulations (solid or liquid), beverages or foodstuffs, and body fluids or tissues (stomach contents, blood, urine, or viscera). As a consequence, it is difficult to describe a single extraction procedure which will encompass all these possibilities.

Furthermore, the extraction of body fluids is complicated by the fact that certain pesticides may be decomposed by acids or alkalis. For example, the substituted ureas are hydrolysed by dilute acid or alkali, and substituted *N*-methylcarbamates decompose in alkaline media. The organophosphorus insecticides are also hydrolysed in alkali and certain members of the class, e.g. azinphos-methyl, diazinon, and malathion, are also unstable in acid.

EXTRACTION SCHEME

The extraction scheme illustrated below is suitable for dealing with formulated products, beverages, foodstuffs, and stomach contents, but would require modification for use with blood, urine, or tissues. These modifications would reflect the quantity of the specimen available, the suspected concentration, and whether the nature of the pesticide is known. The acid or base stability and the likely extent of metabolism must also be considered.

Method. If the sample is a solid or a semi-solid, homogenise it with an equal quantity of water. In the case of foodstuffs or stomach contents, treat the homogenate with saturated calcium chloride solution, allow to stand overnight, and filter.

Extract an aliquot of the sample or of the filtered homogenate with an equal volume of redistilled ether, separate, and retain the ether fraction. Adjust the aqueous fraction to pH 2 by the addition of 2M hydrochloric acid, extract with an equal volume of ether, and combine the two ether fractions. Retain the aqueous fraction for later examination.

Divide the combined ether fractions into two equal portions, evaporate each portion to dryness and retain one of the residues. Treat the other ether residue with about 200 µl of an ethereal solution of diazomethane, allow to stand at room temperature for 30 minutes, and then evaporate to dryness.

Dissolve this residue and the previously retained residue, separately, in 25 µl of ethyl acetate or hexane (do not use ethanol or acetone which can react with the decomposition products of substituted ureas). Examine the underivatised and methylated extracts by gas chromatography using the procedure described below.

Both underivatised and methylated samples are examined because uracil herbicides give a mixture of products on methylation and should be chromatographed in their underivatised forms, whereas carboxylic acid pesticides, e.g. chlorinated phenoxy acid herbicides, are best examined as methyl derivatives.

Scheme for the extraction of pesticides from foodstuffs and stomach contents

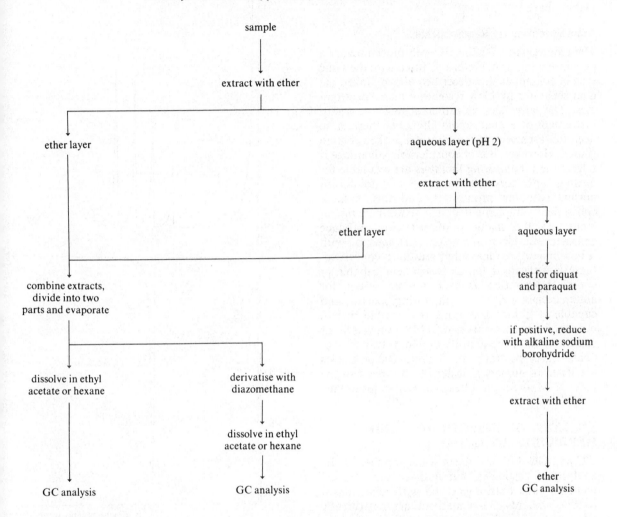

Test a portion of the previously retained aqueous extract for the presence of paraquat and/or diquat, using the Sodium Dithionite test (see p. 144). If this test gives a positive result, adjust the remaining aqueous extract to pH 10 by the addition of *dilute ammonia solution*, add 50 mg of sodium borohydride, allow to stand at room temperature for 30 minutes, and extract with an equal volume of redistilled ether. The ether extract contains the monoene and diene reduction products which can then be confirmed by GC and/or GC–MS.

Gas Chromatography Procedure

Gas chromatography should be carried out with a packed column, using temperature programming, and with an effluent splitter fitted to a dual FID/AFID detection system. System GA (see p. 192) may be used or, preferably, the following system.

System GK

COLUMN. 3% OV-17 on 80–100 mesh Gas Chrom Q, 3 ft × ¼ in internal diameter (1 m × 6 mm).
COLUMN TEMPERATURE. Programmed at 10° per minute from 100° to 260°.
CARRIER GAS. Nitrogen at 50 ml/min.
Inject 1 to 5 μl of the sample extract, together with 1 μl of a solution of caffeine in ethyl acetate containing 1 mg/ml, and determine the relative retention time with respect to this internal standard.
RETENTION DATA. Retention indices for pesticides in System GA, and relative retention times for pesticides in System GK, are given in Table 1

(p. 81) and in the index to Gas Chromatographic Data in Part 3.

Mass Spectrometry Requirements

The requirements for the GC–MS procedure are a gas chromatograph, preferably fitted with the same type of column as that described above, linked via a jet separator to a low resolution mass spectrometer. The latter can be either a magnetic sector instrument or a quadrupole filter, but there is no need for fast scanning facilities if a packed column is used. However, it is of considerable advantage if selected ion monitoring facilities are available for dealing with concentrations too low to permit normal scanning procedures, and this is more conveniently implemented on a quadrupole instrument. As the majority of pesticides produce characteristic electron impact (EI) spectra, with little ambiguity so far as interpretation is concerned, there is little need for an instrument capable of chemical ionisation as well. A data system for automatically acquiring and storing spectra, and capable of library searching, is desirable though not absolutely necessary if GC–MS is only used for confirmation of the identity of one or two components. Mass spectral peaks for over 200 pesticides are listed in numerical order of base peak in the index to Mass Spectral Peaks of Pesticides in Part 3.

ANALYSIS OF INSECTICIDES AND HERBICIDES BY GC–MS

GC and GC–MS have been widely applied in the analysis of pesticides, but most of the reported methods have been concerned with detection of residue amounts. Such methods are not directly relevant to clinical and forensic toxicology where the concentrations encountered are usually several orders of magnitude higher. The mass spectra of a wide range of pesticides have been described comprehensively by Safe and Hutzinger (1973), and further details of fragmentation mechanisms may be found there.

Insecticides

Chlorinated Hydrocarbons

These insecticides, e.g. dicophane and its analogues, isomers of hexachlorocyclohexane, and bridged polycyclic chlorinated compounds, may be chromatographed satisfactorily without prior derivatisation. A typical separation is shown in Fig. 1, using the dual detection system. Although greater sensitivity could be obtained using electron capture

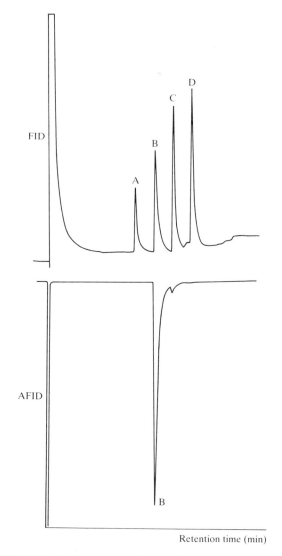

Fig. 1. Gas chromatograms of some chlorinated hydrocarbon insecticides using dual detection (FID/AFID). A, lindane; B, caffeine (internal standard); C, dieldrin; D, dicophane.

detection, this would not normally be required in cases of homicidal or suicidal poisoning because of the large quantities (several grams) usually ingested. In fact, most of the deaths attributed to chlorinated insecticides are due to the solvents, such as kerosene and toluene, in which they are formulated.

Dicophane and its analogues (methoxychlor and dicofol) show interesting mass spectral behaviour. Dicophane and methoxychlor occur in commercial products as a mixture of the *op'* and *pp'* isomers, the latter being the major component. The isomers of dicophane are readily separated by the GC system but their mass spectra are virtually identical. However, the spectra of the analogous isomers of methoxychlor are quite different in respect of the intensity of the ion at m/z 121 which could be due to a methoxy-substituted tropylium ion (Fig. 2).

In general, the fragmentation patterns for 1,1,1-trichlorodiphenylmethane derivatives are dominated by the initial loss of CCl_3, leading to a base peak at m/z 235 for dicophane and at m/z 227 for methoxychlor.

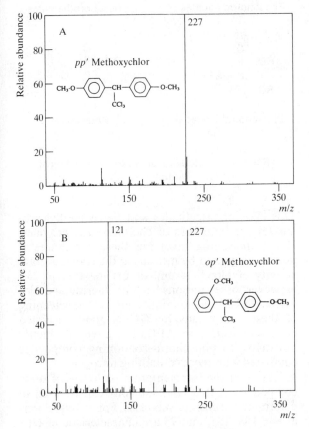

Fig. 2. Electron impact mass spectra of methoxychlor isomers.

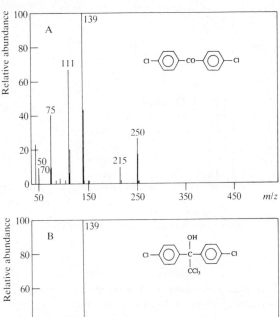

Fig. 3. Electron impact mass spectra of dicofol. A, by GC–MS; B, by direct insertion probe.

The mass spectrum of dicofol (a diphenylmethanol derivative) depends on the type of inlet system used on the mass spectrometer. The spectrum obtained by GC–MS (Fig. 3A) is identical with that of pp'-dichlorobenzophenone, presumably formed by elimination of chloroform from the parent compound in the heated injection port. On the other hand, the direct insertion probe spectrum (Fig. 3B) can be rationalised in terms of the spectrum of dicofol itself (yielding the ion at m/z 251) superimposed on that of pp'-dichlorobenzophenone and chloroform (the ions at m/z 83 and 85 being due to $CHCl_2{}^+$).

The isomeric hexachlorocyclohexanes are the main components of technical benzene hexachloride, the γ-isomer lindane being an important insecticide in its own right. The mass spectrum of lindane features the expulsion of Cl and HCl from both the molecular ion and subsequent fragment ions.

Bridged polycyclic chlorinated hydrocarbon insecticides include the dimethanonaphthalenes and methanoindenes. Their spectra are dominated by retro Diels–Alder fragmentation reactions which are accompanied, or preceded, by expulsion of Cl and/or HCl. A typical dimethanonaphthalene is aldrin, the mass spectrum of which is shown in Fig. 4. The corresponding epoxide of this compound, dieldrin, shows similar features.

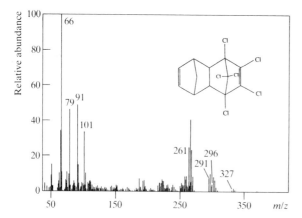

Fig. 4. Electron impact mass spectrum of aldrin.

ORGANOPHOSPHORUS COMPOUNDS

The organophosphorus insecticides are tending to replace the organochlorine compounds. They may be conveniently divided into four main structural groups:

Phosphorodithioates

Phosphorothionates

Phosphorothiolates

Phosphates

(R = alkyl; Z includes a wide variety of chemical structures)

Technical chlordane is a mixture of chlorinated methanoindenes and consists of over 45 components, the identity of some of these being shown in Fig. 5. The multiplicity of components arises as a by-product of its synthesis by the Diels–Alder addition of hexachlorocyclopentadiene with cyclopentadiene to yield chlordene which is then chlorinated.

This class of insecticides and the *N*-methylcarbamates are inhibitors of cholinesterase enzymes. Hence, poisoning involving these substances is usually diagnosed by measuring the cholinesterase activity of blood, serum, or plasma (see p. 23). However, other poisons such as fluoride and also various diseases have a similar effect. The screening of these compounds by GC is greatly assisted because detection by AFID has a ten-fold higher sensitivity to phosphorus-containing compounds compared with those containing nitrogen.

A feature of the fragmentation pathways of these compounds is that common ions can be used to determine the class or sub-class. For example, ions at m/z 158, 125, and 93 are characteristic of *OO*-dimethyl phosphorodithioates, while analogous ions shifted 28 mass units at m/z 186, 153, and 121 are characteristic of the *OO*-diethyl phosphorodithioates. The final identification is given by either the molecular ion (which may vary widely in abundance) or the diagnostic ions reflecting the nature of the Z moiety. However, the picture is complicated by an overlap of the fragmentation pathways and also by thermal isomerisation in the mass spectrometer source, the result of which is that the spectra of the phosphorothiolates and phosphorothionates show common features. This

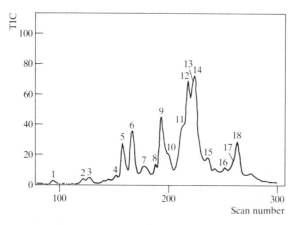

Fig. 5. Total ion current (TIC) trace of technical chlordane. 1, octachlorocyclopentene; 2, and 3, monochloro adduct of tetrachlorocyclopentadiene with cyclopentadiene; 4, chlordene isomer; 5, monochloro adduct of pentachlorocyclopentadiene with cyclopentadiene; 6, heptachlor; 7, unresolved peak consisting of α-chlordene and pentachlor; 8, heptachlor isomer; 9, *p*-chlordene and α-chlordene; 10, chlordane isomer; 11, dihydroheptachlor isomer; 12, *trans*-chlordane; 13, *trans*-nonachlor; 14, *cis*-chlordane; 15, dihydroheptachlor isomer; 16, dihydroheptachlor isomer; 17, *cis*-nonachlor; 18, chlordane isomer.

can also occur during the gas chromatography of these compounds.

CARBAMATES

The carbamate esters fall into two general classes according to their chemical structure and biological activity. The *N*-methylcarbamates are insecticides while the *N*-arylcarbamates are mainly herbicides. Since this classification is not entirely rigorous and they are structurally related, both classes are here considered together.

The differences in chemical structure lead to differences in their thermal stabilities, the *N*-methylcarbamates undergoing thermal decomposition to produce a substituted phenol by the elimination of methyl isocyanate

$$CH_3 \cdot NH \cdot COOR \longrightarrow CH_3 \cdot NCO + ROH$$

The *N*-arylcarbamates are much more thermally stable and are amenable to GC analysis. A wide range of carbamates can be successfully chromatographed intact on a low-loaded Carbowax 20M column, using a modified support and moderate (185°) column and injection port temperatures. However, under the conditions described for System GK, all the *N*-methylcarbamates show extensive decomposition and the mass spectra are dominated by molecular ions arising from their phenolic decomposition products. By contrast, the *N*-arylcarbamates, e.g. propham and chlorpropham, can be analysed on this system without any noticeable decomposition. The *NN*-dimethylcarbamate pirimicarb is also stable under these conditions. The mass spectra of these compounds exhibit molecular ions which are of low intensity but which, together with significant diagnostic ions, permit conclusive identification.

PYRETHRINS

The 'natural' pyrethrin insecticides are esters derived from the alcohols cinerolone, jasmololone, and pyrethrolone (Fig. 6). Extracts of pyrethrum, the dried flowerheads of *Chrysanthemum cinerariae-folium*, contain a mixture of six of these esters (Fig. 6) and are commonly available with the addition of the pyrethrum synergist piperonyl butoxide. Variations on these basic structures have led to the introduction of the closely related synthetic pyrethrin insecticides, the structures of the important ones being shown in Fig. 7. All these compounds can be chromatographed readily, but since they contain only C, H, and O, they do not show selective response to AFID.

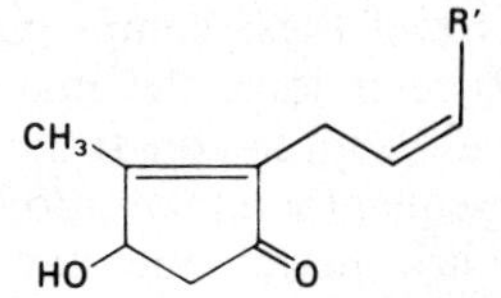

Cinerolone	$R' = CH_3$
Jasmololone	$R' = C_2H_5$
Pyrethrolone	$R' = CH:CH_2$

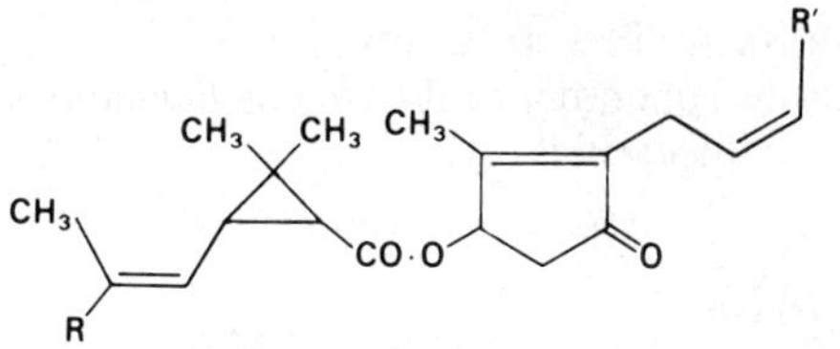

R	R'		
CH_3	CH_3	Cinerin I	Pyrethrin I esters
CH_3	C_2H_5	Jasmolin I	
CH_3	$CH:CH_2$	Pyrethrin I	
$CO \cdot O \cdot CH_3$	CH_3	Cinerin II	Pyrethrin II esters
$CO \cdot O \cdot CH_3$	C_2H_5	Jasmolin II	
$CO \cdot O \cdot CH_3$	$CH:CH_2$	Pyrethrin II	

Fig. 6. Structure of natural pyrethrin insecticides.

R	R'	
$CH:C(CH_3)_2$	CH_3	Allethrin
$CH:CCl_2$	CN	Cypermethrin
$CH:CCl_2$	CH_3	Permethrin
$CH:C(CH_3)_2$		Resmethrin

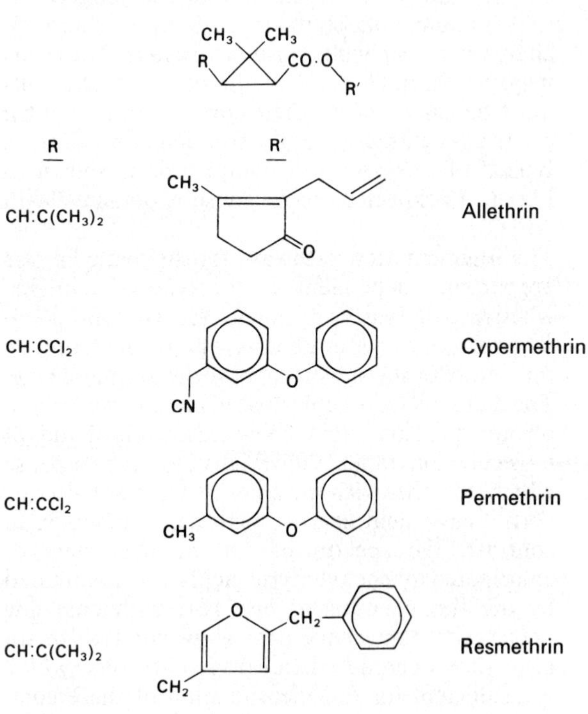

Fig. 7. Structure of synthetic pyrethrin insecticides.

The mass spectra of these compounds show only very weak molecular ions, the major ions being those which result from fission at the ester linkage followed by subsequent fragmentation of these ions. All of the pyrethrin insecticides can be identified using the two characteristic ester fission ions, together with other diagnostic ions in their mass spectra.

Herbicides

CHLORINATED PHENOXY ACIDS

Substituted phenoxy acids used as herbicides have the general formula

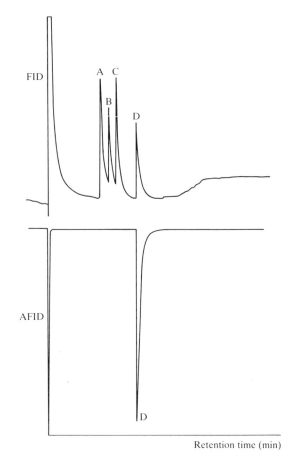

Fig. 8. Gas chromatograms of the methyl esters of some chlorinated phenoxy acids. A, methylchlorophenoxyacetic acid; B, dichlorophenoxyacetic acid; C, trichlorophenoxyacetic acid; D, caffeine (internal standard).

where $n = 1$, 2, or 3 and R_1 and R_2 are CH_3, Cl, or H. They are available in commercial products as salts (sodium, potassium, or alkylamine) or as long-chain esters, particularly iso-octyl esters. The esters may be chromatographed directly, but the salts must be converted to their corresponding methyl esters after extraction of the free acids. A GC trace typical of this group of compounds is shown in Fig. 8. As expected, no response is obtained with AFID.

The fragmentation pathways for the methyl esters are strongly dependent on the type of acid, i.e. whether a derivative of phenoxyacetic acid, phenoxypropionic acid, or phenoxybutyric acid, and on the nature of the substitution of the aromatic ring. The methyl esters of chlorinated phenoxyacetic and phenoxypropionic acids show reasonably abundant molecular ions (about 20% relative to the base peak) which, together with the chlorine isotope patterns, permit easy identification of these compounds. In contrast, the spectra of the methyl esters of chlorinated phenoxybutyric acids are dominated by the fragment ion at m/z 101, with only low abundance of molecular ions. However, the spectra also show characteristic fragment ions which are sufficient for full identification of these compounds.

The derivatives of phenoxyacetic acid containing a chlorine atom in the *ortho* position (i.e. 2,4-D and 2,4,5-T) exhibit a base peak corresponding to the loss of this chlorine atom, whereas the analogous derivatives of phenoxypropionic and phenoxybutyric acids do not. Those compounds with a methyl substituent on the benzene ring, i.e. methylchlorophenoxyacetic acid (MCPA) and its propionic and butyric acid analogues, show abundant ions at m/z 125 and 107; these have been assigned to the chlorotropylium and hydroxytropylium ions, respectively. The iso-octyl esters of the chlorinated phenoxy acid herbicides all show intense ions at m/z 41, 55, 57, 69, 71, and 85, which are typical only of long-chain aliphatic hydrocarbon derivatives, but high-mass ions of significant intensity are also available for their full identification.

SUBSTITUTED UREAS

These herbicides contain nitrogen and respond to both FID and AFID. However, the analysis of these compounds is complicated by their thermal instability. For example, the total ion current trace obtained from the GC–MS of a methanolic solution of monolinuron shows four peaks (Fig. 9). The formation of these peaks is illustrated in Fig. 10. This thermal decomposition appears to be general for the substituted ureas and reaction of substituted phenyl isocyanates with higher alcohols also occurs. As certain substituted alkyl phenylcarbamates are used as pesticides in their own right, inert solvents such as ethyl acetate or hexane should always be used for injection. The mass spectra of the thermal decomposition products show abundant molecular ions with appropriate characteristic isotope patterns which permit conclusive identification of the original substituted urea.

TRIAZINES

Most of the commercial triazine pesticides are trisubstituted 1,3,5-triazines of the general structure

where X = Cl or SCH_3, and Y and Z are usually alkylamino groups.

Since these herbicides contain at least five nitrogen atoms, they show enhanced AFID/FID ratios. With the exception of cyanazine, the spectra of these compounds are characterised by abundant molecular ions and identification is straightforward. Trietazine and aziprotryne are two members of this class of herbicide whose mass spectra differ from those of the main group but they exhibit highly characteristic features.

URACILS

The most commonly used pyrimidine herbicides are the uracils, e.g. bromacil and terbacil, which have the following structures

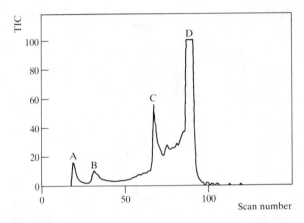

Fig. 9. Total ion current (TIC) trace obtained from a methanolic solution of monolinuron. A, 4-chlorophenyl isocyanate; B, 4-chloroaniline; C, methyl N-(4-chlorophenyl)carbamate; D, monolinuron.

Peak D monolinuron

Peak A 4-chlorophenyl isocyanate

Peak B 4-chloroaniline

Peak C methyl N-(4-chlorophenyl)-carbamate

Fig. 10. Decomposition mechanisms of monolinuron in methanol.

	R_1	R_2	X
Bromacil	H	$CH_3 \cdot CH_2 \cdot CH(CH_3)-$	Br
N-Methylbromacil	CH_3	$CH_3 \cdot CH_2 \cdot CH(CH_3)-$	Br
Terbacil	H	$(CH_3)_3C-$	Cl
N-Methylterbacil	CH_3	$(CH_3)_3C-$	Cl

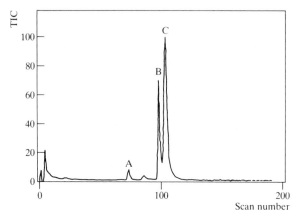

Fig. 11. Total ion current (TIC) trace of methylated terbacil. A, *O*-methylterbacil; B, *N*-methylterbacil; C, terbacil.

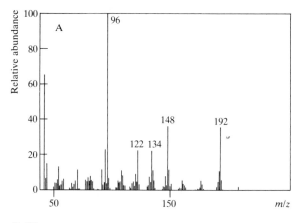

Fig. 12. Reduction of paraquat and diquat with sodium borohydride.

A total ion current trace obtained from the GC–MS of terbacil methylated with diazomethane is shown in Fig. 11. From this it can be seen that derivatisation by this method leads to a mixture of products. It is for this reason that the analytical scheme incorporates an initial gas chromatographic step prior to methylation.

The mass spectra of bromacil and terbacil and their *N*-methyl derivatives show only weak molecular ions, but they have the isotope patterns expected from bromine and chlorine compounds, respectively. The major ions arise from $[M-55]^+$ and $[M-56]^+$ and also reflect the halogen substituent. Less abundant, but highly characteristic ions, corresponding to $[M-99]^+$ and $[M-98]^+$, are formed by retro Diels–Alder fragmentations.

QUATERNARY AMMONIUM HERBICIDES

Paraquat and diquat are the most important members of this class and are readily available in various proprietary formulations. Their analysis is complicated by the fact that they are not extractable by conventional liquid/liquid extraction procedures, nor can they be gas chromatographed in their original form. Ingestion of large amounts (several grams) of paraquat leads rapidly to death, and in these cases ultraviolet spectrophotometry may be used. However, death can occur even with smaller doses (300 mg), and the concentrations in body fluids are consequently much lower. Specific radioimmunoassay methods have been developed (T. Levitt, *Proc. Analyt. Div. Chem. Soc.*, 1979, *16*, 72–76, and D. Fatori and W. M. Hunter, *Clinica chim. Acta*, 1980, *100*, 81–90).

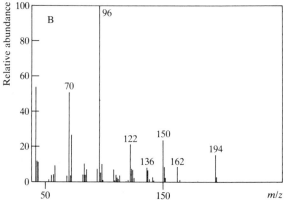

Fig. 13. Electron impact mass spectra of A, paraquat diene and B, paraquat monoene.

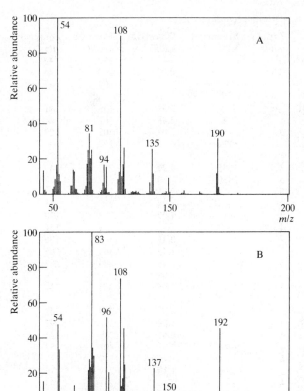

Fig. 14. Electron impact mass spectra of A, diquat diene and B, diquat monoene.

An alternative method, based on gas chromatography, involves the initial reduction of paraquat or diquat by sodium borohydride to produce the diene or monoene, as shown in Fig. 12. These products, which are extractable by ether from alkaline solution, may be gas chromatographed; the limit of detection of the method is 25 ng/ml using AFID. The mass spectra of the monoene and diene formed from paraquat and diquat are shown in Figs 13 and 14, respectively. The spectra of all these products exhibit abundant molecular ions which, together with characteristic fragment ions, readily permit the identification of the original herbicide.

Bibliography

R. Cremlyn, *Pesticides: Preparation and Mode of Action*, New York, Wiley, 1978.
R. E. Gosselin *et al.*, *Clinical Toxicology of Commercial Products*, 5th Edn, Baltimore, Williams and Wilkins, 1984.
P. C. Kearney and D. D. Kaufman, *Herbicides*, New York, Marcel Dekker, Vol. 1 (2nd Edn), 1975; Vol. 2, 1976.
F. Matsumura, *Toxicology of Insecticides*, New York, Plenum Press, 1975.
S. Safe and O. Hutzinger, *Mass Spectrometry of Pesticides and Pollutants*, Boca Raton, Florida, CRC Press, 1973.
The Pesticide Manual, 7th Edn, C. R. Worthing (Ed.), London, British Crop Protection Council, 1983.

Table 1. Classification of pesticides

Abbreviations used in the table		Toxicity rating	Estimated lethal dose (for a 70 kg person)
A	Acaricide	1. Non-toxic	> 1000 g
CB	Carbamate insecticide or herbicide	2. Slightly toxic	500 to 1000 g
CH	Chlorinated hydrocarbon insecticide	3. Moderately toxic	28 to 500 g
CP	Chlorinated phenoxy acid herbicide	4. Very toxic	4 to 28 g
F	Fungicide	5. Extremely toxic	500 mg to 4 g
GCDP	Gas chromatography decomposition product	6. Super toxic	< 500 mg (< 10 drops, a taste)
H	Herbicide		
I	Insecticide		
Misc.	Miscellaneous		
OP	Organophosphorus insecticide		
PY	Pyrethrin insecticide		
QA	Quaternary ammonium herbicide		
RRT	Retention time relative to caffeine		
SU	Substituted urea herbicide		
TR	Triazine herbicide		
UR	Uracil herbicide		
*	Monograph for this pesticide in Part 2		

Table 1. Classification of pesticides (*continued*)

Compound	Use	Class	Toxicity rating	System GA RI	System GK RRT	Molecular weight	Base peak m/z
Acephate	I	OP	3	—	—	183	43
Alachlor	H	CH	3	—	0.95	269	45
Aldicarb	I	CB	6	—	—	190	41
2-Methyl-2-(methylthio)propionaldehyde oxime	—	GCDP	—	—	0.07	133	41
*Aldrin	I	CH	5	1943	0.88	362	66
Allethrin	I	PY	3	—	1.04	302	123
*Ametryne	H	TR	—	1775	—	227	—
*Aminotriazole	H	Misc.	1	—	—	84	84
*Atrazine	H	TR	3	1655	0.79	215	43
*Azinphos-methyl	I	OP	5	2430	1.60	317	77
Aziprotryne	H	TR	3	—	0.85	225	43
Barban	H	CB	3	—	1.24	257	51
Benazolin (methyl ester)	H	Misc.	3	—	1.07	257	170
Bendiocarb	I	CB	4	—	—	223	151
2,2-Dimethyl-1,3-benzodioxol-4-ol	—	GCDP	—	—	0.31	166	126
Benzoylprop-ethyl	H	Misc.	3	—	1.42	365	105
Bromacil	H	UR	3	—	1.15	260	205
Bromacil (*N*-methyl derivative)	—	—	—	—	1.08	274	219
Bromophos	I	OP	3	—	1.05	364	331
2,5-Dichloro-4-bromophenol (Bromophos impurity)	—	—	—	—	0.31	240	242
Bromophos-ethyl	I	OP	4	—	1.09	392	97
Bromoxynil (methyl ether)	H	Misc.	4	—	0.65	289	291
Bromoxynil octanoate	H	Misc.	4	—	1.31	401	57
Captafol	F	Misc.	3	—	1.44	347	79
Captan	F	Misc.	2	2000	1.13	299	79
*Carbaryl	I	CB	4	—	—	201	144
Alphanaphthol	—	GCDP	—	1490	0.47	144	115
Carbendazim	F	Misc.	1	—	—	191	159
Carbetamide	H	Misc.	3	—	—	236	119
Carbofuran	I	CB	5	—	—	221	164
2,3-Dihydro-2,2-dimethylbenzofuran-7-ol	—	GCDP	—	—	0.23	164	164
Chlorbromuron	H	SU	3	—	1.09	292	61
3-Chloro-4-bromoaniline	—	GCDP	—	—	0.54	205	207
3-Chloro-4-bromophenyl isocyanate	—	GCDP	—	—	0.26	231	233
Chlorbufam	H	Misc.	3	—	0.83	223	53
*cis-Chlordane	I	CH	4	—	1.08	406	373
*trans-Chlordane	I	CH	4	—	1.06	406	373
Chlorfenprop-methyl	H	Misc.	3	—	0.55	232	125
Chlorfenvinphos	I	OP	5	—	1.08	358	81
Chloridazon	H	Misc.	3	—	1.10	221	77
Chloroneb	F	Misc.	2	—	0.54	206	191
Chloroxuron	H	SU	3	—	—	290	72
4-(4-Chlorophenoxy)aniline	—	GCDP	—	—	1.01	219	108
4-(4-Chlorophenoxy)phenyl isocyanate	—	GCDP	—	—	0.90	245	245
Chlorpropham	H	CB	3	—	0.63	213	43
Chlorpyrifos	I	OP	4	—	1.00	349	97
Chlorthal dimethyl	H	Misc.	3	—	1.00	332	301
Chlorthiamid	H	Misc.	3	—	—	205	170
Chlortoluron	H	SU	2	—	0.92	212	72
3-Chloro-4-methylaniline	—	GCDP	—	—	0.23	141	141
3-Chloro-4-methylphenyl isocyanate	—	GCDP	—	—	0.13	167	167
Cinerin I	I	PY	3	—	1.17	316	123
Cinerin II	I	PY	3	—	1.50	360	107
Cyanazine	H	TR	4	—	1.10	240	44
Cypermethrin	I	PY	—	—	1.76	415	163
2,4-DB (methyl ester)	H	CP	4	—	0.87	262	101
Dalapon	H	Misc.	3	—	—	142	43
Dazomet	F	Misc.	4	—	0.86	162	162
*Demeton-S-methyl	I	OP	4	1628	0.70	230	88

Table 1. Classification of pesticides (*continued*)

Compound	Use	Class	Toxicity rating	System GA RI	System GK RRT	Molecular weight	Base peak m/z
*Desmetryne	H	TR	3	1795	0.95	213	213
Dialifos	I	OP	6	—	1.61	393	208
Di-allate	H	Misc.	4	—	0.64	269	43
*Diazinon	I	OP	3	1758	0.79	304	137
Dicamba (methyl ester)	H	Misc.	3	—	0.49	234	203
Dichlobenil	H	Misc.	3	—	0.31	171	171
Dichlofenthion	I	OP	4	—	0.88	314	97
Dichlofluanid	F	Misc.	3	—	1.00	332	123
*Dichlorophenoxyacetic acid (2,4-D) (iso-octyl ester)	H	CP	4	—	1.12, 1.18	332	43
*Dichlorophenoxyacetic acid (methyl ester)	H	CP	4	1605	0.65	234	199
Dichlorprop (iso-octyl ester)	H	CP	4	—	1.05, 1.11	346	43
Dichlorprop (methyl ester)	H	CP	4	—	0.48	248	162
Dichlorvos	I	OP	5	—	0.23	220	109
Dicofol	I	CH	3	—	—	368	139
pp-Dichlorobenzophenone	—	GCDP	—	—	1.02	250	139
*Dicophane (op'-DDT)	I	CH	4	2218	1.24	352	235
*Dicophane (pp'-DDT)	I	CH	4	2299	1.32	352	235
*Dieldrin	I	CH	5	2110	1.13	378	79
Dimethirimol (methyl ether)	F	Misc.	3	1725	0.50	223	180
*Dimethoate	I	OP	4	1725	0.86	229	87
Dinitramine	H	Misc.	3	—	0.81	322	305
*Dinitro-orthocresol	I/H	Misc.	5	1617	—	198	—
Dinitro-orthocresol (methyl ether)	I/H	Misc.	—	—	0.74	212	182
Dinobuton	A/F	Misc.	4	—	1.10	326	43
Dinoterb (methyl ether)	H	Misc.	5	—	0.86	254	239
Dioxacarb	I	CB	5	—	—	223	121
2-(1,3-Dioxolan-2-yl)phenol	—	GCDP	—	—	0.28	166	121
Diphenamid	H	Misc.	3	—	1.10	239	72
*Diquat (reduction product I—monoene)	H	QA	4	—	0.40	192	83
*Diquat (reduction product II—diene)	H	QA	4	—	0.49	190	54
Disulfoton	I	OP	5	—	0.86	274	88
*Diuron	H	SU	3	—	—	232	72
3,4-Dichloroaniline	—	GCDP	—	1323	0.36	161	161
3,4-Dichlorophenyl isocyanate	—	GCDP	—	—	0.13	187	187
Dodemorph	F	Misc.	3	—	0.86	281	154
Dodine	F	Misc.	3	—	—	227	43
Drazoxolon	F	Misc.	4	—	—	237	125
*Endosulfan	I	Misc.	4	2085	1.10	404	195
*Endrin	I	CH	5	2183	1.19	378	67
Ethiofencarb	I	CB	4	—	—	225	107
2-Ethylthiomethylphenol	—	GCDP	—	—	0.29	168	107
Ethirimol	F	Misc.	3	—	1.06	209	166
Ethirimol (methyl ether)	F	Misc.	3	—	0.56	223	180
Ethofumesate	H	Misc.	3	—	1.02	286	161
Etrimfos	I	OP	—	—	0.87	292	125
Fenarimol	F	Misc.	3	—	1.58	330	139
Fenitrothion	I	OP	4	—	1.01	277	125
Fenoprop (iso-octyl ester)	H	CP	—	—	1.27	380	57
Fenoprop (methyl ester)	H	CP	—	—	0.72	282	196
Fenpropiomorph	F	Misc.	3	—	0.87	363	128
Fenuron	H	SU	2	—	0.73	164	72
Aniline	—	GCDP	—	1158	0.06	93	93
Phenyl isocyanate	—	GCDP	—	—	0.02	119	119
Flamprop-isopropyl	H	Misc.	3	—	1.26	363	105
Flamprop-methyl	H	Misc.	3	—	1.23	335	105
Fluotrimazole	F	Misc.	—	—	1.38	379	165
Formothion	I	OP	4	—	0.97	257	93
*Heptachlor	I	CH	4	1880	0.85	370	100
Hexazinone	H	Misc.	—	—	1.46	252	171
Iodofenphos	I	OP	3	—	1.18	412	125

Table 1. Classification of pesticides (*continued*)

Compound	Use	Class	Toxicity rating	System GA RI	System GK RRT	Molecular weight	Base peak m/z
Ioxynil (iso-octyl ester)	H	Misc.	4	—	1.54	483	127
Ioxynil (methyl ether)	H	Misc.	4	—	0.75	385	385
Isoproturon	H	SU	3	—	0.99	206	146
Jasmolin I	I	PY	3	—	1.23	330	123
Jasmolin II	I	PY	3	—	1.54	374	107
Lenacil	H	UR	2	—	1.52	234	153
Lenacil (*N*-methyl derivative)	H	UR	2	—	1.41	248	167
*Lindane	I	CH	4	1745	0.76	288	181
Linuron	H	SU	3	—	0.97	248	61
3,4-Dichloroaniline	—	GCDP	—	1323	0.36	161	161
3,4-Dichlorophenyl isocyanate	—	GCDP	—	—	0.13	187	187
MCPB (iso-octyl ester)	H	CP	3	—	1.24, 1.28	340	87
MCPB (methyl ester)	H	CP	3	—	0.79	242	101
*Malathion	I	OP	3	1917	1.03	330	125
Mecoprop (iso-octyl ester)	H	CP	3	—	1.00, 1.05	326	43
Mecoprop (methyl ester)	H	CP	3	—	0.45	228	169
Mephosfolan	I	OP	5	—	1.24	269	41
Metamitron	H	Misc.	—	—	1.36	202	104
Methabenzthiazuron	H	SU	3	—	—	221	164
2-Methylaminobenzthiazole	—	GCDP	—	—	0.72	164	164
Methazole	F	Misc.	3	—	—	260	44
Methidathion	I	OP	5	—	1.19	302	85
Methiocarb	I	CB	4	—	—	225	168
4-Methylthio-3,5-xylenol	—	GCDP	—	—	0.53	168	168
Methomyl	I	CB	5	—	—	162	44
N-Hydroxythioacetimidate	—	GCDP	—	—	0.05	105	45
*Methoprotryne	H	TR	—	2098	—	271	—
*Methoxychlor (*op'*)	I	CH	3	2417	1.40	344	121
*Methoxychlor (*pp'*)	I	CH	3	—	1.46	344	227
*Methylchlorophenoxyacetic acid (MCPA) (methyl ester)	H	CP	3	—	0.54	214	141
Metobromuron	H	SU	3	—	0.79	258	61
4-Bromoaniline	—	GCDP	—	—	0.20	171	171
4-Bromophenyl isocyanate	—	GCDP	—	—	0.08	197	199
Metoxuron	H	SU	3	—	0.49	228	72
3-Chloro-4-methoxyaniline	—	GCDP	—	—	0.49	157	142
3-Chloro-4-methoxyphenyl isocyanate	—	GCDP	—	—	0.35	183	168
Metribuzin	H	Misc.	3	—	0.75	214	198
*Mevinphos	I	OP	6	1450	0.50	224	127
Monocrotophos	I	OP	5	—	0.90	223	127
Monolinuron	H	SU	3	—	0.78	214	61
4-Chloroaniline	—	GCDP	—	1100	0.19	127	127
4-Chlorophenyl isocyanate	—	GCDP	—	—	0.08	153	90
2-Naphthyloxyacetic acid (methyl ester)	H	Misc.	—	—	0.91	216	216
2-(1-Naphthyl)acetic acid (methyl ester)	H	Misc.	—	—	0.76	200	141
Napropamide	H	Misc.	3	—	1.18	271	72
Naptalam (methyl ester)	H	Misc.	2	—	1.64	305	273
*Nicotine	I	Misc.	6	1348	0.31	162	84
Nitrofen	H	Misc.	3	—	1.24	283	283
Nuarimol	F	Misc.	—	—	1.37	314	107
Omethoate	I	OP	5	—	0.73	213	110
Oxadiazon	H	Misc.	2	—	1.17	344	43
Oxydemeton-methyl	I	OP	5	—	1.10	246	109
*Paraquat (reduction product I—monoene)	H	QA	5	—	0.36	194	96
*Paraquat (reduction product II—diene)	H	QA	5	—	0.58	192	96
*Parathion	I	OP	6	1942	1.04	291	97
Parathion-methyl	I	OP	5	1815	0.96	263	109
Pendimethalin	H	Misc.	—	—	1.06	281	252
Pentanochlor	H	Misc.	2	—	0.94	239	141
Permethrin	I	PY	—	—	1.62	390	183

Table 1. Classification of pesticides (*continued*)

Compound	Use	Class	Toxicity rating	System GA RI	System GK RRT	Molecular weight	Base peak m/z
Phenmedipham	H	CB	2	—	0.52	300	133
3-Methoxycarbonylaminophenol	—	GCDP	—	—	0.91	167	167
m-Tolyl isocyanate	—	GCDP	—	—	0.06	133	133
Phorate	I	OP	6	1675	0.71	260	75
Phosalone	I	OP	5	—	1.52	367	182
Picloram (methyl ester)	H	Misc.	3	—	1.08	254	198
Pirimicarb	I	CB	—	—	0.92	238	72
Pirimiphos-ethyl	I	OP	4	—	1.05	333	168
Pirimiphos-methyl	I	OP	3	—	0.76	305	290
*Prometryne	H	TR	—	1853	—	241	—
Propachlor	H	Misc.	3	—	0.58	212	120
Propanil	H	Misc.	3	—	0.94	218	161
Propham	H	CB	3	—	0.35	179	43
Propoxur	I	CB	4	—	—	209	110
4-Isopropylphenyl isocyanate	—	GCDP	—	—	0.13	161	146
o-Isopropoxyphenol	—	GCDP	—	—	0.09	152	110
Pyrethrin I	I	PY	3	—	1.27	328	123
Pyrethrin II	I	PY	3	—	1.59	372	91
Quinomethionate	A	Misc.	3	—	1.14	234	206
Quintozene	F	Misc.	2	—	0.72	293	142
Resmethrin	I	PY	3	—	1.37	338	123
*Rotenone	I	Misc.	—	3242	—	394	—
*Santonin	A	Misc.	5	2174	1.28	246	41
*Simazine	H	TR	3	1690	0.79	201	201
Tecnazene	F	Misc.	2	—	0.55	259	203
Terbacil	H	UR	3	—	1.02	216	160
Terbacil (*N*-methyl derivative)	H	UR	3	—	0.95	230	56
*Terbutryne	H	TR	3	1940	0.99	241	—
Tetrachlorvinphos	I	OP	3	—	—	366	109
Tetrasul	A	Misc.	2	—	1.28	322	252
*Thiabendazole	F	Misc.	3	2040	1.18	201	201
Thiofanox	I	OP	—	—	0.72	218	57
3,3-Dimethyl-1-(methylthio)butan-2-one oxime	—	GCDP	—	—	0.18	161	42
Thiometon	I	OP	4	—	0.72	246	88
Thiophanate-methyl	I	OP	2	—	—	342	44
Thiram	F	Misc.	3	—	1.19	240	88
Tri-allate	H	Misc.	3	—	0.77	303	43
Trichlorobenzoic acid (2,3,6-TBA) (methyl ester)	H	Misc.	3	—	0.51	238	209
*Trichlorophenoxyacetic acid (2,4,5-T) (iso-octyl ester)	H	CP	3	—	1.24, 1.31	366	43
*Trichlorophenoxyacetic acid (methyl ester)	H	CP	3	1740	0.80	268	233
Trichlorphon	I	OP	3	—	0.27	256	109
Tridemorph	F	Misc.	3	—	0.73	297	128
Trietazine	H	TR	3	—	0.83	229	200
Trifluralin	H	Misc.	2	—	0.58	335	43
Vamidothion	I	OP	4	—	1.26	287	87
Vinclozolin	F	Misc.	—	—	0.88	285	54

Table 2. Ultraviolet absorption of some pesticides

Compound	Solvent	λ max	A_1^1	Compound	Solvent	λ max	A_1^1
*Atrazine	Ethanol	263	195	Chlorpropham	Ethanol	240	700
*Azinphos-methyl	Hexane	285	280			279	45
		302	—			287	44
		315	—	2,4-DB	Ethanol	230	296
Barban	Ethanol	238	880			284	—
		277	—			293 (s)	—
		285	—	*Desmetryne	Aqueous acid	258	450
*Carbaryl	Ethanol	279	310	*Diazinon	Hexane	248	170

Table 2. Ultraviolet absorption of some pesticides (*continued*)

Compound	Solvent	λ max	A_1^1	Compound	Solvent	λ max	A_1^1
*Dichlorophenoxyacetic acid (2,4-D)	Ethanol	284	95	*Methoxychlor	Hexane	276	100
		292	—	*Methylchlorophenoxy-acetic acid (MCPA)	Methanol	280	80
Dichlorprop	Ethanol	231	416			287	—
		286	91	2-(1-Naphthyl)acetic acid	Methanol	281	200
		296 (s)	—			271 (s)	—
Dicofol	Hexane	268	20			292 (s)	—
*Dicophane	Methanol	236	510	*Paraquat dichloride	Aqueous acid	257	693
		267	19	*Parathion	Ethanol	274	343
*Dinitro-orthocresol	Aqueous acid	271	631	Parathion-methyl	Ethanol	273	420
	Aqueous alkali	265	251	Phosalone	Hexane	240	338
Dinobuton	Ethanol	243	457			287	—
*Diquat dibromide	Aqueous acid	310	518			293	—
Disulfoton	Hexane	268	267	Pirimicarb	Ethanol	244	1348
		272	270			306 (s)	—
*Diuron	Ethanol	250	1124	Propham	Ethanol	238	700
		287	—			279	45
Fenitrothion	Hexane	268	245			288	44
MCPB	Ethanol	229	365	*Rotenone	Aqueous acid	235	480
		280	—			292	550
		287 (s)	—	*Simazine	Ethanol	262	162
Methiocarb	Ethanol	266	99	*Trichlorophenoxyacetic acid (2,4,5-T)	Methanol	290	100
						298	—

*Monograph for this pesticide in Part 2   (s) = shoulder

Drug Abuse in Sport

M. S. Moss and D. A. Cowan

Drug abuse in sport is often called doping, the international word 'dope' being used both as a noun and as a verb. The Oxford English Dictionary gives its origin as the Dutch word 'doop' which means 'Christian baptism'. It seems likely that the religious fervour associated with this ceremony resulted in the use of the same word, in a somewhat cynical and contemptuous way, to describe the state of intoxication and euphoria induced by certain drugs. The word does not appear in this context before the 20th Century despite the practice of horse 'nobbling', which was known well before this time. For example, the account of the famous trial of Daniel Dawson, publicly hanged at Cambridge in 1812 for poisoning racehorses with arsenic, reveals that drinking troughs in some stables were padlocked. Dope (described as 'exciting substances') was also banned in races in Worksop in 1666. The word appears to have come into use at the turn of the century, and it is probably associated with the rise of the pharmaceutical industry.

The abuse of drugs in an attempt to enhance performance in human sporting competitions is not new. For example, the Greek authors Phylostratos and Galen commented on the ethics of competitors in the Olympics who would take any preparation to improve their performance. Roman gladiators were often drugged to make their fights more lusty and bloody as demanded by the spectators.

The effect of drugs on performance is often extremely difficult to determine, and there is little published work for any species. The results which have been published are often conflicting, some workers suggesting an increase in the competitor's performance and others suggesting no improvement. Changes in speed of less than 1% cannot be demonstrated with statistical significance because of the many variable and uncontrollable factors, yet an improvement of only 1% represents a lead of about 6 lengths in a horse race over one mile.

Although the toxic side-effects of drugs are less difficult to ascertain, the conclusions drawn from the available data are often circumstantial, e.g. the possible links between taking anabolic steroids and liver cancer. Nevertheless, there is sufficient evidence of the harmful effects when certain drugs are misused to justify their prohibition from sports competitions.

No controlling body in any field of sport has explicitly defined doping, despite banning the practice. Many horse-racing authorities now define a dope by its pharmacological action (Table 1). If any drug (or metabolite) in any of the listed categories is found in a sample of body fluid from a racehorse, this constitutes an offence. The list of prohibited substances used internationally by many racing authorities, including the British Jockey Club, is comprehensive, and the intention is to ban the use of any drug in racehorses at the time of competition.

Table 1. Prohibited substances under the rules of horse racing

Drugs which act on the autonomic system
the cardiovascular system
the central nervous system
Drugs which affect the coagulation of blood
the gastro-intestinal function
the immune system and its responses
Analgesics, antipyretic and anti-inflammatory drugs
Antibiotics, synthetic antibacterial and antiviral drugs
Antihistamines
Antimalarial and other antiparasitic agents
Cytotoxic substances
Diuretics
Endocrine secretions and their synthetic counterparts
Local anaesthetics
Muscle relaxants
Respiratory stimulants
Sex hormones, anabolic steroids and corticosteroids

By contrast, the stated intention of the Medical Commission of the International Olympic Committee is to ban those drugs which are likely to be harmful when misused (Table 2), but with the minimum of interference with the normal therapeutic use of drugs. Thus, a competitor who is undergoing a legitimate course of treatment is not disqualified. However, this creates many problems in deciding which drugs should or should not be prohibited, and whether or not a competitor requiring a particular drug treatment should be allowed to compete. The International Olympic Committee and the International Amateur Athletic

Federation list examples of prohibited drugs according to their pharmacological classification. However, they are often far from explicit, using the phrases 'related compounds' and 'chemically or pharmacologically related compounds'. Some horse-racing authorities take action on a report of the presence of any foreign compound, even if not positively identified.

Table 2. Drugs disallowed by various human sports bodies

Psychomotor Stimulants. Amphetamine, benzphetamine, cathine, chlorphentermine, cocaine, diethylpropion, dimethylamphetamine, ethylamphetamine, fencamfamin, fenproporex, meclofenoxate, methylamphetamine, methylphenidate, pemoline, phendimetrazine, phenmetrazine, phentermine, pipradrol, prolintane, and related compounds.

Sympathomimetic Amines. Clorprenaline, ephedrine, etafedrine, isoetharine, isoprenaline, methoxyphenamine, methylephedrine, and related compounds.

Miscellaneous Central Nervous System Stimulants. Amiphenazole, bemegride, doxapram, ethamivan, nikethamide, pentetrazol, picrotoxin, strychnine, and related compounds.

Narcotic Analgesics. Anileridine, codeine, dextromoramide, diamorphine, dihydrocodeine, dipipanone, ethylmorphine, hydrocodone, hydromorphone, levorphanol, methadone, morphine, oxycodone, oxymorphone, pentazocine, pethidine, phenazocine, piminodine, thebacon, trimeperidine, and related compounds.

Anabolic Steroids. Clostebol, ethyloestrenol, fluoxymesterone, methandienone, methandriol, methenolone, methyltestosterone, nandrolone, oxandrolone, oxymetholone, stanolone, stanozolol, testosterone, and related compounds.

The position regarding excessive quantities of normal nutrients is even more confused. Clearly they cannot be included in a prohibited list, yet there is no doubt that certain vitamins (notably B_1, C, and E) have been used in large doses with the intention of affecting performance. In addition, substances such as caffeine are allowable in human sport since they are ingested in normal beverages. However, because of the possibility of taking massive doses to enhance performance, their prohibition has been considered. In such cases, measurement of the concentration in a body fluid is essential in establishing a malpractice. The situation with these normal nutrients is not unlike that for certain endogenous compounds such as hydrocortisone and testosterone and their respective trophic hormones (see below).

The drugs most often reported in horses by the Association of Official Racing Chemists for the years 1959, 1969, and 1979 are presented in Table 3. The most striking trend is the increasing use of anti-inflammatory drugs throughout this period,

representing for the respective years 14%, 21%, and 28% of all drugs reported. The apparently sudden appearance of fentanyl and butorphanol is the result of the recent introduction of tests for these compounds. There has been no comparable recording of drugs encountered in human sport.

Table 3. Drugs most commonly reported by the Association of Official Racing Chemists as occurring in horses, in order of frequency

1959	1969	1979
Caffeine	Procaine	Phenylbutazone
Procaine	Pentazocine	Flunixin
Amphetamine	Phenylbutazone	Methocarbamol
Dipyrone	Caffeine	Caffeine
Theobromine	Amphetamine	Procaine
Phenylbutazone	Theobromine	Fentanyl
Morphine	Methylphenidate	Butorphanol
Phenobarbitone ⎫	Oxyphenbutazone	Theobromine
Theophylline ⎭	Methylamphetamine	Oxyphenbutazone
Nikethamide ⎫	Dipyrone ⎫	Guaiphenesin
Thiamine ⎪	Prednisolone ⎭	
Lignocaine ⎬		
Mephentermine ⎪		
Atropine ⎭		

Sampling

Sample collecting procedures must take into consideration both scientific and legal aspects. The health of the individual being sampled must be safeguarded; incorrect labelling, contamination, or sample-switching must be avoided; the rights of interested parties, generally the owner and trainer of an animal or the individual or team in human sport, must be safeguarded against error by the analyst.

Most horse-racing authorities in Europe divide samples into two portions at the time of sampling, so that the trainer of the horse can arrange a separate analysis on his own behalf. This is not a general practice and is not used in North America. The International Olympic Committee and the International Amateur Athletic Federation always provide a second portion for defence use. This is to be opened only after the first sample has been found to contain a banned drug, and after the competitor has been notified and invited to attend the second analysis, with his own expert if he so wishes. The practice of sample division has been reviewed (M. S. Moss, 1979).

URINE

This is the preferred body fluid in all species. Its collection is non-invasive, it is generally available in sufficient quantity, and the drugs or their metabolites tend to be present in relatively high concentrations. Disadvantages are that a drug may be present as metabolites or in conjugated form, and the parent drug may be present only in a relatively low concentration. Furthermore, the relationship with the concentration in blood is very imprecise.

Urine is collected almost invariably by voiding naturally. Greyhounds urinate very readily after being released from their transporter; 96% of horses in Britain urinate within one hour of racing; humans can generally urinate at will. However, there is the problem of security. Switching of samples is by no means uncommon, because there is usually a period of waiting before obtaining a sample from a dog or a horse, and because of the desire for privacy on the part of man. Racing cyclists have been reported to have carried a rubber bladder of (negative) urine under their arm, connected by a rubber tube to the appropriate discharge point. Horse handlers responsible for collecting a urine sample from their horses sometimes substitute a urine sample of their own. One laboratory has even received a sample of lager purporting to be horse urine. Incidents such as these emphasise the importance of ensuring that a correct collecting procedure is observed. The odour of urines and of the residues produced after solvent extraction generally form a ready distinction between the species. The presence of appreciable quantities of nicotine, cotinine, caffeine, and uric acid in urine provides good evidence of a human source.

Urine samples from greyhounds are caught directly in a bowl held under the animal. For horses, a container held on the end of an extending handle is generally used, e.g. a net held on a metal ring into which is inserted a polythene bag. Metal ladles are unsuitable because the noise produced by the urine falling into them frequently inhibits the horse from urinating further.

BLOOD

The principal advantage of a blood sample is that its integrity is easier to safeguard because it is usually collected by a doctor or veterinary surgeon who is experienced in the procedure. In addition, drug concentrations in blood are more easily interpreted than those in urine, and certain drugs which are not excreted in urine in detectable quantities (e.g. reserpine) can be detected in blood.

Blood is rarely collected from man or the greyhound because of the relative ease of urine sampling. In pistol shooting a small sample (100 µl) is collected from the competitor in order to confirm the estimated blood-alcohol concentration following a breathalyser measurement; the present limit is 500 µg/ml. Blood is being sampled increasingly in horse racing in much of Europe as a second choice when urine is not obtainable, and in New York State for pre-race testing. The Fédération Equestre Internationale takes blood from all horses in order to monitor plasma concentrations of phenylbutazone when this drug has been detected qualitatively in urine. In some European countries, two 25-ml samples of blood are collected from horses in flat racing and steeplechasing. On the other hand, the Federation Equestre Internationale may order larger volumes than this, up to a total of 150 ml if urine is not available.

SALIVA

The principal disadvantages of saliva are that it is difficult to obtain a useful volume and few drugs are present at a concentration higher than that in plasma. Non-ionised and non-protein-bound drugs in plasma diffuse passively into saliva. Thus, alkaline saliva (as in the horse) tends to concentrate acidic drugs but, because the percentage of unbound acidic drug in plasma is generally very low, concentrations remain lower than the corresponding total plasma concentrations. For drugs of low lipid solubility, and for high salivary flow rates, equilibrium is not established, resulting in concentrations even lower than those predicted on theoretical grounds. The principal value of saliva, therefore, is in the detection of topical contamination resulting from fairly recent oral ingestion.

Saliva is rarely used in any species but the horse. Collection is generally achieved by the use of gauze swabs held in long forceps. Yields rarely exceed 5 g and are often much less. It is essential that only cotton gauze is used for this purpose as certain synthetic fibres contain compounds that may interfere in thin-layer chromatography.

SWEAT

Little information is available on drug secretion into sweat; it is used very little because of the difficulty of excluding topical contamination. It is collected almost exclusively from the horse, the most convenient technique being to use a scraper and absorbent gauze.

VOMIT

This is sometimes used in greyhound racing, and is induced with sodium carbonate.

Analytical Approach

Dope is generally administered at or near the therapeutic dose, and this results in relatively low concentrations in biological fluids. There is usually no evidence as to whether or not a drug has been administered, or what sort of drug it might be. Any drug used in human treatment or in veterinary practice may be found. Furthermore, certain classes of drugs or individual drugs which are not normally associated with acute poisoning in man are often abused in both human and animal sports. Thus, screening procedures must be both sensitive and of wide coverage, and they differ in detail from other analytical schemes. However, the sports chemist enjoys the advantage of examining relatively constant material, usually in fairly fresh condition. He thus has a clearer picture of a normal sample than does the forensic or hospital chemist who may be required to examine a wide variety of materials in various states of decomposition.

METABOLITES

Most screening procedures rely upon the detection of unchanged drug rather than metabolites, despite the fact that many drug concentrations are lower than those of their metabolites. The reason is that drugs are almost always lipophilic and readily extractable from body fluids. Water-solubilisation of drugs is an important process in their detoxification, the most important single reaction being that of metabolic conjugation. In those cases where an unconjugated metabolite is identified, the metabolite itself is often pharmacologically active and also extractable, e.g. theophylline and theobromine from caffeine, and oxyphenbutazone from phenylbutazone. The identification of the corresponding metabolites is often useful supplementary evidence to support the identification of the parent drug.

In addition, the presence of metabolites in the appropriate concentrations relative to the parent drug helps to support the conclusion that a drug has been administered. Conversely, the absence of expected metabolites might be strong evidence that a sample has been contaminated.

Occasionally, the parent drug is not excreted in urine at a detectable concentration, and a knowledge of the metabolic pathways in the particular species is thus essential. An example of this is the identification of 5α-estrane-3β,17α-diol in the urine of horses, or of 19-norandrosterone and 19-noretiocholanolone in the urine of humans, to prove administration of the anabolic steroid nandrolone. A few drugs are notable for being excreted in urine

almost entirely in conjugated form as, for instance, apomorphine, fentanyl, nefopam, and pentazocine in the horse. When the presence of these drugs is suspected, hydrolysis before solvent extraction is essential. The metabolism of drugs in the horse has been reviewed (M. S. Moss, 1977).

Drugs can be used either to improve or to impair athletic performance, though in human sport the latter category of drug is unlikely to be used. In sports such as greyhound racing and horse racing, however, decreasing an animal's speed can be a profitable exercise. Hence, sedative drugs are not uncommon in these events and can occur in the acidic, neutral, and basic group extracts. Thus, in horse and dog samples, it is essential that all groups are covered, and these will include steroids, barbiturates, non-steroidal anti-inflammatory drugs, diuretics, and xanthines.

It is apparent that no single analytical scheme will suffice to cover so many different types of compound. For this reason, two types of analysis have come to be recognised; firstly, the general scheme covering the majority of acidic and basic drugs and secondly, target analyses for special drugs or groups. Target analyses are relatively expensive since they cover a smaller number of compounds. Such analyses, therefore, are generally undertaken to meet a special request, or to cover those cases where abuse is believed to exist.

SOLVENTS FOR EXTRACTION

The choice of solvent is limited by the wide range of drugs to be covered, and relatively polar solvents must be used. The choice, therefore, lies between ether and chlorinated hydrocarbons. Because of the importance of the methylxanthines in horse and greyhound doping, one of the extractions should preferably make use of chloroform. If chloroform is used for both the basic and acidic group extracts, the basic group extraction should be performed first in order to avoid the loss of chloroform-soluble salts (e.g. methadone hydrochloride) in the chloroform used to extract the acids. When the sample is urine, the hydroxylated barbiturate metabolites will not be extracted by this process. However, parent barbiturates should be present in sufficient concentration to be detected by gas chromatography.

The above considerations are reflected in the design of screening procedures. Techniques of general solvent extraction and drug screening are detailed under Hospital Toxicology and Drug Abuse Screening (p. 3) but full details of suitable procedures are described here in order to take account of certain special requirements peculiar to screening for doping agents. The method used for gas chromatographic screening for basic drugs is applicable to all species, though different extraction procedures are used for human samples. The additional procedures necessary for non-human samples are described separately.

GAS CHROMATOGRAPHY

The gas chromatographic procedures referred to below will detect a wide range of compounds in urine samples, at concentrations of the order of 1 µg/ml. They depend on the fact that all the compounds of interest contain at least one nitrogen atom and will produce a signal in an alkali flame ionisation detector. The methods of extraction and the selectivity of the detector ensure minimal interference from other compounds which do not contain nitrogen, although certain plasticisers containing phosphorus, such as tributyl phosphate, may produce signals. In addition, other nitrogen-containing compounds which are not prohibited in human sport (e.g. antihistamines) will produce interfering peaks.

Identification is based on retention index; alternatively retention time (relative to a standard) may be used. Details of retention indices or relative retention times of compounds in the systems described below are given in the index to Gas Chromatographic Data in Part 3.

Data obtained using more than one stationary phase will obviously ensure more certain identification; the use of a non-polar, semi-polar, and polar stationary phase is recommended. The identity of a substance may be confirmed using derivative formation and gas chromatography–mass spectrometry, preferably comparing the data obtained with authentic reference material.

SCREENING METHODS FOR STIMULANTS AND NARCOTIC ANALGESICS

Examination of Human Urine

SCREEN A

Method. To 5 ml of the sample in a 10-ml centrifuge tube add 0.5 ml of 5M potassium hydroxide, 3 g of sodium chloride, and 2 ml of freshly-distilled ether containing 10 µg/ml of diphenylamine as a reference standard. Mix thoroughly for 10 minutes on a rotary mixer. Centrifuge, remove about 1 ml of the

ethereal layer, and dry with 0.1 g of anhydrous sodium sulphate. Examine 3 µl of this extract by gas chromatography using 10% Apiezon L and 2% KOH on 80–100 mesh Chromosorb W HP (System GB, p. 193). System GA may also be used.

The use of sodium chloride to increase the ionic strength of the aqueous phase increases the extraction into the ether of many of the compounds, obviating the need for solvent evaporation. Although some polar compounds such as ephedrine are readily extracted in this procedure, it is best suited to less polar compounds.

SCREEN B

This detects the more polar and less volatile drugs and their metabolites, e.g. morphine and codeine glucuronides. Conjugates are cleaved by hydrochloric acid hydrolysis prior to extraction. An antoxidant, such as mercaptoacetic acid or cysteine, should be added to the acid to minimise oxidation of any sensitive compounds during the hydrolysis. The addition of isopropyl alcohol to the extracting solvent, and buffering the urine at pH 9.2, enables most amphoteric compounds to be extracted.

Method. To 5 ml of the sample in a 10-ml centrifuge tube add 0.5 ml of a mixture of *hydrochloric acid* and mercaptoacetic acid (9:1), stopper the tube, heat at 100° for 30 minutes, cool, and add 0.85 ml of 12M sodium hydroxide to neutralise the excess acid; add 2 g of a mixture of sodium bicarbonate and potassium carbonate (3:2) to adjust the pH to 9.2, and extract the hydrolysed mixture with 2 ml of a mixture of ether and isopropyl alcohol (9:1), both freshly distilled and containing 2.5 µg/ml of phenazine as reference standard. Buffer a further 5 ml of the urine to pH 9.2 and extract in the same manner as above but omitting the hydrolysis. Combine the two extracts and evaporate the solvent at 35° under vacuum using a rotary film evaporator. To the drug extract add 50 µl of ethyl acetate and 50 µl of trifluoroacetic anhydride, heat at 65° for 20 minutes, and again evaporate under vacuum as above. To the residue add 0.5 ml of anhydrous ethyl acetate and examine 3 µl by gas chromatography using 3% OV-17 on 80–100 mesh Chromosorb W HP (System GC, p. 193). System GA (p. 192) may also be used.

The formation of the trifluoroacetyl derivatives of phenolic or alcoholic groups increases the volatility of those compounds. The formation of amides from primary or secondary amines will often provide additional information to help identify the compound present.

Examination of Horse Urine

Two methods are described, one using direct solvent extraction, and the other a solid-liquid extraction.

SOLVENT EXTRACTION

The procedure is illustrated below.

Adjust 100 ml of urine to pH 9.5 with 2M sodium hydroxide, and extract with an equal volume of chloroform by rotation in a separating funnel at about 1 revolution per second, in order to avoid the formation of emulsions; separate the solvent layer by filtering through phase-separating paper, add one drop of *hydrochloric acid* and a sintered glass bead, and evaporate to dryness. Redissolve the

Scheme for the solvent extraction of horse urine

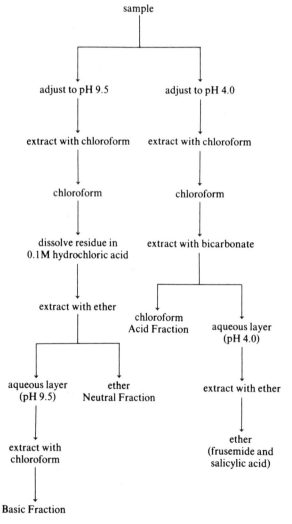

residue in 10 ml of 0.1M hydrochloric acid by warming on a boiling water-bath for about 2 minutes, and then extract with 25 ml of ether to yield the Neutral Fraction.

Adjust the aqueous phase to pH 9.5 by adding 2 g of a mixture of borax and sodium carbonate (20:1), extract with 20 ml of chloroform, filter the chloroform layer through a cotton wool plug, add 1 drop of *hydrochloric acid* and a sintered glass bead to the filtrate, and evaporate to dryness to yield the Basic Fraction.

Adjust 100 ml of urine to pH 4.0 with *dilute sulphuric acid*, extract with 100 ml of chloroform, wash the solvent layer with a 5% solution of sodium bicarbonate, filter the solvent through a phase-separating paper, and evaporate to yield the Acid Fraction. If either frusemide or salicylic acid is suspected, adjust the pH of the sodium bicarbonate layer to 4.0 with *dilute sulphuric acid*, extract with 25 ml of ether, and retain the ether extract for analysis.

SOLID-LIQUID EXTRACTION

An alternative procedure uses the non-ionic resin Amberlite XAD-2 (see Reagent Appendix). Adjust the urine sample to pH 9.5 with 2M sodium hydroxide, add 6 g of XAD-2 for each 100 ml of urine, agitate the mixture for 10 to 15 minutes, and remove the urine. Resuspend the resin in 20 ml of *ammonia buffer (pH 9.5)*, transfer to a column, and pump the resin under vacuum to remove the buffer and to draw air through the resin; partial drying of the resin at this stage reduces the subsequent elution of material which may mask the presence of drugs. Wash the resin with five 5-ml portions of a mixture of ethyl acetate and methylene chloride (1:1), filter the solvent through phase-separating paper, add a drop of *hydrochloric acid*, and evaporate to dryness to yield the Basic Fraction.

Add to the column about 15 ml of a 10% solution of *acetic acid*, allow to stand for about 5 minutes, pump dry under vacuum, and elute with solvent as described above. Evaporate the solvent on a boiling water-bath to yield the Acid Fraction.

TREATMENT OF EXTRACTS OF HORSE URINE
Neutral Fraction

Few doping agents occur in this group, apart from the neutral steroids which are covered by a separate procedure. Benzocaine has occurred occasionally in this group. The neutral sedatives such as carbamates and methyprylone would also be extracted, but these have not been reported as doping agents. Ureides such as carbromal do not present a problem as they are metabolised extremely rapidly in horses, very large doses being tolerated with no apparent effect. This group can be screened by gas chromatography using 2.5 % SE-30 on 80–100 mesh Chromosorb G (System GA, p. 192).

Basic Fraction

The extract is dissolved in methanol and a portion equivalent to about 1 ml of the original urine should be screened by gas chromatography using 10% Apiezon L and 2% KOH on 80–100 mesh Chromosorb W HP (System GB, p. 193), and 3% OV-17 on 80–100 mesh Chromosorb W HP (System GC, p. 193). System GA (p. 192) may also be used.

Examine the methanol extract by thin-layer chromatography using a silica gel G plate and developing with a 100:1.5 mixture of methanol: *strong ammonia solution* (System TA, p. 167). Spray the plate with *acidified iodoplatinate solution* followed 15 minutes later by *Ludy Tenger reagent*; the latter spray is useful for confirming the presence of methylxanthines which may frequently be found in both the acidic and basic fractions. Rf values for compounds in System TA are given in the index to Thin-layer Chromatographic Data in Part 3.

Acid Fraction

This extract contains the very important non-steroidal anti-inflammatory drugs as well as the weak acids theophylline and theobromine. It should be noted that many of the non-steroidal anti-inflammatory drugs are carboxylic acids, which are divided between the bicarbonate extract and the solvent. Despite the loss of an appreciable proportion of this group by the bicarbonate wash, this treatment is essential in removing much of the interfering extraneous matter; phenylbutazone and oxyphenbutazone are not significantly affected. Barbiturates will also be present in this group.

Examine the extract by thin-layer chromatography using two separate silica gel G plates, and develop both with an 8:1:1 mixture of ethyl acetate:methanol:*strong ammonia solution* (System TG, p. 169). Spray the first plate with *chromic acid solution* and the second plate with *Ludy Tenger reagent*.

Details of Rf values and colours of spots are given under System TG.

DRUGS MISUSED IN SPORT

These include the anabolic steroids, the corticosteroids, non-steroidal anti-inflammatory drugs, and the diuretics. Of particular interest are the anabolic steroids and corticosteroids; not only may synthetic analogues be misused but also testosterone or hydrocortisone. This use of a compound that is either indistinguishable, or distinguishable with difficulty, from that which is naturally produced by an individual, presents interesting analytical problems.

Anabolic Steroids

These have come into prominence in the last decade as body-building drugs. In human sport they are used, sometimes in very large quantities, in events such as weight-lifting and shot-putting. In horse-racing their use seems to be more general. They are said to improve a horse's appetite and to produce behavioural changes of a masculinising type in geldings and mares, though they may also be used in stallions. There are broadly two chemical types based upon the androstane and estrane ring systems: those with a 17α-alkyl group which are active orally but possess hepatotoxicity, and 17-nor derivatives administered by injection.

Although steroidal oestrogens and some stilbenes reputedly possess anabolic activity and are employed in beef production, they do not appear to be used as doping agents.

Sampling is carried out at the time of competition and has enabled the misuser to switch from using a preferred synthetic anabolic steroid to testosterone in sufficient time to escape detection.

ANABOLIC STEROIDS IN HUMANS

There are several methods to indicate that testosterone has been administered to a male human. Natural testosterone production is controlled by a feedback mechanism involving the pituitary gland, and administration of testosterone will suppress the natural production of pituitary hormones such as luteinising hormone (LH) and follicle stimulating hormone (FSH).

Radioimmunoassay may be used to measure the urinary ratio of total (free plus conjugated) testosterone to LH. Testosterone is measured in nmol/litre, and LH in International Units of HMG-IR2/litre (Human Menopausal Gonadotropin 2nd International Reference Preparation). A ratio in excess of 200 is abnormal. (R. V. Brooks *et al., J. Steroid Biochem.*, 1979, *11*, 913–917.)

Synthetic anabolic steroids used in man may be readily detected by use of two radioimmunoassay kits which are available, one for nandrolone and one for 17α-methyl substituted anabolic steroids (see Reagent Appendix).

In the human female, whose pituitary hormones may be suppressed by the use of oral contraceptives, the ratio of testosterone to creatinine in urine may be used. Alternatively, a method suitable for both males and females is to measure the ratio of total testosterone to epitestosterone using gas chromatography—mass spectrometry. In this method, the bis(trimethylsilyl) derivative is formed and the intensity of the molecular ions at m/z 432, under electron impact conditions for both of the steroid derivatives, is used to determine the ratio (M. Donike and J. Zimmermann, *J. Chromat.*, 1980, *202*, 483–486). The internationally accepted limit for the ratio is currently 6.

Identification of Anabolic Steroids in Human Urine
(R. J. Ward *et al., Br. J. Sports Med.*, 1975, *9*, 93–97.)
Adjust the urine sample to pH 5 by the addition of *dilute hydrochloric acid*. For each 9 volumes of urine add 1 volume of *acetate buffer (pH 5)* containing 5000 Fishman units/ml of mixed glucuronidase/sulphatase (from *Helix pomatia*), and incubate the mixture at 37° for 24 hours. Centrifuge, pour the supernatant liquid on to a column of Amberlite XAD-2 resin, wash the column with 50 ml of water, and then elute the steroids with 100 ml of ethanol. Evaporate the ethanol using a rotary film evaporator, dissolve the residue in 0.5 ml of ethanol, and add 2 ml of cyclohexane.
Pour the solution on to a column prepared with 6 g of Sephadex LH-20 (see Reagent Appendix), and

fractionate the steroids by elution with a mixture of cyclohexane and ethanol (4:1). Evaporate the solvent from the 10 to 20 ml fraction for the 19-nor steroids, or from the 30 to 40 ml fraction for 17α-methyl substituted steroids. Dissolve the residue in 0.1 ml of dry pyridine.
To the pyridine solution add 0.1 ml of *N*-methyl-*N*-trimethylsilyltrifluoroacetamide and 0.01 ml of tri-methylchlorosilane, and allow to react for 8 hours at room temperature. Remove the reagents under a stream of nitrogen and dissolve the residue in 0.1 ml of cyclohexane. Examine the solution by capillary column gas chromatography–mass spectrometry.
COLUMN. OV-1, 15 m × 0.3 mm internal diameter, connected to a mass spectrometer.
COLUMN TEMPERATURE. Programmed from 100° to 250° at 15° per minute, after the elution of the solvent.
CARRIER GAS. Helium.

ANABOLIC STEROIDS IN THE HORSE
Most of the anabolic steroids used in horses are designed for parenteral use and do not have an alkyl group in position 17. The commonest of these is nandrolone. In addition, boldenone, trenbolone, and testosterone itself, may be used.
Most of the urinary excretion products of these compounds are present as glucuronic acid or sulphate conjugates. The 17α-hydroxy epimers occur mainly as glucuronic acid conjugates, whilst the 17β compounds are mainly sulphate conjugates (Table 4).

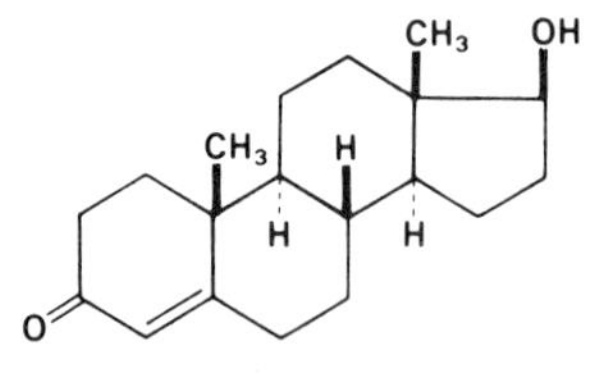

Testosterone

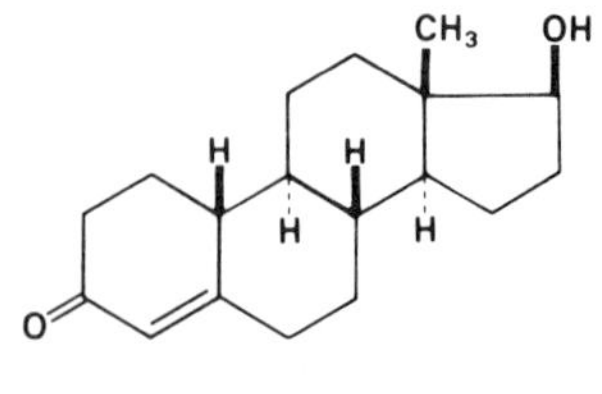

Nandrolone

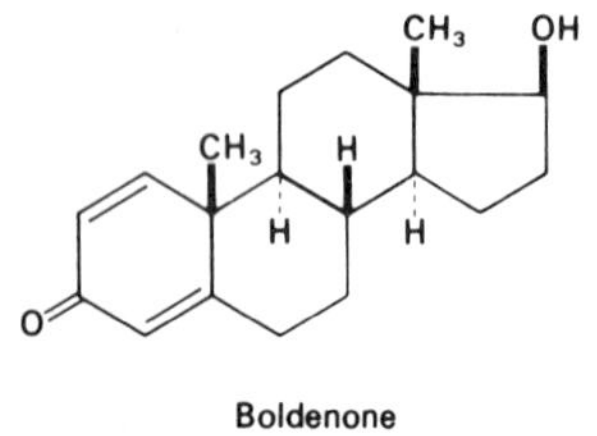

Boldenone

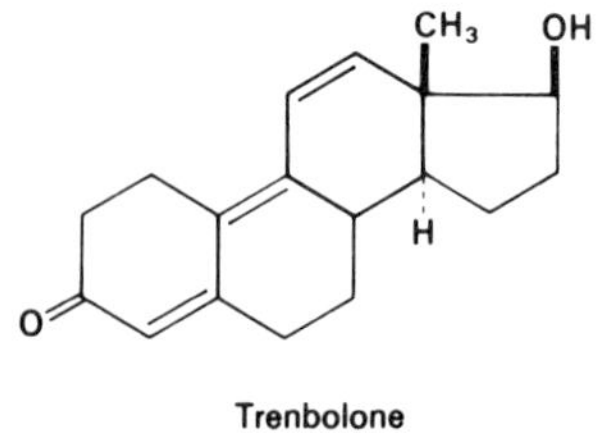

Trenbolone

Table 4. Principal urinary metabolites of anabolic steroids in the horse

Steroid	Major metabolite (glucuronic acid conjugate)	Major metabolite (sulphate conjugate)
Boldenone	17α-Epimer	Boldenone (17β-)
Nandrolone	5α-Estrane-3β,17α-diol	Nandrolone (17β-)
Testosterone	5α-Androstane-3β,17α-diol	Testosterone (17β-)
Trenbolone	17α-Epimer	

(M. C. Dumasia and E. Houghton, *Xenobiotica*, 1981, *11*, 323–331; M. C. Dumasia *et al.*, *Biomed. Mass Spectrom.*, 1983, *10*, 434–440; M. C. Dumasia and E. Houghton, *Xenobiotica*, 1984, *14*, 647–665.)

Although nandrolone has been regarded as exogenous, recent work has shown that it is endogenous to the sexually mature male horse (E. Houghton *et al.*, *Biomed. Mass Spectrom.*, 1984, *11*, 96–99).

In those cases where a suitable antibody for radioimmunoassay is not available, a full multi-component screening procedure is necessary, and also needs to be undertaken as a confirmatory test in cases where the nature of the anabolic steroid is not known.

The full analysis involves the separation of the glucuronic acid and sulphate conjugate fractions and their separate hydrolysis followed by GC–MS of their silyl or methoxime-silyl derivatives. It should be noted that the sulphatase in *Helix pomatia* will not hydrolyse the sulphate conjugates of the 17β-hydroxy steroids, which require mild acid hydrolysis.

Identification of Anabolic Steroids in Horse Urine
Solvate a Sep-Pak C-18 cartridge (see Reagent Appendix) with 5 ml of methanol, followed by a wash with 5 ml of water. Pass 10 ml of the urine sample through the cartridge, wash with 10 ml of water, and elute with 10 ml of methanol. Evaporate the eluate at 50° in a rotary film evaporator and dissolve the residue in 1 to 2 ml of a mixture of chloroform and methanol (17:3).

Prepare a 10 mm internal diameter column of Sephadex LH-20 (see Reagent Appendix) using a slurry of 2 g of the resin in chloroform:methanol (17:3). Apply to the column the dissolved residue obtained above and elute with 30 ml of chloroform:methanol (17:3) to obtain the glucuronic acid conjugates. Carry out a second elution using 50 ml of chloroform:methanol (1:1) to obtain the sulphate conjugates. Evaporate the two eluates separately in a rotary film evaporator.

Hydrolyse the glucuronic acid conjugates by dissolving the residue in 10 ml of *acetate buffer (pH 5)*, adding 5000 Fishman units of mixed glucuronidase/sulphatase (from *Helix pomatia*), and incubating at 37° for 18 hours. Extract the hydrolysate with 10 ml of ethyl acetate.

Hydrolyse the sulphate conjugates by dissolving the residue in 10 ml of ethyl acetate containing 0.1 ml of *sulphuric acid* and incubating at 37° for 18 hours.

The ethyl acetate solutions from both hydrolysates are treated as follows. Wash the ethyl acetate solution with two 5-ml portions of 2M sodium hydroxide, followed by one wash with saturated sodium chloride solution, and evaporate the solutions to dryness in a rotary film evaporator.

In cases where specific anabolic steroids or their metabolites are suspected, and only 17α-hydroxy or 17β-hydroxy compounds are to be tested for, the separation on the Sephadex LH-20 column may be omitted. Hydrolysis is carried out on the residue from the Sep-Pak cartridge, but this will yield somewhat dirtier residues with the possibility of a reduction in sensitivity.

Thin-layer Chromatography. Dissolve the residue in chloroform and apply to a silica gel plate. At the same time apply a solution containing 1 mg/ml of 5α-androstane-3α,17β-diol in methanol as a reference solution. Develop the plate in a mobile phase consisting of ethyl acetate:chloroform (1:1).

Spray the reference solution only with a 10% solution of molybdophosphoric acid in methanol. The reference substance appears as a blue-grey spot on a yellow background.

Elute the corresponding area of the chromatographed extract with methanol, separate the silica gel by centrifugation, and evaporate the methanol to dryness in a reaction tube at 60° in a stream of oxygen-free nitrogen. Testosterone, nandrolone, trenbolone, and 5α-estrane-3β,17α-diol are co-eluted with the standard. Boldenone runs below the other substances; if its presence is suspected, a reference solution should be included in the chromatography.

Gas Chromatography–Mass Spectrometry. Prepare methoxime derivatives by heating the extract from the thin-layer chromatographic plate with 100 μl of an 8% solution of methoxyamine hydrochloride in dry pyridine at 60° for 30 minutes, and evaporate in a rotary film evaporator. Silylate by dissolving the residue in 100 μl of chloroform, adding 100 μl of *N,O*-bis(trimethylsilyl)acetamide and 20 μl of trimethylchlorosilane, then seal, and heat for 2 hours at 60°. When only 5α-estrane-3β,17α-diol is to be confirmed the methoxime formation can be omitted.

Prepare a 2-cm column of Sephadex LH-20 in a Pasteur pipette with a cotton wool plug, using a slurry of the resin in chloroform:hexane (1:1). Transfer the reaction mixture to the column with two 1-ml portions of chloroform:hexane (1:1), add a further 1 ml of the solvent mixture and collect the eluate.

Evaporate the eluate at 60° in a stream of oxygen-free nitrogen, and dissolve the residue in 50 µl of undecane.

Subject this solution to capillary column gas chromatography–mass spectrometry, using the splitless injection technique, and the following chromatographic conditions. Retention indices for these anabolic steroids are given in Table 5.

COLUMN. HP-2100 fused silica, 12.5 m × 0.2 mm internal diameter.

COLUMN TEMPERATURE. Programmed at 20° per minute from 150° to 200°, then at 5° per minute to 260°, and maintained at this temperature for 2 minutes.

CARRIER GAS. Helium.

Table 5. Retention indices of anabolic steroids

Compound	Derivative	RI
Boldenone	Methoxime-trimethylsilyl	2709
Nandrolone	,, ,,	2652
5α-Estrane-3β, 17α-diol	Bis(trimethylsilyl)	2500
Testosterone	Methoxime-trimethylsilyl	2702, 2711*
Trenbolone	,, ,,	2746

*syn and anti isomers

(For further details see E. Houghton et al., Biomed. Mass Spectrom., 1978, 5, 170–173; E. Houghton and P. Teale, ibid., 1981, 8, 358–361.)
Radioimmunoassay. See W. R. Jondorf and M. S. Moss, Xenobiotica, 1978, 8, 197–206; D. I. Chapman et al., Eq. Vet. J., 1982, 14, 213–218; E. Thacker et al., in Proceedings of the 21st International Meeting of the International Association of Forensic Toxicologists, Brighton, England, 1984.

Non-steroidal Anti-inflammatory Drugs

Aspirin and phenylbutazone have been the commonest anti-inflammatory drugs encountered, but a number of other drugs are now used for this purpose. These are mostly carboxylic acids, a few of them non-nitrogenous, and they represent a serious and intractable doping problem in the thoroughbred horse. Their use can result in erratic changes of form of a lame horse from one race to another, and hereditary weakness when breeding from unsound stock may be temporarily masked by them. Some bodies controlling activities such as show-jumping have permitted the use of these

drugs. However, since 1981, the Fédération Equestre Internationale has allowed only phenylbutazone to be used, and this must not exceed a concentration of 4 µg/ml in plasma. The use of phenylbutazone is permitted almost everywhere in the USA.

QUANTIFICATION OF PHENYLBUTAZONE IN HORSE PLASMA OR URINE
(J. Taylor et al., Eq. Vet. J., 1981, 13, 201–203.)
For plasma, acidify 2 ml with 1 ml of a 10% solution of hydrochloric acid. For urine, add 0.25 ml to 2 ml of water.

Extract the solution with 10 ml of a mixture of hexane:tetrahydrofuran (4:1) containing 2.5 µg/ml of hexoestrol as a reference standard. Separate the phases by centrifugation and evaporate 5 ml of the solvent layer at room temperature in an oxygen-free stream of nitrogen.

Dissolve the residue in 150 µl of tetrahydrofuran and examine by high pressure liquid chromatography using the system described below with ultra-violet detection at 240 nm, and applying 10 µl to the column.

COLUMN. Partisil PXS 10/25, 25 cm × 4.6 mm internal diameter.

ELUENT. Hexane:tetrahydrofuran (4:1) to which has been added 20 mg/litre of acetic acid.

Calculate the content of phenylbutazone from a calibration curve prepared by repeating the procedure using appropriate reference solutions of phenylbutazone in plasma or urine.

NOTE. The Fédération Equestre Internationale does not permit the use of oxyphenbutazone but allows it to be present as a metabolite of phenylbutazone. The criteria for deciding this question are not set out in the rules, but would include absolute concentrations and concentrations relative to phenylbutazone and its other metabolites.

IDENTIFICATION OF SALICYLIC ACID IN HORSE URINE
No statutory limit is prescribed for salicylic acid, but it is normally present in horse urine; it is important, therefore, to distinguish between normal concentrations and those arising from medication with aspirin or other salicylates such as topically applied methyl salicylate. Normal urine concentrations rarely exceed 10 µg/ml, but therapeutic doses of aspirin may give concentrations as much as 500 times greater. Addition of 1 ml of freshly prepared ferric chloride solution to 5 ml of urine will give a detectable violet colour when the concentration of salicylic acid exceeds about 100 µg/ml. A positive

result should be followed by an accurate determination of salicylic acid by high pressure liquid chromatography using the system described below with ultraviolet detection at 300 nm.

COLUMN. ODS-silica (Spherisorb-ODS, 10 μm, 25 cm × 4.6 mm internal diameter).

ELUENT. Gradient elution with a mixture of acetonitrile and 0.05M acetic acid, commencing with 10% of acetonitrile and increasing linearly to 90% acetonitrile in 15 minutes.

FLOW RATE. 1.7 ml/min.

IDENTIFICATION OF OTHER NON-STEROIDAL ANTI-INFLAMMATORY DRUGS IN THE HORSE

No one system of analysis is entirely satisfactory for detecting all of these compounds and a combination of techniques is essential. Many of the compounds can be detected by thin-layer chromatography using System TG (p. 169), but the results should be used only as a tentative identification. Systems TD and TF may also be used.

Gas Chromatography. This can be used to detect these compounds using 3% SE-30 on 80–100 mesh Chromosorb G (System GD, p. 194). The compounds should be converted to their methyl derivatives by heating the Acid Fraction obtained from the solvent extraction of horse urine (see above) in a sealed tube at 100° for 30 minutes with 180 μl of iodomethane and 50 mg of potassium carbonate. Trimethylanilinium hydroxide is not recommended for methylating these compounds.

High Pressure Liquid Chromatography. Urine may yield masking compounds on the gas chromatograph, and for complete screening, high pressure liquid chromatography should be used in conjunction with gas chromatography and thin-layer chromatography. The following system is recommended using ultraviolet detection at 280 nm. Systems HD or HW (p. 214) may also be used.

System HV

COLUMN. ODS-silica (Spherisorb-ODS, 5 μm, 20 cm × 4.6 mm internal diameter).

ELUENT. Acetonitrile:0.1M acetic acid (45:55). Elute isocratically for 2 minutes then increase the proportion of acetonitrile by 3% per minute up to 75%, followed by isocratic elution for 6 minutes.

FLOW RATE. 1.7 ml/min.

(For further details see P. Chalmers *et al.,* in *Proceedings of the 21st International Meeting of the International Association of Forensic Toxicologists, Brighton, England,* 1984.)

A list of retention times of anti-inflammatory compounds and other acidic drugs, relative to meclofenamic acid, is given in Table 6.

Table 6. Relative retention times of non-steroidal anti-inflammatory drugs in system HV

Compound	Retention time relative to meclofenamic acid
Alclofenac	0.61
Benoxaprofen	0.98
Bufexamac	*
Clonixin	0.87
Diclofenac	0.85
Diflunisal	0.77
Fenbufen	0.81
Fenclofenac	0.91
Fenoprofen	*
Feprazone	0.92
Flufenamic acid	1.00
Flunixin	0.99
Flurbiprofen	0.89
Frusemide	0.45
Ibuprofen	*
Indomethacin	0.87
Indoprofen	0.52
Ketoprofen	0.66
Meclofenamic acid	1.00
Mefenamic acid	0.95
Naproxen	0.67
Niflumic acid	0.93
Oxyphenbutazone	0.69
Phenylbutazone	0.95
Salsalate	0.69
Sulindac	0.78
Theobromine	†
Theophylline	†
Tolmetin	0.60 and 0.99

*not detected
†elutes with solvent front

Corticosteroids

The term corticosteroids strictly applies only to the steroids of the adrenal cortex. However, it is generally used colloquially as a collective term embracing their synthetic analogues. Only the glucocorticoid steroids are important in doping because of their anti-inflammatory action, and these are abused in the same manner as their non-steroidal counterparts.

In man, hydrocortisone gives mainly 5β metabolites, whereas 11β-hydroxyandrostenedione, which is also secreted by the adrenal cortex, gives mainly 5α metabolites. Thus, if hydrocortisone is administered, it would be expected to decrease the normal ratio of 5α to 5β metabolites. Hence, the ratio of 5α to 5β metabolites in the 11-oxygenated-17-oxo steroid metabolites of hydrocortisone and of 11βhydroxyandrostenedione may be a reliable measure of the administration of hydrocortisone.

A *radioimmunoassay* procedure for urine can be used to detect most synthetic corticosteroids as well as exogenous hydrocortisone (D. I. Chapman *et al.*, *Vet. Rec.*, 1977, *100*, 447–450; M. C. Dumasia *et al.*, *J. Biochem.*, 1973, *133*, 401–404).

High Pressure Liquid Chromatography

High pressure liquid chromatography can be used as a screening procedure instead of radioimmunoassay, although it is less sensitive. Extract 10 ml of urine with 25 ml of methylene chloride, separate the solvent layer, and dry it over anhydrous sodium sulphate. Examine 10 µl of the extract using a silica column (Zorbax SIL, 5 µm) (System HT, p. 219). *k'* Values for corticosteroids are given under System HT.

Gas Chromatography–Mass Spectrometry

Negative-ion chemical ionisation mass spectrometry is the best method to identify a wide range of synthetic corticosteroids in horse urine (E. Houghton *et al.*, *Biomed. Mass Spectrom.*, 1982, *9*, 459–465).

Method. Extract 10 ml of urine with 25 ml of methylene chloride, separate the solvent layer, dry over anhydrous sodium sulphate, and evaporate to dryness in a rotary film evaporator at 30° to 40°. Heat the residue with 100 µl of an 8% solution of methoxyamine hydrochloride in dry pyridine in a reaction tube at 80° for 30 minutes, add 50 µl of trimethylsilylimidazole, and heat at 80° for a further 2 hours.

Prepare a 2-cm column of Sephadex LH-20 in a Pasteur pipette with a cotton wool plug, using a slurry of the resin in chloroform:hexane (1:1). Transfer the reaction mixture to the column with two 1-ml portions of chloroform:hexane (1:1), add a further 1 ml of the solvent mixture and collect the eluate. Evaporate the eluate in a rotary film evaporator at about 30° to 40° and dissolve the residue in 100 µl of dodecane. Subject this solution to capillary column gas chromatography–mass spectrometry using the column and injection technique described under anabolic steroids (p. 95) except that the column temperature is programmed at 20° per minute from 190° to 260°, then at 5° per minute to 280°, and maintained at this temperature for 2 minutes.

Caffeine, Theobromine, and Theophylline

These comprise the most commonly reported horse-doping agents in the United Kingdom, and the use of caffeine is very common world-wide. Theobromine and theophylline are metabolites of caffeine in the horse (M. S. Moss, 1977), and theobromine is frequently ingested with caffeine as a result of the contamination of pelleted horse feed with cocoa husk. Theophylline may also occur as a result of administering aminophylline for respiratory problems. Caffeine appears occasionally in greyhound urine as a result of the widespread practice of giving tea prior to racing. Theobromine, theophylline, and 1,7-dimethylxanthine are all metabolites of caffeine in the horse and man but their proportions vary greatly between the species. In human sport, the upper limit on the urinary concentration of caffeine has recently been set at 15 µg/ml.

Caffeine itself is poorly extracted into ether, though yields can be improved by the addition of sodium chloride or other neutral soluble electrolytes. Chloroform is a much better extracting solvent and its use is essential if theobromine is to be extracted. Although the methylxanthines are often described as alkaloids or as weak bases, the dimethylxanthines are in fact weak acids and are best extracted from acidic solution. They are well separated by high pressure liquid chromatography (A. Aldridge *et al.*, *Clin. Pharmac. Ther.*, 1979, *25*, 447–453), but for gas chromatographic analysis only caffeine can be chromatographed without derivatisation. A convenient technique for distinguishing these dimethylxanthines and the methyluric acid metabolites of caffeine is the gas chromatography–mass spectrometry of their deuteromethyl derivatives, prepared by reaction with deuterodiazomethane, or of their deuterobutyl derivatives (E. Houghton, *Biomed. Mass Spectrom.*, 1982, *9*, 103–107).

Diuretics

Diuretics, and especially frusemide, are widely used in horse racing although the reason is somewhat obscure. They are also used in weight-lifting and other competitions classified by weight. Diuretics are permitted in most of the USA. The dilution of the urine which results from their use can render detection of some other drugs more difficult.

Diuretics can be detected in urine by high pressure liquid chromatography using System HN (p. 217), or by thin-layer chromatography using silica gel G plates and ethyl acetate as the mobile phase (System TF, p. 168). A method applicable to human urine is described under Screening for Abuse of Diuretics, p. 32.

Miscellaneous Substances

ACETYLENE
The use of calcium carbide administered orally in gelatin capsules to horses has been reported in Australia. Acetylene can be detected by head-space gas chromatography of plasma.

ANTHELMINTICS
Thiabendazole, pyrantel tartrate, and phenothiazine are the commonest anthelmintics found in horses.

APOMORPHINE
This has been reported frequently in racehorses in the USA. It has a marked effect on locomotor activity in the horse. Apomorphine is one of a number of compounds which are detected by normal screening procedures only after hydrolysis with β-glucuronidase.

BENZODIAZEPINES
These may be detected in urine using the method described under Hospital Toxicology and Drug Abuse Screening, p. 10.

CAMPHOR
This has the reputation of being a respiratory stimulant in horses and is thought to be usually administered by intramuscular injection. The parent compound is not detectable in horse urine. It undergoes a series of oxidations, one product of which is isoketopinic acid which is found as an acid-labile conjugate. This may be hydrolysed by heating with *hydrochloric acid* at 100° for 10 minutes. The liberated acid can be derivatised to its 2,4-dinitrophenylhydrazone and detected by thin-layer chromatography, using silica gel plates and chloroform as the mobile phase followed by a second development with a mixture of chloroform: methanol (15:1); it occurs as a yellow spot with an Rf of 20.

CHLORBUTOL
This sedative has been found on innumerable occasions in greyhounds and occasionally in horses. Although it can be detected by the Fujiwara Test, p. 135, the concentration in horse urine following its administration is extremely low, and gas chromatography should be used for confirmation (see monograph).

DIMETHYL SULPHOXIDE
This is used as a solvent for the percutaneous administration of certain drugs in the horse. It imparts an odour of rotten cabbage, probably as the result of sulphide formation.

HORDENINE
This has been found occasionally and appears to arise from the presence of sprouting barley in horse feed. It may be detected during gas chromatography of the Basic Fraction.

LUPANINE AND SPARTEINE
These alkaloids appear occasionally in horse and human urine, and may be detected during gas chromatography of the Basic Fraction. Lupins are being used increasingly as a source of dietary protein in horse feed and the compounds may therefore be expected to occur more frequently.

METHYLHYDANTOIN
This arises as a degradation product of urinary creatinine, and occurs only in urine which has aged for several days between voiding and analysis. It may be found during gas chromatography of the Basic Fraction.

4-METHYLTHIAZOL-5-YLETHANOL
This is believed to arise as a metabolite of thiamine and may indicate administration of a vitamin B_1 preparation. Thiamine is thought to have a sedative action in the horse when given in large doses. The metabolite may be detected during gas chromatography of the Basic Fraction. When it occurs the concentration of thiamine should be measured. Urinary concentrations greater than about 100 µg/ml are unusual after oral administration, but much higher concentrations may be found after parenteral administration.

PEMOLINE
This stimulant has been reported frequently in man and occasionally in horses. Although moderate concentrations of pemoline may be detected using Screen B (p. 91), for greater sensitivity the concentration of the metabolite, mandelic acid, should be determined using gas chromatography–mass spectrometry; confirmatory tests for pemoline should also be carried out since mandelic acid is a metabolite of several compounds.

PERLOLINE
This alkaloid, which is a constituent of perennial rye grass, occurs very frequently especially during the summer. It is a troublesome masking agent in ultraviolet spectrophotometry.

POLYETHYLENE GLYCOLS
These compounds, which are mixtures of condensation products of ethylene oxide and water (macrogols), are used as solvents for a variety of pharmaceutical preparations, including some ste-

roid formulations. The presence of polyethylene glycols is considered presumptive evidence of the administration of such a product and is considered to be an offence by some authorities.

Polyethylene glycols are rather poorly extracted by chloroform and not at all by ether. They are detected on paper chromatography systems by their very strong reaction with *acidified iodoplatinate solution*, and with lower sensitivity by thin-layer chromatography. A characteristic of polyethylene glycols is their persistence in several sequential chloroform extracts; extractability at any pH is strongly indicative of these compounds. If they occur in screening procedures based on thin-layer or paper chromatography, it is essential to separate them from the organic bases. This is best done by extracting the bases from the chloroform extract with 0.25M sulphuric acid and back-extracting with several portions of chloroform until the extracts are free from polyethylene glycol, as indicated by the reaction with acidified iodoplatinate solution. The acidic aqueous phase may then be made alkaline and re-extracted to obtain the basic group. The identity of the polyethylene glycols is best established by infra-red spectrophotometry following elution from paper chromatograms. They tend to streak on paper and thin-layer chromatographic systems; the lower molecular weight compounds have higher Rf values.

RESERPINE

This highly potent compound has been used on a number of occasions as a tranquilliser for horses. A dose of only 5 mg has demonstrable effects for several days. The following procedure can be used to detect reserpine in horse plasma following a dose of 1 to 2 mg. (After R. A. Sams and R. Huffman, *J. Chromat.*, 1978, *161*, 410–414.)

Add 2 ml of a saturated solution of borax to 2 ml of plasma, extract with 4 ml of toluene, separate the toluene layer, and evaporate under a stream of nitrogen at 50°. Dissolve the residue in 6 μl of methylene chloride, divide the solution into three 2-μl portions, and examine by thin-layer chromatography using silica gel G plates and the mobile phases shown in Table 7. After development, dry the plates using a hot air blower, expose them to the vapour of *acetic acid* for one hour, and examine under ultraviolet light at 350 nm; reserpine appears as a bright blue spot.

Table 7. Thin-layer chromatography of reserpine

Mobile phase	Rf
Chloroform:acetone (70:30)	15
Chloroform:methanol (95:5)	50
Butanol:water:*acetic acid* (80:20:20)	72

A radioimmunoassay for the detection of reserpine in horses has been described (E. Thacker, *Analyt. Proc.*, 1985, *22*, 136–137).

NOTE. Reserpine is very strongly adsorbed on to glass surfaces and scrupulous cleaning of glassware is essential when analysing this compound.

Bibliography

E. G. C. Clarke, The Doping of Racehorses, *Medicoleg. J.*, 1962, *30*, 180–194.

M. W. Horner, The Passage of Drugs into Horse Saliva and the Suitability of Saliva for Pre-race Testing, *Br. J. Sports Med.*, 1976, *10*, 133–140.

O. R. Idowu and B. Caddy, A Review of the Use of Saliva in the Forensic Detection of Drugs and Other Chemicals, *J. forens. Sci. Soc.*, 1982, *22*, 123–135.

M. S. Moss, The Metabolism and Urinary and Salivary Excretion of Drugs in the Horse and their Relevance to Dope Detection, in *Drug Metabolism—from Microbe to Man*, D. V. Parke and R. L. Smith (Ed.), London, Taylor and Francis, 1977.

M. S. Moss, Role of Referee Samples in European Drug Detection, in *3rd International Symposium on Equine Medication Control*, T. Tobin *et al.* (Ed.), Lexington, Kentucky, 1979.

Therapeutic Drug Monitoring

V. Marks

Drugs have always played an important part in the treatment of diseases, even when few were of proved efficacy and their mode of action was poorly understood. The introduction during the last half century of selective, potent, and potentially dangerous drugs, and the requirement by various regulatory bodies that they are efficacious, has done much to ensure that therapeutic practices that were adequate in a bygone age are no longer acceptable. In order to increase the efficacy and decrease the toxicity of drugs, dosage regimens should take into account the different ways in which different individuals absorb, metabolise, excrete, and respond to drugs. In order to achieve this, the clinician must in many cases tailor his treatment to the individual patient's requirements. Although this is not a new idea, having been practised in digitalis therapy for over two hundred years, its importance as a general principle has been slow to gain acceptance. This has been due to the lack of suitable methods for individualising drug treatment. Usually, both the therapeutic and toxic responses to a drug occur too slowly to permit adjustment of the dose to achieve optimum therapeutic effectiveness, and serious or even irreversible damage can occur because of under- or overtreatment.

It is now recognised that for some drugs (e.g. phenytoin, lithium, procainamide, and theophylline) the therapeutic response correlates better with the concentration in plasma than with the daily dose. This, together with developments in analytical technology that enable measurements to be carried out quickly on small samples of blood, has led to a rapidly developing interest in the possibility of using plasma concentrations as a guide to improving therapeutic efficacy. This chapter examines the conceptual basis of such practices, their usefulness and limitations, and discusses methods for measuring the few drugs for which it has been currently established that clinical monitoring is worthwhile. Non-compliance, i.e. the failure of patients to take their prescribed drugs, is probably the commonest cause of therapeutic failure. The use of blood or urine concentrations has been advocated as a means of detecting and preventing non-compliance, but since the argument is applicable to all drugs it will not be dealt with further here.

Fundamental Concepts

The theoretical basis for therapeutic drug monitoring rests upon three premises. Firstly, that the therapeutic response to a particular drug correlates with its concentration in the blood rather than with the dose. This is clearly inapplicable to drugs which are either not absorbed when given orally (e.g. neomycin) or which exert their effect largely or exclusively at their site of application (e.g. topical steroids, antifungal agents, etc.). Secondly, that there exists an optimum therapeutic range within which the majority of patients experience maximum clinical benefit with minimum toxic or unpleasant side-effects. Thirdly, that by adjusting the dose and the timing of drug administration on the basis of the plasma concentration, the attainment and maintenance of the optimum therapeutic range of a drug leads to a greater patient benefit than can be achieved by the exercise of sound clinical judgement alone.

These premises have so far been established as true for extremely few drugs. In some cases, they are known to be invalid. Drugs whose effects are irreversible and/or exerted through denaturation of intracellular proteins (e.g. the monoamine-oxidase inhibitors) or by depletion of stored materials (e.g. reserpine) belong in this category.

Inherent in the rationale of therapeutic drug monitoring is the assumption that the plasma concentration of the drug reflects its concentration at the cell membrane, and that there is a high degree of correlation between them. This is not necessarily true if the blood supply to the tissue is impaired, as is often the case with poorly vascularised tissues and tumours which have outstripped their blood supply. Also, much of the drug present in the circulation, and measured as such when assays are performed on plasma, is bound to a greater or lesser extent by plasma proteins. The ratio of protein-bound to non-protein-bound drug (free drug) in the plasma is dependent on a number of factors. The most important are the nature of the drug, its molar concentration relative to that of the individual plasma protein (generally albumin), and the presence of competing substances for binding sites (usually other drugs, but occasionally endogenous compounds). Disturbance of the ratio of protein-bound to non-protein-bound drug from the normal by any of these factors can totally invalidate the value of plasma 'total drug' concentration measurements. This occasionally happens in patients with a particular disease, e.g. uraemia, in whom plasma-phenytoin concentrations may be extremely low in the presence of unequivocal phenytoin intoxication.

Another reason for disagreement between plasma-drug concentrations and the biological effects observed is the development of tolerance to the action of the drug at the cellular level as occurs with, for example, morphine and some barbiturates such as phenobarbitone. It can also occur if the cells lose the capacity to respond to the drug, as in the case of the failing heart already maximally stimulated by digoxin.

Therapeutic Response

In practice, there is no advantage in measuring the concentration of drug in the blood if its biological effect can be easily monitored. For example, it is not customary to measure the blood concentration of oral antidiabetic agents such as tolbutamide, chlorpropamide, and other sulphonylureas, since it is more pertinent and simpler to measure the blood-glucose concentration directly. Similarly, it is not often considered necessary to measure the blood concentrations of antihypertensive agents (e.g. propranolol and methyldopa) except as a test of compliance, since it is generally more informative to measure the blood pressure. Also, the control of anticoagulant therapy has long been regulated by reference to the plasma prothrombin time.

In the case of drugs such as the antibacterials, antivirals, antifungals, and antiparasitics, the therapeutic effect is achieved as the result of the differential susceptibility of the parasite and the host's own tissues to the toxic effects of the drug. For some (e.g. the penicillins), the margin between the two is so great that they can be considered as innocuous to humans, but deadly to sensitive organisms. However, with others, e.g. streptomycin, gentamicin, amikacin, and vancomycin, the difference between the concentration that is required to inhibit sensitive parasites, often referred to as the minimum inhibitory concentration, and

that which is toxic to human tissue is so small as to make their use dangerous unless controlled by regular measurements of blood concentration. The same considerations are probably true of antineoplastic agents, e.g. methotrexate and cytarabine, which behave like antibiotics and exert their beneficial effect by virtue of their differential toxicity towards neoplastic and normal tissues. At the present time, too little information is available about the clinical monitoring of this class of compound to make further discussion profitable.

Indications for Measuring Drugs in Blood

The general indications for measuring drugs in blood include the investigation of pharmacokinetics, protein binding, bioavailability, and the comparability of different drug preparations. However, there are a number of specific clinical indications which apply to a greater or lesser extent to all of the drugs for which therapeutic drug monitoring has been established as useful.

The first clinical indication for drug monitoring occurs when the administration of doses that are usually effective in susceptible conditions does not produce a favourable response. The commonest reason for this is non-compliance, but others include reduced bioavailability, non-absorption, more rapid (or slower) metabolism or elimination than normal, reduced access to the drug's site of action, and tissue or organ unresponsiveness.

The second clinical indication for measuring blood-drug concentrations is to provide a guide to the adjustment of drug dosage in order to obtain optimum effectiveness, when no simpler or more directly relevant indicator is available (e.g. phenytoin, theophylline, and gentamicin). This form of therapeutic drug monitoring is better referred to as individualisation of drug therapy.

Coupled with this, but different in concept, is the use of drug measurements to prevent the appearance of severe and irreversible adverse drug reactions when these cannot be predicted by simpler clinical methods. This indication is particularly important when there is co-existing disease (e.g. renal or hepatic failure) which so alters pharmacokinetic behaviour as to render general guidelines on drug usage inappropriate. This is true of anti-arrhythmic drugs such as lignocaine whose half-lives are greatly prolonged by poor liver perfusion. This occurs in patients who have recently suffered myocardial infarction and are the very ones most likely to be treated with drugs of this type.

A fourth reason for measuring drugs in blood is as

an aid to distinguishing between overtreatment and undertreatment when this is difficult on clinical grounds alone. Digoxin measurements are a good example of this situation, since the clinical condition of a patient who has taken an overdose may be indistinguishable from that of a patient who has been prescribed the drug but has not been taking enough. This is the realm of diagnostic biochemistry, and measurements should be made only when there are good clinical indications for them.

Finally, one of the most important indications for measuring blood-drug concentrations occurs during trials of new and established drugs, in order to assess their clinical efficacy and optimum mode of usage. During the first few months of the general release of a new drug, the measurement of blood concentrations would serve to identify those patients in the community who cannot eliminate it normally from their bodies and may, as a consequence, suffer severe or possibly fatal adverse effects.

Choice of Drugs to be Monitored

The blood concentrations of many drugs are measured in clinical laboratories, but it is only for a few that these measurements have been shown unequivocally to provide clinically useful information. This is true in distinguishing between underdosage and overdosage (e.g. digoxin, nortriptyline), and in the adjustment of dosage (e.g. gentamicin, lithium, phenytoin, theophylline).

The features of a drug that make it likely that it will be worth monitoring are best illustrated by reference to lithium. This is almost the perfect example of a drug whose use is only ethically possible because of the ability to measure its concentration in plasma and use the information so obtained to adjust the dosage regimen.

Lithium is used extensively for the prevention of recurrences of symptoms in patients suffering from either manic depression or endogenous depression. The plasma-lithium concentration correlates well, within narrowly defined limits, with therapeutic effectiveness. Plasma concentrations below about 0.5 mmol/litre exert little protective effect against relapse; concentrations above 1.2 mmol/litre are associated with an unacceptably high incidence of side-effects, some of them potentially fatal. The measurement of lithium in plasma is simple, quick, accurate, and precise. Lithium has no metabolites and is relatively free from interference by any other substance ever likely to be present in plasma. It is not protein-bound and has a moderate to long half-life in the body which, though entirely dependent upon renal excretory capacity, can be influenced by dietary factors such as salt content and by concurrent therapy with drugs such as chlorothiazide. The diseases for which lithium therapy is used are serious, economically important, and common. This has enabled both retrospective and prospective clinical trials to be conducted by more than one group of investigators to establish a therapeutic range. For no other drug has such a good case been established for making plasma-drug measurements a part of a drug monitoring programme.

The main drugs for which therapeutic drug monitoring has established itself as useful, are those that affect the metabolism, activity, function, or other attribute of the patient's own tissues, either by reacting with specific receptors in the cell or by interfering with the activity of one or more of its enzymes in a reversible and concentration-dependent manner. This excludes that small group of drugs which appear to bind irreversibly to proteins within the cell, and continue to exert their effects until either the cell dies or the protein to which the drug is attached is replaced by renewed synthesis. Drugs of this kind have been referred to as 'hit and run drugs' and include the alkylating agents, e.g. chlorambucil, melphalan, and cyclophosphamide, and certain enzyme inhibitors, e.g. phenelzine and tranylcypromine. However, it now seems likely that some of the drugs formerly placed in this category (e.g. amiodarone) may need to be reclassified, because more sensitive analytical methods have revealed their continued presence in the blood at extremely low concentrations throughout the period of response.

The Table on p. 107 lists a number of drugs which have been the subject of drug monitoring studies. The clinical value of therapeutic drug monitoring of each of the 25 drugs listed has been classified from well-proved value to no proved value. Included in the table are some drugs which are clearly not worth monitoring but which nevertheless often are, e.g. primidone and phenobarbitone. This is often because the result is generated as a by-product of other reasonably requested assays, e.g. phenytoin, where these are performed by chromatographic techniques.

Choice of Body Fluid for Assay

Most of the developmental work on therapeutic drug monitoring has been carried out using plasma and measuring the total concentration of drug present. However, this does not reflect the concentration of drug at the surfaces of the effector cells as well as would the concentration of the non-protein-bound drug (free drug) measured by ultrafiltration or dialysis. However, the deduction that only free drug is biologically active is unwarranted and denies the possibility that protein binding might facilitate attachment of drug to its receptors on the effector cells. In the absence of conclusive experimental data, the superiority of free over total plasma-drug measurements must still be considered conjectural.

The above situation is also true of measurements carried out on saliva which often, but not invariably, provide a rough estimate of unbound drug concentration. Consequently, despite its greater availability and ease of collection, saliva has not proved to be a clinically useful fluid for therapeutic drug monitoring except in a very limited number of cases, e.g. theophylline whose secretion is relatively uninfluenced by the rate of flow of saliva.

Urine specimens may be received for analysis to check compliance. However, quantitative assays have no advantage over semiquantitative or even simple qualitative methods for this purpose. The result may be extremely difficult to interpret because urinary-drug concentrations, except in the case of alcohol, rarely bear any well-known relationship to those of blood collected at the same time.

Timing of Measurements

Because drugs are usually administered at intervals of time, their concentration in body fluids is subject to fluctuations. The magnitude of the plasma-drug concentration thus depends upon a number of variables, the most important of which are the bioavailability of the product, the frequency of dosing, and the rate of elimination. Therapeutic responses to drugs which act upon the patient's tissues usually correlate better with steady-state rather than with peak plasma-drug concentrations. Toxic effects, on the other hand, often relate more closely to peak than to steady-state plasma-drug concentrations.

When the steady-state concentration is reached, the total body burden of a drug remains more or less constant within relatively narrow limits. In this hypothetical situation there is little or no redistribution between the various body compartments. The maintenance of this ideal state implies that the drug must be administered at regular intervals in an amount equal to the amount eliminated from the body in the interval, and that this interval is long enough to permit complete absorption and distribution through the body compartments.

The steady state is achieved after the lapse of about six biological half-lives of the drug. It can be achieved more quickly, should this be considered clinically necessary, by manipulating the dosing schedule according to the pharmacokinetic behaviour of the drug and by consideration of the patient's own response characteristics. Because of the relatively long interval between altering the dose of a drug and the attainment of a new steady state, little clinical importance can be attached to blood-drug measurements made less than this interval after the last dosage adjustment. This can be as long as a week or more in the case of drugs with very long half-lives.

Once the steady state has been reached, the size and timing of fluctuations about the mean blood-drug concentration are determined by the mode of delivery, the bioavailability, and the interval between dosing, as well as by the pharmacokinetics of the drug itself. Optimum therapeutic ranges for most drugs relate to the blood concentration immediately preceding the next scheduled dose. Thus a blood sample for digoxin would be taken 6 hours after the last dose as it has a half-life of about 36 hours, whilst sodium valproate has a much shorter half-life (11 hours), and samples should be taken earlier. In the case of lithium, a strong case has been made for standardising measurements of the plasma-lithium concentration in the morning, exactly 12 hours after the last dose.

Stages in the Development of a Clinical Assay

The first, and absolutely essential, step in the development of a clinical assay is the production and validation of a suitable analytical technique. The next is to establish that the blood-drug concentration correlates with the therapeutic effectiveness and/or toxicity of the drug. Usually, this can only be achieved by a retrospective study of a large number of subjects over a long period of time, during which many analytical measurements and careful clinical observations have been made and properly documented. If a relationship between plasma concentration and effectiveness does exist, such data should permit a tentative optimum therapeutic range to be derived. During this latter stage it should be possible to establish that when blood-drug measurements are made and are used as the basis of dosage adjustment, the patients fare better than when drug dosage is adjusted empirically or on clinical response alone. The tentative optimum therapeutic range can then be used as the basis for the third stage of development, namely, the prospective clinical trial. Unfortunately, the prospective stage of assay development has been carried out for only a handful of drugs, i.e. lithium, phenytoin, and ethosuximide.

Measurement Techniques

A variety of analytical techniques has been used for measuring the concentration of drugs in body fluids. Some suggested assay methods for therapeutic drug monitoring purposes are given in the Table below. Various published methods and commercial immunoassays are listed to allow the selection of a method according to the instrumentation available. Further methods are given in the monographs in Part 2.

Much of the present pharmacokinetic knowledge, especially that upon which the principles and practice of therapeutic drug monitoring depend, was derived from studies using *colorimetry, spectrophotometry*, and *spectrofluorimetry*. The first two of these techniques are relatively insensitive and susceptible to interference by other substances present in biological fluids. Their use has been virtually abandoned except for the measurement of paracetamol and salicylate in cases of suspected overdose. This susceptibility to interference is also the factor limiting the more general application of spectrofluorimetry to therapeutic drug monitoring. *Bioassay*, which is still often used for measuring antibiotics in biological fluids, is too slow, insensitive, and labour-intensive to justify its widespread application.

Thin-layer chromatography was largely responsible for the upsurge in qualitative analysis of body fluids for drugs, since it separated the drug from its metabolites and interfering compounds. However, it has proved less useful as a quantitative tool, even with the availability of high performance thin-layer chromatography plates and reliable scanning-reflectance spectrophotometers.

Gas chromatography has been the technique of choice for measuring drugs in blood and other biological fluids, although it has the disadvantages that it is relatively slow, labour-intensive, and insufficiently sensitive for many drugs. *High pressure liquid chromatography* has rapidly established itself as adaptable and readily amenable to the rapid measurement of a wide range of drugs although it may lack sensitivity. High pressure liquid chromatographic methods are generally precise and more specific than other analytical techniques. This latter consideration is especially important in the measurement of drugs which undergo extensive metabolism, the products of which may remain in the circulation for longer than the parent compound. The method is quicker to use than gas chromatography and has a wider range of applicability. For both methods, the initial capital costs are often high, but the running costs are usually low.

The growth of clinical interest in the monitoring of therapeutic drug concentrations has been greatly increased by the development and application of *immunoassay* techniques, especially those which dispense with the need for phase separation, i.e. the homogeneous immunoassays. Information on the technique of immunoassay can be found under Immunoassays (p. 148).

Kits for immunoassays are available from a number of commercial sources for measuring most of the drugs for which it has been shown to be worthwhile, as well as for a large number where it has not. Kits seldom require the use of apparatus that is not already generally available in any well-equipped clinical laboratory, though several manufacturers now market pre-programmed microprocessor-controlled instruments designed specifically for use with their own reagents. Homogeneous immunoassay techniques are generally simple, requiring only the addition to the sample of one, two, or three reagents in an orderly, timed sequence. Rarely does the sample size exceed 100 microlitres. Homogeneous immunoassay techniques are generally quick, precise, and sufficiently accurate to make them acceptable in nearly all clinical situations. Commercial reagents do not, at present, have the requisite sensitivity to enable them to be used for measuring drugs whose plasma concentration is much less than 1 ng/ml.

Where exquisite sensitivity is required it is generally still necessary to resort to the use of heterogeneous immunoassay techniques employing radio-, enzyme-, or fluorescent-labelled drugs.

Immunoassays are generally easy to automate, but this is scarcely a real advantage since the nearer the patient and the more rapidly the result can be obtained, the more clinically valuable is the drug measurement likely to be. The most serious objection to immunoassays as a measurement technique for drugs in biological fluids is their susceptibility to interference by metabolites of the drug or its analogues. This generally renders immunoassays unsuitable for use in toxicological diagnosis or in situations in which there is doubt as to the exact nature of the drug being used. Only very rarely does it cause difficulties in therapeutic drug monitoring, since this information is generally available. Another disadvantage in the use of immunoassays occurs in cases where polypharmacy is being practised, as still often happens in the treatment of epilepsy. A separate assay must be performed for each of the drugs it is intended to measure, and it may be impossible to obtain accurate results if the drugs or their metabolites cross-react in the different immunoassays. This is where chromatographic techniques have an advantage, because a separation stage precedes quantification and allows several drugs with similar physicochemical properties to be measured together.

The combination of two different methods of separation and measurement, e.g. HPLC and immunoassay, or GC and mass spectrometry, will increase specificity but is rarely required in therapeutic drug monitoring. Such methods must, however, be used for assessing the analytical reliability of an immunoassay under varying conditions of clinical usage.

Quality Control

Quality control is essential in the performance of therapeutic drug monitoring assays because clinical decisions as to whether the dose should be increased, decreased, or left unchanged are sometimes made exclusively on the basis of the analytical result.

Most externally-organised quality control schemes have revealed that the performance of many participants is unacceptable; this is due mainly to their use of inappropriate methodologies. Other important sources of error are the use of incorrect standards and of inappropriate internal quality controls. Because of the risk of interference by other drugs and metabolites in many analytical techniques, it is vital that external quality control material should be properly prepared. For further information see under Quality Control in Clinical Analysis (p. 118).

Interpretation of Results

It is not uncommon to endow blood-drug measurements with far more predictive or diagnostic importance than they deserve. Apart from analytical errors due to the use of imprecise or inaccurate measurement procedures, the main cause of error in therapeutic drug monitoring is misinterpretation of the data. The commonest reason for this is failure to appreciate the importance of correct timing of specimen collection in relation to dosing and changes in dosing regimen. Another cause of error is to pay too little attention to the effect of other chemical and biological variables upon the physiological and pharmacological significance of a single drug measurement. For example, the concentration of potassium in the plasma is a major determinant of whether a given plasma-digoxin concentration is cardiotoxic. Metabolites which are themselves pharmacologically active should always be considered since the drug:metabolite ratio in the plasma will be quite different at the start of therapy and at steady state (e.g. primidone/phenobarbitone and amitriptyline/nortriptyline). The optimum therapeutic range of one drug in the presence of another with similar biological properties (e.g. anticonvulsants) has rarely been investigated. It is generally assumed to be the same as when the drug in question is given alone. Plasma concentrations commonly associated with optimum therapeutic response for drugs given alone are given in the Table (below) and further information will be found in the monographs for individual drugs.

Analytical technology is no longer the limiting factor to the extension of therapeutic drug monitoring. Instead it is the enormous amount of work that must be put into undertaking retrospective and prospective trials in order to ascertain the optimum therapeutic blood or plasma concentration. Undoubtedly, optimum therapeutic ranges will be established for drugs which are currently available and for those still to be developed. Drugs that are used for the treatment of neoplastic disease and those given prophylactically for relapsing or periodic diseases such as migraine and many psychiatric disorders are especially likely to be improved by our ability to monitor them.

Bibliography

L. Bertilsson, Clinical Pharmacokinetics of Carbamazepine, *Clin. Pharmacokinet.*, 1978, *3*, 128–143.
R. Gugler and G. E. von Unruh, Clinical Pharmacokinetics of Valproic Acid, *Clin. Pharmacokinet.*, 1980, *5*, 67–83.
Individualising Drug Therapy, W. J. Taylor and A. L. Finn (Ed.), New York, Gross, Townsend and Frank, 1981.
S. I. Johannessen, Antiepileptic Drugs: Pharmacokinetic and Clinical Aspects, *Ther. Drug Monit.*, 1981, *3*, 17–37.
F. N. Johnson, *Handbook of Lithium Therapy*, Lancaster, MTP Press, 1980.
E. Karlsson, Clinical Pharmacokinetics of Procainamide, *Clin. Pharmacokinet.*, 1978, *3*, 97–107.

J. Koch-Weser, Drug Therapy: Disopyramide, *New Engl. J. Med.*, 1979, *300*, 957–962.

B. R. Meyers and S. Z. Hirschman, Pharmacologic Studies on Tobramycin and Comparison with Gentamicin, *J. clin. Pharmac.*, 1972, *12*, 321–324.

A. Richens, Clinical Pharmacokinetics of Phenytoin, *Clin. Pharmacokinet.*, 1979, *4*, 153–169.

L. Rivera-Calimlim, Problems in Therapeutic Blood Monitoring of Chlorpromazine, *Ther. Drug Monit.*, 1982, *4*, 41–49.

B. Scoggins, Measurement of Tricyclic Antidepressants. Part II, Applications of Methodology, *Clin. Chem.*, 1980, *26*, 805–815. *Therapeutic Drug Monitoring*, A. Richens and V. Marks (Ed.), Edinburgh, Churchill Livingstone, 1981.

Table. Drugs subjected to therapeutic drug monitoring

Drug	Comments	Suggested assay methods†	Plasma concentrations associated with optimum therapeutic response	Clinical value of therapeutic drug monitoring‡
Amikacin	Plasma concentration must exceed the minimum inhibitory concentration but cannot be accurately predicted from the dose. Toxic effects of overdose are serious. Monitoring is essential to avoid undertreatment and ensure safety.	1. Homogeneous immunoassay* 2. HPLC—J. P. Anhalt and S. D. Brown, *Clin. Chem.*, 1978, *24*, 1940–1947. 3. Bioassay—J. M. Broughall, Aminoglycosides, in *Laboratory Methods in Antimicrobial Chemotherapy*, D. S. Reeves *et al.* (Ed.), Edinburgh, Churchill Livingstone, 1978, pp. 194–207.	Peak, 15–25 µg/ml Trough, 4–6 µg/ml	+ + +
Amitriptyline	Large genetic differences in rate of metabolism; concentrations of drug and metabolite (nortriptyline) cannot be predicted from dosage. Evidence for correlation between plasma concentrations and therapeutic response is mainly negative.	1. HPLC—System HF. 2. GC—S. Dawling and R. A. Braithwaite, *J. Chromat.*, 1978, *146*; *Biomed. Appl.*, 3, 449–456. 3. Radioimmunoassay— G. Mould *et al.*, *Ann. clin. Biochem.*, 1978, *15*, 221–225.	Steady-state, 0.1–0.2 µg/ml	±
Carbamazepine	Retrospective studies suggest linear correlation between sum of plasma carbamazepine and carbamazepine-10,11-epoxide and therapeutic effect.	1. Homogeneous immunoassay* 2. HPLC—J. A. Christofides and D. E. Fry, *Clin. Chem.*, 1980, *26*, 499–501.	Steady-state, 4–12 µg/ml	+ +
Chlorpromazine	Poor response to treatment may be due to impaired absorption, rapid degradation, or insensitivity to the drug. Plasma concentrations can not be predicted from dose.	1. HPLC—J. K. Cooper *et al.*, *J. pharm. Sci.*, 1983, *72*, 1259–1262. 2. GC—D. N. Bailey and J. J. Guba, *Clin. Chem.*, 1979, *25*, 1211–1215. 3. Radioimmunoassay—K. K. Midha *et al.*, *Clin. Chem.*, 1979, *25*, 166–168.	Considerable variation	±
Clonazepam	Correlation between plasma concentration and clinical efficacy not established. Effectiveness decreases with time despite constancy of plasma concentration.	1. HPLC—W. Shaw *et al.*, *J. analyt. Toxicol.*, 1983, 7, 119–122. 2. GC—A. G. de Boer *et al.*, *J. Chromat.*, 1978, *145*; *Biomed. Appl.*, 2, 105–114.	Steady-state, 0.02–0.07 µg/ml	±

† Further methods may be found in individual monographs in Part 2
* Commercial kits are available
‡ Key to the clinical value of therapeutic monitoring
   + + + Well-proved value
   + +   Proved value
   ±   No proved value

Drug	Comments	Suggested assay methods†	Plasma concentrations associated with optimum therapeutic response	Clinical value of therapeutic drug monitoring‡
Diazepam	A well-defined therapeutic range has not been established; development of tolerance to side-effects is common.	1. HPLC—V. A. Raisys et al., J. Chromat., 1980, 183; Biomed. Appl., 9, 441–448. 2. GC—J. L. Valentine, Analyt. Lett. (Part B), 1982, 15, 1665–1683.	Steady-state, 0.1–2.5 µg/ml	±
Digitoxin	Symptoms of overtreatment may be difficult to distinguish from those of undertreatment unless plasma concentrations are measured. No evidence that clinical response is improved by adjusting plasma concentration to optimum therapeutic range in the absence of symptoms.	Radioimmunoassay*	Steady-state, 0.01–0.03 µg/ml	+ + +
Digoxin	As for digitoxin. Low plasma-potassium increases digoxin toxicity which may occur at therapeutic concentrations.	Immunoassay*	Steady-state, 0.001–0.0025 µg/ml	+ + +
Disopyramide	Retrospective studies suggest that plasma concentrations may correlate with clinical effect, but the evidence is weak.	1. Homogeneous immunoassay* 2. HPLC—C. Charette et al., J. Chromat., 1983, 274; Biomed. Appl., 25, 219–230.	Steady-state, 2–5 µg/ml	+ +
Ethosuximide	Retrospective studies and prospective studies reveal good correlation between plasma concentration and therapeutic response. Main use of monitoring is in patients who have failed to respond to conventional doses without side-effects.	1. Homogeneous immunoassay* 2. HPLC—as for Carbamazepine. 3. GC—Supelco Inc. Bull. 779, 1979.	Steady-state, 40–100 µg/ml	+ + +
Gentamicin	Plasma concentration must exceed the minimum inhibitory concentration but cannot be accurately predicted from the dose. Toxic effects of overdose are serious. Retrospective studies suggest that toxic effects correlate better with high trough than with high peak concentrations.	1. Homogeneous immunoassay* 2. HPLC, Bioassay—as for Amikacin.	Peak, 4–12 µg/ml Trough, <2 µg/ml	+ + +
Imipramine	Plasma concentrations correlate positively with clinical improvement but cannot be predicted from dose because of large genetic differences in metabolism.	HPLC, GC—as for Amitriptyline.	Variable, >0.1 µg/ml (imipramine + desipramine)	+ +
Kanamycin	As for Amikacin	1. Radioimmunoassay* 2. Bioassay—as for Amikacin.	Peak, 20–25 µg/ml Trough, 4–6 µg/ml	+ + +
Lignocaine	Retrospective studies suggest that toxic effects are common at plasma concentrations over 6 µg/ml. Concentrations below 2 µg/ml may be ineffective. Concentrations can not be predicted from dose.	1. Homogeneous immunoassay* 2. HPLC—R. Lindberg et al., Clin. Chem., 1983, 29, 1572–1573.	2–5 µg/ml	+ +

Drug	Comments	Suggested assay methods†	Plasma concentrations associated with optimum therapeutic response	Clinical value of therapeutic drug monitoring‡
Lithium	Extensive retrospective and prospective studies have confirmed the value of regulating lithium dosage to maintain plasma concentrations within narrow and well-defined limits. Relapses are common at high plasma concentrations.	1. Emission flame photometry—A. L. Levi and E. M. Katz, *Clin. Chem.*, 1970, *16*, 840–842. 2. Emission flame photometry—R. Robertson *et al.*, *Clinica chim. Acta*, 1973, *45*, 25–31.	0.5–1.2 mmol/litre, 12 hours after the last dose	+ + +
Methotrexate	If high plasma concentrations are maintained for more than 24–48 hours, irreversible bone marrow failure may occur. Toxicity from high blood concentrations can be prevented by administration of antidote (folinic acid) any time before 48 hours after injection.	1. Homogeneous immunoassay* 2. HPLC—G. J. Lawson *et al.*, *J. Chromat.*, 1981, *223*; *Biomed. Appl.*, *12*, 225–231. 3. Radioimmunoassay—G. W. Aherne *et al.*, *Br. J. Cancer*, 1977, *36*, 608–617.	Toxic effects common when concentration > 4.5 µg/ml at 24 hours or > 0.45 µg/ml at 48 hours after injection; folinic acid rescue is indicated.	+ + (acute studies)
Nortriptyline	Large genetic differences in the rate of metabolism preclude reliable estimation of steady-state concentrations from dose. Good, but not undisputed evidence, that high as well as low concentrations are associated with failure to respond. Therapeutic response shows a curvilinear relationship to plasma concentration.	HPLC, GC, Radioimmunoassay—as for Amitriptyline.	Steady-state, 0.05–0.15 µg/ml	+ +
Phenobarbitone	Plasma concentrations relate to dosage but not to therapeutic response.	1. Homogeneous immunoassay* 2. HPLC—as for Carbamazepine. 3. GC—as for Ethosuximide.	Steady-state, 2–30 µg/ml	±
Phenytoin	Retrospective and prospective studies reveal a much better correlation between therapeutic response and plasma concentration than with the dose.	1. Homogeneous immunoassay* 2. HPLC—as for Carbamazepine. 3. GC—as for Ethosuximide.	Steady-state, 10–20 µg/ml	+ + +
Primidone	Metabolised to phenobarbitone and relative plasma concentrations of the two substances change rapidly due to the difference in half-lives. There is no evidence that monitoring the plasma concentration can improve therapeutic response.	1. HPLC—as for Carbamazepine. 2. GC—as for Ethosuximide.	Steady-state, 5–12 µg/ml	±
Procainamide	About 40% of a dose is metabolised to acecainide which accumulates in the blood. Retrospective and prospective studies reveal that therapeutic response correlates better with the plasma concentration of procainamide or of acecainide, than with the dose.	1. Homogeneous immunoassay* 2. HPLC—K. Carr *et al.*, *J. Chromat.*, 1976, *129*, 363–369.	Steady-state, 4–10 µg/ml	+ + +

Drug	Comments	Suggested assay methods†	Plasma concentrations associated with optimum therapeutic response	Clinical value of therapeutic drug monitoring‡
Propranolol	No good evidence that monitoring the plasma concentration improves therapeutic management. Measurement may be used in test for bioavailability when investigating failure to respond.	1. HPLC—R. L. Nation *et al.*, *J. Chromat.*, 1978, *145*; *Biomed. Appl.*, *2*, 429–436. 2. GC—R. E. Kates and C. L. Jones, *J. pharm. Sci.*, 1977, *66*, 1490–1492. 3. Radioimmunoassay— G. P. Mould *et al.*, *Biopharm. Drug Disp.*, 1981, *2*, 49–57.	Steady-state, 0.05–1 μg/ml (variable)	±
Theophylline	Retrospective and prospective studies suggest that improved therapeutic effect is achieved by dose adjustment to achieve optimum plasma concentration rather than by adjustments made according to symptoms.	1. Homogeneous immunoassay* 2. HPLC—S. J. Soldin and J. G. Hill, *Clin. Biochem.*, 1977, *10*, 74–77. 3. GC—H. A. Schwertner, *Clin. Chem.*, 1979, *25*, 212–214.	Steady-state 10–15 μg/ml Toxicity is common above 30 μg/ml	+ + +
Tobramycin	As for Amikacin	1. Homogeneous immunoassay* 2. HPLC, Bioassay—as for Amikacin.	Peak, 4–10 μg/ml Trough, <2 μg/ml	+ + +
Valproic acid	No clear evidence of correlation between plasma concentration and therapeutic response.	1. Homogeneous immunoassay* 2. GC—as for Ethosuximide.	40–100 μg/ml	±

Samples and Sampling

P. A. Toseland

The selection of the correct samples for analysis and their preservation are prerequisites in the investigation of poisoning. Detailed instructions should be given to those who provide the samples so that the integrity of the sample is constantly maintained. The correct labelling of the samples and their transport and storage should all be part of these instructions to ensure that the analyst obtains the right samples in the right condition before he starts his analysis. An appreciation of how drugs may decompose and how contaminants may be introduced is also important, and all these factors are introduced below together with examples of drugs which pose special problems.

COLLECTION

The tissue samples taken for analysis should always be chosen bearing in mind the availability of particular samples and the disposition of the drug or poison concerned. Blood and urine samples are the most usual in clinical cases and to detect doping in athletes; in fatal cases, the pathologist can choose any sample although urine and stomach contents may not always be available. It is essential that all samples are adequately labelled and preserved before being transported to the laboratory, and that as much information as possible surrounding the case is sent to the analyst before he starts his analysis. Labels should include the person's name, the sample identity, the date and time it was taken, etc. Questionnaires of the type used in forensic science laboratories (see p. 39) are ideal and will ensure that analyses are efficiently carried out on the right samples for the right drugs. Any other information, e.g. pathologist's autopsy report or warnings of a hepatitis carrier should also be sent to the laboratory.

The samples most often used are: stomach contents, blood, urine, liver, bile, brain, and kidneys. The requirements for each tissue are given below.

Stomach Contents

The stomach contents (all, however small), stomach washings, vomit, and vomit on clothing should always be submitted. If only a part of the total stomach washings is sent, then a note of the original total volume should be made. Each sample should be packaged separately, preferably in 1-litre plastic buckets.

These samples are essential for use in general screening procedures. Whole capsules or tablets are often present and can be easily recognised. Moreover, the stomach will normally contain the highest concentration of the drug after an oral dose.

A negative result in the screening procedure may indicate that the drug was not taken orally, but it may have been injected. In some cases of smuggling, drugs may be hidden in flexible packages in the rectum of individuals or swallowed. However, if the packaging is damaged, the drug may escape and be absorbed, which can lead to fatal consequences. Conversely, some basic drugs can be secreted into the gastric juices from the blood after an injection so that the detection of a low concentration of such a drug in the stomach contents does not necessarily mean that the drug was taken by mouth.

Blood

This is the most useful sample for identifying drugs and for quantitative analyses. Drug and metabolite concentrations in blood are most useful for the interpretation of the toxicological significance of the data by comparison with previously reported blood concentrations corresponding to therapeutic, toxic, and fatal conditions (see p. 294).

Two samples of blood are needed as a minimum requirement in postmortem cases. One sample is of at least 30 ml, unpreserved, from an identified source in the body, e.g. femoral vein. Fluid scooped from a body cavity must not be used instead. The second sample is 2 to 5 ml preserved with at least 1% of sodium fluoride, and is primarily for alcohol analysis. Blood samples should be thoroughly mixed with the preservative to ensure that it has all dissolved—a quick shake will not do.

The addition of preservative will not ensure a valid measurement of the original alcohol concentration, but it prevents degradation from proceeding further. Thus, the concentration found must be regarded as a minimum.

Samples of free-flowing blood should always be taken, i.e. without the application of a great deal of pressure, or tissue fluid will also be collected which may have a very different drug concentration from that in blood. For example, in a death due to a suspected drug overdose, a sample of free-flowing blood was collected from a femoral vein and found to contain 1.4 µg/ml of amitriptyline and 0.3 µg/ml of nortriptyline (the major metabolite of amitriptyline). However, a second postmortem examination was made later when blood was taken from the same site as the first sample, but with the application of a great deal of pressure in order to obtain sufficient sample. The analysis of this sample gave blood concentrations of 2.4 µg/ml of amitriptyline and 1.1 µg/ml of nortriptyline and all these results were later confirmed by a second laboratory using different assay techniques. Although the relatively high blood concentrations of both drugs and the high amitriptyline:nortriptyline ratio in both blood samples indicated an acute amitriptyline overdose, the differences between the samples shows how the inclusion of tissue fluids in a sample thought only to be blood can cause problems. This effect will always be seen with drugs that are bound to tissues rather than to the proteins in blood.

Blood is a good sample to use in cases of poisoning by gases or volatile compounds provided that it is stored in an airtight container. In a case of fatal nitrous oxide poisoning, the presence of the gas could be demonstrated by head-space gas chromatography even after storage for several weeks at 4°. This is in contrast to the whole lung sample which was stored in several layers of polythene, yet analysis failed to reveal any trace of the nitrous oxide. The use of containers made of a material impervious to the passage of gases is an obvious necessity; in this respect glass containers are best, provided that they have adequate seals (e.g. a PTFE liner).

DISTRIBUTION OF DRUGS IN THE BLOOD

Plasma or serum samples are usually used in clinical analysis because these samples contain fewer interfering substances than whole blood. The vast majority of therapeutic concentrations of drugs reported in the literature are given for either plasma or serum for this reason. However, drugs are usually distributed between erythrocytes and plasma, the ratio varying according to the drug. For this reason, plasma should be separated from the erythrocytes

as soon as possible after the anticoagulant has been added to ensure that haemolysis of the erythrocytes does not interfere with the analysis. For example, the concentration of chlorthalidone in erythrocytes is about 40 times that in the plasma, and even 1% of haemolysis (which cannot easily be seen) will increase the apparent plasma concentration by 25%.

The plasma:erythrocyte ratio can be altered by contaminants in the blood sample. For example, samples collected in an old type of Vacutainer tube leached the plasticiser tris(2-butoxyethyl) phosphate from the rubber. This plasticiser has the ability to displace basic drugs from their binding sites on α_1-acid glycoprotein, which may result in their redistribution into the erythrocytes, depending on the ability of the drug to bind with erythrocytes.

Another feature of the plasma:erythrocyte ratio is the time taken to reach equilibrium. For some drugs, changes in equilibrium may be very quick (a matter of seconds), but for others it may take hours. If terbutaline is added to a sample of whole blood, the free:bound fractions in plasma take seconds to come to equilibrium, but to achieve equilibrium between plasma and erythrocytes can take 8 hours mixing at room temperature. This is an important consideration when spiking blood samples for use as standards which may later have the plasma separated.

The handling of samples of plasma where the free:bound ratio is to be determined is particularly important. With drugs that are highly bound, e.g. phenytoin, 10% higher plasma concentrations can be observed if the sample of blood is equilibrated and centrifuged at 4° rather than at 20°. This is due to the increased binding capacity of plasma proteins at lower temperatures, whilst the binding by the erythrocytes is hardly affected by changes in temperature.

Much of the above also applies to the production of serum samples from whole blood. This should be carried out as quickly as possible in order to prevent any effects due to the lysis of the blood clot.

Whole blood is the sample of choice when trying to detect the presence of a drug in the blood. This ensures that drugs that are concentrated in the erythrocytes or bound to proteins are present in the sample to be analysed. Samples from postmortem examinations are often haemolysed and putrefied, but are the only samples that can be obtained. However, postmortem blood does sometimes separate on standing, and any portion of the sample taken from near the surface may be rich in plasma. The samples should, therefore, be thoroughly mixed to form a homogeneous mixture before a portion is taken for analysis. Ultrasonication for 15 to 30 seconds can be used to disrupt clots of blood when necessary.

Urine

All the available urine should be taken and preserved with sodium fluoride or sodium azide. Phenylmercuric nitrate should not be used because it interferes in immunoassays and in some gas chromatographic methods. The great advantages of using urine are that the concentration of a drug may be about 100 times that in the blood, and that it is free from protein with a consequent low background of interference. Urine has the disadvantage that some drugs are excreted almost entirely as metabolites by this route, e.g. Δ^9-tetrahydrocannabinol and most of the benzodiazepines, so that proving the presence of a particular drug will require the analysis of another fluid or tissue. Also, if death takes place quickly, e.g. from an injected narcotic analgesic or from the inhalation of hydrogen cyanide, then little or none of the drug reaches the urine.

In spite of these disadvantages, urine is still the sample of choice for the detection of doping in athletes because it is easily obtained in reasonably large quantities, and generally contains detectable concentrations of drugs that are given in therapeutic doses.

Liver

Drugs tend to be present in higher concentrations in the liver than in the blood and this, linked with its large size, makes it a very useful sample in postmortem examinations. Liver has been the most important sample for detecting drugs in forensic toxicology cases for the above reasons, but its use is now declining because of the improved sensitivity of the analytical methods used. However, it is particularly useful in cases involving decomposed or exhumed bodies where blood samples are difficult to obtain. A 250-g sample in a 500-ml plastic container is usually sufficient for most purposes. It is essential that the gall bladder is tied off before the sample is taken so that the liver is not contaminated with bile.

Bile

The gall bladder should be tied off and submitted as a separate item. Bile is particularly useful in deaths due to morphine-like compounds because it has such a high concentration of the glucuronides of these drugs.

Brain

This is particularly useful when investigating deaths due to solvent abuse, e.g. toluene or chloroform, because of the high concentrations that these substances attain in the brain and because they are retained after death. This is also true of poisonings due to cyanide. Because the brain is resistant to postmortem putrefaction, samples are very useful for drug analysis when the body has not been found for some days after death.

Lung

Samples of lung are useful where the method of administration of the drug is by inhalation. This is true whether it is a gas such as nitrous oxide, a volatile material such as a solvent (e.g. toluene), or a powder (e.g. cocaine).

Kidney

If heavy metal poisoning is suspected, the kidneys often show histological damage due to the metal, and also the metals causing the damage tend to concentrate in the kidneys. If the metal poisoning is suspected of being a chronic condition, then samples of the hair (with intact roots) and bone should also be submitted to the laboratory.

Injection Sites

If the route of administration is suspected to be intramuscular injection, e.g. in insulin overdose, a 10-cm cube of muscle from the injection site should be taken as well as a control sample of the same size from a similar but uninjected part of the body. Smaller samples should be taken if the injection site is nearer the surface, e.g. as in subcutaneous injections.

Other Tissues

Where a body is severely decomposed, the actual concentration of a drug at the time of death may be difficult to ascertain because of its decomposition by chemical or biological means. In these cases, samples of cerebrospinal fluid and vitreous humour may aid the analyst because these fluids do not have direct blood supplies associated with them and are therefore free from enzymes and the likelihood of microbial contamination.

Although the above gives an outline of what is required, there should always be close liaison between those providing the samples and the analyst. The standing rule for pathologists and clinicians when sending samples must be 'if in doubt, contact the laboratory'.

Containers

Disposable containers should be used whenever possible to reduce the possibility of contamination. Liquid samples (blood, urine, and bile) are best placed in glass containers which are sealed with a liner that is impervious to the sample (e.g. a PTFE liner). Liners made of rubber and similar materials should be avoided since they may absorb drugs or contribute contaminants (e.g. plasticisers) to the sample. Glass may need to be silanised when low concentrations (<10 ng/ml) of drugs are present to avoid adsorption onto the walls.

Plastic containers are useful for solid samples (e.g. liver), since the drug will not come into contact with the walls of the container. The container size should be chosen for each sample such that the container is full, so that loss of volatile components or oxidation of the drug by atmospheric oxygen is reduced to a minimum. Lids should always be airtight and the container must be fully labelled. Each container should be placed in a polythene bag which is then sealed for further security.

When all the samples from one individual are ready, they are best packed in a cardboard box for the protection of the containers, and then placed in a polythene bag to ensure that the box does not get wet during transit to the laboratory. Relevant hazard warning labels should always be placed on the bag. At no time during the sampling procedure should there be any eating, drinking, or smoking.

STORAGE

A drug which is present in a biological sample may decompose during storage and may not be detected when the sample is analysed. In clinical situations, the drug being taken is known and if the drug is not detected it is normally assumed that the drug is not being taken or that it has decomposed. However, the situation is less straightforward in cases where the identity of the drug is not known, or if it is not certain whether a drug was present in the first place.

Examples of drugs which have been found to decompose during the storage of samples of blood or liver at $4°$ are clonazepam, cocaine, isoniazid, lysergide, methadone, methylphenidate, morphine,

nitrazepam, paracetamol, procaine, and triazolam. A sample containing cyanide was found to contain much lower concentrations after storage at $-16°$. In all these cases, the drug was known to have been taken or was measured in fresh portmortem samples. At therapeutic blood concentrations, nitrazepam appears to decompose in samples at a rate of approximately 6% per day at ambient temperature. Other benzodiazepines do not appear to be as unstable. Both nitrazepam and clonazepam appear to be more unstable in blood than in aqueous solution, indicating that the decomposition is enzymatic rather than chemical. The decomposition may be reduced by adding 1% sodium fluoride to the sample. The instability of isoniazid in blood is not surprising in view of its structural similarity to endogenous compounds such as nicotinamide. Factors that must be considered in order to reduce chemical decomposition and putrefaction processes in stored samples are discussed below.

LIGHT

Drugs such as ergot alkaloids and the phenothiazines are photolabile. When present in a solid such as a sample of liver, or in an opaque medium such as blood, the degree of decomposition is reduced. Nevertheless, samples should always be stored protected from light, and the analysis should be carried out away from bright sunlight. Samples of urine and of aqueous standards should be treated with special care, and the containers should preferably be covered with aluminium foil during analysis. For drugs which are extremely photolabile (e.g. lysergide) the analyses are best carried out in a photographic dark room.

OXIDATION

When drugs are known to be easily oxidised, e.g. catecholamines such as adrenaline, all containers should be full and tightly sealed to exclude atmospheric oxygen. In addition, antoxidants such as ascorbic acid or sodium metabisulphite (1% w/v) can be used to remove oxygen from solution. However, these reducing agents can reduce N-oxide metabolites in urine back to the parent amines, e.g. in phenothiazines, thioxanthenes, tricyclic antidepressants, and some antihistamines. Drugs which are phenolic (e.g. paracetamol and morphine) are easily oxidised at $4°$. Drugs containing sulphur groups can be oxidised *in vitro* in alkaline solution. Thus, thiopentone can be converted to pentobarbitone whilst it is being back-extracted from an organic solvent into an aqueous alkaline medium. In addition, thiopentone can be oxidised on standing at room temperature in organic or aqueous solution.

Ion concentration is important in oxidative processes because the metal ions can act as catalysts. The effects of ions in urine can be reduced by the addition of a protein such as bovine serum albumin. Solutions of some labile drugs are more stable in plasma than the same concentration in water.

The decomposition of chlorambucil in urine increases with the concentration of chloride ion.

HYDROLYSIS

Every toxicologist who has had to deal with a case of suspected cocaine administration is well aware of the problems associated with esterase activity. The measurement of cocaine in blood by gas chromatography using alkali flame ionisation detection is a relatively simple exercise if the analysis is made shortly after the suspected consumption of cocaine. However, searching for the compound as an unknown is an entirely different proposition. The esterase activity in blood is high and cocaine is soon hydrolysed via the ester grouping. Similarly, any attempt to extract cocaine from an alkaline solution with a pH greater than 8 will have the same effect.

Many compounds other than local anaesthetics are also esters and can be hydrolysed by storage of the sample at room temperature or during an extraction procedure. Methylphenidate is a compound with similar characteristics as is the narcotic diphenoxylate which is hydrolysed to diphenoxylic acid (a compound with potency equal to the parent). The use of a high concentration of sodium fluoride (at least 1%) is recommended to counteract this esterase activity. The hydrolysis of esters may also be slowed by reducing the pH of the sample to below 4. Two further examples of esters are diamorphine and aspirin. Diamorphine is seldom detected in blood as it is rapidly hydrolysed to 6-monoacetylmorphine and morphine; the monoacetyl derivative is also rarely detected. Similarly, aspirin is rapidly deacetylated in the stomach to salicylic acid. By contrast, drugs such as the sulphonamides and procainamide are metabolised in the liver by acetylation. These amide drugs, although subject to hydrolysis, are not decomposed as easily in blood as are esters.

TEMPERATURE

It is often assumed that the freezing of biological samples is the ideal method for the preservation of drugs. This may be so for many compounds, but there are some notable exceptions, particularly easily oxidised compounds, such as phenothiazines. For example, if plasma containing chlorpromazine is frozen, stored at $-20°$ and thawed, the compound is recovered intact. However, if the same process is applied to a blood sample obtained from a case of chlorpromazine ingestion, then the actual plasma concentration of the parent drug is doubled during the freezing and thawing cycle due to the reduction of sulphoxide and N-oxide metabolites back to the parent compound. Similarly, measurement of the drug after 18 days storage at $4°$ also reveals an increase in the plasma-chlorpromazine concentration.

In general, it is best to store samples that will be analysed within a few days at $4°$. Those that are to be stored longer should be stored at $-20°$, but only thawed once before analysis. For very long-term storage, freeze-drying should be considered, especially for samples that are used for standard solutions or quality assurance standards.

Biological Decomposition

The hydrolysis of esters by esterases in the blood has been considered above, but even more important is the process of putrefaction caused by micro-organisms. Not only will drugs be destroyed by the activity of these micro-organisms, but compounds such as alcohol, hydrogen sulphide, and hydrogen cyanide can be produced, thus confusing the interpretation of analytical results.

It may be necessary to differentiate between antemortem and postmortem production of alcohol in a decomposed body. Little information can be obtained from the analysis of only a single sample of blood. Samples should be taken from several different sites, as well as from the right and left chambers of the heart. These samples should each be divided into two parts, one portion being stored without a preservative and the other preserved with 1% sodium fluoride. If the unpreserved and preserved samples contain different concentrations of alcohol, this is due to the continued destruction or production of alcohol by micro-organisms in the blood. If the results of the analyses are the same, then the decomposition or production of alcohol has either not occurred or has ceased.

Foodstuffs in the stomach of a corpse can ferment and produce alcohol, and this alcohol can diffuse into the tissues close to the gastro-intestinal tract. The overwhelming odour of fermentation on opening the stomach can lead to the assumption that large amounts of alcohol were consumed before death, but this is a most unreliable indication of the quantity of alcohol consumed.

Low concentrations of alcohol can be found after death if ethyl acetate has been inhaled, because ethyl acetate is rapidly broken down by the body esterases to produce alcohol and acetic acid.

It is unfortunate that standard forensic pathology textbooks still speak of the fact that glucose is converted to alcohol after death. In reality the glucose content of an unpreserved sample of blood disappears within a few hours, whereas alcohol production after death requires a minimum of several days and some bacterial presence. Samples of blood for the determination of glucose should not be stored in the normal hospital containers for blood glucose as they only provide a final concentration of 0.1% sodium fluoride in a full tube. The use of 1% is recommended as a universal preservative.

Cyanide can cause poisoning by mouth or by inhalation. It is lost from the blood very quickly on storage so that a low concentration in blood which is a few days old and from a fatal case of poisoning is difficult to interpret. For example, a case of near-fatal overdosage gave a cyanide concentration of 1.4 µg/ml in blood 2 days after the ingestion of the dose, whereas a heavy smoker had a blood-cyanide concentration of 1.6 µg/ml, and a patient receiving a high therapeutic dose of sodium nitroprusside had a concentration of 6.8 µg/ml, the latter two samples having been analysed without delay. The best sample for the analysis of cyanide from a body which has decomposed is a sample from the middle of the brain. Oral cyanide poisoning may be diagnosed by the presence of milligram amounts of cyanide in the stomach, which differentiates it from cyanide formed on smoking or from sodium nitroprusside given by injection.

Preservatives

Reference has already been made to the preservation of biological samples during storage. However, it is worth repeating that the ideal preservatives are either sodium azide (0.1% w/v) or sodium fluoride (1% w/v) with the possible inclusion of potassium oxalate (0.5% w/v) if an anticoagulant is required. Unpreserved blood samples will always be required if investigations into cases of azide, fluoride, or oxalate poisoning are made. In addition, a sample without oxalate is required to investigate delayed deaths due to ethylene glycol poisoning.

Embalming fluids are very good preservatives of dead bodies, but cause considerable interference with analyses other than those for metals and anions. Samples should therefore be taken from the body prior to the embalming process and preserved separately.

CONTAMINANTS

Contamination can arise from compounds produced during the putrefaction of tissues as well as from the containers themselves. The former can be reduced by correct preservation and storage conditions whilst the latter can be reduced by the correct choice of container. Also to be considered are contaminants present in the drugs themselves, since they are not usually 100% pure.

Interferences Caused by Putrefaction

The classic case is phenethylamine produced in a sample that has been inadequately preserved and stored. This compound always gives a very weak (dirty brown) iodoplatinate reaction on a thin-layer chromatographic plate and should be immediately recognisable to most experienced forensic toxicologists. The same poor and indistinct reactions are given in thin-layer chromatography by tyramine and tryptamine which are also produced during the decomposition of tissues.

Contaminants from Containers

Phthalate plasticisers can be leached from plastic containers or from the rubber closures of glass containers as well as deriving from the solvents used for extraction. Their presence in a sample produces an interfering peak on a gas chromatogram when using a flame ionisation or an electron capture detector (see Fig. 1, p. 185). A second container can be used as a control to determine if a peak originated from the container, and a new batch of containers should be checked for the presence of such plasticisers. Interference from phthalate plasticisers can be avoided by using an alkali flame ionisation detector. However, the presence of a trace amount of a volatile phosphate ester produces a large interfering peak with this detector (see Fig. 2, p. 186). These phosphate esters often come from the cap liners of glass containers, and can be removed by using a back-extraction procedure.

Impurities Present in Drugs

Clinical trials and studies of new drugs are usually undertaken with specially purified materials. However, impurities are likely to be present in drugs produced by large-scale manufacture. There is no evidence that such impurities produce an altered clinical response, but they can affect an analysis.

These impurities may be synthetic intermediates, unchanged starting materials, by-products from the reaction process, or decomposition products. In addition, an analyst may be presented with a drug preparation that has been stored at a patient's home for a period well beyond the permitted shelf-life. Some examples of drugs which may contain impurities are given below.

BARBITURATES

Most of the common barbiturates contain a 5-ethyl substituent and some may contain 5,5-diethylbarbituric acid (barbitone) as an impurity. The presence of this compound at a concentration of only 1 to 2% can produce unexpected results. For example, if amylobarbitone containing 1% of barbitone as an impurity caused coma in an overdose complicated by renal failure, the barbitone would form a higher percentage in the blood. This is because amylobarbitone is removed by rapid metabolism in the liver, but barbitone is eliminated more slowly by renal excretion. In the case of coma with renal function being maintained, barbitone would be a major fraction of the barbiturate excreted in the urine; in some cases the concentration has been so high that it has been regarded as a metabolite.

BENZODIAZEPINES

Oxazepam may be present in some pharmaceutical preparations of chlordiazepoxide. Other benzodiazepines may also contain impurities resulting from large-scale manufacture. The differentiation between impurity and drug metabolite is extremely difficult in these cases.

PHENYTOIN

This anticonvulsant has been measured in blood by converting it to benzophenone by permanganate oxidation and then measuring the concentration of the benzophenone. However, benzophenone is also one of the starting materials in the production of phenytoin and its presence has been demonstrated in some preparations. It is therefore important to obtain a sample of the drug thought to have caused the intoxication and analyse it for the presence of the suspected impurities.

PRIMIDONE

Primidone can be manufactured via the intermediate compound phenylethylmalondiamide. This substance is also one of the principal metabolites of primidone in man and, during therapy, it may be present in blood at concentrations comparable to those of primidone.

Toxicologists can often identify an acute overdosage of primidone if the metabolite concentration in the blood is either very small or non-existent because significant metabolism has not occurred. If the drug contained an impurity that was also a metabolite, the analytical data could present a confusing picture because it would not be possible to state whether metabolism had occurred or not.

Bibliography

T. M. Batchelor and H. M. Stevens, Identification Tests for Acidic and Neutral Compounds Extracted from Putrefied Viscera, *J. forens. Sci. Soc.*, 1978, *18*, 209–229.

Blood, Drugs and Other Analytical Challenges, E. Reid (Ed.), Chichester, Ellis Horwood, 1978.

W. E. Cooper *et al.*, *Alcohol, Drugs and Road Traffic*, Cape Town, Juta and Co., 1979.

A. S. Curry, *Poison Detection in Human Organs*, 3rd Edn, Springfield, Illinois, Charles C. Thomas, 1976.

Forensic Toxicology: Proceedings of a Symposium held at the Chemical Defence Establishment, Porton Down, 29–30 June 1972, B. Ballantyne (Ed.), Bristol, John Wright, 1974.

Introduction to Forensic Toxicology, R. H. Cravey and R. C. Baselt (Ed.), Davis, California, Biomedical Publications, 1981.

J. D. Ramsey *et al.*, Gas-liquid Chromatographic Retention Indices of 296 Non-drug Substances on SE-30 or OV-1 Likely to be Encountered in Toxicological Analyses, *J. Chromat.*, 1980, *184*, 185–206.

H. M. Stevens and P. D. Evans, Identification Tests for Bases Formed During the Putrefaction of Visceral Material, *Acta pharmac. tox.*, 1973, *32*, 525–552.

H. M. Stevens, The Stability of Some Drugs and Poisons in Putrefying Human Liver Tissues, *J. forens. Sci. Soc.*, 1984, *24*, 577–589.

Quality Control in Clinical Analysis

D. Burnett and J. Williams

The evaluation of serum-drug concentrations has resulted in a significant improvement in the clinical management of many diseases. This concept of therapeutic drug monitoring has been particularly applied in the field of anticonvulsant, antibiotic, anti-arrhythmic, and antidepressant drugs. It has been reported that 76 to 88% of previously untreated epileptic outpatients could be successfully controlled with a single drug at the appropriate dosage, provided that serum concentrations were regularly monitored. In view of the apparent effectiveness of such an approach, the importance of the accuracy with which the serum determinations are performed becomes self-evident.

When serum-drug concentrations are used as a guide to the adjustment of dosage, the overall impact of an erroneous determination depends on both the patient's actual serum concentration and the therapeutic or optimum range for the drug. Accuracy of measurement within the therapeutic range is perhaps of greatest significance, but it is also important to be able to distinguish clearly between sub-therapeutic, therapeutic, and toxic concentrations. This is important in situations where increasing the dose is likely to induce toxicity; equally, the ability to distinguish between concentrations in the sub-therapeutic range is desirable when monitoring patients on low doses or for evaluating cases of possible non-compliance or enhanced drug metabolism. Quality control is therefore designed to monitor and improve both the precision and accuracy of serum-drug determinations with a view to improving the quality of individual patient care.

There is a certain degree of ambiguity in the terminology which has been used to describe quality control. Because of this ambiguity, some of the more widely used terms are defined below.

The entire procedure of correct patient identification, which includes the collection of the sample from the patient, its analysis, and the return of the data to the requesting physician, is defined by the term *quality assurance*. The long-term continuing assessment of the degree of imprecision of an assay for a particular drug, with the objective of minimising intra-laboratory variation, is defined by the term *internal quality control*.

The terms inter-laboratory quality control, laboratory proficiency testing, or external surveillance surveys are commonly given to the evaluation of the inter-laboratory variation that is expected when the same sample is analysed by a number of laboratories. In view of the substantial time delay that exists between the actual laboratory analysis of the sample and the receipt of the inter-laboratory comparison, there is no immediate opportunity for controlling the method under investigation and for this reason the term *external quality assessment* is more appropriate.

INTERNAL QUALITY CONTROL

Patients' Samples

The repeat analysis of patients' samples is a commonly used method of assessing imprecision between assays. One or more samples from a previous batch are reanalysed in the next batch and the imprecision (standard deviation, s), determined by analysing the difference (d) between pairs using the formula

$$s = \sqrt{(\sum d^2 / 2n)}$$

where n = number of pairs of samples.

A major problem with this approach, which is cheap and simple to operate, is that only two consecutive analytical batches are ever compared, so that the overall between-batch imprecision will be underestimated. In addition, the standard deviation obtained is only an estimate of average imprecision over a wide range of concentrations and is dependent on the range of samples involved, although samples may be grouped in narrow concentration ranges and an average imprecision obtained for each concentration range. Such schemes cannot be recommended for internal quality control on their own as they are insensitive to changes in imprecision and give no indication of the development of systematic errors.

In clinical chemistry, the mean of concentrations of a particular endogenous substance determined each day, e.g. potassium, is sometimes used to assess the development of systematic error. This method, which is applicable to some endogenous substances, cannot be used to control the development of systematic error when the population is variable both in terms of the dose given to individual patients and in the relationship between dose and serum concentration.

If an assay is being used in which it is customary to duplicate the measurement on each sample within the assay (e.g. immunoassay techniques), then precision profiles can be prepared from the duplicate measurements. This is done by calculating the random error for each pair of samples as a coefficient of variation, given by the expression

$$\frac{|x_1 - x_2|}{\frac{1}{2}(x_1 + x_2)} \times 100\%$$

where x_1 and x_2 are the duplicate measurements. The coefficients are then plotted against analyte concentrations.

These profiles can be used to control the day-to-day performance of the assay and also to optimise its design in relation to imprecision at medical decision points relating to underdosage or overdosage of patients.

Pooled Serum

An alternative method to the repeat analysis of individual patient samples is the preparation of a pool of patient sera containing suitable concentrations of the analyte. However, a more practical answer involves the addition of drugs to a drug-free serum of either human or animal origin. The advantage of such an approach is that the operator knows the approximate drug concentration, although a criticism is that such a preparation does not contain drug metabolites which would be present in the clinical situation and which might interfere with the assay. However, the specificity of an assay should have been thoroughly investigated in the developmental stage and it is doubtful whether repeated analysis of a control sample containing an interfering compound would indicate that such interference was occurring unless a target value was available. The major advantage of using a pool system is that the information obtained is cumulative so that indications of change in performance can be obtained relatively quickly even when the number of control specimens per batch is small.

PREPARATION AND USE OF SERUM POOLS

To prepare a quality control pool it is necessary to have a drug-free vehicle and high purity drugs or metabolites. In theory, any desired vehicle can be used, but the literature on this subject deals almost entirely with serum or plasma. Serum pools which contain known concentrations of added drug substance are known as spiked pools. The following comments on the preparation of pooled serum quality control material are also relevant to the preparation of calibration material.

The drug-free material must first be analysed by the relevant analytical technique for which the quality control material is being prepared to ensure that there is no interference from endogenous compounds or contaminants introduced during collection and pooling. For example, serum stored in some plastic containers may become contaminated with a plasticiser which interferes with the assay of phenytoin by gas chromatography.

The weighing operations should be carefully planned to give the desired concentration and, since the drugs are added to the serum as a solution, the solubilities of each drug in ethanol/water mixtures should be investigated. Aqueous solutions are preferable, but it is often necessary to use ethanolic solutions and the solution should then be diluted with water to give a 30% v/v solution of ethanol before addition to serum in order to prevent precipitation of proteins.

The material must be stable for a reasonable length of time and this requirement applies both to the serum and to the drugs or metabolites being measured. Microbial content of the serum can be removed by sterile filtration through membrane filters, and sodium azide can be added provided this does not interfere with the assay. Storage at 4° is desirable because drug-protein binding does not change as it does during freezing or lyophilisation. There is little information in the literature as to the stability of drugs and metabolites under these conditions. Storage at $-20°$ should be suitable for most quality control materials, but some serum components precipitate irreversibly on freezing and thawing. To minimise precipitation due to repeated freezing and thawing, the material should be divided into aliquots before freezing. Lyophilisation has similar disadvantages to freezing, but is the most suitable method for material which has to be distributed between laboratories. Experience indicates that lyophilised serum containing anticonvulsant drugs does not deteriorate when stored for more than 3 years at $-20°$, nor deep-frozen material when stored for one year.

Lyophilised products may be difficult to reconstitute, particularly if stored at room temperature, and storage at 4° is recommended. Thawed or reconstituted lyophilised serum is stable for one to two weeks at 4°.

Quality control materials using serum or urine are commercially available for many drugs which are assayed routinely for therapeutic or toxicological purposes. Such preparations are generally lyophilised and their stability is guaranteed by the manufacturer. The concentration values assigned by the manufacturer should be verified in the user's laboratory before they are used for the construction of control charts.

Ideally, controls should be assayed in duplicate at three concentrations corresponding to below, within, and above the therapeutic range. (Suggested values for some drugs are given in Table 1.)

The advantage of multilevel control is that, if systematic error develops, information may be obtained as to whether the error is proportional to concentration or constant over the assay range. It is also useful to have estimates of imprecision at different concentrations, particularly for methods with non-linear concentration-response relationships.

Table 1. Suggested values for preparing spiked pools

Compound	Low pool	Mid pool	High pool
Amitriptyline	*430 (120)	*650 (180)	*1300 (360)
Carbamazepine	8 (2)	24 (6)	48 (12)
Clonazepam	*90 (25)	*180 (50)	*270 (75)
Desipramine	*560 (150)	*750 (200)	*1500 (400)
Ethosuximide	140 (20)	420 (60)	840 (120)
Imipramine	*550 (155)	*750 (210)	*1500 (420)
Nortriptyline	*190 (50)	*380 (100)	*1520 (400)
Phenobarbitone	20 (5)	60 (15)	180 (45)
Phenytoin	20 (5)	60 (15)	180 (45)
Primidone	15 (3)	45 (9)	90 (18)
Theophylline	55 (10)	82 (15)	165 (30)
Valproic acid	140 (20)	420 (60)	840 (120)

Values are in µmol/litre (approximate µg/ml equivalent) or, when marked with an asterisk, in nmol/litre (approximate ng/ml equivalent)

Unfortunately, quality control of analytical procedures cannot be achieved without increasing the workload, and with batches of less than fifty samples the inclusion of six control samples might be considered excessive. The choice of scheme for smaller batches will depend to a certain extent on the analytical method used. For methods with non-linear concentration-response curves, the inclusion of at least three concentrations is necessary, whereas for methods with linear concentration-response relationships, cutting down to two or even one

concentration might be considered. If single-point calibration is used (for methods with linear calibration curves) it would be wise to run high and low concentrations alternately because a change in the difference between high and low values may be a useful indicator of loss of linearity of the concentration-response relationship.

If only one or two pools are used, it would be sensible to choose concentrations related to medical decision points, i.e. the low and high ends of the appropriate therapeutic range. Whatever the number of pools used, at least one should be analysed in duplicate in each run, as this permits assessment of within- and between-batch imprecision. The control samples should be spread evenly throughout the batch and each should be preceded by a patient sample and not placed in a protected position. Each pool should be large enough to cover at least sixty batches and, preferably, should be a good deal larger as new pools should be overlapped for thirty batches before introduction for quality control purposes. For research projects of short or medium duration the pool(s) should be large enough to last the duration of the project.

Data Collection and Analysis

This section discusses data collection from a multilevel scheme and suggests ways of recording it on a day-to-day basis. In each assay batch, low, mid, and high controls are assayed in duplicate. Fig. 1 shows the form used for data collection using valproic acid as an example with some typical data entered. The results at each level for each drug are designated x_1 and x_2 and the mean of the two results ($\bar{x}$) along with the difference (range) between them (d) can be readily calculated. The target mean ($\bar{x}_T$) for the pool can be established during the overlap period with previous quality control pools and may be calculated from the data in the first twenty to thirty batches together with the target standard deviation (s_T).

If the initial calculation is shown to contain a value more than 3 standard deviations from the mean, the value should be rejected and the mean and standard deviation recalculated. The standard deviation obtained may be used as the target standard deviation (s_T) in preparation of Shewhart charts or a desired standard deviation can be used which might be related to medical need or to a previous period of satisfactory performance. For a practical guide to statistical techniques used in quality control of analytical methods and the

Date of assay	x_1 x_2	Low pool $\bar{x}_T=22.0$ $s_T=2.8\,(2.0)$ $\bar{x}$	d	sI	x_1 x_2	Mid pool $\bar{x}_T=62.0$ $s_T=4.8\,(3.4)$ $\bar{x}$	d	sI	x_1 x_2	High pool $\bar{x}_T=120.0$ $s_T=7.9\,(5.6)$ $\bar{x}$	d	sI
2.4.81	21.1 23.3	22.2	2.2	0.10	63.4 62.9	63.2	0.5	0.35	116.7 118.9	117.8	2.2	−0.39
7.4.81*	25.0 26.0	25.5	1.0	1.75	74.0 74.0	74.0	0	3.53	145.0 154.0	149.5	9.0	5.27
9.4.81	19.1 23.0	21.1	3.9	−0.45	60.4 —	60.4	—	−0.47	119.0 115.5	117.3	3.5	−0.48
14.4.81	24.3 20.6	22.5	3.7	0.25	63.5 60.9	62.2	2.6	0.06	116.3 117.6	117.0	1.3	−0.54
21.4.81	18.4 22.8	20.6	4.4	−0.70	62.6 60.2	61.4	2.4	−0.18	117.8 123.8	120.8	6.0	0.14
23.4.81	21.4 18.6	20.0	2.8	0	64.3 61.3	62.8	3.0	0.24	114.3 120.5	117.4	6.2	−0.46

*Repeated batch

Fig. 1. Form for data collection (duplicate valproate assays), where

$\bar{x}_T$ = target mean
s_T = target standard deviation
　　(value in brackets = $s_T/\sqrt{2}$)
x_1 and x_2 = duplicate assay results (μg/ml)

$\bar{x}$ = mean of x_1 and x_2
d = difference between x_1 and x_2
sI = standard deviation interval = $\dfrac{\bar{x}-\bar{x}_T}{s_T/\sqrt{2}}$

preparation of cusum (cumulative sum) and Shewhart mean and range charts, the reader is referred to the booklet *Quality Control in Clinical Chemistry* (1984).

An example of Shewhart mean and range charts for the three-level pools is given in Fig. 2 for data similar to that shown in Fig. 1. The mean ($\bar{x}$) of the duplicates x_1 and x_2 are plotted on the Shewhart mean chart for each occasion. When plotting the mean of the duplicates the tolerance limits are calculated from the standard error of the mean (SEM), i.e. standard deviation divided by $\sqrt{2}$ when $n=2$. The range chart is less commonly described but is a plot of the differences between replicates (in our case duplicates). It is useful in monitoring the within-batch imprecision of a method, because increasing imprecision may be a first indication of problems in an analytical system. To establish control limits, the range of replicates (d) is measured on 20 to 30 occasions and the mean range calculated. The multiplication factors for control limits for duplicates are 2.45 for the 95% limit and 3.22 for the 99% limit; figures for higher replication are given in *Quality Control in Clinical Chemistry*. A cusum chart for the data in the *high pool* (Fig. 1) is shown in Fig. 3; in this chart, the difference between the target mean and subsequent results is plotted. Small, but definite, changes in slope can imply small trends in the mean value and can act

as a useful early warning system. However, it is not easy with cusum charts to set 'action limits'; they can become unmanageable if the initial mean selected is in error, and when the slope is in excess of 60° it is difficult to see changes in bias. Fig. 3 shows the whole data plotted and the data excluding the value recorded on 7.4.81. Comparison of the two plots shows the major and permanent effect of one aberrant observation on a cusum chart, particularly as reference to Fig. 2 shows that except for the batch on the 7.4.81 the assay was in control throughout the period under consideration.

It is clear that the manual preparation and continual updating of the charts shown in Fig. 2 for a multilevel, multi-analyte quality control system involves a great deal of work. However, it is possible in a multilevel control system to represent all individual values at different levels on one chart which is a variant of the Shewhart mean plot. The difference of an individual value (e.g. x_1) from the target mean ($\bar{x}_T$) is divided by the target standard deviation (s_T) and thus the position of the individual value is represented relative to the target mean in standard deviation intervals (sI), see Fig. 1. The bias of each value, irrespective of its analyte concentration, is therefore represented on the same standard deviation scale. This is very convenient for manual and computer plotting as complex scaling is avoided. Fig. 4 shows an example of this

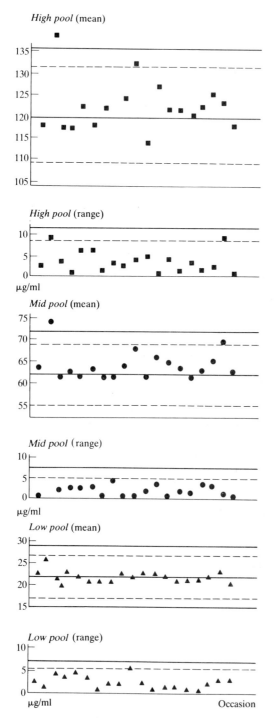

Fig. 2. Shewhart mean and range charts for valproic acid using the data shown in Fig. 1 and similar data from high, mid, and low pools of quality control serum, against occasion of analysis.
----=95% limits   ——=99% limits

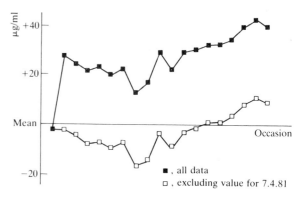

Fig. 3. The cusum chart for valproic acid using the data shown in Fig. 1 and similar data from the high pool of quality control serum, against occasion of analysis.

on the same data as shown in the Shewhart charts of Fig. 2. Care must be taken in interpretation of these charts as bias may change with analyte concentration and these changes are not easily observed by this representation. However, if each level of control is plotted with a different symbol (Fig. 4), interpretation is made easier. If the bias of the mean of the two results (x_1 and x_2) from the target mean is used (as in Fig. 4) then the standard deviation interval must be calculated using the target standard deviation (s_T) divided by $\sqrt{2}$ as described for conventional Shewhart mean charts.

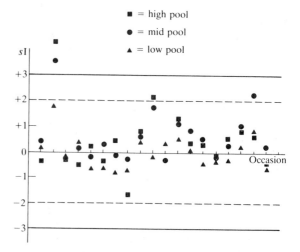

Fig. 4. The mean of paired results for valproic acid (data from Fig. 1) from high, mid, and low pools of quality control serum, plotted in standard deviation intervals against occasion of analysis.

EXTERNAL QUALITY ASSESSMENT

The first external quality assessment scheme for the determination of anticonvulsant drugs was initiated at St. Bartholomew's Hospital, London in 1972 ('BARTSCONTROL') (A. Richens, 1975). Shortly after this, Pippenger set up a similar scheme in New York whereby three pooled sera containing four anticonvulsant drugs were distributed to laboratories in the USA offering a monitoring service (C. E. Pippenger, 1976). The value of regular participation, whereby the participant in the scheme analyses the quality assessment samples and reports the results to the scheme co-ordinator by the appropriate date, is unquestionable. Marked improvement in analytical standards over a period of many months is a consistent finding with many quality assessment schemes.

Inter-laboratory schemes are also organised in The Netherlands by Dijkhuis at the Central Pharmacy, The Hague, and in Scandinavia by Leskinen and Nyberg at Helsinki. These schemes are not restricted to anticonvulsant drugs, recent schemes having been established for other drugs frequently monitored for therapeutic purposes including digoxin, tricyclic antidepressants, lithium, antiarrhythmics, theophylline, and the aminoglycoside antibiotics.

The HEATHCONTROL Scheme

This scheme is a development of the original BARTSCONTROL scheme for external laboratory quality assessment. HEATHCONTROL reference sera are prepared by spiking a homogeneous pool of serum with known amounts of the appropriate drugs. The human serum is prepared from Australia antigen-negative drug-free plasma in the following manner. To 1000 ml of pooled, outdated, blood-bank plasma, 5.55 g (50 mmol) of calcium chloride is added and the pH adjusted to 7.4 with 6M sodium hydroxide. The plasma is incubated at 37° for one hour and the serum allowed to drain by placing the formed clot in a large funnel lined with a fine mesh plastic net. The collected serum is then filtered by passing it under vacuum through a combination of two Carlson-Ford filters, the first being a grade 4 general purpose clarifying sheet with a high output and the second a high purity sterilising grade HP/EK. The filtered serum is then spiked with the appropriate drugs.

Occasionally, serum with a high lipoprotein content becomes cloudy when a lyophilised specimen is reconstituted with water, thus presenting problems for certain enzyme immunoreactive techniques. To overcome this the lipoproteins may be precipitated by adding dextran sulphate 300 mg per litre followed by a 30-minute incubation at 25° and centrifugation prior to the filtration step.

For the antiepileptic scheme, for example, 5-ml aliquots of appropriate spiked serum are withdrawn from the pool and lyophilised. The advantage of lyophilisation is that bacterial growth is impaired thus eliminating the need to add bacteriostatic agents, such as sodium azide, which can interfere with certain immunoassay techniques. During a period of a year, samples spiked with the whole range of drug concentrations are distributed. These samples, for monthly analysis, are posted at three-monthly intervals to the participating laboratories along with the appropriate results forms, which have to be returned to the co-ordinator by a stipulated date. These results are evaluated and a computerised printout of the participant's monthly performance is returned within a month of the results having been received. A typical printout is illustrated in Fig. 5. At the end of the year a summary of the laboratory's performance is supplied, enabling the analyst to evaluate his laboratory's performance over the year and to decide whether any technical change should be implemented.

Analysis and Interpretation of Results

The reports provided to participants in external quality assessment schemes should contain a number of important values. As illustrated in Fig. 5, most schemes include data such as the number of participants accepted in the final analysis, the number rejected, i.e. the outliers, the mean and standard deviation of the accepted results, the spiked value together with the individual participant's value and its standard deviation interval (sI) from the consensus mean. In addition, a computerised frequency distribution histogram is generally provided.

PERFORMANCE INDICES

In an attempt to categorise individual laboratory performance, several schemes have introduced a performance index. The calculation of the performance index varies from one scheme to another. The original BARTSCONTROL performance index was based upon ranking the difference between reported and consensus mean values (without sign). These index values ranged from 1 to 10 with 1 indicating a good performance and constituting the

```
LAB  NO    97

        HEATHCONTROL            SEPTEMBER  1981     *****************************
                                                    OVERALL PERFORMANCE INDEX  7
                                                    *****************************

  SAMPLE:PPC      0981              SAMPLE:PPC      0981             SAMPLE:PPC      0981
  DRUG:PHENYTOIN                    DRUG:PHENOBARBITONE              DRUG:CARBAMAZEPINE
  DRUG   NO.OF                      DRUG   NO.OF                     DRUG   NO.OF
  LEVEL  OBS                        LEVEL  OBS                       LEVEL  OBS

        ***************************       ***************************      ***************************
  36.0   0*                         * 123.0   0*                    *  36.5   0*                      *
  37.0   1*+                        * 127.0   1*+                   *  38.0   0*                      *
  38.0   1*+                        * 131.0   1*+                   *  39.5   2*++                    *
  39.0   0*                         * 135.0   1*+                   *  41.0   0*                      *
  40.0   0*                         * 139.0   0*                    *  42.5   1*+                     *
  41.0   3*+++                      * 143.0   1*+                   *  44.0   2*++                    *
  42.0   2*++                       * 147.0   4*++++                *  45.5   3*++++                  *
  43.0   2*++                       * 151.0   7*+++++++             *  47.0   2*++                    *
  44.0  11*+++++++++++              * 155.0   5*+++++               *  48.5   3*++++                  *
  45.0   4*++++                     * 159.0   3*+++++               *  50.0   2*++                    *
  46.0   5*++++++                   * 163.0  12*++++++++++++        *  51.5   7*++++++++<<<<<<<<<<<<<<<<<<<<*
  47.0   9*+++++++++                * 167.0  11*+++++++++++         *  53.0   9*+++++++++             *
  48.0   7*+++++++                  * 171.0  11*+++++++++++++++     *  54.5  11*+++++++++++           *
  49.0  16*++++++++++++++++         * 175.0   9*+++++++++++         *  56.0  19*+++++++++++++++++++   *
  50.0  18*+++++++++++++++++++      * 179.0  11*+++++++++++         *  57.5  21*+++++++++++++++++++++ *
  51.0  25*+++++++++++++++++++++++++* 183.0  24*++++++++++++++++++++++++* 59.0 24*++++++++++++++++++++++++*
  52.0  14*+++++++++++++            * 187.0  16*++++++++++++++++    *  60.5  12*+++++++++++++         *
  53.0  16*++++++++++++++++         * 191.0  17*+++++++++++++++++   *  62.0  15*++++++++++++++        *
  54.0  12*++++++++++++             * 195.0  11*+++++++++++         *  63.5   8*++++++++              *
  55.0  11*+++++++++++              * 199.0   6*++++++++            *  65.0   8*++++++++              *
  56.0  10*++++++++++               * 203.0   9*+++++++++++         *  66.5   6*++++++                *
  57.0   7*+++++++++                * 207.0   5*+++++++             *  68.0   6*++++++++              *
  58.0   6*+++++++++                * 211.0   5*+++++++             *  69.5   0*                      *
  59.0   3*++++                     * 215.0   6*++++++++            *  71.0   2*++                    *
  60.0   2*++                       * 219.0   1*+                   *  72.5   0*                      *
  61.0   1*+                        * 223.0   2*++                  *  74.0   4*++++++               *
  62.0   2*+++                      * 227.0   0*                    *  75.5   0*                      *
  63.0   1*+                        * 231.0   0*                    *  77.0   3*++++                  *
  64.0   1*+                        * 235.0   0*                    *  78.5   0*                      *
  65.0   0*                         * 239.0   1*+                   *  80.0   0*                      *
        ***************************       ***************************      ***************************

  NUMBER ACCEPTED        190        NUMBER ACCEPTED       188        NUMBER ACCEPTED        170
  NUMBER REJECTED          6        NUMBER REJECTED.        7        NUMBER REJECTED          9
  MEAN                 51.51        MEAN              183.16         MEAN                 59.27
  STANDARD DEVIATION    4.69        STANDARD DEVIATION 18.90        STANDARD DEVIATION    6.69
  COEF. OF VARIATION    9.10%       COEF. OF VARIATION 10.32%       COEF. OF VARIATION   11.28%
  MINIMUM              37.70        MINIMUM           127.50        MINIMUM              40.70
  MAXIMUM              64.00        MAXIMUM           240.00        MAXIMUM              78.30
  MEDIAN               51.50        MEDIAN            183.80        MEDIAN               59.00
  MODE                 51.50        MODE              185.00        MODE                 59.75
  SPIKED VALUE         60.00        SPIKED VALUE      200.80        SPIKED VALUE         61.10
  YOUR VALUE         NO DATA        YOUR VALUE        120.50 REJECTED YOUR VALUE         51.60
                                    NO. SDS FROM MEAN   3.32        NO. SDs FROM MEAN     1.15
                                    ***********************         ***********************
                                    PERFORMANCE INDEX  10           PERFORMANCE INDEX  4
                                    ***********************         ***********************
```

Fig. 5. A typical computerised printout issued on a monthly basis to participants in an external quality assessment scheme; $\langle\langle\langle\langle$ represents the position of the reported value of the individual laboratory in relation to the reported values of other laboratories.

best 10 per cent of participating laboratories. Those with an index of 10 comprised the worst 10 per cent of the participants. However, it is quite possible for a laboratory with a performance index of 10 to be producing clinically satisfactory results. Conversely, if the overall group performance is poor, results could be clinically unacceptable even when the apparent performance index is good. To overcome this limitation, HEATHCONTROL has since re-evaluated the basis for the calculation of its performance index. The index is now calculated by dividing the 3 standard deviation limits either side of the consensus mean, after the elimination of outliers, into 10 zones each of 0.3 standard deviation units in magnitude. Any participant whose reported result falls within ± 0.3 standard deviation units of the consensus mean is awarded a performance index of 1. A participant whose reported result falls within ± 2.8 to 3.0 standard deviation units of the

consensus mean is awarded an index of 10. The categorisation, while still not independent of the performance of the group as a whole, does rank laboratories relative to the overall performance of all participants.

An alternative method for performance index (PI) evaluation has been reported (C. E. Pippenger, 1978) using the formula

$$PI = \frac{\sum_{i=1}^{n} |R_i - S_i|}{\sum_{i=1}^{n} S_i}$$

where R_i represents the reported value for an individual specimen, S_i represents the spiked value for that specimen, and n represents the number of specimens used for the calculation of the index. Based upon experience with performance index patterns, it was stated that a PI of less than 10 was exceptionally good, 10 to 20 satisfactory, and above

20 unacceptable. This interpretation is independent of group performance and, assuming that no systematic error is present, is equivalent to requiring intra-laboratory coefficients of variation of less than 5 per cent for excellent and 5 to 10 per cent for satisfactory performance.

I. E. Dijkhuis (1979) ranked results on the basis of percentage difference from the spiked value into super, excellent, good, moderate, and poor categories. The ratio of deviation within these categories was $1:2:4:8:>8$ and the combined number of results in the super, excellent and good categories was fixed at approximately 70 per cent. This categorisation was therefore dependent on the performance of the group as a whole and consequently subject to the same criticism as the original BARTSCONTROL index.

None of the methods described for the evaluation of the performance index indicate the direction ($+$ or $-$) in which the participant's reported value is different from the mean or spiked value. If this direction were stated and a participant's reported differences were consistently unidirectional, then the recognition of a systematic error would be facilitated.

Further Analysis of Results

If participants in an external quality assessment scheme simply receive the results and check the performance index or some other measure to see if it is satisfactory, a great deal of valuable information is lost. Data from these schemes offer an opportunity to study a laboratory's assay and to assist in the education of laboratory personnel. Simple graphical approaches can be used that do not require complicated calculations. If a laboratory has a computer, more elaborate calculations can be carried out. Basically, the participating laboratory has analysed a sample for a particular analyte and has then to compare the value found with the 'true' value. Possible estimates of the 'true' value include the overall mean for all participants, the method mean, the mean value obtained by designated reference laboratories, or a stated spiked value. Some schemes provide all these values, but the majority provide an overall mean, which will be used in the following discussion. The overall mean has limitations if the technique for elimination of outliers is unsatisfactory or if a particular method, which causes a marked bias at certain concentrations in the overall mean, is used by a significant number of laboratories.

For a day-to-day check on returned results, it is useful to calculate the difference of the value obtained by the participating laboratory (x) from the overall mean value ($\bar{x}$). This is the bias ($x - \bar{x}$); it can either be plotted as such against the date of the sample or divided by the standard deviation of results obtained by all participants (s) to give the standard deviation interval (sI) and then plotted against the sample date.

$$sI = \frac{x - \bar{x}}{s}$$

Fig. 6 is a computer plot of standard deviation interval for phenytoin over two years in one particular laboratory. The method of using bias relative to some measure of imprecision, which was first introduced in discussing internal quality control, is particularly useful if data are to be plotted by computer. It is also useful for manual analysis as a single chart can be prepared with lines at 0 ± 2 and ± 3 sI which can be copied and used for all analytes.

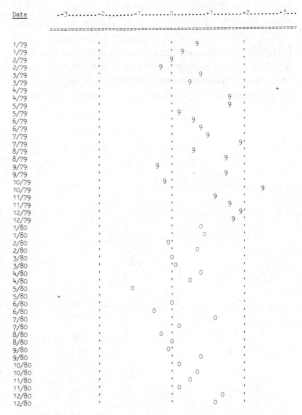

Fig. 6. Standard deviation interval plot for phenytoin. Dotted lines are at 0 and ± 2 standard deviation intervals; '+' marks results outside ± 2.8 standard deviation intervals.

The standard deviation interval approach enables a laboratory to see where its own performance lies in relation to other participants. If a laboratory's performance is equivalent to that of the group (intra-laboratory s = inter-laboratory s) then one would expect a normal distribution about the zero line with nineteen out of twenty points inside ± 2 sI. The limitation of this approach is that it does not analyse bias at different concentrations. If the value obtained by a laboratory is plotted against the overall mean value, this gives a good visual check for linearity of relationship and also an initial indication of the existence of systematic error. Fig. 7 shows data for phenytoin taken from Fig. 6 in which the two years 1979 and 1980 are plotted with different symbols. Fig. 8 shows the same data presented as the bias $(x - \bar{x})$ plotted against the mean $(\bar{x})$. The scale of the y axis can be expanded to show clearly the change in bias with concentration. Fig. 8 confirms that the phenytoin results were biased high relative to the overall mean during 1979, but it is not possible to say whether the difference was constant or additive. There are a number of explanations for this situation; it would occur if, for example, there was a substance interfering with phenytoin in the samples provided in the assessment scheme which did not occur in the material used for calibration of the assay. It is important to realise that, under these circumstances, the assessment scheme could be

indicating that the laboratory was not performing correctly, when in fact the scheme samples were not fully commutable with the routine patient samples. Thus a change may not be called for in the laboratory method, but rather in the samples provided in the assessment scheme. The source of standard for phenytoin was changed at the beginning of 1980 and during that period the performance of the individual laboratory conformed more closely to the overall performance.

Linear regression analysis of the overall mean value against a laboratory's results would be expected to give further information as it provides estimates of slope, intercept, and the standard error of the estimate of bias. These may be used to determine sources of systematic error, proportional (slope), additive (intercept), and random error. However, experience indicates that linear regression analysis is unsuitable for the treatment of such data because the concentration range is limited, the standard error is dependent on the number of laboratories, and analytical precision is not generally constant over the concentration range investigated.

Choice of Method

It would be desirable if scheme co-ordinators could provide newcomers to their particular field with some guidance as to the choice of analytical method, although this has not generally been done. The ability of such schemes to evaluate objectively the suitability of a particular method for a particular drug is unquestionable. Based upon such an evaluation, it has been confirmed that spectrophotometric methods for phenobarbitone, phenytoin,

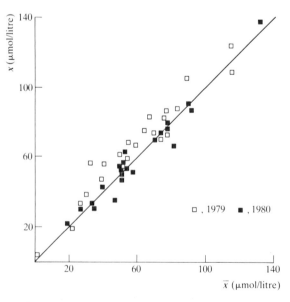

Fig. 7. The value from a participating laboratory (x) plotted against the overall mean value ($\bar{x}$) of data given in Fig. 6.

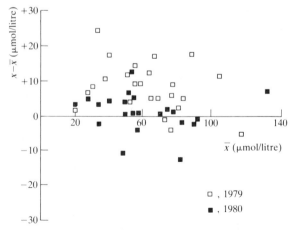

Fig. 8. Bias ($x - \bar{x}$) plotted against the overall mean value ($\bar{x}$) of data given in Fig. 6.

and carbamazepine are totally unsatisfactory. These conclusions were based on the number of outliers obtained and on the large coefficient of variation that persisted even after these outliers were excluded.

If any meaningful recommendations are to be made about the choice of method, then a detailed description of the methods used by each participating laboratory must be examined. At present, method suitability can only be evaluated by grouping laboratories using a particular class of method, e.g. GC, HPLC, etc., and comparing the performance between these groups statistically. Each month, HEATHCONTROL, for example, produces a method analysis for each drug. In time, such method analysis will enable co-ordinators to advise on the suitability of a particular technique although the advice given is rather tentative in view of the extensive variability that exists within any one class of method. Only when these variables are sub-classified and the results re-evaluated can a truly objective suggestion be made as to method suitability.

Bibliography

C. E. Pippenger et al., Antiepileptic Drug Levels Quality Control Program: Interlaboratory Variability, in *Antiepileptic Drugs: Quantitative Analysis and Interpretation*, C. E. Pippenger et al. (Ed.), New York, Raven Press, 1978, pp. 187–197.

C. E. Pippenger et al., Interlaboratory Variability in Determination of Plasma Antiepileptic Drug Concentrations, *Archs Neurol.*, Chicago, 1976, *33*, 351–355.

Quality Control in Clinical Chemistry, Dartford, Kent, Wellcome Diagnostics, 1984.

A. Richens, Results of a Phenytoin Control Scheme, in *Clinical Pharmacology of Antiepileptic Drugs*, H. Schneider et al. (Ed.), Berlin, Springer-Verlag, 1975, pp. 293–303.

Colour Tests

H. M. Stevens

Many substances give distinct colours when brought into contact with various chemical reagents. In some cases, the colour produced with a particular reagent may be specific for the compound under investigation but, more often, the colour reaction is not confined to a single compound but is produced by a number of the compounds in a given class and sometimes by substances not in that class.

The colour tests specified in the monographs are described below. In a number of the tests, the colour responses of drugs are correlated with particular aspects of the drug structures. However, it is not possible to explain the phenomena fully because anomalous responses often occur for no apparent reason. Some anomalous responses are noted in the following tests but these are not necessarily the only ones which may be found. The colour tests included here have been carefully chosen to give a range of tests for particular functional groups (e.g. Folin–Ciocalteu Reagent for phenols), those for groups of drugs (e.g. Forrest Reagent for phenothiazines), and those which have a wide applicability and give useful and diagnostic colours (e.g. Marquis Test).

INTERPRETATION OF COLOUR TESTS

A wide range of colours is produced by reagents in these colour tests and it is not possible to describe the colours with any degree of certainty since any description is open to the vagaries of subjective assessment. Moreover, the colour obtained in any particular test may vary to a greater or lesser extent dependent upon the conditions of the test, the amount of substance present, and the presence of extraneous material in the test sample.

A system has been adopted, therefore, which uses ten basic colours, i.e. the spectral colours red, orange, yellow, green, blue, violet, together with pink, brown, grey, and black. Variations in hue are indicated by combining two colours, e.g. red-brown, the second named colour being considered to be the dominant colour and this is the main colour used in the lists which follow. Hence, red-brown is listed under brown, whereas brown-red is listed under red. When attempting to interpret the result of a test, the lists of colours and drug substances should be consulted and, because of the subjective nature of the assessment of colour, it will often be necessary to search the lists given under two main colours, e.g. for red-brown, the lists under both red and brown should be consulted. An arrow between two colours, e.g. red → brown, indicates that the colour changes during the course of the test. In the monographs, the notation brown/red is used where there are two parts to a test producing two colours. Occasionally, a test solution may display one colour by reflected light and a different colour by transmitted light. Where this occurs, the solution is referred to as being dichroic.

A final decision on the result of a test should be made by comparing the unknown with a reference substance tested under the same conditions.

The colours recorded are usually those obtained with the free acid or base. In the case of a salt, the colour may be modified by the nature of the other radical present. Basic salts of weak acids may give different colours because of the pH change. Hydrochlorides usually give a red colour in Mandelin's Test and a blue colour with Koppanyi–Zwikker reagent (before addition of pyrrolidine). In the case of a compound extracted from biological material no difficulty will arise, as it will be extracted as the base, but care must be taken in applying colour tests directly to pharmaceutical preparations. These may, of course, be converted to the free base. Bromides and iodides can be converted to the nitrate, which gives the same colour as the base, by the following method. To 0.5 ml of a 1% solution of the salt in *dilute acetic acid*, add 1 drop of an 8% solution of silver nitrate followed by 1 drop of a 2% solution of sodium chloride to remove excess silver. Centrifuge in order to separate the precipitated silver halide and use the supernatant liquid, either as a solution or evaporated to dryness where necessary, for the colour tests.

PRACTICAL POINTS

The tests are designed to work on about 1 mg of the solid drug form unless stated otherwise.

When a solution is not stated to be made in a particular solvent it should be made in water. Where an instruction, time, temperature, etc. appears in brackets after the drug name, e.g. (add water), (15 s), or (slowly at 100°), this indicates a change in the test procedure for that particular drug. It is often useful to run a blank test at the same time as the sample test, so that the colours produced by the sample and by the reagent blank may be compared. When more than one drug is present, or the drug itself is coloured, the colour obtained in the test may be a combination of colours. Although the tests are designed as colour tests for use in test-tubes or on white tiles, in many instances they may be used as TLC locating agents, either sprayed or poured on to the plate.

Certain of the tests described here may be carried out by the micro technique (E. G. C. Clarke and M. Williams, *J. Pharm. Pharmac.*, 1955, *7*, 255–262). This applies particularly to Mandelin's Test, Marquis Test, and the Sulphuric Acid test.

Information on the direct application of colour tests to urine, blood, and stomach contents can be found under Hospital Toxicology and Drug Abuse Screening (p. 4).

Where an extraction procedure has been carried out with the production of acidic and basic fractions (see p. 11), the tests below may be applied to the evaporated extracts.

Strong Acid Fraction
Aromaticity
Ferric Chloride
Folin–Ciocalteu Reagent
Liebermann's Test
Millon's Reagent
Nessler's Reagent

Neutral Fraction
Aromaticity
Furfuraldehyde
Koppanyi–Zwikker Test
Liebermann's Test
Mercurous Nitrate
Nessler's Reagent

Weak Acid Fraction
Aromaticity
Coniferyl Alcohol
Diazotisation
Ferric Chloride
Folin–Ciocalteu Reagent
Koppanyi–Zwikker Test
Liebermann's Test
Mercurous Nitrate
Millon's Reagent
Nessler's Reagent

Basic Fraction
Amalic Acid Test
p-Dimethylaminobenz-
    aldehyde
Ferric Chloride
Formaldehyde–Sulphuric
    Acid
Forrest Reagent
FPN Reagent
Liebermann's Test
Mandelin's Test
Marquis Test
Nessler's Reagent
Sulphuric Acid

Tests for inorganic cations and anions will be found in the chapter on Metals and Anions (p. 55).

COLOUR TEST METHODS

Amalic Acid Test

METHOD. Add to the sample a few drops of 10M hydrochloric acid followed by a few crystals of potassium chlorate, and evaporate the mixture to dryness. Observe the colour of the residue and then add 2 or 3 drops of 2M ammonium hydroxide and again observe the colour.

INDICATIONS. A RED, PINK, ORANGE, or YELLOW residue, changing to PINK, RED, or VIOLET after addition of ammonium hydroxide, indicates the presence of a xanthine.

RED (→ violet)	Bufylline
PINK (→ violet)	Oxpentifylline
ORANGE (→ violet)	Acepifylline, bamifylline, caffeine, xanthinol nicotinate
Pink-orange (→ violet)	Fenethylline, pentifylline
YELLOW (→ pink)	Etamiphylline
YELLOW (→ violet)	Diprophylline, proxyphylline, theobromine, theophylline

Ammoniacal Silver Nitrate

REAGENT. To 20 ml of 0.1M silver nitrate add sufficient *strong ammonia solution* to dissolve the initial precipitate.

METHOD. Dissolve the sample in a minimum amount of water, with addition of ethanol if necessary, add an equal volume of the reagent, note any colour which develops, then heat the mixture in a water-bath at 100° for 30 seconds.

INDICATIONS. RED, YELLOW, BROWN, or BLACK colours (especially at room temperature) indicate potent reducing power. This occurs when adjacent carbon atoms in a ring each bear an hydroxyl group. There is no response when the hydroxyl groups are *meta* to each other, but there is some restoration of reducing power when they are *para* to each other. Some colour production is also obtained with ethynyl bonds but not with ethylenic bonds.

Colour at room temperature	Compound	Colour at 100°
RED	Isoetharine	Brown-orange
	Hexoprenaline (→ brown → black)	—
	Isoprenaline (→ red-brown)	Brown
	Rimiterol	Brown
YELLOW	Ethinamate	Brown
	Levodopa (→ brown)	Black
Grey-yellow	Hydroquinone	Brown

Colour at room temperature	Compound	Colour at 100°
BROWN		
Red-brown	Adrenaline	Red-brown
	Methyldopa	Black
Orange-brown	Dopamine	Black
	Methyldopate	Orange-brown
GREY		
Red-grey	Protokylol	Brown
BLACK		
	Ascorbic acid	—
	Benserazide	—
	Dobutamine	—
	Dodecyl gallate	—
	Noradrenaline	—

Ethchlorvynol and ethinyloestradiol both give a white precipitate which turns yellow on heating. Carbidopa gives a silver mirror on heating.

Antimony Pentachloride

REAGENT. Dry some antimony trichloride over phosphorus pentoxide, melt the dried material (m.p. 73°), and pass dry chlorine gas into the melt until a yellow fuming liquid is obtained. Add this liquid to about 10 times its volume of chloroform, filter the solution into a dark glass-stoppered bottle, and store in a desiccator.

METHOD. Place 1 drop of an ethanolic solution of the sample on a filter paper, add 1 drop of the reagent, and dry in a current of warm air. Alternatively, the test may be carried out by adding 1 drop of the reagent to the sample on a white tile.

INDICATIONS. Various colours are obtained with the cardiac glycosides, their aglycones, and certain oestrogens and corticosteroids.

RED	Dienoestrol, stilboestrol
ORANGE	Cholesterol (→ brown), deoxycortone, dydrogesterone, fludrocortisone, hydrocortisone, hydroxyprogesterone, strophanthin-K (→ red)
YELLOW	Alphadolone
(→ brown)	Androsterone, digitoxigenin, digoxigenin
(→ brown → black-violet)	Digitoxin, digoxin, lanatoside C, ouabain (very weak)
Green-yellow	Fluocortolone
GREEN	Betamethasone (→ brown), dexamethasone, mestranol, pancuronium
BROWN	Carbenoxolone, dimethisterone, ethinyl-oestradiol (→ black), fluoxymesterone, norethandrolone, norethisterone, oestradiol, oestriol, oestrone, oxymetholone, rotenone
Orange-brown	Enoxolone (→ violet)
Green-brown	Norethynodrel

No colour is obtained with beclomethasone, cortisone, fluocinolone, flurandrenolone, prednisolone, prednisone, progesterone, testosterone, or triamcinolone.

Aromaticity

METHOD 1. Place a portion of the sample in each of two ignition tubes and to one tube add some solid sodium hydroxide. Heat both tubes carefully, allow water vapour to escape, insert into the vapours in each tube an open capillary tube containing *Marquis reagent*, and observe the colour of the reagent.

INDICATIONS. RED or ORANGE colours indicate that the sample is aromatic in nature. The colours are probably due to the liberation of traces of aromatic hydrocarbons, phenols, etc.

Colours obtained after heating with sodium hydroxide generally indicate the presence of aromatic acids. Colours obtained after heating without sodium hydroxide generally indicate the presence of phenols, phenolic acids, and aldehydes containing more than one hydroxyl group.

A negative result does not necessarily imply that the substance is non-aromatic.

METHOD 2. Add 2 or 3 drops of *nitric acid* to the sample, heat in a water-bath at 100° for 1 minute, cool the mixture, dilute 3 to 4 times with water, and make the solution alkaline by the addition of a 40% solution of sodium hydroxide.

INDICATIONS. A change from COLOURLESS or YELLOW in acid solution to darker colours, e.g. ORANGE or RED-ORANGE, after the addition of sodium hydroxide indicates the presence of a benzene ring in the molecule, probably due to the production of a nitrophenol or other nitro compound.

Certain compounds (e.g. diazepam, methaqualone) give a negative result. ORANGE colours are given by certain non-aromatic corticosteroids (e.g. cortisone), by substances containing sulphur, and by compounds which already contain an aromatic nitro group (e.g. nifursol).

Colourless acid solution changing on addition of alkali to:

RED	Clobazam (heat for 3 min with acid)
ORANGE	Butanilicaine, tolazoline
YELLOW	Amprolium, atropine methobromide, hyoscine butylbromide, hyoscine methobromide, ketoprofen, pipazethate, tetrahydrozoline, tetramisole, trimetaphan
VIOLET	Atropine methonitrate (transient), hyoscine methonitrate (transient)
BROWN	Isopropamide

Yellow acid solution changing on addition of alkali to:

RED	Amethocaine, aminacrine, benzonatate, trimethoprim
Orange-red	Dextromethorphan, haloperidol
ORANGE	Amicarbalide, chromonar, dyclonine, glibenclamide, levallorphan, metocurine, padimate, propanidid, quinuronium, salinazid
BROWN	Dibromopropamidine, dichlorophen, tubocurarine

Dequalinium gives a red solution in acid, changing to brown-violet in alkali.

Note. Certain substances give distinct colours with cold *nitric acid* but the colours fade on heating: RED, aminacrine (15 s), clozapine, dropropizine, medazepam, trimethoprim; BROWN, metocurine; PINK-BROWN, diethylthiambutene, changing to green; BLACK, tubocurarine.

Benedict's Reagent

REAGENT. Dissolve 1.73 g of copper sulphate in 10 ml of water. Dissolve 17.3 g of trisodium citrate and 10 g of anhydrous sodium carbonate in 80 ml of water, with the aid of heat; pour this solution into the copper sulphate solution and dilute the mixture to 100 ml.

METHOD. Add 0.5 ml of the reagent to the sample and heat in a water-bath at 100° for 3 minutes.

INDICATIONS. The formation of RED cuprous oxide occurs with strong reducing agents, e.g. ascorbic acid, dithionites, certain phenolic compounds containing two hydroxyl groups *para* to one another, and compounds containing at least four hydroxyl groups on a non-aromatic ring (e.g. glucose, tetracyclines).

A weak response (ORANGE-BROWN or BROWN colours) is given by streptomycin, hydroxylamine, and substituted hydrazines (e.g. phenelzine). No colour is obtained with beclomethasone, cardiac glycosides, and oestriol (two hydroxyl groups) or clindamycin (three hydroxyl groups).

Carbon Disulphide

METHOD. Mix the sample with 1 ml of water and 0.1 ml of a 1% solution of sodium tetraborate, add 0.2 ml of a 10% v/v solution of carbon disulphide in ethanol, and heat in a water-bath at 100° for 3 minutes; cool the solution and add 3 drops of 0.1M silver nitrate.

INDICATIONS. A BROWN colour indicates the presence of a dithiocarbamate, suggesting that the original substance was an aliphatic or heterocyclic primary or secondary amine. The original sample should be tested to ensure that it does not give a brown colour with silver nitrate alone.

Chromotropic Acid

REAGENT. Dissolve 20 mg of chromotropic acid in 10 ml of *sulphuric acid*.

METHOD. Add a small amount of sample, either solid or in solution, to 1 ml of the reagent. Note any colour which may be produced and then add the solution dropwise to 0.5 ml of water, with cooling. Substances which give a colour with cold *sulphuric acid* must be excluded.

INDICATIONS.

RED (before dilution)	Formaldehyde (paraformaldehyde reacts slowly)
VIOLET (after dilution)	Hydrochlorothiazide, hydroflumethiazide

Coniferyl Alcohol

REAGENT. Warm 0.1 g of coniferyl alcohol until it melts (m.p. 74°), dissolve in 3 ml of ethanol, and dilute to 10 ml with ethanol.

METHOD. Place 1 drop of a solution of the sample on a filter paper, add 1 drop of the reagent, and expose the paper to hydrochloric acid fumes.

INDICATIONS. An ORANGE colour indicates the presence of an aromatic primary amine in which the amino group is attached directly to a benzene ring.

An anomalous reaction is obtained with diphenylamine (bright orange).

Copper Sulphate

METHOD 1. Dissolve the sample in a minimum volume of 0.1M sodium hydroxide and add a 1% solution of copper sulphate, drop by drop, until the colour change is complete.

INDICATIONS. GREEN, BLUE, or BROWN colours indicate the presence of a sulphonamide.

GREEN	Phthalylsulphathiazole, succinylsulphathiazole (→ violet), sulfadoxine, sulfamerazine (→ brown), sulfametopyrazine, sulfaquinoxaline, sulphachlorpyridazine, sulphadimethoxine, sulphadimidine (→ brown), sulphaethidole, sulphamethizole, sulphamethoxazole, sulphapyridine (→ brown-green), sulphasomidine
BLUE	Phthalylsulphacetamide, sulphacetamide, sulphaguanidine, sulphanilamide, sulphaphenazole, sulphaurea, sulphinpyrazone, sulthiame

BROWN	Sulphafurazole
Orange-brown	Sulphasalazine
Green-brown	Sulphamethoxypyridazine, sulphamoxole
Violet-brown	Sulphadiazine, sulphamethoxydiazine, sulphathiazole

METHOD 2. Add 1 or 2 drops of a 1% solution of copper sulphate to the sample on a white tile.
INDICATIONS. A BLUE colour indicates the presence of an alkali salt of a fatty acid, e.g. sodium cromoglycate (1–2 min), sodium valproate. The colours are not produced by a change of pH as negative results are obtained with sodium bicarbonate.

Cyanogen Bromide

REAGENT. (i) Decolorise *bromine solution* by the addition of solid potassium cyanide and then add more *bromine solution* until the solution is pale yellow. (ii) Prepare a saturated solution of aniline in water. These solutions are stable for 1 week. Mix equal volumes of the two solutions immediately prior to the test.
METHOD. Add 1 drop of the mixed reagent to the sample on a white tile.
INDICATIONS. RED, ORANGE, or YELLOW colours indicate the presence of a mono-substituted pyridine ring. Increasing chain-length of the substituent group weakens the response; a delayed response is obtained when the pyridine ring is substituted by nitrogen adjacent to the ring nitrogen; a weak response is obtained where there is a $>C=O$ substituent adjacent to the ring nitrogen. There is no response to the test if the pyridine ring is bound to another ring, nor if it is substituted in more than one position, nor if the nitrogen in the ring is substituted.
Anomalous results are obtained with azatadine (PINK), bisacodyl (no response), and tropicamide (VIOLET-PINK).

RED	Zimeldine (30s)
PINK	Azatadine
Orange-pink	Carbinoxamine, dimethindene, doxylamine, iproniazid, phenyramidol, triprolidine (1–2 min)
Violet-pink	Tropicamide
ORANGE	Azaperone, brompheniramine, chlorpheniramine, isoniazid, metyrapone, nicametate, nicotinamide, nicotine, nicotinic acid, nifenazone, nikethamide, pheniramine, xanthinol nicotinate
Red-orange	Benzyl nicotinate

YELLOW	Halopyramine, mepyramine, tripelennamine

Diazotisation

METHOD. Dissolve the sample in 2M hydrochloric acid, and to 1 drop on a white tile add 1 drop of a 1% solution of sodium nitrite, and 1 drop of a 4% solution of 2-naphthol in 2M sodium hydroxide.
INDICATIONS. A bright RED or ORANGE-RED colour indicates the presence of a primary aromatic amine. Diphenylamine does not give a reaction; aminonitrothiazole (solid) gives a VIOLET colour.

p-Dimethylaminobenzaldehyde

REAGENT. Dissolve 0.5 g of *p*-dimethylaminobenzaldehyde in 50 ml of a mixture containing 60 volumes of ethanol and 40 volumes of *sulphuric acid*. The reagent should be freshly prepared.
METHOD. Add the reagent to the sample in a test-tube, warming if necessary. Observe any colour produced and then carefully dilute with water.
INDICATIONS. Colours are given by a number of substances including ergot alkaloids (VIOLET), cannabinols and certain indoles in which the indole ring is not bonded to another conjugated ring (RED changing to VIOLET on dilution), certain phenols and phenolic amines (RED or ORANGE, usually changing to VIOLET on dilution). Some other types of compound also respond.

RED (changing to VIOLET on dilution)	Cannabinols, phenazone (100°, 5 min), pindolol, tryptamine
RED (no violet on dilution)	Benserazide, cocaine (100°, 3 min), feprazone, harmine, phencyclidine (100°, 3 min)
ORANGE (changing to VIOLET on dilution)	Dobutamine, dopamine, orciprenaline, phenol, terbutaline, tyramine
VIOLET	Dihydroergotamine, ergometrine, ergotamine, ergotoxine, lysergide, methysergide

Diphenylamine Test

REAGENT. A 0.5% solution of diphenylamine in sulphuric acid (60% v/v).
METHOD. Apply the reagent to the sample on a white tile or in a test-tube.
INDICATIONS. A BLUE colour indicates the presence of an oxidising agent such as bromate, chlorate, chromate, dichromate, iodate, lead(IV), manganese (III, IV, VII), nitrate, nitrite, permanganate, or vanadate.

Dragendorff Reagent

REAGENT. Dissolve 1 g of bismuth subnitrate in 3 ml of 10M hydrochloric acid with the aid of heat, dilute to 20 ml with water, and dissolve in the mixture 1 g of potassium iodide. If black bismuth tri-iodide separates, add 2M hydrochloric acid and more potassium iodide to dissolve it.

METHOD. Dissolve the sample in 3 drops of 2M hydrochloric acid, add 2 to 3 ml of the reagent, and dilute to 10 ml with water.

INDICATIONS. An ORANGE, RED-ORANGE, or BROWN-ORANGE precipitate suggests the presence of an alkaloidal base (precipitated as the alkaloidal bismuth iodide). Positive for primary, secondary, tertiary, and quaternary amines.

This reagent is commonly used as a spray for detecting alkaloids on thin-layer chromatographic plates.

Duquenois Reagent

REAGENT. Dissolve 2 g of vanillin and 0.3 ml of acetaldehyde in 100 ml of ethanol. The reagent should be stored in the dark.

METHOD. Place the sample, or an evaporated petroleum ether extract of the sample, in a test-tube and add 0.5 ml of the reagent and an equal volume of 10M hydrochloric acid. Warm gently and note any colour which is produced and then shake the mixture with chloroform and note if the colour is extracted.

INDICATIONS. A colour change from GREY to GREEN through BLUE to VIOLET-BLUE suggests the presence of cannabis but distinction from roasted coffee and patchouli oil is required. The colour change is best with fresh drug material. Only with cannabis is the violet colour extracted into the chloroform layer.

	Initial colour	Colour extracted by chloroform
Cannabis	Violet-blue	Violet
Coffee (roasted)	Violet-brown	nil
Patchouli oil	Violet	nil
Tea (leaves)	Green-blue	nil

No colour is obtained with other natural products, e.g. basil, bay leaf, eucalyptus oil, mace, marjoram, nutmeg, rosemary, sage, thyme, or tobacco.

Ferric Chloride

METHOD. Add *ferric chloride solution* to an ethanolic solution of the sample.

INDICATIONS. RED, ORANGE, GREEN, BLUE, VIOLET, or BROWN colours indicate the presence of a phenolic compound, fatty acid, or a phenylpyrazoline.

RED	Acetates, phenazone
Brown-red	Nifenazone
ORANGE	Hexoprenaline, propyphenazone, sodium valproate
GREEN	Adrenaline, betanaphthol, dobutamine, dopamine, ethamivan, ethylnoradrenaline, hexylresorcinol, hydroquinone, hydroxyquinoline, isoetharine, isoprenaline, levodopa, methyldopa, methyldopate, noradrenaline, paraphenylenediamine, phenothiazine, protokylol, rimiterol
Blue-green	Chlorquinaldol
BLUE	Apomorphine, dodecyl gallate, gallic acid, morphine, paracetamol, parachlorophenol, phenol, tannic acid
VIOLET	Aminosalicylic acid, diflunisal, dipyrone, hexachlorophane (transient), labetalol
Blue-violet	Amidopyrine, salicylamide (after hydrolysis), salicylic acid
BROWN	Aloin, carbidopa
Yellow-brown	Salinazid
Green-brown	Benserazide
BLACK	
Violet-black	Ethyl gallate ($\rightarrow$ blue-black)

Ferrous Sulphate

REAGENT. To 1 volume of a 10% solution of ferrous sulphate ($FeSO_4,7H_2O$) add 5 volumes of *sulphuric acid* with cooling.

METHOD. Add the sample to 0.5 ml of the reagent.

INDICATIONS. A RED or PINK colour is given only by nitrates and nitrites, e.g. glyceryl trinitrate.

Folin–Ciocalteu Reagent

REAGENT. *Stock Solution*. Dissolve 100 g of sodium tungstate and 25 g of sodium molybdate in 800 ml of water in a 1500-ml flask, add 50 ml of *phosphoric acid* and 100 ml of *hydrochloric acid*, and reflux for 10 hours. Cool, add 150 g of lithium sulphate, 50 ml of water, and 4 to 6 drops of bromine, and allow to stand for 2 hours. Boil for 15 minutes to remove the excess of bromine, cool, filter, and dilute to 1000 ml with water.

This stock solution should be stored at a temperature not exceeding 4° and used within 4 months of its preparation; it has a yellow colour and must not be used if any trace of green colour is present.

For use, dilute 1 volume of this stock solution with 2 volumes of water.

METHOD. Add the diluted reagent to the sample and make the mixture alkaline with 2M sodium hydroxide.

INDICATIONS. A BLUE colour indicates the presence of a phenolic compound. The reaction is progressively inhibited with increased halogenation of the phenol nucleus.

Formaldehyde–Sulphuric Acid

REAGENT. To 4 volumes of *sulphuric acid* add 6 volumes of *formaldehyde solution*, using a pipette with the tip below the surface of the acid, with stirring and adequate cooling. When the reagent is warm it will remain clear for about 1 hour. If turbidity develops, it may be dispelled by heating in a water-bath at 100° for about 1 minute.

Note. This reagent is not the same as that used in the Marquis Test.

METHOD. Mix the sample with the reagent and heat at 100° for 1 minute.

INDICATIONS. Benzodiazepines generally give an ORANGE colour with the exception of bromazepam and clozapine (YELLOW), and flurazepam (PINK). Other indications include phenothiazines, tetracyclines, and thioxanthenes. Tryptamine (BROWN) and zomepirac (RED) also react.

RED	*Chlorprothixene, *clopenthixol, fluopromazine, *flupenthixol, fluphenazine, metopimazine, pericyazine, promazine, thiothixene, zomepirac
Brown-red	Lymecycline, oxytetracycline, tolmetin
PINK	Flurazepam, thioproperazine, trifluoperazine
ORANGE	Clonazepam, clorazepic acid, demeclocycline (→ brown-red), demoxepam, diazepam, flunitrazepam, ketazolam, lorazepam, lormetazepam, medazepam (add water), methixene, nitrazepam, nordazepam, oxazepam, prazepam, temazepam, tetrazepam
Red-orange	Methacycline
YELLOW	Bromazepam, clozapine, dimethothiazine, doxycycline
Green-yellow	Rolitetracycline (→ yellow-brown), tetracycline (→ yellow-brown)
GREEN	Thiethylperazine
BLUE	Carphenazine, methotrimeprazine, thioridazine
VIOLET	Mesoridazine, perphenazine
Red-violet	Chlorpromazine, diethazine, ethopropazine, mequitazine, methdilazine, perazine, phenothiazine, prochlorperazine, thiopropazate, trimeprazine
Blue-violet	Acepromazine, acetophenazine, piperacetazine, promethazine, propiomazine
Brown-violet	Thiazinamium
BROWN	Tryptamine
Orange-brown	Chlortetracycline, clomocycline

*Fluoresce ORANGE under ultraviolet light (350 nm)

No response is obtained with chlordiazepoxide, dimethoxanate, or proquamezine.

Forrest Reagent

REAGENT. Mix together equal volumes of a 0.2% solution of potassium dichromate, a 30% v/v solution of *sulphuric acid*, a 20% w/w solution of *perchloric acid*, and a 50% v/v solution of *nitric acid*.

METHOD. Dissolve the sample in a minimum volume of 2M hydrochloric acid and add an equal volume of the reagent.

INDICATIONS. RED, PINK, ORANGE, BLUE, or VIOLET colours are obtained with phenothiazines.

A BLUE colour is obtained with certain dibenzazepines. The blue colour is inhibited by the presence of phenothiazines, and an excess of reagent must be added to overcome this.

RED	Acepromazine, carphenazine, chlorpromazine, diethazine, dimethothiazine, mequitazine, mesoridazine, piperacetazine, prochlorperazine, promethazine, propiomazine, thiazinamium, thiopropazate, thioproperazine
Violet-red	Perphenazine
Brown-red	Trimeprazine
PINK	Ethopropazine
ORANGE	Fluopromazine, fluphenazine, phenothiazine, trifluoperazine
Pink-orange	Acetophenazine
Red-orange	Methdilazine
Brown-orange	Perazine, pericyazine
BLUE	Clomipramine, desipramine, imipramine, opipramol, thiethylperazine, thioridazine, trimipramine
VIOLET	Methotrimeprazine, proquamezine (→ red → orange)
BROWN	Metopimazine
Red-brown	Promazine

FPN Reagent

REAGENT. Mix together 5 ml of *ferric chloride solution*, 45 ml of a 20% w/w solution of *perchloric acid*, and 50 ml of a 50% v/v solution of *nitric acid*.

METHOD. Dissolve the sample in a minimum volume of 2M hydrochloric acid and add an equal volume of the reagent.

INDICATIONS. The indications for this reagent are the same as those stated for Forrest Reagent.

RED	Chlorpromazine, dimethothiazine, mesoridazine, methdilazine, prochlorperazine, thiazinamium, thiopropazate
Orange-red	Mequitazine
Violet-red	Perphenazine, proquamezine ($\rightarrow$ red $\rightarrow$ orange)
Brown-red	Trimeprazine
ORANGE	Acetophenazine, diethazine, ethopropazine ($\rightarrow$ yellow), fluopromazine, fluphenazine, metopimazine, pericyazine, phenothiazine, promethazine, thioproperazine, trifluoperazine
Red-orange	Carphenazine
Pink-orange	Propiomazine ($\rightarrow$ red $\rightarrow$ fades)
Brown-orange	Acepromazine, perazine, piperacetazine
BLUE	Clomipramine, imipramine, thiethylperazine, thioridazine, trimipramine
VIOLET	Methotrimeprazine
BROWN Red-brown	Promazine

Fujiwara Test

REAGENT. Freshly prepared *sodium hydroxide solution*.

METHOD. Mix together 2 ml of the reagent and 1 ml of pyridine, add the sample, and heat in a water-bath at 100° for 2 minutes, with shaking.

INDICATIONS. A RED colour in the pyridine layer indicates the presence of compounds which possess at least two halogen atoms bound to one carbon atom. No colour is given by dicophane; 2,2,2-trichloroethanol gives a yellow colour.

Furfuraldehyde

REAGENT. A 10% solution of furfuraldehyde in ethanol.

METHOD. Dissolve the sample in ethanol, place 1 drop of the solution on a filter paper, add 1 drop of the reagent, and expose the paper to hydrochloric acid fumes for 2 to 3 minutes.

INDICATIONS. A BLACK spot indicates the presence of non-aromatic carbamates. *N*-Substituted carbamates do not react.

Iodine Test

METHOD. Mix the sample with an equal volume of manganese dioxide and heat the mixture carefully to dull redness over a small flame. Repeat the test by heating the sample alone.

INDICATIONS. The appearance of VIOLET vapour indicates the presence of iodine in the molecule. Better results are sometimes obtained when the manganese dioxide is omitted, e.g. amiodarone.

Iodoplatinate Test

REAGENT. Add 2 ml of a 5% solution of platinic chloride and 5 g of potassium iodide to 98 ml of water and shake until dissolved.

METHOD. Dissolve the sample in 2 drops of 2M hydrochloric acid, add 2 to 3 ml of the reagent, and dilute to 10 ml with water.

INDICATIONS. A VIOLET, BLUE-VIOLET, BROWN-VIOLET, or GREY-VIOLET precipitate suggests the presence of an alkaloidal base (precipitated as the alkaloid-iodoplatinate complex). The clearest colours are obtained with tertiary and quaternary amines; primary amines give indistinct colours and amines of small molecular weight do not generally react.

Koppanyi–Zwikker Test

REAGENT. A 1% solution of cobalt nitrate in ethanol.

METHOD. Dissolve the sample in 1 ml of ethanol, add 1 drop of the reagent followed by 10 µl of pyrrolidine, and agitate the mixture.

INDICATIONS. A VIOLET colour is given by substances containing the following structures. *Imides*, in which $>C=O$ and $>NH$ are adjacent in a ring (e.g. barbiturates, glutethimide, oxyphenisatin, saccharin). *Sulphonamides* and other compounds with free $-SO_2 \cdot NH_2$ on a ring (e.g. clopamide, frusemide, sulphanilamide, thiazides), or with $-SO_2 \cdot NH_2$ in a side-chain (e.g. chlorpropamide), or with $-SO_2 \cdot NH_2$ linking a benzene ring with another ring which is other than a pyrazine, pyridazine, pyridine, or pyrimidine ring (e.g. sulphafurazole, sulphamethoxazole). These latter structures give PINK or RED-VIOLET colours (e.g. sulphadiazine, sulphadimethoxine).

No response is obtained with compounds where there are other substituents on the nitrogen atom. Anomalous responses are obtained with paramethadione and theophylline (VIOLET), and with cycloserine, idoxuridine, methoin, niridazole, riboflavine (no response).

Note. Hydrochlorides give a BLUE colour before the addition of pyrrolidine.

Liebermann's Test

REAGENT. Add 5 g of sodium nitrite to 50 ml of *sulphuric acid* with cooling and swirling to absorb the brown fumes.

METHOD. Add 2 or 3 drops of the reagent to the sample on a white tile. Occasionally it is necessary to carry out the test in a tube and heat in a water-bath at 100°.

Many substances give colours with *sulphuric acid* alone, and the test should be repeated using *sulphuric acid* instead of the reagent in order to ascertain that the colour seen is due to the reagent.

INDICATIONS. 1. ORANGE colours are given by substances containing a mono-substituted benzene ring not joined to $>C=O$, $>N-C(=O)-$, or to a ring containing a $>C=N-O-$ grouping.

2. ORANGE or BROWN colours are given by some substances containing two mono-substituted benzene rings (or some di-substituted compounds where fluorine is the second substituent) which are joined either to one carbon atom or to adjacent carbon atoms.

3. A wide range of colours is given by compounds containing $-OH$, $O-$alkyl, or $-O-CH_2 \cdot O-$ groups attached to a benzene ring or to a ring in a polycyclic structure containing a benzene ring. The benzene ring must not bear $-NO_2$, nor be halogenated, nor contain an $-O-$ substituent *ortho* to the oxy groups. Compounds containing ring sulphur give a similar range of colours.

A YELLOW colour is given by a variety of other compounds.

RED	Ajmaline, alprenolol, aminacrine (100°), antazoline, brucine, chlorprothixene, clopenthixol, flupenthixol, mestranol, oxytetracycline, prajmalium, thiazinamium, thiothixene, tolmetin (100°), trifluoperazine, xylazine
Violet-red	Indapamide
Brown-red	Methylchlorophenoxyacetic acid
PINK	Trichlorophenoxyacetic acid (→ brown)
Brown-pink	Prazosin (100° → red-orange)
ORANGE	Aletamine, alverine, ampicillin, atropine methobromide, atropine methonitrate, baclofen, benactyzine (→ brown), bethanidine (→ brown), broxyquinoline, butanilicaine, chloroquine (100°), clidinium (→ brown), cyclandelate, cyclizine, dazomet, decoquinate (slow), diethylthiambutene (100°), dimefline, diuron, doxapram, dyclonine (100°), fenclofenac (100° → brown), fenitrothion, fenpipramide, glibenclamide (100°, 15 s), hyoscine butylbromide, hyoscine methonitrate, linuron, loxapine (50°–60°), methindizate (→ brown), methylphenidate, metolazone (→ green-brown), monolinuron, nomifensine, phenazone (100°), phenelzine, propham, salinazid, sulphinpyrazone, tolazoline, trimetaphan, tripelennamine (→ brown), triprolidine, xipamide, zomepirac (100°)
Red-orange	Acetanilide, amphetamines, aniline, atropine, bamipine, beclamide, benethamine, caramiphen, carbetapentane, chlorcyclizine, cinchophen, cycrimine, diphenylpyraline, doxylamine, dropropizine, ephedrines, famprofazone, fencamfamin, glutethimide, hyoscine, hyoscyamine, isoaminile, isocarboxazid, levamisole, meclozine, mephentermine, methixene, methoin, methyl benzoquate, methylphenobarbitone, metomidate, morazone, nialamide, pentapiperide, pethidine, phenacemide, phenbutrazate, phendimetrazine, phenglutarimide, pheniramine, phenmetrazine, phenobarbitone, phensuximide, phenylmethylbarbituric acid, phenytoin, prolintane, tofenacin, tranylcypromine, triamterene, triphenyltetrazolium, warfarin
Brown-orange	Ambutonium, bumetanide, diphenhydramine, fenuron, feprazone (100° → brown), ibuprofen, labetalol, mepivacaine, methadone, nefopam (→ brown), tetrahydrozoline
YELLOW	Amicarbalide (100°), clonidine (100° → orange), dequalinium (100° → orange), diethylpropion, diloxanide, ethoxzolamide, fenfluramine (100°), flavoxate, gliclazide, metoclopramide, nifenazone (100°), piroxicam, propachlor, tropicamide
Brown-yellow	Amiodarone
GREEN	Bialamicol, chlorotrianisene, colchicine, dextromoramide (100°), diamthazole, hydrastine, mequitazine, naphthols, phenol, phenothiazine, thiocarlide
Blue-green	Hydrochlorothiazide, hydroflumethiazide, pindolol
Brown-green	Cyclopenthiazide
Grey-green	Azapropazone
Black-green	Naproxen
BLUE	Amethocaine (100°), amidopyrine (100°), bendrofluazide, benzonatate (100°), chromonar (100°, 3 min), clomipramine, dipyrone (100°), imipramine, mefenamic acid, mefruside, oxypertine, padimate (100°), procarbazine (100°, 15 s), propyphenazone (100°) (red with water), yohimbine
Green-blue	Amiphenazole (100°)
VIOLET	Methocarbamol, mianserin, paracetamol, penthienate methobromide, phenacetin, propiomazine, resorcinol, timolol (100°), trazodone (100°) (transient)
Red-violet	Chloroxuron
Black-violet	Methoxychlor

BROWN	Acepromazine, acetophenazine, adiphenine, azacyclonol, barban, benzilonium, benzyl nicotinate, biperiden, clemastine, clomiphene, cyclothiazide, dextropropoxyphene, dichlorprop, dicophane, diperodon, diphemanil, diphenidol, emepronium, etenzamide, fenpiprane, flurbiprofen, haloperidol, mepenzolate, methylpiperidyl benzilate, mexiletine, nadolol, penfluridol, phenaglycodol, phenylbutazone (100°), phosalone, pimozide, pipazethate (100°→ red), pipoxolan, pyrrobutamine, rotenone, sotalol (100°), sulindac, veratrine, zimeldine
Red-brown	Benzthiazide, bisacodyl, carphenazine, chlorpromazine, diclofenac, dothiepin, ethopropazine, etisazole, fenbufen, fenoprofen, methapyrilene, perphenazine, polythiazide
Pink-brown	Metoprolol
Orange-brown	Benazolin, diphenadione, maprotiline, methiocarb, piperidolate
Green-brown	Methdilazine, norbormide, promazine, thiopropazate
Violet-brown	Bamethan, clofibrate, dichlorophen
Black-brown	Mecoprop
GREY	Isopropamide
BLACK	Acetomenaphthone, aloin, aminophenols, amodiaquine, apomorphine, atenolol, benorylate, benzquinamide, buprenorphine, butorphanol, carbaryl (→ green), carbidopa, cephaëline, chloroxylenol, chlorphenesin, clomocycline, clorgyline, codeine, cotarnine, cresol, cyclazocine, dextromethorphan, diamorphine, dibromopropamidine, diprenorphine, doxepin, emetine, ethamivan, ethinyloestradiol, etilefrine, frusemide, glycopyrronium, guaiphenesin, hexobendine, hydroxyephedrine, hydroxystilbamidine, ibogaine, indomethacin, levallorphan, mebeverine, mescaline, methylchlorophenoxyacetic acid, methylenedioxyamphetamine, morantel, morphine, naloxone, 1-naphthylacetic acid, narceine, nicergoline, normetanephrine, noscapine, noxiptyline, octaphonium, oestradiol, oestriol, oestrone, oxprenolol, oxyphenisatin, papaverine, pholcodine, pizotifen, practolol, profadol, propanidid, protokylol, pyrantel, rimiterol, ritodrine, rotenone, salbutamol, terbutaline, tetrabenazine, tetracycline, thymol, trimethobenzamide, trimetozine, tubocurarine, verapamil, viloxazine

Mandelin's Test

REAGENT. Dissolve 0.5 g of ammonium vanadate in 1.5 ml of water and dilute to 100 ml with *sulphuric acid*. Filter the solution through glass wool.

METHOD. Add a drop of the reagent to the sample on a white tile.

INDICATIONS. When interpreting the result of this test, account should be taken of the colour given by Sulphuric Acid and by Liebermann's Test. Hydrochlorides give a red colour with this reagent. When the colours differ from those given with Sulphuric Acid or Liebermann's Test, this indicates an aromatic ring together with a saturated 5-, 6-, or 7-membered ring containing only one nitrogen atom. The heterocyclic ring must not contain a second nitrogen atom, nor an oxygen atom, nor must it be substituted, nor bound by —CO·NH— to the aromatic ring. The aromatic ring must not have —CF$_3$ as a substituent. Colours are also produced if sulphur is in a ring, provided that the ring does not contain more than one nitrogen atom.

RED	Ajmaline, azacyclonol, chlorprothixene, diperodon (→ green), dofamium (→ brown), flupenthixol, gelsemine (→ green), indapamide, mequitazine, methotrexate, nialamide, pericyazine, prajmalium, prolintane, sodium cromoglycate, thiothixene, xylometazoline
Brown-red	Nadolol
ORANGE	Dropropizine (slow), ethylnoradrenaline, hydrastinine (→ green), lachesine (→ green), levamisole (→ greygreen), methanthelinium, methixene, methyldopa, methyldopate, methylpiperidyl benzilate (→ brown→ green), noradrenaline, orphenadrine, pipenzolate (→ green), poldine methylsulphate (→ green→ violet), propantheline, proquamezine (→ violet), solanidine (→ violet→ blue), solanine (→ violet→ blue), sulindac, thenalidine (→ brown)
Red-orange	Cotarnine (→ brown)
Green-orange	5-Methyltryptamine
Brown-orange	Mexiletine
YELLOW	Azaperone, benztropine, broxaldine, chelidonine (→ green), conessine, deptropine, desipramine (→ blue), dihydralazine, diphenhydramine, diphenidol, diphenylpyraline, dropropizine (→ orange), halquinol, homidium, lidoflazine, methacycline (→ orange-violet), paraphenylenediamine, penicillamine, protokylol (→ brown), tofenacin, tylosin (→ yellow-brown), veratrine (→ orange→ violet-brown), viprynium
Orange-yellow	Hexoprenaline
Green-yellow	Methoxamine

GREEN   Acepromazine (→ red), adiphenine (→ blue), benorylate, bephenium hydroxynaphthoate, bibenzonium, buclosamide (blue rim), bunamidine, chlorpromazine (→ violet), clefamide (→ brown), codeine, colchicine, cyclazocine, cyclomethycaine (→ brown), debrisoquine, diaveridine, dibenzepin, diethazine (→ violet with excess reagent), diethylthiambutene (→ green-blue), dimethindene, dimethoxanate (→ brown), dimoxyline, dipipanone (→ blue), dothiepin, doxorubicin, doxycycline (→ yellow), ethopropazine (→ violet), fenpiprane, guanoxan, harman, hydroxyephedrine, isoxsuprine, metanephrine, methadone (→ blue), methdilazine (→ violet), methocarbamol, methoxyamphetamine, methylenedioxyamphetamine (→ blue), α-methyltryptamine (→ orange), metopimazine, monocrotaline, niclosamide, nitroxoline, norharman (→ yellow), normetanephrine, obidoxime (→ blue), oleandomycin, oxymetazoline, pecazine (→ violet), pentazocine, perazine (→ violet), phenazone, phenazopyridine, phenformin, phenindamine, phenoxybenzamine (→ violet), phenyltoloxamine, pindolol, piperacetazine (→ red → violet), pipoxolan (→ brown), prenylamine, proflavine, promazine (→ violet), promethazine (→ violet), propranolol, reserpine, ritodrine, thenium, thenyldiamine, thiocarlide (→ yellow), tranylcypromine (→ violet), trifluomeprazine (→ red-violet)

Yellow-green   Normethadone, opipramol

Blue-green   Benzoctamine, berberine (→ brown), edrophonium, hydroxystilbamidine, ketobemidone, methoxyphenamine, phentolamine, profadol (→ green), viloxazine

Brown-green   Benzydamine, chlorphenesin

Grey-green   Alverine, azapropazone, benzhexol, diamphenethide, diethyltryptamine (→ yellow), dihydrocodeine, guaiphenesin, hordenine, levomethadyl acetate, normorphine, oxyphencyclimine, papaverine, terbutaline

BLUE   Bamethan (→ green), clomipramine, deserpidine (→ green), desferrioxamine (→ violet), doxapram, droperidol (→ green), harmine (→ green), imipramine (add water), maprotiline, mebhydrolin, metaraminol, phenaglycodol, phenyramidol, pyridoxine (→ grey-green), salbutamol (blue rim → brown rim), thioridazine (→ violet), trimipramine (add water), triphenyltetrazolium (slow), xipamide, xylazine, yohimbine (→ green)

Green-blue   Chlophedianol, labetalol

VIOLET   Amidephrine, benperidol, bezitramide (→ orange), bisacodyl, captodiame, cephaloridine, chloropyrilene (→ orange), clomiphene (→ orange-brown), clomocycline (→ brown), denatonium, dipyridamole, guanoclor (→ orange → brown-yellow), guanoxan, hexobendine, hydromorphone (→ orange), mepacrine (→ yellow), mepyramine, methisazone (→ yellow), mianserin, morantel, naloxone (→ brown), oxyclozanide (→ orange), oxyphenisatin, oxytetracycline (→ red → orange), penthienate, perphenazine, phenylbutazone, pizotifen (→ green), prilocaine, primaquine (→ orange), propiomazine, pyrantel, pyrrobutamine, rolitetracycline (→ red → orange), strychnine, tetracycline (→ red → orange), thiethylperazine, thiopropazate, triacetyloleandomycin (slow), tridihexethyl, trimeprazine, trimetazidine

Red-violet   Antazoline, carphenazine, dimethothiazine, histapyrrodine, thonzylamine

Blue-violet   Alcuronium, hexocyclium, methotrimeprazine

Brown-violet   Alprenolol, bitoscanate, butaperazine, naphazoline

Grey-violet   Methoserpidine, oxprenolol, tricyclamol

Black-violet   Methapyrilene

BROWN   Amitriptyline (→ green), azapetine, bamipine, carbetapentane (slow), clidinium (→ green), cyclopentolate, diphemanil, dipyrone, doxepin, embutramide, fluanisone, fluphenazine, isoetharine, isometheptene, isoprenaline, methindizate, methyl benzoquate, methysergide, metoclopramide, norpipanone (→ blue), nortriptyline (→ green), phenelzine, phenylephrine, pimozide, piperidolate, prochlorperazine (→ violet), propoxycaine, rescinnamine, salinazid, stanozolol, tetrabenazine, thioproperazine (→ green → violet), tolnaftate, tolpropamine, tramazoline, tubocurarine

Red-brown   Benzthiazide, clioxanide, cycrimine, decoquinate, diclofenac, ethomoxane, fluopromazine, hydrastine (→ red), trifluoperazine

Pink-brown   Metoprolol

Orange-brown   Rifampicin, spiramycin, thebaine

Yellow-brown   Clemastine, clofazimine, physostigmine, rifamycin SV, trimethoprim, tripelennamine

Green-brown   Etenzamide, harmaline, lysergic acid, mesoridazine, narceine, syrosingopine

Violet-brown   Chlortetracycline (→ yellow), cyproheptadine, demeclocycline, dihydroergotamine, ergotamine, lymecycline (→ yellow), methylergometrine, nicergoline (→ brown), octaphonium, oxethazaine, protriptyline, trimethobenzamide

Grey-brown   Dextropropoxyphene, mephenesin carbamate

GREY   Dihydromorphine, diprenorphine, etilefrine (→ green → brown), ibogaine (→ violet), indomethacin, lobeline, lysergide, oxypertine, propranolol, trazodone (→ violet)

Blue-grey   Alphaprodine, diamorphine, morphine

BLACK   Procyclidine

Marquis Test

REAGENT. Mix 1 volume of *formaldehyde solution* with 9 volumes of *sulphuric acid*.

METHOD. Add a drop of the reagent to the sample on a white tile.

INDICATIONS. Various colours representing the whole of the visible spectrum are given by a large number of compounds. Structures which tend to maintain the response to the reagent at the violet end of the spectrum are, in decreasing order of efficacy: ring sulphur (with or without aromatic ring); ring oxygen (with aromatic ring); extra-ring oxygen or sulphur (with aromatic ring); aromatic compounds which consist entirely of C, H, N. Thus, there is a tendency for the response to Marquis reagent to move gradually towards longer wavelength, i.e. through green to orange and red, as the ratio of C, H, N to the other groups in the molecule rises.

RED	Alprenolol, benzylmorphine (→ violet), buphenine, dimethothiazine, etenzamide, etilefrine, fenclofenac (slow), fenpiprane, fluphenazine, flurbiprofen, hexoprenaline, labetalol (→ brown-red), maprotiline, mephenesin carbamate, mequitazine (slow), mesoridazine (→ violet), methoxyphenamine, metopimazine, mexiletine, nadolol, pentazocine (→ green), pericyazine, phenazopyridine, phenoperidine, phenylephrine, piperacetazine, prenylamine, thebaine (→ orange), thiethylperazine (→ green), thioproperazine, thiothixene, tolpropamine, tranylcypromine (→ brown), vinblastine
Orange-red	Alverine, bethanidine, diphemanil, flupenthixol
Violet-red	Thioridazine (→ blue-green)
Brown-red	Alphaprodine
PINK	Fenoprofen, metoprolol
ORANGE	Adrenaline (→ violet), aletamine, amphetamine (→ brown), anileridine (slow), benactyzine (→ green → blue), benzethonium, benzilonium (→ green → blue), benzphetamine, bunamidine (→ red), carbetapentane (slow), carphenazine (→ red-violet), clidinium (→ blue), cyclandelate (slow), cycrimine (→ red), dehydroemetine, dimethyltryptamine, dipyridamole, ethacridine (→ red), ethoheptazine, ethylnoradrenaline (→ brown), famprofazone, fenbufen (→ brown), fencamfamin, fenethylline, fentanyl, harmine, indapamide (→ violet), indomethacin, isothipendyl, ketobemidone, lachesine (→ green → blue), lymecycline, mepenzolate (transient), mephentermine (→ brown), mescaline, metanephrine (→ violet-brown), methacycline, methanthelinium, methindizate (→ green), methylamphetamine, methylpiperidyl benzilate (→ green → blue), 5-methyltryptamine (→ brown), α-methyltryptamine (→ brown), N-methyltryptamine, nefopam (→ brown), nomifensine (slow), normetanephrine (→ violet-brown), oxeladin, oxytetracycline, pentapiperide, pethidine, phenethylamine, phenformin (→ brown), phentermine, piminodine, pipenzolate (→ green → blue), piperidolate, pizotifen (→ red), poldine methylsulphate (→ green → blue), primaquine, profadol (→ red-brown), prolintane (→ brown), propantheline, prothipendyl, psilocybin, rolitetracycline, spiramycin, tetracycline, trimethoprim, trimethoxyamphetamine, tryptamine, veratrine, xylometazoline
Red-orange	Chlorprothixene
Pink-orange	Diuron
Yellow-orange	Orphenadrine, pipradrol
Brown-orange	Amitriptyline
YELLOW	Acriflavine (→ red), amiloride, azacyclonol, benzquinamide, benztropine, bromodiphenhydramine, broxaldine, broxyquinoline, caramiphen, chlordiazepoxide, chlorphenoxamine (→ green), chlortetracycline (→ green), chlorthalidone, cinchophen, clefamide, clemastine (green rim), colchicine, conessine (→ orange), cyclizine, demeclocycline (→ green), deptropine, diethyltryptamine (→ brown), diphenhydramine, diphenidol, diphenylpyraline, DOM, doxycycline, ethoxzolamide, ethylmorphine (→ violet → black), furaltadone, halquinol, hydrocodone (→ brown → violet), hydromorphone (→ red → violet), hydroxyephedrine, isotharine (→ orange), lidoflazine, lorazepam, mepacrine, methyldopa (→ violet), methyldopate (→ violet), norcodeine (→ violet), orciprenaline, oxycodone (→ brown → violet), oxyphenbutazone, phanquone, phenbutrazate (slow), phentolamine, phenyramidol, pindolol (→ brown), pramoxine (→ green), proflavine (→ orange), salbutamol, salinazid, sodium cromoglycate, solanine (→ violet), terbutaline, tetrabenazine, thebacon (→ violet), tofenacin, triamterene, trimetazidine (fades), vancomycin, viprynium embonate, zomepirac (100°, → orange)
Orange-yellow	Stanozolol

GREEN   Berberine, carbaryl, chelidonine, harman, norharman, oleandomycin, propranolol, protriptyline, pseudomorphine, sulindac (slow)

Yellow-green   Acepromazine (→ red), verapamil (→ grey)

Blue-green   Tolnaftate

Brown-green   Harmaline

Grey-green   Cyproheptadine, deserpidine, naphazoline, oxypertine, phenindamine, protokylol, rescinnamine, reserpine (→ brown)

BLUE   Clofibrate, embutramide, nicergoline (→ grey)

Grey-blue   Mebhydrolin, 1-naphthylacetic acid

VIOLET   Apomorphine (→ black), azatadine, benorylate, bisacodyl, buprenorphine, butriptyline, captodiame, chloropyrilene, chlorpromazine, clofazimine, codeine, diamorphine, diethylthiambutene, dihydrocodeine, dimethindene (→ blue), dimethoxanate, doxorubicin, doxylamine, ethopropazine, ethoxazene, guaiphenesin, guanoxan, hexocyclium methylsulphate, mepyramine, 6-monoacetylmorphine, morphine, nalorphine, normorphine, oxprenolol, oxyphenisatin, pecazine, penthienate, perazine, perphenazine, phenoxybenzamine, phenyltoloxamine, pholcodine, pimozide, pipoxolan (→ grey), prochlorperazine, procyclidine, promazine, promethazine, proquamezine, solanidine, thenium, thiopropazate, tricyclamol, trimeprazine, viloxazine

Red-violet   Acetophenazine, benzoctamine, bephenium hydroxynaphthoate, cephaloridine, chlophedianol (→ brown), dihydromorphine, ethomoxane, fluopromazine, isoxsuprine, lobeline, methdilazine, propiomazine, tramazoline, trifluomeprazine, trifluoperazine, trimeperidine

Blue-violet   Methocarbamol, methotrimeprazine, morantel, neopine, noscapine (fades), pyrantel

Brown-violet   Butaperazine, dopamine, tridihexethyl

Grey-violet   Benzhexol, diprenorphine, oxymorphone, pyrrobutamine, thenalidine

Black-violet   Dextropropoxyphene (→ green), methapyrilene, thenyldiamine

BROWN   Bibenzonium, carbidopa, cyclazocine (→ green), diclofenac (slow), dimoxyline, dothiepin, doxepin, ergometrine, ergotamine, erythromycin, hordenine (→ green), ibuprofen (100°, → orange), isoprenaline (→ violet), lysergamide, lysergic acid, naloxone (→ violet), naproxen, narceine (→ green), noradrenaline, phenazocine, rimiterol (→ black), serotonin (slow), syrosingopine, tyramine (→ green)

Red-brown   Biperiden, debrisoquine, methyl benzoquate, oxethazaine, phenprobamate, trimetozine, tripelennamine

Orange-brown   Benethamine (→ brown), clomocycline, nortriptyline

Yellow-brown   Ritodrine, thymoxamine, triacetyloleandomycin, tylosin

Green-brown   Alcuronium, bufotenine, psilocin

Violet-brown   Clomiphene, diethazine, levomethadyl acetate (→ grey-green), methoxamine (→ green)

Grey-brown   Dihydroergotamine, methylergometrine, octaphonium

GREY   Butorphanol, diaveridine (→ violet-brown), ibogaine (→ orange), lysergide, methoserpidine, methysergide, pholedrine (→ green)

Blue-grey   Acetorphine (→ yellow-brown), etorphine (→ yellow-brown)

BLACK
Blue-black   Methylenedioxyamphetamine

McNally's Test

REAGENTS. (i) A 0.5% solution of copper sulphate in 10% acetic acid. (ii) A freshly-prepared 2% solution of sodium nitrite.

METHOD. To the sample in 1 ml of water add 0.2 ml of ethanol or acetone, 3 drops of the copper sulphate solution, and an equal volume of the sodium nitrite solution, shake, and heat in a water-bath at 100° for 3 minutes.

INDICATIONS. A RED colour indicates the presence of free salicylic acid.

Aminosalicylic acid gives a BROWN precipitate; diflunisal gives a VIOLET colour. Certain acids which are produced during the putrefaction of tissues also give RED colours in this test: p-hydroxyphenylacetic acid; p-hydroxyphenylpropionic acid; p-hydroxyphenyl-lactic acid.

Mercurous Nitrate

REAGENT. To a saturated solution of mercurous nitrate add solid sodium bicarbonate until effervescence ceases and the precipitate formed becomes yellow. The precipitate then changes to a biscuit colour. This reagent should be freshly prepared, shaken immediately before use, and should not be kept for more than 1 hour.

METHOD. Dissolve the sample in the minimum amount of ethanol, add 1 drop of the opaque reagent, shake, and examine at intervals during 2 minutes. A blank solution containing only ethanol and reagent should be treated similarly at the same time.

INDICATIONS. A dark GREY or BLACK colour indicates (i) a ring imide group, or (ii) sulphonamides with an additional ring.

The speed and intensity of the reaction varies between different compounds. The following ring imides react in decreasing order of intensity, barbiturates, bemegride, phenytoin > benperidol, cycloserine, pimozide > glutethimide, oxyphenisatin > saccharin, sulphinpyrazone. In the case of sulphonamides, succinylsulphathiazole, sulphamoxole, sulphanilamide, sulphasomidine, and sulphathiazole react with greater intensity than all others. Chlorpropamide and tolbutamide give a moderate response.

Methanolic Potassium Hydroxide

REAGENT. A 20% solution of potassium hydroxide in methanol.

METHOD. Add a few drops of the reagent to a solution of the sample in methanol and heat to develop the colour, if necessary to boiling-point.

INDICATIONS. A change from colourless or from a pale colour to RED, ORANGE, YELLOW, GREEN, or BLUE is given by quinones, diones possessing an aromatic ring, phenols with adjacent hydroxy groups, and by compounds containing nitro groups on a ring. Many of these compounds are coloured already and give pale or colourless solutions in methanol.

RED	Benserazide, isoetharine (→ orange → yellow), metronidazole, nitrofurazone, phenindione
Orange-red	Fenitrothion, quintozene, tecnazene, trifluralin
PINK	Levodopa (→ red-brown)
Orange-pink	Rimiterol
Brown-pink	Dobutamine
ORANGE	Acinitrazole, barban, carbidopa, dinitro-orthocresol (100°), dinobuton, dinoseb, dodecyl gallate, hexoprenaline (→ brown), isoprenaline (→ yellow), nifedipine, nifuratel, nifursol, obidoxime, protokylol (→ yellow)
Pink-orange	Adrenaline (→ brown)
Yellow-orange	Nitrofurantoin
YELLOW	Acebutolol, diphenadione, methyldopa (→ orange), metolazone, niclosamide, niridazole, nitroxoline, nitroxynil, phanquone (→ brown-violet), sodium cromoglycate
Green-yellow	Phytomenadione (→ violet → brown)

GREEN	Apomorphine (→ red), dinitolmide
BLUE	Dopamine (→ orange → brown), methyldopate (→ orange), noradrenaline (→ orange)
VIOLET	Dimetridazole (when boiled)

Millon's Reagent

REAGENT. Dissolve 3 ml of mercury in 27 ml of *fuming nitric acid* and add an equal volume of water with stirring.

METHOD. Add 0.5 ml of reagent to the sample and warm the mixture.

INDICATIONS. A RED or ORANGE-RED colour indicates the presence of a phenolic substance. Primary aryl amines also react. Some basic compounds which contain a phenolic group do not react to this test; a combination of this test with the Folin–Ciocalteu Reagent is therefore advised for phenolic compounds.

Naphthol–Sulphuric Acid

Note. This test should be carried out in conjunction with the Sulphuric Acid test (p. 145).

REAGENT. Mix 1 g of 2-naphthol with 40 ml of *sulphuric acid* and heat in a water-bath at 100°, with occasional stirring, until the 2-naphthol is dissolved.

METHOD. Mix the sample with 1 ml of the reagent, heat in a water-bath at 100° for 2 minutes, and note any colour produced. Cool, add 1 ml of water, and note the colour again.

INDICATIONS. A range of colours is obtained with steroidal structures (see below). A positive response to this test combined with a positive response to the Sulphuric Acid test is indicative of the presence of a steroid.

Compounds other than steroids which give colours with this test include chloral hydrate and chloramphenicol (brown-yellow), starch, and tartaric acid (green).

Colour with hot reagent	Steroid	Colour after dilution
RED	Mestranol	Red
Orange-red	Deoxycortone	Blue-black
	Dydrogesterone	—
	Hydroxy-progesterone	Blue, violet (dichroic)
	Norethynodrel	Brown-red
Brown-red	Ethinyloestradiol	Pink
ORANGE	Norethisterone	Orange-brown
Orange, green (dichroic)	Norethandrolone	Red-orange

Colour with hot reagent	Steroid	Colour after dilution
YELLOW	Stilboestrol	Orange
	Testosterone	Green, brown (dichroic)
Green-yellow	Fluoxymesterone	Yellow
GREEN	Beclomethasone	Brown-yellow
	Fluocinolone	Yellow
Yellow-green	Dexamethasone	Yellow
Green, yellow (dichroic)	Oestriol	Orange
	Oestrone	Orange
	Triamcinolone	Yellow
Green, brown (dichroic)	Flurandrenolone	Yellow
Blue-green, yellow (dichroic)	Oestradiol	Orange
VIOLET	Fludrocortisone	Brown
BROWN	Oxymetholone	Pink-orange
	Prednisolone	Brown
	Prednisone	Orange
	Progesterone	Yellow
Red-brown	Dimethisterone	Brown-green
	Enoxolone	Orange
	Fluocortolone	Red-brown
Orange-brown	Alphadolone	Orange
	Androsterone	Orange
	Cortisone	Orange
	Dienoestrol	Yellow
Yellow-brown	Carbenoxolone	Orange
	Cholesterol	Violet
	Hydrocortisone	Yellow-brown
Green-brown	Betamethasone	Orange-brown

Nessler's Reagent

REAGENT. To a saturated solution of mercuric chloride add solid potassium iodide until the initial red precipitate just dissolves; then add an equal volume of a freshly-prepared 40% solution of sodium hydroxide.

METHOD. Add the reagent to the sample and heat the mixture to 100° in a water-bath, examining it every minute for 10 minutes. A blank solution should be treated similarly at the same time.

INDICATIONS. A BROWN-ORANGE colour is produced quickly by aliphatic amides and thioamides. The presence of an aromatic ring slows the reaction and the nearer the amide group is to the ring, the more the reaction is inhibited. Substituents in the ring may cause a weak reaction.

An immediate BLACK colour is produced by substances containing ortho or para hydroxy groups and by substances containing an —NH—NH— or —NH—NH$_2$ group in an aliphatic side-chain.

Some compounds must be heated to 100° to produce blackening.

ORANGE	Acebutolol (slow), carbidopa (→black), methotrexate
Brown-orange	Acetylcarbromal (slow), bromvaletone, carbromal, chloramphenicol, dinitolmide, etenzamide (weak), ethionamide, fluoroacetamide, nicotinamide, phenacemide (slow), pheneturide (slow), prothionamide, pyrazinamide, salicylamide (weak), urea
YELLOW	Dihydrostreptomycin (→brown), penicillamine
BROWN	Demeclocycline, mebutamate (slow), nadolol, paracetamol (slow)
Yellow-brown	Atenolol (slow)
BLACK (immediate)	Adrenaline, apomorphine, ascorbic acid, benserazide, dihydralazine, dobutamine, dodecyl gallate, dopamine, ethylnoradrenaline, hexoprenaline, hydralazine, iproniazid, isocarboxazid, isoetharine, isoniazid, isoprenaline, levodopa, mebanazine, methyldopa, methyldopate, nialamide, noradrenaline, phenelzine, procarbazine, protokylol, rimiterol
BLACK (at 100°)	Cimetidine, gentamicin, labetalol, meprobamate (grey-black), methallibure, salinazid, thiacetazone

Ninhydrin

REAGENT. Dissolve 0.5 g of ninhydrin in 40 ml of acetone.

METHOD. Dissolve the sample in methanol, place 1 drop of the solution on a filter paper, add 1 drop of the reagent, and dry in a current of hot air.

INDICATIONS. A VIOLET colour, appearing rapidly, indicates the presence of an aliphatic primary amine or an amino acid group.

The presence of an aromatic ring inhibits the response, the inhibition increasing the nearer the amino group is to the ring, e.g. amphetamine (PINK-ORANGE), procainamide and proxymetacaine (both YELLOW). If the amino group is associated with a saturated ring, a positive but weak PINK-VIOLET colour is obtained (amantadine, rimantadine). Gentamicin gives a VIOLET colour after heating for 4 minutes.

Nitric Acid, Fuming

METHOD. Mix the sample with 3 drops of fuming nitric acid, heat at 50° for 30 seconds, and observe any colour produced. Cool the mixture, add 2 drops of it to 2 ml of sulphuric acid, and observe the colour. To the remainder of the cooled mixture, add 2 ml of water followed by 2M sodium hydroxide, dropwise, until a pH of 8 is obtained (use an indicator paper).

INDICATIONS. Chlorinated phenols give a series of colours in the three parts of this test.

ORANGE-RED/ORANGE/ORANGE-BROWN	Hexachlorophane
RED/RED/BROWN-VIOLET	Pentachlorophenol

Nitric–Sulphuric Acid

REAGENT. Mix 1 ml of *nitric acid* with 30 ml of *sulphuric acid*.

METHOD. Dissolve the sample in 1 ml of ethanol, add a pellet of potassium hydroxide, and evaporate to dryness at 100° in a water-bath. To the residue add 0.5 ml of water and 1 ml of carbon tetrachloride, shake, allow to separate, decant the lower carbon tetrachloride layer and shake it with 1 ml of the reagent.

INDICATIONS. A RED colour in the acid layer suggests the presence of dicophane (DDT) or its metabolite, dichlorodiphenyldichloroethylene (DDE). The red colour changes to ORANGE and then to GREEN. Weak PINK colours are given by aldrin, dieldrin, and endrin. A RED colour is also given by dichlorodiphenyldichloroethane (DDD, mitotane) but the colour does not change.

Note. The substance should be tested to ensure that it does not give a colour with *sulphuric acid* alone (p. 145).

Nitrous Acid

METHOD. Dissolve the sample in a minimum volume of water, add an amount of solid sodium nitrite equal in volume to the sample, followed by a few drops of 2M hydrochloric acid, added dropwise. INDICATIONS. ORANGE or YELLOW colours are given by certain sulphonamides and GREEN, BLUE, or VIOLET colours by certain phenylpyrazolines.

ORANGE	Sulphafurazole
YELLOW	Sulfadoxine, sulfametopyrazine, sulphachlorpyridazine, sulphadimidine, sulphaethidole, sulphamethizole, sulphamethoxazole, sulphamethoxydiazine, sulphamethoxypyridazine, sulphamoxole, sulphaphenazole, sulphapyridine, sulphasomidine, sulphathiazole, sulphinpyrazone
GREEN	Phenazone
BLUE	Dipyrone (transient)
VIOLET	Amidopyrine (transient)

No response is obtained with succinylsulphathiazole, sulfamerazine, sulfaquinoxaline, sulphacetamide, sulphadiazine, sulphadimethoxine, sulphaguanidine, and sulthiame, nor with propyphenazone.

Palladium Chloride

REAGENT. Dissolve, with the aid of heat, 0.1 g of palladium chloride in 5 ml of 2M hydrochloric acid and dilute the solution to 100 ml with water. Mix together equal volumes of this solution and of 2M sodium hydroxide. The mixed reagent is stable for several weeks.

METHOD. Mix the sample with 1 ml of the reagent and heat at 100° in a water-bath for 2 minutes. A blank solution should be treated similarly at the same time.

INDICATIONS. RED, ORANGE, YELLOW, BROWN, or BLACK colours are given by aliphatic compounds which have a sulphur atom in the chain, and by aromatic compounds which have a sulphur atom in the side-chain. However, no colour is given when an S-alkyl chain is present, unless the chain is terminated by an halogenated group.

No response is obtained if the sulphur is in a group linking two rings. Reducing agents such as ascorbic acid, chloral hydrate, chloroform, and glucose, and compounds containing a chain with a hydrazine link (—NH—NH—,—NH—NH$_2$), give a translucent dark GREY or BLACK colour, but do not give the gradual yellow to orange to brown colour which is seen with sulphur-containing compounds. Compounds containing adjacent hydroxyl groups on an aromatic ring give ORANGE colours turning BROWN.

RED	Gloxazone
ORANGE	Adrenaline (→ brown), benserazide (→ brown), bitoscanate, captopril, carbidopa (→ brown), carbimazole, disulfiram, dobutamine (→ brown), ecothiopate, isoetharine (→ brown), levodopa (→ brown), methallibure, methimazole, polythiazide, rimiterol, thiacetazone, thiopentone
Brown-orange	Demeton-S
YELLOW	Clindamycin, dazomet, dimercaprol, dimethoate, methisazone (→ orange → brown), penicillamine
Orange-yellow	Thialbarbitone
BROWN	Ambazone, azinphos-methyl, dihydrostreptomycin (slow), ethionamide, malathion, noxythiolin, parathion, phosalone, prothionamide, spironolactone, thiram
Orange-brown	Chlorthiamid, diazinon, disulfoton, fenitrothion, formothion, phorate, vamidothion
Black-brown	Di-allate, dichlofluanid, tri-allate
GREY	Chlorfenvinphos

BLACK	Ascorbic acid, captan, chloral hydrate, chloroform, mebanazine, nifuratel, phenelzine, procarbazine, sulphasalazine, sulphaurea, trichlorfon

Phosphorus Test

METHOD. To the sample add 0.5 ml of *nitric acid* and 0.2 ml of *sulphuric acid*, heat at 100° in a water-bath for 30 minutes, cool, add 1 ml of a 10% solution of ammonium molybdate, and replace in the water-bath at 100° for 5 minutes. A blank solution should be treated at the same time. For some compounds, the reaction may occur after shorter heating times than those stated above.

INDICATIONS. A bright YELLOW solution or precipitate indicates the presence of phosphorus and suggests an organophosphorus pesticide, especially if the sample is a water-immiscible liquid. Cyclophosphamide and triclofos also react.

Potassium Dichromate

METHOD 1. Dissolve the sample in 0.5 ml of 2M hydrochloric acid and add a few crystals of potassium dichromate with shaking.

INDICATIONS. An immediate BROWN colour, or a GREEN colour changing to BROWN, indicates the presence of an aminophenol or of a phenol having two or more hydroxy groups in adjacent positions on the ring. Monophenols, halogenated phenols, and phenols with hydroxyl groups *meta* to each other react more slowly or not at all.

RED	Carbidopa
YELLOW (→ BROWN)	Phenol (2 min)
GREEN (→ BROWN)	Adrenaline, dopamine, hexoprenaline, isoetharine, isoprenaline, levodopa, methyldopa, methyldopate, noradrenaline, rimiterol
Blue-green	Aniline (2 min)
BROWN	Benserazide, o-cresol (30 s), m-cresol (2 min), orciprenaline (slow), protokylol (→ red-brown on warming), terbutaline (slow)
Green-brown	Dobutamine

METHOD 2. If the sample is a liquid, add 1 to 2 drops to 1 ml of water followed by 1 ml of a saturated solution of potassium dichromate in 50% v/v sulphuric acid.

INDICATIONS. A GREEN colour is given by acetaldehyde, ethanol, isopropyl alcohol, methanol, and propanol.

Schiff's Reagent

REAGENT. Dissolve 0.2 g of basic magenta (fuchsin, CI 42510) in 120 ml of hot water, cool, add 20 ml of a 10% solution of sodium hydrogen sulphite and 2 ml of *hydrochloric acid*, and dilute to 200 ml. Store at 4°, protected from light.

METHOD. Add the sample to 1 ml of the reagent.

INDICATIONS. A VIOLET colour indicates the presence of an aliphatic aldehyde. The longer the carbon chain length and especially if it is branched, the weaker the response to the test.

Simon's Test

REAGENT. Dissolve 1 g of sodium nitroprusside in 50 ml of water and add 2 ml of acetaldehyde to the solution with thorough mixing.

METHOD. Add the sample to 1 ml of the reagent.

INDICATIONS. A BLUE colour indicates a secondary aliphatic amine or an unsubstituted heterocyclic amine as its free base.

Sodium Dithionite

REAGENT. A 5% solution of sodium dithionite in a 10% solution of sodium hydroxide.

METHOD. Apply the reagent to the sample either on a white tile or as a solution in a test-tube. A blank solution should be treated similarly at the same time.

INDICATIONS. Colours are produced by bis(pyridyl) compounds.

GREEN	Diquat
BLUE	Paraquat

Dark colours are likely to be given by certain metallic solutions because of reduction.

Sodium Nitroprusside

REAGENT. A 1% solution of sodium nitroprusside.

METHOD 1. Add the sample to 2 ml of the reagent followed by 1 drop of 2M sodium hydroxide.

INDICATIONS. RED or ORANGE-RED colours are given by acetaldehyde and by ketones containing at least one alkyl group.

METHOD 2. Mix the sample with a minimum volume of 2M sodium hydroxide, evaporate to dryness, dissolve the residue in 2 drops of water, and add 0.5 ml of the reagent.

INDICATIONS. A VIOLET colour is given by substances containing labile sulphur in the molecule and by unsubstituted dithiocarbamates.

METHOD 3. Carry out Method 2, above, but after

evaporation to dryness heat the residue until it is yellow or orange in colour before proceeding.

INDICATIONS. A VIOLET colour is given by certain substances containing labile sulphur which do not react to Method 2, e.g. chlormethiazole, lincomycin, and monosulfiram.

Sodium Picrate

REAGENT. To a saturated solution of picric acid add sufficient sodium carbonate to make the solution strongly alkaline.

METHOD. Mix the sample with a little manganese dioxide and heat to dull redness whilst holding a piece of filter paper, impregnated with the reagent, in the vapours issuing from the tube.

INDICATIONS. The yellow colour of the filter paper

changes from ORANGE to BROWN-ORANGE and then to ORANGE-RED or RED in the presence of cyanide. Positive results are given by compounds containing cyanide groups, e.g. cimetidine, diphenoxylate, and isoaminile.

Sulphuric Acid

METHOD. Apply *sulphuric acid* directly to the sample on a white tile or in a test-tube.

INDICATIONS. A range of colours is obtained with compounds of various types. Steroids give ORANGE or YELLOW colours, many of which fluoresce under ultraviolet light (350 nm) either immediately or after dilution (see below). Thioxanthenes give RED or ORANGE colours which fluoresce under ultraviolet light (350 nm).

RED	Caramiphen (when warmed), danthron, fenitrothion, mequitazine (slowly at 100°), methacycline, metopimazine, nuarimol, pipoxolan
Orange-red	*Oxprenolol, quinomethionate
Violet-red	Morantel, oxytetracycline
PINK	Doxylamine, indapamide (slow)
ORANGE	Alprenolol, amitriptyline, benactyzine, benzilonium, benzquinamide, benzyl nicotinate, *chlorprothixene, clidinium, *clopenthixol, cyclothiazide (→ red-brown), diethylthiambutene, diphemanil, diphenhydramine, diphenidol, doxepin, *flupenthixol, indomethacin, mazindol, mebanazine, mecoprop, methapyrilene, methindizate, *methixene, methyclothiazide, methylpiperidyl benzilate, naproxen, nefopam, nifedipine, nortriptyline, orphenadrine, penthienate methobromide, polythiazide, pyrantel (→ violet), rotenone, *thiothixene, tofenacin
YELLOW	Acebutolol, amiloride, amiodarone, benzthiazide, broxaldine, broxyquinoline, cinchophen, clefamide, clemastine (green rim), cyclopenthiazide, diphenadione, doxycycline, enoxolone, fenbufen, frusemide, halquinol, *hydroquinidine, *hydroquinine, lorazepam, methyl benzoquate, 5-methyltryptamine, α-methyltryptamine, N-methyltryptamine, metolazone, minocycline, piperacetazine (→ red), procyclidine, *quinidine, *quinine, rimiterol, salbutamol, salinazid, sodium cromoglycate, trichlormethiazide, veratrine (→ violet), zomepirac
Orange-yellow	Ethyl biscoumacetate, hexoprenaline, pizotifen (→ violet)
GREEN	Phenothiazine, protriptyline
BLUE	
Brown-blue	Chlortetracycline, demeclocycline
VIOLET	Bendrofluazide, chlorotrianisene, *chromonar, clofazimine, cyproheptadine, dothiepin, mesoridazine (→ blue), methylenedioxyamphetamine, nicergoline, perazine, phenindione, rolitetracycline, tetracycline
Red-violet	Trifluomeprazine
BROWN	Chelidonine, sulindac
Red-brown	Lymecycline
Orange-brown	Biperiden, ouabain (slow)
Yellow-brown	Tylosin (slow)
Grey-brown	Octaphonium
BLACK	
Blue-black	Clomocycline

* Fluoresce under ultraviolet light (350 nm)

REACTIONS OF STEROIDS WITH SULPHURIC ACID

Initial colour	Compound	Fluorescence at 350 nm	Fluorescence after dilution
RED			
Orange-red	Dienoestrol	nil	nil
	Dimethisterone	nil	yellow
	Mestranol	yellow	orange (pink in daylight)
PINK			
Orange-pink	Dexamethasone	nil	nil
	Prednisolone	nil	green (red in daylight)
ORANGE	Beclomethasone (slow)	nil	nil
	Cholesterol	nil	white
	Dydrogesterone	green-yellow	green-yellow
	Fludrocortisone	green	green (dichroic in daylight)
	Norethandrolone	green-yellow	—
	Norethisterone	orange	orange (violet in daylight)
	Norethynodrel	orange	orange
	Oxymetholone	nil	nil
	Spironolactone (→ yellow-green)	yellow-green	green
	Stilboestrol	nil	nil
	Triamcinolone	nil	nil → green (slow)
Red-orange	Ethinyloestradiol	orange	orange (red in daylight)
Pink-orange	Betamethasone	nil	nil
Green, orange (dichroic)	Hydrocortisone	green	green
YELLOW	Alphadolone	nil	nil
	Androsterone	nil	white
	Carbenoxolone	nil	yellow
	Cortisone	green	green
	Deoxycortone	green-yellow	yellow (violet in daylight)
	Enoxolone	nil	green-yellow
	Fluocinolone	green	quenched
	Fluoxymesterone	green	quenched
	Flurandrenolone	green	quenched
	Hydroxyprogesterone	green	quenched
	Oestradiol	green	green (orange in daylight)
	Prednisone	green	green
	Progesterone	green	quenched
Orange-yellow	Fluocortolone	(weak)	(weak)
Green-yellow	Oestrone	green	green-yellow (orange in daylight)
NO COLOUR	Oestriol	yellow-green	quenched (orange in daylight)
	Testosterone	green	nil

Sulphuric Acid–Fuming Sulphuric Acid

REAGENT. Mix together 7 ml of *sulphuric acid* and 3 ml of *fuming sulphuric acid*.

METHOD. Dissolve the sample in a minimum volume of toluene and add 1 or 2 drops of the reagent.

INDICATIONS. A RED colour appearing in the lower acid layer indicates the presence of dieldrin (colour develops quickly) or aldrin (colour develops slowly). A PINK-ORANGE colour is obtained with endrin.

Thalleioquin Test

METHOD. Dissolve the sample in a minimum volume of 2M hydrochloric acid, add 2 drops of *bromine solution*, place 1 drop of the mixture on a piece of filter paper, and expose the paper to ammonia fumes.

INDICATIONS. A GREEN colour indicates the presence of a quinine-type structure, e.g. hydroquinidine, hydroquinine, quinidine, and quinine. Cinchonidine and cinchonine do not respond.

Vanillin Reagent

REAGENT. Dissolve 1 g of vanillin in 20 ml of *sulphuric acid*, warming if necessary.

METHOD. Add 2 drops of the reagent to the sample, heat in a water-bath at 100° for 30 seconds, and note any colour which is produced. Dilute the cooled mixture by adding a few drops of water and note any change of colour.

INDICATIONS. Many compounds of different chemical structure react with this reagent. However, for barbiturates, the reaction appears to be a steric phenomenon which depends on the structure of the side-chain at the 5-position. Dark colours which are either dispelled or changed to violet, blue, or green by dilution are produced when either side-chain is greater than 2 carbon atoms in length, or contains a cycloalkene ring. Branching can be proximal to the pyrimidine ring but not distal. No colour is obtained if both side-chains are less than 3 carbon atoms in length, or if either is branched distally or contains an aryl nucleus. Long, straight, saturated chains also appear to hinder reaction. Hydroxy-barbiturates give positive responses, but bemegride, glutethimide, phenytoin, and primidone do not respond.

REACTIONS OF BARBITURATES WITH VANILLIN REAGENT

Colour after heating	Compound	Colour after dilution
RED	3'-Hydroxybuto-barbitone	violet (transient)
Violet-red	Heptabarbitone	colourless
	3'-Hydroxyamylo-barbitone	colourless
Brown-red	Cyclobarbitone	green
	Cyclopentobarbitone	green
	Pentobarbitone	violet
	Quinalbarbitone	violet
	Thiopentone	violet
ORANGE	Butalbital (weak)	colourless
	Secbutobarbitone (weak)	violet

Colour after heating	Compound	Colour after dilution
Brown-orange	Allobarbitone	violet (transient)
	Brallobarbitone	brown-orange
	Talbutal	violet
	Thialbarbitone	violet (transient)
BROWN	Hexobarbitone	violet
Violet-brown	Methohexitone	colourless
	Vinbarbitone	colourless
	3'-Hydroxypento-barbitone	colourless

No response is obtained with amylobarbitone, aprobarbitone, barbitone, butobarbitone, enallyl-propymal, hexethal, ibomal, idobutal, metharbitone, methylphenobarbitone, nealbarbitone, phenobarbitone, or phenylmethylbarbituric acid. With the cold reagent, an ORANGE colour is produced by pentobarbitone, quinalbarbitone, and thiopentone, and a BROWN colour by cyclopentobarbitone.

Bibliography

F. Bamford, *Poisons, Their Isolation and Identification*, 3rd Edn, London, Churchill, 1951.

K. W. Bentley, *The Chemistry of Morphine Alkaloids*, Oxford, Clarendon Press, 1954.

E. G. C. Clarke, The Isolation and Identification of Alkaloids, in *Methods of Forensic Science*, Vol. 1, F. Lundquist (Ed.), London, Wiley, 1962, pp. 1–241.

Drug Identification, C. A. Johnson and A. D. Thornton-Jones (Ed.), London, The Pharmaceutical Press, 1966.

F. Fiegl, *Spot Tests in Organic Analysis*, 7th Edn, Amsterdam, Elsevier, 1966.

T. A. Gonzales *et al.*, Colour Reactions for the Identification of Non-volatile Organic Poisons, in *Legal Medicine, Pathology and Toxicology*, 2nd Edn, New York, Appleton-Century-Crofts, 1954, pp. 1191–1255.

Immunoassays

M. J. Stewart

Immunoassays now have a firm place among routine methods for the analysis of drugs in biological fluids. The popularity of radioimmunoassays has been ensured by the high sensitivity, the lack of necessity for a preliminary extraction stage, and the applicability to the analysis of large numbers of samples. The more recent developments, notably in optical immunoassays, also offer a variety of rapid methods which are suitable for emergency analysis and for therapeutic drug monitoring.

BASIC PRINCIPLES OF IMMUNOASSAYS

The immunoassay technique uses an antibody specific for the drug being assayed, and a labelled form of the same drug. The method depends on the ability of the drug being assayed to compete in the reaction between the antibody and the labelled drug. Ideally the labelled drug should be such that it takes part in the reaction as though it were the unlabelled drug, but this ideal is not always fully satisfied. The label may be a particular radioisotope, an active enzyme, or a fluorescent label, incorporated synthetically.

The basic technique consists of placing a fixed quantity of the antibody in a tube together with a fixed quantity of the labelled drug, and the test sample containing the drug to be assayed. The specific binding sites on the antibody bind both the labelled drug molecules (Drug*), and the unlabelled drug molecules present in the test sample. The proportion of labelled drug molecules bound is inversely proportional to the number of unlabelled drug molecules.

$$\text{Drug*} + \text{Drug} + \text{Antibody} \rightleftharpoons \begin{array}{c} \text{Drug*–Antibody} \\ + \\ \text{Drug–Antibody} \end{array}$$

'Free Drug' 'Bound Drug'

A suitable analytical measurement is then made and the results are compared with a calibration curve.

In radioimmunoassays, the measurement is of radioactivity. However, there is no difference between the signals produced by bound and free labelled-drug so that it is necessary to separate the two before measurement (p. 150). These assays are referred to as *heterogeneous immunoassays*. Since the amount of radiolabelled drug remaining in the solution, or bound to the antibody, depends on the concentration of unlabelled drug, measurement of the radiolabelled drug in either the bound or the free form will give an estimation of the original concentration of unlabelled drug. A calibration curve is constructed in which the percentage of radiolabelled drug bound to the antibody is plotted against the concentration of drug (Fig. 1). Other ways of generating standard curves are described later.

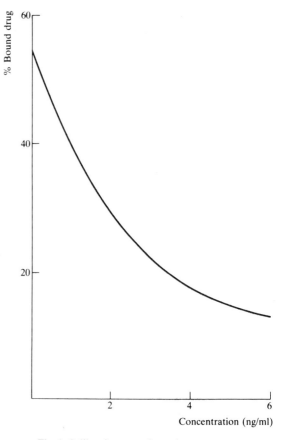

Fig. 1. Calibration curve for an immunoassay.

In assays where the drug is labelled with an enzyme or a fluorescent substance, the measurement is of an optically detected change such as ultraviolet absorption, fluorescence, or luminescence. In these optical immunoassays, there is a difference between the signals generated by the free and the bound labelled-drug. Thus, no separation step is necessary and they are referred to as *homogeneous immunoassays*. The difference between the signals may arise because the signal is suppressed on binding, produced on binding, or altered on binding.

Homogeneous assay systems have obvious advantages over radioimmunoassays, in that no separation stage is necessary and the difficulties of working with radioisotopes are avoided. However, they have the disadvantage of reduced sensitivity because the optical signal is measured in the presence of the original biological fluid, albeit diluted. Consequently, commercial homogeneous optical immunoassays are applicable only to measurements of drugs down to a few ng/ml. For measurement of concentrations below this, radioimmunoassay remains the current method of choice, although heterogeneous optical immunoassays could offer similar sensitivity.

Production of the Antibody

In general, drugs have molecular weights which are too low for them to act as antigens, i.e. to produce antibodies when injected into an animal. It is necessary, therefore, to couple the drug to a larger molecule which is usually a protein. The most commonly used protein is albumin (molecular weight approximately 70 000), taken from a species other than that in which the antibody is to be raised. Before the antigen is prepared and purified, it is necessary to decide on the required specificity. In some cases, there may be advantages in producing an antibody with low specificity in order to detect all of a family of drugs.

The coupling of a drug to a protein such as bovine serum albumin may be carried out by a variety of methods depending on the reactive sites on the drug, and the specificity required. As an example, the production of an antibody to pentobarbitone is shown in Fig. 2. If antigen A is used, the antibody which is produced is insensitive to changes at position 5 and will therefore react, not only with pentobarbitone, but also with other 5,5-disubstituted barbiturates such as barbitone, phenobarbitone, and 5-hydroxy metabolites. However, it will not react with drugs or metabolites which have modifications in positions 1 or 3. If a more specific antibody is required, then a longer chain length between position 5 and the protein must be used, or the protein should be linked to an alternative position on the ring, as illustrated for antigen B.

Injections into the animals are made with the antigen in Freund's complete adjuvant. This adjuvant contains a neutral detergent, paraffin oil, and killed mycobacteria; its purpose is to release the antigen slowly and to speed the production of antibodies by stimulating the immunological response of the animal. Serial multiple injections of small amounts of antigen provide the most satisfactory results. If large quantities of antiserum are required, then large animals such as sheep are preferred. However, some animals provide antisera of a higher titre which may be used at a greater dilution. After about 12 days, samples of blood are

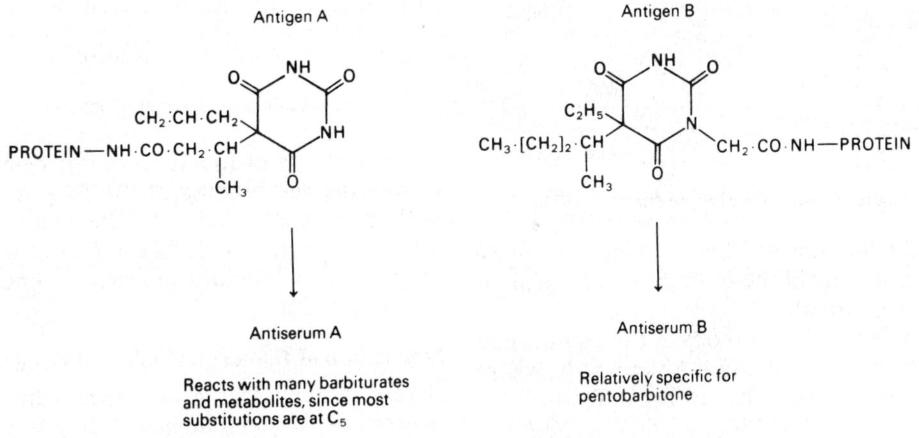

Fig. 2. Different antigens used to produce antisera for pentobarbitone.

withdrawn for testing. When a high concentration of antibody is detected, a large volume of blood is removed and the serum is separated (antiserum).
Determination of Antibody Titre. An appropriate dilution of the serum containing the antibody is used, depending on the quantities of drug to be assayed. The appropriate quantity of labelled drug is chosen, depending on the requirements of sensitivity, accuracy, and ease of sample preparation, and serial dilutions of the original animal serum are made to obtain a titre such that approximately 50% of the labelled drug is bound to the antibody (Fig. 3). This dilution of the serum is then made and used in the immunoassay. If only a low titre is obtained, even after several booster shots have been given, a new batch of animals or different animals can be tried.

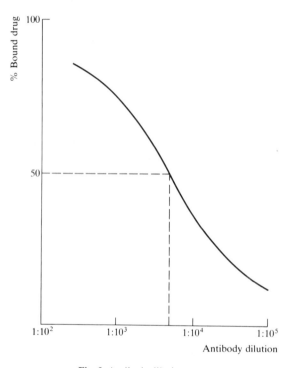

Fig. 3. Antibody dilution curve.

Antibodies vary considerably in their shelf-lives, but they are usually of the order of several years if frozen or freeze-dried.
The avidity (K) of the antibody is the equilibrium constant in the reaction $Ag+Ab \rightleftharpoons AgAb$, where Ag is the drug and Ab is the antibody. Thus

$$K=\frac{[AgAb]}{[Ag][Ab]}$$

It is calculated by the use of a Scatchard plot in which the concentration of bound drug is plotted against the ratio of bound to free drug, after correcting for non-specific binding. The steeper the slope, the lower is K (Fig. 4), and the intercept on the x-axis gives the total concentration of the antibody binding sites (mol/litre).

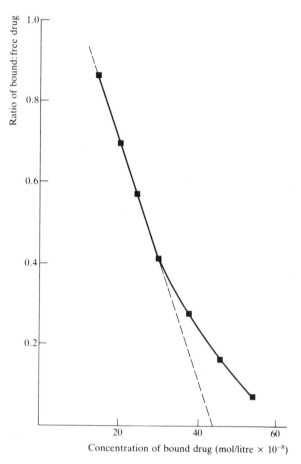

Fig. 4. Scatchard plot of drug bound to antibody.

The specificity of the antiserum is determined by comparing the binding of the drug to which the antiserum is directed with the binding of other drugs and metabolites. The extent to which other drugs and metabolites interfere is known as *cross-reactivity*.

Separation of Bound and Unbound Drug

Before an analytical measurement can be made, it is necessary to separate bound drug from unbound drug in radioimmunoassays and also, if the highest sensitivity is required, in optical immunoassays.

The separation step gives rise to some of the greatest imprecision, and can be greatly influenced by endogenous components in the biological fluid; a system which works well with plasma may not give an efficient separation in urine. These effects can be reduced by the use of high dilutions of the biological fluid but sensitivity is also reduced.

Adsorption with charcoal has been widely used as a separation technique, but a variety of more precise and simpler methods are now available (Table 1). The methods of choice are the double antibody technique, and solid-phase systems. These are also the most easily automated.

Table 1. Methods of separating bound and free drug

Method	Agent used
Adsorption of free drug	Charcoal coated with dextran
	Porous beads
	Filter paper
Precipitation of drug–antibody complex	Ammonium sulphate
	Double antibody
	Polyethylene glycol
Immobilised antibody	Antibody bound to the walls of tubes or to plastic beads or rods
	Magnetic particles

Charcoal Adsorption. This adsorbs the free fraction and the charcoal can be separated by centrifugation or by filtration. Obviously if too strong an adsorbent is used, e.g. activated charcoal, it may also adsorb the bound fraction. To prevent this, the charcoal is often coated with dextran or gelatin.

Double Antibody Technique. Although the drug–antibody complex is large it is still soluble. It can be converted into an insoluble form, which can be centrifuged, by the addition of a second antibody (the precipitating antibody) raised against the globulins of the animal in which the first antibody was raised. The free fraction is then simply decanted out of the tube.

Solid-phase Systems. The antibody to the drug is covalently attached to the inside walls of a plastic tube or to solid particles or rods. After incubation, the drug–antibody complex remains attached to the tube or to the particles (Fig. 5). The free drug may then be discarded and the solid phase washed. It is then possible either to measure the amount of bound labelled drug directly, e.g. by counting gamma emission, or, in the case of optical immunoassays, to dissociate the bound labelled drug, resuspend it in a solution, and measure the optical signal.

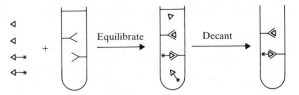

Fig. 5. Solid-phase immunoassay.

Magnetic Particles. Separation may be achieved by using an antibody bound to magnetic particles. This method has been used in fluoroimmunoassays and is described on p. 155.

Techniques for the coupling of antibodies to cellulose particles or tubes were initially unreliable, time-consuming, and hazardous as they involved toxic reagents such as cyanogen bromide. A simple and convenient method is now available which employs 1,1-carbonyldi-imidazole to couple antibody to microcrystalline cellulose.

RADIOIMMUNOASSAY

The principal components in radioimmunoassay (RIA) are a drug labelled with a suitable radioisotope, an antibody specific to that drug, and the assay sample. The drug–antibody complex (bound drug) must be separated from the free drug in the later stages of the assay.

The amounts of antiserum (containing the antibody) and of labelled drug are chosen such that the radioactivity is divided approximately equally between the bound and free fractions. Drug from the sample competes with the radiolabelled drug for the antibody binding sites. After allowing an appropriate time for equilibration (incubation period), the bound and free phases are separated. The radioactivity of either phase may then be measured and plotted as described below. Each assay must include standards covering the range of concentrations being measured, and blank solutions; all assays should be carried out in duplicate.

RADIOISOTOPE-LABELLING OF DRUGS

Tritium (^{3}H), carbon-14 (^{14}C), and iodine-125 (^{125}I) are the three isotopes used in radioimmunoassays; Table 2 gives their radioactive properties and some counting data. The manufacture of ^{3}H- and ^{14}C-labelled drugs can be carried out using the normal synthetic route of the drug or, in the case of tritium, by hydrogenation of the molecule or by exchange with tritiated water.

Table 2. Properties of radioisotopes used in RIA

Element	Symbol	Half-life	Radiation emitted	Energy keV	Counting efficiency %	Back-ground counts/minute
Tritium	^{3}H	12.3 years	Beta	18	60–65	20–30
Carbon-14	^{14}C	5730 years	Beta	155	93–98	20–30
Iodine-125	^{125}I	60 days	X and Gamma	27	60–65	20–30

Since few drugs contain iodine it is necessary to add iodine to the molecule, e.g. *ortho* to a phenolic group, or, if this is not possible, to iodinate a suitable derivative of the drug. For example, a tyrosine derivative of digoxin can be made from digoxigenin (via the 3 position and a succinic acid linkage) and lysergide can be bonded to a synthetic polymer (L-glutamine-L-lysine-L-alanine-L-tyrosine)$_n$. In the above cases the tyrosyl group can then be iodinated in the *ortho* position to the phenol. The iodination is carried out with a solution of radioactive sodium iodide in an aqueous phosphate buffer containing chloramine, and the radiolabelled drug is separated from the components of the reaction mixture by gel filtration, adsorption chromatography, or electrophoresis.

Tritium-labelled assays are more common than carbon-14 assays which are often less sensitive; an exception is the ^{14}C-labelled assay for paraquat (D. Fatori and W. M. Hunter, *Clinica chim. Acta*, 1980, *100*, 81–90; T. Levitt, *Proc. Analyt. Div. Chem. Soc.*, 1979, *16*, 72–76) which has proved useful in emergency cases and has acceptable accuracy despite a very short counting period of 1 minute.

MEASUREMENT OF RADIOACTIVITY

Two methods of measuring radioactivity are used in RIA, namely, liquid-scintillation counting and γ-counting. In liquid-scintillation counting, the radioisotope is placed in a scintillation mixture and the emission of visible light is measured; fresh vials containing the scintillation mixture are required for each measurement. γ-Counting is usually performed in a crystal-scintillation counter; the vial containing the radioisotope is placed directly into the counter and counted for a fixed length of time. β-Radiation can only be measured by means of liquid-scintillation counting whereas γ-radiation may be measured by either crystal-scintillation or liquid-scintillation counting.

The relative advantages of using a β-emitter (^{3}H and ^{14}C), rather than a γ-emitter are:

1. ^{3}H and ^{14}C have long half-lives compared to ^{125}I and thus have relatively long shelf-lives.

2. Radiation hazards from β-emitters with low specific activity are minimal.
3. ^{3}H and ^{14}C may be incorporated into the drug molecule without altering its molecular arrangement. Thus the labelled drug binds to the antibody in an identical manner to the unlabelled drug; this may not be true if the iodinated form of the drug is used.
4. The radioisotopes may be incorporated into the molecule during synthesis, avoiding further manipulation (as in iodination) which may damage it.

The advantages of using a γ-emitter, e.g. ^{125}I, are:

1. Measurement of γ-rays by crystal-scintillation counting is much cheaper and quicker than liquid-scintillation counting.
2. Extraction and purification of the sample containing ^{125}I is not required as γ-rays penetrate coloured solutions and soft tissue with negligible loss of energy. In the case of β-emitters, the scintillation solution must be colourless or quenching corrections must be applied.
3. Higher specific activities can be obtained with ^{125}I labels and therefore the counting time can be reduced, e.g. from 20 minutes to 1 minute. (Specific activity is the radioactivity per unit mass of drug, e.g. MBq/μg, where 1 Bq = 1 disintegration/second = 2.7×10^{-11} Ci.) Approximately 5000 atoms, 100 atoms, and 1 atom of ^{14}C, ^{3}H, and ^{125}I, respectively, are needed to produce the same number of disintegrations per minute because of the different half-lives.

OPTICAL IMMUNOASSAY

Optical immunoassays have a number of advantages over radioimmunoassays (Table 3), mainly because the reagents are stable and homogeneous assays can be produced simply. Various labels can

Table 3. Comparison of radioimmunoassays and homogeneous optical immunoassays

	Radio-immunoassay	Optical immunoassay
Special safety precautions	yes	no
Simple labelling procedures	yes	yes
Limited shelf-life of labelled drug	yes	no
Separation step necessary	yes	no
Measurement time	moderate	short
Precision	moderate	high
Sensitivity	1 pg/ml	1 ng/ml
Automation	partial	full
Signal susceptible to interference	no	yes

be used including enzymes, and fluorescent or chemiluminescent labels.

Commercial optical immunoassays are usually homogeneous, but for the highest sensitivity, separation of bound drug from unbound drug is required.

Enzyme Immunoassays

The principal components in enzyme immuno-assays are a drug labelled with a specific enzyme, an antibody specific to the drug, a substrate capable of producing a measurable optical signal when catalysed by the enzyme, and the sample for assay. When the enzyme-labelled drug is bound to the antibody, the activity of the enzyme is inhibited or reduced (Fig. 6). The drug in the sample displaces a proportion of the enzyme-labelled drug from the antibody, thus activating the enzyme which then acts on the substrate and changes its optical properties (ultraviolet absorption, turbidity, etc.). The change in enzyme activity and hence the change in the optical signal is proportional to the amount of free drug added to the drug–enzyme–antibody complex. The optical signal produced is amplified because the displaced enzyme catalyses numerous conversions of the substrate.

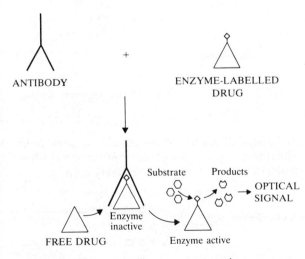

Fig. 6. Mechanism for a homogeneous enzyme immunoassay.

Enzyme immunoassays are also amenable to kinetic measurement. The rate of substrate conversion is proportional to the enzyme activity. Hence an analysis, for example, of the rate of change of ultraviolet absorption may be useful for samples which have a high background absorption.

ENZYME-LABELLING OF DRUGS

The addition of an enzyme molecule to a drug increases the molecular weight considerably but, despite this, it is possible to produce enzyme-labelled drugs which bind to the antibody in a similar manner to the unlabelled drug within a period of only one or two minutes. The simplest linkages are made through —COOH or —NH$_2$ groups on the drug molecule.

A variety of enzymes is employed, such as horse-radish peroxidase, bacterial glucose-6-phosphate dehydrogenase (G6PDH), and muramidase (lyso-zyme). The choice of enzyme depends on the reaction and hence the signal to be measured. Interference from endogenous enzyme activity must be avoided. This may be done by simply ensuring that enzymes of similar substrate-specificity as the label are not present in the sample. Another approach is illustrated by the use of G6PDH as the label. The enzyme is derived from bacteria and requires nicotinamide-adenine dinucleotide (NAD) as the coenzyme. Interference from human G6PDH in serum is avoided because that requires nicotinamide-adenine dinucleotide phosphate (NADP) as the coenzyme.

The method of linking the enzyme to the drug must also be chosen carefully. Antibodies raised by the injection of a drug–protein conjugate may be directed to the drug–protein linkage as well as to the drug. If the enzyme is linked to the drug in the same manner, the enzyme-labelled drug will bind more avidly to the antibody than the unlabelled drug, thus invalidating the assumption that the binding characteristics of the labelled and un-labelled drug are similar. In order to overcome this problem, different linkages should be used for binding drug to protein and drug to enzyme.

Enzyme immunoassays have been widely adopted because the method is extremely rapid and simple, and therefore enables drug analyses to be carried out in a variety of locations. The sample volume required is about 10 to 50 μl, thus making analyses possible on capillary specimens or on samples from neonates. The technique is available in kit form, with high quality reagents and all the necessary standard solutions, thus reducing the requirements for operator skill. In cases where large numbers of analyses are required, the assays may be carried out on a variety of automated analysers.

The disadvantages of enzyme immunoassays lie in their cost and relative insensitivity compared to radioimmunoassays.

Enzyme immunoassays which utilise ultraviolet

absorbance as the measured end-point may be given increased sensitivity if the end-point is converted to a fluorescent measurement.

Fluoroimmunoassays

A variety of immunoassay techniques employ changes in the fluorescent properties of molecules to measure drug concentrations. Labelling of drugs with such molecules avoids the hazards of working with radioisotopes. Fluoroimmunoassays (FIA) also offer enhanced sensitivity in comparison to enzyme immunoassays; they may be homogeneous or heterogeneous.

The choice of fluorophore has a considerable effect upon the sensitivity of the assay, and depends on the assay conditions. Ideally, the fluorophore should have a large Stokes shift (p. 233), it should be easily differentiated from endogenous fluorophores, and should be capable of being coupled simply to the drug. Fluorescein satisfies all these requirements and is the most popular fluorophore used.

Homogeneous Fluoroimmunoassays

In commercial *substrate-labelled fluoroimmunoassay* an enzyme is used to release the fluorophore from the labelled drug molecule. Fig. 7 illustrates the mechanism. One such technique requires a drug labelled with the fluorogen β-galactosyl-umbelliferone (enzyme substrate), a drug-specific antibody, the enzyme β-galactosidase, and the sample. The enzyme hydrolyses the β-galactosyl-umbelliferone linkage to yield a fluorescent species. However, the enzyme cannot gain access to the labelled drug when it is bound to the antibody. Drug from the sample competes with the labelled drug for the antibody binding sites and any unbound labelled drug is hydrolysed by the enzyme. The intensity of fluorescence is therefore proportional to the amount of drug present in the sample.

Another technique, called *fluorescence polarisation immunoassay*, exploits the difference in rotation of bound and free fluorophore-labelled drug. Polarised light incident on a fluorophore-labelled molecule produces emission of plane-polarised light. However, as the labelled drug molecule rotates during the period between absorption and emission of light, the amount of polarised light emitted in any given plane is reduced. Binding of the molecule to antibody reduces the rotation and this increases the intensity of polarised light emitted in a particular plane.

The assay requires the use of a polarising attachment to the fluorimeter, containing liquid crystal

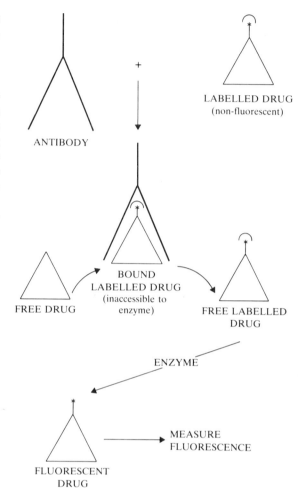

Fig. 7. Mechanism for a substrate-labelled fluoroimmunoassay.

polarising filters which are capable of measuring the emitted light in two planes at 90° to one another. Polarisation is measured in arbitrary units.

$$\text{Polarisation} = \frac{\begin{array}{c}\text{Vertically polarised light} \\ - \text{horizontally polarised light}\end{array}}{\begin{array}{c}\text{Vertically polarised light} \\ + \text{horizontally polarised light}\end{array}}$$

Thus polarisation is directly proportional to the amount of bound labelled drug and inversely proportional to the amount of free drug present. Since a change in the polarisation of the light is measured, the interference from non-specific fluorescence is minimised. However, a blank correction may be needed for drugs present in low concentrations e.g. digoxin.

All of the homogeneous fluoroimmunoassay systems suffer from the possibility of background interference from other drugs and metabolites. Enzyme labels may be inhibited by endogenous molecules, and there may be fluorescence enhancement or quenching from the same sources. This may be overcome by careful choice of assay conditions and the use of high dilutions of the biological sample.

Heterogeneous Fluoroimmunoassays

The most effective method of removing background interference is to use a heterogeneous assay such as that shown in Fig. 8. The assay uses a fluorophore-labelled drug, an antibody bound to magnetic particles, and the assay sample. Drug in the sample competes with the labelled drug for binding to the antibody. The proportion of labelled free drug is related to the amount of drug in the sample. Antibody-bound drug is separated from the free drug by applying a magnetic field. The free drug (labelled and unlabelled) in the supernatant liquid is decanted and discarded. The bound drug is eluted with a buffer, resuspended to separate the bound drug from the antibody, the antibody is sedimented by application of the magnetic field, and the fluorescence in the supernatant liquid is determined. Fluorescence intensity is inversely related to the amount of drug in the sample.

Separation of bound and free drug using antibody bound to magnetic particles avoids centrifugation, is quicker, and allows direct measurement of fluorescence in the supernatant liquid by simply sedimenting the antibody at the bottom of the assay tube by means of a magnetic field.

Other means of separation, such as ammonium sulphate precipitation and bonding of the antibody to cellulose beads may also be used for heterogeneous fluoroimmunoassays.

Fluoroimmunoassays have a number of advantages. There is a wide variety of assay types with choice of fluorophores with different wavelengths of excitation and emission. The instrumentation is simple, there is high precision of measurement of the signal, and the sensitivity is high. The reagents are economical and stable, and the method is applicable to homogeneous and heterogeneous systems.

Disadvantages of fluoroimmunoassays include interference from endogenous fluorophores, quenching of signals, and non-specific binding.

Luminescence Immunoassays

Immunoassays which employ drugs labelled with a substance which emits light when activated have been developed. The basic principles of these assays are similar to those of fluoroimmunoassays. The use of luminescent labels, however, has the advantage that light is not introduced into the system, so giving an increase in sensitivity.

Luminescence is produced chemically by molecules such as luminol following treatment with a peroxide, or enzymatically from luciferon after reaction with luciferase. Two typical reactions are given in Fig. 9. The coupling of luminescent molecules to drugs is similar to the procedure employed for fluorescent labels.

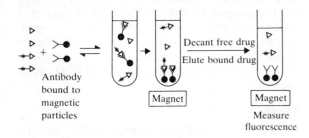

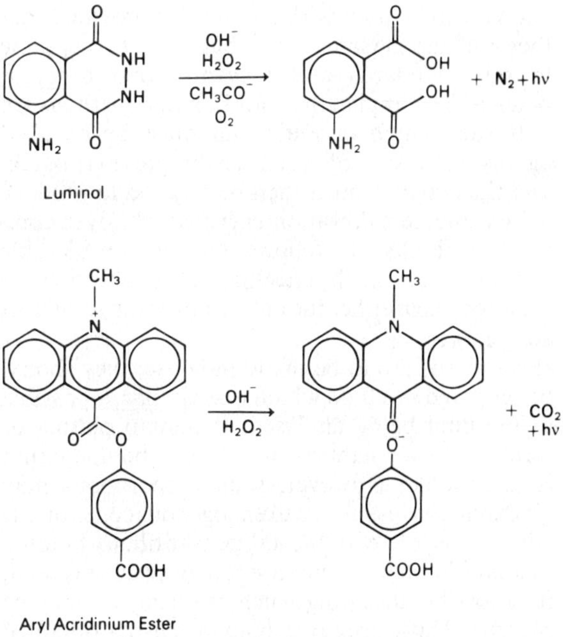

Fig. 8. Heterogeneous fluoroimmunoassay using magnetic particle separation.

Fig. 9. Typical chemiluminescence reactions used in immunoassays.

The quantum yield of luminol is relatively low and developments now in progress use the luminescent light source to excite a secondary fluorescent molecule. Luminescence, like fluorescence, is susceptible to quenching by a variety of drugs and endogenous compounds.

Luminescence is produced rapidly over a very short time-scale (300 ns), and instrumentation is required to allow reproducible and rapid mixing, coupled with accurate integration of the signal over a short time interval. Sensitivities of the order of fg/ml are theoretically possible, allowing the assay of highly diluted specimens and thus minimising interference.

Enzymes and fluorophores represent the most popular optical labels at present, but there is a wide range of alternative labels such as metal atoms and proteins, which provide alternative methods of quantification.

QUANTIFICATION OF IMMUNOASSAYS

Standardisation

Standard solutions covering the range of expected concentrations should be prepared for each assay. The shape of the calibration curve obtained will differ between batches of antisera. For this reason, manufacturers of kits provide matched standards with each kit. Standards and other reagents from one kit can be used with another kit provided that they are from the same batch, but it is not acceptable to mix standards and reagents from different batches. The implications for in-house methods are that each batch of antiserum must be checked against the standards used for the previous batch, and the reagents must then be tailored to produce an acceptable calibration curve which gives comparable results. It follows that a considerable overlap, and much checking of calibration, is required when either the antiserum or the standards are renewed.

If standards are to be made in-house, they should be prepared in a fluid which is as similar as possible to the fluid being analysed. If human plasma or serum is not available then equine or bovine serum is acceptable. However, such preparations may give spurious results due to endogenous constituents which interfere with the antigen–antibody binding reaction. If pooled human serum or plasma is used, it is possible that drugs such as diazepam may be present. Thus, drug-free human plasma obtained from volunteers is the best medium. Pooled plasma should always be checked for cross-reactivity before being used in the production of standards or quality control materials.

The weighed amount of drug should be dissolved in a suitable solvent, and then mixed with the serum or plasma; care must be taken to ensure complete mixing before packing into vials for storage. Standard solutions which have been stored frozen should be thawed gently and mixed thoroughly before use. On no account should standard solutions in biological fluids be frozen and thawed on more than one occasion as this can result in the formation of particulate matter which may cause considerable errors. The stability of the drug when stored at different temperatures should be studied, and arrangements should be made to replace expired standards.

As a final consideration, the possibility of the presence of non-specific binding of drugs by plasma proteins and the specific binding by endogenous drug-specific antibodies should be borne in mind when unexpected results are obtained from an immunoassay.

Calculation of Results

The analysis of a series of standards in an optimised immunoassay will give a calibration curve which is sigmoid in shape when binding is plotted against concentration. Such curves are difficult to plot accurately by hand, and reading from them can lead to errors. There are a number of approaches which have been adopted in order to simplify the work of the operator. The curve may be 'linearised' by plotting appropriate functions of the concentration and the measured signal, or a best-fit curve may be generated by means of a computer.

In optical immunoassays, where signal errors are minimised, the tendency has been towards one of a variety of linearised presentations employing specially designed semilogarithmic graph paper. The disadvantage of this technique is that a specific batch of graph paper is required for each batch of reagents. These charts tend to conceal the fact that the precision at the low and high ends of the line is much lower than that at the mid-point. Microprocessors, with curve storage, are now available for several immunoassay systems. These not only save on reagents and operator time, but also minimise errors.

Quality Control

Antisera from different sources differ greatly, depending on the antigen against which they were raised. Antisera produced by a standard method can be adjusted so as to provide similar reactivity, but material obtained from different manufacturers may show marked differences in specificity. Thus, although an internal quality control scheme may show excellent precision when one set of reagents is employed, comparison with other immunoassays or with non-immunoassay methods may give results which differ markedly.

The assessment of the specificity of an antiserum is the responsibility of those who raise the antiserum and develop the assay. As a basic minimum, it is necessary to check the values obtained from a wide variety of drug-free biological fluids and the cross-reactivity of metabolites and similar drugs. In addition, the effect of pathological concentrations of endogenous metabolites should be assessed; they may not cross-react with the antibody but they may have a significant effect on the binding of the drug to the antibody.

Most commercial kits contain data on cross-reactivity, but some metabolites may not be available for this assessment. In particular, water-soluble conjugates, such as glucuronides and sulphates, are seldom studied. These may not be present in the plasma of healthy persons, but in renal failure they may be present at concentrations which are sufficiently high to give a significant error even if the cross-reactivity is considerably lower than that of the parent drug. For the same reason, reagents prepared and assessed for use in plasma should not be used uncritically for the determination of drugs in urine where concentrations of metabolites may exceed those of the parent drug.

Users of immunoassays should participate in external quality assurance schemes, preferably those using samples obtained from populations of patients (see Quality Control in Clinical Analysis, p. 118). Commercial quality control sera are prepared by adding pure drugs to drug-free serum and therefore do not contain metabolites, etc., which could reveal problems associated with non-specificity.

Assuming that accuracy is satisfactory and that interfering factors are minimal, the major problem is the optimisation of precision. The major factors affecting the precision of an immunoassay are shown in Table 4. The problems relating to the initial dilution and sampling are significant and demand the use of partial automation. A range of pipetter-diluters are available which can minimise this source of error. It is useful if all additions and dilutions can be made at only one setting of the syringe. Where changes have to be made, instru-

ments with clearly marked stepped volumes are preferable to those with continuously variable settings.

Table 4. Factors contributing to imprecision in immunoassays

Factor	Comment
Dispensing errors	Affects all methods; reduced by automation
Binding kinetics	Precision is proportional to the concentration of the drug
Separation of bound and free labelled drug	Applies only to heterogeneous methods
Final measurement of labelled drug	Reproducibility is in the order optical > γ-emitter > β-emitter
Method of plotting curve	Affects all methods; precision lower at the ends of the curves

The effect of temperature on enzyme immunoassays should not be overlooked, and adequate thermostatic control is mandatory. This problem is not met with in other optical immunoassays which gives the latter some advantages.

The final measurement can contribute considerably to imprecision and for optical immunoassays is instrument-related. For radioimmunoassays, considerable improvements in both time and precision may be made by employing γ-labelled drugs and counting in a 16-head γ-counter. Scintillation counters have an accuracy of measurement which is approximately the square root of the total number of counts, e.g. about 1% counting error when measuring 10 000 counts.

The measurement of fluorescence offers potentially the most stable end-point but, since fluorescence is related to the intensity of incident light (unlike absorbance), an instrument which continually measures the ratio of emitted to incident light is necessary for the highest precision. Under these circumstances the precision of the final measurement may approach $\pm 1\%$.

Improvements in automation up to and including the final calculation step are leading to continued improvements in precision, both in large batches and for single assays.

Automation

Automated methods have advantages, in that higher precision is often possible by the elimination of operator bias. Semi-automated techniques are, however, widely used in immunoassays in order to reduce the errors associated with dispensing small volumes of viscous solutions.

A range of pipetter-diluters are available for radioimmunoassays and these are used almost universally, even for small batches. Fully automated RIA systems are available but are only economically viable in major central laboratories. Fully automated systems have the advantage that there is a standardised treatment of tubes at the critical stage of separation of bound and free drug.

Continuous flow systems are also available for RIA. One such system employs an antibody bound to cellulose-coated iron particles which may be removed using a magnetic field. In another, the antibody is bound to the walls of a mixing chamber which is reused after washing. Other continuous flow systems use resin filters which absorb the free drug and allow the bound drug to pass through, or they may use resin beads which bind the antibody–drug complex and are separated from the free drug by filtration.

Homogeneous optical immunoassays are easily automated, and instruments specifically designed for enzyme and fluoroimmunoassay are available. These instruments are capable of rapid analysis of batches as well as of single assays, with standardisation and quality control data held in microprocessors.

APPLICATIONS OF IMMUNOASSAYS

Radioimmunoassay is the method of choice for cardiac glycosides, insulin, lysergide, cannabinoids, and opiates where blood concentrations and/or sample volumes are low. Other applications include screening for drug abuse, the investigation of cases of poisoning, and therapeutic drug monitoring.

Screening for Drug Abuse

Although gas chromatographic methods exist for amphetamines and narcotic alkaloids in urine, quantitative measurement in plasma is a difficult analytical problem. Radioimmunoassay and optical immunoassay methods are available for a variety of these drugs in urine, but there is a wide range of antibodies with different cross-reactivities. Methods for the measurement of these compounds in plasma are restricted to radioimmunoassay because the majority of optical assays are not sufficiently sensitive. Assays employing antibodies of wide specificity are often employed as a means of determining whether one or more of a group of drugs is present. Such assays can be adapted to the measurement of individual drugs and their metabolites by using fractions collected from an HPLC separation.

Investigation of Poisoning

Most of the commercial immunoassays currently available are designed for the analysis of drugs at concentrations up to 2 or 3 times the therapeutic concentration. These kits may be used on diluted samples from poisoned patients in which there may be concentrations up to 10 or 20 times the therapeutic concentration. However, care should be taken when interpreting results because high concentrations of other drugs or metabolites may be present and these may cross-react. For example, an enzyme immunoassay for benzodiazepines may be used for screening for this group of drugs in cases of overdose, but the presence of up to four pharmacologically active metabolites from one parent drug, each with different cross-reactivities, makes interpretation difficult.

Sometimes a relatively non-specific assay for a group of compounds, e.g. barbiturates, can be used and, if a positive result is obtained, it can be followed by specific analyses for individual barbiturates.

Therapeutic Drug Monitoring

Homogeneous optical immunoassays are ideal for use in therapeutic drug monitoring because their speed and simplicity allow the analysis to be performed sufficiently quickly to permit clinical decisions to be made. This type of analysis has proved most beneficial for the aminoglycoside antibiotics gentamicin, and tobramycin, for methotrexate when used in high dosage, and for theophylline in neonates. For these drugs, the rapid return of accurate results can make a major contribution to patient care.

Those drugs for which immunoassays are specifically advocated in therapeutic drug monitoring are indicated in the Table on p. 107.

Bibliography

T. Chard, *An Introduction to Radioimmunoassay and Related Techniques*, Amsterdam, Elsevier, North-Holland, 1981.

L. Edwards, Product Guide for Radioassays and Non-Isotopic Ligand Assays, 3rd Edn, *Clin. Chem.*, 1983, *29*, 891–986.

Immunoassays for Clinical Chemistry, W. M. Hunter and J. J. Corrie (Ed.), 2nd Edn, Edinburgh, Churchill Livingstone, 1983.

Linscott's Catalog of Immunological and Biological Reagents, 1st Edn, Mid Valley, Ca., W. D. Linscott and N. C. Linscott, 1980.

J. Landon and A. C. Moffat, The Radioimmunoassay of Drugs, *Analyst, Lond.*, 1976, *101*, 225–243.

V. Marks, Immunoassay for Drugs, in *Therapeutic Drug Monitoring*, A. Richens and V. Marks (Ed.), Edinburgh, Churchill Livingstone, 1981.

M. J. O'Sullivan *et al.*, Enzyme Immunoassay—a Review, *Ann. clin. Biochem.*, 1979, *16*, 221–240.

C. W. Parker, Radioimmunoassay, *Ann. Rev. Pharmac. Toxicol.*, 1981, *21*, 113–132.

R. F. Schall and H. J. Tenoso, Alternatives to Radioimmunoassay: Labels and Methods, *Clin. Chem.*, 1981, *27*, 1157–1164.

D. S. Smith *et al.*, A Review of Fluoroimmunoassay using Immunofluorometric Assay, *Ann. clin. Biochem.*, 1981, *18*, 253–274.

R. V. Smith and J. T. Stewart, *Textbook of Biopharmaceutic Analysis*, Philadelphia, Lea and Febiger, 1981.

Therapeutic Drug Monitoring, B. Widdop (Ed.), Contemporary Issues in Clinical Biochemistry, Edinburgh, Churchill Livingstone, 1985.

Thin-layer Chromatography

A. C. Moffat

Thin-layer chromatography (TLC) is one of the most widely used techniques for the separation and identification of drugs. It is equally applicable to drugs in their pure state, to those extracted from pharmaceutical formulations, to illicitly manufactured materials, and to biological samples. It has retained favour as an analytical method primarily because of its simplicity, reliability, low cost, and selectivity of detection through the use of various location procedures.

It is a method of chromatography in which a mobile phase moves by capillary action across a uniform thin layer of finely divided stationary phase (adsorbent) bonded on to a plate. When a mixture of drugs is applied to the plate and developed with the mobile phase, the drugs move across the plate at different rates depending on their solubilities, pK_a values, and capability of hydrogen bonding, and so become separated. Although TLC is primarily a separation technique, under controlled conditions it can be used for identification and quantification. TLC has a number of advantages over gas chromatography (GC) and high pressure liquid chromatography (HPLC). The apparatus is cheap and simple and can be used instantly with no warm-up time, a number of samples can be run simultaneously, and there is great flexibility in the choice of the stationary and the mobile phases. It also has the advantage that a substance placed on a plate will remain there, avoiding detection problems associated with non-elution, thermal instability, and masking by the solvent front. TLC has lower sensitivity and resolution than GC and HPLC, although the advent of high performance TLC (HPTLC) has greatly reduced these disadvantages.

MATERIALS

Stationary Phase

A thin layer of the appropriate stationary phase is bonded to a suitable plate made of glass, aluminium foil, or plastic (polyethylene terephthalate). Adherence to the plate is usually assured by mixing a binding agent such as calcium sulphate with the stationary phase. Glass is the most popular plate material, but the others have the advantage that they can be cut easily to make smaller plates and can be stored conveniently because they are flexible. Most stationary phases are adsorbents (e.g. silica and alumina) and the separation achieved is due to interactions between the drugs and the surface of the stationary phase. Other stationary phases (e.g. cellulose) operate primarily by a partition process between the stationary and mobile phases, although there is often a complex interaction between adsorptive and partition processes. Where the stationary phase is more polar than the mobile phase the system is called a normal-phase system (e.g. silica with non-polar organic solvents), whilst when the mobile phase is the more polar the system is termed a reversed-phase system (e.g. a paraffin-impregnated plate using a water-based mobile phase). Those stationary phases that are widely used are given below.

Silica Gel

Silica gel is hydrated silicic acid and is therefore weakly acidic in nature. It is probably the most popular TLC adsorbent. The adsorbent layer is generally very hard and the plates can therefore withstand being stacked on top of each other and being knocked. When calcium sulphate (gypsum) is used as the binder, the plates are termed silica gel G; the hardest plates use an organic binder. The plates have a uniform distribution of particle size, normally about 20 µm in diameter.

Alumina

Alumina (aluminium oxide) is a weakly basic adsorbent. It has fewer applications than silica and needs to be activated to obtain the best separations.

Kieselguhr

This is naturally occurring amorphous silicic acid from the skeletons of diatoms and hence is often referred to as diatomaceous earth. It has less adsorptive properties than silica.

Magnesium Silicate

This material (Florisil) is usually used only for specialised separations when other adsorbents have failed.

Cellulose

This uses partition processes for separation, and cellulose plates mimic paper chromatography very well. Although plates made from cellulose fibres are still available, those made from 50 μm spherical particles are preferred. Cellulose plates generally run much more slowly than silica plates of the same thickness.

Reversed Phases

Silica plates have been impregnated with materials, such as heavy oils, liquid paraffin, silicone oil, and fats, to form reversed-phase partition TLC systems that use mobile phases containing water. These systems give good separations for a wide range of drugs, but have the disadvantages of being slow running, having poor reproducibility, and giving messy extracts when drugs are eluted from the plates. Plates coated with silica particles which have hydrocarbon chains of various lengths chemically bonded to the hydroxyl groups give stationary phases with high resolving power that can be reproducibly manufactured. The most popular phase is that bonded with a C_{18} (octadecyl) chain of up to 12% w/w loading on the silica. If the loading is higher than 12%, the stationary phase may collapse when the percentage of water in the mobile phase is high ($>10\%$). Methanol:water or acetonitrile:water can be used as the mobile phase and the chromatographic properties of these TLC systems correlate well with HPLC systems using similar stationary phases.

Ion-exchange Resins

These TLC plates have cation- or anion-exchange resins bonded to their surfaces. The resins are materials such as styrene–divinylbenzene copolymers having either quaternary ammonium or sulphonic acid groupings for ion exchange. They are particularly useful for substances of high molecular weight and for amphoteric materials. Strong acids or alkalis are usually used as mobile phases.

Mobile Phase

The choice of the mobile phase, either a single solvent or a mixture, will depend on the compounds to be separated and the stationary phase to be used. When a stationary phase has been chosen, solvents of increasing elution strength (see p. 206) can be tried until a particular separation is achieved. Drugs which are strong anions or cations are often best run using ion-pairing agents in the mobile phase.

Solvents should be cheap and easily obtainable in a pure form. They should be stable in air or when mixed with acids or alkalis, capable of being easily removed from the plate after a chromatographic run, non-toxic, and should not react with the substances to be separated.

TECHNIQUE

The technique of TLC involves a number of different stages, namely preparing the plate, applying the sample, running the plate, and locating the spots. These stages are described below.

Preparation of Plates

Prepared TLC plates can be purchased, but they may be prepared easily in the laboratory.
Silica gel G plates. Mix 30 g of silica gel G (sufficient for five 20 × 20 cm plates) with 60 ml of water, stir well to remove all air bubbles, and quickly apply in a layer 250 μm thick to the plates which have been previously cleaned with acetone to remove grease. Allow the plates to dry in air. Commercial slurry-spreading equipment is available.

When complicated or difficult separations are required it is advisable to use plates 20 cm long, otherwise plates of sizes down to 7.5 × 2.5 cm may be used to save time and materials. The conventional thickness for TLC plates used for analytical work is 250 μm, although plates up to 2 mm thick are used for preparative work.

The chromatographic properties of a TLC plate may be modified by treating the stationary phase with various agents. They may be added by spraying or dipping the plate in an appropriate solution or by adding the modifier at the same time as the plates are being prepared. Simple changes in pH can be effective, e.g. treating silica plates with potassium hydroxide decreases retention and gives more rounded spots for basic drugs. Buffered plates also allow the application of salts or free acids or free bases to the plate. Another example is the use of silver nitrate which can increase the separation of certain compounds, particularly those with carbon-carbon double bonds (this is known as argentation TLC). Other materials that can be useful include ion-pairing agents and fluorescent indicators. Alternatively, an adsorbent stationary phase can be activated by heating at 110° for 1 hour to increase its adsorptive effects and so increase retention.

Plates may be scored along their length (by pressing hard with a pencil) to form discrete strips of adsorbent along which the solvent will run. A 20×20 cm plate can give up to 20 such strips, each separated by 2 mm of clear glass. This can improve poor chromatography by allowing the mobile phase to flow up the strip only in straight lines.

Application of Samples

A line is drawn with a pencil parallel to, and 2 cm from, the bottom of the plate. The samples are spotted on to this line, called the origin, starting 2 cm from the side of the plate and at least 1 cm from each other. The sample, normally 1 to 10 μg of material depending on the thickness of the plate, is applied in as small a volume of solvent as possible (usually 1 to 10 μl). It may be applied by a micropipette (commercially available products deliver a known volume with an accuracy of $\pm 2\%$), by a capillary tube drawn out to a fine point, or by a calibrated micro-syringe. Whichever way it is applied, it is vital that the spot is no more than 4 mm in diameter or resolution will be lost. The plate surface must not be cut or gouged by the applicator. The solvent used to apply the spot should be volatile and have low polarity so that the spot does not diffuse too much. The solvent may be applied to the plate in aliquots, and dried off naturally or by use of a hot air blower. It is essential that the spot is dry at the end of application, especially if the solution contains water. Even a small amount of a polar solvent adsorbed on the plate can drastically alter chromatographic properties.

When a large number of samples are to be applied, the use of a template to position the spots accurately is often helpful. Alternatively, automated spotting equipment can be used to apply precise amounts of sample in the position required, either in spots or bands. These devices have the disadvantage of being expensive, difficult to clean, and usually requiring pre-concentration of the sample. Another approach to sample application involves the evaporation of measured volumes of the sample in depressions in a non-wettable polymer film. When dry, the residues are transferred to the plate by pressing the film on to it. It is a very good procedure where the solution is viscous or where it needs to be concentrated.

Some commercial TLC plates have pre-concentration zones. These plates consist of two zones of different adsorbents with a sharply defined boundary, but with the two merging into each other so that the mobile phase does not encounter any resistance in passing from one zone to the other.

One zone is normally kieselguhr, 3 cm long and 150 μm thick, which has comparatively poor adsorptive properties. Thus, any size of spot placed on this layer and run in the mobile phase will become a sharp band before it gets to the analytical silica gel layer. Another form of plate for special applications is one with a pre-concentration zone of octadecyl-silica and an analytical layer of silica. These plates simplify sample application and improve sensitivity, but are very expensive compared with conventional plates. Approximately the same effect can be obtained using conventional plates and running them first in methanol for 0.5 cm. This converts all the spots to thin bands which can then be run in the solvent of choice.

Running the Plates

A saturated developing chamber is normally used. It consists of a glass tank which normally has ground edges at the top to make an airtight seal with the glass lid when coated with soft paraffin. The tank is lined with filter paper on 3 sides and the mobile phase (usually 100 ml for 20×20 cm plates) is added. The tank is then allowed to equilibrate with its vapour for at least 30 minutes.

When the vapours in the tank have equilibrated, the TLC plate is placed in a vertical position in the tank so that the application line is above the level of mobile phase. Special racks are available that allow up to 5 plates to be held vertically and developed simultaneously.

Another type of tank is the sandwich unit in which the TLC plate is clamped horizontally between two glass plates separated by gaskets. A wick at one edge of the TLC plate provides the solvent reservoir to develop the plate. The advantage of this system is that it uses less mobile phase, provides a more quickly saturated vapour system, and gives shorter running times.

When either type of tank is used, it is important to flush the tank with nitrogen if the drugs are easily oxidised and to develop in the dark if they are photolabile. These considerations should also be borne in mind when applying the sample and evaporating the solvent from the plate, especially if the drug is also thermolabile.

It is conventional to develop 20-cm plates for a distance of 10 or 15 cm although this may involve waiting for up to 2 hours for a viscous mobile phase on a cold day. However, the development time can be considerably reduced if the plates are run for only 5 cm, since there is an exponential increase in development time with increasing development distance. For example, a 5-cm run using methanol on silica takes 15 minutes, whereas it takes 45 minutes for a 10-cm run. The other advantages of shorter running distances are an increase in sensitivity (because spots do not diffuse so far) and a saving on materials. The major disadvantage is that resolution is lost, e.g. about a 20% decrease in going from a 10-cm to a 5-cm development distance.

Once the plate has been developed for the predetermined distance, it is removed from the tank and the position of the solvent front quickly marked before any solvent evaporates. The solvent can then be allowed to evaporate naturally or removed with a hot air blower.

CONTINUOUS AND MULTIPLE DEVELOPMENT

Although it is possible to separate completely up to 10 compounds using a 10-cm run, a single run will not always separate all the compounds of interest. In these cases, continuous development may be used by running the mobile phase up the plate and removing it from the top by means of a wick, or by evaporating it using an infra-red lamp.

Although the above procedure is relatively simple, it is better to use a form of multiple development. The plate is run in one mobile phase, dried, and then run again in the same direction using either the same mobile phase or a more polar one, or one with a different pH. This procedure may be repeated a number of times to achieve the desired separations. It is especially useful when separating compounds of very different polarities.

Two-dimensional TLC can be useful when particular separations are needed. The plate is run in one direction with the first mobile phase, dried, turned through 90°, and run again using a different mobile phase. This method is better than linear development since all the plate is used for separating the components of a sample. However, only one sample can be separated on each plate.

Location Procedures

As most organic compounds are colourless, they must be made visible, preferably by a non-destructive technique. Many compounds can be located by examining a plate containing a fluorescent indicator under short wavelength (254 nm) ultraviolet light; absorbing compounds are seen as dark spots on a green background. If long wavelength (350 nm) ultraviolet light is also used, drugs which naturally fluoresce will be seen, e.g. quinine gives a bright blue spot. Any spots visualised with

these procedures should be ringed in pencil. Some drugs will not absorb ultraviolet light because they are in the wrong ionic form on the plate due to the pH of the buffered plate or solvent system used. For example, barbiturates are not visible if the plate is acidic, but are readily seen when ammonia fumes are blown over the plate. Similarly, some bases may be seen more easily if hydrochloric acid fumes are used to change the pH of the plate.

Further non-destructive tests can be performed, such as putting the plate in a tank of iodine vapour to see if brown spots appear. Another example is the use of photographic film for determining the position of radioactive drugs and metabolites in metabolic studies. In addition, pH indicators can be sprayed on the plate, e.g. bromothymol blue which is yellow in an acidic medium and blue in an alkaline medium. Reagent sprays should be applied to the plate as fine aerosols using a hand pump, compressed air line, or propellent cartridge. The spray should be moved backwards and forwards quickly to cover the whole plate but not applying so much that the plate looks wet.

Another very useful general, but destructive, test is to pour *sulphuric acid* on the plate and gently warm it. Organic materials char to produce black or brown spots. Alternatively, the plate can be heated in an atmosphere of ammonium bicarbonate when many compounds give fluorescent derivatives, the sensitivity of detection of which is about ten times that of the sulphuric acid treatment.

Spray reagents may be used either as general locating agents for the visualisation of any drug present (e.g. iodine in methanol) or to pick out one specific class of drug (e.g. *FPN reagent* for phenothiazines). In between these types of reagents are those that can be used as functional group tests (e.g. fluorescamine for primary amines) and others that react with general groups of compounds (e.g. *Dragendorff spray* for alkaloids). In addition, there are reagents such as *Marquis reagent* and *Mandelin's reagent* that give a wide range of colours and can be very useful in identification procedures. In many cases, spray reagents can be sprayed on top of each other on the plate, provided that the drugs are not destroyed or the pH of the plate is not altered too much by the previous spray.

Suitable locating reagents are listed under the TLC systems described at the end of this chapter, and details of their composition are given in the Reagent Appendix. The reagents described under Colour Tests (p. 128) may also be used as TLC location reagents.

STORAGE OF CHROMATOGRAMS

Aluminium and plastic TLC plates are flexible and can easily be mounted with glue or adhesive tape in case books. Glass plates can be stored flat, but quickly become a storage problem in a busy laboratory. It is therefore better to trace the chromatogram on paper, indicating the colours of the spots. Alternatively, the TLC plate can be photographed (preferably with a camera that gives instant prints) or photocopied. In either case, colour reproductions are much more useful than black and white pictures. The actual layer on a glass plate can be preserved and removed by spraying with a solution of a polymer, e.g. polyvinyl propionate, which sets to a clear pliable plastic film. This film can be stripped off the glass plate under water with the adhering TLC layer, dried, and mounted as for a plastic TLC plate.

Rf VALUES

The basic chromatographic measurement of a substance in TLC is the Rf value, defined as

$$Rf = \frac{\text{Distance the substance travels from the origin}}{\text{Distance the solvent front travels from the origin}}$$

This value varies from 0 to 1. However, it is more usual to quote $Rf \times 100$ values to avoid the use of decimals. These $Rf \times 100$ values are sometimes referred to as hRf values, but for simplicity they are subsequently referred to in this chapter and elsewhere as Rf values. The distance travelled by the substance is measured from the centre of the spot, which is easily determined if the spot is round, but with tailing spots it should be measured from the middle of the most dense area.

Rf values are affected by a number of factors and therefore an authentic sample of the suspected drug should be run at the same time on the same plate as the test sample whenever possible. If this is not possible, a reference compound can be run at the same time and the relative Rf value quoted as the ratio of the distances moved by the test substance and the stated reference compound (Rr or RRf value). By far the best approach is to run simultaneously a number of reference compounds whose Rf values are accurately known and then correct the Rf value of the test substance (Rfc value).

Factors Affecting the Reproducibility of Rf Values

Since Rf values are often used in identification procedures, it is important to recognise those factors affecting reproducibility. The most important factors are given below.

Stationary Phase

The quality of the adsorbent and binder, presence of impurities, and uniformity of thickness must be carefully maintained or batch to batch variations will occur. If the plates are to be activated, the procedure should be the same on each occasion. Plates should be stored over silica gel in a desiccator before use and the sample should be applied quickly so that the water vapour in the atmosphere is not adsorbed by the plate. Because of the difficulties associated with activation procedures it is far better to use plates stored at room temperature and not to activate them. The spots must be at least 2 cm from the side of the plate and the solvent used for applying the sample must be completely removed before the plate is run.

Mobile Phase

This should be prepared accurately from pure solvents, and made freshly for each run if one of the solvents is very volatile or hygroscopic, e.g. acetone.

Developing Tank

It is important that saturated conditions are attained for running TLC plates. This is best accomplished by using small tanks with filter paper liners and sufficient solvent, and by leaving the tank to equilibrate for at least 30 minutes before running the plates. A well-fitting lid is essential.

Temperature

Although precise control of temperature is not necessary, the tank should be kept away from draughts, sources of heat, direct sunlight, etc. As the temperature is increased, volatile solvents evaporate more quickly, solvents run faster, and Rf values generally decrease slightly.

Development Distance

There are no great changes in corrected Rf values with changes in development distance provided that the system is kept saturated. If it is not, there is an apparent increase in Rf value with increase in running distance due to the increased evaporation of the solvent from the upper parts of the plate.

Mass of Sample

Increasing the mass of sample on the plate will often increase the Rf of a drug, especially if it normally tails in the system. For example, using a silica gel plate and chloroform:acetone (4:1) as mobile phase, 5 μg of benzoic acid has an Rf of 26, but 20 μg has an Rf of 34. However, if a plate is grossly overloaded, this too will give a tailing spot and will have the effect of apparently decreasing the Rf value. The two situations are normally easy to distinguish by the intensity of the spot.

In general, Rf values are less reproducible in the middle of a chromatogram than at high or low Rf values. However, these differences in reproducibility are not very dramatic and for practical purposes reproducibility can be regarded as independent of the magnitude of the Rf values.

From the above, it is obvious that the standard deviation of measurements of Rf values can be considerable even if all due care is taken. The best way to increase reproducibility is to run an authentic sample at the same time, or to use corrected Rf values. This involves running, at the same time as the test sample, a number of reference compounds (usually 4), the Rf values of which are accurately known. The Rf value of the test substance can then be corrected by a graphical method or by linear regression analysis. Thus, a 6-point correction graph can be drawn by plotting the experimentally determined Rf values of the four reference compounds against their accurately known values, together with the 0,0 (origin) and 100,100 (solvent front) points. The requirements for the reference compounds are that they produce round and distinct spots, and are equally spaced across the chromatographic range. This procedure can reduce the inter-laboratory standard deviation from about 6 Rf units to about 3 Rf units.

SPECIAL TECHNIQUES

Preparative TLC

One of the major uses of TLC is as a separative or purification technique. Preparative TLC is very useful to isolate components in a mixture, either for further analytical studies or to obtain pure materials for use as standards. An analytical TLC plate is normally 100 to 250 μm thick, whilst preparative plates are from 0.5 to 2 mm thick. They can accept from 10 to 100 mg of material depending on the number of components and their chemical nature. As a general rule, the amount that can be applied to a TLC plate without overloading it (the capacity) increases as the square root of the thickness of the adsorbent layer. It is generally better to apply the sample as a band rather than a spot, so that the maximum amount of sample can be chromatographed at the same time.

It is often easier to elute drugs from silica than from either cellulose or alumina, and only bonded stationary phases should be used in reversed-phase systems or else the organic stationary phase will also be eluted. These points should be considered when choosing the stationary phase.

After the plate has been run, non-destructive locating procedures such as the use of ultraviolet light or iodine vapour should be used. If a reagent spray must be used, it should be sprayed only on a small strip of the chromatogram to allow the maximum use of the rest of the material, although not all spray reagents have irreversible effects. For example, the complex formed when basic drugs are sprayed with potassium iodoplatinate solution can be decomposed by aqueous acid containing 10% w/v sodium sulphite.

Once the area containing the drug of interest has been located, it should be scraped off and eluted in a Pasteur pipette or in a funnel, using glass wool to trap the stationary phase. Alternatively, elution can be accomplished in a test-tube followed by centrifugation to separate the phases. A solvent of high eluting power, such as methanol, should be used. Highly adsorbed substances (those with low Rf values) may take several minutes to be eluted from the stationary phase. Often it is better to wet the stationary phase before extracting with the organic solvent, or better still elute with aqueous acid or alkali and then extract the aqueous phase with an organic solvent after changing the pH. It is always useful to treat an area of equal size, scraped from another part of the plate where no drug is present, to act as a control.

Using one of the above procedures, a recovery of 50 to 80% is relatively easy, although devices are available which elute directly from the plate and which claim better than 99% efficiency. These devices fit directly over the spot, after scraping away a ring of stationary phase, and solvent is pumped in from one side of the device and collected at the other side.

Thin-layer Rods

The Iatroscan TH-10 analyser combines TLC with a flame ionisation detector to give the benefits of simple chromatography with a universal detector. It uses rods which are about 150 mm long and 0.9 mm in diameter with a coating of silica 75 μm thick. The sample is applied near one end of the rod, and developed in a conventional TLC tank. The rod is then dried and scanned using a flame ionisation detector (which takes only 20 seconds).

The sensitivity can be as good as 200 ng, but 1 to 20 µg is the optimum working range. Although developed primarily for quantitative work the method has a coefficient of variation of 10% for quantification. It is also difficult to remove the background signal when using a mobile phase of low volatility and, if the rod is heated enough to remove the solvent, volatile drugs can be lost. These features, linked with the destructive nature of the detector, limit the usefulness of the method.

High Performance Thin-layer Chromatography

The availability of new materials, methods, and instrumentation over the last 10 years has so greatly altered TLC, that the new form is now called high performance TLC (HPTLC). The HPTLC plates are far superior to the conventional type, having much smaller particles (2 to 7 µm) as well as a very narrow particle size distribution. This makes HPTLC faster, more reproducible, more sensitive, and more accurate for quantitative work. Its growth in drug applications has been greatly speeded by the use of automated sample application devices and accurate densitometers. A comparison of HPTLC and TLC is given below.

Typical conditions	TLC	HPTLC
Plate dimensions (cm)	20 × 20	10 × 10
Particle size (silica) (µm)	about 20	about 5
Layer thickness (analytical) (µm)	100–250	150–200
Sample volume (µl)	1–10	<0.1
Spot diameter before running (mm)	<4	<1.5
Spot diameter after running (mm)	5–10	2–5
Running distance (cm)	10–15	3–6
Running time (min)	30–120	5–15
Number of samples per plate	10–15	30–40
Detection limit (absorption)* (ng)	10–100	0.5–5
Detection limit (fluorescence)* (ng)	0.1–1	0.01–0.1
Reproducibility of Rf values	about 3%	about 1%
Reproducibility of quantification	about 5%	2–3%

*For strongly absorbent or fluorescent drugs

The main disadvantages of HPTLC are the inability to use another identification technique after eluting a separated sample (since so little sample is used) and the interference of co-extracted material in tissue extracts.

SELECTION OF TLC SYSTEMS

The selection of the best system for a particular application will depend on the use to which it is to be put. For quantification it is most important that both the drug to be measured and the internal standard produce round spots of reproducible magnitude and that they are adequately separated.

However, for identification purposes, the Rf values must be as reproducible as possible and there must be as much separation between drugs as possible.

If a drug is to be separated from unwanted materials, a series of solvents of increasing eluting strength (see p. 206) can be tried until the necessary separation is achieved. When a large number of compounds are to be separated, e.g. for a screening or identification procedure, there are three main features of a TLC system to be considered. Firstly, the system should have a good distribution of Rf values across the plate for the compounds of interest to ensure the maximum probability of separation. Secondly, the Rf values should be as reproducible as possible. Lastly, the correlation of chromatographic properties between systems should be low, so that extra information is obtained when more than one system is used for identification purposes. Features such as sensitivity and speed of running are generally similar whichever TLC system is chosen.

Discriminating Power

To compare the ability of TLC systems to achieve a particular separation, a mathematical method of comparison is needed. A simple method is to use discriminating power measurements. Discriminating power is defined as the probability that two drugs selected at random would be separated by the TLC system. It has a number of advantages over other methods of evaluation in that it is easy to calculate, it can account for the different reproducibilities of systems, it can easily be used for combinations of systems, and it has a simple range of values, i.e. 0 to 1.

Discriminating power is calculated by running the drugs of interest in the TLC system to be evaluated and comparing the measured Rf values for each drug in turn with Rf values for each of all the other drugs. If the Rf values are within a predetermined error factor they are considered to be undiscriminated (or matched) and the total number of matches from all the drugs is designated M. The total number of possible matches is

$$\frac{N(N-1)}{2}$$

(where N = total number of drugs) and therefore the probability of two drugs selected at random being matched is

$$\frac{2M}{N(N-1)}$$

Hence,

$$\text{discriminating power} = 1 - \frac{2M}{N(N-1)}$$

It should be noted that the concept of discriminating power can be applied to GC and HPLC as well as TLC.

QUANTIFICATION

Recent advances in densitometers and data processing devices have brought quantitative TLC into the same accuracy range (2–5% coefficient of variation) as GC and HPLC. Sample application is still a very critical part of quantitative TLC, although calibrated micro-pipettes, micro-syringes, and the use of internal standards, have solved most of the problems. Densitometers can work in transmittance, fluorescence quenching, or reflectance modes for measuring absorbance, and can also measure fluorescence, which is more sensitive for those drugs that do fluoresce. The plates can be read with a high degree of resolution (12 µm) and spots can be scanned many times in order to improve the signal-to-noise ratio by averaging the signals.

When quantitative measurements are made using internal standards, the calibration curves of concentration versus peak-height ratios or peak-area ratios are normally non-linear. Whilst this is a disadvantage, a data processor linked to a densitometer will ensure that accuracy is not lost. The ability of HPTLC to run up to 40 samples simultaneously can make the use of densitometry a viable proposition for therapeutic drug monitoring programmes or for pharmacokinetic studies where large numbers of similar samples are being analysed together.

Although less popular, the use of radioactivity scanners for TLC plates still has a useful role to play in the analysis of radioactive drugs and metabolites. Alternatively, the spot can be scraped off and counted in a scintillation counter.

SYSTEMS FOR THIN-LAYER CHROMATOGRAPHY

The TLC systems given below are general screening methods for nitrogenous bases (Systems TA, TB, and TC) and for acids and neutral compounds (Systems TD, TE, and TF) together with 17 other systems for specific groups of drugs. The drugs are divided into chemical or pharmacological groups but some other drugs are included with certain groups if they are chemically similar and would be extracted with that group.

There may not be one best system for a particular separation and a number of systems can be applied from those suggested. However, each of the systems described has been selected because it gives a good spread of Rf values, has high reproducibility, and has low correlation with the other systems selected for that group of drugs. These systems have proved useful for a large number of groups of drugs over the years and are robust and dependable. At least three systems are given for each group, where possible. The Rf values of the reference compounds suggested for the six general screening systems have been derived using 5 to 10 µg of the substance.

Fluorescent plates should always be used and the absorption or fluorescence of the drug under ultraviolet light (both 254 and 350 nm) should be used as a location procedure. The suggested locating agents include general ones to visualise any drug that might be present as well as more specific ones to pick out individual classes of drugs.

NOTE. In the tables of Rf values, a dash indicates that no value is available for the compound.

BASIC NITROGENOUS DRUGS, GENERAL SCREEN

A. H. Stead et al., Analyst, Lond., 1982, 107, 1106–1168.

System TA

PLATES. Silica gel G, 250 µm thick, dipped in, or sprayed with, 0.1M potassium hydroxide in methanol, and dried.

MOBILE PHASE. Methanol : strong ammonia solution (100 : 1.5).

REFERENCE COMPOUNDS. Diazepam Rf 75, chlorprothixene Rf 56, codeine Rf 33, atropine Rf 18.

System TB

PLATES. This system uses the same plates as System TA with which it may be used because of the low correlation of Rf values.

MOBILE PHASE. Cyclohexane : toluene : diethylamine (75 : 15 : 10).

REFERENCE COMPOUNDS. Dipipanone Rf 66, pethidine Rf 37, desipramine Rf 20, codeine Rf 06.

System TC

PLATES. This system uses the same plates as Systems TA and TB with which it may be used because of the low correlation of Rf values.

MOBILE PHASE. Chloroform : methanol (90 : 10).

REFERENCE COMPOUNDS. Meclozine Rf 79, caffeine Rf 58, dipipanone Rf 33, desipramine Rf 11.

LOCATION REAGENTS. For Systems TA, TB, and TC.

Ninhydrin spray. Spray the plate with the reagent and then heat in an oven at 100° for 5 minutes. Violet or pink spots are given by primary amines and yellow colours by secondary amines.

FPN reagent. Red or brown-red spots are given by phenothiazines and blue spots by dibenzazepines. This reagent may be used to overspray a plate which has been previously sprayed with *ninhydrin spray.*

Dragendorff spray. Yellow, orange, red-orange, or brown-orange spots are given by tertiary alkaloids. This reagent may be used to overspray a plate which has been previously sprayed with *ninhydrin spray* and *FPN reagent.*

Acidified iodoplatinate solution. Violet, blue-violet, grey-violet, or brown-violet spots on a pink background are given by tertiary amines and quaternary ammonium compounds. Primary and secondary amines give dirtier colours. This solution may be used to overspray a plate which has been previously sprayed with *ninhydrin spray, FPN reagent,* and *Dragendorff spray.*

Mandelin's reagent. This reagent is preferably poured on to the plate because of the danger of spraying concentrated acid. Many different colours are given with a variety of drugs (see under Colour Tests, p. 137).

Marquis reagent. This reagent is preferably poured on to the plate because of the danger of spraying concentrated acid. Black or violet spots are given by alkaloids related to morphine. Many different colours are given with a variety of drugs (see under Colour Tests, p. 139).

Acidified potassium permanganate solution. Yellow-brown spots on a violet background are given by drugs with unsaturated aliphatic bonds.

Rf VALUES. Rf values for drugs in these systems will be found in drug monographs and in the indexes to Analytical Data in Part 3; they are also included in the systems for specific groups of drugs which follow.

ACIDIC AND NEUTRAL DRUGS, GENERAL SCREEN

A. H. Stead *et al., Analyst, Lond.,* 1982, *107,* 1106–1168.

System TD

PLATES. Silica gel G, 250 μm thick.
MOBILE PHASE. Chloroform:acetone (4:1).

REFERENCE COMPOUNDS. Methohexitone Rf 73, quinalbarbitone Rf 55, clonazepam Rf 35, paracetamol Rf 15.

System TE

PLATES. This system uses the same plates as System TD with which it may be used because of the low correlation of Rf values.
MOBILE PHASE. Ethyl acetate:methanol:*strong ammonia solution* (85:10:5).
REFERENCE COMPOUNDS. Prazepam Rf 81, temazepam Rf 63, hydrochlorothiazide Rf 34, sulphadimidine Rf 13.

System TF

PLATES. This system uses the same plates as Systems TD and TE with which it may be used because of the low correlation of Rf values.
MOBILE PHASE. Ethyl acetate.
REFERENCE COMPOUNDS. Quinalbarbitone Rf 68, salicylamide Rf 55, phenacetin Rf 38, sulphathiazole Rf 20.

LOCATION REAGENTS. For Systems TD, TE, and TF.

For acidic drugs:

Van Urk reagent. Spray the plate with the reagent and then heat in an oven at 100° for 5 minutes. Yellow spots are given by sulphonamides and by meprobamate, blue spots are given by ergot alkaloids, and pink or violet spots are given by some other compounds, e.g. phenazone.

Ferric chloride solution. Blue or violet spots are given by phenols. This solution may be used to overspray a plate which has been previously sprayed with *Van Urk reagent.*

Mercurous nitrate spray. Barbiturates give dark spots which fade slowly; with some dilute solutions the spots fade rapidly.

Acidified potassium permanganate solution. Yellow-brown spots on a violet background are given by drugs with unsaturated aliphatic bonds, e.g. quinalbarbitone. This solution may be used to overspray a plate which has been previously sprayed with *mercurous nitrate spray.*

For neutral drugs:

Furfuraldehyde reagent. Violet to blue-black spots are given by some neutral compounds, e.g. carbamates.

Acidified iodoplatinate solution. This solution may be used to overspray a plate which has been previously sprayed with *furfuraldehyde reagent.*

Acidified potassium permanganate solution.

Rf VALUES. Rf values for drugs in these systems will be found in drug monographs and in the indexes to Analytical Data in Part 3; they are also included in the systems for specific groups of drugs which follow.

AMPHETAMINES, OTHER STIMULANTS, AND ANORECTICS

Systems TA, TB, or TC, previously described, may be used together with the associated location reagents.

Rf VALUES

	System		
	TA	TB	TC
Adrenaline	00	00	01
Amiphenazole	61	02	33
Amphetamine	43	15	09
Benzphetamine	73	67	70
Caffeine	52	03	58
Cathine	42	25	05
Chlorphentermine	44	18	17
Clorprenaline	57	18	15
Cyclopentamine	20	32	10
Diethylpropion	76	62	63
Dimefline	59	15	48
Doxapram	64	20	70
Ephedrine	30	05	05
Etafedrine	44	35	09
Fencamfamin	54	62	34
Fenfluramine	48	41	16
Heptaminol	23	01	02
Hydroxyamphetamine	35	02	02
Isoprenaline	40	00	01
Lobeline	61	17	35
Mazindol	63	06	13
Meclofenoxate	77	26	42
Mephentermine	25	34	08
Mescaline	20	04	10
Methoxyamphetamine	73	36	77
Methoxyphenamine	23	24	04
Methylamphetamine	31	28	13
Methylenedioxyamphetamine	39	17	12
Methylphenidate	57	34	34
Naphazoline	14	03	06
Nicotine	54	39	35
Nikethamide	59	15	56
Oxedrine	25	04	01
Pemoline	60	00	23
Pentetrazol	72	07	64
Phenbutrazate	72	47	78
Phendimetrazine	57	36	51
Phenelzine	77	37	12
Phenethylamine	49	28	28
Phenmetrazine	50	14	21
Phentermine	46	26	31
Phenylephrine	33	01	01
Phenylpropanolamine	44	04	04
Pipradrol	54	59	38
Prolintane	50	66	32
Pseudoephedrine	33	54	04
Tranylcypromine	54	33	33
Trimethoxyamphetamine	33	08	11
Tuaminoheptane	33	01	07

ANALGESICS, NON-STEROIDAL ANTI-INFLAMMATORY DRUGS, AND OTHER STRONGLY ACIDIC DRUGS

Systems TD or TF, previously described, may be used or System TG, below, which gives good separations.

System TG

PLATES. Silica gel G, 250 μm thick.

MOBILE PHASE. Ethyl acetate:methanol:*strong ammonia solution* (80:10:10).

LOCATION REAGENTS. The reagents given for Systems TD, TE, and TF can be used as well as those given below.

Chromic acid solution. A variety of colours are given by certain substances (see below).

Ludy Tenger reagent. Orange or orange-brown spots are given by certain substances (see below).

Rf VALUES

	System			Chromic	Ludy
	TD	TF	TG	acid	Tenger
Alclofenac	18	28	12		orange
Amidopyrine	25	15	—		
Aspirin	18	30	—		
Baclofen	01	00	—		
Benoxaprofen	—	—	14		orange
Bufexamac	11	19	36		
Clonixin	—	—	30		orange
Diclofenac	25	40	29	red	
Diflunisal	08	10	37	blue-grey	
Fenbufen	18	30	09		
Fenclofenac	—	—	20		
Fenoprofen	42	53	16		orange
Feprazone	—	—	45	yellow	orange
Flufenamic acid	—	—	37	blue	
Flunixin	—	—	33		orange
Flurbiprofen	30	41	16		orange
Frusemide	01	12	19		

	System			Chromic	Ludy
	TD	TF	TG	acid	Tenger
Ibuprofen	46	54	18		
Indomethacin	16	20	20	grey-brown	
Indoprofen	—	—	08		brown-black
Ketoprofen	27	40	14		orange
Meclofenamic acid	—	—	38	violet	
Mefenamic acid	41	54	32	green	
Naproxen	33	45	14		orange
Niflumic acid	—	—	28		orange-brown
Oxyphenbutazone	52	62	25	yellow	orange
Paracetamol	15	34	—		
Phenacetin	38	38	—		
Phenazone	18	14	—		
Phenylbutazone	78	68	23	brown	orange
Salicylic acid	07	25	—		
Salsalate	—	—	23	brown	
Sulindac	14	10	13	white	orange-brown
Theobromine*	—	—	47		orange
Theophylline*	—	—	33		orange
Tolmetin	13	20	10		black
Zomepirac	12	12	—		

*Often extracted with this group of drugs

ANTICONVULSANTS

Systems TD, TE, or TF, previously described, may be used together with the associated location reagents.

Rf VALUES

	System		
	TD	TE	TF
Clonazepam	35	60	45
Ethosuximide	50	57	56
Ethotoin	53	—	—
Methoin	62	76	58
Methsuximide	76	—	—
Paramethadione	00	07	60
Phenacemide	22	65	40
Pheneturide	38	71	53
Phenobarbitone	47	28	65
Phensuximide	71	77	59
Phenytoin	33	36	53
Primidone	08	39	26
Sulthiame	23	53	43
Valproic acid	00	00	00

ANTIDEPRESSANTS

Systems TA, TB, or TC, previously described, may be used together with the associated location reagents. System TB gives the best separations.

Rf VALUES

	System		
	TA	TB	TC
Amitriptyline	51	55	32
Butriptyline	59	61	48
Clomipramine	51	54	34
Clorgyline	67	42	70
Desipramine	26	20	11
Dibenzepin	54	20	35
Dothiepin	51	50	42
Doxepin	51	52	37
Imipramine	48	49	23
Iprindole	47	49	34
Iproniazid	69	01	23
Isocarboxazid	71	17	74
Maprotiline	15	17	05
Mebanazine	70	48	69
Mianserin	58	39	58
Nialamide	70	02	25
Nomifensine	56	08	29
Nortriptyline	34	27	16
Noxiptyline	53	43	35
Opipramol	54	06	22
Phenelzine	77	37	12
Protriptyline	19	17	07
Tofenacin	45	25	21
Tranylcypromine	54	33	33
Trazodone	63	09	58
Trimipramine	59	62	54
Viloxazine	42	07	23
Zimeldine	47	27	25

ANTIHISTAMINES

Systems TA, TB, or TC, previously described, may be used together with the associated location reagents. System TC gives the best separations.

Rf VALUES

	System		
	TA	TB	TC
Antazoline	31	07	07
Bamipine	49	40	43
Bromodiphenhydramine	54	44	43
Brompheniramine	45	33	16
Buclizine	75	61	83
Carbinoxamine	48	25	19
Chlorcyclizine	57	42	46
Chlorpheniramine	45	33	18
Cimetidine	54	00	09

	System		
	TA	TB	TC
Cinnarizine	76	51	78
Clemastine	46	48	25
Clemizole	78	31	69
Cyclizine	57	49	41
Cyproheptadine	51	45	44
Deptropine	13	24	04
Dimethindene	42	36	13
Dimethothiazine	56	13	48
Diphenhydramine	55	45	33
Diphenylpyraline	46	37	28
Doxylamine	48	41	10
Halopyramine	52	41	28
Isothipendyl	52	41	30
Mebhydrolin	57	28	45
Meclozine	76	58	79
Mepyramine	51	39	25
Mequitazine	10	06	06
Methapyrilene	52	43	26
Methdilazine	29	32	15
Phenindamine	63	45	57
Pheniramine	45	35	13
Phenyltoloxamine	53	39	48
Promethazine	50	37	35
Propiomazine	55	34	42
Pyrrobutamine	54	55	37
Thenalidine	50	38	44
Thenyldiamine	53	42	25
Thonzylamine	55	38	28
Tolpropamine	51	52	32
Trimeprazine	58	55	39
Tripelennamine	55	44	27
Triprolidine	51	39	20

BARBITURATES

Systems TD or TE, previously described, may be used or System TH, below, which gives the best separations.

System TH

PLATES. Silica gel G, 250 μm thick.
MOBILE PHASE. Isopropyl alcohol:chloroform: *strong ammonia solution* (90:90:20).

LOCATION REAGENTS. For Systems TD, TE, and TH.
Mercuric chloride–diphenylcarbazone reagent. White spots on a violet background are given in neutral systems, and violet spots on a pink background are given if the plate is alkaline.
Acidified potassium permanganate solution. Yellow-brown spots on a violet background are given by drugs with unsaturated aliphatic bonds.
Zwikker's reagent. Pink spots are given by 5,5-disubstituted barbiturates, green spots are given by thiobarbiturates, and faint pink spots are given by bromobarbiturates and by 1,5,5-trisubstituted barbiturates. The test is not very sensitive.
Fluorescein solution. Spray the plates with a 10% solution of sodium hydroxide and heat at 100° in an oven for 5 minutes before applying the reagent. Pink spots are given by bromobarbiturates.
Mercurous nitrate spray. Barbiturates give dark spots which fade slowly; with some dilute solutions the spots fade rapidly.

Rf VALUES

	System		
	TD	TE	TH
Allobarbitone	50	31	53
Amylobarbitone	52	36	74
Aprobarbitone	48	36	66
Barbitone	41	31	51
Barbituric acid	00	00	03
Brallobarbitone	52	30	47
Butalbital	54	38	67
Butobarbitone	50	38	68
Cyclobarbitone	50	35	59
Cyclopentobarbitone	50	37	62
Enallylpropymal	71	58	87
Heptabarbitone	50	30	62
Hexethal	53	44	74
Hexobarbitone	65	48	85
Ibomal	50	31	61
Idobutal	55	41	71
Metharbitone	66	53	86
Methohexitone	73	58	93
Methylphenobarbitone	70	43	72
Nealbarbitone	58	39	78
Pentobarbitone	55	45	76
Phenobarbitone	47	28	38
Phenylmethylbarbituric acid	29	24	27
Quinalbarbitone	55	44	78
Secbutobarbitone	50	41	69
Talbutal	53	41	71
Thialbarbitone	77	44	75
Thiopentone	77	49	80
Vinbarbitone	50	32	56

BENZODIAZEPINES

Systems TD, TE, or TF, previously described, may be used together with the associated location reagents.

Rf VALUES

	System		
	TD	*TE*	*TF*
Bromazepam	13	62	20
Chlordiazepoxide	10	51	11
Clobazam	53	73	49
Clonazepam	35	60	45
Clorazepic acid	34	63	45
Clozapine	04	63	05
Demoxepam	15	44	22
Diazepam	58	77	48
Flunitrazepam	54	77	48
Flurazepam	03	74	03
Ketazolam	45	73	45
Lorazepam	23	45	39
Lormetazepam	43	61	47
Medazepam	56	79	40
Nitrazepam	35	59	45
Nordazepam	34	67	45
Oxazepam	22	44	37
Prazepam	64	81	55
Temazepam	51	63	47
Triazolam	05	45	02

CANNABINOIDS

These systems may be used for extracts of both cannabis and cannabis resin.

System TI

PLATES. Silica gel G, 250 μm thick, dipped in, or sprayed with, a 10% solution of silver nitrate, and dried.
MOBILE PHASE. Toluene, using unsaturated (open tank) conditions.

System TJ

PLATES. Silica gel G, 250 μm thick, sprayed with diethylamine immediately before use.
MOBILE PHASE. Xylene:hexane:diethylamine (25:10:1).

LOCATION REAGENTS. For Systems TI and TJ.
Fast blue B solution. Cannabidiol gives an orange colour, cannabinol gives a violet colour, and Δ^9-tetrahydrocannabinol gives a red colour. The colours may be intensified by overspraying with M sodium hydroxide or by exposing the plate to ammonia fumes.
Duquenois reagent. After spraying with the reagent, overspray the plate with *hydrochloric acid*. Blue to violet colours are given by cannabinoids.

Rf VALUES

	System	
	TI	*TJ*
Cannabidiol	05	36
Cannabinol	52	20
Δ^9-Tetrahydrocannabinol	30	29

CARDIAC GLYCOSIDES

System TK

E. J. Johnston and A. L. Jacobs, *J. pharm. Sci.*, 1966, *55*, 531–532.
PLATES. Silica gel G, 250 μm thick, activated at 120° for 45 minutes. They should be stored in a desiccator.
MOBILE PHASE. Benzene:ethanol (7:3).

LOCATION REAGENTS
Perchloric acid solution. This gives spots which fluoresce under ultraviolet light (350 nm); a charring effect is produced after the sprayed plate has been heated in an oven at 100° for a few minutes.
p-*Anisaldehyde reagent.* After spraying with the reagent, heat in an oven at 100° for a few minutes. Blue spots are given by cardiac glycosides except for ouabain which gives a yellow spot.

Rf VALUES

	System TK
Acetyldigitoxin	82
Deslanoside	27
Digitoxin	72
Digoxin	62
Lanatoside C	36
Ouabain	09

DIURETICS

Systems TD, TE, or TF, previously described, may be used. System TF gives the best separations.

LOCATION REAGENTS. The reagents given for Systems TD, TE, and TF can be used as well as that given below.
N-*(1-Naphthyl)ethylenediamine solution.* Spray the plate with *dilute sulphuric acid*, expose it to *nitrogen dioxide vapour* for 15 minutes and then spray with the reagent.

Rf VALUES

	System		
	TD	*TE*	*TF*
Acetazolamide	04	03	31
Bendrofluazide	25	52	71

	System		
	TD	*TE*	*TF*
Benzthiazide	14	09	51
Bumetanide	01	03	10
Chlorothiazide	02	02	16
Chlorthalidone	04	42	43
Clopamide	19	52	38
Clorexolone	31	58	51
Cyclopenthiazide	21	66	62
Cyclothiazide	18	59	60
Dichlorphenamide	14	33	64
Ethacrynic acid	03	04	06
Ethiazide	11	50	50
Frusemide	01	07	12
Hydrochlorothiazide	04	34	39
Hydroflumethiazide	07	40	47
Indapamide	38	67	61
Mefruside	45	65	58
Methyclothiazide	19	53	50
Metolazone	23	57	51
Polythiazide	22	63	60
Quinethazone	04	41	21
Spironolactone	66	79	51
Trichlormethiazide	15	14	60
Xipamide	38	11	64

ERGOT ALKALOIDS

Systems TL and TM

R. E. Ardrey and A. C. Moffat, *J. forens. Sci. Soc.*, 1979, *19*, 253–282.

These systems can be run in a single tank as they use the same mobile phase and have low correlation of Rf values.

System TL

PLATES. Silica gel G, 250 μm thick, dipped in, or sprayed with, 0.1M potassium hydroxide in methanol, and dried.
MOBILE PHASE. Acetone.
REFERENCE COMPOUNDS. Meclozine Rf 70, mepivacaine Rf 48, procaine Rf 30, amitriptyline Rf 15.

System TM

PLATES. Aluminium oxide, 250 μm thick.
MOBILE PHASE. Acetone.
REFERENCE COMPOUNDS. Lysergide Rf 70, ergotamine Rf 48, ergometrine Rf 26.

LOCATION REAGENTS. For Systems TL and TM.
Naphthoquinone sulphonate solution. Spray the plate with the reagent, then spray with a 10% v/v solution of *hydrochloric acid* and heat at 110° for 20 minutes.

Red-violet spots on a light pink background are given by ergot alkaloids.
Nitroso–naphthol solution. Spray the plate with the reagent, then spray with a 10% v/v solution of *hydrochloric acid* and heat at 110° for 20 minutes. Blue-black spots on a yellow background are given by ergot alkaloids.
Van Urk reagent. After spraying the plate, heat in an oven at 100° for 5 minutes. Blue spots are given by ergot alkaloids.

Rf VALUES

	System	
	TL	*TM*
Co-dergocrine	29	64
Dihydroergotamine	14	40
Ergometrine	08	26
Ergotamine	23	48
Ergotoxine	48	67
Lysergamide	06	27
Lysergic acid	00	00
Lysergide	24	70
Methylergometrine	12	31
Methysergide	12	33

LOCAL ANAESTHETICS

Systems TA, TB, TC, or TL, previously described, may be used, together with the location reagents listed for Systems TA, TB, and TC. System TL gives the best separations.

Rf VALUES

	System			
	TA	*TB*	*TC*	*TL*
Amethocaine	57	15	32	16
Benzocaine	67	06	57	66
Bupivacaine	69	42	73	65
Butacaine	71	09	30	64
Butanilicaine	76	14	54	61
Chloroprocaine	59	05	23	37
Cinchocaine	63	25	34	35
Cocaine	65	47	47	54
Cyclomethycaine	58	55	36	25
Dimethisoquin	61	55	46	28
Diperodon	70	15	58	66
Dyclonine	60	49	40	25
Lignocaine	70	35	73	63
Mepivacaine	65	27	62	48
Oxethazaine	52	10	07	15
Oxybuprocaine	62	23	41	36
Piperocaine	55	53	37	27
Pramoxine	70	43	55	41

	System			
	TA	TB	TC	TL
Prilocaine	77	29	64	60
Procaine	54	06	31	30
Propoxycaine	58	03	33	28
Proxymetacaine	62	26	41	35

NARCOTIC ANALGESICS

Systems TA, TB, or TC, previously described, may be used together with the associated location reagents.

Rf VALUES

	System		
	TA	TB	TC
Alphaprodine	50	30	35
Anileridine	73	—	—
Apomorphine	83	00	21
Benzylmorphine	41	06	23
Buprenorphine	76	09	68
Codeine	33	06	18
Dextromethorphan	34	44	17
Dextromoramide	76	40	71
Dextropropoxyphene	68	59	55
Dextrorphan	35	13	07
Diamorphine	47	15	38
Dihydrocodeine	26	08	13
Dihydromorphine	25	01	03
Diphenoxylate	74	42	81
Dipipanone	66	66	33
Ethoheptazine	40	45	19
Ethylmorphine	40	07	22
Etorphine	73	07	61
Fentanyl	70	45	74
Hydrocodone	25	04	20
Hydromorphone	23	03	09
Ketobemidone	47	02	09
Levallorphan	67	19	24
Levorphanol	35	13	07
Methadone	48	61	20
6-Monoacetylmorphine	46	06	19
Morphine	37	00	09
Nalorphine	59	01	23
Naloxone	65	09	66
Norcodeine	13	00	05
Normethadone	56	40	34
Normorphine	17	—	—
Norpipanone	68	59	50
Noscapine	64	22	74
Oxeladin	50	51	22
Oxycodone	50	23	51
Oxymorphone	48	10	37

	System		
	TA	TB	TC
Papaverine	61	08	65
Pentazocine	61	15	12
Pethidine	52	37	34
Phenazocine	68	16	39
Phenoperidine	71	26	64
Pholcodine	36	03	18
Piminodine	67	—	—
Pipazethate	47	15	13
Piritramide	70	01	45
Thebacon	45	19	34
Thebaine	45	23	37

PHENOTHIAZINES AND OTHER TRANQUILLISERS

Systems TA, TB, or TC, previously described, may be used together with the associated location reagents.

Rf VALUES

	System		
	TA	TB	TC
Acepromazine	48	26	24
Acetophenazine	53	03	25
Azacyclonol	10	00	03
Benactyzine	66	40	53
Benzoctamine	59	57	52
Butaperazine	53	24	37
Carphenazine	54	05	27
Chlormezanone	66	01	63
Chlorpromazine	49	49	35
Chlorprothixene	56	51	51
Clopenthixol	56	07	32
Clothiapine	59	41	59
Diethazine	58	57	51
Dimethothiazine	56	13	48
Dimethoxanate	39	18	24
Droperidol	67	02	48
Ethopropazine	67	64	47
Fluopromazine	54	49	35
Flupenthixol	62	05	33
Fluphenazine	63	06	23
Fluspirilene	69	04	59
Haloperidol	67	10	27
Hydroxyzine	68	09	54
Mesoridazine	38	03	06
Methdilazine	29	32	15
Methotrimeprazine	57	49	38
Metopimazine	56	00	11
Oxypertine	68	04	65
Pecazine	53	46	44

	System		
	TA	TB	TC
Penfluridol	76	17	60
Pericyazine	58	03	16
Perphenazine	55	07	29
Pimozide	71	04	60
Pipamperone	56	01	12
Piperacetazine	56	06	19
Prochlorperazine	49	33	37
Promazine	44	41	30
Promethazine	50	37	35
Propiomazine	55	34	42
Prothipendyl	47	45	23
Tetrabenazine	69	41	78
Thiethylperazine	51	30	41
Thiopropazate	61	35	53
Thioproperazine	46	07	34
Thioridazine	48	43	30
Thiothixene	49	09	40
Trifluoperazine	53	33	30
Trimeprazine	58	55	39
Trimetozine	61	11	72

QUATERNARY AMMONIUM COMPOUNDS

Systems TN and TO

H. M. Stevens and A. C. Moffat, *J. forens. Sci. Soc.*, 1974, *14*, 141–148.

System TN

PLATES. Cellulose, 250 µm thick.
MOBILE PHASE. Ammonium formate:formic acid: water:tetrahydrofuran (1:5:95:233).

System TO

PLATES. Silica gel (without gypsum), 250 µm thick.
MOBILE PHASE. Methanol:0.2M hydrochloric acid (80:20).

LOCATION REAGENTS. For Systems TN and TO.
Acidified iodoplatinate solution. Violet, blue-violet, grey-violet, or brown-violet spots on a pink background are given by quaternary ammonium compounds.
Cobalt thiocyanate solution. Blue spots are given by quaternary ammonium compounds.

Rf VALUES

	System	
	TN	TO
Acetylcholine chloride	70	60
Atropine methonitrate	95	35
Bretylium tosylate	94	40
Cetrimide	100	50

	System	
	TN	TO
Choline	60	60
Decamethonium bromide	56	16
Gallamine triethiodide	34	05
Guanethidine	56	50
Hexamethonium bromide	36	10
Pancuronium bromide	80	—
Paraquat dichloride	22	10
Suxamethonium chloride	35	10
Suxethonium bromide	40	23
Tubocurarine chloride	85	40

STEROIDS

Systems TP, TQ, TR, and TS

Pharmaceutical Codex, 11th Edn, London, Pharmaceutical Press, 1979, p. 940.

System TP

PLATES. Silica gel G, 250 µm thick.
MOBILE PHASE. Methylene chloride:ether: methanol:water (77:15:8:1.2).

System TQ

PLATES. Silica gel G, 250 µm thick.
MOBILE PHASE. Dichloroethane:methanol:water (95:5:0.2).

System TR

PLATES. Kieselguhr, 250 µm thick, impregnated with a mixture of acetone:formamide (9:1).
MOBILE PHASE. Toluene:chloroform (3:1).

System TS

PLATES. Kieselguhr, 250 µm thick, impregnated with a mixture of acetone:propylene glycol (9:1).
MOBILE PHASE. Cyclohexane:toluene (1:1).

LOCATION REAGENTS. For Systems TP, TQ, TR, and TS.
DPST solution.
Sulphuric acid–ethanol reagent. Spray the plate and then heat at 105° for 10 minutes.
p-*Toluenesulphonic acid solution.* Heat the plate at 120° for 15 minutes, cool, spray with the reagent, heat again at 120° for 10 minutes, and respray.

Rf VALUES

	System			
	TP	TQ	TR	TS
Alphadolone acetate	59	22	80	45s
Alphaxalone	60	22	90	72s

	System			
	TP	TQ	TR	TS
Beclomethasone dipropionate	75	38	89	42s
Betamethasone	30	00	00	00
Betamethasone sodium phosphate	00	00	00	00
Betamethasone valerate	58	27	20	02s
Chlorotrianisene	88	77	98	92
Cortisone acetate	72	28	55	00
Deoxycortone acetate	86	52	98	95
Dexamethasone	32	08	00	00
Dienoestrol	72	25	34	05s
Dimethisterone	80	42	91	95
Dydrogesterone	86	53	96	98
Ethinyloestradiol	72	30	40	40s
Ethisterone	78	39	80	00
Ethyloestrenol	79	50	94	99
Ethynodiol diacetate	83	61	95	99
Fludrocortisone acetate	58	12	30	00
Fluocinolone acetonide	42	08	10	01
Fluocortolone hexanoate	79	39	88	00
Fluocortolone pivalate	78	35	89	58
Fluoxymesterone	51	09	38	16s
Hydrocortisone	27	02	08	00
Hydrocortisone acetate	51	11	38	00
Hydrocortisone hydrogen succinate	08	00	00	00
Hydrocortisone sodium phosphate	00	00	00	00
Hydroxyprogesterone hexanoate	81	55	99	90
Lynoestrenol	77	55	99	97
Medroxyprogesterone acetate	80	50	98	85s
Megestrol acetate	80	50	98	85s
Mestranol	86	52	90	90
Methallenoestril	79	18	70	54s
Methandienone	65	10	87	61
Methylprednisolone	23	80	03	00
Methyltestosterone	70	16	91	71
Nandrolone decanoate	88	49	97	95
Nandrolone phenylpropionate	87	48	97	95
Norethandrolone	71	20	95	78
Norethisterone	71	22	87	63s
Norethisterone acetate	87	39	98	90
Norethynodrel	79	32	91	71
Oestradiol benzoate	79	32	96	79
Oxymetholone	69	23	85	82
Prednisolone	20	00	02s	00
Prednisolone pivalate	69	04	44	00

	System			
	TP	TQ	TR	TS
Prednisolone sodium phosphate	00	00	00	00
Prednisone	41	00	10	00
Progesterone	81	20	99	95
Stanolone	78	11	90	72
Stilboestrol	65s	10s	18s	03
Testosterone	60	07	90	63
Testosterone phenylpropionate	86	28	99	98
Testosterone propionate	78	12	99	98
Triamcinolone	09	00	00	00
Triamcinolone acetonide	32	00	20	06

s = streaking may occur

SULPHONAMIDES
Systems TT, TU, and TV

H. De Clercq *et al.*, *J. pharm. Sci.*, 1977, *66*, 1269–1275.

Sulphonamides are difficult to separate, but these systems are effective and may be used in combination. System TF, previously described, may also be used.

System TT

PLATES. Silica gel G, 250 μm thick.
MOBILE PHASE. Hexanol.

System TU

PLATES. Aluminium oxide, 250 μm thick.
MOBILE PHASE. Acetone:ammonia solution 25% (80:15).

System TV

PLATES. Aluminium oxide, 250 μm thick.
MOBILE PHASE. Chloroform:methanol (70:30).

LOCATION REAGENTS. For Systems TF, TT, TU, and TV.
Acidified potassium permanganate solution. Yellow-brown spots on a violet background are given by sulphonamides.
Copper sulphate solution. This detects *N*-substituted sulphonamides.
Mercuric chloride–diphenylcarbazone reagent. Blue spots are given by sulphonamides.
Van Urk reagent. After spraying, heat the plates in an oven at 100° for 5 minutes. Yellow spots are given by sulphonamides.

Rf VALUES

		System		
	TF	TT	TU	TV
Carbutamide	—	90	27	07
Chlorpropamide	43	84	43	03
Mafenide	01	—	—	—
Phthalylsulphacetamide	00	—	—	—
Phthalylsulphathiazole	00	02	04	04
Succinylsulphathiazole	00	02	01	01
Sulfamerazine	41	33	18	07
Sulfametopyrazine	50	—	—	—
Sulphacetamide	42	53	37	04
Sulphadiazine	39	24	22	03
Sulphadimethoxine	51	85	52	34
Sulphadimidine	45	50	27	62
Sulphaethidole	35	—	—	—
Sulphafurazole	52	74	48	04
Sulphaguanidine	06	21	90	48
Sulphamethizole	23	46	36	02
Sulphamethoxazole	54	88	33	02
Sulphamethoxydiazine	43	55	17	15
Sulphamethoxypyridazine	39	53	26	50
Sulphanilamide	46	61	96	66
Sulphaphenazole	51	89	70	13
Sulphapyridine	42	47	43	73
Sulphasalazine	00	—	—	—
Sulphasomidine	16	11	49	20
Sulphathiazole	20	53	40	05
Tolbutamide	55	98	35	04

PESTICIDES

System TW

M. E. Getz and H. G. Wheeler, *J. Ass. off. analyt. Chem.*, 1968, *51*, 1101–1107.

PLATES. Silica gel, 250 μm thick.

MOBILE PHASE. Cyclohexane:acetone:chloroform (70:25:5).

LOCATION REAGENT. Allow the plate to dry in air, heat at 110° for 2 hours, allow to cool, spray with *molybdate–antimony reagent*, and then lightly overspray with *ascorbic acid reagent*.

Rf VALUES

	System TW
Azinphos-methyl	57
Diazinon	82
Dichlorvos	42
Dimethoate	19
Disulfoton	100
Malathion	74
Mevinphos	23
Oxydemeton-methyl	00
Parathion	81
Parathion-methyl	77
Phorate	100
Trichlorphon	09

Bibliography

Advances in Thin-layer Chromatography: Clinical and Environmental Applications, J. C. Touchstone (Ed.), New York, Wiley, 1982.

A. Baerheim-Svendsen and R. Verpoorte, *Chromatography of Alkaloids, Part A: Thin-layer Chromatography*, Amsterdam, Elsevier, 1983.

Chromatographic and Electrophoretic Techniques, Vol. I, Paper and Thin-layer Chromatography, I. Smith and J. W. T. Seakins (Ed.), 4th Edn, London, Heinemann, 1976.

Densitometry in Thin-layer Chromatography: Practice and Applications, J. C. Touchstone and J. Sherma (Ed.), New York, Wiley, 1979.

Handbook of Chromatography, G. Zweig and J. Sherma (Ed.), Vols I and II, Boca Raton, Florida, CRC Press, 1972.

High Performance Thin-layer Chromatography, A. Zlatkis and R. E. Kaiser (Ed.), Amsterdam, Elsevier, 1977.

Quantitative Paper and Thin-layer Chromatography, E. J. Shellard (Ed.), London, Academic Press, 1975.

Thin-layer Chromatography: Quantitative Environmental and Clinical Applications, J. C. Touchstone and D. Rogers (Ed.), New York, Wiley, 1980.

J. C. Touchstone and M. F. Dobbins, *Practice of Thin-layer Chromatography*, 2nd Edn, New York, Wiley, 1983.

Gas Chromatography

H. Leach and J. D. Ramsey

Gas chromatography, like other forms of chromatography, is a method of separating mixtures of substances of analytical interest either from each other or from an extraction residue. The equipment may be simple or complex, but the principle is a simple one and is analogous to other forms of chromatography.

The separation is performed on a column containing the stationary phase, either solid or liquid, which is maintained at a defined temperature in an oven and has a constant flow of carrier gas (mobile phase). When a mixture of substances is injected at the inlet, each component is swept towards the detector and is partitioned between the stationary phase and the gas phase. Molecules with the greatest affinity for the stationary phase spend more time in that phase and consequently take longer to reach the detector. The detector produces a signal dependent on the mass of substance passing through it and this signal is processed and fed to a chart recorder and perhaps to an integrator. Each substance passing through the column will have a characteristic *retention time* which is defined as the time (minutes) from injection to peak maximum at the detector.

Most gas chromatography (other than capillary chromatography, see page 181) is performed on packed columns of glass [$\frac{1}{4}$ in (6.4 mm) outside diameter and 4 mm internal diameter] or stainless steel [$\frac{1}{8}$ in (3.2 mm) outside diameter and 2 mm internal diameter], 0.5 to 4 metres long. Glass is more inert than stainless steel, and has the advantage that the packing is visible.

Gas chromatography may be divided into gas–solid chromatography (mainly adsorptive processes) and gas–liquid chromatography (mainly partition) depending on whether the stationary phase is a solid or a liquid at its operating temperature. If the stationary phase is a liquid it must be coated on a support for packed column chromatography. For capillary column chromatography, the stationary phase may be coated directly on to the walls of the column, or on to a support which is bonded to the glass walls.

GAS–SOLID CHROMATOGRAPHY

Stationary Phases

In gas–solid chromatography, the stationary phase is an active solid. These solids may be inorganic materials, e.g. synthetic zeolite molecular sieve, carbon molecular sieve, silica gel, or graphitised carbon, or they may be organic polymers. They are generally used for the separation of low molecular weight materials, i.e. gases and liquids.

Molecular Sieve (4A, 5A, 13X) gives good general separation of inorganic gases. Carbon dioxide is irreversibly adsorbed below 160°. Oxygen and nitrogen are well separated. Carbon monoxide in blood is commonly measured using molecular sieve 5A. Carbosieve is a granular carbon molecular sieve useful for the separation of C_1 to C_3 hydrocarbons.

Silica Gel gives good separation of inorganic gases. Porasil is porous silica with a surface area between 1.5 and 500 m^2/g and may be used as conventional silica gel or may be coated. Carbon dioxide, carbon monoxide, hydrogen, and nitrogen are all separated. Oxygen and nitrogen are not resolved.

Molecular sieve and silica gel columns can be used in parallel for the analysis of respiratory gases where resolution of oxygen, nitrogen, and carbon dioxide is of importance.

Chromosorb and *Porapak* series are divinylbenzene cross-linked polystyrene copolymers. Different members of the series vary in surface area and average pore diameter. Separations range from free fatty acids to free amines. Alcohols from methanol to pentanol can be separated on Porapak Q or Chromosorb 102. The maximum operating temperature is about 250°.

Tenax–GC is a porous polymer of 2,6-diphenyl-*p*-phenylene oxide. This material is used both as a chromatographic phase and as a trap for volatile substances prior to analysis.

Carbopak B and *C* are graphitised carbon black, having surface areas of 12 and 100 m^2/g, respectively. They are usually modified with a light coating of a polar stationary phase. Difficult separations of the C_1 to C_{10} hydrocarbons can be achieved rapidly. Carbopak C with 0.2% Carbowax 20M has been used to resolve substances abused by 'glue-sniffers'. Carbopak C modified with 0.2% Carbowax 1500 is the phase of choice for the analysis of ethanol in blood. Carbopak C with 0.8% tetrahydroxyethylenediamine (THEED) is useful for the determination of ethylene glycol in blood. They give approximately the same order of elution of compounds as the Porapak and Chromosorb series, but generally with better resolution.

GAS–LIQUID CHROMATOGRAPHY

In gas–liquid chromatography, the stationary (liquid) phase is coated on a support material.

Support Materials

The behaviour of the column is largely dependent on the stationary phase but the support material can also play a very important role, particularly when a low concentration of liquid phase is used. A good support material should have a very large surface area and a uniform particle size, free from fines and sufficiently robust so that it does not break up into powder with normal handling. It should be chemically inert, without adsorptive effects, and, when coated with stationary phase, should pack easily and uniformly into the column.

The raw material for the most commonly used supports is diatomaceous earth, calcined, usually with a flux, then crushed and graded into a number of particle sizes. The sizes in general use are 60–80, 80–100, and 100–120 mesh.

Chromosorb P is a red diatomaceous earth which has the advantage of resistance to the formation of fines, but it is now rarely used. It is a relatively dense preparation with a packed density of 0.5 g/cm^3, and a surface area of 4 m^2/g. The 'P' denotes the pink colour.

Chromosorb W is a diatomaceous earth calcined with the addition of sodium carbonate. It is less dense than Chromosorb P, with a packed density of approximately 0.3 g/cm^3, and is softer with a greater tendency to produce fines. The surface area is about 1 m^2/g. *Celite 545* is similar to Chromosorb W.

Chromosorb G is a calcined diatomaceous earth with a density similar to that of Chromosorb P but the surface area is much less, about 0.5 m^2/g, and it is the least reactive of the Chromosorbs. The high resistance to mechanical damage together with the density and inertness make it very suitable for low-loaded columns. The amount of stationary phase should not exceed 5% w/w, which is equivalent to 12.5% w/w on other supports.

DEACTIVATION

Various deactivation procedures are applied to support materials. These include acid- or base-washing to remove impurities and fine particles, and treatment with a silanising agent which reacts with surface hydroxyl groups and reduces adsorptive effects. A very light coating of a polar stationary phase may also be used to increase deactivation. Commercial support materials which have been treated by these procedures are available and are usually designated by a suffix to the name, e.g. AW (acid washed) and AW HMDS (acid washed, hexamethyldisilazane treated). Deactivated supports are nearly always to be preferred, but it should be noted that the deactivation procedure may impose an upper temperature limit and may modify the polarity of the stationary phase.

Support materials which have the liquid phase chemically bonded to them are available. These offer decreased bleed rates of stationary phase, an advantage when operating a temperature programme or when using a mass spectrometer as the detector.

Choice of Stationary Phases

Over seven hundred substances have been used as stationary phases. The choice of stationary phase for a particular separation is often a matter of serendipity, depending on a combination of experience, prejudice, intuition, and the desire to use an existing system if it will do the job.

It has been shown that the retention behaviour of benzene, butanol, pentan-2-one, nitropropane, and pyridine can be used to classify stationary phases in terms of their polarity (W. O. McReynolds, *J. chromatogr. Sci.*, 1970, 8, 685–691). The retention indices of each of these five reference compounds are measured, first on the stationary phase being tested and then on a standard phase (squalane). The differences in retention index between the two phases (ΔI) for the five reference compounds are added together to give a constant which is a measure of the polarity of the stationary phase. This constant is known as the *McReynolds Constant* and can be used to compare the ability of stationary phases to separate different classes of compounds (see below). However, this constant gives no information about peak shape, temperature limits, or the suitability for use in capillary columns.

McReynolds Constants of some liquid phases

Liquid phase (maximum temperature)	McReynolds Constant (increasing order of polarity)
Squalane (150°) (reference phase)	0
Apolane-87 (260°)	71
Apiezon L (300°)	143
SE-30 (300°)	217
OV-1 (350°)	222
OV-101 (350°)	229
Apiezon L/KOH (225°)	301
OV-7 (350°)	592
OV-17 (350°)	886
Versamid 900 (275°)	986
Poly A103 (275°)	1072
Carbowax 20M/KOH (225°)	1296
OV-225 (250°)	1813
CHDMS (cyclohexanedimethyl succinate) (250°)	2017
Carbowax 20M (225°)	2308

A system for assessing the effectiveness of chromatographic systems by calculating the discriminating power has been described (A. C. Moffat *et al.*, *J. Chromat.*, 1974, *90*, 1–7). Using this method, a number of stationary phases commonly used in toxicology have been examined (A. C. Moffat *et al.*, *J. Chromat.*, 1974, *90*, 19–33). It was shown that SE-30 columns eluted all the drugs studied and that for screening purposes a single column, either SE-30 (or its more modern equivalents) or OV-17, was sufficient for the identification of drugs. There is little to be gained by using a series of columns of increasing polarity, and high polarity columns are of marginal utility since many drugs which elute from low polarity stationary phases do not elute from high polarity phases. Thus the use of a multiplicity of columns gives little additional evidence of identification and in most cases is counter-productive.

The choice of phases for capillary columns is less than for packed columns, particularly for silica columns. However, the high efficiency available with a capillary column will often more than compensate for the lack of selectivity obtainable with a different phase.

NON-POLAR PHASES

Apiezon L is a hydrocarbon grease which is used for the separation of barbiturates. It has the advantage over the silicone phases that it is stable when coated with alkali to reduce the tailing of strongly basic compounds. The amphetamines may be separated on a column of 10% Apiezon L with 2% potassium hydroxide.

SE-30, OV-1, and *OV-101* are dimethyl silicone polymers which may be regarded as equivalent as far as retention data are concerned. SE-30 is preferred by some workers as a stationary phase for capillary columns although it has a lower maximum operating temperature. OV-1 is preferred for packed columns and has a maximum operating temperature of 350°. Separations on these phases are largely on the basis of molecular weight. A new separation should be attempted first on one of these phases, and only if it is unsuccessful or if a poor peak shape results should a more polar phase be tried. In general, non-polar compounds chromatograph best on non-polar phases and polar compounds on polar phases.

Apolane-87 (24,24-diethyl-19,29-dioctadecylheptatetracontane) is a high temperature non-chiral hydrocarbon phase, which could replace squalane as the standard non-polar phase against which others are compared. It has a useful temperature range of 30–260° but is very expensive.

POLAR PHASES

Carbowax 20M is polyethylene glycol (average molecular weight 20 000) with general characteristics broadly similar to those of the polyethylene glycols of lower molecular weight. It has a maximum operating temperature of 225°. Carbowax 20M can be used for alkaloids and other basic drug separations. Peak shape of bases, e.g. amphetamine, can be improved by pre-coating the support with about 5% of potassium hydroxide.

Very durable and efficient capillary columns can be made from this phase. It is also used to deactivate capillary columns; it may be applied as a thin coating before the main stationary phase or vaporised into an already coated column from a small pre-column heated above the normal maximum operating temperature in the injection port.

OV-17 is phenylmethyl silicone, a useful, moderately polar, silicone phase with a high maximum operating temperature (350°). It is more oxygen-sensitive than most silicone phases and is available in capillary columns. A considerable amount of retention data for drugs on this phase has been published.

XE-60 is cyanoethyl silicone, a phase which was much favoured for steroid analysis and is widely used for capillary columns. It has a maximum operating temperature of 250°.

OV-225 is cyanopropyl phenylmethyl silicone; it is the modern counterpart of XE-60.

Polyesters. A large number of polyester phases have been used, particularly for the separation of fatty acid esters. These phases include neopentyl glycol succinate, adipate, and sebacate; cyclohexanedimethyl adipate; and cyclohexanedimethyl succinate (CHDMS). This latter phase has been recommended for the analysis of underivatised barbiturates.

Polyamides. Poly A103 is useful for the separation of barbiturates and of the tertiary amine tricyclic antidepressants.

Chirasil-Val is a unique chiral phase used in capillary columns for the separation of optical enantiomers. Most amino acids and many drugs containing polar functional groups may be resolved.

Mixed Phases. Mixtures of phases are sometimes used to tailor a column to solve a particular problem. The simultaneous separation of 11 of the commonly used anticonvulsant drugs and associated internal standards can be achieved using a mixture of *SP-2110* and *SP-2510-DA* which is commercially available.

Coating the Support Material

The two basic methods of applying the stationary phase material to the support material use either evaporation or filtration.

EVAPORATION

The support material is weighed into a flask which is sufficiently robust to withstand a vacuum. The amount of stationary phase to give the desired loading is dissolved in a suitable solvent and added to the support material in the flask. The choice of solvent is important and advice is given by most suppliers. A gentle vacuum is applied and the flask agitated, very gently, in a hot water-bath until the material is dry. This requires careful attention in the early stages to avoid foaming and loss of solution. With loadings up to 10%, the packing material should appear as a free-flowing powder. When dry, the powder is transferred to a dish and final drying is done overnight at 100°, with the exception of some oxygen-sensitive phases. If a rotary vacuum evaporator is used, the speed of rotation should be kept low to avoid mechanical damage to the particles of support material.

FILTRATION

The support material (usually 25 g) is weighed and suspended in a solution of stationary phase, the concentration of which should be approximately half the desired loading on the support material. A vacuum is applied to assist penetration, and after standing for a few minutes, the slurry is filtered on a Buchner funnel. The cake of coated support material is transferred to a dish and dried slowly initially, then at 100°. If 25 g of support material and 100 ml of solution are used, the concentration on the support will be approximately twice that of the solution when Celite or Chromosorb W is used as support.

The exact amount can be determined either by evaporating the filtered solution and weighing the residue or by taking a small portion of the coated material and exhaustively extracting it. This method of coating is only for low-loaded supports and, with coatings of the order of 1 or 2%, generally gives a more even thin film than can be produced by the evaporation method.

Packing the Column

The empty column should be cleaned with detergent, dried, treated with 10% dichlorodimethylsilane in toluene, rinsed with toluene and then with methanol, and dried again. A silanised glass wool plug is inserted in the detector end of the column and a vacuum line attached. Portions of packing material are gently poured into the injector end of the column through a funnel attached via a piece of rubber tubing. The column bed is built up gradually, about 10 cm at a time, by tapping with a pencil to consolidate the bed. The process is continued until the packing reaches the injection point, and a plug of silanised glass wool is added to secure the bed.

Capillary Columns

Capillary columns are available in glass (both soda and borosilicate), stainless steel, and silica (or natural quartz). Tubing of outside diameter of the order of 0.5 mm, internal diameter 0.2 to 0.4 mm, and 10 to 50 metres long is commonly used. Glass and silica are the materials of choice, stainless steel mainly finding application in the analysis of hydrocarbons. Silica columns are inherently straight and have the advantage of flexibility and strength, as long as the outside surface remains intact. A coating of heat-resistant polymer, usually polyimide, is applied to prevent damage. Silica columns may be threaded through complex pipework to emerge at the detector jet or mass spectrometer ion source. Capillary columns offer advantages, but are more demanding on instrumental design, and cannot be made in the laboratory without the purchase of a glass drawing machine to produce the tubing. The superior resolution available can be used to separate complex mixtures or to increase the certainty that a single compound is correctly identified. The high efficiency results in tall narrow peaks which considerably enhance the signal-to-noise ratio and consequently the detection limits. Short columns (2–10 m) can be used to give similar resolution to packed columns, but in a shorter time.

It is usually necessary to modify the inside surface to assist wetting, e.g. by etching. If the glass surface itself is coated the column is referred to as a wall-coated open tubular (WCOT) column, whereas support-coated open tubular (SCOT) columns have a support bonded on to the glass walls, e.g. microcrystals of sodium or barium chloride.

Coating techniques aim to produce a uniform film 0.1 to 1.5 μm thick. High efficiency columns have a thin film, but at the cost of lower capacity and the risk of higher adsorptive activity of the column walls. Coating can be achieved either by a dynamic or by a static technique. The dynamic technique consists of forcing a concentrated solution (approximately 100 g/litre) of stationary phase in a suitable solvent through the column by gas pressure. Care is taken to ensure that the solution flows through the whole length of the column at a uniform velocity of 1 to 2 cm/sec. The gas flow is continued until all the solution has been voided and the temperature is then increased to evaporate the remaining solvent. If viscous solutions are used, a small amount of mercury may be added after the coating solution to prevent a thick film being deposited.

In the static technique, a dilute solution (approximately 10 g/litre) of the stationary phase is used to fill the column completely. One end is sealed, the column is placed in a water-bath and a vacuum line is attached to the other end to evaporate the solvent. It is important that no air bubbles or gaps exist in the column and that the solution is degassed, otherwise bumping takes place. There is much debate as to which method gives superior results, but each has its advocates. The dynamic technique is faster and is consequently used commercially.

Support-coated open tubular (SCOT) columns are prepared by similar techniques using a suspension of the support in the stationary phase solution.

INSTALLATION OF CAPILLARY COLUMNS

Glass columns, which are coiled when purchased, must have straight ends to allow them to fit into unions at the injector and detector. A device is commercially available to straighten capillary ends, but it is more usual to use a small butane flame. The column is suspended on a clamp stand and a supply of carrier gas is provided via a length of silicone rubber tubing to produce a flow of about 0.5 ml/min. A cool, small butane flame is used to apply heat, starting a few centimetres from the end and working towards the open end. Gravity is allowed to perform the straightening while the gas flow sweeps pyrolysis products and mobilised stationary phase out of the column. The straightened portion should be inspected with a magnifying glass for constrictions or blockages. Some workers prefer to wash the stationary phase out of the column with solvent before straightening and to deactivate afterwards with silanising reagent.

Having straightened both ends, they may be presented to the fittings, when lengths and angles may be adjusted as necessary. Various fittings are available, but either graphite or Vespel (polyimide) ferrules are recommended. The injector end of the column should be fitted first, tightening the fittings just enough to prevent leakage when tested with a proprietary leak-testing fluid (not soap solution which leaves a residue). A low-volume (0.5 ml) bubble meter is used to check flow to ensure that the column is intact and not blocked. The detector end is then attached and checked for leaks. The column may lie or hang in the oven, but care should be taken to avoid cold spots. The detector is lit and the column tested at room temperature with an injection of 1 or 2 μl of methane, when a needle-sharp peak should be obtained. When the carrier gas pressure has been adjusted to give a velocity of approximately 15 cm/sec for nitrogen or approximately 30 cm/sec for helium, the column may be heated and a test mixture injected. Commercial columns are often supplied with a test mixture and a chromatogram obtained with the mixture. It should be possible to obtain performance equal to or better than the supplied chromatogram.

Various test mixtures are used, including a mixture of dimethylphenol and dimethylaniline with straight-chain paraffins. Any acidity or alkalinity of the column is apparent by loss of peak shape of the amine or phenol. The efficiency obtained will be a function of the entire chromatographic system. Poor efficiency or peak shape is often due to non-swept volume somewhere in the system. It may be necessary to add additional gas to the column outlet to ensure that the detector is effectively purged because most detectors are designed to operate with packed columns and a flow rate of about 30 ml/min, as opposed to the 1 or 2 ml/min delivered by a capillary column.

Column Conditioning

A new column requires conditioning before use. Volatile impurities remaining from the deactivation of the support, and the coating and packing processes must be removed before the column is put into service. The detector should be disconnected and, with the column at room temperature, a flow of carrier gas of 10–20 ml/min should be maintained for an hour to purge oxygen from the system. The temperature may then be raised by about 25° every 30 minutes if an isothermal oven is used, or by 1°/min if a temperature programmer is available. When a temperature about 20° above the desired operating temperature has been reached the column is left for 12 hours. Care must be taken not to exceed the maximum operating temperature. Some phases (e.g. OV-17) are particularly oxygen-sensitive and can be ruined by careless conditioning. A constrictor fitted to the detector end of the column will help prevent back diffusion of oxygen.

Maximum Operating Temperatures

Maximum operating temperatures are usually quoted assuming isothermal operation with a flame ionisation detector. Other detectors may impose different limits, the mass spectrometer being much more susceptible to bleeding of the stationary phase than the thermal conductivity detector. All phases will bleed very slightly at high temperatures although normally this is not noticeable. Operating temperature has a profound effect on column life, particularly for capillary columns. Loss of stationary phase, or breakdown of the thin film into pools of the phase, expose the tubing surface resulting in serious loss of performance. The temperature limit of a column may be determined by the deactivation procedure used in production, rather than by the stationary phase itself. The newer silica columns have a very low metal oxide content, thought to act as a catalyst for the degradation of both sample and stationary phase, thus enabling phases to be run at higher temperatures. These columns have a protective external coating of polyimide which is slowly degraded at elevated temperatures and this can also limit column life. However, separations are usually achieved at lower temperatures on capillary columns than on packed columns.

Detectors

THERMAL CONDUCTIVITY DETECTOR (TCD)

This consists of a pair of heated filaments, each as the arm of a Wheatstone bridge, over which the column effluent and a reference gas stream flow. When a compound reaches the filament, the thermal conductivity is changed and the resulting change in temperature of the wire causes a change in resistance. This change unbalances the bridge to provide the signal. This detector is used for the analysis of permanent gases and in cases where the amount of sample is not limited. The detector will respond to all gases and vapours with a thermal conductivity different from that of the carrier. The disadvantages include a rather low sensitivity and a critical dependence on temperature stability and gas flow.

FLAME IONISATION DETECTOR (FID)

This detector is probably the most widely used of all detectors since it responds to nearly all classes of compound.

The effluent from the column is mixed with hydrogen and the mixture burnt at a small jet in a flow of air. Above the jet is the collector electrode (a wire or ring around the jet) and a polarising potential of about 150 volts is applied between the jet and the electrode. When a component elutes from the column it is burnt in the flame and the resulting ions carry a current between the electrodes which provides the signal.

The detector need not be physically small since the effective volume is approximately that of the flame and is usually only a few microlitres. The background current is very low (10^{-12} amp) as is the noise level (10^{-14} amp). Any of the usual carrier gases can be used and minor changes in gas flow are without effect. The flow of hydrogen should be approximately equal to the carrier flow and an air supply of about 20 times the carrier flow is necessary to purge the detector adequately. Sensitivity is very high and less than 10^{-12} g per ml of carrier gas can be detected. Linearity is remarkable, as high as six orders of magnitude.

The response of the flame ionisation detector is roughly dependent on the number of carbon atoms in the molecule, but the response is lower if oxygen or nitrogen are also present in the molecule. It will respond to all organic compounds containing carbon–hydrogen bonds with the exception of formic acid. The insensitivity of the detector to water is a most useful feature which allows aqueous solutions to be used.

ALKALI FLAME IONISATION DETECTOR (AFID)

The introduction of alkali metal vapours into the flame of a flame ionisation detector confers an enhanced response to compounds containing phosphorus and nitrogen. By adjustment of operating conditions the detector can be made virtually specific for phosphorus compounds, e.g. a phosphorus:carbon response ratio of 50 000:1 and a phosphorus:nitrogen response ratio of 100:1. Even when optimised for nitrogen compounds it retains its response to phosphorus, e.g. a nitrogen:carbon response ratio of 5000:1 and a nitrogen:phosphorus response ratio of 10:1.

Modern versions of this detector have an electrically heated rubidium silicate source of metal ions. The detector is particularly useful for drug analysis since most drugs contain nitrogen, while the solvent and the bulk of the co-extracted material from a biological sample do not.

This detector is especially useful for the detection of pesticides containing phosphorus. The extreme sensitivity to compounds containing phosphorus can be further exploited by the preparation of derivatives containing this element.

ELECTRON CAPTURE DETECTOR (ECD)

This is a selective detector which is very highly sensitive to compounds with a high affinity for electrons. Compounds containing a halogen, nitro group, or a carbonyl group are detected at very low concentrations.

The early form of this detector consisted of a small chamber with two electrodes parallel to each other and a radioactive source, usually ^{63}Ni, placed close to the cathode to ionise the carrier gas. A potential (2–30 volts) applied to the electrodes produces a steady background current. When an electron-capturing substance appears in the chamber some of the electrons are removed and a fall in the detector current results. The response of the detector is therefore a loss of signal rather than an increase in signal as given by most other detectors. More recent designs use concentric electrodes instead of parallel plates. Although the electron capture detector can be polarised from a suitable low voltage direct current supply, it is more sensitive when a pulsed power supply is used. The voltage is applied for a period of 0.5 to 10 microseconds, with an interval between the pulses of 5 to 500 microseconds.

Unfortunately the detector is markedly non-linear when operated in either pulsed or direct current mode. However, modern detectors can be operated in a constant current mode, the polarising pulses being modulated to maintain a constant current. A voltage dependent on the modulation frequency is generated as the output signal. Linearity is markedly improved, typically by 10^4.

If a small amount of a quench gas such as methane is added to the carrier the stability and linearity of the detector are increased. If argon or helium is used the addition of a quenching agent is essential. Additional carrier gas, usually referred to as 'make-up gas', can be added at the detector end of the column. With low column flow rates, as with capillary columns, 'make-up gas' may be necessary to purge the detector adequately and thus avoid peak broadening and distortion.

The selectivity of the electron capture detector, coupled with its extreme sensitivity (down to 1 pg), makes it very useful for compounds such as the benzodiazepines or halogenated pesticides. Alternatively, the great sensitivity of the detector may be utilised by preparing derivatives with reagents such as heptafluorobutyric anhydride. For some compounds the sensitivity of this detector may exceed that of the mass spectrometer.

PHOTOIONISATION DETECTOR (PID)

This uses ultraviolet radiation to produce ionised species which can be collected and detected as a current. Lamps of various energies (8.3, 9.5, 10.2, 11.7 eV) can be used to change the selectivity of the detector. Sensitivity is of the same order as the flame ionisation detector for amenable compounds, although it can be as low as 2 pg for benzene, with a dynamic range of 7 orders of magnitude.

The 11.7 eV lamp gives an almost universal response to hydrocarbons, whereas lamps of lower energy give some degree of selectivity. Compounds with an ionisation potential below that of the lamp will not be detected. Substances such as formaldehyde, hydrogen sulphide, nitrous oxide, tetraethyl lead, phosphine, and ammonia can be detected at better sensitivities and wider dynamic range than with other detectors. The barbiturates can be detected at lower levels than with the flame ionisation detector.

FLAME PHOTOMETRIC DETECTOR (FPD)

This detector burns the column effluent in a hydrogen-rich (reducing) flame and the optical emission is monitored by photomultiplier tubes through interference filters. A filter of 394 nm makes the detector almost totally specific for sulphur, while a filter of 526 nm confers selectivity for phosphorus. For example, with a 394 nm filter the sulphur:phosphorus response ratio is 10 000:1, and with a 526 nm filter the phosphorus:sulphur response ratio is 10:1.

Two photomultiplier filter combinations can be used to obtain the phosphorus and sulphur outputs simultaneously. However, its use for phosphorus is rendered obsolete by the more robust alkali flame ionisation detector, although it is still used for sulphur. In the sulphur mode the output is proportional to the square of the sulphur concentration, although modern electronics can linearise this output.

ELECTROLYTIC CONDUCTIVITY DETECTOR

In this detector, column effluent is mixed with a reaction gas (air or hydrogen) and passed into a reactor at $800°$ containing a catalyst to convert eluting components into conducting species. Interferences are removed by a scrubber placed between the reactor and the conductivity cell. The gas stream then enters a conductivity cell where components dissolve in the circulating electrolyte. The conductivity of this solution is compared with that of the electrolyte alone and the difference provides the output of the detector.

The detector is truly specific for halogens (unlike the electron capture detector), the chlorine:carbon response ratio being $1 \times 10^6 : 1$; it is also specific for nitrogen (unlike the alkali flame ionisation detector), the nitrogen:carbon response ratio also being $1 \times 10^6 : 1$.

For sulphur the detector is of the same order of sensitivity as the flame photometric detector but gives a linear output, the sulphur:carbon (except carbon dioxide) response ratio being $1 \times 10^5 : 1$.

It is comparable in sensitivity to the thermal energy analyser for low molecular weight nitrosamines, the nitrosamines:other nitrogenous compounds response ratio being 500:1. The detection of nitrosamines and the specificity for halogens ensure the continued use of this detector.

MASS SPECTROMETRY

The quadrupole or dodecapole mass spectrometer is an ideal detector as the chromatograph is an almost ideal inlet device for the mass spectrometer. The ability to scan a spectrum rapidly (typically 2 s for a mass range of 50 to 500 mass units), and the tolerance to relatively high source pressure (1×10^{-5} torr) make interfacing quite simple (see under Mass Spectrometry, p. 252).

DUAL DETECTOR SYSTEMS

The use of detectors such as the electron capture detector (ECD) for the identification of amenable compounds and the alkali flame ionisation detector (AFID) for the detection of compounds containing phosphorus and nitrogen, removes many of the extraneous peaks frequently observed when non-selective detectors such as the flame ionisation detector (FID) are used. However, although the use of these selective detectors has increased the

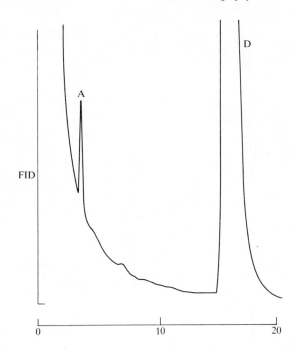

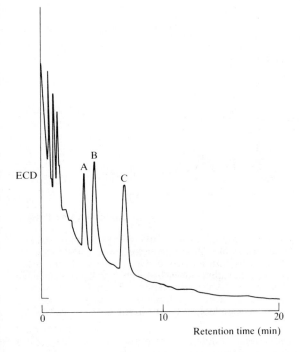

Fig. 1. Chromatograms, using both FID and ECD, of an extract of a blood sample from a patient taking flurazepam who had a blood transfusion. A, di(2-ethylhexyl) phthalate from the polyvinyl chloride transfusion bag; B, N^1-desalkylflurazepam; C, prazepam (internal standard); D, cholesterol.

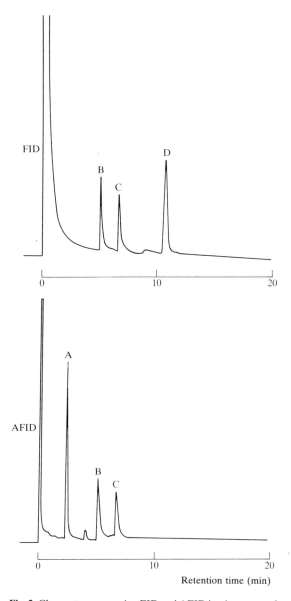

Fig. 2. Chromatograms, using FID and AFID in nitrogen mode, of an extract of a blood sample containing barbiturates. The attenuations were adjusted to give approximately equal-sized peaks for the barbiturates on both detectors. The contamination from tri-isobutyl phosphate introduced from the filter paper is apparent. A, tri-isobutyl phosphate; B, amylobarbitone; C, quinalbarbitone; D, $C_{19}H_{40}$ (retention index marker).

sensitivity of detection of many drug groups, it has exchanged one set of problems for another. Hitherto undetected non-drug substances are now observed which interfere in many toxicological analyses.

The simultaneous use of a combination of a universal detector (FID) and a specific detector to monitor the effluent of a column can provide useful information about the properties of functional groups and substituents in a molecule. The FID response is roughly dependent on the number of carbon atoms in a molecule and is quite predictable. However, the ECD response varies widely for different compounds, is dependent on the electron-deficient part of the compound, and is difficult to predict. The AFID response of a compound depends to some extent on the number of phosphorus or nitrogen atoms in a molecule, but it also depends on their environment. Thus, by using the FID as a reference and measuring the ECD or AFID response relative to it, another characteristic for identification is obtained in addition to retention behaviour.

The ECD is very sensitive to phthalate esters, for example di(2-ethylhexyl) phthalate which is a common contaminant of blood stored in polyvinyl chloride containers (Fig. 1). The AFID can be made virtually specific for phosphorus-containing compounds, but retains its capability to detect phosphorus even when optimised for nitrogen compounds. The contaminant tri-isobutyl phosphate from filter paper is not apparent when using the FID, but produces the largest peak on the chromatogram with the AFID in the nitrogen mode (Fig. 2).

Introduction of Samples

PACKED COLUMNS

Injection of the sample is usually made by means of a syringe and needle through a silicone-rubber septum. The sample may be injected either directly on to the column or into a heated zone in the gas stream before it enters the column. In the latter case the inlet port can be fitted with a removable glass liner to prevent non-volatile material contaminating the column. Unstable materials may be decomposed by the temperature of the injection system, particularly if the system is constructed of metal. For labile substances, the most satisfactory method is on-column injection. The injection port and the column must be in a straight line so that a long syringe needle can just enter the top of the column packing. This is the method of choice for many drugs, but clean extracts should be used to minimise column contamination.

Solids may be dissolved in a suitable solvent and injected with a microsyringe. It is better to keep the solution as concentrated as possible to reduce the size of the solvent peak. The small glass conical-bottomed tubes used for bacteriological agglutination tests (Dreyer tubes) are very cheap and will allow a large number of injections to be made from 0.05 ml of solution.

Liquids can be injected using a microsyringe of 1 to 10 μl capacity, but, with sensitive detection systems, it is necessary to dissolve the sample in a suitable solvent to reduce the sample size and avoid overloading the detector.

Gases and vapours may be introduced by injection through the inlet port septum using a gas-tight syringe. Usual volumes are in the range 0.2 to 10 ml. A gas sampling valve is the method of choice for quantitative work or if much qualitative work is contemplated.

Head-space Analysis

This technique permits the detection of volatile substances in a liquid sample and minimises contamination of the column. A small volume (0.2 to 0.5 ml) of the sample is placed in a small vial (typically 7 ml) sealed with a septum disk which is faced with polytetrafluoroethylene, and the vial is equilibrated at an appropriate elevated temperature for about ten minutes. A sample of the vapour is removed with a syringe, taking care that no liquid is withdrawn, and is then injected on to the column. This technique is used in the assay of ethanol and other solvents in blood and for complex household preparations such as polishes, which contain volatile substances.

CAPILLARY COLUMNS

The low flow rate (about 2 ml/min) through open tubular columns poses constraints on injector design. To overcome this, either the volume of the injector must be decreased or the flow rate through it must be increased.

Split Injection

An inlet splitter allows a high flow through the injector while maintaining a low flow through the column, the excess gas and associated sample components being vented to the atmosphere. The ratio of these two flows (the split ratio) is the proportion of injected sample that reaches the column. The function of the splitter is not to reduce sample volume, but to ensure that the sample enters the column as a plug and is not exponentially diluted. The total flow through the injector may be from 10 to 400 ml/min giving split ratios of 10:1 to 500:1. A good splitter should be linear, that is it should split high- and low-boiling point compounds equally. However, it is rare to meet a sample with a large volatility range in drug analysis. At high split

ratios, large volumes of carrier gas flow through the splitter and care must be taken to ensure that it is adequately pre-heated. Choice of solvent and injector temperature are both important considerations.

Splitless Injection

Splitless injection may be either on-column, using a needle fine enough to enter the column bore, or off-column using a low-volume heated block. In either case the top of the column is held at a temperature low enough for the solvent containing the sample to condense. The solvent temporarily swamps the stationary phase and ensures that the sample components concentrate in a narrow band. Any solvent or sample remaining in the injector is back-flushed with carrier gas, often by automatic valves. The proximal end of the column is then rapidly brought to the operating temperature, when the solvent vaporises and chromatography begins. Care is necessary to select a suitable solvent with regard to boiling point, stationary phase, and sample composition. On-column injection syringes have stainless steel or silica needles which are too fine to penetrate a septum, and, in order to minimise carrier gas loss, valve assemblies are used which grip the needle or which only open when the needle is in the narrow entrance channel.

SOLID INJECTION

When solvent interference is serious the sample may be injected as a solid. The 'moving needle' injector has found application in steroid analysis and for the determination of anticonvulsant drugs. A solution of the material to be injected is placed on the tip of the glass needle with a syringe. A small flow of carrier gas sweeps the solvent out of the top of the device to waste. The dry residue is then introduced by moving the needle into the heated injection zone of the chromatograph with a magnet. This form of injection can only be used with drugs which will not volatilise with the solvent.

Temperature Programming

For complex mixtures with components of widely varying retention characteristics, it is sometimes very difficult or impractical to choose a column temperature which will allow all the components to be resolved. It is therefore necessary to vary the column temperature throughout the analysis. Most instruments are available with a temperature programming option, a multi-ramp programmer being particularly useful for capillary chromatography. The first ramp can be used during splitless injection to bring the column rapidly up to the initial chromatography temperature, followed by a slower analytical ramp to perform the separation. One problem with temperature programming is that the back-pressure increases with temperature and will reduce flow if a flow controller is not used. Column bleed will also increase, resulting in an increasing baseline. For this reason the column should be well conditioned at the upper temperature limit.

Gas Pressure and Flow Control

In order to perform accurate and reproducible gas chromatography it is necessary to maintain a constant carrier gas flow. Some detectors need additional gases which also require flow or pressure control. Under isothermal conditions simple pressure control is adequate for packed or capillary columns. However, the added convenience of a digital flow controller may be considered worthwhile. A pressure gauge between the flow controller and the injector will enable the back-pressure to be monitored, a decrease being symptomatic of a leaking septum and an increase suggesting contamination of the top of the column. It also serves to ensure that the flow controller is performing correctly. If the back-pressure rises to equal the supply pressure, then flow will become pressure controlled.

Flow control is highly desirable if not essential during temperature programming with packed columns and can be used to advantage with on-column injectors on capillary columns. Pressure control, with metal diaphragms, is the only practical means of gas control for capillary work with split injection.

Adequate gas control for flame ionisation detector gases is usually achieved by pressure regulators supplying gas via constrictors. Some alkali flame ionisation detectors require very precise control of hydrogen flow, best achieved by mass flow control.

Derivative Formation

The preparation of derivatives may be used to give additional evidence of identity or to improve gas chromatography characteristics. For identification purposes, the indication that specific functional groups are present and that derivative formation is possible may provide useful information. Although the retention characteristics are changed, the order of elution of a series of derivatives will be the same as for the parent compounds.

Derivative preparation can be used to shorten or lengthen the retention time of a substance and this can be helpful to remove the substance peak away from interfering material or to speed the analysis. For instance, hydroxylated compounds often have long retention times and low sensitivity, and tailing may result. However, they readily form silyl ethers and these derivatives behave similarly to hydrocarbons.

Derivatives may also be used to make the molecule capable of detection by selective detectors.

The reaction may be carried out during extraction (e.g. extractive methylation), on the dry residue (e.g. silylation), or during injection (e.g. methylation). If a compound requires derivatisation in order to reduce its polarity, the use of high pressure liquid chromatography should be considered instead of GLC, assuming that sensitivity is not the limiting factor.

SILYLATION

Most alcohols and phenols will form silyl ethers when treated with trimethylsilyl reagents at room temperature. Some compounds with sterically-hindered hydroxy groups require heating. Since the reagents and the reaction products are very easily hydrolysed, it is essential that the glassware is dry and that water vapour is rigorously excluded. Hexamethyldisilazane will silylate many compounds, although N,O-bis(trimethylsilyl)trifluoro-acetamide is a more powerful reagent, especially when catalysed by 1% trimethylchlorosilane. *tert*-Butyldimethylsilylimidazole reacts in a similar manner to the other reagents, but forms ethers which are much more resistant to hydrolysis.

FORMATION OF IMINES (SCHIFF'S BASES)

Primary amines condense with aldehydes and ketones to form imines, and while many aldehydes and ketones can be used, those of large molecular weight usually give a poorer yield of the derivative. Acetone, isobutyl methyl ketone, and benzaldehyde usually form stable derivatives. Carbon disulphide can be used as a reagent to form isothiocyanate derivatives with primary amines. If a cyclic ketone such as cyclohexanone is used, the carbinolamine derivative will be formed. Ephedrine and other beta-hydroxylated secondary amines form oxazolidines when treated with ketones.

ACYLATION

Primary and secondary amines can be acylated readily by treatment with acid anhydrides and heat. Acetic anhydride, propionic anhydride, and trifluoroacetic anhydride react readily. Direct extractive acetylation using *N*-methylimidazole as catalyst has been reported for a number of drugs including paracetamol. Reagents for preparing electron-capturing derivatives include trifluoroacetic anhydride, heptafluorobutyric anhydride, and pentafluorobenzoic anhydride.

METHYLATION

On-column methylation of barbiturates, hydantoins, and some carboxylic acids can be achieved by injecting the sample mixed with 0.2M trimethylanilinium hydroxide in methanol. For carboxylic acids, the sample can be dissolved in 14% boron trifluoride in methanol and heated at 60 to 100° for 30 minutes. After evaporation of the bulk of the methanol, the mixture is diluted with a few millilitres of water and the methyl derivative extracted with a small volume of hexane.

The use of trimethylanilinium hydroxide can cause a problem. Highly polar material which has not been fully methylated can lie dormant on a column for a long period of time, but can be released by a subsequent injection of trimethylanilinium hydroxide, thus yielding a false positive result.

The toxic and potentially explosive diazomethane may be used for the methylation of drugs, including the barbiturates. The reaction is rapid and can be carried out by dissolving the compound in a few hundred microlitres of an ethereal solution of diazomethane and removing excess reagent with a stream of nitrogen. Diazomethane has the advantage of being clean and fast.

Evaluation of Chromatographic Performance

The evaluation of the performance of the column, whether capillary or packed, is made on the basis of its efficiency (the narrowness of a peak) and the peak shape (i.e. whether it tails or fronts). A well packed column in a well designed system should give symmetrical peaks, as tailing or fronting will adversely affect resolution. Tailing may result from non-swept volume in the system or from component/stationary phase or component/support interactions. The tailing of polar compounds can often be remedied by the use of a more polar stationary phase. Fronting usually results from overloading, particularly with capillary columns.

Peak shape is usually expressed by the peak asymmetry (A_s). In Fig. 3, the peak asymmetry factor for substance B is given by

$$A_s = \frac{YZ}{XY}$$

where a vertical line is drawn through the peak maximum and XYZ is drawn at 10% of the peak height. A symmetrical peak has $A_s = 1$.

Efficiency is dependent on the degree of band broadening relative to the time taken to elute. It is measured in theoretical plates (N) by analogy with distillation. For a particular substance, this can be calculated by

$$N = 16\left[\frac{t_R}{W}\right]^2 \quad or \quad N = 5.54\left[\frac{t_R}{W_{1/2}}\right]^2$$

where t_R = time from injection to peak maximum for the substance, W = idealised peak width at base, $W_{1/2}$ = peak width at half height.

Since N is dimensionless, any units can be used to measure t_R, W, or $W_{1/2}$ as long as they are consistent. Efficiency is usually quoted in plates per metre, or as height equivalent to a theoretical plate (HETP) (h), i.e. the length of column required to generate one plate. It is defined by

$$h = \frac{L}{N}$$

where L is the length of the column.

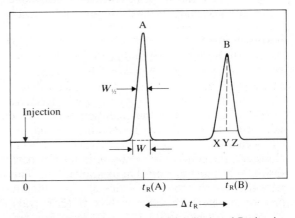

Fig. 3. Chromatogram for two compounds, A and B, showing measurement of significant parameters. W, width at the base of the peak; $W_{1/2}$, width at half peak-height; $t_R(A)$ and $t_R(B)$, retention times of A and B, respectively; Δt_R, the difference in retention time between A and B; XYZ, a line drawn at 10% of the peak height.

With long and very efficient columns, the time taken for a non-retained compound to reach the end of the column after injection (dead-time) can be several minutes. It is determined by injecting a compound such as methane for a flame ionisation detector or methylene chloride for an electron capture detector. Retention times should really compensate for the dead-time rather than being measured from the time of injection, and this is especially important when measuring efficiency, which should be measured using a compound with a retention time at least four times the dead-time.

A useful concept is the separation number (TZ), after Trennzahl who formulated it. It is a measure of how many resolved peaks can be accommodated between adjacent members of an homologous series; any series can be used.

The separation number for A and B which are two members of an homologous series differing by one methylene group (Fig. 3) is given by

$$TZ = \frac{\Delta t_R}{W_{1/2}(A) + W_{1/2}(B)} - 1$$

where Δt_R is the difference in retention time between A and B, and $W_{1/2}(A)$ and $W_{1/2}(B)$ are their peak widths at half height respectively. If $TZ = 0$, no other peak will fit between the two homologues; if $TZ = 1$, then one peak will fit.

For most applications in drug analysis the chromatogram will only contain two or three compounds of interest, but an efficient column will maximise the probability that a peak consists of only one compound and that it is the compound of interest.

Retention Index

In order to be able to communicate gas chromatographic retention data between laboratories, it is necessary to use a means of recording data that is independent of the instrument used. Relative retention time, that is the retention time of the sample relative to that of a reference compound, has been used.

However, the concept of retention index has been shown to be more universal in its application. This system uses a homologous series of *n*-paraffins to provide the reference points on the scale (E. Kovats, *Z. analyt. Chem.*, 1961, *181*, 351–366). For any column temperature and stationary phase, the elution times of members of a series of *n*-paraffin homologues are assumed to increase by an index of 100 for each additional methylene unit. On this scale, H_2 has an index of zero, methane has an index of 100, ethane of 200, and so on up the scale of paraffins. This method produces a scale against which unknown substances are measured, and the variations in retention time, which are frequently very considerable, are obviated. The method is illustrated in Fig. 4, where phenobarbitone has a retention time of 4.5 minutes and a retention index of 1957.

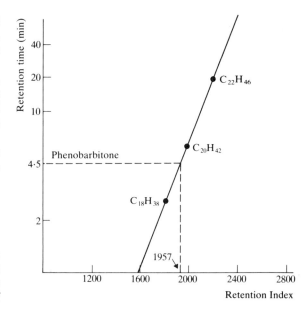

Fig. 4. The determination of the retention index of phenobarbitone from a plot of an homologous series of *n*-paraffins.

Retention indices collected from many sources (R. E. Ardrey *et al., J. Chromat.*, 1981, *220*, 195–252) show remarkable agreement, even when measurements were made on different (though equivalent) phases and at different temperatures. As is to be expected, there is better agreement for non-polar (most hydrocarbon-like) compounds than for polar compounds.

In practice, for isothermal chromatography, the retention index (RI) is found by logarithmic interpolation between *n*-paraffins that bracket the compound. Retention index =

$$100(P_{z+n} - P_z) \times \frac{\log t_R(x) - \log t_R(P_z)}{\log t_R(P_{z+n}) - \log t_R(P_z)} + 100P_z$$

where P_z = carbon number of small paraffin, P_{z+n} = carbon number of large paraffin, t_R = retention time, and x = unknown compound. There is an approximately linear relationship between the retention time and chain length during linear temperature programming if all peaks elute on the same ramp, and this can be used to calculate RI.

Quantitative Determinations

Quantitative work usually requires some form of sample preparation to isolate the drug from the bulk of the sample and some degree of concentration or, more rarely, dilution. These processes will inevitably introduce some degree of analytical error. A further difficulty is caused by the non-reproducibility of injected volumes. In order to compensate for these errors, it is usual to compare the response of the unknown with the response of an added internal standard. The internal standard should be added as early as possible in the assay process and should have chromatographic properties as close as possible to the drug, preferably with a longer retention time. It is often possible to obtain unmarketed analogues of drugs, or compounds specially synthesised for use as internal standards. However, the internal standard will not behave exactly as the drug and careful control of variables, such as pH, is necessary. If a derivative is to be prepared, the standard should also be derivatisable. An inappropriate internal standard can seriously affect precision (K. H. Dudley, Trace Organic Sample Handling, in *Methodological Surveys Sub-series (A)*, Vol. 10, E. Reid (Ed.), Chichester U.K., Ellis Horwood, 1980, p. 336).

If a mass spectrometer is being used as the detector, then the ideal internal standard is a ^{13}C analogue of the drug.

Calibration should include points of higher and lower concentrations than the sample, and quality assessment samples should be included at appropriate concentrations in frequently run assays. Peak measurement may be by peak height or by the peak area obtained by integration. The plot of the ratio of peak height (or area) of the drug to internal standard versus concentration will be a straight line with most detectors.

Practical Points

Carrier gas flow should be optimised for a particular column and a particular carrier gas. This is most important for open tubular columns. Fig. 5 shows the relationship between efficiency expressed as the height equivalent of a theoretical plate versus carrier gas velocity (Van Deemter plot) for a 28 m by 0.25 mm internal diameter wall-coated open tubular column of Carbowax 20M.

It is unwise to assume that published conditions will be correct for any chromatographic system. They may be accurate; on the other hand they may be no more accurate than the calibration of the oven controller or flow meter on the particular instrument. In general, retention times double with a decrease in temperature of 20°.

For a particular separation, the lowest temperature compatible with a reasonable analysis time should be used. If the time is excessive, it is generally

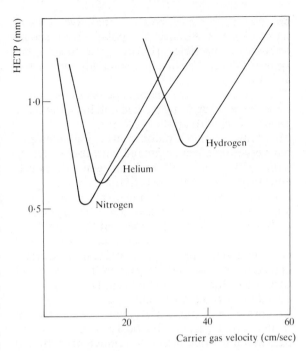

Fig. 5. Van Deemter plots for a 28 m by 0.25 mm internal diameter wall-coated open tubular column coated with Carbowax 20M run with different carrier gases.

better to reduce the stationary phase loading than to increase the column temperature.

There is a maximum temperature at which a column can be operated and there is also a minimum temperature below which the efficiency will drop sharply. The stationary phase must be a liquid at the temperature of operation, and if a column is run at too low a temperature to obtain longer retention times the stationary phase may still be in the solid or semi-solid form.

To ensure even packing of the column the particle size should not exceed 1/20th of the column diameter or there may be some loss of efficiency. The particle size distribution should be as small as possible.

If trace impurities are sought in the presence of a preponderant component, a number of stationary phases of differing polarities should be tried. Trace impurities are easily seen if they emerge before the main component of a mixture, while they may be completely lost in the tail if they come just after the large peak. Early peaks are also sharper and thus, for the same peak area, will be higher, and this effect can contribute enormously to the successful detection of trace substances.

The solvent used for the sample can sometimes

produce unexpected derivatives that give different retention times. An inert non-polar solvent should be used if possible. However, acetone, other ketones, and carbon disulphide readily form derivatives with primary amines.

The gas used as the mobile phase is of minor importance when using packed columns, but has a greater effect with capillary columns.

Modifying the mobile phase in gas chromatography has very little effect compared with that observed with HPLC or TLC and, in general, affects efficiency rather than selectivity. Nitrogen gives higher efficiency, but at the expense of longer analysis time, while the less dense but hazardous hydrogen gives lower efficiency but faster analysis. In practice, nitrogen is usually used for packed columns and helium for capillary columns. Certain detectors impose restrictions on the choice of carrier gas, but an additional supply of gas can be added to the column effluent to purge the detector.

The presence of traces of oxygen or water vapour in the carrier gas will drastically shorten column life. Metal hydride filters (to remove oxygen) and molecular sieves (to remove water vapour) are strongly recommended.

If dirty samples have been injected, the top of the column may show marked deterioration. The top few centimetres of packing should then be replaced with fresh packing, the glass wool should be replaced with new material, and the column reconditioned. Similarly, after continual use a capillary column may often have its former performance restored by removing the first coil with no significant loss of efficiency.

GAS CHROMATOGRAPHY SYSTEMS

The systems given below have been chosen because of their applicability to routine screening, separating, and identifying drugs. The drugs are divided into chemical or pharmacological groups, but some other drugs are also included if they are chemically similar and would be extracted with that group, e.g. apomorphine and naloxone are included in the narcotic analgesics. References to specific systems for the quantification of individual drugs or groups of drugs are given in the monographs in Part 2.

The most general screening system is one using a dimethylsilicone stationary phase such as SE-30, OV-1, or OV-101. This should always be used for screening purposes since it has the greatest chance of eluting any compound of interest. The support should always be a high performance support to eliminate any of its adsorptive effects. Treatment

of the support with potassium hydroxide will ensure that amines give better peak shapes, but at the expense of not being able to elute acids and phenols. If an untreated column is used for chromatographing basic extracts, then acidic compounds such as barbiturates will not be eluted because a small amount of alkaline hydroxide will accumulate at the beginning of the column.

Most of the data are for the drugs themselves, but thermal decomposition may occur and the peak observed may be for the decomposition product rather than the original drug. Where the drug is known to chromatograph badly, or to decompose, data are given for the derivatives, e.g. methyl esters for the sulphonamides.

Wherever possible the retention index of the drug is given. This is a more reproducible retention parameter than retention time or relative retention time and is practically independent of support, loading of phase, and temperature. However, if a laboratory routinely prefers to use these parameters, the retention index data can easily be converted by chromatographing a few representative drugs and using a calibration graph or linear regression analysis of retention indices against retention times or relative retention times. The retention indices on low polarity stationary phases are very similar, so that those for SE-30 can often also be used for Apiezon L etc. Retention indices for non-drug substances that may interfere with toxicological analyses, but are not included in this book, may be found in R. E. Ardrey and A. C. Moffat, *J. Chromat.*, 1981, *220*, 195–252 and J. Ramsey *et al.*, *J. Chromat.*, 1980, *184*, 185–206.

An alkali flame ionisation detector is the best detector for nitrogenous drugs, but a flame ionisation detector should always be used as well, since many drugs do not contain nitrogen, e.g. some anti-inflammatory agents. Electron capture detectors are excellent for benzodiazepines and halogen-containing compounds such as the phenothiazines. Extra selectivity can always be obtained by using element-specific detectors, e.g. those for phosphorus and sulphur for compounds containing those elements.

NOTE. In the tables of retention indices, a dash indicates that no value is available for the compound, not that it does not elute.

GENERAL SCREEN

System GA

R. E. Ardrey and A. C. Moffat, *J. Chromat.*, 1981, *220*, 195–252.

This system may be used for most thermally stable drugs. Because the stated values for drugs are retention indices, the operating conditions for the SE-30 column may be varied to suit particular laboratory situations.

COLUMN. 2.5% SE-30 on 80–100 mesh Chromosorb G (acid-washed and dimethyldichlorosilane-treated), 2 m × 4 mm internal diameter glass column. It is essential that the support is fully deactivated.

COLUMN TEMPERATURE. Normally between 100° and 300°. As an approximate guide, the temperature to use is the retention index ÷ 10.

CARRIER GAS. Nitrogen at 45 ml/min.

REFERENCE COMPOUNDS. n-Alkanes with an even number of carbon atoms.

RETENTION INDICES. Values for drugs in this system will be found in drug monographs and in the indexes to Analytical Data in Part 3; they are also included in the systems for specific groups of drugs which follow.

AMPHETAMINES, OTHER STIMULANTS, AND ANORECTICS

System GA, previously described, may be used, or Systems GB or GC, below. System GA produces tailing peaks with these compounds.

System GB

D. A. Cowan, personal communication.

COLUMN. 10% Apiezon L and 2% KOH on 80–100 mesh Chromosorb W HP, 2 m × 3 mm internal diameter glass column.

COLUMN TEMPERATURE. Programmed at 16° per minute from 170° to 260° and held for 8 minutes.

CARRIER GAS. Nitrogen at 30 ml/min.

REFERENCE COMPOUNDS. n-Alkanes with an even number of carbon atoms, or use retention times relative to diphenylamine (RI 1680).

System GC

D. A. Cowan, personal communication.

In this system, the drugs are chromatographed as tertiary bases or trifluoroacetyl derivatives (see p. 188).

COLUMN. 3% OV-17 on 80–100 mesh Chromosorb W HP, 2 m × 3 mm internal diameter glass column.

COLUMN TEMPERATURE. 170° for 2 minutes and then programmed at 16° per minute to 270° and held for 8 minutes.

CARRIER GAS. Nitrogen at 30 ml/min.

REFERENCE COMPOUNDS. n-Alkanes with an even number of carbon atoms.

RETENTION INDICES. The retention indices given for System GC are those of the tertiary bases or of trifluoroacetyl derivatives.

	System GA	GB	GC
Amiphenazole	—	1150	2563
Amphetamine	1123	1134	1536
Bemegride	1373	—	1253
Benzphetamine	1855	1895	2172
Caffeine	1810	1862	2376
Cathine	1302	1362	1383
Chlorphentermine	1342	1410	1725
Clorprenaline	1604	1614	1880
Cyclopentamine	1087	1095	—
Diethylpropion	1486	1507	1715
Dimefline	2555	—	—
Dimethylamphetamine	1236	1261	1429
Doxapram	2906	—	2230
Ephedrine	1363	1386	1467
Etafedrine	1519	1510	1737
Ethamivan	—	—	2409
Fencamfamin	1677	1745	2180
Fenfluramine	1222	1158	1621
Heptaminol	1118	1084	—
Hydroxyamphetamine	1320	—	—
Isometheptene	1052	994	—
Isoprenaline	1730	—	—
Lobeline	1780	—	—
Mazindol	2355	—	—
Meclofenoxate	1770	1804	2200
Mephentermine	1239	1278	1668
Mescaline	1688	—	—
Methoxamine	1726	1735	—
Methoxyamphetamine	1385	—	—
Methoxyphenamine	1361	1370	1670
Methylamphetamine	1176	1200	1722
Methylenedioxy-amphetamine	1472	—	—
Methylephedrine	1400	1440	1480
Methylphenidate	1737	—	2200
Naphazoline	2057	2122	2457
Nicotine	1348	1375	1573
Nikethamide	1525	1513	1852
Pargyline	1214	1218	1440
Pemoline	2160	—	—
Pentetrazol	1552	1578	2021
Phenbutrazate	2670	—	—
Phendimetrazine	1444	1513	1735
Phenelzine	1335	—	1460
Phenethylamine	1031	—	—
Phenmetrazine	1431	1473	1873
Phentermine	1147	1182	1450

	System		
	GA	GB	GC
Phenylephrine	—	—	1934
Phenylpropanolamine	1313	1353	1383
Pipradrol	2145	2215	2478
Prolintane	1634	1675	1849
Propylhexedrine	1169	1186	1500
Pseudoephedrine	1354	1399	1543
Tranylcypromine	1223	1245	1759
Trimethoxyamphetamine	1748	—	—
Tuaminoheptane	888	849	1287

ANALGESICS, NON-STEROIDAL ANTI-INFLAMMATORY DRUGS, AND OTHER STRONGLY ACIDIC DRUGS

System GA, previously described, may be used, or System GD, below.

System GD

In this system, the substances are chromatographed as their methyl derivatives (see p. 189).

COLUMN. 3% SE-30 on 80–100 mesh Chromosorb G (acid-washed and dimethyldichlorosilane-treated), 2 m × 3 mm internal diameter glass column.

COLUMN TEMPERATURE. 120° for 2 minutes and then programmed at 10° per minute to 260° and held for 5 minutes.

CARRIER GAS. Nitrogen at 40 ml/min.

REFERENCE COMPOUND. Hexadecane (n-$C_{16}H_{34}$).

Note. Free carboxylic acids and phenols will not generally give peaks although large quantities may give tailing peaks.

RETENTION INDICES AND RELATIVE RETENTION TIMES. The values given for System GD are retention times of methyl derivatives relative to n-$C_{16}H_{34}$.

	System	
	GA	GD
Alclofenac	—	1.13
Aletamine	1293	—
Amidopyrine	1903	—
Aspirin	1309	—
Baclofen	2010	—
Benoxaprofen	—	1.98
Bufexamac	—	1.12
Clonixin	—	1.61
Diclofenac	2271	1.42
Diflunisal	—	1.20
Fenbufen	—	1.79
Fenclofenac	—	1.55 and 1.26
Fenoprofen	2021	1.31

	System	
	GA	GD
Feprazone	2380	1.81
Flufenamic acid	1950	1.26
Flunixin	—	1.39
Flurbiprofen	2032	1.30
Frusemide	—	2.64
Ibuprofen	—	0.89
Indomethacin	2685	1.55 and 0.49
Indoprofen	—	2.27 and 2.07
Ketoprofen	—	1.45
Meclofenamic acid	2420	1.62
Mefenamic acid	2201	1.45
Naproxen	2130	1.37 and 1.18
Niflumic acid	—	1.38
Oxyphenbutazone	1630	2.11
Paracetamol	1687	—
Phenacetin	1675	—
Phenazone	1848	—
Phenylbutazone	2365	2.05 and 1.81
Salicylic acid	1309	—
Salsalate	—	0.6 and 0.4
Sulindac	2690, 2750, 2820	0.49
Theophylline	1999	—
Tolmetin	—	1.77 and 1.36
Zomepirac	2048, 1870	—

ANTICONVULSANTS

System GA, previously described, may be used, or System GE, below.

System GE

Quantitative Analysis of Underivatised Antiepileptic Drugs, Supelco Bulletin 779, 1979, Supelco Inc., Bellefonte, Pennsylvania 16823.

COLUMN. 2% SP-2110 and 1% SP-2510-DA on 100–120 mesh Supelcoport, 1 m × 2 mm internal diameter glass column.

COLUMN TEMPERATURE. Programmed at 16° per minute from 120° to 250°.

CARRIER GAS. Nitrogen at 50 ml/min.

REFERENCE COMPOUND. Phenytoin.

Note. This system separates cholesterol from all drugs in the group.

RETENTION INDICES AND RELATIVE RETENTION TIMES. The values given for System GE are retention times relative to phenytoin.

	System	
	GA	GE
Beclamide	1480, 1678	—
Carbamazepine	2290	0.83

	System	
	GA	GE
Cholesterol	3086	1.35
Clonazepam	2885	—
Ethosuximide	1206	0.18
Ethotoin	1800	0.57
Methoin	1791	0.55
Methsuximide	1622	0.35
Paramethadione	1120	0.06
Phenacemide	1473	—
Pheneturide	1465	—
Phenobarbitone	1957	0.74
Phensuximide	1634	0.39
Phenytoin	2330	1.00
Primidone	2247	0.89
Troxidone	1100	0.04
Valproic acid	—	0.09

ANTIDEPRESSANTS

System GA, previously described, may be used, or System GF, below.

System GF

R. J. Flanagan and D. J. Berry, *J. Chromat.*, 1977, *131*, 131–146.

COLUMN. 3% Poly A103 on 80–100 mesh Chromosorb W HP, 1 m × 4 mm internal diameter glass column.

COLUMN TEMPERATURE. 200°.

CARRIER GAS. Nitrogen at 60 ml/min.

REFERENCE COMPOUNDS. *n*-Alkanes with an even number of carbon atoms.

RETENTION INDICES

	System	
	GA	GF
Amitriptyline	2196	2510
Butriptyline	2181	2465
Clomipramine	2406	2795
Clorgyline	1883	—
Desipramine	2242	—
Dibenzepin	2443	2885
Dothiepin	2380	2770
Doxepin	2217	2570
Imipramine	2223	2540
Iprindole	2335	—
Iproniazid	1593	—
Isocarboxazid	1949	—
Maprotiline	2356	—
Mebanazine	1240	—
Mianserin	2211	2595
Nomifensine	2122	2670
Nortriptyline	2210	—

	System	
	GA	GF
Noxiptyline	2267	—
Phenelzine	1335	—
Protriptyline	2261	2590
Tranylcypromine	1223	1455
Trazodone	3250	—
Trimipramine	2201	2505
Zimeldine	2213	—

ANTIHISTAMINES

Systems GA, GB, GC, or GF, previously described, may be used.

RETENTION INDICES

	System			
	GA	GB	GC	GF
Antazoline	2328	—	2749	—
Azatadine	2415	—	—	—
Bamipine	2211	—	—	—
Bromodiphen-hydramine	2155	—	—	2480
Brompheniramine	2096	2159	2457	2470
Buclizine	3286	—	—	—
Carbinoxamine	2080	2090	2430	—
Chlorcyclizine	2225	—	—	2560
Chlorpheniramine	2002	2038	2586	2335
Cinnarizine	3065	—	—	—
Clemastine	2415	—	—	2710
Clemizole	2675	—	—	—
Cyclizine	2020	2081	2348	2320
Cyproheptadine	2366	—	2307	2710
Deptropine	2615	—	—	—
Dimenhydrinate	1844	1875	—	—
Dimethindene	2258	—	2669	—
Dimethothiazine	3078	—	—	—
Diphenhydramine	1873	1872	2378	2105
Diphenylpyraline	2099	2136	2447	2405
Doxylamine	1906	—	—	2170
Halopyramine	2234	—	—	—
Isothipendyl	2267	—	—	—
Mebhydrolin	2465	—	2739	2920
Meclozine	3033	—	—	—
Mepyramine	2220	—	—	2560
Methapyrilene	1981	—	—	2305
Methdilazine	2467	—	—	2920
Phenindamine	2167	—	2926	2515
Pheniramine	1804	1826	—	2100
Phenyltoloxamine	1938	—	—	—
Promethazine	2259	—	2546	2675
Propiomazine	2738	—	—	—
Pyrrobutamine	2419	—	—	2815
Thenalidine	2318	—	—	—

	System			
	GA	GB	GC	GF
Thenyldiamine	1999	2034	2300	2340
Thonzylamine	2203	—	2576	—
Trimeprazine	2309	—	2646	2715
Tripelennamine	1980	—	—	—
Triprolidine	2253	—	2954	2600

BARBITURATES

Systems GA or GF, previously described, may be used.

RETENTION INDICES

	System	
	GA	GF
Allobarbitone	1606	2340
Amylobarbitone	1718	2430
Aprobarbitone	1622	—
Barbitone	1497	2230
Brallobarbitone	1858	2765
Butalbital	1668	2395
Butobarbitone	1665	2390
Cyclobarbitone	1963	2825
Cyclopentobarbitone	1862	—
Enallylpropymal	1561	—
Heptabarbitone	2058	2940
Hexethal	1858	—
Hexobarbitone	1857	2380
Ibomal	1883	—
Idobutal	1698	—
Metharbitone	1472	—
Methohexitone	1766	—
Methylphenobarbitone	1891	—
Nealbarbitone	1720	2460
Pentobarbitone	1740	2465
Phenobarbitone	1957	2960
Phenylmethylbarbituric acid	1880	—
Quinalbarbitone	1791	2510
Secbutobarbitone	1662	—
Talbutal	1701	—
Thialbarbitone	2116	—
Thiopentone	1859	2600
Vinbarbitone	1740	2495
Vinylbitone	1720	—

BENZODIAZEPINES

System GA, previously described, may be used, or System GG, below.

System GG

M. Möller, personal communication.

COLUMN. 2.5% OV-17 on 80–100 mesh Chromosorb G, treatment and dimensions as for System GA.

COLUMN TEMPERATURE, CARRIER GAS, REFERENCE COMPOUNDS. As for System GA.

RETENTION INDICES. The retention indices of benzodiazepines have been shown to be dependent on column temperature (H. Schuetz and V. Westenberger, Z. Rechtsmed., 1978, 82, 43–53 and J. Chromat., 1979, 169, 409–411). The values given by these authors are about 50 retention index units above those generally quoted. The values given below should therefore be checked before use by chromatographing a few sample compounds.

	System	
	GA	GG
Bromazepam	2663	3280
Chlordiazepoxide	2453, 2530, 2799	3065
Clobazam	2694	3174
Clonazepam	2885	3600
Clorazepic acid	2457	3125
Clozapine	2967	3455
Demoxepam	2529	3043
Diazepam	2425	2940
Flunitrazepam	2645	3190
Flurazepam	2785	3220
Ketazolam	2425	2940
Lorazepam	2402	2910
Lormetazepam	2674	—
Medazepam	2226	2620
Nitrazepam	2750	3450
Nordazepam	2496	3041
Oxazepam	2336	2803
Prazepam	2641	3145
Temazepam	2633	3125
Triazolam	2965	—

Hydrolysis products of benzodiazepines and their metabolites

	System GA RI	Parent compound
2-(2-Amino-5-bromobenzoyl)pyridine	2210	Bromazepam
2-Amino-5-chlorobenzophenone	2039	Chlordiazepoxide, clorazepic acid, demoxepam, desmethyl-chlordiazepoxide, nordazepam, oxazepam

	System GA RI	Parent compound
2-Amino-5-chlorodiphenylamine	2028	Desmethylclobazam
2-Amino-5-chloro-2′-fluorobenzophenone	1980	N^1-Desalkylflurazepam
2-Amino-2′-chloro-5-nitrobenzophenone	2516	Clonazepam
2-Amino-5,2′-dichlorobenzophenone	2120	Lorazepam
5-Amino-2′-fluoro-2-methylaminobenzophenone	2653	7-Acetamidoflunitrazepam, 7-aminoflunitrazepam
2-Amino-2′-fluoro-5-nitrobenzophenone	2330	Desmethylflunitrazepam
2-Amino-5-nitrobenzophenone	2388	Nitrazepam
2-Cyclopropylmethylamino-5-chlorobenzophenone	2385	3-Hydroxyprazepam, prazepam
2,5-Diaminobenzophenone	2175	7-Acetamidonitrazepam, 7-aminonitrazepam
2,5-Diamino-2′-chlorobenzophenone	2305	7-Acetamidoclonazepam, 7-aminoclonazepam
2,5-Diamino-2′-fluorobenzophenone	2175	7-Aminodesmethylflunitrazepam
2-Diethylaminoethylamino-5-chloro-2′-fluorobenzophenone	2505	Flurazepam
2-Hydroxyethylamino-5-chloro-2′-fluorobenzophenone	2440	N^1-(2-Hydroxyethyl)flurazepam
2-Methylamino-5-chlorobenzophenone	2105	Diazepam, ketazolam, temazepam
2-Methylamino-5-chlorodiphenylamine	2220	Clobazam
2-Methylamino-5-nitro-2′-fluorobenzophenone	2385	Flunitrazepam

CANNABINOIDS

System GH

D. J. Harvey and W. D. M. Paton, *J. Chromat.*, 1975, *109*, 73–80 and also personal communication. In this system, the substances are chromatographed as their trimethylsilyl derivatives (see p. 188).

COLUMN. 3% SE-30 on 100–120 mesh Gas-Chrom Q, 2 m × 2 mm internal diameter glass column.

COLUMN TEMPERATURE. Programmed at 4° per minute from 100° to 320°.

CARRIER GAS. Nitrogen at 30 ml/min.

REFERENCE COMPOUNDS. *n*-Alkanes with an even number of carbon atoms.

RETENTION INDICES. The values given for System GH are of the trimethylsilyl esters or ethers.

	System	
	GA	GH
Cannabis constituents		
Cannabicyclol	—	2280
Cannabidiol	2382	2270
Cannabigerol	—	2440
Cannabinol	2520	2430
Propylcannabidiol	—	2110
Propyl-Δ^9-THC	—	2170
Δ^9-THC	2473	2350
Metabolites of Δ^9-THC		
8α,11-Dihydroxy-Δ^9-THC	—	2710

	System	
Metabolites of Δ^9-THC (*continued*)	GA	GH
8α-Hydroxy-Δ^9-THC	—	2580
11-Hydroxy-Δ^9-THC	—	2620
11-Nor-Δ^9-THC-9-carboxylic acid	—	2756

DIURETICS

System GA, previously described, may be used.

RETENTION INDICES

	System GA
Benzthiazide	2680
Chlorthalidone	2145
Methazolamide	2187
Polythiazide	2380
Spironolactone	3280
Trometamol	1645

LOCAL ANAESTHETICS

System GA, previously described, may be used.

RETENTION INDICES

	System GA
Amethocaine	2219
Benzocaine	1555
Bupivacaine	2273

	System GA
Butacaine	2457
Butanilicaine	2025
Chloroprocaine	2229
Cinchocaine	2701
Cocaine	2187
Dimethisoquin	2030
Diperodon	2370
Dyclonine	1678
Hexylcaine	1965
Lignocaine	1870
Mepivacaine	2071
Oxethazaine	2525
Oxybuprocaine	2471
Piperocaine	1980
Pramoxine	2281
Prilocaine	1825
Procaine	2018
Propoxycaine	2335
Proxymetacaine	2323

NARCOTIC ANALGESICS

Systems GA, GB, GC, or GF, previously described, may be used.

System GA gives poor peak shapes with some compounds, especially morphine. Phenols such as morphine do not elute in System GB.

RETENTION INDICES. The retention indices given for System GC are those of the tertiary bases or of trifluoroacetyl derivatives (see p. 188).

	System			
	GA	GB	GC	GF
Acetylcodeine	2510	—	—	—
Alphaprodine	1792	—	—	—
Anileridine	2850	—	3469	—
Apomorphine	2530	—	—	—
Benzylmorphine	3015	—	—	—
Codeine	2376	1600	2681	2860
Dextromethorphan	2140	—	—	—
Dextromoramide	2940	—	3625	—
Dextropropoxyphene	2188	1938	2173	2370
Dextrorphan	2230	—	—	—
Diamorphine	2614	—	—	—
Dihydrocodeine	2363	—	2702	2840
Dihydromorphine	2451	—	2504	—
Diphenoxylate	2443	—	—	—
Dipipanone	2474	—	2894	2710
Ethoheptazine	1857	1882	1630	2110
Ethylmorphine	2411	—	—	—
Fentanyl	2650	—	—	—
Hydrocodone	2440	—	3028	2930

	System			
	GA	GB	GC	GF
Hydromorphone	2467	—	—	—
Ketobemidone	2035	—	—	—
Levallorphan	2359	—	—	—
Levorphanol	2230	—	2230	—
Methadone	2148	2124	2470	2370
6-Monoacetyl-morphine	2537	—	—	—
Morphine	2454	—	2542	—
Nalorphine	2577	—	—	—
Naloxone	2640	—	—	—
Norcodeine	2388	—	—	—
Normethadone	2091	—	—	—
Normorphine	2438	—	—	—
Norpipanone	2488	—	—	—
Noscapine	3120	—	—	—
Oxycodone	2524	—	—	—
Oxymorphone	2532	—	—	—
Papaverine	2825	—	—	—
Pentazocine	2275	1528	2225	3030
Pethidine	1751	1753	2025	1995
Phenazocine	2684	—	—	—
Phenoperidine	2872	—	—	—
Pholcodine	3018	—	—	—
Pipazethate	2037	—	—	—
Thebacon	2533	—	—	—
Thebaine	2517	—	—	—
Tilidate	1840	—	—	—

PESTICIDES

A comprehensive system for screening pesticides, System GK, will be found on p. 73.

Retention indices for certain pesticides in System GA, and relative retention times for System GK will be found in Table 1, p. 81, and also in the indexes to Analytical Data in Part 3.

PHENOTHIAZINES AND OTHER TRANQUILLISERS

Systems GA or GF, previously described, may be used.

RETENTION INDICES

	System	
	GA	GF
Acepromazine	2694	3230
Azacyclonol	2243	—
Benactyzine	2248	—
Benzoctamine	2082	2445
Carphenazine	3590	—
Chlormezanone	2238	—
Chlorpromazine	2486	2940

	System	
	GA	GF
Chlorprothixene	2487	2910
Clopenthixol	2274	—
Diethazine	2377	—
Dimethothiazine	3078	—
Dimethoxanate	2029	—
Droperidol	3430	—
Ethopropazine	2357	2775
Fluopromazine	2211	2550
Fluphenazine	3065	—
Fluspirilene	1017	—
Haloperidol	2942	—
Hydroxyzine	2849	—
Methdilazine	2467	—
Methotrimeprazine	2514	2965
Oxypertine	2355	—
Pecazine	2524	—
Penfluridol	3380	—
Pericyazine	3285	—
Perphenazine	2207	—
Phenothiazine	—	2845
Pipamperone	3070	—
Prochlorperazine	2954	—
Promazine	2316	2745
Promethazine	2339	2675
Propiomazine	2738	—
Prothipendyl	2339	—
Thiethylperazine	3247	—
Thiopropazate	3465	—
Thioridazine	3114	—
Thiothixene	3060	—
Trifluoperazine	2683	3050
Trimeprazine	—	2715
Trimetozine	2198	—

PLASTICISERS AND CONTAMINANTS

System GA, previously described, may be used.

RETENTION INDICES

	System
	GA
Cholesterol	3086
Dibutyl phthalate	1913
Diethyl phthalate	1564
Di(2-ethylhexyl) phthalate	2507
Indole	1276
Phenethylamine	1111
Tributyl citrate	2150
Tri-isobutyl phosphate	1483
Trisbutoxyethyl phosphate	2363
Tryptamine	1742

SOLVENTS AND OTHER VOLATILE COMPOUNDS

System GA, previously described, may be used, or System GI, below.

System GI

J. D. Ramsey and R. J. Flanagan, *J. Chromat.*, 1982, *240*, 423–444.

COLUMN. 0.3% Carbowax 20M on 80–100 mesh Carbopak C, 2 m × 2 mm internal diameter glass column.

COLUMN TEMPERATURE. 35° for 2 minutes and then programmed at 5° per minute to 175° and hold for at least 8 minutes.

CARRIER GAS. Nitrogen at 30 ml/min.

RETENTION INDICES AND RETENTION TIMES (min)

	System	
	GA (RI)	GI (RT)
Acetaldehyde	372	0.70
Acetone	469	2.5
Amyl nitrite	680	20.3
Benzaldehyde	947	34.2
Benzene	660	14.8
Bromochlorodifluoro-methane	405	1.6
Butane	400	2.3
Camphor	1136	38.2
Carbon tetrachloride	659	8.6
Chloral hydrate	695	12.5t
Chlorbutol	949	29.8
Chloroform	605	6.2
Dichlorodifluoromethane	305	0.90
Dichlorotetrafluoroethane	361	2.0
Enflurane	462	8.3
Ethanol	421	1.9
Ethchlorvynol	1030	35.2
Ether	515	5.9
Ethyl acetate	596	9.4
Ethylbenzene	849	29.5
Ethylene glycol	798	17.0t
Halothane	533	8.5
Hexane	600	17.4
Isobutyl methyl ketone	724	21.1
Isopropyl alcohol	530	4.0
Isopropyl nitrate	693	12.0
Methanol	491	0.7
Methoxyflurane	701	17.6
Methyl ethyl ketone	579	7.3
Methylene chloride	515	1.9
Methylpentynol	715	20.1
Paraldehyde	786	23.2

	System	
	GA	GI
	(RI)	(RT)
Propane	300	0.6
Propanol	571	5.5
Tetrachloroethane	910	24.9
Tetrachloroethylene	789	24.3
Toluene	756	24.8
1,1,1-Trichloroethane	634	8.2
1,1,2-Trichloroethane	748	16.4
Trichloroethanol	857	25.5
Trichloroethylene	710	14.8
Trichlorofluoromethane	484	3.0
m-Xylene	863	33.2
o-Xylene	884	34.5
p-Xylene	860	34.2

t = tailing peak

SULPHONAMIDES

System GJ

O. Gyllenhaal *et al.*, *J. Chromat.*, 1978, *156*, 275–283.

In this system, the substances are chromatographed as their methyl derivatives (see p. 189).

COLUMN. 5% OV-17 on 80–100 mesh Gas-Chrom Q, 1.5 m × 2 mm internal diameter glass column.

COLUMN TEMPERATURE. 250°.

CARRIER GAS. Nitrogen at 30 ml/min.

REFERENCE COMPOUND. Griseofulvin.

RELATIVE RETENTION TIMES. The values given are retention times of methyl derivatives relative to griseofulvin.

	System GJ
Glymidine	0.53
Sulfamerazine	0.69
Sulphacetamide	0.16
Sulphadiazine	0.66
Sulphadimidine	0.71
Sulphafurazole	0.42
Sulphamethizole	0.98
Sulphamethoxazole	0.40
Sulphamethoxydiazine	1.38
Sulphamethoxypyridazine	0.93
Sulphamoxole	0.40
Sulphaphenazole	1.71
Sulphapyridine	0.47
Sulphathiazole	0.49

Bibliography

W. Jennings, *Gas Chromatography with Glass Capillary Columns*, 2nd Edn, London, Academic Press, 1980.

Handbook of Derivatives for Chromatography, K. Blau and G. S. King (Ed.), Chichester, Heyden, 1977.

W. R. Supina, *The Packed Column in Gas Chromatography*, Bellefonte, Pennsylvania, Supelco, 1974.

J. Q. Walker *et al.*, *Chromatographic Systems, Maintenance and Trouble-shooting*, 2nd Edn, London, Academic Press, 1977.

High Pressure Liquid Chromatography

R. Gill

The modern form of column liquid chromatography has been called high-performance, high-pressure, high-resolution, and high-speed liquid chromatography. However, the abbreviation HPLC is now universally understood to describe the technique that separates mixtures on columns filled with small particles (typically 10 μm or less diameter) by elution with a liquid under high pressure. The essential equipment consists of an eluent reservoir, a high-pressure pump, an injector for introducing the sample, a stainless steel column containing the packing material, a detector, and a chart recorder. Thus, HPLC is similar to other types of chromatography in having a stationary phase (packing material) and a mobile phase (eluent).

HPLC equipment can be obtained as a complete system or assembled from individual modules (pump, injector, detector, etc.). Modular systems are generally more convenient because units (especially detectors) can be interchanged between chromatographs and new modules can be added to update the equipment. Modules are usually linked with standard stainless steel tubing of $\frac{1}{16}$ in (about 1.6 mm) outside diameter so that the coupling of units from different manufacturers is straightforward. However, tubing between the column and detector can be either stainless steel or polytetrafluoroethylene (PTFE). Various compression fittings (using nuts and ferrules) are available for making connections.

Columns

The columns are usually constructed from straight stainless steel tubing having a polished inner surface. Columns 10 to 30 cm long with an internal diameter of 4.5 to 5 mm and an outside diameter of $\frac{1}{4}$ in (6.3 mm) are normally used. The outlet is terminated by a stainless steel mesh disk to retain the packing material. The mesh disk is held in position by the 'end-fitting' with the end of the tubing to the detector flush against the centre. This tubing should have an internal diameter of 0.25 mm or less and be as short as possible to minimise peak broadening.

Injection Systems

Valve injectors consist of switching valves connected to a loop of stainless steel tubing (sample loop). A short tube (0.25 mm or less internal diameter) connects the injector with the top of the column where the end-fitting is identical with that at the bottom. The sample is introduced into the loop when the valve is in the 'load' position, while the eluent flows from the pump to the column through another passage within the valve. When the valve is switched to 'inject', the loop is connected into the line of flow between pump and column. The best quantitative reproducibility is achieved by using a loop of the required volume which is completely filled with sample. However, the sample can be loaded with a graduated syringe to partially fill the loop.

When *syringe injection* is used, the top 5 to 10 mm depth of packing is removed from the column, a stainless steel mesh is placed in position, and the remaining space filled with glass beads (typically 200 μm diameter). The top of the column is then connected directly to the injection device. Such injectors allow the sample to be deposited in the layer of glass beads when the tip of the syringe needle is centrally positioned just above the upper mesh. There are two types of injector used for syringe injection. In a 'stop-flow' injector the pump is switched off and the eluent flow is allowed to subside. A valve is then opened and the syringe needle inserted through a needle guide to deposit the sample. After closing the valve the pump is restarted. A second type of syringe injector allows the sample to be injected without stopping the pump, the syringe needle being inserted through a rubber septum.

Syringe injectors can achieve slightly better column efficiencies than valve injectors and they also cost less. Nevertheless, syringe injectors have several disadvantages. In septum injection, pieces of rubber are often deposited in the glass bead layer which can lead to blockage of syringe needles. Furthermore, the septa have a pressure limitation of about 1500 lb/in^2 (10.3 MPa). This pressure limit can be overcome by using the 'stop-flow' method; however, stopping the pump can lead to disturbances of the baseline. Valve injectors are more robust, require less maintenance, and are generally preferred for routine drug analysis.

Pumps

The flow rate through the column is generally between 1 and 3 ml/min, with pressures ranging from 500 to 4000 lb/in^2 (3.4 to 27.6 MPa). The pumps must show minimum fluctuations within these ranges to achieve maximum stability of the detector response and reproducible retention data. Pumps are either 'constant-pressure' or 'constant-flow', the constant-flow pumps being generally more convenient as changes in column resistance or eluent viscosity are compensated by changes in operating pressure.

The most simple 'pump' consists of the direct application of gas pressure (from a cylinder of compressed nitrogen or air) on to the surface of the eluent contained in a pressure bottle or holding coil. Such devices are relatively cheap but have the disadvantages that the pressure limit is low (typically 1500 lb/in^2, 10.3 MPa), the gas dissolved in the eluent may reappear as bubbles in the detector flow-cell, and a change of eluent requires the apparatus to be dismantled, washed, and refilled. Commercial HPLC pumps use pistons or diaphragms to displace eluent, hence avoiding the problem of dissolved gas. Syringe pumps are of the constant-flow type and have a large piston which is moved at a constant speed by an electric motor. They produce a very smooth flow but the syringe has limited capacity and needs to be manually refilled at the end of each piston stroke. Pneumatic amplifier pumps are of the constant-pressure type with the piston driven by compressed gas. Check valves allow the piston to return to its starting position at the end of each stroke, drawing eluent from a solvent reservoir into the pump.

The most widely used pumps are electrical reciprocating pumps. They are constant-flow pumps with small piston displacements (typically 100 µl) and with check valves to allow eluent to be drawn from a reservoir. Flow rate can be controlled by having a constant speed motor with mechanical adjustment of the piston stroke length, or by having a variable speed motor with constant stroke length. The small internal volume allows a rapid change from one eluent to another. Such single piston pumps produce a pulsating flow and, although the column itself causes considerable damping, other damping devices are generally included. Nevertheless, the smooth flow necessary for detection at very high sensitivities generally requires a pump with 2 or 3 piston heads working out of phase.

Detectors

Four detectors have found widespread application. These are the ultraviolet–visible detector, the fluorescence detector, the refractive index detector, and the electrochemical detector. Only the refractive index detector can be considered as a 'universal' detector as virtually all compounds cause a change in refractive index when dissolved in an eluent. The other three types depend upon the specific properties of the solute rather than changes in the bulk properties of the eluent. Hence, these detectors can confer various degrees of selectivity to the analysis.

An important factor in the choice of a detector is the amount of peak broadening which occurs as the eluted compounds pass through. This is largely controlled by the volume and geometry of the detector flow-cell but is also influenced by the connecting tubing between the column and the detector.

ULTRAVIOLET–VISIBLE DETECTORS

Most applications in drug analysis use detectors which respond to the absorption of ultraviolet radiation (or visible light) by the solute as it passes through the flow-cell. Absorption changes are proportional to concentration following the Beer–Lambert Law. Flow-cells generally have path-lengths of 5 to 10 mm with volumes between 5 and 10 µl. These detectors give good sensitivities with many compounds, are not affected by slight fluctuations in flow rate and temperature, and are non-destructive, thus allowing solutes to be collected.

The simplest detectors are of the fixed-wavelength type and usually contain low-pressure mercury lamps which have an intense emission line at 254 nm. Some instruments offer conversion kits which allow the energy at 254 nm to excite a suitable phosphor to give a new detection wavelength (e.g. 280 nm). Variable-wavelength detectors have a deuterium lamp with a continuous emission from 180 to 400 nm and use a manually operated diffraction grating to select the required wavelength. Tungsten lamps (400–700 nm) are used for the visible region.

Many organic compounds absorb at 254 nm and hence a fixed-wavelength detector has many uses. However, a variable-wavelength detector can be invaluable to increase the sensitivity of detection by using the wavelength of maximum absorption. This can also increase the selectivity of detection by enhancing the peak of interest relative to interfering peaks. Most drugs show some absorption at very low wavelengths (220 nm or less), but as selectivity is low such detection wavelengths should only be used to enhance sensitivity in the analysis of samples known to contain a particular drug (e.g. therapeutic drug monitoring).

Eluents must have sufficient transparency at the selected detection wavelength and Fig. 1 shows the absorption spectra of several solvents commonly employed. The spectra were recorded in 1-cm cells with water as the reference. These represent purified solvents; reagent grade solvents contain impurities which can limit their use to even longer wavelengths. Buffer salts can also limit transparency.

The spectra of some drugs change with pH and the

sensitivity and selectivity of an assay can sometimes be controlled by changing the eluent pH. The influence of such changes on the chromatography must also be considered.

FLUORESCENCE DETECTORS

In this detector, the solute is excited with ultraviolet radiation and emits radiation at a longer wavelength. Some detectors allow for selection of both excitation and emission wavelengths either by the insertion of appropriate filters or by the use of monochromators.

There are only a few drugs which have strong natural fluorescence (e.g. ergot alkaloids), and for such drugs fluorescence detection can achieve better sensitivities than ultraviolet detection. However, many drugs can be converted into fluorescent derivatives. The selectivity of fluorescence detection can be extremely valuable for the identification of drugs since the excitation and emission information can be used in addition to the retention data (L. A. King, *J. Chromat.*, 1981, *208*, 113–117).

Eluents chosen for fluorescence detection should not fluoresce nor should they absorb at the excitation or emission wavelengths used. The pH may also be important because some drugs only show fluorescence in particular ionic forms.

REFRACTIVE INDEX DETECTORS

These detectors respond to changes in refractive index (positive or negative) arising from the presence of a compound in the eluent. All the factors which can affect refractive index must be carefully controlled (e.g. temperature, eluent composition, pressure) otherwise noise and drift will limit the sensitivity. Thus the chromatograph is best placed in a thermostatically-controlled cabinet and good pumps are desirable to minimise pressure fluctuations. Changes in eluent composition will also cause spurious changes in refractive index.

The refractive index detector is inherently insensitive (as much as 100 times less sensitive than UV detectors) and this severely limits its use in drug analysis. However, it can be used when the compounds of interest do not have a suitable ultraviolet chromophore and are present in high concentration, e.g. sugars in drug preparations (B. B. Wheals and P. C. White, *J. Chromat.*, 1979, *176*, 421–426).

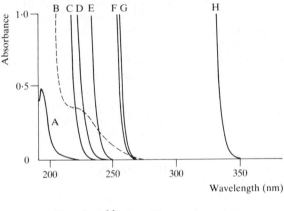

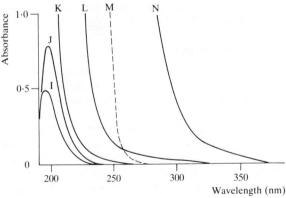

Fig. 1. Ultraviolet absorption of solvents (HPLC grade unless otherwise stated). A, acetonitrile (far-UV grade); B, methyl *tert*-butyl ether; C, acetonitrile; D, 1-chlorobutane; E, methylene chloride; F, acetic acid (AR grade); G, ethyl acetate; H, acetone; I, hexane; J, iso-octane; K, methanol; L, tetrahydrofuran; M, chloroform; N, diethylamine (AR grade).

ELECTROCHEMICAL DETECTORS

In this detector, solutes undergo electrolytic oxidation or reduction at the surface of an electrode, with measurement of the resulting current. Two types of detector are available. The *coulometric detector* has a large electrode surface and the electrochemical reaction of each solute is taken to completion, while the *amperometric detector* has a small electrode with a low degree of conversion (typically $<10\%$). The larger current response of coulometric detectors would be expected to make them more sensitive than amperometric detectors but in practice the difference is very small (P. T. Kissinger, *Analyt. Chem.*, 1977, *49*, 447A–456A).

The major problem with electrochemical detection is the contamination of the electrode surface during operation. Various electrode materials have been used but glassy carbon finds widespread application. Flow-cells with a dropping mercury electrode have the advantage of avoiding contamination by continuous replacement of the electrode surface but they can only be used in the reduction mode.

Eluents for electrochemical detection must be electrically conductive, which is achieved by the addition of inert electrolytes at concentrations between 0.05 and 0.1M. Potassium nitrate is often used for aqueous eluents while tetra-alkylammonium perchlorates can be used for organic eluents. All solvents and buffers used in the preparation of an eluent must be pure, and chosen so that they do not undergo electrochemical changes at the applied potential.

Electrochemical detectors can be used in the oxidative mode for a wide range of drugs, including cannabinoids, haloperidol, morphine, paracetamol, phenothiazines, salicylic acid, and tricyclic antidepressants. Operation in the reductive mode is more difficult as dissolved oxygen must be removed from the eluent (K. Bratin *et al.*, *J. liq. Chromat.*, 1981, *4*, 1777–1795). Reductive applications include chloramphenicol and benzodiazepines.

MISCELLANEOUS DETECTORS

Other detection principles have been applied to HPLC, e.g. conductivity, radioactivity, infra-red, and photoconductivity detectors. Such detectors are not widely used in drug analysis but can find application in special circumstances (e.g. the identification of drug metabolites arising from a radiolabelled drug by radioactivity detection).

Practical Aspects of HPLC Theory

The practical application of HPLC is aided by an awareness of the concepts of chromatographic theory, in particular the measurement of chromatographic retention and the factors which influence resolution.

CHROMATOGRAPHIC RETENTION

The retention of a drug with a given packing material and eluent can be expressed as a retention time or retention volume but both of these are dependent on flow rate, column length, and column diameter. The retention is best described as a column capacity ratio (k') which is independent of these factors. The column capacity ratio of a compound (A) is defined by

$$k'_A = \frac{V_A - V_0}{V_0} = \frac{t_A - t_0}{t_0}$$

where V_A is the elution volume of A and V_0 is the elution volume of a non-retained compound (i.e. void volume). At constant flow rate, retention times (t_A and t_0) can be used instead of retention volumes. The injection of a solvent or salt solution can be used to measure V_0, but the solute used should always be recorded along with reported k' data. The importance of selecting suitable solutes for the measurement of V_0 has been discussed (M. J. M. Wells and C. R. Clark, *Analyt. Chem.*, 1981, *53*, 1341–1345).

It is sometimes convenient to express retention data relative to a known internal standard (B). The ratio of retention times (t_A/t_B) can be used, but the ratio of adjusted retention times $(t_A - t_0)/(t_B - t_0)$ is better when wishing to transfer data between different chromatographs (L. S. Ettre, *J. Chromat.*, 1980, *198*, 229–234).

EVALUATION OF CHROMATOGRAPHIC PERFORMANCE

For information on the evaluation of the performance of chromatographic columns, see under Gas Chromatography, p. 189.

Stationary Phases and Eluents

The systems used are often described as belonging to one of four mechanistic types, adsorption, partition, ion-exchange, and size exclusion. *Adsorption chromatography* arises from interactions between solutes and the surface of the solid stationary phase. Generally, the eluents used for adsorption chromatography are less polar than the stationary phases and such systems are described as 'normal-phase'. *Partition chromatography* involves a liquid stationary phase which is immiscible with the eluent and coated on an inert support. Partition systems can be normal-phase (stationary phase more polar than eluent) or reversed-phase (stationary phase less polar than eluent). *Ion-exchange chromatography* involves a solid stationary phase with anionic or cationic groups on the surface to which solute molecules of opposite charge are attracted. *Size-exclusion chromatography* involves a solid stationary phase with controlled pore size. Solutes are separated according to their molecular size, the large molecules unable to enter the pores eluting first. However, this concept of four separation modes is an over-simplification. In reality there are no distinct boundaries and several different mechanisms often operate simultaneously.

COLUMN PACKING MATERIALS

The most widely used materials are rigid, totally porous particles with diameters in the range 3 to 10 μm. These allow rapid diffusion of solutes between the mobile and stationary phases and give columns of good efficiency with back pressures within the capabilities of modern HPLC pumps. Spherical particles are preferred as these give lower back pressures. It is particularly important that very small particles (fines) are not present as these can block meshes and tubing.

Silica-based Packing Materials

Silica (SiO_2, xH_2O) is the most widely used substance for the manufacture of packing materials. It consists of a network of siloxane linkages (Si—O—Si) in a rigid three-dimensional structure containing interconnecting pores. The size of the pores and the concentration of silanol groups (Si—OH) which line the pores can be controlled in the manufacturing process. Thus a wide range of commercial products is available with surface areas ranging from 100 to 800 m^2/g and average pore sizes from 4 to 33 nm.

The silanol groups on the surface of silica give it a polar character which is exploited in adsorption chromatography using organic eluents. Silanol groups are also slightly acidic and hence basic compounds are particularly strongly adsorbed. Unmodified silicas can thus be used with aqueous eluents for the chromatography of basic drugs.

Silica can be drastically altered by reaction with organochlorosilanes or organoalkoxysilanes giving Si—O—Si—R linkages with the surface. The attachment of hydrocarbon chains to silica produces a non-polar surface suitable for reversed-phase chromatography where mixtures of water and organic solvents are used as eluents. The most popular material is octadecyl-silica (ODS-silica) which contains C_{18} chains, but materials with C_2, C_6, C_8, and C_{22} chains are also available.

During manufacture such materials may be reacted with a small monofunctional silane (e.g. tri-methylchlorosilane) to reduce further the number of silanol groups remaining on the surface (end-capping). Variations in elution order on different commercial packing materials of the same type (e.g. ODS-silica) are often attributed to differences in surface coverage and the presence of residual silanol groups. There is a vast range of materials which have intermediate surface polarities arising from the bonding to silica of other organic compounds which contain groups such as phenyl, cyano, nitro, amino, and hydroxyl. Strong ion-exchangers are also available in which sulphonic acid groups or quaternary ammonium groups are bonded to silica.

For size-exclusion chromatography, a special type of silica is available which has a narrow range of pore diameters. Size-exclusion chromatography can be complicated by adsorption but this can be reduced by treating the surface with trimethyl-chlorosilane.

The useful pH range for columns is 2 to 8 since siloxane linkages are cleaved below pH 2 while at pH values above 8 silica may dissolve. However, the pH range may be extended above 8 if a precolumn packed with microparticulate silica is included between pump and injector to saturate the eluent before it enters the analytical column.

Polymer-based Packing Materials

Several packing materials are available which are based on organic polymers. For example, unmodified styrene-divinylbenzene copolymers have a hydrophobic character and can be used for reversed-phase chromatography. Although they can give lower column efficiencies than ODS-silica they have the advantage of being stable over a wide pH range. They also avoid problems associated with residual silanol groups (e.g. peak tailing). Ion-exchange materials of the styrene-divinylbenzene type are also available in which sulphonic acids, carboxylic acids, or quaternary ammonium groups are incorporated in the polymeric matrix.

PACKING THE COLUMN

Column packing is very straightforward provided that a packing pump, slurry reservoir, and ultra-sonic bath are available. Such equipment rapidly pays for itself as prepacked columns are very expensive. High flow rates and high pressures (up to 10 000 lb/in^2, 69 MPa) are required and pneumatic amplifier pumps are most suitable. A multiple switch valve should be fitted to the solvent inlet line and connected to a series of solvent containers so that solvent changes can be made rapidly without stopping the pump. The pump outlet is connected to the slurry reservoir which in turn is connected to the empty column. This last union should be made with a connector having an internal diameter comparable to that of the column. The slurry reservoir should have a capacity of 30 to 40 ml for packing analytical columns and must obviously be capable of withstanding the packing pressures.

The following procedures are recommended for packing silica and ODS-silica into 100×5 mm internal diameter columns.

Silica. Clean an empty column and fit it with a stainless steel mesh disk at the outlet end. Prime the pump with methanol and set it to deliver a pressure of 7500 lb/in^2 (52 MPa). Clamp the slurry reservoir in a vertical position with the bottom connected to the pump outlet. Weigh 1.8 g of silica into a glass-stoppered flask (50 ml) and add 30 ml of methanol. Shake vigorously until a homogeneous suspension is produced and then place the flask in an ultrasonic bath for 5 minutes. Pour the slurry into the reservoir, connect the empty column to the reservoir (outlet upwards), and switch on the pump. These manipulations must be conducted as rapidly as possible. Allow 100 ml of solvent to pass through the column then invert the whole column-reservoir assembly so that the top of the column is upwards. Pump a further 50 ml of methanol through the column then switch off the pump and allow the pressure to subside (10 minutes). Disconnect the column from the reservoir, remove excess packing material, and fit a stainless steel mesh and end fitting. For normal-phase chromatography, the column must be activated by passing through it a series of solvents with decreasing polarity, finally using dry hexane.

ODS-Silica. The general procedure is similar to that described above. Suspend 1.8 g of ODS-silica in 30 ml of isopropyl alcohol and pack the column in an upward direction using hexane as the pressurising solvent. Allow 100 ml of solvent to pass, then invert the assembly and pass a further 50 ml. Pump 50 ml of methanol through the column followed by 75 ml of a 50:50 (v/v) mixture of methanol and water. Remove the column from the reservoir as above.

All new columns should be tested to check the success of the packing. The test can then be repeated at a later date to monitor the performance of the column with use. If the column has been packed for a particular assay involving the separation of a group of drugs, these compounds can be used as the test mixture. Alternatively, a standard test mixture can be used (P. A. Bristow and J. H. Knox, *Chromatographia*, 1977, *10*, 279–289).

SYSTEMS FOR DRUG ANALYSIS

A large number of eluent/packing material combinations have been used for drug analysis. However, most drug analyses are currently performed on silica or one of the hydrocarbon-bonded silicas (usually ODS-silica). Other types of packing are only employed when these conventional materials fail. The majority of drug analyses can be carried out with the following four types of system.

Silica with Non-polar Eluents

Here the principal mechanism is adsorption chromatography. Separation is controlled by the competition between solute molecules and molecules of the mobile phase for the adsorption sites on the silica surface. Polar groups are most strongly attracted to these sites and hence polar compounds are more strongly retained than non-polar ones. Retention can be decreased by increasing the polarity of the eluent.

Adsorption energies of numerous solvents on alumina (ε° values, see below) have been measured and this scale can be used as a good guide to the elution strengths of eluents on silica as well as alumina (L. R. Snyder, *Principles of Adsorption Chromatography*, New York, Marcel Dekker, 1968, pp. 194–195).

Pentane	0.00	Acetone	0.56
Hexane	0.01	Ethyl acetate	0.58
Iso-octane	0.01	Diethylamine	0.63
Cyclohexane	0.04	Acetonitrile	0.65
Toluene	0.29	Isopropyl alcohol	0.82
1-Chlorobutane	0.30	Ethanol	0.88
Ether	0.38	Methanol	0.95
Chloroform	0.40	Acetic acid	large
Methylene chloride	0.42	Water	large
Tetrahydrofuran	0.45		

Mixtures of solvents can be employed giving elution strengths in between those of the pure solvents. Furthermore, different solvent mixtures having the same ε° value will often give different separations of a group of compounds.

Water is strongly bound to silica and thus the water content of the eluent must be strictly controlled to maintain constant activity of the silica surface and hence reproducible retention times. This is most critical when the eluent is of very low polarity. However, because anhydrous systems are difficult to maintain, a low concentration of water can be used in the eluent, sufficient to deactivate the most active sites without deactivating the whole surface.

Typical water concentrations range from 0.01 to 0.2% v/v. The most satisfactory method of preparing a solvent of known water content is to mix anhydrous and water-saturated solvent in known proportions. Anhydrous hydrocarbon or halohydrocarbon solvents can be prepared by passing them through a bed of activated silica or alumina (200 μm) in a glass column. Because of the problems associated with the control of water concentration, alcohols such as methanol (0.01 to 0.5% v/v) are commonly employed to moderate the silica surface (H. Engelhardt, *J. chromatogr. Sci.*, 1977, *15*, 380–384).

Silica with Polar Eluents
Several systems have been described which involve the use of silica with eluents of moderate to high polarity containing alcohols and/or water as major components. With such eluents, adsorption chromatography is most probably not the principal mechanism. The mechanisms are poorly understood, making the prediction of retention behaviour difficult; nevertheless, many of these systems are very useful for drug analysis.

An eluent consisting of methanol:ammonium nitrate buffer (90:10) (see System HC) is suitable for a wide range of basic drugs (e.g. amphetamines and opiates—see Fig. 2). Retention can be controlled by changes to the pH, ionic strength, or methanol/water ratio, or by addition of other organic solvents such as methylene chloride. With these alkaline eluents the silica surface must bear a negative charge and the principal mechanism is probably cation-exchange.

Benzodiazepines can be chromatographed with methanolic eluents containing perchloric acid (typically 0.001M). Retention can be modified by the addition of other organic solvents (e.g. ether) or by changes to the acid concentration.

Both acidic and basic drugs can be chromatographed on silica using aqueous methanolic eluents containing cetyltrimethylammonium bromide (S. H. Hansen, *J. Chromat.*, 1981, *209*, 203–210). Hydrophobic quaternary ammonium ions are strongly adsorbed on silica giving a dynamically coated stationary phase. Retention may be controlled by varying the concentration or nature of the quaternary ammonium ion, changing the ionic strength or pH of the buffer, or changing the concentration or nature of the organic component.

ODS-Silica with Polar Eluents
Eluents for reversed-phase chromatography on ODS-silica are usually mixtures of methanol or acetonitrile with an aqueous buffer solution. Retention is mainly controlled by the hydrophobic interactions between the drugs and the alkyl chains on the packing material. Retention increases as the solutes decrease in polarity, i.e. polar species are eluted first (Fig. 3). Hence, elution time is increased by increasing the polarity of the eluent (i.e. increasing the water content). The pH of the eluent and the pK_a of the drug are also important since it is the non-ionised species that shows greater retention. Thus, acids show an increase in retention as the pH is reduced while bases show a decrease. It is important to use a buffer of sufficient capacity to cope with any injected sample size otherwise

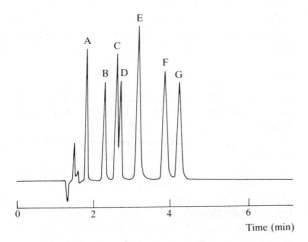

Fig. 2. Separation of some basic drugs using System HC. A, phendimetrazine; B, phenylpropanolamine; C, phentermine; D, amphetamine; E, morphine; F, ephedrine; G, methylamphetamine.

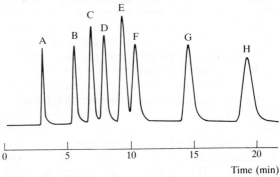

Fig. 3. Separation of some benzodiazepines using System HI. A, clorazepic acid; B, nitrazepam; C, clobazam; D, oxazepam; E, temazepam; F, chlordiazepoxide; G, diazepam; H, ketazolam.

tailing peaks can arise from changes in ionic form during chromatography. Phosphate buffers (0.05 to 0.2M) are widely used as they have a good pH range and low ultraviolet absorbance.

Drugs containing basic nitrogen atoms sometimes show poor efficiencies and give tailing peaks due to interactions with residual silanol groups on the packing material. This can often be improved by the addition of an amine or quaternary ammonium compound to the eluent which competes with the solutes for adsorption sites on the silica. Amines of small molecular weight (e.g. diethylamine) can be used as part of the buffer system. Alternatively, low concentrations (0.001M perhaps) of long-chain hydrophobic modifiers (e.g. NN-dimethyloctylamine) can be added to eluents together with conventional buffers.

Other hydrocarbon-bonded packing materials can be used in reversed-phase chromatography. A decrease in retention is associated with a decrease in the alkyl chain length.

ODS-Silica with Polar Eluents containing Hydrophobic Cations or Anions

Drugs bearing positive or negative charges are poorly retained in reversed-phase systems. If the pH of the eluent cannot be changed to convert the drug to its non-ionised form, a hydrophobic ion of opposite charge can be added to form a neutral ion pair and increase retention. Hence, for a basic drug an acidic eluent is chosen and a hydrophobic anion added. This technique is referred to as reversed-phase ion-pair chromatography.

The sodium salts of alkylsulphonic acids ($RSO_3^- Na^+$ where R = pentyl, hexyl, heptyl, or octyl) are widely used as ion-pair reagents for basic drugs, while quaternary ammonium compounds (e.g. tetrabutylammonium salts) are used for acidic drugs. Ion-pair reagents are generally added to eluents in the concentration range 0.001 to 0.005M and within this range an increase in concentration leads to an increase in retention. When detergents such as sodium lauryl sulphate or cetyltrimethylammonium bromide are used as the ion-pair reagents, the method is sometimes referred to as 'soap chromatography'. With these salts, ions build up on the surface of the packing material and produce a stationary phase which behaves like an ion-exchanger. This type of mechanism has been described as 'dynamic ion-exchange' and probably also occurs with less hydrophobic ion-pair reagents. It is virtually impossible to remove completely an ion-pair reagent from a hydrocarbon-bonded phase

and such columns should not therefore be reused with other reversed-phase eluents.

SELECTION OF CHROMATOGRAPHIC SYSTEMS
There may be many different combinations of packing material and eluent which are suitable for the analysis of a particular compound or group of compounds, and the final choice can be influenced by many factors. The time required for development of a new system can be shortened if it is possible to predict the way in which changes in eluent composition will influence chromatographic retention. Systems using hydrocarbon-bonded phases are particularly attractive from this viewpoint as a large range of parameters can be adjusted (pH, organic solvent, ionic strength, ion-pair reagents) with largely foreseeable consequences. Predictions for silica are generally less reliable. Silica is good for separating drugs belonging to different chemical classes, while hydrocarbon-bonded silicas are preferred for separations of drugs with closely related structures, e.g. barbiturates.

Most of the endogenous material in biological extracts which can interfere with the analysis of a drug is fairly polar. In reversed-phase systems this material generally elutes before the drug and can obscure the drug peak. In these circumstances, reversed-phase ion-pair chromatography can be valuable to increase selectively the retention of the drug relative to the interfering peaks. Normal-phase systems using silica do not generally suffer from this problem as most of the endogenous material usually elutes after the drug. However, these slow eluting compounds can lead to a noisy baseline or may remain adsorbed to the packing material and thus eventually lead to a loss in column performance.

Quantitative Analysis

The methods of quantitative analysis are essentially those inherited from gas chromatography. Peak height or peak area can be measured, either manually or with electronic devices. Peak height measurements have the advantage of simplicity but are sensitive to changes in peak shape; peak area measurements should always be used where peaks are broad and tailing.

For a given system, a calibration graph must be constructed for each compound to be analysed because the detector response to each will be different. This graph of peak height (or area) against drug concentration can then be used to quantify the unknown sample. Such external calibration requires careful control of injection volumes, and valve injection should be used. However, external calibration is still susceptible to errors arising from fluctuations in column performance, and the internal standard technique gives better precision. This involves the addition of a fixed amount of a substance (internal standard) to the sample before injection. Quantification is carried out using peak height (or area) ratios of drug to internal standard. In this case, calibration graphs are prepared by injecting solutions containing known amounts of drug together with the same fixed quantity of internal standard. For the analysis of drugs in complex samples, the internal standard should be added to the mixture before extraction to compensate for extraction losses.

Eluent Preparation

The quality of solvents and inorganic salts is an important consideration. Soluble impurities can give noisy baselines and spurious peaks or can build up on the surface of the packing material, eventually changing chromatographic retentions. Furthermore, the eluate may need to be collected for further analysis (e.g. mass spectrometry) and all contamination must be avoided. In addition, particulate matter should be removed, otherwise pump filters, meshes, and tubing can become blocked.

A wide range of HPLC-grade solvents is now commercially available which are free from particulate matter, have low residues on evaporation, and have guaranteed upper limits of ultraviolet-absorbing and fluorescent impurities. However, if a detector is not to be operated at its maximum sensitivity, analytical grade solvents may be used. Acetonitrile is a particularly difficult solvent to purify and two grades are generally offered; the purer grade is essential for ultraviolet detection at wavelengths around 200 nm. Water should be distilled from glass and should not be stored in plastic containers, which can cause organic contamination.

Air dissolved in the mobile phase can lead to problems. The formation of a bubble in a pump head usually reduces or stops eluent flow, while bubbles formed in the detector can give spurious peaks. The remedy is to degas the eluent by refluxing or by applying a weak vacuum to the eluent in a container placed in an ultrasonic bath. Eluents can also be degassed by purging with helium which has a very low solubility and drives the air out. Care must always be taken when degassing eluents containing volatile components to avoid changing the composition.

It is convenient to prepare eluents as volume plus volume mixtures of solvents, i.e. the volume of each solvent is measured separately and then mixed. Volume changes can occur when solvents are mixed (e.g. methanol and water show a contraction) and this must be remembered if the volume of only one solvent is measured and the second solvent added to make up to volume (v/v).

True pH values can only be measured in aqueous solutions and any measurements made with a pH meter in aqueous–organic solvents should be described as 'apparent pH'. In general, the apparent pH of a buffer solution rises as the proportion of organic solvent in the aqueous mixture increases. When preparing an eluent it is usually best to dissolve the required buffer salts in water at the appropriate concentrations, adjust the pH, then mix this solution (v/v) with the organic solvents.

Column Maintenance

The life of a column can be considerably extended if a few basic precautions are taken. The importance of choosing non-corrosive eluents (e.g. suitable pH values for silica packing materials) and the use of solvents and salts of high purity have already been discussed. In addition, a column should not be subjected to rapid changes in pressure or to flow rates outside of the normal operating range. Eluents can sometimes be left in the column overnight, but aqueous eluents containing inorganic salts should always be removed to prevent crystallisation, bacterial growth, or corrosion. For long-term storage the column must be thoroughly washed with suitable solvents and the ends tightly capped keeping the column wet to prevent the packing bed from cracking. Aqueous methanol (50% v/v) can be used to store ODS-silica columns, while methanol or hexane can be used for silica columns. Columns should be stored at room temperature away from physical disturbance.

A repeat of the test procedure normally applied to a column immediately after packing can quickly reveal any changes in performance. An increase in back pressure probably indicates that the top mesh or the top of the packing bed is blocked with particulate matter. Changes in the chromatographic retention of the test compounds suggest that the column has been contaminated with impurities adsorbed on the packing material. It is sometimes possible to remove such impurities by making large injections (1 ml perhaps) of a solvent with high elution strength. The cleaning of hydro-carbon-bonded silicas should always include a wash with dilute acid (0.1M sulphuric acid), which is effective in removing impurities from residual silanol groups.

If washing fails to restore a column, the contaminated packing material at the top of the column should be replaced. This procedure should also be applied if the packing bed has sunk, leaving a void. Such voids generally manifest themselves by a drop in efficiency, poor peak shape, or even the appearance of two peaks for a single compound. The column should be clamped vertically and the visibly contaminated packing material removed. A perfectly level surface must be left on the top of the packing bed. The space is filled with a thick paste of the packing material in methanol. Once the column has been pressurised on a pump it is sometimes necessary to top up with packing material again. Successful repacking to a depth of about 10 mm is feasible.

Sample Injection

Ideally, samples should be dissolved in the eluent prior to injection. However, if the sample has low solubility, it is sometimes necessary to use a more powerful solvent and in such cases only small injection volumes should be used otherwise broad peaks with shoulders can arise. Injection solvents of lower elution strength than the eluent can be useful for dilute samples, as the material concentrates on the top of the column during the injection. Nevertheless, large injections of any liquid other than eluent can cause serious detector disturbances.

Special Techniques

GRADIENT ELUTION

HPLC can be performed with a single eluent (isocratic elution) or with changes in composition (gradient elution). The elution strength of the eluent is increased during the gradient run by changing polarity, pH, or ionic strength. Gradient elution can be a powerful tool for separating mixtures of compounds with widely differing retention. A direct comparison can be drawn with temperature programming in gas chromatography.

Eluent gradients are usually generated by combining the pressurised flows from two pumps and changing their individual flow rates with an electronic programmer while maintaining the overall flow rate constant. Alternatively, a single pump with a low sweep volume can be used in combination with a gradient generator which controls the ratio of two liquids entering the pump from two liquid reservoirs. Equipment is available which allows the gradient to take almost any conceivable form including a reverse gradient to return the system to the original eluent.

Gradient elution does have several drawbacks. The extra equipment is usually very costly and the technique can be very time-consuming as the column must be reconditioned with the initial eluent between runs. In addition, drifting of the detector response and the appearance of spurious peaks arising from solvent impurities may occur. Although gradient elution should be avoided wherever possible it may be necessary for the analysis of complex mixtures where the components have wide-ranging polarities.

DERIVATIVE FORMATION

Derivatisation of a drug is seldom necessary to achieve satisfactory chromatography. This applies for compounds of all polarities and molecular weights and is an important advantage of HPLC over gas chromatography. Derivatisation is used to enhance the sensitivity and selectivity of detection when available detectors are not satisfactory for the underivatised compounds. Both ultraviolet-absorbing and fluorescent derivatives have been widely used. Ultraviolet derivatisation reagents include N-succinimidyl p-nitrophenylacetate (SNPA), phenylhydrazine, and 3,5-dinitrobenzoyl chloride (DNBC), while fluorescent derivatives can be formed with reagents such as dansyl chloride (DNS-Cl), 4-bromomethyl-7-methoxycoumarin (BMC), and fluorescamine.

Derivative formation can be carried out before the sample is injected on to the column (pre-column) or by on-line chemical reactions between the column outlet and the detector. Such post-column reactions generally involve the addition of reagents to the eluent. With pre-column derivatisation there are no restrictions on reaction conditions (e.g. solvent, temperature) and a large excess of reagent can be used, as this can be separated from the derivatives during the chromatography. The major drawback of pre-column reactions is the need to obtain reproducible yields for accurate quantification, and this is best achieved when the reactions proceed to completion. Furthermore, it is important that the products of pre-column derivatisation reactions are fully characterised. With post-column derivatisation the reaction is well controlled by the flow rates of eluate and reagents, temperature, etc. Hence, it is not necessary for the reaction to proceed to completion or even for the chemistry to be understood as the system is calibrated by the injection of known quantities of the reference standards.

The techniques and applications of derivatisation for drug analysis have been reviewed: J. F. Lawrence and R. W. Frei, *Chemical Derivatization in Liquid Chromatography*, Amsterdam, Elsevier, 1976; R. W. Frei, *J. Chromat.*, 1979, *165*, 75–86; S. Ahuja, *J. chromatogr. Sci.*, 1979, *17*, 168–172; R. W. Frei and J. F. Lawrence, *Chemical Derivatisation in Analytical Chemistry*, New York, Plenum Press, Vol. 1, 1981; Vol. 2, 1982.

DETECTION BY IMMUNOASSAY

Immunoassay techniques (see p. 148) can often be very useful for off-line detection. This involves the collection of the eluate in small fractions (1 ml perhaps) and the performance of a drug assay on each fraction. A chromatogram is then constructed by plotting the assay results against the fraction numbers. Such detection methods are clearly time-consuming but often achieve sensitivities and selectivities much higher than conventional detectors. In many cases biological fluids can be injected directly on to the column.

HPLC with immunoassay detection is useful for the analysis of those metabolites which are difficult to isolate from biological fluids by extraction (e.g. glucuronides). Such polar compounds cannot be observed at low concentrations with conventional detectors as they are obscured by endogenous compounds. HPLC with immunoassay detection can be applied to the determination of cannabinoids, opiates, lysergide, and cardiac glycosides in biological fluids (A. C. Moffat, *Analyt. Proc.*, 1981, *18*, 115–116).

MULTIWAVELENGTH ULTRAVIOLET–VISIBLE DETECTION

It is clearly useful to obtain structural information about the compounds eluting from a column to aid the identification of unknown peaks. For ultraviolet–visible detection this can involve the use of two detectors in series to give a ratio of absorbances at two wavelengths. Alternatively, full absorption spectra may be obtained. The simplest method involves collecting the eluate corresponding to each peak and transferring this to a scanning spectrophotometer. Alternatively, the eluent flow can be stopped as each peak passes through the flow-cell of a variable-wavelength detector, and the spectrum constructed either by recording the absorbance at known wavelength intervals (e.g. 10 nm) or by the

use of equipment with automatic wavelength scan facilities.

These methods of obtaining complete ultraviolet–visible spectra can be very time-consuming. However, rapid scanning spectrophotometers based on optical diode array detectors are now commercially available and are capable of recording complete spectra in very short time intervals (1 second or less). They can therefore be used to obtain spectra of separated components without stopping eluent flow or to detect at several wavelengths simultaneously.

DETECTION BY MASS SPECTROMETRY

The use of a mass spectrometer as a detector (HPLC–MS) can provide much information concerning the structures of the compounds being separated. Interfaces are available (see under Mass Spectrometry, p. 253).

Applications

HPLC complements rather than supplants paper, thin-layer, and gas chromatography. Paper and thin-layer chromatography require only relatively simple and cheap apparatus and are particularly useful as general screening methods, as an unknown compound must appear somewhere between the origin and the solvent front after development. In contrast, a compound may fail to elute at all in gas chromatography or HPLC.

Nevertheless, paper and thin-layer chromatography can rarely compete with the high resolution, sensitivity, and ease of quantification of HPLC and gas chromatography; the latter is the method of choice for compounds which are very volatile (e.g. anaesthetic gases, organic solvents, and alcohol) but is less suitable for compounds of low volatility arising from large molecular weight (e.g. insulin) or the presence of polar functional groups (e.g. quaternary ammonium drugs, drug metabolites, and conjugates). It is also unsuitable for thermally unstable compounds. In these cases HPLC is clearly the method of choice. Between these extremes are a large number of drugs where satisfactory analyses can be performed by gas chromatography or HPLC and the choice of method depends on the availability of suitable equipment (e.g. detectors) and the ability to separate the compounds of interest.

An important difference between HPLC and gas chromatography concerns the methods by which retention and resolution may be controlled. In gas chromatography only stationary phase and temperature have any significant effect, while in HPLC the composition of the mobile phase can also be altered with dramatic effects. The extra flexibility in HPLC can be extremely important, enabling difficult separations to be achieved. This enables a member of a particular drug group to be readily identified, but makes general screening for drugs difficult because there is no universal elution system, universal detector, or unified retention scale. Gas chromatography has these in the form of low polarity stationary phases, the flame ionisation detector, and the retention index scale, respectively. Hence, the major role of HPLC in drug analysis is the identification and quantification of specific drugs and poisons in body fluids and tissues or in pharmaceutical preparations.

Analysis of Drugs in Preparations

HPLC has found widespread use for the quantitative analysis of drugs in preparations of pharmaceutical and illicit manufacture. Drug concentrations are generally high enough to allow dissolution of the sample (tablet, powder, ointment, etc.) in a suitable solvent followed by injection. Ultraviolet–visible, fluorescence, or refractive index detection is normally used.

Within the pharmaceutical industry, HPLC is used at various stages of drug development, e.g. the optimisation of synthetic reactions and stability testing. Furthermore, it is extensively used for quality control during production to monitor the purity of drugs and excipients. HPLC systems can easily be automated (including injection and data handling), allowing large numbers of samples to be analysed rapidly and economically. HPLC is particularly valuable for the analysis of drugs which are polar (e.g. aspirin), thermally unstable (e.g. benzodiazepines), or are present in oil-based formulations where analysis by gas chromatography can be very difficult. Similarly, HPLC can be used for the forensic analysis of illicit preparations to aid the identification of an unknown drug by the measurement of retention times. Furthermore, as the technique is non-destructive, the eluted compounds can be collected for further analysis. HPLC can also be applied to natural materials such as cannabis resin and opium which contain numerous components and give complex chromatograms (Fig. 4). Although not all peaks may be identified, comparison of these 'fingerprint-patterns' can indicate whether two samples have a common origin. A similar approach may be applied to semi-synthetic materials such as illicit diamorphine

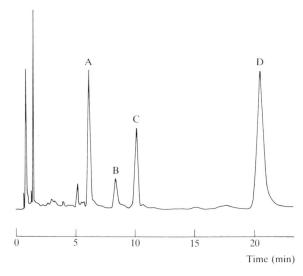

Fig. 4. Chromatogram of cannabis resin using System HL. Resin extracted with methanol:chloroform (4:1). A, cannabidiolic acid; B, cannabinol; C, Δ^9-tetrahydrocannabinol; D, Δ^9-tetrahydrocannabinolic acid.

which may also contain added components (e.g. caffeine, strychnine, or procaine).

Analysis of Drugs in Biological Fluids and Tissues

Several factors determine the ability of HPLC to detect a drug amongst the endogenous compounds present in biological material. Clearly, selective detection of the drug relative to the endogenous material is advantageous. Also the stationary phase and/or mobile phase can be altered to separate the drug peak from interfering peaks (e.g. using ion-pair reagents). Finally, the sample may be extracted before HPLC to concentrate the drug relative to the endogenous material.

The chromatographic system and detector should always be chosen to minimise the time needed for sample preparation. The complexity of the sample preparation procedure is controlled by several factors including the nature of the sample (urine, blood, liver, etc.), the condition of the sample, and the concentration of the drug. Interference from endogenous compounds is most acute when drug concentrations are low (e.g. therapeutic drug monitoring), and extensive sample preparation is often required. Such assays can be very susceptible to changes in the condition of the sample (e.g. a method developed for fresh blood may not be satisfactory for haemolysed samples) and this can present severe difficulties in forensic toxicology.

Thus, methods must be tested with the most difficult samples that may be encountered. In contrast, the analysis of biological samples containing high drug concentrations (e.g. fatal drug overdose) by HPLC generally requires much less sample preparation and is less susceptible to changes in sample condition.

Sample preparation for HPLC is essentially the same as for other methods of drug analysis. A drug which is physically trapped within solid tissue (e.g. liver), or chemically bound to the surface of proteins, must be released; then the protein is precipitated to leave the drug in aqueous solution. The protein may be degraded by strong acids or enzymes, precipitated by various chemicals (e.g. tungstic acid, ammonium sulphate), or removed by ultrafiltration. Some drugs are destroyed by protein degradation methods while ultrafiltration and precipitation can lead to drug losses through protein binding. No single procedure works well for all drugs and the method should be selected to give maximum recovery of the drug being analysed.

When drug concentrations are high (typically µg/ml) and systems with polar mobile phases are used, the direct injection of deproteinised solutions may be acceptable. Proteins must be removed to protect the column from irreversible contamination. A rapid procedure is to mix the biological fluid with at least two volumes of methanol or acetonitrile, centrifuge to remove the precipitated protein, and inject the supernatant liquid. Urine can be similarly treated to guard against the precipitation of salts on the column. It is good policy to use a guard column between the injector and analytical column. This is packed with the same material as the analytical column and replaced at frequent intervals. The ratio of guard-column volume to analytical-column volume should be around 1:20, which keeps band broadening to a minimum while providing sufficient capacity to retain impurities.

When drug concentrations in biological fluids are low and detectors of high selectivity are not available, extraction procedures are generally required. Solvent extraction remains the most popular approach, as many factors can be modified to optimise the extraction. These modifications include changing the polarity of the organic solvent, the pH and ionic strength of the aqueous phase, and the use of ion-pairing agents. The organic extract may be directly injected on to the column, if it is miscible with the eluent, or evaporated to dryness and the residue dissolved in a suitable solvent before injection. Care must be taken that volatile drugs are not lost by evaporation and that lipid material in the residue does not prevent the drug from dissolving in the new solvent.

Drugs can also be extracted by passing the biological fluid through short columns filled with solid adsorbents (e.g. XAD-resin, silica, ODS-silica). The column is washed with suitable solvents to remove endogenous material before the drug is removed by passing a solvent of higher elution strength. Such columns are usually attached to Luer lock syringes or suction devices to facilitate the passage of solvents. Extraction selectivity can be controlled by adjustments to the biological fluid before extraction (e.g. pH, ionic strength) and the choice of washing solvents. Although home-made columns can be used, disposable columns of this type can be purchased.

HPLC SYSTEMS FOR DRUG GROUPS

The following section contains a list of HPLC systems suitable for the chromatography of particular drug groups. The systems have been selected from the chromatographic literature and from systems used by the author, taking account of their suitability for routine applications.

The drugs are divided into chemical or pharmacological groups but some other drugs are included in certain groups if they are chemically similar and would be extracted with that group. In addition, a general screening system for basic drugs is included. The systems are not necessarily those which would be chosen for the quantitative analysis of any particular drug in a biological sample as such procedures require the consideration of other factors such as the method of detection, the type of biological material, the drug concentration, and the sample preparation technique. Nevertheless, the present systems can be used for biological fluid assays in many instances. References to specific HPLC methods for the quantification of drugs in biological samples are given in the individual drug monographs.

Generally, reversed-phase systems using ODS-silica and silica systems using polar eluents have been chosen. Only two systems use materials other than silica or ODS-silica, which demonstrates their wide versatility.

Most chromatographic retention data are presented as k' values; where data have been published as retention times, retention volumes, or relative retention times, these have been converted into k' values with the aid of other information presented in the publication or by experimental measurements.

NOTE. In the tables of k' values, a dash indicates that no value is available for the compound, not that it does not elute.

BASIC NITROGENOUS DRUGS, GENERAL SCREEN

System HA

I. Jane *et al.*, *J. Chromat.*, 1985, *323*, 191–225.
COLUMN. Silica (Spherisorb S5W, 5 µm, 12.5 cm × 4.9 mm internal diameter).
ELUENT. A solution containing 1.175 g (0.01M) of ammonium perchlorate in 1000 ml of methanol; adjust to pH 6.7 by the addition of 1 ml of 0.1M sodium hydroxide in methanol.
k' VALUES. Values for drugs in this system will be found in drug monographs and in the indexes to Analytical Data in Part 3; they are also included in the systems for specific groups of drugs which follow.

AMPHETAMINES, OTHER STIMULANTS, AND ANORECTICS

System HA, previously described, may be used, or Systems HB or HC, below.

System HB

R. Gill *et al.*, *J. Chromat.*, 1981, *218*, 639–646.
COLUMN. ODS-silica (ODS-Hypersil, 5 µm, 25 cm × 5 mm internal diameter).
ELUENT. A solution containing 19.60 g (0.2M) of *phosphoric acid* and 7.314 g (0.1M) of diethylamine in 1000 ml of a 10% v/v solution of methanol; adjust the pH to 3.15 by the addition of *sodium hydroxide solution*.

System HC

B. Law *et al.*, *J. Chromat.*, 1984, *301*, 165–172.
COLUMN. Silica (Spherisorb, 5 µm, 25 cm × 5 mm internal diameter).
ELUENT. Methanol:ammonium nitrate buffer solution (90:10). To prepare the buffer solution add 94 ml of *strong ammonia solution* and 21.5 ml of *nitric acid* to 884 ml of water and adjust to pH 10 by the addition of *strong ammonia solution*.

k' VALUES

	System		
	HA	HB	HC
Adrenaline	—	—	0.63
Amphetamine	0.9	8.48	0.98
Benzphetamine	1.2	—	0.15
Caffeine	0.2	—	0.26
Cathine	1.0	4.39	0.83
Chlorphentermine	0.9	—	0.82
Diethylpropion	1.7	—	0.16
Dimethylamphetamine	—	11.08	1.89
DOM	—	—	1.13
Ephedrine	1.0	5.68	1.79
Fencamfamin	1.3	—	0.72
Fenethylline	—	—	0.27
Fenfluramine	1.3	—	0.88
Hordenine	—	2.00	—
Hydroxyamphetamine	—	2.24	1.11
Hydroxyephedrine	—	0.73	—
Mazindol	1.8	—	0.20
Mephentermine	1.5	—	2.48
Mescaline	1.3	16.82	2.17
Methoxyamphetamine	—	14.95	—
Methoxyphenamine	1.7	32.17	—
Methylamphetamine	2.0	10.52	2.07
Methylenedioxyamphetamine	—	—	0.98
Methylephedrine	2.3	—	1.83
Methylphenidate	1.7	—	0.36
Noradrenaline	—	0.10	—
Normetanephrine	—	—	1.08
Oxedrine	—	0.27	—
Pemoline	0.2	—	0.14
Phendimetrazine	0.9	—	0.32
Phenelzine	1.0	5.91	0.37
Phenethylamine	1.2	3.64	1.31
Phentermine	0.6	19.46	0.86
Phenylephrine	1.3	—	1.64
Phenylpropanolamine	0.9	3.87	0.70
Pipradrol	1.2	—	0.69
Prolintane	2.0	—	1.26
Pseudoephedrine	1.2	5.90	1.77
Tranylcypromine	1.0	—	0.26
Trimethoxyamphetamine	—	—	1.48
Tyramine	1.2	0.81	1.47

ANALGESICS, NON-STEROIDAL ANTI-INFLAMMATORY DRUGS

System HD

H. M. Stevens and R. Gill, unpublished data.
COLUMN. ODS-silica (ODS-Hypersil, 5 µm, 16 cm × 5 mm internal diameter).
ELUENT. Isopropyl alcohol:formic acid:0.1M potassium dihydrogen phosphate (13.61 g/litre) (540:1:1000).

System HW

H. M. Stevens and R. Gill, unpublished data.
COLUMN. As for System HD, above.
ELUENT. Isopropyl alcohol:formic acid:0.1M potassium dihydrogen phosphate (13.61 g/litre) (176:1:1000).

k' VALUES

| | System | |
	HD	HW
Acetanilide	0.5	2.3
Alclofenac	2.6	—
Amidopyrine	0.2	0.32
Aspirin	0.5	2.7
Benorylate	0.7	22.4
Benoxaprofen	11.3	—
Bufexamac	1.95	—
Choline salicylate	0.7	4.8
Diclofenac	11.5	—
Diflunisal	4.1	—
Dipyrone	0.1	0.45
Etenzamide	0.55	4.6
Famprofazone	2.5	—
Fenbufen	4.0	—
Fenoprofen	7.9	—
Flufenamic acid	19.7	—
Ibuprofen	15.1	—
Indomethacin	6.95	—
Indoprofen	1.2	—
Ketoprofen	2.4	—
Mefenamic acid	21.2	—
Methyl salicylate	3.9	—
Morazone	0.4	2.05
Naproxen	3.3	—
Nifenazone	0.1	0.45
Oxyphenbutazone	1.95	—
Paracetamol	0.1	0.32
Phenacetin	0.6	4.4
Phenazone	0.1	0.95
Phenylbutazone	6.5	—
Piroxicam	0.6	7.7
Propyphenazone	1.25	11.0
Salicylamide	0.4	2.5
Salicylic acid	0.7	4.6
Salsalate	3.6	—
Sulindac	1.25	—
Tolmetin	2.05	—
Zomepirac	3.7	—

ANTICONVULSANTS

System HE

J. A. Christofides and D. E. Fry, *Clin. Chem.*, 1980, *26*, 499–501.

COLUMN. Alkyl-silica (SAS-Hypersil, 5 μm, 12.5 cm × 4.5 mm internal diameter).
ELUENT. Acetonitrile:*tetrabutylammonium phosphate, 0.005M, pH 7.5* (20:80).

k' VALUES

	System HE
Carbamazepine	8.30
Ethosuximide	0.91
Ethotoin	2.81
Glutethimide	7.97
Methsuximide	6.02
Pheneturide	6.84
Phenobarbitone	2.76
Phenytoin	9.71
Primidone	1.35
Sulthiame	1.57

ANTIDEPRESSANTS

System HA, previously described, may be used or System HF, below.

System HF

R. Gill, unpublished data after P. M. Kabra *et al.*, *Clinica chim. Acta*, 1981, *111*, 123–132.
COLUMN. ODS-silica (ODS-Hypersil, 5 μm, 16 cm × 5 mm internal diameter).
ELUENT. Acetonitrile:phosphate buffer (pH 3.0) (30:70). To prepare the phosphate buffer, add 0.6 ml of nonylamine to 1000 ml of 0.01M sodium dihydrogen phosphate (1.1998 g/litre) and adjust the pH to 3.0 by the addition of *phosphoric acid*.

k' VALUES

| | System | |
	HA	HF
Amitriptyline	3.3	5.42
Butriptyline	2.7	7.33
Clomipramine	3.4	9.92
Desipramine	2.1	3.60
Dibenzepin	2.8	0.50
Dothiepin	3.2	3.60
Doxepin	3.7	2.27
Imipramine	4.2	4.17
Iprindole	4.1	10.83
Maprotiline	2.2	4.92
Mianserin	1.8	1.92
Nomifensine	0.9	0.42
Nortriptyline	2.0	4.58
Noxiptyline	—	1.63
Opipramol	2.2	1.63
Oxypertine	0.7	1.33
Protriptyline	2.1	3.60
Trimipramine	2.7	6.17

	System	
	HA	*HF*
Viloxazine	2.7	0.17
Zimeldine	3.2t	0.67

t = tailing peak

ANTIHISTAMINES

System HA, previously described, may be used.

k' VALUES

	System HA
Antazoline	1.8
Bromodiphenhydramine	2.7
Brompheniramine	4.1
Buclizine	0.7
Chlorcyclizine	2.3
Chlorpheniramine	3.9
Cinnarizine	0.8
Clemastine	3.7
Cyclizine	2.9
Cyproheptadine	3.2
Deptropine	5.0t
Dimethindene	5.1
Dimethothiazine	2.1
Halopyramine	4.2
Histapyrrodine	3.0
Isothipendyl	3.8
Mebhydrolin	3.0t
Meclozine	0.7
Mepyramine	3.9
Methapyrilene	4.1
Phenindamine	2.5
Pheniramine	4.1
Phenyltoloxamine	3.1
Promethazine	5.0
Pyrrobutamine	2.8
Thenalidine	3.5
Thenyldiamine	4.0
Thonzylamine	3.2
Tolpropamine	2.9
Trimethobenzamide	4.7
Tripelennamine	3.6
Triprolidine	3.2

t = tailing peak

BARBITURATES

System HG

R. Gill *et al.*, *J. Chromat.*, 1981, *204*, 275–284.
COLUMN. ODS-silica (ODS-Hypersil, 5 μm, 15 cm × 4.6 mm internal diameter).
ELUENT. Methanol:0.1M sodium dihydrogen phos-

phate (11.998 g/litre) (40:60); adjust to pH 3.5 by the addition of *phosphoric acid*.

System HH

R. Gill *et al.*, *J. Chromat.*, 1981, *226*; *Biomed. Appl.*, *15*, 117–123.
COLUMN. As for System HG, above.
ELUENT. As for System HG except that the mixture is adjusted to pH 8.5 by the addition of *sodium hydroxide solution*.

k' VALUES

	System	
	HG	*HH*
Allobarbitone	2.46	1.33
Amylobarbitone	10.91	7.05
Aprobarbitone	3.42	2.22
Barbitone	1.11	0.63
Brallobarbitone	3.09	1.72
Butalbital	6.17	3.48
Butobarbitone	5.43	3.42
Cyclobarbitone	5.25	2.61
Cyclopentobarbitone	6.00	3.84
Enallylpropymal	8.65	6.96
Heptabarbitone	9.90	4.93
Hexethal	34.28	20.39
Hexobarbitone	7.37	5.67
Ibomal	4.01	2.58
Idobutal	8.12	4.77
Metharbitone	2.69	1.99
Methohexitone	27.61	20.48
Methylphenobarbitone	7.27	3.84
Nealbarbitone	10.22	6.19
Pentobarbitone	10.96	8.07
Phenobarbitone	3.09	1.23
Phenylmethylbarbituric acid	1.48	0.94
Quinalbarbitone	16.28	11.47
Secbutobarbitone	4.89	3.32
Talbutal	7.25	4.67
Vinbarbitone	4.83	2.32

BENZODIAZEPINES

System HI

R. Gill, unpublished data.
COLUMN. ODS-silica (ODS-Hypersil, 5 μm, 20 cm × 5 mm internal diameter).
ELUENT. Methanol:water:phosphate buffer (55:25:20). To prepare the phosphate buffer dissolve 11.038 g (0.092M) of sodium dihydrogen phosphate and 1.136 g (0.008M) of disodium hydrogen phosphate in sufficient water to produce 1000 ml.

System HJ

R. Gill, unpublished data.
COLUMN. As for System HI, above.
ELUENT. Methanol:water:phosphate buffer (as in System HI), (70:10:20).

System HK

R. Gill, unpublished data after R. J. Flanagan *et al.*, *J. Chromat.*, 1980, *187*, 391–398.
COLUMN. Silica (Spherisorb, 5 µm, 25 cm × 5 mm internal diameter).
ELUENT. Methanol to which has been added 100 µl of *perchloric acid* per litre.

k' VALUES

| | System | | |
	HI	HJ	HK
Alprazolam	4.70	—	2.79
Bromazepam	2.32	—	2.99
Chlordiazepoxide	6.41	—	2.87
Clobazam	3.91	—	0.03
Clonazepam	2.85	—	0.35
Clorazepic acid	1.17	—	2.00
Demoxepam	2.42	—	0.03
Diazepam	9.47	2.29	2.49
Flunitrazepam	3.15	—	0.47
Flurazepam	—	3.19	6.50
Ketazolam	12.81	2.45	0.04
Lorazepam	4.60	—	0.14
Lormetazepam	6.32	—	0.08
Medazepam	—	7.05	4.44
Midazolam	9.75	2.10	5.90
Nitrazepam	2.96	—	1.49
Nordazepam	8.00	—	1.99
Oxazepam	4.62	—	0.73
Prazepam	—	4.60	2.19
Temazepam	5.68	—	0.60
Triazolam	4.38	—	1.83

CANNABINOIDS

System HL

P. B. Baker *et al.*, *J. analyt. Toxicol.*, 1980, *4*, 145–152.
COLUMN. ODS-silica (Spherisorb-ODS, 5 µm, 25 cm × 4.6 mm internal diameter).
ELUENT. 0.01M sulphuric acid:methanol:acetonitrile (7:8:9).

k' VALUES

	System HL
Cannabichromene	19.09
Cannabicyclol	14.78
Cannabidiol	7.47
Cannabidiolic acid	8.76
Cannabigerol	8.18
Cannabinol	11.77
Cannabivarin	7.47
Δ^8-Tetrahydrocannabinol	14.07
Δ^9-Tetrahydrocannabinol	13.35
Tetrahydrocannabinolic acid	25.83
Tetrahydrocannabivaric acid	14.64
Tetrahydrocannabivarin	8.18

CARDIAC GLYCOSIDES

System HM

P. H. Cobb, *Analyst, Lond.*, 1976, *101*, 768–776.
COLUMN. Silica (LiChrosorb SI60, 10 µm, 25 cm × 4 mm internal diameter).
ELUENT. Cyclohexane:ethanol:*acetic acid*(60:9:1).

k' VALUES

	System HM
Digitoxigenin	2.0
Digitoxigenin bisdigitoxoside	3.9
Digitoxigenin monodigitoxoside	2.8
Digitoxin	5.4
Digoxigenin	4.5
Digoxigenin bisdigitoxoside	8.2
Digoxigenin monodigitoxoside	5.5
Digoxin	11.3
Gitaloxin	6.8
Gitoxigenin	3.7
Gitoxigenin bisdigitoxoside	6.5
Gitoxigenin monodigitoxoside	4.5
Gitoxin	8.6
Lanatoside A	17.9
Lanatoside B	31.8
Lanatoside C	39.5

DIURETICS

System HN

R. Gill *et al.*, unpublished data, after P. A. Tisdall *et al.*, *Clin. Chem.*, 1980, *26*, 702–706.
COLUMN. ODS-silica (ODS-Hypersil, 5 µm, 16 cm × 5 mm internal diameter).
ELUENT. Acetonitrile:water containing 10 ml/litre of *acetic acid* (30:70).

k' VALUES

	System HN
Bendrofluazide	15.35
Benzthiazide	9.32
Chlorothiazide	0.54
Chlorthalidone	1.28

	System HN
Clopamide	4.01
Clorexolone	7.26
Cyclopenthiazide	16.45
Cyclothiazide	10.78, 11.91, 12.81
Hydrochlorothiazide	0.70
Hydroflumethiazide	1.30
Mefruside	8.67
Methyclothiazide	3.82
Metolazone	4.89
Polythiazide	15.09
Quinethazone	0.67
Trichlormethiazide	3.10

ERGOT ALKALOIDS

System HA, previously described, may be used or System HP, below.

System HP

R. Gill *et al.*, unpublished data, after P. J. Twitchett *et al.*, *J. Chromat.*, 1978, *150*, 73–84.
COLUMN. ODS-silica (ODS-Hypersil, 5 μm, 10 cm × 5 mm internal diameter).
ELUENT. Methanol:phosphate buffer (60:40). To prepare the phosphate buffer dissolve 3.43 g (0.022M) of sodium dihydrogen phosphate and 10.03 g (0.028M) of disodium hydrogen phosphate in sufficient water to produce 1000 ml.

k' VALUES

	System	
	HA	*HP*
Bromocriptine	—	44.3
Dihydroergocristine	—	18.3
Dihydroergocryptine	—	15.9
Dihydroergotamine	0.6	11.4
Ergocornine	0.4	10.2
Ergocristine	0.3	17.3
Ergocryptine	0.4	15.2
Ergometrine	0.4	0.50
Ergosine	0.3	7.08
Ergosinine	0.3	17.7
Ergotamine	0.4	9.58
Iso-lysergic acid	—	0.83
Iso-lysergide	2.6	0.0
Lysergamide	0.5	0.33
Lysergic acid	0.8t	0.0
Lysergic acid methyl-propylamide	—	1.98
Lysergide	0.7	1.83
Lysergol	1.1	0.83
Methylergometrine	0.4	0.83

	System	
	HA	*HP*
Methysergide	0.4	2.33
2-Oxylysergide	—	0.92

t = tailing peak

LOCAL ANAESTHETICS
System HQ

R. Gill *et al.*, *J. Chromat.*, 1984, *301*, 155–163.
COLUMN.   ODS-silica   (ODS-Hypersil,   5 μm, 16 cm × 5 mm internal diameter).
ELUENT. Methanol:water:1% v/v solution of *phosphoric acid*:hexylamine (30:70:100:1.4).

System HR

R. Gill *et al.*, *ibid*.
COLUMN. As for System HQ, above.
ELUENT. Methanol:1% v/v solution of *phosphoric acid*:hexylamine (100:100:1.4).

k' VALUES

		System	
	HA	*HQ*	*HR*
Amethocaine	2.0	16.25	1.33
Benzocaine	0.1	20.06	1.61
Benzoylecgonine	0.9t	5.68	—
Bupivacaine	0.9	7.19	0.86
Butacaine	1.2	8.97	—
Butanilicaine	—	4.42	—
Chloroprocaine	—	0.24	—
Cinchocaine	1.9	—	5.51
Cocaine	2.8	2.68	—
Cyclomethycaine	—	—	10.31
Dimethisoquin	2.2	—	11.24
Diperodon	—	—	2.48
Dyclonine	—	—	2.78
Lignocaine	0.6	0.79	—
Mepivacaine	0.9	1.09	—
Oxethazaine	—	—	4.14
Oxybuprocaine	—	16.25	0.86
Piperocaine	—	4.59	—
Pramoxine	0.6	—	2.48
Prilocaine	1.0	1.38	—
Procaine	1.9	0.00	—
Propoxycaine	—	1.09	—
Proxymetacaine	2.1	1.38	—

t = tailing peak

NARCOTIC ANALGESICS

Systems HA or HC, previously described, may be used or System HS, below.

System HS

P. B. Baker and T. A. Gough, *J. chromatogr. Sci.*, 1981, *19*, 483–489.

COLUMN. Amino-propyl bonded silica (Spherisorb S5NH$_2$, 5 μm, 25 cm × 4 mm internal diameter).

ELUENT. Acetonitrile: *tetrabutylammonium phosphate, 0.005M, pH 7.5* (85:15).

k′ VALUES

| | System | | |
	HA	HC	HS
Acetylcodeine	—	0.78	0.50
Benzylmorphine	4.4t	1.03	—
Buprenorphine	0.4	0.05	—
Caffeine	0.2	—	0.21
Codeine	4.8t	1.21	1.90
Dextromethorphan	5.6t	—	—
Dextromoramide	0.7	0.09	—
Dextropropoxyphene	1.9	0.19	—
Diamorphine	3.0t	0.66	0.35
Dihydrocodeine	7.2t	2.50	—
Dihydromorphine	5.7t	2.75	—
Diphenoxylate	0.2	—	—
Dipipanone	2.2	1.61	—
Ethoheptazine	3.3	1.55	—
Ethylmorphine	3.7t	1.06	1.45
Etorphine	0.6	1.11	—
Fentanyl	0.8	1.11	—
Hydrocodone	7.1t	2.17	—
Hydromorphone	7.9t	—	—
Ketobemidone	2.8t	—	—
Levallorphan	1.9t	1.46	—
Levorphanol	4.4t	3.20	—
Methadone	2.2	1.03	—
6-Monoacetylmorphine	3.6t	0.80	1.00
Morphine	3.8t	1.30	5.16
Nalorphine	1.0	0.29	—
Naloxone	1.4	0.17	—
Norcodeine	3.1t	3.51	—
Normethadone	—	0.53	—
Normorphine	2.9t	3.92	—
Norpipanone	—	0.35	—
Noscapine	0.3	0.15	0.01
Oxycodone	6.9t	0.85	—
Oxymorphone	6.7t	—	—
Papaverine	0.3	0.16	0.04
Pentazocine	1.8	0.67	—
Pethidine	2.8t	0.55	—
Phenazocine	1.3	0.30	—
Phenoperidine	0.8	0.10	—
Pholcodine	6.0t	1.63	—
Piritramide	0.6	0.14	—
Quinine	2.4	—	2.02

| | System | | |
	HA	HC	HS
Strychnine	13.0t	—	2.43
Thebacon	3.7t	0.85	—
Thebaine	4.6t	0.94	0.79

t = tailing peak

PHENOTHIAZINES

System HA, previously described, may be used.

k′ VALUES

	System HA
Acetophenazine	1.9
Butaperazine	3.4
Carphenazine	1.7
Chlorpromazine	4.1
Diethazine	3.4
Dimethothiazine	2.1
Dimethoxanate	5.8t
Fluopromazine	2.7
Fluphenazine	1.2
Mesoridazine	5.0
Methdilazine	6.0
Methotrimeprazine	3.2
Metopimazine	1.4
Pecazine	3.9
Pericyazine	1.3
Perphenazine	1.9
Piperacetazine	1.9
Prochlorperazine	3.9
Promazine	5.9
Propiomazine	2.1
Thiethylperazine	3.8
Thiopropazate	1.0
Thioproperazine	4.1
Thioridazine	5.2
Trifluoperazine	3.0
Trimeprazine	3.1

t = tailing peak

CORTICOSTEROIDS

System HT

J. Q. Rose and W. J. Jusko, *J. Chromat.*, 1979, *162*; *Biomed. Appl.*, *4*, 273–280.

COLUMN. Silica (Zorbax SIL, 5 μm, 25 cm × 4.6 mm internal diameter).

ELUENT. Methylene chloride: methanol (97:3).

k′ VALUES

	System HT
Beclomethasone	4.2
Cortisone	2.4
Dexamethasone	4.8

	System HT
Hydrocortisone	5.8
Methylprednisolone	7.5
Prednisolone	8.4
Prednisone	3.4
Triamcinolone acetonide	2.5

SULPHONAMIDES

System HU

P. H. Cobb and G. T. Hill, *J. Chromat.*, 1976, *123*, 444–447.

COLUMN. Silica (Spherisorb, 5 μm, 25 cm × 4 mm internal diameter).

ELUENT.   Cyclohexane:ethanol:*acetic   acid* (85.7:11.4:2.9).

k' VALUES

	System HU
Phthalylsulphathiazole	14.0
Succinylsulphathiazole	16.8
Sulfadoxine	4.4
Sulfamerazine	8.1
Sulfaquinoxaline	4.8
Sulphacetamide	7.7
Sulphachlorpyridazine	3.3
Sulphadiazine	8.7
Sulphadimidine	7.1
Sulphafurazole	6.0
Sulphamethoxazole	4.8
Sulphamethoxydiazine	8.2
Sulphamethoxypyridazine	7.5
Sulphamoxole	12.6
Sulphanilamide	8.9
Sulphapyridine	3.8
Sulphathiazole	13.4

NOTE. **System HV** for analgesics and non-steroidal anti-inflammatory drugs is described on p. 97. **System HW**, also for this group of drugs, is described on p. 215.

Bibliography

P. A. Bristow, *Liquid Chromatography in Practice*, Wilmslow, Florida, Laboratory Data Control, 1976.

Chromatography: Fundamentals and Applications of Chromatographic and Electrophoretic Methods (Parts A and B), E. Heftmann (Ed.), Amsterdam, Elsevier, 1983.

H. Engelhardt, High Performance Liquid Chromatography, *Chemical Laboratory Practice Series*, Heidelberg, Springer-Verlag, 1979.

L. Fishbein, *Chromatography of Environmental Hazards*, Vol. 4: Drugs of Abuse, Amsterdam, Elsevier, 1982.

R. W. Giese, Technical Considerations in the Use of 'High-Performance' Liquid Chromatography in Therapeutic Drug Monitoring, *Clin. Chem.*, 1983, *29*, 1331–1343.

GLC & HPLC: Determination of Therapeutic Agents (Parts 1–3), *Chromatographic Science Series*, K. Tsuji and W. Morozowich (Ed.), Vol. 9, New York, Marcel Dekker, Parts 1 & 2, 1978; Part 3, 1979.

T. A. Gough and P. B. Baker, Identification of Major Drugs of Abuse Using Chromatography, *J. chromatogr. Sci.*, 1982, *20*, 289–329.

T. A. Gough and P. B. Baker, Identification of Major Drugs of Abuse Using Chromatography: An Update, *J. chromatogr. Sci.*, 1983, *21*, 145–153.

R. J. Hamilton and P. A. Sewell, *Introduction to High Performance Liquid Chromatography*, 2nd Edn, London, Chapman and Hall, 1982.

High-Performance Liquid Chromatography: Advances & Perspectives, C. Horvath (Ed.), London, Academic Press, Vols 1 & 2, 1980; Vol. 3, 1983.

High-Performance Liquid Chromatography in Forensic Chemistry, I. S. Lurie and J. D. Wittwer (Ed.), New York, Marcel Dekker, 1983.

J. F. Lawrence, *Organic Trace Analysis by Liquid Chromatography*, London, Academic Press, 1981.

N. A. Parris, *Instrumental Liquid Chromatography*, 2nd Edn, Amsterdam, Elsevier, 1984.

A. Pryde and M. T. Gilbert, *Applications of High Performance Liquid Chromatography*, London, Chapman and Hall, 1979.

K. K. Unger, *Porous Silica: Its Properties and Use as Support in Column Liquid Chromatography*, Amsterdam, Elsevier, 1979.

B. B. Wheals and I. Jane, Analysis of Drugs and their Metabolites by High-performance Liquid Chromatography: A Review, *Analyst, Lond.*, 1977, *102*, 625–644.

Ultraviolet, Visible, and Fluorescence Spectrophotometry

A. F. Fell

Analytical absorption spectroscopy in the ultraviolet and visible regions of the electromagnetic spectrum has been widely used in pharmaceutical and biomedical analysis for quantitative purposes and, with certain limitations, for the characterisation of drugs, impurities, metabolites, and related substances. By contrast, luminescence methods, and fluorescence spectroscopy in particular, have been less widely exploited, despite the undoubted advantages of greater specificity and sensitivity commonly observed for fluorescent species. However, the wider availability of spectrofluorimeters capable of presenting corrected excitation and emission spectra, coupled with the fact that reliable fluorogenic reactions now permit non-fluorescent species to be examined fluorimetrically, has led to a renaissance of interest in fluorimetric methods in biomedical analysis.

Ultraviolet and Visible Spectrophotometry

Molecular absorption in the ultraviolet (UV) and visible region arises from energy transitions involving the outer orbital or valency electrons. Spectra in liquid media are usually broad, relatively featureless bands, due to the large number of closely-spaced vibrational and rotational transitions. The fundamental band shape approximates Gaussian or log-normal Gaussian curves. Given the broad, overlapping profiles commonly encountered, the shape and precise location of individual bands are of limited usefulness in qualitative analysis. However, any fine structure detected in the spectra, coupled with solvent and pH effects, can be of diagnostic value. More informative spectra can be obtained for some volatile molecules of toxicological interest, such as benzene and polynuclear aromatic hydrocarbons; when examined in the vapour phase, vibrational and rotational fine structure can be readily seen superimposed on the broad spectral profiles. However, most drugs, metabolites, and related compounds are relatively non-volatile; their spectra are necessarily observed in solution, or possibly in the solid phase by reflectance, or by compression to form a KBr disk, as used in infra-red spectrophotometry.

Ultraviolet and visible spectrophotometry finds its primary application in quantitative analysis. The scope of absorption spectroscopy can be significantly extended by the use of colour reactions, often with a concomitant increase in sensitivity and/or selectivity. Such reactions are used to modify the spectrum of an absorbing molecule so that it can be detected in the visible region, well separated from other interfering components in the ultraviolet spectrum. Moreover, chemical modification can be used to transform an otherwise non-absorbing molecule to a stable derivative possessing significant absorption.

Spectral selectivity can be further enhanced by a number of chemical or instrumental techniques including difference, higher-derivative, and dual-wavelength spectrophotometry. Such methods, and certain graphical techniques such as the Morton–Stubbs method, can contribute in different ways to reducing the general problem of spectral interference in quantitative spectroscopy. Spectral interference can arise from so-called 'irrelevant' non-specific absorption, and also from absorption by other materials and impurities which may be present. When interference arises specifically from the spectral overlap of two or more well-defined components, a number of methods can be applied to measure the individual concentrations. These methods include the Vierordt multi-wavelength technique, least squares deconvolution, and second or higher derivative spectrophotometry, as discussed below.

Spectral selectivity, and in some cases detection sensitivity, can be significantly enhanced by the various chemical and instrumental techniques outlined above. Such methods should of course be validated by applying the conventional analytical criteria of accuracy (against a reference method), linearity, precision, and independence from interfering substances.

The scope of ultraviolet and visible spectrophotometry can be further extended when combined with a chromatographic separation step such as HPLC. The development of rapid-scanning detectors based on the linear photodiode array permits spectra to be acquired during the elution of peaks. Computer-aided manipulation of these spectra has led to new strategies for the examination of chromatographic peak homogeneity, based on classical techniques in spectroscopy. The use of microcomputers enables the development of archive retrieval methods for spectral characterisation (A. F. Fell *et al.*, *J. Chromat.*, 1984, *316*, 423–440).

Nomenclature

In the ultraviolet and visible spectrum, the energy of protons associated with electronic transitions lies in the range 147 to 630 kJ/mol. This energy (ΔE) can be expressed in terms of the principal parameters that define electromagnetic radiation, i.e. frequency v (Hz), wavelength λ (nm), and wavenumber $\tilde{v}$ (cm^{-1})

$$\Delta E = hv = \frac{hc}{\lambda} = hc\tilde{v}$$

where h is Planck's constant, and c is the velocity of radiation *in vacuo*.

The positions of peaks are sometimes described in terms of wavenumber, which has the advantage of being a linear function of energy but this term is much more frequently used in infra-red spectrophotometry. The practical unit most often used in ultraviolet and visible spectrophotometry is wavelength, usually expressed in nanometres (nm). The older units of wavelength, millimicron (mμ) and ångström (Å), are not recommended terms. The position of maximum absorbance of a peak is designated λ_{max}.

The wavelength span is conventionally divided into two ranges: the ultraviolet extends from 200 nm to about 400 nm; the visible range extends from about 400 nm to 800 nm. Outside these limits, the 'far ultraviolet' or 'vacuum ultraviolet' extends from 100 nm to 200 nm, and the 'near infra-red' from 1 μm to about 3 μm.

A molecular grouping which is specifically responsible for absorption is described as a chromophore, usually a conjugated system with extensive delocal-

isation of electron density. Any saturated group which has little or no intrinsic absorption of its own, but which modifies the absorption spectrum when attached directly to a chromophore, is described as an auxochrome, examples being —OR, —NR$_2$, —SR. Auxochromes are considered to exert their effect through partial conjugation of their polarisable lone-pair electrons with those of the adjacent chromophore. If, however, the lone-pair of electrons is involved in bonding as, for example, in the case of a protonated quaternary ammonium group, the auxochromic effect vanishes. This property can be used for molecular characterisation, as discussed below.

Laws of Absorption

The extent of absorption of radiation by an absorbing system at a given monochromatic wavelength is described by the two classical laws of absorptiometry which relate the intensity of radiation incident on the absorbing system (I_0), to the transmitted intensity (I) (Fig. 1). Lambert's (or Bouguer's) Law concerns instrumental factors, and states that at a given concentration (c) of a homogeneous absorbing system, the transmitted intensity (I) decreases exponentially with increase in path-length (b). The complementary Beer's Law deals with concentration and states that for a layer of defined path-length (b), the transmitted intensity (I) decreases exponentially with increase in concentration (c) of a homogeneous absorbing system.

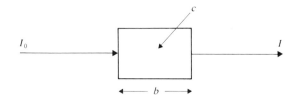

Fig. 1. Diagrammatic representation of energy relationships in absorption spectroscopy. I_0, intensity of incident radiation; I, intensity of transmitted radiation; b, path-length; c, concentration of the absorbing species.

Combination of these observations gives the familiar Beer–Lambert Law

$$\log \frac{I_0}{I} = kcb$$

where k is the absorptivity of the system.

The logarithmic term is linearly related to concentration and path-length and is referred to as absorbance (A). The older terms, extinction (E)

and optical density (*OD*) are not recommended although often found in the literature. Transmittance $(T=I/I_0)$ and percentage transmittance $[\%T=100\,(I/I_0)]$ are not linear functions of concentration and path-length and can be readily related to absorbance

$$A=\log\frac{I_0}{I}=\log\frac{1}{T}=2-\log\,(\%T)$$

The absorptivity (*k*) is a fundamental property of a molecule at a specified monochromatic wavelength. It has two connotations in European usage, and a third according to American convention. If the concentration is expressed in mol/litre, then *k* is described as the molar absorptivity $(\varepsilon,\text{litre/mol/cm})$, and defined as 'the absorbance of a one molar solution in a cell of 1 cm path-length'. It may also be quoted as the logarithm (base 10), the values being in the range 1 to 5.

When concentration is expressed in g/100 ml, *k* is described as the specific absorbance and given the symbol $A_{1\,cm}^{1\,\%}$ or A(1%, 1 cm), defined as 'the absorbance of a 1% w/v solution in a cell of 1 cm path-length'. It is usually written in the shortened form A_1^1 and is widely used in analytical chemistry. It was formerly known as the 'specific extinction coefficient', symbol $E_{1\,cm}^{1\,\%}$ or E(1%, 1 cm).

American convention recognises the constant *k* as 'absorptivity' (*a*, litre/g/cm) defined as 'the absorbance of a 1 g/litre solution in a cell of 1 cm path-length'.

These terms for absorptivity can be readily interconverted, as follows

$$a=\frac{A_1^1}{10}=\frac{\varepsilon}{\text{mol. wt}}$$

Thus a compound with a molecular weight of 100 whose absorptivity $a=20$ at wavelength λ, in a particular solvent at a defined pH (if aqueous) and at a specified temperature, would have a corresponding specific absorbance $A_1^1=200$ and a molar absorptivity $\varepsilon=2000$.

Absorbance and absorptivity are often expressed in logarithmic form in cases where spectra are to be compared. The logarithmic form of the Beer–Lambert Law expresses the effects of absorptivity (*k*), concentration (*c*), and path-length (*b*) as additive terms

$$\log A=\log k+\log c+\log b$$

Since only the absorptivity (*k*) is a function of λ, the shape of a logarithmic absorption curve is independent of concentration and path-length. Their only effect is to shift the log *A* spectrum along the log *A* axis. A disadvantage of the log *A* plot is that fine structure near the top of the peak is compressed.

The practical usefulness of specific absorbance values (A_1^1) clearly depends on a number of factors. These include the state of purity of the substance, the solvent conditions originally used to establish the reference data, the precise conditions employed in the reference instrument, and the extent to which they correspond with those of a particular test laboratory. It is therefore wise to ascertain the status of any absorptivity data in the literature. In the monographs in Part 2, the reliability of all A_1^1 values has been assessed and indicated (see General Notices). However, if a sample of the drug concerned is available in pure form, it is good practice to establish periodically a 'local' value of the absorptivity and to use this in calculating sample concentrations.

VALIDITY OF THE BEER–LAMBERT LAW

The validity of the Beer–Lambert Law is affected by a number of factors. If the radiation is non-monochromatic, i.e. its spectral bandwidth is greater than about 10 per cent of the drug absorption bandwidth at half-height, the observed absorbance will be lower than the 'true' limiting value for monochromatic radiation. Thus, sharp bands are more susceptible than broad bands to absorbance error on this account. Moreover, if the absorbing species is non-homogeneous, or if it undergoes association, dissociation, photodegradation, solvation, complexation or adsorption, or if it emits fluorescence, then positive or negative deviations from the Beer–Lambert Law may be observed. Stray-light effects and the type of solvent used may also lead to non-compliance with the Beer–Lambert Law.

It follows that the validity of the Beer–Lambert Law should be established for each drug under the measurement conditions to be used over an appropriate concentration range. For single-beam instruments, the absorbance range for precise measurements is between about 0.3 and 0.6 absorbance unit, the optimum being at 0.43 absorbance unit. For double-beam spectrophotometers, the optimum range lies between 0.6 and 1.2 absorbance unit. Five or more standard solutions, whose absorbances span the working range, should be measured in duplicate in a matched pair of cells against the solvent as reference; the residual absorbance difference between the cells when filled with solvent (the cell constant) should be subtracted from each individual measurement and should be checked regularly. The graph of absorbance (A) versus concentration (c) should indicate whether any systematic positive or negative deviation is apparent; if so, then additional points should be inserted and the linear working range established. Another test for linearity is to plot the function A/bc (the absorptivity) against concentration of drug, when a horizontal graph indicates compliance with the Beer–Lambert Law.

Stray-light Effects

Stray light is radiation at wavelengths different from those desired. It may arise from light-scattering or other defects within the instrument, or it may be caused by external radiation. If the stray light is not absorbed, the observed absorbance will tend to a constant value as the concentration of drug is increased, thereby yielding a negative deviation from the Beer–Lambert Law.

Stray-light errors are more likely to be observed near the wavelength limits of an instrument, where the radiation intensity of the source and the efficiency of the optical system are reduced, especially below 220 nm and at the crossover point between the ultraviolet and the visible lamps (about 320 to 400 nm). Errors may become serious where the solvent absorbs strongly or where a strongly-absorbing sample is measured by difference spectrophotometry.

The Influence of Solvent

The solvent often exerts a profound influence on the quality and shape of the spectrum. For example, many aromatic chromophores display vibrational fine structure in non-polar solvents, whereas in more polar solvents this fine structure is absent due to solute-solvent interaction effects. A classic case is phenol and related compounds which have different spectra in cyclohexane and in neutral aqueous solution. In aqueous solutions, the pH exerts a profound effect on ionisable chromophores due to the differing extent of conjugation in the ionised and the non-ionised chromophore. In phenolic compounds, for example, addition of alkali to two pH units above the pK_a leads to the classical 'red' or *bathochromic shift* to longer wavelength, a loss of any fine structure, and an increase in molar absorptivity (*hyperchromic effect*). The bathochromic shift is often large (>10 nm) and can be of great diagnostic value.

This effect has been exploited, both for qualitative and quantitative purposes, for the analysis of barbiturates. In acidic or neutral solution, barbiturates show little absorption above 230 nm (Fig. 2), but in 0.05M borax buffer (pH 9.2), ionisation yields an intense conjugated chromophore (Fig. 3) with a well-defined maximum near 240 nm ($A_1^1 = 400$ to 450). In sodium hydroxide solution (pH 13), a second stage of ionisation occurs (except in N-substituted derivatives) to extend further the conjugation, giving a peak maximum near 255 nm (Figs 2 and 3). However, solutions in alkali are unstable due to ring-opening so that measurements must be made rapidly.

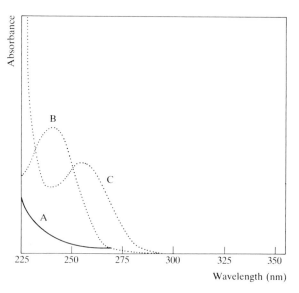

Fig. 2. Effect of pH on the ultraviolet spectrum of phenobarbitone. A, non-ionised barbiturate in 0.1M hydrochloric acid; B, mono-anion in 0.05M borax buffer (pH 9.2); C, di-anion in 0.5M sodium hydroxide (pH 13).

Fig. 3. Dissociation of C_5-substituted barbituric acids. A, undissociated free acid; B, mono-anion; C, di-anion.

The 'blue' or *hypsochromic shift* to shorter wavelengths is shown by aromatic amines. On acidification, the protonated quaternary ammonium group no longer participates in the chromophore so that the spectrum is shifted to lower wavelengths, sometimes by as much as 30 nm, with a sharp fall in absorptivity (*hypochromic effect*).

In addition to their use for characterising a chromophore, pH-induced shifts can also be exploited to shift a spectrum along the wavelength scale to obtain an interference-free window for measurement of an ionisable species in a mixture.

The quality of spectral measurement is directly affected by the type and purity of the solvent used. Each solvent has a cut-off wavelength (corresponding to about 10% transmittance) and this varies with solvent purity (Table 1). A solvent should not be used below its cut-off wavelength even though reference cell compensation is employed, because of the greater risk of stray-light effects. The ultraviolet spectra of some solvents are illustrated on p. 203.

Table 1. Cut-off points equivalent to 10% transmittance for spectroscopic solvents

Solvent	Wavelength nm
Water (distilled) or dilute inorganic acid	190
Acetonitrile	210
Butyl alcohol	210
Cyclohexane	210
Ethanol (96% v/v)	210
Heptane	210
Hexane	210
Isopropyl alcohol	210
Methanol	210
Ether	220
Sodium hydroxide (0.2M)	225
Ethylene dichloride	230
Methylene chloride	235
Chloroform (stabilised with ethanol)	245
Carbon tetrachloride	265
NN-Dimethylformamide	270
Benzene	280
Pyridine	305
Acetone	330

Some cautionary comments may be appropriate at this point. It is better to use single- or double-distilled water, and to avoid deionised water, which can be contaminated with absorptive fragments of ion-exchange resin or contain bacterial metabolites; these can contribute significantly to non-specific absorption at low wavelengths. Ethanol is normally used as the 96% v/v strength, since dehydrated alcohol is usually contaminated with traces of benzene added to form the azeotropic mixture for distillation. Acetonitrile can vary noticeably in quality, depending on the supplier; the grade supplied for use in HPLC is usually to be

recommended. Acetone, sometimes used to clean cells, is highly absorptive and not always easily removed, despite its volatility and aqueous solubility. Chloroform and carbon tetrachloride absorb strongly at about 250 nm and should therefore only be used for measurements at wavelengths above about 280 nm. Ether, although transparent down to 220 nm, presents particular problems due to its volatility (unstable standard solutions) and inflammability. Although absorptivity is considered to be relatively insensitive to temperature changes, organic solvents in general suffer from high temperature coefficients of expansion, so that for ultimate precision a cell provided with a thermostat may be required.

Instrumentation

Colorimeters. These usually employ a single tungsten radiation source in combination with broad-band (~ 30 nm) optical filters of nominal wavelength, or narrow bandwidth interference filters with a defined wavelength for use in the visible range. The range of linearity of the colorimeter may be constrained by the relatively broad spectral bandwidths employed, and therefore should be carefully checked for each type of assay.

Single-beam Spectrophotometers. These differ from the colorimeter in using a prism or a high quality diffraction grating monochromator, together with an additional intense source of ultraviolet radiation, usually a deuterium (or hydrogen) lamp. They are capable of high precision, particularly in the optimum absorbance range (0.3 to 0.6 absorbance units). The reference and sample cells must be manually moved in and out of the radiation beam at each wavelength, and it is not practicable, therefore, to scan a spectrum using this device.

Double-beam Spectrophotometers. These use similar high quality optical components to those in the single-beam instrument. However, the radiation from the monochromator is split into two identical beams by a rotating mirror. One beam passes through the sample and the other through the reference cell, before being recombined to focus on the detector. Each signal is processed appropriately by the detector electronics to measure the absorbance 10 to 20 times per second, which gives full compensation for cell and solvent absorption. A scan motor drives the monochromator to give a constant wavelength change per second, and this is synchronised with a recorder or digital plotter to present the spectrum. For broad bands, scan speeds up to 2 nm/s can be employed. However, some computer-controlled spectrophotometers with fast data-processing capabilities can scan at rates approaching 20 nm/s, while maintaining spectral fidelity even for sharp peaks.

Rapid-scanning Spectrophotometers. These employ multi-channel detectors. The most commonly encountered detector of this type is the linear photodiode array. The reversed-optics mode is employed, so that radiation is passed through the sample or reference cell, then dispersed by a diffraction grating polychromator and detected by a device which comprises several hundred diodes. Each photodiode registers the integrated intensity of radiation incident on it which is determined by the spectral dispersion:photodiode ratio. If, for example, a 200-nm bandwidth of radiation were dispersed across 256 photodiodes, the nominal resolution per photodiode would be 0.78 nm.

A spectrum in a specified range is acquired within 20 milliseconds. The analogue signals from each photodiode are digitised and transferred to a computer, where they are corrected for dark current response and transformed to absorbance. A number of digital techniques are available to increase sensitivity and to extend the use of rapid-scanning detectors to multicomponent analysis, reaction kinetics, tablet dissolution tests, process control, and detection in HPLC (A. F. Fell *et al.*, *Chromatographia*, 1982, *16*, 69–78).

Absorption Cells

In the visible region, a matched pair of glass cells can be used, but they are inappropriate for the ultraviolet region, due to the poor transmission properties of glass in this range. Fused silica or quartz cells have high transmittance from 190 to 1000 nm, and are therefore the cells of choice. The path-length employed is usually 1.00 cm; longer path-length cells are used for poorly absorptive drugs and/or where the concentration is low. Flow cells designed to minimise turbulent flow through the cell are used for monitoring changes in absorbance during a reaction, for tablet dissolution studies, or for HPLC; care should be taken that the cell walls do not block the radiation beam, otherwise variable errors are introduced. Cells provided with a thermostat are used for studies on enzymatic and other processes where temperature is a key parameter.

The meticulous handling and care of cells is a necessary condition for precise and accurate measurement. Cells should be carefully cleaned, filled with an appropriate solvent, and matched for absorbance to less than 1%. Each pair of cells should be marked on the base in soft pencil to identify the set and its normal orientation. It is convenient to designate the more strongly absorbing cell as the 'sample' cell, the other cell being coded as 'reference'. In this way the cell constant (i.e. the difference in absorbance at the measurement wavelength when filled with solvent) will be positive and can thus be subtracted from each absorbance reading. Moreover, the possibility of 'oscillating error' introduced by randomly changing the cell orientation during a series of measurements is eliminated. The 'cell constant' should be regularly checked at the measurement wavelength when filled with an appropriate solvent, or by scanning the baseline over the wavelength range.

Cells should be scrupulously cleaned after use. If they have contained aqueous solutions, they can be readily cleaned by repeated rinsing with distilled water or by soaking overnight in a very dilute solution of detergent; special detergents should be used for the cleaning of cells contaminated with biological material. Periodically, it is good practice to soak cells and stoppers thoroughly in a fresh solution of chromic acid, followed by copious rinsing with distilled water, in order to restore their matched performance. Cells that have been used with organic solvents require special care, a sequence of solvents ending in spectroscopic ether being convenient for obtaining dry, clean cells. In all cases, the manufacturer's instructions should be followed, when available. Sharp glass or metal objects should not be introduced into a cell, lest the internal surface be scratched. The outside optical surfaces should be polished before use with a soft cloth or photographic lens tissue. Cells should be stored in pairs, dry, and in a protective container.

Standardisation

Standards for calibration of absorbance and wavelength are necessary. Certified nichrome metal film filters can be used in the ultraviolet range but usually a solution of pure potassium dichromate is used, for which accepted specific absorbance values are known (Table 2). Other standards which have been proposed for the ultraviolet range are potassium nitrate in water and potassium chromate in dilute potassium hydroxide solution; for the visible range, copper sulphate and ammonium sulphate have been used.

Table 2. Calibration standards

Standard solution	Wave-length nm	Specific absorbance A_1^1 at 20°
Potassium dichromate 60 mg/litre in 0.005M sulphuric acid	235	124.5 ($\pm$1.6)*
	257	144.0 ($\pm$1.6)*
	313	48.6 ($\pm$1.6)*
	350	106.6 ($\pm$1.6)*
Potassium chromate 25 mg/litre in 0.04M potassium hydroxide	373	248.5 ($\pm$1.0)†
Potassium nitrate 10 g/litre in water	262.5	0.148
	302	0.705 ($\pm$0.005)†

*British Pharmacopoeia, London , HMSO, 1980, Appendix IIB.
†J. R. Edisbury, Practical Hints on Absorption Spectrometry, London, Hilger, 1966.

For the wavelength scale, the British Pharmacopoeia (1980) permits a tolerance of $\pm$1 nm in the range 200 to 400 nm and $\pm$3 nm in the range 400 to 600 nm, based on calibration with either holmium perchlorate solution or the emission lines of mercury, deuterium, or hydrogen discharge lamps. However, the most widely used standard is the holmium oxide glass filter (principal peaks at 241.5, 279.4, 287.5, 333.7, 360.9, 418.4, 453.2, 536.2, and 637.5 nm). Neodymium glass filters are also used for additional data in the visible region.

In some assays it is necessary to specify the minimum desirable resolution, since changes in the spectral bandwidth (or monochromator slit-width) can seriously affect the observed absorbance of sharp peaks. The British Pharmacopoeia (1980) requires that the spectral bandwidth employed should be such that further reduction does not lead to an increase in measured absorbance. This is particularly important for drugs that have aromatic or strongly-conjugated systems, e.g. diphenhydramine, phenoxymethylpenicillin, and amphotericin A and B. In such cases, a spectral bandwidth of more than 1 nm leads to a reduction in observed absorbance at the peak maximum (and conversely an increase in absorbance at a peak minimum), since the recorded absorbance is the mean of that over the whole bandwidth at that wavelength. Although increasing the slit-width gives a better signal-to-noise ratio, a slit-width of 2 nm is adequate for most bands, with 1 nm or 0.5 nm being used for very sharp peaks.

The level of stray light should be assessed since it increases with instrument age. The British Pharmacopoeia (1980) requires that the absorbance at 200 nm of a 1.2% w/v solution of potassium chloride should exceed 2 absorbance units with respect to water as reference. Alternatively a glass Vycor filter can be used, since its absorption increases sharply at the cut-off wavelength of 210 nm; any reading below this is attributable to stray light.

The United States Pharmacopeial Convention distributes certified reference standards for comparative analysis of a sample. The use of reference materials eliminates local differences in spectrophotometric performance but requires a considerable effort to ensure the continued validity of the standards.

QUANTITATIVE APPLICATIONS

Pharmacopoeial applications include assays for single drugs and mixtures of drugs, analyses involving colour reactions (colorimetric methods), tests for tablet dissolution, limit tests for impurities, and assays of bulk drugs or an extract thereof. Further applications are for physicochemical measurements, such as pK_a or velocity constants in enzymatic reactions. The scope of such applications has been significantly extended by methods which can confer additional specificity, namely difference spectrophotometry and derivative spectrophotometry.

SINGLE COMPONENTS
Where only one component in the sample absorbs significantly, the wavelength is chosen to coincide with the centre of a broad maximum in the spectrum to minimise wavelength-setting errors. If the spectrum has no suitable maximum, a flat absorption minimum can be used, provided that the consequent loss of sensitivity is acceptable. Wavelengths near the extremities of the ultraviolet and visible ranges must be avoided, because of the danger of stray-light errors.

Assuming that the linear range for compliance with the Beer–Lambert Law has been established and that the drug concentration has been adjusted within the optimum range for the type of instrument concerned, then two approaches to quantification may be employed. If an acceptable reference standard of the drug is available, and if the calibration graph passes through zero, measurement of replicates of the standard (at a comparable concentration) and of the tests are performed in bracketing sequence (i.e. each group of samples is preceded and followed by the standard), under identical conditions of solvent and temperature and using the same pair of matched cells. Each result should be corrected for the cell constant; the concentration of the test sample is then found by reference to the results from the standards.

Alternatively, the specific absorbance is used to calculate the sample concentration, using the absorbance measured in the specified solvent. A check on the accuracy of the absorbance scale is clearly essential. Wavelength accuracy is not so important.

Accurate measurements of a drug in solution may be difficult due to non-specific absorption. In these circumstances, the geometric correction devised by Morton and Stubbs is sometimes applied. This assumes that the non-specific absorption varies linearly with wavelength over the range measured. Taking a solution of pure drug, two equi-absorptive points are selected, one at a lower wavelength (λ_1) and the other at a higher wavelength (λ_3) than that of the peak maximum (λ_2). Any irrelevant absorption in the sample increases the observed absorbance of one equi-absorptive point (usually λ_1) more than the other (λ_3). A simple geometrical calculation involving absorbances at λ_1 and λ_3 enables the absorbance at λ_2 to be corrected for the non-specific absorption (M. Donbrow, *Instrumental Methods in Analytical Chemistry*, Vol. II—Optical Methods, London, Pitman, 1967). The assumption of linearity of the irrelevant absorption can be tested by subtracting the theoretical curve for the calculated quantity of pure material and inspecting the residual difference spectrum.

The classic example of a pharmacopoeial assay based on the Morton–Stubbs correction is that for vitamin A alcohol and the ester. Other techniques proposed for the correction of non-specific absorption include difference spectrophotometry, second derivative spectrophotometry, the use of orthogonal polynomials, and chemical or physical transformation of the drug to give absorption at a longer wavelength.

MULTICOMPONENT SYSTEMS

The absorption spectra of two or more drugs of interest often overlap. Subject to certain conditions, the Vierordt method of simultaneous equations can be employed to obtain the individual concentrations (A. L. Glenn, *J. Pharm. Pharmac.*, 1960, *12*, 598–608). If each of n drugs obeys the Beer–Lambert Law over the concentration range of interest, and if the law of additivity of absorbances applies, then the total absorbance, A_T^λ, observed at any wavelength λ is given by the sum

$$A_T^\lambda = \sum_{i=1}^{n} A_i^\lambda = \sum_{i=1}^{n} k_i^\lambda . c_i . b$$

where the subscript i denotes each component in the system. The term k_i^λ represents the absorptivity a (litre/g/cm), the specific absorbance ($A_{1\,cm}^{1\,\%}$), or

the molar absorptivity ε (litre/mol/cm), as determined by the units selected for concentration c_i.

For a two-component system, two wavelengths λ_1 and λ_2 are selected (as discussed below) and two corresponding simultaneous equations set up

$$A_T^{\lambda_1}/b = k_1^{\lambda_1} . c_1 + k_2^{\lambda_1} . c_2$$
$$A_T^{\lambda_2}/b = k_1^{\lambda_2} . c_1 + k_2^{\lambda_2} . c_2$$

These readily yield the concentration of each component, c_1 and c_2, by conventional algebra.

The selection of appropriate wavelengths and the use of accurate absorptivity values are clearly crucial. Generally λ_1 is the λ_{max} for component 1, while λ_2 is the λ_{max} for component 2, provided that at these wavelengths the absorptivity of the overlapping component is small. If the spectra of both components are very similar, the errors of the method increase appreciably as the difference between the absorptivity ratios tends to zero.

Although this method should apply to the analysis of three or more components, in practice it is often difficult to select wavelengths which fulfil all the requisite conditions. However, computer-aided spectrophotometers exploit the 'principle of overdetermination', where the number (m) of observation wavelengths exceeds the number (n) of components known to be present. This gives an $n \times m$ matrix of data which can be readily solved by standard matrix algebra.

The limit test for amphotericin A (a tetraene, λ_{max} 300 nm) in the antifungal antibiotic amphotericin (consisting primarily of amphotericin B, a heptaene, λ_{max} 380 nm) is an example of such a two-component analysis (British Pharmacopoeia, 1980).

Colorimetric Measurements

Colorimetric methods can selectively transform a drug, its impurity, or a metabolite so that the spectrum is shifted to the visible region and away from interference caused by another drug, formulation components, or biological substances, thereby conferring a further degree of specificity. Moreover, a drug with little or no useful absorption can be more sensitively determined by modifying it to a more highly-absorptive chromophore.

There are several parameters which require critical consideration. Firstly, the colour reagent should be selective for the drug molecule itself, discriminating against degradation products, impurities, and formulation excipients likely to be present. Secondly, the effect and control of any parameters likely to affect the colour reaction should be established, i.e.

solvent, pH, temperature, reagent excess, order of mixing reagents, ageing of reagents, and related factors. Moreover, the time required to establish a stable absorbance plateau and the stability of the chromophore generated, should be carefully assessed. Finally, the analytical performance should be established in terms of recovery, precision, sensitivity, linear range, and robust behaviour.

An interesting example is the assay of clonidine hydrochloride in injections and tablets (British Pharmacopoeia, 1980). In 0.01 M hydrochloric acid, clonidine exhibits two sharp maxima near 272 nm and 279 nm, which are not suitable for precise measurement. However, clonidine forms an ion pair with bromothymol blue, and this can be readily extracted into chloroform for subsequent measurement of the broad maximum near 420 nm. Because of the intrinsic variability of reagents used in such methods, a pharmacopoeial reference standard is employed for calibration. A similar policy is adopted for assays involving chemical modification of the drug, as in the tetrazolium assay for corticosteroids, the assay for folic acid involving hydrolysis, diazotisation, and coupling with N-(1-naphthyl)ethylenediamine, and the reaction of penicillins with imidazole and mercuric salts.

Difference Spectrophotometry

Difference spectrophotometry is a method of compensating for the presence of extraneous materials in a sample which would otherwise interfere with the spectrum of the drug being determined. It involves the measurement of the absorbance difference, at a defined wavelength, between two samples in one of which a physical or chemical property of the drug has been changed. It is assumed that the spectrum of the drug can be changed without affecting the spectrum of the interfering material. Alternatively, the absorbance difference may be measured between the sample and an equivalent solution without the drug. Difference spectrophotometry is sometimes described as 'differential spectrophotometry', but this term is not recommended because of its possible confusion with derivative spectrophotometry.

Many suitable methods for physical and chemical modification of the drug absorbance have been reported. For example, the bathochromic effect is used in the difference spectrophotometric assay of barbiturates. The absorbance of the sample at about pH 10 (A_{10}), where the mono-anionic species contributes (A_B), is used to compensate for the absorption of interfering endogenous materials (A_M) which have been carried through the extraction procedure. The sample absorbance at pH 13 (A_{13}), where the di-anionic species (A_D) contributes, is measured at about 260 nm with reference to the sample absorbance at pH 10 (A_{10}), so that

$$A_{13} = A_D + A_M$$

$$A_{10} = A_B + A_M$$

thus

$$\Delta A = A_{13} - A_{10} = A_D - A_B$$

if

$$\Delta\varepsilon = (\varepsilon_D - \varepsilon_B)$$

$$\Delta A = \Delta\varepsilon bc$$

Thus the difference absorbance can be readily related to concentration by prior calibration of the constant, $\Delta\varepsilon$, or the concentration may be found by simple proportion

$$\Delta A_{test}/\Delta A_{standard} = c_{test}/c_{standard}$$

It should, however, be established that ΔA is a linear function of concentration (c) over the range required. It is convenient to select for the analytical wavelength a value corresponding to a maximum in the difference spectrum, obtained by scanning the sample and reference solution over an appropriate wavelength range.

Difference spectrophotometry can be used for quality control in cases where the interfering material is well-defined, because an appropriate dilution of a suitable reference solution can be used in the reference cell. The difference absorbance is, however, susceptible to systematic error when there is uncertainty in the concentration of interfering materials in the samples to be assayed. This error increases in proportion to the ratio of the molar absorptivity of the interference to that of the drug.

A further technique to correct for absorptive interferences by difference measurement is based on *dual-wavelength spectrophotometry*. In this method, two monochromatic beams at different wavelengths are passed through the same sample. One wavelength (λ_1) is generally characteristic of the drug, while the other (λ_2) is carefully selected so that the absorbance is equivalent to the level of absorptive interference ($A_m^{\lambda_1}$) anticipated at the analytical wavelength (λ_1). Thus, the second radiation beam is analogous to the reference cell employed in conventional difference spectrophotometry, and the difference in absorbance at the two wavelengths (ΔA) represents the absorption of drug ($A_n^{\lambda_1}$) corrected for interference

$$A^{\lambda_1} = A_n^{\lambda_1} + A_m^{\lambda_1}$$

and since

$$A^{\lambda_2} = A_m^{\lambda_1}$$

then

$$\Delta A = A^{\lambda_1} - A^{\lambda_2} = A_n^{\lambda_1}$$

A classic application of this method is the correction of Rayleigh scatter in samples of biological origin.

Derivative Spectrophotometry

In derivative spectrophotometry the absorbance (A) of a sample is differentiated with respect to wavelength (λ) to generate the first, second, or higher order derivatives

$$A = f(\lambda) \qquad dA/d\lambda = f'(\lambda)$$
zero order   first derivative

$$d^2A/d\lambda^2 = f''(\lambda), \text{ etc.}$$
second derivative

Derivative spectra often yield a characteristic profile, where subtle changes of gradient and curvature in the normal (zero order) spectrum are observed as distinctive bipolar features (Fig. 4).

The first derivative of an absorption spectrum, represents the gradient at all points of the spectrum and can be used to locate 'hidden' peaks, since $dA/d\lambda = 0$ at peak maxima (Fig. 4). However, second and higher even-order derivatives are potentially more useful in analysis.

The even-order derivatives are bipolar functions of alternating sign at the centroid (i.e. negative for 2nd, positive for 4th, etc.), whose position coincides with that of the original peak maximum (Fig. 4). To this extent, even-derivative spectra bear a similarity to the original spectrum, although the presence of satellite peaks flanking the centroid adds a degree of complexity to the derivative profile. A key feature is that the derivative centroid peak width of a Gaussian peak decreases to 53%, 41%, and 34% of the original peak width, in the second, fourth, and sixth orders respectively. This feature can increase the resolution of overlapping peaks. However, the increasingly complex satellite patterns detract from resolution enhancement in higher derivative spectra.

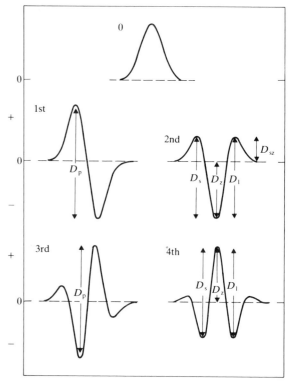

Fig. 4. First to fourth derivatives of a Gaussian peak, and some graphical measures of derivative amplitude (D). D_p, peak-to-peak; D_s, peak-to-satellite at short wavelength; D_z, peak-to-derivative zero; D_l, peak-to-satellite at long wavelength; D_{sz}, satellite peak-to-derivative zero.

An important property of the derivative process is that broad bands are suppressed relative to sharp bands. This effect increases with increasing order of the derivative since the amplitude (D_n) of a Gaussian peak in the nth derivative is inversely related to the original peak width (W), raised to the nth degree

$$D_n \propto (W)^{-n}$$

Thus, for two coincident peaks of equal intensity, the nth derivative amplitude of the sharper peak (X) is greater than that of the broader peak (Y) by a factor which increases with derivative order

$$\frac{D_{n,\,X}}{D_{n,\,Y}} = \left[\frac{W_Y}{W_X}\right]^n$$

This property leads to the selective rejection of broad, additive, spectral interferences such as Rayleigh scattering.

If the Beer–Lambert Law is obeyed, i.e.

$$A = \varepsilon b c$$

then

$$\frac{\mathrm{d}A}{\mathrm{d}\lambda} = \frac{\mathrm{d}\varepsilon}{\mathrm{d}\lambda} . b . c$$

$$\frac{\mathrm{d}^2 A}{\mathrm{d}\lambda^2} = \frac{\mathrm{d}^2\varepsilon}{\mathrm{d}\lambda^2} . b . c$$

and similarly for higher derivatives, where ε = molar absorptivity (litre/mol/cm), b = cell path-length (cm), and c = concentration (mol/litre).

For quantitative work, the amplitude of a derivative peak can be measured in various ways (Fig. 4). Although the true derivative amplitude is that measured with respect to the derivative zero, the most common practice is to record the amplitude with respect to a satellite in the spectrum which affords an extra degree of suppression of interference from extraneous substances. It is essential to run standards in bracketing sequence with samples, thus subjecting both to the same experimental conditions. It should be established that the graphical derivative adopted fulfils the analytical criteria of linear response with concentration, regression through or close to the origin, independence from interfering substances, and optimum precision.

In general, methods for generating derivative spectra fall into two classes. These are optical methods, which operate on the radiation beam itself, and electronic or digital methods operating on the photometric detector output. The electronic analogue device generates the required derivative as a function of time as the spectrum is scanned at constant speed ($\mathrm{d}\lambda/\mathrm{d}t$) and therefore the derivative amplitude varies with the scan speed, slit-width, and gain. Moreover, the signal-to-noise ratio has been reported to degrade by approximately a factor of two in each successive derivative order.

Alternatively, a microcomputer can be used, employing one of a number of digital algorithms to produce smoothed derivative spectra. This is done in real time or by post-run processing of the digitised spectrum. The digital approach is increasingly employed in contemporary spectrophotometers, due to the widespread adoption of microprocessors for instrument control and data handling, coupled with the addition of dedicated microcomputers for further data processing capability.

Although transformation of a spectrum to its second or higher order derivative often yields a more highly characteristic profile than the zero order spectrum, the intrinsic information content of the data is not increased; indeed, some data, such as constant 'offset' factors, are lost. However, the derivative method tends to emphasise subtle spectral features by presenting them in a new and visually more accessible way. The method is generally applicable in analytical chemistry and can be used equally for resolution enhancement of electrochemical, chromatographic, or thermal analysis data.

Derivative spectrophotometry has found significant application in clinical, forensic, and biomedical analysis. In forensic toxicology the suppression of the absorbance due to interfering substances by second derivative spectrophotometry is well demonstrated in studies on amphetamine in an homogenised liver extract (Fig. 5). Transformation of the zero order spectrum (A) to its second derivative (B) using a rapid-scanning multi-channel spectrophotometer permits the characteristically sharp benzenoid peaks of amphetamine to be detected and compared with an authentic standard (D), while the interfering background absorption is substantially reduced. The second and fourth derivative method for biological background correction can give a ten-fold increase in the detection limit of serum paraquat in cases of poisoning (A. F. Fell *et al.*, *Clin. Chem.*, 1981, **27**, 286–292). The derivative method can be successfully combined with difference spectrophotometry, to give second derivative–difference spectra, when enhanced discrimination against interfering substances and sharpened fine structural features are observed.

QUALITATIVE APPLICATIONS

Specific identification of a compound can rarely be made on the basis of spectral evidence alone. Often the spectrum serves as confirmatory evidence of identity, in support of other analytical data. The general approach usually followed in qualitative applications is first to establish by independent means (e.g. chromatography) that the material consists of substantially one absorbing component. Spectra are then recorded in aqueous acidic, basic, and in ethanolic or methanolic solution. The wavelengths of the principal peaks and the corresponding absorptivity values are noted for each solvent system. By comparison with data tabulated in ascending wavelength order (see the index of Ultraviolet Absorption Maxima in Part 3), a number of compounds with absorbing properties

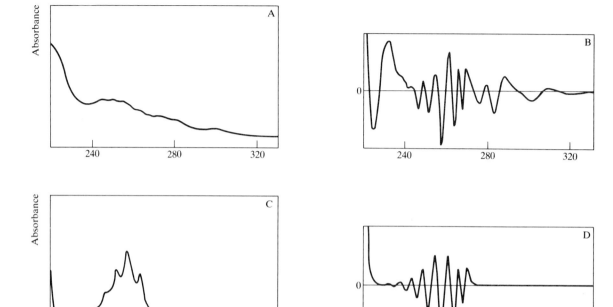

Fig. 5. Detection of amphetamine in homogenised liver extract. Standard zero order (A), and second derivative (B) spectra of the liver extract, compared with the standard zero order (C) and second derivative (D) spectra of amphetamine; solutions were in 0.1 M sulphuric acid. (From R. Gill *et al.*, *J. forens. Sci. Soc.*, 1982, *22*, 165–171.)

similar to the test substance are selected (using a wavelength window of ± 2 nm).

Further evidence can be deduced from the absorptivity ratios of peaks within a spectrum; moreover, the change in these ratios together with the shift in peak positions as the pH is changed can be diagnostic. If a drug molecule ionises reversibly (i.e. without degradation), the family of curves for a constant concentration in acidic and basic solvents will display one or more isosbestic points at characteristic wavelengths, where the absorbance is constant at all values of pH.

Spectral shifts are among the most useful diagnostic features in drug molecules possessing ionisable groups. A marked bathochromic shift in alkaline solution is observed not only for most of the phenolic drugs such as the phenolic oestrogens, but also in the case of hydroxypyridines, ketones, benzodiazepines, pyridones, and nitro-compounds. The barbiturates display a marked bathochromic shift in alkaline solution to give characteristic maxima at about 240 nm (pH 9.2) and 255 nm (pH 13), as discussed above. The hypsochromic shift is

shown by aromatic amines in acid solution and is highly characteristic for many drugs. Further diagnostic detail can also be obtained by reducing the solvent polarity for compounds which form hydrogen bonds in aqueous solvents.

Fluorescence Spectrophotometry

Fluorescence radiation, emitted by a sample which is illuminated at a defined excitation wavelength, is one of several types of luminescence phenomena. Fluorescence spectrophotometry is by far the most widely used luminescence technique in practice, primarily because of its intrinsic sensitivity and selectivity. The sensitivity is generally greater than that achieved by absorption spectrophotometry in which, at low drug concentrations, accurate and precise measurement of the difference in intensity of the two similar beams of radiation, I_0 and I, becomes progressively more difficult. By contrast, the intensity of fluorescence is essentially measured against a 'dark' background, or at least a background with relatively low fluorescence emission.

Although in biological samples the fluorescence intensity of interfering substances may be relatively high, the sensitivity and selectivity of the method is generally such that fluorescent drugs and their metabolites can be analysed more readily than by conventional spectrophotometry.

The selectivity arises from the requirement that two wavelengths are involved—the excitation wavelength (λ_{ex}) and the fluorescence emission wavelength (λ_f). Moreover, the ability of a molecule to fluoresce is in itself a characteristic which discriminates it from the many compounds which do not display significant fluorescence. The fluorescence phenomenon involves the absorption of excitation radiation by a molecule which then loses energy by internal conversion processes, before emitting a photon of radiation at lower energy. The excitation wavelength maximum (λ_{ex}) is lower than the wavelength of maximum fluorescence emission (λ_f), from which it is separated by a characteristic interval described as the *Stokes shift*.

The variety of sampling methods available in spectrofluorimetry makes it a very versatile technique. The most frequent mode of sample presentation is as a dilute solution, although gases, suspensions, and solid surfaces can also be examined. Combinations of spectrofluorimetry with thin-layer chromatography and high pressure liquid chromatography are particularly advantageous for sensitive and selective detection of fluorophores.

Instrumentation

In most conventional single-beam spectrofluorimeters, fluorescence is observed at right angles to the axis of the excitation radiation, to provide a convenient means for optical discrimination between λ_{ex} and λ_f (Fig. 6). Simple filter instruments employ an intense source of radiation (usually a mercury or a xenon lamp) with primary (excitation) and secondary (emission) filters in the right-angle configuration, a cylindrical or oblong clear quartz cell, and a photomultiplier detector. More complex spectrofluorimeters employ two diffraction gratings (or prisms) to select λ_{ex} and λ_f, together with a high-intensity xenon source, scanning motors, and electronic compensation for variations in source intensity as the wavelength is varied.

An excitation spectrum is obtained by monitoring the fluorescence at a convenient fixed wavelength (λ_f) while scanning the excitation monochromator at a fixed speed up to a wavelength no higher than λ_f (Fig. 7). The excitation spectrum should, in principle, be comparable with the absorption spectrum; however, differences arise due principally to the distortion imposed by the instrumental response characteristic of the spectrofluorimeter.

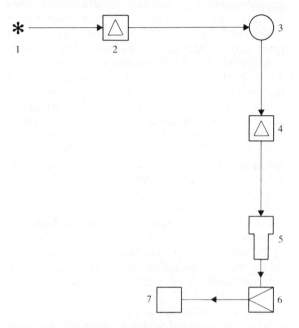

Fig. 6. Diagrammatic representation of a spectrofluorimeter. 1, radiation source; 2, excitation monochromator (filter, prism, or diffraction grating); 3, quartz sample cell; 4, emission monochromator; 5, photomultiplier tube detector; 6, amplifier; 7, recorder.

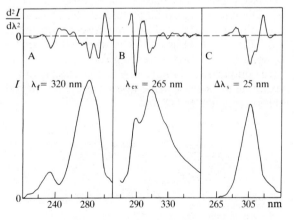

Fig. 7. Excitation, fluorescence, and synchronously-scanned spectra of oestrone in ethanol, and their second derivatives. A, excitation spectrum monitored at a fluorescence wavelength, λ_f; B, fluorescence spectrum obtained at an excitation wavelength, λ_{ex}; C, synchronously-scanned spectrum obtained with a constant interval, $\Delta\lambda_s$, between the excitation and emission monochromators. (From A. F. Fell, in *Proc. 1st Symp. Anal. Steroids, Eger, Hungary*, S. Görög (Ed.), Amsterdam, Elsevier Press, 1982, pp. 495–510.)

The fluorescence spectrum is obtained by illuminating the sample at a convenient fixed excitation wavelength (λ_{ex}) and scanning the emission monochromator at a fixed speed over a wavelength range no lower than λ_{ex} (Fig. 7). For interlaboratory comparisons, corrected fluorescence and excitation spectra should be obtained using one of the generally available digital or instrumental techniques.

Some spectrofluorimeters are capable of scanning the excitation and the emission monochromators synchronously (synchronous-scanning or synchronous-excitation fluorimetry) to yield fluorescence spectra which are generally simpler and considerably sharper than the conventional fluorescence spectrum as indicated in Fig. 7. With computer-aided spectrofluorimetry, the acquisition and digital storage of fluorescence spectra are possible. These can then be manipulated in various ways to give the derivative spectrum where fine structure is accentuated (Fig. 7), the difference spectrum, or multi-wavelength spectral deconvolution for calculating the concentration of known overlapping components (S. A. Winfield *et al.*, *J. pharm. biomed. Analysis*, 1984, *2*, 561–566).

In another digital technique, a series of fluorescence spectra are acquired while sequentially stepping the excitation wavelength. When these spectra are combined to give a matrix of (I_f, λ_f, λ_{ex}), a three-dimensional isometric projection is presented. This type of graphical presentation is described as an 'emission-excitation matrix' or 'fluorogram' (Fig. 8). The data can also be plotted as the equivalent two-dimensional plot of isointensity contours in the (λ_f, λ_{ex}) plane (Fig. 9). The three-dimensional graphics are finding increasing use for the qualitative comparison of fluorescent molecules, as in the example of promethazine and its principal degradation product (Figs 8 and 9).

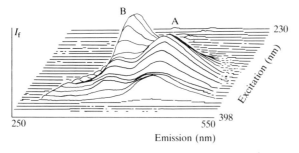

Fig. 8. Isometric projection of emission-excitation matrix ('fluorogram') of fluorescence intensity (I_f) for promethazine hydrochloride (A) and promethazine sulphoxide (B) in buffer at pH 3.0. (From A. F. Fell *et al.*, *J. pharm. biomed. Analysis*, 1983, *1*, 557–572.)

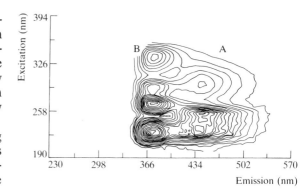

Fig. 9. Contour plot of emission-excitation matrix of promethazine hydrochloride (A) and promethazine sulphoxide (B) in buffer at pH 3.0. (From B. J. Clark *et al.*, *Analytica chim. Acta*, 1985, *170*, 35–44.)

Instrument Standardisation

The calibration of excitation and emission monochromator wavelengths should be checked regularly by the use of sharp lines from the instrument's own radiation source (e.g. xenon lines at 450.1, 462.4, 467.1, and 473.4 nm), or the use of sharp fluorescence peaks in solutions or glasses of trivalent lanthanide ions (Te^{III}, Eu^{III}). Other fluorescence standards in common use are ovulene, and other polycyclic aromatic hydrocarbons with fine vibrational structure, such as naphthalene and anthracene. In practice it is necessary only to calibrate one monochromator, since the other can then be calibrated by the Rayleigh scattered radiation using a sample of colloidal silica in the sample position. The use of an auxiliary light source, such as a mercury light pen, is the least satisfactory method for wavelength calibration.

SIGNAL INTENSITY

Fluorescence is generally more sensitive to environmental factors than absorbance measurements. Signal intensity may be affected by pH, temperature, quenching, interfering substances, solvent, or interference from Rayleigh and Raman scattering. Many fluorescent species contain ionisable groups whose fluorescent properties are sensitive to pH. In some cases only one of the ionised species may be fluorescent. An example is the barbiturates which only fluoresce at elevated pH in the di-anionic form. The relationship of fluorescence intensity with pH should always be examined as part of the development of the method.

An increase in temperature leads to a decrease in the observed fluorescence in dilute solutions due to increased collisional quenching. Since a rise of one degree can give a decrease of 1 to 2% in fluorescence intensity, it is essential to use a sample cell provided with a thermostat when high precision measurements are required.

Quenching occurs if species are present that can reduce the observed fluorescence by forming complexes with either the ground state or the excited state of the fluorescent molecule. It can be described by the Stern–Volmer Law

$$I_f/I_{f(q)} = 1 + k[Q]$$

where I_f represents the fluorescence intensity in the absence of quenching agent and $I_{f(q)}$ denotes the fluorescence intensity observed in the presence of quencher concentration $[Q]$. This relationship can be used for quantitative analysis, e.g. the analysis of sulphonamides by quenching with 9-chloroacridine.

Generally, the fluorescence due to interfering substances in samples of biological origin limits the ultimate sensitivity of a method. Interference can be reduced by suitable sample pre-treatment, the use of spectroscopically pure solvents, triple-distilled water, and scrupulously clean glass-ware. However, when working near the sensitivity limits of an instrument, the variability of the interfering fluorescence detracts significantly from the precision and accuracy of a method. Interference from Rayleigh and Raman scatter is a particular problem when analysing dilute solutions.

Rayleigh scatter results in emission of radiation at the same wavelength as the light source. The intensity of Rayleigh scatter varies inversely with λ^4, so that its effect is more troublesome at lower wavelengths and when the excitation and emission wavelengths are close.

Raman scatter involves a shift in wavelength which depends on the solvent used, and may thus be confused with fluorescence. Its presence may be detected by changing the excitation wavelength; the wavelength of a Raman peak will change in the same direction, whereas a fluorescence peak will remain at the same wavelength. Interference by a Raman peak can therefore be displaced from an emission band by using an excitation wavelength lower than the excitation maximum, with a consequent loss in sensitivity.

QUANTITATIVE APPLICATIONS

In dilute solution, the fluorescence intensity (I_f) for defined values of λ_{ex} and λ_f, is linearly related to molar concentration (c), according to the approximate relationship

$$I_f = k\phi I_0 \varepsilon bc \quad \text{at } \lambda_{ex}, \lambda_f$$

where k = instrumental constant, ϕ = quantum efficiency of fluorescence, I_0 = radiation intensity of source, ε = molar absorptivity, and b = cell pathlength. These constants can be collectively represented as K, under constant instrumental conditions where

$$I_f = Kc \quad \text{at } \lambda_{ex}, \lambda_f$$

A necessary condition is that the total absorbance ($= \varepsilon bc$) of the system should not exceed 0.05 absorbance units, otherwise progressively greater negative deviations from linearity are observed. At high drug concentrations, fluorescence intensity reaches a plateau. Beyond this, fluorescence intensity actually decreases with increasing concentration, due to inner-filter effects, where ground-state molecules absorb the fluorescence emitted by excited molecules.

It is essential to establish the range of linearity of the calibration curve of I_f versus c, using at least five standard solutions, for which the condition that absorbance at the wavelength of maximum excitation is <0.05 absorbance units holds. Samples are usually analysed by single-point bracketing, taking a standard conveniently close to the anticipated sample value and calculating the result by simple proportion.

The sequence of standard measurements before and after measuring the sample permits any baseline drift to be compensated. For additional assay security, two-point bracketing can be employed, where two standard solutions, one higher and the other lower than the concentration observed for the sample are used in bracketing sequence.

Spectrofluorimetry differs from absorption spectrophotometry in not yielding an absolute scale of values. For this reason it is essential to employ a reference standard for quantitative measurements. For example, some pharmacopoeial tests, such as the test for uniformity of content for digitoxin tablets, employ a spectrofluorimetric assay and comparison with an official reference standard. Quantitative spectrofluorimetry has been proposed for a number of naturally fluorescent compounds, including ergometrine, riboflavine, the catecholamines, phenothiazines, the barbiturates (at pH 13), and certain antibiotics such as chlortetracycline and oxytetracycline.

The sensitivity and selectivity of spectrofluorimetry have been well-exemplified in forensic and toxicological studies on lysergide. In the case of weakly fluorescent or non-fluorescent drugs, a number of well-characterised derivatisation reactions are available. These include dansyl chloride (5-dimethylaminonaphthalene-1-sulphonyl chloride) for primary and secondary amines and phenolic hydroxyl groups, fluorescamine (4-phenylspiro-[furan - 2(3H), 1' - isobenzofuran] - 3, 3'-dione), and o-phthalaldehyde for primary amines.

Derivatisation reactions of this type have significantly extended the scope of fluorescence detection in HPLC. Such developments, coupled with the wider use of laser sources for increased sensitivity and the advent of rapid-scanning fluorimetric detectors, further emphasise the considerable contribution which hybrid detection systems can make in liquid chromatography.

Bibliography

M. Donbrow, *Instrumental Methods in Analytical Chemistry*, Vol. 2, Optical Methods, London, Pitman, 1967.

A. Martin *et al.*, *Physical Pharmacy*, 3rd Edn, Philadelphia, Lea and Febiger, 1983.

Modern Fluorescence Spectroscopy, E. L. Wehry (Ed.), Vols 3 and 4, New York, Plenum Press, 1981.

Multichannel Image Detectors, ACS Symposium Series, No. 102, Y. Talmi (Ed.), Washington D.C., American Chemical Society, 1979.

M. Pesez and J. Bartos, Colorimetric and Fluorimetric Analysis of Organic Compounds and Drugs, *Clinical and Biochemical Series*, Vol. 1, New York, Marcel Dekker, 1974.

Practical Absorption Spectrometry, A. Knowles and C. Burgess (Ed.), London, Chapman and Hall, 1984.

Standards in Absorption Spectrometry, C. Burgess and A. Knowles (Ed.), London, Chapman and Hall, 1984.

Standards in Fluorescence Spectrometry, J. N. Miller (Ed.), London, Chapman and Hall, 1981.

S. Udenfriend, *Fluorescence Assays in Biology and Medicine*, New York, Academic Press, Vol. 1, 1964; Vol. 2, 1970.

Infra-red Spectrophotometry

D. I. Chapman

Infra-red spectrophotometry is the study of the reflected, absorbed, or transmitted radiant energy in that region of the electromagnetic spectrum from wavelength (λ) 0.8 to 500 µm. A more commonly used measurement than wavelength is the frequency (the number of waves per unit length). This is expressed in wavenumbers ($\tilde{v}$), the units of which are cm^{-1}. The relationship between wavenumber in cm^{-1} and wavelength in µm is given by

$$\tilde{v} = \frac{10^4}{\lambda}$$

The infra-red spectrum is usually divided into three regions, 12 500 to 4000 cm^{-1} (0.8 to 2.5 µm) ('near infra-red'), 4000 to 400 cm^{-1} (2.5 to 25 µm) ('mid infra-red'), and 400 to 20 cm^{-1} (25 to 500 µm) ('far infra-red'). Only the mid infra-red region (usually referred to simply as 'infra-red') is considered here because it is the region which is widely used in the analysis of drugs and pesticides. However, some dispersive instruments scan from 5000 to about 200 cm^{-1} and this extension to the far infra-red is useful for halogenated compounds and for inorganic substances.

When a molecule is subjected to infra-red radiation, transitions take place between rotational and vibrational energy levels in the ground electronic state. These transitions give rise to an absorption spectrum characteristic of the compound. This is in contrast to ultraviolet radiation which also causes transitions between rotational and vibrational energy levels, but because of its greater energy these transitions occur at higher energy states. In the infra-red, absorption occurs only where a change of the dipole moment of a molecule can take place. This means that diatomic molecules without dipoles, such as hydrogen, nitrogen, and oxygen, do not absorb in the infra-red. Total symmetry about an absorption band will eliminate certain absorptions, e.g. the symmetrical ethane molecule gives no carbon-carbon stretching absorption bands.

Three main types of absorption occur, namely fundamental, overtone, and combination. Fundamental bands are the primary absorption bands for each mode of vibration, overtone bands occur at multiples of the fundamental band wavelength, and combination bands occur at wavelengths which are the sum or difference of two or more fundamental bands. Overtone and combination bands are usually much weaker than fundamental bands.

Particular bonds or functional groups in a molecule have specific absorption bands at given wavenumbers. Changes in the wavenumber of a band have been correlated with changes in either the structural environment or the physical state of the molecule. These correlations form the basis of qualitative analytical work in infra-red spectrophotometry (L. J. Bellamy, 1965). However, many bands in the complex region from 1600 to 400 cm^{-1}, which is usually referred to as the 'fingerprint region', are still of unconfirmed origin. A proportion of the bands are characteristic of the molecule as a whole and cannot be assigned to particular functional groups.

INSTRUMENTATION

Dispersive Spectrophotometers

The basic components of a dispersive infra-red spectrophotometer are shown in Fig. 1. The source of infra-red radiation is an electrically conducting element, such as a Globar or Opperman source, which is maintained at about 1000°.

Infra-red spectrophotometers can be single- or double-beam instruments, or both facilities may be available. In the double-beam mode, the beam of radiation passes through both the sample and a reference path (or reference cell). The use of a reference cell enables compensation to be made for unwanted absorption, e.g. from solvents. Alternatively, an instrument fitted with computing facilities can record and remember the solvent spectrum and then subtract it from a subsequent spectrum obtained with the same cell.

In optical null instruments, radiation is passed through the sample and reference paths simultaneously or the instrument may be designed to pass the radiation through each path alternately (pre-sample chopping). A wedge or comb attenuator is moved in or out of the reference beam until absorption in both beams is equal. The movement of the

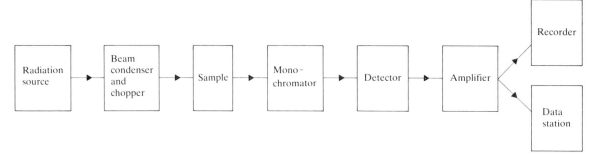

Fig. 1. Schematic diagram of a dispersive infra-red spectrophotometer.

attenuator is linked to the recorder pen which records the spectrum directly. These instruments lack sensitivity when the sample absorption is high, because of the lack of energy to activate the system. Thus, measurements made at below about 15% transmittance are imprecise. This problem is overcome with ratio-recording instruments in which the ratio of the intensities of the sample and reference beams is measured; the pen response remains constant, so enabling precise and reproducible values of the ordinate to be obtained, even at very small transmission values.

The detector may be a thermocouple, a Golay cell (which senses the change of pressure in a gas, caused by the heating effect), or a pyroelectric compound such as triglycine sulphate, and the response is amplified and fed to a recorder and/or data processor.

Infra-red spectrophotometers may not always record the correct frequency of the absorption bands because of various errors. Such errors may be inherent in the instrument, errors of adjustment, errors in fitting the paper to the recorder, or in the printing of the paper. The error in the frequency is greater at higher wavenumbers than at lower ones. For older dispersive instruments, the error at 5000 cm^{-1} inherent in the instrument alone can be as large as $\pm 50 \text{ cm}^{-1}$, and it is essential to calibrate each spectrum before it is removed from the recorder. With modern dispersive instruments, the error should be $\pm 5 \text{ cm}^{-1}$ or less at 5000 cm^{-1}, and within $\pm 1 \text{ cm}^{-1}$ below 2000 cm^{-1}. However, the occasional calibration ensures that the instrument is up to specification.

To calibrate the wavenumber scale, first record the spectrum of the sample and then place a polystyrene film in the sample beam and record a few of the main bands whose frequency is known and which do not coincide with the main bands in the spectrum

of the sample. The spectrum of bromvaletone calibrated with polystyrene is shown in Fig. 2. The differences between the recorded and correct frequency of the polystyrene bands are then calculated for each region of the spectrum and used in tabular or graphical form to correct the observed band positions of the sample.

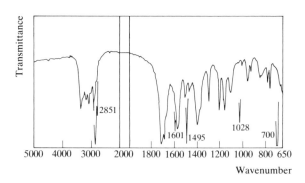

Fig. 2. Infra-red spectrum of bromvaletone calibrated with polystyrene.

Interferometric Spectrophotometers

The Fourier transform infra-red spectrophotometer incorporates an interferometer (Fig. 3). Its basic components are a beam splitter and two mirrors, perpendicular to each other, one fixed and one which can be moved backwards and forwards at right angles to its plane. Approximately half of the radiation from the source is reflected to the fixed mirror where it is reflected back to the beam splitter which transmits about half (i.e. a quarter of the original) to the detector. The other half of the original radiation passes through the beam splitter to the movable mirror where it is reflected back to the beam splitter and about half (i.e. a quarter of the original) is reflected to the detector. When the two mirrors are equidistant from the beam splitter,

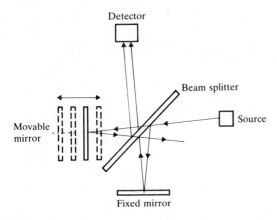

Fig. 3. Schematic diagram of the optics of an interferometer.

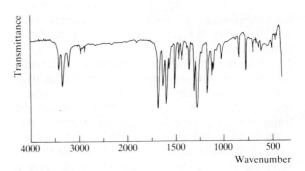

Fig. 5. Infra-red spectrum obtained from the interferogram of benzocaine shown in Fig. 4. (Courtesy of Nicolet Instruments Ltd.)

the two beams are said to interfere constructively. When the movable mirror is displaced in either direction by a quarter of a wavelength ($\lambda/4$), the two beams are said to interfere destructively. With monochromatic light, the detector records a beam whose intensity varies as a sine wave as the mirror moves. However, with polychromatic light the detector records the sum of all the sine waves; when both mirrors are equidistant from the beam splitter, all the sine waves are in phase (they interfere constructively) and a strong central peak is recorded in the interferogram. A sample placed in the beam will absorb light of certain wavelengths and therefore the recorded interferogram will be the sum of all the waves except those absorbed by the sample. The interferogram of benzocaine is shown in Fig. 4. This can be transformed mathematically (by the Fourier transform) to give its infra-red spectrum (Fig. 5). For the mid infra-red region, the

source is usually a Globar operated at about 1500°, and the beam splitter is germanium-coated potassium bromide. The detector is either a pyroelectric bolometer which can be operated at room temperature or a photon detector operating in liquid nitrogen.

Fourier transform infra-red spectrophotometers have a number of advantages over dispersive instruments. Firstly, they can scan quickly (as fast as 10 scans per second), and can therefore be used with gas or liquid chromatography for recording spectra as compounds are eluted. Secondly, all the frequencies are detected simultaneously, rather than sequentially, thus obtaining a much better signal-to-noise ratio and a resultant increase in sensitivity (the Felgett or Multiplex advantage). Also, the level of stray light is low, typically less than 0.02% transmittance. This means that the absorbance values remain linear beyond three absorbance units. This in turn leads to more accurate quantitative measurements even with strongly absorbing bands.

Data Processing

The use of data-processing equipment in conjunction with infra-red spectrophotometers, both dispersive and interferometric, produces three advantages, namely instrument control, spectrum manipulation, and spectrum identification and interpretation.

Firstly, the control of the instrument is simplified and the reproducibility and accuracy of wavelength and transmission (or absorbance) are greatly enhanced. For example, one commercial Fourier transform instrument uses a helium–neon laser to obtain an accuracy of better than 0.01 cm^{-1} at 4000 cm^{-1}, whereas older dispersive instruments could have an error of 50 cm^{-1}. The accuracy of

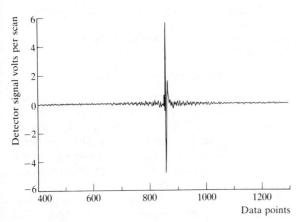

Fig. 4. Interferogram of benzocaine. (Courtesy of Nicolet Instruments Ltd.)

the transmittance of Fourier transform instruments is better than 0.1% in the range 0.1 to 100% transmittance.

The infra-red spectrum of a compound represents the variation of absorption, or transmittance, with changing wavenumber. It is customary to present the ordinate of an infra-red spectrum as percent transmittance and most collections of spectra made in the past have been recorded in this way. However, logarithmic conversion to absorbance is now readily achieved and modern instruments usually give a choice for presentation of spectra.

The second advantage, which is based upon the fact that spectra can be recorded in digital form, is the ability to accumulate spectra and to manipulate them. Solvent and impurity spectra can be recorded and subtracted from the sample spectrum, which can then be levelled, smoothed, and converted from transmittance to absorbance or vice versa. The absorbance scale can also be expanded considerably. The spectrum of a weak sample can be scanned repeatedly which, together with averaging of the signal, can reduce noise appreciably. This leads to a dramatic improvement in sensitivity. For example, there is little difference between the spectra of carbon disulphide and of benzocaine in carbon disulphide shown in Fig. 6, but with spectrum manipulation, a good spectrum of benzocaine is readily obtained (Fig. 7). The amount of benzocaine in the cell was approximately 4 µg but only about one quarter of this was in the infra-red

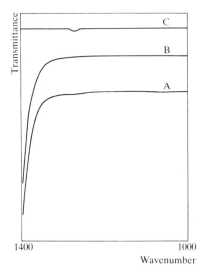

Fig. 6. Infra-red spectra of A, benzocaine in carbon disulphide; B, carbon disulphide; C, the difference spectrum (A − B). (Courtesy of Perkin-Elmer Ltd.)

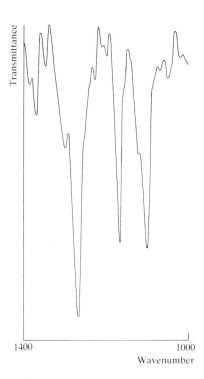

Fig. 7. The difference spectrum of benzocaine shown in Fig. 6, smoothed, corrected for baseline contribution, and absorbance expanded approximately 200 times. (Courtesy of Perkin-Elmer Ltd.)

beam. Each spectrum was recorded in less than 30 seconds.

The third major advantage afforded by data processing of spectra in digital form is in the identification and interpretation of spectra. The spectrum of a sample can be compared readily with a library of spectra and a list of the compounds of best fit can be either displayed on a screen or printed out. The presence of certain functional groups can also be recorded. These aspects are discussed more fully in later sections.

PURIFICATION OF SAMPLES

It is essential to use pure samples for infra-red spectrophotometry. The main difficulty is that of purifying and handling a few micrograms of material without substantial losses, although these problems have largely been overcome by linking gas or liquid chromatography with Fourier transform spectrophotometry.

This section gives practical advice on the purification of microgram amounts of a sample. It is assumed that the starting material is a residue from the evaporation of a solvent extract of urine, blood, tissue, or other material. For the toxicologist, the most suitable method of purification is some form of chromatography.

Paper and Thin-layer Chromatography.

Suitable systems for thin-layer chromatography are described on pp. 167 to 177. Any of these systems is potentially useful where it is required to elute a spot, but reversed-phase systems should be avoided because it is difficult to remove the spot without the stationary phase, which would interfere with the infra-red spectrum. Furthermore, location reagents must be chosen with care, and a destructive reagent such as the Marquis reagent for alkaloids, should not be used. Non-destructive reagents such as iodoplatinate solution can be used because the colour complex is decomposable to yield the original compound. However, even this procedure may introduce extraneous peaks into the spectrum and, ideally, location reagents are best avoided. If the compound cannot be detected under ultraviolet light, it could be applied to the paper or thin-layer plate twice and only a portion of the chromatogram sprayed, thus allowing the unsprayed portion to be eluted.

Elution from cellulose thin-layer and paper chromatograms is generally more efficient than from silica gel thin-layer chromatograms; quantitative recoveries from silica gel are rarely attainable. However, thin-layer chromatographic systems produce results more quickly than paper chromatographic systems and will often give better resolution of spots. Thin-layer plates are available with fluorescent additives which facilitate location of spots without altering them chemically. Only experience can determine the best chromatographic system and eluting solvent for any particular compound.

The use of aqueous acid or alkali to elute the compound from the thin-layer plate or paper chromatogram, followed by solvent extraction of the aqueous solution, is more efficient than direct solvent extraction of the adsorbent.

In one method of direct extraction, the adsorbent is scraped from around the spot, the glass adjacent to the spot is carefully cleaned, and the adsorbent is eluted *in situ* directly on to a wall of potassium bromide built around the tip of the spot. The potassium bromide is then pressed into a disk. This technique is only suitable for well-resolved spots. Elution of the spot sideways will reduce contamination from compounds that are not as well resolved. The recovery of material from chromato-

grams varies from nil to over 70%. Compounds containing hydroxyl and carboxyl groups, which can readily form hydrogen bonds with the solid support, tend to be recovered in low yield. Considerable interference in the 1100 cm^{-1} region is found with some adsorbents and compounds.

In a variation of this method, the thin-layer adsorbent is placed in the bottom of a glass vessel together with a triangular 'wick' of compressed potassium bromide. Solvent is added and it rises up the wick and evaporates from the upper region. The compound is conveyed up the wick by the solvent and accumulates at the tip of the triangle which is then cut off, dried, and used to prepare a disk. About $10 \, \mu g$ of compound is required to produce a satisfactory spectrum. The advantage of this technique is that the lower part of the potassium bromide wick acts as a filter and removes finely divided adsorbent which can give rise to spurious peaks.

In a further method, the thin-layer adsorbent is scraped onto a small amount of potassium bromide powder in the hub of an 18-gauge metal hypodermic needle. A 1-ml glass syringe is filled with pure solvent and connected to the needle, and the compound is eluted dropwise onto a mound (10 mg) of dry potassium bromide powder. Each drop of solvent is allowed to evaporate completely before the elution of the next drop. The powder and solute are then mixed and pressed into a disk.

Eluted material almost always includes unwanted extraneous matter co-extracted from the paper or thin-layer chromatogram. Thus it is advisable to use the eluent from a 'blank' area as a reference solution. Contamination from plasticisers, solvents, and dirty glassware can also be a serious problem when a spectrum has to be obtained from a few micrograms of a compound. Even momentary contact of dry adsorbent with plastic tubing can remove appreciable quantities of plasticisers. Hence the following precautions should be taken: (a) use the minimum amount of the purest adsorbent available; (b) elute with less than 1 ml of a solvent containing less than 0.0001% (1 ppm) of non-volatile residue; (c) keep sample handling to a minimum; (d) clean all glassware with an efficient detergent in an ultrasonic bath; (e) avoid contact of materials and samples with plastics.

Gas Chromatography

Gas chromatography can provide a very convenient method of obtaining pure samples for infra-red spectrophotometry. However, the sample can still be contaminated with impurities eluted from the stationary phase. The effluent from the chromatograph is a hot vapour and the problem is to obtain small quantities in a form suitable for presentation to the spectrophotometer. The spectrum of the vapour can be recorded directly or the compound can be trapped and then its spectrum recorded. Unfortunately, there is no entirely satisfactory method for the direct coupling of a gas chromatograph to a standard dispersive infra-red spectrophotometer. The outlet of the gas chromatograph can be split and one part connected to a heated cell (or light pipe) placed in the beam of an infra-red spectrophotometer. The gas flow is then stopped, trapping the sample in the cell, and the spectrum is recorded in the vapour phase. This technique can provide acceptable spectra of volatile compounds such as butyl acetate, which has a strong carbonyl band, but spectra of less volatile compounds such as caffeine and phenylbutazone are more difficult to obtain. The temperatures of the connecting pipe and cell are clearly of great importance to keep the compounds as vapours. The coupling of a gas chromatograph to a Fourier transform instrument is much more satisfactory because the speed of scanning is sufficiently rapid to enable the spectrum of a compound to be recorded as it is eluted. Nevertheless, the temperatures of the cell and pipework are still of critical importance.

The method used for trapping a compound will depend on whether it is a solid or a liquid and, if the latter, on its volatility. Ways in which small samples can be obtained from a gas chromatograph in a form suitable for presentation to the spectrophotometer are given below.

Cooled Tubes
Most techniques of collecting the effluent employ cooled tubes of glass or metal, but it is difficult to obtain good recoveries of a few micrograms of compounds of differing volatilities by any one technique. Drugs such as barbiturates and phenothiazines can be recovered in 50 to 70% yields in glass or metal capillary tubes held at room temperature, whereas more volatile drugs such as amphetamines require cooling in liquid nitrogen or solid carbon dioxide (A. S. Curry *et al.*, *J. Chromat.*, 1968, *38*, 200–208; A. De Leenheer, *J. Chromat.*, 1972, *74*, 35–41).

Silver Chloride Microcells
Microcells extruded from silver chloride and known as 'Extrocells' can be fitted with a silicon rubber serum cap and connected to the outlet of the gas chromatograph by means of a hypodermic needle. The sample collects in the neck of the cell which is then centrifuged in order to force the sample into the main body of the cell. Solvents can be added if solution spectra are required and are, of course, necessary if the compound is a solid. The cells can be used at room temperature or they can be cooled in freezing mixtures or in liquid nitrogen; they can be used many times provided that they are stored in the dark. The cells are available with pathlengths from 0.1 to 0.01 mm and volumes of 2 to 0.2 µl. The main disadvantage is that they have to be centrifuged for cleaning as well as for filling and emptying.

Membrane Filters
Membrane filters composed of cellulose esters can be used to collect samples. The filters, about 25 µm thick, are supplied in matched pairs to compensate for their absorption in a double-beam instrument. The filter is placed in a specially designed metal and PTFE holder. The PTFE inlet section reduces condensation of the effluent before it reaches the filter and the metal outlet section allows the filter to be cooled. The filter holder is connected to the outlet of the chromatograph by a Luer fitting just before the sample emerges. When the sample has been collected, the filter is removed and placed in the spectrophotometer. The method is simple and easy to use and is capable of giving extremely good results.

Alkali Halide Tubes
A straight tube containing a plug of powdered alkali halide is connected to the outlet of the chromatograph. The effluent condenses on the halide which can then be pressed into a disk. This technique is most useful for compounds which are solid at room temperature.

The main difficulty, common to all these methods of collecting fractions, is to determine the optimum temperature of the outlet tube from the chromatograph and the temperature of the collecting device. This problem can only be solved by trial and error.

High Pressure Liquid Chromatography

High pressure liquid chromatography provides a very convenient method of purification, particularly where gas chromatography is either inapplicable or where derivatisation of the compound is necessary. Unlike gas chromatographs, liquid chromatographs are usually operated at or slightly above ambient temperature, and most types of detector are non-destructive. Thus, the appropriate fraction of eluate can be collected by holding a test-tube under the exit port.

The method used to retrieve the sample from the eluate for presentation to the spectrophotometer will depend upon whether the compound is a solid or a liquid and, if the latter, on its volatility as well as the quantity present. All the common solvents absorb in the infra-red region. However, with the data processing facilities of modern infra-red spectrophotometers, this is not a great disadvantage. The spectrum of the solvent can be recorded and then subtracted from the combined spectra of the compound and solvent to give a difference spectrum. If the concentration of the sample is low, the difference spectrum can be enhanced either by repetitive scanning and signal averaging or by expansion of the ordinate scale (see Figs 6 and 7). In many cases, however, the amount of material will be too small to enable the compound to be collected and transferred to standard cells. The use of microcells such as 'Extrocells' may be advantageous.

Alternatively, the compound can be recovered by evaporation of the solvent. However, evaporation will also concentrate any non-volatile impurities in the solvent and the use of pure solvents is essential. Another possible source of contamination is the packing material used in liquid chromatography columns. Many of these materials are based on silica gel and appreciable amounts of silica may be dissolved by certain solvents.

Microsublimation

This simple technique can be highly effective in purifying certain compounds (Fig. 8). Drugs may be sublimed from an evaporated solvent extract in the tube on to the cold finger of the apparatus, and the sublimate transferred by grinding the potassium bromide powder gently with the cold finger.

SAMPLE PREPARATION

Infra-red spectra can be determined in the vapour, liquid, and solid phases, but most compounds of interest to the toxicologist are solid at room temperature and the determination of spectra in this phase has been used most widely. However, it is all too easy to rush for the potassium bromide and prepare a disk, and to forget some of the problems that may arise with this technique. The advantages of determining the spectrum of a solid as a solution in a suitable solvent should not be overlooked.

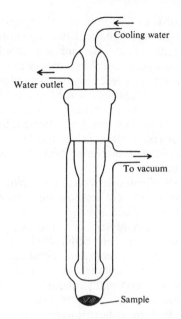

Fig. 8. Apparatus for microsublimation.

The physical state of a drug may have a marked effect on its infra-red spectrum and a suggested hierarchy of sample preparation procedures for liquids is: (1) solution; (2) if insoluble, undiluted in a thin cell; (3) liquid film between salt plates. For solids: (1) solution; (2) mineral-oil mull; (3) potassium bromide disk; (4) pyrolysate.

An infra-red spectrum can be obtained from as little as 1 µg or less of a compound, but greater sensitivity is obtained by placing the maximum number of molecules of the sample in the infra-red beam. Thus, where the amount of sample is limited, the area of the infra-red beam must be reduced by using a beam condenser and expanding the transmittance scale.

Gases

Infra-red spectra in the vapour phase are rarely determined with dispersive spectrophotometers unless the substance is a gas at room temperature. Special long-path, airtight gas cells are required. The technique has become more widely used with the advent of Fourier transform infra-red spectrophotometers coupled directly to gas chromatographs.

Liquids and Solutions

A wide range of types of cell is available for determining the spectra in the liquid phase. These cells usually consist of two parallel transparent windows (0.1 to 0.01 mm apart) separated by a spacing gasket and fitted with inlet and outlet ports. Variable path-length cells are also available, in which one window on a piston moves in relation to the other window. These cells are particularly useful for concentrated solutions since the solvent can be placed in the reference beam of the spectrophotometer and the solvent peaks neutralised. Spectra of viscous non-volatile liquids can also be determined by sandwiching a thin film between two alkali halide plates.

The number of suitable solvents is limited and the most widely used are carbon tetrachloride and carbon disulphide because they have relatively few absorption bands in the infra-red region. Other solvents which may be used include chloroform, ethylene dichloride, methylene chloride, benzene, cyclohexane, and heptane. The concentration of the compound is usually about 5 to 10%, but concentrations up to 20% w/v can be employed. With these high concentrations, hydroxyl and amino compounds often exhibit bands due to intermolecular hydrogen bonding.

A disadvantage of this method is that interactions between the compound and the solvent can occur. This may result in quite considerable changes in the frequency of certain bands in different solvents. Also, the heat of infra-red radiation can cause evaporation of volatile solvents to give changes in concentrations.

Solids

Solids are generally examined either as thin films or as dispersions in either liquids or solids, since finely packed solids scatter infra-red radiation.

MULLS

Solid compounds are dispersed in a liquid, e.g. liquid paraffin (Nujol). The finely powdered compound (about 0.2 mg) is mixed with one drop of the liquid and ground in an agate mortar. Sufficient liquid is then added so that the final mull is the consistency of a thin cream. The mull is spread on an alkali halide plate, usually sodium chloride or potassium bromide, and another plate placed on top, taking care to exclude air bubbles. A disadvantage of this method is that the spectrum of the liquid will be superimposed upon that of the sample. Consequently, liquid paraffin cannot be used if the carbon-hydrogen stretching frequencies are to be examined and a halogenated liquid such as 'Fluorolube' (a fluorinated hydrocarbon) or hexachlorobutadiene must be employed. Changes in

polymorphic forms and consequent changes in spectra may occur with this method.

ALKALI HALIDE DISKS

The technique of dispersing the compound in an alkali halide has been used widely in the identification of drugs. Originally, potassium bromide was used and the technique is still often referred to as the 'KBr technique'. However, potassium chloride is superior to potassium bromide because it is less hygroscopic. The finely powdered dry compound (about 1 mg) is mixed with the alkali halide (about 250 mg), ground either mechanically in an agate ball mill or by hand in an agate mortar, and pressed into a thin disk. If the sample is insufficiently ground, asymmetrical bands may be formed which vary in position and intensity from the accepted values (the Christiansen effect) and may give the impression of impurities in the sample. If only small quantities of the compound are available (about 200 µg), a thin cardboard mask with a slot in the centre can be used. The mask is placed in the die and the slot filled with the mixture before pressing. A mask is often employed routinely because it provides a support for the alkali halide and so enables the disk to be handled more easily.

Microdisks of diameter down to 0.5 mm can be prepared by using metal (lead or stainless steel) disks of 13 mm diameter with the appropriate size hole in the centre. The hole is filled with potassium bromide (about 1 mg) containing from 0.05 to 0.2% of the sample, which is then pressed in the usual way. The metal disks should be washed before use in both polar and non-polar solvents and finally in good quality acetone to remove traces of oil and grease, which may produce artefacts in the C—H region of the spectrum. The method may fail if excessive pressure is used, causing deformation of the lead disk.

Another useful technique consists of dissolving the compound in a small volume of chloroform and drawing it into a Hamilton-type syringe held in a repeater holder. A small cluster of fine potassium bromide particles is picked up on the end of the needle by a trace of chloroform expressed from the needle. The solvent is evaporated under a table lamp and the rest of the solution is fed into the potassium bromide from the syringe as it evaporates. A disk is then made from the powder. It is important that the end of the needle is cut at right angles to the shaft and ground flat; those supplied for use with liquid chromatographs are suitable. For bases one must decide whether to evaporate solvents without the addition of hydrochloric acid, and accept the consequent loss of certain amines by volatilisation, or to add hydrochloric acid and accept the reduced solubility of the amine hydrochlorides in chloroform. Considerable losses of the sample by evaporation may occur for other types of compound (e.g. phenols), particularly when dilute solutions are used. It is essential to use dry hydrophobic solvents, since water can cause artefacts in the spectra, particularly when scale expansion is used.

Because potassium bromide is hygroscopic and it is sometimes difficult to remove the last trace of water, silver chloride may be used instead. An indentation about 0.8 mm deep and slightly wider is made in the centre of a small piece of silver chloride sheet, and a solution (about 0.1 μl) containing as little as 500 ng of substance is placed in the indentation and gently warmed to evaporate the solvent. The sheet is then placed in a die which produces a cone of silver chloride with the sample embedded in it. A similar cone of plain silver chloride is mounted in the reference beam. Excellent spectra can be obtained with this technique.

The alkali halide disks can be stored in cellophane envelopes and give good spectra several years after preparation. A well-prepared disk should have over 80% transmittance in regions where the sample does not absorb, although it will not necessarily be visually clear. It is not always easy to obtain a good disk when a very small amount of a recovered drug is available. In these circumstances, attenuation of the reference beam can 'sharpen' the spectrum. Another technique is to heat the alkali halide disk to about 80° for 30 to 60 minutes with an infra-red lamp to evaporate any absorbed water. However, the high temperature accentuates the disadvantages of the alkali halide disk technique. In addition, the following artefacts have been observed: (i) formation of anhydrides from carboxylic acids, (ii) ketals and cyanohydrins reverting to the parent ketone, and (iii) loss of water from secondary alcohols.

There are several disadvantages inherent in the alkali halide disk technique. The alkali halides which are generally used are hygroscopic and it is very difficult to exclude all traces of water. This often results in a hydroxyl band in the spectrum. A number of compounds containing hydroxyl groups either form hydrogen bonds with the alkali halide or are adsorbed on its surface, so the method is unsuitable if the hydroxyl band is to be examined. In such cases, polytetrafluoroethylene (PTFE) powder can sometimes be used in place of the alkali halide. Polymorphism occurs in many compounds and the grinding and pressing can alter the crystal form and consequently the spectrum. Splitting of bands also frequently occurs. Another disadvantage is the possibility of chemical changes occurring during the preparation of the disk. For example, double decomposition can occur:

$$\text{Base HCl} + \text{KBr} \rightarrow \text{Base HBr} + \text{KCl}$$

Hence, hydrochlorides should preferably be examined in potassium chloride. Bromide may be oxidised to bromine by some compounds, particularly strong oxidising agents, and this may lead to a disk becoming either discoloured or having yellow-brown spots.

If the sample is a potential oxidising agent, other techniques of sample preparation should also be used in order to check the reliability of the spectra obtained from the alkali disk.

Organic compounds that contain nitrogen in a functional group should not be used with plates which are made of thallium bromide and thallium iodide (KRS-5 plates) as they appear to react with the plates.

Despite these disadvantages, the technique is still a most useful one for solid drugs. The advantages are that, besides being easy to use, the absorption of the alkali halide is very low and the quantity of compound required is small. The disks can easily be stored for reference purposes or the compound can be recovered if required.

Thin Films

This method is of use where it is necessary to obtain spectra free from dispersing media. The film can be prepared either by melting the solid and pouring it on to a suitable surface or by evaporation of a solution. This method is not widely used.

Attenuated Total Reflectance

This method can be used to identify solid drugs but is only of use where relatively large amounts of compounds are available. The finely-ground sample is spread as a thin layer onto the sticky side of a piece of self-adhesive tape, and the tape is placed against the reflecting surface of the instrument with the sample side in contact. Sufficient sample is required to cover the surface of the tape completely, otherwise the spectrum of the tape will be recorded in addition to that of the sample. The technique is of use when the acid and salt forms need to be differentiated.

IDENTIFICATION OF SPECTRA

In recent years, much work has been devoted to the identification and interpretation of infra-red spectra by computer. Collections of spectra on paper can be converted into a numerical form (digitised) and recorded on a disk or tape, and many modern infra-red spectrophotometers record the spectra directly in digital form. The use of a data station coupled to an infra-red spectrophotometer enables the spectrum to be matched automatically against those in the library collection, and the names of compounds giving the closest fit displayed. An indication of the closeness of fit may also be given. It is important that the identification is checked by a careful comparison of the spectrum with a printed copy of that of the compound(s) indicated.

With some data systems the spectrum retrieved from the library can be displayed at the same time as that of the sample and the two spectra may even be superimposed, so allowing easy comparison and the identification of any differences.

The method employed to identify the spectrum will depend very largely on how much other information about the compound is already available, e.g. Rf values and colour reactions. If the identity of the compound is suspected, the spectrum should be compared with that obtained from an authentic sample of the substance.

If this procedure fails and in cases where the type of compound is unknown or can only be allocated to a certain class, e.g. a phenothiazine or a barbiturate, then reference may be made to the

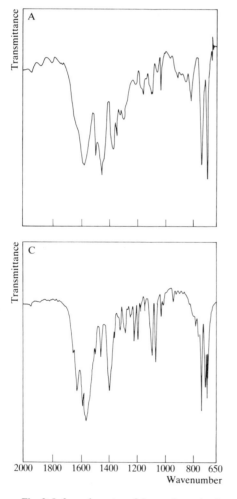
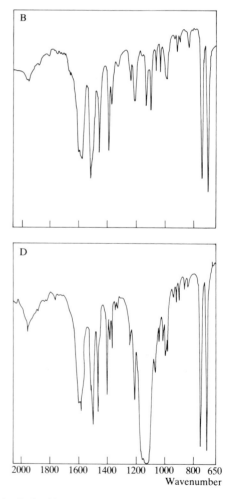

Fig. 9. Infra-red spectra of A, amphetamine base; B, amphetamine hydrochloride; C, amphetamine mandelate; D, amphetamine sulphate.

index of Infra-red Peaks in Part 3 and to the information in the individual monographs. Comparison of the spectrum of the unknown with that of the suspected compound should either confirm or disprove the tentative identification. If the two spectra have been recorded under similar conditions on the same type of instrument then they should be very similar in appearance. If the spectra have been recorded on different instruments then they may, superficially at least, appear very different. In this case a more detailed study of band frequencies and relative intensities must be undertaken.

It must also be remembered that different forms of the same compound will give different infra-red spectra. For example, the spectra for amphetamine base and the hydrochloride have many similarities, but the hydrochloride spectrum shows much finer detail (Figs 9A and 9B). Also the spectra for the hydrochloride and mandelate salts show differences (Figs 9B and 9C) due to the absorption of the mandelic acid. However, the spectra of the hydrochloride and sulphate (Figs. 9B and 9D) are very similar since they are both inorganic salts, the only major difference being the absorption band due to the sulphate at $1110 \, cm^{-1}$.

If the spectrum does not agree with any of the available spectra and the type of compound is known, then the appropriate collections of spectra can be consulted.

Spurious bands can occur readily in infra-red spectra, particularly when a biological sample has undergone several purification procedures. Traces of plasticisers, surfactants, and oils left on glassware can all give rise to artefacts; some spurious infra-red bands are given below (after H. A. Szymanski, *A Systematic Approach to the Interpretation of Infra-red Spectra*, Buffalo, New York, Hertillon Press, 1971).

Wavenumber cm^{-1}	Assignment	Comments
3800–2500	H_2O	Bound or unbound water in a molecule can give rise to sharp or broad bands. In alkali halide disks a water band at $3350 \, cm^{-1}$ may appear
3300–3000	NH_3^+	Lens tissues
1810–1600	$C=O$	Impurities containing the carbonyl group, e.g. phosgene in chloroform, plasticisers
1750–1500	H_2O	Bound or unbound water can give rise to sharp or broad bands
1610–1515	COO^-	Alkali salts (which also have a weaker band at $1425 \, cm^{-1}$) can be produced from alkali halides
1400	NH_3^+	Lens tissues

Wavenumber	Assignment	Comments
1265	$Si-CH_3$	Stopcock grease or silicone oil
1110–1050	$Si-O-Si$	Glass or hydrolysed Si compounds
730 & 720	Polyethylene	Polyethylene laboratory ware
700	Polystyrene	Polystyrene laboratory ware

The final stage in the process of identification is, ideally, the comparison of the spectrum of the unknown with that of the pure drug obtained under as near identical conditions as possible and on the same instrument. This is particularly important where the identity of the spectrum has been determined automatically. The data station can only select spectra that are in its library and if the spectrum of the compound under investigation is absent, then it will select those giving the next best fit.

INTERPRETATION OF SPECTRA

When a suitable fit for an identity cannot be obtained for a spectrum, it must be interpreted from first principles.

Most types of functional group exhibit absorption bands in particular regions of the spectrum. For example, the hydroxyl groups of alcohols, phenols, and acids exhibit an O—H stretching band in the region from 3700 to $2500 \, cm^{-1}$. The carbonyl groups of ketones, aldehydes, acids, and esters exhibit a C=O stretching band in the region from 1870 to $1535 \, cm^{-1}$. The precise location of the band will often give an indication of the structural environment of the group. The correlation of frequency with functional groups is discussed in detail by L. J. Bellamy (1975).

The approach to the interpretation of the infra-red spectrum of an unknown drug is illustrated by reference to the barbiturates. These are derivatives of malonylurea (barbituric acid) and all of them have two substituents at position 5. In addition, some of them are also substituted at position 1 and in others the oxygen atom attached to position 2 is replaced by sulphur to form thiobarbiturates.

The barbiturates can be classified chemically into three classes: 5,5-disubstituted barbituric acids, 1,5,5-trisubstituted barbituric acids, and 5,5-disubstituted thiobarbituric acids.

These classes can be further divided depending on whether the substituents in position 5 are alkyl, alkenyl, aryl, or cycloalkenyl. In most common barbiturates, one of the 5-substituents is either ethyl or allyl and the other is either a straight- or branched-chain alkyl or alkenyl group with five or fewer carbon atoms. Some barbiturates are marketed as sodium salts. The infra-red spectrum of a barbiturate will therefore depend on the class of compound, the nature of the substituents, and whether it is the free acid or the sodium salt.

The various polymorphs of a compound often exhibit different infra-red spectra. Among drugs, the barbiturates are most notable for the extent to which they exhibit polymorphism, including many metastable forms found only in mixtures. Spectral differences between polymorphs are associated with different types of hydrogen bonding, and there is a correlation between hydrogen bond strength and duration of action of the barbiturates on the central nervous system. The crystalline structure of barbiturates can be affected by grinding with an alkali halide or in preparing a mull, but if precautions are taken to ensure reproducibility, the spectra of the barbiturates are sufficiently different to be used for identification purposes.

With the exception of phenobarbitone and barbituric acid, the free barbiturates do not absorb appreciably above 3300 cm^{-1} (e.g. barbitone, Fig. 10A), a feature which distinguishes them from the ureides; a weak band of unknown origin occurs sometimes between 3500 and 3400 cm^{-1}. All the barbiturates have two bands which occur near 3200 and 3100 cm^{-1} and are due to N—H stretching vibrations. In the 5,5-disubstituted compounds, the relative intensity of the two bands is similar although that at 3100 cm^{-1} is usually slightly less intense. In compounds substituted on the nitrogen atom at position 1, the intensity of the band at 3100 cm^{-1} may be greatly reduced and is often present only as a shoulder on the band at 3200 cm^{-1}, e.g. metharbitone. Methylphenobarbitone appears to be an exception in that the band at 3100 cm^{-1} is the most intense one in the region. A similar phenomenon occurs with the sodium salts since here again one of the hydrogen atoms in either position 1 or 3 has been replaced.

A series of up to four medium to intense bands occurs in the region 3000 to 2800 cm^{-1}, and is due to alkyl C—H stretching vibrations of the substituents in positions 1 and 5. The intensity of the bands gives a very approximate indication of the number of C—H bonds and hence the number of

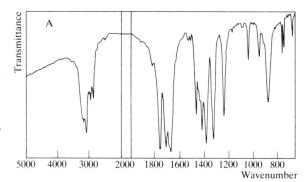

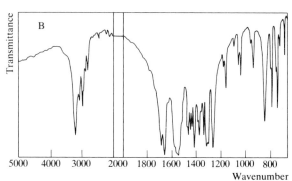

Fig. 10. Infra-red spectra of A, barbitone and B, barbitone sodium.

carbon atoms in the chain. This does not appear to apply to the sodium salts, in which the band occurring at 3000 to 2950 cm^{-1} is usually increased in intensity, compared to that of the free acid, and becomes the strongest band. Compare, for example, the spectra of barbitone (Fig. 10A) and barbitone sodium (Fig. 10B).

The barbiturates have up to three strongly absorbing bands in the region 1765 to 1670 cm^{-1} which are due to C=O stretching vibrations. A knowledge of the origin of these bands is useful in helping to understand the differences in the spectra of the various types of barbiturate.

In symmetrical molecules, the three bands are all of similar intensity. In asymmetrical molecules, the band at the highest frequency is often less intense than the other two, and this is particularly so when the molecule is substituted in position 1. The sodium salts of the barbiturates have only two bands in this region, since the molecule is no longer symmetrical, and these occur at a lower frequency, between 1700 and 1650 cm^{-1}. In addition, a broad strongly absorbing band occurs between 1600 and 1550 cm^{-1}; the free barbiturates show practically no absorption in this region. The sodium salts of the thiobarbiturates exhibit only the lowest of the three C=O vibrations in the region 1700 to 1680 cm^{-1}. They do, however, exhibit the broad, strongly absorbing band which occurs between 1650 and 1600 cm^{-1}. Therefore, the number, position and intensity of the bands between 1800 and 1500 cm^{-1} give a very good indication of whether the barbiturate is the free acid, the salt, or a thiobarbiturate.

Most barbiturates have a number of strongly absorbing bands between 1460 and 1250 cm^{-1}, and some of these are due to C—H deformation and C—N stretching vibrations. The sodium salts of the thiobarbiturates have a broad strongly absorbing band between 1500 and 1480 cm^{-1} which is believed to be due to C—N stretching vibrations of the carbon atom attached to sulphur. This band is not present in the ordinary barbiturates and therefore provides another means of distinguishing those containing sulphur. Many barbiturates exhibit a few weak to medium intensity absorption bands in the region 1150 to 900 cm^{-1}. The 1-substituted barbiturates exhibit a greater number of sharp bands of medium intensity. Those compounds which contain an allyl group exhibit bands at about 1000 to 960 cm^{-1} which are due probably to C—H deformation vibrations. The sodium salts of the thiobarbiturates show a band of medium intensity between 1020 and 1000 cm^{-1}. Finally, many barbiturates, but not the thiobarbiturates, exhibit a broad band of medium to strong intensity between 900 and 800 cm^{-1}.

Infra-red Data in Monographs

It has been shown (A. S. Curry et al., J. Pharm. Pharmac., 1969, 21, 224–231; P. H. B. Ingle and D. W. Mathieson, Pharm. J., 1976, 216, 73) that an infra-red spectrum of a particular substance can be retrieved from a collection, with some degree of confidence, by reference to its six major absorption bands. This forms the basis for a system of identification.

Data consisting of six major absorption bands which have been selected from the recorded spectrum over the range 2000 to 650 cm^{-1} (5 to 15 µm) are included in the monographs in Part 2. In many cases, the spectrum is also reproduced in a reduced size. The selected peaks are the six most intense peaks, except that peaks in the region where Nujol absorbs (1490 to 1320 cm^{-1}, 6.7 to 7.6 µm) have been omitted. The peaks are arranged in descending order of amplitude. It should be noted that, because of variations in instruments and conditions, other determinations of the spectrum may not give peaks with the same relative intensities.

All the spectra are included in the index of Infra-red Peaks in Part 3. Details of how to use the infra-red data are given in the index.

Published Spectra

GENERAL COLLECTIONS

Sadtler Collection. The most comprehensive collection of published spectra is that of the Sadtler Research Laboratories. In the solid and liquid phases, over 63 000 spectra of pure compounds including 600 spectra of commonly abused drugs, 600 spectra of prepared drugs, 1200 spectra of pharmaceuticals, 750 spectra of steroids, and 700 spectra of toxic chemicals have been published, in addition to 36 000 spectra of commercial products. There are also 7400 spectra in the vapour phase. Many are, or will be, available in numerical form so that they can be searched automatically by an appropriate Fourier transform spectrophotometer.

Chemical Rubber Company Collection. An atlas of 12 000 spectra: J. G. Grasselli and W. M. Ritchey, CRC Atlas of Spectral Data and Physical Constants for Organic Compounds, 2nd Edn, Cleveland, USA, CRC Press Inc, 1975.

Aldrich Collection. A library of over 12 000 spectra: C. J. Pouchert, The Aldrich Library of Infra-red Spectra, 3rd Edn, Milwaukee, USA, Aldrich Chemical Co. Inc., 1981.

Coblentz Society Collection. A library of over 800 spectra: The Coblentz Society Desk Book of Infra-red Spectra, C. D. Craver (Ed.), Kirkwood, Mo., USA, The Coblentz Society.

British Pharmacopoeia Collection. A collection of 394 spectra together with detailed methods of sample preparation: Infra-red Reference Spectra, British Pharmacopoeia Commission, London, HMSO, 1980; First Supplement 1981; Second Supplement 1982; Third Supplement 1984.

SPECIALISED COLLECTIONS

Alkaloids. 1000 spectra with other physical data: J. Holubek and O. Strouf, Spectral Data and Physical Constants of Alkaloids, London, Heyden and Sons Ltd, 1965–1973.

Antibiotics. A comprehensive collection published by the International Centre of Information on

Antibiotics: C. Lenzen and L. Delcambe, *ICIA Inf. Bull.*, 1972, *10*, 78–160; 1973, *11*, 1–157; 1975, *12*, 1–178; 1976, *13*, 1–178; 1977, *15*, 1–208; 1977, *16*, 1–212; 1978, *17*, 1–248; 1979, *18*, 1–268.

Barbiturates. Solution spectra of 41 barbiturates: A. Sucharda-Sobczyk, *Roczn. Chem.*, 1970, *44*, 1435–1445; also R. J. Mesley, *Spectrochim. Acta*, 1970, *26A*, 1427–1448.

Carbohydrates. Spectra of 79 carbohydrates: L. P. Kuhn, *Analyt. Chem.*, 1950, *22*, 276–283.

Narcotics and related bases. L. Levi *et al.*, *Bull. Narcot.*, 1955, *7*, 42–84; C. G. Farmilo and K. Genest, Narcotics and Related Bases, in *Progress in Chemical Toxicology*, Vol. 1, A. Stolman (Ed.), London, Academic Press Inc., 1963, pp. 199–295.

Natural products. Spectra of alkaloids, amino acids, carbohydrates, carotenoids, steroids, and terpenes: K. Yamaguchi, *Spectral Data of Natural Products*, Vol. 1, Amsterdam, Elsevier, 1970.

Organophosphorus compounds. R. R. Shagidullin *et al.*, *Atlas of IR Spectra of Organophosphorus Compounds*, Moscow, Nauka, 1977.

Pesticides and related compounds. Spectra of 76 pesticides: R. C. Gore *et al.*, *J. Ass. off. analyt. Chem.*, 1971, *54*, 1040–1082. Spectra of 478 pesticides, disinfectants, fumigants, fungicides, etc.: P. Giang, Spectroscopic Methods of Analysis, in *Analytical Methods for Pesticides and Plant Growth Regulators*, Vol. 9, G. Zweig (Ed.), London, Academic Press Inc., 1977, pp. 153–290. Spectra for 68 substances which may occur as impurities, residues, or adjuvants in commercial pesticides: R. R. Collerson *et al.*, *NPL Report Chem. 48*, National Physical Laboratory, Division of Chemical Standards, 1976.

Pharmaceutical spectra of 335 substances: O. R. Sammul *et al.*, *J. Ass. off. agric. Chem.*, 1964, *47*, 918–991.

Phenothiazines. Spectra of 19 phenothiazines: G. Scapini and G. P. Gardini, *Ateneo parmense*, 1964, *35*, 328–334. Phenothiazines and their sulph-oxides: B. Kreyenbuhl *et al.*, *Pharm. Acta Helv.*, 1979, *54*, 197–205; L. K. Turner, *J. forens. Sci. Soc.*, 1963, *4*, 39–49.

Plasticisers. Spectra of 284 plasticisers and additives: *Plasticisers and Other Additives*, C. D. Craver (Ed.), Kirkwood, Mo., USA, The Coblentz Society, 1977.

Steroids. Spectra of 900 steroids: W. Neudert and H. Roepke, *Atlas of Steroid Spectra*, Berlin, Springer-Verlag, 1965. Also A. P. Arzamastsev and D. S. Yashkina, *Ultraviolet and Infra-red Spectra of Drugs, No. 1, Steroids*, Moscow, Meditsina, 1975. Ketosteroids: F. Hodosan *et al.*, *Studii Cerc. Chim.*, 1971, *19*, 191–210; Yu. N. Levchuck *et al.*, *Zh. prikl. spektrosk.*, 1971, *14*, 735–738. Corticosteroids and contraceptive steroids: R. J. Mesley, *Spectrochim. Acta*, 1966, *22*, 889–917. Fluorinated corticosteroids: G. Bellomonte, *Ann. Ist. Super Sanita*, 1973, *9*, 121–128.

Surfactants. Spectra of 466 surfactants: D. Hummel, *Identification and Analysis for Surface-Active Agents by Infra-red and Chemical Methods*, Vols 1 & 2, trans. E. A. Wilkow, London, Interscience Publishers, 1962.

Sulphonamides. Spectra of 10 sulphonamides: D. Edwards, *J. Pharm. Pharmac.*, 1971, *23*, 956–962.

Bibliography

L. J. Bellamy, *Infra-red Spectra of Complex Molecules*, London, Chapman and Hall, Vol. I, 3rd Edn, 1975; Vol. II, 2nd Edn, 1980.
M. J. de Faubert Maunder, *Practical Hints on Infra-red Spectrometry with Particular Reference to Forensic Analysis*, London, Adam Hilger, 1971.
R. G. J. Miller and B. C. Stace, *Laboratory Methods in Infra-red Spectroscopy*, Chichester, Heyden, 1972.
R. A. Nyquist and R. O. Kagel, *Infra-red Spectra of Inorganic Compounds*, New York, Academic Press, 1972.
A. L. Smith, *Applied Infra-red Spectroscopy: Fundamentals, Techniques and Analytical Problem-solving*, New York, Wiley, 1979.
H. A. Szymanski, *A Systematic Approach to the Interpretation of Infra-red Spectra*, New York, Hertillon Press, 1971.
D. Welti, *Infra-red Vapour Spectra*, London, Heyden, 1970.

Mass Spectrometry

R. E. Ardrey

Mass spectrometry is concerned with the electron ionisation and subsequent fragmentation of molecules, and with the determination of the mass to charge ratios (m/z) and the relative abundances of the ions which are produced. Functional groups in the molecule direct the fragmentation in such a way that, knowing the structure of the molecule, it is possible to predict the fragmentation pattern. Conversely, knowing the fragmentation pattern, a plausible structure of the original molecule can often be suggested. In addition, the technique allows the molecular weight to be determined and this is probably the most important piece of information available from a mass spectrum. If the appropriate spectrometer is available a unique formula may be obtained.

The advantage of mass spectrometry over other commonly used analytical techniques lies in the wide range of samples that may be examined and the amount of information that may be obtained. In many cases a single mass spectrum allows an unambiguous identification to be made. The sensitivity and specificity of the technique allow minor components of mixtures to be quantified down to the picogram level. The main disadvantages lie in its complexity and cost. The interrelationship of the component electronic modules makes fault-finding an expert task and the best results are usually obtained by having an operator dedicated to the operation and maintenance of the instrument. This is not quite so important in the case of bench-top machines which are designed for multi-operator use and are more easily maintained.

A mass spectrometer may be very costly depending on the facilities available and the data handling which is provided. Taking into account depreciation, maintenance, spares, etc., the minimum operating cost (1985) is around £25 per hour. As it is possible to analyse only about 6 solid samples (or 2 or 3 samples from a gas chromatographic column) per hour, the technique is fairly expensive. This must be equated with the results that may be obtained and therefore mass spectrometry should not be used for routine analyses that can be carried out using less costly techniques.

Mass spectrometry, either alone or in combination with a chromatographic separation, is probably the most effective method for the identification of drugs and their metabolites. The specificity and sensitivity of the technique allow a full mass spectrum, and, in many cases, an unambiguous identification to be obtained from less than 50 ng of material. Quantitative measurements can be carried out at the picogram or even femtogram levels. The limit of detection is governed by the level of the background spectrum obtained rather than by the inherent sensitivity of the technique. Theoretical calculations show that 20 pg of material entering the ion source of a mass spectrometer is sufficient to enable a full spectrum to be obtained and this has been demonstrated. Similar calculations show that quantification should be possible down to the 1 fg level.

INSTRUMENTATION

A mass spectrometer may be conveniently divided into five basic components: sample inlet system, ionisation, ion separation, ion detection and amplification, and presentation of results (Fig. 1).

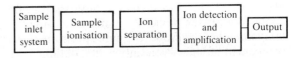

Fig. 1. Schematic diagram of a mass spectrometer.

Sample Inlet System

The interior of a mass spectrometer is under high vacuum (10^{-6} torr) in order to minimise the number of collisions undergone by ions and thereby maximise the number of ions reaching the detector. Sample inlet systems must enable the sample to be introduced without loss of the vacuum and must be capable of handling samples as gases, liquids, or solids, either as single components or as multi-component mixtures.

For solids, a direct insertion probe is used. The sample, either as a solid or as a solution in a volatile

UNIVERSITY OF GREENWICH LIBRARY

solvent, is placed in a small glass crucible at the end of the probe. The whole probe assembly is then inserted through a vacuum lock and positioned close to the ion source. The sample is vaporised directly into the ion beam, either by the heat associated with the source or by external heating. Thermal decomposition may take place; for example, methyprylone (molecular weight 183) decomposes in the ion source of the mass spectrometer at 200°, producing the spectrum shown in Fig. 2A. If the source temperature is approximately 150° the true spectrum is obtained (Fig. 2B). In some cases the sample vapour pressure cannot reach 10^{-6} torr and conversion to a more volatile chemical derivative is necessary.

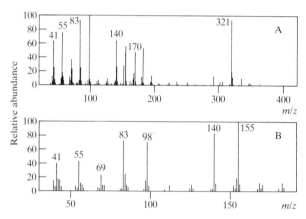

Fig. 2. Mass spectrum obtained by probe analysis of methyprylone, molecular weight 183, with mass spectrometer source at A, 200° and B, 150°.

Mixtures of solids of different volatilities may be analysed using the probe. By gently increasing the temperature of the probe, the pure spectrum of the component of higher volatility is first obtained; as the temperature is slowly increased, the more volatile component distils off and the spectrum of the less volatile component appears. This technique can sometimes be utilised in the analysis of materials eluted in thin-layer or paper chromatography to reduce the effect of the background spectrum. The probe allows rapid analysis but this must be balanced against the possibility of interference from the background spectrum and/or thermal decomposition making the spectrum difficult to interpret.

Gases and volatile liquids may be studied by using a heated evacuated vessel. This is linked to the ion source usually by a glass capillary which allows the sample to enter the source at a constant rate.

Mixtures are best studied by the combination of mass spectrometry with a chromatographic separation. This may be by paper or thin-layer chromatography, but more importantly, by the direct linking of gas chromatography or high pressure liquid chromatography with the mass spectrometer (GC–MS and HPLC–MS).

INTERFACES FOR GAS CHROMATOGRAPHY

Two types of gas chromatographic column, capillary and packed, are in routine use (see page 178). However, the width of the chromatographic peak places limitations on the performance of the mass spectrometer, and the difference in flow rates affects the way in which each type of column must be interfaced to the mass spectrometer.

Capillary columns operate at carrier gas flow rates of about 1 to 2 ml/min and the mass spectrometer can accept all the effluent from the column without loss of performance. Packed columns operate at much greater flow rates (around 30 ml/min) and in order to maintain the vacuum an enriching device, or separator, must be used to prevent all of the effluent entering the ion source. Three types of separator are in common use and each relies on the difference in physical properties of the carrier gas and the sample.

Jet Separator

This is available in two forms, the single-stage or the two-stage jet. The single-stage jet separator consists of a series of aligned orifices, the gap between the orifices being evacuated by a rotary pump (10^{-2} torr). As the effluent from the chromatographic column passes through the first orifice the lighter molecules of carrier gas (usually helium) have less momentum and tend to diverge and are pumped away. Those with higher momentum have less opportunity to spread out and so pass into the next orifice. The two-stage jet separator consists of two single-stage separators in series, the volume around the second set of orifices being evacuated with a diffusion pump. The separator is usually constructed of glass or stainless steel to minimise decomposition of the sample and is kept at a suitably high temperature to prevent condensation of less volatile organic components.

The efficiency of this device depends on several factors. (i) The molecular weight of the carrier gas should be as low as possible and helium, molecular weight 4, is preferred. This is especially important if the carrier gas is being used as a reagent gas for chemical ionisation and a compromise between chemical ionisation and separator efficiency has sometimes to be reached. (ii) The physical dimensions of the jets and the gap(s) between them are critical because if the gap is too great, sample molecules are pumped away, while if the gap is too small, the amount of carrier gas removed is reduced. (iii) The optimum carrier gas flow rate is related to the dimensions of the separator, and the relationship should be determined experimentally for each particular interface.

Membrane Separator

This separator relies on the fact that the conductance of a silicone rubber film, a few micrometres thick, is several orders of magnitude greater for organic molecules than for the carrier gas. The column effluent is passed over this membrane, the other side of which is directly attached to the ion source of the mass spectrometer, which is at high vacuum. Transfer of sample occurs with high efficiency.

Glass Frit Separator

The chromatographic column is connected to the ion source of the mass spectrometer by means of a porous tube, the outside of which is maintained at low pressure. The smaller molecules of carrier gas diffuse through the porous tube and are pumped away whilst the enriched stream of sample molecules passes into the mass spectrometer.

The relative performance of particular examples of these devices will depend on many instrumental features but a comparison of their characteristics is given below.

Interface	Proportion transferred	Temperature limitations	Lag time
Single-stage jet	about 40%	350°	none
Two-stage jet	up to 60%	350°	none
Membrane	up to 95%	250°	noticeable
Glass frit	about 50%	350°	negligible

INTERFACES FOR HIGH PRESSURE LIQUID CHROMATOGRAPHY

The use of high pressure liquid chromatography enables many compounds to be studied which are not amenable to gas chromatographic analysis, for example those that are thermally labile. Eluent flow rates of between 0.5 and 2.0 ml/min are commonly used, whilst the maximum input the mass spectrometer can accommodate is about 1 to 4 ml/min of gas at standard temperature and pressure (s.t.p.). Simple calculations show that 1 ml of liquid hexane gives 172 ml of gas at s.t.p., 1 ml of chloroform gives 285 ml, 1 ml of methanol 550 ml, and 1 ml of

water 1200 ml. In the low pressure environment of the mass spectrometer ion source these volumes are much greater. The problems of maintaining a satisfactory vacuum when interfacing a high pressure liquid chromatograph with a mass spectrometer are therefore much greater than those associated with a gas chromatography interface.

There are three possible ways of making high pressure liquid chromatography compatible with mass spectrometry. They are increasing the pumping capability of the mass spectrometer, reducing the flow through the chromatographic column, and developing an interface.

The first method imposes too many limitations on the system to make it viable in practice, while low-flow high pressure liquid chromatography is still being developed and has only been reported for the separation of mixtures of pure compounds.

Two types of interface are available, one of which uses direct liquid insertion and the other uses a moving belt. In the *direct liquid insertion interface*, the total effluent from the column passes through the interface and past a pinhole orifice adjacent to the ion source of the mass spectrometer; the size of the orifice can be altered. A small volume of effluent passes through the pinhole and into the mass spectrometer. Coolant must be provided to prevent vaporisation of the solvent which would otherwise increase the ion source pressure to an unacceptable level. When electron impact mass spectra are required, the ion source pressure must be low and, therefore, only 0.1% of the effluent can be allowed into the source. Chemical ionisation allows a much larger proportion of the effluent to be used (up to 10%) and hence the use of this interface is restricted, on the grounds of sensitivity, to chemical ionisation only. The main disadvantages of the direct liquid insertion interface are that pre-evaporation of sample in the interface degrades chromatographic performance and that the very small orifice tends to become blocked.

In the *moving belt interface*, effluent from the column is brought into contact with the belt, and the film of effluent is carried under an infra-red lamp evaporator which rapidly removes most of the solvent. The solute and residual solvent then pass through two vacuum locks, where remaining solvent is removed, and into the ion source of the mass spectrometer where the sample is flash vaporised. The belt then travels over a clean-up heater which removes any residual solute.

The solvent capacity of this system ranges from about 0.2 ml/min for solutions containing large amounts of water, e.g. water: methanol (90:10), to about 1.5 ml/min for volatile non-polar solvents. If solutions with a large proportion of water are used, the solvent tends to form droplets on the belt rather than an even film. This leads to distortion of the mass spectra, but this may be alleviated by dropping a small amount of detergent or alcohol on to the belt just before the application of the column effluent. An alternative approach is the use of post-column liquid/liquid extraction to remove the aqueous phase and this can give 99% separation.

The advantage of the belt interface is that it may be used to obtain electron impact spectra, although in practice the background spectrum renders the low mass range ($m/z < 100$) useless for interpretation purposes. This background is even greater if volatile buffers are used in the chromatographic system. Non-volatile buffers or ion-pair reagents tend to be deposited on the belt impairing the performance of the interface and are normally removed by use of a belt wiper. The belt interface also tends to degrade the column performance slightly.

Ionisation

The most widely used method of ionisation is by *electron impact* (EI) in which the vaporised sample molecules are bombarded with a stream of high energy electrons. Usually, electrons of 70 eV energy are used although only 10 eV is required for ionisation. The excess energy absorbed (up to 10 eV) causes fragmentation of the molecule to produce both negative and positive ions.

POSITIVE IONS

The simplest process which may initially occur is the removal of a single electron from the intact molecule to give the positively charged 'molecular ion'. The abundance of this molecular ion varies according to the structure concerned. For example, lysergide (mol. wt 323) contains a stable ring structure and the molecular ion is the most intense ion (Fig. 3) whereas it is totally absent in the spectrum of amphetamine (mol. wt 135) in which a

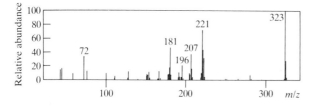

Fig. 3. Electron impact mass spectrum of lysergide, molecular weight 323.

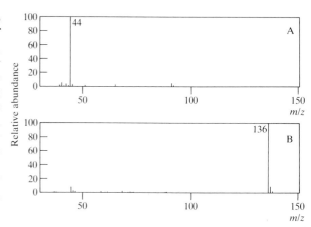

Fig. 4. Electron impact (A) and chemical ionisation (B) mass spectra of amphetamine.

very labile bond exists (Fig. 4A). The molecular ion may rearrange and/or fragment into ions of lower mass to charge ratio (m/z) which may fragment further.

The very short-lived ions ($< 10^{-6}$ s) will decompose in the source of the mass spectrometer and will not be detected as such, while long-lived ions ($> 10^{-5}$ s) are accelerated through the mass spectrometer to reach the detector intact. The ions of intermediate lifetime (10^{-5} to 10^{-6} s) are accelerated from the source with mass m_1 but before reaching the mass analyser decompose to give a smaller ion of mass m_2. In the case of a magnetic sector instrument a broad 'metastable ion' peak (m^*) is observed at a non-integral m/z value given by the relationship

$$m^* = \frac{(m_2)^2}{m_1}$$

for $m_1^+ \rightarrow m_2^+ + m$ (neutral)

These ions are of diagnostic use, for their presence shows that a certain fragmentation occurs although their absence does not necessarily signify that it does not.

The most important piece of information which may be obtained from a mass spectrum is the molecular weight. However, certain classes of compounds do not show molecular ions and in other cases it is not always possible to identify unequivocally the molecular ion. Therefore a family of so called 'soft ionisation' techniques has been developed. These generate a molecular ion or 'quasi-molecular ion' and fragmentation is kept to a minimum. The most commonly used technique is *chemical ionisation* (CI) in which the sample is mixed with a large excess of a reagent gas such as isobutane or methane. The mixture is then bombarded with high energy electrons, as in electron impact ionisation. The reagent gas undergoes preferential ionisation and the primary ions so produced react with further reagent gas molecules to produce a number of chemically reactive species such as CH_5^+ and $C_2H_5^+$ in the case of methane, and $C_4H_9^+$ in the case of isobutane. These secondary ions subsequently react with the sample molecules to produce new ions predominantly with a mass one greater than the molecular weight by transfer of a proton. Usually, few fragmentation/rearrangement ions are observed and this quasi-molecular ion is the most intense ion in the spectrum (base peak). Fig. 4 shows the electron impact and chemical ionisation spectra of amphetamine.

An alternative method which may be used to depress fragmentation and enhance the molecular ion is to reduce the energy of the bombarding electron beam from 70 eV to a value just above the so-called 'appearance potential' of the molecular ion. In this case, sufficient energy is available to ionise the molecule, but not to cause fragmentation. This technique suffers from a very low sensitivity and in many cases still does not give a recognisable molecular ion.

Electron impact and chemical ionisation are complementary techniques and it is possible to obtain instrumentation which allows spectra of both types to be collected alternately throughout lengthy analyses, thus providing both molecular weight and fragmentation information from a single determination. For qualitative work this approach is adequate, but more critical conditions are required to obtain the best and most consistent performance from chemical ionisation, and it is recommended that a spectrometer is devoted solely to the production of chemical ionisation spectra. Continued use of chemical ionisation also contaminates the source and reduces electron impact performance. Under normal circumstances chemical ionisation is slightly less sensitive than electron impact although this does depend on the material under consideration. Chemical ionisation is more susceptible to source conditions and, in order to maximise the proton transfer process, a gas-tight source is essential. Any factor which reduces this, such as chipped interface jets, results in loss of sensitivity.

In addition to the confirmation of molecular weight, chemical ionisation may be used to indicate the presence of a mixture, the spectrum usually containing a single intense ion from each component. This may be used to advantage in the analysis of thin-layer chromatography spots when the background spectrum, often prominent under electron impact conditions, is usually suppressed.

NEGATIVE IONS

The study of negative ions is more difficult because their abundance is usually 3 or 4 orders of magnitude less than that of positive ions. Also, they usually occur in the low mass range and are therefore of little structural significance. However, if the bombardment is carried out under chemical ionisation conditions using a reagent gas which, on electron impact, yields anions, e.g. methylene chloride, these combine with sample molecules to form negative cluster ions e.g. $(M+Cl)^-$. Under these conditions the sensitivity of certain classes of compounds is several orders of magnitude greater than when using positive ion techniques. The types of compounds amenable to this type of analysis are those with high electron affinity, i.e. those often detected by electron capture in gas chromatography. It is, therefore, worthwhile considering the use of chemical derivatives such as pentafluorobenzoyl, heptafluorobutyryl, etc. to enhance the electron-capturing ability of the compounds under consideration.

Other soft ionisation techniques include field desorption, field ionisation, atmospheric pressure ionisation, and fast atom bombardment and each increases the range of molecules which may be studied by mass spectrometry. Vitamins of molecular weight around 1400 may now be studied and the molecular ion identified. These techniques are at present useful for confirmation of structure or molecular weight but because of the production of cluster ions such as $(M+Na)^+$, $(M+2Na)^+$, $2M^+$, etc., they are not used in the investigation of unknowns.

Ion Separation

The collimated ion beam, having left the source, is separated into groups of ions of different mass to charge ratio (m/z) usually by employing a *magnetic sector* or a *quadrupole filter*. The ability of the mass spectrometer to separate these ions is termed the resolution, and mass spectrometers may be of low, medium, or high resolution.

Low resolution mass spectrometers essentially have resolution of the order of 1000 (i.e. they are able to differentiate between m/z 1000 and 1001 or between m/z 100.0 and 100.1) and have a single mass separation stage. Medium and high or ultra-high resolution mass spectrometers have resolutions ranging from about 10 000 to about 150 000. They employ two separation/focussing stages and allow an m/z value to be determined to four decimal places and accurate atomic compositions to be obtained.

Ions, when subjected to an accelerating voltage, take up a circular path in a magnetic field. In a magnetic sector instrument, ions of different m/z may be brought to focus at a detector by variation of the magnetic field. Laminated magnets allow faster scan speeds than solid magnets because of their low hysteresis characteristics.

The quadrupole filter comprises four symmetrically arranged parallel rods. A field is set up in the space between the rods by the use of a radiofrequency field and a d.c. voltage which may be varied to allow ions of different m/z to reach the detector.

The main advantage of the quadrupole filter is its fast scan speed (scan speeds in the millisecond range are possible), since only a change in voltage is involved and problems associated with magnet hysteresis are not encountered. The ion source of a quadrupole mass spectrometer is maintained at very low voltages (typically tens of volts) while magnetic sector instruments require high voltages (typically 3 to 4 kV). Magnetic sector instruments are therefore much more susceptible to leaks, pressure fluctuations, and flashovers caused by dirty sources, etc. The mass range of a quadrupole filter is more limited than that of a magnetic sector instrument, commercial instruments being limited to ion masses below about 1200. However, this is not a practical problem since the vast majority of drugs have molecular weights below this limit. The intensity of an ion above about m/z 300 obtained using a quadrupole filter is usually less than that obtained from the same sample using a magnetic sector instrument, and this discrimination effect should be taken into account when spectra from quadrupole and magnetic sector instruments are compared. Further disadvantages of the quadrupole filter are that it is not capable of high resolution and that metastable peaks are not observed.

For most routine applications quadrupole instruments and single focussing magnetic sector instruments are of comparable performance. However, quadrupole instruments are much more compact.

Double Focussing Mass Spectrometers. Two factors that limit the resolution of a single focussing mass spectrometer to a maximum of about 5000 are the angular divergence and the spread of the kinetic energies of the ions as they leave the source. To correct for these, an electrostatic analyser (ESA) is introduced, usually before the magnetic sector. The radius of curvature of an ion passing through an electrostatic analyser is determined by its kinetic energy. The beam of ions emerging from the source of a mass spectrometer is therefore brought to a focus at a series of points, each representing a common kinetic energy. These are then passed into the magnetic sector and the separate beams are refocussed at one point for each m/z ratio.

In this way, resolution of up to 150 000 and a mass-measurement accuracy of 0.3 ppm may be obtained. Thus the accurate molecular weight of a compound can be measured to ± 0.0002 mass units and an unambiguous assignment of the elemental composition of an ion may be made. For example, although dibutyl phthalate and triprolidine each have a nominal molecular weight of 278 their accurate molecular weights of 278.1556 and 278.1862 reflect their differing atomic compositions, $C_{16}H_{22}O_4$ and $C_{19}H_{22}N_2$, respectively.

The double focussing mass spectrometer also allows the use of a series of 'linked scanning' techniques. In conventional double focussing mass spectrometry, the electrostatic analyser voltage (E) is held constant while the magnetic field (B) is varied to generate the mass spectrum. If, however, B and E are linked in a specific way, various modes of ion decomposition may be studied. If the ratio B/E is kept constant, the daughter ions formed by decomposition of an individual ion may be studied. This may be used as an aid to structural determination since ions with the same atomic composition, but different structures, will fragment differently (the B/E linked scan of m/z 73 from $CH_3 \cdot CO \cdot O \cdot CH_2$ will be different from that obtained from $CH_2 \cdot CH_2 \cdot COOH$). This technique may also be used to obtain a fingerprint mass spectrum for identification purposes. By monitoring the molecular ion of a compound which may be present as a minor component of a mixture, only the fragmentation of this ion will be observed. Thus a characteristic mass spectrum will be obtained for that minor component and the background spectrum will be effectively removed.

Another application is the differentiation of closely related isomers. The conventional mass spectra of butobarbitone and secbutobarbitone are qualitatively identical (Figs 5A and 5B). The B/E linked scans of their $(M-29)^+$ ions (m/z 183) shown in

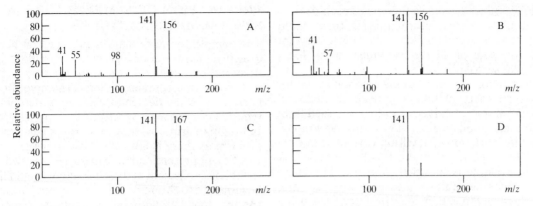

Fig. 5. Electron impact mass spectra of butobarbitone (A) and secbutobarbitone (B), and daughter-ion linked spectra of m/z 183 from butobarbitone (C) and secbutobarbitone (D).

Figs 5C and 5D are clearly different, thus allowing ready discrimination.

A similar technique applicable to reverse geometry mass spectrometers (magnetic sector before electrostatic analyser) is that of mass-analysed ion kinetic energy spectrometry (MIKES). In this technique the ion to be studied is 'isolated' by the magnet and induced to fragment by collision activation in a small chamber filled with a gas such as helium. The product ions are then detected by scanning the electrostatic analyser voltage.

If the electrostatic analyser voltage and magnetic field are scanned such that B^2/E is constant, all precursor ions of a selected daughter ion may be observed. The main use of this technique is in structure determinations to investigate the interrelationships of ions.

A third scanning mode, in which the ratio $B/E\sqrt{(1-E)}$ is kept constant, allows ions arising by a specific neutral loss to be observed. This permits ions containing a common functional group to be identified and related compounds in a mixture to be picked out. Similar results may be obtained by the use of a triple quadrupole arrangement in which the first quadrupole is used to isolate the ion of interest, the second as a collision cell to induce fragmentation, and the third to monitor the selected decomposition mode.

Ion Detection and Amplification

The beam of ions is directed through a set of resolving slits to a detector, usually an electron multiplier. The current generated is amplified, typically by a factor of 10^6, so that it may be observed using an oscilloscope and may be recorded using some device which allows a permanent record to be obtained.

Presentation of Results

The recording device must accept the data generated by the mass spectrometer at a range of scan speeds. It must also allow the ready comparison of the intensities of both major and minor ion peaks within a single scan. A chart recorder equipped with ultraviolet-sensitive paper and using a light beam instead of a pen is capable of producing simultaneous traces at different sensitivities and thus satisfies the requirements. However, a computer equipped with some sort of data storage device (data system) is now more common. Its advantage is that data may be stored permanently and manipulated in many sophisticated ways (background subtraction, library matching, etc.). Depending on the size of the storage device (magnetic tape, floppy or cartridge disk) either all scans or selected scans are stored. Simple systems allow data to be acquired, then processed only when data acquisition is complete. More complex systems include those in which one set of data may be acquired at the same time as a second set of data, either from the current run or from a previous run, is being manipulated (Foreground/Background). Other systems control several mass spectrometers at the same time as data processing is being carried out.

The data system detects ions occurring during a mass spectrometer scan and measures their intensities. The signal obtained is proportional to the number of ions of the particular m/z produced. Comparison with known masses obtained from a reference material, allows the m/z of each peak to be calculated. This information is then stored together with other data such as the total ion current (TIC, the sum of all the individual ions), for a particular scan.

These data for successive scans are then stored for subsequent manipulation. The reconstructed total ion current trace, equivalent to that obtained from a flame ionisation detector in gas chromatography, shows the variation of total ion current with time and allows spectra of interest to be identified. A typical example is shown in Fig. 6A. The background may be subtracted to give clean spectra, and their identification may be attempted using libraries of standard spectra. If a composite spectrum is obtained from two unresolved peaks, complex subtraction routines may be used to obtain a pure spectrum of each of the components. These may be separately submitted for library searching. The spectra may then be plotted or obtained as a mass versus intensity listing.

Single ion chromatograms, i.e. the variation in intensity of a single ion with time, may be generated to identify particular components in a complex mixture or to identify particular structural fragments and thereby draw attention to peaks of special interest (Fig. 6B).

The data system therefore allows manipulations that are impracticable or impossible without the use of a computer and offers the great advantage that it is possible to re-examine the data at a later date.

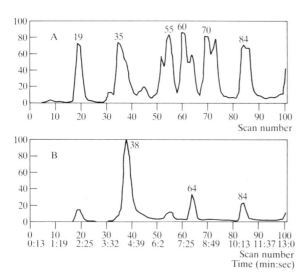

Fig. 6. Reconstructed total ion current trace (A) and a single ion chromatogram from m/z 91 (B) for a typical GC–MS run.

PREPARATION OF SAMPLES FOR MASS SPECTROMETRIC ANALYSIS

The sample for examination may be the parent drug in a pharmaceutical preparation or illicit drug preparation, or may be the drug together with a metabolite in a complex biological sample. In the latter case, some degree of clean-up/separation is required prior to mass spectrometric analysis.

In drug preparations, sensitivity is not a particular problem as there is always sufficient of the active constituent present. Suitable extraction procedures should be carried out and each fraction should then be subjected to chromatographic analysis. The mass spectra, together with the appropriate retention parameters, may then be used for identification purposes. In many cases mass spectrometric analysis is undertaken as confirmation of an identification based on the physical characteristics such as size, colour, markings, etc., of the tablet or capsule.

Mass spectrometry may be used not only to identify the major components but also the trace impurities. This information may be used for quality control purposes, and may enable the route of manufacture of certain drugs to be determined.

The analysis of drugs in biological materials presents more of a problem since the amounts of material encountered are much smaller and they are in a much more complex sample. In most cases therefore, some type of clean-up procedure is carried out prior to chromatographic separation and mass spectrometric analysis. It is not usual to analyse this type of sample by use of the probe because of the excessive background spectrum that is obtained. However, this background may be reduced using the mass spectrometer in the chemical ionisation mode, and probe analysis can then be used as a screening technique. This can give significant information concerning compounds present, but will not usually allow discrimination between compounds with the same molecular weight. Chromatographic separation may be carried out to isolate the substance(s) of interest before analysis using thin-layer chromatography, paper chromatography, or preparative gas chromatography, or using 'on-line' chromatographic techniques (GC, HPLC) in which the separated substances pass directly into the mass spectrometer for analysis.

Thin-layer Chromatography and Paper Chromatography

The major problems encountered with these techniques are co-extraction of contaminants from the chromatographic paper or plate, or from the solvents used for extraction.

The simplest method of transferring the material for analysis to the insertion probe of the mass spectrometer involves scraping off the relevant portion of the thin-layer plate or cutting the chromatographic paper and placing it in a micro test-tube. The drug is extracted by shaking with the minimum amount of a volatile solvent such as methanol, separating the supernatant liquid by centrifugation, transferring to the insertion probe, and then evaporating. Alternatively, the adsorbent from a thin-layer plate can be placed in a Pasteur pipette in which the constriction is packed with clean cotton wool and the material of interest eluted with about 50 µl of an appropriate solvent directly into the probe.

The problem of background spectra may be overcome by carrying out the above extraction procedure using a portion from an equivalent position on the plate or paper which has been run in the same solvent but with no sample. This spectrum may then be subtracted to give a clean spectrum of the sample. Thin-layer plates may be precleaned by running them in solvents before attempting to run a sample. The background spectra most often encountered, arising from solvent contaminants, is characterised by an intense ion of m/z 149 due to phthalate ester plasticisers.

Gas Chromatography

The interfaces which allow compatibility between the widely different pressure requirements of gas chromatography and mass spectrometry have been discussed previously. The main modification is the use of helium as the carrier gas in the chromatographic column. Since the carrier gas is ionised within the source of the mass spectrometer this will always contribute to the total ion current and will result in a high standing current. The use of a carrier gas having a high ionisation potential is therefore advocated to reduce this standing current. This may be further reduced by decreasing the energy of the bombarding electrons to a value which is below the relevant ionisation potential of the carrier gas but still allows efficient ionisation of the organic sample molecules. A value of 24 eV, compared with the more usual 70 eV, is normally used.

Problems caused by column bleed include elevated background in total ion current traces, contamination of the separator and/or ion source, and contamination of the spectra. These problems may be overcome by using silicone polymer type stationary phases, which are thermally stable and inert. They are conditioned at their maximum operating temperature for several days, and then used at lower temperatures to reduce the level of bleed. Alternatively, a background spectrum may be obtained and then subtracted from the spectrum of interest in the same way as described for thin-layer and paper chromatography.

Capillary and packed columns impose different operating criteria upon the mass spectrometer. Packed columns usually give peaks with a width of about 20 to 30 seconds at half height, whereas capillary columns give peak widths of about 5 seconds. The scan speed of the mass spectrometer must be fast enough to ensure that spectra are not grossly distorted by the variation in concentration of the drug during the scan. If a computer is used, at least three scans must be obtained and averaged. This is not a problem with packed columns, when scan rates of 10 seconds/decade may be used to give high accuracy mass measurements. For capillary columns, a cycle time of less than 1 second is required and, in the past, this necessitated the use of quadrupole mass spectrometers with their inherently faster scan speeds. However, the development of laminated magnets has made it possible to scan at cycle times of about 0.5 seconds using a magnetic sector instrument. This is perfectly adequate to obtain high resolution data from the highest performance capillary columns. For overlapping peaks, examination of a series of consecutively obtained spectra enables the analyst to identify the ions associated with each component of the mixture. In each of the above cases which cause distortion of spectra, removal of background and deconvolution of overlapping peaks are most easily dealt with by use of a data system.

A restriction to the operation of GC–MS can be caused by solvent peaks. If the solvent injected onto a packed column flows via a separator into the ion source of the mass spectrometer, it results in an unacceptable increase in pressure which causes the built-in pressure protection devices to shut the mass spectrometer down. It also much reduces the lifetime of source components such as filaments and heaters. Therefore a valve is fitted at the end of the column, which allows effluent to be vented to a pump or to the atmosphere until the solvent has passed. The flow rates associated with the use of capillary columns are such that the pressure generated by the solvent is not as great as with a packed column. The total effluent may therefore be passed directly into the source of the mass spectrometer, but in order to prolong the life of filaments etc. the mass spectrometer is usually turned off until the solvent elutes.

The temperature of the interface is of great importance. If it is too low the chromatographic performance is degraded or the material of interest simply condenses and is not observed, whilst if the temperature is too high, thermal decomposition or even pyrolysis may occur. The gas lines, if constructed of glass-lined tubing, should be uniformly heated, of the minimum possible length, and should not contain any sharp bends. These tend to crack after temperature cycling and lead to active sites in the tubing which again degrade performance and may result in small quantities of material being lost altogether. It should also be remembered that the mass spectrometer, in its qualitative mode, is equivalent to the flame ionisation detector in gas chromatography and, unless multiple ion detection or single ion monitoring is used, does not function as a selective detector.

Chemical derivatives may be used to improve the chromatographic characteristics of polar compounds, e.g. acids may be converted to their methyl esters and barbiturates to their methyl derivatives. This technique may also provide information concerning the number of active sites in a molecule by noting the increase in molecular weight on methylation. In many cases the mass spectrum of the derivative may be of more use for identification purposes.

High Pressure Liquid Chromatography

The use of HPLC–MS is far from routine. The fast scanning limitation is removed since peak widths are of the order of those associated with packed gas chromatography columns. Much greater spectrum background is encountered, however, to the extent that details below m/z 100 are completely obscured.

COMPOUND IDENTIFICATION

The identification of a compound from its mass spectrum may be achieved by matching the spectrum against libraries of spectra. However, if the compound is not already known, e.g. a drug intermediate or an unknown metabolite which is not in the library collections, the fragmentation pattern must be interpreted from first principles using as much other analytical information (UV, IR, NMR, etc.) as may be available.

Reference Collections

The most efficient way to use reference collections of mass spectra is to build up a collection of spectra containing the compounds most likely to be encountered. Experience shows that a library of approximately 2000 spectra enables more than 80% of samples analysed to be identified.

With the advent of dedicated data systems it is now possible to store relatively large numbers of full spectra efficiently. However, for efficient searching it is necessary to abbreviate the spectra. For those without data systems it is also necessary to abbreviate the spectra in order to construct hardcopy indexes for manual searching.

Two equally efficient types of spectral abbreviation are in use, these being based on either the n (usually 8) most intense ions in the mass spectrum or the n in m range system in which the n largest ions in each m mass range are used (e.g. 1 in 7, 1 in 14, or 2 in 14). The main disadvantage of the n most intense ions system is that the ions could all be of low m/z and have little structural significance. This can result in library matches being obtained which are similar only in the ions due to the hydrocarbon moieties (m/z 57, 71, 85, etc.). A modification of this procedure involves the assignment of a 'significance factor' for the mass number in which ions of higher m/z are considered to be more significant than those of lower m/z. The intensity of each ion is then multiplied by this factor and the n most intense or most significant ions are used in the abbreviation. The advantage of the range system is that the significant high mass ions are always used. The n in m range system also allows ready coding of spectra using binary notation and leads to the identification of homologous series of ions.

Having decided on the format of a library of spectra, one must then consider how the data will be searched. Manually, the analyst extracts the relevant data from the spectrum of the 'unknown', orders them according to the format of the hard copy listing, and carries out the search. The analyst compares the similar spectra and uses his experience to judge which is the best match. It is possible for an experienced analyst to conclude that the mass spectrum is not a single component but a mixture since, although all ions in the library spectrum are present, there are also other significant ions present. These other ions are then used as the basis of a further search. Searches using data systems are carried out in a similar way but much more rapidly. Most computer programs list library matches in order of 'fit factor', a measure of the similarity between the library spectrum and the 'unknown' spectrum. It is usually calculated using a formula involving the differences in intensities of matching ions in the two spectra. Two main types of search are used, the so-called forward and reverse searches.

In the forward search, all of the ions in both the library spectrum and the unknown spectrum are used in the calculation of the fit factor, while in the reverse search only the ions in the library spectrum are used in this calculation. Forward searches work well only for pure compounds, while the reverse search is admirably suited for dealing with the composite spectra from mixtures.

When small mass spectral collections do not identify an unknown, use is usually made of large, commercially available collections. The strength of these collections is their size, but it is also their weakness because manual searches take a considerable time and a large number of entries are irrelevant to some analysts. This weakness is of minor importance if the collection can be searched by a computer. Two major collections exist one of which, the EPA/NIH Mass Spectral Data Base, is available on a worldwide commercial time-share computer by the National Bureau of Standards, Washington, U.S.A. This data-base is accessible via a telephone and a suitable terminal. The collection contains around 34 000 spectra which may be searched in a variety of ways.

The simplest method is termed the 'peak' search in which a series of ions, within an intensity range, are input to the computer one by one. The file is then searched and the output consists of those spectra containing the required ion(s) with the correct intensity. Additional ions are then input and the first set of spectra is further reduced until eventually it contains only those entries which incorporate all of the ions required. When the subset has been reduced to a manageable number, a list of the relevant spectra may be produced, including information such as molecular weight, molecular formula, and reference number. A full listing of the peaks of these spectra is also available. The bar chart representation of this complete collection of spectra may be obtained in book form, arranged in order of molecular weight. Other computer searches which are available include molecular weight, peak and molecular weight, molecular formula, and peak and molecular formula. This collection is also available on commercially available data systems to allow interactive searching.

The second collection available, both in book form and on magnetic tape for computer searching, is 'The Eight Peak Index of Mass Spectra', published by the Mass Spectrometry Data Centre (MSDC) Nottingham. This differs from the previous collection in that it contains only the eight most intense peaks, with intensities; the 1983 edition contains data for over 60 000 spectra.

Interpretation of Mass Spectra

If it is not possible to identify a mass spectrum from library collections it is necessary to attempt the interpretation of the mass spectrum. However, before consideration of the mass spectrum all other available data should be collected together. For example, the method of extraction using acidic or basic conditions, should rule out a large number of possibilities. If possible, infra-red and ultraviolet spectra should be examined and chromatographic retention values should be determined. Armed with this information the mass spectrum can be examined. Firstly, the molecular ion (M^+) must be identified. This will probably be the ion of highest m/z in the spectrum, but this is not always the case. The molecular ion must be capable of yielding the other high mass ions observed in the spectrum by loss of convenient neutral species (losses of 4 to 14, 21 to 25, 33, 37, and 38 are highly unlikely). If possible, the molecular weight should be confirmed by use of a soft ionisation technique. If high resolution facilities are available, the accurate molecular composition may be determined from the molecular ion.

Even if only low resolution data are available, a great deal of information may be obtained. If the molecule has an odd mass it must contain an odd number of nitrogen atoms. If, however, it is of even mass it either contains no nitrogen or an even number of atoms of the element. This is a consequence of the even atomic weight and odd valency of nitrogen. The intensity of the molecular ion gives an indication of the structure. An intense M^+ indicates the presence of a stable ring structure. Chain branching substantially decreases the stability of M^+. The presence of a multiplet in the M^+ region is often indicative of the presence of heteroatoms possessing characteristic isotopic patterns. The elements which are commonly identified in this way are silicon, sulphur, chlorine, and bromine, each of which gives characteristic contributions at $(M+2)$ (^{28}Si:^{29}Si:^{30}Si—to give peaks in the ratio 100:5:3, ^{32}S:^{34}S ratio 100:4, ^{35}Cl:^{37}Cl ratio 3:1, and ^{79}Br:^{81}Br ratio 1:1).

The high mass end of the spectrum is then examined for characteristic losses, and the low mass end for characteristic ions which may be rationalised in terms of the structure. The presence of metastable ions, not usually detected by data systems, gives information regarding the fragmentation pathways, this type of information being supplemented by that available from linked scanning experiments if a double focussing instrument is available. By examination of the interrelationships between the ions observed in a mass spectrum it is possible to work out a complete breakdown scheme and then by piecing together all the available information it is often possible to arrive at an unambiguous assignment of structure.

The information extracted and deduced in the steps above may be used in a different way in an attempt to identify an unknown compound. This utilises a file of known chemical structures stored in a computer-compatible form known as the Wiswesser Line Notation (WLN). This notation retains substructural information and forms the basis of a search system (R. E. Ardrey and C. Brown, *J. forens. Sci. Soc.*, 1977, *17*, 63–71). The types of information available from the mass spectrum, i.e. molecular weight, accurate atomic composition, structural groups, presence of heteroatoms with characteristic isotopic patterns, etc., are supplemented with the information from other analytical techniques. The ultraviolet spectrum may suggest, for example, a barbiturate, and the infra-red spectrum may, for example, exclude the presence of certain chemical groupings. When these data are entered into the search program via an interactive input, the output consists of a list of all structures which fulfil the required analytical criteria. The analyst must then consider each structure in the light of the evidence at his disposal. Certain aspects of the analytical data may not seem significant on first consideration but, when taken in the light of a possible structure, may assume greater importance. Having reduced the list of possible structures to manageable numbers, hopefully only one or two, it is best to obtain a genuine sample of the material and compare analytical data.

QUANTIFICATION

The technique known variously as multiple ion detection (MID), selected ion recording (SIR), and selected ion monitoring (SIM) employs the mass spectrometer to monitor only a few significant ions. In this way both the sensitivity and selectivity are increased markedly, the former by a factor approaching 100 due to the increased amount of time spent monitoring each particular ion. For the successful quantitative estimation of a compound its mass spectrum should contain at least two reasonably intense ions at the high mass end of the spectrum. By using two ions of known relative abundance from the parent compound, contributions at these masses from extraneous material present can be ruled out and thereby increase the precision of the determination.

It is also advantageous to have access to a substance which may be used as an internal standard. This should be chemically similar to the material under investigation, should possess two ions capable of being monitored, but should not have significant ion contributions at the masses previously chosen for monitoring. Ideally, a deuterated derivative or homologue of the material to be determined is used. The internal standard should be added prior to any clean-up/extraction procedure so that any losses will apply equally to both the internal standard and the drug under investigation. Using a calibration graph of relative peak heights/areas of particular ions from solutions containing a fixed amount of internal standard plotted against different amounts of the drug of interest, a direct determination of the amount in an unknown solution can be made. It is possible to measure picogram concentrations of materials from biological extracts, although the detection limit is set not by the sensitivity of the mass spectrometer but by the interference generated by co-extracted materials, etc. If a double focussing instrument is available, the selectivity may be increased further by monitoring the accurate mass corresponding to a particular atomic composition rather than the nominal integer mass.

Double focussing instrumentation also allows the monitoring of metastable transitions. This technique increases the sensitivity and specificity because metastable ions are observed at non-integer m/z values where there are no other ions.

MASS SPECTRAL DATA

Many of the monographs in Part 2 contain mass spectral data in the form of the eight most intense ions, in descending order of intensity. These values have also been used to compile an 8-peak index in Part 3 for rapid searching for an unknown.

The complete mass spectra for about 1000 drugs, metabolites, and other compounds of forensic and pharmaceutical interest are reproduced in *Pharmaceutical Mass Spectra*, London, Pharmaceutical Press, 1985. This collection also contains three 8-

peak indexes in which substances appear alphabetically by name, in numerical order of base peak, and in order of molecular weight.

Bibliography

R. E. Ardrey *et al.*, *Pharmaceutical Mass Spectra*, London, Pharmaceutical Press, 1985.

Biochemical Applications of Mass Spectrometry, G. R. Waller (Ed.), New York, Wiley-Interscience, 1972, and Suppl., 1980.

J. R. Chapman, *Computers in Mass Spectrometry*, London, Academic Press, 1978.

Fundamentals of Integrated GC-MS (Parts 1–3), *Chromatographic Science Series*, B. J. Gudzinowicz *et al.* (Ed.), Vol. 7, New York, Marcel Dekker, Parts 1 & 2, 1976; Part 3, 1977.

Handbook of Analytical Derivatization Reactions, D. R. Knapp (Ed.), New York, Wiley, 1979.

S. R. Heller and G. W. A. Milne, *EPA/NIH Mass Spectral Data Base*, Washington, U.S. Dept of Commerce, 1978, and 1st Suppl., 1980.

Mass Spectrometry in Drug Metabolism, A. Frigerio and E. L. Ghisalberti (Ed.), New York, Plenum Press, 1977.

W. H. McFadden, Liquid Chromatography/Mass Spectrometry, Systems and Applications, *J. chromatogr. Sci.*, 1980, *18*, 97–102.

W. H. McFadden, *Techniques of Combined Gas Chromatography/Mass Spectrometry—Applications in Organic Analysis*, New York, Wiley, 1973.

F. W. McLafferty, *Interpretation of Mass Spectra*, 3rd Edn, Reading, Massachusetts, W. A. Benjamin, 1980.

B. J. Millard, *Quantitative Mass Spectrometry*, London, Heyden, 1978.

Recent Developments in Mass Spectrometry in Biochemistry and Medicine, A. Frigerio (Ed.), New York, Plenum Press, Vol. 1, 1978; Vol. 2, 1979.

U. P. Schlunegger, *Advanced Mass Spectrometry: Applications in Organic and Analytical Chemistry*, Oxford, Pergamon Press, 1980.

Nuclear Magnetic Resonance Spectroscopy

G. P. Carr

Nuclear magnetic resonance spectroscopy (NMR) is based on the fact that when nuclei of NMR-active species are placed in a magnetic field they distribute themselves into a number of quantised orientations with respect to this field. Each orientation corresponds to an energy level and if the nucleus is then subjected to an oscillating radiofrequency field of the correct frequency, energy is absorbed and transitions between these energy levels are induced. NMR spectroscopy involves detecting the absorption of energy with a radiofrequency receiver and observing the frequencies at which such transitions occur.

The number of orientations available to a nucleus varies depending on its type, in accordance with the following principle. The nuclei of all atoms carry a positive charge and, in the case of some isotopes, possess spin. These nuclei therefore have an angular momentum defined by $I(I+1)h/2\pi$, where I is the spin quantum number and h is Planck's constant. The value of I varies for different nuclei and may be $0, \frac{1}{2}, 1, \frac{3}{2} \ldots$ Nuclei for which $I=0$ are not NMR-active and some important atoms are included in this category, e.g. ^{12}C and ^{16}O, all of which have mass numbers which are divisible by four. Examples of NMR-active nuclei are ^{1}H, ^{13}C and ^{19}F $(I=\frac{1}{2})$, ^{14}N and ^{2}H $(I=1)$, and ^{11}B $(I=\frac{3}{2})$.

Detailed descriptions of the theory and instrumentation of nuclear magnetic resonance spectroscopy can be found elsewhere (see Bibliography). In this chapter the important features of the NMR spectrum and their use in the interpretation of spectra are described, together with details of certain special procedures which assist interpretation.

THE NMR SPECTRUM

Chemical Shift

Nuclei are brought to resonance as a result of the absorption of energy from a radiofrequency oscillator of the correct frequency. The value of this frequency is dependent on the intensity of the magnetic field being experienced by the nucleus, which in turn is dependent on various factors. Firstly, there is the operating field strength of the spectrometer. Various instruments are available in this respect, e.g. with an operating field strength of 1.41 T (14 100 gauss) in which the proton comes to resonance at 60 MHz, or of 2.35 T (23 500 gauss) for which the resonance frequency for the proton is 100 MHz. Instruments containing magnets with field strengths up to about 9.4 T (94 000 gauss) are available but spectrometers operating at frequencies (v) of about 60 MHz to 220 MHz for protons are probably the most widely used.

The second feature that influences this magnetic field is the environment of the nucleus within the molecule. The distribution of electrons around the nucleus, or around neighbouring atoms within the molecule, serves to screen it from the magnetic field so that the field actually experienced by each individual nucleus in the molecule may be different. Thus the frequency at which they come to resonance is also different. This effect is known as *shielding*. Nuclei surrounded by a relatively high level of electron density are referred to as *shielded* and those with a relatively low level of electron density as *deshielded*. As a result of shielding, nuclei come to resonance at frequencies which are characteristic of the functional groups associated with them and the different positions of these resonance lines are called chemical shifts.

This is demonstrated in Fig. 1 which illustrates the proton spectrum of 1,4-bis(2-oxopropyloxy)-benzene. Spectra are conventionally scanned from low field to high field with the low field end on the left. The aromatic protons are the least shielded followed by the methylene protons and then the methyl protons which are the most shielded.

It is not necessary to know the absolute value of resonance frequencies. It is sufficient and far more convenient to determine chemical shifts relative to

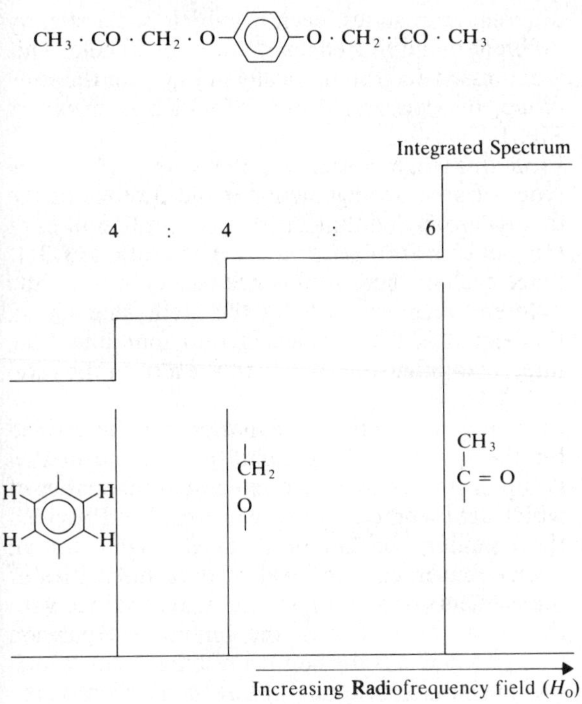

$CH_3 \cdot CO \cdot CH_2 \cdot O$—⬡—$O \cdot CH_2 \cdot CO \cdot CH_3$

Integrated Spectrum

4 : 4 : 6

H—⬡—H (benzene with H substituents)

CH_2
O

CH_3
$C = O$

Increasing **Radio**frequency field (H_0)

Fig. 1. Diagram of the proton spectrum of 1,4-bis(2-oxopropyl-oxy)benzene.

a standard reference substance. The reference substance used for samples in organic solvents, in both proton magnetic resonance (PMR) and ^{13}C spectroscopy, is tetramethylsilane (TMS). Since silicon is less electronegative than carbon, the four methyl groups are strongly shielded by the high electron density surrounding them. This leads to readily identifiable proton and ^{13}C signals which are at higher fields than the resonances of most organic molecules commonly encountered. Tetramethylsilane is not soluble in water and the usual standard for deuterium oxide (D_2O) solutions is sodium 3-(trimethylsilyl)propanesulphonate (TSS). Since the operating frequency of a spectrometer is dependent on the field strength of its magnet, the frequency at which a particular sample comes to resonance will be different in instruments containing magnets of different field strengths. Chemical shift data are therefore expressed in a form which is independent of the operating frequency of the instrument, i.e. δ parts per million, where

$$\delta = \frac{\text{Difference in resonance frequency between sample and TMS}}{\text{Operating frequency of the spectrometer}} \times 10^6 \text{ ppm}$$

The ratio is multiplied by 10^6 so that the data are in a more convenient form. Thus if tetramethyl-silane is arbitrarily set at $\delta 0.00$, the majority of proton resonances occur in the range 0 to 10 ppm. An alternative scale is the τ scale which is defined as $10 - \delta$ ppm so that tetramethylsilane is set at $\tau 10.00$ ppm. This scale is only really of value for proton spectroscopy and all further data in this chapter will be expressed on the δ scale.

Although their resonance frequencies may be different, the transitions undergone by protons in different groups represent the same energy change. As a result, the ratio of the integrated intensities of signals is equal to the ratio of the number of protons in each group.

In Fig. 1 there are four aromatic protons, four methylene protons, and six methyl protons so that the ratio of the integrated intensities of these three signals is 4:4:6. This is very useful since it provides information on the relative numbers of protons responsible for resonance signals thereby assisting in the interpretation of spectra. This proportionality does not occur so readily in ^{13}C spectroscopy. Since chemical shifts are dependent on the nature of the functional groups associated with the nucleus, tables have been compiled to correlate this data (see Bibliography).

Spin-spin Coupling

On a high-resolution spectrometer, the resonance lines corresponding to groups of equivalent nuclei frequently exhibit fine structure. Thus, under certain circumstances, resonance signals may be split into doublets, triplets, quartets, etc. This splitting is known as spin-spin coupling.

In Fig. 2 protons H_1 and H_2 resonate at quite different chemical shifts and are both split into doublets with the spacings between the two elements of both doublets being equal. This spacing is called the *coupling constant*. Coupling constants are measured in Hz, their values are characteristic of

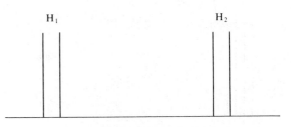

H_1 H_2

Fig. 2. Diagram of the proton spectrum of CHR_1R_2—CHR_3R_4 showing spin-spin coupling.

certain molecular features and are independent of the field strength of the spectrometer. They are conventionally referred to as values of J with appropriate subscripts to define the particular couplings of interest. So in Fig. 2, having assigned one of the protons as H_1 and the other as H_2, the coupling constant may be written as

$$J_{1,2} = x \, \text{Hz}$$

The multiplicity of a coupling system depends essentially on two factors—the number of equivalent nuclei with which the nucleus of interest is coupling (n), and their spin quantum numbers (I). These two factors may be combined by the expression

$$\text{number of observed lines} = 2nI + 1$$

Thus in Fig. 2 for each proton, $n = 1$ and $I = \frac{1}{2}$ and there are, therefore, two lines. In the example CH_3—CH_2—X, where X is a functional group such that the chemical shifts of the methyl and methylene protons are very different, the multiplicity of observed lines is greater. For the methyl group, $n = 2$ and for the methylene group $n = 3$, so the methyl group is split into a triplet and the methylene group into a quartet (Fig. 3). Once again the spacings between the elements of the multiplets (coupling constants) are the same in both groups.

These splittings are explained by considering the factors that cause nuclei in different environments to resonate at different chemical shifts. One of these factors is that the magnetic field experienced by the nucleus is influenced by adjacent NMR-active nuclei. However, these adjacent nuclei can exist in different spin states, each of which has a slightly different modifying effect on the applied field. This is expressed diagrammatically in Fig. 4 for the ethyl group, the coupling system of which is shown in Fig. 3.

From this it can be seen that there are four possible types of spin arrangement for the protons of the methyl group and that the relative probabilities of the four spin arrangements are in the ratio $1:3:3:1$. Since each of these spin states results in a slightly different chemical shift for the methylene signal, this signal is then dispersed into four lines, the integrated intensities of which are also in the ratio $1:3:3:1$.

From Fig. 4, a similar explanation may be derived for the splitting of the signal due to the methyl group into three lines, the integrated intensities of which are theoretically in the ratio $1:2:1$. Provided the coupling constant remains the same for all nuclei concerned, the ideal relative intensities of the elements of a multiplet are in accordance with the coefficients of x in the binomial expansion $(1 + x)^n$ where n is the number of nuclei with which the nucleus is coupling. More conveniently the multiplet may be considered as lying symmetrically about the centre of the resonance band with the relative intensities of the lines in accordance with a Pascal triangle, i.e., $n = 0$, no split; $n = 1$, lines split 1–1; $n = 2$, lines split 1–2–1; $n = 3$, lines split 1–3–3–1, etc. The chemical shift of the resonance concerned is theoretically the centre of the multiplet.

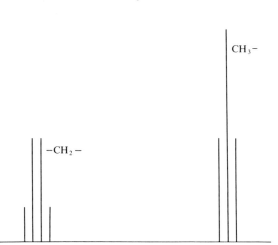

Fig. 3. Diagram of the proton spectrum of CH_3—CH_2—X showing spin-spin coupling.

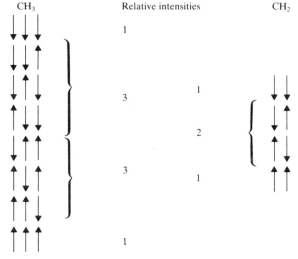

Fig. 4. Diagram of the spin states which give rise to spin-spin coupling between the protons of an ethyl group.

Spin-spin coupling does not usually occur between nuclei which are separated by more than three bonds, except in conjugated systems where couplings may be observed between nuclei separated by up to five bonds. The magnitude of the coupling constants in such 'long-range' systems is, however, very low. Thus, whereas coupling constants between protons on neighbouring carbon atoms of a freely-rotating hydrocarbon chain have values of about 6 to 7 Hz, the coupling constants between protons *para* to each other in a phenyl ring have values of about 0 to 1 Hz. Coupling constants between protons may be as high as 18 Hz for *gem*-protons or *trans*-olefinic protons. Much higher coupling constants, however, occur with other nuclei; for example values of up to about 80 Hz may be observed between protons and ^{19}F and up to about 200 Hz between protons and ^{13}C.

Coupling systems in which the number and relative intensities of observed lines are in accordance with that predicted from the principles outlined above are rarely obtained in practice. To obtain such a spectrum, it would be necessary for the difference in chemical shift of the two resonances to be at least ten times their coupling constant, i.e. for two sets of coupled, equivalent nuclei for which $J_{1,2} = 5$ Hz they should come to resonance with chemical shifts at least 50 Hz from each other. When this condition is satisfied the spectrum is described as first order. As the chemical shift difference becomes smaller, spectra gradually diverge from first order. This first becomes apparent when the integrated intensities of the lines of coupling systems show deviations from the predicted intensities. This is demonstrated for the methyl and methylene coupling system in an ethyl group in Fig. 5.

The inner lines of the coupling system increase in intensity at the expense of the outer lines. Thus, although the overall integrated intensities of the methyl and methylene groups retain their 3:2 ratio, the elements of the triplet and quartet do not retain their predicted values. This phenomenon is referred to as *roofing* and often assists in the interpretation of spectra containing several coupling systems. Since the elements of a coupling system tend to 'roof' towards each other it provides a means of identifying which groups of resonances are associated with each other. This loss of first order characteristics can therefore be of great advantage and in practice it is very rare to obtain spectra which do not show some evidence of roofing.

When the chemical shifts of nuclei are very close together, the number of lines observed often

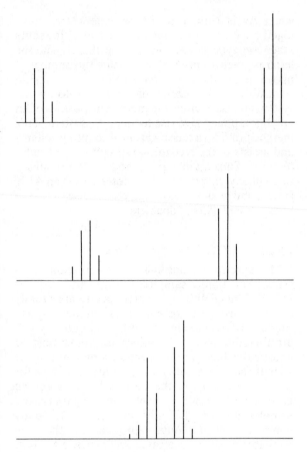

Fig. 5. Diagram of the spin-spin coupling between the protons of an ethyl group showing loss of first-order character as the ratio $\Delta v/J$ decreases.

becomes greater than expected which can cause considerable difficulties in interpretation. An advantage of using spectrometers with higher operating frequencies is that they are more likely to produce spectra of greater first order character. Finally, when the chemical shifts of the nuclei concerned are almost identical, the coupling system completely collapses, degenerating to a single line. Alternatively when a coupling system consists of more than two interacting groups, the overall multiplicity obtained is the sum of those expected from each coupling.

In order to define different types of spin system, the participating nuclei are designated letters of the alphabet such that when their chemical shift difference Δv is much greater than their coupling constant J the letters are widely separated and when Δv is similar to J, the letters are closer together. When more than one nucleus of the same magnetic type is responsible for the signal, the letter is given a subscript to indicate the number of nuclei. Thus the two *ortho* protons of a 1,2,3,4-tetrasubstituted benzene may give rise to an AB system and the methyl and methylene protons of an ethyl group may give rise to an A_2X_3 system. This method provides a classification of coupling systems and assists in the recognition of certain molecular features. Thus a vinyl group and a 1,2,4-trisubstituted phenyl ring may both be described as an ABX system and would be expected to give rise to twelve lines as three pairs of doublets.

PREPARATION OF SPECTRA

NMR spectra are normally prepared using solutions. For liquid samples the spectra may be recorded 'neat' although better spectra are usually obtained using a solvent since viscous liquids produce resonance signals with broad lines which are therefore less well resolved. Solvents must be chemically inert and exhibit minimal resonance signals (both in number and amplitude). Thus, for proton spectroscopy the ideal solvent might be carbon tetrachloride, its limitation being that many samples are insufficiently soluble in it. Many common solvents contain protons but they are available as their deuterated analogues, e.g. D_2O, $CDCl_3$, $(CD_3)_2CO$, etc.

One of the main drawbacks of NMR is its lack of sensitivity. For a continuous wave proton spectrum, about 0.25 to 0.5 ml of solution containing about 20 mg of sample is preferred, but this may be reduced to about 5 mg if the instrument is operated at its maximum sensitivity. Microcells are available which allow spectra to be acquired with only about 25 µl of solution and hence about 1 mg of sample.

Another technique for increasing sensitivity is by use of a Computer of Average Transients (CAT). This may be used to collect several scans of the spectrum of a sample and improves sensitivity because sample signals are accumulated whereas random noise signals are averaged. This, however, only leads to an increase of sensitivity equal to the square root of the number of scans. Since a single scan takes about five minutes it would therefore require about eight hours to gain a ten times increase in sensitivity. By using a CAT together with a microcell it is feasible to obtain a spectrum with 100 µg of sample.

The spectral accumulation approach is also used in Fourier Transform Spectrometers. In this case spectral data are collected far more rapidly and spectra may be obtained in a reasonable period of time from about 20 µg of sample. However, these instruments are much more expensive than continuous wave spectrometers although they may also be used to prepare ^{13}C spectra.

Sample solutions should be free from solid particles for maximum resolution and placed in glass sample tubes. For proton spectra, tubes of about 5 mm outside diameter are used, although for ^{13}C spectroscopy, tubes of wider bore are generally used to increase sensitivity. The tube is inserted between the poles of the magnet of the spectrometer and spun at about 30 Hz in order to average out any inhomogeneities of the applied field in different parts of the tube. Having selected suitable settings for the amplitude of the irradiating frequency and amplification of detected signals, the spectrum is recorded over a suitable sweep width using a scan speed of about 2 Hz per second.

Although NMR is relatively insensitive, it is also non-destructive and so valuable samples may be subsequently recovered for further experimental work.

INTERPRETATION OF SPECTRA

The following procedure provides a convenient method for the interpretation of proton spectra and it is useful to tabulate these data.

1. Determine the chemical shifts for each resonance.
2. Determine the relative numbers of protons responsible for each resonance from their integrated intensities.
3. Determine the multiplicities and coupling constants for each resonance.

From chemical shift tables it should be possible to identify possible functional groups that may be associated with the observed resonances. At this point, other analytical information becomes very useful e.g. the elements which are present and infrared or ultraviolet data, especially for functional groups. Using integrated intensities, multiplicities, and coupling constants, considerable information is provided on how the groups responsible for resonances fit in the molecule, relative to each other.

The use of this procedure is demonstrated for a simple example, benzocaine, the proton spectrum of which is shown in Fig. 6 and in Table 1.

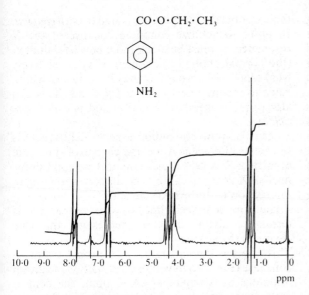

$CO \cdot O \cdot CH_2 \cdot CH_3$

NH_2

Fig. 6. PMR spectrum of benzocaine (10% solution in deuterochloroform).

Table 1. Data from proton magnetic resonance spectrum of benzocaine

Chemical shift δ ppm	Relative number of protons	Multiplicity	Coupling constants Hz
1.35	3	Triplet	7
4.15	Total of 4 for $\delta 4.15$ and	Very broad	—
4.36	$\delta 4.36$ signals	Quartet	7
6.68	2	Doublet with some fine coupling	9
7.90	2	Doublet with some fine coupling	9

A signal also appears at about $\delta 7.30$ ppm and this can be identified as an impurity since its integrated intensity corresponds to only about 0.2 protons. It is due to the proton of chloroform which is present as a trace impurity in the solvent, deuterochloroform ($CDCl_3$).

The $\delta 1.35$ ppm signal is assignable to the three methyl protons. In a straight-chain hydrocarbon, methyl protons would be expected to resonate at about $\delta 0.9$ ppm but the oxygen atom of the ester group β to the $-CH_3$ causes slight deshielding which would be expected to add about 0.4 ppm to the chemical shift. Furthermore, the integrated intensity of the signal corresponds to three protons and its multiplicity, a triplet with a coupling constant of 7 Hz, is consistent with the $-CH_3$ of an ethyl group.

The $\delta 4.36$ ppm signal is assignable to the two methylene protons. The methylene protons of a straight-chain hydrocarbon are expected to resonate at about $\delta 1.25$ ppm. However, oxygen has a very strong deshielding effect and a methylene group attached to the oxygen atom of an aromatic ester group is expected to show a signal at about $\delta 4.3$ ppm. When comparing calculated with observed chemical shifts, a fit to within 0.1 ppm is generally expected, but it may sometimes degenerate to ± 0.2 ppm when there are several substituents influencing the final result. Another cause of error occurs when the resonance is split into a multiplet. Here the true chemical shift is rarely at the centre of the multiplet as account must be taken of the 'roofing' effect so that the chemical shift is the 'centre of gravity' of the multiplet. The integrated intensity of the $\delta 4.36$ ppm signal corresponds to two protons and the multiplicity, a quartet with a coupling constant of 7 Hz, is consistent with the $-CH_2-$ of an ethyl group. This quartet and triplet pattern is typical of an A_2X_3 spin system in which the two methylene protons are the A_2 protons and the X_3 represents the three methyl protons.

The broad signal centred at about $\delta 4.15$ ppm, due to the two amino protons, is of interest. ^{14}N is an NMR-active nucleus for which $I = 1$. Using the formula of $(2nI + 1)$, this signal would be expected to be a triplet. However, like many other nuclei for which I is greater than $\frac{1}{2}$, ^{14}N possesses a quadrupole moment. This is capable of providing an efficient relaxation mechanism for this nucleus and the broad resonance observed represents the resulting collapse of the $^{14}N-^{1}H$ coupling. In many cases, this collapse is sufficient to provide a fairly sharp signal. The position of amino signals is very variable, probably being dependent on the basicity of the nitrogen, i.e. the greater the basicity, the more available are the lone pair of electrons for shielding the attached protons, so that the resonance is observed at higher fields. Typically, amino resonances are observed in the range $\delta 1$ ppm to $\delta 4$ ppm. In this case, therefore, the signal, at $\delta 4.15$ ppm is at a particularly low field. This is probably due to the electron-withdrawing effect of the *para* ester function on the lone pair of electrons on the nitrogen thus deshielding its attached protons.

The resonances at $\delta 6.68$ ppm and $\delta 7.90$ ppm are assignable to aromatic protons. The positions of aromatic protons are very strongly influenced by substituents. As a general rule, activating substituents lead to shielding, especially of the *ortho* and *para* protons, and therefore to chemical shifts at higher fields than $\delta 7.27$ ppm (the chemical shift of the protons of benzene) whereas, deactivating substituents lead to deshielding and chemical shifts at lower fields than $\delta 7.27$ ppm. Expected chemical shifts are calculated from the sum of the shielding or deshielding effects of all substituents. Thus, in this case, for each resonance we must take account of an *ortho* and *meta* substituent. For the protons on C_2 and C_6 there is an *ortho* ester group for which 0.75 ppm should be added and a *meta* amino group for which 0.25 ppm should be subtracted, leading to an expected value of $\delta 7.77$ ppm. For the protons on C_3 and C_5 there is an *ortho* amino group for which 0.75 ppm should be subtracted and a *meta* ester group for which 0.15 ppm should be added, leading to an expected value of $\delta 6.67$ ppm.

These calculations are generally expected to provide agreement with observed values to within about 0.2 ppm but variations may occur due to complex substituents and interactions between substituents. Since the protons on the aromatic ring resonate at different chemical shifts, the degeneracy of the signal is removed and coupling systems are set up which can exhibit long range coupling. For phenyl systems, the coupling constants are 7 to 10 Hz for *ortho* protons, 2 to 3 Hz for *meta* protons, and 0 to 1 Hz for *para* protons. In this case the coupling constant is 8.5 Hz and therefore characteristic of an *ortho* coupling as expected but showing some fine splitting. Thus although the pairs of protons on C_2 and C_6 and those on C_3 and C_5 are chemically equivalent it is incorrect to refer to this as an A_2B_2 system as this would show simply a pair of doublets with no fine coupling. It is more correct to consider this system as $AA'BB'$ to account for the weak *para* couplings.

It is often found that spectra cannot be readily interpreted due to complications that may arise because of, for instance, overlap of the coupling system of two or more resonances or multiplets caused by several couplings. Under these circumstances it is useful to simplify the spectrum in order to assist with interpretation, and there are various means available for this including spin decoupling techniques and the use of lanthanide shift reagents.

Spin Decoupling

An AX spin system is expected to show a pair of doublets (assuming that both A and X were nuclei for which $I = \frac{1}{2}$). If a second radiofrequency v_2 is then applied at the resonance frequency of nucleus A, the signal corresponding to X will collapse to a singlet. This process is called *spin decoupling* and in this example the X resonance is said to be *decoupled*. In order to achieve complete collapse of the X resonance, v_2 must be much more powerful than v_1 (the normal applied frequency). If v_2 is relatively weaker, partial decoupling may be achieved which leads to incompletely collapsed systems. This can also provide useful information and is called *spin tickling*.

Since v_2 is a powerful radiofrequency field, it causes *saturation* of nucleus A, i.e. the change of spin state of nucleus A is very rapid. Under these conditions, nucleus X does not exhibit signals corresponding to interaction with the two spin states of A but only a single time-averaged line is observed and this resonance signal therefore represents the true chemical shift of nucleus X.

This effect is demonstrated with propyl hydroxybenzoate (Fig. 7A) in which the α-methylene group resonates as a triplet at $\delta 4.32$ ppm, the central methylene group as a sextet centred at $\delta 1.84$ ppm, and the methyl group as a triplet at $\delta 1.00$ ppm. Irradiation of the $\delta 1.84$ ppm signal collapses both triplets to singlets (Fig. 7B). Irradiation of the $\delta 4.32$ ppm triplet collapses the $\delta 1.84$ ppm signal to a quartet (Fig. 7C) and this signal collapses to a triplet when the $\delta 1.00$ ppm resonance is irradiated (Fig. 7D). Irradiation of the $\delta 4.32$ ppm signal has no effect on the $\delta 1.00$ ppm triplet and vice versa (Fig. 7C and 7D, respectively).

Lanthanide Shift Reagents

If a paramagnetic metal complex is added to a sample the chemical shifts may be altered very significantly; certain lanthanide complexes can produce good shifted spectra without causing the unacceptable line broadening which is often observed when first row transition elements are used. Probably the lanthanide most used for this purpose is europium, usually in the form of a β-diketone complex such as tris(1,1,1,2,2,3,3-heptafluoro-7,7-dimethyloctan-4,5-dionato)europium (known as $Eu(FOD)_3$).

Lanthanide shift reagents are weak Lewis acids and, on addition to a substrate, are coordinated to basic sites. The ability of basic sites to coordinate decreases in the following order:

amines > hydroxyls > ketones > aldehydes > ethers > esters > nitriles

The shift reagent is added in incremental portions and the spectrum scanned after each addition. Coordination of the metal to basic sites is a reversible process and time-averaged chemical

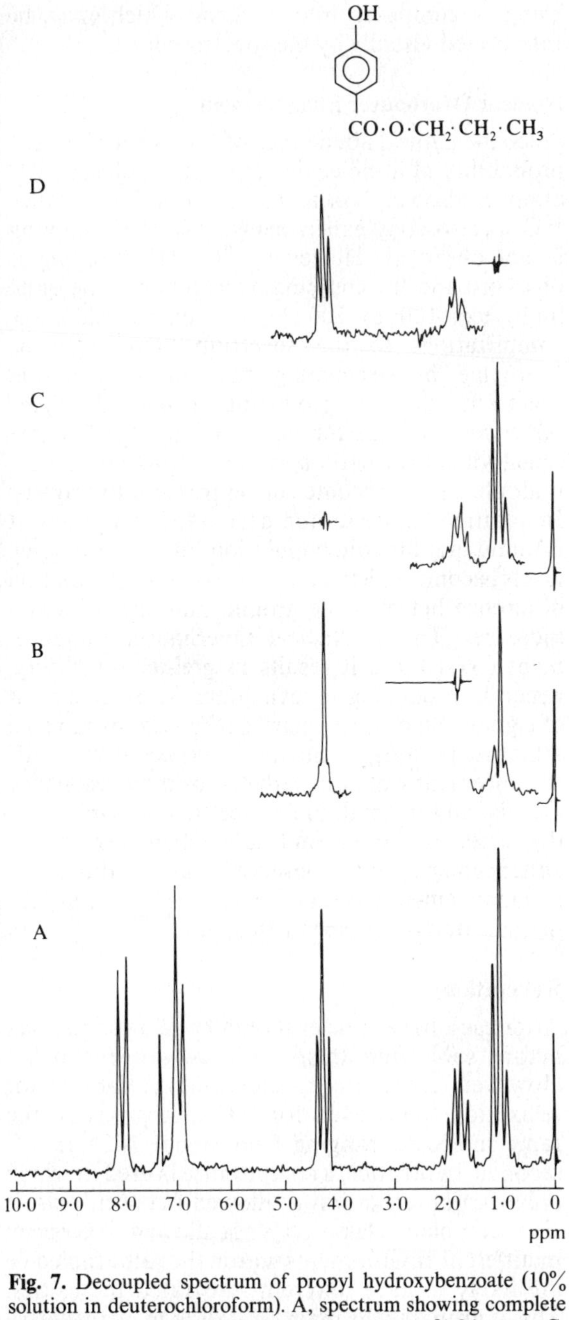

OH

CO·O·CH$_2$·CH$_2$·CH$_3$

D

C

B

A

space, to the metal ion (for pseudocontact shifts) are most affected, valuable information on structure may be established from the extent that resonance signals are shifted.

The effect of a shift reagent is demonstrated in Fig. 8 using 2-aminoheptane. Spectrum A is the proton spectrum of 2-aminoheptane before adding the shift reagent. It shows a broadened multiplet centred at about $\delta2.9$ ppm. This may be assigned to the methine proton on C_2 and should show as a sextet. It is probably broadened because of the proximity of the nitrogen atom. A clear methyl triplet is seen centred at $\delta1.0$ ppm which may be assigned to the protons on C_7 and the remaining 13 protons are in the broad resonance at $\delta1.1$ to $\delta1.5$ ppm.

After addition of 0.35 mole equivalents of Eu(FOD)$_3$, spectrum B is obtained. The C_2 methine proton has now shifted to $\delta7.8$ ppm but the outside lines of the sextet structure are very poorly resolved. The C_1 methyl doublet shows at $\delta5.3$ ppm but now

NH$_2$

CH$_3$ · **CH$_2$** · CH$_2$ · CH$_2$ · CH$_2$ · CH · CH$_3$

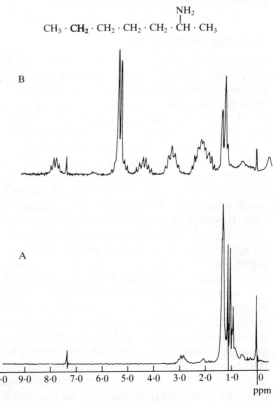

B

A

10·0 9·0 8·0 7·0 6·0 5·0 4·0 3·0 2·0 1·0 0
ppm

Fig. 8. Lanthanide-shifted spectrum of 2-aminoheptane (10% solution in deuterochloroform). A, before adding Eu(FOD)$_3$; B, after adding Eu(FOD)$_3$.

10·0 9·0 8·0 7·0 6·0 5·0 4·0 3·0 2·0 1·0 0
ppm

Fig. 7. Decoupled spectrum of propyl hydroxybenzoate (10% solution in deuterochloroform). A, spectrum showing complete couplings; B, decoupling frequency set at $\delta1.84$ ppm; C, decoupling frequency set at $\delta4.32$ ppm; D, decoupling frequency set at $\delta1.00$ ppm.

shifts are observed, the affected nuclei being shifted further on successive additions of reagent. Since nuclei which are closest, via bonds, to the coordination sites (for contact shifts) or closest, through

another sextet has become resolved centred at $\delta4.35$ ppm. The only other sextet normally expected for 2-aminoheptane would be due to the C_6 methylene protons but this resonance would not be expected to be so strongly influenced by the shift reagent. A more likely explanation is that this signal is due to the C_3 methylene group and that the presence of the large europium-containing molecule is preventing free rotation of this group so that the two methylene protons are not equivalent. Each proton therefore produces a separate signal, one at around $\delta4.3$ ppm and the other at around $\delta4.5$ ppm. These then couple as usual with the neighbouring methine and methylene protons on C_2 and C_4 and also with each other and this would be expected to provide a pair of overlapping quintets. The quintet centred at $\delta3.3$ ppm is almost certainly due to the C_4 methylene protons. The elements of this quintet appear rather broad and this could be due to slightly different coupling constants for the two couplings with the non-equivalent protons on C_3. The C_5 and C_6 methylene protons are not resolved from each other.

^{13}C SPECTROSCOPY

The most abundant isotope of carbon, ^{12}C, is a nucleus for which $I=0$ and it is therefore NMR-inactive. This is probably very desirable since if it were not the case, proton spectra would include C—H coupling, leading to very complicated coupling systems and making interpretation extremely difficult. However, ^{13}C is NMR-active ($I=\frac{1}{2}$).

Carbon spectroscopy has the problem of low sensitivity because the natural abundance of ^{13}C is only about 1.1%, the energy difference between the two spin states is very low, and relaxation times are long. However, the sensitivity problems have been overcome to a large extent by the development of pulsed spectrometers and by the introduction of stable wide-bore magnets which allow the use of wider sample tubes and thereby increase the amount of material being sampled between the poles of the magnet.

In a pulsed NMR experiment, the sample is irradiated with a strong, wide band radiofrequency pulse. As a result of this, all the nuclei precess with the Larmor frequencies characteristic of their environments generating a transverse magnetic field which decays exponentially. This is called *free induction decay* and contains all the information of a conventional frequency spectrum except that it requires conversion by Fourier transformation using a computer into a form which may be interpreted visually by the spectroscopist.

Nuclear Overhauser Enhancement

Since the natural abundance of ^{13}C is very low, the probability of a molecule containing adjacent ^{13}C atoms is also very low and so in natural abundance ^{13}C spectroscopy experiments, ^{13}C—^{13}C coupling is not observed. However, ^{13}C—^{1}H coupling is observed and the coupling constants may be quite high, e.g. 120 to 200 Hz, causing considerable complications to the spectrum. This may be overcome by decoupling the complete proton spectrum, thereby producing a *noise-decoupled spectrum*. This has the added advantage that the sensitivity of the carbon lines is improved because multiplets have become concentrated into singlets. In addition, under proton decoupled conditions, it is found that the spin populations of the ^{13}C energy levels become redistributed such that the population difference between the ground and excited states increases. This is Nuclear Overhauser Enhancement (NOE) and it results in greater sensitivity, generally producing about a threefold enhancement of signals. Since quaternary carbon atoms have no attached protons, it might be expected that this enhancement would be reduced in their resonance signals, and in small molecules this is found to be the case. In larger molecules, however, a full enhancement is often observed, but this difference in enhancement is one of the reasons for limitations in quantitative ^{13}C spectroscopy.

Relaxation

After each pulse, nuclei should be allowed to relax before subjecting them to a subsequent pulse. However, there are considerable variations for relaxation times even for ^{13}C atoms within the same molecule, ranging from about 10^{-2} to 10^3 seconds. In practice, a compromise is used in which only partial relaxation is allowed between pulses; since complete relaxation is not allowed, ^{13}C nuclei in different environments within the same molecule are likely to have different integrated intensities. This is probably the main limitation to quantitative ^{13}C spectroscopy.

Off-resonance Decoupling

Although proton coupling can cause considerable complications to the spectrum, it is often very helpful to have some information on ^{13}C—^{1}H couplings to assist interpretation. If the multiplicity of the coupling system is known, it is possible to identify the primary, secondary, tertiary, and quaternary ^{13}C atoms of the molecule. This is achieved by using off-resonance decoupling. Off-resonance decoupled spectra are produced by irradiating the sample at a frequency which is just outside the proton spectral range while acquiring the ^{13}C spectrum. Under these conditions, partial proton decoupling results so that multiplicities may be observed, but the spacings between the lines of multiplets are reduced. Protons which resonate closer to the decoupling frequency show greater reduction of these spacings, which also provides useful structural information.

Fig. 9A shows a fully noise-decoupled spectrum of pilocarpine nitrate. One feature of the noise-decoupled spectrum which makes ^{13}C spectroscopy so valuable is that each carbon atom of the sample gives a separate line. Unlike ^{1}H spectroscopy, overlap of resonance signals is less frequently observed because, whereas the chemical shift range for ^{1}H is about 10 ppm, the chemical shift range for ^{13}C is about 230 ppm. By making use of the multiplicities of the off-resonance decoupled spectrum (Fig. 9B) and taking account of shielding effects of functional groups, all the signals in the spectrum can be assigned (Table 2).

Table 2. Assignments of ^{13}C spectrum of pilocarpine nitrate

Chemical shift relative to TMS δ ppm	Multiplicity	Assignment carbon number
14.2	quartet	11
20.6	triplet	10
23.5	triplet	5
36.1	quartet	1
38.8	doublet	6
47.2	doublet	9
73.9	triplet	7
119.5	doublet	3
135.1	singlet	4
137.9	doublet	2
184.6	singlet	8

APPLICATIONS

Nuclear magnetic resonance spectroscopy is complementary to infra-red and ultraviolet spectrophotometry, and mass spectrometry, as a method for identification of drugs. Infra-red and ultraviolet spectrophotometry are used to identify functional groups but NMR is mainly used to study the molecular structure around the functional groups. Differences in chemical shifts are often due to the influence of the substituents on their surrounding hydrocarbon skeleton and, by studying coupling systems, much valuable information is obtained on how the various parts of this skeleton fit together.

Drug Metabolism Studies

The concentration of metabolites in samples of body fluids is usually low but, in spite of its low sensitivity, NMR has made a valuable contribution to the study of drug metabolism.

However, conjugation reactions, especially glucuronide formation, have not been studied as much as other routes of metabolism, mainly because of the poor solubility of these conjugates in commonly used solvents. Aromatic and aliphatic hydroxylations are processes which are very common during the metabolism of drugs and NMR can often provide a means of identifying the position of the hydroxyl group on a molecule by analysing the coupling systems of the remaining aromatic protons thus revealing the substitution pattern of the metabolite.

This is illustrated in a study of 4-chlorobiphenyl, which produced two metabolites. They were shown by mass spectrometry to contain one and two phenolic groups, respectively, and NMR was used to determine their positions. In one case the aromatic protons appeared as four sets of doublets with the same coupling constants, which is typical of an *ortho* coupling, and one metabolite was

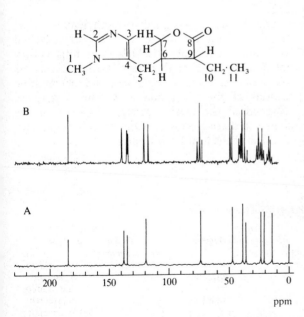

Fig. 9. ^{13}C spectrum of pilocarpine nitrate (10% solution in deuterium oxide). A, fully noise-decoupled; B, off-resonance noise-decoupled.

therefore identified as 4'-chlorobiphenyl-4-ol. The other metabolite contained two hydroxyl groups and gave a signal due to a proton indicating an *ortho* coupling, another signal due to a proton indicating a *meta* coupling, and a third signal due to a proton indicating an *ortho* and a *meta* coupling. This helped to identify the second metabolite as 4'-chlorobiphenyl-3,4-diol (S. Safe *et al.*, *J. Chem. Soc.*, *Perkin Transactions I*, 1976, 357–359).

Identification

Nuclear magnetic resonance spectroscopy can be used to distinguish between the phosphate esters of steroids. The free steroids can be distinguished by infra-red spectrophotometry, but the phosphate esters are sufficiently polar to give rise to absorption bands that dominate the IR spectra and make distinction difficult. The NMR spectra of these steroid esters are not subject to this interference, and although they may be very difficult to interpret, they do provide the necessary distinction.

A similar situation arises in the case of the aminoglycoside antibiotics framycetin sulphate, kanamycin sulphate and acid sulphate, gentamicin sulphate, and tobramycin. Their infra-red spectra are dominated by hydroxyl and amino absorptions of the amino sugar and, except for tobramycin, by sulphate absorptions. The proton spectra however contain sufficient differences to distinguish them.

Determination of Water Content

NMR may also be used as a test for the water content of a drug such as cloprostenol, since water shows a resonance signal at $\delta4.72$ ppm. However, cloprostenol contains three hydroxyl groups and when the spectrum is recorded in deuterium oxide, the protons of these hydroxyl groups rapidly exchange with deuterium of the solvent and therefore contribute to this $\delta4.72$ ppm resonance.

To compensate for this contribution the olefinic resonances are used as an internal standard. Cloprostenol possesses four olefinic protons, two from the 5-*cis*-olefin and two from the 13-*trans*-olefin which give rise to an overlapping multiplet between $\delta5.2$ and $\delta5.8$ ppm. The integrated intensity of this multiplet is equivalent to four protons and so by subtracting 0.75 of this value from the integrated intensity of the $\delta4.72$ ppm peak the three hydroxyl groups are accounted for and the remainder is due to water.

Forensic Applications

NMR has become established as a useful tool in forensic science and some references to this application are cited in the Bibliography.

An example of the use of NMR in forensic science is the identification of four 5-ethyl-5-alkyl substituted barbiturates, butobarbitone, pentobarbitone, secbutobarbitone, and amylobarbitone. The proton spectra of all four barbiturates show a very broad signal at around $\delta8$ ppm to $\delta10$ ppm which is characteristic of amido protons. The useful region of the spectrum for the differentiation of these barbiturates lies between $\delta0.5$ and $\delta2.5$ ppm due to the substituents on C_5. There are three groups of multiplets in this region and the data for these groups for the four barbiturates are presented in Table 3.

Group 1 may be assigned to methylene and (or) methine protons on carbon atoms directly attached to C_5 and are the most deshielded protons as they are β to two carbonyl groups. Group 2 may be assigned to the central methylene and (or) methine protons of the alkyl chains. Group 3 may be assigned to the methyl groups. Analysis of the signals in these groups provides unequivocal identification of the four barbiturates.

Table 3. Data from NMR spectra of barbiturates

	Group 1 $\delta1.6$ ppm to $\delta2.5$ ppm		Group 2 $\delta1.2$ ppm to $\delta1.6$ ppm		Group 3 $\delta0.5$ ppm to $\delta1.2$ ppm	
	Relative number of protons	Multiplicity	Relative number of protons	Multiplicity	Relative number of protons	Multiplicity
Butobarbitone	4	skewed quartet	4	multiplet	6	triplet with fine coupling
Pentobarbitone	3	quartet	4	multiplet	9	quartet with fine coupling
Secbutobarbitone	3	quartet	2	multiplet	9	quartet with fine coupling
Amylobarbitone	4	skewed quartet	3	multiplet	9	triplet

Bibliography

S. Alm et al., The use of ^{13}C NMR Spectroscopy in Forensic Drug Analysis, *Forens. Sci. Int.*, 1982, *19*, 271–280.

British Pharmacopoeia, Vols I and II, London, HMSO, 1980 (Identification of Steroid Esters and the Examination of Aminoglycoside Antibiotics).

British Pharmacopoeia (Veterinary), London, HMSO, 1977 (Determination of Water in Cloprostenol Sodium).

I.C. Calder, The Applications of Nuclear Magnetic Resonance Spectroscopy in Drug Metabolism, in *Progress in Drug Metabolism*, Vol. 3, J.W. Bridges and L.F. Chasseaud (Ed.), Chichester, Wiley, 1979, pp. 303–340.

A.F. Cockerill et al., Lanthanide Shift Reagents for Nuclear Magnetic Resonance Spectroscopy, *Chem. Rev.*, 1973, *73*, 553–588.

T.C. Kram, Analysis of Illicit Drug Exhibits by Hydrogen-1 Nuclear Magnetic Resonance Spectroscopy, *J. forens. Sci.*, 1978, *23*, 456–469.

Nuclear Magnetic Resonance for Organic Chemists, D.W. Mathieson (Ed.), London, Academic Press, 1967.

R.T. Parfitt, Nuclear Magnetic Resonance Spectroscopy, in *Practical Pharmaceutical Chemistry*, Part 2, A.H. Beckett and J.B. Stenlake (Ed.), 3rd Edn, London, Athlone Press, 1976, pp. 361–416.

F.W. Wehrli and T. Wirthlin, *Interpretation of Carbon-13 NMR Spectra*, Chichester, Heyden, 1976.

Pharmacokinetics, Metabolism, and the Interpretation of Results

W. J. Tilstone and A. H. Stead

In order to interpret the analytical results in a toxicological investigation, it is necessary to have a knowledge of drug disposition and metabolism. A variety of questions may be put to the toxicologist, including 'What drug was taken?', 'What was its dose?', 'By which route and when was it taken?', 'Was the observed pharmacological response a result of chronic or acute exposure to the drug?', and 'Can the response be explained in terms of the drug concentration found?'. A knowledge of the aspects of anatomy and physiology which determine the absorption, distribution, and elimination of drugs from the body, together with an understanding of drug metabolism, will allow these questions to be answered with a fair degree of confidence.

Basic Concepts of Pharmacokinetics

The onset, duration, and intensity of action of a drug after administration are controlled by the rate at which the drug reaches its site of action and by the concentration of the drug at the receptor. The physiological disposition of a drug is controlled by the three major processes of absorption, distribution into and within tissues, and elimination. Pharmacokinetics is a mathematical consideration of these processes which relates the dose given, the concentration in the blood, and the pharmacological response.

Most drugs given by intravenous injection or by mouth will give blood (or plasma) concentration-time curves of the type shown in Fig. 1A and Fig. 1B, respectively. Following intravenous administration, there is a rapid decrease in plasma-drug concentration in the early period (α-phase) when distribution is the major process, followed by a slower, constant rate of decrease in the elimination phase (β-phase). After oral administration, plasma concentrations initially increase whilst the drug is being absorbed and then decrease when elimination becomes the major process.

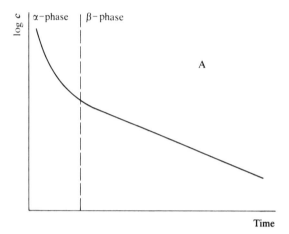

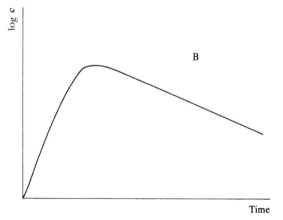

Fig. 1. Typical semilogarithmic plots of plasma concentration (c) versus time for a drug given A, by intravenous injection, and B, orally. The terminal rate of decline of plasma concentrations is the same irrespective of the route of administration.

ABSORPTION

To produce an effect, a drug must first enter the blood stream and be carried to the target organ. With the exception of intravenous injection, the first process is that of absorption, either from the gastro-intestinal tract, from an injection site, or

276

from the lungs. The route of administration is an important factor in determining the rate and extent of absorption. For example, absorption after an oral dose can be relatively slow and erratic, whilst absorption from the lungs is usually fast because of the good blood supply. Most drugs are administered orally, and an understanding of the mechanism of absorption by this route is by far the most important for the toxicologist.

Absorption from the Gastro-intestinal Tract

The traditional way of describing drug absorption is by the pH-partition hypothesis. This hypothesis regards the passage of a drug into the blood as being by passive diffusion of non-ionised molecules across the lipoid barrier of the cells of the gut lining and into the blood. Complex factors control the release of a drug from a pharmaceutical preparation, but apart from this the hypothesis is an over-simplification because the gastro-intestinal wall is not a single lipoid membrane but rather a layer of cells.

According to the hypothesis, an acid drug such as aspirin (pK_a 3.5) is absorbed in the stomach at about pH 2 when the drug is non-ionised. The drug diffuses passively across a single barrier into the capillaries and is taken up by the plasma at pH 7.4. Here, it ionises and is therefore unable to return to the stomach because there is a net concentration gradient of 25 000 to 1, stomach to plasma, of the non-ionised species. In practice, aspirin is not totally absorbed in the stomach due to the poor blood supply and small surface area. Basic drugs such as ephedrine (pK_a 9.6) are only slightly absorbed in the stomach, the major part being absorbed from the upper section of the small intestine (pH 5 to 7), the lower section (pH 7 to 8), or from the colon (pH 7 to 8).

However, contrary to the hypothesis, the absorption of ionised species also occurs. For example, paraquat is highly ionised but appears to be absorbed slowly from the gastro-intestinal tract throughout its length and over a considerable period of time from the moment of ingestion. Poisoning with such compounds can be treated effectively by the prompt administration of an oral adsorbent which prevents further absorption of the drug.

Absorption generally depends very much on the large difference in drug concentration between the gastro-intestinal tract and the blood. A knowledge of the blood flow to the different parts of the gastro-intestinal tract and of the pH of its contents is therefore important. These factors, together with the surface areas available for absorption and the gastro-intestinal transit times are shown in Fig. 2. Absorption is possible throughout the gastro-intestinal tract, from stomach to rectum, although the major site is the upper small intestine. This has high peristalsis, a high surface area, high blood flow, and optimal pH for the absorption of most drugs, all of which result in a high absorption rate. Drug absorption tends to be much less rapid from other parts of the tract.

Bioavailability

The extent to which a drug is absorbed from its site of administration into the systemic circulation is known as its (absolute or systemic) bioavailability (F). It is determined experimentally from the ratio

$$F = \frac{\text{AUC (extravascular)}}{\text{AUC (intravenous)}}$$

where AUC (the area under the plasma concentration–time curve) represents the amount of drug entering the systemic circulation during t_0 to t_∞ for a single dose, or at steady state, within a given dose interval. The bioavailability is simply the fraction of the drug dose which is absorbed intact by any given route compared with intravenous administration, which gives the equivalent of 100% absorption. Although absolute bioavailability requires reference to an intravenous standard, the relative bioavailabilities of formulations can be determined using other routes of administration. The effects of the first passage of a drug through the liver (first-pass metabolism) are explained on p. 281.

Enterohepatic Circulation

Drugs and metabolites which are eliminated from the liver into the bile subsequently pass into the lumen of the gastro-intestinal tract. Such compounds, usually of relatively high molecular weight (>500), and containing a hydrophilic residue in the molecule (e.g. digitoxin), may then be reabsorbed either directly or indirectly following further metabolism. This recycling of drugs is known as enterohepatic circulation. Glucuronide conjugates of drugs which are excreted in significant amounts in the bile, such as morphine, may be hydrolysed by the intestinal microflora and reabsorbed. Enterohepatic circulation thus prolongs the persistence of a drug in the body and may lead to delayed toxicity, or to toxicity arising from the absorption of a drug metabolite produced by intestinal bacteria. Drugs which undergo enterohepatic circulation may be detected in the faeces in unchanged form even if they have been administered by a parenteral route.

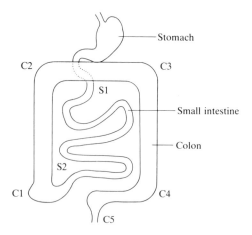

Organ	pH	Surface area	Blood flow*	Motility and transit time of contents
Stomach†	1–3	<5 m²	Rises on stimulation of gastric secretions	Relatively 'quiet'. Transit time of contents depends on their chemical and physical nature, including pH and osmotic pressure. Placed in order of increasing transit times, liquids < solids; carbohydrates < proteins < fats. Times vary from 0.5 h for a small amount of liquid carbohydrate to 20 h for a large fatty meal.
Small intestine, S	S1, 5–7 S2, 7–8	200 m²	Very fast counter-current flow in villi. Blood transit time— 1 s after meals; 5 s resting; 30 s in shock	Food churned, and propelled by very active movements in waves, by both peristalsis and by segmentation. Transit time—about 2 h.
Colon, C	7–8	<5 m²	Average	Residues of meals found at C1 after 4 h, C2 after 6 h, C3 after 9 h, and C4 after 12 h. Residues are held up in the rectum (C5) and then egested in faeces over a period of time. Earliest traces may be egested within 6 h, the last may take 1 week. On average 75% of residues are egested by the 3rd day.

*Average is 36 ml/min per 100 g intestine, 50–75% of which circulates in the mucosal layers
† The volume of the stomach can change markedly: 50 ml during fasting and up to 2 litres when full

Fig. 2. Factors which influence the passage and absorption of drugs in the gastro-intestinal tract.

DISTRIBUTION

After a drug has been absorbed, i.e. after it has passed from the gastro-intestinal tract, through the liver, and into the systemic circulation, it is then distributed throughout the body. Distribution depends on a number of factors. These include the blood flow to the tissues, the partition coefficient of the drug between blood and the tissue, the degree of ionisation of the drug at the pH of plasma, the molecular size of the drug, and the extent of tissue and plasma protein binding. For example, the distribution of plasma protein-bound drugs such as the warfarin-type anticoagulants is restricted to plasma and extracellular fluid, whereas alcohol distributes equally into the total body water.
The approximate volumes of the body water

compartments for a person of average weight are: intracellular water 25 litres and extracellular water 17 litres (of which 3 litres is plasma water). An intravenous dose of a drug which is distributed immediately into the total body water (approximately 42 litres) would give an initial plasma concentration (dose divided by 42) approximately two-fifths of that obtained if the same dose was distributed only into extracellular water (dose divided by 17). If the drug is extensively bound to tissue proteins, an even lower initial plasma concentration would be obtained, and the volume term relating the dose to the plasma concentration could exceed the volume of the body. The approximate proportions of weights and water contents of the various body tissues are given in Tables 1 and 2.

Table 1. Comparison of weights of tissues and water content in the average adult male

	% Body weight	% Water
Muscle	40	76
Fat	10	10
Liver	2.5	68
Brain	2	75
Lungs	0.7	79
Kidneys	0.4	83

Table 2. Total body water

	% Body weight	
Age	Male	Female
10–18	59	57
18–40	61	51
40–60	55	47
>60	52	46

Volume of Distribution

A full description of drug distribution can be complex, whether it is based on a knowledge of tissue perfusion and partition of drug from plasma to tissue, or whether it is based on a kinetic analysis of plasma concentration–time curves. One of the major descriptive parameters, which is probably of most interest to the toxicologist, is the volume of distribution (V_d). This is the amount of drug in the body (A) divided by the plasma concentration (c) after distribution equilibrium has been established,

$$V_d = \frac{A}{c}$$

The drug concentration in body fluids other than plasma may be used, e.g. whole blood, but different values for V_d are obtained for each; it is extremely important, therefore, to note which fluid is being used. In the monographs in Part 2, volumes of distribution, unless otherwise stated, are based on plasma concentrations.

The value of the volume of distribution is determined mainly by the physiological processes of perfusion and protein binding, but it seldom has a true physiological meaning. For example, the volume of distribution of frusemide, a drug which is highly bound to plasma albumin, is of the order of 15 litres, and that of alcohol is about 35 litres; however, the value for digoxin, which is extensively distributed and bound in extravascular tissues, is of the order of 450 litres.

After distribution equilibrium has been established, a knowledge of the volume of distribution allows the amount of drug in the body to be estimated from a single measured blood concentration

$$A = V_d c$$

If the time elapsed since drug administration (t) is known, together with some pharmacokinetic data for the drug, then it should be possible to estimate the original dose (D) of the drug. Thus, for a drug given by intravenous injection,

$$D = V_d c \, e^{k_{el} t}$$

where k_{el} is the elimination rate constant (see p. 281). However, if the drug is given orally, a much more complex relationship applies. It is necessary to know the bioavailability (F), and the absorption rate constant (k_a). Then the dose is given by the expression

$$D = \frac{V_d c (k_a - k_{el})}{F k_a} \cdot \frac{1}{e^{-k_{el} t} - e^{-k_a t}}$$

If a drug were distributed instantaneously throughout the body, then the volume of distribution would be constant at all times and the decrease in plasma concentration could be attributed solely to elimination of the drug. However, in practice there is a rapid initial decrease in plasma concentration largely due to distribution of the drug into the tissues. This distribution phase (α-phase) lasts approximately 30 minutes to 2 hours for most drugs. During this phase, although the total amount of drug in the body remains virtually constant, the volume of distribution changes continually. It only remains constant when the decrease in plasma concentration is due only to elimination because distribution is complete. The elimination phase (β-phase) is characterised by a slower decline in plasma concentration which is accompanied by a parallel decline in tissue concentrations.

It is generally assumed that absorption, metabolism, and elimination follow first-order kinetics, i.e. the rate at which the process proceeds is dependent solely on the concentration of the drug. Occasionally, the rate is limited by saturation of the body's capacity to process the drug. An increase in the drug concentration does not affect the rate in such cases and the process is said to follow zero-order kinetics.

When it is assumed that the equilibrium between concentrations of the drug throughout the body and plasma is attained instantaneously, the body is regarded as a single homogeneous entity. The use of this one-compartmental model of the body (and assuming first-order kinetics) simplifies the mathematics involved in describing the pharmacokinetics of a drug. When distribution is not instantaneous throughout the body, more complex multi-compartmental models are required to describe adequately the fate of the drug. Fig. 1A illustrates a biphasic plasma concentration–time curve and it would be appropriate to use the two-compartmental model of the body in this case. In general, only highly perfused tissues such as the liver and kidneys have tissue drug concentrations in instantaneous equilibrium with those in plasma. Distribution of a drug into and out of poorly perfused tissues such as muscle and fat is discernible in the plasma concentration–time curve of the drug, and requires a separate compartment for adequate pharmacokinetic treatment. Less frequently, further subdivision into rapidly- and slowly-distributing tissues is also required.

Evaluation of the volume of distribution becomes difficult in the case of a drug which requires a model with two or more compartments to describe its disposition. One method of determining the final volume of distribution is to extrapolate the terminal linear part of a semilogarithmic plot of plasma concentration–time to the point $t = 0$, but this treatment yields an inaccurate figure. One of the best ways to determine the volume of distribution when the drug is in the β-phase (V_β) is to use the relationship

$$V_\beta = \frac{D}{\beta \int_{t=0}^{\infty} c \cdot dt}$$

where β is the terminal elimination rate constant. This expression, sometimes known as V_{area}, may be used to relate plasma-drug concentration to the amount of drug in the body for a two-compartmental drug which is in the β-phase, or indeed at any time for the one-compartmental model when β is replaced by the elimination rate constant k_{el} in the above expression.

Distribution of Drugs to Tissues

The instantaneous equilibrium of drug concentrations throughout the body as considered above does not necessarily require that the concentrations are equal throughout the body. In fact, drug concentrations in tissues are rarely equal to those in plasma. For example, the tissue : plasma concentration ratio will be very low immediately following intravenous administration. As time progresses, the amount of drug in the tissue compartment will increase and,

like that in the plasma compartment, will eventually reach a plateau. If the drug is actively stored in a particular tissue compartment, then the ultimate concentration ratio between the tissue and plasma will be relatively high. It should also be noted that the tissue : plasma concentration ratio depends not only on the processes of distribution, but also to a large extent on the route of drug administration, and on whether single or multiple doses have been given.

ELIMINATION

Most drugs are eliminated from the body by metabolism in the liver and/or by excretion of the drug and its metabolites by the kidneys. However, metabolism and elimination by other tissues such as the lungs may occur, as well as excretion of drugs and metabolites in the bile.

Clearance

The elimination of drugs from the body can be described quantitatively using the concept of clearance, and this can be related to physiological events.

Overall, the efficiency of elimination by an organ can be expressed as the proportion of drug entering the organ which is eliminated from the plasma in a single passage; this is called the *extraction ratio*. The other major factor which controls the overall ability of an organ to remove drug from the body is the rate of delivery of the drug (i.e. blood flow) to the organ. Drug elimination can be represented as the product of this rate of delivery and the extraction ratio. This product gives the volume of plasma from which drug is completely removed per unit time and is given the name clearance (Cl). Clearances by different organs are additive. Although the reference fluid normally used is plasma, whole blood may also be used.

In the monographs in Part 2, clearance has been included where possible and usually refers to the total plasma clearance (or total whole blood clearance) after intravenous administration. In some instances, the total clearance calculated after oral administration has been included if the drug is known to be well absorbed and is not subject to significant first-pass metabolism.

The concept of clearance has found particular application in clinical work as it offers a simple relationship between dose rate (dose divided by the time interval between doses, D/τ), and the average plasma concentration ($\bar{c}$) of the drug

$$\bar{c} = \frac{D/\tau}{Cl}$$

The efficiency of an eliminating organ in removing drug from plasma depends on the health of the organ. Thus, diseased kidneys operate less efficiently, and the net change in clearance is proportional to the extent of renal impairment.

Despite its clinical utility, the concept of clearance has certain limitations for the forensic toxicologist because it does not give an immediate indication of the persistence of a drug in the body. For example, although gentamicin and digoxin have similar clearances (about 100 ml/min), digoxin will stay in the body much longer than gentamicin. This is because the volume of distribution of digoxin is several times that of gentamicin, and there is therefore a much greater volume of fluid from which the drug must be cleared before it is all eliminated. It is therefore of some advantage to the toxicologist to be able to relate clearance to the persistence of a drug in the body. This can be done by expressing clearance as a fractional clearance, i.e. clearance divided by the volume of distribution. Fractional clearance (Cl/V_d) has the dimension reciprocal time and represents the proportion of drug removed from the body per unit time, i.e. it is a first-order rate constant for drug elimination (k_{el}). This rate constant is given by the gradient of the terminal part of the concentration–time curves shown in Fig. 1.

Half-life

The half-life of a drug $(t_{1/2})$ is the time required for plasma concentrations to decline by 50%, provided that elimination occurs by a first-order process (Fig. 3). It is related to the elimination rate constant (k_{el}) by the equation

$$t_{1/2} = \frac{0.693}{k_{el}}$$

The half-life of a drug provides a measure of the rate of irreversible drug loss from the blood. If the dose is known, the half-life of a drug can be used together with information on the volume of distribution, and bioavailability where necessary, to estimate the time elapsed since administration. Conversely, if the elapsed time is known, the half-life can be used to estimate the drug dose. The half-life is a function of both volume of distribution and clearance, the proportion of drug elimination in unit time depending on both the extent of its distribution and on the efficiency of its elimination.

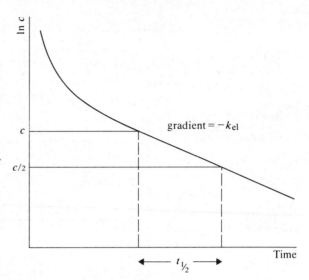

Fig. 3. Plot of natural logarithm of plasma drug concentration (ln c) versus time (t) following intravenous administration. The gradient of the linear part of the curve is equal to the elimination rate constant (k_{el}).

Thus the half-life of a drug may differ between children and adults because of size and weight, even though the clearances are equivalent.

Elimination by the Liver

The principal pathways of drug elimination involving the liver are shown in Fig. 4. The drug may enter the liver from the general circulation via the hepatic artery (approximately 300 ml of blood per minute), or via the portal vein (approximately 1000 ml of blood per minute) from the gastro-intestinal tract. The concentration of drug in the hepatic artery during the absorption phase can be several orders of magnitude less than that in the portal vein. Drugs in the liver are immediately exposed to the metabolic enzyme systems. Thus, drugs which are absorbed from the gastro-intestinal tract into the portal vein may undergo metabolism in the liver before reaching the general circulation. The effect is known as *first-pass metabolism*. It results in a low and extremely variable fraction of an oral dose reaching the systemic circulation. First-pass metabolism is responsible for much of the inter- and intra-individual variations in blood concentrations and in the pharmacological responses observed for many drugs of clinical and forensic interest (e.g. aspirin, dextropropoxyphene, imipramine, morphine, paracetamol, and propranolol).

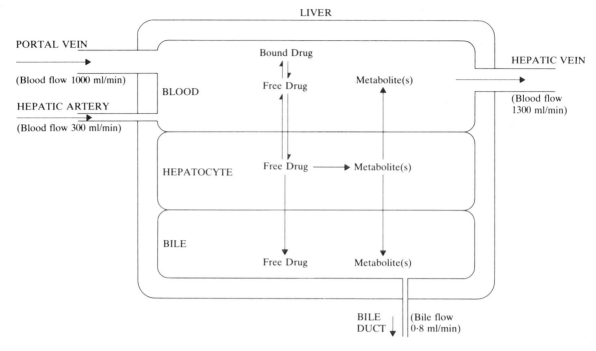

Fig. 4. Drug elimination by the liver.

Drugs are removed from the liver as metabolites or as unchanged drug, either by biliary secretion (flow rate approximately 0.8 ml/min), or in the hepatic vein (approximately 1300 ml of blood per minute). Some drugs and metabolites, e.g. morphine glucuronide, are excreted in the bile in high concentrations.

Elimination by the Kidneys

The significant factors in renal drug elimination are shown in Fig. 5. The drug is brought to the kidneys with a total plasma flow for both kidneys of approximately 1400 ml/min. The plasma is filtered at the rate of 125 ml/min in the glomeruli, which are the principal site of excretion. Filtration is passive and only non-protein-bound drug in the plasma is eliminated by this pathway. A considerable amount of filtered drug may be reabsorbed into the plasma by diffusion back across the tubule wall (which is permeable to non-ionised, lipid-soluble species). This is because the drug concentration in the filtrate in the lower parts of the tubule is higher than that in the plasma. The filtrate (125 ml/min) is gradually concentrated as it passes down the tubule to give a final production of urine of about 1 ml/min. About 575 ml/min of plasma circulates in intimate contact with the proximal and distal renal tubules.

The renal tubule may contribute to elimination by active secretion, and in such cases protein-bound drug may also be eliminated from the plasma.

The extent of elimination by the kidneys can be extremely variable depending on which of the three processes of filtration, secretion, or reabsorption predominates for the drug in question. Thus, procainamide is eliminated partly by metabolism and partly as unchanged drug through the kidney. Its renal clearance is of the order of 450 ml/min, indicating major involvement of tubular secretion. By contrast, digoxin has a renal clearance of about 120 ml/min, and this could be explained by either filtration alone, or by the fact that secretion is balanced by reabsorption. In practice, it is known that filtration accounts for almost all of the renal clearance of digoxin. A further example is methaqualone, which has a renal clearance of about 1 ml/min, clearly indicating extensive reabsorption of filtered drug.

The principal factor which determines the variability in the rate of drug excretion into the urine, other than organ function and blood flow, is the pH of the urine. Only non-ionised species are available

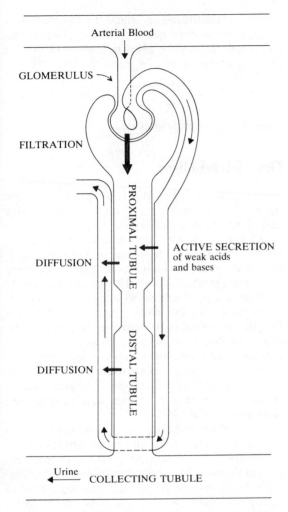

Arterial Blood

GLOMERULUS

FILTRATION

PROXIMAL TUBULE

DIFFUSION

ACTIVE SECRETION
of weak acids
and bases

DISTAL TUBULE

DIFFUSION

Urine

COLLECTING TUBULE

Fig. 5. Drug elimination by the kidneys. Schematic diagram of a nephron to illustrate the sites of filtration, diffusion, and active secretion of drugs.

for reabsorption by the tubules along the concentration gradient. Thus, acidic drugs (e.g. barbiturates, salicylates) are excreted more rapidly at high pH than basic drugs (e.g. amphetamines). Conversely, basic drugs are excreted more rapidly at low pH. For example, about 85% of a dose of aspirin is excreted as free salicylic acid in alkaline urine, but only about 5% is excreted when the urine is acidic. Conversely, about 75% of a dose of amphetamine is excreted unchanged in acidic urine but less than 5% if the urine is alkaline.

The effect of varying urinary pH has been used in the treatment of drug overdose by applying forced alkaline diuresis as an adjunct to the treatment of salicylate or phenobarbitone poisoning. The success of the treatment is limited by the extent to which these drugs are distributed, and by the presence of alternative pathways of elimination. There is a general limitation to the success of treating an overdose by increasing drug clearance because a highly-distributed drug will have a relatively long half-life; any increase in clearance will not make much difference to its persistence.

Persons who abuse amphetamines have used the effect of urinary pH on excretion by simultaneously ingesting bicarbonate. This produces an alkaline urine which delays elimination of the amphetamine and therefore prolongs its stimulant effect. Conversely, substances which acidify urine have been taken by athletes to enhance elimination of amphetamine-like stimulants in the hope of avoiding detection in routine dope-screening procedures. Exercise in itself can also decrease urinary pH and thus increase the renal clearance of basic drugs. Where pH is known to have a significant effect on the disposition and elimination of a drug, this has been noted in the monographs in Part 2.

Despite these complications, there is in general a relationship between the concentration of a drug in plasma, its plasma clearance, and its excretion rate by any particular mechanism. The relationship is one of simple proportion, in that the excretion rate is equal to the product of the plasma concentration and the renal clearance. The higher the plasma concentration and the greater the clearance by a particular mechanism, the greater will be the excretion rate of a drug by that mechanism. Thus, the quantity of drug in a urine sample is the product of the renal clearance of the drug, the average plasma concentration of the drug during the interval that the urine was produced, and the duration of that interval. This relationship is one of the fundamental principles of pharmacokinetics, and shows that if a drug has a constant renal clearance, there is no direct relationship between the plasma concentration and the urine concentration because urinary flow rate must also be considered. However, for drugs which are extensively reabsorbed, renal clearance may not be constant but will tend to vary with the urine flow. In these cases, there is a relationship between the concentration in urine and the concentration in plasma.

In general, the interpretation of urine data in terms of plasma concentrations is a difficult procedure. An approximate working relationship can be determined because the daily urine output is usually fairly constant at about 1500 ml per day (1 ml/min), in healthy adults. Under these circumstances, the amount of drug in a urine sample collected over a short interval will be equal to the product of the renal clearance of the drug and its average concentration in plasma during that interval. If the renal clearance is known, the approximate plasma concentration can be calculated from the urine concentration (or vice versa). As most drugs normally have a renal clearance greater than 1 ml/min, average drug concentrations in urine for any time interval will exceed those in plasma. For such drugs, urine is a relatively good sample for drug screening procedures. However, for drugs which are eliminated very rapidly, the mean plasma concentration over a day would be negligible. The mean urine concentration would also be low, and the collection of urine over 24 hours would be pointless.

If the renal clearance of a drug varies with urine flow, as with an extensively reabsorbed neutral drug such as methaqualone, then there may be a random sequence of positive and negative findings during the analysis of consecutive urine samples.

In view of these difficulties, the interpretation of analytical data from urine samples alone should not be attempted unless urine is the only fluid available and there is some other information which will allow an estimate of the dose to be made.

Drug Accumulation

Drugs accumulate in plasma or tissues if more than one dose is administered and the interval between doses is less than the time taken to eliminate the previous dose. Under these circumstances, there will also be a change in the shapes of the plasma concentration–time and the tissue concentration–time curves. In all cases, accumulation is controlled by the size of the dose, the dose interval, and the first-order elimination rate constant for loss of drug from the body (k_{el}). The problems of drug accumulation are of particular interest to the toxicologist because the resulting high drug concentrations may lead to a progressive and insidious toxicity.

The extent to which a drug will accumulate in multiple dosing can be estimated. After each successive dose, the maximum, minimum, and average plasma concentrations will be higher than those for the previous dose. This is so in the early stages, but since drug elimination is a first-order rate process, the total amount of drug in the body will increase until the amount eliminated during a dose interval equals the amount taken in (total injected dose or the net absorbed dose after oral dosing). At this so-called *steady state*, the average

plasma concentration is equal to the dose rate divided by the clearance of the drug. The accumulation ratio relates the average amount of drug in the body at steady state (A_{ss}) and the dose (D)

$$\frac{A_{ss}}{D} = \frac{1.44\,t_{1/2}}{\tau}$$

where τ is the dosage interval.

Drug Metabolism

Metabolism is an integral part of drug elimination. As well as facilitating excretion of a drug, it may also affect the pharmacological response of a drug by altering its potency and/or duration of action. When a lipid-insoluble, polar, or ionised drug is absorbed into the body it is largely excreted unchanged by the kidneys. However, the majority of drugs are lipid-soluble to some extent and are reabsorbed into the blood from the glomerular filtrate. They need to be converted to a more polar (water-soluble) form before they can be excreted in the urine. Such compounds often undergo extensive metabolism. Metabolites are usually excreted in the urine although large proportions of the glucuronides of some drugs (e.g. morphine and codeine) are eliminated in the bile.

Although the metabolic process is usually regarded as one of detoxification, this is not always so and metabolites which are more toxic than the parent drug are known. Metabolites may be pharmacologically inactive (e.g. the hydroxylated derivative of phenobarbitone) or they may be active with different pharmacokinetic properties but similar modes of action to the parent drug. This is the case with many psychotropic drugs. For example, hydroxylation and demethylation of the tranquilliser diazepam gives the metabolites temazepam and oxazepam, both of which are also marketed as drugs in their own right. Similarly, amitriptyline, a tricyclic antidepressant, is demethylated to yield another antidepressant, nortriptyline. Active metabolites may also have different modes of action or different potencies; thus dealkylation of the antidepressant drug iproniazid gives the tuberculostatic drug isoniazid, while the anticonvulsant drug primidone is metabolised to phenobarbitone, another anticonvulsant which has a much longer duration of action.

Pathways of drug metabolism are conventionally divided into two groups, non-synthetic and synthetic. The *non-synthetic routes* are principally oxidation (including hydroxylation, *N*- and *O*-dealkylation, and sulphoxide formation) and to a lesser extent reduction and hydrolysis. These are generally referred to as Phase I reactions. The *synthetic routes* mainly involve conjugation with glucuronic acid, but acetylation, methylation, and conjugation with amino acids and sulphate also occur. These are usually referred to as Phase II reactions. Phase II reactions remove or mask functional groups (e.g. amino, carboxyl, hydroxyl, sulphydryl, etc.) on the drug or Phase I metabolite by the addition of an endogenous substrate. In this way Phase I and Phase II reactions are frequently associated with each other, although this is by no means a prerequisite. The major Phase II reaction is conjugation of glucuronic acid with the phenolic or alcoholic hydroxyl groups which are common products of Phase I reactions. Conjugation reactions usually result in a reduction of toxicity and can therefore be referred to as genuine detoxification mechanisms.

Despite the extensive range of reactions which a drug molecule can undergo, the majority are catalysed by microsomal membrane-bound enzymes in the hepatocytes (parenchymal cells of the liver). For example, the cytochrome P-450 mixed function oxidase system which catalyses oxidations, and glucuronyl transferase, the enzyme responsible for conjugation with glucuronic acid, are both located on microsomal membranes. However, some metabolic pathways employ non-microsomal enzymes or those which are not bound to membranes. For example, oxidative deamination of a number of drugs is performed by monoamine oxidases which are widely distributed in the mitochondria; acetylation, an important metabolic pathway for some drugs, is carried out by the non membrane-bound acetyltransferase found in intracellular fluids. Metabolism can occur in tissues other than the liver; the gastro-intestinal tract, kidneys, and lungs may have a significant effect on the metabolism of a drug depending on its route of administration. For example, many metabolic reactions occur in the gastro-intestinal tract before an orally-administered drug is absorbed, carried out by enzymes in the mucosal lining or by microflora. Most of these reactions involve reduction and hydrolysis because of the anaerobic environment. Plasma esterases cause extensive hydrolysis of drugs such as cocaine and procaine.

An individual drug may be extensively metabolised, and may undergo several completely different reactions. Thus, chlorpromazine gives rise to at least twenty metabolites by its three major routes of metabolism, i.e. hydroxylation, *N*-demethylation, and sulphoxidation. Fortunately, such complicated patterns of metabolism are not a major problem to the analyst since most metabolites occur only in very small amounts.

Using drugs principally of forensic interest, a number of examples are given below to illustrate the variety of metabolic routes which can be followed in man and the effects that these might have on disposition and pharmacological activity. The list is not intended to be exhaustive with regard to either the pathways or the drugs covered. Oxidation reactions are emphasised as these occur most frequently, yielding metabolites which are commonly conjugated before excretion.

Oxidation Reactions

All the major oxidative mechanisms can be illustrated by considering the metabolism of the barbiturates, benzodiazepines, amphetamines, tricyclic antidepressants, phenothiazines, and opiates.

BARBITURATES

The barbiturates are derivatives of barbituric acid and have the general structure given below. The nitrogen atom at position 1 may be methylated. Substitution of sulphur for oxygen at position 2 gives the thiobarbiturates.

The barbiturates can be metabolised by five major routes: (1) hydroxylation of alkyl and aryl substituents at C_5 (e.g. pentobarbitone and phenobarbitone); (2) *N*-dealkylation at the N^1-position (e.g. methohexitone); (3) oxidation of alkyl groups at C_5 to give carboxylic acids (e.g. thiopentone); (4) desulphuration at C_2 (e.g. thiopentone); and (5) oxidative ring fission at the 1:6 position (e.g. amylobarbitone).

The major metabolic pathway of the 5,5-disubstituted barbiturates is hydroxylation, usually of the larger of the two substituents, e.g. the phenyl group in phenobarbitone, the 1-methylbutyl group in pentobarbitone, and the alicyclic group in cyclobarbitone. Hydroxylation of aliphatic groups at the C_5 position is usually at the $\omega-1$ (penultimate) position, giving oxygenated products which are further oxidised to ketones. Hydroxylation of aliphatic groups at the ω position can also occur, usually giving products which undergo further oxidation to the corresponding carboxylic acid. With the exception of 3'-hydroxyamylobarbitone, all hydroxylated metabolites have little or no hypnotic activity. Desulphuration to the ketone and N-dealkylation are general routes of metabolism of thiobarbiturates and N-alkyl barbiturates, respectively; both reactions occur to a variable extent. Ring fission of barbiturates to give substituted malonylureas appears to be only a minor reaction.

Most barbiturates are extensively metabolised; for example, less than 5% of a dose of amylobarbitone, quinalbarbitone, or pentobarbitone is excreted unchanged in urine. However, with phenobarbitone (the least lipid-soluble of the common barbiturates) about 25% of a dose is excreted unchanged, and the highly water-soluble barbitone is excreted almost entirely unchanged.

The metabolism of amylobarbitone is illustrated below; $\omega - 1$ hydroxylation is the major metabolic reaction producing 3'-hydroxyamylobarbitone which can be detected in urine five days after administration of a 100-mg dose. This is in contrast to the unchanged drug which can only be detected

for the first two to three days. Practically none of the hydroxy metabolite is excreted as the glucuronide or other conjugate.

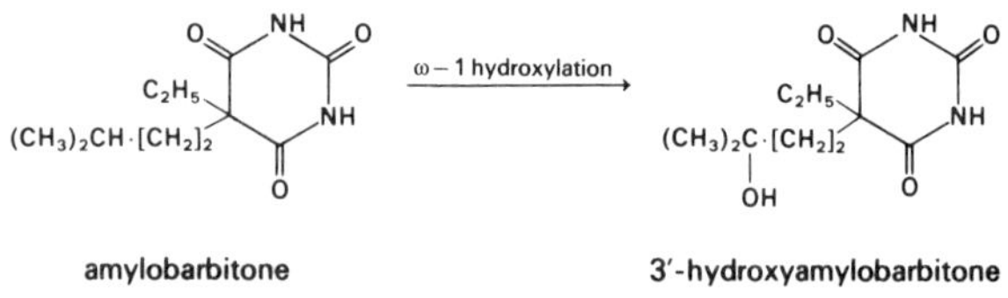

amylobarbitone   3'-hydroxyamylobarbitone

Hexobarbitone illustrates a variety of the metabolic transformations which the barbiturates undergo, including 1:6 ring fission (see below).

BENZODIAZEPINES

The benzodiazepines, one of the most widely prescribed groups of drugs, undergo extensive metabolism by routes already described for the barbiturates, namely N-dealkylation and hydroxylation. However, unlike the barbiturates, metabolic conversion yields derivatives which have similar pharmacological activities and potencies to those of the parent compounds. For example, the three major metabolites of diazepam are desmethyldiazepam (nordazepam), 3-hydroxydiazepam (temazepam), and desmethyl-3-hydroxydiazepam

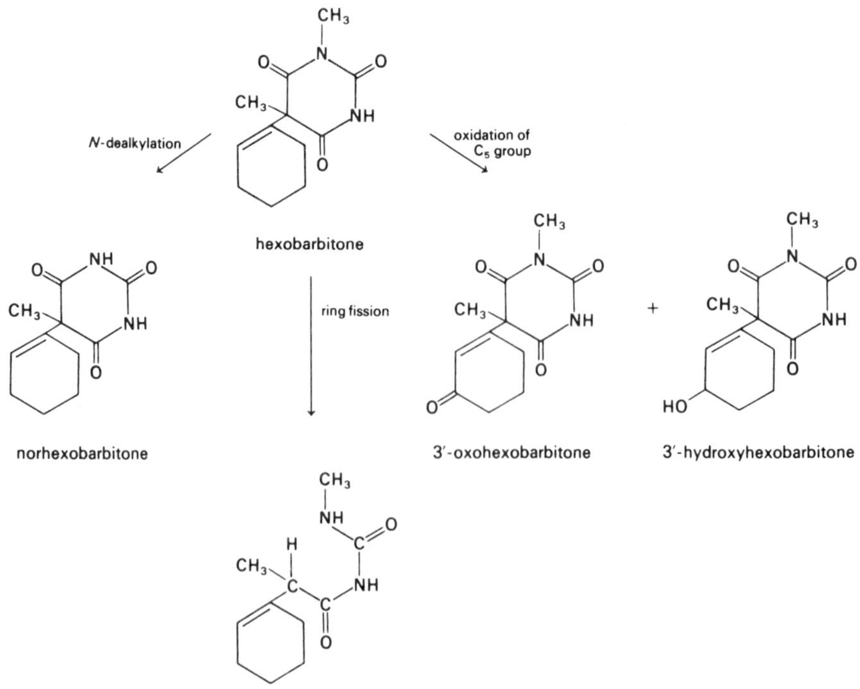

norhexobarbitone   hexobarbitone   3'-oxohexobarbitone   +   3'-hydroxyhexobarbitone

medazepam $\xrightarrow{\text{oxidation}}$ diazepam

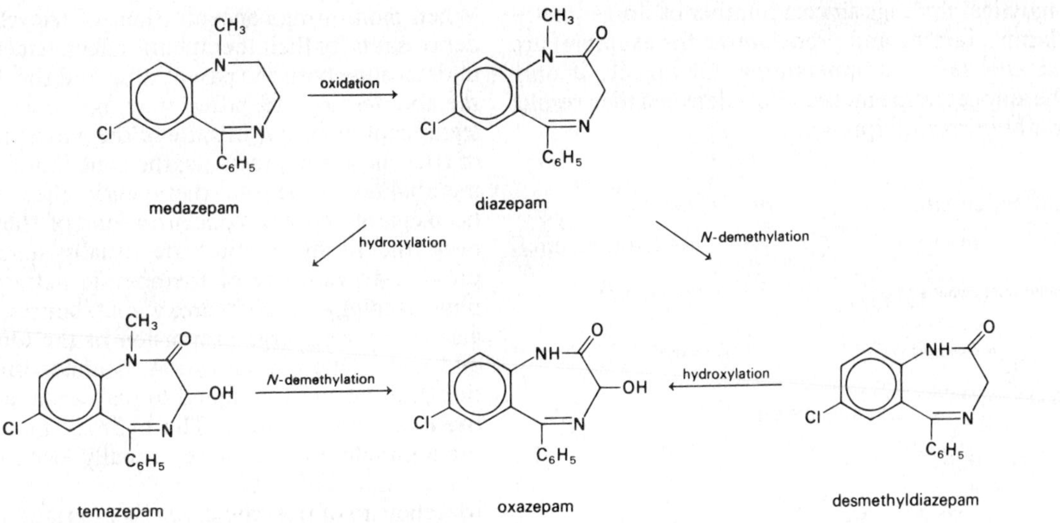

hydroxylation   N-demethylation

temazepam $\xrightarrow{\text{N-demethylation}}$ oxazepam $\xleftarrow{\text{hydroxylation}}$ desmethyldiazepam

(oxazepam), the hydroxylated derivatives being marketed as drugs in their own right. Diazepam itself is a metabolite of another benzodiazepine, medazepam.

After chronic administration of diazepam, i.e. at steady state, plasma concentrations of desmethyldiazepam (the major metabolite in blood) are similar to those of diazepam. The hydroxylated metabolites of the benzodiazepines, together with benzodiazepines which have an hydroxyl group at the C_3 position (e.g. lorazepam), are conjugated with glucuronic acid and it is these derivatives which account for the major fraction of the dose excreted in the urine.

AMPHETAMINES

Amphetamines can be metabolised by (1) oxidative deamination followed by oxidation or reduction of the ketone and conjugation of the resulting acid and alcohol products; (2) N-oxidation; (3) hydroxylation of the aromatic ring and of the alkyl side-chain at the β-position; and (4) N-dealkylation.

Amphetamine is converted by oxidative deamination to phenylacetone which is further oxidised to benzoic acid; this latter product is excreted as its glycine conjugate, hippuric acid.

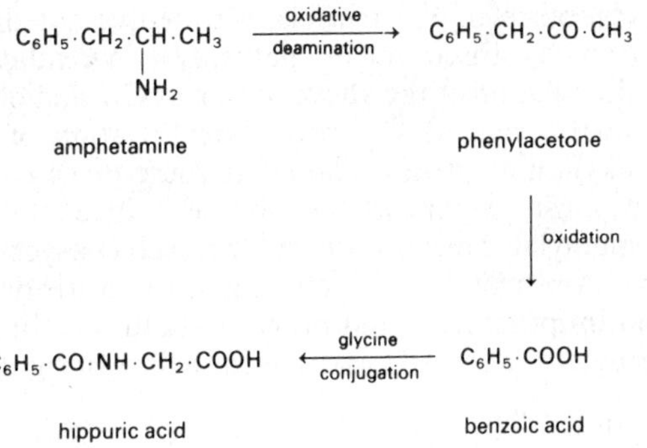

Although reduction of ketones is possible, it does not seem to be a very important route of metabolism in man. Oxidative deamination (following N-dealkylation where appropriate) appears to be the major pathway for those drugs which are extensively metabolised. N-Oxidation of amphetamines gives rise to hydroxylamines and nitro derivatives,

$$C_6H_5 \cdot CH_2 \cdot CH \cdot CH_3 \quad \xrightarrow[\text{deamination}]{\text{oxidative}} \quad C_6H_5 \cdot CH_2 \cdot CO \cdot CH_3$$
$$| $$
$$NH_2$$

amphetamine   phenylacetone

oxidation

$$C_6H_5 \cdot CO \cdot NH \cdot CH_2 \cdot COOH \quad \xleftarrow[\text{conjugation}]{\text{glycine}} \quad C_6H_5 \cdot COOH$$

hippuric acid   benzoic acid

but these products are rarely excreted in the urine in large quantities; hydroxylamines are generally excreted as conjugates or as free and conjugated oximes after further rearrangement of the molecule.

Aromatic hydroxylation to yield phenolic derivatives varies with different amphetamines. For some (e.g. methylamphetamine) it is a relatively important route of metabolism (accounting for up to 15% of the dose excreted) whereas for others (e.g. fenfluramine and amphetamine) it is insignificant. β-Hydroxylation of the alkyl side-chain accounts for only a relatively small proportion of the total metabolism of most amphetamines; less than 5% of amphetamine is excreted as norephedrine (phenylpropanolamine).

The extent of N-dealkylation of phenethylamine drugs may be important in the interpretation of analytical findings since a number of drugs (methylamphetamine and prenylamine for example) are metabolised to amphetamine. Obviously, if only the amphetamine metabolite is detected then results might be misinterpreted.

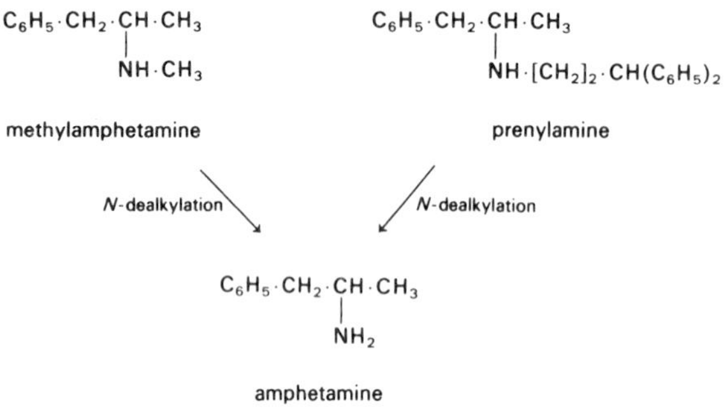

$C_6H_5 \cdot CH_2 \cdot CH \cdot CH_3$
|
$NH \cdot CH_3$

methylamphetamine

$C_6H_5 \cdot CH_2 \cdot CH \cdot CH_3$
|
$NH \cdot [CH_2]_2 \cdot CH(C_6H_5)_2$

prenylamine

N-dealkylation   *N*-dealkylation

$C_6H_5 \cdot CH_2 \cdot CH \cdot CH_3$
|
NH_2

amphetamine

TRICYCLIC ANTIDEPRESSANTS

Metabolism of the tricyclic antidepressant drugs occurs by three major pathways: *N*-oxidation, hydroxylation of the alicyclic ring at C_{10} and of the aromatic ring at C_2, and *N*-dealkylation of the dialkylamino group. The latter route gives rise to the most important metabolites since the *N*-demethylated metabolites are themselves psychoactive. Amitriptyline is metabolised to nortriptyline, and imipramine to desipramine, both metabolites being used clinically as drugs in their own right.

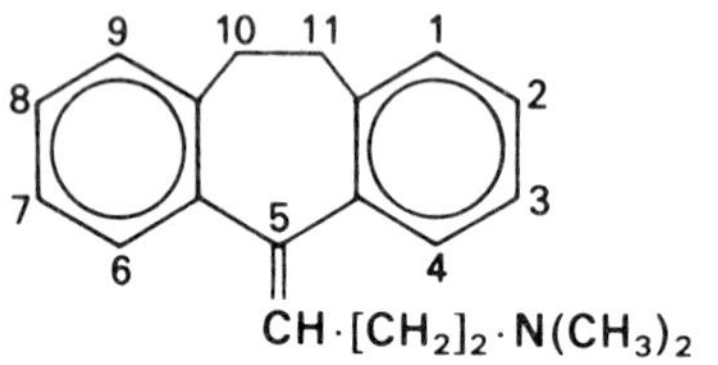

$CH \cdot [CH_2]_2 \cdot N(CH_3)_2$

amitriptyline

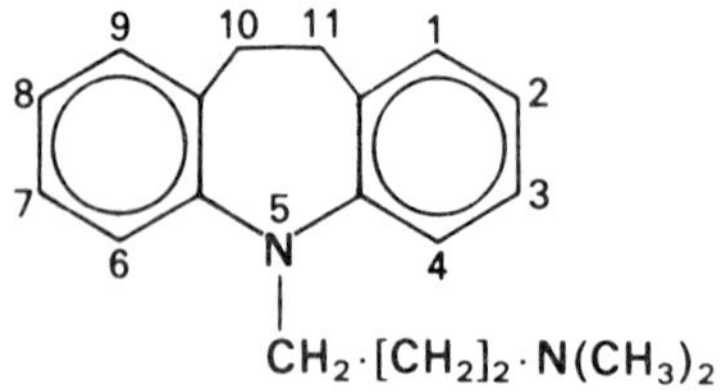

$CH_2 \cdot [CH_2]_2 \cdot N(CH_3)_2$

imipramine

When monitoring concentrations of tricyclic antidepressants for their therapeutic effect, it is essential to determine both the parent drug and the desalkyl metabolites as the latter may be present in a significant quantity. In spite of the widespread use of tricyclic antidepressants, the contribution of the metabolites to the total therapeutic effect has not been quantified and concentrations of the parent drug and its metabolites are usually summed to provide an estimate of therapeutic activity. The pharmacology of 10-hydroxy metabolites, which also make up a large proportion of the total drug and metabolite concentration, is under investigation and they may be found to play a major role in the total clinical effect. The hydroxy metabolites predominate in the urine, usually occurring as glucuronide conjugates.

Metabolism of tricyclic drugs by aromatic hydroxylation and *N*-oxidation is of minor importance.

PHENOTHIAZINES

The phenothiazines have the general formula

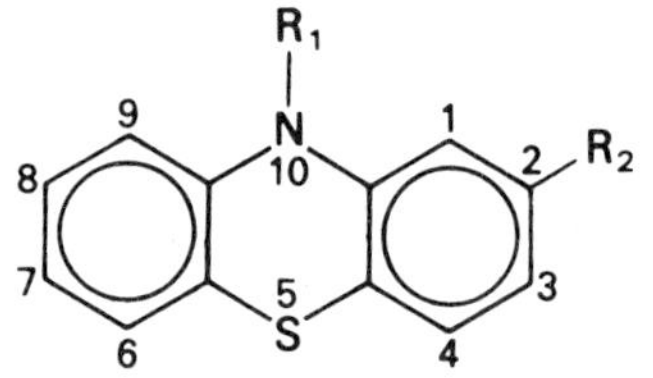

They provide examples of drugs which undergo sulphoxidation to yield sulphoxides and sulphones. In addition, *N*-oxidation (at the N^{10}-position), hydroxylation of one or both of the aromatic rings, *N*-dealkylation of the N^{10}-side-chain, and fission of the N^{10}-side-chain may also occur. The phenolic metabolites are then conjugated with glucuronic acid or sulphate; the metabolites are excreted in both the urine and the bile.

The number of different metabolic routes which are possible results in a complex mixture of metabolites for many phenothiazines. For example, many of the drugs which contain an *NN*-dimethylaminoalkyl side-chain (e.g. chlorpromazine) are extensively metabolised by *N*-oxidation, together with hydroxylation, sulphoxidation, and *N*-dealkylation.

OPIATES

The opiates are metabolised by a wide variety of pathways even within a single compound. These include hydrolysis followed by conjugation, *O*-dealkylation, as well as the more common *N*-

Chlorpromazine – Major Metabolic Routes

dealkylation. Thus diamorphine (heroin) is rapidly hydrolysed in the body to 6-monoacetylmorphine, which is further and more slowly hydrolysed to morphine. The morphine so formed is excreted

largely as the 3-glucuronide together with some free morphine.

Morphine may also be metabolised by N-demethylation to normorphine. Alkylation to produce codeine (the 3-O-methyl derivative) has also been suggested but more recent work indicates that codeine arises due to the presence of codeine or acetylcodeine as contaminants in morphine or illicit diamorphine preparations. Codeine can be metabolised by the reverse reaction, O-demethylation, to yield morphine, as well as by conjugation with glucuronic acid and N-demethylation.

Reduction Reactions

Aldehydes and ketones undergo reduction to primary and secondary alcohols (e.g. chloral is converted to trichloroethanol and prednisone is reduced to prednisolone).

$$CCl_3 \cdot CHO \xrightarrow{\text{reduction}} CCl_3 \cdot CH_2OH$$

chloral   trichloroethanol

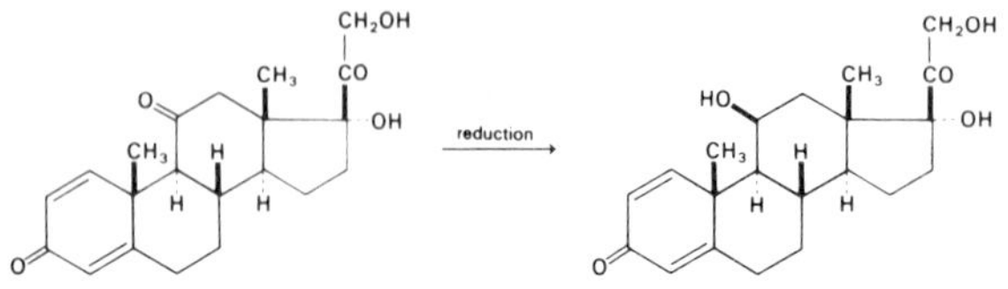

prednisone   prednisolone

Nitro and azo compounds are reduced to amines (e.g. nitrofurantoin is reduced to its amino derivative and sulphasalazine is reduced to sulphapyridine).

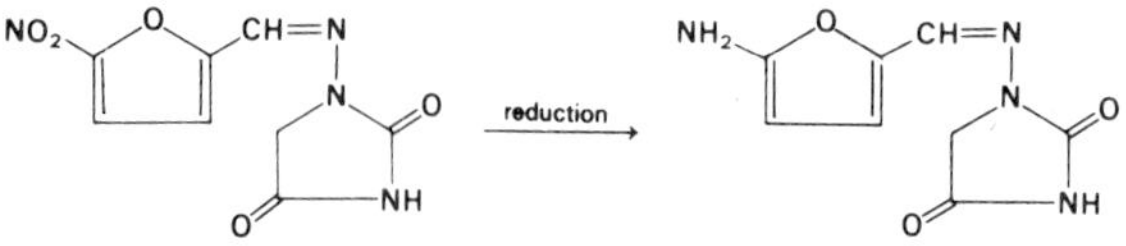

nitrofurantoin   aminonitrofurantoin

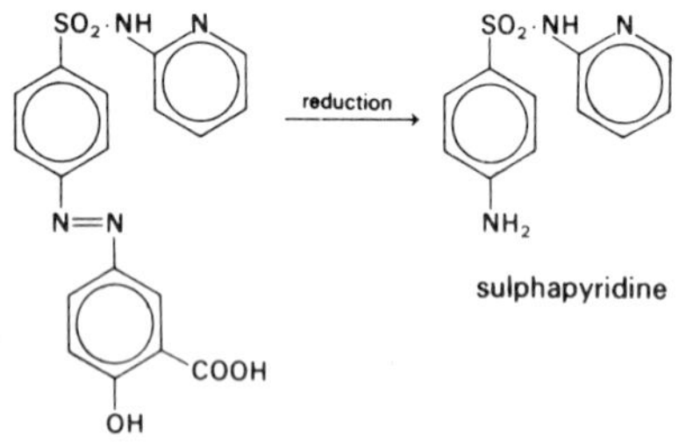

sulphapyridine

sulphasalazine

Another example is the reduction of disulphides to thiols (e.g. disulfiram is converted to diethyldithiocarbamic acid).

$$(C_2H_5)_2N \cdot CS \cdot S \cdot S \cdot CS \cdot N(C_2H_5)_2 \xrightarrow{\text{reduction}} (C_2H_5)_2N \cdot CS \cdot SH$$

disulfiram   diethyldithiocarbamic acid

Hydrolysis

Hydrolysis is an important route of metabolism for esters, amides, carbamates, and acyl hydrazines. Aspirin is rapidly converted to salicylic acid; this may be further metabolised to gentisic acid (5-hydroxysalicylic acid), conjugated with glucuronic acid or glycine, or excreted unchanged.

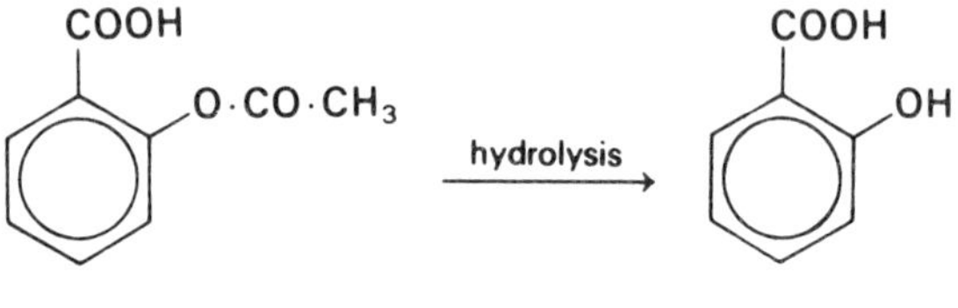

aspirin   salicylic acid

Procaine is hydrolysed by plasma esterases to 4-aminobenzoic acid and diethylaminoethanol.

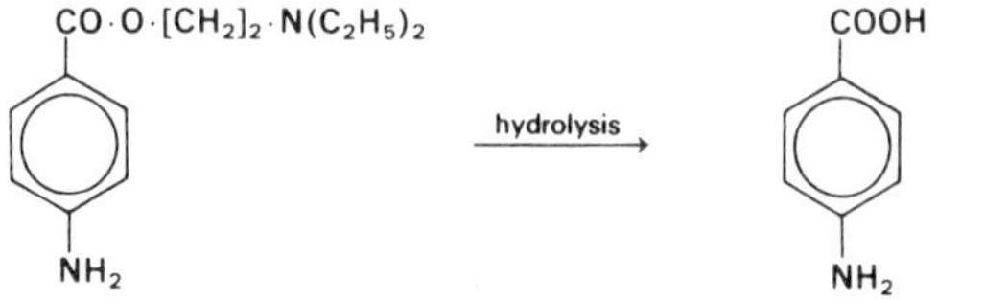

procaine   4-aminobenzoic acid

Hydrolysis of isoniazid gives isonicotinic acid which is further metabolised to its glycine conjugate.

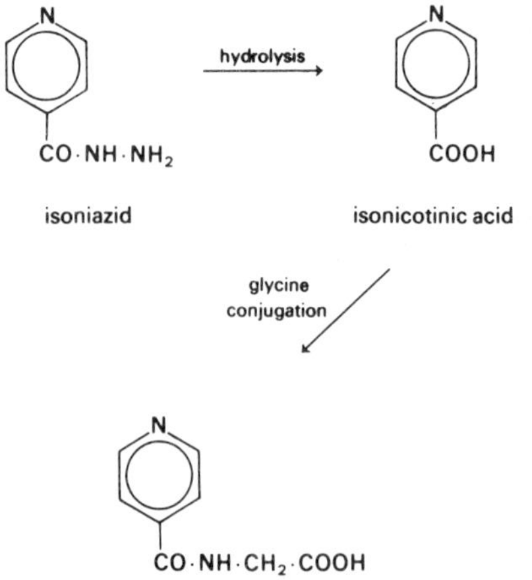

isoniazid   isonicotinic acid

glycine conjugate of isonicotinic acid

The major pathway for chlordiazepoxide metabolism involves hydrolysis of the 2-methylamino substituent to yield the lactam derivative, demoxepam. This is excreted in the urine unchanged or undergoes further cleavage to the corresponding acid before excretion.

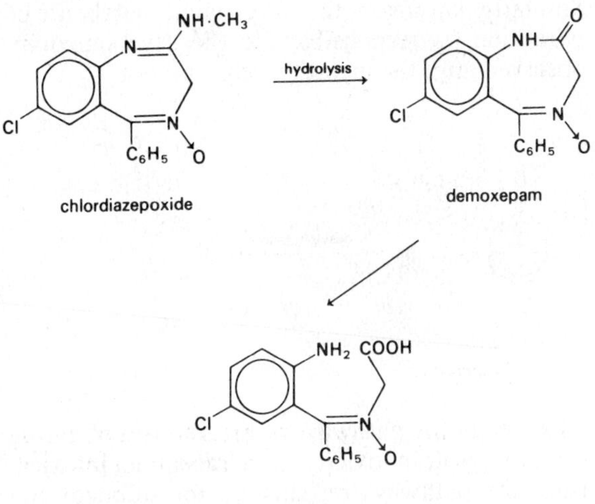

chlordiazepoxide

hydrolysis →

demoxepam

Conjugation Reactions

Oxidation, reduction, and hydrolysis usually produce metabolites which have a reactive functional group. Several of the more common conjugation reactions which mask these functional groups have been mentioned above and are now described in more detail.

GLUCURONIDE FORMATION

Glucuronic acid can be conjugated with a wide variety of functional groups to form either an ester (as with carboxylic acids such as phenylacetic acid), or an ether (as with phenolic or alcoholic groups, e.g. morphine or trichloroethanol). O-Glucuronides may be formed with primary, secondary, and tertiary alcohols. Analogous N- and S-glucuronides may also be produced (e.g. meprobamate and

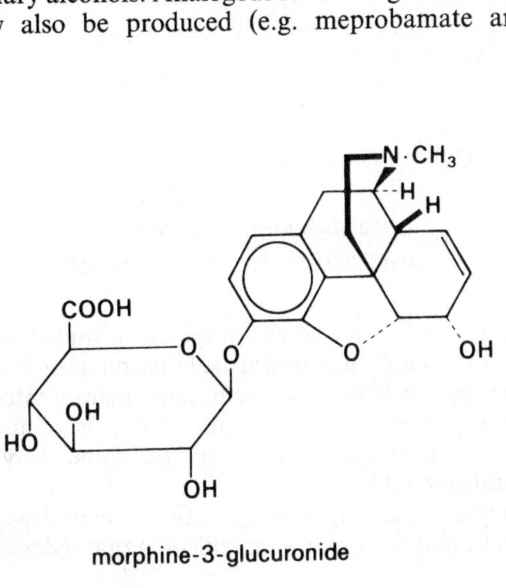

morphine-3-glucuronide

diethyldithiocarbamic acid), and a C—C linked glucuronide is formed with phenylbutazone.

Although the different glucuronides all facilitate drug elimination either by the kidney or the liver, they differ quite markedly in their stability. Thus, N-glucuronides of aromatic amines and sulphonamides tend to be unstable while, at the other extreme, ether glucuronides require hot concentrated acid to effect hydrolysis of the conjugate. It has been suggested that artefactual N-glucuronides of some drugs may be produced in urine on long standing.

SULPHATE FORMATION

Sulphate conjugates are formed with hydroxy compounds (e.g. alcohols and phenols) or aromatic amines. For example, morphine-3-O-ethereal sulphate is a minor metabolite of morphine and N-phenylsulphamic acid is a metabolite of aniline. Sulphate conjugates are strong acids and are readily excreted in the urine; they are of relatively little importance in drug metabolism.

ACETYLATION

Acetylation by N-acetyltransferase occurs frequently with primary and secondary amines (e.g. sulphadiazine) and substituted hydrazines (e.g. isoniazid and hydralazine); the N-monoacetyl derivatives are usually produced.

METHYLATION

Methylation is a common feature of the metabolism of phenols and N-heterocyclic compounds. Thus, phenolic steroids, adrenaline, and some other catecholamines undergo O-methylation, while pyridine, nicotinic acid, and normorphine undergo N-methylation. The reaction occurs under the influence of S-adenosylmethionine and a non-specific methyl transferase.

CONJUGATION WITH AMINO ACIDS

Following the activation of drugs and metabolites by acetyl-coenzyme A, conjugation with glutamine (in particular of arylacetic acids such as phenylacetic acid) and glycine (of carboxylic and aromatic acids such as salicylic acid) is common. Glutamine conjugation occurs less frequently than conjugation with glycine.

CONJUGATION WITH GLUTATHIONE

Reactive electrophiles produced by oxidative reactions conjugate with the tripeptide glutathione (glutamylcysteinylglycine) with the aid of a series of glutathione-S-transferases. Paracetamol, which is largely excreted as ethereal sulphate and glucu-

phenylacetic acid activated with acetyl-coenzyme A   +   glutamine   →   glutamine conjugate of phenylacetic acid

salicylic acid   +   glycine   →   salicyluric acid

ronide conjugates, also undergoes metabolism to an active intermediate which is then conjugated with glutathione. This conjugate is rapidly hydrolysed and excreted in the urine as the mercapturic acid (*N*-acetylcysteine) derivative.

mercapturic acid conjugate of paracetamol

DRUG METABOLISM AND TOXICITY

Toxic metabolites can occur in the same way that pharmacologically active and/or inactive metabolites are produced. For example, deacetylation of phenacetin yields *p*-phenetidine, the precursor of substances believed to be responsible for methaemoglobinaemia.

phenacetin   —deacetylation→   *p*-phenetidine

Similarly, paraoxon, the oxygenated metabolite of parathion, is responsible for the severe toxicity observed after the ingestion of parathion.

parathion   —desulphuration→   paraoxon

Changes in the pathways of metabolism of a drug can also result in toxicity. In paracetamol intoxication, the pathways responsible for sulphate and glucuronide conjugation become saturated and the concentrations of cysteine and mercapturic acid metabolites increase. When the production of the two latter metabolites increases sufficiently to deplete stores of glutathione, the active intermediate can no longer be conjugated and is thought to bind irreversibly to cellular macromolecules such as DNA, RNA, and proteins, resulting in a dose-related hepatic necrosis. Initial theories suggested that an epoxide metabolite was responsible for the tissue damage, but this metabolite has not been isolated. It is now believed that the toxic molecule arises from the oxidation of paracetamol to acetyl-imino-*p*-benzoquinone.

acetylimino-*p*-benzoquinone
(oxidation product of paracetamol)

Whatever the actual pathway, the administration of compounds containing sulphydryl groups has been shown to be effective in paracetamol intoxication, presumably because they are able to bind to the electrophilic species in the same way as glutathione.

Another example of drug toxicity related to the extent and nature of metabolism is that associated with acetylation. The rate of acetylation is controlled by an *N*-acetyltransferase which shows genetic polymorphism; about 60% of Caucasians are classified as 'slow' acetylators. The extent of acetylation is related to the toxic effects of certain drugs. For example, the *N*-hydroxy metabolite of acetylated isoniazid is thought to cause isoniazid-related hepatotoxicity. This toxicity is more severe in 'rapid' acetylators than in 'slow' acetylators but, as with paracetamol, some protection can be given by sulphydryl compounds.

In contrast, 'slow' acetylators appear to show a greater incidence of systemic lupus erythematosus following administration of hydrazine drugs than do 'rapid' acetylators as this toxic reaction is related to the parent drug.

Drug Concentration and Pharmacological Response

For most drugs there is a correlation between the dose given, the concentration of the drug in blood, and the duration and intensity of the biological effect. In general, as blood concentrations rise above those associated with a therapeutic effect, the frequency and severity of toxic side-effects increase.

The relationship between drug action and the processes of absorption, distribution, and elimination has been successfully applied in clinical pharmacology for the optimisation and individualisation of therapy. In clinical and forensic toxicology, similar relationships are applied in the interpretation of analytical results.

The significance of toxicological data is assessed by attempting to explain the clinical or toxicological effects in terms of the drug concentrations found. Before this can be done the toxicologist must be satisfied that the clinical and analytical data are valid.

VALIDITY OF TOXICOLOGICAL DATA

A number of factors affect the validity of toxicological findings and the interpretation of them. It is important to ensure that the measured concentration of the drug and any active metabolites can be related directly to the concentration at the receptor. This is obviously dependent on the sample and the sampling procedure, the distribution of drugs and metabolites in the sample, the analytical method-

ology, and the rational interpretation of the pharmacological response.

Samples

The choice of the sample is of paramount importance if the clinical condition is to be interpreted in terms of the analytical result. Blood and urine are the samples most commonly used for analysis, but the concentration in blood is generally considered to provide the best possible estimate of the amount of drug at the receptor site. If blood is provided, care must be taken to ensure that the sample has not been contaminated during autopsy by other fluids such as stomach washings or urine. The origin of a blood sample must be established, as blood from different parts of the body can have very different drug concentrations.

Whenever possible, it is advantageous to measure the drug concentration in two or more independent samples; the value of a result from a single sample will always be limited unless the distribution of the drug is known. Tissues which selectively take up a particular drug may have a much higher concentration than that found in blood. For example, solvents and other lipid-soluble substances are preferentially absorbed into the fatty tissues of the brain; digoxin and other cardiac glycosides are taken up by cardiac muscle; biliary concentrations of drugs which are excreted from the liver as glucuronides (e.g. morphine) may be considerably higher than their concentrations in blood.

In addition to being distributed unevenly throughout the body, a drug may not be distributed evenly within the separate parts of a single tissue. In blood, drugs may tend to be concentrated either in the plasma or in the erythrocytes. Thus, it may prove to be of little value to examine a plasma sample in a case where the drug involved is known to be concentrated in the erythrocytes (e.g. acetazolamide). It is usual to examine whole blood in forensic cases whereas plasma is usually examined in clinical situations, and there could be a significant difference in the concentrations when measured in the two situations. The whole blood concentration and the plasma concentration cannot be compared until one or the other has been corrected by reference to the plasma:whole blood ratio.

Analytical Methodology

The techniques used to extract and quantify a drug may also lead to problems in relating the measured drug concentration to the observed clinical condition. Different extraction procedures may lead to different results, so much so that the amount of drug recovered from the sample may bear little relation to the amount actually present. Similarly, it is futile to try to interpret a drug concentration which has been measured by a technique which is not sufficiently selective to exclude all metabolites, other drugs, and endogenous materials which might interfere with the analysis. For example, radioimmunoassay (RIA) techniques are being increasingly used to screen for the presence of as many individual drugs from within a pharmacological or chemical group as is possible. Hence, drug concentrations measured by RIA are often higher than those obtained by a more specific method, e.g. phenobarbitone concentrations measured by HPLC may be only 10% of those measured by RIA. This illustrates the obvious dangers of trying to interpret drug concentrations which have been obtained using an RIA designed for screening purposes.

An accurate interpretation of analytical results requires the use of a specific immunoassay, or identification and quantification with a chromatographic technique.

Similarly, it is pointless to determine the concentration of a drug which has been identified only as a member of a large pharmacological group, especially when that group has a wide range of biological potencies (e.g. barbiturates). In such cases, the drug concentration cannot be related to the pharmacological response. For example, a blood-barbiturate concentration of 15 µg/ml may represent a therapeutic concentration of phenobarbitone, a toxic concentration of amylobarbitone, or a fatal concentration of thiopentone.

Pharmacological Response

Even when it has been established that the measured drug concentration in the blood accurately represents the concentration of drug at the receptor site, it must also be established that the clinical response is a primary consequence of the presence of the drug. For example, drugs with an irreversible biochemical effect, such as reserpine and monoamine oxidase inhibitors, still have clinical effects long after drug administration has stopped, and when plasma concentrations of the drug are negligible. Similarly, unless the time of ingestion is known with reasonable accuracy, it is almost impossible to relate drug concentrations measured post mortem with the secondary and potentially fatal responses to substances such as paracetamol (liver damage), and paraquat (lung necrosis). Incorporation of drugs or chemicals into endogenous metabolic cycles may result in a toxicity (lethal synthesis) which is not related to blood concentrations of the drug. Finally, interpretation is made difficult or impossible when underlying disease has altered the pharmacological action of the drug, or when a patient has died of asphyxia following inhalation of vomit.

Active Metabolites

When an active metabolite makes an important contribution to the overall pharmacological response, the interpretation of toxicological data is further complicated. Toxicological situations involving such metabolites (e.g. oxazepam, nortriptyline, desipramine, and phenobarbitone, derived from diazepam, amitriptyline, imipramine, and methylphenobarbitone, respectively) can be misinterpreted if only the parent drugs are assayed. The concentrations of active metabolites must be taken into account. Although there is controversy over the best way to evaluate the contribution of metabolites, the individual concentrations of drug and metabolites are often added together to provide an estimate of the total amount of active drug species present in the sample. This assumes that their relative pharmacological activities are equal, which is not generally true.

THERAPEUTIC, TOXIC, AND FATAL DRUG CONCENTRATIONS

Reliable assessments of the significance of analytical findings can be made only by comparing the results with information on drug concentrations and associated clinical responses which have been reported in other cases. Comprehensive collections of reference data which present the relationship between concentration and effect (i.e. therapeutic, toxic, and fatal concentrations) are an essential aid in determining whether or not a measured drug concentration might explain the observed response. Wherever possible, appropriate data have been included in the monographs in Part 2.

In order that a concentration–effect relationship can be more easily recognised, analytical data should be expressed in a form which allows an accurate assessment of the significance of results to be made. Concentration–response curves, which are analogous to the dose–response curves used in experimental pharmacology, can be used in clinical and forensic toxicology. Curves of this type are illustrated in Fig. 6 which shows the cumulative

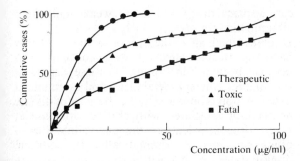

Fig. 6. Cumulative plots of percentage of cases versus blood concentrations of phenobarbitone in therapeutic, toxic, and fatal categories (A. H. Stead and A. C. Moffat, *J. forens. Sci. Soc.*, 1982, *22*, 47–56).

plots of blood-phenobarbitone concentrations measured in subjects showing a therapeutic, toxic, or fatal response to the drug. The curve shows that a phenobarbitone concentration of 50 µg/ml includes all of the subjects in the therapeutic category, about 75% of toxic (hospital emergency) cases, and about 50% of the fatalities. The curves present all available data in a clear and concise way and give a good indication of the likelihood of a measured drug concentration giving rise to the observed response. As well as dividing data into the three clinical categories, it may also be useful to subdivide results further by age, acute or chronic use, etc.

Concentration ranges derived from concentration–response curves can also be used to describe the relationship between concentration and effect. The blood concentration which accounts for 50% of patients within each clinical category (median effective concentration, EC50 value) can be compared with the concentrations which account for 10% (EC10 values), and 90% (EC90 values) of the patients. The range of concentrations into which most data are known to fall (EC10 to EC90) is analogous to the linear part of the classic dose–response curve used in pharmacology, the full curve being sigmoid in shape.

It is clear that visual or numerical representations of drug concentrations derived from different sources can only be compared if the clinical or toxicological responses with which they are associated are rigorously defined. For example, the description of an observed pharmacological response as 'toxic' is often totally inadequate since toxic effects can range for instance from drowsiness to severe coma.

FACTORS WHICH AFFECT PHARMACOLOGICAL RESPONSE

Similar drug concentrations will not produce the same response in all subjects. Some may respond at drug concentrations which might be considered subtherapeutic, whilst others may not respond with blood concentrations which are normally associated with toxic side-effects; concentrations found in chronic drug users or in drug abusers and addicts may be much higher than in normal subjects because of tolerance to pharmacological effects; the half-life of a drug in elderly subjects may be increased because of a decreased rate of metabolism and excretion. Differences in the capacity to eliminate drugs probably account for the major part of individual variability, but many other factors, both physiological and pharmacological, can influence drug concentrations and their associated clinical responses.

The combined effect of all of these factors is to make the task of interpreting analytical results even more difficult. Pharmacokinetic and toxicological data, such as that given in the monographs in Part 2, must be used circumspectly when a specific case is being examined because there is always the possibility of misinterpretation if consideration is not given to the special circumstances of the case.

Physiological Factors

AGE

Young children and elderly people generally have a lower metabolic capacity compared with subjects between these extremes of age. The enhanced sensitivity of the very young to drugs can be accounted for by the fact that the microsomal enzymes which are responsible for metabolism (especially conjugation with glucuronic acid) are not fully active until several months after birth. Further, very young children do not have the necessary plasma-binding proteins which help to compartmentalise drugs. Older children (over 5 years old) usually metabolise drugs at similar rates and by similar routes to adults, but they require lower doses to produce comparable effects because the drugs are distributed into a smaller volume.

In elderly subjects (over 60 years old) there appears to be a decreasing capacity for drug metabolism as a consequence of a gradual decline in overall physiological efficiency. In addition, the amount of protein binding may decrease and the renal excretion may be reduced. The resulting higher blood-drug concentrations per dose (Fig. 7), and increased

drug:metabolite concentration ratios (Fig. 8), together with a wider range of therapeutic drug
concentrations usually found in the elderly, will
obviously complicate the interpretation of data. A
further complication is that subjects tend to show
an increased susceptibility and/or reduced tolerance
to drug action with increasing age.

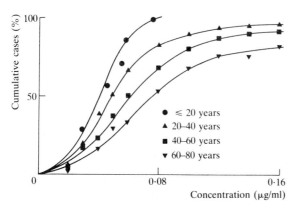

Fig. 7. Cumulative plots of the percentage of cases versus blood
concentrations of amitriptyline (normalised to a dose of 100 mg)
associated with different age groups.

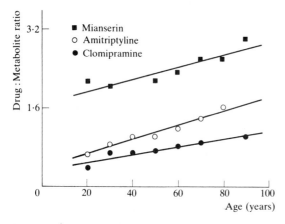

Fig. 8. Variation of blood drug:metabolite concentration ratios
with increasing age.

DISEASE

Diseases can affect all the processes by which a
drug is absorbed, distributed, and eliminated from
the body. A drug may be poorly absorbed during
gastro-intestinal disturbance; the rate of uptake of
drugs which rapidly cross tissue membranes may
be altered in cardiovascular diseases which alter
peripheral blood flow; endogenous free fatty acids
which are released into the plasma during trauma
can displace drugs which are weak acids from
albumin binding sites.

Diseases which affect the liver or kidneys probably
have the greatest effect on drug concentrations
because normal functioning of these organs is
essential for efficient metabolism and excretion. If
liver function is impaired, either because of disease
or necrosis associated with chronic drug use or
severe drug intoxication, the bioavailabilities of
drugs can increase dramatically. In addition,
disease states which lower plasma protein concentrations are believed to increase free concentrations
of highly bound drugs and subsequently lead to an
increase in the frequency of adverse effects associated with such drugs. However, this is seldom a
problem in long-term therapy as it is the unbound
drug which is eliminated.

Renal disease leads to a decreased ability to excrete
drugs and/or their metabolites. A drug will accumulate in plasma or tissues if the interval between
doses is such that not all of the previously
administered drug is removed before the next dose.
Even for those drugs where excretion into the urine
does not normally appear to be an important route
of elimination, there can be a risk of increased
toxicity during disease if significant drug accumulation takes place. This is especially true where
potentially serious interactions can occur with the
accumulated drug or metabolite. For example,
metabolites can displace their parent drugs from
binding sites on plasma and tissue proteins if their
concentrations build up sufficiently.

WEIGHT

The weight of an individual obviously affects
concentrations of drug in the blood as it determines
the volume into which the drug is distributed.
Absolute body size may account for some of the
variations in drug handling which are observed
between males and females, although differences in
the ratio of fat:body water (greater in females), or
in the rate of drug metabolism (higher in males)
probably have a greater influence. However, such
differences are usually small and probably have
little forensic significance.

GENETIC FACTORS

The genetic control of the number of receptor sites,
and genetic variations in the extent of protein
binding or the rate and extent of drug metabolism,
can make a marked contribution to variations in
drug concentrations and responses. Polymorphic
drug metabolism, caused by either missing enzymes
or enzymes with reduced activity, can result in high

drug concentrations and, particularly for drugs with a low therapeutic index, abnormal clinical responses. Drugs which undergo *p*-hydroxylation (debrisoquine), acetylation (isoniazid), and oxidative dealkylation (phenacetin), provide good examples of polymorphic metabolism. Inefficient drug metabolism can lead to increased bioavailability, accumulation of the drug, and therefore to increased toxicity. For example, with some hydrazine monoamine-oxidase inhibitors, the incidence of side-effects and toxicity is increased in slow acetylators. The inability to oxidise tolbutamide has been related to an increased incidence of cardiovascular toxicity with the drug.

Pharmacological Factors

ROUTE OF ADMINISTRATION

The route of drug administration, together with the nature of the dosage form, determines the rate and extent of absorption. Administration by inhalation or intravenous injection leads to relatively high but transient blood concentrations, whilst administration orally or by intramuscular injection produces lower concentrations of longer duration.

If proprietary preparations are given by the recommended route it may be possible to make predictions of the dose from blood concentrations because comparable data are usually available. However, when illicit drugs or preparations are involved, prediction is much more difficult. Volatile solvents which are encountered in glue-sniffing are inhaled under a wide variety of conditions; variable amounts of cannabinoids are absorbed from the lung during smoking of cannabis; there may be considerable variations in the amount of lysergide administered by mouth from paper tabs impregnated with a solution of the drug.

The majority of overdoses and poisonings encountered by the toxicologist involve drugs which have been administered orally. Compared with administration of drugs given by intravenous injection, where absorption can be considered as total and almost instantaneous, administration by mouth often leads to reduced and variable bioavailability. This can be attributed to a number of factors: drugs may be unstable in the acidic conditions of the stomach or in the alkaline conditions of the small intestine; they may be metabolised by bacteria in the gastro-intestinal tract or by enzymes in the mucosal lining of the gut prior to absorption; they may become adsorbed onto the stomach contents; they may be absorbed in varying amounts if the gut motility and/or the blood flow in the gut wall are

disordered. Finally, and probably the most important, the individual's capacity to metabolise drugs during the first pass of the drug through the liver has an enormous effect on the fraction of drug absorbed and which remains for further distribution to peripheral tissues, especially if the drug is extensively metabolised by the liver.

As well as affecting the amount of a drug which gets into the blood, the route of administration also affects the rate of entry. In some respects this rate may be more important than the final blood concentration in determining the severity of the observed clinical response. Thus, a fatal drug dose given intravenously is often much smaller than a fatal dose given by mouth because the injected drug is able to reach the site of action very rapidly.

DOSE AND DURATION OF THERAPY

The concentration of a drug in the body is mainly determined by the size of the dose and the frequency of dosing. In general, the concentration following administration of multiple doses is higher than that observed after a single dose. If a drug with a long half-life is given in multiple doses with a sufficiently small dose interval, the drug will accumulate in the body, and this may lead to progressively serious toxicity. This is a particular problem with some tranquillisers and hypnotics which are slowly eliminated and it may result in unwanted daytime sedation and impaired performance.

Clinical and forensic toxicologists are involved most often with drugs which have been taken in large single doses rather than with drugs which have been administered regularly in small doses over a long period. In the normal dosage range, the rates of absorption, distribution, metabolism, and excretion of most drugs are generally considered to be proportional to the dose or concentration of the drug in blood (i.e. the processes are first-order). However, a very large dose of some drugs (e.g. barbiturates, glutethimide, and related hypnotics) can reduce gastric motility with the consequence that absorption is prolonged over several days. Overdose with slow-release preparations presents similar problems. If the dose or concentration reaches a sufficiently high level, the processes involved in drug clearance may become saturated and reduced to zero-order functions. High drug doses, therefore, have pharmacokinetic consequences as well as the more obvious pharmacological results, and the assumption of first-order kinetic behaviour may not be appropriate in cases of overdose (Fig. 9). As the eliminating systems

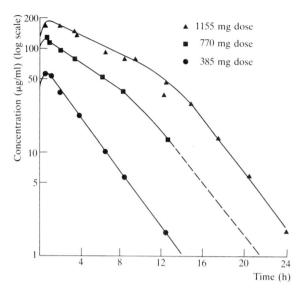

▲ 1155 mg dose

■ 770 mg dose

● 385 mg dose

Fig. 9. Semilogarithmic plots of plasma concentrations versus time for 3 doses of salicylate administered to the same subject, illustrating capacity-limited elimination. At low plasma concentrations, parallel straight lines are obtained from which the first-order elimination rate constant can be estimated. As long as concentrations remain sufficiently high to saturate the process, elimination follows zero-order kinetics (C. A. M. van Ginneken *et al.*, *J. Pharmacokinet. Biopharm.*, 1974, **2**, 395–415).

become saturated, the half-life of the drug will increase. In addition, the relationship between dose and blood concentrations may become non-linear, with drug concentrations increasing disproportionately more rapidly than the increase in dose.

Several drugs, including salicylate (in overdose), alcohol, and possibly some hydrazines and other drugs which are metabolised by acetylation, have saturable elimination kinetics, but the only significant clinical example is phenytoin. With this drug, capacity-limited elimination is complicated further by its low therapeutic index. A 50% increase in the dose of phenytoin can result in a 600% increase in the steady-state blood concentration, and thus expose the patient to potential toxicity.

Capacity-limited pathways of elimination lead to plasma concentrations of drugs which can be described by a form of the Michaelis–Menten equation. In such cases, the plasma concentration at steady state is given by

$$\frac{K_m R}{V_{max} - R}$$

where V_{max} is the maximum rate of metabolism, K_m is a constant equal to the plasma concentration at which the rate of metabolism is one-half the maximum, and R is the rate of metabolism.

Other pathways will continue to operate but, for plasma concentrations of the order of K_m, an apparently linear decrease in concentration with time will be seen. Thus, for alcohol in healthy adult males, K_m has an average value of 82 µg/ml, and V_{max} an average value of 202 µg/ml/hour. About 90% of alcohol elimination is usually by the capacity-limited alcohol dehydrogenase (oxidative) pathway, the remainder being by the kidneys and other routes of excretion. The renal clearance of alcohol depends on urine flow, and is approximately equal to urine flow rate, i.e. about 1 ml/min; only a trace is eliminated via the lungs. For blood-alcohol concentrations of 100, 350, 1000, and 3500 µg/ml, the elimination of alcohol will be as shown in Table 3. As the concentration rises, so the elimination rate increases (but not proportionately) to reach a value of approximately V_{max}. The contribution of the kidneys to elimination is negligible at low concentrations, but is about 5% of the total at 3500 µg/ml.

Table 3. Elimination of alcohol from blood at various concentrations

Concentration of alcohol in blood µg/ml	Total elimination from blood µg/ml/h	Excretion of unchanged alcohol in urine µg/ml/h	% total
100	111	0.3	0.25
350	165	1.0	0.6
1000*	195	3.0	1.5
3500*	207	10.0	4.8

*The concentration–time curve will appear linear at these concentrations, but it is only at the higher concentration that the enzyme-mediated pathway is truly zero-order.

When repeated doses of a drug are given, tolerance to the drug may arise if it affects its own disposition or response. Enzyme activities can be enhanced, which leads to an increased capacity for metabolism (e.g. patients on chronic therapy with barbiturates metabolise the drugs more rapidly than patients who have not previously taken the drugs). Alternatively, the receptor sensitivity may be modified so that the effect of a particular concentration of a drug is reduced after chronic use (e.g. the sedative effects of benzodiazepines).

Increasing tolerance results in a progressively decreasing drug effect, and the need for an increased dose; habituation and addiction may be the final clinical outcome. Thus, addicts can tolerate doses of morphine which might be considered toxic or even fatal in non-addicts. Similarly, rapidly developing tolerance to the sedative effects of phenobarbitone is a common feature of prolonged therapy with the drug. Epileptic patients treated with phenobarbitone are often free from any adverse effects despite having blood-drug concentrations normally associated with serious toxicity in patients not accustomed to taking the drug.

Tolerance invariably extends the upper limit of the therapeutic range of drugs, and there is a more marked overlap between concentrations associated with different clinical responses. When tolerance is suspected, some of the problems of interpreting data can best be resolved by reference to previous results from the same patient (e.g. results of a therapeutic drug monitoring programme). Unfortunately, in most forensic cases such background information is not available and in these instances blood concentrations alone are of little value. A more reliable interpretation of analytical data can only be made by comparison of blood concentrations with those measured in urine, bile, or liver (where concentrations can be much higher in addicts), and/or by measuring the relative amounts of unchanged drug and its metabolite(s).

PROTEIN BINDING AND DISTRIBUTION IN BLOOD

After absorption, a drug is distributed non-uniformly around the body, including binding to plasma proteins, distribution between plasma and erythrocytes, and binding to peripheral tissues. The extent of this binding and distribution in the blood has a considerable influence on the blood concentration, and on the intensity and duration of its pharmacological effect, because only the free (unbound) drug can be cleared from the body by metabolism and excretion. Furthermore, only the free fraction can diffuse across biological membranes and equilibrate with the receptor site.

It has been proposed that measurement of the concentration of free drug in the plasma (i.e. that fraction of the drug which is available to cause a response) may be more relevant than measurement of the concentration of total drug (i.e. free plus bound) in whole blood or plasma. However, this is not always practicable, and neither clinical nor forensic toxicologists do so routinely. It is generally assumed that the total concentration of drug in the blood is proportional to its free concentration. This may be true for low concentrations of drugs, or for drugs whose binding is not capacity-limited. However, for those drugs whose binding to plasma proteins is saturable, free concentrations will increase proportionately more rapidly than increases in total concentrations, for any given increase in dose. For example, the free concentration of a drug which is 90% bound at the point of saturation of the protein binding will be 10% of the total drug concentration. If the total concentration is doubled, no more drug will be bound to proteins, and the free concentration will increase by a factor of 11 to over 50% of the total concentration. The extent of the binding of a drug to plasma proteins, and also its distribution between plasma and erythrocytes, are important factors in establishing the concentration–effect relationship in an individual.

Some drugs are only poorly protein-bound (e.g. codeine, digoxin, meprobamate, paracetamol), whilst others are highly bound (e.g. amitriptyline, chlorpromazine, medazepam), although the percentage of bound drug can vary between individuals. Similarly, some drugs are only poorly taken up by erythrocytes (e.g. digitoxin, promethazine, warfarin), whilst uptake can be extensive for others (e.g. acetazolamide, chlorthalidone).

Information about the extent of protein binding, and about the plasma:whole blood ratio provides an invaluable guide to the interpretation of drug concentrations in unfractionated blood samples. Using such data, total blood concentrations can be related to the unbound drug concentrations which are responsible for the observed condition. These data have been included, wherever possible, in the monographs in Part 2.

The degree of binding or of distribution of a drug in the blood is influenced by a number of factors of which disease, dose, and competition for binding sites between two drugs are the most important. The low concentrations of plasma proteins associated with some disease states can lead to the saturation of binding sites even with therapeutic doses. Similarly, if the concentration of plasma proteins is normal, binding sites can become saturated if sufficiently large doses are given, as with an overdose. This is especially true of most weakly acidic drugs which are almost completely ionised at the pH of plasma and therefore have a high affinity for albumin.

In general, the competition for binding sites between two drugs is only of toxicological significance if the displaced drug is normally extensively bound (i.e. more than 75%), and if its volume of distribution is low (i.e. less than about 0.07 litres/kg), so that a small percentage change in binding has a relatively large effect on free drug concentrations in blood. For example, if warfarin and phenylbutazone are administered simultaneously, competition for the same binding sites (on albumin) can increase the concentration of unbound warfarin (which has the lower affinity for protein) resulting in enhanced anticoagulant activity.

Thus, any disturbance of the binding of a drug, or of its distribution in the blood, changes its pharmacokinetic characteristics. These changes are predominantly associated with the apparent volume of distribution and the half-life of the drug, both of which decrease with decreased binding. Consequently, as the free drug fraction increases, so its total clearance also increases. However, the intrinsic clearance (the maximum attainable clearance of the unbound drug) remains constant as it is only a measure of the drug-eliminating capacity of a particular organ. When it is suspected that there has been some change in the binding of a drug or in its distribution in the blood, and especially for drugs which are highly bound or are concentrated in the erythrocytes, literature values for volume of distribution and half-life must be used with caution.

DRUG INTERACTIONS

In the majority of cases in clinical and forensic toxicology, there is more than one drug involved. Multi-drug therapy and abuse is prevalent and this, together with the added problems of self-medication with over-the-counter drugs and the widespread use of alcohol, makes interpretation of data even more complicated. The pharmacokinetic and other data in the monographs in Part 2 refer to drug concentrations and responses observed following the administration of the drug alone. In practice, when comparing these data with analytical results involving several drugs, it must be remembered that the clinical response is often a consequence of the combined actions of more than one drug. If the significance of the results is to be assessed correctly, it is essential to consider the quantitative effects of any interactions which might occur between drugs taken in combination.

Drug interactions can be divided into two types: those which affect the drug concentration (i.e. which alter the processes of absorption, distribution, and elimination) and those which affect the response (by changing its duration and severity). The consequences of most drug combinations can be predicted relatively accurately with a knowledge of their pharmacology and pharmacokinetics.

Drugs with opposite pharmacological activities (e.g. barbiturates and amphetamines) may have an antagonistic effect. Conversely, the additive effects or side-effects of two drugs with the same pharmacological action (e.g. central nervous system depressants) may prove fatal even though the individual drug concentrations are not toxic themselves. Further, a drug with a high affinity for tissue proteins might displace a second drug from binding sites, while a drug which changes urinary pH or which competes for the same active transport system in the proximal tubules of the kidney might inhibit renal excretion. Other important mechanisms for drug interactions include: interference with absorption of other drugs; modification of rates and routes of metabolism; and changing the accessibility of receptors and tissue sites.

Unfortunately, although a number of excellent texts discuss the mechanisms of drug interactions and their pharmacological implications in detail, very little is understood about their quantitative effects. In most cases, these effects can only be ascertained by an examination of previous findings where the

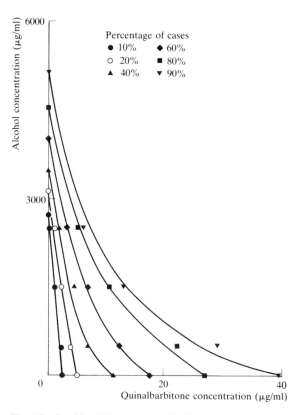

Fig. 10. Combined blood alcohol-barbiturate concentration curves in reported cases of fatal quinalbarbitone poisoning. The various lines connect those concentration pairs which would account for the percentage of cases shown (A. H. Stead and A. C. Moffat, *Human Toxicol.*, 1983, **2**, 5–14).

same combination of drugs has been used. Combined drug–drug concentration curves which connect those pairs of drug concentrations which are equally effective in causing a defined clinical condition (e.g. driving impairment, death, etc.) offer the most effective way of quantifying drug interactions. For example, the likelihood of a fatality occurring with any given combination of alcohol and quinalbarbitone can be estimated relatively easily from curves such as those shown in Fig. 10. This shows that, for instance, an alcohol concentration of 1500 µg/ml (alone accounting for 2 to 3% of fatalities) when combined with a quinalbarbitone concentration of 10 µg/ml (alone accounting for 35% of fatalities) will account for more than 75% of fatalities, where both alcohol and barbiturate were found together in such concentrations.

The Interpretation of Analytical Results

The qualitative or semi-quantitative analysis of a biological sample provides the clinical pharmacologist and the forensic toxicologist with evidence of drug intake. Such analyses may be used, for example, to confirm that a patient has or has not been complying with a therapeutic regimen, or to indicate that a controlled drug is being abused. Further, the detection of metabolites in a biological sample can show that a drug has been absorbed into the body and then eliminated (either wholly or partly) from it. Such evidence might be used to refute an allegation that a sample had been tampered with, or contaminated, after it had been taken. Quantitative analysis, on the other hand, is essential if the toxicologist is to show that sufficient drug has been administered to account for the observed clinical or toxicological condition of the patient. In addition, where several drugs have common metabolic pathways, quantification of the parent compound and any major metabolite(s) can show which drug was taken. Finally, the drug and metabolite concentrations, together with the pharmacokinetic parameters of the drug, might be used to estimate when and how much of a drug was administered, and by which route it was taken.

IDENTIFYING THE DRUG

In most cases, qualitative analysis is sufficient to show that a particular drug has been administered. However, problems arise when a drug is rapidly and extensively metabolised so that there is none,

or very little, of the parent compound in the sample. An example of this is the difficulty of distinguishing between the use of benzphetamine alone, methylamphetamine alone, and amphetamine and methylamphetamine together, by the analysis of urine. Benzphetamine is extensively metabolised to methylamphetamine which is itself converted to amphetamine. Unless subject to chronic abuse, benzphetamine is not detected in urine following oral ingestion.

Another example involves codeine, diamorphine, and morphine. After a single therapeutic dose of codeine, the morphine concentration in urine represents about 10% of the codeine concentration for 2 to 8 hours after dosing; 24 to 30 hours after dosing, only morphine (largely as the glucuronide) is readily detectable in urine. Diamorphine is also converted to morphine in the body. The situation is further complicated by the fact that codeine is often found in the urine of persons taking illicit diamorphine despite the fact that it is not a normal metabolite. This codeine is thought to be the result of deacetylation of acetylcodeine, present as an impurity in illicit diamorphine. In this case, the codeine produced represents about 10% of the administered diamorphine. Urinary concentrations of the various drugs and metabolites can be used to differentiate between consumption of crude or pure diamorphine, and illicit or pharmaceutical preparations of morphine or codeine. However, results should be interpreted with great caution, particularly if the time between dosing and collection of a urine sample is prolonged.

In most cases, urine analysis can provide valuable information on the identity of a drug, for example in screening for drugs of abuse or in emergency toxicology. However, it is quite clear that the analysis of a blood sample obtained at the same time is essential for the identification of those compounds which are not excreted by the kidneys. Drug concentrations are generally much lower in blood than in urine but, with the appropriate choice of analytical technique, it is more likely that the parent compound will be detected rather than its metabolite.

In cases where the only evidence of drug intake is the presence of an inactive metabolite in the urine or bile, there is a further restraint in making a direct link between the drug and the clinical condition of the patient. If the drug has been completely metabolised, then the body probably withstood the primary action of the drug. The real cause of the pharmacological response may be a secondary effect or it may be some other unidentified drug.

ESTIMATING THE TIME AFTER ADMINISTRATION

The time between ingestion and taking the sample, or the survival time following a fatal dose, can be estimated in a variety of ways. Simple indications include the presence of unabsorbed drug in the stomach or further down the gastro-intestinal tract. Unfortunately, such simple approaches are not always appropriate and can be unreliable. The measurement of drug and metabolite concentrations in various tissues usually provides more useful information.

When a drug has a relatively rapid rate of metabolism, the relationship between time and drug or metabolite concentrations can help to indicate whether the drug was taken recently or in the more distant past. Diamorphine is rapidly metabolised to morphine via 6-monoacetylmorphine. Following intravenous injection, neither diamorphine nor 6-monoacetylmorphine can be detected in postmortem tissues if the survival time is prolonged. Thus, even if only traces of 6-monoacetylmorphine are detected in a postmortem sample of blood, this indicates intravenous use of diamorphine in the very recent past. No matter how rapidly death occurs, diamorphine itself is never detected because of the hydrolytic action of the plasma esterases.

The blood concentration of free morphine as a metabolite of diamorphine also correlates well with the survival time, at least over 24 hours. Average blood concentrations of morphine observed in cases where death has occurred from circulatory shock and respiratory arrest less than 3 hours after administration are 3 to 10 times greater than those seen after deaths following prolonged coma (3 to 24 hours).

Cannabis provides a similar example. The detection of Δ^9-tetrahydrocannabinol in blood indicates very recent use of the drug (within 8 hours). Further, the concentrations of 11-nor-Δ^9-tetrahydrocannabinol-9-carboxylic acid and its glucuronide increase with time, the ratio of the acid to Δ^9-tetrahydrocannabinol increasing to over 50 after about 3 hours.

Concentration ratios of drug:metabolite or metabolite:metabolite of the above type often provide better estimates of the time since ingestion than the individual blood concentrations, especially when

the time involved is relatively long. Unless a drug is very rapidly metabolised (as is the case with diamorphine and cannabis), only very low blood concentrations of metabolites are present a short time after a single dose. Consequently, a relatively high drug:metabolite ratio can be expected in cases of very rapid death following acute overdose.

In fatalities due to overdoses of paracetamol and dextropropoxyphene, the postmortem blood concentrations of dextropropoxyphene are generally high compared with those of the major metabolite, norpropoxyphene, the dextropropoxyphene:norpropoxyphene ratio being greater than 5. This indicates that death is relatively rapid (less than 1 hour). Dextropropoxyphene is assumed to be the cause of death if total blood concentrations of drug and metabolite are in excess of 2 µg/ml. As survival time is increased, the drug:metabolite concentration ratio decreases. Thus, when an individual survives the initial phase of acute respiratory depression associated with dextropropoxyphene, the drug:metabolite ratio falls dramatically to about 0.33 at 6 hours, and to 0.1 at 12 to 24 hours.

The majority of examples mentioned above deal with fatal cases and with the estimation of survival time. In non-fatal cases, it can be no less important to differentiate between recent drug use (up to 24 hours) and use in the distant past. When metabolism is extensive, and when drug and/or metabolite concentrations in the blood are very low, it can be profitable to compare the urinary concentration of one metabolite with another. For example, diazepam is metabolised either by N-demethylation to desmethyldiazepam which then undergoes 3-hydroxylation to yield oxazepam, or by hydroxylation to temazepam (N-methyloxazepam) which is then demethylated to oxazepam. All the urinary metabolites appear as their glucuronides. After administration of a single oral dose of diazepam, the concentration of desmethyldiazepam in the urine reaches a maximum 6 to 12 hours after ingestion, the temazepam concentration reaches its maximum after 12 to 24 hours, and the oxazepam concentration reaches a maximum after 1 to 3 days. From the second day, oxazepam is the major urinary metabolite. Up to 24 hours after ingestion, the oxazepam:desmethyldiazepam concentration ratio is 1 or less, with a corresponding oxazepam:temazepam ratio of less than 0.7. Beyond 24 hours, the ratios cover a wider range of times, and estimates of the time since ingestion can only be made by comparing metabolite:metabolite ratios with absolute metabolite concentrations.

As well as relating drug and metabolite concentrations in the same biological sample, the concentration of the drug in one tissue can be related to a concentration in another. For example, if a fatality occurs shortly after the oral ingestion of a drug, then the liver:blood concentration ratio is higher than if death had occurred after a more prolonged period. Relatively high urine:blood or bile:blood concentration ratios in association with low total drug concentrations indicate that the time since drug administration is relatively long.

If a reasonable estimate of the dose is available, pharmacokinetic data can be used to estimate the survival time or the time (t) since drug administration

$$t = \frac{1}{k_{el}} \ln\left[\frac{D}{V_d c}\right]$$

This equation is for an intravenous dose. For drugs given by mouth, the equation must be modified as shown previously for estimating the dose from the time and k_{el}, and would need knowledge of the absorption rate constant (k_a), and the bioavailability (F).

$$t = \frac{1}{k_{el}} \ln\left[\frac{DFk_a}{V_d c(k_a - k_{el})}\right]$$

If two or more drugs are administered at the same time in a single pharmaceutical preparation, pharmacokinetic data can be applied to estimate the time since ingestion, even in those cases where an estimate of the dose is not available. In such situations, the determination of the relative concentrations of each drug allows the solution of simultaneous equations for concentration versus time. This approach has been used to estimate the survival time following ingestion of an overdose of a mixture of amylobarbitone and quinalbarbitone. The measurement of barbiturate concentrations in body tissues indicated an average ratio of amylobarbitone to quinalbarbitone of 1.02. Using a value of 29 hours for the half-life of amylobarbitone and 26.5 hours for the half-life of quinalbarbitone, and knowing that the preparation contained equal amounts of the two barbiturates, it was possible to estimate that death had taken place 6 to 10 hours after ingestion.

ESTIMATING THE DOSE

Estimates of how much of a drug has been taken are necessary to indicate whether an overdose has been taken and whether it was accidental or suicidal.

Measurement of a blood concentration may not always allow the differentiation of multiple therapeutic doses from large accidental or suicidal doses. Thus, thioridazine concentrations after the administration of multiple doses may show a marked overlap with those seen in fatal poisonings. However, fatal drug concentrations in the liver are at least $2\frac{1}{2}$ times greater than those seen after chronic therapy. Hence, measurement of liver concentrations as well as blood concentrations may help to evaluate the toxicological situation.

In the same way that drug and metabolite concentrations can be linked to time, they can also be related to dose regimens. Thus, steady-state drug:metabolite concentration ratios are sometimes used to check drug compliance. Also, since the extent of drug metabolism tends to decrease with increasing dose, the ratio of unchanged drug to metabolite will increase with increasing dose. Examination of the relative concentrations of parent drug and its major metabolite(s) in blood, or in other tissues as necessary, can provide invaluable information as to the size of the dose given. Thus, an amitriptyline:nortriptyline concentration ratio of less than 2 is consistent with steady-state drug concentrations following administration of therapeutic doses, while a ratio greater than 2 is more consistent with the ingestion of larger, potentially toxic doses.

When a drug is extensively metabolised, large acute doses can result in metabolic profiles significantly different from those seen after therapeutic doses. Thus, following administration of normal single doses of phenylbutazone, the ratio of the blood concentrations of its major metabolites oxyphenbutazone and 3'-hydroxyphenylbutazone may be as high as 10:1. In overdose, the pattern of metabolism can be reversed, giving ratios as low as 1:5. Similarly, the metabolic profile of diazepam in urine changes dramatically with dose, and the ratio of desmethyldiazepam to oxazepam concentrations can provide useful information regarding the relative size of an ingested dose of the drug. When doses are low, demethylation of diazepam appears to be more important than hydroxylation, while hydroxylation becomes more important at higher doses.

Once tissue-drug concentrations or drug:metabolite concentration ratios have established that an overdose was or was not administered, the actual amount of drug ingested may be estimated. Ideally, the dose should be determined by measuring the total amount of drug remaining in the body (including any unabsorbed drug in the gastro-intestinal tract) and adding to this the amount which has been metabolised and/or excreted. Obviously this is not always practical as it is often difficult to account for the amount of drug which has been eliminated. A compromise is usually made by estimating the minimum amount of drug ingested. This can be attempted in a number of ways.

Analytical results may be compared with previously recorded data in fatal cases for which drug doses are known. The next best method is the direct comparison of peripheral blood concentrations with clinical data, i.e. blood concentrations following the administration of therapeutic doses. Finally, drug doses can be estimated using pharmacokinetic data. The half-life of the drug ($t_{1/2}$) and a reasonable estimate of the time elapsed between administration and sampling (t), together with the blood concentration (c), allow the calculation of a theoretical drug concentration at time zero (c_0) which, for intravenous administration is

$$\ln c_0 = \ln c + \frac{0.693}{t_{1/2}} t$$

This concentration can be used to estimate the dose if the volume of distribution of the drug (V_d) is known (p. 279), or it may be compared with clinical data as described above.

This pharmacokinetic approach probably gives a better estimate of the actual dose administered since it takes some account of the amount of drug eliminated. However, the use of pharmacokinetic equations may not always be appropriate, especially if relatively accurate survival times are not available and if the kinetic characteristics of the drug following administration of large acute doses are significantly different from those observed following therapeutic doses. Some of these problems can be overcome in the clinical situation if sufficient samples are available to characterise the terminal elimination kinetics of a drug taken in overdose. For example, the area under the plasma concentration–time curve of one of the major metabolites of carbamazepine (trans-10,11-dihydro-10,11-dihydroxycarbamazepine) has been used to estimate the amount of parent drug absorbed. Although estimates of the amount of carbamazepine administered are not always totally accurate, the approach has much to offer the clinical and forensic toxicologist.

IDENTIFYING THE ROUTE OF ADMINISTRATION

The rate at which a drug reaches its site of action is a critical factor governing the duration and the severity of the pharmacological response. If analytical findings are to be interpreted correctly, the route by which a drug is given should therefore always be considered. In a case of criminal poisoning it may be essential to establish the route of drug administration in order to corroborate evidence.

In some cases, simple facts give a clear indication of the route. Thus, residual drug in the stomach contents or gastro-intestinal tract points to oral ingestion, a needle mark in the arm indicates intravenous injection, and high concentrations in muscle tissue point to intramuscular injection. However, in the majority of cases the situation is more complex.

When there is no direct evidence to indicate how the drug entered the body, drug:metabolite concentration ratios can be particularly helpful because rates and pathways of metabolism can vary markedly with the route of administration. Thus, drug:metabolite concentration ratios in the blood are high if a drug is given intravenously, because it is distributed widely around the systemic circulation before reaching the liver. Conversely, concentration ratios can be low where the drug is given by mouth because of immediate transport to the liver (and the major metabolic sites) following absorption from the gut. Thus, more than 90% of orally administered fluphenazine is oxidised in the liver before it even reaches the systemic circulation. If the drug is metabolised in the gut itself (e.g. isoprenaline), a large fraction of the parent compound may be lost before it can be absorbed. Isoprenaline is metabolised by O-methylation and by conjugation of both the parent drug and its methylated derivative with sulphate. Following oral administration (and after inhalation where much of the drug appears to be swallowed) the metabolic profile is very different from that obtained following intravenous administration. Given orally, the drug is largely transformed to its sulphate conjugate at sites at or in the gut wall; very little of the drug is methylated and the conjugate is rapidly excreted. After intravenous injection, most of the drug is eliminated as the O-methylated derivative, either free or conjugated with sulphate. Thus, if the urinary concentration ratio of 3-O-methylisoprenaline sulphate:isoprenaline is greater than 2, and/or if the isoprenaline sulphate:isoprenaline ratio is less than about 10, it is reasonable to suppose that administration of the drug was by the intravenous route.

The route-dependent variability of drug disposition into tissues may also provide useful information relating to the route of administration. Because of the physiological processes involved, substantially smaller amounts of an intravenously administered drug are partitioned into the liver than when the same drug is given orally. If death results rapidly following a large overdose by intravenous injection, the liver- to blood-drug concentration ratio would therefore be lower than that observed had the drug been given by mouth. Thus, liver:blood ratios of 2.50 and 5.01 have been observed in pentobarbitone fatalities involving intravenous and oral administration respectively, and ratios of 1.27 and 4.21 have been found for intravenous and oral fatalities involving morphine.

Bibliography

S. H. Curry, *Drug Disposition and Pharmacokinetics*, 3rd Edn, Oxford, Blackwell, 1980.

Drug Metabolism: From Microbe to Man, D. V. Parke and R. L. Smith (Ed.), 4th Edn, London, Kimpton, 1979.

M. Gibaldi and D. Perrier, Pharmacokinetics, 2nd Edn, *Drugs and the Pharmaceutical Sciences*, J. Swarbrick (Ed.), Vol. 15, New York, Marcel Dekker, 1982.

P. D. Hansten, *Drug Interactions*, 5th Edn, Philadelphia, Lea and Febiger, 1985.

M. Rowland and T. N. Tozer, *Clinical Pharmacokinetics: Concepts and Applications*, Philadelphia, Lea and Febiger, 1980.

A. H. Stead, The Use of Pharmacokinetic and Drug Metabolism Data in Forensic Toxicology, in *Progress in Drug Metabolism*, Vol. 9, J. W. Bridges and L. F. Chasseaud (Ed.), London, Taylor and Francis, 1985.

A. H. Stead and A. C. Moffat, A Collection of Therapeutic, Toxic and Fatal Blood Drug Concentrations in Man, *Human Toxicol.*, 1983, 3, 437–464.

J. B. Stenlake, The Chemical Basis of Drug Action, *Foundations of Molecular Pharmacology*, Vol. 2, London, Athlone Press, 1979.

I. H. Stockley, *Drug Interactions*, London, Blackwell, 1981.

B. Testa and P. Jenner, Drug Metabolism: Chemical and Biochemical Aspects, *Drugs and the Pharmaceutical Sciences*, J. Swarbrick (Ed.), Vol. 4, New York, Marcel Dekker, 1976.

PART 2: Monographs
Analytical and Toxicological Data

Ultraviolet Absorption Data

In the reproductions of ultraviolet spectra,
the following notation has been used:

——————— acid solution

· · · · · · · · · · · alkaline solution

– – – – – – – – – neutral solution

The A_1^1 values are divided into three categories in
order to provide an indication of reliability:

The letter 'a' after a figure indicates that the value
is a mean value based on several reported figures
all of which lie within a range of $\pm 10\%$ of the
mean.

The letter 'b' after a figure indicates that the value
is a single reported value of unknown reliability.

The letter 'c' after a figure indicates that the value
is a mean value based on several reported figures
some of which lie outside $\pm 10\%$ of the mean.

Acebutolol

Beta-adrenoceptor Blocking Agent

($\pm$) - 3' - Acetyl - 4' - (2 - hydroxy - 3 - isopropylamino-propoxy)butyranilide

$C_{18}H_{28}N_2O_4 = 336.4$

CAS—37517-30-9

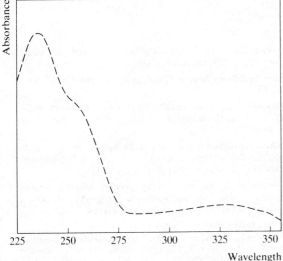

Crystals. M.p. 119° to 123°.

Acebutolol Hydrochloride

Proprietary Names. Neptall; Prent; Sectral. It is an ingredient of Secadrex.

$C_{18}H_{28}N_2O_4$,HCl = 372.9

CAS—34381-68-5

A white or slightly cream-coloured powder. M.p. 141° to 144°.

Dissociation Constant. pK_a 9.4.

Colour Tests. Methanolic Potassium Hydroxide—yellow; Nessler's Reagent—orange (slow); Sulphuric Acid—yellow.

Thin-layer Chromatography. *System TA*—Rf 47; *system TB*—Rf 00; *system TC*—Rf 03.

Gas Chromatography. *System GA*—RI 2440 and 2775.

High Pressure Liquid Chromatography. *System HA*—k' 1.4.

Ultraviolet Spectrum. Aqueous acid—234 nm ($A_1^1 = 655$ b), 320 nm ($A_1^1 = 75$ b); methanol—235 nm ($A_1^1 = 866$ a), 328 nm.

Infra-red Spectrum. Principal peaks at wavenumbers 1665, 1245, 1525, 1495, 1217, 1285 (acebutolol hydrochloride, KBr disk).

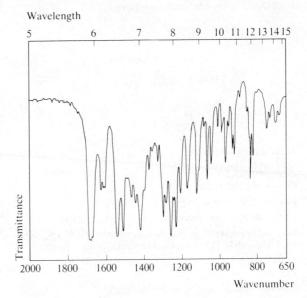

Mass Spectrum. Principal peaks at *m/z* 72, 43, 30, 56, 151, 221, 41, 98.

Quantification. HIGH PRESSURE LIQUID CHROMATOGRAPHY. In plasma or urine: acebutolol and metabolites, sensitivity 20 ng/ml in plasma, UV detection—J. N. Buskin *et al., J. Chromat.,* 1982, *230*; *Biomed. Appl., 19*, 438–442.

RADIOIMMUNOASSAY. In plasma: detection limit 10 pg—B. Gourmel *et al., Clinica chim. Acta,* 1980, *108*, 229–237. In plasma: diacetalol—B. Gourmel *et al., Clinica chim. Acta,* 1981, *115*, 229–234.

Disposition in the Body. Absorbed after oral administration; bioavailability about 40%. The major metabolite is the acetyl derivative, diacetalol, which is active. After an oral dose, about 20 to 40% of the dose is excreted in the urine in 24 hours, about 9 to 12% of the dose as unchanged drug and about 12 to 24% as diacetalol. Up to about 60% of the dose is eliminated in the faeces as unchanged drug and diacetalol. After an intravenous dose, relatively more is excreted in the urine than in the faeces, and the proportion of unchanged drug in the urine is greater than after an oral dose.

THERAPEUTIC CONCENTRATION.

After a single oral dose of 400 mg, administered to 8 subjects, a mean peak plasma concentration of 0.7 µg/ml was attained in 2 hours; a mean peak concentration of diacetalol of 0.8 µg/ml was attained in 4 hours (A. A. Gulaid *et al., Biopharm. Drug Disp.,* 1981, *2*, 103–114).

Steady-state concentrations of 0.51 to 1.23 µg/ml (mean 0.7) were reported during chronic oral administration of 300 mg every 6 to 8 hours to 6 subjects; the concentration of diacetalol was 0.63 to 4.43 µg/ml (mean 2.2) (R. A. Winkle *et al., Br. J. clin. Pharmac.,* 1977, *4*, 519–522).

HALF-LIFE. Plasma half-life, acebutolol about 7 to 11 hours, diacetalol about 12 hours.

VOLUME OF DISTRIBUTION. About 1 to 3 litres/kg.

DISTRIBUTION IN BLOOD. Plasma: whole blood ratio, about 0.8.

PROTEIN BINDING. In plasma, about 20%.

Dose. The equivalent of 0.2 to 1.2 g of acebutolol daily.

Acecainide

Anti-arrhythmic

Synonym. N-Acetylprocainamide
4'-[(2-Diethylaminoethyl)carbamoyl]acetanilide
$C_{15}H_{23}N_3O_2 = 277.4$
CAS—32795-44-1

CO·NH·CH₂·CH₂·N(C₂H₅)₂

NH·CO·CH₃

Acecainide Hydrochloride
$C_{15}H_{23}N_3O_2,HCl = 313.8$
CAS—34118-92-8
Crystals. M.p. 190° to 193°.

Gas Chromatography. *System GA* —RI 2698.

Ultraviolet Spectrum. Aqueous acid or alkali—266 nm.

Infra-red Spectrum. Principal peaks at wavenumbers 1639, 1509, 1527, 1696, 1600, 1259 (acecainide hydrochloride, KBr disk).

Mass Spectrum. Principal peaks at *m/z* 86, 58, 99, 56, 162, 132, 149, 205.

Quantification. See also under Procainamide.

GAS CHROMATOGRAPHY–MASS SPECTROMETRY. In plasma: sensitivity 500 ng/ml—J. M. Strong *et al., J. Pharmacokinet. Biopharm.*, 1975, *3*, 223–235.

Disposition in the Body. Readily absorbed after oral administration; bioavailability about 85%. Up to 85% of a dose is excreted in the urine as unchanged drug in 48 hours, with only 2 to 3% excreted as procainamide and less than 1% as the monodesethyl metabolite.
Acecainide is the principal active metabolite of procainamide.

THERAPEUTIC CONCENTRATION. In plasma, usually in the range 10 to 30 µg/ml.

After a single oral dose of 1.5 g to 9 subjects, peak plasma concentrations of 7.4 to 17.2 µg/ml (mean 12), were attained in 1.5 to 4 hours (W. K. Lee *et al., Clin. Pharmac. Ther.*, 1976, *19*, 508–514).

Following oral administration of 1 g four times a day to 8 subjects, steady-state plasma concentrations of 9.3 to 25.5 µg/ml (mean 18) were reported (A. J. Atkinson *et al., Clin. Pharmac. Ther.*, 1977, *21*, 575–587).

TOXICITY. Toxic effects may occur at plasma concentrations within the therapeutic range.

HALF-LIFE. Plasma half-life, about 6 to 9 hours in normal subjects; increased in subjects with heart disease or renal impairment.

VOLUME OF DISTRIBUTION. About 1.5 litres/kg.

CLEARANCE. Plasma clearance, about 3 ml/min/kg.

PROTEIN BINDING. In plasma, about 10%.

NOTE. For a review of the pharmacokinetics of acecainide see S. J. Connolly and R. E. Kates, *Clin. Pharmacokinet.*, 1982, *7*, 206–220.

Dose. Acecainide has been given in doses of 2 to 6 g daily.

Acepifylline

Xanthine Bronchodilator

Synonyms. Acefylline Piperazine; Piperazine Theophylline Ethanoate.
Proprietary Names. Dynaphylline; Etaphylline; Etophylate.

Piperazine bis(theophyllin-7-ylacetate)
$(C_9H_{10}N_4O_4)_2,C_4H_{10}N_2 = 562.5$
CAS—18833-13-1

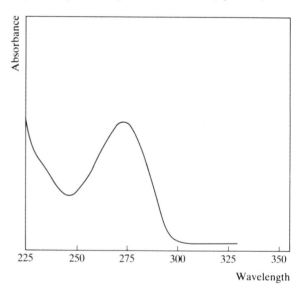

A white crystalline powder. M.p. 260°.
Freely **soluble** in water; slightly soluble in ethanol.

Colour Test. Amalic Acid Test—orange/violet.

Thin-layer Chromatography. *System TA*—Rf 04; *system TB*—Rf 01; *system TC*—Rf 01. (*Acidified iodoplatinate solution*, positive.)

Gas Chromatography. *System GA*—RI 1000.

Ultraviolet Spectrum. Aqueous acid—274 nm ($A_1^1 = 317$ a).

Absorbance

225   250   275   300   325   350
Wavelength

Infra-red Spectrum. Principal peaks at wavenumbers 1700, 1660, 1612, 1538, 1298, 1219 (KBr disk).

Mass Spectrum. Principal peaks at *m/z* 44, 194, 109, 67, 86, 238, 56, 85.

Quantification. GAS CHROMATOGRAPHY. In urine: FID—J. Zuidema and H. Hilbers, *J. Chromat.*, 1980, *182; Biomed. Appl.*, *8*, 445–447.

HIGH PRESSURE LIQUID CHROMATOGRAPHY. In plasma: theophylline-7-acetic acid, sensitivity 25 ng/ml, UV detection—S. Sved *et al., Biopharm. Drug Disp.*, 1981, *2*, 177–184.

Disposition in the Body. Very poorly absorbed after oral administration. It is metabolised to theophylline-7-acetic acid but does not appear to be converted to theophylline.

THERAPEUTIC CONCENTRATION.
Following a single oral dose of 1 g to 2 subjects, peak plasma concentrations of 0.28 and 0.14 µg/ml of theophylline-7-acetic acid were attained in 1.5 and 2 hours, respectively (S. Sved *et al., ibid.*).

Wavelength

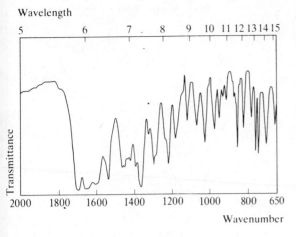

HALF-LIFE. Plasma half-life, theophylline-7-acetic acid about 1 to 2 hours.

VOLUME OF DISTRIBUTION. Theophylline-7-acetic acid 0.5 litre/kg (single subject).

CLEARANCE. Plasma clearance, theophylline-7-acetic acid 7 ml/min/kg (single subject).

REFERENCE. S. Sved *et al., ibid.*

Dose. 1.5 to 3 g daily.

Acepromazine   *Tranquilliser*

Synonym. Acetylpromazine
Proprietary Name. Plégicil
10-(3-Dimethylaminopropyl)phenothiazin-2-yl methyl ketone
$C_{19}H_{22}N_2OS = 326.5$
CAS—61-00-7

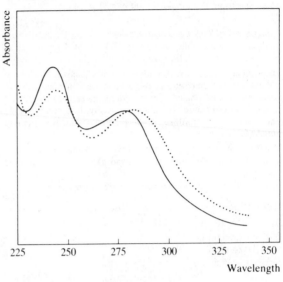

An orange-coloured oil.

Acepromazine Maleate
Proprietary Names. Plégicil. It is an ingredient of Immobilon (for large animals).
$C_{19}H_{22}N_2OS,C_4H_4O_4 = 442.5$
CAS—3598-37-6
A yellow crystalline powder. M.p. 136° to 139°.
Soluble 1 in 27 of water, 1 in 13 of ethanol, and 1 in 3 of chloroform; slightly soluble in ether and light petroleum.

Dissociation Constant. pK_a 9.3.

Partition Coefficient. Log *P* (octanol/pH 7.4), 2.3.

Colour Tests. Formaldehyde–Sulphuric Acid—blue-violet; Forrest Reagent—red; FPN Reagent—brown-orange; Liebermann's Test—brown; Mandelin's Test—green → red; Marquis Test—yellow-green → red.

Thin-layer Chromatography. *System TA*—Rf 48; *system TB*—Rf 26; *system TC*—Rf 24. (*Acidified iodoplatinate solution, positive.*)

Gas Chromatography. *System GA*—RI 2694; *system GF*—RI 3230.

High Pressure Liquid Chromatography. *System HA*—k′ 4.1.

Ultraviolet Spectrum. Aqueous acid—243 nm ($A_1^1 = 765$ a), 279 nm; aqueous alkali—245 nm, 283 nm.

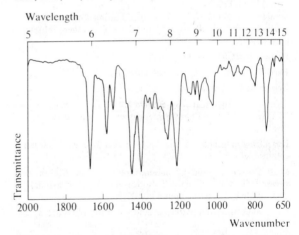

Infra-red Spectrum. Principal peaks at wavenumbers 1675, 1220, 1265, 1587, 746, 1562 (KBr disk).

Wavelength

Mass Spectrum. Principal peaks at *m/z* 100, 72, 240, 340, 44, 197, 254, 43 (acepromazine maleate).

Dose. Acepromazine has been given in doses of 6 to 60 mg daily.

Acetaldehyde

Synonyms. Acetic Aldehyde; Aldehyde; Ethanal; Ethyl Aldehyde.
$CH_3 \cdot CHO = 44.05$
CAS—75-07-0
A colourless inflammable liquid. F.p. −123.5°. B.p. 20.2°.
Refractive index, at 20°, 1.3316.
Miscible with water, ethanol, and ether.

Colour Tests. Potassium Dichromate (Method 2)—green; Schiff's Reagent—violet; Sodium Nitroprusside (Method 2)—red.

Gas Chromatography. *System GA*—RI 372; *system GI*—retention time 0.7 min.

Mass Spectrum. Principal peaks at m/z 29, 44, 43, 42, 26, 41, 28, 27.

Quantification. GAS CHROMATOGRAPHY. In blood: head-space analysis, detection limit 18 ng/ml, FID—J. M. Christensen *et al., Clinica chim. Acta*, 1981, *116*, 389–395.

Disposition in the Body. Acetaldehyde is a major intermediate metabolite of ethanol and is also a metabolite of metaldehyde, paraldehyde, and phenacetin. It undergoes further metabolism by oxidation to acetic acid and, eventually, to carbon dioxide and water. A minor pathway involves condensation with pyruvic acid to form acetoin.

TOXICITY. Acetaldehyde is more toxic than ethanol or acetic acid. The maximum permissible atmospheric concentration is 100 ppm.

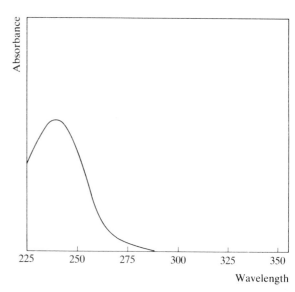

Acetanilide   *Analgesic*

Synonym. Antifebrin
N-Phenylacetamide
$C_8H_9NO = 135.2$
CAS—103-84-4

$$C_6H_5 \cdot NH \cdot CO \cdot CH_3$$

Colourless shining lamellar crystals or white crystalline powder. M.p. 113° to 115°.

Soluble 1 in 200 of water, 1 in 20 of boiling water, 1 in 3.5 of ethanol, 1 in 8 of chloroform, and 1 in 50 of ether; soluble in acetone.

Dissociation Constant. pK_a 0.6 (25°).

Partition Coefficient. Log P (octanol), 1.2.

Colour Test. Liebermann's Test—red-orange.

Thin-layer Chromatography. *System TD*—Rf 45; *system TE*—Rf 70; *system TF*—Rf 45. (*Acidified potassium permanganate solution*, positive.)

Gas Chromatography. *System GA*—acetanilide RI 1358, paracetamol RI 1687.

High Pressure Liquid Chromatography. *System HA*—k′ 0.1; *system HD*—acetanilide k′ 0.5, paracetamol k′ 0.1; *system HW*—acetanilide k′ 2.3, paracetamol k′ 0.32.

Ultraviolet Spectrum. Aqueous acid—239 nm ($A_1^1 = 815$ a). No alkaline shift.

Infra-red Spectrum. Principal peaks at wavenumbers 1660, 1598, 752, 1538, 1315, 1500 (KBr disk).

Mass Spectrum. Principal peaks at m/z 93, 135, 43, 66, 65, 39, 94, 92; paracetamol 109, 151, 43, 80, 108, 81, 53, 52.

Quantification. GAS CHROMATOGRAPHY. In plasma: FID—N. Buchanan *et al., Br. J. clin. Pharmac.*, 1980, *9*, 525–526.

Disposition in the Body. Rapidly and completely absorbed after oral administration, with maximum plasma concentrations achieved after one to two hours. It is distributed throughout the body. The main metabolic reaction is oxidation to paracetamol through which the analgesic and antipyretic effects of the drug are chiefly exerted; paracetamol is then conjugated with glucuronic acid or sulphate. A minor reaction is deacetylation of

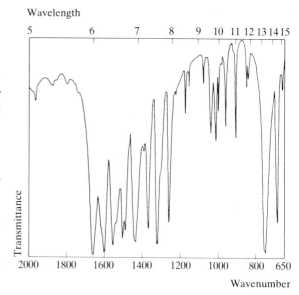

acetanilide to aniline. About 0.1% of an oral dose is excreted unchanged in the urine in 24 hours, about 4% as free paracetamol, 80% as paracetamol conjugates, and 0.05% as aniline. About 0.1% of an oral dose may be eliminated in the faeces.

TOXICITY. The main toxic effect is the formation of methaemoglobin due to the production of aniline or other toxic metabolites.

HALF-LIFE. Plasma half-life, about 1.5 hours.

VOLUME OF DISTRIBUTION. About 0.7 litre/kg.

CLEARANCE. Plasma clearance, about 6 ml/min/kg.

PROTEIN BINDING. In plasma, not significantly bound.

Dose. Acetanilide was formerly given in doses of 0.36 to 1.2 g daily.

Acetarsol   *Antiprotozoal*

Synonyms. Acetarsone; Acetphenarsinum; Osarsolum.
Proprietary Names. Stovarsol; SVC.
3-Acetamido-4-hydroxyphenylarsonic acid
$C_8H_{10}AsNO_5 = 275.1$
CAS—97-44-9

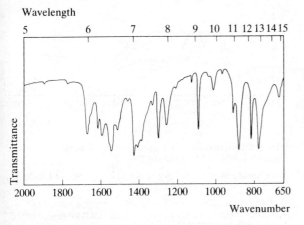

A white crystalline powder. M.p. about 240°, with decomposition.
Practically **insoluble** in cold water, moderately soluble in boiling water; practically insoluble in ethanol; soluble in dilute alkalis.

Acetarsol Sodium

$C_8H_9AsNNaO_5,5H_2O = 387.2$
CAS—5892-48-8 (anhydrous)
White crystals or crystalline powder.
Soluble 1 in 7 of water; practically insoluble in ethanol, chloroform, and ether.

Dissociation Constant. pK_a 3.7, 7.9, 9.3.

Ultraviolet Spectrum. Aqueous acid—281 nm $(A_1^1 = 94$ b); aqueous alkali—250 nm $(A_1^1 = 567$ b), 299 nm $(A_1^1 = 177$ b).

Infra-red Spectrum. Principal peaks at wavenumbers 887, 1538, 784, 823, 1297, 1584 (KBr disk).

Wavelength

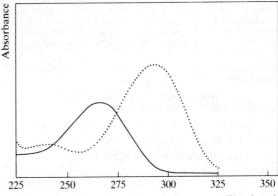

Dose. Up to 500 mg daily, for 10 days.

Acetazolamide   *Carbonic Anhydrase Inhibitor*

Synonyms. Acetazolam; Acetazoleamide.
Proprietary Names. Défiltran; Diamox; Diuriwas; Glaucomide; Glaupax; Inidrase.
N-(5-Sulphamoyl-1,3,4-thiadiazol-2-yl)acetamide
$C_4H_6N_4O_3S_2 = 222.2$
CAS—59-66-5
A fine, white to yellowish-white, crystalline powder. M.p. about 260°, with decomposition.

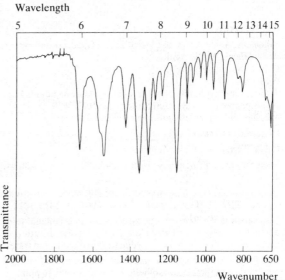

Soluble 1 in 1400 of water, 1 in 400 of ethanol, and 1 in 100 of acetone; practically insoluble in carbon tetrachloride, chloroform, and ether.

Acetazolamide Sodium

Proprietary Name. Diamox Sodium
$C_4H_5N_4NaO_3S_2 = 244.2$
CAS—1424-27-7
Soluble in water.

Dissociation Constant. pK_a 7.2, 9.0 (25°).

Colour Test. Koppanyi–Zwikker Test—red-violet (transient).

Thin-layer Chromatography. *System TD*—Rf 04; *system TE*—Rf 03; *system TF*—Rf 31.

High Pressure Liquid Chromatography. *System HA*—k′ 0.1.

Ultraviolet Spectrum. Aqueous acid—265 nm $(A_1^1 = 475$ a); aqueous alkali—240 nm, 291 nm.

Infra-red Spectrum. Principal peaks at wavenumbers 1167, 1548, 1316, 1665, 671, 1115 (KBr disk).

Wavelength

Mass Spectrum. Principal peaks at m/z 43, 180, 42, 45, 44, 64, 100, 222.

Quantification. GAS CHROMATOGRAPHY. In blood, plasma or saliva: detection limit 10 ng, ECD—S. M. Wallace *et al., J. pharm. Sci.,* 1977, *66,* 527–530.

GAS CHROMATOGRAPHY—MASS SPECTROMETRY. In blood or saliva: detection limit 25 pg—K. Kishida *et al., Analyt. Lett. (Part B),* 1981, *14,* 335–347.

HIGH PRESSURE LIQUID CHROMATOGRAPHY. In blood, plasma, or urine: sensitivity 50 ng/ml, UV detection—D. J. Chapron and L. B. White, *J. pharm. Sci.,* 1984, *73,* 985–989.

Disposition in the Body. Readily absorbed after oral administration. Acetazolamide binds tightly to carbonic anhydrase and will accumulate in tissues in which this enzyme is present, particularly in red blood cells and the renal cortex. About 70 to 90% of a dose is excreted in the urine as unchanged drug in 24 hours but the renal clearance is increased if the urine is alkaline; small amounts of unchanged drug are excreted in the bile.

THERAPEUTIC CONCENTRATION. In plasma, usually in the range 10 to 15 µg/ml.

Following a single oral dose of 250 mg to 5 subjects, peak plasma concentrations of 10 to 18 µg/ml (mean 14) were attained in 1 to 3 hours; peak erythrocyte concentrations of 13 to 29 µg/ml were reached about 1 hour after the peak plasma concentrations (S. M. Wallace *et al., J. pharm. Sci.,* 1977, *66,* 527–530).

TOXICITY. Fatal cases of agranulocytosis, aplastic anaemia, and thrombocytopenia have been reported.

HALF-LIFE. Plasma half-life, about 13 hours; blood and erythrocyte concentrations decrease more slowly.

VOLUME OF DISTRIBUTION. About 0.2 litre/kg.

SALIVA. Plasma: saliva ratio, about 100.

PROTEIN BINDING. In plasma, about 90 to 95%.

Dose. In the treatment of glaucoma 0.25 to 1 g daily.

Acetic Acid

Synonyms. Acide Acetique Cristallisable; Concentrated Acetic Acid; Glacial Acetic Acid.

$CH_3 \cdot COOH = 60.05$

CAS—64-19-7

A translucent crystalline mass or a clear colourless liquid. M.p. 15°. B.p. about 117°. Refractive index, at 20°, 1.3718.

Miscible with water, ethanol, chloroform, and ether.

Dissociation Constant. pK_a 4.8 (25°).

Colour Test. Ferric Chloride—red.

Mass Spectrum. Principal peaks at m/z 45, 29, 43, 60, 42, 28, 44, 41.

Quantification. GAS CHROMATOGRAPHY. In blood: sensitivity 1 µg/ml, FID—D. Lester, *Analyt. Chem.,* 1964, *36,* 1810–1812.

Disposition in the Body. Acetic acid occurs as a metabolite of ethanol and also of paraldehyde after its depolymerisation to acetaldehyde. It is further oxidised to carbon dioxide and water.

TOXICITY. The estimated minimum lethal dose is 5 ml and the maximum permissible atmospheric concentration is 10 ppm.

Acetohexamide

Antidiabetic

Proprietary Names. Dimelor; Dymelor; Ordimel.

1-(4-Acetylbenzenesulphonyl)-3-cyclohexylurea

$C_{15}H_{20}N_2O_4S = 324.4$

CAS—968-81-0

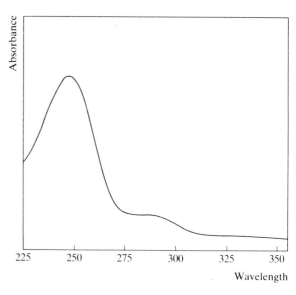

A white crystalline powder. M.p. 182° to 187°.

Practically **insoluble** in water and ether; soluble 1 in 230 of ethanol and 1 in 210 of chloroform; soluble in pyridine and in dilute solutions of alkali hydroxides.

Colour Test. Koppanyi–Zwikker Test—violet.

Thin-layer Chromatography. *System TD*—Rf 39; *system TE*—Rf 12; *system TF*—Rf 43.

Ultraviolet Spectrum. Aqueous acid—247 nm ($A_1^1 = 508$ b); aqueous alkali—249 nm ($A_1^1 = 427$ a).

Infra-red Spectrum. Principal peaks at wavenumbers 1165, 1031, 1681, 1531, 905, 1264 (Nujol mull).

Mass Spectrum. Principal peaks at m/z 210, 56, 43, 184, 211, 75, 99, 76.

Quantification. SPECTROFLUORIMETRY. In plasma: limit of detection 200 ng—P. Girgis-Takla and I. Chroneos, *Analyst, Lond.,* 1979, *104,* 117–123.

GAS CHROMATOGRAPHY. In biological fluids: FID—J. W. Kleber *et al., J. pharm. Sci.,* 1977, *66,* 635–638.

Disposition in the Body. Readily absorbed after oral administration and rapidly metabolised to (−)-1-hydroxyhexamide which has about 2.5 times the hypoglycaemic activity of the unchanged drug. Minor metabolites include 4'-*trans*-hydroxyacetohexamide, 4'-*trans*-hydroxy-1-hydroxyhexamide and, to a lesser extent, the 4'-*cis*-, 3'-*cis*-, and 3'-*trans*-isomers. About 80% of a dose is excreted in the urine in 24 hours, mainly as metabolites.

THERAPEUTIC CONCENTRATION. In plasma, usually in the range 20 to 60 µg/ml.

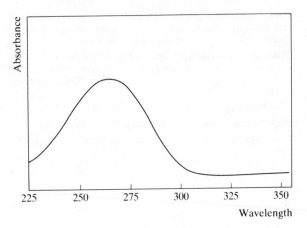

Following oral administration of 750 mg of three different tablet formulations to 8 subjects, mean peak plasma-acetohexamide concentrations of about 28, 40, and 44 µg/ml were attained 2 hours after a dose; mean peak plasma concentrations of (−)-1-hydroxyhexamide averaged about 30 µg/ml (J. W. Kleber et al., J. pharm. Sci., 1977, 66, 635–638).

After daily oral doses of 0.5 g to 18 subjects, an average serum concentration of 42 µg/ml was reported 3 to 5 hours after the dose (J. Sheldon et al., Diabetes, 1965, 14, 362–367).

TOXICITY. Prolonged hypoglycaemia has been reported.

HALF-LIFE. Plasma half-life, acetohexamide about 1.3 hours, (−)-1-hydroxyhexamide about 5 hours.

PROTEIN BINDING. In plasma, about 96%.

NOTE. For a review of the pharmacokinetics of oral hypoglycaemic agents see L. Balant, Clin. Pharmacokinet., 1981, 6, 215–241.

Dose. 0.25 to 1.5 g daily.

Acetomenaphthone   *Vitamin K Activity*

Synonyms. Acetomenadione; Menadiol Diacetate.
Proprietary Name. It is an ingredient of Pernivit.
2-Methylnaphthalene-1,4-diyl diacetate
$C_{15}H_{14}O_4 = 258.3$
CAS—573-20-6

A white crystalline powder. M.p. 112° to 115°.
Practically **insoluble** in water; slightly soluble in cold ethanol; soluble 1 in 3.3 of boiling ethanol; soluble in acetic acid.

Colour Test. Liebermann's Test—black.

Ultraviolet Spectrum. Dehydrated alcohol—285 nm ($A_1^1 = 245$ b), 322 nm ($A_1^1 = 37$ b).

Infra-red Spectrum. Principal peaks at wavenumbers 1210, 1760, 1163, 1070, 775, 1030 (KBr disk).

Dose. 5 to 20 mg daily.

Acetone   *Solvent*

Synonyms. Cetona; Dimethyl Ketone; 2-Propanone.
$CH_3 \cdot CO \cdot CH_3 = 58.08$
CAS—67-64-1
A clear, colourless, volatile, mobile, inflammable liquid. F.p. −94°. B.p. about 56°. Refractive index 1.3591.
Miscible with water, ethanol, chloroform, and ether.

Partition Coefficient. Log P (octanol), −0.2.

Colour Test. Sodium Nitroprusside (Method 1)—red.

Gas Chromatography. System GA—RI 469; system GI—retention time 2.5 min.

Ultraviolet Spectrum. Aqueous acid—265 nm.

Mass Spectrum. Principal peaks at m/z 43, 58, 59, 27, 42, 26, 39, 29.

Quantification. GAS CHROMATOGRAPHY. In plasma or breath: FID—M. D. Trotter et al., Clinica chim. Acta, 1971, 35, 137–143.

Disposition in the Body. Absorbed through the lungs and skin. It is excreted in the urine and through the lungs; large amounts are mainly excreted unchanged but small doses may be oxidised to carbon dioxide or utilised in the body as acetate or formate.
Acetone is the main metabolite of isopropyl alcohol; it occurs naturally in the blood and urine of diabetics.

TOXICITY. Acetone is one of the solvents abused in 'glue-sniffing'. Severe toxic effects have been associated with blood concentrations of 200 to 300 µg/ml; a blood concentration of 550 µg/ml has been reported in a fatality. The maximum permissible atmospheric concentration is 1000 ppm. Exposure to 1600 ppm for about 15 minutes causes irritation to the eyes and nose. Up to 20 ml has been ingested without ill-effect.

Acetophenazine   *Tranquilliser*

Synonym. Acephenazine
10-{3-[4-(2-Hydroxyethyl)piperazin-1-yl]propyl}phenothiazin-2-yl methyl ketone
$C_{23}H_{29}N_3O_2S = 411.6$
CAS—2751-68-0

Acetophenazine Maleate

Synonym. Acetophenazine Dimaleate
Proprietary Name. Tindal
$C_{23}H_{29}N_3O_2S, 2C_4H_4O_4 = 643.7$
CAS—5714-00-1
A fine yellow powder. M.p. about 165°, with decomposition.
Soluble 1 in 10 of water, 1 in 260 of ethanol, 1 in 370 of acetone, 1 in 2850 of chloroform, 1 in 6000 of ether, and 1 in 11 of propylene glycol.

Colour Tests. Formaldehyde–Sulphuric Acid—blue-violet; Forrest Reagent—pink-orange; FPN Reagent—orange; Liebermann's Test—brown; Marquis Test—red-violet.

Thin-layer Chromatography. *System TA*—Rf 53; *system TB*—Rf 03; *system TC*—Rf 25. (*Dragendorff spray*, positive; *FPN reagent*, pink; *acidified iodoplatinate solution*, positive; *Marquis reagent*, orange.)

Gas Chromatography. *System GA*—not eluted.

High Pressure Liquid Chromatography. *System HA*—k′ 1.9.

Ultraviolet Spectrum. Aqueous acid—243 nm ($A_1^1 = 500$ a), 278 nm.

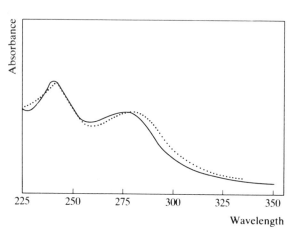

Infra-red Spectrum. Principal peaks at wavenumbers 1670, 1220, 1265, 1587, 746, 1149 (KBr disk).

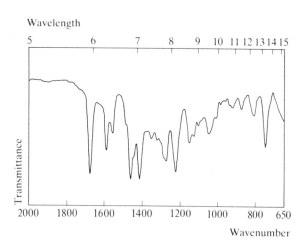

Mass Spectrum. Principal peaks at *m/z* 254, 143, 42, 70, 411, 113, 56, 157.

Dose. 40 to 120 mg of acetophenazine maleate daily; up to 600 mg daily has been given.

Acetorphine

Narcotic Analgesic

(6R,7R,14R) - 3 - O - Acetyl - 7,8 - dihydro - 7 - (1 - hydroxy - 1 - methylbutyl)-6-O-methyl-6,14-ethenomorphine
$C_{27}H_{35}NO_5 = 453.6$
CAS—25333-77-1

M.p. 193°.

Soluble 1 in 4000 of water; freely soluble in ethanol, chloroform, and ether.

Caution. It is dangerous to smell or taste this substance.

Acetorphine Hydrochloride

Synonym. M183
$C_{27}H_{35}NO_5,HCl = 490.0$
CAS—25333-78-2
A white, crystalline, hygroscopic powder. M.p. 204°. It is hydrolysed in solution to etorphine and acetic acid.
Soluble 1 in 50 of water and 1 in 10 of ethanol.

Colour Test. Marquis Test—blue-grey → yellow-brown.

Thin-layer Chromatography. *System TA*—Rf 72. (*Acidified iodoplatinate solution*, positive; *Marquis reagent*, grey; *acidified potassium permanganate solution*, positive.)

High Pressure Liquid Chromatography. *System HA*—k′ 0.4.

Ultraviolet Spectrum. Aqueous acid—284 nm ($A_1^1 = 45$ b).

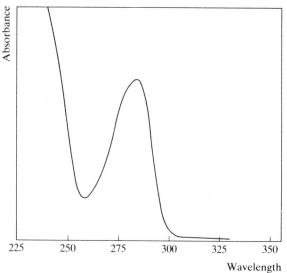

Infra-red Spectrum. Principal peaks at wavenumbers 1200, 1218, 1168, 1760, 1150, 1122 (acetorphine hydrochloride, KBr disk).

Wavelength

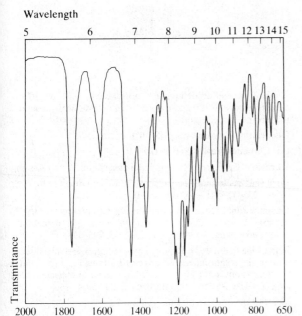

$[CH_3 \cdot CO \cdot O \cdot CH_2 \cdot CH_2 \cdot \overset{+}{N}(CH_3)_3] Cl^-$

A white, very hygroscopic, crystalline powder. M.p. about 150°. Very **soluble** in water yielding unstable solutions; very soluble in ethanol and propylene glycol; freely soluble in chloroform; practically insoluble in ether.

Acetylcholine Bromide

$C_7H_{16}BrNO_2 = 226.1$
CAS—66-23-9
Deliquescent colourless crystals or white crystalline powder. Hydrolysed by hot water and alkalis. M.p. 143°.
Freely **soluble** in water; soluble in ethanol; practically insoluble in ether.

Thin-layer Chromatography. *System TA*—Rf 02; *system TN*—Rf 70; *system TO*—Rf 60. (*Acidified iodoplatinate solution*, positive.)

Infra-red Spectrum. Principal peaks at wavenumbers 949, 1089, 869, 1231, 1000, 1740 (KBr disk).

Wavelength

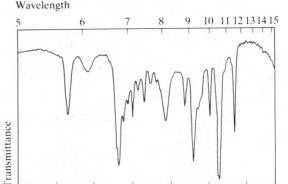

Mass Spectrum. Principal peaks at m/z 58, 43, 57, 149, 71, 42, 41, 55.

Dose. Acetylcholine chloride is used as a 1% ophthalmic solution; it was formerly given parenterally in doses of 20 to 200 mg.

Acetylcarbromal   *Sedative*

Synonyms. Acecarbromal; Acetcarbromal.
Proprietary Names. Abasin; Sedamyl.
1-Acetyl-3-(2-bromo-2-ethylbutyryl)urea
$C_9H_{15}BrN_2O_3 = 279.1$
CAS—77-66-7

$$Br \cdot \underset{\underset{C_2H_5}{|}}{\overset{\overset{C_2H_5}{|}}{C}} \cdot CO \cdot NH \cdot CO \cdot NH \cdot CO \cdot CH_3$$

Colourless crystals or white crystalline powder. M.p. 109°.
Soluble 1 in 1000 of water; soluble in ethanol, chloroform, and ether.

Colour Test. Nessler's Reagent—brown-orange (slow).

Thin-layer Chromatography. *System TD*—Rf 49; *system TE*—Rf 57; *system TF*—Rf 48.

Gas Chromatography. *System GA*—RI 1215.

Infra-red Spectrum. Principal peaks at wavenumbers 1776, 1730, 1183, 1267, 1149, 1236 (Nujol mull).

Mass Spectrum. Principal peaks at m/z 43, 129, 69, 41, 86, 97, 55, 44.

Dose. 0.75 to 1.5 g daily.

Acetylcholine Chloride   *Parasympathomimetic*

Proprietary Name. Miochol
(2-Acetoxyethyl)trimethylammonium chloride
$C_7H_{16}ClNO_2 = 181.7$
CAS—51-84-3 (acetylcholine); *60-31-1* (chloride)

Acetylcodeine

3-*O*-Methyl-6-*O*-acetylmorphine
$C_{20}H_{23}NO_4 = 341.4$
CAS—6703-27-1

M.p. 134° to 135°.
It is a contaminant of codeine and up to 12% may be found in illicit heroin.

Gas Chromatography. *System GA*—RI 2510.

High Pressure Liquid Chromatography. *System HC*—k' 0.78; *system HS*—k' 0.50.

Ultraviolet Spectrum. Aqueous acid—284 nm ($A_1^1 = 37$ b).

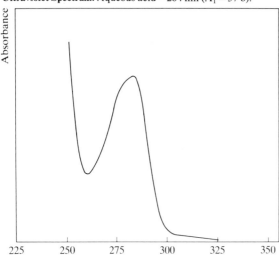

Infra-red Spectrum. Principal peaks at wavenumbers 1233, 1731, 1272, 1042, 1055, 1501.

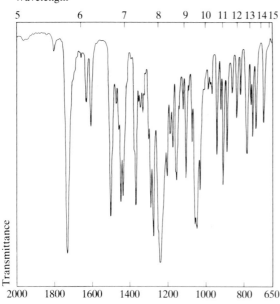

Mass Spectrum. Principal peaks at m/z 341, 282, 229, 42, 43, 59, 342, 204.

Acetylcysteine   *Mucolytic/Paracetamol Antidote*

Synonym. N-Acetylcysteine

Proprietary Names. Airbron; Fabrol; Fluimucil; Mucolyticum; Mucomyst; Nac; Parvolex.
N-Acetyl-L-cysteine
$C_5H_9NO_3S = 163.2$
CAS—616-91-1

A white, crystalline, deliquescent powder. M.p. 104° to 110°. **Soluble** 1 in 8 of water and 1 in 2 of ethanol; practically insoluble in chloroform and ether.

Dissociation Constant. pK_a 9.5 (30°).

Gas Chromatography. *System GA*—RI 1547.

Ultraviolet Spectrum. No significant absorption, 230 to 360 nm.

Infra-red Spectrum. Principal peaks at wavenumbers 1530, 1300, 1230, 1275, 1580, 1715 (Nujol mull).

Quantification. HIGH PRESSURE LIQUID CHROMATOGRAPHY. In plasma or urine: detection limit 50 ng/ml, UV detection— P. A. Lewis *et al.*, *J. pharm. Sci.*, 1984, *73*, 996–998.

Disposition in the Body. Readily absorbed after oral administration, peak plasma concentrations being attained in 2 to 3 hours; concentrations in the lung are similar to those in plasma. About 20% of a dose is excreted in the urine in 24 hours.

PROTEIN BINDING. In plasma, about 78%.

REFERENCE. D. Rodenstein *et al.*, *Clin. Pharmacokinet.*, 1978, *3*, 247–254.

Dose. As a mucolytic, 600 mg daily by mouth. In the treatment of paracetamol overdosage, initially 150 mg/kg by rapid intravenous infusion.

Acetyldigitoxin   *Cardiac Glycoside*

Synonyms. Acetyldigitoxoside; α-Digitoxin Monoacetate.
Proprietary Name. Acylanid(e)
3β-[(O-3-O-Acetyl-2,6-dideoxy-β-D-*ribo*-hexopyranosyl-(1 → 4)-O-2,6-dideoxy-β-D-*ribo*-hexopyranosyl-(1 → 4)-2,6-dideoxy-β-D-*ribo*-hexopyranosyl)oxy]-14-hydroxy-5β,14β-card-20(22)-enolide
$C_{43}H_{66}O_{14} = 807.0$
CAS—1111-39-3

A white hygroscopic crystalline powder. M.p. 217° to 221°.

Soluble 1 in 6100 of water, 1 in 63 of ethanol, and 1 in 12 of chloroform; practically insoluble in ether and light petroleum; soluble in methanol.

Thin-layer Chromatography. *System TK*—Rf 82. (p-*Anisaldehyde reagent*, blue; *perchloric acid solution*, followed by examination under ultraviolet light, red fluorescence.)

Ultraviolet Spectrum. No significant absorption, 230 to 360 nm.

Disposition in the Body. About 65% of a dose is absorbed after oral administration. It is slowly excreted in the urine, about 20% of a dose being excreted in 6 days; digitoxin accounts for about 60% of the urinary material. About 15 to 20% of a dose is eliminated in the faeces over a period of 18 days.

HALF-LIFE. Plasma half-life, about 8 to 9 days.

PROTEIN BINDING. In plasma, about 80%.

REFERENCE. G. Bodem *et al., Arzneimittel-Forsch.*, 1975, *25*, 1448–1452.

Dose. Maintenance, 100 to 200 µg daily.

Acinitrazole   *Antiprotozoal*

Synonyms. Aminitrozole; Nithiamide.
Proprietary Names. Tricosil; Trigamma.
N-(5-Nitrothiazol-2-yl)acetamide
$C_5H_5N_3O_3S = 187.2$
CAS—140-40-9

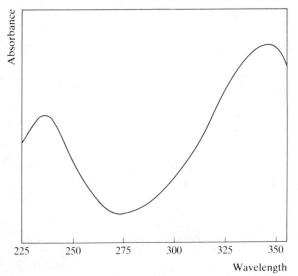

A buff or yellowish-buff powder. M.p. 264° to 265°; slight decomposition may occur.

Very slightly **soluble** in water; soluble 1 in 300 of ethanol and 1 in 900 of chloroform; slightly soluble in ether; soluble in aqueous solutions of sodium hydroxide and ammonia.

Colour Test. Methanolic Potassium Hydroxide—orange.

Thin-layer Chromatography. *System TA*—Rf 80. (*Acidified potassium permanganate solution*, positive.)

Ultraviolet Spectrum. Aqueous acid—237 nm, 345 nm ($A_1^1 = 435$ b).

Infra-red Spectrum. Principal peaks at wavenumbers 1314, 1176, 1709, 1215, 818, 740.

Dose. Acinitrazole has been given in doses of 200 to 400 mg daily.

Aconitine   *Alkaloid*

Synonym. Acetylbenzoylaconine
8-Acetoxy-3,11,18-trihydroxy-16-ethyl-1,6,19-trimethoxy-4-methoxymethylaconitan-10-yl benzoate
$C_{34}H_{47}NO_{11} = 645.7$
CAS—302-27-2
An alkaloid present in species of *Aconitum*, including *A. napellus* agg. (Ranunculaceae).
Colourless crystals or white crystalline powder. M.p. 196°, with decomposition.
Soluble 1 in 4500 of water, 1 in 40 of ethanol (90%), 1 in 3 of chloroform, 1 in 70 of ether, and 1 in 2800 of light petroleum.

Aconitine Nitrate
$C_{34}H_{47}NO_{11},HNO_3 = 708.8$
CAS—6509-18-8
Colourless crystals or white crystalline powder. M.p. about 200°, with decomposition.
Soluble in water and ethanol.

Dissociation Constant. pK_a 8.1 (25°).

Partition Coefficient. Log *P* (ether), 0.8.

Thin-layer Chromatography. *System TA*—Rf 68; *system TB*—Rf 08; *system TC*—Rf 39. (*Acidified iodoplatinate solution*, positive.)

Ultraviolet Spectrum. Aqueous acid—234 nm ($A_1^1 = 233$ a), 275 nm.

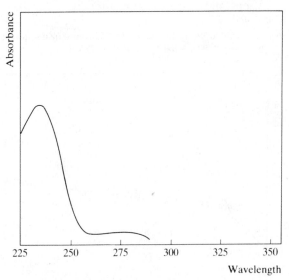

Infra-red Spectrum. Principal peaks at wavenumbers 1092, 1273, 1713, 1235, 710, 1020 (KBr disk). (See below)

Mass Spectrum. Principal peaks at *m/z* 105, 554, 540, 43, 45, 77, 31, 29.

Wavelength

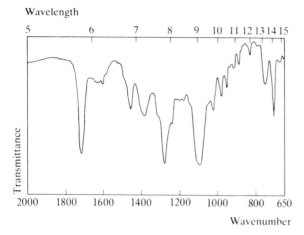

Disposition in the Body.

TOXICITY. Aconitine affects both the heart and the central nervous system and is one of the most potent and quick-acting poisons. It is well absorbed from the gastro-intestinal tract and death may occur within a few minutes. The estimated minimum lethal dose is 2 mg of aconitine, 5 ml of aconite tincture (25% v/v) or 1 g of aconite root, although recovery after ingestion of 10 mg of aconitine has been reported.

Acriflavine
Antiseptic

Synonym. Acriflavine Hydrochloride
Proprietary Names. Diacrid; Panflavin.

A mixture of 3,6-diamino-10-methylacridinium chloride hydrochloride and 3,6-diaminoacridine dihydrochloride, the latter being present to the extent of approximately one-third.
$C_{14}H_{14}ClN_3,HCl = 296.2$; $C_{13}H_{11}N_3,2HCl = 282.2$
CAS—8063-24-9

An orange-red to red crystalline powder. A precipitate may form in aqueous solutions on dilution or on standing.

Soluble 1 in about 3 of water and 1 in 40 of ethanol; practically insoluble in chloroform and ether.

Dissociation Constant. pK_a 9.1 (25°).

Colour Test. Marquis Test—yellow → red.

Thin-layer Chromatography. *System TA*—four spots at Rf 07, 22, 28, and 62. (Location under ultraviolet light, yellow-green fluorescence.)

Ultraviolet Spectrum. Aqueous acid—262 nm ($A_1^1 = 1515$ a). No alkaline shift.

Infra-red Spectrum. Principal peaks at wavenumbers 1631, 1590, 1171, 1181, 1316, 1242.

Adiphenine
Anticholinergic

2-Diethylaminoethyl diphenylacetate
$C_{20}H_{25}NO_2 = 311.4$
CAS—64-95-9

$$C_6H_5 \cdot CH \cdot CO \cdot O \cdot [CH_2]_2 \cdot N(C_2H_5)_2 \overset{C_6H_5}{|}$$

Adiphenine Hydrochloride

Synonym. Spasmolytine
$C_{20}H_{25}NO_2,HCl = 347.9$
CAS—50-42-0
A white crystalline powder. M.p. 112° to 115°.
Soluble in water, ethanol, and chloroform; practically insoluble in ether.

Colour Tests. Liebermann's Test—brown; Mandelin's Test—green → blue.

Thin-layer Chromatography. *System TA*—Rf 64; *system TB*—Rf 56; *system TC*—Rf 60. (*Acidified iodoplatinate solution*, positive.)

Gas Chromatography. *System GA*—RI 2186.

High Pressure Liquid Chromatography. *System HA*—k' 1.8.

Ultraviolet Spectrum. Aqueous acid—253 nm, 258 nm ($A_1^1 = 14.5$ a), 264 nm.

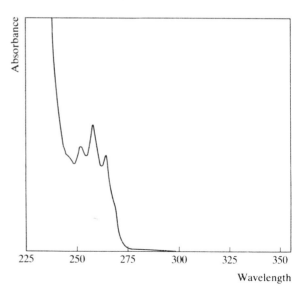

Infra-red Spectrum. Principal peaks at wavenumbers 1736, 1145, 700, 1190, 1500, 746 (KBr disk).

Mass Spectrum. Principal peaks at m/z 86, 30, 167, 99, 87, 58, 165, 29.

Dose. Adiphenine hydrochloride has been given in doses of 225 to 450 mg daily.

Adrenaline   *Sympathomimetic*

Synonyms. Epinephrine; Epirenamine; Levorenin; Suprarenin.
Proprietary Names. Bronkaid Mistometer; Dyspné-Inhal; Epiglaufrin; Epinal; Eppy; Glauposine; Simplene; Sus-Phrine; Vaponefrin. It is an ingredient of Asma-Vydrin, Brovon, Ganda, Isopto Epinal, Riddovydrin Inhalant, and Rybarvin.
(R)-1-(3,4-Dihydroxyphenyl)-2-methylaminoethanol
$C_9H_{13}NO_3 = 183.2$
CAS—51-43-4

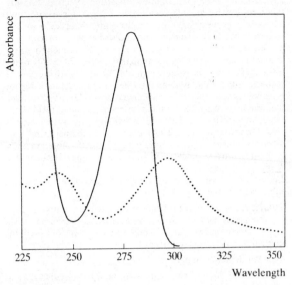

A white or creamy-white crystalline powder or granules. It darkens in colour on exposure to air and light. It is unstable in neutral or alkaline solution. M.p. about 212°, with decomposition.

Sparingly **soluble** in water; practically insoluble in ethanol, chloroform, ether, and light petroleum; freely soluble in solutions of mineral acids and boric acid solution, and in solutions of sodium or potassium hydroxide.

Adrenaline Acid Tartrate

Synonyms. Adrenaline Bitartrate; Adrenaline Tartrate; Epinephrine Bitartrate.
Proprietary Names. E1; E2; Epitrate; Liadren; Lyophrin; Medihaler Epi. It is an ingredient of E-Pilo, Mydricaine, PE, and Welder's Flash Drops.
$C_9H_{13}NO_3, C_4H_6O_6 = 333.3$
CAS—51-42-3
A white to greyish-white or light brownish-grey, crystalline powder. It slowly darkens on exposure to air and light. Incompatible with alkalis. M.p. 147° to 152°, with decomposition.
Soluble 1 in 3 of water and 1 in 520 of ethanol; practically insoluble in chloroform and ether.

Adrenaline Hydrochloride

Proprietary Names. Epifrin; Glaucon; Glycirenan. It is an ingredient of Riddobron Inhalant and Riddofan.
$C_9H_{13}NO_3, HCl = 219.7$
CAS—55-31-2

Dissociation Constant. pK_a 8.7, 10.2, 12.0 (20°).

Colour Tests. Ammoniacal Silver Nitrate—red-brown/red-brown; Ferric Chloride—green; Folin–Ciocalteu Reagent—blue; Marquis Test—orange → violet; Methanolic Potassium Hydroxide—pink-orange → brown; Nessler's Reagent—black; Palladium Chloride—orange → brown; Potassium Dichromate (Method 1)—green → brown.

Thin-layer Chromatography. *System TA*—Rf 00; *system TB*—Rf 00; *system TC*—Rf 01. (*Acidified potassium permanganate solution*, positive.)

High Pressure Liquid Chromatography. *System HC*—k' 0.63.

Ultraviolet Spectrum. Aqueous acid—280 nm ($A_1^1 = 155$ a); aqueous alkali—242 nm, 297 nm.

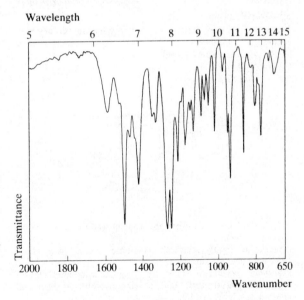

Infra-red Spectrum. Principal peaks at wavenumbers 1253, 1274, 1500, 945, 1224, 871 (KBr disk).

Mass Spectrum. Principal peaks at m/z 44, 42, 124, 165, 163, 123, 93, 65.

Quantification. SPECTROFLUORIMETRY. In plasma: adrenaline and noradrenaline—J. F. O'Hanlon *et al.*, *Analyt. Biochem.*, 1970, *34*, 568–581.

GAS CHROMATOGRAPHY. In plasma, erythrocytes, serum, or urine: adrenaline and noradrenaline, detection limit $10^{-7}\mu g$, FID—H. G. Lovelady and L. L. Foster, *J. Chromat.*, 1975, *108*, 43–52.

Disposition in the Body. Rapidly destroyed in the gastro-intestinal tract after oral administration; the effects of adrenaline after subcutaneous injection are produced within 5 minutes and appear more slowly than after intramuscular injection. Rapidly taken up by the heart, spleen, several glandular tissues, and adrenergic nerves; only metabolites are detectable in the cerebrospinal fluid. The major metabolic reactions are oxidative deamination and *O*-methylation followed by reduction or by glucuronic acid or sulphate conjugation. About 70 to 95% of an intravenous dose is excreted in the urine; of the excreted material about 80% is *O*-methyl metabolites, 2% is catechol metabolites, and only 1% is unchanged drug. The major urinary metabolite is 4-hydroxy-3-methoxymandelic acid (HMMA); other metabolites include 4-hydroxy-3-methoxyphenylacetic acid (homovanillic acid, HVA), conjugated metanephrine, and 4-hydroxy-3-methoxyphenylglycol together with minor amounts of 3,4-dihydroxymandelic acid in free or conjugated form and *N*-methyladrenaline.

Endogenous plasma concentrations of adrenaline in normal subjects are in the range 30 to 160 pg/ml.

TOXICITY. The minimum subcutaneous lethal dose is about 4 mg, but recoveries have occurred after accidental overdosage with 16 mg subcutaneously and 30 mg intravenously, followed by immediate supportive treatment.

PROTEIN BINDING. In plasma, about 50%.

Dose. 200 to 500 µg, subcutaneously or intramuscularly, as a single dose which may be repeated.

Ajmaline   *Anti-arrhythmic*

Synonym. Rauwolfine

Proprietary Names. Aritmina; Cardiorythmine; Gilurytmal; Ritmos.

(17*R*,21*R*)-Ajmalan-17,21-diol

$C_{20}H_{26}N_2O_2 = 326.4$

CAS—4360-12-7

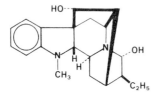

An alkaloid obtained from the root of *Rauwolfia serpentina* (Apocynaceae).

A white or slightly yellowish crystalline powder. M.p. about 195°, with decomposition.

Practically **insoluble** in water; freely soluble in ethanol, chloroform, and glacial acetic acid; sparingly soluble in ether and methanol; soluble in dilute hydrochloric acid.

Ajmaline Hydrochloride

Proprietary Name. Cardiorythmine

$C_{20}H_{26}N_2O_2,2HCl,2H_2O = 435.4$

Crystals. M.p. 140°.

Soluble 1 in 40 of water.

Ajmaline Monoethanolate

$C_{20}H_{26}N_2O_2,C_2H_6O = 372.5$

CAS—60991-48-2

A white or slightly yellowish crystalline powder.

Practically **insoluble** in water; freely soluble in ethanol, chloroform, and glacial acetic acid; sparingly soluble in ether and methanol.

Dissociation Constant. pK_a 8.2.

Colour Tests. Liebermann's Test—red; Mandelin's Test—red; Marquis Test—violet.

Thin-layer Chromatography. *System TA*—Rf 62. (*Acidified potassium permanganate solution*, positive.)

Gas Chromatography. *System GA*—RI 2705.

High Pressure Liquid Chromatography. *System HA*—k' 2.8 (tailing peak).

Ultraviolet Spectrum. Aqueous acid—245 nm ($A_1^1 = 223$ a), 289 nm. No alkaline shift.

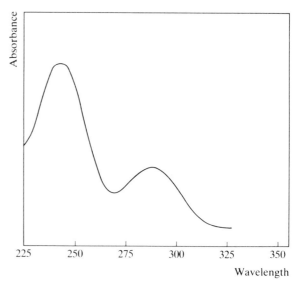

Infra-red Spectrum. Principal peaks at wavenumbers 756, 741, 1103, 1092, 1046, 1280.

Quantification. SPECTROFLUORIMETRY. In plasma—E. Welman *et al., Br. J. clin. Pharmac.*, 1977, **4**, 549–551.

GAS CHROMATOGRAPHY–MASS SPECTROMETRY. In blood—D. St. Clemans *et al., Arzneimittel-Forsch.*, 1977, **27**, 1128–1130.

THIN-LAYER CHROMATOGRAPHY. In plasma—L. J. Drombowski *et al., J. pharm. Sci.*, 1975, **64**, 643–645.

Disposition in the Body. Variably absorbed after oral administration, and mainly metabolised by the liver.

THERAPEUTIC CONCENTRATION.

After intravenous injection of 50 mg to 1 subject, a plasma concentration of about 1.7 µg/ml was reported at 1 minute (E. Welman *et al., Br. J. clin. Pharmac.*, 1977, **4**, 549–551).

TOXICITY.

In a fatality due to the ingestion of 2.5 g of ajmaline and 300 mg of diazepam the following postmortem tissue concentrations of ajmaline were reported: blood 10 µg/ml, liver 50 µg/g, urine 44 µg/ml; a blood-alcohol concentration of 1590 µg/ml was also reported (A. R. Alha 1966—personal communication).

Dose. Maintenance, 200 to 300 mg daily.

Albendazole

Anthelmintic (Veterinary)

Proprietary Name. Valbazen
Methyl 5-propylthio-1*H*-benzimidazol-2-ylcarbamate
$C_{12}H_{15}N_3O_2S = 265.3$
CAS—54965-21-8

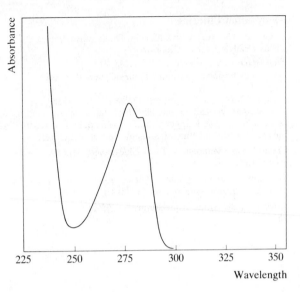

Colourless crystals. M.p. 208° to 210°.

Ultraviolet Spectrum. Aqueous acid—292 nm ($A_1^1 = 370$ b);
aqueous alkali—309 nm ($A_1^1 = 742$ b).

Alclofenac

Analgesic

Proprietary Names. Mervan; Zumaril.
(4-Allyloxy-3-chlorophenyl)acetic acid
$C_{11}H_{11}ClO_3 = 226.7$
CAS—22131-79-9

A white or slightly yellowish-white crystalline powder. M.p.
about 91°.
Slightly **soluble** in water; soluble 1 in 3 of ethanol, 1 in 4 of
chloroform, and 1 in 6 of ether.

Dissociation Constant. pK_a 4.6.

Thin-layer Chromatography. *System TD*—Rf 18; *system TE*—Rf
04; *system TF*—Rf 28; *system TG*—Rf 12. (*Ludy Tenger reagent*,
orange.)

Gas Chromatography. *System GD*—retention time of methyl
derivative 1.13 relative to n-$C_{16}H_{34}$.

High Pressure Liquid Chromatography. *System HD*—k' 2.6;
system HV—retention time 0.61 relative to meclofenamic acid.

Ultraviolet Spectrum. Aqueous acid—277 nm ($A_1^1 = 77$ b);
dehydrated alcohol—282 nm ($A_1^1 = 88$ a), 290 nm ($A_1^1 = 78$ a).

Infra-red Spectrum. Principal peaks at wavenumbers 1258, 1689,
1235, 933, 1016, 1500 (KBr disk).

Mass Spectrum. Principal peaks at *m/z* 41, 226, 77, 143, 181,
141, 39, 145.

Quantification. GAS CHROMATOGRAPHY. In plasma or urine:
alclofenac and two metabolites, FID—R. Roncucci *et al., J.
Chromat.,* 1971, *62*, 135–137.

Disposition in the Body. Variably absorbed after oral or rectal
administration and distributed into the synovial fluid. Metabolised by glucuronic acid conjugation, some conjugation with
glycine, deallylation to form 3-chloro-4-hydroxyphenylacetic
acid, and hydroxylation to form 3-chloro-4-(2,3-dihydroxypro-
pyloxy)phenylacetic acid, which may be methylated; an epoxide

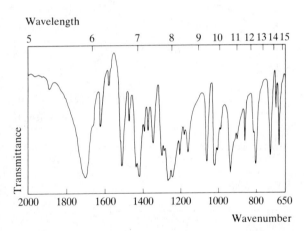

metabolite has also been identified. Up to about 90% of an oral
dose is excreted in the urine in 24 hours, mostly as unchanged
drug and the glucuronide conjugate.

THERAPEUTIC CONCENTRATION.

After an oral dose of 1 g to 10 subjects, a mean peak plasma concentration
of 136 μg/ml was attained in about 1 hour; concentrations in the synovial
fluid reached a mean peak of 32 μg/ml in 2 hours (G. M. Thomas *et al.,
Curr. med. Res. Opinion,* 1975, *3*, 264–267).

HALF-LIFE. Plasma half-life, 1.5 to 5.5 hours (mean 2.5).

VOLUME OF DISTRIBUTION. About 0.1 litre/kg.

PROTEIN BINDING. In plasma, about 99%.

NOTE. For a review of the pharmacokinetics of alclofenac see
R. N. Brogden *et al., Drugs,* 1977, *14*, 241–259.

Dose. Alclofenac has been given in doses of 1.5 to 3 g daily.

Alcuronium Chloride   *Muscle Relaxant*

Synonyms. Allnortoxiferin Chloride; Diallylnortoxiferine Dichloride; Diallyltoxiferine Chloride.
Proprietary Name. Alloferin
NN'-Diallylbisnortoxiferinium dichloride pentahydrate
$C_{44}H_{50}Cl_2N_4O_2,5H_2O = 827.9$
CAS—23214-96-2 (alcuronium); *15180-03-7* (chloride)
A colourless crystalline powder. No characteristic melting-point; a brown colour appears at 220°; still not melted at 350°.
Soluble in water and ethanol; soluble 1 in 5 of methanol.

Colour Tests. Mandelin's Test—blue-violet; Marquis Test—green-brown.

Thin-layer Chromatography. *System TA*—Rf 01. (*Acidified potassium permanganate solution,* positive.)

Ultraviolet Spectrum. Aqueous acid—255 nm, 291 nm ($A_1^1 = 185$ b).

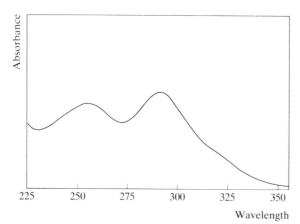

Infra-red Spectrum. Principal peaks at wavenumbers 1495, 1592, 1283, 1650, 1030, 757 (KBr disk).

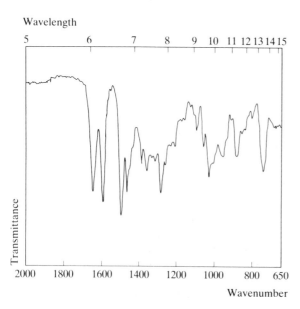

Quantification. SPECTROFLUORIMETRY. In plasma—J. Walker *et al., Eur. J. clin. Pharmac.,* 1980, *17,* 449–457.

HIGH PRESSURE LIQUID CHROMATOGRAPHY. In plasma: sensitivity 100 ng/ml, electrochemical detection—C. Tovey *et al., J. Chromat.,* 1983, *278; Biomed. Appl., 29,* 216–219.

Disposition in the Body. After intravenous administration it is widely distributed throughout the tissues. About 80 to 85% of a dose is excreted in the urine as unchanged drug and about 10 to 15% is secreted in the bile and eliminated in the faeces.

THERAPEUTIC CONCENTRATION.
Following intravenous administration of 0.25 mg/kg to 17 subjects, plasma concentrations of 0.74 to 2.25 µg/ml (mean 1.4) were reported after 3 to 30 minutes (J. Walker *et al., idem.*).

HALF-LIFE. Plasma half-life, about 3 hours; increased in subjects with renal failure.

VOLUME OF DISTRIBUTION. About 0.4 litre/kg.

CLEARANCE. Plasma clearance, about 1.3 ml/min/kg.

PROTEIN BINDING. In plasma, about 40%.

NOTE. For a review of the pharmacokinetics of alcuronium chloride and other muscle relaxants, see M. I. Ramzan *et al., Clin. Pharmacokinet.,* 1981, *6,* 25–60.

Dose. Initially 200 to 300 µg/kg intravenously.

Aldosterone   *Corticosteroid*

Synonym. Electrocortin
Proprietary Name. Aldocorten
11β,18-Epoxy-18,21-dihydroxypregn-4-ene-3,20-dione
$C_{21}H_{28}O_5 = 360.4$
CAS—52-39-1 (+)

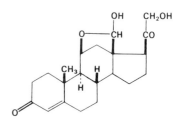

M.p. 164°.

Ultraviolet Spectrum. Methanol—241 nm ($A_1^1 = 437$ b).

Infra-red Spectrum. Principal peaks at wavenumbers 1650, 986, 1020, 999, 1062, 1075 (KBr disk).

Dose. Aldosterone has been given in doses of 500 µg intravenously, repeated several times a day.

Aldrin   *Insecticide*

Synonym. HHDN
Proprietary Names. Alderstan; Aldrex.
Aldrin usually contains 95% w/w of 1,2,3,4,10,10-hexachloro-1,4,4a,5,8,8a-hexahydro-1,4:5,8-dimethanonaphthalene (HHDN) together with 5% w/w of active related compounds.
$C_{12}H_8Cl_6 = 364.9$
CAS—309-00-2

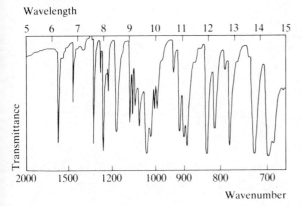

White crystals. When heated to decomposition it evolves highly toxic fumes of phosgene and hydrogen chloride. The technical grade is a tan to dark brown solid containing 85% or more of HHDN. M.p. 104° (pure grade), 49° to 60° (technical grade). Practically **insoluble** in water; soluble 1 in 20 of ethanol, 1 in 1 of acetone, 1 in 0.55 of benzene, and 1 in 0.33 of carbon tetrachloride; soluble in ether.

Partition Coefficient. Log P (octanol), 3.0.

Colour Tests. Nitric–Sulphuric Acid—pink; Sulphuric Acid–Fuming Sulphuric Acid—red (slow).

Gas Chromatography. *System GA*—aldrin RI 1943, dieldrin RI 2110; *system GK*—aldrin retention time 0.88, dieldrin retention time 1.13, both relative to caffeine.

Ultraviolet Spectrum. No significant absorption, 230 to 360 nm.

Infra-red Spectrum. Principal peaks at wavenumbers 696, 1036, 835, 723, 1255, 893 (KBr disk).

Wavelength

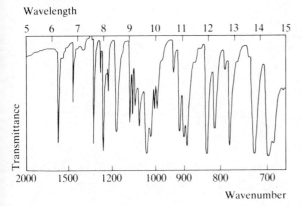

Mass Spectrum. Principal peaks at m/z 66, 91, 79, 263, 65, 101, 261, 265; dieldrin 79, 82, 81, 263, 77, 108, 265, 80.

Disposition in the Body. Poorly absorbed after oral ingestion but when dissolved in oils or other lipids it is readily absorbed by the skin and gastro-intestinal tract. It is rapidly metabolised in the body by epoxidation to dieldrin; dieldrin is stored in the body fat and persists for several weeks after the cessation of exposure. It is slowly eliminated in the faeces, mainly as unknown hydrophilic metabolites; a small amount is excreted in the urine as metabolites.

BLOOD CONCENTRATION. Blood concentrations of dieldrin averaging 0.001 µg/ml have been reported in 10 subjects with no occupational exposure to insecticides. Serum concentrations in subjects with low to high occupational exposure averaged 0.001 to 0.002 µg/ml for aldrin and 0.009 to 0.027 µg/ml for dieldrin.

TOXICITY. Severe symptoms may follow absorption of 1 to 3 g; the estimated minimum lethal dose is 5 g. The maximum permissible atmospheric concentration is 0.25 mg/m³ and the maximum permissible concentration in food is 0.1 ppm.

The body fat of a 23-year-old man poisoned by aldrin whilst working in a formulating plant, contained 60 µg/g of dieldrin 15 days after the last exposure; a blood concentration of 0.1 µg/ml was reported 4 months later. The blood concentrations of two men exposed to aldrin in the same plant and showing symptoms of poisoning were 0.28 and 0.13 µg/ml of dieldrin 1 month after the last exposure. In 2 further cases of poisoning, the concentrations of dieldrin in the body fat 3 and 5 weeks after exposure were 149 and 44 µg/g respectively; the corresponding blood concentrations were 0.53 and 0.13 µg/ml (G. Kazantzis *et al., Br. J. ind. Med.,* 1964, *21,* 46–51).

HALF-LIFE. Blood half-life, dieldrin 50 to 170 days (mean 97).

DISTRIBUTION IN BLOOD. Plasma: whole blood ratio, dieldrin about 1.5.

Aletamine   *Analgesic*

Synonym. Alfetamine
α-Allylphenethylamine
$C_{11}H_{15}N = 161.2$
CAS—4255-23-6

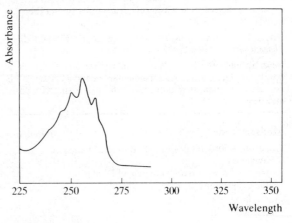

Aletamine Hydrochloride
$C_{11}H_{15}N,HCl = 197.7$
CAS—4255-24-7
White crystals.
Soluble in water.

Colour Tests. Liebermann's Test—orange; Marquis Test—orange.

Thin-layer Chromatography. *System TA*—Rf 59; *system TB*—Rf 37; *system TC*—Rf 40. (*Acidified iodoplatinate solution,* positive; *acidified potassium permanganate solution,* positive.)

Gas Chromatography. *System GA*—RI 1293.

Ultraviolet Spectrum. Aqueous acid—251 nm, 257 nm ($A_1^1 = 10$ b), 263 nm.

Mass Spectrum. Principal peaks at m/z 70, 120, 43, 91, 39, 103, 71, 65.

Dose. Aletamine hydrochloride has been given in doses of 375 to 750 mg daily.

Alfentanil
Narcotic Analgesic

N-{1-[2-(4-Ethyl-5-oxo-2-tetrazolin-1-yl)ethyl]-4-(methoxy-methyl)-4-piperidyl}propionanilide
$C_{21}H_{32}N_6O_3 = 416.5$
CAS—71195-58-9

Alfentanil Hydrochloride
Proprietary Name. Rapifen
$C_{21}H_{32}N_6O_3$, HCl, $H_2O = 471.0$
CAS—69049-06-5 (anhydrous); *70879-28-6* (monohydrate)
A white powder. M.p. 135° to 140°.
Readily **soluble** in water; soluble 1 in 5 of ethanol, 1 in less than 2 of chloroform, and 1 in less than 2 of methanol; practically insoluble in ether.

Dissociation Constant. pK_a 6.5.

Ultraviolet Spectrum. Isopropyl alcohol—258 nm ($A_1^1 = 6.3$ b), 264 nm ($A_1^1 = 4.5$ b), 268 nm ($A_1^1 = 3.1$ b).

Infra-red Spectrum. Principal peaks at wavenumbers 1722, 1654, 1252, 1109, 715, 967 (alfentanil hydrochloride, KBr disk).

Quantification. GAS CHROMATOGRAPHY. In plasma: sensitivity 1 ng/ml, AFID—R. Woestenborghs *et al., J. Chromat.,* 1981, *224*; *Biomed. Appl., 13,* 122-127.

RADIOIMMUNOASSAY. In plasma: sensitivity <50 pg/ml—M. Michiels *et al., J. Pharm. Pharmac.,* 1983, *35,* 86–93.

Disposition in the Body.

THERAPEUTIC CONCENTRATION.
Following an intravenous injection of 50 µg/kg to 2 subjects, a mean plasma concentration of 0.54 µg/ml was reported at 1 minute, decreasing to 0.038 µg/ml at 1 hour (M. Michiels *et al., ibid.*).

HALF-LIFE. Plasma half-life, about 1.5 hours.

VOLUME OF DISTRIBUTION. About 0.5 to 1.0 litre/kg.

CLEARANCE. Plasma clearance, about 3 to 8 ml/min/kg.

DISTRIBUTION IN BLOOD. Plasma: whole blood ratio, 1.6.

PROTEIN BINDING. In plasma, about 90% (concentration-dependent; decreases at plasma concentrations greater than 0.1 µg/ml).

NOTE. For a review of alfentanil see L. E. Mather, *Clin. Pharmacokinet.,* 1983, *8,* 422–446.

Dose. Initially the equivalent of up to 500 µg of alfentanil intravenously, followed by supplementary doses of 250 µg. With assisted ventilation, an initial dose of 30 to 50 µg/kg intravenously may be given.

Allobarbitone
Barbiturate

Synonyms. Allobarbital; Diallylbarbitone; Diallylmalonylurea; Diallymalum.
Proprietary Name. It is an ingredient of Dialog.

5,5-Diallylbarbituric acid
$C_{10}H_{12}N_2O_3 = 208.2$
CAS—52-43-7

A white crystalline powder. M.p. about 173°.
Soluble 1 in 700 of water, 1 in 15 of ethanol, and 1 in 20 of ether; soluble in solutions of alkalis.

Dissociation Constant. pK_a 7.8 (25°).

Colour Tests. Koppanyi–Zwikker Test—violet; Mercurous Nitrate—black; Vanillin Reagent—brown-orange/violet (transient).

Thin-layer Chromatography. *System TD*—Rf 50; *system TE*—Rf 31; *system TF*—Rf 66; *system TH*—Rf 53. (*Mercurous nitrate spray,* black; *acidified potassium permanganate solution,* yellow-brown.)

Gas Chromatography. *System GA*—RI 1606; *system GF*—RI 2340.

High Pressure Liquid Chromatography. *System HG*—k' 2.46; *system HH*—k' 1.33.

Ultraviolet Spectrum. *Borax buffer 0.05M* (pH 9.2)—241 nm ($A_1^1 = 460$ a); M sodium hydroxide (pH 13)—256 nm ($A_1^1 = 356$ b).

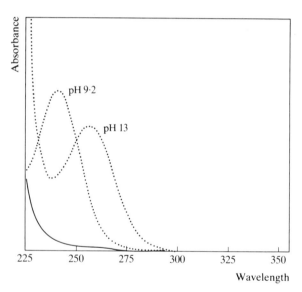

Infra-red Spectrum. Principal peaks at wavenumbers 1687, 1315, 925, 1219, 847, 1640 (KBr disk).

Mass Spectrum. Principal peaks at m/z 41, 167, 124, 39, 80, 53, 68, 141.

Quantification. See under Amylobarbitone.

Disposition in the Body. Absorbed after oral administration. It may persist unchanged in the body for up to one week; about 10 to 35% of a dose is slowly excreted in the urine unchanged.

THERAPEUTIC CONCENTRATION. In plasma, usually in the range 15 to 40 µg/ml.

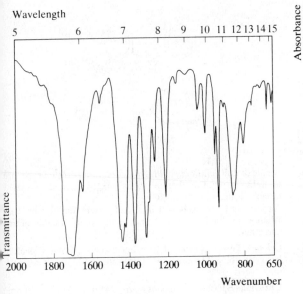

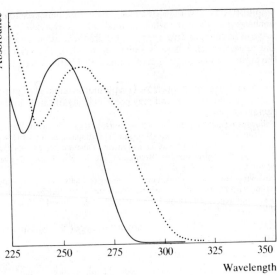

Infra-red Spectrum. Principal peaks at wavenumbers 1692, 1587, 916, 1224, 1235, 956 (KBr disk).

TOXICITY. The estimated minimum lethal dose is 2 g. Plasma concentrations of 50 μg/ml or more are usually toxic.

Dose. Allobarbitone has been given in doses of 90 to 200 mg daily.

Allopurinol   *Xanthine-oxidase Inhibitor*

Synonyms. HPP; Isopurinol.

Proprietary Names. Alloprin; Allopur; Aluline; Apurin; Caplenal; Capurate; Cosuric; Foligan; Lopurin; Progout; Purinol; Uriscel; Zyloprim; Zyloric.

1*H*-Pyrazolo[3,4-*d*]pyrimidin-4-ol
$C_5H_4N_4O = 136.1$
CAS—315-30-0

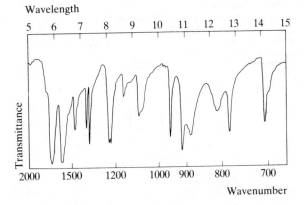

A white microcrystalline powder. No characteristic melting point; it is unchanged up to 300°, after which it begins to darken and at an indefinite high temperature it chars and decomposes. Very slightly **soluble** in water and ethanol; practically insoluble in chloroform and ether; soluble in dimethylformamide and in dilute solutions of alkali hydroxides.

Dissociation Constant. pK_a 9.4.

Colour Test. Folin–Ciocalteu Reagent—grey-blue.

Gas Chromatography. *System GA*—RI 882.

Ultraviolet Spectrum. Aqueous acid (prepared by dissolving in alkali and diluting with acid)—250 nm ($A_1^1 = 563$ a); aqueous alkali—257 nm ($A_1^1 = 523$ a).

Mass Spectrum. Principal peaks at *m/z* 136, 135, 52, 28, 137, 109, 29, 18.

Quantification. GAS CHROMATOGRAPHY–MASS SPECTROMETRY. In serum or urine: allopurinol and oxypurinol, sensitivity 25 ng/ ml for allopurinol—C. Lartigue-Mattei *et al., J. Chromat.,* 1982, *229; Biomed. Appl., 18,* 211–216.

HIGH PRESSURE LIQUID CHROMATOGRAPHY. In plasma or urine: allopurinol and oxypurinol, detection limit 100 ng/ml, UV detection—H. Breithaupt and G. Goebel, *J. Chromat.,* 1981, *226; Biomed. Appl., 15,* 237–242.

Disposition in the Body. Rapidly absorbed after oral administration; bioavailability about 90%. The major metabolite, oxypurinol (alloxanthine), is active but less potent than allopurinol. Subjects with a genetic deficiency of xanthine oxidase are unable to metabolise allopurinol to oxypurinol. The excretion of unchanged drug appears to vary with acute or chronic administration, less than 10% of a single dose being excreted unchanged in the urine whereas about 30% is excreted in the urine as unchanged drug after chronic administration. Most of the remainder of a dose is slowly excreted in the urine as oxypurinol; about 20% of a dose is eliminated in the faeces in 72 hours.

THERAPEUTIC CONCENTRATION. Oxypurinol accumulates during chronic administration and may contribute significantly to the therapeutic effect.

Following a single oral dose of 300 mg given to 6 subjects, peak plasma concentrations of 1.4 to 2.6 µg/ml (mean 2) of allopurinol and 4.4 to 7.8 µg/ml (mean 6.3) of oxypurinol were attained in about 0.5 to 2 hours and 2 to 5 hours respectively (H. Breithaupt and M. Tittel, *Eur. J. clin. Pharmac.,* 1982, *22,* 77–84).

Following daily oral administration of 300 mg to 7 subjects, steady-state serum concentrations of oxypurinol, determined immediately prior to a dose, were reported to range from 3.4 to 19.4 µg/ml (mean 9.7) (G. P. Rodnan *et al., J. Am. med. Ass.,* 1975, *231,* 1143–1147).

HALF-LIFE. Plasma half-life, allopurinol about 0.5 to 2 hours, oxypurinol 12 to 40 hours.

VOLUME OF DISTRIBUTION. About 0.6 litre/kg.

CLEARANCE. Plasma clearance, about 11 ml/min/kg.

PROTEIN BINDING. In plasma, allopurinol less than 5%, oxypurinol about 17%.

Dose. 100 to 600 mg daily.

Allyloestrenol   *Progestational Steroid*

Synonym. Allylestrenol
Proprietary Names. Gestanin; Gestanon.
17α-Allylestr-4-en-17β-ol
$C_{21}H_{32}O = 300.5$
CAS—432-60-0

Crystals. M.p. 80°.
Practically **insoluble** in water; soluble in ethanol, chloroform, and ether.

Ultraviolet Spectrum. No significant absorption, 230 to 360 nm.

Infra-red Spectrum. Principal peaks at wavenumbers 905, 1008, 999, 1020, 1101, 985 (Nujol mull).

Dose. Allyloestrenol has been given in doses of 5 to 20 mg daily.

Aloin   *Purgative*

A crystalline substance extracted from aloes and consisting almost entirely of barbaloin, 10-β-D-glucopyranosyl-1,8-dihydroxy-3-hydroxymethylanthrone.
$C_{21}H_{22}O_9 = 418.4$
CAS—8015-61-0; 1415-73-2 (barbaloin)

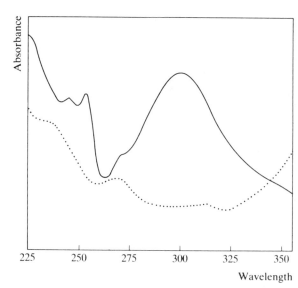

A pale or dull yellow crystalline powder. It darkens on exposure to light. M.p. of barbaloin about 148°. It quickly forms a monohydrate, m.p. 70° to 80°.
Almost completely **soluble** 1 in 130 of water; soluble 1 in 20 of ethanol; soluble in acetone; very slightly soluble in chloroform and ether.

Colour Tests. Ferric Chloride—brown; Folin–Ciocalteu Reagent—blue; Liebermann's Test—black; Millon's Reagent—pink → red.

Ultraviolet Spectrum. Aqueous acid—245 nm, 253 nm, 300 nm; aqueous alkali—268 nm.

Dose. Aloin has been given in doses of 13 to 60 mg.

Aloxiprin   *Analgesic*

Proprietary Names. Palaprin Forte; Rumatral.
A polymeric condensation product of aluminium oxide and aspirin which contains about 83% of total salicylates.
CAS—9014-67-9
A fine white or slightly pink powder.
Practically **insoluble** in water, ethanol, and ether; soluble 1 in 200 of chloroform.

Thin-layer Chromatography. *System TD*—Rf 04; *system TE*—Rf 09; *system TF*—Rf 10.

Ultraviolet Spectrum. Aqueous acid—231 nm; aqueous alkali—298 nm.

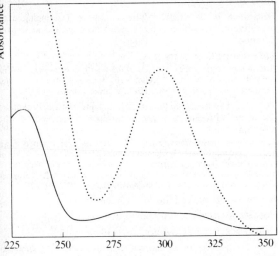

Infra-red Spectrum. Principal peaks at wavenumbers 1597, 1198, 1562, 1220, 1745, 760 (KBr disk).

Mass Spectrum. Principal peaks at m/z 43, 45, 60, 120, 42, 92, 138, 44.

Disposition in the Body. Aloxiprin is hydrolysed to aspirin in the gastro-intestinal tract.

Dose. Up to 100 mg/kg daily, by mouth.

Alpha Tocopheryl Acetate

Vitamin E Activity

Synonyms. α-Tocopherol Acetate; *dl*-α-Tocopherol Acetate; α-Tocopheryl Acetate; Vitamin E Acetate.
Proprietary Names. Aquasol E; Ephynal; Evion; Tocomine; Tokols (*d*); Vita-E (*d*).

$(\pm)$-α-Tocopherol acetate
$C_{31}H_{52}O_3 = 472.8$
CAS—7695-91-2

A clear, slightly greenish-yellow, viscous, oily liquid. Relative density 0.952 to 0.966.
Practically **insoluble** in water; soluble in ethanol; freely soluble in dehydrated alcohol, chloroform, and ether.

Ultraviolet Spectrum. Methanol—284 nm ($A_1^1 = 43$ a).

Infra-red Spectrum. Principal peaks at wavenumbers 1210, 1755, 1075, 1105, 1160, 1250 (thin film).

Alphadolone

General Anaesthetic

Synonym. Alfadolone
3α,21-Dihydroxy-5α-pregnane-11,20-dione
$C_{21}H_{32}O_4 = 348.5$
CAS—14107-37-0

M.p. 167° to 170°.

Alphadolone Acetate

Synonym. It is an ingredient of Alphadione (with alphaxalone).
Proprietary Names. It is an ingredient of Alfatesin(e), Alfathesin, Althesin, and Saffan (vet.).
$C_{23}H_{34}O_5 = 390.5$
CAS—23930-37-2
A white to creamy-white powder. M.p. 175° to 181°.
Practically **insoluble** in water; soluble 1 in 15 of ethanol and 1 in 2 of chloroform.

Colour Tests. Antimony Pentachloride—yellow; Naphthol–Sulphuric Acid—orange-brown/orange; Sulphuric Acid—yellow.

Thin-layer Chromatography. Alphadolone acetate: *system TD*—Rf 35; *system TE*—Rf 71; *system TF*—Rf 40; *system TP*—Rf 59; *system TQ*—Rf 22; *system TR*—Rf 80; *system TS*—Rf 45, streaking may occur. (p-*Toluenesulphonic acid solution*, positive.)

Ultraviolet Spectrum. Alphadolone acetate: methanol—290 nm ($A_1^1 = $ about 2).

Infra-red Spectrum. Principal peaks at wavenumbers 1228, 1758, 1710, 1278, 1010, 1043 (alphadolone acetate, KBr disk).

Mass Spectrum. Principal peaks at m/z 317, 43, 271, 147, 289, 390, 95, 81 (alphadolone acetate).

Quantification. GAS CHROMATOGRAPHY. In plasma: sensitivity 10 ng/ml, ECD—A. J. Pateman, *J. Chromat.*, 1981, *226*; *Biomed. Appl.*, *15*, 213–218.

Disposition in the Body. Rapidly and widely distributed after injection. Alphadolone acetate is metabolised in the liver to alphadolone and alphadolone glucuronide which are excreted in the urine. Alphadolone is considered to be about 50% as potent an anaesthetic as alphaxalone.

PROTEIN BINDING. In plasma, 20 to 40%.

Dose. See under Alphaxalone.

Alphaprodine

Narcotic Analgesic

Synonym. Prisilidene
$(\pm)$-*cis*-1,3-Dimethyl-4-phenyl-4-piperidyl propionate
$C_{16}H_{23}NO_2 = 261.4$
CAS—77-20-3; 15867-21-7 ($\pm$)

Practically **insoluble** in water; soluble in chloroform.

Alphaprodine Hydrochloride

Proprietary Name. Nisentil
$C_{16}H_{23}NO_2,HCl = 297.8$
CAS—561-78-4 $(\pm)$
A white crystalline powder. M.p. 218° to 220°.
Soluble 1 in 2 of water, 1 in 7 of ethanol, 1 in 47 of acetone, and 1 in 3 of chloroform; very slightly soluble in ether.

Dissociation Constant. pK_a 8.7 (20°).

Colour Tests. Mandelin's Test—blue-grey; Marquis Test—brown-red.

Thin-layer Chromatography. *System TA*—Rf 50; *system TB*—Rf 30; *system TC*—Rf 35. (*Dragendorff spray*, positive; *acidified iodoplatinate solution*, positive; *Marquis reagent*, red-brown.)

Gas Chromatography. *System GA*—RI 1792.

High Pressure Liquid Chromatography. *System HA*—k' 2.8 (tailing peak).

Ultraviolet Spectrum. Aqueous acid—251 nm, 257 nm ($A_1^1 = 9$ a), 263 nm. No alkaline shift.

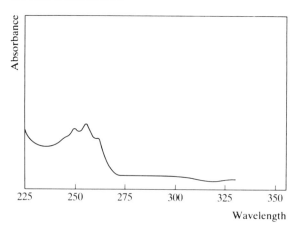

Infra-red Spectrum. Principal peaks at wavenumbers 1740, 1178, 1134, 694, 1030, 1055 (KBr disk).

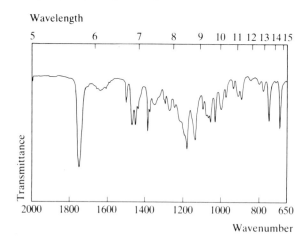

Mass Spectrum. Principal peaks at *m/z* 172, 187, 84, 57, 42, 188, 44, 43.

Quantification. GAS CHROMATOGRAPHY. In plasma: sensitivity 30 ng/ml, FID—D. L. Fung *et al., J. clin. Pharmac.,* 1980, *20,* 37–41.

Disposition in the Body. Alphaprodine is a homologue of pethidine but its action is more rapid in onset and of shorter duration.

THERAPEUTIC CONCENTRATION.

After a rapid intravenous injection of 0.5 mg/kg to 6 subjects, plasma concentrations of about 0.8 μg/ml were measured after 5 minutes, declining to 0.07 μg/ml at 5 hours (D. L. Fung *et al., ibid.*).

TOXICITY. The estimated minimum lethal dose is 0.1 g. Prolonged use of alphaprodine is liable to produce dependence of the morphine type.

The following postmortem tissue concentrations were reported in an accidental fatality caused by the intravenous administration of 40 mg of alphaprodine: blood 0.62 μg/ml, liver 0.97 μg/g, urine 0.30 μg/ml; a blood-alcohol concentration of 1.7 μg/ml was also reported (E. Griesemer and G. R. Nakamura, *Bull. int. Ass. forens. Toxicol.,* 1973, *9* (1–2), 5).

HALF-LIFE. Plasma half-life, about 2 hours.

VOLUME OF DISTRIBUTION. About 2 litres/kg.

CLEARANCE. Plasma clearance, about 10 ml/min/kg.

Dose. 20 to 60 mg of alphaprodine hydrochloride by subcutaneous injection, or 10 to 30 mg intravenously.

Alphaxalone   *General Anaesthetic*

Synonyms. Alfaxalone. It is an ingredient of Alphadione (with alphadolone acetate).

Proprietary Names. It is an ingredient of Alfatesin(e), Alfathesin, Althesin, and Saffan (vet.).

3α-Hydroxy-5α-pregnane-11,20-dione
$C_{21}H_{32}O_3 = 332.5$
CAS—23930-19-0

A white to creamy-white powder. M.p. 165° to 171°.
Practically **insoluble** in water; soluble 1 in 10 of ethanol and 1 in 2 of chloroform.

Thin-layer Chromatography. *System TP*—Rf 60; *system TQ*—Rf 22; *system TR*—Rf 90; *system TS*—Rf 72, streaking may occur. (p-*Toluenesulphonic acid solution*, positive.)

Ultraviolet Spectrum. Methanol—290 nm ($A_1^1 =$ about 2).

Infra-red Spectrum. Principal peaks at wavenumbers 1695, 1148, 1220, 1267, 1000, 1252 (KBr disk).

Quantification. GAS CHROMATOGRAPHY. In plasma: sensitivity 10 ng/ml, AFID—J. W. Sear *et al., J. Pharm. Pharmac.,* 1980, *32,* 349–352.

Disposition in the Body. Rapidly and widely distributed following injection. It undergoes almost 100% first-pass metabolism by reduction of the 20-oxo group and conjugation with glucuronic acid, and is excreted in the urine. About 60% of a dose is excreted in the urine in 24 hours and 80% in 5 days.

THERAPEUTIC CONCENTRATION.
During constant intravenous infusion of 18, 52, and 90 μg/min/kg, to 22 subjects, mean steady-state plasma concentrations of 1.9, 2.9, and 3.9 μg/ml, respectively, were reported (J. W. Sear and C. Prys-Roberts, *Br. J. Anaesth.*, 1979, *51*, 861–865).

HALF-LIFE. Plasma half-life, about 0.5 hour.

VOLUME OF DISTRIBUTION. About 0.8 litre/kg.

CLEARANCE. Plasma clearance, about 20 ml/min/kg.

PROTEIN BINDING. In plasma, 20 to 50%.

NOTE. For a review of the pharmacokinetics of intravenous anaesthetic agents see P. Duvaldestin, *Clin. Pharmacokinet.*, 1981, *6*, 61–82.

Dose. A solution containing alphaxalone 9 mg and alphadolone acetate 3 mg/ml has been administered intravenously; doses of 0.05 to 0.075 ml/kg and 10 to 20 ml/hour have been given to induce and maintain anaesthesia, respectively.

Alprazolam   *Tranquilliser*

Proprietary Name. Xanax

8 - Chloro - 1 - methyl - 6 - phenyl - 4*H* - 1,2,4 - triazolo[4,3 - *a*]-[1,4]benzodiazepine
$C_{17}H_{13}ClN_4 = 308.8$
CAS—28981-97-7

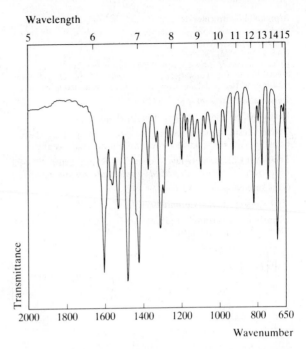

A white crystalline powder. M.p. 225° to 231°.
Practically **insoluble** in water; soluble in ethanol and methanol; freely soluble in chloroform.

Dissociation Constant. pK_a 2.4.

High Pressure Liquid Chromatography. *System HI*—k′ 4.70; *system HK*—k′ 2.79.

Ultraviolet Spectrum. Aqueous acid—260 nm.

Infra-red Spectrum. Principal peaks at wavenumbers 1490, 1610, 697, 1316, 1540, 827 (KBr disk). Three polymorphic forms may occur.

Mass Spectrum. Principal peaks at *m/z* 308, 279, 204, 273, 77, 307, 310, 309.

Quantification. GAS CHROMATOGRAPHY. In plasma: sensitivity 250 pg/ml, ECD—D. J. Greenblatt *et al., J. Chromat.,* 1981, *225*; *Biomed. Appl., 14*, 202–207.

Disposition in the Body. Readily absorbed after oral administration and undergoes extensive metabolism. The major metabolites are α-hydroxyalprazolam (active) and a benzophenone derivative of alprazolam. About 80% of a dose is excreted in the urine in 72 hours of which 11% is unchanged drug, 15% is α-hydroxyalprazolam, and 9% is the benzophenone metabolite.

Small amounts of desmethylalprazolam and 4-hydroxyalprazolam are also excreted in the urine. About 7% of a dose is eliminated in the faeces.

THERAPEUTIC CONCENTRATION.
After a single oral dose of 1 mg given to 10 subjects, peak plasma concentrations of 0.011 to 0.020 μg/ml (mean 0.015) were attained in about 1.75 hours. Following daily oral doses of 0.5 mg three times a day to the same subjects, minimum steady-state plasma concentrations of 0.006 to 0.017 μg/ml (mean 0.011) and a mean maximum steady-state plasma concentration of 0.018 μg/ml were reported (R. B. Smith *et al., Clin. Pharm.,* 1983, *2*, 139–143).

HALF-LIFE. Plasma half-life, 6 to 20 hours (mean 12).

VOLUME OF DISTRIBUTION. About 1 litre/kg.

CLEARANCE. Plasma clearance, about 1 ml/min/kg.

PROTEIN BINDING. In plasma, about 70%.

NOTE. For a review of alprazolam, see G. W. Dawson *et al., Drugs,* 1984, *27*, 132–147.

Dose. 1 to 3 mg daily.

Alprenolol   *Beta-adrenoceptor Blocking Agent*

(±)-1-(2-Allylphenoxy)-3-isopropylaminopropan-2-ol
$C_{15}H_{23}NO_2 = 249.4$
CAS—13655-52-2; 23846-70-0 (±)

M.p. 57° to 59°.

Alprenolol Hydrochloride

Proprietary Names. Aptin(e); Betacard; Gubernal.

$C_{15}H_{23}NO_2$,HCl = 285.8

CAS—13707-88-5; 13678-97-2 (±)

Colourless crystals or a white crystalline powder. M.p. 108° to 111°.

Soluble 1 in less than 1 of water, 1 in 2 of ethanol, and 1 in 3 of chloroform; soluble in acetone and dilute acetic acid; practically insoluble in ether.

Dissociation Constant. pK_a 9.5 (20°).

Partition Coefficient. Log P (octanol/pH 7.0), 0.5.

Colour Tests. Liebermann's Test—red; Mandelin's Test—brown-violet; Marquis Test—red; Sulphuric Acid—orange.

Thin-layer Chromatography. *System TA*—Rf 52; *system TB*—Rf 11; *system TC*—Rf 12. (*Acidified iodoplatinate solution,* positive.)

Gas Chromatography. *System GA*—RI 1760.

High Pressure Liquid Chromatography. *System HA*—k' 1.2.

Ultraviolet Spectrum. Aqueous acid—270 nm ($A_1^1 = 69$ b), 276 nm. No alkaline shift.

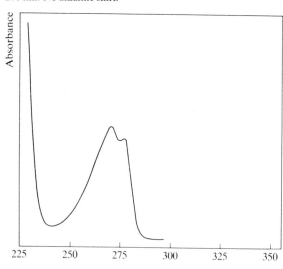

Infra-red Spectrum. Principal peaks at wavenumbers 1242, 746, 1031, 1492, 1079, 916 (KBr disk).

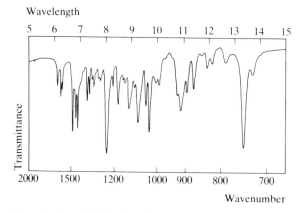

Mass Spectrum. Principal peaks at *m/z* 72, 30, 56, 73, 249, 98, 234, 102.

Quantification. GAS CHROMATOGRAPHY. In plasma: detection limit 2.5 ng/ml, ECD—C. F. Poole *et al., J. Chromat.,* 1980, *194,* 365–377. In serum: detection limit 2 pg, ECD—D. DeBruyne *et al., J. pharm. Sci.,* 1979, *68,* 511–512.

Disposition in the Body. Rapidly and almost completely absorbed after oral administration but undergoes extensive first-pass metabolism; bioavailability about 5 to 10%. About 90% of an oral dose is excreted in the urine in 24 hours with about 40% as the glucuronide conjugate of the active metabolite 4-hydroxy-alprenolol, 5% as free 4-hydroxyalprenolol, 20 to 30% as alprenolol glucuronide, 1% as desisopropylalprenolol, and less than 1% as unchanged drug; unknown metabolites account for the remainder of the dose.

THERAPEUTIC CONCENTRATION. There is considerable intersubject variation in plasma concentrations and in the ratio of 4-hydroxyalprenolol to alprenolol.

After oral administration of 200 mg to 2 subjects, peak plasma-alprenolol concentrations of 0.07 and 0.22 μg/ml were reported; peak plasma concentrations of the 4-hydroxy metabolite were 0.04 and 0.06 μg/ml (G. Alvan *et al., J. Pharmacokinet. Biopharm.,* 1977, *5,* 193–205).

Following oral administration of 200 mg three times a day to 16 subjects, average steady-state plasma-alprenolol concentrations of 0.01 to 0.14 μg/ml (mean 0.04) were reported (P. Collste *et al., Eur. J. clin. Pharmac.,* 1976, *10,* 85–88).

TOXICITY.

In 2 fatalities due to the ingestion of about 4 g and 20 g, respectively, the following postmortem tissue-alprenolol concentrations were reported: blood 40 and 43 μg/ml, liver 72 and 91 μg/g (S. J. Dickson *et al., J. analyt. Toxicol.,* 1978, *2,* 242–244).

HALF-LIFE. Plasma half-life, alprenolol and 4-hydroxyalprenolol about 2 to 3 hours.

VOLUME OF DISTRIBUTION. About 3 litres/kg.

CLEARANCE. Plasma clearance, about 15 ml/min/kg.

DISTRIBUTION IN BLOOD. Plasma : whole blood ratio, about 1.6.

PROTEIN BINDING. In plasma, 80 to 90%.

Dose. 200 to 800 mg of alprenolol hydrochloride daily.

Alverine
Antispasmodic

Synonyms. Dipropyline; Phenpropamine.

N-Ethyl-3,3'-diphenyldipropylamine

$C_{20}H_{27}N = 281.4$

CAS—150-59-4

$$C_6H_5 \cdot [CH_2]_3 \cdot \overset{\overset{\displaystyle C_2H_5}{|}}{N} \cdot [CH_2]_3 \cdot C_6H_5$$

Alverine Citrate

Proprietary Names. Profenil; Spasmavérine; Spasmonal.

$C_{20}H_{27}N,C_6H_8O_7 = 473.6$

CAS—5560-59-8

A white powder. M.p. 100° to 103°.

Slightly **soluble** in water and chloroform; sparingly soluble in ethanol; very slightly soluble in ether.

Colour Tests. Liebermann's Test—orange; Mandelin's Test—grey-green; Marquis Test—orange-red.

Thin-layer Chromatography. *System TA*—Rf 66; *system TB*—Rf 65; *system TC*—Rf 39. (*Acidified potassium permanganate solution,* positive.)

Gas Chromatography. *System GA*—RI 2142.

High Pressure Liquid Chromatography. *System HA*—k' 1.8.

Ultraviolet Spectrum. Aqueous acid—253 nm, 259 nm (A_1^1 = 14.4 b), 264 nm, 268 nm.

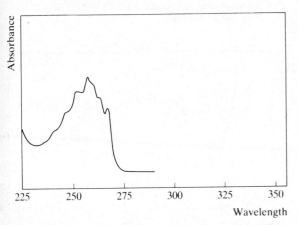

Infra-red Spectrum. Principal peaks at wavenumbers 694, 1190, 740, 1075, 1020, 1694 (KBr disk).

Wavelength

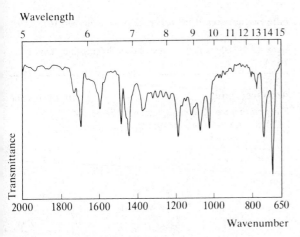

Mass Spectrum. Principal peaks at m/z 72, 176, 91, 58, 177, 41, 42, 30.

Dose. The equivalent of 40 to 240 mg of alverine daily.

Amantadine   *Antiviral/Antiparkinsonian*

Synonym. 1-Adamantanamine
Tricyclo[3.3.1.1^{3,7}]dec-1-ylamine
$C_{10}H_{17}N$ = 151.3
CAS—768-94-5

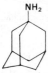

Crystals.
Sparingly **soluble** in water; soluble in chloroform.

Amantadine Hydrochloride
Proprietary Names. Antadine; Mantadix; Symmetrel; Virofral.
$C_{10}H_{17}N,HCl$ = 187.7
CAS—665-66-7
A white crystalline powder. M.p. 360°, with decomposition.
Soluble 1 in 2.5 of water, 1 in about 5 of ethanol, and 1 in 18 of chloroform; practically insoluble in ether.

Amantadine Sulphate
Proprietary Names. Contenton; PK-Merz; Trivaline.
$C_{10}H_{17}N,\frac{1}{2}H_2SO_4$ = 200.3
CAS—31377-23-8

Dissociation Constant. pK_a 10.4.

Partition Coefficient. Log P (octanol/pH 7.4), −0.4.

Colour Test. Ninhydrin—pink-violet.

Thin-layer Chromatography. *System TA*—Rf 23; *system TB*—Rf 19; *system TC*—Rf 07. (*Acidified iodoplatinate solution*, positive.)

Gas Chromatography. *System GA*—RI 1257.

Ultraviolet Spectrum. No significant absorption, 230 to 360 nm.

Infra-red Spectrum. Principal peaks at wavenumbers 1503, 1497, 1316, 1603, 1089, 1517 (amantadine hydrochloride, KBr disk).

Wavelength

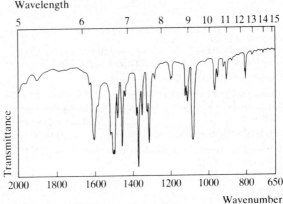

Mass Spectrum. Principal peaks at m/z 94, 151, 57, 95, 40, 41, 58, 108.

Quantification. GAS CHROMATOGRAPHY. In plasma or urine: sensitivity 100 ng/ml in plasma and 4 μg/ml in urine, FID—P. M. Bélanger and O. Grech-Bélanger, *J. Chromat.*, 1982, *228*; *Biomed. Appl.*, 17, 327–332. In plasma or urine: detection limit 10 ng/ml, ECD—A. Sioufi and F. Pommier, *J. Chromat.*, 1980, *183*; *Biomed. Appl., 9,* 33–39.

Disposition in the Body. Slowly but almost completely absorbed after oral administration. It does not appear to be metabolised in the body, about 56% of a dose being excreted in the urine unchanged in 24 hours and about 86% in 4 days.

THERAPEUTIC CONCENTRATION.
Following a single oral dose of 150 mg given to 6 subjects, peak plasma concentrations of 0.32 to 0.56 μg/ml (mean 0.4) were attained in about 3 to 4 hours (F. Y. Aoki *et al., Clin. Pharmac. Ther.*, 1979, 26, 729–736).
After oral administration of 100 mg twice daily, steady-state plasma concentrations of 0.1 to 1.1 μg/ml (mean 0.5) were observed in 22 patients (D. J. Greenblatt *et al., J. clin. Pharmac.*, 1977, 17, 704–708).

TOXICITY.
In a fatality involving the ingestion of amantadine, the following postmortem tissue concentrations were reported: blood 21 μg/ml, bile

418.6 µg/ml, liver 135.4 µg/g, urine 1330 µg/ml (P. C. Reynolds and S. Van Meter, *J. analyt. Toxicol.*, 1984, *8*, 100).

HALF-LIFE. Plasma half-life, 10 to 30 hours (mean 15).

Dose. Usually 100 to 200 mg of amantadine hydrochloride daily.

Ambazone   *Bacteriostat*

Proprietary Names. Bridal; Iversal; Primal(s).
4-Amidinohydrazonocyclohexa-2,5-dien-1-one thiosemicarbazone monohydrate
$C_8H_{11}N_7S,H_2O = 255.3$
CAS—6011-12-7

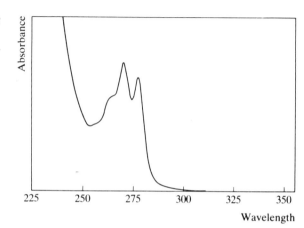

A brown microcrystalline powder. M.p. 192° to 194°, with decomposition.
Practically **insoluble** in water; very slightly soluble in ethanol; soluble in solutions of acids and of alkali hydroxides.

Colour Test. Palladium Chloride—brown.

Thin-layer Chromatography. *System TA*—Rf 55; *system TB*—Rf 00; *system TC*—Rf 04. (*Acidified potassium permanganate solution*, positive.)

Ultraviolet Spectrum. No significant absorption, 230 to 360 nm.

Infra-red Spectrum. Principal peaks at wavenumbers 1130, 1515, 1587, 1612, 1639, 1315.

Dose. Ambazone is given as 10-mg lozenges in doses of 30 to 50 mg daily.

Ambenonium Chloride   *Anticholinesterase*

Synonyms. Ambestigmini Chloridum; Oxazyl.
Proprietary Names. Mysuran; Mytelase.
NN' - [Oxalylbis(iminoethylene)]bis[(2 - chlorobenzyl)diethylammonium] dichloride
$C_{28}H_{42}Cl_4N_4O_2 = 608.5$
CAS—7648-98-8 (ambenonium); *115-79-7* (chloride, anhydrous); *52022-31-8* (chloride, tetrahydrate)

A white powder. M.p. about 200°.
Soluble 1 in 5 of water and 1 in 20 of ethanol; slightly soluble in chloroform; practically insoluble in acetone and ether.

Thin-layer Chromatography. *System TA*—Rf 02. (*Acidified iodoplatinate solution*, positive.)

Ultraviolet Spectrum. Aqueous acid—271 nm ($A_1^1 = 30$ c), 277 nm ($A_1^1 = 29$ c). No alkaline shift.

Infra-red Spectrum. Principal peaks at wavenumbers 1675, 1505, 767, 806, 1136, 1190 (KBr disk).

Dose. 15 to 100 mg daily; doses of over 200 mg daily have been given.

Ambucetamide   *Antispasmodic*

Proprietary Name. It is an ingredient of Femerital.
2-Dibutylamino-2-(4-methoxyphenyl)acetamide
$C_{17}H_{28}N_2O_2 = 292.4$
CAS—519-88-0

A white crystalline powder. M.p. 134°.
Practically **insoluble** in water; soluble in ethanol, chloroform, glacial acetic acid, and isopropyl alcohol.

Thin-layer Chromatography. *System TA*—Rf 73; *system TB*—Rf 05; *system TC*—Rf 68. (*Acidified iodoplatinate solution*, positive.)

Gas Chromatography. *System GA*—RI 2235.

Ultraviolet Spectrum. Aqueous acid—235 nm; aqueous alkali—279 nm, 286 nm.

Infra-red Spectrum. Principal peaks at wavenumbers 1656, 1513, 1176, 1250, 1026, 820 (KBr disk).

Mass Spectrum. Principal peaks at *m/z* 248, 44, 249, 121, 136, 29, 164, 192.

Dose. 300 to 600 mg daily.

Ambutonium Bromide

Anticholinergic

Proprietary Name. It is an ingredient of Aludrox SA.
(3 - Carbamoyl - 3,3 - diphenylpropyl)ethyldimethyl-ammonium bromide
$C_{20}H_{27}BrN_2O = 391.4$
CAS—14007-49-9 (ambutonium); *115-51-5* (bromide)

$$\left[CH_3 \cdot CH_2 \cdot \overset{\overset{CH_3}{|}}{\underset{\underset{CH_3}{|}}{N^+}} [CH_2]_2 \cdot \overset{\overset{C_6H_5}{|}}{\underset{\underset{C_6H_5}{|}}{C}} \cdot CO \cdot NH_2 \right] Br^-$$

White crystals. M.p. 228° to 229°, with decomposition.
Soluble 1 in 1.4 of water, 1 in 27 of ethanol, 1 in 500 of acetone, and 1 in 3.5 of chloroform.

Colour Test. Liebermann's Test—brown-orange.

Thin-layer Chromatography. *System TA*—Rf 03. (*Acidified iodoplatinate solution*, positive.)

Ultraviolet Spectrum. Aqueous acid—253 nm, 259 nm ($A_1^1 =$ 11.5 b), 265 nm.

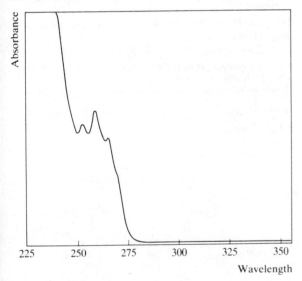

Infra-red Spectrum. Principal peaks at wavenumbers 700, 1664, 764, 1590, 1315, 979.

Dose. 7.5 to 20 mg daily.

Ametazole

Diagnostic Agent (Gastric Secretion)

Synonym. Betazole
2-(Pyrazol-3-yl)ethylamine
$C_5H_9N_3 = 111.1$
CAS—105-20-4

A viscous liquid.

Ametazole Hydrochloride

Proprietary Names. Betazol; Histalog.
$C_5H_9N_3,2HCl = 184.1$
CAS—138-92-1
A white, hygroscopic, crystalline powder. M.p. about 240° after softening at about 215°.
Soluble 1 in 3 of water and 1 in 50 of ethanol; practically insoluble in chloroform; very slightly soluble in ether.

Dissociation Constant. pK_a 2.2, 9.6 (20°).

Thin-layer Chromatography. *System TA*—Rf 26; *system TB*—Rf 11; *system TC*—Rf 00. (*Dragendorff spray*, positive; *acidified iodoplatinate solution*, positive; *Marquis reagent*, brown; *ninhydrin spray*, positive; *acidified potassium permanganate solution*, positive.)

Gas Chromatography. *System GA*—RI 1390.

Ultraviolet Spectrum. No significant absorption, 230 to 360 nm.

Infra-red Spectrum. Principal peaks at wavenumbers 1563, 1316, 1647, 775, 928, 1044.

Mass Spectrum. Principal peaks at m/z 82, 30, 81, 83, 55, 54, 42, 27.

Dose. 500 µg/kg of ametazole hydrochloride by subcutaneous or intramuscular injection.

Amethocaine

Local Anaesthetic

Synonym. Tetracaine
Proprietary Name. It is an ingredient of Locan.
2-Dimethylaminoethyl 4-butylaminobenzoate
$C_{15}H_{24}N_2O_2 = 264.4$
CAS—94-24-6

$$CO \cdot O \cdot [CH_2]_2 \cdot N(CH_3)_2$$

$$NH \cdot [CH_2]_3 \cdot CH_3$$

A white or light yellow, waxy solid. M.p. 41° to 46°.
Very slightly **soluble** in water; soluble 1 in 5 of ethanol, 1 in 2 of chloroform, and 1 in 2 of ether.

Amethocaine Hydrochloride

Synonyms. Butethanol; Dicainum.
Proprietary Names. Anethaine; Contralgine; Decicain; Pantocain; Pontocaine Hydrochloride. It is an ingredient of Biosone GA, Eludril (spray), Norgotin, and Riddofan.
$C_{15}H_{24}N_2O_2,HCl = 300.8$
CAS—136-47-0
A white, hygroscopic, crystalline powder. It melts at about 148° or may occur in either of two polymorphic modifications which melt at about 134° and 139°. Mixtures of the forms may melt within the range 134° to 147°.
Soluble 1 in 7.5 of water, 1 in 40 of ethanol, and 1 in 30 of chloroform; practically insoluble in acetone and ether.

Dissociation Constant. pK_a 8.5 (20°).

Colour Tests. Aromaticity (Method 2)—yellow/red; Liebermann's Test (100°)—blue.

Thin-layer Chromatography. *System TA*—Rf 57; *system TB*—Rf 15; *system TC*—Rf 32; *system TL*—Rf 16. (*Dragendorff spray*, positive; *acidified iodoplatinate solution*, positive.)

Gas Chromatography. *System GA*—amethocaine RI 2219, 4-aminobenzoic acid RI 1547; *system GF*—RI 2715.

High Pressure Liquid Chromatography. *System HA*—k′ 2.0; *system HQ*—k′ 16.25; *system HR*—k′ 1.33.

Ultraviolet Spectrum. Aqueous acid—229 nm ($A_1^1 = 561$ a), 281 nm, 312 nm; aqueous alkali—227 nm, 303 nm.

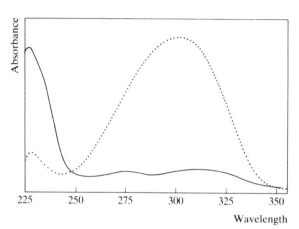

Infra-red Spectrum. Principal peaks at wavenumbers 1600, 1286, 1174, 1688, 1126, 1532 (amethocaine hydrochloride, KBr disk).

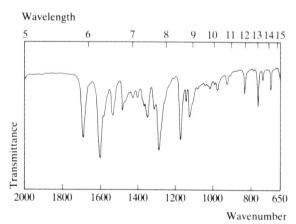

Mass Spectrum. Principal peaks at *m/z* 58, 71, 150, 176, 72, 193, 105, 59 (no peaks above 200); 4-aminobenzoic acid 137, 120, 92, 65, 39, 138, 121, 63.

Disposition in the Body. Amethocaine is rapidly hydrolysed in the blood to 4-aminobenzoic acid; it is completely metabolised within one hour of injection. It can rarely be isolated from blood even within a few minutes of administration. The maximum amount that may be safely administered by injection is probably 50 mg.

Dose. 5 to 20 mg of amethocaine hydrochloride (0.5% solution) is injected for spinal anaesthesia; 0.5 to 2% solutions have been used for surface anaesthesia.

Ametryne   *Herbicide*

Synonym. Ametryn
Proprietary Name. Gesapax
2-Ethylamino-4-isopropylamino-6-methylthio-1,3,5-triazine
$C_9H_{17}N_5S = 227.3$
CAS—834-12-8

Colourless crystals. M.p. 84° to 86°.
Very slightly **soluble** in water; soluble in chloroform and methanol.

Thin-layer Chromatography. *System TA*—Rf 76. (*Dragendorff spray*, positive.)

Gas Chromatography. *System GA*—RI 1775.

Infra-red Spectrum. Principal peaks at wavenumbers 1515, 1595, 1294, 1166, 806, 1140 (KBr disk).

Amicarbalide   *Antiprotozoal (Veterinary)*

1,3-Bis(3-amidinophenyl)urea
$C_{15}H_{16}N_6O = 296.3$
CAS—3459-96-9

Amicarbalide Isethionate
Proprietary Name. Diampron
$C_{19}H_{28}N_6O_9S_2 = 548.6$
CAS—3671-72-5
A white or slightly cream-coloured powder. M.p. 200° to 204°.
Soluble 1 in less than 1 of water and 1 in 250 of ethanol; practically insoluble in chloroform and ether.

Colour Tests. Aromaticity (Method 2)—yellow/orange; Liebermann's Test (100°)—yellow.

Thin-layer Chromatography. *System TA*—Rf 05, streaking. (*Acidified iodoplatinate solution*, positive.)

Ultraviolet Spectrum. Aqueous acid—231 nm ($A_1^1 = 1236$ a), inflexion at 256 nm.

Infra-red Spectrum. Principal peaks at wavenumbers 1195, 1590, 1672, 1250, 1562, 1052 (KBr disk).

Amidephrine

Sympathomimetic

Synonym. Amidefrine
3-(1-Hydroxy-2-methylaminoethyl)methanesulphonanilide
$C_{10}H_{16}N_2O_3S = 244.3$
CAS—3354-67-4

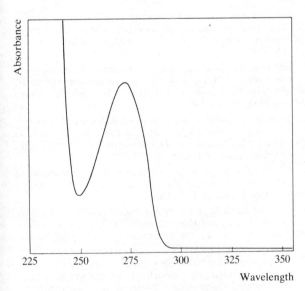

Crystals. M.p. 159° to 161°.

Amidephrine Mesylate
$C_{10}H_{16}N_2O_3S,CH_4O_3S = 340.4$
CAS—1421-68-7
A white crystalline solid. M.p. 207° to 209°.
Soluble 1 in about 5 of water; very slightly soluble in chloroform.

Dissociation Constant. pK_a 9.1.

Colour Test. Mandelin's Test—violet.

Thin-layer Chromatography. *System TA*—Rf 15; *system TB*—Rf 00; *system TC*—Rf 01. (*Acidified potassium permanganate solution,* positive.)

Gas Chromatography. *System GA*—not eluted.

Ultraviolet Spectrum. Aqueous acid—272 nm ($A_1^1 = 22$ a).

Infra-red Spectrum. Principal peaks at wavenumbers 1101, 1153, 1270, 799, 1207, 1316.

Mass Spectrum. Principal peaks at *m/z* 44, 42, 147, 120, 65, 43, 45, 39.

Use. A 0.1% solution of amidephrine mesylate has been used as a nasal decongestant.

Amidopyrine

Analgesic

Synonyms. Amidazofen; Amidopyrine-Pyramidon; Amino-phenazone; Aminopyrine; Dimethylaminoantipyrine; Dimethylaminophenazone.
4-Dimethylamino-1,5-dimethyl-2-phenyl-4-pyrazolin-3-one
$C_{13}H_{17}N_3O = 231.3$
CAS—58-15-1

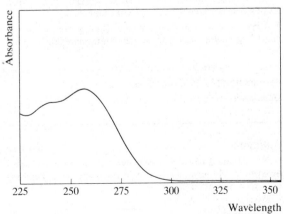

Small colourless crystals or white crystalline powder. M.p. about 108°.
Soluble 1 in 20 of water, 1 in 2 of ethanol, 1 in 1 of chloroform, and 1 in 13 of ether.
A number of salts of amidopyrine have been used including the ascorbate, gentisate, hydroxyisophthalate and salicylate.

Dissociation Constant. pK_a 5.0 (20°).

Partition Coefficient. Log *P* (octanol/pH 7.4), 1.0.

Colour Tests. Ferric Chloride—blue-violet; Liebermann's Test (100°)—blue; Nitrous Acid—violet (transient).

Thin-layer Chromatography. *System TA*—Rf 66; *system TD*—Rf 25; *system TE*—Rf 63; *system TF*—Rf 15. (*Acidified iodoplatinate solution,* positive.)

Gas Chromatography. *System GA*—RI 1903; *system GB*—RI 1666; *system GC*—RI 2370; *system GF*—RI 2265.

High Pressure Liquid Chromatography. *System HA*—k′ 0.3; *system HD*—k′ 0.2; *system HW*—k′ 0.32.

Ultraviolet Spectrum. Aqueous acid—257 nm ($A_1^1 = 443$ c); aqueous alkali—264 nm ($A_1^1 = 353$ b).

Infra-red Spectrum. Principal peaks at wavenumbers 1660, 1315, 1126, 750, 700, 1620 (KBr disk).

Wavelength

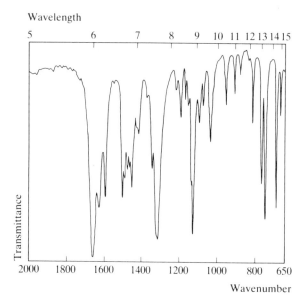

Mass Spectrum. Principal peaks at m/z 56, 231, 97, 111, 112, 42, 77, 71.

Quantification. GAS CHROMATOGRAPHY. In plasma: detection limit 100 ng/ml, FID—A. Sioufi and D. Colussi, *J. Chromat.*, 1978, *146*; *Biomed. Appl.*, *3*, 503–507.

HIGH PRESSURE LIQUID CHROMATOGRAPHY. In urine: detection limits 120 ng for amidopyrine, 25 ng for 4-acetamidophenazone and 50 ng for 4-aminophenazone, UV detection—K. Shimada and Y. Nagase, *J. Chromat.*, 1980, *181*; *Biomed. Appl.*, *7*, 51–57.

Disposition in the Body. Absorbed after oral administration. It is rapidly and extensively metabolised. About 30 to 50% of a dose is excreted in the urine in 3 days as 4-aminophenazone and its acetyl derivative 4-acetamidophenazone which is the major urinary metabolite; other metabolites found in the urine include two red pigments, rubazonic acid and methylrubazonic acid; dimethylnitrosamine may be formed in the stomach. Less than 5% of a dose is excreted in the urine unchanged.

TOXICITY. The use of amidopyrine is discouraged due to the risk of fatal agranulocytosis. The estimated minimum lethal dose is 5 g.

HALF-LIFE. Plasma half-life, about 2 to 3 hours.

PROTEIN BINDING. In plasma, 25 to 30%.

Dose. Amidopyrine was formerly given in doses of up to 1.5 g in 24 hours.

Amikacin
Antibiotic

6-*O*-(3-Amino-3-deoxy-α-D-glucopyranosyl)-4-*O*-(6-amino-6-deoxy-α-D-glucopyranosyl)-1-*N*-[(2*S*)-4-amino-2-hydroxy-butyryl]-2-deoxy-D-streptamine
$C_{22}H_{43}N_5O_{13} = 585.6$
CAS—37517-28-5

A white crystalline powder. M.p. 201° to 204°, with decomposition.
Sparingly **soluble** in water.

Amikacin Sulphate
Proprietary Names. Amikin; Biklin.
$C_{22}H_{43}N_5O_{13},2H_2SO_4 = 781.8$
CAS—39831-55-5
Freely **soluble** in water.

Ultraviolet Spectrum. No significant absorption, 230 to 360 nm.

Infra-red Spectrum. Principal peaks at wavenumbers 1050, 1630, 1120, 1145, 1545, 940 (KBr disk).

Quantification. GAS CHROMATOGRAPHY. In serum: amikacin, gentamicin, and tobramycin, sensitivity 600 ng/ml, ECD—J. W. Mayhew and S. L. Gorbach, *J. Chromat.*, 1978, *151*, 133–146.

HIGH PRESSURE LIQUID CHROMATOGRAPHY. In serum: amikacin, gentamicin, and tobramycin, sensitivity 1 µg/ml, fluorescence detection—J. P. Anhalt and S. D. Brown, *Clin. Chem.*, 1978, *24*, 1940–1947.

IMMUNOASSAY. In serum: radioimmunoassay—C. Ashby *et al.*, *Clin. Chem.*, 1978, *24*, 1734–1737. In serum: fluoroimmunoassay—S. G. Thompson and J. F. Burd, *Antimicrob. Ag. Chemother.*, 1980, *18*, 264–268.

BIOASSAY. Aminoglycoside antibiotics in biological fluids—J. M. Broughall, Aminoglycosides, in *Laboratory Methods in Antimicrobial Chemotherapy*, D. S. Reeves *et al.* (Ed.), Edinburgh, Churchill Livingstone, 1978, pp. 194–207.

REVIEW. For a review of methods for the determination of aminoglycoside antibiotics in biological fluids, see S. K. Maitra *et al.*, *Clin. Chem.*, 1979, *25*, 1361–1367.

Disposition in the Body. Poorly absorbed after oral administration but rapidly absorbed after intramuscular injection. About 90% of a dose is excreted in the urine unchanged in 24 hours.

THERAPEUTIC CONCENTRATION. During treatment, the serum concentration should be in the range 15 to 25 µg/ml and should be monitored regularly, especially in patients who have renal insufficiency. During multiple dosing, the trough concentration immediately preceding a dose should not exceed 10 µg/ml.
A single intramuscular dose of 500 mg given to 6 subjects, produced a mean peak serum concentration of 20 µg/ml in 1.5 hours (R. A. Yates *et al.*, *J. antimicrob. Chemother.*, 1978, *4*, 335–341).

TOXICITY. Toxic effects may be produced at serum concentrations of 30 µg/ml or more or, during chronic treatment, if the trough serum concentration exceeds 10 µg/ml.
The following postmortem tissue concentrations were reported in a patient who died 5 days after discontinuation of amikacin treatment:

serum 2.2 µg/ml, heart 20 µg/g, kidney 794 µg/g, liver 30 µg/g, lungs 48 µg/g, muscle 11 µg/g (M. A. French *et al., Antimicrob. Ag. Chemother.,* 1981, *19,* 147–152).

HALF-LIFE. Plasma half-life, 2 to 3 hours.

VOLUME OF DISTRIBUTION. About 0.2 litre/kg.

CLEARANCE. Plasma clearance, about 1 ml/min/kg.

PROTEIN BINDING. In plasma, less than 10%.

NOTE. For a review of the pharmacokinetics of amikacin see D. Andrews, *Can. J. hosp. Pharm.,* 1977, *30,* 146–148.

Dose. The equivalent of 15 mg of amikacin/kg daily, given parenterally; maximum of 1.5 g daily. The total dose should not exceed 15 g.

Amiloride   *Diuretic*

N-Amidino-3,5-diamino-6-chloropyrazine-2-carboxamide
$C_6H_8ClN_7O = 229.6$
CAS—2609-46-3

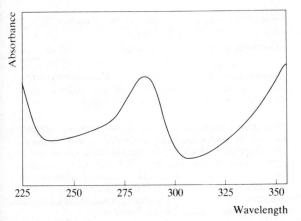

M.p. 240° to 242°.

Amiloride Hydrochloride

Synonym. Amipramizide
Proprietary Names. Arumil; Midamor; Modamide. It is an ingredient of Amilco, Frumil, Moducren, and Moduretic.
$C_6H_8ClN_7O,HCl,2H_2O = 302.1$
CAS—2016-88-8 (anhydrous)
A pale yellow to greenish-yellow powder. M.p. 285° to 288°, with decomposition.
Soluble in water and ethyl acetate; soluble 1 in 350 of ethanol; practically insoluble in chloroform and ether.

Dissociation Constant. pK_a 8.7.

Colour Tests. Marquis Test—yellow; Sulphuric Acid—yellow.

Thin-layer Chromatography. *System TA*—Rf 24; *system TB*—Rf 00; *system TC*—Rf 01. (*Acidified iodoplatinate solution,* strong reaction.)

Ultraviolet Spectrum. Aqueous acid—285 nm ($A_1^1 = 731$ a), 361 nm ($A_1^1 = 802$ a).

Infra-red Spectrum. Principal peaks at wavenumbers 1634, 1602, 1504, 1686, 1238, 1538 (amiloride hydrochloride, K Br disk).

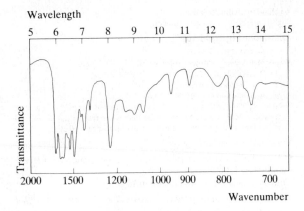

Mass Spectrum. Principal peaks at *m/z* 43, 187, 42, 171, 229, 86, 144, 170.

Quantification. SPECTROFLUORIMETRY. In plasma, serum, or urine—J. E. Baer *et al., J. Pharmac. exp. Ther.,* 1967, *157,* 472–485.

THIN-LAYER CHROMATOGRAPHY–SPECTROFLUORIMETRY. In plasma—K. Reuter *et al., J. Chromat.,* 1982, *233; Biomed. Appl., 22,* 432–436.

Disposition in the Body. Incompletely absorbed after oral administration; it does not appear to be metabolised. About 50% of an oral dose is excreted unchanged in the urine and 40% is eliminated in the faeces in 72 hours.

THERAPEUTIC CONCENTRATION.

After a single oral dose of 20 mg to 6 subjects, peak serum concentrations of about 0.05 µg/ml were attained in 4 hours (A. J. Smith and R. N. Smith, *Br. J. Pharmac.,* 1973, *48,* 646–649).

HALF-LIFE. Plasma half-life, 6 to 10 hours.

VOLUME OF DISTRIBUTION. About 5 litres/kg.

PROTEIN BINDING. In plasma, not significantly bound.

Dose. 5 to 20 mg of amiloride hydrochloride daily.

Aminacrine   *Disinfectant*

Synonym. Aminoacridine
9-Aminoacridine
$C_{13}H_{10}N_2 = 194.2$
CAS—90-45-9

Yellow needles. M.p. 241°.
Freely **soluble** in ethanol; soluble in acetone; slightly soluble in chloroform.

Aminacrine Hexylresorcinate

Synonyms. Acrisorcin; Aminacrine 4-Hexylresorcinate.
$C_{13}H_{10}N_2,C_{12}H_{18}O_2 = 388.5$
CAS—7527-91-5
A yellow crystalline powder.
Slightly **soluble** in water and ethanol.

Aminacrine Hydrochloride

Synonym. Acramine Yellow
Proprietary Names. Aminopt; Monacrin.
$C_{13}H_{10}N_2,HCl,H_2O = 248.7$
CAS—134-50-9 (anhydrous)
A yellow crystalline powder. M.p. about 235°.
Soluble 1 in 300 of water; a saturated solution in water is pale yellow with a greenish-blue fluorescence, becoming blue when freely diluted. Soluble 1 in 150 of ethanol; practically insoluble in chloroform and ether.

Dissociation Constant. pK_a 9.5 (25°).

Colour Tests. Aromaticity (Method 2)—yellow/red; Liebermann's Test (100°)—red.
Cold *nitric acid* gives a red colour in 15 seconds.

Thin-layer Chromatography. *System TA*—Rf 54. (*Acidified iodoplatinate solution*, positive.)

Gas Chromatography. *System GA*—RI 2240.

Ultraviolet Spectrum. Aqueous acid—260 nm ($A_1^1 = 4442$ a), 313 nm ($A_1^1 = 74$ b), 326 nm ($A_1^1 = 81$ b); methanol—260 nm ($A_1^1 = 4480$ b), 311 nm, 325 nm.

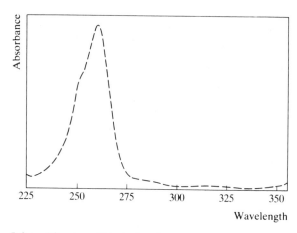

Infra-red Spectrum. Principal peaks at wavenumbers 760, 1556, 1645, 1655, 750, 1612 (KBr disk).

Aminobenzoic Acid   *Sunscreen Agent*

Synonyms. Amben; PAB; PABA; Pabacidum; Para-aminobenzoic Acid; Vitamin H'.
Proprietary Names. Hill-Shade; Pabagel; Pabanol; Paraminan; Presun 8; RVPaba.
4-Aminobenzoic acid
$C_7H_7NO_2 = 137.1$
CAS—150-13-0

White or slightly yellow crystals or crystalline powder. It gradually darkens on exposure to air and light. M.p. 186° to 189°.
Soluble 1 in 200 of water, 1 in 10 of boiling water, 1 in 8 of ethanol, and 1 in 50 of ether; slightly soluble in chloroform; freely soluble in solutions of alkali hydroxides and carbonates.

Potassium Aminobenzoate

Proprietary Name. Potaba
$C_7H_6KNO_2 = 175.2$
CAS—138-84-1
A crystalline powder.
Very **soluble** in water; less soluble in ethanol; practically insoluble in ether.

Dissociation Constant. pK_a 2.4, 4.9 (25°).

Colour Tests. Coniferyl Alcohol—orange; Diazotisation—red.

Thin-layer Chromatography. *System TA*—Rf 58; *system TD*—Rf 19; *system TE*—Rf 01; *system TF*—Rf 43. (*Acidified potassium permanganate solution*, positive; *Van Urk reagent*, yellow.)

Gas Chromatography. *System GA*—RI 1547.

Ultraviolet Spectrum. Aqueous acid—270 nm ($A_1^1 = 95$ b); aqueous alkali—265 nm ($A_1^1 = 1063$ a).

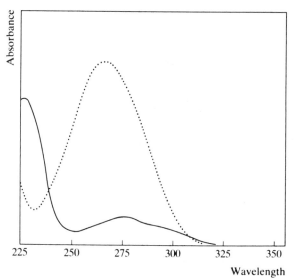

Infra-red Spectrum. Principal peaks at wavenumbers 1597, 1168, 1290, 1665, 1305, 1625 (KBr disk).

Mass Spectrum. Principal peaks at m/z 137, 120, 92, 65, 39, 138, 121, 63.

Quantification. HIGH PRESSURE LIQUID CHROMATOGRAPHY. In serum or urine: aminobenzoic acid and metabolites, UV detection—N. D. Brown and E. J. Michalski, *J. Chromat.*, 1976, *121*, 76–78.

Disposition in the Body. Readily absorbed after oral administration. It is conjugated with aminoacetic acid to form *p*-aminohippuric acid which is excreted in the urine together with a small amount of *p*-aminobenzoyl glucuronide, *p*-acetamidobenzoyl glucuronide, and traces of *p*-acetamidohippuric acid, *p*-acetamidobenzoic acid, and unchanged aminobenzoic acid. Aminobenzoic acid may be detected in the urine as a metabolite of amethocaine, benzocaine, and procaine.

Wavelength

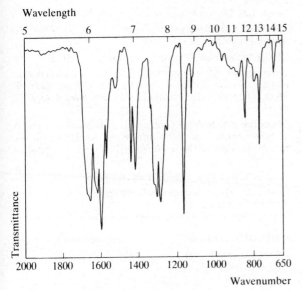

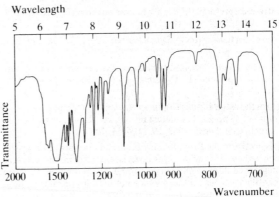

REFERENCE. For a review of aminocaproic acid see *Aust. J. Pharm.*, 1981, *62*, 403–407.

Dose. 3 to 6 g may be given 4 to 6 times daily.

TOXICITY. Toxic effects are infrequent and are usually associated with plasma concentrations greater than about 600 µg/ml.

Uses. Aminobenzoic acid is used topically as a 5% solution; potassium aminobenzoate has been given orally, in doses of 12 g daily.

Aminocaproic Acid
Haemostatic

Synonyms. EACA; Epsilon Aminocaproic Acid.
Proprietary Names. Amicar; Capralense; Capramol; Ekaprol; Epsikapron; Hemocaprol.
6-Aminohexanoic acid
$C_6H_{13}NO_2 = 131.2$
CAS—60-32-2

$$NH_2 \cdot [CH_2]_5 \cdot COOH$$

Colourless crystals or white crystalline powder. M.p. about 204°, with decomposition.
Soluble 1 in 1.5 of water; slightly soluble in ethanol; practically insoluble in chloroform and ether; freely soluble in solutions of acids and alkalis.

Dissociation Constant. pK_a 4.4, 10.8 (25°).

Infra-red Spectrum. Principal peaks at wavenumbers 1538, 1613, 1098, 1319, 1258, 1203 (KBr disk).

Quantification. HIGH PRESSURE LIQUID CHROMATOGRAPHY. In serum: detection limits 10 pg and 3 ng for fluorescence or UV detection, respectively—N. A. Farid, *J. pharm. Sci.*, 1979, *68*, 249–252.

Disposition in the Body. Readily absorbed after oral administration and widely distributed throughout the body fluids. About 70 to 80% of a dose is excreted in the urine unchanged in 12 hours.

THERAPEUTIC CONCENTRATION. In plasma, usually in the range 100 to 400 µg/ml.

HALF-LIFE. Plasma half-life, about 2 to 5 hours.

VOLUME OF DISTRIBUTION. About 0.4 litre/kg.

Aminoglutethimide
Antineoplastic

Proprietary Name. Orimeten
3-(4-Aminophenyl)-3-ethylpiperidine-2,6-dione
$C_{13}H_{16}N_2O_2 = 232.3$
CAS—125-84-8

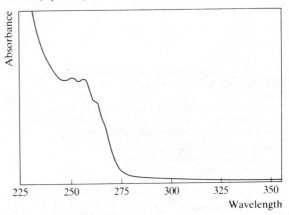

A white crystalline powder. M.p. about 151°.
Very slightly **soluble** in water; freely soluble in organic solvents.

Colour Tests. Coniferyl Alcohol—yellow; Koppanyi-Zwikker Test—violet; Mercurous Nitrate—black.

Thin-layer Chromatography. *System TD*—Rf 32; *system TE*—Rf 65; *system TF*—Rf 47.

Gas Chromatography. *System GA*—RI 2227.

Ultraviolet Spectrum. Aqueous acid—251 nm $(A_1^1 = 18 \text{ b})$, 257 nm $(A_1^1 = 18 \text{ b})$.

Infra-red Spectrum. Principal peaks at wavenumbers 1695, 1185, 1200, 1515, 1623, 1267 (KCl disk).

Mass Spectrum. Principal peaks at m/z 203, 232, 132, 175, 204, 233, 160, 118.

Quantification. COLORIMETRY. In plasma or urine: sensitivity 2 µg/ml in plasma—F. T. Murray *et al.*, *J. clin. Pharmac.*, 1979, *19*, 704–711.

HIGH PRESSURE LIQUID CHROMATOGRAPHY. In plasma: detection limit < 230 ng/ml, UV detection—B. A. Robinson and F. N. Cornell, *Clin. Chem.*, 1983, *29*, 1104–1105.

Disposition in the Body. Readily absorbed after oral administration. About 10% of an oral dose is excreted in the urine as unchanged drug in 48 hours; acetamidoglutethimide has been identified as a metabolite. Aminoglutethimide appears to induce its own metabolism.

THERAPEUTIC CONCENTRATION.
After a single oral dose of 500 mg given to 6 subjects, peak plasma concentrations of 5.8 to 6.3 µg/ml (mean 5.9) were attained in 1.3 hours (T. A. Thompson *et al.*, *J. pharm. Sci.*, 1981, *70*, 1040–1043).
Steady-state serum concentrations of 4.7 to 32.4 µg/ml (mean 11.5) were reported in 7 subjects receiving chronic treatment with oral doses of 1 g daily (F. T. Murray *et al.*, *J. clin. Pharmac.*, 1979, *19*, 704–711).

TOXICITY. The estimated minimum lethal dose is 5 g.

HALF-LIFE. Plasma half-life, about 13 hours following a single dose but appears to decrease during chronic treatment.

VOLUME OF DISTRIBUTION. About 1.4 litre/kg.

CLEARANCE. Plasma clearance, about 1.3 ml/min/kg.

DISTRIBUTION IN BLOOD. Plasma:whole blood ratio, about 0.7.

PROTEIN BINDING. In plasma, about 25%.

Dose. 0.5 to 1 g daily.

Aminohippuric Acid   *Diagnostic Agent (Renal Function)*

Synonyms. *p*-Aminobenzoylglycine; PAHA; Para-aminohippuric Acid.
N-4-Aminobenzoylaminoacetic acid
$C_9H_{10}N_2O_3 = 194.2$
CAS—61-78-9

A white crystalline powder, which discolours on exposure to light. M.p. about 195°, with decomposition.
Soluble 1 in 45 of water, 1 in 50 of ethanol, and 1 in 5 of dilute hydrochloric acid; very slightly soluble in carbon tetrachloride, chloroform, and ether; freely soluble, with decomposition, in solutions of alkali hydroxides and carbonates.

Sodium Aminohippurate
Proprietary Name. Nephrotest
$C_9H_9N_2NaO_3 = 216.2$
CAS—94-16-6
Soluble in water.

Dissociation Constant. pK_a 3.6.

Colour Test. Diazotisation—red.

Thin-layer Chromatography. *System TA*—Rf 55. (*Van Urk reagent*, yellow.)

Ultraviolet Spectrum. Methanol—280 nm ($A_1^1 = 880$ b).

Quantification. HIGH PRESSURE LIQUID CHROMATOGRAPHY. In plasma or urine: detection limit 1 µg/ml, UV detection—T. Prueksaritanont *et al.*, *J. Chromat.*, 1984, *306*; *Biomed. Appl.*, *31*, 89–97.

Disposition in the Body. Aminohippuric acid is a major metabolite of aminobenzoic acid. After intravenous administration it is rapidly excreted in the urine in subjects with normal renal function.

HALF-LIFE. Biological half-life, about 0.2 hour.

Dose. 2 to 30 g of sodium aminohippurate intravenously, to measure renal function.

Aminonitrothiazole   *Antiprotozoal (Veterinary)*

2-Amino-5-nitrothiazole
$C_3H_3N_3O_2S = 145.1$
CAS—1320-42-9

A greenish-yellow to orange-yellow light powder. M.p. 200°, with decomposition.
Slightly **soluble** in water; soluble 1 in 250 of ethanol and of ether; practically insoluble in chloroform; soluble in dilute mineral acids and propylene glycol.

Colour Test. Diazotisation—violet.

Thin-layer Chromatography. *System TA*—Rf 75. (Visible yellow spot; *acidified iodoplatinate solution*, strong reaction.)

Gas Chromatography. *System GA*—not eluted.

Ultraviolet Spectrum. Water—386 nm ($A_1^1 = 1060$ a).

Infra-red Spectrum. Principal peaks at wavenumbers 1200, 1623, 1176, 1504, 1515, 1252 (KBr disk).

4-Aminophenol

Synonyms. *p*-Aminophenol; *p*-Hydroxyaniline.
$C_6H_7NO = 109.1$
CAS—123-30-8

Crystals. M.p. about 190°. The commercial product is usually pink; m.p. 186°.
Slightly **soluble** in water; soluble in dehydrated alcohol; practically insoluble in chloroform.

Colour Test. Liebermann's Test—black.

Thin-layer Chromatography. *System TD*—Rf 21; *system TE*—Rf 59; *system TF*—Rf 40. (*Ferric chloride solution,* violet; *acidified potassium permanganate solution,* positive; *Van Urk reagent,* yellow.)

Gas Chromatography. *System GA*—RI 1265.

Ultraviolet Spectrum. Aqueous acid—271 nm ($A_1^1 = 133$ b); aqueous alkali—266 nm (broad) ($A_1^1 = 731$ b); methanol—233 nm ($A_1^1 = 587$ b), 303 nm ($A_1^1 = 177$ b).

Mass Spectrum. Principal peaks at *m/z* 109, 80, 53, 81, 108, 52, 54, 110.

Disposition in the Body. 4-Aminophenol is a metabolite of aniline, nitrobenzene, and phenazopyridine.

Aminosalicylic Acid   *Antituberculous Agent*

Synonyms. Aminosalylum; Para-aminosalicylic Acid; PAS; Pasalicylum.

Proprietary Names. Nemasol; Parasal; Teebacin Acid.

4-Amino-2-hydroxybenzoic acid
$C_7H_7NO_3 = 153.1$
CAS—65-49-6

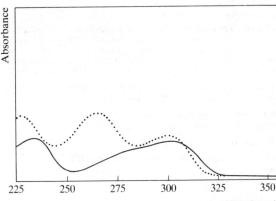

A white bulky powder, which darkens on exposure to air and light. Aqueous solutions are unstable. M.p. 150° to 151°, with effervescence.

Soluble 1 in about 600 of water, 1 in about 20 of ethanol, 1 in 6 of acetone, 1 in 4000 of chloroform, and 1 in 50 of ether.

Calcium Aminosalicylate

Synonym. Aminosalicylate Calcium
$(C_7H_6NO_3)_2Ca,3H_2O = 398.4$
CAS—133-15-3 (anhydrous)
A white or slightly yellow, hygroscopic, crystalline powder. Aqueous solutions are unstable and darken in colour.
Soluble 1 in 7 to 1 in 10 of water; slightly soluble in ethanol.

Phenyl Aminosalicylate

Synonym. Fenamisal
$C_{13}H_{11}NO_3 = 229.2$
CAS—133-11-9
A white crystalline solid. M.p. 153°.
Practically **insoluble** in water.

Potassium Aminosalicylate

Synonym. Aminosalicylate Potassium
Proprietary Name. Teebacin Kalium
$C_7H_6KNO_3 = 191.2$
CAS—133-09-5
A white to cream-coloured crystalline powder. Aqueous solutions are unstable.
Freely **soluble** in water; sparingly soluble in ethanol; very slightly soluble in chloroform and ether.

Sodium Aminosalicylate

Synonyms. Aminosalicylate Sodium; Pasalicylum Solubile.
Proprietary Names. Eupasal Sodico; Italpas Sodico; Parasal Sodium; Pasalba; Teebacin.
$C_7H_6NNaO_3,2H_2O = 211.1$
CAS—133-10-8 (anhydrous); *6018-19-5* (dihydrate)

White or cream-coloured crystals or crystalline powder. Aqueous solutions are unstable.
Soluble 1 in 2 of water; sparingly soluble in ethanol; practically insoluble in chloroform and ether.

Dissociation Constant. pK_a 1.8 (—NH_2), 3.6 (—COOH).

Partition Coefficient. Log *P* (octanol), 0.87.

Colour Tests. Coniferyl Alcohol—orange; Ferric Chloride—violet; Folin–Ciocalteu Reagent—blue; McNally's Test—brown precipitate.

Thin-layer Chromatography. *System TA*—Rf 70; *system TD*—Rf 05; *system TE*—Rf 07; *system TF*—Rf 24. (Location under ultraviolet light, blue fluorescence; *ferric chloride solution,* violet; *acidified potassium permanganate solution,* positive; *Van Urk reagent,* yellow.)

Gas Chromatography. *System GA*—RI 1309.

Ultraviolet Spectrum. Aqueous acid—234 nm ($A_1^1 = 496$ a), 300 nm ($A_1^1 = 330$ a); aqueous alkali—265 nm ($A_1^1 = 846$ a), 300 nm ($A_1^1 = 532$ a).

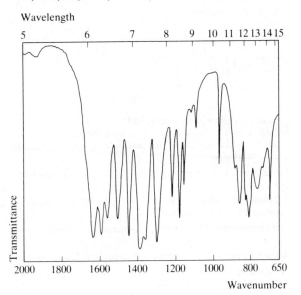

Infra-red Spectrum. Principal peaks at wavenumbers 1301, 1638, 1595, 1510, 805, 1180 (KBr disk).

Mass Spectrum. Principal peaks at m/z 109, 80, 44, 81, 53, 39, 52, 54.

Quantification. HIGH PRESSURE LIQUID CHROMATOGRAPHY. In plasma or urine: aminosalicylic acid and p-acetamidosalicylic acid, sensitivity 500 ng/ml in plasma, fluorescence detection—R. G. Stoll *et al.*, *Res. Commun. chem. Path. Pharmac.*, 1972, *4*, 327–338. In plasma: limit of detection 0.5 ng, fluorescence detection—I. L. Honigberg *et al.*, *J. Chromat.*, 1980, *181*; *Biomed. Appl.*, 7, 266–271.

Disposition in the Body. Readily absorbed after oral administration and widely distributed throughout the body with high concentrations in the kidneys, lungs, and liver. It is metabolised by acetylation to p-acetamidosalicylic acid and by conjugation with glycine, producing p-aminosalicyluric acid; both metabolites are inactive. More than 80% of a dose is excreted in the urine in 24 hours with about 50% of the dose consisting of p-acetamidosalicylic acid; up to 25% of the dose may be excreted as free and acetylated p-aminosalicyluric acid, and the remainder is mostly unchanged drug with small amounts of 2,4-dihydroxybenzoic acid.

THERAPEUTIC CONCENTRATION.

Following a single oral dose of 4 g of aminosalicylic acid to 12 subjects, a mean peak plasma concentration of 50 µg/ml was attained in 3.5 hours; after oral administration of 4 g of sodium aminosalicylate to the same subjects, a mean peak plasma concentration of 155 µg/ml was attained in about 0.8 hour (S. H. Wan *et al.*, *J. pharm. Sci.*, 1974, *63*, 708–711).

TOXICITY. Prolonged administration may give rise to toxic symptoms characteristic of the salicylates.

HALF-LIFE. Plasma half-life, aminosalicylic acid about 0.5 to 1 hour, p-acetamidosalicylic acid about 1.5 hours.

PROTEIN BINDING. In plasma, 60 to 70%.

Dose. 12 g of sodium aminosalicylate daily; up to 20 g daily has been given.

Aminotriazole   *Herbicide*

Synonyms. Amitrole; ATA.
Proprietary Names. Weedazol. It is an ingredient of a number of proprietary weed-killers.
3-Amino-1,2,4-triazole
$C_2H_4N_4 = 84.1$
CAS—61-82-5

A white crystalline powder. M.p. 159°.
Soluble 1 in 3.5 of water and 1 in 4 of ethanol; practically insoluble in acetone, ether, and non-polar solvents; sparingly soluble in ethyl acetate.

Colour Test. Add *sodium hypobromite solution* to the sample—orange-red.

Thin-layer Chromatography. *System TA*—Rf 68. (*Acidified iodoplatinate solution*, positive.)

Gas Chromatography. *System GA*—not eluted; *system GK*—not eluted.

Ultraviolet Spectrum. No significant absorption, 230 to 360 nm.

Infra-red Spectrum. Principal peaks at wavenumbers 1639, 1047, 1534, 1595, 1211, 971 (KBr disk).

Mass Spectrum. Principal peaks at m/z 84, 58, 43, 44, 42, 53, 55, 86.

Amiodarone   *Anti-arrhythmic*

2 - Butylbenzofuran - 3 - yl 4 - (2 - diethylaminoethoxy) - 3,5 - di - iodophenyl ketone
$C_{25}H_{29}I_2NO_3 = 645.3$
CAS—1951-25-3

Amiodarone Hydrochloride
Proprietary Names. Cordarone; Cordarone X.
$C_{25}H_{29}I_2NO_3,HCl = 681.8$
CAS—19774-82-4
A white crystalline powder. M.p. about 161°.
Very slightly **soluble** in water; soluble in ethanol; freely soluble in chloroform.

Dissociation Constant. pK_a 5.6.

Colour Tests. Iodine Test (omitting MnO_2)—positive; Liebermann's Test—brown-yellow; Sulphuric Acid—yellow.

Thin-layer Chromatography. System TA—Rf 72; system TB—Rf 62; system TC—Rf 68. (*Dragendorff spray*, positive; *acidified iodoplatinate solution*, positive; *Marquis reagent*, yellow.)

Gas Chromatography. System GA—RI 3335; decomposition on column produces two major products, RI 2590 and 2780.

High Pressure Liquid Chromatography. System HA—amiodarone k' 2.4, monodesethylamiodarone k' 1.8.

Ultraviolet Spectrum. Aqueous acid—241 nm; aqueous alkali—251 nm.

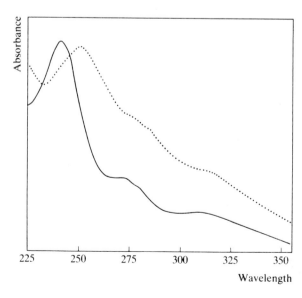

Infra-red Spectrum. Principal peaks at wavenumbers 1630, 748, 1245, 1558, 1170, 998 (amiodarone hydrochloride, KBr disk).

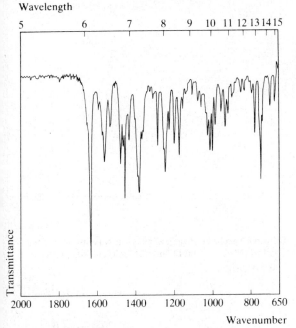

Wavelength

Wavenumber

Mass Spectrum. Principal peaks at m/z 86, 36, 87, 84, 58, 56, 44, 38.

Quantification. HIGH PRESSURE LIQUID CHROMATOGRAPHY. In plasma: amiodarone and monodesethylamiodarone, sensitivity 100 ng/ml, UV detection—G. C. A. Storey *et al.*, *Ther. Drug Monit.*, 1982, *4*, 385–388. In plasma, urine or tissues: amiodarone and monodesethylamiodarone, sensitivity 25 ng/ml in plasma, UV detection—T. A. Plomp *et al.*, *J. Chromat.*, 1983, *273*; *Biomed. Appl.*, *24*, 379–392.

Disposition in the Body. Slowly and incompletely absorbed after oral administration; distributed to the tissues where it is strongly bound. Metabolised by N-dealkylation to monodesethylamiodarone which is the major plasma metabolite during chronic dosing. High concentrations of amiodarone and monodesethylamiodarone are found in the liver, lungs, and adipose tissue. Enterohepatic circulation may occur. Only a small amount is excreted in the urine as unchanged drug.

THERAPEUTIC CONCENTRATION. Accumulates on chronic administration; steady-state plasma concentrations are attained in about one month.
Following oral administration of 400 mg to 7 subjects, peak plasma concentrations of about 0.5 to 1 μg/ml were attained in about 7 hours. After administration of 200 mg 8-hourly to 6 subjects for one month, plasma concentrations determined immediately before the morning dose ranged from 0.75 to 2.8 μg/ml (mean 1.5) (F. Andreasen *et al.*, *Eur. J. clin. Pharmac.*, 1981, *19*, 293–299).
During chronic treatment with 400 mg daily to 33 subjects, mean steady-state plasma concentrations of 2.2 μg/ml of amiodarone and 2.0 μg/ml of monodesethylamiodarone were reported (R. J. Flanagan *et al.*, *J. Pharm. Pharmac.*, 1982, *34*, 638–643).

HALF-LIFE. Plasma half-life during chronic dosing, 14 to 107 days (mean 50).

DISTRIBUTION IN BLOOD. Plasma: whole blood ratio, 1.3.

PROTEIN BINDING. In plasma, extensively bound.

NOTE. For a review of the pharmacokinetics of amiodarone see R. Latini *et al.*, *Clin. Pharmacokinet.*, 1984, *9*, 136–156.

Dose. Initially 600 mg of amiodarone hydrochloride daily; maintenance, 200 to 400 mg daily.

Amiphenazole   *Respiratory Stimulant*

Synonym. DAPT
5-Phenylthiazole-2,4-diamine
$C_9H_9N_3S = 191.3$
CAS—490-55-1

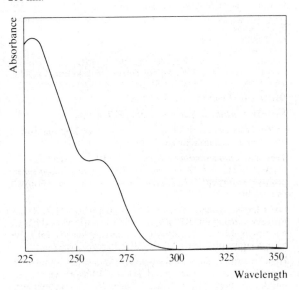

Flakes which turn brown on exposure to light and air. M.p. 163° to 164°, with decomposition.

Amiphenazole Hydrochloride
Synonym. Amiphenazole Chloride
Proprietary Names. Daptazile; Daptazole.
$C_9H_9N_3S,HCl = 227.7$
CAS—942-31-4
A white, fine crystalline or granular, mobile powder. Aqueous solutions hydrolyse slowly. M.p. 236°.
Soluble 1 in 16 of water and 1 in 50 of ethanol; slightly soluble in acetone, chloroform, and ether.

Colour Test. Liebermann's Test (100°)—green-blue.

Thin-layer Chromatography. *System TA*—Rf 61; *system TB*—Rf 02; *system TC*—Rf 33. (*Acidified iodoplatinate solution*, positive.)

Gas Chromatography. *System GB*—RI 1150; *system GC*—RI 2563.

Ultraviolet Spectrum. Aqueous acid—230 nm ($A_1^1 = 998$ a), 261 nm.

Wavelength

Infra-red Spectrum. Principal peaks at wavenumbers 1495, 1637, 688, 750, 1665, 1050 (KBr disk).

Mass Spectrum. Principal peaks at m/z 191, 121, 77, 104, 122, 43, 51, 192.

Dose. Amiphenazole hydrochloride has been given parenterally in doses of 100 to 150 mg.

Amitriptyline   *Antidepressant*

3-(10,11-Dihydro-5H-dibenzo[a,d]cyclohepten-5-ylidene)-NN-dimethylpropylamine
$C_{20}H_{23}N = 277.4$
CAS—50-48-6

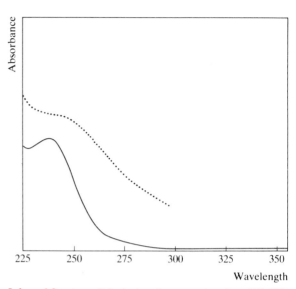

A colourless oil, which becomes yellow on standing due to oxidation to a ketonic product.

Amitriptyline Embonate
Proprietary Name. Tryptizol (syrup)
$(C_{20}H_{23}N)_2,C_{23}H_{16}O_6 = 943.2$
CAS—17086-03-2
A pale yellow to brownish-yellow powder. M.p. about 140°.
Practically **insoluble** in water; soluble 1 in 120 of ethanol, 1 in 6 of acetone, and 1 in 8 of chloroform.

Amitriptyline Hydrochloride
Proprietary Names. Adepril; Amavil; Amiline; Amitid; Amitril; Deprex; Domical; Elavil; Endep; Laroxyl; Lentizol; Levate; Meravil; Novotriptyn; Saroten; Sarotex; Tryptanol; Tryptizol. It is an ingredient of Etrafon, Limbatril, Limbitrol, Triavil, and Triptafen.
Note. Deprex is also used as a proprietary name for dibenzepin hydrochloride.
$C_{20}H_{23}N,HCl = 313.9$
CAS—549-18-8
Colourless crystals or white powder. M.p. 195° to 199°.
Soluble 1 in 1 of water, 1 in 1.5 of ethanol, 1 in 56 of acetone, 1 in 1.2 of chloroform, and 1 in 1 of methanol; practically insoluble in ether.

Dissociation Constant. pK_a 9.4 (25°).

Partition Coefficient. Log P (octanol/pH 7.4), 3.0.

Colour Tests. Mandelin's Test—brown → green; Marquis Test—brown-orange; Sulphuric Acid—orange.

Thin-layer Chromatography. *System TA*—Rf 51; *system TB*—Rf 55; *system TC*—Rf 32; *system TL*—Rf 15. (*Dragendorff spray*, positive; *acidified iodoplatinate solution*, positive; *Marquis reagent*, brown.)

Gas Chromatography. *System GA*—amitriptyline RI 2196, 10-hydroxyamitriptyline RI 2360, 10-hydroxynortriptyline RI 2385, nortriptyline RI 2210; *system GF*—amitriptyline RI 2510, 10-hydroxyamitriptyline RI 2830 or 2880 (stereoisomers).

High Pressure Liquid Chromatography. *System HA*—amitriptyline k′ 3.3, 10-hydroxyamitriptyline k′ 2.9, 10-hydroxynortriptyline k′ 1.8, nortriptyline k′ 2.0; *system HF*—amitriptyline k′ 5.42, nortriptyline k′ 4.58.

Ultraviolet Spectrum. Aqueous acid—239 nm ($A_1^1 = 504$ a).

Infra-red Spectrum. Principal peaks at wavenumbers 756, 770, 746, 969, 1014, 1258 (amitriptyline hydrochloride, KBr disk).

Mass Spectrum. Principal peaks at m/z 58, 59, 202, 42, 203, 214, 217, –; 10-hydroxyamitriptyline 58, 42, 69, 41, 30, 215, 202, 59; 10-hydroxynortriptyline 44, 45, 26, 218, 215, 203, 202, 42; nortriptyline 44, 202, 45, 220, 218, 215, 91, –.

Quantification. GAS CHROMATOGRAPHY. In plasma: amitriptyline and nortriptyline, detection limit 10 ng/ml, AFID—S. Dawling and R. A. Braithwaite, *J. Chromat.*, 1978, *146*; *Biomed. Appl.*, *3*, 449–456.

HIGH PRESSURE LIQUID CHROMATOGRAPHY. In plasma: amitriptyline and nortriptyline, UV detection—B. Mellström and R. Braithwaite, *J. Chromat.*, 1978, *157*, 379–385. In plasma or serum: amitriptyline and nortriptyline, sensitivity 5 ng/ml, UV detection—P. M. Kabra *et al.*, *Clinica chim. Acta*, 1981, *111*, 123–132. In urine: amitriptyline and major metabolites, detection limit 100 ng/ml, UV detection—S. R. Biggs *et al.*, *Drug Met. Disp.*, 1979, *7*, 233–236.

RADIOIMMUNOASSAY. In serum, saliva, or urine: amitriptyline and nortriptyline, sensitivity 500 pg/ml—G. P. Mould *et al.*, *Ann. clin. Biochem.*, 1978, *15*, 221–225.

REVIEW. For a review of analytical methods see B. A. Scoggins *et al.*, *Clin. Chem.*, 1980, *26*, 5–17.

Disposition in the Body. Readily absorbed after oral administration and rapidly taken up by the tissues; bioavailability 30 to 60%. The main metabolic reaction is demethylation together with hydroxylation and conjugation with glucuronic acid. The major active metabolite is nortriptyline together with didesmethylamitriptyline and their 10-hydroxy derivatives and conjugates; some amitriptyline N-oxide may also be formed. It is mainly excreted in the urine as free and conjugated metabolites, up to about 35% of a single dose being excreted in 24 hours. About 50% of the excreted material is 10-hydroxynortriptyline and its glucuronide conjugate, up to 27% is 10-hydroxyamitriptyline (mainly conjugated); unchanged drug and nortriptyline each account for less than 5% of the excreted material. About 8% of a dose may be eliminated in the faeces as unchanged drug. There appears to be polymorphic variation in the metabolite pattern.

THERAPEUTIC CONCENTRATION. In plasma, usually in the range 0.1 to 0.2 µg/ml (combined amitriptyline and nortriptyline).

After a single oral dose of 50 mg to 3 subjects, peak plasma concentrations for amitriptyline of 0.02 to 0.04 µg/ml (mean 0.025) and for nortriptyline of about 0.01 µg/ml were attained in 2 to 4 hours (W. A. Garland, *J. pharm. Sci.*, 1977, *66*, 77–81).

Following daily oral doses of 150 mg to 14 subjects for 3 weeks, steady-state serum concentrations of 0.05 to 0.24 µg/ml (mean 0.13) of amitriptyline, 0.04 to 0.26 µg/ml (mean 0.11) of nortriptyline, 0.05 to 0.25 µg/ml (mean 0.13) of E-10-hydroxynortriptyline, and 0.005 to 0.04 µg/ml (mean 0.02) of 10-hydroxyamitriptyline were reported (P. M. Edelbroek *et al.*, *Clin. Pharmac. Ther.*, 1984, *35*, 467–473).

TOXICITY. Moderate intoxication is associated with plasma concentrations of 0.05 to **0.17** to 0.43 µg/ml and severe toxic symptoms with concentrations greater than 0.3 µg/ml. The fatal blood concentration range is 0.55 to **3.3** to 16.1 µg/ml. Corresponding toxic doses are greater than 1 g (moderate intoxication) and greater than 2 g (severe or fatal).

In 7 fatalities attributed to amitriptyline overdose, postmortem concentrations, µg/ml or µg/g (mean), were:

	Amitriptyline	Nortriptyline
Blood	0.43–8.30 (3.4)	0.29–6.50 (1.6)
Liver	10.4–243 (92)	4.2–456 (94)

(D. N. Bailey and R. F. Shaw, *J. analyt. Toxicol.*, 1980, *4*, 232–236).

In 3 fatalities attributed to amitriptyline overdose, tissue concentrations, µg/ml or µg/g, were:

	Amitriptyline	Nortriptyline
Blood	6, 18, 3	5, —, 2
Liver	72, 66, 58	98, 24, 60
Urine	6, 28, 7	10, 12, 7

(E. C. Munksgaard, *Acta pharmac. Tox.*, 1969, *27*, 129–134).

HALF-LIFE. Plasma half-life, 8 to 51 hours (mean 28), increased in overdosage.

DISTRIBUTION IN BLOOD. Plasma: whole blood ratio, 1.2.

SALIVA. Plasma: saliva ratio, 3.

PROTEIN BINDING. In plasma, 91 to 97%.

NOTE. For a review of the pharmacokinetics of tricyclic antidepressants see G. Molnar and R. N. Gupta, *Biopharm. Drug Disp.*, 1980, *1*, 283–305.

Dose. 50 to 150 mg of amitriptyline hydrochloride daily; up to 300 mg daily has been given.

Amodiaquine   *Antimalarial*

Synonym. Amodiachin
Proprietary Name. Basoquin
4-(7-Chloro-4-quinolylamino)-2-(diethylaminomethyl)phenol
$C_{20}H_{22}ClN_3O = 355.9$
CAS—86-42-0

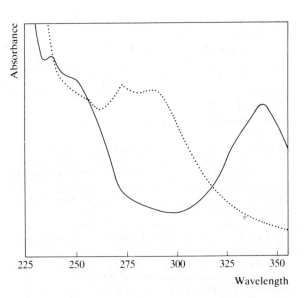

White crystals. M.p. 208°.

Amodiaquine Hydrochloride

Proprietary Names. Camoquin; Flavoquine.
$C_{20}H_{22}ClN_3O,2HCl,2H_2O = 464.8$
CAS—69-44-3 (anhydrous); *6398-98-7* (dihydrate)
A yellow crystalline powder. M.p. about 158°.
Soluble 1 in about 22 of water and 1 in about 70 of ethanol; practically insoluble in chloroform and ether.

Colour Tests. Folin–Ciocalteu Reagent—blue; Liebermann's Test—black; Millon's Reagent—orange.

Thin-layer Chromatography. *System TA*—Rf 62; *system TB*—Rf 08; *system TC*—Rf 40. (*Acidified iodoplatinate solution*, positive.)

Gas Chromatography. *System GA*—not eluted.

Ultraviolet Spectrum. Aqueous acid—237 nm ($A_1^1 = 600$ b), 343 nm; aqueous alkali—273 nm, 287 nm.

Infra-red Spectrum. Principal peaks at wavenumbers 1565, 815, 1535, 1255, 869, 847 (KBr disk).

Mass Spectrum. Principal peaks at *m/z* 58, 282, 30, 284, 355, 73, 283, 44.

Quantification. SPECTROFLUORIMETRY. In plasma or serum: sensitivity 50 ng/ml—G. M. Trenholme *et al.*, *Bull. Wld Hlth Org.*, 1974, *51*, 431–434.

Disposition in the Body. Readily absorbed after oral administration and widely distributed throughout the tissues. After absorption it is slowly released into the blood and excreted in the urine for at least 7 days after a single dose; the rate of excretion is increased in acid urine.

THERAPEUTIC CONCENTRATION.

Following a single oral dose of 10 mg/kg to 5 subjects, serum concentrations of 0.30 to 0.68 µg/ml (mean 0.5) were reported after 4 hours; the ratio of erythrocyte to serum concentration varied with time and between individuals, but erythrocyte concentrations were generally higher than serum concentrations after 48 hours (G. M. Trenholme *et al.*, *ibid.*).

Dose. For an acute attack, the equivalent of 1.5 g of amodiaquine in 48 hours (1.2 g in the first 24 hours); for suppression, the equivalent of 300 to 600 mg every 7 days.

Amoxapine   *Antidepressant*

2-Chloro-11-(piperazin-1-yl)dibenz[*b,f*][1,4]oxazepine
$C_{17}H_{16}ClN_3O = 313.8$
CAS—14028-44-5

Crystals. M.p. 175° to 176°.

Gas Chromatography. *System GA*—RI 2659.

Ultraviolet Spectrum. Aqueous acid—252 nm ($A_1^1 = 362$ a), 293 nm ($A_1^1 = 315$ a); aqueous alkali—250 nm, 299 nm.

Infra-red Spectrum. Principal peaks at wavenumbers 1604, 1592, 752, 1181, 1246, 1107.

Mass Spectrum. Principal peaks at *m/z* 245, 257, 247, 193, 56, 246, 228, 259.

Quantification. GAS CHROMATOGRAPHY. In serum or urine: amoxapine and metabolites, ECD for serum and FID for urine—T. B. Cooper and R. G. Kelly, *J. pharm. Sci.*, 1979, *68*, 216–219.

HIGH PRESSURE LIQUID CHROMATOGRAPHY. In serum: amoxapine and 8-hydroxyamoxapine, detection limit 50 ng/ml, UV detection—J. J. Tasset and F. M. Hassan, *Clin. Chem.*, 1982, *28*, 2154–2157. In plasma: amoxapine and metabolites, sensitivity 25 ng/ml, UV detection—S. M. Johnson *et al.*, *J. pharm. Sci.*, 1984, *73*, 696–699.

Disposition in the Body. Rapidly and almost completely absorbed after oral administration. It is metabolised by hydroxylation to 7-hydroxyamoxapine and 8-hydroxyamoxapine which are both active. The hydroxylated metabolites are excreted in the urine as glucuronide conjugates and are also eliminated in the faeces in unconjugated form. Less than 5% of a dose is excreted in the urine as unchanged drug.
Amoxapine is a metabolite of loxapine.

THERAPEUTIC CONCENTRATION.

After a single oral dose of 50 mg to 26 subjects, a mean peak serum-amoxapine concentration of 0.03 µg/ml was attained in 1 to 2 hours; the peak concentration of 8-hydroxyamoxapine was of a similar order (T. B. Cooper and R. G. Kelly, *idem.*).

Following oral administration of 300 mg daily in divided doses to 10 subjects, steady-state serum concentrations of 0.02 to 0.09 µg/ml of amoxapine and 0.16 to 0.51 µg/ml of 8-hydroxyamoxapine were reported (W. E. Boutelle, *Neuropharmacology*, 1980, *19*, 1229–1231).

TOXICITY.

The following postmortem concentrations were reported in 3 fatalities due to amoxapine overdose: blood 11.5, 2.8, 0.89 µg/ml, bile 1264.5, 69.1, 14.3 µg/ml, liver 112.2, 40.1, 16.8 µg/g; in the first case brain and urine concentrations of 2.5 µg/g and 28.3 µg/ml, respectively, were also reported (C. L. Winek *et al.*, *Forens. Sci. Int.*, 1984, *26*, 33–38).

In a review of 33 cases of amoxapine overdose, 3 subjects had no toxic symptoms, 10 suffered mild toxic reactions, 15 developed severe toxicity, and 5 died. Postmortem blood concentrations of 0.26 to 6.70 µg/ml (mean 2.8) of amoxapine plus 8-hydroxyamoxapine were reported in 4 of the 5 fatalities (T. L. Litovitz and K. G. Troutman, *J. Am. med. Ass.*, 1983, *250*, 1069–1071).

The following postmortem tissue concentrations were reported in a fatality due to ingestion of 2 g of amoxapine: blood 7.2 µg/ml, bile 823 µg/ml, liver 36 µg/g; a blood-alcohol concentration of 280 µg/ml was also reported. In a further 2 cases where amoxapine was a contributory cause of death, postmortem concentrations were: blood 1.66 and 2.95 µg/ml, bile 75, – µg/ml, liver –, 23.2 µg/g, urine 22, – µg/ml (N.B. Wu Chen *et al.*, *J. forens. Sci.*, 1983, *28*, 116–121).

HALF-LIFE. Plasma half-life, amoxapine about 8 hours, 7-hydroxyamoxapine about 6 hours, 8-hydroxyamoxapine about 30 hours.

PROTEIN BINDING. In plasma, about 90%.

NOTE. For a review of the pharmacokinetics of amoxapine see S. G. Jue *et al.*, *Drugs*, 1982, *24*, 1–23.

Dose. 150 to 600 mg daily.

Amoxycillin   *Antibiotic*

Synonyms. D(−)-α-Amino-*p*-hydroxybenzylpenicillin; Amoxicillin; Amoxicilline.

(6R)-6-[α-D-(4-Hydroxyphenyl)glycylamino]penicillanic acid
$C_{16}H_{19}N_3O_5S = 365.4$
CAS—26787-78-0

Amoxycillin Sodium

Proprietary Names. Amoxil (injection); Clamoxyl (injection).
$C_{16}H_{18}N_3NaO_5S = 387.4$
CAS—34642-77-8
A white powder.
Soluble 1 in less than 1 of water.

Amoxycillin Trihydrate

Synonym. Amoxicillin

Proprietary Names. Amoxican; Amoxil; Amoxypen; Clamoxyl; Imacillin; Larotid; Moxacin; Moxilean; Novamoxin; Penamox; Polymox; Robamox; Trimox; Utimox; Wymox. It is an ingredient of Augmentin.
$C_{16}H_{19}N_3O_5S, 3H_2O = 419.4$
CAS—61336-70-7
A white crystalline powder.
Soluble 1 in 400 of water, 1 in 1000 of ethanol, and 1 in 200 of methanol; practically insoluble in chloroform and ether.

Dissociation Constant. pK_a 2.4, 7.4, 9.6.

Partition Coefficient. Log *P* (octanol), 0.87.

Ultraviolet Spectrum. Amoxycillin trihydrate: aqueous acid—230 nm ($A_1^1 = 225$ a), 272 nm ($A_1^1 = 26$ a); aqueous alkali—247 nm ($A_1^1 = 286$ b), 291 nm ($A_1^1 = 62$ a).

Infra-red Spectrum. Principal peaks at wavenumbers 1775, 1583, 1684, 1248, 1613, 1313 (amoxycillin trihydrate, KBr disk).

Quantification. HIGH PRESSURE LIQUID CHROMATOGRAPHY. In urine: amoxycillin and penicilloic acid, sensitivity 2.5 µg/ml, fluorescence detection—T. L. Lee, *J. pharm. Sci.*, 1979, *68*, 454–458. In plasma: sensitivity 500 ng/ml, UV detection—T. L. Lee and M. A. Brooks, *J. Chromat.*, 1984, *306*; *Biomed. Appl.*, *31*, 429–435.

Disposition in the Body. Rapidly absorbed after oral administration. About 60% of an oral dose is excreted in the urine as unchanged drug in 6 hours and 20% as the inactive metabolite, penicilloic acid, in the same period. After parenteral administration, up to 75% of a dose is excreted in the urine unchanged in 6 hours.

THERAPEUTIC CONCENTRATION.
Following an oral dose of 500 mg to 8 subjects, peak plasma concentrations of 6.0 to 15.3 µg/ml (mean 10) were attained in 1 to 2 hours (A. Arancibia *et al., Antimicrob. Ag. Chemother.*, 1980, *17*, 199–202).

HALF-LIFE. Plasma half-life, about 1 hour, increased in renal failure.

VOLUME OF DISTRIBUTION. About 0.2 to 0.4 litre/kg.

CLEARANCE. Plasma clearance, 3 to 5 ml/min/kg.

PROTEIN BINDING. In plasma, about 20%.

NOTE. For reviews of the pharmacokinetics of amoxycillin see R. N. Brogden *et al., Drugs*, 1975, *9*, 88–140 and R. N. Brogden *et al., Drugs*, 1979, *18*, 169–184 (amoxycillin injectable).

Dose. The equivalent of 0.75 to 1.5 g of amoxycillin daily. One-day courses of 3 to 6 g are also given.

Amphetamine   *Central Stimulant*

Synonym. Racemic Desoxynorephedrine
Proprietary Names. It is an ingredient of Biphetamine and Durophet.
($\pm$)-α-Methylphenethylamine
$C_9H_{13}N = 135.2$
CAS—300-62-9

$$C_6H_5 \cdot CH_2 \cdot \overset{\overset{\textstyle NH_2}{|}}{CH} \cdot CH_3$$

A colourless, mobile, slowly volatile liquid. It absorbs carbon dioxide from the air forming a volatile carbonate. B.p. 200° to 203°.
Soluble 1 in 50 of water; very soluble in ethanol, chloroform, and ether; freely soluble in acids.

Amphetamine Phosphate
Synonyms. Benzpropaminum Phosphoricum; Monobasic Racemic Amphetamine Phosphate.
$C_9H_{13}N,H_3PO_4 = 233.2$
CAS—139-10-6
A white crystalline powder with no characteristic melting-point; it sinters at about 150° and decomposes at about 300°.
Freely **soluble** in water; slightly soluble in ethanol; practically insoluble in chloroform and ether.

Amphetamine Sulphate
Synonyms. Phenaminum; Phenopromini Sulphas; Phenylaminopropanum Racemicum Sulfuricum; Psychedrinum.

Proprietary Name. Benzedrine
$(C_9H_{13}N)_2,H_2SO_4 = 368.5$
CAS—60-13-9
A white crystalline powder. M.p. about 300°, with decomposition.
Soluble 1 in 9 of water and 1 in 515 of ethanol; practically insoluble in chloroform and ether.

Dissociation Constant. pK_a 9.9 (20°).

Partition Coefficient. Log P (octanol), 1.8.

Colour Tests. Liebermann's Test—red-orange; Marquis Test—orange → brown; Ninhydrin—pink-orange.

Thin-layer Chromatography. System *TA*—Rf 43; system *TB*—Rf 15; system *TC*—Rf 09. (*Dragendorff spray*, positive; *FPN reagent*, pink; *acidified iodoplatinate solution*, positive; *Marquis reagent*, brown; *ninhydrin spray*, positive; *acidified potassium permanganate solution*, positive.)

Gas Chromatography. System *GA*—RI 1123; system *GB*—RI 1134; system *GC*—RI 1536; system *GF*—RI 1315.

High Pressure Liquid Chromatography. System *HA*—k′ 0.9; system *HB*—k′ 8.48; system *HC*—k′ 0.98.

Ultraviolet Spectrum. Aqueous acid—251 nm, 257 nm ($A_1^1 = 14$ a), 263 nm.

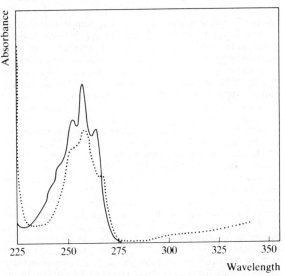

Infra-red Spectrum. Principal peaks at wavenumbers 700, 740, 1495, 1090, 1605, 825 (thin film). (See below)

Mass Spectrum. Principal peaks at *m/z* 44, 91, 40, 42, 65, 45, 39, 43; phenylacetone 43, 91, 134, 92, 65, 39, 63, 135.

Quantification. GAS CHROMATOGRAPHY. In urine: amphetamine and methylamphetamine, detection limit 10 ng/ml, ECD—M. Terada *et al., J. Chromat.*, 1982, *237*, 285–292.

GAS CHROMATOGRAPHY–MASS SPECTROMETRY. In plasma or cerebrospinal fluid—N. Narasimhachari *et al., J. Chromat.*, 1979, *164*; *Biomed. Appl.*, *6*, 386–393.

HIGH PRESSURE LIQUID CHROMATOGRAPHY. In plasma or urine: sensitivity 20 ng/ml and 4 ng/ml, respectively, UV detection—B. M. Farrell and T. M. Jeffries, *J. Chromat.*, 1983, *272*; *Biomed. Appl.*, *23*, 111–128.

Disposition in the Body. Readily absorbed after oral or rectal administration; rapidly distributed extravascularly and taken up, to some extent, by red blood cells. The main metabolic

Wavelength

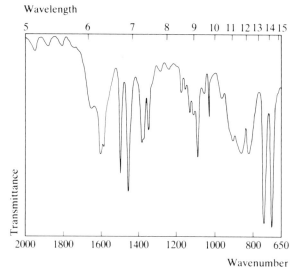

reaction is oxidative deamination to form phenylacetone, which is then oxidised to benzoic acid and conjugated with glycine to form hippuric acid; minor reactions include aromatic hydroxylation to form 4-hydroxyamphetamine (an active metabolite), β-hydroxylation which is stereoselective for the (+)-isomer of amphetamine, to form norephedrine (phenylpropanolamine), and N-oxidation to form a hydroxylamine derivative. The products of aromatic hydroxylation and N-oxidation may be conjugated with sulphate or glucuronic acid.

Excretion of amphetamine is markedly dependent on urinary pH, being greatly increased in acid urine. After large doses, amphetamine may be detected in urine for several days. Under uncontrolled urinary pH conditions, about 30% of the dose is excreted unchanged in the urine in 24 hours and a total of about 90% of the dose is excreted in 3 to 4 days. The amount excreted unchanged in 24 hours may increase to 74% of the dose in acid urine and decrease to 1 to 4% in alkaline urine; under alkaline conditions, hippuric acid and benzoic acid account for about 50% of the urinary material. Under normal conditions 16 to 28% is excreted as hippuric acid, about 4% as benzoylglucuronide, 2 to 4% as 4-hydroxyamphetamine and about 2% as norephedrine in 24 hours; small amounts of conjugated 4-hydroxynorephedrine and phenylacetone are also excreted. No elimination in the faeces has been detected.

Amphetamine is a metabolite of benzphetamine, methylamphetamine, and selegiline.

THERAPEUTIC CONCENTRATION. After normal therapeutic doses the plasma concentration is usually below 0.1 µg/ml. However, continued use of amphetamine may cause addiction, and ingestion of 10 times the usual therapeutic dose is common among addicts; in such cases the plasma concentration may be up to 3 µg/ml.

After a single oral dose containing 10 mg of amphetamine to 4 subjects, peak plasma concentrations of about 0.02 µg/ml were attained (S. H. Wan et al., Clin. Pharmac. Ther., 1978, 23, 585–590).

Steady-state blood concentrations of 2 to 3 µg/ml were observed in a regular user who ingested about 1 g a day (R. H. Cravey and N. C. Jain, Trauma, 1973, 15, 49–94).

The intravenous administration of 160 mg of amphetamine to a regular user resulted in a plasma concentration of 0.59 µg/ml after 1 hour (E. Anggard et al., Scand J. clin. Lab. Invest., 1970, 26, 137–143).

TOXICITY. The estimated minimum lethal dose in non-addicted adults is 200 mg. Toxic effects may be produced with blood concentrations of 0.2 to 3 µg/ml, and fatalities with concentrations greater than 0.5 µg/ml. Deaths from overdosage are comparatively rare.

The following postmortem tissue concentrations were reported in 3 fatalities due to amphetamine (route of administration intravenous in cases 1 and 3, unknown in case 2): blood 0.5, 6, 7 µg/ml, kidney 4, –, 8 µg/g, liver 45, 35, 12 µg/g, urine –, 700, – µg/ml (S. Orrenius and A. C. Maehly, Z. Rechtsmed., 1970, 67, 184–189).

In a fatality due to intravenous administration of amphetamine, the following postmortem tissue concentrations were reported: blood 41 µg/ml, liver 23 µg/g, urine 39 µg/ml (G. Adjutantis et al., Medicine, Sci. Law, 1975, 15, 62–63).

Urine concentrations of <0.5 to 320 µg/ml (mean 76) were reported in 11 fatalities due to amphetamine (P. Holmgren and O. Lindquist, Z. Rechtsmed., 1975, 75, 265–273).

HALF-LIFE. Plasma half-life, 4 to 8 hours when the urine is acidic and about 12 hours in subjects whose urinary pH values are uncontrolled.

VOLUME OF DISTRIBUTION. About 3 to 4 litres/kg.

SALIVA. Plasma: saliva ratio, about 0.35.

PROTEIN BINDING. In plasma, 15 to 40%.

Dose. 20 to 100 mg of amphetamine sulphate daily.

Amphetericin   *Antifungal*

Synonyms. Amphotericin B; Anfotericina B.
Proprietary Names. Ampho-Moronal; Fungilin; Fungizone. It is an ingredient of Mysteclin (syrup).

A mixture of antifungal polyenes produced by the growth of certain strains of *Streptomyces nodosus* or by any other means. $C_{47}H_{73}NO_{17} = 924.1$
CAS—1397-89-3

A yellow to orange powder. It gradually decomposes above 170°. Practically **insoluble** in water, ethanol, chloroform, and ether; soluble 1 in 200 of dimethylformamide and 1 in 20 of dimethyl sulphoxide; soluble in propylene glycol.

Dissociation Constant. pK$_a$ 5.5, 10.0.

Infra-red Spectrum. Principal peaks at wavenumbers 1010, 1065, 1038, 1103, 1183, 1126 (KBr disk).

Quantification. HIGH PRESSURE LIQUID CHROMATOGRAPHY. In serum or cerebrospinal fluid: sensitivity 20 ng/ml, UV detection—I. Nilsson-Ehle et al., J. infect. Dis., 1977, 135, 414–422.

Disposition in the Body. Poorly absorbed after oral, intramuscular, or subcutaneous administration. It is slowly excreted in the urine, less than 10% of a dose being excreted unchanged in 24 hours; up to 40% of a dose is excreted in the urine in 7 days and traces are still detectable in urine 2 months after cessation of treatment.

THERAPEUTIC CONCENTRATION.

A mean serum concentration of 1.2 µg/ml was reported in 20 subjects 1 hour after an intravenous infusion of 50 mg (B. T. Fields et al., Appl. Microbiol., 1970, 19, 955–959).

HALF-LIFE. Plasma half-life, about 24 to 48 hours; a longer terminal elimination phase of about 15 days has also been reported.

VOLUME OF DISTRIBUTION. About 4 litres/kg.

CLEARANCE. Plasma clearance, about 0.4 ml/min/kg.

PROTEIN BINDING. In plasma, 90 to 97%.

NOTE. For a review of amphotericin see T. K. Daneshead and D. W. Warnock, *Clin. Pharmacokinet.*, 1983, *8*, 19–23.

Dose. Up to 800 mg daily by mouth. Doses of 0.25 to 1 mg/kg daily are given intravenously.

Ampicillin   *Antibiotic*

Synonyms. Aminobenzylpenicillin; Anhydrous Ampicillin.
Proprietary Names of Ampicillin, Ampicillin Sodium and Ampicillin Trihydrate. A-Cillin; Alpen; Amblosin; Amcill; Amfipen; Amperil; Ampilar; Ampilean; Binotal; Biosan; Britcin; D-Amp; Omnipen; Pen A; Penbritin(e); Pensyn; Pentrexyl; Polycillin; Principen; Robamox; Supen; Totacillin; Vidopen.

(6*R*)-6-(α-D-Phenylglycylamino)penicillanic acid
$C_{16}H_{19}N_3O_4S = 349.4$
CAS—69-53-4

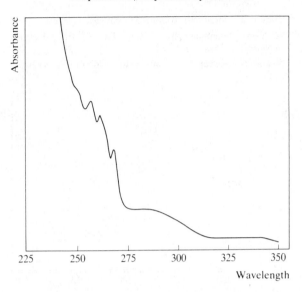

A white crystalline powder. M.p. about 200°.
Soluble 1 in 170 of water; practically insoluble in ethanol, acetone, carbon tetrachloride, chloroform, and ether.

Ampicillin Sodium
$C_{16}H_{18}N_3NaO_4S = 371.4$
CAS—69-52-3
A white, hygroscopic, crystalline or amorphous powder. Aqueous solutions containing 10% or more deteriorate rapidly on storage. M.p. about 205°, with decomposition.
Soluble 1 in 2 of water and 1 in 50 of acetone; slightly soluble in chloroform; practically insoluble in ether. With ethanol, ampicillin sodium forms a colloidal dispersion which gels on standing.

Ampicillin Trihydrate
$C_{16}H_{19}N_3O_4S,3H_2O = 403.4$
CAS—7177-48-2
A white crystalline powder.
Soluble 1 in 150 of water; practically insoluble in ethanol, acetone, carbon tetrachloride, chloroform, and ether.

Dissociation Constant. pK_a 2.5 (—COOH), 7.3 (—NH₂), (25°).

Colour Tests. Liebermann's Test—orange.
Suspend 10 mg in 1 ml of water and add 2 ml of a mixture of 2 ml of *potassium cupri-tartrate solution* and 6 ml of water—red-violet.

Ultraviolet Spectrum. Aqueous acid—257 nm ($A_1^1 = 9.2$ a), 262 nm, 268 nm.

Infra-red Spectrum. Principal peaks at wavenumbers 1775, 1693, 1526, 1308, 1497, 1583 (KBr disk).

Quantification. SPECTROFLUORIMETRY. In serum: sensitivity 50 ng/ml—H. J. H. Keshavan *et al.*, *Clin. Chem.*, 1979, *25*, 1674–1675.

HIGH PRESSURE LIQUID CHROMATOGRAPHY. In plasma, saliva or urine: sensitivity 500 ng/ml, UV detection—T. B. Vree *et al.*, *J. Chromat.*, 1978, *145*; *Biomed. Appl.*, *2*, 496–501.

POLAROGRAPHY. In serum or urine—S. Schroeder *et al.*, *Pharmazie*, 1978, *33*, 432–434.

Disposition in the Body. Readily but incompletely absorbed after oral administration. About 30% of an oral dose is excreted in the urine in 6 hours as unchanged drug and about 10% as penicilloic acid; after parenteral administration about 75% is excreted unchanged in 6 hours. High concentrations of ampicillin are attained in the bile.

THERAPEUTIC CONCENTRATION.
After an oral dose of 500 mg given to 6 young subjects, peak plasma concentrations of 2.65 to 4.0 µg/ml (mean 3.4) were attained in about 2 hours; higher concentrations were reported when a similar dose was given to 6 elderly subjects (E. J. Triggs *et al.*, *Eur. J. clin. Pharmac.*, 1980, *18*, 195–198).

HALF-LIFE. Plasma half-life, about 1 to 2 hours.

VOLUME OF DISTRIBUTION. About 0.2 to 0.5 litre/kg.

CLEARANCE. Plasma clearance, about 3 to 4 ml/min/kg.

DISTRIBUTION IN BLOOD. Plasma: whole blood ratio, 1.8.

PROTEIN BINDING. In plasma, about 20%.

NOTE. For a review of the pharmacokinetics of penicillins see M. Barza and L. Weinstein, *Clin. Pharmacokinet.*, 1976, *1*, 297–308.

Dose. 1 to 8 g daily.

Amprolium Hydrochloride   *Coccidiostat (Veterinary)*

Proprietary Names. It is an ingredient of Amprolmix-UK, Amprol-Plus, Pancoxin, and Supacox.

1-(4-Amino-2-propylpyrimidin-5-ylmethyl)-2-methylpyridin-iumchloride hydrochloride
$C_{14}H_{19}ClN_4,HCl = 315.2$
CAS—121-25-5 (amprolium); *137-88-2* (hydrochloride)

A white powder. M.p. 247°, with decomposition.
Soluble 1 in 2 of water and 1 in 170 of ethanol; practically insoluble in chloroform; very slightly soluble in ether.

Colour Test. Aromaticity (Method 2)—colourless/yellow.

Thin-layer Chromatography. *System TA*—Rf 02. (*Acidified iodoplatinate solution*, positive.)

Ultraviolet Spectrum. Aqueous acid—246 nm ($A_1^1 = 420$ b), 262 nm.

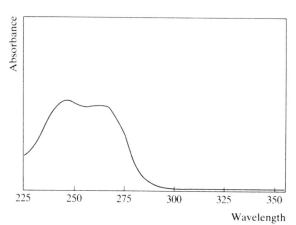

Infra-red Spectrum. Principal peaks at wavenumbers 1638, 1522, 1593, 787, 1562, 1149 (amprolium, KBr disk).

Amygdalin

Synonym. Amygdaloside

Note. The name 'laetrile' is frequently used to describe amygdalin but it has also been used to describe *l*-mandelonitrile-β-glucuronide, a substance which may be derived from amygdalin.

O-(6-O-β-D-Glucopyranosyl-β-D-glucopyranosyl)-D-mandelonitrile

$C_{20}H_{27}NO_{11} = 457.4$

CAS—29883-15-6

A colourless, crystalline, cyanogenic, glycoside present in bitter almond seeds, *Prunus amygdalus* var. *amara*, apricot kernels and other seeds of the Rosaceae. M.p. about 220°; after solidifying the substance remelts at 125° to 130°.

Soluble 1 in 12 of water and 1 in 900 of ethanol; practically insoluble in ether.

Infra-red Spectrum. Principal peaks at wavenumbers 1065, 1025, 695, 758, 1272, 890 (KCl disk).

Mass Spectrum. Principal peaks at *m/z* 43, 31, 57, 73, 60, 29, 55, 44.

Quantification. GAS CHROMATOGRAPHY. In plasma: sensitivity 2 µg/ml, FID—J. F. Stobaugh, *Analyt. Lett. (Part B)*, 1978, *11*, 753–764.

HIGH PRESSURE LIQUID CHROMATOGRAPHY. In plasma or urine: amygdalin and prunasin, sensitivity 1 µg/ml, UV detection—A. G. Rauws *et al.*, *Pharm. Weekbl. (Sci. Edn)*, 1982, *4*, 172–175.

Disposition in the Body. Poorly absorbed after ingestion and slowly hydrolysed in the gastro-intestinal tract to mandelonitrile-β-glucoside (prunasin), mandelonitrile, and glucose, and finally to benzaldehyde and hydrogen cyanide. After ingestion, about 8 to 32% of a dose is excreted unchanged in the urine; after parenteral administration, only small amounts are hydrolysed and most of a dose is excreted unchanged in the urine. Urinary cyanide and thiocyanate concentrations are not significantly elevated after oral or intravenous administration.

BLOOD CONCENTRATION.

In 6 subjects ingesting 500 mg of amygdalin three times a day, peak plasma concentrations of <1 µg/ml of amygdalin were attained in 30 to 60 minutes; peak plasma-cyanide concentrations of 0.4 to 2.1 µg/ml (mean 1.0) were reported 1.5 to 2 hours after a dose on the second day; plasma-thiocyanate concentrations accumulated on repeated administration of amygdalin to about 25 µg/ml on the last day of ingestion (C. G. Moertel *et al.*, *J. Am. med. Ass.*, 1981, *245*, 591–594).

Following an intramuscular injection of 6 g to 1 subject, a peak plasma concentration of 180 µg/ml was attained in 1.25 hours (M. M. Ames *et al.*, *Res. Commun. chem. Path. Pharmac.*, 1978, *22*, 175–185).

TOXICITY. Several reports of cyanide poisoning following administration of amygdalin have been recorded, mostly involving the ingestion of apricot or other fruit kernels. Cyanide release from amygdalin is known to occur in the presence of β-glucosidase enzymes which are present in some raw fruits and vegetables. Toxic effects or fatalities have been associated with blood-cyanide concentrations greater than 2 µg/ml.

A blood-cyanide concentration of 10 µg/ml was reported in one subject with toxic effects following daily ingestion of 1500 mg of amygdalin (F. P. Smith *et al.*, *J. Am. med. Ass.*, 1977, *238*, 1361).

In a fatality involving amygdalin ingestion, a postmortem blood-cyanide concentration of 2.18 µg/ml was reported (S. N. Vogel *et al.*, *Clin. Toxicol.*, 1981, *18*, 367–383).

NOTE. For a review of the literature on amygdalin see R. F. Chandler *et al.*, *Pharm. J.*, 1984, *232*, 330–332.

Amyl Acetate   *Solvent*

A mixture of isomers, principally isoamyl acetate (3-methylbutyl acetate), *sec*-amyl acetate (2-methylbutyl acetate), and *n*-amyl acetate.

$C_7H_{14}O_2 = 130.2$

CAS—123-92-2 (iso); *53496-15-4* (sec); *628-63-7* (n)

A colourless, mobile, inflammable liquid. B.p. about 140°. Refractive index 1.1400.

Slightly **soluble** in water; miscible with ethanol and ether.

Mass Spectrum. Principal peaks at *m/z* 43, 70, 55, 42, 41, 73, 61, 87.

Disposition in the Body.

TOXICITY. The estimated minimum lethal dose is 50 g and the maximum permissible atmospheric concentration is 100 ppm for iso- or *n*-amyl acetate and 125 ppm for *sec*-amyl acetate.

Amyl Alcohol   *Solvent*

Synonym. Amylic Alcohol

A mixture of mainly 3-methylbutan-1-ol (primary isoamyl alcohol) [$(CH_3)_2CH \cdot CH_2 \cdot CH_2OH$] with some 2-methylbutan-1-ol (primary amyl alcohol) [$CH_3 \cdot CH_2 \cdot CH(CH_3) \cdot CH_2OH$].

$C_5H_{12}O = 88.15$

CAS—123-51-3 (3-methylbutan-1-ol); *137-32-6* (2-methylbutan-1-ol)

A colourless liquid obtained by purifying fusel oil. B.p. 128° to 132°. Refractive index 1.4075.
Slightly **soluble** in water; miscible with ethanol, chloroform, and ether.

Mass Spectrum. Principal peaks at m/z 55, 41, 42, 43, 70, 57, 29, 31.

Disposition in the Body.

TOXICITY. It is toxic after ingestion. The estimated minimum lethal dose is 30 g and the maximum permissible atmospheric concentration is 100 ppm.

Amyl Nitrite   *Anti-anginal Vasodilator*

Synonyms. Isoamyl Nitrite; Isopentyl Nitrite.
It consists of the nitrites of 3-methylbutan-1-ol $[(CH_3)_2CH \cdot CH_2 \cdot CH_2OH]$ and 2-methylbutan-1-ol $[CH_3 \cdot CH_2 \cdot CH(CH_3) \cdot CH_2OH]$, with other nitrites of the homologous series.
$C_5H_{11}NO_2 = 117.1$
CAS—8017-89-8; 110-46-3
A clear, yellow, volatile, inflammable liquid, with a fragrant odour. Incompatible with ethanol. Store in a cool place in airtight containers; protect from light. Wt per ml 0.868 to 0.878 g. B.p. 96°. Refractive index 1.3871.
Practically **insoluble** in water; miscible with ethanol, chloroform, and ether.
Caution. Amyl nitrite forms an explosive mixture with air or oxygen. It is very inflammable and must not be used where it may be ignited.

Colour Tests. To 0.2 ml add 2 ml of a 2% ferrous sulphate solution and 5 ml of *dilute hydrochloric acid*—green-brown; to 0.2 ml add 0.5 ml of aniline and 5 ml of *acetic acid*—orange-red.

Gas Chromatography. *System GA*—RI 680; *system GI*—retention time 20.3 min.

Mass Spectrum. Principal peaks at m/z 70, 43, 55, 41, 57, 42, 71, -.

Disposition in the Body. Absorbed from the mucous membranes after inhalation but rapidly inactivated by hydrolysis. Inactive after ingestion due to hydrolysis in the gastro-intestinal tract.

TOXICITY. Recovery has occurred after the ingestion of 12 ml.

Dose. 0.12 to 0.3 ml, by inhalation.

Amylmetacresol   *Antiseptic*

Synonym. 6-Pentyl-*m*-cresol
Proprietary Name. It is an ingredient of Strepsils.
5-Methyl-2-pentylphenol
$C_{12}H_{18}O = 178.3$
CAS—1300-94-3

A colourless or slightly yellow, clear liquid or solid crystalline mass, which darkens on keeping. M.p. 24°.
Practically **insoluble** in water; soluble in ethanol and ether.

Ultraviolet Spectrum. Acidified dehydrated alcohol—278 nm ($A_1^1 = 132$ a), 286 nm.

Infra-red Spectrum. Principal peaks at wavenumbers 1120, 1225, 1272, 805, 1584, 938 (thin film).

Amylobarbitone   *Barbiturate*

Synonyms. Amobarbital; Pentymalum.
Proprietary Names. Amal; Amylbarb; Amytal; Etamyl; Eunoctal; Neur-Amyl; Stadadorm. It is an ingredient of Dexamyl.
5-Ethyl-5-isopentylbarbituric acid
$C_{11}H_{18}N_2O_3 = 226.3$
CAS—57-43-2

A white crystalline powder. M.p. 155° to 161°.
Soluble 1 in 1500 of water, 1 in 5 of ethanol, 1 in 20 of chloroform, and 1 in 6 of ether; soluble in aqueous solutions of alkali hydroxides and carbonates.

Amylobarbitone Sodium

Synonyms. Amobarbital Sodium; Barbamylum; Soluble Amylobarbitone.
Proprietary Names. Amylbarb Sodium; Amylobeta; Neur-Amyl Sodium; Sodium Amytal. It is an ingredient of Tuinal.
$C_{11}H_{17}N_2NaO_3 = 248.3$
CAS—64-43-7
A white, hygroscopic, granular powder. M.p. about 156°.
Soluble 1 in less than 1 of water and 1 in 2 of ethanol; practically insoluble in chloroform and ether. Solutions in water decompose on standing.

Dissociation Constant. pK_a 7.9 (25°).

Partition Coefficient. Log P (octanol/pH 7.4), 1.6.

Colour Tests. Koppanyi–Zwikker Test—violet; Mercurous Nitrate—black.

Thin-layer Chromatography. *System TD*—Rf 52; *system TE*—Rf 36; *system TF*—Rf 65; *system TH*—Rf 74. (*Mercuric chloride-diphenylcarbazone reagent*, positive; *mercurous nitrate spray*, black; *Zwikker's reagent*, pink.)

Gas Chromatography. *System GA*—amylobarbitone RI 1718, 3'-hydroxyamylobarbitone RI 1632; *system GF*—RI 2430.

High Pressure Liquid Chromatography. *System HG*—k' 10.91; *system HH*—k' 7.05.

Ultraviolet Spectrum. *Borax buffer 0.05M* (pH 9.2)—240 nm ($A_1^1 = 445$ a); *M sodium hydroxide* (pH 13)—255 nm ($A_1^1 = 364$ b). (See below)

Infra-red Spectrum. Principal peaks at wavenumbers 1725, 1696, 1758, 1317, 1240, 850 (KBr disk) (See below).

Mass Spectrum. Principal peaks at m/z 156, 141, 157, 41, 55, 142, 98, 39; 3'-hydroxyamylobarbitone 59, 157, 156, 141, 43, 41, 71, 69.

Quantification. The following are general methods for most barbiturates.

GAS CHROMATOGRAPHY. In plasma or urine: detection limit <500 pg/ml, AFID—T. Villén and I. Petters, *J. Chromat.*, 1983, *258*, 267–270. In plasma: sensitivity <500 ng/ml, AFID—A. Turcant *et al.*, *J. Chromat.*, 1982, *229*; *Biomed. Appl.*, *18*, 222–

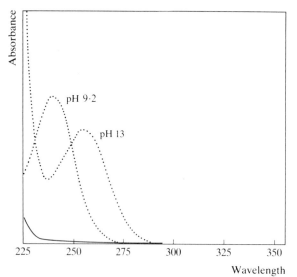

Wavelength

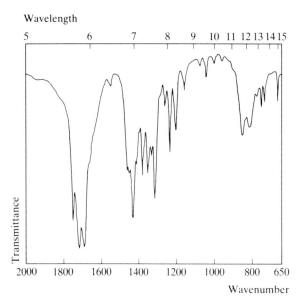

Wavenumber

226. For a review of gas chromatographic methods see D. N. Pillai and S. Dilli, *J. Chromat.*, 1981, *220*; *Chromatogr. Rev.*, *25*, 253–274.

HIGH PRESSURE LIQUID CHROMATOGRAPHY. In blood: detection limit < 1 µg/ml, UV detection—R. Gill *et al.*, *J. Chromat.*, 1981, *226*; *Biomed. Appl.*, *25*, 117–123.

IMMUNOASSAY. In urine: barbiturates and metabolites, sensitivity 2 µg/ml for quinalbarbitone using EMIT and 10 ng/ml using RIA—B. Law and A. C. Moffat, *J. forens. Sci. Soc.*, 1981, *21*, 55–66.

Disposition in the Body. Readily and almost completely absorbed after oral administration; bioavailability about 95%. It is metabolised by hydroxylation to give the major metabolite 3'-hydroxyamylobarbitone, which has about one-third of the

activity of the parent substance. About 80 to 90% of a dose is excreted in the urine in 6 days, of which 30 to 50% is 3'-hydroxyamylobarbitone, up to 30% is *N*-β-D-glucopyranosylamylobarbitone, and about 1% is unchanged drug. The metabolite pattern appears to be genetically determined. 5-(3'-Carboxybutyl)-5-ethylbarbituric acid has also been identified as a metabolite in urine. About 5% of a dose is eliminated in the faeces in 6 days.

THERAPEUTIC CONCENTRATION. In plasma, usually in the range 2 to 12 µg/ml.

TOXICITY. The estimated minimum lethal dose is 1.5 g. Toxic effects are associated with plasma concentrations greater than 9 µg/ml and fatalities with postmortem blood concentrations of 9 to **26** to 72 µg/ml.

In a review of 55 cases of fatal overdosage, postmortem blood concentrations were in the range 13 to 96 µg/ml (R. C. Gupta and J. Kofoed, *Can. med. Ass. J.*, 1966, *94*, 863–865).

In 3 fatalities attributed to amylobarbitone overdose, the following postmortem tissue concentrations, µg/ml or µg/g, were reported:

	Amylo-barbitone	3'-Hydroxyamylo-barbitone
Blood	36, 35, 25	2, —, 2
Bile	198, 178, —	6, —, —
Kidney	32, 59, 87	—, 2, 4
Liver	71, 79, 224	1, 2, 2
Lung	43, 40, 84	—, 2, 4
Spleen	77, 63, 104	—, 1, —
Urine	12, 12, —	9, —, —

(A. E. Robinson and R. D. McDowall, *J. Pharm. Pharmac.*, 1979, *31*, 357–365).

HALF-LIFE. Plasma half-life, 8 to 40 hours (mean 24).

VOLUME OF DISTRIBUTION. About 1 litre/kg.

CLEARANCE. Plasma clearance, about 0.5 ml/min/kg.

SALIVA. Plasma: saliva ratio, about 2.8.

PROTEIN BINDING. In plasma, 40 to 60%.

NOTE. For a review of the clinical pharmacokinetics of barbiturates see D. D. Breimer, *Clin. Pharmacokinet.*, 1977, *2*, 93–109.

Dose. 30 to 240 mg daily; up to 600 mg daily has been given.

Androsterone   *Androgen*

3α-Hydroxy-5α-androstan-17-one
$C_{19}H_{30}O_2 = 290.4$
CAS—53-41-8

A white crystalline powder. M.p. about 185°.

Practically **insoluble** in water; soluble in ethanol, ether, and in most organic solvents.

Colour Tests. Antimony Pentachloride—yellow → brown; Naphthol–Sulphuric Acid—orange-brown/orange; Sulphuric Acid—yellow.

Gas Chromatography. *System GA*—RI 2488.

Ultraviolet Spectrum. No significant absorption, 230 to 360 nm.

Infra-red Spectrum. Principal peaks at wavenumbers 1724, 1000, 1031, 1062, 1242, 1282 (Nujol mull).

Mass Spectrum. Principal peaks at m/z 290, 67, 108, 107, 79, 55, 41, 93.

Disposition in the Body. Androsterone is a naturally occurring androgen which may be isolated from male urine. It is a major metabolite of testosterone.

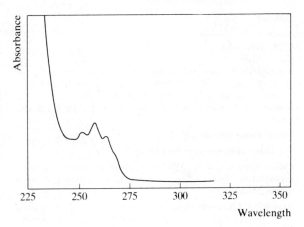

Wavelength

Anileridine   *Narcotic Analgesic*

Ethyl 1-(4-aminophenethyl)-4-phenylpiperidine-4-carboxylate
$C_{22}H_{28}N_2O_2 = 352.5$
CAS—144-14-9

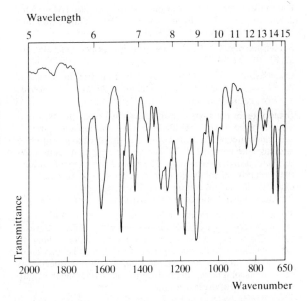

Wavelength

Wavenumber

A white to yellowish-white crystalline powder. When exposed to light and air it oxidises and darkens in colour. There are 2 crystalline forms which melt at about 80° and about 89°.
Very slightly **soluble** in water; soluble 1 in 2 of ethanol and 1 in 1 of chloroform; soluble in ether but solutions may be turbid.

Anileridine Hydrochloride
Proprietary Name. Leritine (tablets)
$C_{22}H_{28}N_2O_2,2HCl = 425.4$
CAS—126-12-5
A white crystalline powder. M.p. about 270°, with decomposition.
Soluble 1 in 5 of water and 1 in 80 of ethanol; practically insoluble in chloroform and ether.

Anileridine Phosphate
Proprietary Name. Leritine (injection)
$C_{22}H_{28}N_2O_2,H_3PO_4 = 450.5$
CAS—4268-37-5
A white crystalline powder.
Very **soluble** in water. Solutions are unstable above pH 4.

Dissociation Constant. pK_a 3.7, 7.5.

Colour Tests. Diazotisation—red; Marquis Test—orange (slow).

Thin-layer Chromatography. *System TA*—Rf 73. (*Acidified iodoplatinate solution*, positive).

Gas Chromatography. *System GA*—RI 2850; *system GC*—RI 3469.

High Pressure Liquid Chromatography. *System HA*—k' 1.1.

Ultraviolet Spectrum. Aqueous acid—252 nm, 258 nm, 264 nm.

Infra-red Spectrum. Principal peaks at wavenumbers 1700, 1120, 1179, 1512, 1219, 1620 (KCl disk).

Mass Spectrum. Principal peaks at m/z 246, 247, 42, 120, 218, 172, 106, 91.

Disposition in the Body. Readily absorbed after oral administration. Metabolised by hydrolysis to anileridinic acid followed by acetylation to acetylanileridinic acid; conjugation with acetic

acid followed by partial de-esterification to acetylanileridinic acid also occurs. After oral administration, 5% of the dose is excreted in the urine as unchanged drug, with 7 to 14% as free anileridinic acid, 1 to 2% as acetylanileridinic acid, 0.5 to 2% as acetylanileridine, and 15 to 35% as diazotisable metabolites, tentatively identified as *p*-acetylaminophenylacetic acid; norpethidine has also been detected in urine.

TOXICITY. The estimated minimum lethal dose is 0.5 g but it may be up to 5 g in addicts.

The following postmortem concentrations were reported in a fatality attributed to oral overdosage of anileridine: blood 0.9 µg/ml, bile 2.4 µg/ml, urine 11.4 µg/ml, vitreous humour 0.07 µg/ml; diazepam was also detected (M. A. Peat and L. Kopjak, *Bull. int. Ass. forens. Toxicol.*, 1979, *14*(3), 19).

Dose. Up to the equivalent of 200 mg of anileridine daily.

Aniline

Synonym. Phenylamine
$C_6H_5 \cdot NH_2 = 93.13$
CAS—62-53-3

A colourless or pale yellow, oily liquid, with a characteristic odour. It readily darkens to brown on exposure to air and light. F.p. $-6°$. B.p. about $183°$. Refractive index 1.5863.

Soluble 1 in 30 of water; miscible with ethanol, chloroform, and ether.

Dissociation Constant. pK_a 4.6 (25°).

Partition Coefficient. Log P (octanol), 0.9.

Colour Tests. Coniferyl Alcohol—orange; Diazotisation—red; Liebermann's Test—red-orange; Potassium Dichromate—blue-green (2 min).

Thin-layer Chromatography. *System TA*—Rf 72. (*Acidified potassium permanganate solution*, positive; *Van Urk reagent*, bright yellow.)

Gas Chromatography. *System GA*—aniline RI 1158, 4-aminophenol RI 1265.

Ultraviolet Spectrum. Aqueous acid—249 nm ($A_1^1 = 13$ b), 255 nm ($A_1^1 = 16$ b), 261 nm ($A_1^1 = 12.5$ b); ethanol—235 nm ($A_1^1 = 1007$ b), 286 nm ($A_1^1 = 179$ b).

Mass Spectrum. 4-Aminophenol: principal peaks at m/z 109, 80, 53, 81, 108, 52, 54, 110.

Quantification. GAS CHROMATOGRAPHY. In postmortem tissues: AFID—J. S. Oliver and D. J. Williams, *Bull. int. Ass. forens. Toxicol.*, 1974, *10*(2), 6–7.

Disposition in the Body. Readily absorbed from the skin and mucous membranes. Metabolised to 4-aminophenol and 4-acetamidophenol which are excreted in the urine as glucuronide and sulphate conjugates. *N*-Phenylsulphamic acid (aniline *N*-sulphate) is also a metabolite. The main toxic effect of aniline, the formation of methaemoglobin, is thought to be due to an oxidation product of aniline, phenylhydroxylamine. Aniline is a metabolite of phenazopyridine.

TOXICITY. The minimum lethal dose may be as low as 1 g although recovery has followed the ingestion of 30 g. Serious toxic effects may occur after exposure for about 1 hour to atmospheric concentrations of 100 to 160 ppm. The maximum permissible atmospheric concentration is 2 ppm. Urinary concentrations of greater than 10 μg/ml of 4-aminophenol may indicate toxic exposure to aniline.

The following postmortem tissue concentrations were reported in a fatality attributed to ingestion of an aniline-based ink: blood 6.3 μg/ml, liver 20 μg/g, urine 40 μg/ml (J. S. Oliver and D. J. Williams, *ibid.*).

Anisindione   *Anticoagulant*

Proprietary Names. Miradon; Unidone.
2-(4-Methoxyphenyl)indan-1,3-dione
$C_{16}H_{12}O_3 = 252.3$
CAS—117-37-3

A white or creamy-white powder. M.p. 152° to 158°. Practically **insoluble** in water; soluble in ether and methanol.

Dissociation Constant. pK_a 4.1.

Gas Chromatography. *System GA*—RI 2273.

Ultraviolet Spectrum. Aqueous acid—273 nm; ethanol—286 nm ($A_1^1 = 1400$ b), 340 nm.

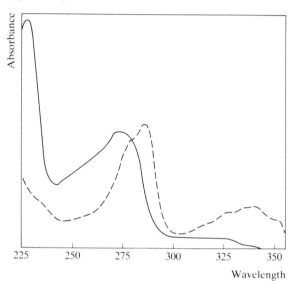

Mass Spectrum. Principal peaks at m/z 252, 237, 253, 181, 238, 77, 76, 209.

Dose. Maintenance, 25 to 250 mg daily.

Antazoline   *Antihistamine*

Synonyms. Imidamin; Phenazoline.
N-Benzyl-*N*-(2-imidazolin-2-ylmethyl)aniline
$C_{17}H_{19}N_3 = 265.4$
CAS—91-75-8

Crystals. M.p. about 121°.

Antazoline Hydrochloride

Synonym. Phenazolinum
Proprietary Name. Antistin(e) (tablets)
$C_{17}H_{19}N_3, HCl = 301.8$
CAS—2508-72-7

A white crystalline powder. M.p. about 240°, with decomposition.
Soluble 1 in 50 of water and 1 in 16 of ethanol; slightly soluble in chloroform; practically insoluble in ether.

Antazoline Mesylate

Synonym. Antazoline Methanesulphonate
Proprietary Name. Antistin (injection)
$C_{17}H_{19}N_3, CH_3SO_3H = 361.5$
CAS—3131-32-6

A white, slightly hygroscopic powder. M.p. 165° to 168°.
Soluble 1 in 6 of water, 1 in 7 of ethanol, and 1 in 12 of chloroform; practically insoluble in ether.

Antazoline Phosphate

Proprietary Name. It is an ingredient of Vasocon A.
$C_{17}H_{19}N_3,H_3PO_4 = 363.4$
CAS—154-68-7
A white crystalline powder. M.p. 194° to 198°, with decomposition.
Soluble in water; sparingly soluble in methanol; practically insoluble in ether.

Dissociation Constant. pK_a 2.5, 10.1 (25°).

Colour Tests. Liebermann's Test—red; Mandelin's Test—red-violet.

Thin-layer Chromatography. *System TA*—Rf 31; *system TB*—Rf 07; *system TC*—Rf 07. (*Dragendorff spray*, positive; *FPN reagent*, pink; *acidified iodoplatinate solution*, positive.)

Gas Chromatography. *System GA*—RI 2328; *system GC*—RI 2749.

High Pressure Liquid Chromatography. *System HA*—k' 1.8.

Ultraviolet Spectrum. Aqueous acid—241 nm ($A_1^1 = 578$ a), 291 nm; aqueous alkali—247 nm, 295 nm.

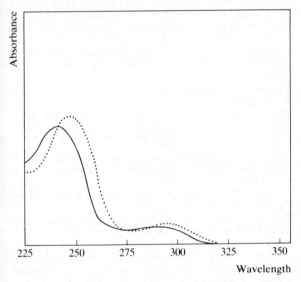

Infra-red Spectrum. Principal peaks at wavenumbers 1164, 1599, 1042, 1508, 750, 700 (antazoline mesylate, KBr disk).

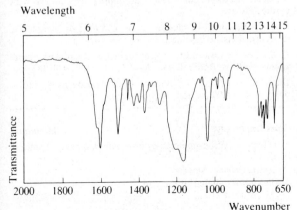

Mass Spectrum. Principal peaks at *m/z* 84, 91, 77, 55, 182, 85, 65, 104.

Quantification. COLORIMETRY. In urine—N. Wahba *et al.*, *Pharmazie*, 1974, *29*, 790–791.

Disposition in the Body. Readily absorbed after oral or parenteral administration. About 2% of an oral dose is excreted unchanged in the urine in 24 hours.

Dose. Antazoline hydrochloride has been given in doses of 100 to 600 mg daily.

Apomorphine   *Emetic*

(6a*R*) - 5,6,6a,7 - Tetrahydro - 6 - methyl - 4*H* - dibenzo-[*de,g*]quinoline-10,11-diol
$C_{17}H_{17}NO_2 = 267.3$
CAS—58-00-4

Crystals. M.p. about 195°, with decomposition. The crystals and aqueous solutions oxidise rapidly in light and air, turning green. Slightly **soluble** in water and ether; soluble in ethanol and chloroform.

Apomorphine Hydrochloride

$C_{17}H_{17}NO_2,HCl,\frac{1}{2}H_2O = 312.8$
CAS—314-19-2 (anhydrous); *41372-20-7* (hemihydrate)
White or greyish-white glistening crystals or microcrystalline powder. Decomposes between 225° and 236°.
Soluble 1 in 50 of water and 1 in 20 of water at 80°; soluble 1 in 50 of ethanol; very slightly soluble in chloroform and ether.

Dissociation Constant. pK_a 7.2, 8.9 (15°).

Colour Tests. Ferric Chloride—blue; Liebermann's Test—black; Marquis Test—violet → black; Methanolic Potassium Hydroxide—green → red; Nessler's Reagent—black.

Thin-layer Chromatography. *System TA*—Rf 83; *system TB*—Rf 00; *system TC*—Rf 21. (*Acidified iodoplatinate solution*, positive.)

Gas Chromatography. *System GA*—RI 2530.

High Pressure Liquid Chromatography. *System HA*—k' 3.7 (tailing peak).

Ultraviolet Spectrum. Aqueous acid—272 nm ($A_1^1 = 626$ a); aqueous alkali—253 nm. (See below)

Infra-red Spectrum. Principal peaks at wavenumbers 1265, 1298, 1204, 752, 985, 790 (KBr disk).

Mass Spectrum. Principal peaks at *m/z* 266, 267, 224, 220, 268, 44, 250, 248.

Quantification. GAS CHROMATOGRAPHY. In plasma: sensitivity 1 µg/ml, FID—D. M. Baaske *et al.*, *J. Chromat.*, 1977, *140*, 57–64.

HIGH PRESSURE LIQUID CHROMATOGRAPHY. In plasma: sensitivity 100 ng/ml, fluorescence detection—R. V. Smith and M. R. De Moreno, *J. Chromat.*, 1983, *274*; *Biomed. Appl.*, *25*, 376–380.

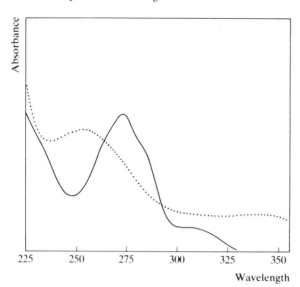

Dose. 100 µg/kg of apomorphine hydrochloride subcutaneously, as a single dose.

Aprindine

Anti-arrhythmic

N-(3-Diethylaminopropyl)-*N*-indan-2-ylaniline
$C_{22}H_{30}N_2 = 322.5$
CAS—37640-71-4

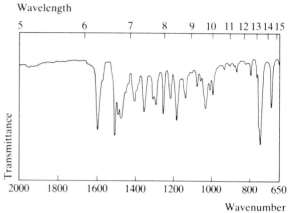

Aprindine Hydrochloride

Proprietary Names. Amidonal; Fibocil; Fiboran.

$C_{22}H_{30}N_2,HCl = 359.0$
CAS—33237-74-0

A white to yellowish-white microcrystalline powder. M.p. 127° to 130°.
Very **soluble** in water; freely soluble in ethanol and chloroform; practically insoluble in ether.

Dissociation Constant. pK_a 10.1.

Gas Chromatography. *System GA*—RI 2475.

Ultraviolet Spectrum. Aqueous acid—260 nm, 266 nm ($A_1^1 = 38$ a), 272 nm; ethanol—258 nm ($A_1^1 = 389$ a), 296 nm ($A_1^1 = 47$ a).

Infra-red Spectrum. Principal peaks at wavenumbers 745, 1510, 1602, 1187, 1258, 1035 (aprindine hydrochloride, KBr disk).

Mass Spectrum. Principal peaks at *m/z* 113, 86, 116, 98, 117, 115, 58, 84.

Quantification. GAS CHROMATOGRAPHY. In plasma: sensitivity 20 ng/ml, AFID—J. F. Nash and R. H. Carmichael, *J. pharm. Sci.*, 1980, *69*, 1094–1096.

HIGH PRESSURE LIQUID CHROMATOGRAPHY. In plasma: aprindine and monodesethylaprindine, sensitivity 20 ng/ml and 50 ng/ml, respectively, UV detection—T. Kobari *et al.*, *J. Chromat.*, 1983, *278*; *Biomed. Appl.*, *29*, 220–224.

Disposition in the Body. Almost completely absorbed after oral administration; bioavailability about 75%. Extensively meta-

bolised by aromatic hydroxylation and *N*-dealkylation followed by glucuronic acid conjugation; the monodesethyl metabolite, which can be detected in plasma after chronic administration, is active. Less than 1% of a dose is excreted in the urine as unchanged drug and about 40 to 65% as conjugated metabolites; 35 to 60% of the dose is eliminated in the faeces over a period of 5 days.

THERAPEUTIC CONCENTRATION. In plasma, usually in the range 0.7 to 2 µg/ml.

After a single oral dose of 200 mg to 12 subjects, peak plasma concentrations of 0.6 to 2 µg/ml (mean 0.9) were attained in 2 hours (A. F. Fasola and R. Carmichael, *Acta Cardiol.*, 1974, *Suppl.*, *18*, 317–333).

Following daily oral doses of 100 to 150 mg, plasma concentrations in 28 patients ranged from 0.73 to 2.55 µg/ml (J. P. Van Durme *et al.*, *Eur. J. clin. Pharmac.*, 1974, *7*, 343–346).

TOXICITY. Toxic effects are usually associated with plasma concentrations greater than 2 µg/ml.

Toxic effects were found in 9 patients whose plasma concentrations ranged from 1.2 to 4.9 µg/ml (mean 2.6) (J. P. Van Durme *et al.*, *ibid.*).

HALF-LIFE. Plasma half-life, 12 to 66 hours (mean 30) in normal subjects but the half-life is apparently longer in patients with chronic ventricular arrhythmias and myocardial infarction (average, about 50 hours).

VOLUME OF DISTRIBUTION. About 4 litres/kg.

CLEARANCE. Plasma clearance, about 2.5 ml/min/kg in normal subjects; decreased to about 1 ml/min/kg in patients with cardiac disease.

PROTEIN BINDING. In plasma, more than 95% at therapeutic concentrations, decreasing at higher concentrations.

NOTE. For a review of the pharmacokinetics of anti-arrhythmic agents see R. A. Ronfeld, *Am. Heart J.*, 1980, *100*, 978–983.

Dose. 50 to 100 mg of aprindine hydrochloride daily; initial doses of up to 200 mg daily may be given.

Aprobarbitone

Barbiturate

Synonyms. Allylisopropylmalonylurea; Allypropymal; Aprobarbital.

Proprietary Name. Alurate

5-Allyl-5-isopropylbarbituric acid
$C_{10}H_{14}N_2O_3 = 210.2$
CAS—77-02-1

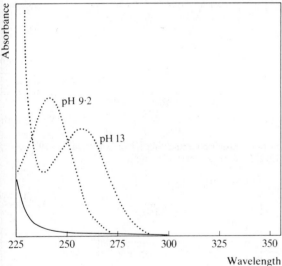

A white crystalline powder. M.p. about 142°.

Soluble 1 in 350 of water, 1 in 30 of boiling water, 1 in 2.5 of ethanol, 1 in 40 of chloroform, and 1 in 5 of ether; soluble in aqueous solutions of alkali hydroxides and carbonates.

Aprobarbitone Sodium

$C_{10}H_{13}N_2NaO_3 = 232.2$

CAS—125-88-2

A white, hygroscopic, microcrystalline powder.

Very **soluble** in water; very slightly soluble in ethanol; practically insoluble in ether.

Dissociation Constant. pK_a 8.0 (25°).

Colour Test. Koppanyi–Zwikker Test—violet.

Thin-layer Chromatography. *System TD*—Rf 48; *system TE*—Rf 36; *system TF*—Rf 65; *system TH*—Rf 66. (*Mercurous nitrate spray*, black; *acidified potassium permanganate solution*, yellow-brown; *Zwikker's reagent*, pink.)

Gas Chromatography. *System GA*—RI 1622.

High Pressure Liquid Chromatography. *System HG*—k′ 3.42; *system HH*—k′ 2.22.

Ultraviolet Spectrum. *Borax buffer 0.05M* (pH 9.2)—241 nm ($A_1^1 = 451$ a); M *sodium hydroxide* (pH 13)—257 nm ($A_1^1 = 331$ b).

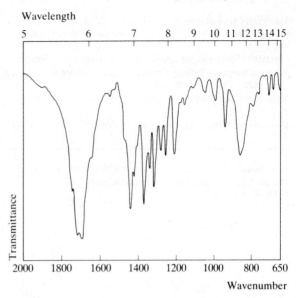

Wavelength

Wavenumber

Infra-red Spectrum. Principal peaks at wavenumbers 1693, 1720, 1745, 1316, 1255, 860 (KBr disk).

Mass Spectrum. Principal peaks at *m/z* 167, 41, 124, 168, 97, 39, 169, 45; *N*-hydroxyaprobarbitone 41, 43, 183, 167, 140, 184, 124, 109.

Quantification. See also under Amylobarbitone.

GAS CHROMATOGRAPHY–MASS SPECTROMETRY. In urine: aprobarbitone, *N*-hydroxyaprobarbitone and aprobarbitone diol— J. N. T. Gilbert *et al.*, *J. Pharm. Pharmac.*, 1978, *30*, 173–175.

Disposition in the Body. Absorbed after oral administration and slowly excreted in the urine, mainly as metabolites, less than 3% of a dose being excreted as unchanged drug in 24 hours. About 12% of a dose is excreted in the urine as the diol derivative and 4% as *N*-hydroxyaprobarbitone in 3 days, together with 9% as unchanged drug.

THERAPEUTIC CONCENTRATION. In plasma, usually in the range 10 to 40 µg/ml.

TOXICITY. The estimated minimum lethal dose is 2 g. Plasma concentrations greater than 40 µg/ml are usually associated with toxic effects; concentrations greater than 50 µg/ml may be fatal.

In 4 cases of death attributed to overdoses ranging from 2.5 to 7.7 g, antemortem serum concentrations ranged from 120 to 150 µg/ml. In 44 cases of overdose in which the patients subsequently recovered, the serum concentrations 24 hours after ingestion were in the range 40 to 130 µg/ml (P. Lous, *Acta pharmac. tox.*, 1954, *10*, 261–280).

In a number of fatalities attributed to aprobarbitone, a mean postmortem blood concentration of 50 µg/ml in 9 cases and a mean postmortem liver concentration of 83 µg/g in 12 cases were reported (R. Bonnichsen *et al.*, *J. forens. Sci.*, 1961, *6*, 411–443).

HALF-LIFE. Plasma half-life, 0.5 to 1.5 days.

PROTEIN BINDING. In plasma, 55 to 70%.

Dose. 40 to 160 mg daily.

Apronal
Hypnotic/Sedative

Synonyms. Allylisopropylacetylurea; Apronalide.

N-(2-Isopropylpent-4-enoyl)urea

$C_9H_{16}N_2O_2 = 184.2$

CAS—528-92-7

$$CH_2 \cdot CH:CH_2$$
$$(CH_3)_2CH \cdot CH \cdot CO \cdot NH \cdot CO \cdot NH_2$$

Colourless crystals or white crystalline powder. M.p. 194°.

Soluble 1 in 4000 of water, 1 in 50 of ethanol, 1 in 45 of chloroform, and 1 in 100 of ether.

Thin-layer Chromatography. *System TD*—Rf 33; *system TE*—Rf 67; *system TF*—Rf 64. (*Acidified potassium permanganate solution*, positive.)

Ultraviolet Spectrum. No significant absorption, 230 to 360 nm.

Infra-red Spectrum. Principal peaks at wavenumbers 1676, 1704, 1092, 1620, 1185, 750 (KBr disk).

Mass Spectrum. Principal peaks at *m/z* 55, 44, 142, 141, 41, 61, 81, 82.

Dose. Apronal was formerly given in doses of 250 to 750 mg daily.

Arecoline   *Purgative/Taenifuge (Veterinary)*

Methyl 1,2,5,6-tetrahydro-1-methylnicotinate
$C_8H_{13}NO_2 = 155.2$
CAS—63-75-2

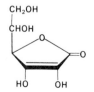

Arecoline is an alkaloid which is obtained from the seeds of *Areca catechu* (Palmae).

An oily liquid which is a strong base. B.p. 209°.

Miscible with water, ethanol, chloroform, and ether.

Arecoline Hydrobromide

$C_8H_{13}NO_2,HBr = 236.1$
CAS—300-08-3

A white crystalline powder. Unstable in light. M.p. 172° to 175°.

Soluble 1 in 1 of water and 1 in 10 of ethanol; very slightly soluble in chloroform and ether.

Dissociation Constant. pK_a 7.4 (20°).

Thin-layer Chromatography. *System TA*—Rf 53. (*Acidified potassium permanganate solution*, positive.)

Ultraviolet Spectrum. No significant absorption, 230 to 360 nm.

Infra-red Spectrum. Principal peaks at wavenumbers 1712, 1262, 1135, 1282, 1020, 1650 (KCl disk).

Mass Spectrum. Principal peaks at *m/z* 155, 96, 140, 43, 42, 81, 94, 53.

Ascorbic Acid   *Vitamin*

Synonyms. L-Ascorbic Acid; Cevitamic Acid; Vitamin C.

Proprietary Names of Ascorbic Acid or Sodium Ascorbate. Adenex; Alba-Ce; Ascorbef; Ascorbicap; CC-Kaps; Cebion(e); Cecon; Cemill; Cenolate; Cetane; Cevalin; Cevi-Bid; Ce-Vi-Sol; C-Long; Duoscorb; Megascorb; Redoxon; Roscorbic; Vitascorb; Viterra C. Ascorbic acid is an ingredient of Ce-Cobalin, Oralcer, and Reactivan.

The enolic form of 3-oxo-L-gulofuranolactone
$C_6H_8O_6 = 176.1$
CAS—50-81-7

Colourless crystals or white or very pale yellow crystalline powder. Solutions, especially when made alkaline, deteriorate rapidly in air. M.p. about 190°, with decomposition.

Soluble 1 in 3 to 1 in 3.5 of water, 1 in 25 of ethanol, and 1 in 10 of methanol; soluble in acetone; practically insoluble in chloroform and ether.

Sodium Ascorbate

$C_6H_7NaO_6 = 198.1$
CAS—134-03-2

White or very faintly yellow crystals or crystalline powder. It gradually darkens on exposure to light.

Soluble 1 in 1.3 of water; very slightly soluble in ethanol; practically insoluble in chloroform and ether.

Dissociation Constant. pK_a 4.2, 11.6 (25°).

Colour Tests. Ammoniacal Silver Nitrate—black; Benedict's Reagent—red; Nessler's Reagent—black; Palladium Chloride—black.

Ultraviolet Spectrum. Aqueous acid—243 nm ($A_1^1 = 556$ a).

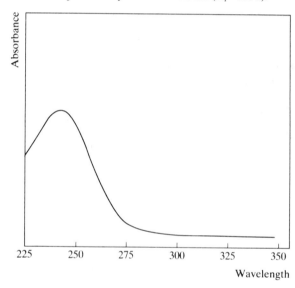

Wavelength

Infra-red Spectrum. Principal peaks at wavenumbers 1026, 1111, 1312, 1136, 1653, 990 (Nujol mull).

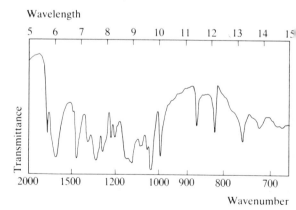

Mass Spectrum. Principal peaks at *m/z* 29, 41, 39, 42, 69, 116, 167, 168.

Quantification. HIGH PRESSURE LIQUID CHROMATOGRAPHY. In serum or urine: electrochemical detection—L. A. Pachla and P. T. Kissinger, *Analyt. Chem.*, 1976, *48*, 364–367. In urine: UV detection—E. S. Wagner *et al.*, *J. Chromat.*, 1979, *163*; *Biomed. Appl.*, *5*, 225–229. In postmortem tissues: UV detection—W. J. Allender, *J. analyt. Toxicol.*, 1982, *6*, 202–204.

Disposition in the Body. Readily absorbed after oral administration; the proportion of a dose absorbed tends to decrease with increasing dose; it is widely distributed in the body tissues. The concentration of ascorbic acid is higher in leucocytes and platelets than in erythrocytes and plasma. Ascorbic acid is metabolised to dehydroascorbic acid, 2,3-diketogulonic acid, oxalate, and carbon dioxide; some conjugation with sulphate occurs to form ascorbate-3-sulphate. Ascorbic acid in excess of the body's requirements is rapidly eliminated in the urine. About 85% of an intravenous dose, given to subjects previously saturated with the vitamin, is excreted in the urine in 24 hours, with about 70% of the dose excreted unchanged and 15% as dehydroascorbic acid and diketogulonic acid. The amount normally present in the body is in excess of 1.5 g.

BLOOD CONCENTRATION. Concentrations in plasma and in leucocytes are normally about 5 to 12 µg/ml and 25 to 30 µg/10^8 cells respectively; these concentrations exhibit circadian and seasonal rhythms.

PROTEIN BINDING. In plasma, about 25%.

Dose. 0.2 to 3 g daily.

Aspirin   *Analgesic*

Synonyms. Acetylsalicylic Acid; Salicylic Acid Acetate.
Proprietary Names. Alka-Seltzer; Angiers; Aspro; Claradin; Disprin; Genasprin; Solprin.
Aspirin is an ingredient of many proprietary preparations—see *Martindale, The Extra Pharmacopoeia*, 28th Edn.

O-Acetylsalicylic acid
$C_9H_8O_4 = 180.2$
CAS—50-78-2

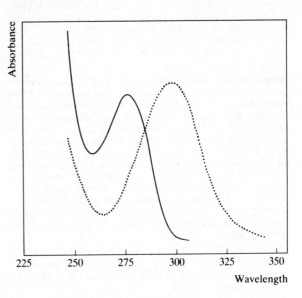

Colourless or white crystals or white crystalline powder or granules. It is stable in dry air but gradually hydrolyses in contact with moisture to acetic and salicylic acids. M.p. about 143°.
Soluble 1 in 300 of water, 1 in 6 of ethanol, 1 in 17 of chloroform, and 1 in 20 of ether; soluble in solutions of acetates and citrates and, with decomposition, in solutions of alkali hydroxides and carbonates.

Dissociation Constant. pK$_a$ 3.5 (25°).

Partition Coefficient. Log *P* (octanol/pH 7.4), −1.1.

Colour Test. McNally's Test—red (after hydrolysis).

Thin-layer Chromatography. *System TD*—aspirin Rf 18, salicylic acid Rf 07, salicyluric acid Rf 00; *system TE*—aspirin Rf 16, salicylic acid Rf 11, salicyluric acid Rf 00; *system TF*—aspirin Rf 30, salicylic acid Rf 25, salicyluric acid Rf 00.

Gas Chromatography. *System GA*—RI 1309.

High Pressure Liquid Chromatography. *System HD*—aspirin k′ 0.5, salicylic acid k′ 0.7; *system HW*—aspirin k′ 2.7, salicylic acid k′ 4.6.

Ultraviolet Spectrum. Aqueous acid—230 nm (A$_1^1$ = 466 a), 278 nm (A$_1^1$ = 68 a); aqueous alkali—231 nm (A$_1^1$ = 409 b), 298 nm (A$_1^1$ = 190 b).

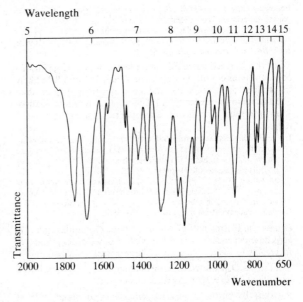

Infra-red Spectrum. Principal peaks at wavenumbers 1183, 1688, 1305, 1755, 925, 1219 (KBr disk).

Mass Spectrum. Principal peaks at *m/z* 120, 43, 138, 92, 121, 39, 64, 63; salicylic acid 120, 92, 138, 64, 39, 63, 121, 65; salicyluric acid 121, 120, 69, 92, 195, 39, 93, 45.

Quantification. GAS CHROMATOGRAPHY. In plasma: aspirin, salicylic acid, and salicylamide, detection limit 200 to 500 ng/ml for all three compounds, FID—M. J. Rance *et al.*, *J. Pharm. Pharmac.*, 1975, *27*, 425–429.

HIGH PRESSURE LIQUID CHROMATOGRAPHY. In plasma: aspirin, salicylic acid, and salicyluric acid, sensitivity 50 ng/ml for aspirin in plasma; also aspirin metabolites in urine, UV detection—J. N. Buskin et al., Clin. Chem., 1982, 28, 1200–1203. In plasma or urine: aspirin and its major metabolites, detection limits in plasma 100 ng/ml for aspirin and salicyluric acid, 500 ng/ml for salicylic acid, and 200 ng/ml for gentisic acid, UV detection—R. H. Rumble et al., J. Chromat., 1981, 225; Biomed. Appl., 14, 252–260.

Disposition in the Body. Readily absorbed after oral administration and rapidly hydrolysed to salicylic acid which is the active agent. Salicylic acid is conjugated with glucuronic acid and glycine to form acyl and ether glucuronides and salicyluric acid; some hydroxylation also occurs to give dihydroxy and trihydroxy derivatives of salicylic acid. Aspirin is excreted almost entirely in the urine with about 50 to 80% of a dose as salicyluric acid, 10 to 30% as salicyl O-glucuronide, 5% as salicyl ester glucuronide, and 5 to 10% as free salicylic acid, together with small amounts of gentisic acid, gentisuric acid, and unchanged drug; salicylates are reabsorbed by the renal tubules from acid urine and thus alkaline diuresis increases the rate of salicylate elimination; about 85% of a dose is excreted as free salicylic acid if the urine is made alkaline.
Aspirin is a metabolite of aloxiprin and benorylate.

THERAPEUTIC CONCENTRATION. In plasma, salicylic acid usually in the range 20 to 100 µg/ml for analgesia and 150 to 300 µg/ml for anti-inflammatory effect.

After a single oral dose of 900 mg given to 5 subjects, peak plasma-aspirin concentrations of 16 to 50 µg/ml (mean 37) were attained in about 14 minutes, and peak plasma-salicylic acid concentrations of 47 to 113 µg/ml (mean 78) were reported at 0.5 to 1 hour (B. E. Cham et al., Ther. Drug Monit., 1980, 2, 365–372).

Following daily oral doses of 3.9 g to 8 subjects for 8 days, steady-state plasma-salicylic acid concentrations of 105 to 227 µg/ml (mean 173) were reported; by the 36th day of treatment the steady-state plasma concentrations had declined to 45 to 208 µg/ml (mean 129) (R. H. Rumble et al., Br. J. clin. Pharmac., 1980, 9, 41–45).

TOXICITY. The estimated minimum lethal dose is 15 g. Plasma concentrations of salicylic acid greater than 300 µg/ml are likely to produce toxic reactions and concentrations greater than 500 µg/ml are associated with moderate to severe intoxication. The maximum permissible atmospheric concentration is 5 mg/m³.

In a review of 62 fatalities attributed to salicylate poisoning, the following postmortem tissue concentrations were reported: blood 61 to 7320 µg/ml (mean 661, 52 cases), brain 22 to 700 µg/g (mean 218, 20 cases), kidney 19 to 1200 µg/g (mean 408, 21 cases), liver 13 to 1000 µg/g (mean 437, 24 cases), spleen 103 to 1230 µg/g (mean 421, 16 cases), urine 180 to 1350 µg/ml (mean 593, 15 cases) (C. J. Rehling, Poison Residues in Human Tissues, in Progress in Chemical Toxicology, Vol. 3, A. Stolman (Ed.), London, Academic Press Inc., 1967, pp. 363–386).

HALF-LIFE. Plasma half-life, aspirin about 17 minutes, salicylic acid dose-dependent (2 to 4 hours after doses of less than 3 g, increasing to about 19 hours after large doses).

VOLUME OF DISTRIBUTION. Aspirin about 0.15 litre/kg, salicylic acid about 0.1 to 0.2 litre/kg (dose-dependent).

PROTEIN BINDING. In plasma, salicylic acid about 90% at concentrations below 100 µg/ml, decreasing to 50% at concentrations above 400 µg/ml.

NOTE. For reviews of the pharmacokinetics of salicylates see M. Mandelli and G. Tognoni, Clin. Pharmacokinet., 1980, 5, 424–440, and G. Levy, Pediatrics, 1978, 62, Suppl., 865–872.

Dose. Usually 1.2 to 4 g daily; doses of up to 8 g daily are given in acute rheumatic disorders.

Atenolol
Beta-adrenoceptor Blocking Agent

Proprietary Names. Tenormin(e). It is an ingredient of Tenoret(ic).

2-[4-(2-Hydroxy-3-isopropylaminopropoxy)phenyl]acetamide
$C_{14}H_{22}N_2O_3 = 266.3$
CAS—29122-68-7

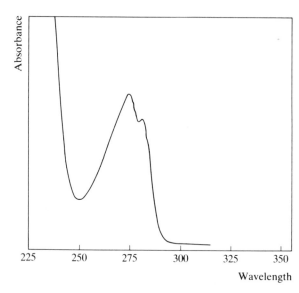

Crystals. M.p. 146° to 148°.

Dissociation Constant. pK_a 9.6 (24°).

Partition Coefficient. Log P (octanol), 0.23.

Colour Tests. Liebermann's Test—black; Nessler's Reagent—yellow-brown (slow).

Thin-layer Chromatography. System TA—Rf 45; system TB—Rf 00; system TC—Rf 02.

Gas Chromatography. System GA—RI 2355.

High Pressure Liquid Chromatography. System HA—k′ 1.3.

Ultraviolet Spectrum. Aqueous acid—274 nm ($A_1^1 = 48$ b), 280 nm. No alkaline shift.

Infra-red Spectrum. Principal peaks at wavenumbers 1633, 1245, 1510, 1184, 805, 820.

Mass Spectrum. Principal peaks at m/z 72, 30, 56, 98, 43, 107, 41, 73.

Quantification. GAS CHROMATOGRAPHY. In plasma or urine: sensitivity 5 ng/ml, ECD—M. Ervik et al., J. Chromat., 1980, 182; Biomed. Appl., 8, 341–347.

Wavelength

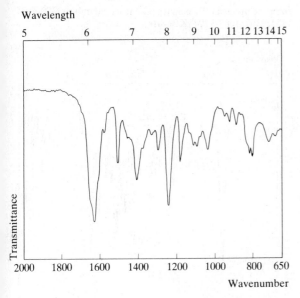

Transmittance

Wavenumber

HIGH PRESSURE LIQUID CHROMATOGRAPHY. In plasma or whole blood: sensitivity 2 ng/ml, fluorescence detection—Y. G. Yee *et al.*, *J. Chromat.*, 1979, *171*, 357–362. In plasma, urine, or breast-milk: sensitivity < 50 ng/ml, fluorescence detection—D. W. Holt *et al.*, *Br. J. clin. Pharmac.*, 1982, *14*, 148P–149P.

THIN-LAYER CHROMATOGRAPHY. In plasma or urine: detection limits 5 ng/ml in plasma and 500 ng/ml in urine, fluorescence detection—M. Schaefer and E. Mutschler, *J. Chromat.*, 1979, *169*, 477–481.

Disposition in the Body. Rapidly but incompletely absorbed after oral administration; bioavailability about 50%. It is excreted almost entirely as unchanged drug, 35 to 50% of an oral dose being excreted in the urine and 30 to 50% in the faeces, in 24 hours; small amounts of 2-hydroxyatenolol and atenolol glucuronide are excreted in the urine.

THERAPEUTIC CONCENTRATION.

After a single oral dose of 100 mg given to 12 subjects, peak plasma concentrations of 0.41 to 0.87 µg/ml (mean 0.6) were attained in about 3 hours (J. McAinsh *et al.*, *Biopharm. Drug Disp.*, 1980, *1*, 323–332).

Following daily oral doses of 25, 50 and 100 mg to 7, 7, and 6 subjects respectively, mean maximum steady-state plasma concentrations of 0.12, 0.22, and 0.39 µg/ml were reported 4 hours after a dose; the corresponding mean trough concentrations were 0.02, 0.04, and 0.07 µg/ml (T. Ishizaki *et al.*, *Br. J. clin. Pharmac.*, 1983, *16*, 17–25).

TOXICITY. Atenolol is relatively non-toxic; a case of ingestion of 1.2 g with subsequent recovery has been reported.

HALF-LIFE. Plasma half-life, 4 to 14 hours (mean 7).

VOLUME OF DISTRIBUTION. About 0.5 to 1.5 litre/kg.

CLEARANCE. Plasma clearance, about 2 ml/min/kg.

DISTRIBUTION IN BLOOD. Plasma: whole blood ratio, about 0.8 to 0.9.

PROTEIN BINDING. In plasma, less than 5%.

NOTE. For reviews of the pharmacokinetics of atenolol see R. C. Heel *et al.*, *Drugs*, 1979, *17*, 425–460, and W. Kirch and K. G. Görg, *Eur. J. drug Met. Pharmacokinet.*, 1982, *7*, 81–91.

Dose. 50 to 100 mg daily.

Atrazine   *Herbicide*

2-Chloro-4-ethylamino-6-isopropylamino-1,3,5-triazine
$C_8H_{14}ClN_5 = 215.7$
CAS—1912-24-9

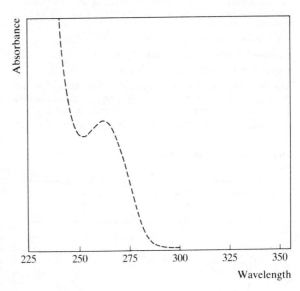

Colourless crystals. M.p. 173° to 175°.
Practically **insoluble** in water; soluble 1 in 20 of chloroform, 1 in 80 of ether, and 1 in 55 of methanol.

Thin-layer Chromatography. *System TA*—Rf 77.

Gas Chromatography. *System GA*—RI 1655; *system GK*—retention time 0.79 relative to caffeine.

Ultraviolet Spectrum. Ethanol—263 nm ($A_1^1 = 195$ b).

Absorbance

Wavelength

Infra-red Spectrum. Principal peaks at wavenumbers 1539, 1612, 1295; 804, 1161, 1121 (KBr disk).

Mass Spectrum. Principal peaks at *m/z* 43, 58, 44, 200, 68, 215, 41, 42.

Atropine   *Anticholinergic*

Synonym. (±)-Hyoscyamine
Proprietary Names. Atropinol. It is an ingredient of Riddofan and Riddovydrin.

(1*R*,3*r*,5*S*)-Tropan-3-yl (±)-tropate
$C_{17}H_{23}NO_3 = 289.4$
CAS—51-55-8

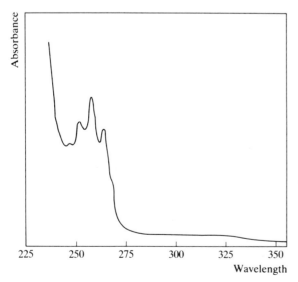

An alkaloid obtained from *Duboisia* spp. and other solanaceous plants, or prepared by synthesis.

Colourless crystals or white crystalline powder. M.p. 114° to 118°.

Soluble 1 in 400 of water, 1 in 50 of boiling water, 1 in 3 of ethanol, 1 in 1 of chloroform, and 1 in 60 of ether.

Atropine Sulphate

Proprietary Names. Atropisol; Atropt; Dosatropine; Liotropina. It is an ingredient of Antrocol, Enuretrol, Mydrapred, Mydricaine, and Taumasthman.

$(C_{17}H_{23}NO_3)_2,H_2SO_4,H_2O = 694.8$
CAS—55-48-1 (anhydrous); *5908-99-6* (monohydrate)

Colourless crystals or white crystalline powder. It effloresces in dry air. M.p. about 190°, with decomposition, after drying at 135° for 15 minutes.

Soluble 1 in less than 1 of water and 1 in 4 of ethanol; practically insoluble in chloroform and ether.

Dissociation Constant. pK_a 9.9 (20°).

Partition Coefficient. Log P (octanol), 1.8.

Colour Test. Liebermann's Test—red-orange.

Thin-layer Chromatography. *System TA*—Rf 18; *system TB*—Rf 06; *system TC*—Rf 03. (*Dragendorff spray*, positive; *acidified iodoplatinate solution*, positive; *Marquis reagent*, pink.)

Gas Chromatography. *System GA*—RI 2199; *system GF*—RI 2660.

High Pressure Liquid Chromatography. *System HA*—k' 3.9 (tailing peak).

Ultraviolet Spectrum. Aqueous acid—252 nm, 258 nm ($A_1^1 = 6.3$ c), 264 nm. No alkaline shift.

Infra-red Spectrum. Principal peaks at wavenumbers 1720, 1035, 1153, 1163, 1063, 1204 (KBr disk).

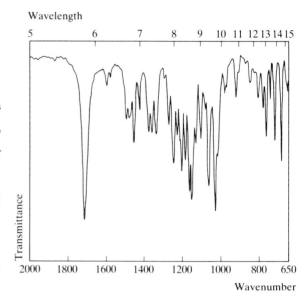

Mass Spectrum. Principal peaks at *m/z* 124, 82, 94, 83, 42, 96, 103, 67.

Quantification. RADIOIMMUNOASSAY. In plasma or serum: atropine and hyoscyamine, detection limit 2.5 ng/ml for both compounds—R. Virtanen *et al.*, *Acta pharmac. tox.*, 1980, *47*, 208–212.

Disposition in the Body. Readily absorbed from mucous membranes, skin and the gastro-intestinal tract but not from the stomach. About 80 to 90% of a dose is excreted in the urine in 24 hours, 50% of the dose as unchanged drug, less than 2% as tropic acid and tropine, and about 30% as unknown metabolites. Traces of the dose are eliminated in the faeces.

THERAPEUTIC CONCENTRATION.

Following an intravenous dose of 1 mg to 6 subjects, plasma concentrations of about 0.25 µg/ml were observed at 2 minutes decreasing to 0.005 µg/ml at 20 minutes; following an intramuscular dose of 1 mg to 4 subjects, peak plasma concentrations of about 0.003 µg/ml were attained in 30 minutes (L. Berghem *et al.*, *Br. J. Anaesth.*, 1980, *52*, 597–601).

TOXICITY. The amount of a toxic dose appears to vary considerably with individuals. Fatalities are reported to have occurred with doses of 50 to 100 mg but recovery has occurred after administration of 1 g; doses of 10 mg or less may be lethal in children or in susceptible individuals.

A man was found dead after having ingested an unknown amount of atropine sulphate tablets. The blood contained 0.2 µg/ml and the urine 1.5 µg/ml of atropine (B. W. Corbett and A. J. McBay, *Bull. int. Ass. forens. Toxicol.*, 1978, *14*(1), 36–37).

HALF-LIFE. Plasma half-life, about 2 to 4 hours; a longer terminal phase of 13 to 38 hours has also been reported.

VOLUME OF DISTRIBUTION. About 2 to 3 litres/kg.

CLEARANCE. Plasma clearance, about 8 ml/min/kg.

PROTEIN BINDING. In plasma, about 50%.

Dose. Usually 0.25 to 2 mg of atropine sulphate daily.

Atropine Methobromide

Anticholinergic

Synonyms. Atropine Methylbromide; Methylatropine Bromide; Mydriasine.

(1R,3r,5S)-8-Methyl-3-[($\pm$)-tropoyloxy]tropanium bromide
$C_{18}H_{26}BrNO_3 = 384.3$
CAS—2870-71-5

Colourless crystals or a white crystalline powder. M.p. about 215°, with decomposition.

Soluble 1 in 1 of water and 1 in 20 of ethanol; very slightly soluble in dehydrated alcohol; practically insoluble in chloroform and ether.

Colour Tests. Aromaticity (Method 2)—colourless/yellow; Liebermann's Test—orange.

Atropine Methonitrate

Anticholinergic

Synonym. Methylatropine Nitrate

Proprietary Names. Eumydrin. It is an ingredient of Asma-Vydrin, Brovon, PIB, Riddobron and Rybarvin.

(1R,3r,5S)-8-Methyl-3-[($\pm$)-tropoyloxy]tropanium nitrate
$C_{18}H_{26}N_2O_6 = 366.4$
CAS—52-88-0

Colourless crystals or a white crystalline powder. M.p. about 167°.

Soluble 1 in less than 1 of water and 1 in 13 of ethanol; practically insoluble in chloroform and ether. Aqueous solutions are unstable.

Colour Tests. Aromaticity (Method 2)—colourless/violet (transient); Liebermann's Test—orange.

Thin-layer Chromatography. *System TA*—Rf 02; *system TN*—Rf 95; *system TO*—Rf 35. (*Acidified iodoplatinate solution*, positive.)

Ultraviolet Spectrum. Aqueous acid—252 nm (A_1^1 = about 5), 258 nm (A_1^1 = about 5), 264 nm (A_1^1 = about 4).

Infra-red Spectrum. Principal peaks at wavenumbers 1159, 1045, 1718, 1176, 700, 1212 (Nujol mull).

Atropine Oxide

Anticholinergic

Atropine *N*-oxide
$C_{17}H_{23}NO_4 = 305.4$
CAS—4438-22-6

A very hygroscopic, crystalline powder. M.p. 127° to 128°; it decomposes at 135°.

Soluble in ethanol and chloroform; practically insoluble in ether.

Atropine Oxide Hydrochloride
Proprietary Names. Génatropine; X-tro.
$C_{17}H_{23}NO_4,HCl = 341.8$
CAS—4574-60-1
Crystals. M.p. 192° to 193°.

Thin-layer Chromatography. *System TA*—Rf 21. (*Acidified iodoplatinate solution*, positive.)

Infra-red Spectrum. Principal peaks at wavenumbers 1164, 1730, 1118, 1026, 1056, 1195.

Azacyclonol

Tranquilliser

α-Phenyl-α-4-piperidylbenzyl alcohol
$C_{18}H_{21}NO = 267.4$
CAS—115-46-8

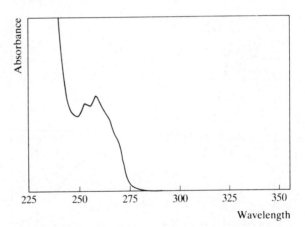

Crystals. M.p. 160° to 161°.

Azacyclonol Hydrochloride
Synonym. Azacyclonolium Chloride
Proprietary Name. Frenquel
$C_{18}H_{21}NO,HCl = 303.8$
CAS—1798-50-1
Small white crystals or crystalline powder. M.p. 270° to 281°.

Soluble 1 in 200 of water and 1 in 1000 of ethanol; practically insoluble in acetone, chloroform, ether, and light petroleum.

Colour Tests. Liebermann's Test—brown; Mandelin's Test—red; Marquis Test—yellow.

Thin-layer Chromatography. *System TA*—Rf 10; *system TB*—Rf 00; *system TC*—Rf 03. (*Acidified iodoplatinate solution*, positive.)

Gas Chromatography. *System GA*—RI 2243.

High Pressure Liquid Chromatography. *System HA*—k' 1.2.

Ultraviolet Spectrum. Aqueous acid—253 nm, 259 nm (A_1^1 = 17.4 a).

Infra-red Spectrum. Principal peaks at wavenumbers 702, 745, 1316, 1063, 971, 1155 (KBr disk).

Mass Spectrum. Principal peaks at m/z 85, 84, 183, 105, 56, 77, 55, 30.

Dose. Azacyclonol hydrochloride has been given in doses of 100 to 800 mg daily.

Azaperone

Tranquilliser (Veterinary)

Proprietary Name. Suicalm
4'-Fluoro-4-[4-(2-pyridyl)piperazin-1-yl]butyrophenone
$C_{19}H_{22}FN_3O = 327.4$
CAS—1649-18-9

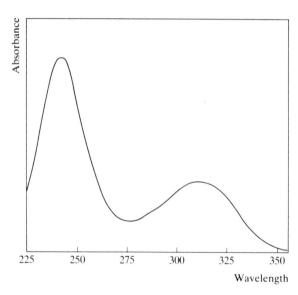

A white to yellowish-white microcrystalline powder. M.p. 90° to 95°.

Practically **insoluble** in water; soluble 1 in 29 of ethanol, 1 in 4 of chloroform, and 1 in 31 of ether; soluble in dilute organic acids.

Partition Coefficient. Log P (octanol), 3.3.

Colour Tests. Cyanogen Bromide—orange; Mandelin's Test—yellow.

Thin-layer Chromatography. *System TA*—Rf 66. (*Acidified iodoplatinate solution*, positive.)

Gas Chromatography. *System GA*—RI 2705.

Ultraviolet Spectrum. Aqueous acid—242 nm ($A_1^1 = 800$ a), 312 nm; methanol—247 nm ($A_1^1 = 1260$ b), 300 nm ($A_1^1 = 200$ b).

Infra-red Spectrum. Principal peaks at wavenumbers 1587, 1669, 775, 1236, 1222, 1152 (KBr disk).

Mass Spectrum. Principal peaks at m/z 107, 165, 123, 95, 121, –, –, –.

Azapetine   *Vasodilator*

Synonym. Azepine
6-Allyl-6,7-dihydro-5H-dibenz[c,e]azepine
$C_{17}H_{17}N = 235.3$
CAS—146-36-1

Azapetine Phosphate

Proprietary Name. Ilidar
$C_{17}H_{17}N,H_3PO_4 = 333.3$
CAS—130-83-6
Crystals. M.p. 211° to 215°, with decomposition.
Soluble at least 1 in 100 of water.

Colour Test. Mandelin's Test—brown.

Thin-layer Chromatography. *System TA*—Rf 70; *system TB*—Rf 57; *system TC*—Rf 67. (*Acidified iodoplatinate solution*, positive.)

Gas Chromatography. *System GA*—RI 1939.

Ultraviolet Spectrum. Aqueous acid—248 nm.

Infra-red Spectrum. Principal peaks at wavenumbers 748, 918, 1063, 990, 1111, 1639 (KBr disk).

Mass Spectrum. Principal peaks at m/z 165, 234, 194, 235, 193, 196, 166, 179.

Dose. The equivalent of 75 to 225 mg of azapetine has been given daily.

Azapropazone   *Analgesic*

Synonym. Apazone
Proprietary Names. Prolixan; Rheumox.
5 - Dimethylamino - 9 - methyl - 2 - propylpyrazolo[1,2 - a][1,2,4]benzotriazine-1,3($2H$)-dione dihydrate
$C_{16}H_{20}N_4O_2,2H_2O = 336.4$
CAS—13539-59-8 (anhydrous)

Almost colourless crystals. M.p. 228° (anhydrous); 247° to 248° (dihydrate).

Partition Coefficient. Log P (octanol/pH 7.4), 1.0.

Colour Tests. Liebermann's Test—grey-green; Mandelin's Test—grey-green.

Thin-layer Chromatography. *System TA*—Rf 68; *system TB*—Rf 53; *system TC*—Rf 05.

Gas Chromatography. *System GA*—RI 2461; *system GF*—RI 3010.

Ultraviolet Spectrum. Azapropazone dihydrate: aqueous acid— 250 nm ($A_1^1 = 1040$ b); aqueous alkali—255 nm ($A_1^1 = 1080$ b), 325 nm.

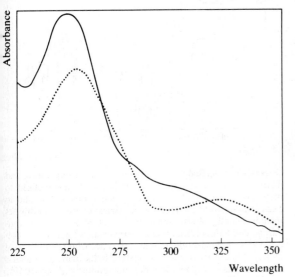

Infra-red Spectrum. Principal peaks at wavenumbers 1590, 1640, 1500, 1133, 1270, 1695.

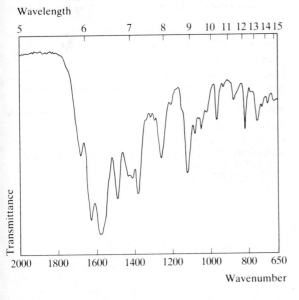

Mass Spectrum. Principal peaks at m/z 160, 300, 189, 145, 188, 301, 161, 42.

Quantification. COLORIMETRY. In serum: sensitivity 10 µg/ml— D. S. Farrier, *Arzneimittel-Forsch.*, 1974, *24*, 747–751.

ULTRAVIOLET SPECTROPHOTOMETRY. In plasma: comparison with gas chromatographic and colorimetric methods—H. Leach, *Curr. med. Res. Opinion*, 1976, *4*, 35–43.

HIGH PRESSURE LIQUID CHROMATOGRAPHY. In plasma or urine: detection limits 400 ng/ml for azapropazone and 1.5 to 3 µg/ml for 6-hydroxyazapropazone, UV detection—B. J. Kline *et al.*, *Arzneimittel-Forsch.*, 1983, *33*, 504–506.

Disposition in the Body. Readily absorbed after oral administration. About 95% of a dose is excreted in the urine, of which about 60% is unchanged drug and about 20% is the inactive metabolite, 6-hydroxyazapropazone.

THERAPEUTIC CONCENTRATION.
After a single oral dose of 600 mg, administered to 6 subjects, plasma concentrations of 34 to 54 µg/ml (mean 43) were attained in 4 hours (A. E. S. Ritch *et al.*, *Br. J. clin. Pharmac.*, 1982, *14*, 116–119).
Steady-state plasma concentrations of 32 to 89 µg/ml (mean 57) were reported during the daily administration of 800 mg to 10 subjects (S. Thune, *Curr. med. Res. Opinion*, 1976, *4*, 70–75).

HALF-LIFE. Plasma half-life, 8 to 24 hours (mean 15), increased in elderly subjects and in subjects with impaired renal or liver function.

VOLUME OF DISTRIBUTION. About 0.2 litre/kg.

CLEARANCE. Plasma clearance, 0.1 to 0.2 ml/min/kg.

PROTEIN BINDING. In plasma, about 99%.

Dose. 0.6 to 1.2 g daily.

Azatadine   *Antihistamine*

6,11 - Dihydro - 11 - (1 - methyl - 4 - piperidylidene) - 5*H* - benzo-[5,6]cyclohepta[1,2-*b*]pyridine
$C_{20}H_{22}N_2 = 290.4$
CAS—3964-81-6

Azatadine Maleate
Proprietary Names. Idulian; Optimine; Zadine. It is an ingredient of Congesteze.
$C_{20}H_{22}N_2,2C_4H_4O_4 = 522.6$
CAS—3978-86-7
A white crystalline powder. M.p. 145° to 154°.
Soluble in water, ethanol, chloroform, dimethylformamide, and methanol; practically insoluble in ether.

Colour Tests. Cyanogen Bromide—pink; Marquis Test—violet.

Thin-layer Chromatography. *System TA*—Rf 39. (*Acidified potassium permanganate solution*, strong reaction.)

Gas Chromatography. *System GA*—RI 2415.

Ultraviolet Spectrum. Aqueous acid—283 nm ($A_1^1 = 330$ b).

Infra-red Spectrum. Principal peaks at wavenumbers 752, 1271, 1124, 803, 984, 795 (KBr disk).

Dose. 2 to 4 mg of azatadine maleate daily.

Azathioprine

Immunosuppressant

Proprietary Names. Azamune; Imuran; Imurek; Imurel.
6-(1-Methyl-4-nitroimidazol-5-ylthio)purine
$C_9H_7N_7O_2S = 277.3$
CAS—446-86-6

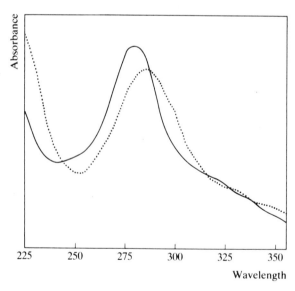

A pale yellow powder. M.p. about 238°, with decomposition.
Practically **insoluble** in water; very slightly soluble in ethanol
and chloroform; sparingly soluble in dilute mineral acids; soluble
in dilute solutions of alkali hydroxides but decomposes in
stronger solutions.

Dissociation Constant. pK_a 8.2 (25°).

Thin-layer Chromatography. *System TA*—Rf 53; *system TB*—Rf
03; *system TC*—Rf 08.

Ultraviolet Spectrum. Aqueous acid—280 nm ($A_1^1 = 600$ a);
aqueous alkali—285 nm.

Infra-red Spectrum. Principal peaks at wavenumbers 1237, 1306,
1580, 832, 1500, 1531 (KBr disk).

Mass Spectrum. Principal peaks at *m/z* 231, 42, 119, 232, 92, 65,
67, 74.

Quantification. SPECTROFLUORIMETRY. In plasma: azathioprine
and mercaptopurine, sensitivity 10 ng/ml—J. L. Maddocks, *Br.
J. clin. Pharmac.*, 1979, *8*, 273–278.

HIGH PRESSURE LIQUID CHROMATOGRAPHY. In plasma: azathioprine and mercaptopurine, sensitivity 40 ng/ml for azathioprine
and 5 ng/ml for mercaptopurine, UV detection—T. L. Ding and
L. Z. Benet, *J. Chromat.*, 1979, *163*; *Biomed. Appl.*, *5*, 281–288.

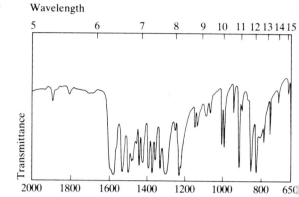

Disposition in the Body. Absorbed after oral administration and
distributed throughout the body. It is readily metabolised to
mercaptopurine, which is the major active metabolite, and to
1-methyl-4-nitro-5-(*S*-glutathionyl)imidazole; other metabolites
include 1-methyl-4-nitroimidazole, 1-methyl-4-nitro-5-thioimi-
dazole, and 6-thiouric acid; mercaptopurine is further metabolised to its ribonucleotide, thioinosinic acid, which is the active
moiety. About 50% of a dose is excreted in the urine in 24 hours,
mainly as thiouric acid and other metabolites with about 10%
consisting of unchanged drug; about 12% of a dose is eliminated
in the faeces in 48 hours.

THERAPEUTIC CONCENTRATION.

After daily oral doses of 50 to 100 mg to 3 renal transplant patients, peak
steady-state plasma concentrations of 0.05 to 0.08 µg/ml of mercaptopurine were reported 1 hour after a dose (T. L. Ding and L. Z. Benet,
ibid.).

HALF-LIFE. Plasma half-life, azathioprine about 3 hours, mercaptopurine about 0.5 to 1.5 hours.

PROTEIN BINDING. In plasma, about 30%.

Dose. 1 to 5 mg/kg daily, by mouth.

Azinphos-methyl

Pesticide

Synonym. DBD
Proprietary Name. Gusathion
S-(3,4-Dihydro-4-oxobenzo[*d*][1,2,3]-triazin-3-ylmethyl) *OO*-
dimethyl phosphorodithioate
$C_{10}H_{12}N_3O_3PS_2 = 317.3$
CAS—86-50-0

Colourless crystals. It is rapidly hydrolysed in alkaline or acid
media. M.p. 73° to 74°.

Soluble 1 in 30 000 of water; soluble in ethanol, methanol, and
propylene glycol.

Colour Tests. Palladium Chloride—brown; Phosphorus Test—
yellow.

Thin-layer Chromatography. *System TW*—Rf 68.

Gas Chromatography. *System GA*—RI 2430; *system GK*—retention time 1.60 relative to caffeine.

Ultraviolet Spectrum. Hexane—285 nm ($A_1^1 = 280$ b), 302 nm, 315 nm.

Infra-red Spectrum. Principal peaks at wavenumbers 1000, 1666, 833, 781, 1041, 775.

Mass Spectrum. Principal peaks at m/z 77, 160, 132, 44, 105, 104, 93, 76.

Disposition in the Body.

TOXICITY. Azinphos-methyl is less toxic than mevinphos or parathion. The maximum permissible atmospheric concentration is 0.2 mg/m³.

Bacampicillin   *Antibiotic*

Synonym. Carampicillin

1-(Ethoxycarbonyloxy)ethyl   (6R)-6-(α-D-phenylglycylamino)-penicillanate

$C_{21}H_{27}N_3O_7S = 465.5$

CAS—50972-17-3

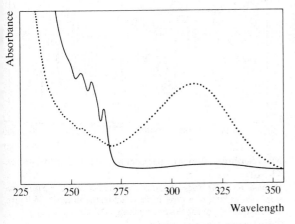

Bacampicillin Hydrochloride

Proprietary Names. Ambaxin; Penglobe; Spectrobid.

$C_{21}H_{27}N_3O_7S,HCl = 502.0$

CAS—37661-08-8

A white crystalline powder.

Soluble 1 in 15 of water, 1 in 7 of ethanol, and 1 in 10 of chloroform; practically insoluble in ether.

Ultraviolet Spectrum. Water—258 nm, 263 nm ($A_1^1 = 13$ b), 269 nm; aqueous alkali—310 nm.

Infra-red Spectrum. Principal peaks at wavenumbers 1770, 1075, 1788, 1263, 1687, 1744 (bacampicillin hydrochloride, K Br disk).

Dose. 0.8 to 2.4 g of bacampicillin hydrochloride daily.

Bacitracin   *Antibiotic*

Proprietary Names. Baciguent; Bacitin. It is an ingredient of Ototrips and Polybactrin Soluble GU.

CAS—1405-87-4

Bacitracin is a polypeptide produced by the growth of an organism of the *licheniformis* group of *Bacillus subtilis*. A white to pale buff hygroscopic powder.

Freely **soluble** in water; soluble in ethanol; practically insoluble in chloroform and ether.

Bacitracin Zinc

Synonyms. Bacitracins Zinc Complex; Zinc Bacitracin.

Proprietary Names. It is an ingredient of Cicatrene, Cicatrex, Cicatrin, Dispray Antibiotic, Polyfax and Tribiotic.

CAS—1405-89-6

A white, pale buff or tan, hygroscopic powder.

Soluble 1 in 900 of water and 1 in 500 of ethanol; very slightly soluble in ether; practically insoluble in chloroform.

Ultraviolet Spectrum. Bacitracin zinc: aqueous acid—252 nm ($A_1^1 = 18$ b).

Baclofen   *Muscle Relaxant*

Synonym. Aminomethyl Chlorohydrocinnamic Acid

Proprietary Name. Lioresal

4-Amino-3-(4-chlorophenyl)butyric acid

$C_{10}H_{12}ClNO_2 = 213.7$

CAS—1134-47-0

A white crystalline solid. M.p. about 207°.

Slightly **soluble** in water; poorly soluble in organic solvents.

Dissociation Constant. pK_a 3.9, 9.6.

Colour Test. Liebermann's Test—orange.

Thin-layer Chromatography. *System TD*—Rf 01; *system TE*—Rf 00; *system TF*—Rf 00.

Gas Chromatography. *System GA*—RI 2010.

Ultraviolet Spectrum. Aqueous acid—259 nm, 266 nm ($A_1^1 = 11.3$ a), 274 nm. No alkaline shift.

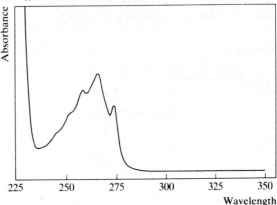

Infra-red Spectrum. Principal peaks at wavenumbers 1527, 835, 1574, 1495, 1624, 1095 (KBr disk).

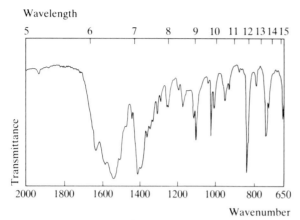

Mass Spectrum. Principal peaks at m/z 30, 138, 195, 140, 103, 197, 77, 196.

Quantification. GAS CHROMATOGRAPHY. In plasma or urine: sensitivity 50 ng/ml, ECD—P. H. Degen and W. Riess, *J. Chromat.*, 1976, *117*, 399–405.

GAS CHROMATOGRAPHY–MASS SPECTROMETRY. In serum or cerebrospinal fluid: sensitivity 5 ng/ml—C. G. Swahn *et al.*, *J. Chromat.*, 1979, *162*; *Biomed Appl.*, *4*, 433–438.

Disposition in the Body. Rapidly absorbed after oral administration. About 80% of a dose is excreted in the urine in 24 hours, mostly as unchanged drug. About 15% of a dose is metabolised, mainly to the deaminated derivative; about 20% of a dose may be eliminated in the faeces as unchanged drug and metabolites.

THERAPEUTIC CONCENTRATION.

After an oral dose of 40 mg to 1 subject, a peak plasma concentration of unchanged drug of about 0.6 µg/ml was attained in 2 hours; a peak concentration of metabolites of about 0.1 µg/ml was attained in about 4 hours (J. W. Faigle and H. Keberle, *Postgrad. med. J.*, 1972, *48* (Oct.), Suppl., 9–13).

TOXICITY. Recovery has occurred after the ingestion of 1.5 g.

Coma, respiratory failure and severe seizures occurred in a 39-year-old female subject after ingestion of 450 mg; following treatment, the patient regained consciousness within 36 hours, at which time a plasma concentration of 0.2 µg/ml was reported; the plasma half-life was found to be 35 hours (K. Ghose *et al.*, *Postgrad. med. J.*, 1980, *56*, 865–867).

HALF-LIFE. Plasma half-life, about 2 to 4 hours.

PROTEIN BINDING. In plasma, about 30%.

Dose. 15 to 60 mg daily; maximum of 100 mg daily.

Bamethan   *Vasodilator*

2-Butylamino-1-(4-hydroxyphenyl)ethanol
$C_{12}H_{19}NO_2 = 209.3$
CAS—3703-79-5

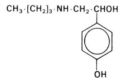

Crystals. M.p. 123.5° to 125°.

Bamethan Sulphate

Proprietary Names. Vasculat; Vasculit.
$(C_{12}H_{19}NO_2)_2,H_2SO_4 = 516.6$
CAS—5716-20-1
Soluble in water.

Dissociation Constant. pK_a 9.0, 10.2 (25°).

Colour Tests. Folin–Ciocalteu Reagent—blue; Liebermann's Test—violet-brown; Mandelin's Test—blue → green.

Thin-layer Chromatography. *System TA*—Rf 55; *system TB*—Rf 04; *system TC*—Rf 06. (*Acidified potassium permanganate solution, positive.*)

Gas Chromatography. *System GA*—RI 1920.

High Pressure Liquid Chromatography. *System HA*—k' 0.9.

Ultraviolet Spectrum. Aqueous acid—275 nm ($A_1^1 = 64$ a); aqueous alkali—242 nm, 290 nm.

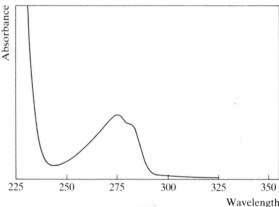

Infra-red Spectrum. Principal peaks at wavenumbers 832, 1228, 1066, 1264, 1494, 1108 (KBr disk).

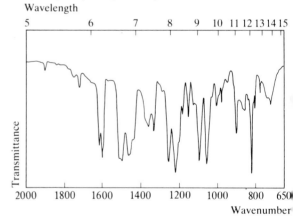

Mass Spectrum. Principal peaks at m/z 86, 30, 57, 108, 44, 29, 84, 41.

Disposition in the Body. Rapidly absorbed after oral administration. About 80% of a dose is excreted in the urine in 24 hours, with about 30% of the dose as unchanged drug.

THERAPEUTIC CONCENTRATION.

After a single oral dose of 25 mg given to 5 subjects, peak serum concentrations of 0.04 to 0.11 µg/ml (mean 0.07) were attained in 0.5 to 1 hour (J. H. Hengstmann and B. Steinkamp, *Arzneimittel-Forsch.*, 1981, *31*, 843–848).

HALF-LIFE. Plasma half-life, about 2.5 hours.

VOLUME OF DISTRIBUTION. 2.5 to 5 litres/kg (mean 3.7).

CLEARANCE. Plasma clearance, 12 to 20 ml/min/kg (mean 16).

REFERENCE. J. H. Hengstmann and B. Steinkamp, *ibid.*

Dose. 100 mg of bamethan sulphate daily.

Bamifylline
Xanthine Bronchodilator

8 - Benzyl - 7 - [2 - (*N* - ethyl - 2 - hydroxyethylamino)ethyl]-theophylline
$C_{20}H_{27}N_5O_3 = 385.5$
CAS—2016-63-9

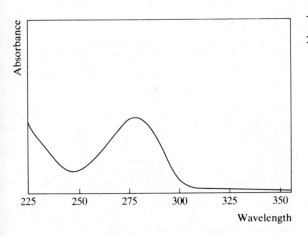

Crystals. M.p. 80°.

Bamifylline Hydrochloride
Proprietary Name. Trentadil
$C_{20}H_{27}N_5O_3,HCl = 421.9$
CAS—20684-06-4
A crystalline solid. M.p. about 185°.
Soluble in water.

Colour Test. Amalic Acid Test—orange/violet.

Thin-layer Chromatography. *System TA*—Rf 65; *system TB*—Rf 00; *system TC*—Rf 54. (*Acidified iodoplatinate solution*, positive.)

Ultraviolet Spectrum. Aqueous acid—278 nm $(A_1^1 = 310$ a); methanol—277 nm $(A_1^1 = 280$ b).

Infra-red Spectrum. Principal peaks at wavenumbers 1650, 1698, 1538, 729, 1041, 1205 (KBr disk).

Mass Spectrum. Principal peaks at *m/z* 102, 84, 58, 56, 42, 30, 103, 91.

Quantification. HIGH PRESSURE LIQUID CHROMATOGRAPHY. In plasma: bamifylline and desalkyl metabolites, sensitivity 10 ng/ml, UV detection—G. Nicot *et al., J. Chromat.,* 1983, *277*; *Biomed. Appl., 28,* 239–249.

Dose. Bamifylline hydrochloride has been given in doses of 0.9 to 1.8 g daily.

Bamipine
Antihistamine

N - Benzyl - *N* - (1 - methyl - 4 - piperidyl)aniline
$C_{19}H_{24}N_2 = 280.4$
CAS—4945-47-5

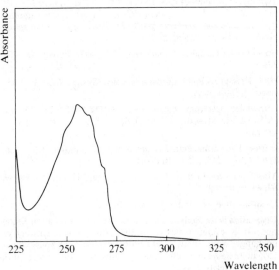

Crystals. M.p. about 115°.
Soluble 1 in 75 of water.

Bamipine Hydrochloride
Proprietary Names. Soventol; Taumidrine.
$C_{19}H_{24}N_2,2HCl = 353.3$
CAS—61732-85-2
A white crystalline powder. M.p. 208° to 209°.

Colour Tests. Liebermann's Test—red-orange; Mandelin's Test—brown.

Thin-layer Chromatography. *System TA*—Rf 49; *system TB*—Rf 40; *system TC*—Rf 43. (*Acidified iodoplatinate solution*, positive.)

Gas Chromatography. *System GA*—RI 2211.

Ultraviolet Spectrum. Aqueous acid—257 nm $(A_1^1 = 16$ b); methanol—251 nm $(A_1^1 = 439$ b), 298 nm $(A_1^1 = 62$ b).

Infra-red Spectrum. Principal peaks at wavenumbers 745, 1593, 725, 1495, 690, 1275 (KBr disk).

Mass Spectrum. Principal peaks at m/z 97, 43, 71, 70, 96, 91, 98, 42.

Dose. Bamipine hydrochloride has been given in doses of 75 to 400 mg daily.

Barbitone   *Barbiturate*

Synonyms. Barb; Barbital; Diemalum; Diethylmalonylurea; Malonal.
5,5-Diethylbarbituric acid
$C_8H_{12}N_2O_3 = 184.2$
CAS—57-44-3

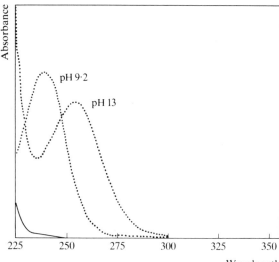

Colourless crystals or white crystalline powder. M.p. 188° to 192°.

Soluble 1 in 160 of water, 1 in 13 of boiling water, 1 in 15 of ethanol, 1 in 6 of acetone, 1 in 75 of chloroform, and 1 in 40 of ether; soluble in ethyl acetate and in solutions of alkali carbonates and hydroxides.

Barbitone Sodium

Synonyms. Diemalnatrium; Soluble Barbitone.
$C_8H_{11}N_2NaO_3 = 206.2$
CAS—144-02-5
A white crystalline powder. A solution in water slowly decomposes. M.p. about 190°.
Soluble 1 in 5 of water and 1 in 600 of ethanol; practically insoluble in chloroform and ether.

Dissociation Constant. pK_a 8.0 (25°).

Colour Tests. Koppanyi–Zwikker Test—violet; Mercurous Nitrate—black.

Thin-layer Chromatography. *System TD*—Rf 41; *system TE*—Rf 31; *system TF*—Rf 61; *system TH*—Rf 51. (*Mercuric chloride-diphenylcarbazone reagent*, positive; *mercurous nitrate spray*, black; *Zwikker's reagent*, pink.)

Gas Chromatography. *System GA*—RI 1497; *system GF*—RI 2230.

High Pressure Liquid Chromatography. *System HG*—k' 1.11; *system HH*—k' 0.63.

Ultraviolet Spectrum. *Borax buffer 0.05M* (pH 9.2)—239 nm ($A_1^1 = 549$ a); M sodium hydroxide (pH 13)—254 nm ($A_1^1 = 427$ b).

Infra-red Spectrum. Principal peaks at wavenumbers 1680, 1720, 1767, 1320, 1245, 875 (KBr disk).

Mass Spectrum. Principal peaks at m/z 156, 141, 55, 155, 98, 39, 82, 43.

Quantification. See under Amylobarbitone.

Disposition in the Body. Readily absorbed after oral administration. It is excreted slowly in the urine almost entirely as unchanged drug; about 2% of a dose is excreted in 8 hours, about 16% in 32 hours and detectable amounts may still be present in the urine after 16 days.
Barbitone is a metabolite of metharbitone.

THERAPEUTIC CONCENTRATION. In plasma, usually in the range 5 to 30 µg/ml.

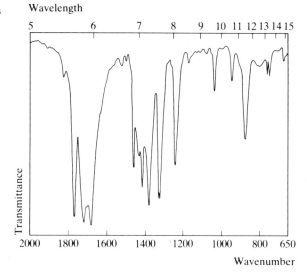

TOXICITY. The estimated minimum lethal dose is 2 g. Toxic effects may be produced with blood concentrations of about 20 µg/ml or more and concentrations greater than 90 µg/ml may be lethal.

In 6 cases of acute poisoning, the amounts ingested ranged from 5 to about 25 g. In 2 cases, death ensued after 150 and 160 hours when the serum concentrations were about 100 and 170 µg/ml respectively. In the other 4 cases, the serum concentrations on awakening from coma were 70 to 150 µg/ml (P. Lous, *Acta pharmac. tox.*, 1954, *10*. 147–165 and 261–280).

HALF-LIFE. Plasma half-life, about 2 days.

VOLUME OF DISTRIBUTION. About 0.5 litre/kg.

SALIVA. Plasma : saliva ratio, about 1.

PROTEIN BINDING. In plasma, less than 20%.

Dose. Barbitone has been given in a dose of 300 to 600 mg.

Barbituric Acid

Synonym. Malonylurea
Pyrimidine-2,4,6-trione
$C_4H_4N_2O_3 = 128.1$
CAS—67-52-7

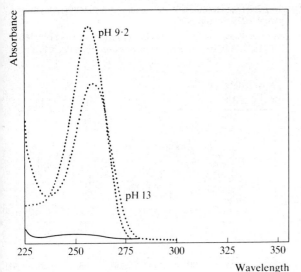

Crystals. M.p. about 248°, with some decomposition.

Dissociation Constant. pK_a 4.0.

Thin-layer Chromatography. *System TD*—Rf 00; *system TE*—Rf 00; *system TF*—Rf 00; *system TH*—Rf 03.

Ultraviolet Spectrum. *Borax buffer 0.05M* (pH 9.2)—257 nm; M sodium hydroxide (pH 13)—259 nm.

Infra-red Spectrum. Principal peaks at wavenumbers 1710, 1734, 1750, 1225, 775, 1190 (KBr disk).

Mass Spectrum. Principal peaks at m/z 42, 128, 85, 43, 44, 41, 70, 69.

Beclamide
Anticonvulsant

Synonyms. Benzchlorpropamide; Chloroethylphenamide.
Proprietary Names. Neuracen; Nydrane; Posedrine.
N-Benzyl-3-chloropropionamide
$C_{10}H_{12}ClNO = 197.7$
CAS—501-68-8

$CH_2 \cdot NH \cdot CO \cdot CH_2 \cdot CH_2 \cdot Cl$

Colourless crystals. M.p. 91° to 94°.
Practically **insoluble** in water; soluble 1 in 14 of ethanol, 1 in 5 of chloroform, and 1 in less than 100 of ether.

Colour Test. Liebermann's Test—red-orange.

Thin-layer Chromatography. *System TA*—Rf 65; *system TB*—Rf 08; *system TC*—Rf 65. (*Acidified potassium permanganate solution*, positive, developing slowly.)

Gas Chromatography. *System GA*—RI 1480 and 1678.

Ultraviolet Spectrum. Aqueous acid—252 nm, 258 nm, 264 nm; methanol—252 nm, 258 nm ($A_1^1 = 9.6$ b), 264 nm, 268 nm.

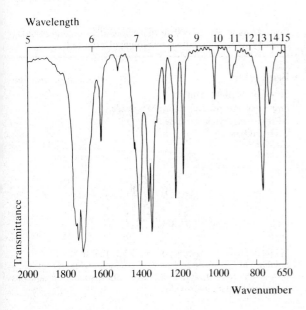

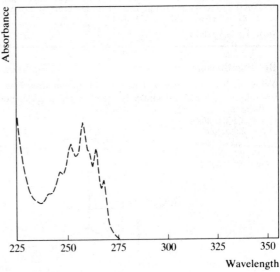

Infra-red Spectrum. Principal peaks at wavenumbers 1640, 696, 736, 1558, 1275, 1290 (KBr disk).

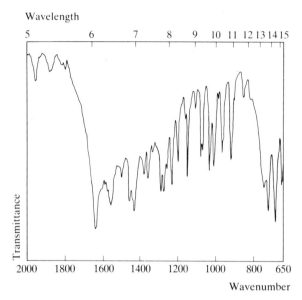

Wavelength

Mass Spectrum. Principal peaks at m/z 91, 106, 197, 162, 107, 148, 27, 63.

Quantification. GAS CHROMATOGRAPHY. In plasma: sensitivity 200 ng/ml, FID—O. P. Jones et al., *Br. J. clin. Pharmac.*, 1975, 2, 364–365.

Disposition in the Body. Absorbed after oral administration. Less than 0.5% of a dose is excreted in the urine as unchanged drug in 24 hours; a metabolite, tentatively identified as an *N*-hydroxybenzyl-3-chloropropionamide, has been detected in the urine as a glucuronide conjugate.

THERAPEUTIC CONCENTRATION.

Following a single oral dose of 1 g to 6 subjects, peak plasma concentrations of 8.7 to 18.9 µg/ml (mean 13) were attained in 1 to 4 hours (H. Leach *et al.*, *Br. J. clin. Pharmac.*, 1975, 2, 377P–378P).

Dose. 1.5 to 4 g daily.

Beclomethasone   *Corticosteroid*

Synonyms. Beclometasone; 9α-Chloro-16β-methylprednisolone.
9α-Chloro-11β,17α,21-trihydroxy-16β-methylpregna-1,4-diene-3,20-dione
$C_{22}H_{29}ClO_5 = 408.9$
CAS—4419-39-0

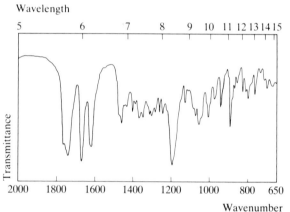

Beclomethasone Dipropionate

Proprietary Names. Aldecin; Becloforte; Beclovent; Beconase; Becotide; Clenil; Propaderm; Sanasthmyl; Turbinal; Vanceril; Vanceril; Viarox. It is an ingredient of Ventide.
$C_{28}H_{37}ClO_7 = 521.0$
CAS—5534-09-8
A white to creamy-white powder. M.p. about 212°, with decomposition. Practically **insoluble** in water; soluble 1 in 60 of ethanol and 1 in 8 of chloroform; freely soluble in acetone.

Colour Tests. Naphthol–Sulphuric Acid—green/brown-yellow; Sulphuric Acid—orange (slow).

Thin-layer Chromatography. Beclomethasone dipropionate: *system TP*—Rf 75; *system TQ*—Rf 38; *system TR*—Rf 89; *system TS*—Rf 42, streaking may occur. (p-*Toluenesulphonic acid solution*, positive.)

High Pressure Liquid Chromatography. *System HT*—k′ 4.2.

Ultraviolet Spectrum. Beclomethasone dipropionate: dehydrated alcohol—239 nm ($A_1^1 = 292$ a).

Infra-red Spectrum. Principal peaks at wavenumbers 1190, 1658, 1730, 1608, 890, 1053 (beclomethasone dipropionate, KBr disk).

Wavelength

Dose. Usually 300 to 400 µg of beclomethasone dipropionate daily, by aerosol inhalation; maximum of 2 mg daily.

Bemegride   *Respiratory Stimulant*

Synonym. Methetharimide.
Proprietary Names. Eukraton; Megimide.
3-Ethyl-3-methylglutarimide
$C_8H_{13}NO_2 = 155.2$
CAS—64-65-3

White flakes or crystalline powder. M.p. 126° to 128°.
Soluble 1 in 170 of water, 1 in 30 of ethanol, 1 in 12 of acetone, 1 in 4 of chloroform, and 1 in 100 of ether; soluble in aqueous solutions of alkali hydroxides.

Bemegride Sodium

$C_8H_{12}NNaO_2 = 177.2$
CAS—25334-00-3
A fine white powder.
Soluble 1 in 11 of water and 1 in 20 of ethanol; practically insoluble in acetone and ether.

Dissociation Constant. pK_a 11.6.

Colour Tests. Koppanyi–Zwikker Test—violet; Mercurous Nitrate—black.

Thin-layer Chromatography. *System TD*—Rf 52; *system TE*—Rf 68; *system TF*—Rf 53. (*Mercuric chloride–diphenylcarbazone reagent*, positive; *mercurous nitrate spray*, black.)

Gas Chromatography. *System GA*—RI 1373; *system GC*—RI 1253.

Ultraviolet Spectrum. No significant absorption, 230 to 360 nm.

Infra-red Spectrum. Principal peaks at wavenumbers 1680, 1277, 1730, 860, 1160, 1145 (KBr disk).

Mass Spectrum. Principal peaks at m/z 55, 83, 82, 41, 113, 70, 29, 69.

Disposition in the Body. Metabolised by hydroxylation of the ethyl side-chain and excreted in the urine as unchanged drug and as the hydroxy metabolite.

Dose. Bemegride has been given in doses of 25 to 50 mg intravenously, repeated as necessary.

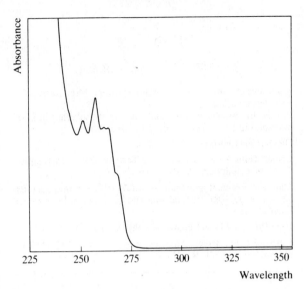

Wavelength

Benactyzine   *Tranquilliser*

2-Diethylaminoethyl benzilate
$C_{20}H_{25}NO_3 = 327.4$
CAS—302-40-9

$$HO \cdot \underset{\underset{C_6H_5}{|}}{\overset{\overset{C_6H_5}{|}}{C}} \cdot CO \cdot O \cdot [CH_2]_2 \cdot N(C_2H_5)_2$$

Crystals. M.p. 51°.

Benactyzine Hydrochloride

Proprietary Name. It is an ingredient of Deprol.
$C_{20}H_{25}NO_3,HCl = 363.9$
CAS—57-37-4
A white crystalline powder. M.p. 177° to 181°.
Soluble 1 in 14 of water and 1 in 22 of ethanol; very slightly soluble in ether.

Dissociation Constant. pK_a 6.6.

Colour Tests. Liebermann's Test—orange → brown; Marquis Test—orange → green → blue; Sulphuric Acid—orange.

Thin-layer Chromatography. *System TA*—Rf 66; *system TB*—Rf 40; *system TC*—Rf 53. (*Acidified iodoplatinate solution*, positive.)

Gas Chromatography. *System GA*—RI 2248.

High Pressure Liquid Chromatography. *System HA*—k' 1.7.

Ultraviolet Spectrum. Aqueous acid—252 nm, 258 nm ($A_1^1 = 14$ a), 262 nm, 264 nm.

Infra-red Spectrum. Principal peaks at wavenumbers 695, 1723, 1231, 1054, 1162, 751 (KBr disk).

Mass Spectrum. Principal peaks at m/z 86, 105, 77, 87, 182, 99, 183, 58.

Disposition in the Body. Rapidly metabolised and excreted.

Dose. 3 to 9 mg of benactyzine hydrochloride daily.

Benapryzine   *Anticholinergic*

Synonym. Benaprizine
2-(*N*-Ethylpropylamino)ethyl benzilate
$C_{21}H_{27}NO_3 = 341.4$
CAS—22487-42-9

$$HO \cdot \underset{\underset{C_6H_5}{|}}{\overset{\overset{C_6H_5}{|}}{C}} \cdot CO \cdot O \cdot CH_2 \cdot CH_2 \cdot \underset{}{\overset{\overset{C_2H_5}{|}}{N}} \cdot CH_2 \cdot CH_2 \cdot CH_3$$

Benapryzine Hydrochloride

$C_{21}H_{27}NO_3,HCl = 377.9$
CAS—3202-55-9
A white crystalline powder. M.p. about 166°.
Soluble 1 in 35 of water, 1 in 56 of dehydrated alcohol, 1 in 120 of acetone, and 1 in 8 of chloroform.

Ultraviolet Spectrum. Aqueous acid—251 nm, 257 nm, 261 nm, 264 nm.

Infra-red Spectrum. Principal peaks at wavenumbers 1753, 1215, 700, 690, 1180, 1020 (benapryzine hydrochloride, KCl disk).

Dose. 150 to 200 mg of benapryzine hydrochloride daily.

Bendrofluazide   *Diuretic*

Synonyms. Bendroflumethiazide; Benzydroflumethiazide.
Proprietary Names. Aprinox; Berkozide; Centyl; Naturetin; Neo-NaClex; Pluryl; Polidiuril; Salural; Sinesalin; Urizide. It is an ingredient of Abicol, Corgaretic, Inderetic, Inderex, Prestim, Rauzide, and Tenavoid.
3-Benzyl-3,4-dihydro-6-trifluoromethyl-2*H*-1,2,4-benzothia-diazine-7-sulphonamide 1,1-dioxide
$C_{15}H_{14}F_3N_3O_4S_2 = 421.4$
CAS—73-48-3

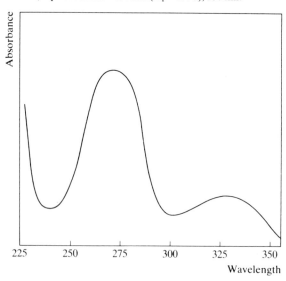

A white or cream-coloured crystalline powder. M.p. about 220°, with decomposition.

Practically **insoluble** in water and chloroform; soluble 1 in 17 of ethanol, 1 in 1.5 of acetone, and 1 in 500 of ether.

Dissociation Constant. pK$_a$ 8.5 (25°).

Colour Tests. Koppanyi–Zwikker Test—violet; Liebermann's Test—blue; Sulphuric Acid—violet.

Thin-layer Chromatography. *System TD*—Rf 25; *system TE*—Rf 52; *system TF*—Rf 71. (Location under ultraviolet light, violet fluorescence.)

High Pressure Liquid Chromatography. *System HN*—k′ 15.35.

Ultraviolet Spectrum. Aqueous acid—273 nm (A$_1^1$ = 585 a), 325 nm; aqueous alkali—273 nm (A$_1^1$ = 410 a), 330 nm.

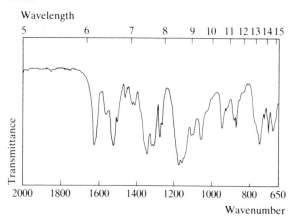

Infra-red Spectrum. Principal peaks at wavenumbers 1170, 1155, 1306, 1518, 1621, 750 (KBr disk). There are 2 polymorphic forms.

Mass Spectrum. Principal peaks at *m/z* 330, 118, 91, 319, 219, 64, 92, 421.

Quantification. GAS CHROMATOGRAPHY. In plasma: sensitivity 5 ng/ml, ECD—B. Beerman *et al.*, *Eur. J. clin. Pharmac.*, 1976, *10*, 293–295.

Disposition in the Body. Readily and almost completely absorbed after oral administration. Up to about 30% of a dose is excreted unchanged in the urine in 48 hours; the remainder is excreted as unidentified metabolites.

THERAPEUTIC CONCENTRATION.

A single oral dose of 10 mg given to 9 subjects, produced peak plasma concentrations of 0.07 to 0.10 μg/ml in 1.6 to 2.4 hours (B. Beerman *et al.*, *Clin. Pharmac. Ther.*, 1977, *22*, 385–388).

Peak plasma concentrations of 0.04 to 0.06 μg/ml (mean 0.05) were reported 2 hours after a dose, following administration of 5 mg daily to 8 hypertensive patients (B. Beerman *et al.*, *Eur. J. clin. Pharmac.*, 1978, *13*, 119–124).

HALF-LIFE. Plasma half-life, about 9 hours.

VOLUME OF DISTRIBUTION. About 1.5 litres/kg.

PROTEIN BINDING. In plasma, about 94%.

NOTE. For a review of the clinical pharmacokinetics of diuretics see B. Beerman and M. Groschinsky–Grind, *Clin. Pharmacokinet.*, 1980, *5*, 221–245.

Dose. 2.5 to 10 mg daily.

Benethamine   *Pharmaceutical Adjuvant*

N-Benzylphenethylamine
C$_{15}$H$_{17}$N = 211.3

$$C_6H_5 \cdot CH_2 \cdot CH_2 \cdot NH \cdot CH_2 \cdot C_6H_5$$

Soluble in chloroform.

Colour Tests. Liebermann's Test—red-orange; Marquis Test—orange-brown → brown.

Thin-layer Chromatography. *System TA*—Rf 64; *system TB*—Rf 48; *system TC*—Rf 59. (*Acidified iodoplatinate solution*, positive.)

Gas Chromatography. *System GA*—RI 1798.

Ultraviolet Spectrum. Water—258 nm (A$_1^1$ = 12 b).

Infra-red Spectrum. Principal peaks at wavenumbers 696, 745, 1111, 1022, 1592, 1067 (KBr disk).

Mass Spectrum. Principal peaks at *m/z* 91, 120, 65, 121, 92, 105, 77, 118.

Benorylate   *Analgesic*

Synonyms. Benorilate; Fenasprate.
Proprietary Names. Benoral; Benortan; Salipran.
4-Acetamidophenyl *O*-acetylsalicylate
C$_{17}$H$_{15}$NO$_5$ = 313.3
CAS—5003-48-5

A white crystalline powder. M.p. 178° to 181°.
Practically **insoluble** in water; soluble 1 in 88 of ethanol, 1 in 22 of acetone, 1 in 18 of chloroform, and 1 in 900 of ether.

Colour Tests. Liebermann's Test—black; Mandelin's Test—green; Marquis Test—violet.

Thin-layer Chromatography. *System TA*—Rf 67; *system TB*—Rf 00; *system TC*—Rf 51. (*Marquis reagent*, positive.)

Gas Chromatography. *System GA*—benorylate RI 1840, aspirin RI 1309, paracetamol RI 1687.

High Pressure Liquid Chromatography. *System HD*—benorylate k' 0.7, aspirin k' 0.5, paracetamol k' 0.1; *system HW*—benorylate k' 22.4, aspirin k' 2.7, paracetamol k' 0.32.

Ultraviolet Spectrum. Dehydrated alcohol—240 nm $(A_1^1 = 740$ a).

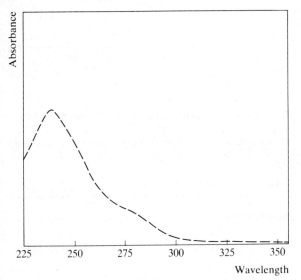

Infra-red Spectrum. Principal peaks at wavenumbers 1182, 1050, 1661, 1730, 1248, 1194, (KBr disk).

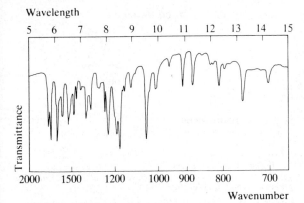

Mass Spectrum. Principal peaks at *m/z* 121, 163, 151, 109, 43, 122, 108, 65; aspirin 120, 43, 138, 92, 121, 39, 64, 63; paracetamol 109, 151, 43, 80, 108, 81, 53, 52.

Quantification. See also under Aspirin and Paracetamol.

GAS CHROMATOGRAPHY. In plasma: aspirin and salicylic acid, sensitivity 2 μg/ml for aspirin, FID—A. Cailleux *et al.*, *Therapie*, 1979, *34*, 73–79.

HIGH PRESSURE LIQUID CHROMATOGRAPHY. In plasma: benory-late and paracetamol, sensitivity 200 ng/ml for benorylate and 400 ng/ml for paracetamol, UV detection—A. Cailleux *et al.*, *ibid.*

Disposition in the Body. Readily absorbed after oral administration. It is hydrolysed in the blood to aspirin and paracetamol, and about 85% of a dose is excreted in the urine in 72 hours by the normal metabolic routes for these substances. About 15% of a dose is eliminated in the faeces.

THERAPEUTIC CONCENTRATION.
Following oral administration of 4 g as a suspension to 20 subjects, mean peak plasma concentrations of 2.2 μg/ml of benorylate and about 120 μg/ml of salicylate were attained in 0.5 and 3 hours respectively (M. Aylward *et al.*, *Scand. J. Rheumatol.*, 1976, *Suppl.* 13, 9–12).

HALF-LIFE. Plasma half-life, about 1 hour.

Dose. 4.5 to 8 g daily.

Benoxaprofen   *Analgesic*

Proprietary Names. Opren; Oraflex.
2-[2-(4-Chlorophenyl)benzoxazol-5-yl]propionic acid
$C_{16}H_{12}ClNO_3 = 301.7$
CAS—51234-28-7

A cream-coloured solid. M.p. 189° to 190°.

Dissociation Constant. pK_a 3.5.

Thin-layer Chromatography. *System TG*—Rf 14. (*Ludy Tenger reagent*, orange.)

Gas Chromatography. *System GD*—retention time of methyl derivative 1.98 relative to $n\text{-}C_{16}H_{34}$.

High Pressure Liquid Chromatography. *System HD*—k' 11.3; *system HV*—retention time 0.98 relative to meclofenamic acid.

Ultraviolet Spectrum. Aqueous alkali—244 nm $(A_1^1 = 295$ b), 309 nm $(A_1^1 = 900$ b).

Infra-red Spectrum. Principal peaks at wavenumbers 728, 1695, 833, 1086, 1050, 1010 (KBr disk). (See below)

Mass Spectrum. Principal peaks at *m/z* 256, 301, 91, 258, 119, 65, 257, 303.

Quantification. GAS CHROMATOGRAPHY. In plasma or urine: sensitivity 10 ng/ml, ECD—D. H. Chatfield and T. J. Woodage, *J. Chromat.*, 1978, *153*, 101–106.

HIGH PRESSURE LIQUID CHROMATOGRAPHY. In plasma or urine: detection limit 25 ng/ml, UV detection—L. Ekman *et al.*, *J. Chromat.*, 1980, *182*; *Biomed. Appl.*, *8*, 478–481.

Disposition in the Body. Readily absorbed after oral administration. About 15% of a dose is excreted in the urine in 24 hours, mainly as the glucuronic acid conjugate, together with small

Wavelength

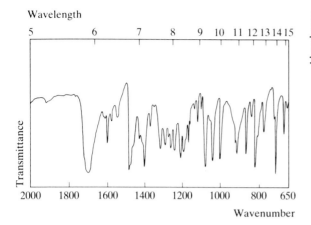

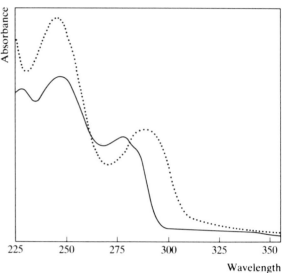

Wavelength

amounts of unchanged drug. In 5 days about 60% of a dose is excreted in the urine and 40% is eliminated in the faeces.

THERAPEUTIC CONCENTRATION.
After a single oral dose of 400 mg, administered to 4 subjects, a mean peak plasma concentration of 45 µg/ml was attained in 2 to 4 hours (G. L. Smith *et al.*, *Br. J. clin. Pharmac.*, 1977, *4*, 585–590).

TOXICITY. Because of reports of adverse reactions and fatalities, benoxaprofen was withdrawn worldwide in 1982.

HALF-LIFE. Plasma half-life, about 30 to 35 hours; increased in renal impairment.

PROTEIN BINDING. In plasma, more than 99%.

Dose. Benoxaprofen has been given in doses of 600 mg daily.

Benperidol   *Tranquilliser*

Synonym. Benzperidol
Proprietary Names. Anquil; Frenactil; Glianimon.
1-{1-[3-(4-Fluorobenzoyl)propyl]-4-piperidyl}benzimidazolin-2-one
$C_{22}H_{24}FN_3O_2 = 381.4$
CAS—2062-84-2

An off-white amorphous powder or crystals. It darkens slowly on exposure to light. M.p. 170° to 175°.
Practically **insoluble** in water; soluble 1 in 1000 of ethanol, 1 in 4 of chloroform, and 1 in 625 of ether; sparingly soluble in dilute mineral acids.

Colour Tests. Koppanyi–Zwikker Test—violet; Mandelin's Test—violet; Mercurous Nitrate—black.

High Pressure Liquid Chromatography. *System HA*—k' 1.1.

Ultraviolet Spectrum. Aqueous acid—231 nm, 249 nm ($A_1^1 =$ 348 b), 279 nm; aqueous alkali—248 nm ($A_1^1 = 445$ b), 288 nm.

Infra-red Spectrum. Principal peaks at wavenumbers 1694, 757, 1587, 1162, 1204, 1219.

Mass Spectrum. Principal peaks at *m/z* 230, 109, 82, 187, 243, 363, 42, 123.

Quantification. GAS CHROMATOGRAPHY. In plasma: sensitivity 30 ng/ml, FID—M. P. Quaglio *et al.*, *Boll. chim.-farm.*, 1982, *121*, 276–284.

Dose. 0.25 to 1.5 mg daily.

Benserazide   *Dopa-decarboxylase Inhibitor*

Synonym. Serazide
DL-2-Amino-3-hydroxy-2'-(2,3,4-trihydroxybenzyl)propiono-hydrazide
$C_{10}H_{15}N_3O_5 = 257.2$
CAS—322-35-0

Benserazide Hydrochloride
Proprietary Names. It is an ingredient of Madopar and Prolopa.
$C_{10}H_{15}N_3O_5,HCl = 293.7$
CAS—14919-77-8; 14046-64-1
An off-white crystalline powder.
Soluble 1 in 3 of water, 1 in 118 of ethanol, 1 in 66 of acetone, 1 in 180 of chloroform, and 1 in 455 of ether.

Colour Tests. Ammoniacal Silver Nitrate—black; *p*-Dimethyl-aminobenzaldehyde—red/–; Ferric Chloride—green-brown; Folin–Ciocalteu Reagent—blue; Methanolic Potassium Hydroxide—red; Millon's Reagent—red-orange; Nessler's Reagent—black; Palladium Chloride—orange → brown; Potassium Dichromate—brown.

Thin-layer Chromatography. *System TA*—Rf 01; *system TB*—Rf 00; *system TC*—Rf 01.

Ultraviolet Spectrum. Aqueous acid—272 nm ($A_1^1 = 36.5$ b).

Infra-red Spectrum. Principal peaks at wavenumbers 1500, 1665, 1593, 1195, 1570, 1265 (KBr disk).

Wavelength

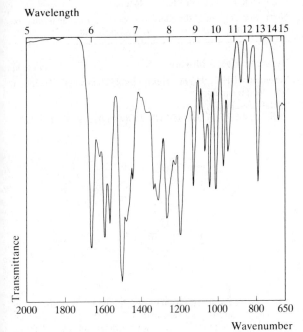

Mass Spectrum. Principal peaks at *m/z* 60, 42, 88, 30, 31, 43, 29, 70.

Disposition in the Body. Rapidly absorbed after oral administration and appears to be rapidly metabolised. About 50 to 60% of an oral dose and 80% of an intravenous dose is excreted in the urine in 24 hours, and about 30% and 10% of the respective doses are eliminated in the faeces in 7 days.

THERAPEUTIC CONCENTRATION.
After an oral dose of 50 mg of ^{14}C-benserazide hydrochloride, peak plasma concentrations of about 1 µg/ml were attained in 1 hour (D. E. Schwartz *et al.*, *Eur. J. clin. Pharmac.*, 1974, *7*, 39–45).

Dose. Usually the equivalent of 50 mg of benserazide daily, increasing to 100 to 250 mg daily (given in combination with levodopa in the treatment of parkinsonism).

Benzaldehyde   *Flavouring Agent*

Synonym. Artificial Essential Oil of Almond
$C_6H_5 \cdot CHO = 106.1$
CAS—100-52-7
A clear, colourless, strongly refractive liquid, with a characteristic odour of bitter almonds. It becomes yellowish on storage and oxidises in air to benzoic acid. B.p. about 179°. Refractive index, at 20°, 1.544 to 1.5465.
Soluble 1 in 350 of water; miscible with ethanol and ether.

Gas Chromatography. *System GA*—RI 947; *system GI*—retention time 34.2 min.

Ultraviolet Spectrum. Ethanol—245 nm ($A_1^1 = 1294$ b), 279 nm ($A_1^1 = 126$ b), 289 nm ($A_1^1 = 105$ b).

Infra-red Spectrum. Principal peaks at wavenumbers 1700, 1210, 1601, 1175, 1318, 753 (thin film).

Mass Spectrum. Principal peaks at *m/z* 77, 106, 105, 51, 50, 78, 52, 39.

Quantification. GAS CHROMATOGRAPHY. In blood: detection and identification of volatile compounds using head-space analysis and FID—J. D. Ramsey and R. J. Flanagan, *J. Chromat.*, 1982, *240*, 423–444.

GAS CHROMATOGRAPHY–MASS SPECTROMETRY. In serum: headspace analysis—A. Zlatkis *et al.*, *J. Chromat.*, 1974, *91*, 379–383.

Benzalkonium Chloride   *Cationic Disinfectant*

Proprietary Names. Benzalchlor-50; Cetal Conc. A and B; Empigen BAC; Hyamine 3500; Laudamonium; Morpan BC; Ovules Pharmatex; Quartamon; Roccal; Sabol; Silquat B10; Silquat B50; Vantoc CL; Zephiran. It is an ingredient of Polycide, Stomosol, and Timodine.

A mixture of alkylbenzyldimethylammonium chlorides of the general formula $[C_6H_5 \cdot CH_2 \cdot N(CH_3)_2 \cdot R]Cl$, in which R represents a mixture of the alkyls from C_8H_{17} to $C_{18}H_{37}$.
CAS—8001-54-5
A white or yellowish-white amorphous powder, thick gel, or gelatinous pieces. A solution in water gives a clear, colourless or pale yellow, syrupy liquid, which foams strongly when shaken.
Very **soluble** in water, ethanol, and acetone; practically insoluble in ether.

Ultraviolet Spectrum. Water—256 nm ($A_1^1 = 4.9$ b), 262 nm ($A_1^1 = 5.8$ b), 268 nm ($A_1^1 = 4.6$ b).

Infra-red Spectrum. Principal peaks at wavenumbers 702, 726, 780, 875, 1618, 1211 (thin film).

Benzbromarone   *Uricosuric*

Proprietary Names. Desuric; Narcaricin; Normurat; Uricovac M.
3,5-Dibromo-4-hydroxyphenyl 2-ethylbenzofuran-3-yl ketone
$C_{17}H_{12}Br_2O_3 = 424.1$
CAS—3562-84-3

Yellowish crystals. M.p. 151°.

Ultraviolet Spectrum. Methanolic acid—237 nm ($A_1^1 = 666$ b), 274 nm (inflexion), 281 nm ($A_1^1 = 314$ b); aqueous alkali—240 nm ($A_1^1 = 440$ b), 281 nm (inflexion), 355 nm ($A_1^1 = 513$ b).

Quantification. HIGH PRESSURE LIQUID CHROMATOGRAPHY. In serum: benzbromarone and benzarone, detection limits 140 and 90 ng/ml, respectively, UV detection—H. Vergin and G. Bishop, *J. Chromat.*, 1980, *183*; *Biomed. Appl.*, *9*, 383–386.

Disposition in the Body. Incompletely absorbed after oral administration. It is metabolised by debromination to bromobenzarone and benzarone which are both active metabolites. About 50% of a dose is excreted in the bile as free and conjugated (glucuronide) metabolites and less than 10% of a dose is excreted in the urine.

THERAPEUTIC CONCENTRATION.

Following a single oral dose of 100 mg to 7 subjects, peak plasma concentrations of 1.4 to 2.9 µg/ml (mean 2.2) of benzbromarone and 0.6 to 1.2 µg/ml (mean 0.8) of benzarone were attained in about 3 and 6 hours respectively (H. Ferber *et al.*, *Eur. J. clin. Pharmac.*, 1981, *19*, 431–435).

HALF-LIFE. Plasma half-life, benzbromarone about 3 hours, benzarone about 13 hours.

NOTE. For a review of benzbromarone see R. C. Heel *et al.*, *Drugs*, 1977, *14*, 349–366.

Dose. Usually 100 mg daily; up to 300 mg daily has been given.

Benzene   *Solvent*

Synonym. Phenyl Hydride
$C_6H_6 = 78.11$
CAS—71-43-2

A clear, colourless, mobile, inflammable liquid, with a characteristic aromatic odour, which burns with a smoky flame. B.p. 80°. It solidifies when cooled to 0°.

Practically **immiscible** with water; miscible with dehydrated alcohol, acetone, ether, and glacial acetic acid.

Gas Chromatography. *System GA*—RI 660; *system GI*—retention time 14.8 min.

Ultraviolet Spectrum. Ethanol—255 nm ($A_1^1 = 28$ b).

Mass Spectrum. Principal peaks at *m/z* 78, 77, 52, 51, 50, 39, 79, 74.

Quantification. GAS CHROMATOGRAPHY. In blood or tissues: head-space analysis, FID—W. D. Collom and C. L. Winek, *Clin. Toxicol.*, 1970, *3*, 125–130. In tissues—C. A. Snyder *et al.*, *Am. ind. Hyg. Ass. J.*, 1977, *38*, 272–276. In urine: phenol, detection limit 10 ng/ml, FID—D. L. Rick *et al.*, *J. analyt. Toxicol.*, 1982, *6*, 297–300.

Disposition in the Body. Benzene is absorbed from the gastro-intestinal tract, through the skin, and from the lungs. About 50% of inhaled benzene is retained in the body; eventually up to 50% of the retained benzene may be eliminated via the lungs, only very small amounts (approximately 0.1%) appearing unchanged in the urine. The remainder of the retained benzene is excreted in the urine, mainly as phenol together with small amounts of catechol and quinol. The excretion of phenol is highest in the first 24 hours and is complete within 48 hours of exposure. The phenolic metabolites are excreted mainly in the conjugated form as ethereal sulphates and glucuronides.

TOXICITY. The maximum permissible atmospheric concentration is 10 ppm or 30 mg/m³. Chronic poisoning may result from exposure to low concentrations over a period of time; 1500 ppm for an hour causes marked depression of the central nervous system and 7500 ppm for half an hour or 20000 ppm for a few minutes may cause death; chronic inhalation of as little as 100 ppm is likely to cause severe bone marrow depression. The ingestion of 10 ml has caused death.

In a death attributed to inhalation of benzene vapours (glue sniffing), the postmortem concentration of benzene in the blood was 0.94 µg/ml and in the kidney 5.5 µg/g (W. D. Collom and C. L. Winek, *Clin. Toxicol.*, 1970, *3*, 125–130).

The following postmortem tissue concentrations were reported in a fatality due to the ingestion of benzene: blood 38 µg/ml, brain 253 µg/g, kidney 21 µg/g, liver 105 µg/g, urine 20 µg/ml (A. Alha *et al.*, *Bull. int. Ass. forens. Toxicol.*, 1975, *11*(3), 9).

A 3-year-old child drank some benzene and died 2 hours later; postmortem concentrations were: brain 250 µg/g, kidney 20 µg/g, liver 800 µg/g (A. Heyndrickx *et al.*, *J. Pharm. Belg.*, 1966, *21*, 406–408).

HALF-LIFE. Plasma half-life, 9 to 24 hours.

NOTE. For a review of the effects on health of benzene inhalation see T. J. Haley, *Clin. Toxicol.*, 1977, *11*, 531–548.

Benzene Hexachloride   *Pesticide*

Synonyms. BHC; HCH; Hexachlorocyclohexane; Technical Benzene Hexachloride.
$C_6H_6Cl_6 = 290.8$
CAS—319-84-6 (α); *319-85-7* (β); *58-89-9* (γ); *319-86-8* (δ); *6108-10-7* (ε)

A mixture of the several isomers of 1,2,3,4,5,6-hexachlorocyclohexane; it contains not less than 12% of the gamma isomer. Benzene hexachloride has five known isomers designated alpha, beta, gamma, delta, and epsilon; of these only the gamma isomer (see Lindane) is outstandingly active as an insecticide.

White to light brown granules, flakes or powder, with a characteristic musty odour. M.p. α 159°, β 312°, γ 112°, δ 138°, ε 219°.

Practically **insoluble** in water; its solubility in organic solvents depends on the proportions of the various isomers present.

Gas Chromatography. *System GA*—α-isomer RI 1690, β-isomer RI 1710, δ-isomer RI 1755, γ-isomer RI 1745.

Infra-red Spectrum. Principal peaks at wavenumbers 688, 855, 704, 781, 917, 957 (Nujol mull).

Quantification. See under Lindane.

Disposition in the Body. Absorbed after ingestion, inhalation or through the skin. It is stored in the body fat and adrenal glands. The β-isomer accumulates on chronic exposure (see under Lindane).

TOXICITY. Benzene hexachloride has a greater chronic toxicity than lindane. Ingestion of 20 to 30 g may produce serious toxic effects but death is unlikely unless it is dissolved in an organic solvent.

Benzethonium Chloride   *Cationic Disinfectant*

Proprietary Names. Hyamine 1622; Phemerol Chloride.
Benzyldimethyl(2 - {2 - [4 - (1,1,3,3 - tetramethylbutyl)-phenoxy]ethoxy}ethyl)ammonium chloride
$C_{27}H_{42}ClNO_2 = 448.1$
CAS—121-54-0

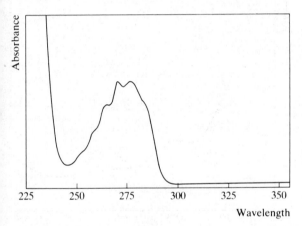

White crystals. A solution in water foams strongly when shaken. M.p. after drying, 158° to 163°.

Soluble 1 in 0.6 of water, 1 in 0.6 of ethanol, and 1 in 1 of chloroform; slightly soluble in ether; practically insoluble in light petroleum.

Colour Test. Marquis Test—orange.

Thin-layer Chromatography. *System TA*—Rf 03. (*Acidified iodoplatinate solution*, positive.)

Ultraviolet Spectrum. Aqueous acid—263 nm, 269 nm ($A_1^1 = 29$ c), 274 nm ($A_1^1 = 28$ c). No alkaline shift.

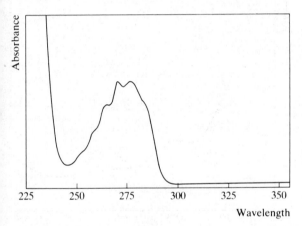

Infra-red Spectrum. Principal peaks at wavenumbers 1240, 1505, 1120, 826, 1063, 769 (KBr disk).

Use. Used as 0.1 to 0.2% solutions.

Benzhexol   *Anticholinergic*

Synonym. Trihexyphenidyl
1-Cyclohexyl-1-phenyl-3-piperidinopropan-1-ol
$C_{20}H_{31}NO = 301.5$
CAS—144-11-6

M.p. 114°.

Benzhexol Hydrochloride

Synonyms. Cyclodolum; Trihexyphenidylium Chloride.

Proprietary Names. Anti-Spas; Aparkane; Artane; Artilan; Broflex; Novohexidyl; Parkinane; Peragit; Pipanol; Tremin, Trixyl.
$C_{20}H_{31}NO,HCl = 337.9$
CAS—52-49-3
A white or creamy-white crystalline powder. M.p. about 250°, with decomposition.
Soluble 1 in 100 of water, 1 in 22 of ethanol, 1 in 15 of chloroform, and 1 in 10 of methanol; practically insoluble in ether.

Colour Tests. Mandelin's Test—grey-green; Marquis Test—grey-violet.

Thin-layer Chromatography. *System TA*—Rf 68; *system TB*—Rf 65; *system TC*—Rf 61. (*Acidified iodoplatinate solution*, positive.)

Gas Chromatography. *System GA*—RI 2219.

High Pressure Liquid Chromatography. *System HA*—k' 1.8.

Ultraviolet Spectrum. Aqueous acid—252 nm ($A_1^1 = 6$ c), 258 nm ($A_1^1 = 7$ c), 264 nm ($A_1^1 = 6$ c).

Infra-red Spectrum. Principal peaks at wavenumbers 702, 756, 973, 1206, 1196, 935 (benzhexol hydrochloride, KBr disk).

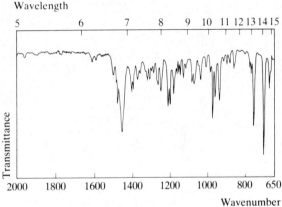

Mass Spectrum. Principal peaks at *m/z* 98, 105, 55, 41, 99, 77, 218, 84.

Disposition in the Body. Absorbed after oral administration; disappears rapidly from the tissues.

TOXICITY. In some patients, doses of more than 12 mg daily may produce severe mental disturbance and excitement.

The following postmortem concentrations were observed in a 16-year-old youth who experienced hallucinations and was found dead in a nearby lake 2 days after the ingestion of 20 mg of benzhexol: blood 0.03 µg/ml, urine 0.38 µg/ml (L. Kopjak and T. A. Jennison, *Bull. int. Ass. forens. Toxicol*, 1976, *12*(1), 8).

Dose. 1 to 15 mg of benzhexol hydrochloride daily.

Benzilonium Bromide   *Anticholinergic*

Proprietary Names. Portyn; Ulcoban.
3-Benziloyloxy-1,1-diethylpyrrolidinium bromide
$C_{22}H_{28}BrNO_3 = 434.4$
CAS—1050-48-2

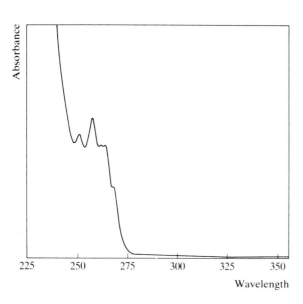

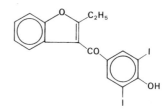

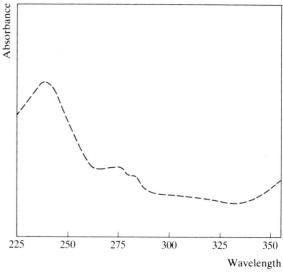

A white crystalline powder. M.p. 203° to 204°.
Soluble in water.

Colour Tests. The following tests are performed on benzilonium nitrate (see page 128): Liebermann's Test—brown; Marquis Test—orange → green → blue; Sulphuric Acid—orange.

Thin-layer Chromatography. *System TA*—Rf 03. (*Acidified iodoplatinate solution*, positive.)

Ultraviolet Spectrum. Aqueous acid—252 nm, 258 nm ($A_1^1 = 11$ a), 264 nm.

Infra-red Spectrum. Principal peaks at wavenumbers 1728, 1220, 1190, 1162, 690, 1052 (KBr disk).

Quantification. GAS CHROMATOGRAPHY–MASS SPECTROMETRY. In plasma: sensitivity 5 ng/ml—H. Dahlström *et al.*, *J. Chromat.*, 1980, *183*; *Biomed. Appl.*, *9*, 511–513.

Dose. 30 to 70 mg daily.

Benziodarone   *Anti-anginal Vasodilator*

Proprietary Name. Amplivix
2-Ethylbenzofuran-3-yl 4-hydroxy-3,5-di-iodophenyl ketone
$C_{17}H_{12}I_2O_3 = 518.1$
CAS—68-90-6

A yellowish powder. M.p. 167°.
Soluble 1 in about 500 of water at 25°, and 1 in about 100 of water at 45°; soluble in acetone and chloroform.

Thin-layer Chromatography. *System TD*—Rf 62; *system TE*—Rf 23; *system TF*—Rf 58.

Ultraviolet Spectrum. Methanol—240 nm ($A_1^1 = 1280$ b), 275 nm, 357 nm.

Infra-red Spectrum. Principal peaks at wavenumbers 1618, 756, 1577, 1135, 1293, 1176 (Nujol mull).

Mass Spectrum. Principal peaks at *m/z* 518, 173, 264, 519, 373, 376, 520, 249.

Dose. Benziodarone has been given in initial doses of 600 mg daily and maintenance doses of 300 to 400 mg daily.

Benzocaine   *Local Anaesthetic*

Synonyms. Anaesthesinum; Anesthamine; Éthoforme; Ethyl Aminobenzoate.
Proprietary Names. Americaine; Anaesthesin. It is an ingredient of AAA, Audicort, Auralgan, Auralgicin, Auraltone, Merocaine, Transvasin, Tyrosolven, and Tyrozets.
Ethyl 4-aminobenzoate
$C_9H_{11}NO_2 = 165.2$
CAS—94-09-7

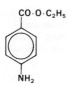

Colourless crystals or white crystalline powder. M.p. 88° to 92°.
Soluble 1 in 2500 of water, 1 in 8 of ethanol, 1 in 2 of chloroform, and 1 in 4 of ether; soluble in dilute acids.

Dissociation Constant. pK_a 2.8 (25°).

Colour Test. Diazotisation—red.

Thin-layer Chromatography. *System TA*—Rf 67; *system TB*—Rf 06; *system TC*—Rf 57; *system TD*—Rf 56; *system TE*—Rf 77; *system TF*—Rf 62; *system TL*—Rf 66. (*Ninhydrin spray*, positive; *acidified potassium permanganate solution*, positive; *Van Urk reagent*, bright yellow.)

Gas Chromatography. *System GA*—benzocaine RI 1555, 4-aminobenzoic acid RI 1547; *system GF*—RI 2100.

High Pressure Liquid Chromatography. *System HA*—k' 0.1; *system HQ*—k' 20.06; *system HR*—k' 1.61.

Ultraviolet Spectrum. Aqueous acid—272 nm ($A_1^1 = 90$ c), 278 nm; aqueous alkali—285 nm ($A_1^1 = 930$ a); ethanol—293 nm ($A_1^1 = 1238$ a).

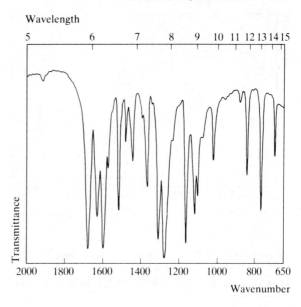

Wavelength

Wavenumber

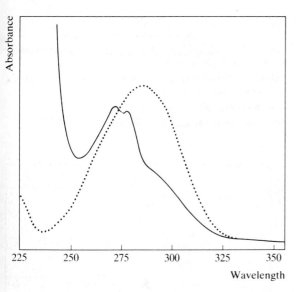

Wavelength

Infra-red Spectrum. Principal peaks at wavenumbers 1280, 1680, 1598, 1170, 1315, 1634 (KBr disk).

Mass Spectrum. Principal peaks at m/z 120, 165, 92, 65, 137, 39, 121, 93; 4-aminobenzoic acid 137, 120, 92, 65, 39, 138, 121, 63.

Disposition in the Body. Benzocaine is metabolised by hydrolysis to 4-aminobenzoic acid. At the concentrations normally used (2 to 10%) it is comparatively non-irritant and non-toxic, having only about one-tenth the toxicity of cocaine. The maximum safe amount for topical use is 5000 mg (25 ml of a 20% w/v solution).

Benzoctamine   *Tranquilliser*

N - (9,10 - Dihydro - 9,10 - ethanoanthracen - 9 - ylmethyl)-methylamine
$C_{18}H_{19}N = 249.4$
CAS—17243-39-9

Benzoctamine Hydrochloride
Proprietary Name. Tacitin(e)
$C_{18}H_{19}N,HCl = 285.8$
CAS—10085-81-1
A white crystalline powder. M.p. about 315°, with decomposition.

Soluble in water, ethanol, and chloroform; sparingly soluble in acetone and ether.

Colour Tests. Mandelin's Test—blue-green; Marquis Test—red-violet.

Thin-layer Chromatography. *System TA*—Rf 59; *system TB*—Rf 57; *system TC*—Rf 52. (*Acidified iodoplatinate solution*, positive.)

Gas Chromatography. *System GA*—RI 2082; *system GF*—RI 2445.

High Pressure Liquid Chromatography. *System HA*—k' 1.7.

Ultraviolet Spectrum. Aqueous acid—264 nm, 271 nm ($A_1^1 = 57$ a). (See below)

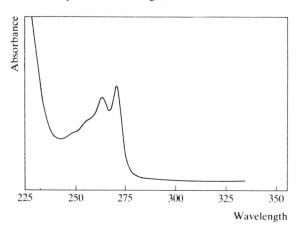

Infra-red Spectrum. Principal peaks at wavenumbers 757, 743, 732, 1134, 1060, 1020 (KBr disk).

Mass Spectrum. Principal peaks at m/z 218, 44, 191, 221, 219, 178, 42, 180.

Dose. 30 to 60 mg of benzoctamine hydrochloride daily.

Benzoic Acid   *Preservative*

Synonyms. Benzenecarboxylic Acid; Phenylformic Acid.
Proprietary Names. It is an ingredient of Aserbine and Malatex.
$C_6H_5 \cdot COOH = 122.1$
CAS—65-85-0
Colourless, light feathery crystals or white scales or powder. M.p. 121° to 124°. It sublimes on heating.
Soluble 1 in about 350 of water, 1 in 20 of boiling water, 1 in 3 of ethanol, 1 in 5 of chloroform, and 1 in 3 of ether; freely soluble in acetone.

Sodium Benzoate
$C_6H_5 \cdot CO_2Na = 144.1$
CAS—532-32-1
A white, amorphous, granular, flaky or crystalline powder.
Soluble 1 in 2 of water and 1 in 90 of ethanol.

Dissociation Constant. pK_a 4.2 (25°).

Partition Coefficient. Log P (octanol), 1.9.

Thin-layer Chromatography. *System TD*—Rf 26; *system TE*—Rf 07; *system TF*—Rf 39.

Gas Chromatography. *System GA*—RI 1180.

Ultraviolet Spectrum. Aqueous acid—230 nm ($A_1^1 = 923$ a), 273 nm ($A_1^1 \doteq 85$ a); methanol—227 nm ($A_1^1 = 895$ a), 272 nm ($A_1^1 = 73$ a), 280 nm ($A_1^1 = 61$ b).

Infra-red Spectrum. Principal peaks at wavenumbers 709, 1689, 1296, 667, 935, 685 (KBr disk).

Mass Spectrum. Principal peaks at m/z 105, 77, 51, 122, 50, 39, 74, 76; hippuric acid 105, 135, 51, 134, 77, 106, 50, 78.

Quantification. GAS CHROMATOGRAPHY. In plasma or urine: sensitivity 10 ng/ml, ECD—A. Sioufi and F. Pommier, *J. Chromat.*, 1980, *181*; *Biomed. Appl.*, 7, 161–168.

Disposition in the Body. Benzoic acid is metabolised in the liver by conjugation with glycine and is rapidly and completely excreted in the urine as hippuric acid. Normal urinary excretion of hippuric acid is 1 to 2.5 g daily, equivalent to 0.7 to 1.7 g of benzoic acid. When taken in large doses, a proportion may be excreted as benzoylglucuronic acid.
Benzoic acid may be found in the urine as a metabolite of benzaldehyde, and is also a metabolite of numerous other compounds.

Uses. Benzoic acid is used as a preservative in a concentration of 0.1%. Sodium benzoate is given by mouth in a dose of 6 g, to test liver function.

Benzonatate   *Cough Suppressant*

Synonyms. Benzonatine; Benzononatine.
Proprietary Name. Tessalon
3,6,9,12,15,18,21,24,27-Nonaoxaoctacosyl 4-butylaminobenzoate
$C_{13}H_{18}NO_2(OCH_2CH_2)_nOCH_3$, where n has an average value of 8.
CAS—104-31-4 (where $n = 8$)

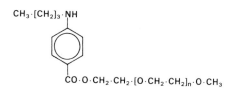

A clear, pale yellow, viscous liquid.
Miscible with water, ethanol, chloroform, and ether.

Colour Tests. Aromaticity (Method 2)—yellow/red; Liebermann's Test (at 100°)—blue.

Thin-layer Chromatography. *System TA*—Rf 61. (*Acidified iodoplatinate solution*, positive.)

Gas Chromatography. *System GA*—not eluted.

Ultraviolet Spectrum. Ethanol—308 nm ($A_1^1 = 473$ c).

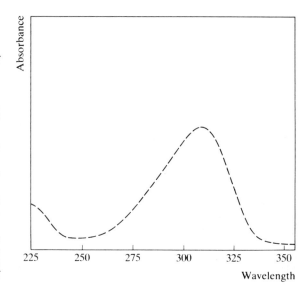

Infra-red Spectrum. Principal peaks at wavenumbers 1095, 1605, 1266, 1172, 1698, 1527 (KBr disk).

Mass Spectrum. Principal peaks at m/z 176, 59, 132, 150, 45, 193, 105, 29.

Dose. 300 to 600 mg daily.

Benzoylecgonine

Alkaloid

Synonym. Ecgonine Benzoate

$(1R,2R,3s,5S)$-2-Carboxytropan-3-yl benzoate

$C_{16}H_{19}NO_4 = 289.3$

CAS—519-09-5

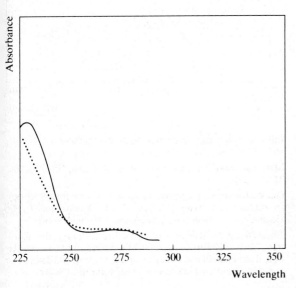

An alkaloid obtained from coca leaves, *Erythroxylum coca* (Erythroxylaceae) and its varieties.

The hydrated form occurs as crystals and melts at 86°. The anhydrous form melts at 195°, with decomposition.

Very **soluble** in hot water; soluble in ethanol; practically insoluble in ether; soluble in dilute acids and alkalis.

Thin-layer Chromatography. *System TA*—Rf 21; *system TB*—Rf 00; *system TC*—Rf 01. (*Acidified iodoplatinate solution*, positive.)

Gas Chromatography. *System GA*—RI 2570.

High Pressure Liquid Chromatography. *System HA*—k′ 0.9 (tailing peak); *system HQ*—k′ 5.68.

Ultraviolet Spectrum. Aqueous acid—234 nm ($A_1^1 = 376$ a), 274 nm.

Infra-red Spectrum. Principal peaks at wavenumbers 1275, 1720, 1618, 717, 1116, 1316.

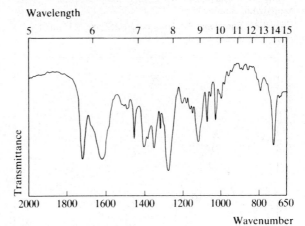

Mass Spectrum. Principal peaks at m/z 124, 82, 168, 77, 105, 42, 94, 83.

Quantification. See under Cocaine.

Disposition in the Body. Benzoylecgonine is the first hydrolysis product formed in the metabolism of cocaine; it is then further hydrolysed to ecgonine.

Benzphetamine

Anorectic

$(+)$-*N*-Benzyl-*N*α-dimethylphenethylamine

$C_{17}H_{21}N = 239.4$

CAS—156-08-1

$$C_6H_5 \cdot CH_2 \cdot CH \cdot N \cdot CH_2 \cdot C_6H_5$$

with CH₃ substituents: $\overset{CH_3}{\underset{CH_3}{}}$

A liquid.

Practically **immiscible** with water; miscible with ethanol, chloroform, and ether.

Benzphetamine Hydrochloride

Proprietary Names. Didrex; Inapétyl.

$C_{17}H_{21}N,HCl = 275.8$

CAS—5411-22-3

A white crystalline powder. M.p. about 131°.

Freely **soluble** in water, ethanol, and chloroform; slightly soluble in ether.

Dissociation Constant. pK$_a$ 6.6.

Colour Test. Marquis Test—orange.

Thin-layer Chromatography. *System TA*—Rf 73; *system TB*—Rf 67; *system TC*—Rf 70. (*Dragendorff spray*, positive; *acidified iodoplatinate solution*, positive; *Marquis reagent*, brown.)

Gas Chromatography. *System GA*—benzphetamine RI 1855, amphetamine RI 1123, methylamphetamine RI 1176; *system GB*—benzphetamine RI 1895, amphetamine RI 1134, methylamphetamine RI 1200; *system GC*—benzphetamine RI 2172, amphetamine RI 1536, methylamphetamine RI 1722; *system GF*—benzphetamine RI 2050, amphetamine RI 1315, methylamphetamine RI 1335.

High Pressure Liquid Chromatography. *System HA*—benzphetamine k' 1.2, amphetamine k' 0.9, methylamphetamine k' 2.0; *system HC*—benzphetamine k' 0.15, amphetamine k' 0.98, methylamphetamine k' 2.07.

Ultraviolet Spectrum. Aqueous acid—252 nm, 258 nm ($A_1^1 = 19$ c), 262 nm, 268 nm.

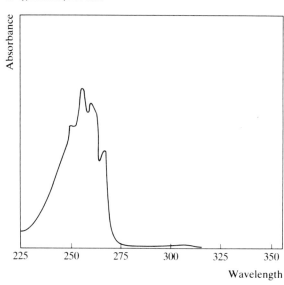

Infra-red Spectrum. Principal peaks at wavenumbers 1497, 740, 698, 1028, 1125, 1220 (KBr disk).

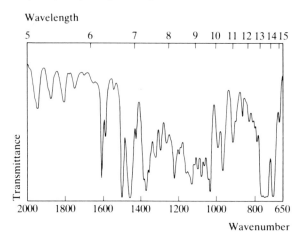

Mass Spectrum. Principal peaks at m/z 91, 148, 149, 65, 92, 42, 56, 39.

Quantification. ENZYME IMMUNOASSAY–GAS CHROMATOGRAPHY. In urine: benzphetamine, amphetamine, and methylamphetamine, sensitivity 150 ng/ml for benzphetamine and 50 ng/ml for amphetamine and methylamphetamine—R. D. Budd and N. C. Jain, *J. analyt. Toxicol.*, 1978, *2*, 241.

Disposition in the Body. Readily absorbed after oral administration and mainly excreted in the urine as amphetamine and methylamphetamine; very little is excreted as unchanged drug.

Dose. 25 to 150 mg of benzphetamine hydrochloride daily.

Benzquinamide   *Anti-emetic*

3-Diethylcarbamoyl-1,3,4,6,7,11b-hexahydro-9,10-dimethoxy-2H-benzo[a]quinolizin-2-yl acetate
$C_{22}H_{32}N_2O_5 = 404.5$
CAS—63-12-7

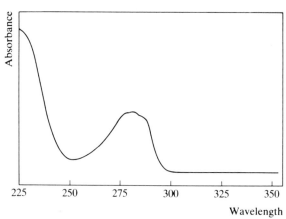

A yellowish crystalline powder. M.p. 130° to 131.5°.
Soluble in dilute acetic acid.

Benzquinamide Hydrochloride
Proprietary Name. Emete-con
$C_{22}H_{32}N_2O_5,HCl = 441.0$
CAS—113-69-9

Dissociation Constant. pK_a 5.9.

Colour Tests. Liebermann's Test—black; Marquis Test—yellow; Sulphuric Acid—orange.

Thin-layer Chromatography. *System TA*—Rf 65; *system TB*—Rf 07; *system TC*—Rf 69. (*Acidified iodoplatinate solution*, positive.)

High Pressure Liquid Chromatography. *System HA*—k' 0.3.

Ultraviolet Spectrum. Aqueous acid—282 nm ($A_1^1 = 95$ b). No alkaline shift.

Infra-red Spectrum. Principal peaks at wavenumbers 1244, 1733, 1633, 1204, 1515, 1123 (KBr disk).

Mass Spectrum. Principal peaks at m/z 205, 244, 191, 345, 206, 72, 272, 246.

Quantification. GAS CHROMATOGRAPHY–MASS SPECTROMETRY. In plasma: sensitivity 10 ng/ml—D. C. Hobbs and A. G. Connolly, *J. Pharmacokinet. Biopharm.*, 1978, *6*, 477–485.

Disposition in the Body. Readily absorbed after oral administration; bioavailability about 35%. Metabolised by O-demethylation, deacetylation and N-dealkylation. After an oral dose, up to about 7% is excreted unchanged in the urine in 24 hours.

THERAPEUTIC CONCENTRATION.
Following oral administration of 200 mg to 20 subjects, a mean peak plasma concentration of 0.6 µg/ml was attained in 1.2 hours. Following intramuscular injection of 50 mg to 20 subjects, a mean peak plasma concentration of 0.7 µg/ml was attained in 0.26 hour (D. C. Hobbs and A. G. Connolly, *ibid.*).

HALF-LIFE. Plasma half-life, about 1 hour.

VOLUME OF DISTRIBUTION. About 1 litre/kg.

REFERENCE. D. C. Hobbs and A. G. Connolly, *ibid.*

Dose. The equivalent of 50 mg of benzquinamide by intramuscular injection, repeated as necessary.

Benzthiazide   *Diuretic*

Proprietary Names. Aquatag; Exna; Hydrex. It is an ingredient of Decaserpyl Plus and Dytide.

3-Benzylthiomethyl-6-chloro-2*H*-1,2,4-benzothiadiazine-7-sulphonamide 1,1-dioxide
$C_{15}H_{14}ClN_3O_4S_3 = 431.9$
CAS—91-33-8

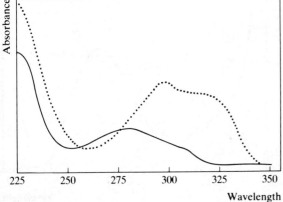

A white crystalline powder. M.p. about 240°.
Practically **insoluble** in water, chloroform, and ether; slightly soluble in ethanol; soluble 1 in 100 of acetone; freely soluble in dimethylformamide and in solutions of alkalis.

Colour Tests. Koppanyi–Zwikker Test—violet; Liebermann's Test—red-brown; Sulphuric Acid—yellow.

Thin-layer Chromatography. *System TD*—Rf 14; *system TE*—Rf 09; *system TF*—Rf 51.

Gas Chromatography. *System GA*—RI 2680.

High Pressure Liquid Chromatography. *System HN*—k' 9.32.

Ultraviolet Spectrum. Aqueous acid—283 nm ($A_1^1 = 292$ a); aqueous alkali—297 nm ($A_1^1 = 310$ b).

Infra-red Spectrum. Principal peaks at wavenumbers 1180, 1160, 1310, 1502, 1620, 1590 (KBr disk).

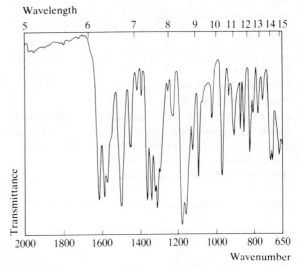

Mass Spectrum. Principal peaks at *m/z* 91, 121, 65, 122, 309, 64, 230, 123.

Quantification. HIGH PRESSURE LIQUID CHROMATOGRAPHY. In plasma, urine or faeces: sensitivity 10 ng/ml in plasma and 50 ng/ml in urine, UV detection—M. C. Meyer *et al.*, *Biopharm. Drug Disp.*, 1982, **3**, 1–9.

Disposition in the Body. Poorly absorbed after oral administration. Less than 10% of a dose is excreted in the urine as unchanged drug in 48 hours, and about 80% of a dose is eliminated in the faeces.

THERAPEUTIC CONCENTRATION.
Following an oral dose of 50 mg to 4 subjects, peak plasma concentrations of about 0.008 and 0.02 µg/ml were attained in 3 hours in 2 subjects; in the remaining 2 subjects benzthiazide was not detectable in the plasma (M. C. Meyer *et al.*, *ibid.*).

HALF-LIFE. Derived from urinary excretion data, about 10 to 15 hours.

REFERENCE. M. C. Meyer *et al.*, *ibid.*

Dose. 50 to 200 mg daily.

Benztropine   *Anticholinergic*

Synonym. Benzatropine
(1*R*,3*r*,5*S*)-3-Benzhydryloxytropane
$C_{21}H_{25}NO = 307.4$
CAS—86-13-5

Soluble in chloroform.

Benztropine Mesylate

Synonyms. Benztropine Methanesulphonate; Tropine Diphenylmethyl Ether.

Proprietary Names. Bensylate; Cogentin.

$C_{21}H_{25}NO,CH_4O_3S = 403.5$

CAS—132-17-2

A white, slightly hygroscopic, crystalline powder. M.p. 141° to 145°.

Soluble 1 in 0.7 of water, 1 in 1.5 of ethanol, and 1 in 2 of chloroform; practically insoluble in ether.

Dissociation Constant. pK_a 10.0 (20°).

Partition Coefficient. Log P (heptane), 0.4.

Colour Tests. Mandelin's Test—yellow; Marquis Test—yellow.

Thin-layer Chromatography. *System TA*—Rf 13; *system TB*—Rf 26; *system TC*—Rf 06. (*Acidified iodoplatinate solution*, positive.)

Gas Chromatography. *System GA*—RI 2314.

High Pressure Liquid Chromatography. *System HA*—k' 3.7 (tailing peak).

Ultraviolet Spectrum. Aqueous acid—253 nm, 259 nm ($A_1^1 = 14.5$ a).

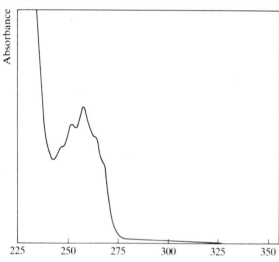

Infra-red Spectrum. Principal peaks at wavenumbers 1054, 700, 742, 1191, 1204, 1075 (KBr disk).

Mass Spectrum. Principal peaks at *m/z* 83, 140, 82, 124, 96, 97, 42, 125.

Disposition in the Body. Absorbed after oral administration.

TOXICITY.

In a fatality attributed to the ingestion of an unknown quantity of benztropine tablets, the following postmortem concentrations were reported: blood 0.7 µg/ml, liver 1.6 µg/g, urine 0.8 µg/ml. In a second case a liver concentration of 2.3 µg/g was found (G. del Villar and M. Liddy, *Bull. int. Ass. forens. Toxicol.*, 1976, *12*(2), 11–12).

Dose. 0.5 to 6 mg of benztropine mesylate daily.

Benzydamine   *Analgesic*

Synonym. Benzindamine

3-(1-Benzyl-1*H*-indazol-3-yloxy)-*NN*-dimethylpropylamine

$C_{19}H_{23}N_3O = 309.4$

CAS—642-72-8

M.p. 38° to 39°.

Benzydamine Hydrochloride

Proprietary Names. Afloben; A-Termadol; Difflam; Imotryl; Multum; Tantum; Verax.

$C_{19}H_{23}N_3O,HCl = 345.9$

CAS—132-69-4

A white crystalline powder. M.p. about 159°.

Soluble 1 in 1 of water, 1 in 8 of ethanol, and 1 in 4 of chloroform; practically insoluble in ether.

Colour Test. Mandelin's Test—brown-green.

Thin-layer Chromatography. *System TA*—Rf 44; *system TB*—Rf 36; *system TC*—Rf 22. (*Acidified iodoplatinate solution*, positive.)

Gas Chromatography. *System GA*—RI 2368.

Ultraviolet Spectrum. Aqueous acid—307 nm ($A_1^1 = 144$ c). No alkaline shift.

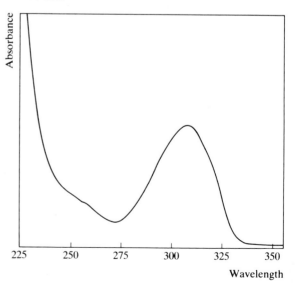

Infra-red Spectrum. Principal peaks at wavenumbers 1529, 740, 1491, 1613, 1182, 1141 (KBr disk).

Mass Spectrum. Principal peaks at m/z 85, 58, 86, 91, 84, 70, 42, 225.

Quantification. ULTRAVIOLET SPECTROPHOTOMETRY. In plasma or urine—K. Andersson and H. Larsson, *Arzneimittel-Forsch.*, 1974, *24*, 1686–1688.

Disposition in the Body. Absorbed after oral administration. About 50% of a dose is excreted unchanged in the urine.

THERAPEUTIC CONCENTRATION.

An oral dose of 1 mg/kg produced a blood concentration of about 0.8 µg/ml within 2 hours and a significant concentration was maintained for several hours (B. Catanese *et al.*, *Arzneimittel-Forsch.*, 1966, *16*, 1354–1357).

PROTEIN BINDING. A fraction of benzydamine is bound to proteins in the blood.

REFERENCE. B. Catanese *et al.*, *ibid*.

Dose. 150 to 200 mg of benzydamine hydrochloride daily.

Benzyl Alcohol

Local Anaesthetic/Disinfectant

Synonyms. Phenylcarbinol; Phenylmethanol.
$C_6H_5 \cdot CH_2OH = 108.1$
CAS—100-51-6
A colourless liquid with a faint aromatic odour. Wt per ml 1.043 to 1.046 g. B.p. 203° to 208°.
Soluble 1 in 25 of water; miscible with ethanol, chloroform, and ether.

Gas Chromatography. *System GA*—RI 1046.

Ultraviolet Spectrum. Methanol—252 nm ($A_1^1 = 14$ b), 258 nm ($A_1^1 = 17$ b), 264 nm ($A_1^1 = 13$ b).

Mass Spectrum. Principal peaks at m/z 79, 77, 108, 101, 51, 50, 39, 40.

Use. Topically in concentrations of up to 10%.

Benzyl Benzoate

Acaricide

Proprietary Names. Antiscabiosum Mago; Ascabiol; Benzemul; Scabanca.
$C_6H_5 \cdot CO \cdot O \cdot CH_2 \cdot C_6H_5 = 212.2$
CAS—120-51-4
Colourless crystals or a clear colourless oily liquid. B.p. about 320°.
Practically **insoluble** in water; miscible with ethanol, acetone, carbon disulphide, chloroform, and ether.

Gas Chromatography. *System GA*—RI 1738.

Ultraviolet Spectrum. Ethanol—230 nm ($A_1^1 = 843$ b).

Infra-red Spectrum. Principal peaks at wavenumbers 1263, 1706, 1106, 713, 698, 1067 (thin film).

Mass Spectrum. Principal peaks at m/z 77, 105, 91, 51, 65, 212, 50, 78.

Disposition in the Body. Rapidly hydrolysed to benzoic acid and benzyl alcohol; benzyl alcohol then undergoes further oxidation to benzoic acid followed by conjugation with glycine to form hippuric acid. Excreted in the urine mainly as hippuric acid.

Uses. Topically as a 25% application; a 5% solution is used as an insect repellent.

Benzyl Nicotinate

Topical Vasodilator

Proprietary Names. Rubriment. It is an ingredient of Bayolin.
$C_{13}H_{11}NO_2 = 213.2$
CAS—94-44-0

A liquid.

Colour Tests. Cyanogen Bromide—red-orange; Liebermann's Test—brown; Sulphuric Acid—orange.

Thin-layer Chromatography. *System TA*—Rf 63; *system TB*—Rf 42; *system TC*—Rf 71. (*Acidified potassium permanganate solution, positive.*)

Ultraviolet Spectrum. Methanol—262 nm ($A_1^1 = 152$ b).

Infra-red Spectrum. Principal peaks at wavenumbers 1278, 1724, 1108, 740, 699, 1587 (KCl disk).

Use. Topically in a concentration of 2.5%.

Benzylmorphine

Narcotic Analgesic/Antitussive

3-*O*-Benzylmorphine
$C_{24}H_{25}NO_3 = 375.5$
CAS—14297-87-1

A colourless crystalline powder. M.p. 132°.
Soluble 1 in 2500 of water.

Benzylmorphine Hydrochloride
$C_{24}H_{25}NO_3,HCl = 411.9$
CAS—630-86-4
A colourless microcrystalline powder.
Soluble 1 in 200 of water and 1 in 160 of ethanol; practically insoluble in chloroform and ether.

Dissociation Constant. pK_a 8.1 (20°).

Colour Test. Marquis Test—red → violet.

Thin-layer Chromatography. *System TA*—Rf 41; *system TB*—Rf 06; *system TC*—Rf 23. (*Acidified iodoplatinate solution, positive.*)

Gas Chromatography. *System GA*—RI 3015.

High Pressure Liquid Chromatography. *System* ?? ? ? ? ? (tailing peak), *system HC*—κ 1.03.

Ultraviolet Spectrum. Aqueous acid—284 nm ($A_1^1 = 48$ b). (See below)

Infra-red Spectrum. Principal peaks at wavenumbers 1274, 1040, 1502, 1017, 763, 1056.

Mass Spectrum. Principal peaks at m/z 284, 91, 375, 81, 42, 36, 285, 175.

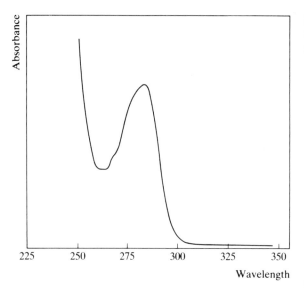

Wavelength

Dose. Benzylmorphine hydrochloride was formerly given in doses of 8 to 30 mg.

Benzylpenicillin   *Antibiotic*

Synonyms. Crystalline Penicillin G; Penicillin; Penicillin G.

Note. The name 'benzylpenicillin' and its synonyms are commonly used to describe either benzylpenicillin potassium or benzylpenicillin sodium.

(6R)-6-(2-Phenylacetamido)penicillanic acid
$C_{16}H_{18}N_2O_4S = 334.4$
CAS—61-33-6

An antimicrobial acid produced by the growth of certain strains of *Penicillium notatum*.

Benzylpenicillin Potassium

Proprietary Names. Abbocillin-G; Crystapen G; Falapen; Hyasorb; M-Cillin B; Megacillin; Novopen; P-50; Paclin G; Pentids; Pfizerpen; Sugracillin.

Note. Megacillin is also used as a proprietary name for clemizole penicillin, phenoxymethylpenicillin, and procaine penicillin.

$C_{16}H_{17}KN_2O_4S = 372.5$
CAS—113-98-4

A white, finely crystalline powder. M.p. 214° to 217°, with decomposition. Very **soluble** in water; soluble in ethanol; practically insoluble in chloroform and ether.

Benzylpenicillin Sodium

Proprietary Names. Crystapen; Gonopen; Spécilline G. It is an ingredient of Bicillin and Triplopen.

Note. Bicillin is also used as a proprietary name for benzathine penicillin.

$C_{16}H_{17}N_2NaO_4S = 356.4$
CAS—69-57-8

A white to slightly yellow, finely crystalline powder. Very **soluble** in water; soluble in ethanol; practically insoluble in chloroform and ether.

Dissociation Constant. pK_a 2.8 (25°).

Ultraviolet Spectrum. Benzylpenicillin sodium: water—257 nm ($A_1^1 = 7$ b), 264 nm, 325 nm.

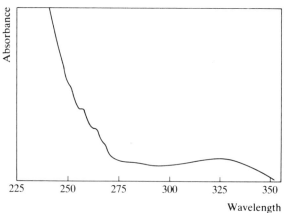

Wavelength

Infra-red Spectrum. Principal peaks at wavenumbers 1620, 1777, 1500, 1310, 1700, 703 (benzylpenicillin sodium, KBr disk).

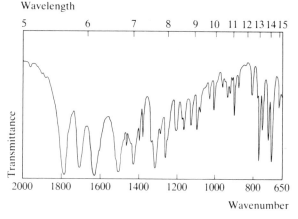

Disposition in the Body. About 30% of an oral dose is absorbed, the remainder being inactivated by gastric acid; maximum concentrations are attained about 1 hour after oral administration. After intramuscular injection it is rapidly absorbed, peak concentrations being attained in 15 to 30 minutes. About 60 to 90% of an intramuscular dose is excreted in the urine, mainly in the first few hours; the urinary material consists of unchanged drug and penicilloic acid (about 20% of the dose). Biliary excretion also occurs.

THERAPEUTIC CONCENTRATION. In plasma, minimum inhibitory concentration 0.006 to 2 μg/ml.

HALF-LIFE. Plasma half-life, about 0.5 to 1 hour; increased in infants, elderly subjects and in renal impairment.

DISTRIBUTION IN BLOOD. Plasma: whole blood ratio, 1.6.

PROTEIN BINDING. In plasma, 45 to 65%.

NOTE. For a review of the pharmacokinetics of penicillin antibiotics see M. Barza and L. Weinstein, *Clin. Pharmacokinet.*, 1976, *1*, 297–308.

Dose. 0.6 to 2.4 g daily, given parenterally; up to 24 g daily in severe infections.

Bephenium Hydroxynaphthoate   *Anthelmintic*

Synonym. Naphthammonum
Proprietary Name. Alcopar(a)
Benzyldimethyl(2-phenoxyethyl)ammonium 3-hydroxy-2-naph-
thoate
$C_{28}H_{29}NO_4 = 443.5$
CAS—7181-73-9 (bephenium); *3818-50-6* (hydroxynaphthoate)

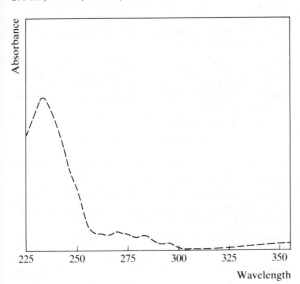

A yellow to greenish-yellow crystalline powder, which gives a
green fluorescence when examined under ultraviolet light. M.p.
168° to 173°, with decomposition.
Practically **insoluble** in water; soluble 1 in 50 of ethanol.

Colour Tests. Mandelin's Test—green; Marquis Test—red-
violet.

Thin-layer Chromatography. *System TA*—Rf 77. (*Acidified
potassium permanganate solution*, positive.)

Ultraviolet Spectrum. Methanol—234 nm ($A_1^1 = 1300$ b), 263 nm,
270 nm, 283 nm, 295 nm, 352 nm.

Infra-red Spectrum. Principal peaks at wavenumbers 1233, 768,
1653, 1590, 858, 726 (KBr disk).

Quantification. COLORIMETRY. In urine—E. W. Rogers, *Br. med.
J.*, 1958, *2*, 1576–1577.

Disposition in the Body. Poorly absorbed after oral administration; less than 1% of a dose is excreted in the urine in 24 hours.

Dose. The equivalent of 2.5 g of bephenium, as a single dose.

Berberine   *Alkaloid*

5,6 - Dihydro - 9,10 - dimethoxybenzo[*g*] - 1,3 - benzodioxolo[5,
6-*a*]quinolizinium hydroxide
$C_{20}H_{19}NO_5 = 353.4$
CAS—2086-83-1 ($C_{20}H_{18}NO_4^+$); *117-74-8* ($C_{20}H_{18}NO_4 \cdot OH$)

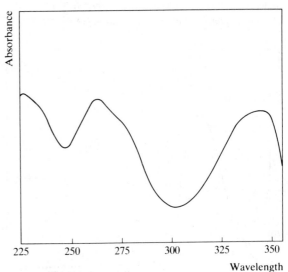

A quaternary alkaloid present in hydrastis, in various species of
Berberis, and in many other plants.
Yellow crystals. M.p. 144°.
Soluble 1 in 4.5 of water and 1 in 100 of ethanol; very slightly
soluble in ether.

Berberine Hydrochloride
Synonym. Berberine Chloride
$C_{20}H_{18}ClNO_4,2H_2O = 407.8$
CAS—633-65-8 (anhydrous); *5956-60-5* (dihydrate)
Bright yellow acicular crystals or powder.
Soluble 1 in 400 of water; freely soluble in boiling water; soluble in
ethanol; practically insoluble in chloroform and ether.

Berberine Sulphate
Synonyms. Berberine Acid Sulphate; Berberine Bisulphate.
$C_{20}H_{18}NO_4,HSO_4 = 433.4$
CAS—633-66-9
Bright yellow acicular crystals or dark yellow powder.
Soluble 1 in about 150 of water; slightly soluble in ethanol.

Partition Coefficient. Log *P* (octanol), −2.1.

Colour Tests. Mandelin's Test—blue-green → brown; Marquis
Test—green.

Thin-layer Chromatography. *System TA*—Rf 07. (*Acidified
iodoplatinate solution*, positive.)

Gas Chromatography. *System GA*—RI 2070.

Ultraviolet Spectrum. Aqueous acid—264 nm ($A_1^1 = 554$ b),
345 nm.

Infra-red Spectrum. Principal peaks at wavenumbers 1505, 1271,
1234, 1030, 1587, 1098 (KBr disk).

Mass Spectrum. Principal peaks at *m/z* 321, 278, 320, 292, 306, 191, 322, 304.

Quantification. GAS CHROMATOGRAPHY–MASS SPECTROMETRY. In urine: sensitivity 1 ng/ml—H. Miyazaki *et al.*, *J. Chromat.*, 1978, *152*, 79–86.

Disposition in the Body. After oral administration, less than 0.1% of a dose is excreted in the urine unchanged in 24 hours.

Dose. Berberine sulphate has been given in doses of 150 mg daily.

Betahistine   *Vasodilator*

N-Methyl-2-(2-pyridyl)ethylamine
$C_8H_{12}N_2 = 136.2$
CAS—5638-76-6

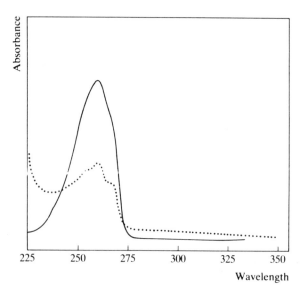

A liquid. B.p. about 114°.
Miscible with water, ethanol, chloroform, and ether.

Betahistine Hydrochloride
Proprietary Names. Betaserc; Microser; Serc; Vasomotal.
$C_8H_{12}N_2,2HCl = 209.1$
CAS—5579-84-0
A white or creamy-white, hygroscopic, crystalline powder. M.p. about 152°.
Freely **soluble** in water; soluble in ethanol and methanol; practically insoluble in carbon tetrachloride, chloroform, and ether.

Dissociation Constant. pK_a 3.5, 9.7.

Thin-layer Chromatography. *System TA*—Rf 10. (*Acidified iodoplatinate solution*, strong reaction.)

Gas Chromatography. *System GA*—RI 1235.

High Pressure Liquid Chromatography. *System HA*—k' 3.1.

Ultraviolet Spectrum. Aqueous acid—261 nm ($A_1^1 = 358$ b).

Infra-red Spectrum. Principal peaks at wavenumbers 1585, 1560, 1290, 762, 1238, 1145 (KBr disk).

Mass Spectrum. Principal peaks at *m/z* 79, 105, 104, 51, 78, 52, 50, 77.

Quantification. GAS CHROMATOGRAPHY. In serum: sensitivity 600 ng/ml, FID—J. F. Douglas and T. L. Hohing, *Experientia*, 1978, *34*, 499–500.

Disposition in the Body. Readily absorbed after oral administration; peak plasma concentrations of the metabolites are attained in 3 to 5 hours. Most of a dose is excreted in the urine as metabolites.

Dose. 24 to 48 mg of betahistine hydrochloride daily.

Betaine   *Treatment of Hypochlorhydria*

Synonyms. Glycine Betaine; Glycocoll Betaine; Lycine; Oxy-neurine; Trimethylglycine.
(Carboxymethyl)trimethylammonium hydroxide inner salt
$C_5H_{11}NO_2 = 117.1$
CAS—107-43-7

$$(CH_3)_3N^+ \cdot CH_2 \cdot COO^-$$

Deliquescent crystals. M.p. about 310°, with decomposition.
Soluble 1 in 0.6 of water and 1 in 11 of ethanol; sparingly soluble in ether; soluble 1 in 2 of methanol.

Betaine Hydrochloride
Proprietary Names. It is an ingredient of Acidol-Pepsin and Kloref.
$C_5H_{11}NO_2,HCl = 153.6$
CAS—590-46-5
Colourless crystals or white crystalline powder. When dissolved in water betaine hydrochloride hydrolyses and almost 25% of its weight of hydrochloric acid is formed. M.p. about 230°, with decomposition.
Soluble 1 in 2 of water and 1 in 20 of ethanol (90%); practically insoluble in chloroform and ether.

Dissociation Constant. pK_a 1.8 (25°).

Colour Test. To an aqueous solution add *iodine solution*—red precipitate.

Thin-layer Chromatography. *System TA*—Rf 23. (*Acidified iodoplatinate solution*, positive.)

Ultraviolet Spectrum. No significant absorption, 230 to 360 nm.

Infra-red Spectrum. Principal peaks at wavenumbers 1731, 1206, 885, 994, 902, 1250 (KBr disk).

Dose. 0.18 to 3.5 g of betaine hydrochloride daily.

Betamethasone   *Corticosteroid*

Synonyms. Flubenisolonum; 9α-Fluoro-16β-methylprednis-olone.

Proprietary Names. Betnelan; Betnesol; Celeston(e); Desacort-Beta; Minisone; No-Reumar; Pertene.

9α-Fluoro-11β,17α,21-trihydroxy-16β-methylpregna-1,4-diene-3,20-dione
$C_{22}H_{29}FO_5 = 392.5$
CAS—378-44-9

Absorbance (y-axis) vs Wavelength (x-axis: 225, 250, 275, 300, 325, 350)

Betamethasone is a synthetic glucocorticoid and an isomer of dexamethasone.

A white to creamy-white crystalline powder. M.p. about 240°, with decomposition. A solution in dioxan is dextrorotatory.

Practically **insoluble** in water; soluble 1 in 75 of ethanol, 1 in 15 of warm ethanol, and 1 in 1100 of chloroform; very slightly soluble in ether; sparingly soluble in acetone and methanol.

Betamethasone Acetate

$C_{24}H_{31}FO_6 = 434.5$
CAS—987-24-6

A white to creamy-white powder. M.p. about 165° and, with decomposition, 200° to 220°.

Practically **insoluble** in water; soluble 1 in 9 of ethanol and 1 in 16 of chloroform; freely soluble in acetone.

Betamethasone Benzoate

Proprietary Names. Beben; Benisone; Uticort.
$C_{29}H_{33}FO_6 = 496.6$
CAS—22298-29-9

A white powder. M.p. about 220°, with decomposition.

Practically **insoluble** in water; soluble in ethanol, chloroform, and methanol.

Betamethasone Dipropionate

Proprietary Name. Diprosone
$C_{28}H_{37}FO_7 = 504.6$
CAS—5593-20-4

A white or creamy-white powder. M.p. 170° to 179°, with decomposition. Practically **insoluble** in water; sparingly soluble in ethanol; freely soluble in acetone and chloroform.

Betamethasone Sodium Phosphate

Synonym. Betamethasone Disodium Phosphate
Proprietary Names. Bentelan; Betameson; Betnesol; Celeston(e); Emilan; Paucisone; Vista-Methasone.
$C_{22}H_{28}FNa_2O_8P = 516.4$
CAS—151-73-5

A white hygroscopic powder.
Soluble 1 in 2 of water and 1 in 350 of dehydrated alcohol; freely soluble in methanol; practically insoluble in acetone, chloroform, and ether.

Betamethasone Valerate

Synonym. 9α-Fluoro-16β-methylprednisolone 17-Valerate
Proprietary Names. Bedermin; Betacort; Betaderm; Betnelan-V; Betnesol-V; Betneval; Betnovat(e); Bextasol; Celestoderm(-V); Celestone-V; Dermovaleas; Ecoval; Valisone.
$C_{27}H_{37}FO_6 = 476.6$
CAS—2152-44-5

A white to creamy-white powder. M.p. about 190°, with decomposition. Practically **insoluble** in water; soluble 1 in 12 to 1 in 16 of ethanol, 1 in 2 of chloroform, and 1 in 50 of isopropyl alcohol; freely soluble in acetone; slightly soluble in ether.

Note. In alkaline media betamethasone 17-valerate undergoes a rearrangement to betamethasone 21-valerate.

Colour Tests. Antimony Pentachloride—green → brown; Naphthol–Sulphuric Acid—green-brown/orange-brown; Sulphuric Acid—pink-orange.

Thin-layer Chromatography. Betamethasone: *system TP*—Rf 30; *system TQ*—Rf 00; *system TR*—Rf 00; *system TS*—Rf 00. (*DPST solution.*) Betamethasone valerate: *system TP*—Rf 58; *system TQ*—Rf 27; *system TR*—Rf 20; *system TS*—Rf 02, streaking may occur. (*DPST solution.*) Betamethasone sodium phosphate remains on the baseline in all systems.

Ultraviolet Spectrum. Betamethasone: ethanol—240 nm ($A_1^1 = 390$ a). Betamethasone sodium phosphate: water—241 nm ($A_1^1 = 296$ a).

Infra-red Spectrum. Principal peaks at wavenumbers 1660, 1617, 1606, 1710, 1056, 907 (KBr disk).

Wavelength

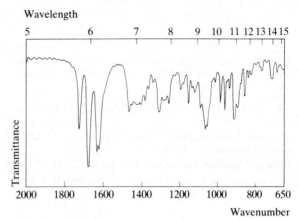

Mass Spectrum. Principal peaks at *m/z* 121, 43, 122, 223, 147, 91, 41, 135.

Dose. 0.5 to 9 mg daily.

Betanaphthol   *Parasiticide*

Synonyms. β-Naftol; Naphthol.
2-Naphthol
$C_{10}H_8O = 144.2$
CAS—135-19-3

White crystalline leaflets or powder; stable in air but darkens on exposure to light. M.p. 121° to 123°. B.p. 285° to 286°.

Soluble 1 in 1000 of cold water, 1 in 80 of boiling water, 1 in 2 of ethanol, and 1 in 1.5 of ether; soluble in chloroform and in solutions of alkali hydroxides.

Colour Tests. Ferric Chloride—green; Liebermann's Test—green.

To 200 mg add 2 ml of an 8% sodium hydroxide solution and 1 drop of chloroform, then warm—blue.

Ultraviolet Spectrum. Ethanol—274 nm ($A_1^1 = 326$ b), 285 nm ($A_1^1 = 230$ b), 322 nm ($A_1^1 = 120$ b), 330 nm ($A_1^1 = 140$ b).

Disposition in the Body. Rapidly absorbed from the gastrointestinal tract and may be absorbed through intact skin. It is excreted mainly as the glucuronide and gives a reddish tint to the urine.

TOXICITY. The estimated minimum lethal dose is 2 g. Severe nephritis and fatalities have occurred following its absorption through intact skin.

Bethanechol Chloride   *Parasympathomimetic*

Synonym. Carbamylmethylcholine Chloride
Proprietary Names. Duvoid; Mechothane; Myotonachol; Myotonine Chloride; Urecholine; Urocarb; Vesicholine.
(2-Carbamoyloxypropyl)trimethylammonium chloride
$C_7H_{17}ClN_2O_2 = 196.7$
CAS—674-38-4 (bethanechol); *590-63-6* (chloride)

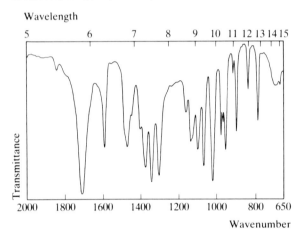

Colourless or white hygroscopic crystals, or white crystalline powder. There are two crystalline forms, one melts at about 211° and the other at about 219°.

Soluble 1 in 1 of water and 1 in 10 of ethanol, less soluble in dehydrated alcohol; practically insoluble in chloroform and ether.

Thin-layer Chromatography. *System TA*—Rf 02. (*Acidified iodoplatinate solution*, positive.)

Ultraviolet Spectrum. No significant absorption, 230 to 360 nm.

Infra-red Spectrum. Principal peaks at wavenumbers 1712, 1014, 1300, 1062, 1094, 946 (KBr disk).

Mass Spectrum. Principal peaks at m/z 43, 58, 42, 143, 85, 171, 157, 102.

Dose. 15 to 200 mg daily.

Bethanidine   *Antihypertensive*

Synonym. Betanidine
1-Benzyl-2,3-dimethylguanidine
$C_{10}H_{15}N_3 = 177.2$
CAS—55-73-2

Crystals. M.p. 195° to 197°.

Bethanidine Sulphate

Proprietary Names. Esbaloid; Esbatal; Regulin.
$(C_{10}H_{15}N_3)_2, H_2SO_4 = 452.6$
CAS—114-85-2
A white crystalline powder. M.p. about 280°.

Soluble 1 in 1 of water and 1 in 30 of ethanol; practically insoluble in ether.

Dissociation Constant. pK_a 12 (20°).

Colour Tests. Liebermann's Test—orange → brown; Marquis Test—orange-red.

Thin-layer Chromatography. *System TA*—Rf 01; *system TB*—Rf 00; *system TC*—Rf 00. (*Dragendorff spray*, positive.)

Gas Chromatography. *System GA*—RI 1925.

Ultraviolet Spectrum. Aqueous acid—252 nm, 258 nm ($A_1^1 = 11$ a), 264 nm. No alkaline shift.

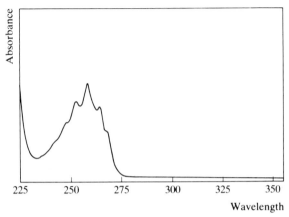

Infra-red Spectrum. Principal peaks at wavenumbers 1630, 1111, 1174, 701, 1192, 1066 (bethanidine sulphate, KBr disk).

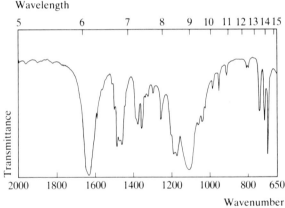

Mass Spectrum. Principal peaks at m/z 71, 91, 106, 177, 57, 72, 65, 30.

Quantification. SPECTROFLUORIMETRY. In plasma: sensitivity 4 ng/ml—C. N. Corder *et al., J. pharm. Sci.,* 1975, *64,* 785–788.

GAS CHROMATOGRAPHY–MASS SPECTROMETRY. In plasma or urine: guanethidine and other guanido-containing drugs, sensitivity 1 ng/ml—J. H. Hengstmann *et al., Analyt. Chem.,* 1974, *46,* 34–39.

HIGH PRESSURE LIQUID CHROMATOGRAPHY. In plasma: detection limit 20 ng/ml, UV detection—J. R. Shipe *et al., Clin. Chem.,* 1983, *29,* 1793–1795.

Disposition in the Body. Readily but incompletely absorbed after oral administration. It does not appear to be metabolised. After an intravenous dose, about 90% is excreted unchanged in the urine in 3 to 4 days; after an oral dose, 50 to 85% is excreted in the urine and up to about 50% is eliminated in the faeces.

THERAPEUTIC CONCENTRATION. In plasma, usually in the range 0.02 to 0.5 µg/ml.

After a single oral dose of 10 mg to 3 subjects, peak plasma concentrations of about 0.02 to 0.15 µg/ml were attained in 2 hours (C. N. Corder *et al.*, *J. pharm. Sci.*, 1975, *64*, 785–788).

After daily oral administration of 30 to 150 mg in divided doses to 12 subjects, steady-state plasma concentrations of 0.02 to 0.5 µg/ml (mean 0.12) were reported (C. N. Corder *et al.*, *J. clin. Pharmac.*, 1978, *18*, 249–258).

HALF-LIFE. The plasma half-life is multiphasic and there is considerable intersubject variation; after intravenous administration, plasma half-lives of about 2 to 6 hours and terminal half-lives of several days have been reported.

PROTEIN BINDING. In plasma, not significantly bound.

Dose. 20 to 200 mg of bethanidine sulphate daily.

Bezafibrate   *Lipid Regulating Agent*

Proprietary Names. Bezalip; Cedur.

2 - [4 - (2 - *p* - Chlorobenzamidoethyl)phenoxy] - 2 - methylpropionic acid
$C_{19}H_{20}ClNO_4 = 361.8$
CAS—41859-67-0

An off-white crystalline powder. M.p. 183° to 186°.
Practically **insoluble** in water; slightly soluble in ethanol, acetone, and methanol; soluble in dimethylformamide.

Ultraviolet Spectrum. Methanol—230 nm ($A_1^1 = 644$ b).

Infra-red Spectrum. Principal peaks at wavenumbers 1715, 1540, 1610, 1140, 1500, 1220 (KBr disk).

Dose. 400 to 600 mg daily.

Bezitramide   *Narcotic Analgesic*

Synonym. Burgodin

4 - [4 - (2,3 - Dihydro - 2 - oxo - 3 - propionyl - 1*H* - benzimidazol - 1 - yl)piperidino]-2,2-diphenylbutyronitrile
$C_{31}H_{32}N_4O_2 = 492.6$
CAS—15301-48-1

A white, amorphous or crystalline powder. M.p. 145° to 149°.
Practically **insoluble** in water and ethanol; soluble 1 in 45 of acetone, 1 in 2 of chloroform, and 1 in 400 of ether.

Colour Test. Mandelin's Test—violet → orange.

Thin-layer Chromatography. *System TA*—Rf 71; *system TB*—Rf 41; *system TC*—Rf 79. (*Acidified iodoplatinate solution*, positive.)

High Pressure Liquid Chromatography. *System HA*—k′ 0.2.

Ultraviolet Spectrum. After solution in chloroform and dilution with acid isopropyl alcohol—251 nm ($A_1^1 = 118$ b), inflexion at 274 nm.

Infra-red Spectrum. Principal peaks at wavenumbers 1733, 755, 1708, 700, 1286, 1054 (KBr disk).

Mass Spectrum. Principal peaks at *m/z* 286, 300, 96, 42, 244, 230, 301, 82.

Quantification. GAS CHROMATOGRAPHY. In urine: 3-cyano-3,3-diphenylpropionic acid, sensitivity 600 ng/ml, AFID—H. H. van Rooy *et al.*, *J. Chromat.*, 1978, *148*, 447–452.

HIGH PRESSURE LIQUID CHROMATOGRAPHY. In urine: 1,3-dihydro-1-(piperidin-4-yl)benzimidazol-2-one, sensitivity 150 ng/ml, UV detection—H. H. van Rooy and C. Soe-Agnie, *J. Chromat.*, 1978, *156*, 189–195.

Disposition in the Body. Absorbed after oral administration. It is metabolised by hydrolysis to 3-cyano-3,3-diphenylpropionic acid and 1,3-dihydro-1-(piperidin-4-yl)benzimidazol-2-one which are excreted in the urine.

THERAPEUTIC CONCENTRATION.

Following a single oral dose of 5 mg to 7 subjects, peak plasma concentrations (bezitramide plus major metabolite) of about 0.005 µg/ml were attained in about 3 hours; in 3 of the subjects, plasma concentrations remained fairly constant over a period of 7 hours; in a further 2 subjects, distinct secondary peak plasma concentrations were observed (D. K. F. Meijer *et al.*, *Eur. J. clin. Pharmac.*, 1984, *27*, 615–618).

Dose. Bezitramide has been given in doses of 5 mg; maximum of 30 mg in 24 hours.

Bialamicol   *Anti-amoebic*

Synonyms. Biallylamicol; Biethylamicol.
3,3′-Diallyl-5,5′-bis(diethylaminomethyl)biphenyl-4,4′-diol
$C_{28}H_{40}N_2O_2 = 436.6$
CAS—493-75-4

Bialamicol Hydrochloride
Proprietary Name. Camoform
$C_{28}H_{40}N_2O_2,2HCl = 509.6$
CAS—3624-96-2
A white crystalline powder. M.p. about 210°.
Soluble 1 in 5 of water, 1 in 40 of ethanol, and 1 in 150 of chloroform; slightly soluble in ether.

Colour Tests. Folin–Ciocalteu Reagent—blue; Liebermann's Test—green.

Dissolve 100 mg in 2 ml of water and add 2 ml of *nitric acid*—intense orange-red.

Thin-layer Chromatography. *System TA*—Rf 74; *system TB*—Rf 62; *system TC*—Rf 80.

Ultraviolet Spectrum. Aqueous acid—266 nm ($A_1^1 = 440$ a).

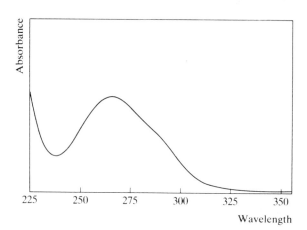

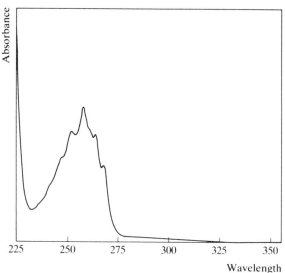

Mass Spectrum. Principal peaks at *m/z* 58, 30, 363, 44, 72, 29, 27, 364.

Disposition in the Body. Rapidly absorbed from the gastrointestinal tract and stored in high concentrations in the liver, lungs and tissues. Slowly excreted in the bile and eliminated in the faeces.

Dose. Bialamicol hydrochloride has been given in doses of 0.75 to 1.5 g daily.

Bibenzonium Bromide   *Cough Suppressant*

Synonym. Diphenetholine Bromide
Proprietary Name. Lysobex
[2-(1,2-Diphenylethoxy)ethyl]trimethylammonium bromide
$C_{19}H_{26}BrNO = 364.3$
CAS—59866-76-1 (bibenzonium); *15585-70-3* (bromide)

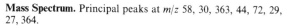

Crystals. M.p. 142° to 144°.
Very **soluble** in water and ethanol; practically insoluble in ether.

Colour Tests. The following tests are performed on bibenzonium nitrate (see page 128): Mandelin's Test—green; Marquis Test—brown.

Thin-layer Chromatography. *System TA*—Rf 02. (*Acidified iodoplatinate solution*, positive.)

Gas Chromatography. *System GA*—RI 1923.

Ultraviolet Spectrum. Aqueous acid—253 nm, 258 nm ($A_1^1 = 11.4$ b), 264 nm, 268 nm.

Infra-red Spectrum. Principal peaks at wavenumbers 705, 1095, 749, 759, 1020, 952 (KBr disk).

Dose. 40 to 120 mg daily.

Biperiden   *Anticholinergic*

1-(Bicyclo[2.2.1]hept-5-en-2-yl)-1-phenyl-3-piperidinopropan-1-ol
$C_{21}H_{29}NO = 311.5$
CAS—514-65-8

A white crystalline powder. M.p. 112° to 116°.
Practically **insoluble** in water; soluble 1 in 75 of ethanol, 1 in 2 of chloroform, and 1 in 14 of ether.

Biperiden Hydrochloride
Proprietary Names. Akineton (tablets); Akinophyl.
$C_{21}H_{29}NO,HCl = 347.9$
CAS—1235-82-1
A white crystalline powder. M.p. about 275°, with decomposition.
Slightly **soluble** in water, ethanol, chloroform, and ether; sparingly soluble in methanol.

Biperiden Lactate
Proprietary Name. Akineton (injection)
$C_{21}H_{29}NO,C_3H_6O_3 = 401.5$
CAS—7085-45-2

Colour Tests. Liebermann's Test—brown; Marquis Test—red-brown; Sulphuric Acid—orange-brown.

Thin-layer Chromatography. *System TA*—Rf 64; *system TB*—Rf 68; *system TC*—Rf 64. (*Acidified iodoplatinate solution*, positive.)

Gas Chromatography. *System GA*—RI 2266.

Ultraviolet Spectrum. Aqueous acid—252 nm, 259 nm ($A_1^1 =$ 5.6 b), 264 nm.

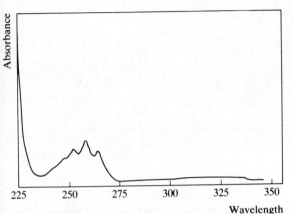

Infra-red Spectrum. Principal peaks at wavenumbers 702, 735, 1121, 997, 760, 1153 (Nujol mull).

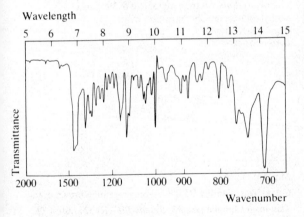

Mass Spectrum. Principal peaks at m/z 98, 218, 99, 55, 41, 42, 77, 84.

Quantification. GAS CHROMATOGRAPHY (CAPILLARY COLUMN). In plasma: sensitivity 250 pg/ml, AFID–Th. Le Bris and E. Brode, *Arzneimittel-Forsch.*, 1985, *35*, 149–151.

Disposition in the Body. Rapidly absorbed after oral administration.

THERAPEUTIC CONCENTRATION.
Following a single oral dose of 4 mg to 6 subjects, peak plasma concentrations of 0.004 to 0.006 µg/ml were attained in 1.5 hours (M. Hollman *et al.*, *Eur. J. clin. Pharmac.*, 1984, *27*, 619–621).

HALF-LIFE. Plasma half-life, about 18 hours.

Dose. 2 to 12 mg of biperiden hydrochloride daily, by mouth. Biperiden lactate is given parenterally in doses of 5 to 20 mg daily.

Bisacodyl   *Purgative*

Proprietary Names. Bisacolax; Biscolax; Contlax; Deficol; Delco-Lax; Dulcolax; Laco; Laxbene; Perilax; Theralax; Toilax. It is an ingredient of Dulcodos.
4,4′-(2-Pyridylmethylene)di(phenyl acetate)
$C_{22}H_{19}NO_4 = 361.4$
CAS—603-50-9

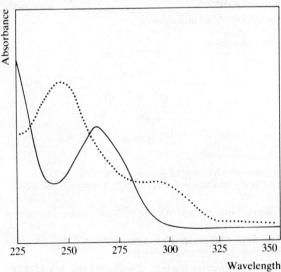

A white crystalline powder. M.p. 131° to 135°.
Very slightly **soluble** in water; soluble 1 in 100 of ethanol, 1 in 35 of chloroform, and 1 in 170 of ether; sparingly soluble in methanol; soluble in dilute acids.

Colour Tests. Liebermann's Test—red-brown; Mandelin's Test—violet; Marquis Test—violet.

Thin-layer Chromatography. *System TA*—Rf 74; *system TB*—Rf 15; *system TC*—Rf 76. (*Acidified iodoplatinate solution*, positive.)

Gas Chromatography. *System GA*—RI 2820.

Ultraviolet Spectrum. Aqueous acid—264 nm ($A_1^1 = 270$ a); methanolic potassium hydroxide—248 nm ($A_1^1 = 650$ a).

Infra-red Spectrum. Principal peaks at wavenumbers 1212, 1198, 1754, 1162, 1500, 909 (KBr disk). (See below)

Mass Spectrum. Principal peaks at m/z 361, 277, 319, 276, 199, 318, 362, 43.

Quantification. HIGH PRESSURE LIQUID CHROMATOGRAPHY. In urine: bisacodyl diphenol, sensitivity 1 µg/ml, UV detection— L. Loof *et al.*, *Ther. Drug Monit.*, 1980, *2*, 345–349.

Wavelength

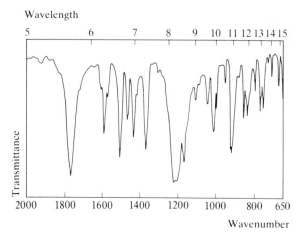

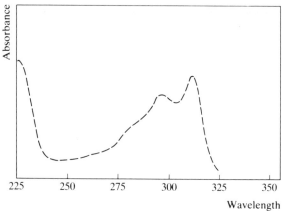

Wavenumber

Wavelength

THIN-LAYER CHROMATOGRAPHY–COLORIMETRY. In urine: bisa-codyl diphenol—R. Jauch *et al.*, *Arzneimittel-Forsch.*, 1975, *25*, 1796–1800.

Disposition in the Body. Variably absorbed after oral administra-tion and metabolised by deacetylation to the active metabolite, bis(4-hydroxyphenyl)-2-pyridylmethane (bisacodyl diphenol). Up to about 30% of a dose is excreted in the urine in 48 hours as bisacodyl diphenol glucuronide; about 50% of a dose is eliminated in the faeces as unconjugated bisacodyl diphenol.

Dose. 5 to 10 mg daily.

Bitoscanate   *Anthelmintic*

Phenylene-1,4-bisisothiocyanate
$C_8H_4N_2S_2 = 192.3$
CAS—4044-65-9

A yellowish-white crystalline powder. M.p. 130° to 132°.
Practically **insoluble** in water; soluble in ethanol, chloroform, and ether.

Colour Tests. Mandelin's Test—brown-violet; Palladium Chloride—orange.

Thin-layer Chromatography. *System TA*—Rf 65. (*Acidified potassium permanganate solution*, positive.)

Ultraviolet Spectrum. Ethanol—296 nm, 311 nm ($A_1^1 = 1795$ a).

Disposition in the Body. Partly absorbed after oral administration. About 28% of a dose is excreted in the urine in 30 days and 55% is eliminated in the faeces, mainly in the first week.

THERAPEUTIC CONCENTRATION.

Following a single oral dose of 100 mg of ^{14}C-labelled bitoscanate to 6 subjects, peak blood concentrations of total radioactivity equivalent to 0.58 to 2.1 µg/ml (mean 1.4) of bitoscanate were reported at about 24 hours (O. E. Christ *et al.*, *Arzneimittel-Forsch.*, 1970, *20*, 756–762).

HALF-LIFE. Plasma half-life (total radioactivity), about 26 hours.
REFERENCE. O. E. Christ *et al.*, *ibid.*

Dose. 100 mg at 12-hourly intervals for 3 doses.

Brallobarbitone   *Barbiturate*

Synonym. Brallobarbital
Proprietary Name. It is an ingredient of Vesparax.
5-Allyl-5-(2-bromoallyl)barbituric acid
$C_{10}H_{11}BrN_2O_3 = 287.1$
CAS—561-86-4

M.p. 168° to 169°.

Colour Test. Vanillin Reagent—brown-orange/brown-orange.

Thin-layer Chromatography. *System TD*—Rf 52; *system TE*—Rf 30; *system TF*—Rf 69; *system TH*—Rf 47.

Gas Chromatography. *System GA*—brallobarbitone RI 1858, 5-acetonyl-5-allylbarbituric acid RI 1795; *system GF*—RI 2765.

High Pressure Liquid Chromatography. *System HG*—k' 3.09; *system HH*—k' 1.72.

Ultraviolet Spectrum. *Borax buffer 0.05M* (pH 9.2)—240 nm ($A_1^1 = 304$ b); M sodium hydroxide (pH 13)—256 nm ($A_1^1 = 236$ b).

Mass Spectrum. Principal peaks at *m/z* 207, 41, 39, 124, 91, 165, 122, 44.

Quantification. See under Amylobarbitone.

Disposition in the Body. Absorbed after oral administration. About 5% of a dose is excreted in the urine as unchanged drug, 9% as 5-acetonyl-5-allylbarbituric acid and less than 1% each as 5-acetonyl-5-(2-bromoallyl)barbituric acid and 5-allyl-5-(2-hydroxypropyl)barbituric acid.

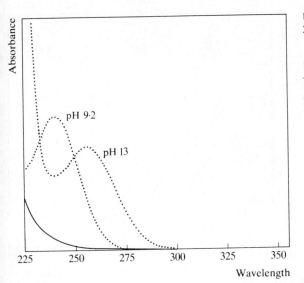

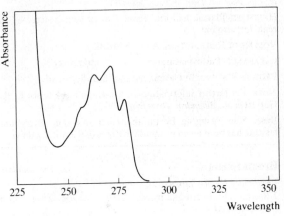

Ultraviolet Spectrum. Aqueous acid—263 nm, 272 nm ($A_1^1 =$ 22 a), 278 nm. No alkaline shift.

Infra-red Spectrum. Principal peaks at wavenumbers 1188, 1012, 1032, 1120, 680, 815 (KBr disk).

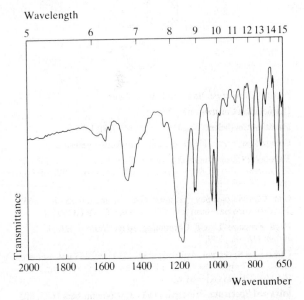

TOXICITY.

In 10 fatalities involving the ingestion of a preparation containing brallobarbitone, quinalbarbitone and hydroxyzine, the following post-mortem concentrations, $\mu g/g$ (mean, n) were reported:

	Brallobarbitone	Quinalbarbitone
Blood	9.8–25 (16.3, 9)	10–33.4 (17.7, 9)
Brain	1.9–24.1 (12.7, 10)	8.6–50 (29.3, 10)
Kidney	8.9–28.1 (20.4, 10)	14.5–83.4 (30.6, 10)
Liver	14.9–241 (50.2, 10)	23.1–231 (95.7, 10)
Urine	1.8–201 (40.8, 6)	1.0–7.1 (4.0, 6)

(G. Sticht and H. Kaferstein, *Z. Rechtsmed.*, 1980, *85*, 169–175).

In an overdose involving the ingestion of more than 3 g of brallobarbitone (in combination with quinalbarbitone), plasma concentrations of 106 μg/ml of brallobarbitone and 57 μg/ml of quinalbarbitone were reported 6 hours and 4 hours, respectively, after ingestion; the subject slowly recovered after treatment by haemoperfusion (G. de Groot *et al.*, *Vet. Hum. Toxicol.*, 1979, *21*, 8–11).

Bretylium Tosylate   *Anti-arrhythmic/Antihypertensive*

Synonym. Bretylium Tosilate

Proprietary Names. Bretylate; Bretylol.

(2-Bromobenzyl)ethyldimethylammonium toluene-4-sulphonate $C_{11}H_{17}BrN,C_7H_7O_3S = 414.4$

CAS—59-41-6 (bretylium); *61-75-6* (tosylate).

A white crystalline powder. M.p. about 98°.

Soluble 1 in 1 of water and 1 in 0.4 of ethanol; practically insoluble in ether.

Thin-layer Chromatography. *System TA*—Rf 01; *system TN*—Rf 94; *system TO*—Rf 40. (*Acidified iodoplatinate solution*, positive.)

High Pressure Liquid Chromatography. *System HA*—k' 4.3 (tailing peak).

Quantification. GAS CHROMATOGRAPHY. In plasma or urine: sensitivity 5 ng/ml, ECD—C.-M. Lai *et al.*, *J. pharm. Sci.*, 1980, *69*, 681–683. In plasma, urine or myocardial tissue: sensitivity 1 ng/ml, ECD—E. Patterson *et al.*, *J. Chromat.*, 1980, *181*; *Biomed. Appl.*, 7, 33–39.

Disposition in the Body. Poorly absorbed after oral administration; bioavailability about 25%. Excreted mainly in the urine as unchanged drug but a high proportion of bretylium is also excreted into the bile. After intravenous infusion about 70% of the dose is excreted in the urine in 24 hours and 90% in 48 hours. After chronic oral dosing about 20% of a dose is excreted in the 24-hour urine.

THERAPEUTIC CONCENTRATION.

After a single oral dose of 5 mg/kg to 10 subjects, peak serum concentrations of 0.04 to 0.14 μg/ml (mean 0.08) were attained in 1 to 8 hours; following intravenous infusion of 5 mg/kg over 30 minutes to the same subjects, serum concentrations at the end of the infusion were reported to be in the range 1.1 to 2.4 µg/ml (mean 1.9) (J. L. Anderson *et al.*, *Clin. Pharmac. Ther.*, 1980, *28*, 468–478).

HALF-LIFE. Plasma half-life, about 7 to 10 hours, increased in renal impairment.

VOLUME OF DISTRIBUTION. About 8 litres/kg.

CLEARANCE. Plasma clearance, about 11 ml/min/kg.

PROTEIN BINDING. In plasma, not significantly bound.

NOTE. For further information on bretylium tosylate see E. R. Garrett *et al.*, *Biopharm. Drug Disp.*, 1982, *3*, 129–164.

Dose. 5 to 10 mg/kg by intramuscular injection. Bretylium tosylate has been given by mouth in doses of 0.3 to 1.2 g daily.

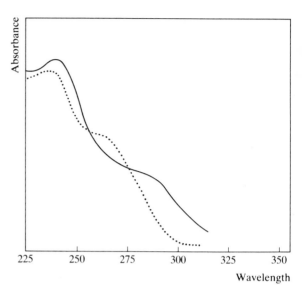

Bromazepam   *Tranquilliser*

Proprietary Names. Lexotan; Lexotanil.
7-Bromo-1,3-dihydro-5-(2-pyridyl)-2H-1,4-benzodiazepin-2-one
$C_{14}H_{10}BrN_3O = 316.2$
CAS—1812-30-2

A pale yellow crystalline solid. M.p. about 247°.

Dissociation Constant. pK_a 2.9, 11.0.

Partition Coefficient. Log P (octanol/pH 7.4), 1.6.

Colour Test. Formaldehyde–Sulphuric Acid—yellow.

Thin-layer Chromatography. *System TA*—Rf 61; *system TB*—Rf 12; *system TC*—Rf 41; *system TD*—Rf 13; *system TE*—Rf 62; *system TF*—Rf 20.

Gas Chromatography. *System GA*—bromazepam RI 2663, 3-hydroxybromazepam RI 2537; *system GG*—RI 3280.

High Pressure Liquid Chromatography. *System HI*—k' 2.32; *system HK*—k' 2.99.

Ultraviolet Spectrum. Aqueous acid—239 nm, 345 nm; aqueous alkali—237 nm ($A_1^1 = 920$ b), 348 nm; methanol—233 nm ($A_1^1 = 1050$ b), 320 nm ($A_1^1 = 61$ b).

Infra-red Spectrum. Principal peaks at wavenumbers 1685, 825, 750, 802, 1315, 1230.

Mass Spectrum. Principal peaks at *m/z* 236, 317, 315, 288, 316, 286, 208, 78; 3-hydroxybromazepam 79, 78, 52, 105, 304, 314, 316, 51.

Quantification. GAS CHROMATOGRAPHY. In plasma: sensitivity 5 ng/ml, ECD—U. Klotz, *J. Chromat.*, 1981, *222*; *Biomed. Appl.*, *11*, 501–506.

HIGH PRESSURE LIQUID CHROMATOGRAPHY. In plasma: sensitivity 5 ng/ml, UV detection–H. Hirayama *et al.*, *J. Chromat.*, 1983, *277*; *Biomed. Appl.*, *28*, 414–418.

Disposition in the Body. Well absorbed after oral administration. About 70% of a dose is excreted in the urine in 72 hours, including about 2% of the dose as unchanged bromazepam, about 28% as the glucuronide of 3-hydroxybromazepam, about

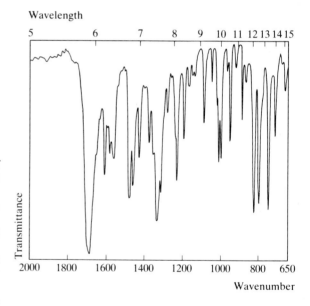

39% as the glucuronide of 2-amino-3-hydroxy-5-bromobenzoyl-pyridine, and less than 1% as 2-(2-amino-5-bromobenz-oyl)pyridine.

THERAPEUTIC CONCENTRATION.

After a single oral dose of 12 mg, administered to 10 subjects, peak plasma concentrations of 0.11 to 0.17 µg/ml (mean 0.13) were attained in 1 to 4 hours. Steady-state concentrations of 0.08 to 0.15 µg/ml (mean 0.12) were measured during dosing of 6 subjects with 9 mg daily (S. A. Kaplan *et al.*, *J. Pharmacokinet. Biopharm.*, 1976, *4*, 1–16).

HALF-LIFE. Plasma half-life, 8 to 19 hours (mean 12).

VOLUME OF DISTRIBUTION. About 0.9 litre/kg.

PROTEIN BINDING. In plasma, 40 to 70%.

Dose. Usually 6 to 9 mg daily; up to 36 mg daily has been given.

Bromhexine
Mucolytic Expectorant

N-(2-Amino-3,5-dibromobenzyl)-*N*-cyclohexylmethylamine
$C_{14}H_{20}Br_2N_2 = 376.1$
CAS—3572-43-8

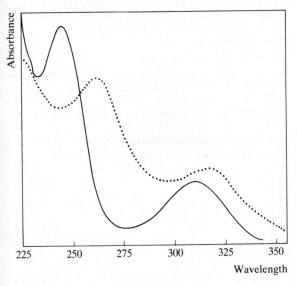

Bromhexine Hydrochloride
Proprietary Names. Bisolvon; Broncokin; Dakryo Biciron; Ophtosol. It is an ingredient of Alupent Expectorant and Bisolvomycin.

$C_{14}H_{20}Br_2N_2,HCl = 412.6$
CAS—611-75-6
A white crystalline powder. M.p. about 235°.
Soluble 1 in 250 of water, 1 in 100 of ethanol, 1 in 300 of chloroform, and 1 in 50 of methanol; practically insoluble in acetone; soluble in glacial acetic acid.

Thin-layer Chromatography. *System TA*—Rf 75; *system TB*—Rf 67; *system TC*—Rf 79. (*Acidified iodoplatinate solution*, positive.)

Gas Chromatography. *System GA*—RI 2337.

High Pressure Liquid Chromatography. *System HA*—k' 0.4.

Ultraviolet Spectrum. Aqueous acid—245 nm ($A_1^1 = 259$ a), 310 nm; aqueous alkali—262 nm, 317 nm.

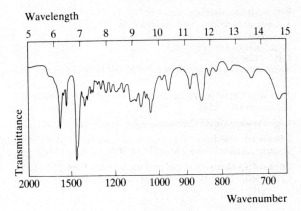

Infra-red Spectrum. Principal peaks at wavenumbers 1602, 1031, 1074, 1548, 1122, 857 (KBr disk).

Mass Spectrum. Principal peaks at *m/z* 70, 112, 293, 264, 44, 42, 305, 41.

Quantification. GAS CHROMATOGRAPHY. In plasma: sensitivity 1 ng/ml, ECD—A. P. DeLeenheer and L. M. R. Vandecasteele-Thienpont, *J. pharm. Sci.*, 1980, *69*, 99–100.

HIGH PRESSURE LIQUID CHROMATOGRAPHY. In plasma or urine: detection limit 4 ng/ml in plasma and 2 ng/ml in urine, UV detection—E. Bechgaard and A. Nielsen, *J. Chromat.*, 1982, *228*; *Biomed. Appl.*, *17*, 392–397.

Disposition in the Body. Well absorbed after oral administration but undergoes considerable first-pass metabolism including conjugation with glucuronic acid or sulphate; ambroxol, *trans*-4-(2-amino-3,5-dibromobenzylamino)cyclohexanol, is an active metabolite of bromhexine. About 70% of an oral dose is excreted in the urine in 24 hours as metabolites with less than 1% as unchanged drug.

THERAPEUTIC CONCENTRATION.

Following single oral doses of 32 mg to 10 subjects, peak plasma concentrations of 0.01 to 0.14 µg/ml (mean 0.04) were attained in 0.5 to 2.5 hours (E. Bechgaard and A. Nielsen, *Biopharm. Drug Disp.*, 1982, *3*, 337–344).

HALF-LIFE. Derived from plasma and urinary data, about 6 hours.

REFERENCE. E. Bechgaard and A. Nielsen, *ibid.*

Dose. 24 to 64 mg of bromhexine hydrochloride daily.

Bromocriptine
Dopaminergic Agent

Synonyms. 2-Bromo-alpha-ergocryptine; Bromocryptine; 2-Bromoergocryptine.
2 - Bromo - 12′ - hydroxy - 5′α - isobutyl - 2′ - isopropylergotaman - 3′,6′,18-trione
$C_{32}H_{40}BrN_5O_5 = 654.6$
CAS—25614-03-3

Crystals. M.p. 215° to 218°, with decomposition.

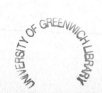

Bromocriptine Mesylate

Synonym. Bromocriptine Methanesulphonate
Proprietary Names. Parlodel; Pravidel.
$C_{32}H_{40}BrN_5O_5,CH_4O_3S = 750.7$
CAS—22260-51-1
A yellowish-white crystalline powder. M.p. 192° to 196°, with decomposition.

Thin-layer Chromatography. *System TA*—Rf 72; *system TB*—Rf 00; *system TC*—Rf 69.

High Pressure Liquid Chromatography. *System HP*—k' 44.3.

Ultraviolet Spectrum. Aqueous acid—306 nm $(A_1^1 = 138 \text{ b})$; aqueous alkali—239 nm $(A_1^1 = 373 \text{ b})$, 300 nm $(A_1^1 = 144 \text{ b})$.

Infra-red Spectrum. Principal peaks at wavenumbers 1170, 1633, 1217, 1660, 1715, 1045 (bromocriptine mesylate).

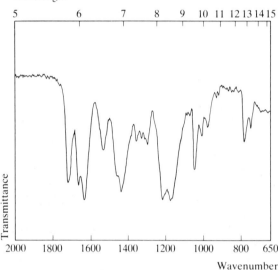

Mass Spectrum. Principal peaks at *m/z* 70, 43, 154, 71, 41, 209, 86, 195.

Quantification. GAS CHROMATOGRAPHY. In plasma: comparison with GC-MS and HPLC, sensitivity 500 pg/ml for GC and 1 ng/ml for GC-MS and HPLC—N. E. Larsen *et al.*, *J. Chromat.*, 1979, *174*, 341–349.

RADIOIMMUNOASSAY. In plasma: sensitivity 100 pg/ml—H. F. Schran *et al.*, *Clin. Chem.*, 1979, *25*, 1928–1933.

Disposition in the Body. Rapidly absorbed after oral administration. It undergoes extensive first-pass metabolism by hydrolysis and isomerisation to 2-bromolysergic acid and 2-bromoisolysergic acid, and by hydroxylation, further oxidation and conjugation to produce a large number of metabolites. About 7% of a dose is excreted in the urine as metabolites together with a small fraction as unchanged drug. About 70% of a dose is eliminated in the faeces via the bile within 5 days of a single oral dose.

THERAPEUTIC CONCENTRATION.
Following a single oral dose of 25 mg to 9 subjects, peak plasma concentrations of 0.001 to 0.004 µg/ml were attained in about 90 minutes; after single doses of 50 and 100 mg to 7 and 5 subjects, respectively, peak plasma concentrations of 0.003 to 0.020 µg/ml (mean 0.01) and 0.006 to 0.025 µg/ml (mean 0.01) were attained in about 90 to 120 minutes (P. Price *et al.*, *Br. J. clin. Pharmac.*, 1978, *6*, 303–309).

Following daily oral administration of 60 to 150 mg in divided doses to 4 subjects, minimum steady-state plasma concentrations of 0.009 to 0.054 µg/ml (mean 0.03) and saliva concentrations of 0.0001 to 0.0004 µg/ml were reported (M. L. Friis *et al.*, *Eur. J. clin. Pharmac.*, 1980, *18*, 171–174).

HALF-LIFE. Plasma half-life, about 3 hours.

VOLUME OF DISTRIBUTION. About 3 litres/kg.

PROTEIN BINDING. In plasma, 90 to 96%.

Dose. The equivalent of 1.25 to 30 mg of bromocriptine daily. In parkinsonism, the usual maintenance dose is the equivalent of 40 to 100 mg daily, but up to 300 mg daily has been given.

Bromodiphenhydramine   *Antihistamine*

Synonyms. Bromazine; Bromdiphenhydramine; Histabromamine.

2-(4-Bromobenzhydryloxy)-*NN*-dimethylethylamine
$C_{17}H_{20}BrNO = 334.3$
CAS—118-23-0

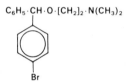

Bromodiphenhydramine Hydrochloride

Proprietary Name. Ambodryl
$C_{17}H_{20}BrNO,HCl = 370.7$
CAS—1808-12-4
A white to pale buff-coloured crystalline powder. M.p. 148° to 152°.
Soluble 1 in less than 1 of water, 1 in 2 of ethanol, 1 in 2 of chloroform, and 1 in 31 of isopropyl alcohol; practically insoluble in ether.

Dissociation Constant. pK_a 8.6 (25°).

Colour Test. Marquis Test—yellow.

Thin-layer Chromatography. *System TA*—Rf 54; *system TB*—Rf 44; *system TC*—Rf 43. (*Dragendorff spray*, positive; *acidified iodoplatinate solution*, positive; *Marquis reagent*, yellow.)

Gas Chromatography. *System GA*—RI 2155; *system GF*—RI 2480.

High Pressure Liquid Chromatography. *System HA*—k' 2.7.

Ultraviolet Spectrum. Aqueous acid—230 nm $(A_1^1 = 465 \text{ a})$.

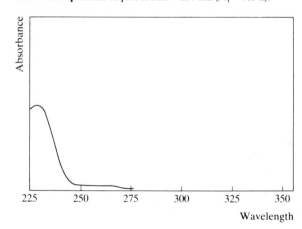

Infra-red Spectrum. Principal peaks at wavenumbers 1067, 1094, 1007, 696, 1041, 746 (KBr disk).

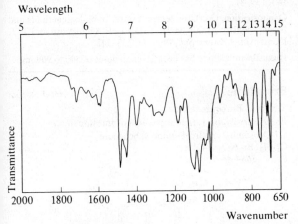

Wavelength

Mass Spectrum. Principal peaks at m/z 58, 73, 45, 165, 59, 42, 166, 149.

Disposition in the Body. Absorbed after oral administration. A number of metabolites have been identified in the urine including the N-oxide, monodesmethyl and didesmethyl derivatives, 4-bromobenzhydrol, 4-bromobenzophenone, and 4-hydroxybenzophenone; glucuronide conjugates of some of these metabolites have also been reported. Unchanged drug is also excreted in the urine.

Dose. 75 to 100 mg of bromodiphenhydramine hydrochloride daily.

Brompheniramine   *Antihistamine*

Synonym. Parabromdylamine
(±)-3-(4-Bromophenyl)-*NN*-dimethyl-3-(2-pyridyl)propylamine
$C_{16}H_{19}BrN_2 = 319.2$
CAS—86-22-6

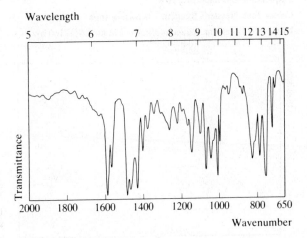

A slightly yellow, oily liquid.
Miscible with dilute acids.

Brompheniramine Maleate
Proprietary Names. Antial; Dimegan; Dimetane; Dimotane; Drauxin; Ebalin; Gammistin; Ilvin; Veltane. It is an ingredient of Dimotapp and Exyphen.
$C_{16}H_{19}BrN_2,C_4H_4O_4 = 435.3$
CAS—980-71-2; 32865-01-3 (±)
A white crystalline powder. M.p. 130° to 135°.

Soluble 1 in 5 of water, 1 in 15 of ethanol, and 1 in 15 of chloroform; slightly soluble in ether.

Dissociation Constant. pK_a 3.9, 9.2.

Colour Test. Cyanogen Bromide—orange.

Thin-layer Chromatography. *System TA*—Rf 45; *system TB*—Rf 33; *system TC*—Rf 16. (*Acidified iodoplatinate solution,* positive.)

Gas Chromatography. *System GA*—RI 2096; *system GB*—RI 2159; *system GC*—RI 2457; *system GF*—RI 2470.

High Pressure Liquid Chromatography. *System HA*—k′ 4.1.

Ultraviolet Spectrum. Aqueous acid—265 nm ($A_1^1 = 272$ a); aqueous alkali—262 nm ($A_1^1 = 177$ a), 269 nm.

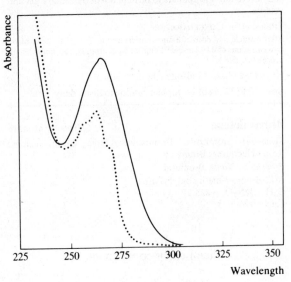

Infra-red Spectrum. Principal peaks at wavenumbers 1585, 750, 1003, 1067, 1565, 1040 (KBr disk).

Wavelength

Mass Spectrum. Principal peaks at m/z 247, 249, 58, 72, 248, 167, 250, 168.

Quantification. GAS CHROMATOGRAPHY. In blood or urine: sensitivity 10 ng/ml in blood, ECD—R. B. Bruce *et al.*, *Analyt. Chem.*, 1968, *40*, 1246–1250.

Disposition in the Body. Absorbed after oral administration; accumulates in the body during chronic daily dosing. The main metabolic reactions are *N*-demethylation and deamination. About 50% of a ^{14}C-labelled dose is excreted in the urine in 5 days, with 10% of the dose as unchanged brompheniramine, 11% as monodesmethylbrompheniramine, 10% as didesmethyl-brompheniramine, 4% as 3-(4-bromophenyl)-3-(2-pyridyl)-propionic acid, and 2% as its glycine conjugate; other unidentified polar metabolites are also present. Less than 3% of the dose is eliminated in the faeces. Under steady-state conditions the daily excretion rate appears to be dependent on urinary pH and volume.

THERAPEUTIC CONCENTRATION.

After a single oral dose of 8 mg administered to 2 subjects, peak blood concentrations of 0.012 and 0.017 µg/ml were attained in 3 hours (R. B. Bruce *et al.*, *ibid.*).

HALF-LIFE. Plasma half-life, about 15 hours.

Dose. 12 to 32 mg of brompheniramine maleate daily.

Bromvaletone

Hypnotic/Sedative

Synonyms. Bromisoval; Bromisovalerylurea; Bromisovalum; Bromvalerylurea; Bromylum.
Proprietary Name. Bromural
N-(2-Bromo-3-methylbutyryl)urea
$C_6H_{11}BrN_2O_2 = 223.1$
CAS—496-67-3

$$(CH_3)_2CH \cdot \overset{\overset{\displaystyle Br}{|}}{CH} \cdot CO \cdot NH \cdot CO \cdot NH_2$$

Small, white, acicular or scale-like crystals, which sublime on heating. M.p. about 150°.
Soluble 1 in 500 of water, 1 in 15 of ethanol, 1 in 6 of chloroform, and 1 in 25 of ether; soluble in solutions of alkali hydroxides.

Dissociation Constant. pK_a 10.8.

Colour Test. Nessler's Reagent—brown-orange.

Ultraviolet Spectrum. Aqueous alkali—233 nm ($A_1^1 = 160$ b).

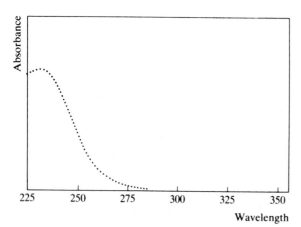

Wavelength

Infra-red Spectrum. Principal peaks at wavenumbers 1720, 1700, 1581, 1210, 1170, 1300 (KBr disk). Polymorphism may occur.

Mass Spectrum. Principal peaks at *m/z* 44, 83, 180, 182, 137, 143, 139, 41.

Quantification. GAS CHROMATOGRAPHY. In biological fluids and tissues: sensitivity 200 ng/ml, FID—L. R. Goldbaum and T. J. Domanski, *J. forens. Sci.*, 1966, *11*, 233–242.

Dose. Bromvaletone has been given in doses of 300 to 900 mg.

Broxaldine

Antiprotozoal

Synonym. Brobenzoxaldine
Proprietary Name. It is an ingredient of Intestopan.
5,7-Dibromo-2-methyl-8-quinolyl benzoate
$C_{17}H_{11}Br_2NO_2 = 421.1$
CAS—3684-46-6

An off-white powder.
Practically **insoluble** in water; soluble in ether.

Colour Tests. Mandelin's Test—yellow; Marquis Test—yellow; Sulphuric Acid—yellow.

Thin-layer Chromatography. *System TA*—Rf 74; *system TB*—Rf 52; *system TC*—Rf 79. (*Acidified iodoplatinate solution, strong reaction.*)

Gas Chromatography. *System GA*—RI 2686.

Mass Spectrum. Principal peaks at *m/z* 105, 77, 106, 44, 51, 128, 78, 40.

Dose. 120 to 300 mg daily, usually in combination with broxyquinoline.

Broxyquinoline

Antiprotozoal

Synonym. Broxichinolinum
Proprietary Name. It is an ingredient of Intestopan.
5,7-Dibromoquinolin-8-ol
$C_9H_5Br_2NO = 303.0$
CAS—521-74-4

A cream-coloured powder. M.p. 196°.
Practically **insoluble** in water; soluble in chloroform.

Colour Tests. Liebermann's Test—orange; Marquis Test—yellow; Millon's Reagent—red; Sulphuric Acid—yellow.

Thin-layer Chromatography. *System TA*—Rf 51; *system TB*—Rf 00; *system TC*—Rf 06. (*Acidified potassium permanganate solution, positive.*)

Ultraviolet Spectrum. Aqueous acid—263 nm ($A_1^1 = 800$ b); ethanol—249 nm ($A_1^1 = 1525$ b), 325 nm ($A_1^1 = 125$ b).

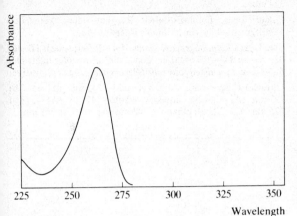

Infra-red Spectrum. Principal peaks at wavenumbers 1316, 1190, 930, 806, 1258, 782 (KBr disk).

Mass Spectrum. Principal peaks at m/z 303, 301, 305, 115, 194, 196, 114, 87.

Quantification. COLORIMETRY. In urine—L. Berggren and O. Hansson, *Clin. Pharmac. Ther.*, 1968, *9*, 67–70. In urine—L. A. M. Rodriguez and J. A. Close, *Biochem. Pharmac.*, 1968, *17*, 1647–1653.

Disposition in the Body. Absorbed after oral administration. About 36% of a dose is excreted in the urine in 24 hours, mainly as the glucuronide conjugate; very little unchanged drug is excreted and 8-hydroxyquinoline accounts for less than 2% of the dose.

REFERENCE. L. A. M. Rodriguez and J. A. Close, *ibid.*

Dose. 0.6 to 1.5 g daily, usually in combination with broxaldine.

Brucine   *Alkaloid*

Synonym. Dimethoxystrychnine
10,11-Dimethoxystrychnine
$C_{23}H_{26}N_2O_4,4H_2O = 466.5$
CAS—357-57-3 (anhydrous)

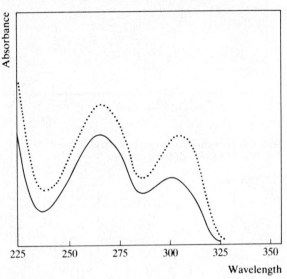

An alkaloid present in the seeds of *Strychnos nux-vomica* and other species of *Strychnos* (Loganiaceae).
Small white crystals. M.p. of the anhydrous base, 178° and of the hydrated form, 105°.
Soluble 1 in 1320 of water, 1 in 1.3 of ethanol, 1 in 5 of chloroform, and 1 in 187 of ether.

Brucine Sulphate
$(C_{23}H_{26}N_2O_4)_2,H_2SO_4,7H_2O = 1013$
CAS—4845-99-2 (anhydrous); *60583-39-3* (heptahydrate)

Small white crystals or powder.
Soluble 1 in 75 of cold water, 1 in about 10 of boiling water, 1 in 105 of ethanol, and 1 in 170 of chloroform.

Dissociation Constant. pK_a 2.3, 8.0 (25°).

Colour Test. Liebermann's Test—red.

Thin-layer Chromatography. *System TA*—Rf 16; *system TB*—Rf 00; *system TC*—Rf 17. (*Acidified iodoplatinate solution*, positive.)

Gas Chromatography. *System GA*—RI 3280.

High Pressure Liquid Chromatography. *System HA*—k' 11.1 (tailing peak).

Ultraviolet Spectrum. Aqueous acid—265 nm ($A_1^1 = 330$ a), 300 nm; aqueous alkali—266 nm ($A_1^1 = 320$ a), 304 nm.

Infra-red Spectrum. Principal peaks at wavenumbers 1500, 1660, 1280, 1195, 1120, 1212 (KBr disk).

Mass Spectrum. Principal peaks at m/z 394, 395, 379, 392, 120, 197, 203, 393.

Buclizine   *Antihistamine*

1-(4-*tert*-Butylbenzyl)-4-(4-chlorobenzhydryl)piperazine
$C_{28}H_{33}ClN_2 = 433.0$
CAS—82-95-1

Buclizine Hydrochloride
Proprietary Names. Aphilan R; Bucladin-S; Longifene. It is an ingredient of Equivert and Migraleve (pink tablets).
$C_{28}H_{33}ClN_2,2HCl = 506.0$
CAS—129-74-8
A white crystalline powder. M.p. 230° to 240°.
Slightly **soluble** in water.

Thin-layer Chromatography. *System TA*—Rf 75; *system TB*—Rf 61; *system TC*—Rf 83. (*Acidified iodoplatinate solution*, positive.)

Gas Chromatography. *System GA*—RI 3286.

High Pressure Liquid Chromatography. *System HA*—k′ 0.7.

Ultraviolet Spectrum. Methanol—255 nm, 260 nm ($A_1^1 = 19$ b).

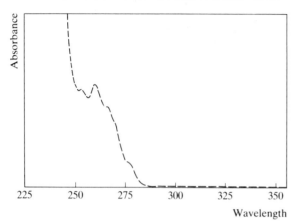

Wavelength

Infra-red Spectrum. Principal peaks at wavenumbers 1002, 1131, 754, 800, 1075, 694 (KBr disk).

Wavelength

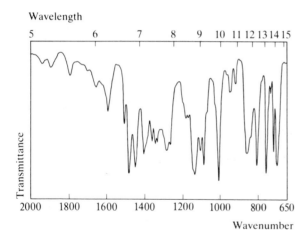

Wavenumber

Mass Spectrum. Principal peaks at *m/z* 231, 147, 285, 232, 201, 132, 165, 166.

Dose. 25 to 150 mg of buclizine hydrochloride daily.

Buclosamide   *Antifungal*

N-Butyl-4-chlorosalicylamide
$C_{11}H_{14}ClNO_2 = 227.7$
CAS—575-74-6

A white crystalline powder. M.p. about 91°.
Practically **insoluble** in water; soluble 1 in 3 of ethanol, and 1 in 3 of ether.

Colour Tests. Folin–Ciocalteu Reagent—blue; Mandelin's Test—green → blue rim; Millon's Reagent—red.

Thin-layer Chromatography. *System TA*—Rf 90; *system TB*—Rf 02; *system TC*—Rf 67. (Location under ultraviolet light, blue fluorescence; *acidified potassium permanganate solution*, positive.)

Ultraviolet Spectrum. Aqueous acid—245 nm ($A_1^1 = 532$ b), 297 nm ($A_1^1 = 204$ b); aqueous alkali—247 nm ($A_1^1 = 391$ b), 325 nm ($A_1^1 = 323$ a); ethanol—243 nm ($A_1^1 = 497$ a), 301 nm.

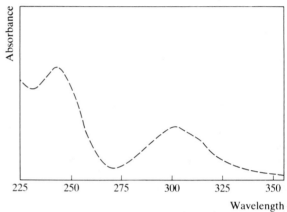

Wavelength

Infra-red Spectrum. Principal peaks at wavenumbers 1543, 898, 1190, 1590, 1201, 1506 (KBr disk).

Mass Spectrum. Principal peaks at *m/z* 155, 157, 227, 154, 185, 44, 30, 156.

Use. Buclosamide has been applied topically in a concentration of 10%.

Bufexamac   *Analgesic*

Proprietary Names. Droxaryl; Norfemac; Paraderm; Parfenac.
2-(4-Butoxyphenyl)acetohydroxamic acid
$C_{12}H_{17}NO_3 = 223.3$
CAS—2438-72-4

$CH_3 \cdot [CH_2]_3 \cdot O$—⟨phenyl ring⟩—$CH_2 \cdot CO \cdot NHOH$

Almost colourless pearly flakes. M.p. 158° to 160°, with decomposition.
Practically **insoluble** in water.

Thin-layer Chromatography. *System TD*—Rf 11; *system TE*—Rf 18; *system TF*—Rf 19; *system TG*—Rf 36.

Gas Chromatography. *System GD*—retention time of methyl derivative 1.12 relative to *n*-$C_{16}H_{34}$.

High Pressure Liquid Chromatography. *System HD*—k′ 1.95.

Ultraviolet Spectrum. Aqueous alkali—275 nm ($A_1^1 = 72$ b).

Infra-red Spectrum. Principal peaks at wavenumbers 1612, 1234, 1515, 980, 1052, 1176.

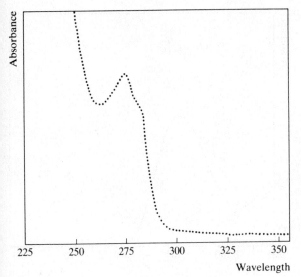

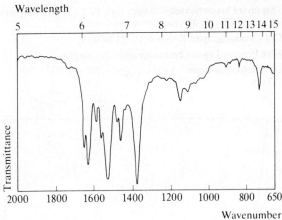

Mass Spectrum. Principal peaks at m/z 107, 163, 223, 108, 29, 164, 41, 57.

Dose. 0.75 to 1.5 g daily.

Buformin   *Antidiabetic*

1-Butylbiguanide
$C_6H_{15}N_5 = 157.2$
CAS—692-13-7

$$CH_3 \cdot [CH_2]_3 \cdot NH \cdot \overset{NH}{\underset{||}{C}} \cdot NH \cdot \overset{NH}{\underset{||}{C}} \cdot NH_2$$

Buformin Hydrochloride
Proprietary Names. Silubin; Sindiatil.
$C_6H_{15}N_5,HCl = 193.7$
CAS—1190-53-0
A fine white crystalline powder. M.p. 174° to 177°.
Soluble in water and ethanol.

Thin-layer Chromatography. System *TA*—Rf 02; *system TB*—Rf 00; *system TC*—Rf 00.

Ultraviolet Spectrum. Aqueous alkali—230 nm ($A_1^1 = 919$ b).

Infra-red Spectrum. Principal peaks at wavenumbers 1530, 1634, 1666, 1562, 1587, 1149 (KBr disk).

Mass Spectrum. Principal peaks at m/z 43, 114, 85, 30, 101, 86, 44, 72.

Quantification. ULTRAVIOLET SPECTROPHOTOMETRY. In urine—E. R. Garrett and J. Tsau, *J. pharm. Sci.*, 1972, *61*, 1404–1410. In plasma or whole blood—E. R. Garrett *et al.*, *ibid.*, 1411–1418.

GAS CHROMATOGRAPHY. In biological fluids or tissues: AFID—G. de Groot *et al.*, *J. analyt. Toxicol.*, 1980, *4*, 281–285. In plasma or urine: sensitivity 1 ng/ml, ECD—S. B. Matin *et al.*, *Analyt. Chem.*, 1975, *47*, 545–548.

Disposition in the Body. Absorbed after oral administration. About 35% of an oral dose is excreted in the urine as unchanged drug in 24 hours and up to 30% is eliminated in the faeces; after intravenous administration about 90% is excreted unchanged in the urine in 12 hours.

THERAPEUTIC CONCENTRATION. In plasma, usually in the range 0.2 to 0.6 µg/ml.
Following a single oral dose of 100 mg to 6 subjects, a mean peak plasma concentration of 0.4 µg/ml was reported after 2.5 hours; plasma concentrations greater than 0.2 µg/ml were maintained up to 8 hours after the dose (H. Gutsche *et al.*, *Arzneimittel-Forsch.*, 1976, *26*, 1227–1229).

TOXICITY. Lactic acidosis is associated with plasma concentrations greater than 1 µg/ml.
An 84-year-old diabetic died 6 hours after admission to hospital with severe lactic acidosis caused by buformin. The plasma concentration on admission was 5.5 µg/ml. Postmortem tissue concentrations were: plasma 3.2 µg/ml, bile 6.3 µg/ml, heart 3.0 µg/g, kidney 98 µg/g, liver 5.2 µg/g, lung 2.8 µg/g (G. de Groot *et al.*, *J. analyt. Toxicol.*, 1980, *4*, 281–285).

HALF-LIFE. Plasma half-life, about 2 to 6 hours.

VOLUME OF DISTRIBUTION. About 2 litres/kg.

PROTEIN BINDING. In plasma, about 10%.

Dose. 100 to 300 mg of buformin hydrochloride daily.

Bufotenine   *Hallucinogen*

Synonyms. *NN*-Dimethylserotonin; 5-Hydroxy-*NN*-dimethyltryptamine; Mappine.
3-(2-Dimethylaminoethyl)indol-5-ol
$C_{12}H_{16}N_2O = 204.3$
CAS—487-93-4

An indole alkaloid obtained from the seeds and leaves of *Piptadenia peregrina* and *P. macrocarpa* (Mimosaceae). It has also been isolated from species of *Amanita* (Agaricaceae) and from the skin glands of toads (*Bufo* spp.).
A white crystalline powder. M.p. 138° to 140°.
Practically **insoluble** in water; freely soluble in ethanol; slightly soluble in ether; soluble in dilute acids and alkalis.

Colour Test. Marquis Test—green-brown.

Thin-layer Chromatography. *System TA*—Rf 35; *system TB*—Rf 00; *system TC*—Rf 01. (*Van Urk reagent*, violet.)

Gas Chromatography. *System GA*—RI 2030.

High Pressure Liquid Chromatography. *System HA*—k′ 3.1.

Ultraviolet Spectrum. Aqueous acid—278 nm (A$_1^1$ = 269 b), 297 nm.

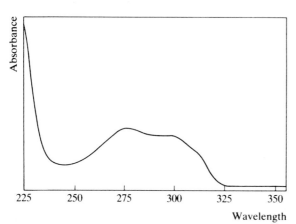

Infra-red Spectrum. Principal peaks at wavenumbers 1232, 824, 1493, 1615, 792, 1052 (KBr disk).

Mass Spectrum. Principal peaks at *m/z* 58, 204, 146, 59, 42, 160, 43, 159.

Quantification. GAS CHROMATOGRAPHY–MASS SPECTROMETRY. In urine: detection limit 300 pg/ml—M. Räisänen and J. Kärrkkäinen, *J. Chromat.*, 1979, *162*; *Biomed. Appl.*, *4*, 579–584.

Bufylline   *Xanthine Bronchodilator*

Synonyms. Ambuphylline; Theophylline-aminoisobutanol.
Proprietary Names. Butaphyllamine; Buthoid. It is an ingredient of Nethaprin and Nethaprin Dospan.

2-Amino-2-methylpropan-1-ol theophyllinate
C$_{11}$H$_{19}$N$_5$O$_3$ = 269.3
CAS—5634-34-4

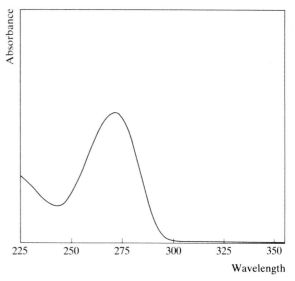

A white crystalline powder. M.p. about 255°.
Slightly **soluble** in water.

Colour Test. Amalic Acid Test—red/violet.

Gas Chromatography. *System GA*—RI 2301.

Ultraviolet Spectrum. Aqueous acid—271 nm (A$_1^1$ = 350 b).

Infra-red Spectrum. Principal peaks at wavenumbers 1665, 1712, 1636, 1562, 740, 1180 (KBr disk).

Mass Spectrum. Principal peaks at *m/z* 180, 95, 68, 41, 58, 53, 123, 96.

Dose. 60 to 120 mg every 3 to 4 hours.

Bumetanide   *Diuretic*

Proprietary Names. Burinex; Fordiuran.
3-Butylamino-4-phenoxy-5-sulphamoylbenzoic acid
C$_{17}$H$_{20}$N$_2$O$_5$S = 364.4
CAS—28395-03-1

A white crystalline powder. M.p. about 230°.

Colour Tests. Koppanyi–Zwikker Test—violet; Liebermann's Test—brown-orange; Mercurous Nitrate—black.

Thin-layer Chromatography. *System TD*—Rf 01; *system TE*—Rf 03; *system TF*—Rf 10.

Ultraviolet Spectrum. Aqueous acid—340 nm (A$_1^1$ = 80 b); aqueous alkali—317 nm (A$_1^1$ = 87 b).

Infra-red Spectrum. Principal peaks at wavenumbers 1695, 1215, 1199, 1153, 1587, 1280 (KBr disk).

Mass Spectrum. Principal peaks at *m/z* 321, 364, 304, 240, 168, 91, 322, 365.

Quantification. GAS CHROMATOGRAPHY. In serum or urine: sensitivity 1 ng/ml, FID—D. L. Davies *et al.*, *Clin. Pharmac. Ther.*, 1974, *15*, 141–155.

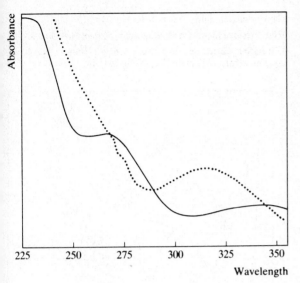

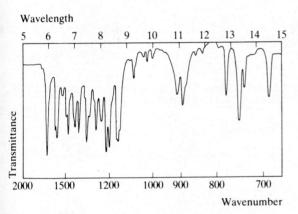

HIGH PRESSURE LIQUID CHROMATOGRAPHY. In plasma or urine: detection limit in plasma 5 ng/ml, fluorescence detection—D. E. Smith, *J. pharm. Sci.*, 1982, *71*, 520–523.

RADIOIMMUNOASSAY. In plasma or urine: sensitivity 1 ng/ml— W. R. Dixon *et al.*, *J. pharm. Sci.*, 1976, *65*, 701–704.

Disposition in the Body. Rapidly and completely absorbed after oral administration. Metabolised to some extent by hydroxylation of the butyl side-chain to give the 2′-, 3′-, and 4′-alcohols; the 3′-carboxylic acid and desbutyl metabolites have also been reported. About 50% of a dose is excreted in the urine as unchanged drug in 24 hours together with 4 to 6% as the 3′-alcohol. A total of about 80% of a dose is excreted in the urine and 10% to 15% is eliminated in the faeces in 48 hours.

THERAPEUTIC CONCENTRATION.
After a single dose of 1 mg given to 12 subjects, a mean peak plasma concentration of 0.03 μg/ml was attained in 1 to 8 hours (A. A. Holazo *et al.*, *J. pharm. Sci.*, 1984, *73*, 1108–1113).

HALF-LIFE. Plasma half-life, about 1 hour.

VOLUME OF DISTRIBUTION. About 0.2 litre/kg.

CLEARANCE. Plasma clearance about 3 ml/min/kg.

PROTEIN BINDING. In plasma, about 96%.

NOTE. For a review of bumetanide see A. Ward and R. C. Heel, *Drugs*, 1984, *28*, 426–464.

Dose. Usually 1 to 2 mg daily; doses of 20 mg or more daily have been given.

Bunamidine   *Anthelmintic (Veterinary)*

NN-Dibutyl-4-hexyloxy-1-naphthamidine
$C_{25}H_{38}N_2O = 382.6$
CAS—3748-77-4

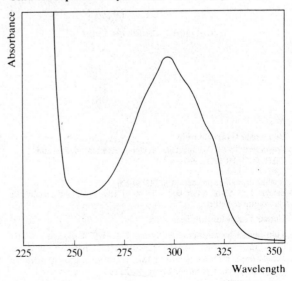

Bunamidine Hydrochloride
Proprietary Name. Scolaban
$C_{25}H_{38}N_2O,HCl = 419.0$
CAS—1055-55-6
A white crystalline powder. M.p. about 210°.
Soluble 1 in 200 of water, 1 in 2 of ethanol, and 1 in 2 of chloroform; practically insoluble in ether.
Caution. Bunamidine hydrochloride is irritant, especially to the eyes, and should be handled with care.

Bunamidine Hydroxynaphthoate
$C_{36}H_{46}N_2O_4 = 570.8$
CAS—13501-04-7
A pale yellow crystalline powder. M.p. 170° to 175°.
Practically **insoluble** in water; soluble 1 in 35 of ethanol, 1 in 3 of chloroform, and 1 in 300 of ether.

Colour Tests. Mandelin's Test—green; Marquis Test—orange→red.

Thin-layer Chromatography. *System TA*—Rf 64. (*Acidified iodoplatinate solution*, positive.)

Gas Chromatography. *System GA*—not eluted.

Ultraviolet Spectrum. Aqueous acid—298 nm ($A_1^1 = 240$ a).

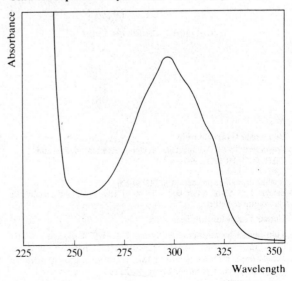

Infra-red Spectrum. Principal peaks at wavenumbers 1572, 1079, 1263, 1234, 763, 1511 (KBr disk).

Bunitrolol
Beta-adrenoceptor Blocking Agent

Proprietary Name. Stresson (hydrochloride)
2-(3-*tert*-Butylamino-2-hydroxypropoxy)benzonitrile
$C_{14}H_{20}N_2O_2 = 248.3$
CAS—34915-68-9

$$CN$$

O·CH₂·CH·CH₂·NH·C(CH₃)₃ with OH

A crystalline solid. M.p. about 164°.

Ultraviolet Spectrum. Aqueous acid—232 nm ($A_1^1 = 332$ b), 292 nm ($A_1^1 = 142$ b).

Quantification. HIGH PRESSURE LIQUID CHROMATOGRAPHY. In plasma or urine: bunitrolol and 4-hydroxybunitrolol, sensitivity 2.5 ng/ml in plasma and 250 pg/ml in urine, fluorescence detection—A. Nagakura and H. Kohei, *J. Chromat.*, 1982, *232*; *Biomed. Appl.*, *21*, 137–143.

Disposition in the Body. Absorbed after oral administration and metabolised by *p*-hydroxylation followed by conjugation with glucuronic acid. About 1% of a dose is excreted in the urine as unchanged drug and 5% as the *p*-hydroxy metabolite, in 6 hours.

REFERENCE. A. Nagakura and H. Kohei, *ibid.*

Dose. Bunitrolol hydrochloride has been given in doses of 20 to 40 mg daily.

Buphenine
Vasodilator

Synonym. Nylidrin
1 - (4 - Hydroxyphenyl) - 2 - (1 - methyl - 3 - phenylpropyl-amino)propan-1-ol
$C_{19}H_{25}NO_2 = 299.4$
CAS—447-41-6

CH₃   CH₃
C₆H₅·[CH₂]₂·CH·NH·CH·CHOH with OH

M.p. 111° to 112°.

Buphenine Hydrochloride
Proprietary Names. Arlidin; Dilatol; Opino; Penitardon; Pervadil.
$C_{19}H_{25}NO_2,HCl = 335.9$
CAS—849-55-8
A white crystalline powder. M.p. 223° to 226°.
Soluble 1 in 65 of water and 1 in 40 of ethanol; slightly soluble in chloroform and ether.

Colour Test. Marquis Test—red.

Thin-layer Chromatography. *System TA*—Rf 74; *system TB*—Rf 03; *system TC*—Rf 14. (*Dragendorff spray*, positive; *acidified iodoplatinate solution*, positive; *Marquis reagent*, brown; *acidified potassium permanganate solution*, positive.)

Gas Chromatography. *System GA*—RI 2314.

High Pressure Liquid Chromatography. *System HA*—k′ 0.9.

Ultraviolet Spectrum. Aqueous acid—273 nm ($A_1^1 = 40$ a); aqueous alkali—242 nm ($A_1^1 = 390$ b), 291 nm.

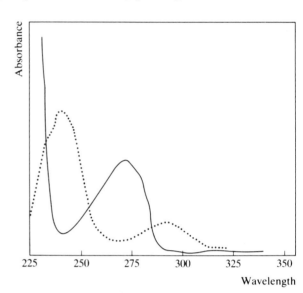

Infra-red Spectrum. Principal peaks at wavenumbers 1512, 1220, 750, 695, 1182, 837 (KBr disk).

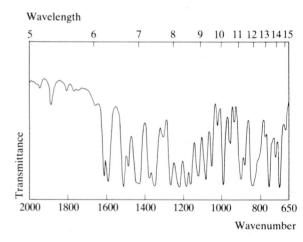

Mass Spectrum. Principal peaks at *m/z* 91, 133, 176, 174, 44, 107, 92, 177.

Quantification. GAS CHROMATOGRAPHY. In urine: FID—H. Li and P. Cervoni, *J. pharm. Sci.*, 1976, *65*, 1352–1356.

Disposition in the Body. Readily absorbed after oral administration. About 5% of a single dose is excreted in the urine as unchanged drug in 24 hours.

TOXICITY. The estimated minimum lethal dose in adults is 2 g and in children 200 mg.

Dose. 18 to 48 mg of buphenine hydrochloride daily.

Bupivacaine

Local Anaesthetic

($\pm$)-(1-Butyl-2-piperidyl)formo-2',6'-xylidide
$C_{18}H_{28}N_2O = 288.4$
CAS—2180-92-9

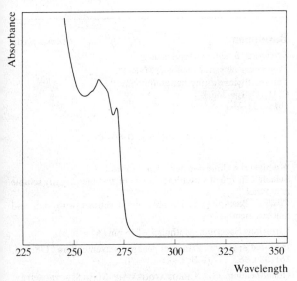

M.p. 107° to 108°.

Bupivacaine Hydrochloride

Proprietary Names. Carbostesin; Marcain(e).

$C_{18}H_{28}N_2O,HCl,H_2O = 342.9$
CAS—18010-40-7 (anhydrous); *14252-80-3* (monohydrate)
A white crystalline powder. M.p. about 248° to 250°, with decomposition.
Soluble 1 in 25 of water and 1 in 8 of ethanol; slightly soluble in acetone, chloroform, and ether.

Dissociation Constant. pK_a 8.1.

Thin-layer Chromatography. *System TA*—Rf 69; *system TB*—Rf 42; *system TC*—Rf 73; *system TL*—Rf 65. (*Acidified iodoplatinate solution*, positive.)

Gas Chromatography. *System GA*—RI 2273.

High Pressure Liquid Chromatography. *System HA*—k' 0.9; *system HQ*—k' 7.19; *system HR*—k' 0.86.

Ultraviolet Spectrum. Aqueous acid—263 nm ($A_1^1 = 16$ a), 271 nm.

Infra-red Spectrum. Principal peaks at wavenumbers 1667, 1522, 1279, 1222, 787, 944 (bupivacaine hydrochloride, KBr disk).

Mass Spectrum. Principal peaks at m/z 140, 141, 84, 41, 29, 96, 56, 55.

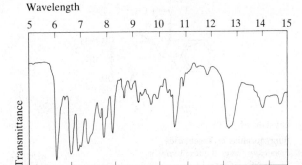

Quantification. GAS CHROMATOGRAPHY. In serum: bupivacaine and 2',6'-pipecoloxylidide, sensitivity 50 ng/ml for both compounds, AFID—L. J. Lesko *et al.*, *J. Chromat.*, 1980, *182*; *Biomed. Appl.*, *8*, 226–231. In blood: sensitivity 15 ng/ml, FID— A. Berlin *et al.*, *J. Pharm. Pharmac.*, 1973, *25*, 466–469.

Disposition in the Body. Bupivacaine is metabolised in the liver by oxidative dealkylation to 2',6'-pipecoloxylidide (PPX); 3'- and 4'-hydroxylation also occur. Less than 10% of a dose is excreted in the urine as unchanged drug in 24 hours.

THERAPEUTIC CONCENTRATION.

After slow intravenous infusion of 1.35 mg/kg to 3 subjects, peak venous-plasma concentrations of 2.6 to 4.5 µg/ml were reported 3 to 17 minutes after completion of the infusion (L. E. Mather *et al.*, *Clin Pharmac. Ther.*, 1971, *12*, 935–943).

After epidural administration of 150 mg with adrenaline to 12 subjects, mean peak plasma concentrations of 1.1 µg/ml were reported at 0.3 hour and peak cerebrospinal fluid concentrations averaged 30 µg/ml at 0.5 hour (G. R. Wilkinson and P. C. Lund, *Anesthesiology*, 1970, *2*, 482–486).

TOXICITY. Bupivacaine is several times more toxic than lignocaine. Muscular rigidity has been reported in 2 subjects having blood concentrations of 9 and 12 µg/ml following the administration of approximately 210 mg, and convulsions have been reported at plasma concentrations greater than 4 µg/ml.

HALF-LIFE. Plasma half-life, about 1 to 3 hours, increased in neonates.

VOLUME OF DISTRIBUTION. About 1 litre/kg.

CLEARANCE. Plasma clearance, about 8 ml/min/kg.

DISTRIBUTION IN BLOOD. Plasma: whole blood ratio, about 1.4.

PROTEIN BINDING. In plasma, about 90%.

NOTE. For a review of the clinical pharmacokinetics of local anaesthetics see G. T. Tucker and L. E. Mather, *Clin. Pharmacokinet.*, 1979, *4*, 241–278.

Dose. Bupivacaine hydrochloride is given by injection as a 0.25 or 0.5% solution (calculated as the anhydrous hydrochloride); maximum recommended dose is 2 mg/kg in any 4-hour period.

Buprenorphine

Narcotic Analgesic

(6*R*,7*R*,14*S*)-17-Cyclopropylmethyl-7,8-dihydro-7-[(1*S*)-1-hydroxy-1,2,2-trimethylpropyl]-6-*O*-methyl-6,14-ethano-17-normorphine
$C_{29}H_{41}NO_4 = 467.6$
CAS—52485-79-7

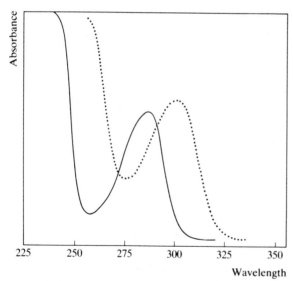

Crystals. M.p. 209°.

Buprenorphine Hydrochloride
Proprietary Names. Buprex; Temgesic.
$C_{29}H_{41}NO_4,HCl = 504.1$
CAS—53152-21-9
A white crystalline powder.

Dissociation Constant. pK_a 8.5, 10.0.

Colour Tests. Liebermann's Test—black; Marquis Test—violet.

Thin-layer Chromatography. *System TA*—Rf 76; *system TB*—Rf 09; *system TC*—Rf 68.

High Pressure Liquid Chromatography. *System HA*—k' 0.4; *system HC*—k' 0.05.

Ultraviolet Spectrum. Aqueous acid—286 nm ($A_1^1 = 33$ b); aqueous alkali—300 nm.

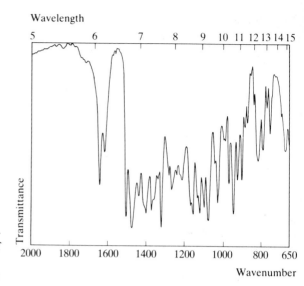

Infra-red Spectrum. Principal peaks at wavenumbers 1320, 1077, 1503, 1155, 1120, 947 (buprenorphine hydrochloride, KCl disk).

Mass Spectrum. Principal peaks at m/z 55, 378, 43, 29, 57, 410, 379, 84.

Quantification. RADIOIMMUNOASSAY. In plasma: sensitivity 50 pg/ml—A. J. Bartlett *et al.*, *Eur. J. clin. Pharmac.*, 1980, *18*, 339–345.

Disposition in the Body. Absorbed after parenteral or sublingual administration and metabolised mainly by *N*-dealkylation and conjugation. It is eliminated mainly in the faeces with a small proportion excreted in the urine, as metabolites.

THERAPEUTIC CONCENTRATION.
Peak plasma concentrations of 0.0005 to 0.0009 μg/ml (mean 0.0007) were reported in 5 subjects about 3 hours after a sublingual dose of 0.4 mg (administered 3 hours after a 0.3 mg intravenous dose) (R. E. S. Bullingham *et al.*, *Br. J. clin. Pharmac.*, 1982, *13*, 665–673).

HALF-LIFE. Plasma half-life, 4 to 6 hours.

VOLUME OF DISTRIBUTION. About 2.5 litres/kg.

PROTEIN BINDING. In plasma, about 96%.

Dose. The equivalent of 300 to 600 μg of buprenorphine given parenterally, or 200 to 400 μg by the sublingual route, every 6 to 8 hours.

Busulphan
Antineoplastic

Synonyms. Busulfan; Myelosan.
Proprietary Names. Misulban; Myleran.
Tetramethylene di(methanesulphonate)
$C_6H_{14}O_6S_2 = 246.3$
CAS—55-98-1

$$CH_3 \cdot SO_2 \cdot O \cdot [CH_2]_4 \cdot O \cdot SO_2 \cdot CH_3$$

A white crystalline powder. M.p. 115° to 118°.
Soluble 1 in 750 of water and 1 in 25 of acetone; slightly soluble in ethanol.
Caution. Busulphan is irritant; avoid contact with skin and mucous membranes.

Ultraviolet Spectrum. Methanol—256 nm ($A_1^1 = 20$ b).

Infra-red Spectrum. Principal peaks at wavenumbers 1178, 934, 861, 980, 962, 773 (KBr disk).

Quantification. GAS CHROMATOGRAPHY–MASS SPECTROMETRY. In plasma: sensitivity 10 ng/ml—H. Ehrsson and M. Hassan, *J. pharm. Sci.*, 1983, *72*, 1203–1205.

Disposition in the Body. Readily absorbed after oral administration. It is mainly excreted in the urine as metabolites; about 1% of a dose is excreted in the urine unchanged in 24 hours.

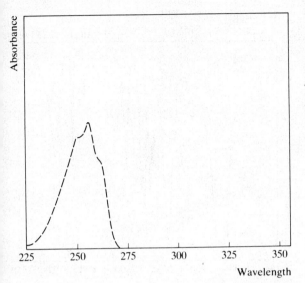

Ultraviolet Spectrum. Aqueous acid—272 nm, 278 nm (A_1^1 = 72 b); aqueous alkali—282 nm.

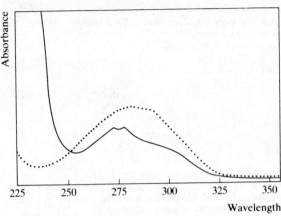

Wavelength

Infra-red Spectrum. Principal peaks at wavenumbers 1275, 1165, 1598, 1694, 1639, 1111 (KBr disk).

Mass Spectrum. Principal peaks at m/z 120, 263, 142, 178, 100, 264, 41, 29.

Use. A 2% solution of butacaine sulphate has been used for surface anaesthesia.

THERAPEUTIC CONCENTRATION.
Following single oral doses of 6 mg to 5 subjects, peak plasma concentrations of 0.05 to 0.13 µg/ml (mean 0.08) were reported (H. Ehrsson et al., Clin. Pharmac. Ther., 1983, 34, 86–89).

HALF-LIFE. Plasma half-life, about 2 to 3 hours.

Dose. Usually 2 to 4 mg daily; maintenance, 0.5 to 2 mg daily.

Butalamine   *Vasodilator*

NN - Dibutyl - N' - (3 - phenyl - 1,2,4 - oxadiazol - 5 - yl)-ethylenediamine
$C_{18}H_{28}N_4O = 316.4$
CAS—22131-35-7

Butacaine   *Local Anaesthetic*

3-Dibutylaminopropyl 4-aminobenzoate
$C_{18}H_{30}N_2O_2 = 306.4$
CAS—149-16-6

A liquid.

Butacaine Sulphate
Proprietary Name. It is an ingredient of Rhinamid.
$(C_{18}H_{30}N_2O_2)_2,H_2SO_4 = 711.0$
CAS—149-15-5
A white, very hygroscopic, crystalline powder. Unstable to light and moisture. M.p. about 100°.
Soluble 1 in 1.5 of water, 1 in 2 of ethanol, 1 in 2.5 of chloroform, and 1 in 2000 of ether; slightly soluble in acetone.

Dissociation Constant. pK_a 9.0.

Colour Test. Diazotisation—red.

Thin-layer Chromatography. *System TA*—Rf 71; *system TB*—Rf 09; *system TC*—Rf 30; *system TL*—Rf 64. (*Dragendorff spray*, positive; *acidified iodoplatinate solution*, positive; *ninhydrin spray*, positive; *Van Urk reagent*, bright yellow.)

Gas Chromatography. *System GA*—RI 2457.

High Pressure Liquid Chromatography. *System HA*—k' 1.2; *system HQ*—k' 8.97.

Butalamine Hydrochloride
Proprietary Names. Adrevil; Surheme.
$C_{18}H_{28}N_4O,HCl = 352.9$
CAS—56974-46-0
A white crystalline powder. M.p. 135° to 141°.
Soluble 1 in 7 of water, 1 in 10 of ethanol, and 1 in 2.5 of chloroform.

Thin-layer Chromatography. *System TA*—Rf 68; *system TD*—Rf 11; *system TE*—Rf 86; *system TF*—Rf 29. (*Acidified iodoplatinate solution*, positive.)

Gas Chromatography. *System GA*—RI 2490.

Ultraviolet Spectrum. Aqueous acid—228 nm ($A_1^1 = 812$ a).

Infra-red Spectrum. Principal peaks at wavenumbers 1639, 751, 1603, 694, 1492, 1170.

Mass Spectrum. Principal peaks at m/z 142, 143, 100, 155, 44, 112, 57, 29.

Dose. Butalamine hydrochloride has been given in doses of 160 to 320 mg daily.

Butalbital
Barbiturate

Synonyms. Alisobumalum; Allylbarbituric Acid; Itobarbital; Tetrallobarbital.

Proprietary Names. Sandoptal. It is an ingredient of Fiorinal.

Note. The name Butalbital has also been applied to talbutal, the *sec*-butyl analogue.

5-Allyl-5-isobutylbarbituric acid
$C_{11}H_{16}N_2O_3 = 224.3$
CAS—77-26-9

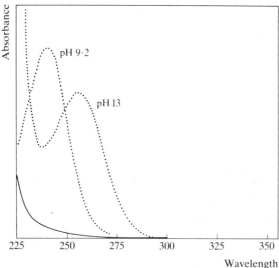

A white crystalline powder. M.p. 138° to 141°.

Slightly **soluble** in cold water; soluble in boiling water; freely soluble in ethanol, chloroform, and ether; soluble in aqueous solutions of alkali hydroxides and carbonates.

Dissociation Constant. pK_a 7.6 (20°).

Colour Tests. Koppanyi–Zwikker Test—violet; Vanillin Reagent—orange/colourless.

Thin-layer Chromatography. *System TD*—Rf 54; *system TE*—Rf 38; *system TF*—Rf 67; *system TH*—Rf 67. (*Mercurous nitrate spray*, black; *acidified potassium permanganate solution*, yellow-brown.)

Gas Chromatography. *System GA*—RI 1668; *system GF*—RI 2395.

High Pressure Liquid Chromatography. *System HG*—k' 6.17; *system HH*—k' 3.48.

Ultraviolet Spectrum. *Borax buffer 0.05M* (pH 9.2)—240 nm $(A_1^1 = 439 \, a)$; M sodium hydroxide (pH 13)—255 nm $(A_1^1 = 329 \, b)$.

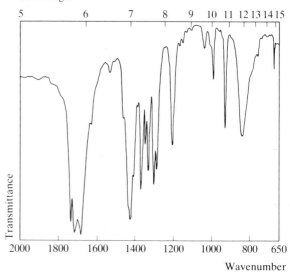

Wavelength

Infra-red Spectrum. Principal peaks at wavenumbers 1690, 1720, 1740, 1310, 1290, 1200 (KBr disk).

Mass Spectrum. Principal peaks at *m/z* 41, 167, 168, 39, 124, 97, 141, 181.

Quantification. See under Amylobarbitone.

Disposition in the Body. Absorbed after oral administration. About 5% of a dose is excreted in the urine as unchanged drug in 96 hours and 20 to 60% as 5-(2,3-dihydroxypropyl)-5-isobutylbarbituric acid.

THERAPEUTIC CONCENTRATION. In plasma, usually in the range 1 to 10 µg/ml.

TOXICITY. Plasma concentrations of 10 to 25 µg/ml are usually associated with toxic effects.

The following concentrations were reported in one fatality attributed to butalbital overdose: blood 26 µg/ml, liver 50 µg/g (R. C. Baselt and R. H. Cravey, *J. analyt. Toxicol.*, 1977, *1*, 81–103).

HALF-LIFE. Derived from urinary excretion data, about 30 to 40 hours.

Dose. 200 mg as a hypnotic; 150 to 400 mg daily as a sedative.

Butanilicaine
Local Anaesthetic

2-Butylamino-6'-chloroaceto-*o*-toluidide
$C_{13}H_{19}ClN_2O = 254.8$
CAS—3785-21-5

Crystals. M.p. 45° to 46°.

Butanilicaine Phosphate

Proprietary Name. Hostacain (also as hydrochloride).
$C_{13}H_{19}ClN_2O, H_3PO_4 = 352.8$
CAS—2081-65-4
Crystals. M.p. 126° to 127°.

Colour Tests. Aromaticity (Method 2)—colourless/orange; Koppanyi–Zwikker Test—violet; Liebermann's Test—orange.

Thin-layer Chromatography. *System TA*—Rf 76; *system TB*—Rf 14; *system TC*—Rf 54; *system TL*—Rf 61. (*Acidified iodoplatinate solution*, positive.)

Gas Chromatography. *System GA*—RI 2025.

High Pressure Liquid Chromatography. *System HQ*—k' 4.42.

Ultraviolet Spectrum. Aqueous acid—267 nm ($A_1^1 = 15$ b), 275 nm.

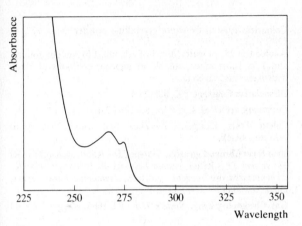

Infra-red Spectrum. Principal peaks at wavenumbers 1495, 1694, 770, 1136, 1562, 1587.

Mass Spectrum. Principal peaks at *m/z* 86, 30, 72, 44, 141, 42, 29, 57.

Quantification. GAS CHROMATOGRAPHY. In horse plasma or urine: sensitivity 5 ng/ml, AFID—F. T. Delbeke and M. Debackere, *J. Chromat.*, 1982, *237*, 344–349.

Dose. Butanilicaine phosphate has been administered by injection, as a 0.5 to 3% solution.

Butaperazine   *Tranquilliser*

Synonym. Butyrylperazine

1-{10-[3-(4-Methylpiperazin-1-yl)propyl]phenothiazin-2-yl}-butan-1-one

$C_{24}H_{31}N_3OS = 409.6$

CAS—653-03-2

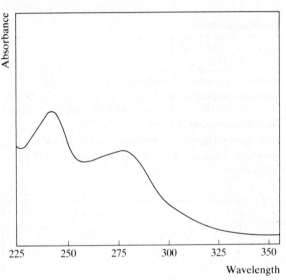

A yellow oil. B.p. 195° to 210°.

Butaperazine Maleate

Synonym. Butaperazine Dimaleate

Proprietary Name. Repoise

$C_{24}H_{31}N_3OS,2C_4H_4O_4 = 641.7$

CAS—1063-55-4

A yellow crystalline powder. M.p. about 195°.

Soluble in water; practically insoluble in chloroform and ether.

Butaperazine Phosphate

Synonym. Butaperazine Diphosphate

$C_{24}H_{31}N_3OS,2H_3PO_4 = 605.6$

CAS—7389-45-9

A yellow crystalline powder. M.p. 161° to 162°.

Soluble in water; practically insoluble in chloroform and ether.

Colour Tests. Mandelin's Test—brown-violet; Marquis Test—brown-violet.

Thin-layer Chromatography. *System TA*—Rf 53; *system TB*—Rf 24; *system TC*—Rf 37. (*Acidified potassium permanganate solution*, positive.)

High Pressure Liquid Chromatography. *System HA*—k' 3.4.

Ultraviolet Spectrum. Aqueous acid—242 nm ($A_1^1 = 609$ a), 277 nm.

Infra-red Spectrum. Principal peaks at wavenumbers 1675, 749, 1279, 1193, 1163, 1143.

Mass Spectrum. Principal peaks at *m/z* 113, 70, 409, 43, 141, 283, 42, 127.

Quantification. SPECTROFLUORIMETRY. In plasma—D. H. Manier *et al.*, *Clinica chim. Acta*, 1974, *57*, 225–230.

GAS CHROMATOGRAPHY. In biological fluids: sensitivity 5 ng/ml, AFID—J. I. Javaid *et al.*, *J. chromatogr. Sci.*, 1979, *17*, 666–670.

Disposition in the Body. Readily absorbed after oral administration. Metabolised to the sulphoxide and sulphone; other unidentified metabolites have been detected in plasma.

THERAPEUTIC CONCENTRATION.

Following oral administration of 40 mg as a single dose to 13 subjects, peak plasma concentrations of 0.07 to 0.69 µg/ml (mean 0.28) were attained in 2 to 4 hours; peak erythrocyte concentrations of 0.01 to 0.52 µg/ml (mean 0.11) were also reported (D. L. Garver *et al.*, *Archs gen. Psychiat.*, 1976, *33*, 862–866).

Following oral administration of 20 mg twice a day to 9 subjects, minimum steady-state plasma concentrations of 0.02 to 0.20 µg/ml (mean 0.09), and erythrocyte concentrations of 0.01 to 0.06 µg/ml (mean 0.03) were reported; therapeutic effect appeared to correlate with erythrocyte concentrations in the range 0.03 to 0.06 µg/ml (R. Casper *et al.*, *Archs gen. Psychiat.*, 1980, *37*, 301–305).

HALF-LIFE. Plasma half-life, 5 to 30 hours (mean 12).

Dose. Usually the equivalent of 15 to 30 mg of butaperazine daily; maximum of 100 mg daily.

Butethamate

Antispasmodic/Bronchodilator

Synonym. Butetamate
2-Diethylaminoethyl 2-phenylbutyrate
$C_{16}H_{25}NO_2 = 263.4$
CAS—14007-64-8

$$CH_3 \cdot CH_2 \cdot \overset{\overset{\displaystyle C_6H_5}{|}}{CH} \cdot CO \cdot O \cdot [CH_2]_2 \cdot N(C_2H_5)_2$$

Butethamate Citrate

Proprietary Name. It is an ingredient of CAM.
$C_{16}H_{25}NO_2, C_6H_8O_7 = 455.5$
CAS—13900-12-4
Colourless crystals. M.p. 107° to 110°.
Soluble 1 in 10 of water and 1 in 40 of ethanol.

Thin-layer Chromatography. *System TA*—Rf 69; *system TB*—Rf 59; *system TC*—Rf 57. (*Acidified iodoplatinate solution,* positive.)

Gas Chromatography. *System GA*—RI 1754.

High Pressure Liquid Chromatography. *System HA*—k' 1.7.

Ultraviolet Spectrum. Aqueous acid—253 nm, 258 nm (A_1^1 = 7.6 b), 264 nm.

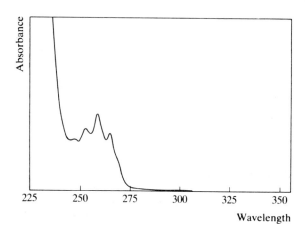

Infra-red Spectrum. Principal peaks at wavenumbers 1730, 1158, 1194, 694, 1265, 1219 (KBr disk).

Mass Spectrum. Principal peaks at *m/z* 86, 99, 91, 191, 87, 119, 58, 248.

Dose. Butethamate citrate has been given in doses of 18 to 90 mg daily.

Butobarbitone

Barbiturate

Synonyms. Butethal; Butobarbital (distinguish from Butabarbital).
Proprietary Names. Sonabarb; Soneryl.

5-Butyl-5-ethylbarbituric acid
$C_{10}H_{16}N_2O_3 = 212.2$
CAS—77-28-1

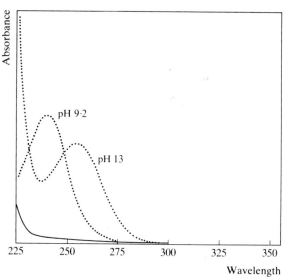

Colourless crystals or white crystalline powder. M.p. 122° to 127°.

Soluble 1 in 250 of water, 1 in 1 of ethanol, 1 in 3 of chloroform, and 1 in 10 of ether; soluble in aqueous solutions of alkali hydroxides and carbonates.

Dissociation Constant. pK$_a$ 8.0 (25°).

Partition Coefficient. Log *P* (octanol/pH 7.4), 1.7.

Colour Tests. Koppanyi–Zwikker Test—violet; Mercurous Nitrate—black.

Thin-layer Chromatography. *System TD*—Rf 50; *system TE*—Rf 38; *system TF*—Rf 65; *system TH*—Rf 68. (*Mercuric chloride-diphenylcarbazone reagent,* positive; *mercurous nitrate spray,* black; *Zwikker's reagent,* pink.)

Gas Chromatography. *System GA*—RI 1665; *system GF*—RI 2390.

High Pressure Liquid Chromatography. *System HG*—k' 5.43; *system HH*—k' 3.42.

Ultraviolet Spectrum. *Borax buffer 0.05M (pH 9.2)*—239 nm (A_1^1 = 477 a); M sodium hydroxide (pH 13)—254 nm (A_1^1 = 388 b).

Infra-red Spectrum. Principal peaks at wavenumbers 1696, 1727, 1760, 1242, 850, 1215 (KBr disk).

Mass Spectrum. Principal peaks at *m/z* 141, 156, 41, 55, 98, 39, 142, 155; 3'-hydroxybutobarbitone 156, 141, 45, 157, 41, 29, 55, 27.

Quantification. See also under Amylobarbitone.

Wavelength

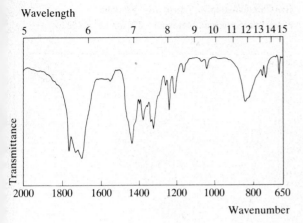

GAS CHROMATOGRAPHY–MASS SPECTROMETRY. In urine: butobarbitone and metabolites—J. N. T. Gilbert and J. W. Powell, *Eur. J. drug Met. Pharmacokinet.*, 1976, *1*, 188–193.

Disposition in the Body. Readily absorbed after oral administration. Metabolic reactions include side-chain oxidation to form the 3'-hydroxy, 3'-oxo, and 3'-carboxypropyl metabolites. About 5 to 9% of an oral dose is excreted in the urine unchanged, 22 to 28% as 3'-hydroxybutobarbitone, 14 to 18% as 3'-oxobutobarbitone, and 4 to 8% as 5-(3'-carboxypropyl)-5-ethylbarbituric acid.

THERAPEUTIC CONCENTRATION. In plasma, usually in the range 2 to 15 µg/ml.

A single oral dose of 200 mg given to 5 subjects, produced peak plasma concentrations of 2.9 to 4.1 µg/ml (mean 3.6) in 0.6 to 2 hours; following oral doses of 200 mg daily for 3 days to 2 subjects, plasma concentrations of 6.5 and 6.4 µg/ml were observed 9 hours after the last dose (D. D. Breimer, *Eur. J. clin. Pharmac.*, 1976, *10*, 263–271).

TOXICITY. The estimated minimum lethal dose is 2 g. Toxic effects are associated with plasma concentrations of 14 to 32 to 98 µg/ml and fatalities with blood concentrations of 11 to 30 to 75 µg/ml.

In 3 fatalities attributed to butobarbitone overdose, the following postmortem tissue concentrations, µg/ml or µg/g, were reported:

	Butobarbitone	3'-Hydroxybutobarbitone
Blood	18, 22, 49	—, 3, —
Bile	49, 27, 131	204, 4, 312
Kidney	31, 23, 72	—, 8, 12
Liver	47, 58, 83	2, 10, 17
Lung	26, 19, 52	—, 8, 19
Urine	4, 26, 38	259, —, 5

(A. E. Robinson and R. D. McDowall, *J. Pharm. Pharmac.*, 1979, *31*, 357–365).

HALF-LIFE. Plasma half-life, about 40 hours following single doses, but may be reduced to about 30 hours after multiple dosing.

VOLUME OF DISTRIBUTION. About 0.8 litre/kg.

PROTEIN BINDING. In plasma, about 26%.

Dose. 100 to 200 mg, as a hypnotic.

Butorphanol   *Narcotic Analgesic*

Synonym. Levo-BC-2627

(−)-9a-Cyclobutylmethylmorphinan-3,14-diol

$C_{21}H_{29}NO_2 = 327.5$

CAS—42408-82-2

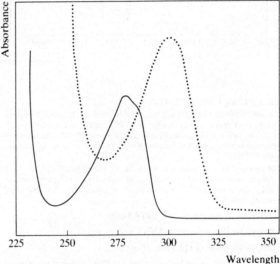

Butorphanol Tartrate

Proprietary Name. Stadol

$C_{21}H_{29}NO_2,C_4H_6O_6 = 477.6$

CAS—58786-99-5

A white crystalline powder. M.p. 217° to 219°, with decomposition. Sparingly **soluble** in water; slightly soluble in methanol; practically insoluble in ethanol, chloroform, and ether; soluble in dilute acids.

Colour Tests. Liebermann's Test—black; Marquis Test—grey.

Ultraviolet Spectrum. Aqueous acid—278 nm $(A_1^1 = 62\,b)$; aqueous alkali—299 nm.

Infra-red Spectrum. Principal peaks at wavenumbers 1269, 1130, 1233, 1575, 1249, 1303 (butorphanol tartrate, KBr disk). (See below)

Mass Spectrum. Principal peaks at *m/z* 272, 273, 41, 327, 145, 76, 42, 29.

Quantification. GAS CHROMATOGRAPHY. In serum: sensitivity 2 ng/ml, ECD—M. Pfeffer *et al.*, *J. pharm. Sci.*, 1980, *69*, 801–803.

RADIOIMMUNOASSAY. In serum: sensitivity < 25 pg—K. A. Pittman *et al.*, *J. pharm. Sci.*, 1980, *69*, 160–163.

Disposition in the Body. Well absorbed after oral or intramuscular administration; bioavailability about 17%. It undergoes extensive first-pass metabolism, mainly by hydroxylation, dealkylation and conjugation. The major metabolite is 3'-hydroxybutorphanol. About 70% of a dose is excreted in the urine and 13% eliminated in the faeces in 5 days. In 24 hours, 5 to 10% of a dose is excreted in the urine as unchanged drug, 5 to 10% as free and conjugated norbutorphanol, and about 50% as 3'-hydroxybutorphanol.

Wavelength

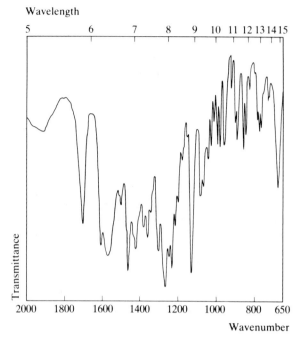

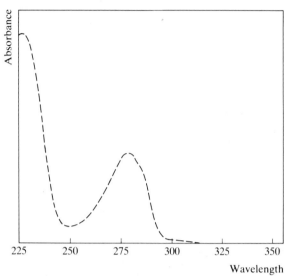

Gas Chromatography. *System GA*—RI 1640.

Ultraviolet Spectrum. Methanol—279 nm ($A_1^1 = 152$ b).

Infra-red Spectrum. Principal peaks at wavenumbers 1282, 1724, 1111, 740, 1020, 1587.

Use. Topically in a concentration of 2.5%.

Butriptyline *Antidepressant*

($\pm$) - 3 - (10,11 - Dihydro - 5*H* - dibenzo[*a*,*d*]cyclohepten - 5 - yl) - 2,*N*,*N*-trimethylpropylamine

$C_{21}H_{27}N = 293.5$

CAS—*35941-65-2*

An oil.

Butriptyline Hydrochloride

Proprietary Name. Evadyne

$C_{21}H_{27}N,HCl = 329.9$

CAS—*5585-73-9*

A white crystalline powder. M.p. about 186°.

Soluble in water, ethanol, and chloroform; practically insoluble in ether.

Colour Test. Marquis Test—violet.

Thin-layer Chromatography. *System TA*—Rf 59; *system TB*—Rf 61; *system TC*—Rf 48. (*Acidified iodoplatinate solution*, positive.)

Gas Chromatography. *System GA*—RI 2181; *system GF*—RI 2465.

High Pressure Liquid Chromatography. *System HA*—butriptyline k′ 2.7, norbutriptyline k′ 1.7; *system HF*—k′ 7.33.

Ultraviolet Spectrum. Aqueous acid—265 nm.

THERAPEUTIC CONCENTRATION.

A single intramuscular dose of 2 mg, administered to 6 subjects, produced a mean peak plasma concentration of 0.002 μg/ml of butorphanol in 0.5 to 1 hour, and a mean peak plasma concentration of 0.001 μg/ml of 3′-hydroxybutorphanol in 4 to 6 hours (R. C. Gaver *et al.*, *Drug Met. Disp.*, 1980, *8*, 230–235).

Following oral administration of 16 mg of butorphanol tartrate to 4 subjects, peak serum concentrations of 0.0003 to 0.003 μg/ml (mean 0.001) were attained in 2 to 4 hours (K. A. Pittman *et al.*, *J. pharm. Sci.*, 1980, *69*, 160–163).

HALF-LIFE. Plasma half-life, 2 to 4 hours.

VOLUME OF DISTRIBUTION. About 5 litres/kg.

PROTEIN BINDING. In plasma, about 80%.

NOTE. For a review of butorphanol see R. C. Heel *et al.*, *Drugs*, 1978, *16*, 473–505.

Dose. 1 to 4 mg of butorphanol tartrate every 4 hours by intramuscular injection; doses of 4 to 16 mg have been given by mouth.

Butoxyethyl Nicotinate *Topical Vasodilator*

Proprietary Names. It is an ingredient of Actinac and Finalgon.

2-Butoxyethyl nicotinate

$C_{12}H_{17}NO_3 = 223.3$

CAS—*13912-80-6*

Soluble in ether; slightly soluble in dilute acetic acid.

Thin-layer Chromatography. *System TA*—Rf 63; *system TB*—Rf 45; *system TC*—Rf 69. (*Acidified iodoplatinate solution*, positive.)

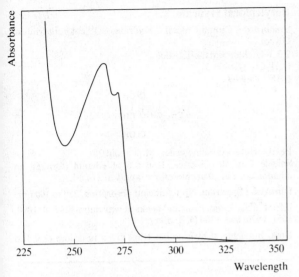

Infra-red Spectrum. Principal peaks at wavenumbers 757, 1033, 1265, 740, 1098, 1149 (KCl disk).

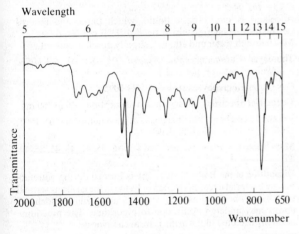

Mass Spectrum. Principal peaks at m/z 58, 293, 45, 59, 193, 100, 178, 294.

Quantification. GAS CHROMATOGRAPHY. In plasma: sensitivity 10 ng/ml, FID—T. R. Norman *et al., J. Chromat.*, 1977, *134*, 524–528.

Disposition in the Body. Readily absorbed after oral administration. It is rapidly metabolised, and the metabolites are thought to undergo enterohepatic circulation; the major metabolite is norbutriptyline. Butriptyline is slowly excreted in the urine mainly as metabolites; up to 25% of a dose is excreted in the urine in 24 hours with less than 2% of the dose as unchanged drug, and about 4% as glucuronide conjugates; about 1 to 2% of a dose is eliminated in the faeces in 24 hours.

THERAPEUTIC CONCENTRATION.

After a single oral dose of 75 mg to 14 subjects, peak plasma concentrations of 0.024 to 0.11 µg/ml (mean 0.05) were attained in about 3 hours (J. Bourgouin *et al., Biopharm. Drug Disp.*, 1981, *2*, 123–130).

Following oral administration of 50 mg three times a day to 9 subjects, steady-state plasma-butriptyline concentrations of 0.06 to 0.28 µg/ml (mean 0.15) were reported 6 hours after the final dose; plasma concentrations of norbutriptyline were of a similar order (G. D. Burrows *et al., Med. J. Aust.*, 1977, *2*, 604–606).

HALF-LIFE. Plasma half-life, about 20 hours.

PROTEIN BINDING. In plasma, more than 90%.

Dose. The equivalent of 75 to 150 mg of butriptyline daily.

Butyl Aminobenzoate   *Local Anaesthetic*

Synonyms. Butamben; Butoforme; Scuroforme.
Butyl 4-aminobenzoate
$C_{11}H_{15}NO_2 = 193.2$
CAS—94-25-7

A white crystalline powder. It slowly hydrolyses when boiled with water. M.p. 57° to 59°.
Very slightly **soluble** in water; soluble 1 in 3 of ethanol, and 1 in 2 of ether; soluble in chloroform and in dilute mineral acids.

Butyl Aminobenzoate Picrate
Proprietary Name. Butesin Picrate
$(C_{11}H_{15}NO_2)_2, C_6H_3N_3O_7 = 615.6$
CAS—577-48-0
A yellow powder. M.p. 109° to 110°.
Very slightly **soluble** in water; soluble in ethanol, chloroform, and ether.

Colour Test. Diazotisation—red.

Gas Chromatography. *System GA*—RI 1742.

Ultraviolet Spectrum. Aqueous acid—279 nm; aqueous alkali—285 nm; ethanol—294 nm ($A_1^1 = 1065$ a).

Infra-red Spectrum. Principal peaks at wavenumbers 1273, 1595, 1681, 1630, 1111, 1163.

Mass Spectrum. Principal peaks at m/z 120, 137, 193, 92, 65, 121, 138, 41.

Dose. The maximum safe dose for topical use is estimated to be 5 g.

Butylated Hydroxyanisole   *Antoxidant*

Synonym. BHA
Proprietary Names. Embanox BHA; Nipantiox 1-F; Tenox BHA.
2-*tert*-Butyl-4-methoxyphenol
$C_{11}H_{16}O_2 = 180.2$
CAS—25013-16-5

A white crystalline powder or a yellowish-white waxy solid. M.p. 62° to 65°.

It contains a variable proportion of 3-*tert*-butyl-4-methoxyphenol.

Practically **insoluble** in water; soluble 1 in 4 of ethanol, 1 in 2 of chloroform, 1 in 1.2 of ether, and 1 in 2 of propylene glycol; soluble in solutions of alkali hydroxides.

Colour Tests. Dissolve 0.1 g in 10 ml of ethanol, add 2 ml of a 2% solution of borax and a few crystals of 2,6-dichloroquinonechloroimide—blue (compare blue colour produced by butylated hydroxytoluene).

Dissolve a few crystals in 10 ml of ethanol and add 0.5 ml of a 0.2% solution of ferric ammonium sulphate in 0.5M sulphuric acid—green-blue.

Gas Chromatography. *System GA*—RI 1462.

Ultraviolet Spectrum. Acid ethanol—228 nm $(A_1^1 = 340 \text{ a})$, 292 nm $(A_1^1 = 205 \text{ a})$.

Infra-red Spectrum. Principal peaks at wavenumbers 1202, 1220, 1050, 805, 1185, 1294 (KBr disk).

Quantification. GAS CHROMATOGRAPHY. In plasma or urine: detection limit < 100 ng/ml, FID—R. El-Rashidy and S. Niazi, *J. pharm. Sci.*, 1979, *68*, 103–104.

Disposition in the Body. Absorbed after oral administration and may be stored in body fat after large doses. Metabolised by *O*-demethylation and conjugation with glucuronic acid and sulphate. Less than 1% of a dose is excreted in the urine unchanged in 24 hours together with 44% as the glucuronide, 26% as the sulphate and about 22% each as the glucuronide and sulphate conjugates of the desmethyl metabolite.

PROTEIN BINDING. In plasma, highly bound.

REFERENCE. R. El-Rashidy and S. Niazi, *Biopharm. Drug Disp.*, 1983, *4*, 389–396.

Butylated Hydroxytoluene   *Antoxidant*

Synonyms. BHT; DBPC.

Proprietary Names. Anullex BHT; Embanox BHT.

2,6-Di-*tert*-butyl-*p*-cresol

$C_{15}H_{24}O = 220.4$

CAS—128-37-0

Colourless crystals or white crystalline powder.

Practically **insoluble** in water; soluble 1 in 4 of ethanol, 1 in 1.1 of chloroform, and 1 in 0.5 of ether; practically insoluble in propylene glycol and in solutions of alkali hydroxides.

Colour Test. Dissolve 0.1 g in 10 ml of ethanol, add 2 ml of a 2% solution of borax and a few crystals of 2,6-dichloroquinonechloroimide—faint blue (compare blue colour produced by butylated hydroxyanisole).

Gas Chromatography. *System GA*—RI 1490.

Ultraviolet Spectrum. Dehydrated alcohol—278 nm $(A_1^1 = 85 \text{ a})$.

Disposition in the Body. Readily absorbed after oral administration. About 50% of a dose is excreted in the urine in 24 hours mainly as glucuronide conjugates of oxidation products.

Butylchloral Hydrate   *Hypnotic*

Synonyms. Croton-Chloral Hydrate; Trichlorobutylidene Glycol.

2,2,3-Trichlorobutane-1,1-diol

$C_4H_7Cl_3O_2 = 193.5$

CAS—76-40-4

Pearly-white crystalline scales. M.p. about 78°.

Soluble 1 in 40 of water, 1 in 0.6 of ethanol (forming an ethanolate), 1 in 20 of chloroform, and 1 in 2 of ether.

Ultraviolet Spectrum. No significant absorption, 230 to 360 nm.

Infra-red Spectrum. Principal peaks at wavenumbers 830, 1090, 1051, 1020, 690, 1300 (KBr disk).

Dose. Butylchloral hydrate has been given in a dose of 0.3 to 1.2 g.

Cadaverine   *Putrefactive Base*

Synonym. Pentamethylenediamine

Pentane-1,5-diamine

$NH_2 \cdot [CH_2]_5 \cdot NH_2 = 102.2$

CAS—462-94-2

A colourless syrupy basic liquid, which fumes and absorbs carbon dioxide on exposure to air. F.p. 9°. B.p. 178° to 180°.

Miscible with water and ethanol; slightly miscible with ether.

Thin-layer Chromatography. *System TA*—Rf 02. (*Acidified iodoplatinate solution*, positive.)

Gas Chromatography. *System GA*—RI 1035.

Ultraviolet Spectrum. No significant absorption, 230 to 360 nm.

Infra-red Spectrum. Principal peaks at wavenumbers 1565, 1508, 1600, 1120, 1173, 923 (KBr disk).

Mass Spectrum. Principal peaks at m/z 56, 55, 41, 43, 45, 85, 42, 84.

Disposition in the Body. Cadaverine is formed during putrefaction by bacterial decarboxylation of lysine in the gastro-intestinal tract. It may be deaminated to yield ammonia and an aldehyde, and it may undergo cyclisation to piperidine. The piperidine normally excreted in the urine is from cadaverine.

Caffeine   *Xanthine Stimulant*

Synonyms. Anhydrous Caffeine; Coffeinum; Guaranine; Methyltheobromine; Théine.

Proprietary Names. No Doz; Pro-Plus.

Caffeine is an ingredient of many proprietary preparations—see *Martindale, The Extra Pharmacopoeia*, 28th Edn.

7-Methyltheophylline

$C_8H_{10}N_4O_2 = 194.2$

CAS—58-08-2

An alkaloid obtained from tea waste, or coffee, or from the dried leaves of *Camellia sinensis* (Theaceae), or prepared synthetically; it is also present in guarana, maté, and kola.

Silky white crystals, usually matted together, or a white crystalline powder. It sublimes at about 180°. M.p. 234° to 239°. When crystallised from water, caffeine contains 1 molecule of water of crystallisation, but it is anhydrous when crystallised from ethanol, chloroform, or ether. It is decomposed by strong solutions of caustic alkalis.

Soluble 1 in 60 of water, 1 in 1 of boiling water, 1 in 130 of ethanol, and 1 in 7 of chloroform; slightly soluble in ether; soluble in dilute acids.

Caffeine Citrate

Synonym. Citrated Caffeine
Proprietary Names. It is an ingredient of Antoin, Cojene, and Myolgin.
$C_8H_{10}N_4O_2,C_6H_8O_7 = 386.3$
CAS—69-22-7
A mixture of caffeine and citric acid containing 47 to 50% of anhydrous caffeine.
A white powder which is decomposed by water.
Soluble 1 in 4 of hot water, dissociating on further dilution with the separation of caffeine on cooling which redissolves in about 32 of water; soluble 1 in 25 of ethanol.

Caffeine Hydrate

Synonym. Caffeine Monohydrate
Proprietary Names. It is an ingredient of Migril and Pardale.
$C_8H_{10}N_4O_2,H_2O = 212.2$
CAS—5743-12-4
Silky white crystals, usually matted together, or a white crystalline powder. It effloresces in dry air and loses its water of crystallisation when heated, becoming anhydrous at 100°. It sublimes at about 180°. M.p. 234° to 239°.
Soluble 1 in 60 of water and 1 in 110 of ethanol; soluble in chloroform with the separation of water; slightly soluble in ether.

Dissociation Constant. pK_a 14.0 (25°).

Partition Coefficient. Log P (octanol/pH 7.4), 0.0.

Colour Test. Amalic Acid Test—orange/violet.

Thin-layer Chromatography. *System TA*—Rf 52; *system TB*—Rf 03; *system TC*—Rf 58. (*Dragendorff spray*, positive; *acidified iodoplatinate solution*, positive.)

Gas Chromatography. *System GA*—RI 1810; *system GB*—RI 1862; *system GC*—RI 2376; *system GF*—RI 2340.

High Pressure Liquid Chromatography. *System HA*—k' 0.2; *system HC*—k' 0.26; *system HS*—k' 0.21.

Ultraviolet Spectrum. Aqueous acid—273 nm ($A_1^1 = 504$ a). No alkaline shift.

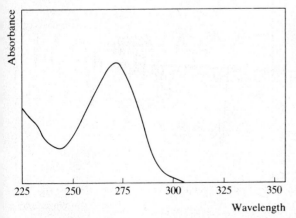

Infra-red Spectrum. Principal peaks at wavenumbers 1658, 1698, 747, 1548, 1242, 760 (KBr disk).

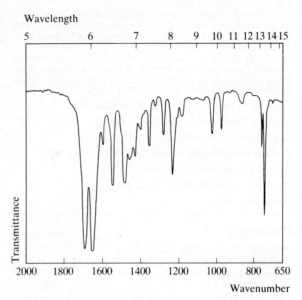

Mass Spectrum. Principal peaks at *m/z* 194, 109, 55, 67, 82, 195, 42, 110.

Quantification. GAS CHROMATOGRAPHY. In plasma: detection limit 50 ng/ml, AFID—I. D. Bradbrook *et al.*, *J. Chromat.*, 1979, *163*; *Biomed. Appl.*, *5*, 118–122.

HIGH PRESSURE LIQUID CHROMATOGRAPHY. In plasma, serum or saliva: detection limit 100 ng/ml, UV detection—D. B. Haughey *et al.*, *J. Chromat.*, 1982, *229*; *Biomed. Appl.*, *18*, 387–395. In plasma: sensitivity 100 ng/ml, UV detection—S. E. O'Connell and F. J. Zurzola, *J. pharm. Sci.*, 1984, *73*, 1009–1011.

Disposition in the Body. Rapidly absorbed after oral administration; bioavailability almost 100%. Metabolic reactions include *N*-demethylation and oxidation to uric acid derivatives. About 85% of a dose is excreted in the urine in 48 hours with up to 40% of the dose as 1-methyluric acid, 10 to 15% as 1-methylxanthine and up to 35% as 5-acetylamino-6-formylamino-3-methyluracil and 5-acetylamino-6-amino-3-methyluracil; other metabolites excreted in the urine include theophylline, 1,7-dimethylxanthine (paraxanthine), 7-methylxanthine, and 1,3-dimethyluric acid. Less than 10% is excreted in the urine as unchanged drug. The extent of *N*-acetylation is genetically determined. Caffeine, theophylline, theobromine, and paraxanthine are found in plasma from dietary sources especially coffee, tea and cocoa. An average cup of coffee or tea contains approximately 100 mg of caffeine.

THERAPEUTIC CONCENTRATION.

Following a single dose of 130 mg to 36 subjects, peak plasma concentrations of 2.5 to 6.8 µg/ml (mean 4.0) were attained in 20 to 40 minutes (S. E. O'Connell and F. J. Zurzola, *J. pharm. Sci.*, 1984, *73*, 1009–1011).

Following a single oral dose of 5 mg/kg to 10 subjects, peak plasma concentrations of 6.9 to 16.1 µg/ml (mean 10) were attained in about 0.5 hour (J. Blanchard and S. J. A. Sawers, *Eur. J. clin. Pharmac.*, 1983, *24*, 93–98).

TOXICITY. Fatalities have occurred after the ingestion of 5 to 50 g of caffeine, but recovery following the ingestion of 30 g has been reported. Toxic effects are associated with blood concentrations greater than 15 µg/ml and fatalities with blood concentrations greater than 80 µg/ml.

The following postmortem tissue concentrations were reported in a fatality due to the ingestion of 5.3 g of caffeine by a 5-year-old child: blood 159 µg/ml, kidney 230 µg/g, liver 198 µg/g, urine 114 µg/ml (V. J. M. DiMaio and J. G. Garriott, *Forens. Sci.*, 1974, *3*, 275–278).

In a fatality due to the ingestion of 50 g of caffeine, the following postmortem tissue concentrations were reported: blood 79 µg/ml, brain 105 µg/g, kidney 145 µg/g, liver 214 µg/g, urine 280 µg/ml (E. Grusz-Harday, *Bull. int. Ass. forens. Toxicol.*, 1973, *9*(1–2), 6–7).

HALF-LIFE. Plasma half-life, 2 to 10 hours (mean 4).

VOLUME OF DISTRIBUTION. About 0.5 litre/kg.

CLEARANCE. Plasma clearance, 1 to 2 ml/min/kg.

DISTRIBUTION IN BLOOD. Plasma: whole blood ratio, 0.93.

SALIVA. Plasma: saliva ratio, about 1.3.

PROTEIN BINDING. In plasma, about 35%.

Dose. 100 to 300 mg.

Camazepam   *Tranquilliser*

Proprietary Names. Albego; Limpidon.

7 - Chloro - 2,3 - dihydro - 1 - methyl - 2 - oxo - 5 - phenyl - 1*H* - 1,4 -benzodiazepin-3-yl dimethylcarbamate
$C_{19}H_{18}ClN_3O_3 = 371.8$
CAS—36104-80-0

A white crystalline powder. M.p. 173° to 174°.
Soluble in water and ethanol.

Gas Chromatography. *System GA*—RI 2954.

Ultraviolet Spectrum. Methanol—231 nm ($A_1^1 = 937$ b), 315 nm ($A_1^1 = 67$ b).

Infra-red Spectrum. Principal peaks at wavenumbers 1680, 1718, 1193, 1318, 1110, 703.

Mass Spectrum. Principal peaks at *m/z* 58, 72, 43, 78, 271, 57, 44, 77.

Quantification. GAS CHROMATOGRAPHY. In plasma: limit of detection 1 ng/ml, ECD—G. Cuisinaud *et al.*, *J. Chromat.*, 1979, *178*, 314–319.

Dose. 20 to 60 mg daily.

Cambendazole   *Anthelmintic*

Proprietary Names. Bovicam (vet.). It is an ingredient of Porcam (vet.).

Isopropyl 2-(thiazol-4-yl)-1*H*-benzimidazol-5-ylcarbamate
$C_{14}H_{14}N_4O_2S = 302.4$
CAS—26097-80-3

A white crystalline powder. M.p. 238° to 240°, with decomposition.

Practically **insoluble** in water; soluble in ethanol and dimethylformamide; sparingly soluble in acetone.

Ultraviolet Spectrum. Aqueous acid—235 nm ($A_1^1 = 620$ b), 319 nm ($A_1^1 = 689$ b); aqueous alkali—237 nm ($A_1^1 = 936$ b), 314 nm ($A_1^1 = 649$ b).

Mass Spectrum. Principal peaks at *m/z* 260, 302, 216, 215, 243, 189, 242, 188.

Camphor   *Rubefacient*

Synonyms. Alcanfor; 2-Camphanone; Camphre Droit (natural); Camphre du Japon (natural); Cânfora.
Proprietary Name. It is an ingredient of Pernomol.

Bornan-2-one
$C_{10}H_{16}O = 152.2$
CAS—76-22-2; 464-49-3 (+)

Camphor is obtained by distillation from the wood of *Cinnamomum camphora* (Lauraceae) and purified by sublimation, or it may be prepared synthetically. Natural camphor is dextrorotatory; the synthetic product is optically inactive.

Colourless transparent or white crystals, crystalline masses, blocks, or powdery masses known as 'flowers of camphor'. M.p. 174° to 181°.

Soluble 1 in 700 to 1 in 800 of water, 1 in 1 of ethanol, 1 in 0.25 of chloroform, and 1 in 1 of ether.

Gas Chromatography. *System GA*—RI 1136; *system GI*—retention time 38.2 min.

Ultraviolet Spectrum. Methanol—289 nm ($A_1^1 =$ about 2 b).

Infra-red Spectrum. Principal peaks at wavenumbers 1730, 1047, 1025, 1277, 1095, 755 (KCl disk).

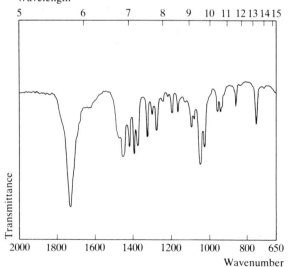

Mass Spectrum. Principal peaks at *m/z* 95, 81, 41, 69, 55, 83, 67, 137.

Quantification. GAS CHROMATOGRAPHY. In plasma: detection limit 100 ng/ml, FID—R. C. Kelly *et al.*, *J. analyt. Toxicol.*, 1979, *3*, 76–77.

Disposition in the Body. Absorbed after ingestion, through the mucous membranes and through the skin. Metabolised by hydroxylation and excreted in the urine mainly as the glucuronides of 2-hydroxy- and 3-hydroxycamphor. Oxidation also occurs at the 7-position yielding a small amount of a carboxylic acid.

TOXICITY. Poisoning by camphor has usually been due to ingestion of camphorated oil. The fatal dose in a one-year-old child is stated to be about 1 g of camphor although some children have survived the ingestion of 5 g. In adults, doses in the region of 2 g are likely to produce toxic symptoms and a dose of 4 g or more may be lethal, although a man has survived after ingestion of as much as 30 g in the form of 150 ml of camphorated oil. The maximum permissible atmospheric concentration is 2 ppm.

A plasma concentration of 1.7 µg/ml was reported in a severely intoxicated subject, 12 hours after the ingestion of about 18 g of camphor; the patient recovered after treatment by resin haemoperfusion (R. Kopelman *et al.*, *J. Am. med. Ass.*, 1979, *241*, 727–728).

A serum concentration of 19.5 µg/ml was observed 7 hours after the ingestion of 0.7 g of camphor in a moderately intoxicated 3-year-old child (W. J. Phelan, *Pediatrics*, 1976, *57*, 428–431).

Dose. Camphor was formerly given by mouth in doses of 120 to 300 mg.

Cannabis   *Psychomimetic*

Synonyms. Bhang; Cannabis Indica; Chanvre; Charas; Dagga; Ganja; Guaza; Hashish; Indian Hemp; Kif; Maconha; Marihuana.

Marihuana usually refers to a mixture of the leaves and flowering tops. *Bhang, dagga, ganja, kif,* and *maconha* are commonly used in various countries to describe similar preparations. *Hashish* and *charas* are names often applied to the resin, although in some countries hashish is applied to any cannabis preparation.

Note. Many other synonyms and approximate synonyms for cannabis and cannabis resin have been used—see *Martindale, The Extra Pharmacopoeia*, 28th Edn.

CAS—8063-14-7

The dried flowering or fruiting tops of the pistillate plant of *Cannabis sativa (Cannabinaceae)*. In some countries, the legal definition includes the leaves and roots.

The active principles of the drug are present in the resin which contains about 30 derivatives of 2-(2-isopropyl-5-methylphenyl)-5-pentylresorcinol, known as cannabinoids. Considerable confusion exists in the nomenclature, depending on whether they are numbered as substituted monoterpenes or dibenzopyrans. To avoid confusion the dibenzofuran system is used in this volume.

dibenzofuran numbering:

Where appropriate, the alternative numbering system based on a substituted monoterpene structure is given in parentheses.

monoterpenoid numbering:

The most important cannabinoids are cannabidiol (CBD), cannabinol (CBN), (−)-*trans*-Δ^9-tetrahydrocannabinol [Δ^9-THC (Δ^1-THC)], (−)-*trans*-Δ^8-tetrahydrocannabinol [Δ^8-THC (Δ^{1-6}-THC)], and Δ^9-tetrahydrocannabinolic acid.

Cannabidiol

Synonym. CBD
$C_{21}H_{30}O_2 = 314.5$
CAS—13956-29-1

White crystals. M.p. 66° to 67°.
Practically **insoluble** in water; readily soluble in chloroform and light petroleum.

Cannabinol

Synonym. CBN
$C_{21}H_{26}O_2 = 310.4$
CAS—521-35-7

White crystals. M.p. 76° to 77°.
Practically **insoluble** in water; readily soluble in chloroform and light petroleum.

Δ^9-Tetrahydrocannabinol

Synonyms. Δ^1-THC; Δ^9-THC; (−)-*trans*-Δ^9-Tetrahydrocannabinol.
$C_{21}H_{30}O_2 = 314.5$
CAS—1972-08-3

A viscous oil.
Practically **insoluble** in water; soluble 1 in 1 of ethanol and 1 in 1 of acetone; readily soluble in chloroform and light petroleum.

Δ^8-Tetrahydrocannabinol

Synonyms. Δ^{1-6}-THC; Δ^8-THC; $(-)$-*trans*-Δ^8-Tetrahydrocannabinol
$C_{21}H_{30}O_2 = 314.5$
CAS—5957-75-5

Practically **insoluble** in water; readily soluble in chloroform and light petroleum.

Δ^9-Tetrahydrocannabinolic Acid

$C_{22}H_{30}O_4 = 358.5$
CAS—23978-85-0

The amount of the major constituents in various samples of cannabis varies between about 5% and zero, depending on climatic and genetic factors. Almost all the psychomimetic activity of the plant is associated with the Δ^9-THC content, which is usually twenty times as great as that of Δ^8-THC. The Δ^9-THC content may average 1, 3, and 5% in marihuana, ganja, and hashish, respectively. Δ^9-Tetrahydrocannabinolic acid, which is present in abundance in some cannabis samples, is itself inactive but it is converted by smoking into active Δ^9-THC. Cannabinol and cannabidiol may be present in large amounts but have little activity.

Dissociation Constant. Δ^9-THC, pK$_a$ 10.6.

Colour Tests. *p*-Dimethylaminobenzaldehyde—red/violet (cannabinols); Duquenois Test—violet-blue/violet.

Thin-layer Chromatography. For information on the constituents of cannabis resin see Systems TI and TJ, p. 172.

Gas Chromatography. For information on the constituents of cannabis resin and on metabolites of Δ^9-THC see Systems GA and GH, p. 197.

High Pressure Liquid Chromatography. For information on the constituents of cannabis resin see System HL, p. 217.

Ultraviolet Spectrum. Ethanol—cannabidiol 278 nm, cannabinol 285 nm, Δ^9-THC 278 nm, Δ^9-tetrahydrocannabinolic acid 278 nm and 283 nm.

Infra-red Spectrum. Main components have principal peaks at the following wavenumbers (all thin films):
Cannabidiol—1585, 1630, 1020, 1210, 1240, 1050
Cannabinol—1620, 1050, 1580, 1030, 1120, 1228
Δ^8-THC—1580, 1030, 1620, 1180, 1080, 1260
Δ^9-THC—1580, 1040, 1620, 1180, 1130, 1050

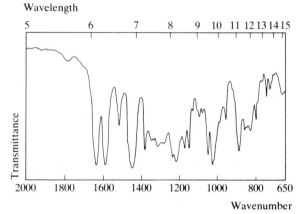

Cannabidiol

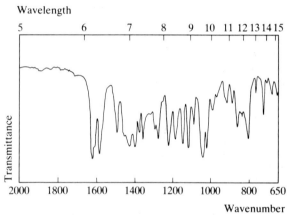

Cannabinol

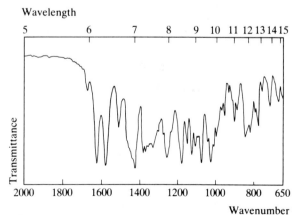

Δ^8-Tetrahydrocannabinol

Wavelength

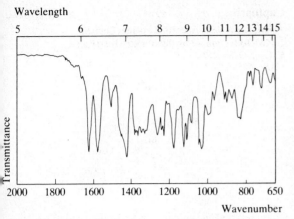

Δ^9-Tetrahydrocannabinol

Mass Spectrum. Main components and metabolites have principal peaks at the following m/z:
Cannabidiol—231, 246, 314, 232, 121, 193, 74, 174
Cannabinol—295, 296, 238, 310, 119, 43, 251, 239
Δ^8-THC—221, 314, 248, 261, 193, 236, 222, 315
Δ^9-THC—299, 231, 314, 43, 41, 295, 55, 271
8α-Hydroxy-Δ^9-THC—271, 43, 41, 311, 295, 312, 297, 91
8β-Hydroxy-Δ^9-THC—271, 43, 295, 41, 297, 29, 330, 272
11-Hydroxy-Δ^9-THC—299, 43, 41, 67, 300, 69, 231, 29
Δ^9-THC-11-oic acid—41, 229, 43, 329, 69, 344, 29, 283

Quantification. GAS CHROMATOGRAPHY. In blood or brain tissues: Δ^9-THC, detection limit 200 to 300 pg/ml in blood and 2.5 ng/g in brain samples, FID—N. K. McCallum and S. M. Shaw, *J. analyt. Toxicol.*, 1981, *5*, 148–149.

GAS CHROMATOGRAPHY–MASS SPECTROMETRY. In blood: Δ^9-THC, initial screening by radioimmunoassay, detection limit 1 ng/ml—R. A. Bergman *et al.*, *J. analyt. Toxicol.*, 1981, *5*, 85–89.

HIGH PRESSURE LIQUID CHROMATOGRAPHY–MASS SPECTROMETRY. In plasma: Δ^9-THC, detection limit 2.5 ng/ml—J. L. Valentine *et al.*, *J. pharm. Sci.*, 1977, *66*, 1263–1266.

HIGH PRESSURE LIQUID CHROMATOGRAPHY–RADIOIMMUNOASSAY. In blood, plasma, serum, or urine: Δ^9-THC and metabolites, sensitivity 6.5 ng/ml for plasma and 3.3 ng/ml for urine—B. Law *et al.*, *J. analyt. Toxicol.*, 1984, *8*, 19–22.

RADIOIMMUNOASSAY. In body fluids: cannabinoid metabolites, sensitivity 10 ng/ml for blood and 2 ng/ml for urine—*idem*, 14–18.

Disposition in the Body. Δ^9-THC is absorbed from the gastrointestinal tract but absorption is slow and irregular; bioavailability after ingestion is about 6 to 20% and during smoking is about 18%. Δ^9-THC is lipophilic and is widely distributed in the body. It is oxidised to the active metabolites 11-hydroxy-Δ^9-THC and 8β-hydroxy-Δ^9-THC. The inactive substances 8α-hydroxy-Δ^9-THC and 8α,11-dihydroxy-Δ^9-THC are also formed. 11-Hydroxy-Δ^9-THC is further oxidised to 11-nor-Δ^9-THC-9-carboxylic acid (Δ^9-THC-11-oic acid), and many other polar mono- and di-carboxylic acids are formed; these are conjugated with glucuronic acid to a variable extent. Enterohepatic circulation of metabolites may occur. Up to about 25% of a dose is excreted in the urine in 3 days, mainly as 11-nor-Δ^9-THC-9-carboxylic acid glucuronide, together with the other carboxylic acids in free and conjugated form. Δ^9-THC-*O*-glucuronide has

also been detected in urine. The major excretion route is via the faeces, up to about 65% of a dose being excreted in 5 days, mainly as 11-hydroxy-Δ^9-THC and the carboxylic acids in conjugated form. Δ^9-THC metabolites have been detected in urine for up to 12 days following a single oral dose.

BLOOD CONCENTRATION.
After 11 subjects had smoked 11.6 to 15.6 mg (mean 13.0) of Δ^9-THC from a cigarette over a period of 5 to 7 minutes, peak plasma concentrations of 0.03 to 0.12 µg/ml (mean 0.08) of Δ^9-THC were observed within 3 minutes after termination of smoking; the concentration fell rapidly to 0.003 to 0.01 µg/ml (mean 0.007) at 1 hour and to 0.0006 to 0.003 µg/ml (mean 0.0016) at 4 hours, after smoking. When 20 mg of Δ^9-THC was given orally to the same subjects, peak plasma concentrations of 0.004 to 0.01 µg/ml of Δ^9-THC were produced between 60 and 300 minutes after ingestion (A. Ohlsson *et al.*, *Clin. Pharmac. Ther.*, 1980, *28*, 409–416).

TOXICITY. Cannabis or Δ^9-THC intoxication may result in loss of consciousness or even death, but reports of fatalities are rare. In one case of fatal poisoning by Δ^9-THC, the following postmortem concentrations of Δ^9-THC in tissues were reported: liver 37.5 µg/g, kidney 42 µg/g, and spleen 12 µg/g (S. N. Tewari and J. D. Sharma, *Toxicol. Lett.*, 1980, *5*, 279–281).

HALF-LIFE. Plasma half-life, Δ^9-THC about 20 to 36 hours.

VOLUME OF DISTRIBUTION. Δ^9-THC about 10 litres/kg.

DISTRIBUTION IN BLOOD. Plasma : whole blood ratio, Δ^9-THC 1.8.

PROTEIN BINDING. In plasma, Δ^9-THC and 11-hydroxy-Δ^9-THC 94 to 99%.

NOTE. For a review of Δ^9-THC metabolism and disposition see M. E. Wall and M. Perez-Reyes, *J. clin. Pharmac.*, 1981, *21*, 178s–189s. See also M. E. Wall *et al.*, *Clin. Pharmac. Ther.*, 1983, *34*, 352–363, and B. Law *et al.*, *J. Pharm. Pharmac.*, 1984, *36*, 289–294.

Further references. Determination of the distribution of cannabinoids in cannabis resin—P. B. Baker *et al.*, *J. analyt. Toxicol.*, 1980, *4*, 145–152. The Δ^9-THC and Δ^9-tetrahydrocannabinolic acid content of cannabis products—P. B. Baker *et al.*, *J. Pharm. Pharmac.*, 1981, *33*, 369–372. Detection of cannabinoids in saliva and in breath—J. L. Valentine and P. Psaltis, *Analyt. Lett. (Part B)*, 1979, *12*, 855–866 and 867–880. Swabbing the hands for traces of marihuana—R. Thibault *et al.*, *J. forens Sci.*, 1983, *28*, 15–17.

Cantharidin   *Vesicant*

Proprietary Name. Cantharone
Hexahydro-3aα,7aα-dimethyl-4β,7β-epoxyisobenzofuran-1,3-dione
$C_{10}H_{12}O_4 = 196.2$
CAS—56-25-7

Cantharidin is obtained from cantharides, the dried beetle *Cantharis vesicatoria* (= *Lytta vesicatoria*) (Meloidae) or other spp., containing not less than 0.6%, or from mylabris, the dried beetles *Mylabris sidae* (= *M. phalerata*), *M. cichorii* and *M. pustulata* (Meloidae), containing not less than 1%.

Colourless, glistening crystals, which sublime at about 120°. M.p. 216° to 218°.

Very slightly **soluble** in water; soluble 1 in about 1100 of ethanol, 1 in 40 of acetone, 1 in 55 of chloroform, and 1 in 700 of ether.

Gas Chromatography. *System GA*—RI 1490.

Infra-red Spectrum. Principal peaks at wavenumbers 1242, 962, 900, 1786, 1852, 1002 (Nujol mull).

Mass Spectrum. Principal peaks at m/z 128, 96, 70, 39, 41, 27, 42, 29.

Disposition in the Body. Readily absorbed from the skin and mucous membranes. It does not appear to be metabolised.

TOXICITY. When taken orally it causes great pain as well as blistering and gross inflammation of the gastro-intestinal tract, the kidneys and the bladder. The lethal dose is between 10 and 60 mg although a crystal weighing not more than 0.5 mg lodged in the mucosa might produce a blister which could be fatal.

A 27-year-old woman died about 17 hours after she had eaten coconut ice into which a small quantity of cantharidin had been introduced by a fellow employee. The postmortem findings revealed that between 65 and 130 mg of cantharidin was circulating in the organs. At the same time as the above incident a 19-year-old girl also ate a piece of the cantharidin-impregnated coconut ice. She died 26 hours later. The postmortem level of cantharidin in the organs was somewhat less than in the former case (L. C. Nickolls and D. Teare, *Br. med. J.*, 1954, **2**, 1384).

Captodiame
Tranquilliser

Synonym. Captodiamine

2-(4-Butylthiobenzhydrylthio)-*NN*-dimethylethylamine

$C_{21}H_{29}NS_2 = 359.6$

CAS—486-17-9

$$C_6H_5 \cdot CH \cdot S \cdot [CH_2]_2 \cdot N(CH_3)_2$$

$$S \cdot [CH_2]_3 \cdot CH_3$$

Captodiame Hydrochloride

Proprietary Name. Covatine

$C_{21}H_{29}NS_2, HCl = 396.0$

CAS—904-04-1

Crystals. M.p. 131° to 132°.

Colour Tests. Mandelin's Test—violet; Marquis Test—violet.

Thin-layer Chromatography. *System TA*—Rf 66. (*Acidified iodoplatinate solution*, positive.)

Gas Chromatography. *System GA*—RI 2774.

Ultraviolet Spectrum. Aqueous acid—266 nm ($A_1^1 = 370$ b); aqueous alkali—273 nm.

Infra-red Spectrum. Principal peaks at wavenumbers 694, 751, 1086, 1041, 1010, 714 (KBr disk).

Mass Spectrum. Principal peaks at m/z 58, 165, 255, 359, 166, 73, 199, 45.

Dose. Captodiame hydrochloride has been given in doses of 150 mg daily.

Captopril
Antihypertensive

Proprietary Names. Acepril; Capoten; Lopirin.

1-[(2*S*)-3-Mercapto-2-methylpropionyl]-L-proline

$C_9H_{15}NO_3S = 217.3$

CAS—62571-86-2

$$SH \cdot CH_2 \cdot \overset{H}{\underset{CH_3}{C}} \cdot CO \cdot N \underset{}{\overset{}{\bigcirc}} \cdot COOH$$

A white crystalline powder. M.p. about 106°.

Freely **soluble** in water, ethanol, chloroform, and methanol.

Dissociation Constant. pK_a 3.7, 9.8.

Colour Tests. Palladium Chloride—orange; Sodium Nitroprusside (Method 2)—violet.

Thin-layer Chromatography. *System TD*—Rf 05; *system TE*—Rf 02; *system TF*—Rf 02. (*Ferric chloride solution*, yellow; *mercuric chloride–diphenylcarbazone reagent*, violet, turns pink on heating; *acidified potassium permanganate solution*, yellow; *Van Urk reagent*, yellow, fades on heating.)

Gas Chromatography. Decomposition occurs giving a single, broad and severely tailing peak.

Ultraviolet Spectrum. Aqueous acid—no significant absorption, 230 to 360 nm; aqueous alkali—238 nm ($A_1^1 = 235$ c).

Infra-red Spectrum. Principal peaks at wavenumbers 1589, 1742, 1202, 1192, 1229, 1245 (KBr disk). Polymorphism may occur.

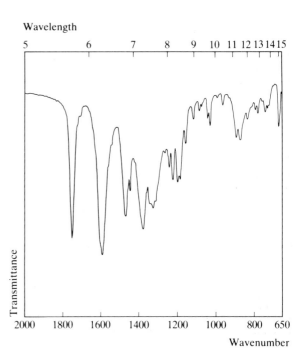

Wavelength

Transmittance

Wavenumber

Mass Spectrum. Principal peaks at *m/z* 70, 41, 69, 75, 114, 42, 217, 68.

Quantification. GAS CHROMATOGRAPHY. In plasma or blood: sensitivity 20 ng/ml for captopril in blood, 50 ng/ml for captopril and metabolites in plasma, ECD—M. S. Bathala *et al.*, *J. pharm. Sci.*, 1984, *73*, 340–344.

GAS CHROMATOGRAPHY–MASS SPECTROMETRY. In plasma or urine: detection limits 1 ng/ml for captopril, 25 ng/ml for captopril disulphide—O. H. Drummer *et al.*, *J. Chromat.*, 1984, *305*; *Biomed. Appl.*, *30*, 83–93.

HIGH PRESSURE LIQUID CHROMATOGRAPHY. In blood or urine: sensitivity 5 ng/ml in blood and 100 ng/ml in urine, UV detection—Y. Kawahara *et al.*, *Chem. pharm. Bull.*, 1981, *29*, 150–157. In plasma: detection limit 30 ng/ml, fluorescence detection—B. Jarrott *et al.*, *J. pharm. Sci.*, 1981, *70*, 665–667.

RADIOIMMUNOASSAY. In plasma: sensitivity 2 ng/ml—F. M. Duncan *et al.*, *Clinica chim. Acta*, 1983, *131*, 295–303.

Disposition in the Body. Readily absorbed after oral administration; about 75% of the dose is absorbed. Up to 40% of an oral dose is excreted in the urine as unchanged drug, about 3% as captopril disulphide and about 30% as polar metabolites. Excretion in the urine is rapid, about half the dose being excreted within the first 4 hours. An *S*-methyl metabolite has been identified in plasma and urine.

THERAPEUTIC CONCENTRATION.

After a single oral dose of 100 mg of ^{35}S-labelled captopril to 10 subjects, peak blood concentrations of 0.51 to 1.31 µg/ml (mean 0.8) of captopril and 0.11 to 0.49 µg/ml (mean 0.23) of captopril disulphide, were attained in 0.5 to 1.5 hours (K. J. Kripalani *et al.*, *Clin. Pharmac. Ther.*, 1980, *27*, 636–641).

Following oral administration of 25 mg, three times a day to 12 subjects, a mean maximum steady-state blood concentration of 0.14 µg/ml of captopril was reported 0.9 hour after a dose (R. J. Cody *et al.*, *Clin. Pharmac. Ther.*, 1982, *32*, 721–726).

HALF-LIFE. Blood half-life, about 1 to 2 hours.

VOLUME OF DISTRIBUTION. In blood, about 0.7 litre/kg.

CLEARANCE. Blood clearance, about 13 ml/min/kg.

PROTEIN BINDING. In plasma, about 30%.

NOTE. For a review of captopril see J. A. Romankiewicz *et al.*, *Drugs*, 1983, *25*, 6–40.

Dose. 75 to 150 mg daily; maximum of 450 mg daily.

Caramiphen   *Anticholinergic*

2-Diethylaminoethyl 1-phenylcyclopentane-1-carboxylate
$C_{18}H_{27}NO_2 = 289.4$
CAS—77-22-5

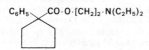

A liquid.

Caramiphen Edisylate

Synonym. Caramiphen Ethanedisulphonate
$C_{18}H_{27}NO_2, \frac{1}{2}C_2H_6O_6S_2 = 384.5$
CAS—125-86-0
Crystals. M.p. 115° to 116°.
Soluble in water and ethanol.

Caramiphen Hydrochloride

$C_{18}H_{27}NO_2, HCl = 325.9$
CAS—125-85-9
White crystals or crystalline powder. M.p. 142° to 146°.
Soluble 1 in 4 of water and 1 in 8 of ethanol; practically insoluble in ether.

Partition Coefficient. Log *P* (octanol), 2.3.

Colour Tests. Liebermann's Test—red-orange; Marquis Test—yellow; Sulphuric Acid (when warmed)—red.

Thin-layer Chromatography. *System TA*—Rf 66. (*Acidified iodoplatinate solution*, positive.)

Gas Chromatography. *System GA*—RI 1971.

Ultraviolet Spectrum. Aqueous acid—252 nm ($A_1^1 = 7.9$ b), 259 nm ($A_1^1 = 7.9$ b), 265 nm.

Infra-red Spectrum. Principal peaks at wavenumbers 1718, 1154, 694, 1173, 1220, 1060 (KBr disk).

Mass Spectrum. Principal peaks at *m/z* 86, 99, 91, 144, 58, 56, 41, 87.

Quantification. GAS CHROMATOGRAPHY. In blood: sensitivity <2.5 ng/ml, AFID—P. Levandoski and T. Flanagan, *J. pharm. Sci.*, 1980, *69*, 1353–1354.

Disposition in the Body.

THERAPEUTIC CONCENTRATION.

Following daily oral administration of 20 mg of caramiphen edisylate at 0, 4, and 8 hours to 11 subjects for 4 days, peak blood concentrations of 0.018 to 0.078 µg/ml (mean 0.046) were reported 1 to 2 hours after a dose (P. Levandoski and T. Flanagan, *ibid.*).

Dose. Caramiphen hydrochloride has been given in doses of 50 to 600 mg daily.

Carbachol   *Parasympathomimetic*

Synonyms. Carbacholine; Carbamoylcholine Chloride; Carbamylcholine Chloride; Choline Chloride Carbamate.
Proprietary Names. Carbyl; Doryl; Miostat.
(2-Carbamoyloxyethyl)trimethylammonium chloride
$C_6H_{15}ClN_2O_2 = 182.6$
CAS—51-83-2

$$[NH_2 \cdot CO \cdot O \cdot [CH_2]_2 \cdot N^+(CH_3)_3] \, Cl^-$$

White or faintly yellow, hygroscopic, crystals or crystalline powder. M.p. 200° to 204°, with decomposition.
Soluble 1 in 1 of water and 1 in 50 of ethanol; very slightly soluble in dehydrated alcohol, more readily soluble on boiling; practically insoluble in acetone, chloroform, and ether.

Dissociation Constant. pK_a 4.8.

Thin-layer Chromatography. *System TA*—Rf 01. (*Acidified iodoplatinate solution*, positive.)

Ultraviolet Spectrum. No significant absorption, 230 to 360 nm.

Infra-red Spectrum. Principal peaks at wavenumbers 1730, 1083, 1056, 930, 1102, 1200 (KBr disk).

Mass Spectrum. Principal peaks at *m/z* 43, 58, 42, 44, 30, 129, 36, 143.

Dose. 6 mg daily by mouth. For acute symptoms, 250 µg by subcutaneous injection, repeated if necessary.

Carbamazepine

Anticonvulsant

Proprietary Names. Convuline; Tegretol; Timonil.
5*H*-Dibenz[*b,f*]azepine-5-carboxamide
$C_{15}H_{12}N_2O = 236.3$
CAS—298-46-4

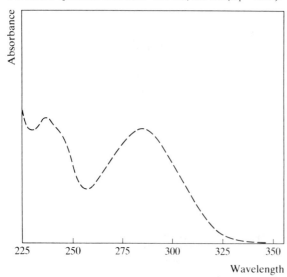

A white or yellowish-white crystalline powder. M.p. 189° to 193°.

Practically **insoluble** in water and ether; soluble 1 in 10 of ethanol and 1 in 10 of chloroform; soluble in acetone.

Colour Test. Dissolve the sample in 1 ml of chloroform, add 0.2 ml of *sodium hypobromite solution* and mix for 1 minute—blue-violet (detection limit 250 μg/ml).

Thin-layer Chromatography. *System TA*—Rf 60; *system TB*—Rf 04; *system TC*—Rf 56. (*Acidified potassium permanganate solution*, positive.)

Gas Chromatography. *System GA*—carbamazepine RI 2290, carbamazepine-10,11-epoxide RI 2030, iminostilbene RI 1930; *system GE*—carbamazepine retention time 0.83 relative to phenytoin; *system GF*—carbamazepine RI 2610, carbamazepine-10,11-epoxide RI 2560, iminostilbene RI 2620.

High Pressure Liquid Chromatography. *System HE*—k′ 8.30.

Ultraviolet Spectrum. Methanol—237 nm, 285 nm ($A_1^1 = 490$ a).

Infra-red Spectrum. Principal peaks at wavenumbers 1678, 1594, 800, 769, 787, 1298 (KBr disk).

Mass Spectrum. Principal peaks at *m/z* 193, 192, 236, 191, 194, 165, 190, 237; carbamazepine-10,11-epoxide 180, 179, 178, 152, 44, 181, 223, 51; *trans*-10,11-dihydro-10,11-dihydroxycarbamazepine 180, 77, 181, 44, 179, 51, 209, 167.

Quantification. GAS CHROMATOGRAPHY. In plasma: carbamazepine and carbamazepine-10,11-epoxide, FID—A. Ranise *et al.*, *J. Chromat.*, 1981, *222*; *Biomed. Appl.*, *11*, 120–124. In plasma or urine: carbamazepine and other anticonvulsants,

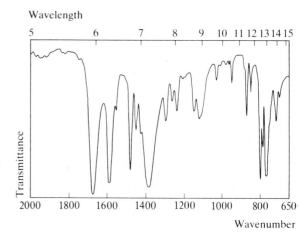

detection limit 1 μg/ml, FID—R. Riva *et al.*, *J. Chromat.*, 1980, *221*; *Biomed. Appl.*, *10*, 75–84.

HIGH PRESSURE LIQUID CHROMATOGRAPHY. In plasma or saliva: carbamazepine and carbamazepine-10,11-epoxide, sensitivity 20 ng/ml for carbamazepine and 120 ng/ml for the metabolite in plasma, UV detection—J. J. MacKichan, *J. Chromat.*, 1980, *181*; *Biomed. Appl.*, *7*, 373–383. In plasma or serum: carbamazepine and other anticonvulsants, sensitivity about 1 μg/ml, UV detection—J. A. Christofides and D. E. Fry, *Clin. Chem.*, 1980, *26*, 499–501.

THIN-LAYER CHROMATOGRAPHY–SPECTROFLUORIMETRY. In serum: carbamazepine and two metabolites, detection limits 100 ng/ml for carbamazepine and 50 ng/ml for its metabolites—H. K. L. Hundt and E. C. Clark, *J. Chromat.*, 1975, *107*, 149–154.

Disposition in the Body. Slowly but almost completely absorbed after oral administration; bioavailability greater than 70%. Metabolic reactions include epoxidation to form the 10,11-epoxide, which is active, followed by hydroxylation to *trans*-10,11-dihydro-10,11-dihydroxycarbamazepine; glucuronic acid conjugation also occurs. The rate of metabolism is higher in children than in adults. About 25% of a dose is excreted in the urine as the dihydroxy metabolite, together with 2% as the 10,11-epoxide and less than 10% as unchanged drug; other metabolites identified in the urine include carbamazepine-*N*-glucuronide, iminostilbene, and several monohydroxy- and trihydroxycarbamazepine isomers. About 30% of a dose is eliminated in the faeces.

THERAPEUTIC CONCENTRATION. In plasma, usually in the range 4 to 12 μg/ml.

Following single oral doses of 200 mg given to 9 subjects, peak plasma concentrations of 7.8 to 14 μg/ml (mean 10) were attained in about 9 hours (M. Anttila *et al.*, *Eur. J. clin. Pharmac.*, 1979, *15*, 421–425).

Steady-state plasma concentrations of 3 to 13 μg/ml (mean 8) for carbamazepine and 0.6 to 5.7 μg/ml (mean 3) for the epoxide metabolite, were reported in 24 subjects receiving daily oral doses of 8 to 30 mg/kg (J. J. MacKichan *et al.*, *Br. J. clin. Pharmac.*, 1981, *12*, 31–37).

TOXICITY. The estimated minimum lethal dose is 5 g. Plasma concentrations of 2.4 to **6.0** to 10.5 μg/ml have been associated with slight toxic effects and concentrations of 3.2 to **10** to 21 μg/ml with severe toxicity.

In a fatality due to carbamazepine and ethanol intoxication, postmortem blood concentrations were: carbamazepine 53 μg/ml, ethanol 1930 μg/ml (M. Rousseau *et al.*, *Bull. int. Ass. forens. Toxicol.*, 1981, *16*(1), 14–15).

In a fatality due to carbamazepine and alcohol, postmortem kidney and liver concentrations of 306 µg/g and 173 µg/g, respectively, of carbamazepine were reported: the blood-alcohol concentration was 1600 µg/ml (T. Borkowski and E. Janowska, *Bull. int. Ass. forens. Toxicol.*, 1983, *17*(2), 16–17).

A 50-year-old man was admitted to hospital comatose 12 hours after the ingestion of an estimated 20 g of carbamazepine; a plasma concentration of 62 µg/ml was reported; he regained consciousness after 45 hours but remained confused for a further 4 days (P. J. Leslie *et al.*, *Br. med. J.*, 1983, *286*, 1018).

HALF-LIFE. Plasma half-life, 18 to 65 hours (mean 35) after single doses; reduced during chronic treatment to about 10 to 30 hours for adults and 8 to 19 hours for children.

VOLUME OF DISTRIBUTION. About 1 litre/kg.

DISTRIBUTION IN BLOOD. Plasma: whole blood ratio, about 1.6.

SALIVA. Plasma: saliva ratio, about 3 to 5.

PROTEIN BINDING. In plasma, carbamazepine about 75% and 10,11-epoxycarbamazepine about 50%.

NOTE. For a review of the pharmacokinetics of carbamazepine see L. Bertilsson, *Clin. Pharmacokinet.*, 1978, *3*, 128–143.

Dose. Initially 100 to 400 mg daily, increasing to 0.4 to 1.6 g daily.

Carbarsone   *Anti-amoebic*

Synonym. Aminarsonum
4-Ureidophenylarsonic acid
$C_7H_9AsN_2O_4 = 260.1$
CAS—121-59-5

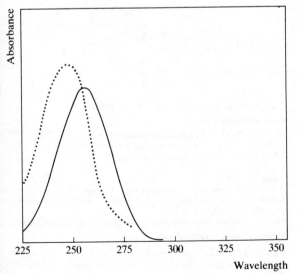

A white powder. M.p. 174°.

Soluble 1 in 330 of water and 1 in 400 of ethanol; very slightly soluble in chloroform and ether; soluble in solutions of alkali hydroxides and carbonates.

Ultraviolet Spectrum. Aqueous acid—257 nm; aqueous alkali—248 nm.

Infra-red Spectrum. Principal peaks at wavenumbers 1508, 1580, 1101, 903, 1681, 1248.

Dose. 500 to 750 mg daily, for 10 days.

Carbaryl   *Insecticide*

Synonym. Carbaril
Proprietary Names. Carylderm; Derbac (shampoo); Murvin; Sevin; Suleo-C.
1-Naphthyl methylcarbamate
$C_{12}H_{11}NO_2 = 201.2$
CAS—63-25-2

A white crystalline solid. M.p. 142°.
Practically **insoluble** in water; soluble in most polar organic solvents.

Colour Tests. Liebermann's Test—black→green; Marquis Test—green.

Gas Chromatography. Alphanaphthol (decomposition product): *system GA*—RI 1490; *system GK*—retention time 0.47 relative to caffeine.

Ultraviolet Spectrum. Ethanol—279 nm ($A_1^1 = 310$ b).

Infra-red Spectrum. Principal peaks at wavenumbers 1724, 1219, 1250, 1111, 781, 1265.

Mass Spectrum. Principal peaks at *m/z* 144, 115, 116, 57, 58, 63, 145, 89.

Quantification. GAS CHROMATOGRAPHY. In animal blood or tissues: detection limit 20 ng/ml for blood, 100 ng/ml for tissues, ECD—M. E. Mount and F. W. Oehme, *J. analyt. Toxicol.* 1980, *4*, 286–292.

Carbazochrome   *Haemostatic*

Synonym. Adrenochrome Monosemicarbazone
Proprietary Names. Adrenoxyl; Cromosil.
5,6-Dihydro-3-hydroxy-1-methylindoline-5,6-dione   5-semi-carbazone
$C_{10}H_{12}N_4O_3 = 236.2$
CAS—69-81-8

An oxidation product of adrenaline.
Yellowish-red or red crystals or crystalline powder. M.p. about 222°, with decomposition.
Very slightly **soluble** in water and ethanol; practically insoluble in ether.

Carbazochrome Salicylate

Proprietary Name. Adrenosem Salicylate
A complex of carbazochrome with sodium salicylate
CAS—13051-01-9
A fine, orange-red, crystalline powder. M.p. 196° to 197.5°, with decomposition.
Soluble in water and ethanol.

Carbazochrome Sodium Sulphonate

Proprietary Names. Adona; Emex.
$C_{10}H_{11}N_4NaO_5S = 322.3$
CAS—51460-26-5
Orange to yellow, fine needle-like crystals. M.p. 227° to 228°, with decomposition.
Soluble 1 in 67 of cold water; slightly soluble in ethanol; practically insoluble in chloroform and ether.

Thin-layer Chromatography. *System TD*—Rf 00; *system TE*—Rf 16; *system TF*—Rf 00.

Ultraviolet Spectrum. Methanol—356 nm ($A_1^1 = 960$ b).

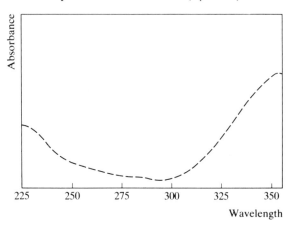

Mass Spectrum. Principal peaks at *m/z* 147, 43, 146, 42, 193, 118, 164, 44.

Dose. The equivalent of 5 to 10 mg of carbazochrome has been given intramuscularly or by mouth.

Carbenicillin   *Antibiotic*

Synonym. α-Carboxybenzylpenicillin
(6R)-6-(2-Carboxy-2-phenylacetamido)penicillanic acid
$C_{17}H_{18}N_2O_6S = 378.4$
CAS—4697-36-3

Carbenicillin Sodium

Proprietary Names. Anabactyl; Carbapen; Fugacillin; Geopen; Microcillin; Pyopen.
$C_{17}H_{16}N_2Na_2O_6S = 422.4$
CAS—4800-94-6
A white, hygroscopic, crystalline powder.
Soluble 1 in 1.2 of water and 1 in 25 of ethanol; practically insoluble in chloroform and ether.

Dissociation Constant. pK_a 2.6, 2.7.

Ultraviolet Spectrum. Aqueous acid—259 nm, 265 nm, 327 nm.

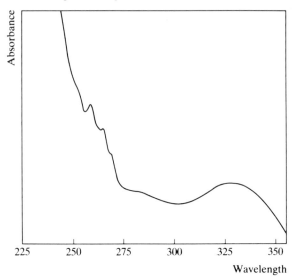

Infra-red Spectrum. Principal peaks at wavenumbers 1612, 1754, 1315, 1123, 1030, 1000.

Dose. The equivalent of 20 to 30 g of carbenicillin daily, intravenously.

Carbenoxolone   *Treatment of Peptic Ulcer*

Synonyms. Glycerrhetic Acid Hydrogen Succinate; Glycyrrhetinic Acid Hydrogen Succinate.
3β-(3-Carboxypropionyloxy)-11-oxo-olean-12-en-30-oic acid
$C_{34}H_{50}O_7 = 570.8$
CAS—5697-56-3

Cream-coloured crystals. M.p. 291° to 294°.

Carbenoxolone Sodium

Synonym. Disodium Enoxolone Succinate
Proprietary Names. Biogastrone; Duogastrone; Gastrausil; Neogel; Ulcus-Tablinen. It is an ingredient of Pyrogastrone.
$C_{34}H_{48}Na_2O_7 = 614.7$
CAS—7421-40-1
A white or pale cream-coloured hygroscopic powder.
Soluble 1 in 6 of water and 1 in 30 of ethanol; practically insoluble in chloroform and ether.
Caution. Carbenoxolone sodium powder is irritating to nasal membranes.

Dissociation Constant. pK_a 6.7, 7.1.

Colour Tests. Antimony Pentachloride—brown; Naphthol-Sulphuric Acid—yellow-brown/orange; Sulphuric Acid—yellow.

Mix 5 mg with 50 mg of resorcinol and 2 ml of 80% v/v sulphuric acid, heat at 200° for 10 minutes, cool, and add to 200 ml of water; make just alkaline with *sodium hydroxide solution*—an intense green fluorescence is produced.

Thin-layer Chromatography. *System TD*—Rf 07; *system TE*—Rf 00; *system TF*—Rf 17. (*Acidified potassium permanganate solution*, positive, faint.)

Ultraviolet Spectrum. Carbenoxolone sodium: aqueous acid—248 nm; aqueous alkali—257 nm ($A_1^1 = 172$ b).

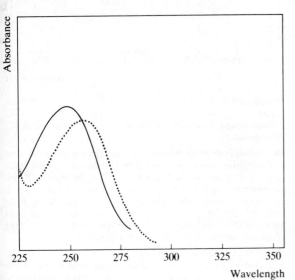

Wavelength

Infra-red Spectrum. Principal peaks at wavenumbers 1562, 1642, 1715, 1289, 1261, 1210 (carbenoxolone sodium, KBr disk).

Quantification. GAS CHROMATOGRAPHY. In serum: sensitivity 5 μg/ml, FID—C. Rhodes and P. A. Wright, *J. Pharm. Pharmac.*, 1974, *26*, 894–898.

RADIOIMMUNOASSAY. In serum: sensitivity 1 ng/ml—B. M. Peskar *et al.*, *J. Pharm. Pharmac.*, 1976, *28*, 720–721.

Disposition in the Body. Rapidly and almost completely absorbed after oral administration; absorption is reduced at gastric pH levels above 2 and delayed after food. It is almost entirely eliminated in the faeces via the bile, less than 5% being excreted in the urine. Carbenoxolone is excreted mainly as the glucuronide conjugate together with small amounts as the sulphate conjugate of β-glycyrrhetic acid (enoxolone).

THERAPEUTIC CONCENTRATION.
After a single oral dose of 200 mg to 10 subjects, peak blood concentrations of 13 to 35 μg/ml (mean 24) were attained in 1 to 2 hours, followed by a second peak of 3 to 32 μg/ml (mean 20) at 3 to 6 hours; in some subjects, the second peak was higher than the first (H. D. Downer *et al.*, *J. Pharm. Pharmac.*, 1970, *22*, 479–487).
Following oral administration of 100 mg to 3 fasting subjects, peak serum concentrations of 15 to 20 μg/ml were attained in 1 to 2 hours; following administration of 100 mg to 2 subjects after meals, peak serum concentrations of 8 to 9 μg/ml were reported at 5 to 6 hours.
After oral doses of 100 mg three times a day to 9 subjects, serum concentrations of 20 to 98 μg/ml (mean 49) were reported on the 8th day (J. H. Baron *et al.*, Factors affecting the Absorption of Carbenoxolone in Patients with Peptic Ulcer, in *4th Symposium on Carbenoxolone*, F. A. Jones and D. V. Parke (Ed.), London, Butterworths, 1975, pp. 115–124).

HALF-LIFE. Plasma half-life 8 to 20 hours (mean 13), increased in elderly subjects.

VOLUME OF DISTRIBUTION. About 0.1 litre/kg.

PROTEIN BINDING. In plasma, more than 99%.

NOTE. For a review of carbenoxolone see R. M. Pinder *et al.*, *Drugs*, 1976, *11*, 245–307.

Dose. 150 to 300 mg of carbenoxolone sodium daily.

Carbetapentane   *Cough Suppressant*

Synonym. Pentoxyverine
2-(2-Diethylaminoethoxy)ethyl 1-phenylcyclopentane-1-carboxylate
$C_{20}H_{31}NO_3 = 333.5$
CAS—77-23-6

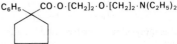

Carbetapentane Citrate
Proprietary Names. Atussil; Germapect; Sedotussin; Toclase; Tuclase; Tussa-Tablinen.
$C_{20}H_{31}NO_3,C_6H_8O_7 = 525.6$
CAS—23142-01-0
A white crystalline powder. M.p. 90° to 95°.
Very **soluble** in water and chloroform; soluble in ethanol; practically insoluble in ether.

Colour Tests. Liebermann's Test—red-orange; Mandelin's Test—brown (slow); Marquis Test—orange (slow).

Thin-layer Chromatography. *System TA*—Rf 48; *system TB*—Rf 48; *system TC*—Rf 22. (*Dragendorff spray*, positive; *acidified iodoplatinate solution*, positive; *Marquis reagent*, brown.)

Gas Chromatography. *System GA*—RI 2232; *system GF*—RI 2455.

Ultraviolet Spectrum. Aqueous acid—252 nm, 258 nm ($A_1^1 = 6.1$ a), 264 nm. No alkaline shift.

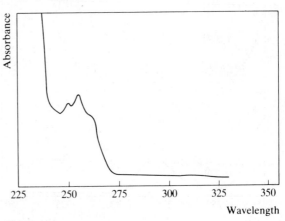

Wavelength

Infra-red Spectrum. Principal peaks at wavenumbers 1725, 1120, 1158, 1176, 694, 1234, (KBr disk).

Mass Spectrum. Principal peaks at *m/z* 86, 91, 87, 145, 58, 144, 30, 44.

Dose. 25 to 150 mg of carbetapentane citrate daily.

Carbidopa

Dopa-decarboxylase Inhibitor

Synonym. (−)-L-α-Methyldopa Hydrazine
Proprietary Name. It is an ingredient of Sinemet.
S-2-(3,4-Dihydroxybenzyl)-2-hydrazinopropionic acid mono-hydrate
$C_{10}H_{14}N_2O_4,H_2O = 244.2$
CAS—28860-95-9 (anhydrous); *38821-49-7* (monohydrate)

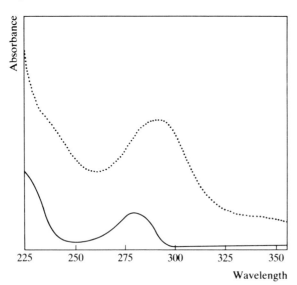

A white or creamy-white powder. M.p. about 210°, with decomposition.
Soluble 1 in 500 of water; practically insoluble in ethanol, chloroform, and ether; freely soluble in 3M hydrochloric acid.

Colour Tests. Ammoniacal Silver Nitrate (on warming)—silver mirror; Ferric Chloride—brown; Folin–Ciocalteu Reagent—blue; Liebermann's Test—black; Marquis Test—brown; Methanolic Potassium Hydroxide—orange; Millon's Reagent (cold)—orange; Nessler's Reagent—orange→black; Palladium Chloride—orange→brown; Potassium Dichromate (Method 1)—red.

Thin-layer Chromatography. *System TD*—Rf 00; *system TE*—Rf 00; *system TF*—Rf 02.

Ultraviolet Spectrum. Methanolic acid—282 nm ($A_1^1 = 130$ a); aqueous alkali—291nm.

Infra-red Spectrum. Principal peaks at wavenumbers 1625, 1121, 1260, 1525, 1290, 875 (KBr disk).

Mass Spectrum. Principal peaks at *m/z* 123, 57, 42, 103, 44, 85, 124, 51.

Wavelength

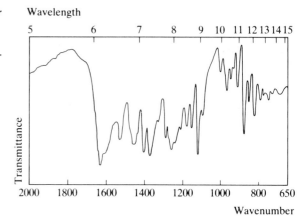

Quantification. HIGH PRESSURE LIQUID CHROMATOGRAPHY. In plasma: sensitivity 15 ng/ml, electrochemical detection—E. Nissinen and J. Taskinen, *J. Chromat.*, 1982, *231*; *Biomed. Appl.*, *20*, 459–462.

Disposition in the Body. Readily but incompletely absorbed after oral administration. About 50% of an oral dose is excreted in the urine in 48 hours and 47% is eliminated in the faeces. Of the urinary material, about 30% is unchanged drug, 10 to 14% is 2-(4-hydroxy-3-methoxybenzyl)propionic acid, 10% is 2-(3,4-dihydroxybenzyl)propionic acid, 5% is 3,4-dihydroxyphenylacetone and 10% is 2-(3-hydroxybenzyl)propionic acid. The metabolites are excreted mainly as glucuronide conjugates.

THERAPEUTIC CONCENTRATION.
Following an oral dose of 50 mg to 10 subjects, a mean peak plasma concentration of 0.2 µg/ml was attained in 2 to 4 hours (S. Vickers *et al.*, *Drug Met. Disp.*, 1974, *2*, 9–22).

HALF-LIFE. Plasma half-life, about 2 hours.

PROTEIN BINDING. In plasma, about 36%.

NOTE. For a review of the pharmacokinetics of carbidopa see R. M. Pinder *et al.*, *Drugs*, 1976, *11*, 329–377.

Dose. Usually the equivalent of 75 to 150 mg of anhydrous carbidopa daily, given in combination with levodopa.

Carbimazole

Antithyroid Agent

Proprietary Names. Carbazole; Carbotiroid; Neo-Mercazole; Neo-Morphazole; Neo-Thyreostat; Neo-Tireol.
Ethyl 3-methyl-2-thioxo-4-imidazoline-1-carboxylate
$C_7H_{10}N_2O_2S = 186.2$
CAS—22232-54-8

A white or creamy-white crystalline powder. M.p. 122° to 125°.
Soluble 1 in 500 of water, 1 in 50 of ethanol, 1 in 17 of acetone, 1 in 3 of chloroform, and 1 in 330 of ether.

Colour Tests. Palladium Chloride—orange.
To a small quantity add 1 drop of *iodobismuthous acid solution*—red.

Thin-layer Chromatography. *System TA*—Rf 72; *system TD*—Rf 63; *system TE*—Rf 47; *system TF*—Rf 48. (*Acidified iodoplatinate solution*, positive; *acidified potassium permanganate solution*, positive.)

Gas Chromatography. *System GA*—carbimazole RI 1678, methimazole RI 1550.

Ultraviolet Spectrum. Aqueous acid—291 nm $(A_1^1 = 557\ a)$; aqueous alkali—244 nm.

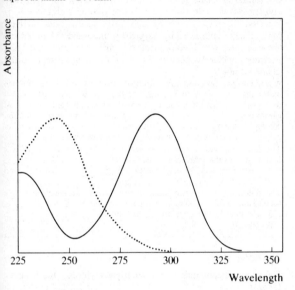

Wavelength

Infra-red Spectrum. Principal peaks at wavenumbers 1574, 1275, 740, 1246, 1150, 767 (KBr disk).

Wavelength

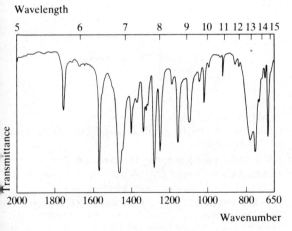

Wavenumber

Mass Spectrum. Principal peaks at *m/z* 186, 114, 29, 72, 42, 113, 27, 109; methimazole 114, 42, 72, 113, 69, 81, 54, 115.

Quantification. GAS CHROMATOGRAPHY. In plasma: methimazole, limit of detection 30 ng/ml, AFID—M. R. Bending and D. Stevenson, *J. Chromat.*, 1978, *154*, 267–271.

GAS CHROMATOGRAPHY–MASS SPECTROMETRY. In plasma: methimazole, sensitivity 2 ng/ml—S. Floberg *et al.*, *J. Chromat.*, 1980, *182*; *Biomed. Appl.*, *8*, 63–70.

HIGH PRESSURE LIQUID CHROMATOGRAPHY. In plasma: methimazole, limit of detection 5 ng/ml, absorbance detection at 405 nm—A. Meulemans *et al.*, *J. liq. Chromat.*, 1980, *3*, 287–298.

Disposition in the Body. Rapidly and almost completely absorbed after oral administration and converted to the active metabolite methimazole. Almost completely excreted in the urine in 24 hours as metabolites; 3-methyl-2-thiohydantoin has been identified as a minor metabolite in urine and plasma. About 3% of a dose is eliminated in the faeces.

THERAPEUTIC CONCENTRATION.
After an oral dose of 60 mg, given to 11 subjects, peak serum concentrations of methimazole of 0.5 to 3.4 µg/ml (mean 0.9) were attained in about 0.7 to 3 hours (A. Melander *et al.*, *Eur. J. clin. Pharmac.*, 1980, *17*, 295–299).

HALF-LIFE. Plasma half-life, methimazole about 3 to 5 hours.

VOLUME OF DISTRIBUTION. Methimazole, about 0.5 litre/kg.

PROTEIN BINDING. In plasma, methimazole, not significantly bound.

NOTE. For a review of the pharmacokinetics of antithyroid drugs, see J. P. Kampmann and J. M. Hansen, *Clin. Pharmacokinet.*, 1981, *6*, 401–428.

Dose. Initially 30 to 60 mg daily; maintenance, 5 to 20 mg daily.

Carbinoxamine   *Antihistamine*

2-[4-Chloro-α-(2-pyridyl)benzyloxy]-*NN*-dimethylethylamine
$C_{16}H_{19}ClN_2O = 290.8$
CAS—486-16-8

Cl — (4-chlorophenyl) — CH·O·[CH₂]₂·N(CH₃)₂ with pyridyl (N)

A liquid.

Carbinoxamine Maleate
Proprietary Names. Allergefon; Clistin; Histex; Ziriton. It is an ingredient of Davenol, Extil, and Rondec.
$C_{16}H_{19}ClN_2O,C_4H_4O_4 = 406.9$
CAS—3505-38-2
A white crystalline powder. M.p. 116° to 121°.
Soluble 1 in less than 1 of water, 1 in 1.5 of ethanol, and 1 in 1.5 of chloroform; very slightly soluble in ether.

Dissociation Constant. pK_a 8.1 (25°).

Colour Test. Cyanogen Bromide—orange-pink.

Thin-layer Chromatography. *System TA*—Rf 48; *system TB*—Rf 25; *system TC*—Rf 19. (*Dragendorff spray*, positive; *acidified iodoplatinate solution*, positive; *Marquis reagent*, pink.)

Gas Chromatography. *System GA*—RI 2080; *system GB*—RI 2090; *system GC*—RI 2430.

High Pressure Liquid Chromatography. *System HA*—k' 4.7 (tailing peak).

Ultraviolet Spectrum. Aqueous acid—263 nm $(A_1^1 = 323\ a)$; aqueous alkali—261 nm $(A_1^1 = 181\ a)$ (See below).

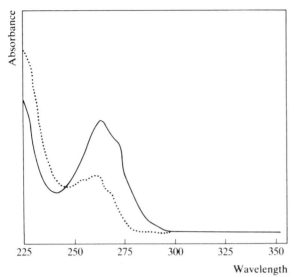

Wavelength

Infra-red Spectrum. Principal peaks at wavenumbers 1084, 1110, 1584, 1041, 763, 1010 (KBr disk).

Mass Spectrum. Principal peaks at m/z 58, 71, 26, 54, 167, 72, 42, 44.

Quantification. GAS CHROMATOGRAPHY (CAPILLARY COLUMN). In plasma: sensitivity 200 pg/ml, AFID—D. J. Hoffman *et al.*, *J. pharm. Sci.*, 1983, *72*, 1342–1344.

Dose. 12 to 32 mg of carbinoxamine maleate daily.

Carbon Tetrachloride   *Anthelmintic (Veterinary)/Solvent*

Synonym. Carboneum Tetrachloratum Medicinale
Tetrachloromethane
$CCl_4 = 153.8$
CAS—56-23-5
A heavy, clear, colourless, volatile liquid, with a chloroform-like odour. It is non-inflammable but in contact with a flame it decomposes and gives rise to toxic products, which have an acrid odour. Wt per ml 1.592 to 1.595 g. B.p. 76° to 78°. Refractive index 1.4607.

Soluble 1 in 1500 of water; miscible with dehydrated alcohol, chloroform, and ether.

Colour Test. Fujiwara Test—red.

Gas Chromatography. *System GA*—RI 659; *system GI*—retention time 8.6 min.

Mass Spectrum. Principal peaks at m/z 117, 119, 47, 35, 121, 82, 84, 49.

Quantification. GAS CHROMATOGRAPHY. In biological material and expired air: simultaneous determination of carbon tetrachloride and chloroform, sensitivity 5 μg by FID, 15 ng by ECD—C. J. Reddrop *et al.*, *J. Chromat.*, 1980, *193*, 71–82.

Disposition in the Body. Readily absorbed after inhalation and also absorbed after ingestion or through the skin; the rate of absorption is increased by the concomitant ingestion of alcohol. It is excreted mainly from the lungs as carbon tetrachloride and carbon dioxide; excretion in the urine as urea and an unidentified metabolite, and elimination in the faeces also occur.

TOXICITY. The minimum lethal dose is 3 to 5 ml but recoveries have occurred following ingestion of 30 to 40 ml. Carbon tetrachloride injures almost all cells of the body including those of the blood, central nervous system, liver and kidney; the kidneys and liver of fatal cases often show marked fatty degeneration. The maximum permissible atmospheric concentration is 10 ppm. Inhalation of concentrations of 1000 ppm, even for short periods, may cause acute toxic reactions. Continued exposure to concentrations of about 100 ppm may give rise to chronic poisoning. When carbon tetrachloride is ingested together or immediately after alcohol, its toxicity, particularly nephrotoxicity, is greatly increased. Toxic effects are associated with blood concentrations of 20 to 50 μg/ml and a postmortem blood concentration of 260 μg/ml has been reported in one fatality.

A middle-aged alcoholic ingested about 30 ml of carbon tetrachloride under the impression that it was alcohol. He was seriously ill but recovered. On his admission to hospital the serum concentration of carbon tetrachloride was 20 μg/ml. The first 24-hour urine collection contained 8 μg/ml and the first peritoneal dialysate contained 1 μg/ml of carbon tetrachloride (S. L. Tompsett, personal communication, 1967).

The following postmortem tissue concentrations were reported in a fatality due to the inhalation of carbon tetrachloride: kidney 32 μg/g, liver 142 μg/g, lung 39 μg/g, muscle 46 μg/g (H. D. Korenke and O. Pribilla, *Arch. Tox.*, 1969, *25*, 109–126).

The following postmortem tissue concentrations were reported in a fatality due to inhalation of carbon tetrachloride: blood 18 μg/ml, brain 175 μg/g, lung 12.5 μg/g (A. Franc, *Bull. int. Ass. forens. Toxicol.*, 1983, *17*(2), 22–25).

Carbromal   *Hypnotic*

Synonyms. Bromadal; Bromodiethylacetylurea; Karbromal; Uradal.
Proprietary Names. Adalin; Mirfudorm.
N-(2-Bromo-2-ethylbutyryl)urea
$C_7H_{13}BrN_2O_2 = 237.1$
CAS—77-65-6

$$CH_3 \cdot CH_2 \cdot \underset{\underset{C_2H_5}{|}}{\overset{\overset{Br}{|}}{C}} \cdot CO \cdot NH \cdot CO \cdot NH_2$$

A white crystalline powder. M.p. 117° to 120°.

Soluble 1 in 3000 of water, 1 in 18 of ethanol, 1 in 2 of chloroform, and 1 in 25 of ether.

Colour Test. Nessler's Reagent—brown-orange.

Thin-layer Chromatography. *System TD*—Rf 53; *system TE*—Rf 74; *system TF*—Rf 56. (*Fluorescein solution*, pink.)

Gas Chromatography. *System GA*—carbromal RI 1513, 2-bromo-2-ethylbutyramide RI 1205, 2-bromo-2-ethyl-3-hydroxybutyramide RI 1340, 2-ethylbutyrylurea RI 1380.

Ultraviolet Spectrum. No significant absorption, 230 to 360 nm.

Infra-red Spectrum. Principal peaks at wavenumbers 1694, 660, 1600, 1094, 1212, 834 (KBr disk).

Mass Spectrum. Principal peaks at m/z 44, 69, 41, 208, 210, 55, 71, 43; 2-bromo-2-ethylbutyramide 69, 43, 41, 44, 71, 167, 165, 55; 2-bromo-2-ethyl-3-hydroxybutyramide 150, 152, 165, 41, 167, 43, 44, 130; 2-ethylbutyrylurea 45, 130, 44, 71, 42, 61, 115, 55.

Wavelength

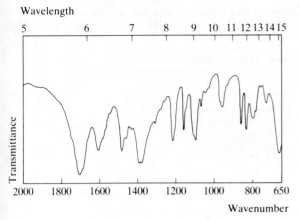

Carbutamide

Antidiabetic

Synonym. Glybutamide

Proprietary Names. Diabetoplex; Dia-Tablinen; Glucidoral; Insoral; Invenol; Nadisan.

Note. Insoral is also used as a proprietary name for phenformin hydrochloride.

1-Butyl-3-sulphanilylurea
$C_{11}H_{17}N_3O_3S = 271.3$
CAS—339-43-5

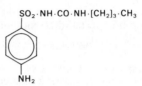

A white finely crystalline powder. M.p. 144° to 145°.
Practically **insoluble** in water, chloroform, and ether; soluble in ethanol and acetone.

Dissociation Constant. pK_a 6.0 (20°).

Thin-layer Chromatography. *System TA*—Rf 78; *system TT*—Rf 90; *system TU*—Rf 27; *system TV*—Rf 07.

Ultraviolet Spectrum. Aqueous acid—266 nm ($A_1^1 = 149$ a); aqueous alkali—255 nm ($A_1^1 = 616$ a).

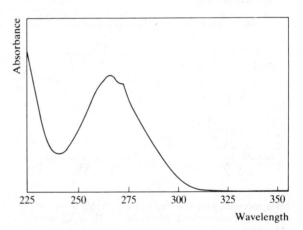

Infra-red Spectrum. Principal peaks at wavenumbers 1661, 1147, 1599, 1089, 1635, 1310 (KBr disk).

Quantification. HIGH PRESSURE LIQUID CHROMATOGRAPHY. In serum: UV detection—F. Saffar *et al.*, *Chem. pharm. Bull.*, 1982, *30*, 679–683.

Disposition in the Body. Absorbed after oral administration. It is excreted in the urine mainly as the acetyl derivative.

THERAPEUTIC CONCENTRATION.

Following an oral dose of 250 mg to 5 subjects, a mean peak serum concentration of 48.8 µg/ml was reported at 2.6 hours (F. Saffar *et al.*, *ibid.*).

HALF-LIFE. Plasma half-life, about 24 hours.

REFERENCE. F. Saffar *et al.*, *ibid.*

Dose. Carbutamide has been given in doses of 0.5 to 1 g daily.

Quantification. GAS CHROMATOGRAPHY. In blood: determined as inorganic bromide, FID—J. Wells and G. Cimbura, *J. forens. Sci.*, 1973, *18*, 437–440.

HIGH PRESSURE LIQUID CHROMATOGRAPHY. In plasma: carbromal, 2-bromo-2-ethylbutyramide and 2-ethylbutyrylurea, sensitivity 200 ng/ml for carbromal, UV detection—M. Eichelbaum *et al.*, *Arch. Tox.*, 1978, *41*, 187–193.

Disposition in the Body. Readily absorbed after oral administration. The major metabolite is free bromide ion; hydrolysis to an active metabolite, 2-bromo-2-ethylbutyramide, also occurs followed by oxidation to 2-bromo-2-ethyl-3-hydroxybutyramide; other metabolites include 2-ethylbutyrylurea and 2-ethyl-2-hydroxybutyric acid. Carbromal is excreted in the urine mainly as bromide ion and partly as 2-ethyl-2-hydroxybutyric acid, with very little as unchanged drug. Peak bromide excretion is attained after about 48 hours.

THERAPEUTIC CONCENTRATION.

Following a single oral dose of 1 g given to 4 subjects, mean peak serum concentrations of about 6 µg/ml of carbromal and 3 µg/ml of 2-bromo-2-ethylbutyramide were attained in 0.5 and 4 hours respectively; the total bromide concentration reached about 12 µg/ml in 9 hours and was still increasing (H. W. Vohland *et al.*, *Arch. Tox.*, 1976, *36*, 31–42).

TOXICITY. Fatalities have occurred in adults following the ingestion of 10 to 25 g but they are rare. Long-term use of carbromal may give rise to symptoms of chronic toxicity resembling bromism. Toxic effects are associated with serum-bromide concentrations of 300 to **1200** to 3200 µg/ml.

In 11 fatalities attributed to carbromal overdose, the following postmortem tissue concentrations, µg/ml or µg/g (mean, *n*), were reported:

	Carbromal	Bromoethylbutyramide
Blood	19.9–26.1 (23, *3*)	0.2–27.2 (15, *10*)
Brain	0.6–120.9 (45, *8*)	23.3–118.4 (66, *11*)
Kidney	0.4–13 (6, *4*)	16.1–79.6 (45, *9*)
Liver	1.1–2.8 (2.3, *4*)	1.75–50.5 (14, *9*)
Urine	0.85–47.4 (24, *5*)	2.5–36.9 (23, *8*)

Total bromide concentrations in the blood ranged from 145 to 1898 µg/ml (mean 536) (H. Kaferstein and G. Sticht, *Z. Rechtsmed.*, 1978, *81*, 269–283).

Postmortem serum-carbromal concentrations of 158 and 71 µg/ml were found in 2 fatalities resulting from acute intoxication (H. Gruska *et al.*, *Arch. Tox.*, 1970, *26*, 149–160, and 1971, *28*, 149–158).

HALF-LIFE. Plasma half-life, carbromal 7 to 15 hours, bromide about 15 days.

Dose. 0.3 to 1 g, as a hypnotic.

Carisoprodol
Muscle Relaxant

Synonym. N-Isopropylmeprobamate

Proprietary Names. Carisoma; Flexartal; Mioxom; Rela; Sanoma; Soma; Somadril.

Note. The name Soma has also been applied to an hallucinogenic fungus.

2-Methyl-2-propyltrimethylene carbamate isopropylcarbamate
$C_{12}H_{24}N_2O_4 = 260.3$
CAS—78-44-4

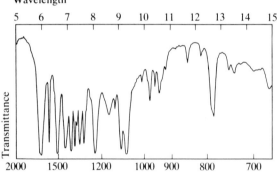

A white crystalline powder. M.p. 92° to 94°.

Soluble 1 in 3300 of water; soluble in most common organic solvents.

Thin-layer Chromatography. *System TD*—Rf 36; *system TE*—Rf 73; *system TF*—Rf 53. (*Furfuraldehyde reagent*, positive.)

Gas Chromatography. *System GA*—carisoprodol RI 1830, meprobamate RI 1796.

Ultraviolet Spectrum. No significant absorption, 230 to 360 nm.

Infra-red Spectrum. Principal peaks at wavenumbers 1695, 1527, 1075, 1246, 1101, 1319 (Nujol mull).

Wavelength

[Infra-red spectrum chart: x-axis Wavenumber from 2000 to 700, y-axis Transmittance; Wavelength axis from 5 to 15]

Mass Spectrum. Principal peaks at *m/z* 55, 57, 43, 97, 41, 56, 158, 44; meprobamate 83, 84, 55, 56, 43, 71, 41, 62 (no peaks above 160).

Quantification. GAS CHROMATOGRAPHY. In serum or urine: carisoprodol and meprobamate, FID—H. R. Adams *et al., J. forens. Sci.*, 1975, *20*, 200–202. In biological fluids and tissues—R. Maes *et al., Eur. J. Toxicol.*, 1970, *3*, 140–143.

Disposition in the Body. Absorbed after oral administration. It is metabolised principally to meprobamate, which is active, and to hydroxymeprobamate and their glucuronide conjugates. Less than 1% of a dose is excreted in the urine as unchanged drug in 24 hours and about 5% is excreted as meprobamate in the same period.

TOXICITY.

The following concentrations were reported 4.5 hours after the ingestion of 3.5 g by a young child: blood, carisoprodol 36.4 µg/ml, meprobamate 15 µg/ml; urine, carisoprodol 24.4 µg/ml, meprobamate 166.4 µg/ml; the child's condition deteriorated and death occurred within 36 hours (H.R. Adams *et al., J. forens. Sci.*, 1975, *20*, 200–202).

The following postmortem tissue concentrations were reported in a suicide case: blood 110 µg/ml, bile 64 µg/ml, kidney 110 µg/g, liver 127 µg/g, urine 165 µg/ml (R. Maes *et al., J. forens. Sci.*, 1969, *14*, 235–254).

Dose. 1.05 to 1.4 g daily.

Carphenazine
Tranquilliser

Synonym. Carfenazine

1-(10-{3-[4-(2-Hydroxyethyl)piperazin-1-yl]propyl}phenothiazin-2-yl)propan-1-one
$C_{24}H_{31}N_3O_2S = 425.6$
CAS—2622-30-2

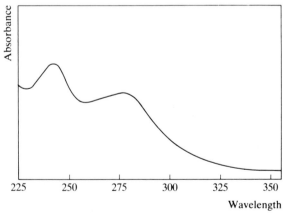

Carphenazine Maleate

Proprietary Name. Proketazine
$C_{24}H_{31}N_3O_2S,2C_4H_4O_4 = 657.7$
CAS—2975-34-0

A fine yellow powder. M.p. 176° to 185°, with decomposition.

Soluble 1 in 600 of water and 1 in 400 of ethanol; practically insoluble in chloroform and ether.

Colour Tests. Formaldehyde–Sulphuric Acid—blue; Forrest Reagent—red; FPN Reagent—red-orange; Liebermann's Test—red-brown; Mandelin's Test—red-violet; Marquis Test—orange → red-violet.

Thin-layer Chromatography. *System TA*—Rf 54; *system TB*—Rf 05; *system TC*—Rf 27. (*Acidified iodoplatinate solution*, positive.)

Gas Chromatography. *System GA*—RI 3590.

High Pressure Liquid Chromatography. *System HA*—k' 1.7.

Ultraviolet Spectrum. Aqueous acid—243 nm ($A_1^1 = 606$ a), 277 nm. No alkaline shift.

[Ultraviolet absorption spectrum chart: x-axis Wavelength from 225 to 350, y-axis Absorbance]

Infra-red Spectrum. Principal peaks at wavenumbers 1585, 1557, 1666, 1204, 751, 1298 (KBr disk).

Mass Spectrum. Principal peaks at *m/z* 268, 143, 425, 70, 269, 42, 394, 157.

Dose. 75 to 400 mg of carphenazine maleate daily.

Cathine

Anorectic

Synonyms. Katine; (+)-Norpseudoephedrine; Pseudonorephedrine.
threo-2-Amino-1-phenylpropan-1-ol
$C_9H_{13}NO = 151.2$
CAS—492-39-7; 36393-56-3

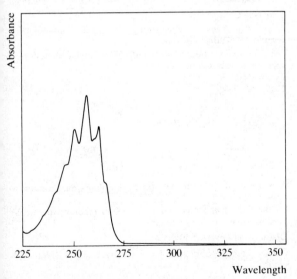

An alkaloid obtained from catha, the fresh or dried leaves of *Catha edulis* (Celastraceae). Catha (also known as Abyssinian, African, or Arabian Tea; Kat; Kath; Khat; Miraa) is used in northern and eastern Africa as a stimulant, the leaves either being chewed or used as an infusion.
Crystals. M.p. 77° to 78°.
Soluble in ethanol, chloroform, and ether.

Cathine Hydrochloride

Proprietary Names. Adiposetten N; Amorphan Depot.
$C_9H_{13}NO,HCl = 187.7$
CAS—2153-98-2
Crystals. M.p. 180° to 181°.
Soluble in water.

Dissociation Constant. pK_a 9.4.

Thin-layer Chromatography. *System TA*—Rf 42; *system TB*—Rf 25; *system TC*—Rf 05. (*Acidified potassium permanganate solution*, positive.)

Gas Chromatography. *System GA*—RI 1302; *system GB*—RI 1362; *system GC*—RI 1383.

High Pressure Liquid Chromatography. *System HA*—k′ 1.0; *system HB*—k′ 4.39; *system HC*—k′ 0.83.

Ultraviolet Spectrum. Aqueous acid—252 nm, 258 nm ($A_1^1 = 10$ a), 263 nm. No alkaline shift.

Infra-red Spectrum. Principal peaks at wavenumbers 1045, 695, 754, 704, 1091, 976 (KBr disk).

Mass Spectrum. Principal peaks at *m/z* 44, 57, 43, 40, 55, 41, 79, 77.

Wavelength

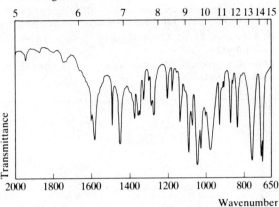

Wavenumber

Disposition in the Body. About 40% of an ingested dose is excreted unchanged in the urine in 6 hours.
Cathine is a metabolite of pseudoephedrine.

THERAPEUTIC CONCENTRATION.
Following a single oral dose of 60 mg to 6 subjects, a mean peak plasma concentration of 0.2 µg/ml was attained in 1.3 hours; cathine could not be detected in the plasma after 24 hours (F. Frosch, *Arzneimittel-Forsch.*, 1977, **27**, 665–668).

TOXICITY. Addiction to catha has been reported.

HALF-LIFE. Plasma half-life, about 3 hours.

Dose. Cathine hydrochloride has been given in doses of 20 to 60 mg daily.

Cephaëline

Emetic/Expectorant

Synonym. Desmethylemetine
7′,10,11-Trimethoxyemetan-6′-ol
$C_{28}H_{38}N_2O_4 = 466.6$
CAS—483-17-0

An alkaloid present in ipecacuanha, the dried root, or rhizome and root, of *Cephaëlis ipecacuanha* (= *Uragoga ipecacuanha*) (Rubiaceae) or *C. acuminata*.
Needles. M.p. 115° to 116°.
Practically **insoluble** in water; soluble in ethanol and chloroform; slightly soluble in ether.

Cephaëline Hydrochloride

$C_{28}H_{38}N_2O_4,2HCl = 539.5$
CAS—5853-29-2
White crystals or crystalline powder. Solutions turn yellow.
Soluble in water, ethanol, acetone, and chloroform.

Colour Test. Liebermann's Test—black.

Thin-layer Chromatography. *System TA*—Rf 53; *system TB*—Rf 01; *system TC*—Rf 19. (*Acidified iodoplatinate solution*, positive.)

High Pressure Liquid Chromatography. *System HA*—k' 7.7 (tailing peak).

Ultraviolet Spectrum. Aqueous acid—283 nm ($A_1^1 = 127$ b); ethanol—235 nm, 276 nm ($A_1^1 = 144$ b).

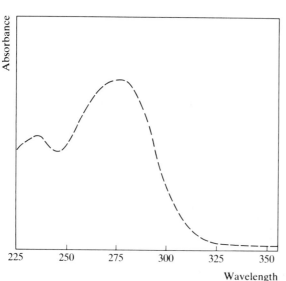

Infra-red Spectrum. Principal peaks at wavenumbers 1264, 1515, 1116, 1229, 1213, 1616 (cephaëline hydrochloride, KBr disk).

Mass Spectrum. Principal peaks at *m/z* 178, 192, 272, 466, 244, 288, 191, 273.

Quantification. See under Emetine.

Dose. Cephaëline hydrochloride has been given in doses of 5 to 10 mg.

Cephalexin   *Antibiotic*

Synonym. Cefalexin

Proprietary Names. Ceporex; Ceporexin(e); Keflex; Keforal; Oracef.

(7*R*)-3-Methyl-7-(α-D-phenylglycylamino)-3-cephem-4-carboxylic acid monohydrate
$C_{16}H_{17}N_3O_4S,H_2O = 365.4$
CAS—15686-71-2 (anhydrous); *23325-78-2* (monohydrate)

A white to cream-coloured, slightly hygroscopic, crystalline powder.

Soluble 1 in 100 of water and 1 in 30 of 0.2% hydrochloric acid; practically insoluble in ethanol, chloroform, and ether; soluble in solutions of dilute alkalis.

Dissociation Constant. pK$_a$ 2.5, 5.2, 7.3.

Ultraviolet Spectrum. Aqueous acid—258 nm; water—260 nm ($A_1^1 = 232$ a).

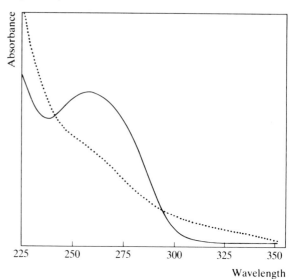

Infra-red Spectrum. Principal peaks at wavenumbers 1754, 1582, 1681, 1271, 695, 1186 (KBr disk).

Quantification. HIGH PRESSURE LIQUID CHROMATOGRAPHY. Review of methods for the analysis of antibiotics in biological fluids—I. Nilsson-Ehle, *J. liq. Chromat.*, 1983, *6*, 251–293.

Dose. 1 to 6 g daily.

Cephaloridine   *Antibiotic*

Synonym. Cefaloridine

Proprietary Names. Cepaloridin; Cepalorin; Ceporan; Ceporin(e); Keflodin; Loridine.

(7*R*)-3-(1-Pyridiniomethyl)-7-[2-(2-thienyl)acetamido]-3-cephem-4-carboxylate
$C_{19}H_{17}N_3O_4S_2 = 415.5$
CAS—50-59-9

A white crystalline powder, which discolours on exposure to light.

Soluble 1 in 5 of water and 1 in 1000 of ethanol; practically insoluble in chloroform and ether.

Dissociation Constant. pK$_a$ 3.4.

Colour Tests. Mandelin's Test—violet; Marquis Test—red-violet.

Thin-layer Chromatography. *System TA*—Rf 73. (*Acidified potassium permanganate solution*, positive.)

Ultraviolet Spectrum. Aqueous acid—241 nm ($A_1^1 = 350$ a), 254 nm ($A_1^1 = 341$ a); aqueous alkali—261 nm ($A_1^1 = 88$ b); methanol—234 nm ($A_1^1 = 372$ a).

Infra-red Spectrum. Principal peaks at wavenumbers 1600, 1764, 1656, 1538, 715, 1143 (KBr disk).

Dose. 1 to 3 g daily, intramuscularly; maximum of 6 g daily.

Cephalothin   *Antibiotic*

Synonym. Cefalotin

(7R)-3-Acetoxymethyl-7-[2-(2-thienyl)acetamido]-3-cephem-4-carboxylic acid

$C_{16}H_{16}N_2O_6S_2 = 396.4$

CAS—153-61-7

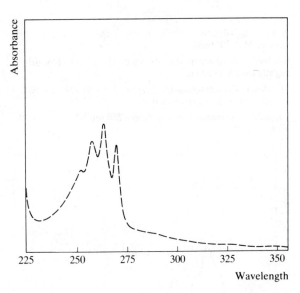

M.p. 160°.

Cephalothin Sodium

Proprietary Names. Ceporacin; Cepovenin; Keflin.

$C_{16}H_{15}N_2NaO_6S_2 = 418.4$

CAS—58-71-9

A white crystalline powder.

Soluble 1 in 3.5 of water and 1 in 700 of ethanol; practically insoluble in chloroform and ether.

Dissociation Constant. pK_a 2.2 (35°).

Ultraviolet Spectrum. Cephalothin sodium: water—237 nm ($A_1^1 = 335$ a), 265 nm ($A_1^1 = 204$ b).

Infra-red Spectrum. Principal peaks at wavenumbers 1704, 1724, 1637, 1600, 1227, 1510 (cephalothin sodium, KBr disk).

Dose. The equivalent of 4 to 12 g of cephalothin daily, intravenously.

Cephradine   *Antibiotic*

Synonym. Cefradine

Proprietary Names. Anspor; Eskacef; Maxisporin; Megacef; Sefril; Velosef.

(7R)-7-(α-D-Cyclohexa-1,4-dienylglycylamino)-3-methyl-3-cephem-4-carboxylic acid

$C_{16}H_{19}N_3O_4S = 349.4$

CAS—38821-53-3

A white to cream-coloured crystalline powder.

Soluble 1 in 100 of water and 1 in 70 of methanol; practically insoluble in ethanol, chloroform, and ether.

Dissociation Constant. pK_a 2.5, 7.3 (35°).

Ultraviolet Spectrum. Aqueous acid—257 nm.

Infra-red Spectrum. Principal peaks at wavenumbers 1754, 1582, 1678, 1271, 1235, 1190 (KBr disk).

Dose. 1 to 4 g daily.

Cetalkonium Chloride   *Cationic Disinfectant*

Proprietary Names. Baktonium. It is an ingredient of AAA, Bonjela, and Teejel.

Benzylhexadecyldimethylammonium chloride

$C_{25}H_{46}ClN = 396.1$

CAS—122-18-9

A white crystalline powder. M.p. 58° to 60°.

Sparingly **soluble** in cold water, soluble in hot water; soluble in ethanol, chloroform, and ether.

Thin-layer Chromatography. *System TA*—Rf 12, streaking. (*Acidified iodoplatinate solution*, positive.)

Ultraviolet Spectrum. Aqueous acid—258 nm ($A_1^1 = 8$ b), 264 nm ($A_1^1 = 10$ b), 270 nm ($A_1^1 = 8$ b); methanol—253 nm, 258 nm, 263 nm ($A_1^1 = 11$ b), 270 nm.

Infra-red Spectrum. Principal peaks at wavenumbers 722, 698, 1612, 1204, 875, 790 (KBr disk).

Use. In a concentration of 0.01% in preparations applied to the mouth or throat.

Cetrimide   *Cationic Disinfectant*

Proprietary Names. Cetavlon; Morpan CHSA; Silquat C100. It is an ingredient of Ceanel, Cetal (liquid), Savloclens, Savlodil, Savlon (liquid), and Travasept.

Consists chiefly of tetradecyltrimethylammonium bromide together with smaller amounts of dodecyl- and hexadecyltrimethylammonium bromides.

CAS—8044-71-1

A white to creamy-white, voluminous, free-flowing, hygroscopic powder. A solution in water foams on shaking. M.p. 232° to 247°.

Soluble 1 in 2 of water; freely soluble in ethanol; soluble in ether.

Thin-layer Chromatography. *System TA*—Rf 02; *system TN*—Rf 100; *system TO*—Rf 50. (*Acidified iodoplatinate solution*, positive.)

Infra-red Spectrum. Principal peaks at wavenumbers 961, 909, 952, 719, 970, 724 (KCl disk).

Cetylpyridinium Chloride   *Cationic Disinfectant*

Proprietary Names. Ceepryn; Cepacol; Dobendan; Merocet(s). It is an ingredient of Merocaine and Tyrosolven.

1-Hexadecylpyridinium chloride monohydrate
$C_{21}H_{38}ClN,H_2O = 358.0$
CAS—7773-52-6 (cetylpyridinium); *123-03-5* (chloride, anhydrous); *6004-24-6* (chloride, monohydrate)

$$\left[\begin{array}{c} CH_2 \cdot [CH_2]_{14} \cdot CH_3 \\ N^+ \\ \end{array} \right] \quad Cl^-, H_2O$$

A white powder. A solution in water foams strongly when shaken. M.p. 79° to 84°.

Soluble 1 in 20 of water; very soluble in ethanol and chloroform; slightly soluble in ether.

Thin-layer Chromatography. *System TA*—Rf 20. (*Acidified iodoplatinate solution*, positive.)

Ultraviolet Spectrum. Aqueous acid—260 nm ($A_1^1 = 123$ a). No alkaline shift.

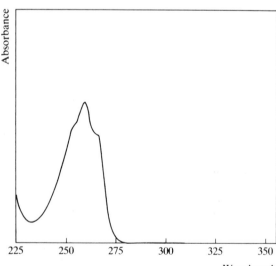

Infra-red Spectrum. Principal peaks at wavenumbers 685, 1629, 776, 1174, 715, 1205.

Use. In concentrations of 0.01 to 1%.

Chelidonine   *Alkaloid*

(+) - [5b*S* - (5bα,6β,12bα)] - 5b,6,7,12b,13,14 - Hexahydro - 13 - methyl[1,3]benzodioxolo[5,6 - *c*] - 1,3 - dioxolo[4,5 - *i*]phenanthridin-6-ol
$C_{20}H_{19}NO_5 = 353.4$
CAS—476-32-4

An alkaloid obtained from the greater celandine, *Chelidonium majus* (Papaveraceae).

A white crystalline powder. M.p. 135° to 136°.

Practically **insoluble** in water; soluble in ethanol, chloroform, and ether.

Colour Tests. Mandelin's Test—yellow → green; Marquis Test—green; Sulphuric Acid—brown.

Thin-layer Chromatography. *System TA*—Rf 72. (*Acidified iodoplatinate solution*, positive.)

Infra-red Spectrum. Principal peaks at wavenumbers 1035, 1257, 1222, 1497, 748, 1070 (KBr disk).

Mass Spectrum. Principal peaks at *m/z* 332, 333, 304, 335, 176, 303, 334, 162.

Chlophedianol   *Cough Suppressant*

Synonym. Clofedanol
2-Chloro-α-(2-dimethylaminoethyl)-α-phenylbenzyl alcohol
$C_{17}H_{20}ClNO = 289.8$
CAS—791-35-5

$$C_6H_5 \cdot \underset{\displaystyle}{\overset{\displaystyle OH}{C}} \cdot [CH_2]_2 \cdot N(CH_3)_2$$

Chlophedianol Hydrochloride
Proprietary Names. Detigon; Pectolitan.
$C_{17}H_{20}ClNO,HCl = 326.3$
CAS—511-13-7
Crystals. M.p. 190° to 191°.
Soluble in water and ethanol; sparingly soluble in ether.

Colour Tests. Mandelin's Test—green-blue; Marquis Test—red-violet → brown.

Thin-layer Chromatography. *System TA*—Rf 52; *system TB*—Rf 41; *system TC*—Rf 37. (*Acidified iodoplatinate solution*, positive.)

Gas Chromatography. *System GA*—RI 2080.

Ultraviolet Spectrum. Aqueous acid—259 nm ($A_1^1 = 14.6$ a), 265 nm. No alkaline shift.

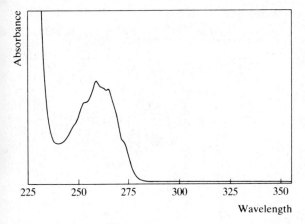

Absorbance

225 250 275 300 325 350

Wavelength

Infra-red Spectrum. Principal peaks at wavenumbers 756, 700, 1035, 770, 1190, 735 (KBr disk).

Mass Spectrum. Principal peaks at m/z 58, 254, 45, 44, 77, 42, 59, 72.

Dose. 75 to 100 mg of chlophedianol hydrochloride daily.

Chloral Betaine

Hypnotic/Sedative

The adduct formed by chloral hydrate, $CCl_3 \cdot CH(OH)_2$, and betaine, $C_5H_{11}NO_2$, containing about 58% of chloral hydrate. $C_7H_{12}Cl_3NO_3, H_2O = 282.6$
CAS—2218-68-0

$$CCl_3 \cdot CH(OH)_2 \cdot (CH_3)_3 N^+ \cdot CH_2 \cdot COO^-$$

A white crystalline powder. M.p. about 124°, with decomposition.
Soluble 1 in 1 of water and 1 in 4 of ethanol; practically insoluble in chloroform and ether.

Ultraviolet Spectrum. No significant absorption, 230 to 360 nm.

Infra-red Spectrum. Principal peaks at wavenumbers 840, 1630, 1085, 1130, 730, 1500 (KBr disk).

Mass Spectrum. Principal peaks at m/z 81, 83, 46, 110, 82, 112, 84, 117.

Dose. Usually 0.87 to 2.61 g daily, but doses of up to 3.5 g may be necessary.

Chloral Hydrate

Hypnotic/Sedative

Synonym. Chloral
Proprietary Names. Aquachloral; Chloradorm; Chloraldurat; Chloralex; Chloralvan; Dormel; Elix-Nocte; Noctec; Novochlorhydrate; Rectules.
2,2,2-Trichloroethane-1,1-diol
$CCl_3 \cdot CH(OH)_2 = 165.4$
CAS—302-17-0
Colourless or white crystals which volatilise slowly on exposure to air and are decomposed by caustic alkalis, liberating chloroform. It liquefies between 50° and 58° and boils at 98° with dissociation into water and trichloroacetaldehyde.
Soluble 1 in 0.3 of water, 1 in 0.2 of ethanol, 1 in 3 of chloroform, and 1 in less than 1 of ether. Ethanolic solutions may deposit crystals of chloral ethanolate.

Dissociation Constant. pK_a 10.0.

Partition Coefficient. Log P (octanol), 0.6.

Colour Tests. Fujiwara Test—red; Palladium Chloride—black.

Gas Chromatography. *System GA*—RI 695 (tailing peak); *system GI*—retention time 12.5 min (tailing peak).

Ultraviolet Spectrum. No significant absorption, 230 to 360 nm.

Infra-red Spectrum. Principal peaks at wavenumbers 835, 1083, 1300, 970, 1620.

Mass Spectrum. Principal peaks at m/z 82, 47, 84, 29, 111, 83, 113, 85; trichloroacetic acid 44, 83, 85, 36, 28, –, –, –; trichloroethanol 31, 49, 77, 113, 115, 82, 51, 117.

Quantification. ULTRAVIOLET SPECTROPHOTOMETRY. In blood or urine: trichloroethanol (modified Fujiwara reaction)—A. J. McBay *et al.*, *J. analyt. Toxicol.*, 1980, *4*, 99–101.

GAS CHROMATOGRAPHY. In plasma or urine: trichloroethanol, ECD—D. J. Berry, *J. Chromat.*, 1975, *107*, 107–114. In blood or urine: chloral hydrate, trichloroethanol and trichloroacetic acid, head-space analysis, detection limit 500 ng/ml for chloral hydrate and trichloroethanol, ECD—D. D. Breimer *et al.*, *J. Chromat.*, 1974, *88*, 55–63.

Disposition in the Body. Readily absorbed following oral administration. It is rapidly metabolised by reduction to trichloroethanol, the major active metabolite, which is further metabolised by conjugation with glucuronic acid to give urochloralic acid and by oxidation to trichloroacetic acid, the major urinary metabolite. About 10 to 30% of a dose is excreted in the urine as urochloralic acid and up to 5% as trichloroethanol in 24 hours. Trichloroacetic acid is slowly excreted in urine over several days; a small amount of urochloralic acid may be excreted in the bile.

THERAPEUTIC CONCENTRATION. Chloral hydrate is difficult to detect in body fluids after normal doses. The plasma concentration of trichloroethanol is usually in the range 1.5 to 15 µg/ml. Trichloroacetic acid and urochloralic acid are present in plasma at concentrations similar to, or greater than, those of trichloroethanol. When alcohol has been taken, peak plasma concentrations of trichloroethanol are increased and remain elevated for about 6 hours after ingestion, and those of trichloroacetic acid are decreased. Trichloroacetic acid accumulates in the plasma during chronic administration of chloral hydrate.

Following a single oral dose of 825 mg to 5 subjects, peak plasma-trichloroethanol concentrations of 7.6 to 12.2 µg/ml (mean 9.7) were attained in 0.5 to 1 hour (D. J. Berry, *J. Chromat.*, 1975, *107*, 107–114).

TOXICITY. Fatalities have occurred following the ingestion of 1.25 and 3 g but recovery has occurred after ingestion of 30 g. Plasma concentrations greater than 40 µg/ml of trichloroethanol are likely to produce toxic effects; fatalities have been reported at blood concentrations of 20 to **155** to 495 µg/ml of trichloroethanol.

In 4 fatalities known to involve the acute ingestion of 15 to 30 g of chloral hydrate, postmortem blood-trichloroethanol concentrations ranged from 100 to 640 µg/ml (mean 265) (R. C. Baselt and R. H. Cravey, *J. analyt. Toxicol.*, 1977, *1*, 81–103).

In a fatality due to the ingestion of chloral hydrate, the following postmortem tissue concentrations of trichloroethanol were reported: blood 55 µg/ml, brain 91 µg/g, liver 200 µg/g, urine 30 µg/ml (A. Poklis *et al.*, *Bull. int. Ass. forens. Toxicol.*, 1973, *9*(3 & 4), 8–9).

HALF-LIFE. Plasma half-life, chloral hydrate about 4 minutes, trichloroethanol about 8 hours, urochloralic acid about 7 hours, trichloroacetic acid about 4 days.

VOLUME OF DISTRIBUTION. Trichloroethanol, about 0.6 litre/kg.

DISTRIBUTION IN BLOOD. Plasma: whole blood ratio, trichloro-ethanol, about 0.9.

PROTEIN BINDING. In plasma, trichloroethanol 35% and tri-chloroacetic acid 94%.

NOTE. For a review of the pharmacokinetics of hypnotic drugs see D. D. Breimer, *Clin. Pharmacokinet.*, 1977, *2*, 93–109.

Dose. 0.5 to 2 g daily.

Chlorambucil   *Antineoplastic*

Synonym. Chlorbutinum
Proprietary Names. Chloraminophène; Leukeran.
4-[4-Bis(2-chloroethyl)aminophenyl]butyric acid
$C_{14}H_{19}Cl_2NO_2 = 304.2$
CAS—305-03-3

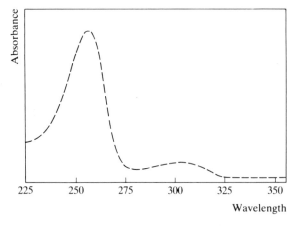

A white crystalline or granular powder. M.p. 64° to 69°.
Practically **insoluble** in water; soluble 1 in 1.5 of ethanol, 1 in 2 of acetone, and 1 in 2.5 of chloroform; soluble in ether.
Caution. Chlorambucil is irritant; avoid contact with skin and mucous membranes.

Dissociation Constant. pK_a 5.8.

Partition Coefficient. Log *P* (octanol/pH 7.4), 1.7.

Thin-layer Chromatography. *System TD*—Rf 33; *system TE*—Rf 06; *system TF*—Rf 40.

Ultraviolet Spectrum. Methanol—258 nm ($A_1^1 = 642$ a), 303 nm. No alkaline shift.

Infra-red Spectrum. Principal peaks at wavenumbers 1695, 1520, 1229, 1610, 1175, 1270 (KBr disk).

Mass Spectrum. Principal peaks at *m/z* 254, 256, 118, 255, 303, 305, 63, 45.

Quantification. GAS CHROMATOGRAPHY–MASS SPECTROMETRY. In plasma: sensitivity < 10 ng/ml—H. Ehrsson *et al.*, *J. pharm. Sci.*, 1980, *69*, 710–712.

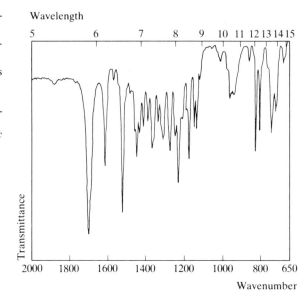

HIGH PRESSURE LIQUID CHROMATOGRAPHY. In plasma: sensitivity 100 ng/ml, UV detection—A. E. Ahmed *et al.*, *J. Chromat.*, 1982, *233*; *Biomed. Appl.*, *22*, 392–397.

Disposition in the Body. Rapidly absorbed after oral administration with peak plasma concentrations being attained in 0.5 to 2 hours. It is extensively metabolised; less than 1% of a dose is excreted in the urine unchanged. Phenylacetic acid mustard is a major metabolite.

HALF-LIFE. Plasma half-life, about 1 to 2 hours.

Dose. Initially 200 µg/kg daily, by mouth; maintenance, 30 to 100 µg/kg daily.

Chloramine   *Disinfectant*

Synonyms. Chloramidum; Chloramine T; Cloramina; Mianin; Natrium Sulfaminochloratum; Tosylchloramide Sodium.
Proprietary Names. Hydroclonazone; Klortee.
Note. The name Chloramin is applied to a preparation of chlorpheniramine maleate.
Sodium *N*-chlorotoluene-*p*-sulphonimidate trihydrate
$C_7H_7ClNNaO_2S,3H_2O = 281.7$
CAS—127-65-1 (anhydrous)

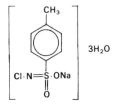

A white or slightly yellow crystalline powder. It effloresces in air, losing chlorine, becoming yellow in colour and less soluble in water.

Soluble 1 in 7 of water and 1 in 2 of boiling water; soluble 1 in 12 of ethanol, with slow decomposition; practically insoluble in chloroform and ether.

Ultraviolet Spectrum. No significant absorption, 230 to 360 nm.

Infra-red Spectrum. Principal peaks at wavenumbers 1165, 1316, 1105, 825, 710, 920 (KCl disk).

Use. As a 2% solution for wound irrigation.

Chloramphenicol   *Antibiotic*

Synonyms. Chloranfenicol; Cloranfenicol; Laevomycetinum.

Proprietary Names. Amphicol; Chloromycetin; Chloroptic; Econochlor; Fenicol; Kemicetine; Novochlorocap; Sno Phenicol.

2,2 - Dichloro - N - [($\alpha R, \beta R$) - β - hydroxy - α - hydroxymethyl - 4 - nitrophenethyl]acetamide
$C_{11}H_{12}Cl_2N_2O_5 = 323.1$
CAS—56-75-7

$$
\begin{array}{c}
CH_2OH \\
| \\
H\text{---}C\text{---}NH\cdot CO\cdot CHCl_2 \\
| \\
HO\text{---}C\text{---}H
\end{array}
$$

NO₂

Fine, white to greyish-white or yellowish-white crystals. M.p. 149° to 153°. A solution in dehydrated alcohol is dextrorotatory and a solution in ethyl acetate is laevorotatory.

Soluble 1 in 400 of water and 1 in 2.5 of ethanol; freely soluble in acetone and ethyl acetate; slightly soluble in chloroform and ether.

Chloramphenicol Cinnamate

$C_{20}H_{18}Cl_2N_2O_6 = 453.3$
CAS—14399-14-5
A white or yellowish-white crystalline powder. M.p. about 119°.
Very slightly **soluble** in water; soluble 1 in 25 of ethanol, 1 in 50 of chloroform, and 1 in 500 of ether.

Chloramphenicol Palmitate

Synonyms. Chloramphenicol α-Palmitate; Palmitylchloramphenicol.
Proprietary Names. Chloromycetin Palmitate Suspension; Globenicol.
$C_{27}H_{42}Cl_2N_2O_6 = 561.5$
CAS—530-43-8
A fine, white, unctuous, crystalline powder. M.p. 87° to 95°.
Practically **insoluble** in water; soluble 1 in 45 of ethanol, 1 in 6 of chloroform, and 1 in 14 of ether; freely soluble in acetone; soluble in ethyl acetate.

Chloramphenicol Sodium Succinate

Synonym. Chloramphenicol α-Sodium Succinate
Proprietary Names. Chloromycetin Succinate; Globenicol; Kemicetine Succinate; Mychel-S.
$C_{15}H_{15}Cl_2N_2NaO_8 = 445.2$
CAS—982-57-0
A white or yellowish-white hygroscopic powder.
Soluble 1 in less than 1 of water and 1 in 1 of ethanol; practically insoluble in chloroform and ether.

Dissociation Constant. pK_a 5.5.

Partition Coefficient. Log *P* (octanol), 1.1.

Colour Tests. Fujiwara Test—red; Nessler's Reagent—brown-orange.

Gas Chromatography. *System GA*—RI 2310.

Ultraviolet Spectrum. Water—278 nm $(A_1^1 = 298\ a)$. Chloramphenicol palmitate: dehydrated alcohol—271 nm $(A_1^1 = 178\ a)$.

Infra-red Spectrum. Principal peaks at wavenumbers 1681, 847, 1072, 1515, 816, 1562 (Nujol mull).

Wavelength

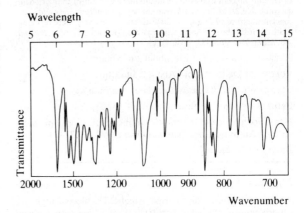

Mass Spectrum. Principal peaks at m/z 70, 150, 151, 153, 77, 51, 118, 60.

Quantification. GAS CHROMATOGRAPHY. In cerebrospinal fluid, plasma or urine: ECD—L. K. Pickering *et al.*, *Clin. Chem.*, 1979, *25*, 300–305. In urine: chloramphenicol or thiamphenicol and their metabolites, FID—T. Nakagawa *et al.*, *J. Chromat.*, 1975, *111*, 355–364.

HIGH PRESSURE LIQUID CHROMATOGRAPHY. In plasma: chloramphenicol and chloramphenicol succinate, detection limits 500 ng/ml for chloramphenicol and 1 µg/ml for the succinate, UV detection—R. Velagapudi *et al.*, *J. Chromat.*, 1982, *228*; *Biomed. Appl.*, *17*, 423–428. In cerebrospinal fluid, plasma or serum: sensitivity 100 to 200 ng/ml, UV detection—R. H. B. Sample *et al.*, *Antimicrob. Ag. Chemother.*, 1979, *15*, 491–493.

Disposition in the Body. Readily absorbed after oral administration. The inactive palmitate ester is hydrolysed to free drug in the gastro-intestinal tract before absorption and the inactive sodium succinate ester, given parenterally, is similarly hydrolysed *in vivo*. It is widely distributed in the body, giving a concentration in the cerebrospinal fluid about 50% of that in the blood. The main metabolic pathway is conjugation with glucuronic acid; chloramphenicol is also hydrolysed to 1-(4-nitrophenyl)-2-aminopropane-1,3-diol. Both metabolites are inactive. Up to about 90% of a dose is excreted in the urine in 24 hours, mainly as the glucuronide, with about 5 to 10% of the dose in unchanged form. About 3% of the dose is excreted in the bile but this is mainly reabsorbed to give about 1% eliminated in the faeces.

THERAPEUTIC CONCENTRATION. In plasma, usually in the range 10 to 20 µg/ml.

Following oral administration of chloramphenicol palmitate, equivalent to 15 to 27 mg/kg of chloramphenicol, four times a day to 18 children, plasma concentrations of 15.2 to 38.9 µg/ml (mean 27.5) were reported 1.5 hours after a dose (R. E. Kauffman *et al.*, *J. Pediat.*, 1981, *99*, 963–967).

TOXICITY. There is an increased incidence of reversible bone marrow depression when plasma concentrations exceed 25 µg/ml. The 'grey' syndrome (cardiovascular collapse, respiratory depression, and coma) has been reported in patients with plasma concentrations in the range 40 to 200 µg/ml.

A 26-year-old woman received an initial 1-g dose followed in 7 and 12 hours by two 10-g doses. A plasma concentration of 201 µg/ml was measured 5½ hours after the last dose while she was in severe shock, but she recovered (W. L. Thompson *et al.*, *J. Am. med. Ass.*, 1975, *234*, 149–150).

In a fatality involving ingestion of an unknown quantity of chloramphenicol (probably 2.5 to 4 g) by a 5-year-old boy, postmortem liver and urine concentrations of 10.7 µg/g and 2090 µg/ml, respectively, were reported; death occurred about 18 hours after ingestion (E. Grusz-Harday, *Bull. int. Ass. forens. Toxicol.*, 1973, *9*(3 & 4), 10–11).

HALF-LIFE. Plasma half-life, about 2 to 5 hours.

VOLUME OF DISTRIBUTION. About 0.5 to 1 litre/kg.

CLEARANCE. Plasma clearance, about 4 ml/min/kg.

PROTEIN BINDING. In plasma, about 40 to 60%.

NOTE. For a review of the pharmacokinetics of chloramphenicol see P. J. Ambrose, *Clin. Pharmacokinet.*, 1984, *9*, 222–238.

Dose. Usually 2 g daily.

Chlorbutol   *Preservative*

Synonyms. Acetone-Chloroforme; Alcohol Trichlorisobutylicus; Chlorbutanol; Chlorbutanolum Hydratum; Chloretone; Chlorobutanol; Trichlorbutanolum.

1,1,1-Trichloro-2-methylpropan-2-ol hemihydrate
$C_4H_7Cl_3O, \frac{1}{2}H_2O = 186.5$
CAS—57-15-8 (anhydrous); *6001-64-5* (hemihydrate)

$$\left[\begin{array}{c} CH_3 \\ CCl_3 \cdot C \cdot OH \\ CH_3 \end{array} \right] \frac{1}{2}H_2O$$

Colourless or white crystals which are volatile at ordinary temperatures. M.p. about 76° to 79°; anhydrous chlorbutol, about 95°. B.p. about 167°.

Soluble 1 in 130 of water, 1 in 0.6 of ethanol, and 1 in 3 of chloroform; very soluble in ether.

Colour Test. Fujiwara Test—red.

Gas Chromatography. *System GA*—RI 949; *system GI*—retention time 29.8 min.

Ultraviolet Spectrum. No significant absorption, 230 to 360 nm.

Infra-red Spectrum. Principal peaks at wavenumbers 790, 833, 1145, 1186, 917, 980 (Nujol mull).

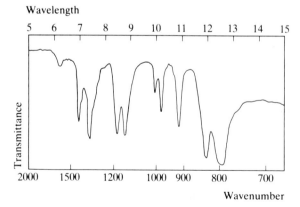

Wavelength

Quantification. GAS CHROMATOGRAPHY. In blood, urine or tissues: limit of detection about 100 ng/ml, ECD—J. C. Valentour and I. Sunshine, *Z. Rechtsmed.*, 1975, *77*, 61–63.

Disposition in the Body. Rapidly absorbed after oral administration, peak plasma concentrations being attained within 0.25 to 1 hour. About 10% of a dose is excreted in the urine in 17 days mostly as the glucuronide and sulphate conjugates.

TOXICITY.

In a non-fatal case of chlorbutol toxicity, a man who had been taking 1 to 1.5 g daily was admitted to hospital. An initial plasma concentration of about 100 µg/ml was reported and the plasma half-life was found to be about 13 days (T. Borody *et al.*, *Med. J. Aust.*, 1979, *1*, 288).

In a fatality due to chlorbutol overdose, the following postmortem tissue concentrations were found: blood 64 µg/ml, bile 123 µg/ml, brain 161 µg/g, kidney 87 µg/g, liver 141 µg/g, spleen 120 µg/g, urine 31 µg/ml (J. C. Valentour and I. Sunshine, *Z. Rechtsmed.*, 1975, *77*, 61–63).

HALF-LIFE. Plasma half-life, about 10 days.

VOLUME OF DISTRIBUTION. About 3 litres/kg.

PROTEIN BINDING. In plasma, about 50 to 60%.

NOTE. For a report on the pharmacokinetics of chlorbutol see C. Tung *et al.*, *Biopharm. Drug Disp.*, 1982, *3*, 371–378.

Uses. Chlorbutol is used in a concentration of 0.5%. It was formerly given as a sedative in doses of 0.3 to 1.2 g.

Chlorcyclizine   *Antihistamine*

Synonym. Histachlorazine

(±)-1-(4-Chlorobenzhydryl)-4-methylpiperazine
$C_{18}H_{21}ClN_2 = 300.8$
CAS—82-93-9

A liquid.

Chlorcyclizine Hydrochloride

Synonym. Chlorcyclizinium Chloride
Proprietary Names. Di-Paralene; Trihistan. It is an ingredient of Fedrazil.
$C_{18}H_{21}ClN_2, HCl = 337.3$
CAS—1620-21-9; 14362-31-3
A white crystalline powder. M.p. about 225°.
Soluble 1 in 2 of water, 1 in 11 of ethanol, and 1 in 4 of chloroform; practically insoluble in ether.

Dissociation Constant. pK_a 2.4, 7.8 (25°).

Colour Test. Liebermann's Test—red-orange.

Thin-layer Chromatography. *System TA*—Rf 57; *system TB*—Rf 42; *system TC*—Rf 46. (*Dragendorff spray*, positive; *acidified iodoplatinate solution*, positive.)

Gas Chromatography. *System GA*—RI 2225; *system GF*—RI 2560.

High Pressure Liquid Chromatography. *System HA*—k' 2.3.

Ultraviolet Spectrum. Aqueous acid—232 nm ($A_1^1 = 581$ a).

Infra-red Spectrum. Principal peaks at wavenumbers 988, 725, 760, 706, 1087, 870 (chlorcyclizine hydrochloride, Nujol mull).

Mass Spectrum. Principal peaks at *m/z* 99, 56, 72, 165, 300, 228, 229, 242.

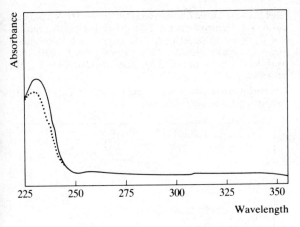

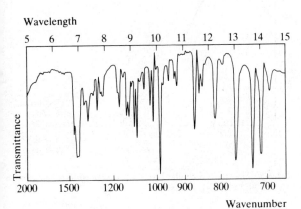

Quantification. COLORIMETRY. In animal plasma or tissues: chlorcyclizine, cyclizine and their metabolites—R. Kuntzman et al., J. Pharmac. exp. Ther., 1965, 149, 29–35.

Disposition in the Body. Readily absorbed after oral administration and widely distributed throughout the body. Metabolised by N-demethylation to form norchlorcyclizine and by N-oxidation. High concentrations of the N-desmethyl metabolite are found in the liver, lungs, kidney, and spleen. Slowly excreted in the urine; measurable amounts of norchlorcyclizine have been detected in the urine for up to 3 weeks after the cessation of chronic oral administration. About 0.5% of a dose is excreted in the urine as the N-oxide.

THERAPEUTIC CONCENTRATION.

After a single oral dose of 2 mg/kg to 4 subjects, average peak plasma concentrations of about 0.05 µg/ml and 0.03 µg/ml were attained in 5 hours for unchanged drug and norchlorcyclizine, respectively. After oral administration of 50 mg 3 times a day for 6 days, plasma concentrations of norchlorcyclizine of 0.05 to 0.11 µg/ml were reported on the first day after the cessation of treatment, and plasma concentrations of 0.02 to 0.04 µg/ml were found on the tenth day after cessation of treatment (R. Kuntzman et al., Ann. N.Y. Acad. Sci., 1973, 226, 131–147).

HALF-LIFE. Plasma half-life, chlorcyclizine about 12 hours, norchlorcyclizine 6 to 9 days.

PROTEIN BINDING. In plasma, norchlorcyclizine, about 85 to 90%.

Dose. 50 to 200 mg of chlorcyclizine hydrochloride daily.

Chlordane   *Pesticide*

Synonym. Chlordan
Proprietary Names. Murphy Ant Killer; Nippon Ant Powder; Sydane. It is an ingredient of Cooper Ant Killer.

1,2,4,5,6,7,8,8 - Octachloro - 2,3,3a,4,7,7a - hexahydro - 4,7 - methanoindene
$C_{10}H_6Cl_8 = 409.8$
CAS—57-47-9; 12789-03-6 (technical grade); *22212-52-8* (*cis*); *5103-74-2* (*trans*)

Technical chlordane is a mixture of chlorinated methanoindenes, the major components being the two stereoisomers *cis*-chlordane and *trans*-chlordane.
The technical grade is an amber viscous liquid which is decomposed by alkalis.
Practically **immiscible** with water, miscible with ethanol, chloroform, and ether.

Gas Chromatography. *System GK—cis*-chlordane and *trans*-chlordane retention times 1.08 and 1.06, respectively, relative to caffeine.

Infra-red Spectrum. Principal peaks at wavenumbers 704, 1265, 1020, 1075, 1612, 826.

Mass Spectrum. Principal peaks at *m/z* 373, 375, 377, 371, 44, 109, 75, 272 (*cis*-chlordane); 373, 375, 377, 371, 272, 237, 75, 65 (*trans*-chlordane).

Quantification. GAS CHROMATOGRAPHY. In blood—W. E. Dale et al., Life Sci., 1966, 5, 46-54.

Disposition in the Body. Readily absorbed from the gastrointestinal tract, lungs, and the skin. It is stored in adipose tissue. Oxychlordane has been detected in adipose tissue and breast milk.

TOXICITY. Severe toxicity may result after ingestion or skin contamination with greater than 1 g, and fatalities have occurred after the ingestion of more than 2 g and after excessive skin contamination. The maximum permissible atmospheric concentration is 0.5 mg/m³.

In a non-fatal poisoning case, a 4-year-old child who ingested an unknown amount of chlordane and developed intermittent convulsions had an initial serum concentration of 3.4 µg/ml which decreased to 0.14 µg/ml after 72 hours; the rate of decline of the serum concentration was non-linear with a terminal half-life of 88 days. Urine samples obtained during the first 3 days after ingestion, showed a decrease from 1.9 µg/ml to 0.05 µg/ml but increased to 0.13 µg/ml on the 35th day (F. D. Aldrich and J. M. Holmes, Archs envir. Hlth, 1969, 19, 129–132).

The following postmortem concentrations were reported in a fatality due to the ingestion of chlordane: blood 4.4 µg/ml, urine 0.24 µg/ml (R. O. Bost and I. Sunshine, Bull. int. Ass. forens. Toxicol., 1978, 14(1), 30).

A 66-year-old man who ingested about 400 ml of a 70% commercial solution and died after 40 hours had the following postmortem tissue concentrations: blood 1.7 µg/ml, fat 378 µg/g, kidney 14 µg/g, liver 43 µg/g, urine 0.6 µg/ml (R. Morano per Disposition of Toxic Drugs and Chemicals in Man, 2nd Edn, R. C. Baselt (Ed.), Davis, California, Biomedical Publications, 1982, pp. 140–142).

Chlordantoin

Antifungal

Synonym. Clodantoin
Proprietary Name. Sporostacin
5 - (1 - Ethylpentyl) - 3 - (trichloromethylthio)imidazolidine - 2,4 - dione
$C_{11}H_{17}Cl_3N_2O_2S = 347.7$
CAS—5588-20-5

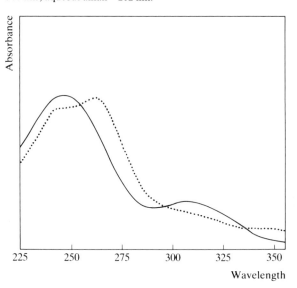

Ultraviolet Spectrum. No significant absorption, 230 to 360 nm.

Infra-red Spectrum. Principal peaks at wavenumbers 1730, 1786, 730, 1059, 766, 1309.

Use. Topically in a concentration of 1%.

Chlordiazepoxide

Tranquilliser

Synonym. Methaminodiazepoxide
Proprietary Names. Libritabs; Librium (tablets); Risolid. It is an ingredient of Libraxin, Limbatril, Limbitrol, and Menrium.
7-Chloro-2-methylamino-5-phenyl-3*H*-1,4-benzodiazepine   4-oxide
$C_{16}H_{14}ClN_3O = 299.8$
CAS—58-25-3

A yellow crystalline powder, sensitive to sunlight. M.p. about 240°.
Practically **insoluble** in water; soluble 1 in 50 of ethanol and 1 in 130 of ether; slightly soluble in chloroform.

Chlordiazepoxide Hydrochloride

Proprietary Names. A-Poxide; Corax; C-Tran; Librium; Medilium; Nack; Novopoxide; Relaxil; SK-Lygen; Solium; Trilium; Tropium. It is an ingredient of Librax.
$C_{16}H_{14}ClN_3O,HCl = 336.2$
CAS—438-41-5
A white or slightly yellowish crystalline powder. M.p. 212° to 218°, with decomposition.
Soluble 1 in 10 of water and 1 in 40 of ethanol; practically insoluble in chloroform and ether.

Dissociation Constant. pK_a 4.6 (20°).

Partition Coefficient. Log P (octanol/pH 7.4), 2.5.

Colour Test. Marquis Test—yellow.

Thin-layer Chromatography. *System TA*—Rf 62; *system TB*—Rf 02; *system TC*—Rf 50; *system TD*—Rf 10; *system TE*—Rf 51; *system TF*—Rf 11. (*Dragendorff spray*, positive; *FPN reagent*, yellow; *acidified iodoplatinate solution*, positive; *Marquis reagent*, yellow.)

Gas Chromatography. *System GA*—chlordiazepoxide RI 2453, 2530, 2799, demoxepam RI 2529, desmethyldiazepam RI 2496, oxazepam RI 2336; *system GG*—chlordiazepoxide RI 3065, desmethyldiazepam RI 3041, oxazepam RI 2803.

High Pressure Liquid Chromatography. *System HI*—chlordiazepoxide k' 6.41, demoxepam k' 2.42, desmethylchlordiazepoxide k' 4.47, desmethyldiazepam k' 8.00, oxazepam k' 4.62; *system HK*—chlordiazepoxide k' 2.87, demoxepam k' 0.03, desmethylchlordiazepoxide k' 2.39, desmethyldiazepam k' 1.99, oxazepam k' 0.73.

Ultraviolet Spectrum. Aqueous acid—246 nm ($A_1^1 = 1112$ a), 308 nm; aqueous alkali—262 nm.

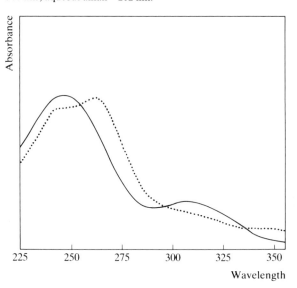

Infra-red Spectrum. Principal peaks at wavenumbers 1625, 760, 1260, 690, 1590, 850 (KBr disk).

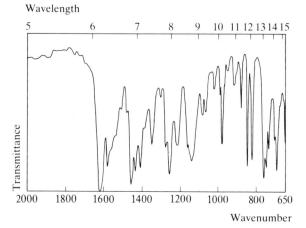

Mass Spectrum. Principal peaks at m/z 282, 299, 284, 283, 241, 56, 301, 253; demoxepam 285, 286, 269, 287, 241, 242, 77, 270; desmethylchlordiazepoxide 285, 268, 284, 77, 286, 42, 287, 233; desmethyldiazepam 242, 269, 270, 241, 243, 271, 244, 272; oxazepam 257, 77, 268, 239, 205, 267, 233, 259.

Quantification. GAS CHROMATOGRAPHY. In serum: chlordiazepoxide and demoxepam, sensitivity 45 ng/ml for chlordiazepoxide, ECD—S. R. Sun and D. J. Hoffman, *J. pharm. Sci.*, 1978, *67*, 1647–1648.

HIGH PRESSURE LIQUID CHROMATOGRAPHY. In plasma or urine: chlordiazepoxide and four metabolites, detection limit 20 ng/ml for all compounds, UV detection—T. B. Vree *et al.*, *J. Chromat.*, 1981, *224*; *Biomed. Appl.*, *13*, 519–525.

RADIOIMMUNOASSAY. In blood, plasma or saliva: sensitivity 50 ng/ml in blood or plasma and 500 pg/ml in saliva—R. Dixon *et al.*, *J. pharm. Sci.*, 1979, *68*, 261.

Disposition in the Body. Readily absorbed after oral administration; bioavailability almost 100%. Metabolised by demethylation and subsequent deamination to the active metabolites desmethylchlordiazepoxide and demoxepam. Demoxepam is further metabolised by hydrolysis with cleavage of the lactam ring and by reduction to desmethyldiazepam (nordazepam) followed by hydroxylation to oxazepam (desmethyldiazepam and oxazepam are also pharmacologically active). About 60% of a dose is excreted in the urine and 10 to 20% is eliminated in the faeces; less than 1% of a dose is excreted in the urine unchanged, about 6% is excreted as demoxepam, and the remainder as ring-opened derivatives and glucuronide conjugates of oxazepam and other hydroxylated metabolites.

THERAPEUTIC CONCENTRATION. In plasma, usually in the range 0.4 to 4 µg/ml. Demoxepam and desmethyldiazepam may accumulate in the plasma of patients on chronic therapy; demoxepam is not normally detectable in plasma after a single dose of chlordiazepoxide.

Following a single oral dose of 20 mg to 6 subjects, peak plasma concentrations of 0.78 to 1.24 µg/ml (mean 1.0) of chlordiazepoxide were attained in 2 to 6 hours; desmethylchlordiazepoxide was detectable 5 hours after the dose and peak plasma concentrations of 0.14 to 0.46 µg/ml (mean 0.3) were attained in 8 to 24 hours (M. A. Schwartz *et al.*, *J. pharm. Sci.*, 1971, *60*, 1500–1503).

Following daily oral administration of 10 mg three times a day to 8 subjects, mean steady-state plasma concentrations were: chlordiazepoxide 0.5 to 1.0 µg/ml (mean 0.8), desmethylchlordiazepoxide 0.3 to 0.8 µg/ml (mean 0.5), demoxepam 0.24 to 0.44 µg/ml (mean 0.36) (H. G. Boxenbaum *et al.*, *J. Pharmacokinet. Biopharm.*, 1977, *5*, 25–39).

TOXICITY. Toxic reactions may be produced by plasma concentrations greater than 3 µg/ml; plasma concentrations in the region of 20 µg/ml may produce coma or death, but fatalities caused by chlordiazepoxide alone are rare. Recoveries have occurred after the ingestion of single doses of about 2 g.

The following postmortem chlordiazepoxide tissue concentrations were reported in a fatality in which death occurred 18 to 20 hours after the ingestion of an unknown quantity of chlordiazepoxide: blood 26.4 µg/ml, bile 39 µg/ml, kidney 11 µg/g, liver 10 µg/g, spleen 9 µg/g, urine 7.8 µg/ml (H. Mohseni, *Bull. int. Ass. forens. Toxicol.*, 1975, *11*(2), 17–18).

The following peak plasma concentrations were observed in a comatose adult subject who had ingested 1 g: chlordiazepoxide 20 µg/ml after 6 hours, desmethylchlordiazepoxide 12 µg/ml after 21 hours, demoxepam 9 µg/ml after 51 hours (J. A. F. de Silva and L. D'Arconte, *J. forens. Sci.*, 1969, *14*, 184–202).

HALF-LIFE. Plasma half-life, chlordiazepoxide 5 to 30 hours (mean 15), demoxepam 14 to 95 hours (mean 40); desmethyldiazepam about 40 to 100 hours, but there is considerable intersubject variation—see under Nordazepam.

VOLUME OF DISTRIBUTION. 0.3 to 0.6 litre/kg.

CLEARANCE. Plasma clearance, about 0.5 ml/min/kg.

SALIVA. Plasma: saliva ratio, about 33.

PROTEIN BINDING. In plasma, about 90 to 97%.

NOTE. For a review of the pharmacokinetics of chlordiazepoxide see D. J. Greenblatt *et al.*, *Clin. Pharmacokinet.*, 1978, *3*, 381–394.

Dose. 30 to 100 mg daily.

Chlorhexidine
Cationic Disinfectant

Proprietary Names. Hexol. It is an ingredient of Cetal (liquid).

1,1′-Hexamethylenebis[5-(4-chlorophenyl)biguanide]

$C_{22}H_{30}Cl_2N_{10} = 505.5$

CAS—55-56-1

Crystals. M.p. 134°.

Chlorhexidine Acetate

Proprietary Names. Hibitane (powder). It is an ingredient of Norgotin and Travasept.

$C_{22}H_{30}Cl_2N_{10}, 2C_2H_4O_2 = 625.6$

CAS—56-95-1

A white to pale cream microcrystalline powder. When heated it decomposes with the production of trace amounts of 4-chloroaniline. Aqueous solutions slowly decompose.

Soluble 1 in 55 of water and 1 in 15 of ethanol; very slightly soluble in propylene glycol.

Chlorhexidine Gluconate Solution

Proprietary Names. Corsodyl; Dispray; Hibicare; Hibiclens; Hibidil; Hibiscrub; Hibisol; Hibitane (solution); pHiso-MED; Rotersept. It is an ingredient of Cyteal, Eludril, Savloclens, Savlodil, Savlon (liquid) and Stomosol.

An aqueous solution containing 19 to 21% of $C_{22}H_{30}Cl_2N_{10}, 2C_6H_{12}O_7$ (= 897.8).

CAS—18472-51-0 (chlorhexidine gluconate)

A colourless to pale straw-coloured liquid which is affected by light. Wt per ml 1.06 to 1.07 g.

Miscible with water, with up to 5 parts of ethanol, and with up to 3 parts of acetone.

Chlorhexidine Hydrochloride

Proprietary Names. Hibitane (powder); Sterilon (powder).

$C_{22}H_{30}Cl_2N_{10}, 2HCl = 578.4$

CAS—3697-42-5

A white crystalline powder, affected by light. M.p. about 255°, with decomposition.

Soluble 1 in 1700 of water, 1 in 450 of ethanol, and 1 in 50 of propylene glycol; slightly soluble in methanol.

Colour Test. Stir a small quantity on a white tile with a drop of *bromine solution* followed by a drop of *sodium hydroxide solution*—red.

Thin-layer Chromatography. *System TA*—Rf 33. (*Acidified iodoplatinate solution*, positive.)

Ultraviolet Spectrum. Aqueous acid—245 nm; aqueous alkali (pH 10)—232 nm, 253 nm. (See below)

Infra-red Spectrum. Principal peaks at wavenumbers 1527, 1628, 1575, 1235, 820, 1080 (KBr disk). (See below)

Quantification. HIGH PRESSURE LIQUID CHROMATOGRAPHY. In blood, serum or urine: sensitivity 1 µg/ml, UV detection—C. E. Huston *et al.*, *J. Chromat.*, 1982, *237*, 457–464.

Use. Chlorhexidine gluconate is used in solutions containing 0.01 to 0.5%.

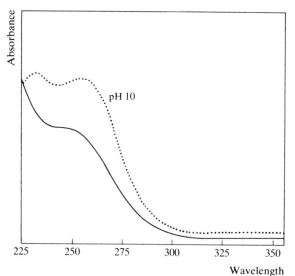

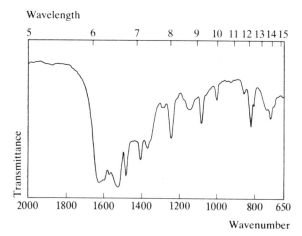

Practically **insoluble** in water; soluble 1 in 160 of ethanol, 1 in 1.5 of chloroform, and 1 in 210 of ether.

Ultraviolet Spectrum. Methanol—285 nm ($A_1^1 = 575$ b).

Infra-red Spectrum. Principal peaks at wavenumbers 1238, 1724, 1646, 1219, 881, 1597 (KBr disk).

Dose. Chlormadinone acetate has been given in doses of 2 to 10 mg daily.

Chlormethiazole
Hypnotic/Sedative

Synonym. Clomethiazole

Proprietary Names of Chlormethiazole and Chlormethiazole Edisylate. Distraneurin(e); Hemineurin(e); Heminevrin.

5-(2-Chloroethyl)-4-methylthiazole

$C_6H_8ClNS = 161.6$

CAS—533-45-9

A colourless to slightly yellow-brown, oily, viscous liquid.

Soluble 1 in 100 of water; miscible with ethanol, chloroform, and ether.

Chlormethiazole Edisylate

Synonym. Chlormethiazole Ethanedisulphonate

$C_{14}H_{22}Cl_2N_2O_6S_4 = 513.5$

CAS—1867-58-9

A white crystalline powder. M.p. 126° to 129°.

Freely **soluble** in water and warm ethanol; practically insoluble in ether.

Dissociation Constant. pK_a 3.2.

Colour Test. Sodium Nitroprusside (Method 3)—violet.

Thin-layer Chromatography. *System TA*—Rf 64; *system TB*—Rf 44; *system TC*—Rf 69. (*Acidified iodoplatinate solution*, positive.)

Gas Chromatography. *System GA*—RI 1230.

High Pressure Liquid Chromatography. *System HA*—k′ 0.1.

Ultraviolet Spectrum. Aqueous acid—258 nm ($A_1^1 = 288$ a); aqueous alkali—250 nm ($A_1^1 = 270$ b).

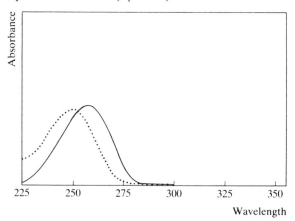

Infra-red Spectrum. Principal peaks at wavenumbers 1190, 1227, 1041, 1031, 779, 823 (chlormethiazole edisylate, KBr disk).

Mass Spectrum. Principal peaks at m/z 112, 161, 85, 45, 163, 113, 114, 59.

Chlormadinone Acetate
Progestational Steroid

Proprietary Names. Gestafortin; Lutéran.

6-Chloro-3,20-dioxopregna-4,6-dien-17α-yl acetate

$C_{23}H_{29}ClO_4 = 404.9$

CAS—1961-77-9 (chlormadinone); *302-22-7* (acetate)

A white to creamy-white, fluffy, crystalline powder. M.p. 208° to 212°.

Wavelength

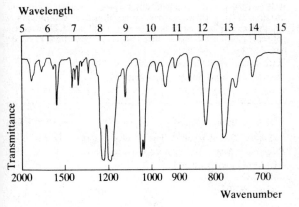

In a report of 2 cases of fatal overdose, postmortem concentrations were: blood 21 and 214 µg/ml, liver blood 21 and 100 µg/ml, bile 38 and 143 µg/ml, urine 5 and 114 µg/ml; in three further cases blood concentrations were reported to be 3.4, 50, and 75 µg/ml (A. E. Robinson and R. D. McDowall, *Forens. Sci. Int.*, 1979, *14*, 49–55).

HALF-LIFE. Plasma half-life, about 3 to 7 hours, increased in elderly subjects and in patients with liver disease.

VOLUME OF DISTRIBUTION. About 3 to 12 litres/kg (mean 8).

CLEARANCE. Plasma clearance, 10 to 25 ml/min/kg.

DISTRIBUTION IN BLOOD. Plasma: whole blood ratio, about 1.2.

PROTEIN BINDING. In plasma, about 60 to 70%.

NOTE. For a review of chlormethiazole toxicity see A. Houston *et al.*, *Human Toxicol.*, 1983, *2*, 361–369.

Dose. Chlormethiazole as Heminevrin (*Astra*) is given in doses of 2 to 3 capsules daily. An initial dose of 12 capsules daily, for 2 days, is given in alcohol withdrawal.

NOTE. Due to variations in bioavailability: for an equivalent therapeutic effect, one capsule (192 mg chlormethiazole base) ≡ 5 ml syrup (250 mg/5 ml chlormethiazole edisylate).

Quantification. GAS CHROMATOGRAPHY. In blood or plasma: chlormethiazole and two metabolites, sensitivity 32 ng for chlormethiazole in plasma, AFID—S. E. Tsuei *et al.*, *J. Chromat.*, 1980, *182*; *Biomed. Appl.*, *8*, 55–62. In plasma or urine: sensitivity 50 ng/ml for chlormethiazole edisylate, FID—R. G. Moore *et al.*, *Eur. J. clin. Pharmac.*, 1975, *8*, 353–357.

GAS CHROMATOGRAPHY-MASS SPECTROMETRY. In blood or plasma: sensitivity 1 ng/ml—K. G. Jostell *et al.*, *Acta pharmac. tox.*, 1978, *43*, 180–189. In plasma: chlormethiazole and two metabolites, sensitivity 1 ng/ml for chlormethiazole—R. L. Nation *et al.*, *Eur. J. clin. Pharmac.*, 1977, *12*, 137–145.

HIGH PRESSURE LIQUID CHROMATOGRAPHY. In plasma: detection limit 200 ng/ml, UV detection—R. Hartley *et al.*, *J. Chromat.*, 1983, *276*; *Biomed. Appl.*, *27*, 471–477.

Disposition in the Body. Rapidly absorbed after oral administration but extensively metabolised. A considerable number of metabolites have been identified in small quantities in urine. Less than 5% of a dose is excreted unchanged in the urine, and up to about 14% is excreted as 4-methylthiazole-5-acetic acid. Other metabolites identified in the urine include 5-(1-hydroxy-2-chloroethyl)-4-methylthiazole and 5-(2-hydroxyethyl)thiazole-4-carbolactone (which appear to be more abundant than 4-methylthiazole-5-acetic acid), together with 5-acetyl-4-methyl-thiazole, 5-(1-hydroxyethyl)-4-methylthiazole, and 5-(2-hydroxy-ethyl)-4-methylthiazole in both free and conjugated forms. 5-Ethyl-2-hydroxy-4-methylthiazole has been found in the tissues following overdoses of chlormethiazole. 5-(1-Hydroxyethyl)-4-methylthiazole and 5-acetyl-4-methylthiazole may be present in the plasma at concentrations similar to, or greater than those of unchanged drug.

THERAPEUTIC CONCENTRATION. In plasma, usually in the range 0.1 to 2.8 µg/ml.

Following single oral doses of 192 mg to 6 subjects, peak plasma concentrations of 0.10 to 0.55 µg/ml (mean 0.27) were attained in about 0.6 hour (P. J. Pentikainen *et al.*, *Eur. J. clin. Pharmac.*, 1980, *17*, 275–284).

TOXICITY. Toxic effects are associated with plasma concentrations of 1.6 to **13** to 26 µg/ml, and fatalities with concentrations of 8 to **50** to 170 µg/ml.

In a report of 9 cases of fatal overdose, in which doses of about 10 to 50 g had been ingested, postmortem blood concentrations of 25 to 80 µg/ml (mean 56) were found; in a further 6 fatalities due to chlormethiazole and alcohol ingestion, postmortem blood concentrations ranged from 5 to 47 µg/ml (mean 21) (S. Jakobsson and M. Möller, *Forens. Sci.*, 1972, *1*, 114).

Chlormezanone   *Tranquilliser*

Synonym. Chlormethazanone

Proprietary Names. Rexan; Rilaquil; Supotran; Tanafol; Trancopal. It is an ingredient of Lobak and Trancoprin.

2-(4-Chlorophenyl)-3-methylperhydro-1,3-thiazin-4-one 1,1-dioxide

$C_{11}H_{12}ClNO_3S = 273.7$

CAS—80-77-3

A white crystalline powder. M.p. about 115°.

Very slightly **soluble** in water; sparingly soluble in ethanol; freely soluble in acetone and chloroform.

Thin-layer Chromatography. *System TA*—Rf 66; *system TB*—Rf 01; *system TC*—Rf 63.

Gas Chromatography. *System GA*—RI 2238.

Ultraviolet Spectrum. Aqueous acid—258 nm, 265 nm ($A_1^1 = 23$ b), 272 nm; aqueous alkali—259 nm. (See below)

Infra-red Spectrum. Principal peaks at wavenumbers 1650, 1150, 1130, 1315, 880, 1090 (KBr disk). (See below)

Mass Spectrum. Principal peaks at *m/z* 98, 152, 154, 42, 69, 174, 208, 153.

Quantification. GAS CHROMATOGRAPHY. In plasma: sensitivity 100 ng/ml, ECD—K. Ohya *et al.*, *J. Chromat.*, 1980, *221*; *Biomed. Appl.*, *10*, 67–74.

Disposition in the Body. Rapidly absorbed after oral administration. Less than 5% of a dose is excreted in the urine as unchanged drug in 48 hours; about 40% of a dose is excreted in the urine in 72 hours as acidic metabolites, mainly 4-chlorohippuric acid.

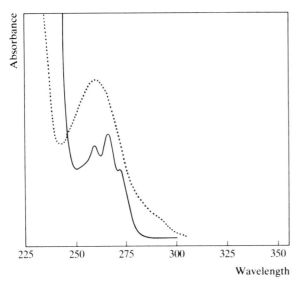

Absorbance

Wavelength

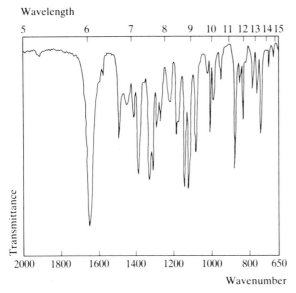

Wavelength

Transmittance

Wavenumber

THERAPEUTIC CONCENTRATION.

After a single oral dose of 200 mg to 5 subjects, peak plasma concentrations of 2.5 to 3.4 µg/ml (mean 2.8) were attained in about 4 hours (K. Ohya *et al.*, *ibid.*).

After a single oral dose of 400 mg to 4 subjects, peak plasma concentrations of 4.9 to 9.9 µg/ml (mean 7) were attained in 1 to 2 hours; following oral doses of 150 mg three times a day for 3 days to 4 subjects, plasma concentrations of 5.8 to 8.4 µg/ml (mean 6.8) were reported 2 hours after the final dose (E. W. McChesney *et al.*, *Biochem. Pharmac.*, 1967, *16*, 813–826).

TOXICITY.

In a fatality due to the combined ingestion of chlormezanone (possibly up to 10 g) and diazepam, the following postmortem tissue concentrations of chlormezanone were reported: blood 53 µg/ml, brain 109 µg/g, liver 88 µg/g, urine 31 µg/ml (J. Kristinsson, *Bull. int. Ass. forens. Toxicol.*, 1980, *15*(2), 6–7).

A 36-year-old woman was admitted to hospital comatose following the ingestion of 7 g of chlormezanone; an initial plasma concentration of 60 µg/ml was reported which declined with a half-life of 29 hours; the patient regained consciousness after 15 hours (D. Armstrong *et al.*, *Br. med. J.*, 1983, *286*, 845–846).

HALF-LIFE. Plasma half-life, about 20 to 30 hours.

PROTEIN BINDING. In plasma, about 50%.

Dose. 300 to 800 mg daily.

Chlorocresol   *Disinfectant*

Synonyms. Chlorkresolum; Parachlorometacresol; PCMC.
Proprietary Name. Wright's Vaporizing Fluid
4-Chloro-3-methylphenol
$C_7H_7ClO = 142.6$
CAS—59-50-7

OH

CH₃

Cl

Colourless crystals or crystalline powder. It is volatile in steam. M.p. 64° to 66°.

Soluble 1 in 260 of water, 1 in 50 of boiling water, and 1 in 0.4 of ethanol; soluble in acetone, chloroform, and ether. Solutions in water acquire a yellowish colour on exposure to light and air.

Dissociation Constant. pK_a 9.2 (20°).

Ultraviolet Spectrum. Aqueous acid—279 nm ($A_1^1 = 105$ a); aqueous alkali—244 nm, 299 nm.

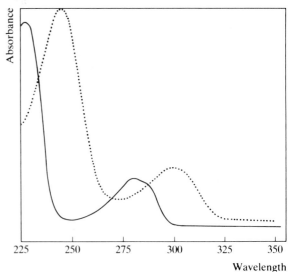

Absorbance

Wavelength

Use. In concentrations of 0.1 to 0.2%.

Chloroform   *General Anaesthetic*

Synonyms. Chloroformium Anaesthesicum; Chloroformum pro Narcosi.
Trichloromethane
$CHCl_3 = 119.4$
CAS—67-66-3

A colourless mobile volatile liquid. Wt per ml 1.474 to 1.479 g. B.p. about 61°. Refractive index 1.4464. Chloroform (*B.P.*) contains 1 to 2% v/v of ethanol.

Soluble 1 in 200 of water; miscible with dehydrated alcohol and ether.

Colour Tests. Fujiwara Test—red; Palladium Chloride—black. Heat with a small amount of resorcinol in 2M sodium hydroxide—red. If the resorcinol is replaced by either alpha- or betanaphthol—blue.

Gas Chromatography. *System GA*—RI 605; *system GI*—retention time 6.2 min.

Infra-red Spectrum. Principal peaks at wavenumbers 714, 787, 1205, 1220, 928, 1515 (thin film).

Mass Spectrum. Principal peaks at m/z 83, 85, 47, 87, 48, 49, 35, 82.

Quantification. GAS CHROMATOGRAPHY. In blood: FID—N. Poobalasingham, *Br. J. Anaesth.*, 1976, *48*, 953–956. In expired air, blood or urine: ECD—B. J. Fry *et al.*, *Archs int. Pharmacodyn. Thér.*, 1972, *196*, 98–111.

Disposition in the Body. Almost completely absorbed after oral administration, rapidly absorbed after inhalation and subject to first-pass metabolism in the liver and lungs. It is rapidly distributed throughout the body and is taken up by adipose tissue. Between 20 and 70% of a dose is exhaled unchanged in 8 hours and up to about 50% is exhaled as carbon dioxide in the same period; less than 0.01% of a dose is excreted in the urine.

BLOOD CONCENTRATION.

After a single oral dose of 500 mg to 2 subjects, peak blood concentrations of about 1 and 5 µg/ml were attained in 1 hour (B. J. Fry *et al.*, *Archs. int. Pharmacodyn. Thér.*, 1972, *196*, 98–111).

A mean chloroform concentration in arterial blood of 173 µg/ml was reported in spontaneously breathing subjects during surgical anaesthesia (N. Poobalasingham and J. P. Payne, *Br. J. Anaesth.*, 1978, *50*, 325–329).

TOXICITY. The minimum lethal dose is 10 ml by ingestion and the maximum permissible atmospheric concentration is 10 ppm. Exposure to air concentrations of 100 to 1000 ppm for short periods may cause discomfort and dizziness and concentrations of 7000 ppm or more will produce rapid loss of consciousness.

The following postmortem tissue concentrations were reported in 7 fatalities: blood 10 to 48 µg/ml (mean 32, 7 cases); brain 50.4 to 156 µg/g (mean 101, 4 cases); kidney 16 to 27 µg/g (mean 20, 3 cases); liver 6 to 86.2 µg/g (mean 43.4, 6 cases); urine 0 to 60 µg/ml (mean 15, 5 cases) (R. Bonnichsen and A. C. Maehly, *J. forens. Sci.*, 1966, *11*, 414–427 and G. V. Giusti and M. Chiarotti, *Medicine, Sci. Law*, 1981, *21*, 2–3).

HALF-LIFE. Blood half-life, about 1.5 hours.

VOLUME OF DISTRIBUTION. In blood, about 2 to 3 litres/kg.

CLEARANCE. Blood clearance, about 20 ml/min/kg.

Dose. Concentrations of 2 to 4% of the vapour have been used for induction and 1 to 2% for maintenance of anaesthesia.

Chloroprocaine

Local Anaesthetic

2-Diethylaminoethyl 4-amino-2-chlorobenzoate
$C_{13}H_{19}ClN_2O_2 = 270.8$
CAS—133-16-4

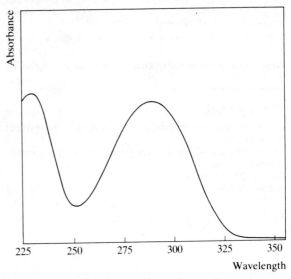

Chloroprocaine Hydrochloride

Proprietary Name. Nesacaine
$C_{13}H_{19}ClN_2O_2,HCl = 307.2$
CAS—3858-89-7

A white crystalline powder. M.p. 173° to 176°.

Soluble 1 in 20 of water and 1 in 100 of ethanol; very slightly soluble in chloroform; practically insoluble in ether.

Dissociation Constant. pK_a 8.7.

Colour Test. Diazotisation—red.

Thin-layer Chromatography. *System TA*—Rf 59; *system TB*—Rf 05; *system TC*—Rf 23; *system TL*—Rf 37. (*Acidified iodoplatinate solution*, positive; *Van Urk reagent*, yellow.)

Gas Chromatography. *System GA*—RI 2229.

High Pressure Liquid Chromatography. *System HQ*—k' 0.24.

Ultraviolet Spectrum. Aqueous acid—230 nm ($A_1^1 = 330$ b), 288 nm ($A_1^1 = 311$ b).

Infra-red Spectrum. Principal peaks at wavenumbers 1595, 1698, 1240, 1625, 1111, 1315 (KBr disk).

Mass Spectrum. Principal peaks at m/z 86, 99, 154, 30, 87, 58, 29, 156.

Quantification. Gas Chromatography. In plasma: sensitivity 10 ng/ml, FID—J. E. O'Brien *et al.*, *J. pharm. Sci.*, 1979, *68*, 75–78.

Gas Chromatography–Mass Spectrometry. In plasma: sensitivity <2 ng/ml—B. R. Kuhnert *et al.*, *J. Chromat.*, 1981, *224*; *Biomed. Appl.*, *13*, 488–491.

Thin-layer Chromatography. In plasma, whole blood or urine: 4-amino-2-chlorobenzoic acid—J. E. O'Brien *et al.*, *J. pharm. Sci.*, 1979, *68*, 75–78.

Disposition in the Body. Rapidly hydrolysed in the plasma to 4-amino-2-chlorobenzoic acid and 2-diethylaminoethanol. About 50% of an intravenous dose is excreted in the urine in 90 minutes, mainly as an unidentified conjugate (possibly the glycine conjugate) of 4-amino-2-chlorobenzoic acid.

Therapeutic Concentration.

After intravenous infusion of 250 mg over a period of 30 minutes to 3 subjects, peak plasma concentrations of 3.5 to 4.3 µg/ml of 4-amino-2-chlorobenzoic acid were attained at the end of the infusion; chloroprocaine was not detectable in the plasma (J. E. O'Brien *et al.*, *ibid.*).

Toxicity. The maximum safe intravenous or topical dose is 750 mg.

Dose. Chloroprocaine hydrochloride is injected as a 0.5 to 3% solution.

Chloropyrilene   *Antihistamine*

Synonyms. Chloromethapyrilene; Chlorothen; Chlorpyrilen; Histachlorylene.

N - (5 - Chloro - 2 - thenyl) - *N′N′* - dimethyl - *N* - (2 - pyridyl)-ethylenediamine

$C_{14}H_{18}ClN_3S = 295.8$

CAS—148-65-2

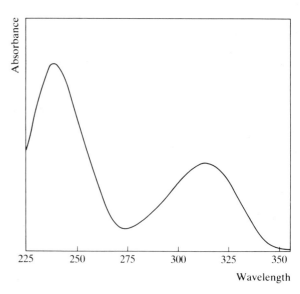

A liquid.

Chloropyrilene Citrate

Proprietary Name. Panta

$C_{14}H_{18}ClN_3S, C_6H_8O_7 = 488.0$

CAS—148-64-1

A white crystalline powder. M.p. 112° to 116°; on further heating it gradually solidifies and remelts at 125° to 140°, with decomposition.

Soluble 1 in 35 of water; sparingly soluble in ethanol; practically insoluble in chloroform and ether.

Dissociation Constant. pK_a 8.4 (25°).

Colour Tests. Mandelin's Test—violet → orange; Marquis Test—violet.

Thin-layer Chromatography. *System TA*—Rf 53. (*Acidified iodoplatinate solution*, positive.)

Gas Chromatography. *System GA*—RI 2133.

High Pressure Liquid Chromatography. *System HA*—k′ 4.0.

Ultraviolet Spectrum. Aqueous acid—237 nm ($A_1^1 = 520$ c), 312 nm; aqueous alkali—243 nm ($A_1^1 = 676$ b), 308 nm ($A_1^1 = 148$ b).

Infra-red Spectrum. Principal peaks at wavenumbers 1595, 767, 990, 1562, 1149, 1234 (KBr disk).

Mass Spectrum. Principal peaks at *m/z* 58, 131, 72, 71, 79, 42, 30, 78.

Dose. Up to 150 mg of chloropyrilene citrate daily.

Chloroquine   *Antimalarial*

Synonym. Cloroquina

7-Chloro-4-(4-diethylamino-1-methylbutylamino)quinoline

$C_{18}H_{26}ClN_3 = 319.9$

CAS—54-05-7

A white or slightly yellow crystalline powder. M.p. 87° to 92°. Very slightly **soluble** in water; soluble in chloroform and ether.

Chloroquine Phosphate

Synonyms. Chingaminum; Chlorochinum Diphosphoricum; Quingamine.

Proprietary Names. Aralen (tablets); Avloclor; Chlorquin; Klorokin; Malarivon; Resochin(e). It is an ingredient of Aralis.

$C_{18}H_{26}ClN_3, 2H_3PO_4 = 515.9$
CAS—50-63-5
A white powder. It discolours on exposure to light. There are 2 forms which melt at 193° to 195° and at 210° to 215°.
Soluble 1 in 4 of water; very slightly soluble in ethanol; practically insoluble in chloroform and ether.

Chloroquine Sulphate

Proprietary Name. Nivaquine
$C_{18}H_{26}ClN_3, H_2SO_4, H_2O = 436.0$
CAS—132-73-0 (anhydrous)
A white crystalline powder. M.p. 205° to 210°.
Soluble 1 in 3 of water; practically insoluble in ethanol and acetone; very sparingly soluble in chloroform and ether.

Dissociation Constant. pK_a 8.4, 10.8 (20°).

Colour Test. Liebermann's Test (100°)—orange.

Thin-layer Chromatography. *System TA*—Rf 38; *system TB*—Rf 14; *system TC*—Rf 04. (*Acidified iodoplatinate solution,* positive.)

Gas Chromatography. *System GA*—RI 2590; *system GF*—RI 3245.

High Pressure Liquid Chromatography. *System HA*—k′ 15.2 (tailing peak).

Ultraviolet Spectrum. Aqueous acid—257 nm, 329 nm ($A_1^1 = 600$ b), 343 nm ($A_1^1 = 625$ b); aqueous alkali—254 nm ($A_1^1 = 555$ b), 330 nm.

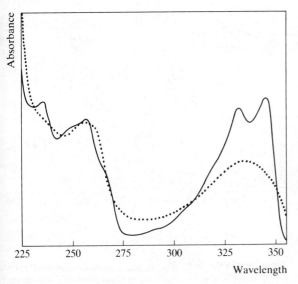

Infra-red Spectrum. Principal peaks at wavenumbers 1573, 1538, 1612, 1155, 800, 870 (KBr disk).

Mass Spectrum. Principal peaks at *m/z* 86, 58, 319, 87, 73, 247, 245, 112.

Quantification. SPECTROFLUORIMETRY. In plasma, erythrocytes or urine: sensitivity 5 ng/ml—S. A. Adelusi and L. A. Salako, *J. Pharm. Pharmac.,* 1980, *32,* 711–712.

GAS CHROMATOGRAPHY (CAPILLARY COLUMN). In plasma or blood: sensitivity 3 ng/ml for chloroquine and monodesethyl-

Wavelength

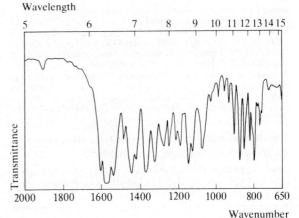

Wavenumber

chloroquine, 10 ng/ml for didesethylchloroquine, AFID—Y. Bergqvist and S. Eckerbom, *J. Chromat.,* 1984, *306;* Biomed. Appl., *31,* 147–153.

HIGH PRESSURE LIQUID CHROMATOGRAPHY. In plasma: chloroquine, monodesethylchloroquine and didesethylchloroquine, sensitivity 5 ng for all compounds, UV detection—N. D. Brown *et al., J. Chromat.,* 1982, *229;* Biomed. Appl., *18,* 248–254. In plasma, erythrocytes or urine: chloroquine and monodesethylchloroquine, detection limits 1 ng/ml for chloroquine and 500 pg/ml for monodesethylchloroquine in plasma, fluorescence detection—G. Alvan *et al., J. Chromat.,* 1982, *229;* Biomed. Appl., *18,* 241–247.

Disposition in the Body. Rapidly absorbed after oral administration; bioavailability about 80 to 90%. Metabolic reactions include *N*-dealkylation and deamination followed by conjugation, possibly with glucuronic acid, of the carboxylic acid metabolites; the metabolites include monodesethyl- and didesethylchloroquine, 4-(7-chloroquinol-4-ylamino)pentan-1-ol, and 4-(7-chloroquinol-4-ylamino)pentanoic acid and its conjugate. Chloroquine is excreted slowly and may persist in the tissues for prolonged periods; about 55% is excreted in the urine and about 10% is eliminated in the faeces in 90 days following therapy with 310 mg of the phosphate daily for 14 days; the urinary excretion of unchanged drug is dependent upon urinary pH and larger amounts are excreted in acid urine than in alkaline urine; of the material excreted in the urine, about 70% is unchanged, 23% is monodesethylchloroquine, 1 to 2% is didesethylchloroquine and an unidentified metabolite, and 1 to 2% is conjugated carboxylic acid metabolites.

THERAPEUTIC CONCENTRATION. In plasma, usually in the range 0.02 to 0.2 µg/ml.

Following a single oral dose of 300 mg to 11 subjects, peak plasma concentrations of 0.056 to 0.10 µg/ml (mean 0.08) of chloroquine and 0.01 to 0.02 µg/ml of monodesethylchloroquine were attained in 1 to 6 hours (L. L. Gustafsson *et al., Br. J. clin. Pharmac.,* 1983, *15,* 471–479).

TOXICITY. Doses as low as 1 g have caused deaths in children and fatalities have occurred in adults after the ingestion of 3 to 44 g. Plasma concentrations greater than 0.6 µg/ml may produce toxic effects and concentrations greater than 3 µg/ml may be fatal.

In a review of 9 fatal cases of overdosage, the following concentrations were reported: brain 2.8 to 50 µg/g (mean 16), kidney 110 to 640 µg/g (mean 303), liver 200 to 750 µg/g (mean 410); in two cases the blood concentration was reported to be 30 µg/ml (F. W. Kiel, *J. Am. med. Ass.,* 1964, *190,* 398–400).

In two fatal cases of overdosage in which about 3 g and 10 g, had been ingested, the postmortem concentrations were: blood 16 and 12.4 µg/ml, kidney 70 and 300 µg/g, liver 175 and 344 µg/g, liver blood 90 and 44 µg/ml, lung 38 and 98 µg/g, urine 20 and 68.4 µg/ml; in the second of these cases the antemortem blood concentration was reported to be 8.6 µg/ml (A. E. Robinson *et al.*, *J. Pharm. Pharmac.*, 1970, *22*, 700–703). A 26-year-old woman died after ingesting an unknown quantity of chloroquine, possibly to induce abortion; postmortem concentrations were: blood 4.2 µg/ml, brain 3.8 µg/g, kidney 32.9 µg/g, liver 71 µg/g; alcohol was also present (A. Noirfalise, *Forens. Sci.*, 1978, *11*, 177–179).

HALF-LIFE. Plasma half-life, about 25 to 60 days.

DISTRIBUTION IN BLOOD. Plasma : whole blood ratio, about 0.3.

PROTEIN BINDING. In plasma, about 50 to 70%.

Dose. For an acute attack, the equivalent of 1.5 g of chloroquine over three days (900 mg on the first day); for suppression, 300 to 600 mg every 7 days.

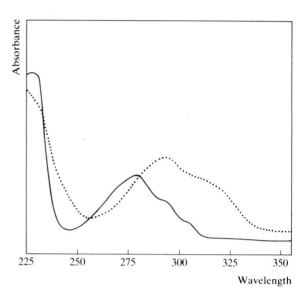

Chlorothiazide   *Diuretic*

Synonym. Clorotiazida
Proprietary Names. Azide; Chlotride; Diubram; Diuret; Diuril; Diurilix; Diurone; Saluric. It is an ingredient of Aldoclor and Diupres.
6-Chloro-2*H*-1,2,4-benzothiadiazine-7-sulphonamide   1,1-dioxide
$C_7H_6ClN_3O_4S_2 = 295.7$
CAS—58-94-6

A white crystalline powder. M.p. about 340°, with decomposition.
Practically **insoluble** in water, chloroform, and ether; soluble 1 in 650 of ethanol and 1 in 100 of acetone; freely soluble in dimethylformamide and dimethyl sulphoxide.

Chlorothiazide Sodium
Synonym. Sodium Chlorothiazide
Proprietary Name. Diuril (injection)
$C_7H_5ClN_3NaO_4S_2 = 317.7$
CAS—7085-44-1
A crystalline solid.
Soluble in water.

Dissociation Constant. pK_a 6.7, 9.5 (20°).

Partition Coefficient. Log P (ether/pH 7.4), −1.9.

Colour Tests. Koppanyi–Zwikker Test—blue; Mercurous Nitrate—black.

Thin-layer Chromatography. *System TD*—Rf 02; *system TE*—Rf 02; *system TF*—Rf 16. (*Mercuric chloride–diphenylcarbazone reagent*, positive.)

High Pressure Liquid Chromatography. *System HN*—k′ 0.54.

Ultraviolet Spectrum. Aqueous acid—278 nm ($A_1^1 = 400$ a); aqueous alkali—292 nm ($A_1^1 = 430$ a).

Infra-red Spectrum. Principal peaks at wavenumbers 1157, 1305, 1595, 1090, 1123, 1620 (KBr disk).

Quantification. HIGH PRESSURE LIQUID CHROMATOGRAPHY. In plasma or urine: chlorothiazide or hydrochlorothiazide, sensitivity 10 ng/ml in plasma and 2 µg/ml in urine, UV detection—R. H. Barbhaiya *et al.*, *J. pharm. Sci.*, 1981, *70*, 291–295.

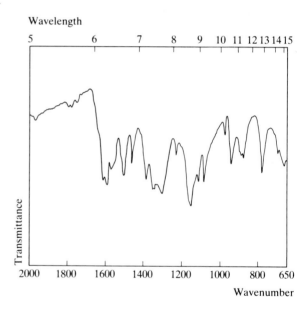

Disposition in the Body. Poorly and erratically absorbed after oral administration; bioavailability, about 20 to 30% after doses of 250 mg, decreasing with increasing dose. Chlorothiazide is not significantly metabolised and is excreted in the urine to a variable extent depending on the extent of absorption.

THERAPEUTIC CONCENTRATION.
Following single oral doses of 125, 250, and 500 mg to 12 subjects, mean peak plasma concentrations of 0.64, 0.92, and 1.3 µg/ml were attained in about 1 hour (P. G. Welling *et al.*, *Curr. ther. Res.*, 1982, *31*, 379–385).

HALF-LIFE. Plasma half-life, about 1.5 hours.

PROTEIN BINDING. In plasma, about 95%.

Dose. 0.5 to 2 g daily.

Chlorotrianisene

Oestrogen

Synonym. Tri-*p*-anisylchloroethylene
Proprietary Names. Anisene; Chlorotrisin; Merbentul; Tace; Triagen.
Chlorotris(4-methoxyphenyl)ethylene
$C_{23}H_{21}ClO_3 = 380.9$
CAS—569-57-3

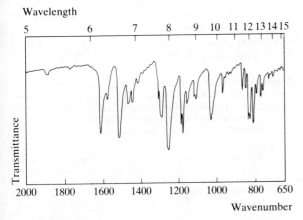

Small white crystals or crystalline powder. M.p. about 118°.
Soluble 1 in 4200 of water, 1 in 360 of ethanol, 1 in 7 of acetone, 1 in 1.5 of chloroform, and 1 in 28 of ether.
Caution. Chlorotrianisene is a powerful oestrogen. Contact with the skin or inhalation should be avoided.

Colour Tests. Liebermann's Test—green; Sulphuric Acid—violet.

Thin-layer Chromatography. *System TP*—Rf 88; *system TQ*—Rf 77; *system TR*—Rf 98; *system TS*—Rf 92.

Ultraviolet Spectrum. Ethanol—247 nm ($A_1^1 = 635$ a), 307 nm ($A_1^1 = 410$ a).

Infra-red Spectrum. Principal peaks at wavenumbers 1250, 1510, 1606, 1174, 813, 1184 (KBr disk).

Wavelength

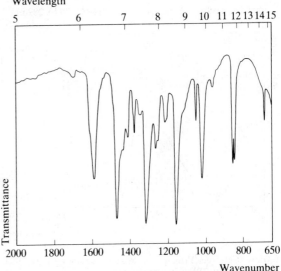

Mass Spectrum. Principal peaks at *m/z* 380, 223, 382, 238, 152, 345, 215, 113.

Dose. 12 to 24 mg daily.

Chloroxylenol

Disinfectant

Synonyms. Parachlorometaxylenol; PCMX.
Proprietary Names. Dettol; Metasep.
4-Chloro-3,5-dimethylphenol
$C_8H_9ClO = 156.6$
CAS—88-04-0

White or cream-coloured crystals or crystalline powder. Volatile in steam. M.p. 114° to 116°.
Soluble 1 in 3000 of water, 1 in 200 of boiling water, and 1 in 1 of ethanol; soluble in ether.

Colour Test. Liebermann's Test—black.

Ultraviolet Spectrum. Aqueous acid—279 nm ($A_1^1 = 83$ a); aqueous alkali—242 nm ($A_1^1 = 650$ a), 296 nm.

Infra-red Spectrum. Principal peaks at wavenumbers 1158, 1317, 1590, 1020, 858, 848 (KCl disk).

Disposition in the Body. About 14% of ingested chloroxylenol is excreted in the urine as a glucuronide conjugate and 17% as the sulphate, together with traces of unchanged chloroxylenol; the amount of unchanged chloroxylenol excreted is increased if the urine is alkaline.

TOXICITY.

In a fatality due to the ingestion of at least 100 ml of a solution containing 4.8% w/v of chloroxylenol, postmortem chloroxylenol concentrations were as follows: blood 23 µg/ml, liver 8 µg/g (A. Coutselinis and D. Boukis, *Medicine, Sci. Law*, 1976, *16*, 180).

A subject who had ingested about 17 g of chloroxylenol in solution was admitted to hospital 30 minutes afterwards and recovered after intensive treatment (P. Joubert *et al.*, *Br. med. J.*, 1978, *1*, 890).

Use. Chloroxylenol is available in concentrations of about 5% w/v; it is further diluted before use.

Chlorphenesin

Antifungal

Synonym. *p*-Chlorophenyl α-Glyceryl Ether
Proprietary Names. Mycil; Soorphenesin.
3-(4-Chlorophenoxy)propane-1,2-diol
$C_9H_{11}ClO_3 = 202.6$
CAS—104-29-0

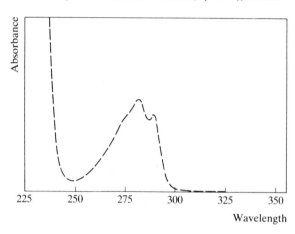

White or pale cream-coloured crystals or crystalline aggregates. M.p. 78° to 81°.

Soluble 1 in 200 of water and 1 in 5 of ethanol; soluble in ether.

Colour Tests. Liebermann's Test—black; Mandelin's Test—brown-green.

Thin-layer Chromatography. *System TA*—Rf 82. (*Acidified iodoplatinate solution*, positive.)

Gas Chromatography. *System GA*—RI 1677.

Ultraviolet Spectrum. Methanol—281 nm ($A_1^1 = 79$ b), 289 nm.

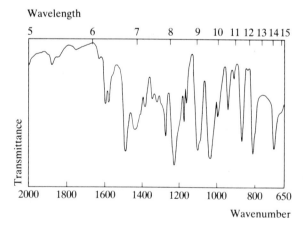

Infra-red Spectrum. Principal peaks at wavenumbers 1232, 1043, 818, 1109, 1490, 710 (KBr disk).

Mass Spectrum. Principal peaks at *m/z* 128, 130, 202, 31, 29, 65, 43, 111.

Use. Topically in concentrations of 0.5 to 1%.

Chlorphenesin Carbamate   *Muscle Relaxant*

Proprietary Name. Maolate

3-(4-Chlorophenoxy)propane-1,2-diol 1-carbamate

$C_{10}H_{12}ClNO_4 = 245.7$

CAS—886-74-8

A white crystalline powder. M.p. about 90°.

Practically **insoluble** in water; soluble in ethanol, acetone, and chloroform.

Thin-layer Chromatography. *System TD*—Rf 11; *system TE*—Rf 53; *system TF*—Rf 34. (*Furfuraldehyde reagent*, positive.)

Ultraviolet Spectrum. Ethanol—280 nm ($A_1^1 = 75$ b), 288 nm ($A_1^1 = 62$ b).

Infra-red Spectrum. Principal peaks at wavenumbers 1724, 1234, 1028, 1692, 1111, 824 (KBr disk).

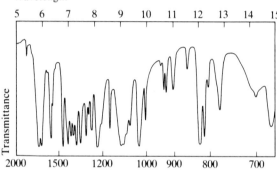

Mass Spectrum. Principal peaks at *m/z* 128, 130, 202, 43, 129, 111, 75, 204.

Quantification. COLORIMETRY. In serum—A. A. Forist and R. W. Judy, *J. pharm. Sci.*, 1971, *60*, 1686–1688.

GAS CHROMATOGRAPHY. In serum: sensitivity 500 ng/ml, FID—D. G. Kaiser and S. R. Shaw, *J. pharm. Sci.*, 1974, *63*, 1094–1097.

Disposition in the Body. Readily absorbed after oral administration. About 85% of a dose is excreted in the urine as a glucuronide conjugate in 24 hours together with small amounts of unchanged drug, and the oxidised metabolites, 4-chlorophenoxylactic acid, 4-chlorophenoxyacetic acid and 4-chlorophenol.

THERAPEUTIC CONCENTRATION.

Following a single oral dose of 800 mg to 10 subjects, peak serum concentrations of 3.9 to 17.0 µg/ml (mean 10) were attained in about 2 hours; after daily oral dosing with 800 mg three times a day for 11 weeks to the same subjects, a mean peak serum concentration of 14.4 µg/ml was reported about 2 hours after the last dose (R. G. Stoll *et al.*, *J. clin. Pharmac.*, 1974, *14*, 520–524).

HALF-LIFE. Plasma half-life, about 2 to 5 hours.

VOLUME OF DISTRIBUTION. About 1 litre/kg.

Dose. Initially 2.4 g daily, reduced to 1.6 g daily or less.

Chlorpheniramine   *Antihistamine*

Synonyms. Chlorphenamine; Chlorprophenpyridamine.

($\pm$)-3-(4-Chlorophenyl)-*NN*-dimethyl-3-(2-pyridyl)propylamine

$C_{16}H_{19}ClN_2 = 274.8$

CAS—132-22-9; 42882-96-2 ($\pm$)

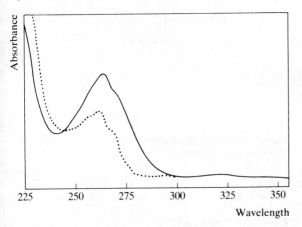

An oily liquid.

Chlorpheniramine Maleate

Proprietary Names. Allergex; AL-R; Alunex; Bramahist; Chlor-100; Chloramin; Chlor-Mal; Chlormene; Chlorspan; Chlortab; Chlor-Trimeton; Chlor-Tripolon; Drize; Histaids; Histalon; Histaspan; Lorphen; Niatron; Novopheniram; Piriton; Teldrin. It is an ingredient of Colrex Compound, Coriforte, CoTylenol, Deconamine, Demazin, Dristan (tablets), Expulin, Fedahist, Haymine, Intensin, Naldecon, Neotep, Sancos Co, Sine-Off, and Triocos.

Note. The name Chloramin has been applied to chloramine.

$C_{16}H_{19}ClN_2,C_4H_4O_4 = 390.9$

CAS—113-92-8

A white crystalline powder. M.p. 130° to 135°.

Soluble 1 in 4 of water, 1 in 10 of ethanol, and 1 in 10 of chloroform; slightly soluble in ether.

Dissociation Constant. pK_a 9.1 (25°).

Colour Test. Cyanogen Bromide—orange.

Thin-layer Chromatography. *System TA*—Rf 45; *system TB*—Rf 33; *system TC*—Rf 18. (*Dragendorff spray*, positive; *FPN reagent*, blue; *acidified iodoplatinate solution*, positive; *Marquis reagent*, violet; *ninhydrin spray*, positive.)

Gas Chromatography. *System GA*—RI 2002; *system GB*—RI 2038; *system GC*—RI 2586; *system GF*—RI 2335.

High Pressure Liquid Chromatography. *System HA*—k' 3.9.

Ultraviolet Spectrum. Aqueous acid—265 nm $(A_1^1 = 302 a)$; aqueous alkali—262 nm $(A_1^1 = 205 a)$.

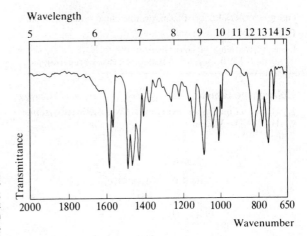

Infra-red Spectrum. Principal peaks at wavenumbers 1585, 1086, 746, 1010, 830, 1562 (KBr disk).

Mass Spectrum. Principal peaks at m/z 203, 58, 44, 205, 54, 204, 72, 202.

Quantification. GAS CHROMATOGRAPHY. In urine: sensitivity <60 ng, FID—H. M. Ali and A. H. Beckett, *J. Chromat.*, 1981, *223*; *Biomed. Appl.*, *12*, 208–212. In serum: sensitivity 0.5 to 1 ng/ml, ECD—J. W. Barnhart and J. D. Johnson, *Analyt. Chem.*, 1977, *49*, 1085–1086.

HIGH PRESSURE LIQUID CHROMATOGRAPHY. In plasma, saliva or urine: chlorpheniramine and two metabolites, sensitivity 2 ng/ml in plasma for chlorpheniramine, UV detection—N. K. Athanikar *et al.*, *J. Chromat.*, 1979, *162*; *Biomed. Appl.*, *4*, 367–376.

RADIOIMMUNOASSAY. In plasma: sensitivity 156 pg/ml—K. K. Midha *et al.*, *J. pharm. Sci.*, 1984, *73*, 1144–1147.

Disposition in the Body. Readily and almost completely absorbed after oral administration, but extensively metabolised to polar and non-polar metabolites; bioavailability about 35%. The major metabolites are monodesmethyl- and didesmethylchlorpheniramine. About 35% of a single dose is excreted in the urine in 48 hours; the 24-hour excretion of unchanged drug accounts for about 3 to 10% of the dose but this is increased by acidification of the urine and increased urinary flow, and decreased when the urine is alkaline; more non-polar metabolites appear to be excreted after intravenous than after oral administration. After daily oral administration, about 20% of a dose is excreted in the 24-hour urine as unchanged drug, 20% as monodesmethylchlorpheniramine, and 5% as didesmethylchlorpheniramine. Less than 1% of a dose is eliminated in the faeces.

THERAPEUTIC CONCENTRATION.

Following a single oral dose of 8 mg to 5 subjects, peak plasma concentrations of 0.01 to 0.04 µg/ml (mean 0.02) were attained in 2 to 3 hours; after repeated oral administration of 6 mg twice a day to 2 subjects, mean plasma steady-state concentrations of 0.02 and 0.03 µg/ml were reported; the plasma concentration of monodesmethylchlorpheniramine averaged 0.008 µg/ml and plasma concentrations of didesmethylchlorpheniramine were less than 0.003 µg/ml (S. M. Huang *et al.*, *Eur. J. clin. Pharmac.*, 1982, *22*, 359–365).

TOXICITY. Toxic effects may be produced by plasma concentrations greater than 20 µg/ml.

The following postmortem tissue concentrations were reported in a fatality due to the ingestion of chlorpheniramine and alcohol: blood 1.1 µg/ml, bile 1.5 µg/ml, brain 2.5 µg/g, kidney 1.4 µg/g, liver 6.6 µg/g, lung 5.2 µg/g; a blood-alcohol concentration of 1200 µg/ml was also reported (D. Reed, *Clin. Toxicol.*, 1981, *18*, 941–943).

HALF-LIFE. Plasma half-life, 18 to 40 hours (mean 25); decreased in children.

VOLUME OF DISTRIBUTION. About 3 litres/kg.

CLEARANCE. Plasma clearance, about 1.5 ml/min/kg.

DISTRIBUTION IN BLOOD. Plasma: whole blood ratio, about 0.83.

PROTEIN BINDING. In plasma, about 70%.

Dose. 12 to 16 mg of chlorpheniramine maleate daily; up to 36 mg daily has been given in sustained-release preparations.

Chlorphenoxamine   *Anticholinergic*

2-(4-Chloro-α-methylbenzhydryloxy)-*NN*-dimethylethylamine
$C_{18}H_{22}ClNO = 303.8$
CAS—77-38-3

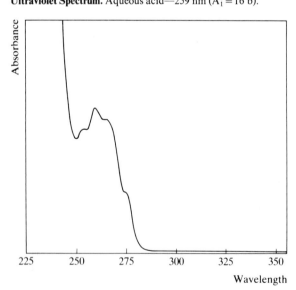

An oil.

Chlorphenoxamine Hydrochloride
Proprietary Names. Phenoxene; Systral.
$C_{18}H_{22}ClNO,HCl = 340.3$
CAS—562-09-4
A white crystalline powder. M.p. 130° to 135°.
Soluble 1 in 2 of water, 1 in 1.8 of ethanol, and 1 in 1.5 of chloroform; practically insoluble in ether.

Colour Test. Marquis Test—yellow → green.

Thin-layer Chromatography. *System TA*—Rf 53; *system TB*—Rf 47; *system TC*—Rf 36. (*Acidified iodoplatinate solution*, positive.)

Gas Chromatography. *System GA*—RI 2072; *system GF*—RI 2365.

High Pressure Liquid Chromatography. *System HA*—k' 2.9.

Ultraviolet Spectrum. Aqueous acid—259 nm ($A_1^1 = 16$ b).

Infra-red Spectrum. Principal peaks at wavenumbers 1088, 1490, 1010, 760, 700, 990 (chlorphenoxamine hydrochloride, KBr disk).

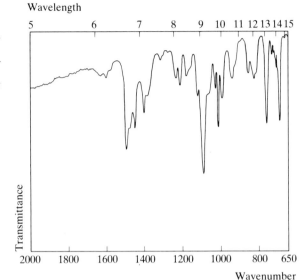

Mass Spectrum. Principal peaks at *m/z* 58, 59, 179, 42, 178, 72, 77, 30.

Dose. 150 to 400 mg of chlorphenoxamine hydrochloride daily.

Chlorphentermine   *Anorectic*

4-Chloro-αα-dimethylphenethylamine
$C_{10}H_{14}ClN = 183.7$
CAS—461-78-9

A liquid.

Chlorphentermine Hydrochloride
Proprietary Name. Pre-Sate
$C_{10}H_{14}ClN,HCl = 220.1$
CAS—151-06-4
A white or off-white crystalline powder. M.p. about 234°.
Soluble in water and ethanol; sparingly soluble in chloroform; practically insoluble in ether.

Dissociation Constant. pK_a 9.6.

Thin-layer Chromatography. *System TA*—Rf 44; *system TB*—Rf 18; *system TC*—Rf 17. (*Dragendorff spray*, positive; *acidified iodoplatinate solution*, positive.)

Gas Chromatography. *System GA*—RI 1342; *system GB*—RI 1410; *system GC*—RI 1725.

High Pressure Liquid Chromatography. *System HA*—k' 0.9; *system HC*—k' 0.82.

Ultraviolet Spectrum. Aqueous acid—259 nm, 267 nm ($A_1^1 =$ 11.6 c), 274 nm. No alkaline shift.

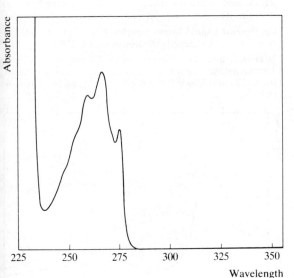

Infra-red Spectrum. Principal peaks at wavenumbers 818, 1493, 1092, 1020, 848, 754 (chlorphentermine hydrochloride, KBr disk).

Mass Spectrum. Principal peaks at m/z 58, 42, 41, 125, 59, 30, 89, 168.

Quantification. GAS CHROMATOGRAPHY. In urine: chlorphentermine and metabolites, FID—A. H. Beckett and P. M. Bélanger, *Br. J. clin. Pharmac.*, 1977, *4*, 193–200. In blood: sensitivity 25 ng/ml, FID—H. W. Jun and E. J. Triggs, *J. pharm. Sci.*, 1970, *59*, 306–309.

Disposition in the Body. Absorbed after oral administration and metabolised mainly by *N*-oxidation and *N*-hydroxylation to nitro, nitroso, and hydroxylamine derivatives. Excretion in the urine is dependent upon urinary pH, a much greater proportion of unchanged drug being excreted when the urine is acidic than when it is alkaline. In normal urine, about 17% of a dose is excreted unchanged and about 50% as *N*-oxidised metabolites in 48 hours. If the urine is maintained at an acid pH, these proportions are approximately reversed, about 70% of a dose being excreted in 24 hours. In alkaline urine less than 12% of a dose is excreted unchanged in 48 hours.

THERAPEUTIC CONCENTRATION.
A single oral dose of 100 mg given to 4 subjects produced a mean peak blood concentration of about 0.32 µg/ml in 4 hours (H. W. Jun and E. J. Triggs, *ibid.*).

HALF-LIFE. Plasma half-life, about 40 hours.

VOLUME OF DISTRIBUTION. About 2 to 3 litres/kg.

Dose. Usually the equivalent of 65 mg of chlorphentermine daily.

Chlorproguanil   *Antimalarial*

1-(3,4-Dichlorophenyl)-5-isopropylbiguanide
$C_{11}H_{15}Cl_2N_5 = 288.2$
CAS—537-21-3

NH   NH
‖   ‖
NH·C·NH·C·NH·CH(CH₃)₂

Chlorproguanil Hydrochloride
Proprietary Name. Lapudrine
$C_{11}H_{15}Cl_2N_5,HCl = 324.6$
CAS—15537-76-5
A white crystalline powder. M.p. 246° to 247°.
Soluble 1 in 140 of water and 1 in 50 of ethanol; practically insoluble in chloroform and ether.

Colour Tests. To 10 ml of a saturated aqueous solution add 1 drop of 10% copper sulphate solution and 2.5 ml of *dilute ammonia solution* and shake well; add 5 ml of toluene and shake again—toluene layer is violet-red. Dissolve 5 mg in 5 ml of a warm 1% solution of cetrimide in water, add 1 ml of *sodium hydroxide solution* and 1 ml of *bromine solution*—red.

Thin-layer Chromatography. *System TA*—Rf 03; *system TB*— Rf 00; *system TC*—Rf 01. (*Acidified potassium permanganate solution*, positive.)

Gas Chromatography. *System GA*—RI 1621.

Ultraviolet Spectrum. Aqueous acid—250 nm ($A_1^1 = 293$ c); methanol—260 nm ($A_1^1 = 755$ b).

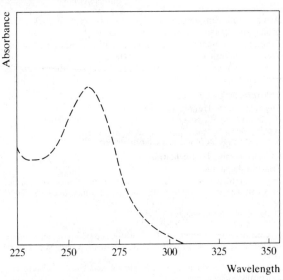

Infra-red Spectrum. Principal peaks at wavenumbers 1520, 1562, 1620, 1600, 1128, 1290 (chlorproguanil hydrochloride, KBr disk). (See below)

Mass Spectrum. Principal peaks at m/z 127, 43, 229, 44, 161, 231, 85, 186.

Dose. 20 mg of chlorproguanil hydrochloride every 7 days.

Wavelength

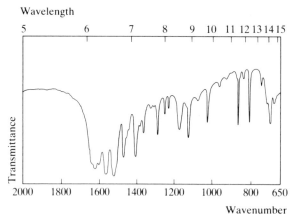

Thin-layer Chromatography. *System TA*—Rf 49; *system TB*—Rf 49; *system TC*—Rf 35. (*Dragendorff spray*, positive; *FPN reagent*, pink; *acidified iodoplatinate solution*, positive; *Marquis reagent*, pink.)

Gas Chromatography. *System GA*—chlorpromazine RI 2486, monodesmethylchlorpromazine RI 2480, didesmethylchlorpromazine RI 2480; *system GF*—RI 2940.

High Pressure Liquid Chromatography. *System HA*—chlorpromazine k′ 4.1, monodesmethylchlorpromazine k′ 2.2.

Ultraviolet Spectrum. Aqueous acid—255 nm $(A_1^1 = 1025$ a). Chlorpromazine sulphoxide: aqueous acid—239 nm $(A_1^1 = 1107$ b), 274 nm $(A_1^1 = 343$ b), 300 nm $(A_1^1 = 232$ b), 341 nm $(A_1^1 = 168$ b).

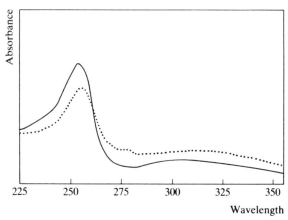

Infra-red Spectrum. Principal peaks at wavenumbers 747, 1240, 1561, 1125, 1095, 1220 (KBr disk).

Wavelength

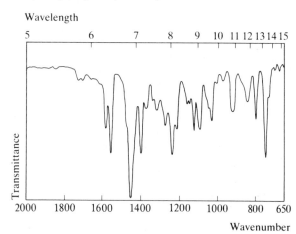

Wavenumber

Mass Spectrum. Principal peaks at m/z 58, 86, 318, 85, 320, 272, 319, 273.

Quantification. GAS CHROMATOGRAPHY. In serum: sensitivity 5 ng/ml for chlorpromazine and chlorpromazine sulphoxide, 20 ng/ml for monodesmethylchlorpromazine and 10 ng/ml for didesmethylchlorpromazine, AFID—D. N. Bailey and J. J. Guba, *Clin. Chem.*, 1979, 25, 1211–1215.

GAS CHROMATOGRAPHY–MASS SPECTROMETRY. In plasma or tissues: limit of detection 1 ng/ml for chlorpromazine, monodes-

---

Chlorpromazine   *Tranquilliser*

Proprietary Names. Largactil (suppositories); Procalm; Thorazine (suppositories).
3-(2-Chlorophenothiazin-10-yl)-*NN*-dimethylpropylamine
$C_{17}H_{19}ClN_2S = 318.9$
CAS—50-53-3

A white to creamy-white powder or waxy solid. It darkens on prolonged exposure to light. M.p. 56° to 60°.
Practically **insoluble** in water; soluble 1 in 2 of ethanol, 1 in less than 1 of chloroform, and 1 in 1 of ether.
Caution. Chlorpromazine may cause severe dermatitis in sensitised persons.

Chlorpromazine Embonate
Proprietary Name. Largactil (suspension)
$(C_{17}H_{19}ClN_2S)_2,C_{23}H_{16}O_6 = 1026$
A pale yellow powder.
Very slightly **soluble** in water; soluble in acetone.

Chlorpromazine Hydrochloride
Synonym. Aminazine
Proprietary Names. Chloractil; Chlorprom; Chlor-Promanyl; Dozine; Largactil; Promachlor; Promacid; Promapar; Protran; Sonazine; Thorazine.
$C_{17}H_{19}ClN_2S,HCl = 355.3$
CAS—69-09-0
A white or creamy-white crystalline powder. It decomposes on exposure to air and light becoming yellow, pink, and finally violet. M.p. 195° to 198°.
Soluble 1 in 0.4 of water, 1 in 1.4 of ethanol, and 1 in 1 of chloroform; practically insoluble in ether.

Dissociation Constant. pK_a 9.3 (20°).

Partition Coefficient. Log *P* (octanol/pH 7.4), 3.4.

Colour Tests. Formaldehyde–Sulphuric Acid—red-violet; Forrest Reagent—red; FPN Reagent—red; Liebermann's Test—red-brown; Mandelin's Test—green → violet; Marquis Test—violet.

methylchlorpromazine and 7-hydroxychlorpromazine in plasma—G. Alfredsson *et al.*, *Psychopharmacology*, 1976, *48*, 123–131.

HIGH PRESSURE LIQUID CHROMATOGRAPHY. In plasma: sensitivity 1 ng/ml, UV detection—K. K. Midha *et al.*, *J. pharm. Sci.*, 1981, *70*, 1043–1046. In plasma: sensitivity 250 pg/ml, electrochemical detection—J. K. Cooper *et al.*, *J. pharm. Sci.*, 1983, *72*, 1259–1262. In postmortem samples: chlorpromazine and metabolites, UV detection—W. J. Allender *et al.*, *J. analyt. Toxicol.*, 1983, *7*, 203–206.

RADIOIMMUNOASSAY. In plasma: sensitivity 200 pg/ml—K. K. Midha *et al.*, *Clin. Chem.*, 1979, *25*, 166–168.

Disposition in the Body. Readily absorbed after oral administration, but extensively metabolised by sulphoxidation, *N*-demethylation, hydroxylation, *N*-oxidation, glucuronic acid conjugation, and possibly ring fission; bioavailability about 20 to 30%, reduced during chronic therapy. A large number of metabolites have been isolated and some of the metabolites are active, particularly 7-hydroxychlorpromazine, although less so than the parent drug; several metabolites may be detected in plasma at concentrations similar to those of chlorpromazine during chronic treatment. Chlorpromazine may stimulate the drug-metabolising enzymes of the liver and may therefore stimulate its own metabolism. About 20 to 70% of an oral dose is excreted in the urine as metabolites, mostly conjugated, with 5% of the dose as the sulphoxide, and less than 1% as unchanged drug; about 5% of a dose is eliminated in the faeces as metabolites. Chlorpromazine metabolites have been detected in urine up to 18 months after discontinuation of long-term treatment. The monodesmethyl, 7-hydroxy, and sulphoxide metabolites are taken up by erythrocytes along with traces of the parent drug and its *N*-oxide.

THERAPEUTIC CONCENTRATION. Plasma concentrations vary considerably between individual subjects.

Peak plasma concentrations of 0.010 to 0.026 µg/ml (mean 0.018) were reported 3 hours after administration of a single oral dose of 150 mg to 6 subjects (L. E. Hollister *et al.*, *Clin. Pharmac. Ther.*, 1970, *11*, 49–59).

Following daily oral doses of 200 to 600 mg to 10 subjects, minimum steady-state plasma concentrations of 0.002 to 0.122 µg/ml (mean 0.03) of chlorpromazine were reported; monodesmethylchlorpromazine and 7-hydroxychlorpromazine plasma concentrations averaged 16% and 30% respectively of the chlorpromazine plasma concentration, but there were considerable intersubject variations (G. Alfredsson *et al.*, *Psychopharmacology*, 1976, *48*, 123–131).

TOXICITY. Severe toxic symptoms have occurred with doses of less than 0.1 g. Overdosage with chlorpromazine is a fairly common occurrence, but fatalities are relatively rare. Blood concentrations in the region of 0.5 to 2 µg/ml are associated with toxic effects and concentrations of 2 µg/ml or greater may be lethal.

In a review of 8 fatal cases, blood concentrations of 3 to 35 µg/ml (mean 17), and liver concentrations of 54 to 2110 µg/g (mean 366) were reported (R. Bonnichsen *et al.*, *Z. Rechtsmed.*, 1970, *67*, 158–169).

The following tissue distribution was reported in 2 fatalities: blood 4.2 and 6.7 µg/ml, brain 126 and 148 µg/g, kidney 134 and 162 µg/g, liver 240 and 280 µg/g, urine 62 and 78 µg/ml (A. Coutselinis *et al.*, *Forens. Sci.*, 1974, *4*, 191–194).

HALF-LIFE. Plasma half-life, 7 to 120 hours; mean values are usually in the range 15 to 30 hours.

PROTEIN BINDING. In plasma, about 95 to 98%.

NOTE. For a review of the pharmacokinetics of antipsychotics see T. B. Cooper, *Clin. Pharmacokinet.*, 1978, *3*, 14–38.

Dose. 75 to 300 mg of chlorpromazine hydrochloride daily; 1 g or more daily has been given to psychotic patients.

Chlorpropamide   *Antidiabetic*

Synonym. Chlorglypropamide

Proprietary Names. Chloromide; Chloronase; Diabetoral; Diabinese; Glymese; Insulase; Melitase; Mellinese; Novopropamide; Promide; Stabinol.

1-(4-Chlorobenzenesulphonyl)-3-propylurea
$C_{10}H_{13}ClN_2O_3S = 276.7$
CAS—94-20-2

SO$_2$·NH·CO·NH·[CH$_2$]$_2$·CH$_3$

Cl

A white crystalline powder. M.p. 126° to 130°.

Practically **insoluble** in water; soluble 1 in 12 of ethanol, 1 in 5 of acetone, 1 in 9 of chloroform, and 1 in 200 of ether.

Dissociation Constant. pK_a 5.0 (20°).

Colour Tests. Koppanyi–Zwikker Test—violet; Mercurous Nitrate—black.

Thin-layer Chromatography. *System TA*—Rf 72; *system TD*—Rf 38; *system TE*—Rf 11; *system TF*—Rf 43; *system TT*—Rf 84; *system TU*—Rf 43; *system TV*—Rf 03.

Gas Chromatography. *System GA*—RI 1791.

Ultraviolet Spectrum. Methanolic acid—232 nm ($A_1^1 = 598$ a).

Infra-red Spectrum. Principal peaks at wavenumbers 1661, 1159, 1553, 757, 1086, 909 (KBr disk).

Wavelength

Wavenumber

Mass Spectrum. Principal peaks at *m/z* 111, 175, 75, 85, 30, 276, 127, 113.

Quantification. GAS CHROMATOGRAPHY. In plasma: chlorpropamide or tolbutamide, detection limit 50 ng/ml, FID—K. K. Midha *et al.*, *J. pharm. Sci.*, 1976, *65*, 576–579. In blood or plasma: chlorpropamide or tolbutamide, sensitivity 1 µg/ml, ECD—S. B. Matin and M. Rowland, *J. Pharm. Pharmac.*, 1973, *25*, 186–187.

HIGH PRESSURE LIQUID CHROMATOGRAPHY. In serum: chlorpropamide or tolbutamide, sensitivity 7 μg/ml for chlorpropamide, UV detection—R. E. Hill and J. Crechiolo, *J. Chromat.*, 1978, *145*; *Biomed. Appl.*, 2, 165–168. In urine: chlorpropamide and metabolites, using initial separation by thin-layer chromatography, UV detection—J. A. Taylor, *Clin. Pharmac. Ther.*, 1972, *13*, 710–718.

Disposition in the Body. Rapidly and completely absorbed after oral administration. The main metabolic reactions are hydroxylation at the 2- and 3- positions of the propyl substituent in the side-chain, *N*-dealkylation, and hydrolysis to form the sulphonamide metabolite. About 80% of a single oral dose is excreted in the urine in 7 days. During chronic therapy, up to 100% of a dose is excreted in the urine in 24 hours, with about 18% of the dose as unchanged drug, 2% as 4-chlorobenzenesulphonamide, 20% as 4-chlorobenzenesulphonylurea, 55% as 2-hydroxychlorpropamide, and 2% as 3-hydroxychlorpropamide.

THERAPEUTIC CONCENTRATION. In plasma, usually in the range 30 to 250 μg/ml.

Following single oral doses of 250 mg to 6 subjects, peak plasma concentrations of 23.9 to 39.4 μg/ml (mean 28) were attained in 1 to 7 hours. After daily oral doses of 250 to 500 mg to 4 subjects, steady-state plasma concentrations of 75.5 to 245.5 μg/ml (mean 142) were reported; plasma concentrations of 4-chlorobenzenesulphonylurea and 2-hydroxychlorpropamide ranged from 3 to 6 μg/ml and <1 to 9 μg/ml, respectively (J. A. Taylor, *Clin. Pharmac. Ther.*, 1972, *13*, 710–718).

TOXICITY. Prolonged hypoglycaemic coma has been reported after overdosage but fatalities are comparatively rare, although some instances of fatal blood dyscrasias have been reported. Peak plasma concentrations of 200 to 750 μg/ml have been observed in comatose subjects.

HALF-LIFE. Plasma half-life, 20 to 45 hours (mean 35); increased in renal impairment.

VOLUME OF DISTRIBUTION. About 0.1 to 0.3 litre/kg.

PROTEIN BINDING. In plasma, 60 to 95%.

Dose. 100 to 500 mg daily.

Chlorprothixene   *Tranquilliser*

Proprietary Names. Taractan; Tarasan; Truxal; Truxaletten.

(*Z*)-3-(2-Chlorothioxanthen-9-ylidene)-*NN*-dimethylpropylamine

$C_{18}H_{18}ClNS = 315.9$

CAS—113-59-7

A yellow crystalline powder. M.p. 96.5° to 101.5°.

Soluble 1 in 1700 of water, 1 in 29 of ethanol, 1 in 18 of acetone, 1 in 2 of chloroform, and 1 in 14 of ether.

Dissociation Constant. pK_a 8.8.

Partition Coefficient. Log *P* (octanol/pH 7.0), 2.7.

Colour Tests. Formaldehyde–Sulphuric Acid—red (orange fluorescence under ultraviolet light); Liebermann's Test—red; Mandelin's Test—red; Marquis Test—red-orange; Sulphuric Acid—orange (fluoresces under ultraviolet light).

Thin-layer Chromatography. *System TA*—Rf 56; *system TB*—Rf 51; *system TC*—Rf 51. (*Acidified iodoplatinate solution*, positive.)

Gas Chromatography. *System GA*—RI 2487; *system GF*—RI 2910.

High Pressure Liquid Chromatography. *System HA*—k′ 3.0.

Ultraviolet Spectrum. Aqueous acid—230 nm ($A_1^1 = 1096$ b), 268 nm, 324 nm.

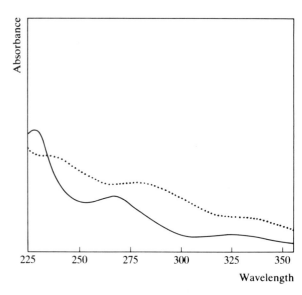

Infra-red Spectrum. Principal peaks at wavenumbers 776, 1104, 832, 746, 1030, 1170 (KBr disk).

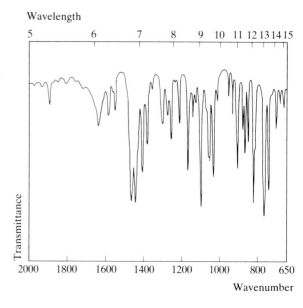

Mass Spectrum. Principal peaks at *m/z* 58, 59, 221, 30, 42, 222, 255, 43.

Quantification. SPECTROFLUORIMETRY. In plasma—T. Mjörndal and L. Oreland, *Acta pharmac. tox.*, 1971, *29*, 295–302. In blood: sensitivity 1 ng/ml—J. Raaflaub, *Experientia*, 1975, *31*, 557–558.

ULTRAVIOLET SPECTROPHOTOMETRY. In blood, liver or urine: chlorprothixene and metabolites, sensitivity 500 ng/g, separation by thin-layer chromatography—H. Christensen, *Acta pharmac. tox.*, 1974, *34*, 16–26.

Disposition in the Body. Readily absorbed after oral administration, but undergoes extensive first-pass metabolism; bioavailability about 40%. The major metabolite is the sulphoxide, but *N*-demethylation and *N*-oxidation also occur. After daily oral doses, up to about 30% is excreted in the urine in 24 hours as chlorprothixene sulphoxide, and up to about 40% is eliminated in the faeces also as the sulphoxide.

THERAPEUTIC CONCENTRATION.
Following a single oral dose of 30 mg to one subject, a peak blood concentration of about 0.01 µg/ml was attained in 4 hours (J. Raaflaub, *Experientia*, 1975, *31*, 557–558).

TOXICITY. The estimated minimum lethal dose is 2.5 g, although recovery has occurred after the ingestion of 12 g.
In 6 fatalities attributed to the ingestion of about 2.5 to 4 g of chlorprothixene, the following postmortem concentrations were reported: blood, chlorprothixene <0.1 to 0.4 µg/ml, total metabolites <0.1 to 0.6 µg/ml; liver, chlorprothixene 5 to 42 µg/g (mean 18), total metabolites 14 to 67 µg/g (mean 25); in 1 case a urine concentration of total thioxanthenes of 15 µg/ml was also reported; desmethylchlorprothixene was the major metabolite in the liver. Alcohol was also detected in 3 cases (H. Christensen, *Acta pharmac. tox.*, 1974, *34*, 16–26).
In a fatality involving the ingestion of up to 4 g of chlorprothixene, the following postmortem tissue concentrations were reported (µg/ml):

	Chlorprothixene	Chlorprothixene sulphoxide
Blood	0.1	0.6
Bile	3.9	7.0
Urine	0.4	3.4

(A. Poklis *et al.*, *J. analyt. Toxicol.*, 1983, *7*, 29–32).

HALF-LIFE. Plasma half-life, about 8 to 12 hours.

VOLUME OF DISTRIBUTION. About 10 to 20 litres/kg.

CLEARANCE. Plasma clearance, about 14 to 20 ml/min/kg.

Dose. 75 to 200 mg daily; up to 600 mg daily has been given.

Chlorquinaldol   *Antibacterial/Antifungal*

Synonyms. Chlorchinaldol; Hydroxydichloroquinaldine.
Proprietary Names. Gyno-Sterosan; Gynothérax; Siogen(o); Siosteran; Sterosan; Steroxin.
5,7-Dichloro-2-methylquinolin-8-ol
$C_{10}H_7Cl_2NO = 228.1$
CAS—72-80-0

A green or yellowish-brown crystalline powder. M.p. about 113°. Practically **insoluble** in water; soluble 1 in 100 of ethanol, 1 in 20 of chloroform, and 1 in 33 of ether; soluble in acetone.

Colour Test. Ferric Chloride—blue-green.

Thin-layer Chromatography. *System TA*—Rf 71. (*Acidified iodoplatinate solution*, positive.)

Gas Chromatography. *System GA*—RI 1802.

Ultraviolet Spectrum. Aqueous acid—263 nm ($A_1^1 = 2100$ b), 330 nm ($A_1^1 = 132$ b); aqueous alkali—263 nm ($A_1^1 = 1410$ b), 345 nm ($A_1^1 = 186$ b); methanol—251 nm ($A_1^1 = 1900$ b), 315 nm ($A_1^1 = 146$ b).

Infra-red Spectrum. Principal peaks at wavenumbers 1656, 1739, 1605, 758, 1111, 1153 (KBr disk).

Uses. Chlorquinaldol is used topically in a concentration of 3%; it has been used as 200-mg vaginal tablets.

Chlortetracycline   *Antibiotic*

7-Chlorotetracycline
$C_{22}H_{23}ClN_2O_8 = 478.9$
CAS—57-62-5

A yellow crystalline powder. M.p. 168° to 169°.
Very slightly **soluble** in water; slightly soluble in ethanol and acetone; practically insoluble in ether.

Chlortetracycline Calcium
CAS—5892-31-9
A white powder.
Practically **insoluble** in water.

Chlortetracycline Hydrochloride
Synonym. Biomycin
Proprietary Names. Aureomycin(e); Chlortet. It is an ingredient of Aureocort and Deteclo.
$C_{22}H_{23}ClN_2O_8,HCl = 515.3$
CAS—64-72-2
Yellow crystals. M.p. about 210°, with decomposition.
Soluble 1 in 75 to 1 in 110 of water and 1 in 250 to 1 in 560 of ethanol; practically insoluble in acetone, chloroform, and ether; soluble in solutions of alkali hydroxides and carbonates.

Dissociation Constant. pK_a 3.3, 7.4, 9.3 (25°).

Partition Coefficient. Log *P* (octanol/pH 7.5), −0.9.

Colour Tests. Benedict's Reagent—red; Formaldehyde–Sulphuric Acid—orange-brown; Mandelin's Test—violet-brown → yellow; Marquis Test—yellow → green; Sulphuric Acid—brown-blue.

Thin-layer Chromatography. *System TA*—Rf 05, streaking. (Location under ultraviolet light, orange fluorescence; *acidified potassium permanganate solution*, positive.)

Ultraviolet Spectrum. Aqueous acid—266 nm ($A_1^1 = 386$ a), 359 nm; aqueous alkali—253 nm, 284 nm, 346 nm. (See below)

Infra-red Spectrum. Principal peaks at wavenumbers 1622, 1580, 1666, 1311, 1041, 1227 (chlortetracycline hydrochloride, KBr disk). Polymorphism may occur.

Disposition in the Body. Readily absorbed after oral administration but rapidly inactivated in the body. It is eliminated mainly by biliary excretion with only about 15% of a dose being excreted in the urine as unchanged drug.

HALF-LIFE. Plasma half-life, about 6 hours.

PROTEIN BINDING. In plasma, about 47%.

Dose. 1 to 2 g of chlortetracycline hydrochloride daily.

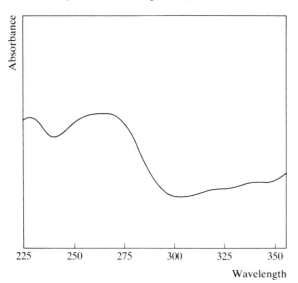

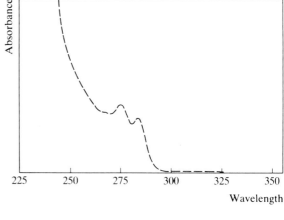

Infra-red Spectrum. Principal peaks at wavenumbers 1685, 1033, 1160, 845, 1190, 1310 (KBr disk).

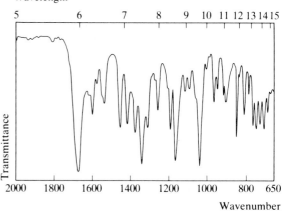

Chlorthalidone

Diuretic

Synonym. Chlortalidone

Proprietary Names. Hydro-long; Hygroton; Igrolina; Novothalidone; Renon; Uridon; Urolin; Zambesil. It is an ingredient of Kalspare, Lopresoretic, Regroton, and Tenoret(ic).

2 - Chloro - 5 - (1 - hydroxy - 3 - oxoisoindolin - 1 - yl)benzenesulphonamide

$C_{14}H_{11}ClN_2O_4S = 338.8$
CAS—77-36-1

A white or yellowish-white crystalline powder. M.p. about 220°, with decomposition.

Practically **insoluble** in water; soluble 1 in 150 of ethanol, 1 in 650 of chloroform, and 1 in 25 of methanol; slightly soluble in ether; soluble in solutions of alkali hydroxides.

Dissociation Constant. pK_a 9.4.

Colour Tests. Koppanyi–Zwikker Test—violet; Marquis Test—yellow.

Thin-layer Chromatography. *System TD*—Rf 04; *system TE*—Rf 42; *system TF*—Rf 43.

Gas Chromatography. *System GA*—RI 2145.

High Pressure Liquid Chromatography. *System HN*—k′ 1.28.

Ultraviolet Spectrum. Ethanol—275 nm ($A_1^1 = 57$ a), 284 nm ($A_1^1 = 45$ a).

Mass Spectrum. Principal peaks at m/z 76, 239, 104, 240, 285, 241, 50, 75.

Quantification. GAS CHROMATOGRAPHY. In plasma, erythrocytes or urine: sensitivity 10 ng/ml in plasma, AFID—H. L. J. Fleuren and J. M. van Rossum, *J. Chromat.*, 1978, *152*, 41–54.

HIGH PRESSURE LIQUID CHROMATOGRAPHY. In blood, plasma or urine: sensitivity 30 ng/ml, UV detection—P. J. M. Guelen *et al.*, *J. Chromat.*, 1980, *181*; *Biomed. Appl.*, 7, 497–503. In blood or urine: sensitivity 100 ng/ml, UV detection—T. R. MacGregor *et al.*, *Ther. Drug Monit.*, 1984, *6*, 83–90.

Disposition in the Body. Readily but incompletely absorbed after oral administration; bioavailability about 65%. It does not appear to be significantly metabolised. After a single dose, about 25 to 40% is excreted in the urine as unchanged drug and about 1% is eliminated in the bile; the quantity excreted in the urine appears to be dose-dependent. During daily therapy, about 50% of the daily dose is excreted unchanged in the urine in 24 hours and about 25% is eliminated in the faeces.

THERAPEUTIC CONCENTRATION.

After single oral doses of 50 to 75 mg given to 7 subjects, peak plasma concentrations of 0.14 to 0.26 μg/ml were attained in 1 to 3 hours (H. L. J. Fleuren *et al.*, *Eur. J. clin. Pharmac.*, 1979, *15*, 35–50).

Following daily oral doses of 50 mg to 10 subjects, steady-state plasma concentrations of 0.2 to 1.4 µg/ml (mean 0.5) were reported (P. Collste *et al.*, *Eur. J. clin. Pharmac.*, 1976, *9*, 319–325).

HALF-LIFE. Plasma half-life, 35 to 70 hours (mean 48), increased in elderly subjects.

VOLUME OF DISTRIBUTION. About 4 litres/kg.

CLEARANCE. Plasma clearance, about 1 to 2 ml/min/kg.

DISTRIBUTION IN BLOOD. Plasma: whole blood ratio, about 0.04 at therapeutic concentrations.

PROTEIN BINDING. In plasma, about 75%.

NOTE. For a review of the pharmacokinetics of diuretics, see B. Beerman and M. Groschinsky-Grind, *Clin. Pharmacokinet.*, 1980, *5*, 221–245.

Dose. Usually 50 mg daily or 100 to 200 mg on alternate days.

Chlorzoxazone
Muscle Relaxant

Synonym. Chlorobenzoxazolinone
Proprietary Names. Biomioran; Paraflex. It is an ingredient of Parafon.

5-Chlorobenzoxazol-2(3*H*)-one
$C_7H_4ClNO_2 = 169.6$
CAS—95-25-0

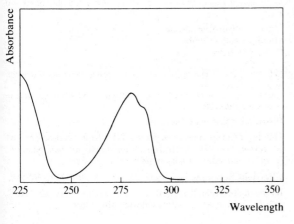

Colourless crystals or white crystalline powder. M.p. 190° to 194°.
Slightly **soluble** in water; soluble 1 in 20 of ethanol, 1 in 250 of chloroform, and 1 in 60 of ether; soluble in acetone and methanol.

Dissociation Constant. pK_a 8.0 (20°).

Colour Test. Koppanyi–Zwikker Test—violet.

Gas Chromatography. *System GA*—RI 1728.

Ultraviolet Spectrum. Aqueous acid—280 nm ($A_1^1 = 306$ a); aqueous alkali—243 nm ($A_1^1 = 580$ a), 287 nm ($A_1^1 = 409$ a).

Infra-red Spectrum. Principal peaks at wavenumbers 1762, 801, 962, 1149, 840, 1300 (KBr disk).

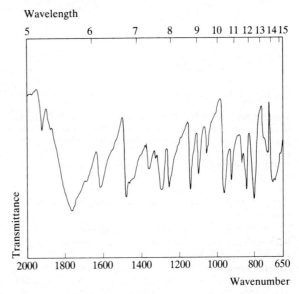

Mass Spectrum. Principal peaks at *m/z* 169, 78, 171, 113, 115, 63, 51, 170.

Quantification. SPECTROFLUORIMETRY. In plasma or urine: detection limits 60 ng/ml in plasma and 130 ng/ml in urine—J. T. Stewart and C. Chan, *J. pharm. Sci.*, 1979, *68*, 910–912.

HIGH PRESSURE LIQUID CHROMATOGRAPHY. In plasma: chlorzoxazone and 6-hydroxychlorzoxazone, sensitivity 80 ng, UV detection—I. L. Honigberg *et al.*, *J. pharm. Sci.*, 1979, *68*, 253–255.

Disposition in the Body. Absorbed after oral administration and rapidly metabolised to 6-hydroxychlorzoxazone. Up to 90% of a dose is excreted in the urine in 48 hours as conjugates of the 6-hydroxy metabolite; less than 1% is excreted as unchanged drug; 5-chloroacetanilide and 6-hydroxybenzoxazol-2(3*H*)-one have also been detected in urine.

THERAPEUTIC CONCENTRATION.
Following a single oral dose of 750 mg of chlorzoxazone and 900 mg of paracetamol, a mean peak plasma concentration of 36.3 µg/ml of chlorzoxazone was attained in 0.7 hour (R. K. Desiraju *et al.*, *J. pharm. Sci.*, 1983, *72*, 991–994).

HALF-LIFE. Plasma half-life, about 1 hour.

Dose. 0.75 to 3 g daily.

Cholecalciferol
Vitamin

Synonyms. Activated 7-Dehydrocholesterol; Colecalciferol; Vitamin D₃.
Proprietary Names. D-Mulsin; D₃-Vicotrat forte; Neo-Dohyfral D₃.

(5Z,7E)-9,10-Secocholesta-5,7,10(19)-trien-3β-ol
$C_{27}H_{44}O = 384.6$
CAS—67-97-0

White crystals. It is affected by air and light and should be stored in a cool place in hermetically sealed containers in which the air has been replaced by an inert gas. Solutions in volatile solvents are unstable. M.p. about 84°.

Practically **insoluble** in water; freely soluble in ethanol, chloroform, and ether.

Colour Test. To a 10% solution in chloroform, add 0.3 ml of acetic anhydride and 0.1 ml of *sulphuric acid*—red → violet → blue-green.

Ultraviolet Spectrum. Ethanol—265 nm ($A_1^1 = 480$ a).

Infra-red Spectrum. Principal peaks at wavenumbers 1052, 894, 901, 967, 862, 1075 (KBr disk).

Quantification. HIGH PRESSURE LIQUID CHROMATOGRAPHY. In plasma: cholecalciferol, ergocalciferol and the 25-hydroxy metabolites, detection limit 500 pg/ml, UV detection—G. Jones, *Clin. Chem.*, 1978, **24**, 287–298.

Disposition in the Body. Well absorbed after oral administration and subject to enterohepatic circulation; decreased absorption may occur in subjects with impaired liver and biliary function. Metabolised by hydroxylation to active metabolites. The major metabolite is 25-hydroxycholecalciferol which is formed in the liver. This is further metabolised by 1α- or 24-hydroxylation in the kidneys. Most of a dose is excreted in the bile and eliminated in the faeces; about 25% of a dose is excreted as conjugates. Unchanged cholecalciferol does not appear to be excreted in the urine.

BLOOD CONCENTRATION. Normal serum concentrations of 25-hydroxycholecalciferol are about 0.015 to 0.040 µg/ml, but there are considerable intersubject and seasonal variations.

HALF-LIFE. Plasma half-life, about 1 to 2 days; after intravenous administration a terminal elimination half-life of about 18 days has been reported.

PROTEIN BINDING. Bound to some extent to globulins and to lipoproteins.

Dose. 0.025 to 5 mg daily.

Cholesterol

Synonym. Cholesterin
Cholest-5-en-3β-ol
$C_{27}H_{46}O = 386.7$
CAS—57-88-5

White or faintly yellow, pearly leaflets, needles, powder or granules. It acquires a yellow to pale tan colour on prolonged exposure to light. M.p. 147° to 150°.

Practically **insoluble** in water; slowly soluble 1 in 100 of ethanol and 1 in 50 of dehydrated alcohol; soluble in acetone, chloroform, dioxan, and ether.

Colour Tests. Antimony Pentachloride—orange → brown; Naphthol–Sulphuric Acid—yellow-brown/violet; Sulphuric Acid—orange.

To a solution of 10 mg in 1 ml of chloroform add 1 ml of *sulphuric acid*; chloroform layer—red, sulphuric acid layer—green fluorescence.

Dissolve about 5 mg in 2 ml of chloroform, add 1 ml of acetic anhydride and 1 drop of *sulphuric acid*—pink → red → blue → green.

Gas Chromatography. *System GA*—RI 3086; *system GE*—retention time 1.35 relative to phenytoin.

Infra-red Spectrum. Principal peaks at wavenumbers 1059, 1022, 800, 959, 952, 839 (Nujol mull).

Mass Spectrum. Principal peaks at *m/z* 386, 368, 43, 55, 275, 81, 57, 95.

Choline

Proprietary Name. Neurotropan
2-Hydroxyethyltrimethylammonium hydroxide
$C_5H_{15}NO_2 = 121.2$
CAS—62-49-7 (cation)

$$[HO \cdot [CH_2]_2 \cdot \overset{+}{N}(CH_3)_3] \, OH^-$$

A colourless, viscid, hygroscopic, strongly alkaline liquid.
Very **soluble** in water and ethanol; practically insoluble in ether.

Choline Bitartrate

Synonym. Choline Acid Tartrate
$C_9H_{19}NO_7 = 253.3$
CAS—87-67-2
A white, hygroscopic, crystalline powder.
Very **soluble** in water; slightly soluble in ethanol; practically insoluble in chloroform and ether.

Choline Chloride

Proprietary Name. Becholine
$C_5H_{14}ClNO = 139.6$
CAS—67-48-1
White, very hygroscopic crystals.
Very **soluble** in water and ethanol; practically insoluble in chloroform and ether.

Choline Dihydrogen Citrate

Synonym. Choline Citrate
$C_{11}H_{21}NO_8 = 295.3$
CAS—77-91-8
Colourless, translucent, hygroscopic crystals or white crystalline powder. M.p. 103° to 108°.
Soluble 1 in 1 of water and 1 in 45 of ethanol; very slightly soluble in chloroform and ether.

Dissociation Constant. pK_a 8.9.

Thin-layer Chromatography. *System TA*—Rf 02; *system TN*—Rf 60; *system TO*—Rf 60. (*Acidified iodoplatinate solution*, positive; *acidified potassium permanganate solution*, positive.)

Ultraviolet Spectrum. No significant absorption, 230 to 360 nm.

Infra-red Spectrum. Principal peaks at wavenumbers 1636, 1620, 953, 1075, 1040, 860 (choline chloride, thin film).

Quantification. COLORIMETRY. In urine—S. Eksborg and B. A. Persson, *Acta pharm. suec.*, 1971, *8*, 605–608.

Disposition in the Body. Choline is a metabolite of suxamethonium chloride and suxethonium bromide.

Dose. Choline has been given in doses of 2 to 4 g daily.

Chromonar
Anti-anginal Vasodilator

Synonym. Carbocromen
Ethyl   3-(2-diethylaminoethyl)-4-methylcoumarin-7-yloxyacetate
$C_{20}H_{27}NO_5 = 361.4$
CAS—804-10-4

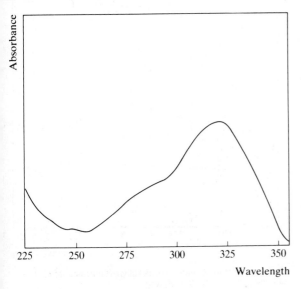

Practically **insoluble** in water; soluble in chloroform and ether.

Chromonar Hydrochloride
Synonym. Cassella 4489
Proprietary Name. Intensain
$C_{20}H_{27}NO_5,HCl = 397.9$
CAS—655-35-6
A white crystalline powder. M.p. about 159°.
Soluble in water, ethanol, and chloroform; sparingly soluble in ether.

Colour Tests. Aromaticity (Method 2)—yellow/orange; Liebermann's Test (100°)—blue (3 min); Sulphuric Acid—violet (blue fluorescence at 350 nm).

Thin-layer Chromatography. *System TA*—Rf 48; *system TB*—Rf 17; *system TC*—Rf 24. (*Acidified iodoplatinate solution*, positive.)

Gas Chromatography. *System GA*—RI 2820.

Ultraviolet Spectrum. Aqueous acid—321 nm ($A_1^1 = 527$ a).

Infra-red Spectrum. Principal peaks at wavenumbers 1708, 1608, 1210, 1755, 1178, 1085 (KBr disk).

Mass Spectrum. Principal peaks at *m/z* 86, 87, 58, 30, 29, 84, 56, 42.

Quantification. SPECTROFLUORIMETRY. In plasma or urine: sensitivity 40 ng/ml—Y. C. Martin and R. G. Wiegand, *J. pharm. Sci.*, 1970, *59*, 1313–1318.

Disposition in the Body. Incompletely absorbed after oral administration (about 35%); rapidly hydrolysed to the corresponding carboxylic acid. About 70% of an intravenous dose and 20% of an oral dose is excreted in the 24-hour urine as the carboxylic acid metabolite.

THERAPEUTIC CONCENTRATION.
Following oral administration of 150 mg three times a day to 6 subjects, a peak plasma concentration of 0.9 µg/ml of the carboxylic acid metabolite was reported, declining to 0.06 µg/ml, 10 hours after the last dose (Y. C. Martin and R. G. Wiegand, *J. pharm. Sci.*, 1970, *59*, 1313–1318).

HALF-LIFE. Plasma half-life, carboxylic acid metabolite about 0.8 hour.

VOLUME OF DISTRIBUTION. Carboxylic acid metabolite, about 0.4 litre/kg.

REFERENCE. Y. C. Martin and R. G. Wiegand, *J. pharm. Sci.*, 1970, *59*, 1313–1318.

Dose. Chromonar hydrochloride has been given in doses of 225 to 675 mg daily.

Cimetidine
Histamine H_2-Receptor Antagonist

Proprietary Name. Tagamet
2-Cyano-1-methyl-3-[2-(5-methylimidazol-4-ylmethylthio)-ethyl]guanidine
$C_{10}H_{16}N_6S = 252.3$
CAS—51481-61-9

A crystalline powder. M.p. about 142°.
Soluble 1 in about 88 of water.

Dissociation Constant. pK_a 6.8.

Colour Tests. Nessler's Reagent (100°)—black; Sodium Picrate—red.

Thin-layer Chromatography. *System TA*—Rf 54; *system TB*—Rf 00; *system TC*—Rf 09.

High Pressure Liquid Chromatography. *System HA*—k' 0.4.

Ultraviolet Spectrum. No significant absorption, 230 to 360 nm.

Infra-red Spectrum. Principal peaks at wavenumbers 1588, 1620, 1208, 1082, 1160, 1503 (KBr disk). Polymorphism may occur. (See below)

Mass Spectrum. Principal peaks at *m/z* 30, 57, 82, 116, 99, 53, 55, 42.

Quantification. HIGH PRESSURE LIQUID CHROMATOGRAPHY. In serum or urine: cimetidine and metabolites, limit of detection 50 ng/ml for cimetidine, UV detection—J. A. Ziemniak *et al.*, *Clin. Chem.*, 1981, *27*, 272–275. In plasma or urine: detection limit 25 ng/ml, UV detection—M. S. Ching *et al.*, *J. pharm. Sci.*, 1984, *73*, 1015.

Disposition in the Body. Rapidly absorbed after oral administration; bioavailability about 70% but there is considerable intersubject variation. About 50 to 80% of an intravenous dose

Wavelength

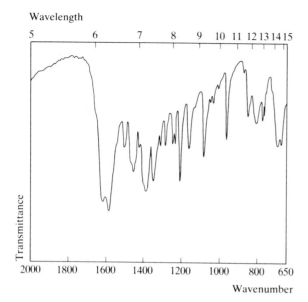

is excreted in the urine as unchanged drug in 24 hours, together with about 10% as the sulphoxide metabolite and about 5% as the 5-hydroxymethyl derivative. Up to about 10% of the dose is eliminated in the faeces.

THERAPEUTIC CONCENTRATION. In plasma, usually in the range 0.5 to 1.5 µg/ml.

A single oral dose of 200 mg administered to 20 subjects, resulted in peak blood concentrations of 0.6 to 1.9 µg/ml (mean 1.1) in 1 to 2 hours (A. Redolfi et al., Eur. J. clin. Pharmac., 1979, 15, 257–261).

Following oral administration of 200 mg five times a day to 10 subjects, minimum steady-state plasma concentrations of 0.26 to 0.80 µg/ml (mean 0.4) were reported; steady-state plasma concentrations of the sulphoxide metabolite ranged from 0.07 to 0.21 µg/ml (mean 0.12) (R. Larsson, Br. J. clin. Pharmac., 1982, 13, 163–170).

TOXICITY. Cimetidine appears to be relatively non-toxic; recovery has occurred after ingestion of 24 g in one dose, and ingestion of 60 g during 5 days caused no untoward effects. During chronic therapy, toxic effects are reportedly associated with trough plasma concentrations greater than 1.3 µg/ml.

In 3 cases of overdose due to the ingestion of 5.2, 16, and 19.6 g of cimetidine, plasma concentrations of 37, 57, and 36 µg/ml, respectively, were reported 2 to 3 hours after ingestion; the subjects all recovered (R. N. Illingworth and D. R. Jarvie, Br. med. J., 1979, 1, 453–454).

In a fatality due to the ingestion of cimetidine and diazepam, postmortem blood concentrations of 110 µg/ml of cimetidine and 5.8 µg/ml of diazepam were reported (J. Hiss et al., Lancet, 1982, 2, 982).

HALF-LIFE. Plasma half-life, 1 to 3 hours.

VOLUME OF DISTRIBUTION. About 1 to 2 litres/kg.

CLEARANCE. Plasma clearance, about 9 ml/min/kg; considerably reduced in elderly patients.

DISTRIBUTION IN BLOOD. Plasma: whole blood ratio, about 1.0.

PROTEIN BINDING. In plasma, 13 to 26%.

NOTE. For a review of the pharmacokinetics of cimetidine see A. Somogyi and R. Gugler, Clin. Pharmacokinet., 1983, 8, 463–495.

Dose. 0.8 to 1.6 g daily; maximum of 2.4 g daily.

Cinchocaine   *Local Anaesthetic*

Synonyms. Cincainum; Dibucaine.
Proprietary Name. It is an ingredient of Biosone GA.
2-Butoxy-N-(2-diethylaminoethyl)quinoline-4-carboxamide
$C_{20}H_{29}N_3O_2 = 343.5$
CAS—85-79-0

A white, somewhat hygroscopic powder. M.p. 62° to 65.5°.
Soluble 1 in 4600 of water, 1 in less than 1 of ethanol and of chloroform, and 1 in 1.5 of ether.

Cinchocaine Hydrochloride

Synonyms. Percainum; Sovcainum.
Proprietary Names. Cincain; Nupercaine.
$C_{20}H_{29}N_3O_2,HCl = 379.9$
CAS—61-12-1
Fine, white, hygroscopic, crystals or white crystalline powder. M.p. 95° to 100°.
Soluble 1 in 0.5 of water; freely soluble in ethanol and acetone; soluble in chloroform; practically insoluble in ether.

Dissociation Constant. pK_a 7.5 (20°).

Colour Test. Mercurous Nitrate—black.

Thin-layer Chromatography. *System TA*—Rf 63; *system TB*—Rf 25; *system TC*—Rf 34; *system TL*—Rf 35. (*Acidified iodoplatinate solution*, positive.)

Gas Chromatography. *System GA*—RI 2701.

High Pressure Liquid Chromatography. *System HA*—k' 1.9; *system HR*—k' 5.51.

Ultraviolet Spectrum. Aqueous acid—247 nm ($A_1^1 = 720$ a), 319 nm ($A_1^1 = 260$ a); aqueous alkali—238 nm, 325 nm.

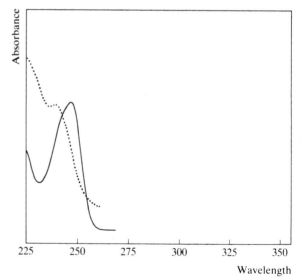

Infra-red Spectrum. Principal peaks at wavenumbers 1598, 1643, 1540, 766, 1236, 1574 (KBr disk).

Mass Spectrum. Principal peaks at m/z 86, 87, 58, 149, 111, 99, 57, 41 (no peaks above 210).

Wavelength

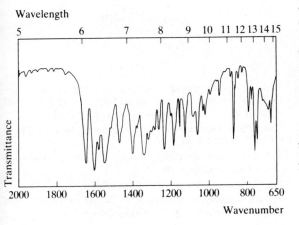

Thin-layer Chromatography. *System TA*—Rf 49; *system TB*—Rf 06; *system TC*—Rf 10. (*Dragendorff* spray, positive; *acidified iodoplatinate solution*, positive.)

Gas Chromatography. *System GA*—RI 2590.

High Pressure Liquid Chromatography. *System HA*—k' 3.1.

Ultraviolet Spectrum. Aqueous acid—236 nm ($A_1^1 = 1208$ a), 316 nm.

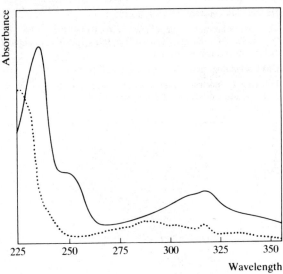

Quantification. GAS CHROMATOGRAPHY–MASS SPECTROMETRY. In serum: sensitivity 1 ng/ml—D. Alkalay *et al.*, *Analyt. Lett.* (*Part B*), 1981, *14*, 1745–1756.

Disposition in the Body.

TOXICITY. Cinchocaine is more toxic than procaine by injection, and more toxic than cocaine by local application.

In a fatality involving the ingestion of cinchocaine, the following postmortem tissue concentrations were reported: blood 0.6 µg/ml, kidney 5.7 µg/g, liver 25 µg/g; ethanol was also detected in blood at a concentration of 1500 µg/ml (T. Borkowski and W. Gubala, *Bull. int. Ass. forens. Toxicol.*, 1976, *12*(3), 18).

HALF-LIFE. Plasma half-life, about 11 hours.

Use. Cinchocaine is used in concentrations of 0.1 to 2%, for surface anaesthesia.

Infra-red Spectrum. Principal peaks at wavenumbers 754, 899, 1090, 800, 877, 1587 (KBr disk).

Mass Spectrum. Principal peaks at *m/z* 136, 81, 137, 42, 41, 55, 130, 128.

Disposition in the Body. Metabolised by 2'-hydroxylation of the quinoline nucleus followed by 2-hydroxylation of the quinuclidine ring; both 2'-hydroxycinchonidine and 2,2'-dihydroxycinchonidine have been detected in urine.

Dose. Cinchonidine sulphate was formerly given in doses of 60 to 600 mg.

Cinchonidine   *Antimalarial*

(8*S*,9*R*)-Cinchonan-9-ol
$C_{19}H_{22}N_2O = 294.4$
CAS—485-71-2

Cinchonine   *Antimalarial*

(8*R*,9*S*)-Cinchonan-9-ol
$C_{19}H_{22}N_2O = 294.4$
CAS—118-10-5

An alkaloid present in the bark of various species of *Cinchona* (Rubiaceae). Cinchonidine is the (−)-stereoisomer of cinchonine; quinine is its (−)-6'-methoxy derivative.
White crystals or powder. M.p. about 210°, with decomposition. Slightly **soluble** in water and ether; soluble 1 in 10 of ethanol.

Cinchonidine Sulphate

$(C_{19}H_{22}N_2O)_2,H_2SO_4,7H_2O = 813.0$
CAS—524-61-8 (anhydrous)
Colourless, shining, silky crystals. M.p. about 207° (anhydrous salt).
Soluble 1 in 100 of water and 1 in 60 of ethanol; practically insoluble in chloroform and ether.

Dissociation Constant. pK$_a$ 4.0, 8.2 (25°).

An alkaloid present in the bark of various species of *Cinchona* (Rubiaceae). Cinchonine is the (+)-stereoisomer of cinchonidine; quinidine is its (+)-6'-methoxy derivative.

White shining prisms or needles. M.p. 264°, subliming at 220°. Practically **insoluble** in water; slightly soluble in ethanol, chloroform, and ether.

Cinchonine Hydrochloride

$C_{19}H_{22}N_2O,HCl,2H_2O = 366.9$
CAS—5949-11-1 (anhydrous)
White microcrystalline flakes or needles. M.p. about 215°, with decomposition (anhydrous salt).
Soluble 1 in 20 of water, 1 in 2 of ethanol, and 1 in 300 of ether.

Dissociation Constant. pK_a 4.1, 8.2 (25°).

Thin-layer Chromatography. *System TA*—Rf 49; *system TB*—Rf 06; *system TC*—Rf 10. (*Dragendorff spray*, positive; *acidified iodoplatinate solution*, positive.)

Gas Chromatography. *System GA*—RI 2590.

Ultraviolet Spectrum. Aqueous acid—235 nm $(A_1^1 = 1208\ a)$, 315 nm; aqueous alkali—288 nm, 302 nm, 315 nm.

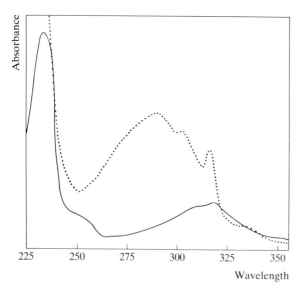

Wavelength

Infra-red Spectrum. Principal peaks at wavenumbers 760, 1110, 1505, 1590, 990, 909 (KBr disk).

Mass Spectrum. Principal peaks at *m/z* 136, 294, 81, 159, 55, 42, 41, 143.

Disposition in the Body. Rapidly and almost completely absorbed from the gastro-intestinal tract, peak plasma concentrations being attained in 1 to 2 hours. Metabolised by 2'-hydroxylation of the quinoline nucleus followed by 2-hydroxylation of the quinuclidine ring. About 55% of a dose is excreted as 2'-hydroxycinchonine, 22% as 2,2'-dihydroxycinchonine, and 5% as unchanged cinchonine.

Dose. Cinchonine hydrochloride was formerly given in doses of 60 to 600 mg.

Cinchophen   *Analgesic*

Synonyms. Acifenokinolin; Phenylcinchoninic Acid; Quinophan.
2-Phenylquinoline-4-carboxylic acid
$C_{16}H_{11}NO_2 = 249.3$
CAS—132-60-5

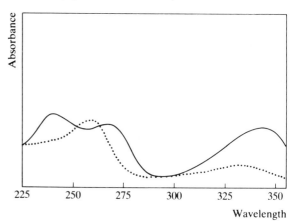

White or yellowish crystals or powder. M.p. 213° to 216°. Practically **insoluble** in water; soluble 1 in 120 of ethanol, 1 in 40 of acetone, 1 in 400 of chloroform, and 1 in 100 of ether.

Colour Tests. Liebermann's Test—red-orange; Marquis Test—yellow; Sulphuric Acid—yellow.

Thin-layer Chromatography. *System TA*—Rf 75. (*Acidified iodoplatinate solution*, positive.)

Gas Chromatography. *System GA*—not eluted.

Ultraviolet Spectrum. Aqueous acid—243 nm $(A_1^1 = 610\ b)$, 268 nm, 344 nm; aqueous alkali—259 nm, 330 nm.

Infra-red Spectrum. Principal peaks at wavenumbers 759, 1250, 1698, 699, 731, 1199 (KBr disk).

Disposition in the Body. Readily absorbed after oral administration and extensively metabolised; less than 5% of a dose is excreted in the urine unchanged.

HALF-LIFE. Plasma half-life, about 4 hours.

Dose. Cinchophen was formerly given in doses of 300 to 600 mg.

Cineole   *Essential Oil*

Synonyms. Cajuputol; Eucalyptol.
1,8-Epoxy-*p*-menthane
$C_{10}H_{18}O = 154.3$
CAS—470-82-6

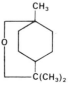

Cineole is obtained from eucalyptus oil, cajuput oil, and other oils.
A colourless liquid with an aromatic camphoraceous odour. Wt per ml 0.922 to 0.924 g. F.p. not lower than 0°. B.p. about 175°.

Refractive index, at 20°, 1.456 to 1.460.
Practically **insoluble** in water; miscible with ethanol, chloroform, ether, and glacial acetic acid.

Infra-red Spectrum. Principal peaks at wavenumbers 980, 1075, 1219, 847, 1162, 1052.

Cinnarizine
Antihistamine

Proprietary Names. Cerepar; Cinnacet; Gigantēn; Midronal; Stugeron.
1-Benzhydryl-4-cinnamylpiperazine
$C_{26}H_{28}N_2 = 368.5$
CAS—298-57-7

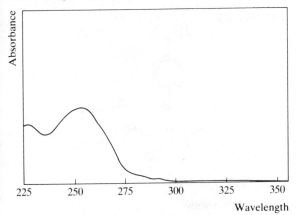

Practically **insoluble** in water; soluble in dilute hydrochloric acid.

Thin-layer Chromatography. *System TA*—Rf 76; *system TB*—Rf 51; *system TC*—Rf 78. (*Acidified iodoplatinate solution*, positive.)

Gas Chromatography. *System GA*—RI 3065.

High Pressure Liquid Chromatography. *System HA*—k' 0.8.

Ultraviolet Spectrum. Aqueous acid—254 nm ($A_1^1 = 584$ a).

Infra-red Spectrum. Principal peaks at wavenumbers 702, 691, 1138, 964, 740, 1000 (K Br disk).

Mass Spectrum. Principal peaks at m/z 201, 117, 167, 202, 251, 165, 118, 115.

Quantification. GAS CHROMATOGRAPHY. In plasma or urine: sensitivity 500 pg/ml, AFID—R. Woestenborghs *et al.*, *J. Chromat.*, 1982, *232*; *Biomed. Appl.*, *21*, 85–91.

HIGH PRESSURE LIQUID CHROMATOGRAPHY. In plasma: sensitivity 20 ng/ml, UV detection—V. Nitsche and H. Mascher, *J. Chromat.*, 1982, *227*; *Biomed. Appl.*, *16*, 521–524.

Disposition in the Body.
THERAPEUTIC CONCENTRATION.
Following a single oral dose of 50 mg to 6 subjects, a mean peak plasma concentration of 0.08 µg/ml was attained in 2.3 hours (H. K. L. Hundt *et al.*, *J. Chromat.*, 1980, *183*; *Biomed. Appl.*, *9*, 378–382).

Wavelength

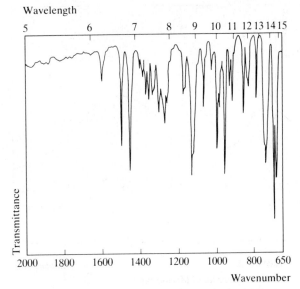

HALF-LIFE. Plasma half-life, about 5 hours.

Dose. Usually 45 to 90 mg daily; doses of 150 to 225 mg daily are given in peripheral arterial disease.

Clefamide
Anti-amoebic

Synonym. Chlorophenoxamide
2,2 - Dichloro - *N* - (2 - hydroxyethyl) - *N* - [4 - (4 - nitrophen-oxy)benzyl]acetamide
$C_{17}H_{16}Cl_2N_2O_5 = 399.2$
CAS—3576-64-5

NO₂ ⟨⟩ O ⟨⟩ CH₂·N·CO·CHCl₂
                              CH₂·CH₂OH

A lemon-yellow crystalline powder. M.p. 134° to 137°.
Practically **insoluble** in water; soluble 1 in 100 of ethanol, 1 in 40 of acetone, and 1 in 80 of chloroform.

Colour Tests. Mandelin's Test—green → brown; Marquis Test—yellow; Sulphuric Acid—yellow.

Thin-layer Chromatography. *System TA*—Rf 69; *system TB*—Rf 00; *system TC*—Rf 56. (*Acidified iodoplatinate solution*, positive.)

Ultraviolet Spectrum. Ethanol—303 nm ($A_1^1 = 310$ b). (See below)

Infra-red Spectrum. Principal peaks at wavenumbers 1244, 1666, 1510, 1595, 1078, 880 (K Br disk).

Mass Spectrum. Principal peaks at m/z 228, 182, 363, 88, 229, 76, 276, 257.

Disposition in the Body. Poorly absorbed after oral administration.

Dose. Clefamide has been given in doses of 1.5 to 2.25 g daily.

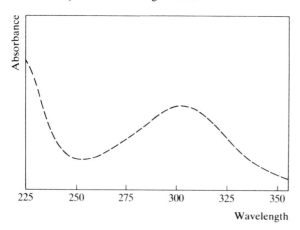

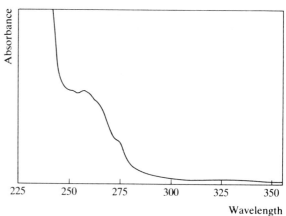

Clemastine   *Antihistamine*

Synonyms. Meclastine; Mecloprodin.
(+)-(2R)-2-{2-[(R)-4-Chloro-α-methylbenzhydryloxy]ethyl}-1-methylpyrrolidine
$C_{21}H_{26}ClNO = 343.9$
CAS—15686-51-8

Soluble in chloroform.

Clemastine Fumarate

Proprietary Names. Aller-eze; Tavegil; Tavegyl; Tavist.
$C_{21}H_{26}ClNO,C_4H_4O_4 = 460.0$
CAS—14976-57-9
A white crystalline powder.
Slightly **soluble** in dilute acetic acid; soluble in methanol.

Colour Tests. Liebermann's Test—brown; Mandelin's Test—yellow-brown; Marquis Test—yellow (green rim); Sulphuric Acid—yellow (green rim).

Thin-layer Chromatography. *System TA*—Rf 46; *system TB*—Rf 48; *system TC*—Rf 25. (*Acidified iodoplatinate solution*, positive.)

Gas Chromatography. *System GA*—RI 2415; *system GF*—RI 2710.

High Pressure Liquid Chromatography. *System HA*—k' 3.7.

Ultraviolet Spectrum. Aqueous acid—257 nm ($A_1^1 = 27$ b).

Infra-red Spectrum. Principal peaks at wavenumbers 1090, 1011, 700, 763, 1121, 1210 (KBr disk).

Mass Spectrum. Principal peaks at *m/z* 84, 128, 179, 42, 85, 178, 214, 98.

Quantification. GAS CHROMATOGRAPHY. In plasma: sensitivity 1 ng/ml, ECD—R. Tham *et al., Arzneimittel-Forsch.*, 1978, *28*, 1017–1020.

Disposition in the Body.

THERAPEUTIC CONCENTRATION.

Following a single oral dose equivalent to 2 mg of clemastine to 12 subjects, peak plasma concentrations of about 0.002 µg/ml were attained in 3 to 5 hours (R. Tham *et al., ibid.*).

Dose. The equivalent of 2 to 6 mg of clemastine daily.

Clemizole   *Antihistamine*

1-(4-Chlorobenzyl)-2-(pyrrolidin-1-ylmethyl)benzimidazole
$C_{19}H_{20}ClN_3 = 325.8$
CAS—442-52-4

Crystals. M.p. 167°.

Clemizole Hydrochloride

Proprietary Name. Allercur
$C_{19}H_{20}ClN_3,HCl = 362.3$
CAS—1163-36-6
A white crystalline powder. M.p. about 246°.
Sparingly **soluble** in water; soluble in ethanol and chloroform; practically insoluble in ether.

Thin-layer Chromatography. *System TA*—Rf 78; *system TB*—Rf 31; *system TC*—Rf 69. (*Dragendorff spray*, positive; *acidified iodoplatinate solution*, positive.)

Gas Chromatography. *System GA*—RI 2675.

High Pressure Liquid Chromatography. *System HA*—k' 4.8 (tailing peak).

Ultraviolet Spectrum. Aqueous acid—275 nm ($A_1^1 = 330$ a); aqueous alkali—254 nm ($A_1^1 = 253$ b), 269 nm, 275 nm, 283 nm.

Infra-red Spectrum. Principal peaks at wavenumbers 748, 765, 740, 833, 1111, 1010 (KBr disk).

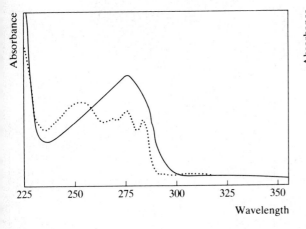

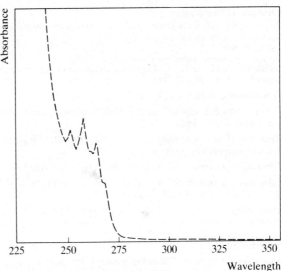

Mass Spectrum. Principal peaks at m/z 131, 256, 125, 42, 255, 89, 258, 257.

Dose. 40 to 160 mg of clemizole hydrochloride daily.

Clidinium Bromide   *Anticholinergic*

Proprietary Names. Quarzan. It is an ingredient of Librax(in).

3-Benziloyloxy-1-methylquinuclidinium bromide
$C_{22}H_{26}BrNO_3 = 432.4$
CAS—7020-55-5 (clidinium); *3485-62-9* (bromide)

A white crystalline powder. M.p. about 242°.
Soluble in water and ethanol; slightly soluble in ether.

Colour Tests. The following tests are performed on the nitrate (see p. 128): Liebermann's Test—orange → brown; Mandelin's Test—brown; Marquis Test—orange → blue; Sulphuric Acid—orange.

Thin-layer Chromatography. *System TA*—Rf 02. (*Acidified iodoplatinate solution,* positive.)

Ultraviolet Spectrum. Aqueous acid—253 nm ($A_1^1 = 10$ b), 259 nm ($A_1^1 = 11$ b); methanol—252 nm, 258 nm ($A_1^1 = 10.4$ a), 264 nm.

Infra-red Spectrum. Principal peaks at wavenumbers 1730, 1240, 769, 1190, 712, 1011.

Mass Spectrum. Principal peaks at m/z 105, 77, 96, 183, 51, 42, 182, 94.

Disposition in the Body. The major metabolite is 3-hydroxy-1-methylquinuclidinium bromide.

Dose. 7.5 to 20 mg daily.

Clindamycin   *Antibiotic*

Synonyms. Chlorodeoxylincomycin; (7S)-Chloro-7-deoxylincomycin.

Note. The name Clinimycin was formerly used for clindamycin and has also been used for a preparation of oxytetracycline.

Methyl 6-amino-7-chloro-6,7,8-trideoxy-*N*-[(2S,4R)-1-methyl-4-propylprolyl]-1-thio-β-L-*threo*-D-*galacto*-octopyranoside
$C_{18}H_{33}ClN_2O_5S = 425.0$
CAS—18323-44-9

A yellow, amorphous solid.

Clindamycin Hydrochloride

Proprietary Names. Cleocin; Dalacin C; Dalacin(e); Sobelin (all as capsules).

$C_{18}H_{33}ClN_2O_5S,HCl,H_2O = 479.5$
CAS—21462-39-5 (anhydrous); *58207-19-5* (monohydrate)
A white crystalline powder. M.p. 141° to 143°.
Soluble 1 in 2 of water and 1 in 200 of ethanol; freely soluble in methanol; very slightly soluble in chloroform.

Clindamycin Palmitate Hydrochloride

Proprietary Names. Cleocin; Dalacin; Dalacin C; Sobelin (all as granules for oral suspension).

$C_{34}H_{63}ClN_2O_6S,HCl = 699.9$
CAS—36688-78-5 (palmitate); *25507-04-4* (palmitate hydrochloride)
A white amorphous powder. It hydrolyses in solutions above pH 6.0.
Freely **soluble** in water, ethanol, chloroform, and ether.

Clindamycin Phosphate

Proprietary Names. Cleocin; Dalacin; Dalacin C; Sobelin (all as injection).
$C_{18}H_{34}ClN_2O_8PS = 505.0$
CAS—24729-96-2
A white, hygroscopic, crystalline powder.
Soluble 1 in 2.5 of water; slightly soluble in dehydrated alcohol; practically insoluble in chloroform and ether.

Dissociation Constant. pK_a 7.7 (25°).

Colour Tests. Palladium Chloride—yellow; Sodium Nitroprusside (Method 2)—violet.

Thin-layer Chromatography. *System TA*—Rf 72. (*Acidified iodoplatinate solution*, positive.)

Ultraviolet Spectrum. No significant absorption, 230 to 360 nm.

Infra-red Spectrum. Principal peaks at wavenumbers 1513, 1664, 1080, 1050, 1302, 1250 (KBr disk).

Dose. The equivalent of 0.6 to 1.8 g of clindamycin daily.

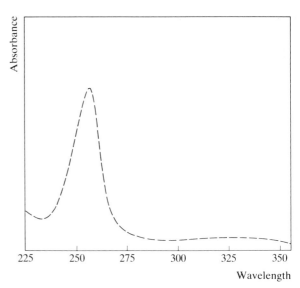

Clioquinol   *Anti-amoebic*

Synonyms. Chinoform; Chloroiodoquine; Cliochinolum; Iodochlorhydroxyquin; Iodochlorhydroxyquinoline; Quiniodochlor; Vioformo.
Proprietary Names. Budoform; Entero-Valodon; Entero-Vioform; Vioform. It is an ingredient of Oralcer and Unidiarea.
5-Chloro-7-iodoquinolin-8-ol
$C_9H_5ClINO = 305.5$
CAS—130-26-7

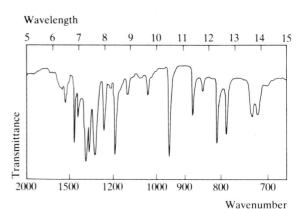

A yellowish-white to brownish-yellow, voluminous powder. It darkens on exposure to light. M.p. about 180°, with decomposition.
Practically **insoluble** in water and ethanol; soluble 1 in 43 of boiling ethanol and 1 in about 120 of chloroform; soluble in dimethylformamide; very slightly soluble in ether.

Thin-layer Chromatography. *System TA*—Rf 56; *system TB*—Rf 00; *system TC*—Rf 05.

Ultraviolet Spectrum. Methanol—255 nm ($A_1^1 = 1196$ a), 325 nm.

Infra-red Spectrum. Principal peaks at wavenumbers 953, 1198, 808, 784, 1266, 728 (KBr disk).

Mass Spectrum. Principal peaks at m/z 305, 150, 307, 115, 152, 114, 306, 123.

Quantification. GAS CHROMATOGRAPHY. In plasma: sensitivity 50 ng/ml, ECD—A. Sioufi and F. Pommier, *J. Chromat.*, 1981, *226*; *Biomed. Appl.*, *15*, 219–223.

HIGH PRESSURE LIQUID CHROMATOGRAPHY. In plasma or urine: detection limit 600 ng/ml, UV detection—K. Hayakawa *et al.*, *J. Chromat.*, 1982, *229*; *Biomed. Appl.*, *18*, 159–165.

Disposition in the Body. Poorly absorbed after oral administration. About 25% of a dose is excreted in the urine in 24 hours as glucuronide and sulphate conjugates.

THERAPEUTIC CONCENTRATION.

Following single oral doses of 250 and 1500 mg to 6 subjects, peak plasma concentrations of 1.7 to 8.3 μg/ml (mean 5.2) and 14.6 to 34.8 μg/ml (mean 23), respectively, were attained in 2 to 4 hours (D. B. Jack and W. Riess, *J. pharm. Sci.*, 1973, *62*, 1929–1932).

HALF-LIFE. Plasma half-life, 11 to 14 hours.

REFERENCE. D. B. Jack and W. Riess, *ibid.*

Dose. Usually 0.75 to 1.5 g daily.

Clioxanide   *Anthelmintic (Veterinary)*

2-(4-Chlorophenylcarbamoyl)-4,6-di-iodophenyl acetate
$C_{15}H_{10}ClI_2NO_3 = 541.5$
CAS—14437-41-3

A white crystalline powder. M.p. 215° to 216°.

Sparingly **soluble** in water; moderately soluble in ethanol and acetone; soluble in chloroform.

Colour Tests. Iodine Test—positive; Mandelin's Test—red-brown.

Thin-layer Chromatography. *System TA*—Rf 79. (*Acidified potassium permanganate solution*, positive.)

Gas Chromatography. *System GA*—not eluted.

Ultraviolet Spectrum. Ethanol—233 nm ($A_1^1 = 625$ b); aqueous alkali—240 nm ($A_1^1 = 561$ b), 282 nm ($A_1^1 = 270$ b), 362 nm ($A_1^1 = 172$ b).

Infra-red Spectrum. Principal peaks at wavenumbers 1190, 1647, 1520, 1309, 1764, 816 (Nujol mull).

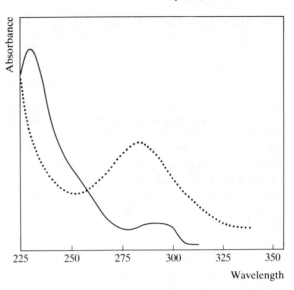

Clobazam   *Tranquilliser*

Proprietary Names. Frisium; Urbadan; Urbanyl.

7 - Chloro - 1 - methyl - 5 - phenyl - 1*H* - 1,5 - benzodiazepine - 2,4(3*H*,5*H*)-dione
$C_{16}H_{13}ClN_2O_2 = 300.7$
CAS—22316-47-8

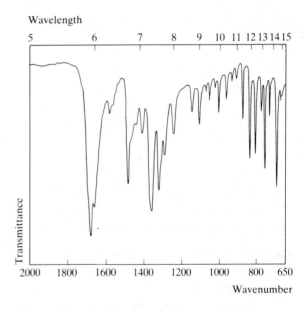

Crystals. M.p. 180° to 182°.

Practically **insoluble** in water; sparingly soluble in ethanol; freely soluble in acetone and chloroform.

Colour Test. Aromaticity (Method 2)—colourless (heat for 3 min)/red.

Thin-layer Chromatography. *System TA*—Rf 62; *system TB*—Rf 09; *system TC*—Rf 70; *system TD*—Rf 53; *system TE*—Rf 73; *system TF*—Rf 49.

Gas Chromatography. *System GA*—clobazam RI 2694, desmethylclobazam RI 2755; *system GG*—RI 3147.

High Pressure Liquid Chromatography. *System HI*—clobazam k' 3.91, desmethylclobazam k' 3.06; *system HK*—clobazam k' 0.03, desmethylclobazam k' 0.01.

Ultraviolet Spectrum. Aqueous acid—230 nm ($A_1^1 = 1373$ b), 289 nm ($A_1^1 = 76$ b); aqueous alkali—286 nm ($A_1^1 = 193$ b).

Infra-red Spectrum. Principal peaks at wavenumbers 1684, 1664, 704, 1490, 764, 845 (KBr disk).

Mass Spectrum. Principal peaks at *m/z* 300, 258, 77, 259, 283, 302, 231, 256; desmethylclobazam 286, 244, 77, 218, 51, 217, 288, 215.

Quantification. GAS CHROMATOGRAPHY. In plasma: limits of detection 3 ng/ml for clobazam and 5 ng/ml for desmethylclobazam, ECD—D. J. Greenblatt, *J. pharm. Sci.*, 1980, *69*, 1351–1352.

HIGH PRESSURE LIQUID CHROMATOGRAPHY. In plasma: sensitivity 50 ng/ml for clobazam and 100 ng/ml for desmethylclobazam, UV detection—A. Brachet-Liermain *et al.*, *Ther. Drug Monit.*, 1982, *4*, 301–305.

Disposition in the Body. Readily absorbed after oral administration. Metabolites found in the serum include desmethylclobazam, which is thought to be active, 4'-hydroxyclobazam, and 4'-hydroxydesmethylclobazam. About 90% of a dose is excreted in the urine in 17 days and about 2% is eliminated in the faeces.

THERAPEUTIC CONCENTRATION.

After a single oral dose of 20 mg, administered to 16 subjects, peak serum concentrations of 0.30 to 0.95 µg/ml (mean 0.57) were attained in about 1.3 hours (H. R. Ochs *et al.*, *Eur. J. clin. Pharmac.*, 1984, *26*, 499–503).

Following daily oral doses of 10 mg to 7 young male and 6 elderly male subjects, the mean steady-state plasma concentrations for the two groups were: clobazam 0.12 to 0.25 µg/ml (mean 0.17) and 0.17 to 0.41 µg/ml (mean 0.3); desmethylclobazam 0.12 to 0.25 µg/ml (mean 0.16) and 0.21 to 12.8 µg/ml (mean 3.9), respectively. The corresponding steady-state plasma concentrations in 5 young female and 6 elderly female subjects, receiving the same dosage schedule, were: clobazam 0.19 to 0.27 µg/ml (mean 0.23) and 0.16 to 0.32 µg/ml (mean 0.23); desmethylclobazam 0.22 to 1.37 µg/ml (mean 0.7) and 0.17 to 4.13 µg/ml (mean 1.0), respectively (D. J. Greenblatt *et al.*, *Clin. Pharmacokinet.*, 1983, *8*, 83–94).

TOXICITY. Up to 300 mg has been ingested without serious toxic effects.

HALF-LIFE. Plasma half-life, clobazam 10 to 58 hours (mean 25), desmethylclobazam, about 40 hours. The half-life may be prolonged considerably in elderly subjects.

VOLUME OF DISTRIBUTION. About 1 litre/kg.

CLEARANCE. Plasma clearance, about 0.5 ml/min/kg.

PROTEIN BINDING. In plasma, about 85%.

NOTE. For a review of the pharmacokinetics of clobazam see R. N. Brogden *et al.*, *Drugs*, 1980, *20*, 161–178.

Dose. 20 to 60 mg daily.

Clobetasol Propionate   *Corticosteroid*

Proprietary Names. Dermoval; Dermovat(e); Dermoxin.
21-Chloro-9α-fluoro-11β,17α-dihydroxy-16β-methylpregna-1,4-diene-3,20-dione 17-propionate
$C_{25}H_{32}ClFO_5 = 467.0$
CAS—25122-41-2 (clobetasol); *25122-46-7* (propionate)

A white to creamy-white, crystalline powder. M.p. about 195°.
Practically **insoluble** in water; soluble 1 in 100 of ethanol and 1 in 1000 of ether; soluble in acetone and chloroform.

Ultraviolet Spectrum. Methanol—239 nm ($A_1^1 = 390$ b).

Infra-red Spectrum. Principal peaks at wavenumbers 1666, 1612, 1724, 884, 1063, 1010.

Use. Topically in a concentration of 0.05%.

Clobetasone Butyrate   *Corticosteroid*

Proprietary Names. Emovat(e); Eumovate. It is an ingredient of Trimovate.
21-Chloro-9α-fluoro-17α-hydroxy-16β-methylpregna-1,4-diene-3,11,20-trione 17-butyrate
$C_{26}H_{32}ClFO_5 = 479.0$
CAS—54063-32-0 (clobetasone); *25122-57-0* (butyrate)

A white crystalline powder. M.p. 90° to 100°.
Practically **insoluble** in water; soluble in many organic solvents.

Ultraviolet Spectrum. Methanol—236 nm ($A_1^1 = 330$ b).

Mass Spectrum. Principal peaks at *m/z* 331, 43, 71, 332, 121, 147, 131, 41 (clobetasone).

Use. Topically in a concentration of 0.05%.

Clofazimine   *Antileprotic*

Synonym. Riminophenazine
Proprietary Name. Lampren(e)
3 - (4 - Chloroanilino) - 10 - (4 - chlorophenyl) - 2,10 - dihydro - 2 - phenazin-2-ylideneisopropylamine
$C_{27}H_{22}Cl_2N_4 = 473.4$
CAS—2030-63-9

Dark red crystals or orange-red microcrystalline powder. M.p. about 215°.
Practically **insoluble** in water; soluble 1 in 700 of ethanol, 1 in 15 of chloroform, and 1 in 1000 of ether; soluble in dilute acetic acid and dimethylformamide.

Colour Tests. Mandelin's Test—yellow-brown; Marquis Test—violet; Sulphuric Acid—violet.

Thin-layer Chromatography. *System TA*—Rf 70; *system TB*—Rf 57; *system TC*—Rf 59. (*Acidified iodoplatinate solution*, positive.)

Gas Chromatography. *System GA*—not eluted.

Ultraviolet Spectrum. Methanolic acid—283 nm ($A_1^1 = 1300$ b).

Infra-red Spectrum. Principal peaks at wavenumbers 1508, 1560, 1295, 1587, 747, 1083 (KBr disk).

Mass Spectrum. Principal peaks at *m/z* 455, 457, 472, 474, 459, 456, 458, 473.

Quantification. HIGH PRESSURE LIQUID CHROMATOGRAPHY. In plasma: sensitivity 10 ng/ml, UV detection—J. H. Peters *et al.*, *J. Chromat.*, 1982, *229*; *Biomed. Appl.*, *18*, 503–508.

THIN-LAYER CHROMATOGRAPHY. In plasma: detection limit 5 ng/ml—Z. Lanyi and J. P. Dubois, *J. Chromat.*, 1982, *232*; *Biomed. Appl.*, *21*, 219–223.

Disposition in the Body. Incompletely absorbed after oral administration. It is stored in body tissues and only very slowly

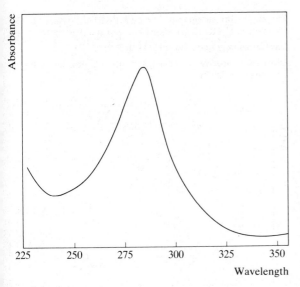

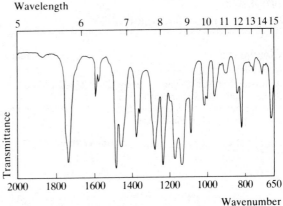

A clear, colourless to pale yellow liquid. Wt per ml 1.138 to 1.144 g.
Practically **immiscible** with water; readily miscible with ethanol, chloroform, and ether.

Dissociation Constant. pK_a 3.0 (clofibric acid).

Colour Tests. Liebermann's Test—violet-brown; Marquis Test—blue (deepening).

Thin-layer Chromatography. *System TD*—Rf 75; *system TE*—Rf 82; *system TF*—Rf 66.

Gas Chromatography. *System GA*—RI 1549.

Ultraviolet Spectrum. Dehydrated alcohol—280 nm ($A_1^1 = 43$ b), 288 nm ($A_1^1 = 31$ b).

Infra-red Spectrum. Principal peaks at wavenumbers 1140, 1238, 1735, 1175, 1282, 1090 (KBr disk).

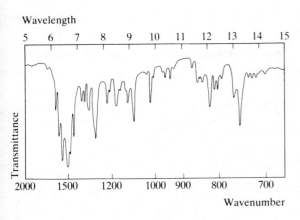

Mass Spectrum. Principal peaks at *m/z* 128, 130, 169, 87, 41, 129, 242, 171.

Quantification. GAS CHROMATOGRAPHY. In plasma: sensitivity 1 µg/ml for clofibrate and clofibric acid, FID—M. S. Wolf and J. J. Zimmerman, *J. pharm. Sci.*, 1980, *69*, 92–93.

HIGH PRESSURE LIQUID CHROMATOGRAPHY. In plasma, saliva or urine: sensitivity 500 ng/ml for clofibric acid, UV detection—T. D. Bjornsson *et al.*, *J. Chromat.*, 1977, *137*, 145–152. In plasma or urine: sensitivity 10 µg/ml for clofibric acid and 1.5 µg/ml for the glucuronide, UV detection—J. R. Veenendaal and P. J. Meffin, *J. Chromat.*, 1981, *223*; *Biomed. Appl.*, *12*, 147–154.

Disposition in the Body. Readily and almost completely absorbed after oral administration. Rapidly hydrolysed by serum enzymes to clofibric acid, 2-(4-chlorophenoxy)-2-methylpropionic acid (active), which is conjugated with glucuronic acid. About 50 to 85% of a dose is excreted in the urine in 48 hours mostly as conjugated clofibric acid.

excreted in the urine. 3-(*p*-Hydroxy)clofazimine and a 3-glucuronide conjugate have been detected in the urine, each accounting for less than 0.5% of a daily dose.

THERAPEUTIC CONCENTRATION.
Following single oral doses of 200 mg and 400 mg to 1 subject, peak plasma concentrations of 0.07 µg/ml and 0.16 µg/ml were attained in 8 and 4 hours respectively; plasma concentrations of clofazimine were still detectable at 264 hours (Z. Lanyi and J. P. Dubois, *ibid.*).

Dose. 50 to 100 mg daily; 300 mg daily for lepra reactions.

Clofibrate   *Lipid Regulating Agent*

Synonyms. Ethyl Chlorophenoxyisobutyrate; Ethyl Clofibrate.
Proprietary Names. Amotril; Atheropront; Atromidin; Atromid-S; Azionyl; Claripex; Clofibral; Clofirem; Lipavlon; Liprin(al); Normolipol; Novofibrate; Regelan; Skleromexe.
Ethyl 2-(4-chlorophenoxy)-2-methylpropionate
$C_{12}H_{15}ClO_3 = 242.7$
CAS—637-07-0

THERAPEUTIC CONCENTRATION.

After a single oral dose of 1 g, given to 8 subjects, peak plasma concentrations of 43 to 79 µg/ml (mean 55) of clofibric acid were attained in 2 to 8 hours (L. F. Chasseaud *et al.*, *J. clin. Pharmac.*, 1974, *14*, 382–386).

After a single oral dose of 2 g, given to 5 subjects, a mean plasma concentration of 151 µg/ml of clofibric acid was attained in 4 to 6 hours; a mean steady-state plasma concentration of 122 µg/ml of clofibric acid was achieved after administering 1 g twice daily to 5 subjects (R. Gugler, *Clin. Pharmac. Ther.*, 1978, *24*, 432–438).

TOXICITY.

A 15-year-old boy who took 24.5 g of clofibrate in a suicide attempt complained of headache, pain in the arms, and inability to walk, but no evidence of toxicity was found in the following 5 days (A. H. Greenhouse, *J. Am. med. Ass.*, 1968, *204*, 402–403).

HALF-LIFE. Plasma half-life, clofibric acid 12 to 25 hours but may be decreased when free fatty acid concentrations are high; longer half-lives have been reported after repeated doses, and in subjects with renal impairment.

VOLUME OF DISTRIBUTION. Clofibric acid, about 0.1 to 0.2 litre/kg.

PROTEIN BINDING. In plasma, clofibric acid, about 95 to 98%. This may be reduced in the presence of high free fatty acid concentrations and is progressively reduced at plasma concentrations greater than 50 µg/ml.

NOTE. For a summary of the clinical pharmacokinetics of clofibrate see L. B. Sheiner *et al.*, *J. Pharmacokinet. Biopharm.*, 1981, *9*, 84–87.

Dose. 20 to 30 mg/kg daily, by mouth.

Clomiphene   *Induction of Ovulation*

Synonyms. Chloramiphene; Clomifene.

A mixture of the *E* and *Z* isomers of 2-[4-(2-Chloro-1,2-diphenylvinyl)phenoxy]triethylamine.

Clomiphene may be separated into its *E* and *Z* isomers, enclomiphene and zuclomiphene.

$C_{26}H_{28}ClNO = 406.0$

CAS—911-45-5; 15690-57-0 (E); 15690-55-8 (Z)

Cl
|
C₆H₅·C:C·C₆H₅

O·[CH₂]₂·N(C₂H₅)₂

A white to pale yellow solid. M.p. 111° to 115°.
Sparingly **soluble** in water and ethanol; slightly soluble in chloroform.

Clomiphene Citrate

Proprietary Names. Clomid; Clomivid; Dyneric; Serophene.

$C_{26}H_{28}ClNO,C_{6}H_{8}O_{7} = 598.1$

CAS—50-41-9; 7599-79-3 (E); 7619-53-6 (Z)

A white to pale yellow powder. M.p. about 145°, with decomposition.

Soluble 1 in 900 of water, 1 in 40 of ethanol, and 1 in 800 of chloroform; freely soluble in glacial acetic acid and methanol; practically insoluble in ether.

Colour Tests. Liebermann's Test—brown; Mandelin's Test—violet → orange-brown; Marquis Test—violet-brown.

Thin-layer Chromatography. *System TA*—Rf 60; *system TB*—Rf 56; *system TC*—Rf 52. (*Acidified iodoplatinate solution*, positive.)

Gas Chromatography. *System GA*—RI 2930.

Ultraviolet Spectrum. Aqueous acid—235 nm ($A_1^1 = 464$ b), 292 nm ($A_1^1 = 259$ b).

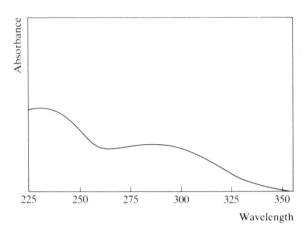

Infra-red Spectrum. Principal peaks at wavenumbers 1590, 1111, 1245, 1505, 700, 1170.

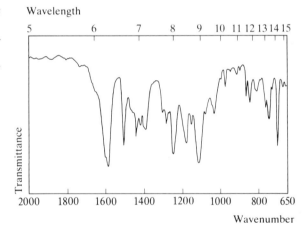

Mass Spectrum. Principal peaks at *m/z* 86, 87, 100, 30, 58, 44, 42, 29.

Quantification. HIGH PRESSURE LIQUID CHROMATOGRAPHY. In plasma: detection limit 350 pg/ml, photolysis and fluorescence detection—P. J. Harman *et al.*, *J. Chromat.*, 1981, *225*; *Biomed. Appl.*, *14*, 131–138.

Disposition in the Body. Absorbed after oral administration and slowly excreted in the bile; enterohepatic circulation occurs.

HALF-LIFE. Biological half-life, about 5 days.

Dose. 50 mg of clomiphene citrate daily, for 5 days; up to 250 mg daily has been given.

Clomipramine
Antidepressant

Synonyms. Chlorimipramine; Monochlorimipramine.
3-(3-Chloro-10,11-dihydro-5*H*-dibenz[*b*,*f*]azepin-5-yl)-*NN*-dimethylpropylamine
$C_{19}H_{23}ClN_2 = 314.9$
CAS—303-49-1

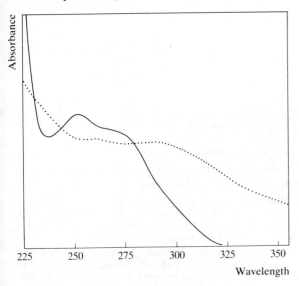

Clomipramine Hydrochloride
Proprietary Name. Anafranil
$C_{19}H_{23}ClN_2,HCl = 351.3$
CAS—17321-77-6
A white or slightly yellow crystalline powder. M.p. about 192°.
Soluble 1 in 8 of water, 1 in 5 of ethanol, 1 in 3 of chloroform, and 1 in 100 of ether.

Partition Coefficient. Log *P* (octanol/pH 7.4), 3.3.

Colour Tests. Forrest Reagent—blue; FPN Reagent—blue; Liebermann's Test—blue; Mandelin's Test—blue.

Thin-layer Chromatography. *System TA*—Rf 51; *system TB*—Rf 54; *system TC*—Rf 34. (*Acidified iodoplatinate solution*, strong reaction.)

Gas Chromatography. *System GA*—RI 2406; *system GF*—RI 2795.

High Pressure Liquid Chromatography. *System HA*—clomipramine k' 3.4, monodesmethylclomipramine k' 2.0; *system HF*—k' 9.92.

Ultraviolet Spectrum. Aqueous acid—251 nm ($A_1^1 = 253$ a).

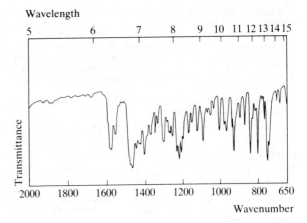

Infra-red Spectrum. Principal peaks at wavenumbers 752, 1225, 805, 842, 1212, 1237 (clomipramine hydrochloride, KBr disk).

Mass Spectrum. Principal peaks at *m/z* 58, 85, 269, 268, 270, 271, 314, 242; monodesmethylclomipramine 44, 71, 268, 227, 193, 42, 269, 229; 8-hydroxyclomipramine 58, 85, 86, 57, 84, 70, 43, 268.

Quantification. GAS CHROMATOGRAPHY. In plasma: detection limit 5 ng, AFID—L. Gifford *et al.*, *J. Chromat.*, 1975, *105*, 107–113.

HIGH PRESSURE LIQUID CHROMATOGRAPHY. In plasma or blood: sensitivity 5 ng/ml for clomipramine and 10 ng/ml for monodesmethylclomipramine, UV detection—J. Godbillon and S. Gauron, *J. Chromat.*, 1981, *204*, 303–311.

RADIOIMMUNOASSAY. In plasma: sensitivity 200 pg/ml—G. F. Read and D. Riad-Fahmy, *Clin. Chem.*, 1978, *24*, 36–40.

REVIEW. For a review of analytical methods see B. A. Scoggins *et al.*, *Clin. Chem.*, 1980, *26*, 5–17.

Disposition in the Body. Rapidly and completely absorbed after oral administration, but undergoes extensive first-pass *N*-demethylation to the major active metabolite, monodesmethylclomipramine. Clomipramine and monodesmethylclomipramine are further metabolised by 8-hydroxylation, *N*-oxidation, and conjugation. About 10 to 15% of a dose is excreted in the urine in 24 hours, of which less than 0.2% is unchanged clomipramine or monodesmethylclomipramine. A total of 45 to 60% of a dose is excreted in the urine over a period of 14 days and about 20 to 30% is slowly eliminated in the faeces.

THERAPEUTIC CONCENTRATION. Plasma concentrations of clomipramine and the desmethyl metabolite vary considerably between individual patients. Steady-state concentrations of clomipramine are usually achieved in about 1 to 2 weeks, but monodesmethylclomipramine may continue to accumulate for 6 weeks or longer. 8-Hydroxyclomipramine and 8-hydroxydesmethylclomipramine have been detected in plasma at significant concentrations during high-dose chronic treatment.

After a single oral dose of 50 mg, given to 5 subjects, peak plasma concentrations of clomipramine of 0.02 to 0.07 µg/ml (mean 0.05) were attained in 2 to 4 hours; peak plasma concentrations of monodesmethylclomipramine of 0.0005 to 0.012 µg/ml (mean 0.005) were attained in 4 to 24 hours (R. Jones and D. Luscombe, *Postgrad. med. J.*, 1976, *52*, Suppl. 3, 62–67).

Steady-state plasma concentrations of 0.10 to 0.48 µg/ml (mean 0.23) were reported after daily oral doses of 150 mg given to 17 subjects; the steady-state concentration of monodesmethylclomipramine was 0.24 to 0.96 µg/ml (mean 0.45) (S. Montgomery *et al.*, *Postgrad. med. J.*, 1980, *56*, Suppl. 1, 130–133).

TOXICITY. Toxic effects have been associated with blood concentrations greater than 0.4 µg/ml of clomipramine plus monodesmethylclomipramine.

In 2 fatalities due to clomipramine, postmortem concentrations were: blood 1 μg/ml, trace; brain –, 4.5 μg/g; liver 30, 22 μg/g; urine 25, – μg/ml (M. T. Haqqani and D. R. Gutteridge, *Forens. Sci.*, 1974, *3*, 83–87).

In a fatality due to clomipramine overdose, the following postmortem concentrations were reported: blood, clomipramine 0.54 μg/ml and monodesmethylclomipramine 0.58 μg/ml; urine, clomipramine 0.35 μg/ml and monodesmethylclomipramine 0.70 μg/ml (R. C. Meatherall *et al.*, *J. analyt. Toxicol.*, 1983, *7*, 168–171).

For details of a fatality involving the ingestion of clomipramine and trimipramine, see under Trimipramine.

HALF-LIFE. Plasma half-life, 20 to 84 hours (mean 36); decreased in children.

DISTRIBUTION IN BLOOD. Plasma: whole blood ratio, 1.2.

PROTEIN BINDING. In plasma, clomipramine 90 to 95%, monodesmethylclomipramine 97 to 99%.

NOTE. For a review of the pharmacokinetics of tricyclic antidepressants see G. Molnar and R. N. Gupta, *Biopharm. Drug Disp.*, 1980, *1*, 283–305.

Dose. 10 to 150 mg of clomipramine hydrochloride daily.

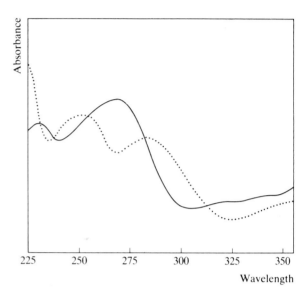

Wavelength

Clomocycline   *Antibiotic*

Synonyms. Chlormethylencycline; N^2-(Hydroxymethyl)chlortetracycline; Methylolchlortetracycline.

7-Chloro-N^2-(hydroxymethyl)tetracycline
$C_{23}H_{25}ClN_2O_9 = 508.9$
CAS—1181-54-0

Clonazepam   *Anticonvulsant*

Proprietary Names. Clonopin; Rivotril.
5-(2-Chlorophenyl)-1,3-dihydro-7-nitro-2H-1,4-benzodiazepin-2-one
$C_{15}H_{10}ClN_3O_3 = 315.7$
CAS—1622-61-3

A yellow powder. It is sensitive to light and air, and undergoes decomposition between 145° and 170° without a definite melting point.

Clomocycline Sodium
Proprietary Name. Megaclor
$C_{23}H_{24}ClN_2NaO_9 = 530.9$
A yellow powder. It is sensitive to light and air, and undergoes decomposition without melting.
Very **soluble** in water; soluble 1 in 250 of ethanol; practically insoluble in chloroform and ether.

Colour Tests. Benedict's Reagent—red; Formaldehyde–Sulphuric Acid—orange-brown; Liebermann's Test—black; Mandelin's Test—violet → brown; Marquis Test—orange-brown; Sulphuric Acid—blue-black.

Thin-layer Chromatography. *System TA*—Rf 05, streaking. (*Acidified potassium permanganate solution*, strong reaction.)

Ultraviolet Spectrum. Aqueous acid—229 nm, 268 nm ($A_1^1 = 350$ b); aqueous alkali—251 nm, 283 nm.

Infra-red Spectrum. Principal peaks at wavenumbers 1600, 1634, 1501, 1307, 1205, 1235 (clomocycline sodium, KBr disk).

Dose. 0.68 to 1.36 g of clomocycline sodium daily.

A light yellow powder. M.p. about 239°.
Practically **insoluble** in water; slightly soluble in ethanol and ether; sparingly soluble in acetone and chloroform.

Dissociation Constant. pK_a 1.5, 10.5.

Partition Coefficient. Log P (octanol/pH 7.4), 2.4.

Colour Test. Formaldehyde–Sulphuric Acid—orange.

Thin-layer Chromatography. *System TA*—Rf 72; *system TB*—Rf 00; *system TC*—Rf 53; *system TD*—Rf 35; *system TE*—Rf 60; *system TF*—Rf 45. (*Acidified iodoplatinate solution*, positive; *acidified potassium permanganate solution*, positive.)

Gas Chromatography. *System GA*—clonazepam RI 2885, 7-acetamidoclonazepam RI 3263, 7-aminoclonazepam RI 2900, 7-amino-3-hydroxyclonazepam RI 2890; *system GG*—RI 3600.

High Pressure Liquid Chromatography. *System HI*—k' 2.85; *system HK*—k' 0.35.

Ultraviolet Spectrum. Aqueous acid—273 nm ($A_1^1 = 645$ b); methanol—245 nm ($A_1^1 = 460$ b), 309 nm ($A_1^1 = 360$ b).

Infra-red Spectrum. Principal peaks at wavenumbers 1685, 1610, 748, 1255, 1578, 1532 (KBr disk).

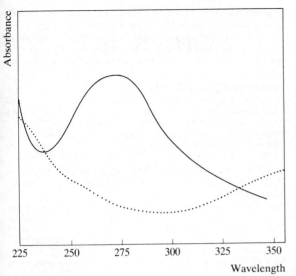

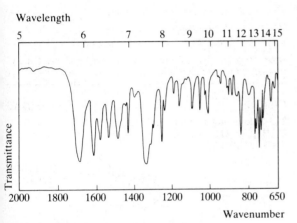

Mass Spectrum. Principal peaks at m/z 280, 314, 315, 286, 234, 288, 316, 240; 7-acetamidoclonazepam 43, 327, 299, 298, 292, 329, 328, 256; 7-aminoclonazepam 285, 256, 257, 258, 44, 287, 110, 220.

Quantification. GAS CHROMATOGRAPHY (CAPILLARY COLUMN). In plasma: detection limit 1 ng/ml, ECD—A. G. de Boer *et al.*, *J. Chromat.*, 1978, *145*; *Biomed. Appl.*, *2*, 105–114. In plasma: sensitivity 5 ng/ml, AFID—A. K. Dhar and H. Kutt, *J. Chromat.*, 1981, *222*; *Biomed. Appl.*, *11*, 203–211.

HIGH PRESSURE LIQUID CHROMATOGRAPHY. In plasma: clonazepam, 7-acetamidoclonazepam, and 7-aminoclonazepam, sensitivity 10 ng/ml, UV detection—I. Petters *et al.*, *J. Chromat.*, 1984, *306*; *Biomed. Appl.*, *31*, 241–248.

RADIOIMMUNOASSAY. In plasma: sensitivity 5 ng/ml—W. Dixon *et al.*, *J. pharm. Sci.*, 1977, *66*, 235–237.

Disposition in the Body. Rapidly absorbed after oral administration; bioavailability greater than 80%. The major metabolic reaction is reduction of the nitro group to 7-aminoclonazepam,

followed by acetylation to 7-acetamidoclonazepam; 7-amino-clonazepam is slightly active and is found in plasma at concentrations similar to those of clonazepam. 3-Hydroxylation of clonazepam and its two metabolites may also occur, followed by conjugation with glucuronic acid or sulphate. Less than 1% of a dose is excreted unchanged in the urine in 24 hours. Urinary excretion accounts for up to 70% of a dose, as both free and conjugated metabolites, over a period of 7 days, of which about 50% consists of 7-aminoclonazepam and 7-acetamido-clonazepam.

THERAPEUTIC CONCENTRATION. In plasma, usually in the range 0.02 to 0.07 µg/ml.

A single oral dose of 2 mg given to 8 subjects produced peak plasma concentrations of 0.007 to 0.024 µg/ml (mean 0.017) in 1 to 4 hours (A. Berlin and H. Dahlström, *Eur. J. clin. Pharmac.*, 1975, *9*, 155–159).

After daily oral dosing of 25 subjects with 6 mg per day, steady-state plasma concentrations of 0.029 to 0.075 µg/ml of clonazepam, 0.023 to 0.137 µg/ml of 7-aminoclonazepam, and <0.003 to 0.013 µg/ml of 7-acetamidoclonazepam were reported (J. Naestoft and N.-E. Larsen, *J. Chromat.*, 1974, *93*, 113–122).

TOXICITY. Toxicity is associated with plasma concentrations greater than 0.1 µg/ml.

HALF-LIFE. Plasma half-life, 18 to 45 hours.

VOLUME OF DISTRIBUTION. About 2 to 4 litres/kg.

CLEARANCE. Plasma clearance, about 1 ml/min/kg.

PROTEIN BINDING. In plasma, about 85%.

NOTE. For a review of the pharmacokinetics of clonazepam, see R. M. Pinder *et al.*, *Drugs*, 1976, *12*, 321–361.

Dose. 4 to 8 mg daily.

Clonidine   *Antihypertensive*

Synonym. Chlophazoline
2,6-Dichloro-*N*-(imidazolidin-2-ylidene)aniline
$C_9H_9Cl_2N_3 = 230.1$
CAS—4205-90-7

A white powder. M.p. 140° to 143°.
Soluble 1 in 8 of chloroform and 1 in 50 of ether.

Clonidine Hydrochloride
Proprietary Names. Catapres(an); Dixarit; Isoglaucon.
$C_9H_9Cl_2N_3,HCl = 266.6$
CAS—4205-91-8
A white crystalline powder. M.p. about 313°.
Soluble 1 in 13 of water, 1 in 25 of ethanol, 1 in 38 of dehydrated alcohol, and 1 in 250 of chloroform; practically insoluble in ether.

Dissociation Constant. pK_a 8.2.

Colour Test. Liebermann's Test—yellow (→ orange at 100°).

Thin-layer Chromatography. *System TA*—Rf 62; *system TB*—Rf 08; *system TC*—Rf 31. (*Acidified iodoplatinate solution, positive.*)

Gas Chromatography. *System GA*—RI 2248.

High Pressure Liquid Chromatography. *System HA*—k′ 1.2.

Ultraviolet Spectrum. Aqueous acid—271 nm ($A_1^1 = 21$ a), 278 nm.

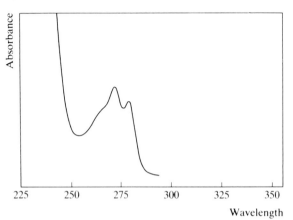

Infra-red Spectrum. Principal peaks at wavenumbers 1653, 1610, 778, 795, 1295, 1568 (clonidine hydrochloride, KBr disk).

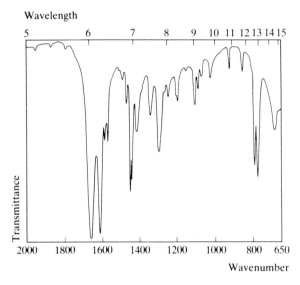

Mass Spectrum. Principal peaks at m/z 229, 30, 231, 172, 194, 174, 200, 230.

Quantification. GAS CHROMATOGRAPHY. In plasma or urine: sensitivity 25 pg/ml in plasma, ECD—L.-C. Chu *et al.*, *J. pharm. Sci.*, 1979, *68*, 72–74.

GAS CHROMATOGRAPHY (CAPILLARY COLUMN). In plasma: sensitivity 100 pg/ml, ECD—P. O. Edlund, *J. Chromat.*, 1980, *187*, 161–169.

GAS CHROMATOGRAPHY–MASS SPECTROMETRY. In plasma or urine: detection limit 100 pg/ml in plasma—S. Murray *et al.*, *Biomed. Mass Spectrom.*, 1981, *8*, 500–502.

RADIOIMMUNOASSAY. In plasma: detection limit 100 pg/ml— D. Arndts *et al.*, *Arzneimittel-Forsch.*, 1979, *29*, 532–538.

Disposition in the Body. Well absorbed after oral administration; bioavailability almost 100%. About 30 to 50% of a single dose is excreted in the urine as unchanged drug in 24 hours, and about 20% of a dose is eliminated in the faeces in 4 days. Several inactive metabolites have been detected in urine in small quantities.

THERAPEUTIC CONCENTRATION.

Peak plasma concentrations of 0.001 to 0.0018 µg/ml (mean 0.0014) were attained 90 minutes after administration of a single dose of 0.3 mg to 5 subjects (D. S. Davies *et al.*, *Br. J. clin. Pharmac.*, 1976, *3*, 348P).

Following oral administration of 0.075 mg three times a day to 8 subjects, steady-state serum concentrations of 0.0003 to 0.00035 µg/ml were reported (A. Keränen *et al.*, *Eur. J. clin. Pharmac.*, 1978, *13*, 97–101).

TOXICITY. Serious toxic effects have been reported after ingestion of doses of 0.4 to 4 mg by children and 4 to 11 mg by adults. However, recovery is usually rapid.

Two women were accidentally given doses of 25 mg instead of 0.025 mg; plasma concentrations of 0.025 and 0.027 µg/ml were reported on admission and at 24 hours, respectively, and decreased with a half-life of 22 hours; the subjects recovered with treatment (J. A. Rotellar *et al.*, *Lancet*, 1981, *1*, 1312).

In a fatality due to clonidine overdose, the following postmortem concentrations were reported: blood 0.023 µg/ml, brain 0.024 µg/g, kidney 0.086 µg/g (I. Lukkari *et al.*, *Bull. int. Ass. forens. Toxicol.*, 1983, *17*(2), 13–14).

HALF-LIFE. Plasma half-life, 10 to 25 hours.

VOLUME OF DISTRIBUTION. 2 to 4 litres/kg.

PROTEIN BINDING. In plasma, about 20 to 40%.

Dose. Usually 0.1 to 1.2 mg of clonidine hydrochloride daily; doses of 1.8 mg or more daily may be given.

Clonixin   *Analgesic*

2-(3-Chloro-*o*-toluidino)nicotinic acid
$C_{13}H_{11}ClN_2O_2 = 262.7$
CAS—17737-65-4

A colourless or cream-coloured solid. M.p. about 234°.

Thin-layer Chromatography. *System TG*—Rf 30. (*Ludy Tenger reagent*, orange.)

Gas Chromatography. *System GD*—retention time of methyl derivative 1.61 relative to *n*-$C_{16}H_{34}$.

High Pressure Liquid Chromatography. *System HV*—retention time 0.87 relative to meclofenamic acid.

Ultraviolet Spectrum. Methanol—289 nm ($A_1^1 = 950$ b), 335 nm.

Disposition in the Body. Rapidly absorbed after oral administration. Metabolised by hydroxylation to 4′-hydroxy-, 5′-hydroxy-, and 2′-hydroxymethyl derivatives. About 60% of a dose is excreted in the urine in 24 hours.

THERAPEUTIC CONCENTRATION.

Following a single oral dose of 750 mg to 12 subjects, peak serum concentrations of 29 to 66 µg/ml (mean 46) were attained in about 1.7

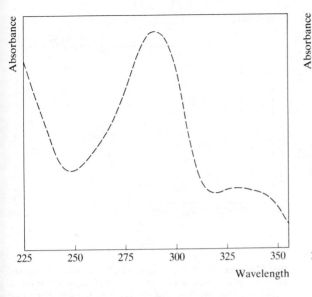

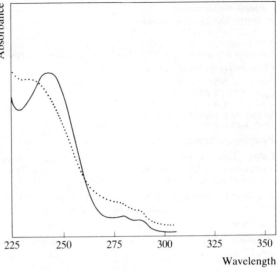

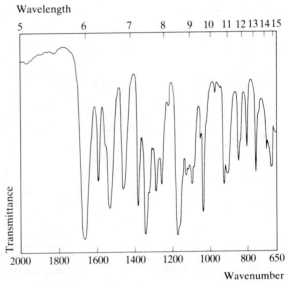

Wavelength

hours (D. E. Furst and H. E. Paulus, *Clin. Pharmac. Ther.*, 1975, *17*, 622–626).

HALF-LIFE. Plasma half-life, about 1.5 hours.

Dose. Clonixin has been given in doses of 600 mg.

Clopamide   *Diuretic*

Synonym. Chlosudimeprimyl
Proprietary Names. Brinaldix. It is an ingredient of Viskaldix.
4-Chloro-*N*-(2,6-dimethylpiperidino)-3-sulphamoylbenzamide
$C_{14}H_{20}ClN_3O_3S = 345.8$
CAS—636-54-4

A white crystalline powder. M.p. about 246°.
Soluble 1 in about 250 of water, 1 in about 100 of dehydrated alcohol, 1 in about 250 of chloroform, and 1 in 35 of methanol.

Colour Tests. Koppanyi–Zwikker Test—violet; Mercurous Nitrate—black.

Thin-layer Chromatography. *System TA*—Rf 79; *system TD*—Rf 19; *system TE*—Rf 52; *system TF*—Rf 38. (*Acidified iodoplatinate solution*, strong reaction.)

High Pressure Liquid Chromatography. *System HN*—k' 4.01.

Ultraviolet Spectrum. Aqueous acid—242 nm ($A_1^1 = 346$ b); methanol—232 nm, 277 nm ($A_1^1 = 48$ b), 286 nm ($A_1^1 = 36$ b).

Infra-red Spectrum. Principal peaks at wavenumbers 1663, 1172, 1038, 1532, 1285, 928.

Mass Spectrum. Principal peaks at *m/z* 111, 127, 55, 83, 59, 41, 112, 42.

Dose. 20 to 60 mg daily.

Clopenthixol   *Tranquilliser*

Synonym. Cloperphenthixan
2-{4-[3-(2-Chlorothioxanthen-9-ylidene)propyl]piperazin-1-yl}-ethanol
$C_{22}H_{25}ClN_2OS = 401.0$
CAS—982-24-1

Clopenthixol Decanoate

Proprietary Name. Clopixol (injection)

$C_{32}H_{43}ClN_2O_2S = 555.2$

A yellowish oily liquid.

Practically **insoluble** in water; soluble in ethanol, chloroform, and ether.

Clopenthixol Hydrochloride

Proprietary Names. Ciatyl; Clopixol (tablets); Sordinol.

$C_{22}H_{25}ClN_2OS,2HCl = 473.9$

CAS—633-59-0

Crystals. M.p. about 257°, with decomposition.

Freely **soluble** in water; sparingly soluble in ethanol.

Partition Coefficient. Log P (octanol/pH 7.0), 2.3.

Colour Tests. Formaldehyde–Sulphuric Acid—red (orange fluorescence under ultraviolet light); Liebermann's Test—red; Sulphuric Acid—orange (fluoresces under ultraviolet light).

Thin-layer Chromatography. *System TA*—Rf 56; *system TB*—Rf 07; *system TC*—Rf 32. (*Acidified iodoplatinate solution*, positive.)

Gas Chromatography. *System GA*—RI 2274.

Ultraviolet Spectrum. Aqueous acid—231 nm ($A_1^1 = 891$ a), 269 nm, 325 nm.

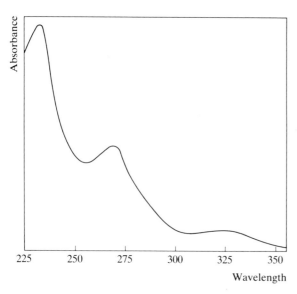

Infra-red Spectrum. Principal peaks at wavenumbers 1150, 1090, 757, 740, 1052, 1123 (KBr disk).

Mass Spectrum. Principal peaks at *m/z* 143, 70, 100, 144, 42, 56, 98, 221.

Quantification. SPECTROFLUORIMETRY. In serum: clopenthixol decanoate, clopenthixol and des-(2-hydroxyethyl)clopenthixol, limit of detection about 3 ng/ml for clopenthixol decanoate and about 2 ng/ml for clopenthixol and the metabolite—K. Overø, *Acta psychiat. scand.*, 1980, *61*, *Suppl.* 279, 92–103.

HIGH PRESSURE LIQUID CHROMATOGRAPHY. In serum: *cis*- and *trans*-clopenthixol and des-(2-hydroxyethyl)clopenthixol, sensitivity 500 pg/ml for clopenthixol and 2.5 ng/ml for the metabolite, UV detection—T. Aaes-Jørgensen, *J. Chromat.*, 1980, *183*; *Biomed. Appl.*, *9*, 239–245.

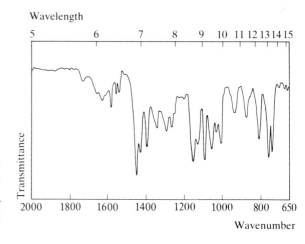

Wavelength

Transmittance

Wavenumber

Disposition in the Body. Clopenthixol decanoate is slowly absorbed after injection to give peak serum concentrations of clopenthixol and the des-(2-hydroxyethyl) metabolite after about 3 to 7 days. Clopenthixol, the des-(2-hydroxyethyl) metabolite, and their sulphoxide metabolites have been detected in urine together with small amounts of clopenthixol glucuronide.

THERAPEUTIC CONCENTRATION.

A mean minimum steady-state serum concentration of 0.004 µg/ml of clopenthixol was reported in 24 subjects, who had been receiving average doses of 200 mg intramuscularly every 4 weeks, for 5 to 6 months (S. J. Dencker *et al.*, *Acta psychiat. scand.*, 1980, *61*, *Suppl.* 279, 55–63).

Following an oral dose of 30 mg of clopenthixol to 1 subject, a peak serum concentration of about 0.005 µg/ml of *cis*-clopenthixol was attained in about 3 hours; the peak concentration of the inactive *trans*-isomer was slightly higher and was attained after 4 hours; the serum concentrations declined slowly and were still measureable after 48 hours; only traces of the des-(2-hydroxyethyl) metabolite were detected (T. Aaes-Jørgensen, *J. Chromat.*, 1980, *183*; *Biomed. Appl.*, *9*, 239–245).

Dose. The equivalent of 20 to 150 mg of clopenthixol daily; up to 250 mg daily has been given.

Clopidol   *Coccidiostat (Veterinary)*

Synonyms. Clopindol; Meticlorpindol.

3,5-Dichloro-2,6-dimethylpyridin-4-ol

$C_7H_7Cl_2NO = 192.0$

CAS—2971-90-6

A white crystalline powder. M.p. greater than 320°.

Practically **insoluble** in water; slightly soluble in ethanol; soluble in methanol.

Ultraviolet Spectrum. Ethanol—269 nm ($A_1^1 = 460$ b).

Infra-red Spectrum. Principal peaks at wavenumbers 1538, 1504, 753, 1618, 762, 1095 (KBr disk).

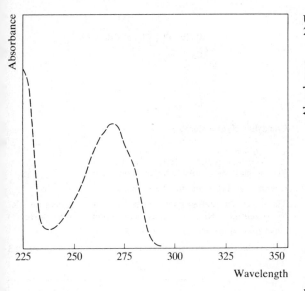

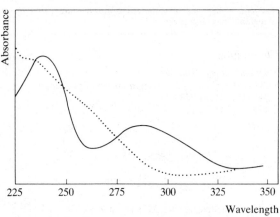

Ultraviolet Spectrum. Clorazepate dipotassium: aqueous acid—237 nm ($A_1^1 = 747$ b), 287 nm.

Clorazepic Acid

Tranquilliser

7-Chloro-2,3-dihydro-2-oxo-5-phenyl-1*H*-1,4-benzodiazepine-3-carboxylic acid

$C_{16}H_{11}ClN_2O_3 = 314.7$

CAS—23887-31-2

Clorazepate Dipotassium

Proprietary Names. Tranxen(e); Tranxilen; Tranxilium.

$C_{16}H_{11}ClK_2N_2O_4 = 408.9$

CAS—57109-90-7

A fine, light yellow powder.

Very **soluble** in water; practically insoluble in organic solvents. In aqueous solution, it converts to the monopotassium salt.

Clorazepate Monopotassium

Proprietary Name. Azene

$C_{16}H_{10}ClKN_2O_3 = 352.8$

CAS—5991-71-9

A fine, off-white powder.

Very **soluble** in water; practically insoluble in organic solvents.

Dissociation Constant. pK_a 3.5, 12.5.

Colour Test. Formaldehyde–Sulphuric Acid—orange.

Thin-layer Chromatography. *System TA*—Rf 84; *system TB*—Rf 03; *system TC*—Rf 56; *system TD*—Rf 34; *system TE*—Rf 63; *system TF*—Rf 45.

Gas Chromatography. *System GA*—clorazepic acid RI 2457, desmethyldiazepam RI 2496, oxazepam RI 2336; *system GG*—clorazepic acid RI 3125, desmethyldiazepam RI 3041, oxazepam RI 2803.

High Pressure Liquid Chromatography. *System HI*—k' 1.17; *system HK*—k' 2.00.

Infra-red Spectrum. Principal peaks at wavenumbers 1597, 1548, 1300, 702, 1230, 830 (clorazepate dipotassium, KBr disk).

Mass Spectrum. Principal peaks at *m/z* 242, 43, 270, 269, 241, 103, 243, 76.

Quantification. GAS CHROMATOGRAPHY. In blood or urine: clorazepic acid and desmethyldiazepam, sensitivity 4 ng/ml in blood and 5 ng/ml in urine, ECD; also oxazepam in urine, sensitivity 25 ng/ml, ECD—M. A. Brooks *et al.*, *J. Chromat.*, 1977, *135*, 123–131.

HIGH PRESSURE LIQUID CHROMATOGRAPHY. In plasma: clorazepate dipotassium and desmethyldiazepam, UV detection—P. Colin *et al.*, *J. Chromat.*, 1983, *273*; *Biomed. Appl.*, 24, 367–377.

Disposition in the Body. Rapidly decarboxylated below pH 4 to the active metabolite desmethyldiazepam (nordazepam), and thus is absorbed mainly as desmethyldiazepam after oral administration; this is then hydroxylated to form oxazepam which is conjugated with glucuronic acid. Up to about 10% of a dose is excreted in urine in 24 hours, mainly as oxazepam glucuronide, together with small amounts of unchanged clorazepate and conjugated desmethyldiazepam. Oxazepam glucuronide is still detectable in urine 12 days after a single dose.

THERAPEUTIC CONCENTRATION.

Following a single oral dose of 15 mg to 4 subjects, peak blood concentrations of desmethyldiazepam of 0.14 to 0.18 µg/ml (mean 0.16) were attained in 0.5 to 1 hour; peak blood-clorazepate concentrations of 0.03 to 0.11 µg/ml (mean 0.06) were reported at about 1 hour (C. W. Abruzzo *et al.*, *J. Pharmacokinet. Biopharm.*, 1977, *5*, 377–390).

Average steady-state serum concentrations of 0.40 to 0.61 µg/ml (mean 0.48) of desmethyldiazepam were reported in 7 patients receiving daily oral doses of 0.6 mg/kg (A. J. Wilensky *et al.*, *Clin. Pharmac. Ther.*, 1978, *24*, 22–30).

TOXICITY. Fatalities from overdosage are rare and recovery from an overdose of 600 mg has been reported.

HALF-LIFE. Plasma half-life, clorazepate about 2 hours, desmethyldiazepam about 40 to 100 hours but there is considerable intersubject variation—see under Nordazepam.

VOLUME OF DISTRIBUTION. Desmethyldiazepam 0.5 to 2.5 litres/kg, increased in elderly subjects.

CLEARANCE. Plasma clearance, desmethyldiazepam about 0.1 to 0.3 ml/min/kg.

DISTRIBUTION IN BLOOD. Plasma: whole blood ratio, desmethyl-diazepam 1.7.

PROTEIN BINDING. In plasma, desmethyldiazepam about 97%.

Dose. 7.5 to 22.5 mg of clorazepate dipotassium daily; up to 60 mg daily has been given.

Clorexolone   *Diuretic*

Proprietary Name. Nefrolan
6-Chloro-2-cyclohexyl-3-oxoisoindoline-5-sulphonamide
$C_{14}H_{17}ClN_2O_3S = 328.8$
CAS—2127-01-7

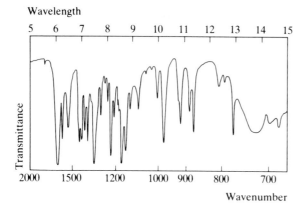

A white crystalline powder. M.p. about 266°.
Very slightly **soluble** in water; soluble in dimethylformamide, methanol, and solutions of alkali hydroxides.

Colour Test. Koppanyi–Zwikker Test—violet.

Thin-layer Chromatography. *System TA*—Rf 76; *system TD*—Rf 31; *system TE*—Rf 58; *system TF*—Rf 51. (*Acidified iodoplatinate solution*, positive.)

High Pressure Liquid Chromatography. *System HN*—k' 7.26.

Ultraviolet Spectrum. Ethanol—252 nm ($A_1^1 = 246$ a).

Infra-red Spectrum. Principal peaks at wavenumbers 1661, 1172, 1234, 1149, 978, 1613 (KBr disk).

Mass Spectrum. Principal peaks at *m/z* 247, 285, 328, 249, 41, 287, 330, 55.

Disposition in the Body. Absorbed after oral administration. It is almost completely excreted in the urine in 48 hours as three cyclohexane ring-hydroxylated metabolites.

Dose. 10 to 100 mg daily.

Clorgyline   *Antidepressant (Monoamine Oxidase Inhibitor)*

Synonym. Clorgiline
N-[3-(2,4-Dichlorophenoxy)propyl]-N-methylprop-2-ynylamine
$C_{13}H_{15}Cl_2NO = 272.2$
CAS—17780-72-2

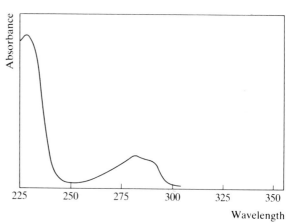

Clorgyline Hydrochloride
$C_{13}H_{15}Cl_2NO,HCl = 308.6$
CAS—17780-75-5
A white crystalline powder. M.p. 102° to 103°.
Very **soluble** in water; soluble in chloroform.

Colour Test. Liebermann's Test—black.

Thin-layer Chromatography. *System TA*—Rf 67; *system TB*—Rf 42; *system TC*—Rf 70. (*Acidified iodoplatinate solution*, positive.)

Gas Chromatography. *System GA*—RI 1883.

Ultraviolet Spectrum. Aqueous acid—228 nm ($A_1^1 = 310$ b), 282 nm.

Infra-red Spectrum. Principal peaks at wavenumbers 1280, 1250, 1055, 1099, 801, 1124.

Dose. Clorgyline hydrochloride has been tried in doses of 10 to 30 mg daily.

Clorprenaline   *Sympathomimetic*

Synonyms. Chlorprenaline; Isoprophenamine.
1-(2-Chlorophenyl)-2-isopropylaminoethanol
$C_{11}H_{16}ClNO = 213.7$
CAS—3811-25-4

$(CH_3)_2CH \cdot NH \cdot CH_2 \cdot CHOH$

Soluble in chloroform.

Clorprenaline Hydrochloride
$C_{11}H_{16}ClNO,HCl,H_2O = 268.2$
CAS—6933-90-0 (anhydrous); *5588-22-7* (monohydrate)
White crystals. M.p. 161° to 162°.
Soluble in water.

Thin-layer Chromatography. *System TA*—Rf 57; *system TB*—Rf 18; *system TC*—Rf 15. (*Acidified potassium permanganate solution, positive.*)

Gas Chromatography. *System GA*—RI 1604; *system GB*—RI 1614; *system GC*—RI 1880.

High Pressure Liquid Chromatography. *System HA*—k′ 1.1.

Ultraviolet Spectrum. Aqueous acid—262 nm, 266 nm ($A_1^1 = 10.1$ b).

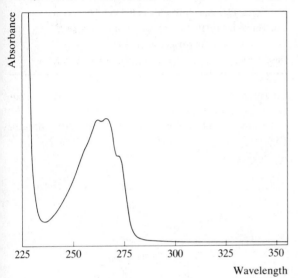

Infra-red Spectrum. Principal peaks at wavenumbers 1075, 775, 1587, 1041, 1030, 1123.

Mass Spectrum. Principal peaks at *m/z* 72, 30, 43, 77, 73, 51, 41, 27.

Dose. Clorprenaline hydrochloride has been given in doses of 30 to 80 mg daily.

Clothiapine   *Tranquilliser*

Synonym. Clotiapine
Proprietary Name. Entumin(e)
2 - Chloro - 11 - (4 - methylpiperazin - 1 - yl)dibenzo[*b,f*]-[1,4]thiazepine
$C_{18}H_{18}ClN_3S = 343.9$
CAS—2058-52-8

Crystals. M.p. 116° to 122°.
Soluble 1 in 10 of hydrochloric acid.

Thin-layer Chromatography. *System TA*—Rf 59; *system TB*—Rf 41; *system TC*—Rf 59. (*Acidified iodoplatinate solution, positive.*)

Ultraviolet Spectrum. No significant absorption, 230 to 360 nm.

Infra-red Spectrum. Principal peaks at wavenumbers 1596, 1570, 1548, 1295, 757, 1234 (KBr disk).

Mass Spectrum. Principal peaks at *m/z* 83, 70, 273, 244, 209, 42, 71, 43.

Dose. Clothiapine has been given in doses of 40 to 120 mg daily.

Clotrimazole   *Antifungal*

Synonym. Chlortritylimidazol
Proprietary Names. Canesten; Eparol; Gyne-Lotrimin; Lotrimin; Mycelex; Trimysten.
1 - (α - 2 - Chlorotrityl)imidazole
$C_{22}H_{17}ClN_2 = 344.8$
CAS—23593-75-1

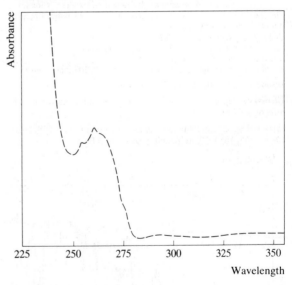

A white to pale yellow crystalline powder. M.p. about 142°, with decomposition.
Practically **insoluble** in water; freely soluble in ethanol and chloroform; slightly soluble in ether.

Gas Chromatography. *System GA*—RI 2100.

Ultraviolet Spectrum. Methanol—254 nm, 260 nm ($A_1^1 = 20$ b).

Infra-red Spectrum. Principal peaks at wavenumbers 765, 752, 708, 1075, 741, 1205 (KBr disk). (See below)

Mass Spectrum. Principal peaks at *m/z* 277, 279, 165, 278, 241, 239, 242, 240.

Uses. Topically in a concentration of 1 or 2% or as vaginal tablets.

Wavelength

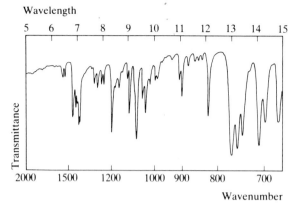

Wavenumber

Cloxacillin   *Antibiotic*

(6R) - 6 - [3 - (2 - Chlorophenyl) - 5 - methylisoxazole - 4 - carbox-amido]penicillanic acid
$C_{19}H_{18}ClN_3O_5S = 435.9$
CAS—61-72-3

Cloxacillin Sodium

Proprietary Names. Austrastaph; Bactopen; Cloxapen; Cloxilean; Cloxypen; Ekvacillin; Novocloxin; Orbenin(e); Staphybiotic; Tegopen. It is an ingredient of Ampiclox.
$C_{19}H_{17}ClN_3NaO_5S, H_2O = 475.9$
CAS—642-78-4 (anhydrous); *7081-44-9* (monohydrate)
A white, hygroscopic, crystalline powder.
Soluble 1 in 2.5 of water, 1 in 30 of ethanol, and 1 in 500 of chloroform.

Dissociation Constant. pK_a 2.7 (25°).

Ultraviolet Spectrum. Cloxacillin sodium: aqueous acid—352 nm ($A_1^1 = 67$ b).

Infra-red Spectrum. Principal peaks at wavenumbers 1598, 1620, 1765, 1495, 1659, 771 (cloxacillin sodium, KBr disk).

Wavelength

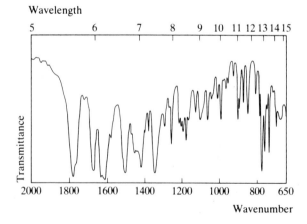

Wavenumber

Quantification. HIGH PRESSURE LIQUID CHROMATOGRAPHY. In serum or urine: sensitivity 50 ng/ml, UV detection—F. W. Teare *et al.*, *J. pharm. Sci.*, 1982, **71**, 938–941. In serum: sensitivity 500 ng/ml, UV detection—S. J. Soldin *et al.*, *Ther. Drug Monit.*, 1980, **2**, 417–422.

Disposition in the Body. Incompletely absorbed after oral administration. About 35% of an oral dose is excreted in the urine unchanged in 12 hours, together with about 11% as penicilloic acid; about 10% of a dose is excreted in the bile.

HALF-LIFE. Plasma half-life, about 0.5 to 1.5 hours.

VOLUME OF DISTRIBUTION. About 0.1 litre/kg.

PROTEIN BINDING. In plasma, about 94%.

Dose. Usually the equivalent of 2 g of cloxacillin daily.

Clozapine   *Tranquilliser*

Proprietary Name. Leponex
8 - Chloro - 11 - (4 - methylpiperazin - 1 - yl) - 5H - dibenzo-[b,e][1,4]diazepine
$C_{18}H_{19}ClN_4 = 326.8$
CAS—5786-21-0

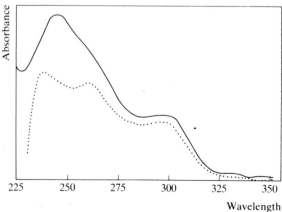

Yellow crystals. M.p. about 183°.

Colour Tests. Formaldehyde–Sulphuric Acid—yellow.
Cold *nitric acid* gives a red colour.

Thin-layer Chromatography. *System TA*—Rf 57; *system TB*—Rf 04; *system TC*—Rf 38; *system TD*—Rf 04; *system TE*—Rf 63; *system TF*—Rf 05.

Gas Chromatography. *System GA*—RI 2967; *system GG*—RI 3455.

Ultraviolet Spectrum. Aqueous acid—245 nm, 297 nm; aqueous alkali—238 nm, 261 nm, 297 nm.

Wavelength

Wavelength

Infra-red Spectrum. Principal peaks at wavenumbers 1600, 1560, 758, 1136, 1101, 1117.

Mass Spectrum. Principal peaks at m/z 243, 256, 70, 245, 192, 227, 258, 326.

Dose. Clozapine has been given in doses of 150 to 600 mg daily.

Cocaine
Local Anaesthetic

Synonyms. Methyl Benzoylecgonine; Neurocaine.
$(1R,2R,3s,5S)$ - 2 - Methoxycarbonyltropan - 3 - yl benzoate
$C_{17}H_{21}NO_4 = 303.4$
CAS—50-36-2

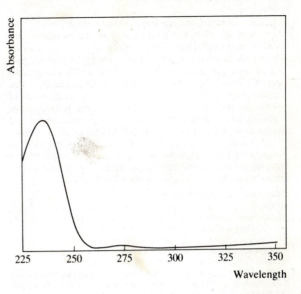

An alkaloid obtained from coca, the dried leaves of *Erythroxylum coca* and other species of *Erythroxylum* (Erythroxylaceae), or by synthesis from ecgonine.
A white crystalline, slightly volatile, powder. M.p. 96° to 98°.
Soluble 1 in 600 of water, 1 in 7 of ethanol, 1 in about 0.5 of chloroform, and 1 in 4 of ether.

Cocaine Hydrochloride
Synonym. Cocainium Chloride
Proprietary Name. It is an ingredient of Mydricaine (injection).
$C_{17}H_{21}NO_4,HCl = 339.8$
CAS—53-21-4
Hygroscopic colourless crystals or white crystalline powder. M.p. about 197°, with decomposition.
Soluble 1 in 0.5 of water, 1 in 3.5 to 1 in 4.5 of ethanol, and 1 in 15 to 1 in 18 of chloroform; practically insoluble in ether.

Dissociation Constant. pK_a 8.6 (20°).

Colour Test. *p*-Dimethylaminobenzaldehyde (100° for 3 min)—red.

Thin-layer Chromatography. *System TA*—Rf 65; *system TB*—Rf 47; *system TC*—Rf 47; *system TL*—Rf 54. (*Dragendorff spray*, positive; *acidified iodoplatinate solution*, positive.)

Gas Chromatography. *System GA*—cocaine RI 2187, benzoylecgonine RI 2570, ecgonine not eluted; *system GF*—RI 2550.

High Pressure Liquid Chromatography. *System HA*—cocaine k′ 2.8, benzoylecgonine k′ 0.9 (tailing peak), ecgonine k′ 1.1; *system HQ*—cocaine k′ 2.68, benzoylecgonine k′ 5.68.

Ultraviolet Spectrum. Aqueous acid—233 nm ($A_1^1 = 430$ a), 275 nm.

Infra-red Spectrum. Principal peaks at wavenumbers 1710, 1738, 1275, 1110, 712, 1037 (KBr disk).

Mass Spectrum. Principal peaks at m/z 82, 182, 83, 105, 303, 77, 94, 96; benzoylecgonine 124, 82, 168, 77, 105, 42, 94, 83.

Quantification. GAS CHROMATOGRAPHY. In plasma, urine or erythrocytes: ECD—J. I. Javaid *et al.*, *J. Chromat.*, 1978, *152*, 105–113. In whole blood or plasma: sensitivity 20 ng/ml, AFID—B. H. Dvorchik *et al.*, *J. Chromat.*, 1977, *135*, 141–148.

GAS CHROMATOGRAPHY–MASS SPECTROMETRY. In biological samples: cocaine, benzoylecgonine and norcocaine, sensitivity 5 ng/ml—D. M. Chinn *et al.*, *J. analyt. Toxicol.*, 1980, *4*, 37–42.

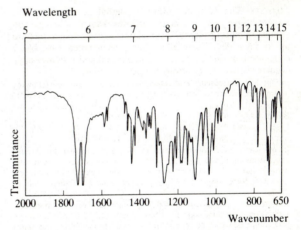

In urine: ecgonine methyl ester, sensitivity 100 ng/ml—J. J. Ambre *et al.*, *J. analyt. Toxicol.*, 1982, *6*, 26–29.

HIGH PRESSURE LIQUID CHROMATOGRAPHY. In plasma or tissues: cocaine and metabolites, limit of detection <1 µg/ml, UV detection—M. A. Evans and T. Morarity, *J. analyt. Toxicol.*, 1980, *4*, 19–22.

RADIOIMMUNOASSAY. In urine: benzoylecgonine (comparison with TLC, GLC and enzyme immunoassay), sensitivity 2 ng/ml—S. J. Mulé *et al.*, *Clin. Chem.*, 1977, *23*, 796–801. In blood or urine: benzoylecgonine (comparison with HPLC), limit of detection 20 ng/ml—K. Robinson and R. N. Smith, *J. Pharm. Pharmac.*, 1984, *36*, 157–162.

REVIEWS. J. E. Wallace *et al.*, *J. analyt. Toxicol.*, 1977, *1*, 20–26 and J. E. Lindgren, *J. Ethnopharmac.*, 1981, *3*, 337–351.

Disposition in the Body. Cocaine is normally only used as a surface anaesthetic in the eye, ear, nose, and throat because of the possibility of systemic toxic effects when given by other routes. Addicts may inject it or use it as a snuff; it is less toxic when taken orally due to hydrolysis in the gastro-intestinal tract.

The main metabolites are benzoylecgonine, ecgonine, and ecgonine methyl ester, all of which are inactive; some norcocaine, an active metabolite, may also be produced; other metabolites which have been reported are ethylecgonine, hydroxycocaine, and methylecgonidine. About 1 to 9% of a daily intravenous dose of 120 mg of cocaine is excreted unchanged in the urine, together with 35 to 55% as benzoylecgonine; the excretion of unchanged drug is increased when the urine is acid; some ecgonine may also be present. After an intranasal dose of 1.5 mg/kg, up to 4% of the dose is excreted in the urine unchanged in 24 hours, and 16 to 36% of the dose is excreted as benzoylecgonine. About 30 to 60% of an oral, intranasal, or intravenous dose is excreted in the urine as ecgonine methyl ester. No unchanged drug is eliminated in the faeces.

THERAPEUTIC CONCENTRATION.

After a dose of 1.5 mg/kg, administered intranasally to 9 subjects, peak plasma concentrations of 0.12 to 0.47 µg/ml were attained in 1 hour (C. Van Dyke et al., Science, 1976, 191, 859–861).

Following a dose of 16 mg, administered intravenously to 10 subjects, peak plasma concentrations of 0.09 to 0.31 µg/ml were reported after 5 minutes (J. I. Javaid et al., Science, 1978, 202, 227–228).

After a dose of 2 mg/kg, administered orally to 3 subjects, peak plasma concentrations of 0.10 to 0.42 µg/ml were attained in 50 to 90 minutes (C. Van Dyke et al., Science, 1978, 200, 211–213).

TOXICITY. The estimated minimum lethal dose is 1.2 g but susceptible persons have died from doses as small as 30 mg when applied to mucous membranes; addicts may be able to tolerate up to 5 g a day. Toxic effects have been noted with blood concentrations in the range 0.25 to 5 µg/ml and fatalities have occurred with concentrations of 1 µg/ml or more.

In 5 fatalities attributed to intravenous overdoses of cocaine, the following postmortem tissue concentrations, µg/ml or µg/g (mean), were reported:

	Cocaine	Benzoylecgonine
Blood	0–7.6 (2.7)	1.0–7.4 (4.4)
Liver	0.04–3.2 (1.2)	1.4–7.1 (4.2)
Urine	38.4–118.6 (76)	15–185 (110)

In one case, brain concentrations of 10.4 and 1.0 µg/g and kidney concentrations of 0.1 and 2.9 µg/g were reported for cocaine and benzoylecgonine, respectively. Norcocaine was detected in low concentrations in some samples (D. M. Chinn et al., J. analyt. Toxicol., 1980, 4, 37–42).

In 4 fatalities due to the ingestion of large amounts of cocaine (more than 1 g), postmortem blood concentrations ranged from 7 to 12.8 µg/ml (mean 8.9), compared with blood concentrations of 0.1 to 11 µg/ml (mean 3) in 6 fatalities due to intravenous cocaine, and 0.3 to 11 µg/ml (mean 4.4) in 4 fatalities due to intranasal overdose (C. V. Wetli and R. K. Wright, J. Am. med. Ass., 1979, 241, 2519–2522).

A known addict was thought to have ingested 2 to 3 g of stolen cocaine whilst being taken into custody; he died about 5 hours later. Postmortem concentrations were: blood 8 µg/ml, kidney 12 µg/g, liver 8 µg/g, urine 50 µg/ml (K. R. Price, J. forens. Sci. Soc., 1974, 14, 329–333).

HALF-LIFE. Plasma half-life, 0.7 to 1.5 hours (dose-dependent).

VOLUME OF DISTRIBUTION. About 1 to 3 litres/kg.

CLEARANCE. Plasma clearance, 10 to 30 ml/min/kg (dose-dependent).

Use. Cocaine hydrochloride is used in concentrations of 1 to 20% for local anaesthesia.

Codeine   Narcotic Analgesic

Synonym. Morphine Methyl Ether
Proprietary Name. Codicept
3 - O - Methylmorphine monohydrate
$C_{18}H_{21}NO_3,H_2O = 317.4$
CAS—76-57-3 (anhydrous); 6059-47-8 (monohydrate)

An alkaloid obtained from opium or prepared by methylation of morphine.
Colourless crystals or white crystalline powder which effloresces slowly in dry air and is affected by light. M.p. 154° to 158°.
Soluble 1 in 120 of water, 1 in 15 of boiling water, 1 in 2 of ethanol, 1 in 0.5 of chloroform, and 1 in 50 of ether.

Codeine Hydrochloride
$C_{18}H_{21}NO_3,HCl,2H_2O = 371.9$
CAS—1422-07-7 (anhydrous)
A white crystalline powder. M.p. about 280°, with some decomposition.
Soluble 1 in 30 of water, 1 in 100 of ethanol (90%), and 1 in 800 of chloroform.

Codeine Phosphate
Synonym. Methylmorphine Phosphate
Proprietary Names. Codlin; Paveral; Tricodein.
Codeine phosphate is an ingredient of many proprietary preparations—see Martindale, The Extra Pharmacopoeia, 28th Edn.
$C_{18}H_{21}NO_3,H_3PO_4,\frac{1}{2}H_2O = 406.4$
CAS—52-28-8 (anhydrous); 41444-62-6 (hemihydrate); 5913-76-8 (sesquihydrate)
Small colourless crystals or white crystalline powder.
Soluble 1 in 4 of water, 1 in 450 of ethanol, and 1 in 125 of boiling ethanol; practically insoluble in chloroform and ether.

Codeine Sulphate
Synonym. Codeine Sulfate
Proprietary Name. It is an ingredient of Bepro.
$(C_{18}H_{21}NO_3)_2,H_2SO_4,3H_2O = 750.9$
CAS—1420-53-7 (anhydrous); 6854-40-6 (trihydrate)
White crystals or crystalline powder.
Soluble 1 in 30 of water and 1 in 1300 of ethanol; practically insoluble in chloroform and ether.

Dissociation Constant. pK_a 8.2 (20°).

Partition Coefficient. Log P (octanol/pH 7.4), 0.6.

Colour Tests. Liebermann's Test—black; Mandelin's Test—green; Marquis Test—violet.

Thin-layer Chromatography. System TA—Rf 33; system TB—Rf 06; system TC—Rf 18. (Dragendorff spray, positive; acidified iodoplatinate solution, positive; Marquis reagent, violet.)

Gas Chromatography. System GA—codeine RI 2376, morphine RI 2454, norcodeine RI 2388; system GB—RI 1600; system GC—codeine RI 2681, morphine RI 2542; system GF—RI 2860.

High Pressure Liquid Chromatography. System HA—codeine k' 4.8 (tailing peak), morphine k' 3.8 (tailing peak), norcodeine k' 3.1 (tailing peak); system HC—codeine k' 1.21, morphine k' 1.30, norcodeine k' 3.51; system HS—codeine k' 1.90, morphine k' 5.16.

Ultraviolet Spectrum. Aqueous acid—285 nm ($A_1^1 = 55$ a). No alkaline shift.

Infra-red Spectrum. Principal peaks at wavenumbers 1052, 1268, 1500, 1111, 793, 934, (KBr disk).

Mass Spectrum. Principal peaks at m/z 299, 42, 162, 124, 229, 59, 300, 69; morphine 285, 162, 42, 215, 286, 124, 44, 284; norcodeine 285, 81, 215, 148, 286, 164, 110, 115.

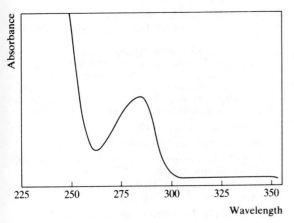

Wavelength

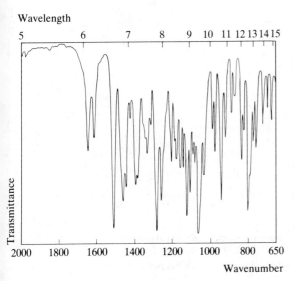

Wavenumber

Quantification. GAS CHROMATOGRAPHY. In blood, urine or tissues: codeine and morphine, sensitivity 20 ng in blood, 500 ng in urine and tissues, FID—G. R. Nakamura and E. L. Way, *Analyt. Chem.*, 1975, *47*, 775–778.

GAS CHROMATOGRAPHY (CAPILLARY COLUMN). In biological fluids: detection limit 5 ng/ml for codeine and 1 ng/ml for morphine, ECD—P. O. Edlund, *J. Chromat.*, 1981, *206*, 109–116.

GAS CHROMATOGRAPHY–MASS SPECTROMETRY. In blood, urine or tissues: sensitivity 13 ng/ml for codeine and morphine—N. B. Wu Chen *et al.*, *J. analyt. Toxicol.*, 1982, *6*, 231–234.

HIGH PRESSURE LIQUID CHROMATOGRAPHY. In plasma: sensitivity 10 ng/ml, UV detection— V. Nitsche and H. Mascher, *J. pharm. Sci.*, 1984, *73*, 1556–1558. In urine: codeine, norcodeine and morphine, sensitivity 25 ng/ml, UV detection—B. L. Posey and S. N. Kimble, *J. analyt. Toxicol.*, 1984, *8*, 68–74.

RADIOIMMUNOASSAY. In plasma: sensitivity <1 ng/ml—J. W. A. Findlay *et al.*, *Life Sci.*, 1976, *19*, 389–394.

Disposition in the Body. Well absorbed after oral administration; bioavailability about 50%. Metabolised in the liver by *O*-demethylation to form morphine, *N*-demethylation to form norcodeine, and conjugation to form glucuronides and sulphates of both unchanged drug and its metabolites. After an oral dose, about 86% is excreted in the urine in 24 hours; of the excreted material, 40 to 70% is free or conjugated codeine, 5 to 15% is free or conjugated morphine, 10 to 20% is free or conjugated norcodeine, and trace amounts may be free or conjugated normorphine; some of the dose is excreted in the bile and trace amounts are found in the faeces; unchanged drug accounts for 6 to 8% of the dose in urine in 24 hours but this may increase to about 10% when the urinary pH is decreased. After an intramuscular dose, 15 to 20% is excreted unchanged in acid urine in 24 hours. Small amounts of hydrocodone, norhydrocodone, 6α-hydrocodol, and 6β-hydrocodol have also been detected in urine.

THERAPEUTIC CONCENTRATION.

After a single oral dose of 60 mg of codeine phosphate in combination with 650 mg of aspirin, administered to 12 subjects, peak plasma concentrations of 0.11 to 0.23 μg/ml (mean 0.16) of codeine were attained in 0.5 to 1.5 hours, and peak plasma concentrations of morphine of 0.0003 to 0.014 μg/ml (mean 0.007) were reported at 1.5 hours (J. W. A. Findlay *et al.*, *Clin. Pharmac. Ther.*, 1978, *24*, 60–68).

TOXICITY. The estimated minimum lethal dose is 800 mg, but codeine is much less toxic than morphine and death directly attributable to codeine is rare; in most fatalities involving codeine, other drugs and/or alcohol are also present. Drug addicts may use doses up to 10 times normal before showing toxic effects, whilst children may show toxicity with only 1/20th of the dose.

Concentrations of codeine in the blood of 1.4 to 5.6 μg/ml (mean 3.6) were found in 8 fatal cases of codeine overdosage (J. A. Wright *et al.*, *Clin. Toxicol.*, 1975, *8*, 457–463).

In 39 fatal cases in which codeine was implicated, the postmortem blood concentrations for codeine ranged from <0.1 μg/ml to 8.8 μg/ml (mean 1.2), and for morphine from <0.1 μg/ml to 0.7 μg/ml (mean 0.16); in 22 of these cases, the following concentrations, μg/ml or μg/g (mean), in other tissues and fluids were reported:

	Codeine	Morphine
Bile	0.5–43 (11)	<0.1–119 (33)
Kidney	<0.1–36.3 (7)	<0.1–12.4 (2)
Liver	<0.1–45 (5)	<0.1–6.4 (2)
Urine	3.2–229 (60)	<0.1–69.8 (20)

In all cases, other drugs were also present (G. R. Nakamura *et al.*, *J. forens. Sci.*, 1976, *21*, 518–524).

In 2 fatalities involving the ingestion of large numbers of codeine tablets, postmortem blood concentrations of codeine of 15 and 48 μg/ml were reported; urine concentrations were 155 and 370 μg/ml; in both cases alcohol had also been ingested and in one case a low concentration of salicylate was also found in the blood (M. A. Peat and A. Sengupta, *Forens. Sci.*, 1977, *9*, 21–32).

HALF-LIFE. Plasma half-life, 2 to 4 hours.

VOLUME OF DISTRIBUTION. About 3.5 litres/kg.

CLEARANCE. Plasma clearance, 10 to 15 ml/min/kg.

PROTEIN BINDING. In plasma, about 7 to 25%.

Dose. 10 to 60 mg up to 6 times a day.

Co-dergocrine Mesylate *Vasodilator*

Synonyms. Co-dergocrine Methanesulphonate; DEA; DHAE; Dihydroergotoxine Mesylate; Dihydrogenated Ergot Alkaloids; Hydrogenated Ergot Alkaloids.

Proprietary Names. Circanol; Deapril-ST; Hydergin(e); Progeril.

A mixture in equal proportions of dihydroergocornine mesylate ($C_{31}H_{41}N_5O_5,CH_4O_3S = 659.8$), dihydroergocristine mesylate ($C_{35}H_{41}N_5O_5,CH_4O_3S = 707.8$), and α- and β-dihydroergocryptine mesylates ($C_{32}H_{43}N_5O_5,CH_4O_3S = 673.8$) in the ratio 2:1. *CAS—11032-41-0 (co-dergocrine); 8067-24-1 (mesylate)*

A white to yellowish-white powder. M.p. 196° to 206°, with decomposition.

Soluble 1 in 50 of water, 1 in 30 of ethanol, 1 in 10 of acetone, and 1 in 100 of chloroform; practically insoluble in ether.

Dissociation Constant. pK_a 6.9 (24°).

Thin-layer Chromatography. Co-dergocrine: *system TA*—Rf 66; *system TB*—Rf 01; *system TC*—Rf 48; *system TL*—Rf 29; *system TM*—Rf 64.

High Pressure Liquid Chromatography. *System HP*—dihydroergocristine k' 18.3, dihydroergocryptine k' 15.9.

Infra-red Spectrum. Principal peaks at the following wavenumbers (all KBr disk):
Dihydroergocornine 1633, 1662, 1720, 1705, 1558, 768
Dihydroergocristine 1635, 1728, 1510, 1215, 760, 1540
Dihydroergocryptine mesylate 1633, 1210, 1172, 1048, 1675, 1732

Mass Spectrum. Principal peaks at the following *m/z*:
Co-dergocrine 70, 154, 125, 41, 43, 155, 42, 225
Dihydroergocornine 70, 71, 269, 154, 195, 55, 59, 57
Dihydroergocristine 125, 70, 91, 153, 41, 244, 43, 71
Dihydroergocryptine 154, 70, 155, 167, 223, 225, 349, 153

Quantification. HIGH PRESSURE LIQUID CHROMATOGRAPHY. In plasma: detection limit 700 pg/ml, fluorescence detection—L. Zecca *et al.*, *J. Chromat.*, 1983, *272*; *Biomed. Appl.*, *23*, 401–405.

RADIOIMMUNOASSAY. In plasma: detection limit 10 pg/ml—W. Loh and B. G. Woodcock, *Arzneimittel-Forsch.*, 1983, *33*, 568–570.

Disposition in the Body. Poorly absorbed after oral administration; bioavailability 5 to 12%.

THERAPEUTIC CONCENTRATION.
Following a single oral dose of 4.5 mg to 8 subjects, peak plasma concentrations of 0.0003 to 0.0011 μg/ml (mean 0.0006) were attained in 0.2 to 1.2 hours (B. G. Woodcock *et al.*, *Clin. Pharmac. Ther.*, 1982, *32*, 622–627).

HALF-LIFE. Plasma half-life, 8 to 25 hours (mean 13).

VOLUME OF DISTRIBUTION. 10 to 20 litres/kg.

CLEARANCE. Plasma clearance, 20 to 30 ml/min/kg.

REFERENCE. B. G. Woodcock *et al.*, *Clin. Pharmac. Ther.*, 1982, *32*, 622–627.

Dose. Up to 4.5 mg daily, by mouth; 0.75 to 3 mg daily, sublingually.

Colchicine   *Gout Suppressant*

Proprietary Names. Colchineos; Colcin; Colgout; Coluric.
(*S*)-*N*-(5,6,7,9-Tetrahydro-1,2,3,10-tetramethoxy-9-oxobenzo[*a*]heptalen-7-yl)acetamide
$C_{22}H_{25}NO_6 = 399.4$
CAS—64-86-8

An alkaloid obtained from the corm and seeds of the meadow saffron, *Colchicum autumnale* (Liliaceae) and other *Colchicum* species.

Pale yellow to greenish-yellow crystals, or amorphous scales or powder, darkening on exposure to light. M.p. about 157°.

Soluble 1 in about 20 of water, but moderately concentrated aqueous solutions may deposit crystals of a sesquihydrate, which is less soluble in cold water than the anhydrous alkaloid. Freely soluble in ethanol and chloroform; soluble 1 in 160 of ether.

Dissociation Constant. pK_a 1.7 (20°).

Partition Coefficient. Log *P* (octanol), 1.0.

Colour Tests. Liebermann's Test—green; Mandelin's Test—green; Marquis Test—yellow.

Thin-layer Chromatography. *System TA*—Rf 55; *system TB*—Rf 00; *system TC*—Rf 37. (*Van Urk reagent*, yellow.)

High Pressure Liquid Chromatography. *System HA*—k' 0.2.

Ultraviolet Spectrum. Ethanol—243 nm ($A_1^1 = 730$ a), 350 nm ($A_1^1 = 425$ a).

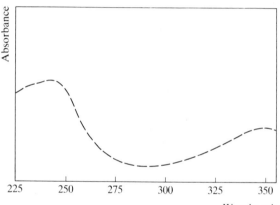

Wavelength

Infra-red Spectrum. Principal peaks at wavenumbers 1250, 1550, 1588, 1610, 1090, 1655 (KBr disk).

Mass Spectrum. Principal peaks at *m/z* 312, 43, 399, 297, 356, 281, 371, 311.

Quantification. SPECTROFLUORIMETRY. In plasma or urine—R. Bourdon and M. Galliot, *Annls Biol. clin.*, 1976, *34*, 393–401.

HIGH PRESSURE LIQUID CHROMATOGRAPHY. In plasma: sensitivity 5 ng/ml, UV detection—D. Jarvie *et al.*, *Clin. Toxicol.*, 1979, *14*, 375–381. In whole blood: sensitivity 10 ng/ml, UV detection—Y. H. Caplan *et al.*, *J. analyt. Toxicol.*, 1980, *4*, 153–155.

RADIOIMMUNOASSAY. In serum: sensitivity 350 pg/ml—J. M. Scherrmann *et al.*, *J. Pharm. Pharmac.*, 1980, *32*, 800–802.

Disposition in the Body. Readily absorbed after oral administration; metabolised by demethylation to desmethylcolchicine. Up to 50% of a dose is excreted in the urine in 48 hours as unchanged drug and metabolites; colchicine is excreted in the bile and undergoes enterohepatic circulation.

THERAPEUTIC CONCENTRATION.
After a single oral dose of 1 mg given to 10 subjects, a mean peak plasma concentration of 0.003 μg/ml was reported at 0.5 to 2 hours (S. L. Wallace and N. H. Ertel, *Metabolism*, 1973, *22*, 749–753).

Steady-state serum concentrations of 0.0003 to 0.0024 μg/ml were reported after daily oral doses of 1 mg given to 8 subjects (H. Halkin *et al.*, *Clin. Pharmac. Ther.*, 1980, *28*, 82–87).

TOXICITY. The minimum lethal dose in man is about 6 mg although recovery has occurred after much larger doses.

In a reported fatality following the ingestion of 7.5 mg of colchicine together with unknown quantities of phenylbutazone and alcohol, a plasma concentration of 0.02 µg/ml was obtained at 6 hours which decreased to less than 0.005 µg/ml at 24 hours; death occurred 45 hours after ingestion (D. Jarvie *et al., ibid.*).

In a fatality due to the ingestion of colchicine, the following postmortem colchicine concentrations were reported: bile 3.2 µg/ml, liver 1 µg/g. In a second fatality, desmethylcolchicine concentrations were: liver 3.3 µg/g, urine 12.5 µg/ml (W. J. Allender, *J. forens. Sci.*, 1982, *27*, 944–947).

A blood concentration of 0.25 µg/ml was reported in 1 subject, 2 hours after the ingestion of 20 mg of colchicine; death occurred after 40 hours and colchicine was not detectable in the postmortem blood (Y. H. Caplan *et al., ibid.*).

HALF-LIFE. Plasma half-life, about 1 hour.

VOLUME OF DISTRIBUTION. About 0.7 to 2 litres/kg.

PROTEIN BINDING. In plasma, about 30 to 50%.

Dose. 1 mg initially, followed by 500 µg every 2 or 3 hours; maximum total dose of 10 mg.

Conessine   *Anti-amoebic*

3β-Dimethylaminocon-5-enine
$C_{24}H_{40}N_2 = 356.6$
CAS—546-06-5

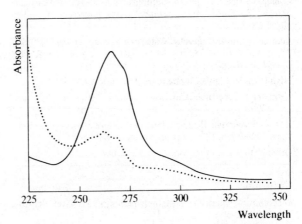

An alkaloid obtained from the seeds of *Holarrhena antidysenterica* (Apocynaceae).
A white crystalline powder. M.p. 127° to 129°.
Sparingly **soluble** in water.

Conessine Hydrobromide
Synonym. Conessine Bromide
$C_{24}H_{40}N_2,2HBr = 518.4$
CAS—5913-82-6
White acicular crystals or microcrystalline powder. M.p. 340°, with decomposition.
Soluble 1 in 5 of water and 1 in 11 of ethanol (90%); very slightly soluble in ether.

Colour Tests. Mandelin's Test—yellow; Marquis Test—yellow → orange.

Thin-layer Chromatography. *System TA*—Rf 28; *system TB*—Rf 49; *system TC*—Rf 03. (*Acidified iodoplatinate solution*, positive.)

Ultraviolet Spectrum. No significant absorption, 230 to 360 nm.

Mass Spectrum. Principal peaks at *m/z* 84, 71, 85, 82, 80, 341, 70, 356.

Dose. Conessine hydrobromide was formerly given in doses of 300 to 500 mg daily.

Coniine   *Alkaloid*

Synonyms. Cicutine; Conicine; Conine.
(*S*)-2-Propylpiperidine
$C_8H_{17}N = 127.2$
CAS—458-88-8

An alkaloid obtained mainly from the fruits and leaves of hemlock, *Conium maculatum* (Umbelliferae).
An almost colourless volatile liquid. F.p. −2°. B.p. 166°.
Soluble 1 in 100 of water; miscible with ethanol and ether; slightly soluble in chloroform.

Coniine Hydrobromide
$C_8H_{17}N,HBr = 208.1$
CAS—637-49-0
Colourless crystals. M.p. about 211°.
Soluble 1 in 2 of water and 1 in 3 of ethanol; soluble in chloroform and ether.

Dissociation Constant. pK_a 11.0 (25°).

Thin-layer Chromatography. *System TA*—Rf 26. (*Acidified iodoplatinate solution*, positive.)

Gas Chromatography. *System GA*—not eluted.

Ultraviolet Spectrum. Aqueous acid—266 nm ($A_1^1 = 6$ b); aqueous alkali—262 nm, 268 nm.

Infra-red Spectrum. Principal peaks at wavenumbers 1033, 1007, 1575, 1300, 1078, 1139 (coniine hydrobromide, Nujol mull).

Mass Spectrum. Principal peaks at *m/z* 84, 82, 80, 56, 43, 28, 30, 41.

Disposition in the Body.

TOXICITY. Coniine is well absorbed from the gastro-intestinal tract and is very poisonous; the estimated minimum lethal dose is 150 mg and toxic symptoms may occur after ingestion of 60 mg. Death may occur within 30 minutes or be delayed 3 to 12 hours. Coniine resembles nicotine in its peripheral action but produces more pronounced paralysis of the central nervous system and of the skeletal muscle nerve-endings.

Cortisone

Corticosteroid

Synonyms. Compound E; 11-Dehydro-17-hydroxycorticoster-one.

17α,21-Dihydroxypregn-4-ene-3,11,20-trione
$C_{21}H_{28}O_5 = 360.4$
CAS—53-06-5

Crystals. M.p. 217° to 224°, with some decomposition.
Very slightly **soluble** in water; soluble in ethanol; sparingly soluble in chloroform and ether.

Cortisone Acetate

Synonym. Cortisone 21-Acetate
Proprietary Names. Adreson; Cortate; Cortelan; Cortisol; Cortison; Cortistab; Cortisyl; Cortone; Cortone Acetate; Sterop.
Note. The name Cortisol is also applied to hydrocortisone.
$C_{23}H_{30}O_6 = 402.5$
CAS—50-04-4
A white crystalline powder. M.p. about 240°, with decomposition.
Soluble 1 in 5000 of water, 1 in 300 to 1 in 350 of ethanol, and 1 in 4 of chloroform; slightly soluble in ether.

Colour Tests. Naphthol–Sulphuric Acid—orange-brown/orange; Sulphuric Acid—yellow (green fluorescence under ultraviolet light).

Thin-layer Chromatography. Cortisone acetate: *system TP*—Rf 72; *system TQ*—Rf 28; *system TR*—Rf 55; *system TS*—Rf 00. (*DPST solution*).

High Pressure Liquid Chromatography. *System HT*—k′ 2.4.

Ultraviolet Spectrum. Cortisone acetate: ethanol—240 nm ($A_1^1 = 390$ a).

Infra-red Spectrum. Principal peaks at wavenumbers 1700, 1660, 1235, 1720, 1275, 1750 (cortisone acetate, KBr disk).

Dose. 25 to 50 mg of cortisone acetate daily.

Cotarnine

Haemostatic

8-Methoxy-2-methyl-6,7-methylenedioxy-1,2,3,4-tetrahydro-isoquinolin-1-ol
$C_{12}H_{15}NO_4 = 237.3$
CAS—82-54-2

An alkaloid obtained by oxidising noscapine with nitric acid.
Crystals. M.p. 132° to 137°, with decomposition.
Slightly **soluble** in water; soluble in ethanol, chloroform, and ether.

Cotarnine Chloride

Synonyms. Cotarnine Hydrochloride; Stypticine.
$C_{12}H_{14}ClNO_3,2H_2O = 291.7$
CAS—10018-19-6 (anhydrous); *16210-52-9* (dihydrate)
A pale yellow deliquescent powder. M.p. 197°. When heated to decomposition, highly toxic fumes are evolved.
Soluble in water, ethanol, and chloroform; practically insoluble in ether.

Colour Tests. Liebermann's Test—black; Mandelin's Test—red-orange→ brown.

Thin-layer Chromatography. *System TA*—Rf 02. (*Acidified iodoplatinate solution*, positive.)

Gas Chromatography. *System GA*—RI 1808.

High Pressure Liquid Chromatography. *System HA*—k′ 8.2 (tailing peak).

Ultraviolet Spectrum. Aqueous acid—253 nm ($A_1^1 = 582$ b), 332 nm ($A_1^1 = 666$ b); aqueous alkali—286 nm, 330 nm.

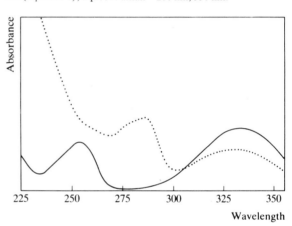

Infra-red Spectrum. Principal peaks at wavenumbers 1605, 1086, 1490, 1655, 1505, 1300 (cotarnine chloride, KCl disk).

Dose. Cotarnine chloride was formerly given in doses of 20 to 100 mg.

Coumatetralyl

Rodenticide

Proprietary Name. Racumin
4-Hydroxy-3-(1,2,3,4-tetrahydro-1-naphthyl)coumarin
$C_{19}H_{16}O_3 = 292.3$
CAS—5836-29-3

A yellowish-white crystalline powder. M.p. 172° to 176°.
Practically **insoluble** in water; soluble in ethanol and acetone; slightly soluble in ether.

Thin-layer Chromatography. *System TD*—Rf 73; *system TE*—Rf 13; *system TF*—Rf 74. (Location under ultraviolet light, pink fluorescence; *acidified potassium permanganate solution*, positive.)

Ultraviolet Spectrum. Aqueous acid—275 nm, 285 nm, 309 nm; aqueous alkali—311 nm.

Infra-red Spectrum. Principal peaks at wavenumbers 1615, 762, 740, 1685, 1250, 1570.

Mass Spectrum. Principal peaks at m/z 292, 121, 188, 130, 115, 91, 128, 129.

Cresol   *Disinfectant*

Synonyms. Cresylic Acid; Tricresol. It is an ingredient of Lysol (Cresol and Soap Solution containing 50% v/v of cresol).
Note. The use of the name Lysol is limited. In some countries it is a trade-mark applied to a product of different composition.
Proprietary Name. It is an ingredient of Lyseptol.
Cresol is a mixture of *o*-, *m*-, and *p*-cresols ($CH_3 \cdot C_6H_4 \cdot OH = 108 \cdot 1$), in which the *m*-isomer predominates, and of other phenols obtained from coal tar.
CAS—1319-77-3; *95-48-7* (*o*-cresol); *108-39-4* (*m*-cresol); *106-44-5* (*p*-cresol)
An almost colourless to pale brownish-yellow liquid, becoming darker with age or on exposure to light. Wt per ml 1.029 to 1.044 g. B.p. 195° to 205°.
Almost completely **soluble** 1 in 50 of water; miscible with ethanol, chloroform, and ether.

Dissociation Constant. pK_a *m*-cresol 10.1, *o*-cresol 10.3, *p*-cresol 10.3 (25°).

Colour Tests. Folin–Ciocalteu Reagent—blue; Liebermann's Test—black; Potassium Dichromate—brown (*o*-cresol—30 s, *m*-cresol—2 min).
Heat with about an equal quantity of phthalic anhydride and a few drops of *sulphuric acid* until the mixture is orange-brown; cool the mixture with a few drops of water and make alkaline with *sodium hydroxide solution*—red with *o*-cresol and blue-violet with *m*-cresol.

Ultraviolet Spectrum. Aqueous alkali—239 nm ($A_1^1 = 949$ b), 290 nm ($A_1^1 = 251$ b); ethanol—275 nm ($A_1^1 = 163$ b), 279 nm ($A_1^1 = 145$ b).

Infra-red Spectrum. Principal peaks at wavenumbers 1209, 816, 1515, 741, 1176, 1105 (*p*-cresol, Nujol mull).

Mass Spectrum. Principal peaks at m/z 107, 108, 77, 79, 51, 39, 53, 50 (*p*-cresol).

Quantification. GAS CHROMATOGRAPHY. In blood, urine or tissues: sensitivity 20 µg/ml, FID—A. M. Bruce *et al.*, *Medicine, Sci. Law*, 1976, *16*, 171–176.

Disposition in the Body. Absorbed after ingestion, and through the skin and mucous membranes. It is metabolised by conjugation and oxidation; *p*-cresol is endogenously produced in normal subjects, and may be present in urine at concentrations of 20 to 200 µg/ml (mainly in conjugated form).

TOXICITY. The estimated minimum lethal dose is 2 g, and the maximum permissible atmospheric concentration is 5 ppm.

In 2 fatalities due to the ingestion of cresol, the following postmortem tissue concentrations were reported: blood 71, 190 µg/ml; brain 2.8, – µg/g; kidney 396, – µg/g; liver 900, 480 µg/g; urine –, 304 µg/ml (A. M. Bruce *et al.*, *ibid.*).

Cropropamide   *Respiratory Stimulant*

Synonym. It is an ingredient of Prethcamide which is a mixture of equal parts by weight of cropropamide and crotethamide.
Proprietary Names. It is an ingredient of Micoren and of Respirot.

NN-Dimethyl-2-(*N*-propylcrotonamido)butyramide
$C_{13}H_{24}N_2O_2 = 240.3$
CAS—633-47-6 (cropropamide); *8015-51-8* (prethcamide)

$$CH_3 \cdot CH\text{:}CH \cdot CO \cdot N \cdot CH \cdot CO \cdot N(CH_3)_2$$

with C_2H_5 and $CH_2 \cdot CH_2 \cdot CH_3$ substituents

A liquid.
Miscible with water, ethanol, and ether.

Thin-layer Chromatography. *System TA*—Rf 64; *system TB*—Rf 29; *system TC*—Rf 69. (*Acidified potassium permanganate solution, positive.*)

Gas Chromatography. *System GA*—RI 1738.

Ultraviolet Spectrum. No significant absorption, 230 to 360 nm.

Infra-red Spectrum. Principal peaks at wavenumbers 1654, 1617, 1219, 1282, 1098, 1123 (K Br disk).

Dose. Prethcamide (cropropamide and crotethamide) is usually given in doses of 1.2 to 1.6 g daily.

Crotamiton   *Acaricide/Antipruritic*

Proprietary Names. Crotamitex; Eurax; Euraxil.
N-Ethylcrotono-*o*-toluidide
$C_{13}H_{17}NO = 203.3$
CAS—483-63-6

$$CH_3 \cdot CH\text{:}CH \cdot CO \cdot N \cdot C_2H_5$$

with CH_3 substituent on ring

A colourless or pale yellow, oily liquid.
Soluble 1 in 400 of water; miscible with ethanol, ether, and methanol.

Thin-layer Chromatography. *System TA*—Rf 83. (*Acidified iodoplatinate solution*, positive.)

Gas Chromatography. *System GA*—RI 1550.

Ultraviolet Spectrum. No significant absorption, 230 to 360 nm.

Infra-red Spectrum. Principal peaks at wavenumbers 1656, 1623, 1235, 1280, 1316, 1590 (thin film).

Use. Topically in a concentration of 10%.

Crotethamide   *Respiratory Stimulant*

Synonyms. Crotetamide. It is an ingredient of Prethcamide which is a mixture of equal parts by weight of cropropamide and crotethamide.
Proprietary Names. It is an ingredient of Micoren and of Respirot.
2-(*N*-Ethylcrotonamido)-*NN*-dimethylbutyramide
$C_{12}H_{22}N_2O_2 = 226.3$
CAS—6168-76-9 (crotethamide); *8015-51-8* (prethcamide)

$$CH_3 \cdot CH\text{:}CH \cdot CO \cdot N \cdot CH \cdot CO \cdot N(CH_3)_2$$

with C_2H_5 substituents

A liquid.

Miscible with water, ethanol, and ether.

Thin-layer Chromatography. *System TA*—Rf 61; *system TB*—Rf 28; *system TC*—Rf 67. (*Acidified potassium permanganate solution, positive.*)

Gas Chromatography. *System GA*—RI 1688.

Ultraviolet Spectrum. No significant absorption, 230 to 360 nm.

Infra-red Spectrum. Principal peaks at wavenumbers 1655, 1617, 1234, 1098, 1282, 1123 (KBr disk).

Dose. See under Cropropamide.

Cyanocobalamin   *Haemopoietic Vitamin*

Synonyms. Cobamin; Cycobemin; Vitamin B_{12}.
Proprietary Names. Anacobin; Bedoz; Berubigen; Betalin 12; Bio-12; Cyanabin; Cytacon; Cytamen; Hepacon-B12; Neo-Rubex; Redisol; Rubesol; Rubion; Rubramin; Ruvite; Sytobex. It is an ingredient of Ce-Cobalin, Hepanorm, and Reactivan.
Coα-[α-(5,6-Dimethylbenzimidazolyl)]-Coβ-cyanocobamide
$C_{63}H_{88}CoN_{14}O_{14}P = 1355$
CAS—68-19-9
Dark red hygroscopic crystals or powder.
Soluble 1 in 80 of water and 1 in 180 of ethanol (90%); practically insoluble in chloroform and ether.

Ultraviolet Spectrum. Water—278 nm ($A_1^1 = 119$ a), 361 nm ($A_1^1 = 207$ a), 550 nm ($A_1^1 = 63$ a).

Infra-red Spectrum. Principal peaks at wavenumbers 1660, 1497, 1575, 1070, 1150, 1220 (KBr disk).

Dose. Initially 0.25 to 1 mg intramuscularly, on alternate days.

Cyclandelate   *Vasodilator*

Proprietary Names. Cyclobral; Cyclospasmol; Spasmocyclon.
3,3,5-Trimethylcyclohexyl mandelate
$C_{17}H_{24}O_3 = 276.4$
CAS—456-59-7

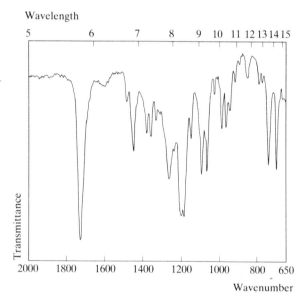

A white amorphous powder, which may sublime on storage into a crystalline form resembling cotton wool. M.p. below 60°.
Practically **insoluble** in water; soluble 1 in about 1 of ethanol; very soluble in ether.

Colour Tests. Liebermann's Test—orange; Marquis Test—orange (slow).

Thin-layer Chromatography. *System TD*—Rf 74; *system TE*—Rf 81; *system TF*—Rf 71.

Gas Chromatography. *System GA*—RI 1903.

Ultraviolet Spectrum. Methanol—252 nm, 258 nm ($A_1^1 = 7.6$ b), 264 nm.

Infra-red Spectrum. Principal peaks at wavenumbers 1734, 1192, 1212, 1274, 1104, 1074 (KBr disk).

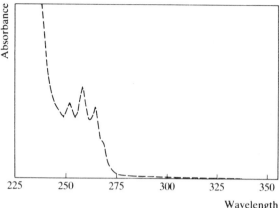

Mass Spectrum. Principal peaks at *m/z* 107, 69, 125, 83, 79, 55, 41, 77.

Dose. 1.6 g daily.

Cyclazocine   *Narcotic Antagonist*

3-Cyclopropylmethyl-1,2,3,4,5,6-hexahydro-6,11-dimethyl-2,6-methano-3-benzazocin-8-ol
$C_{18}H_{25}NO = 271.4$
CAS—3572-80-3

Crystals. M.p. 201° to 204°.
Soluble in chloroform and dilute acetic acid.

Partition Coefficient. Log P (octanol/pH 7.4), 1.3.

Colour Tests. Liebermann's Test—black; Mandelin's Test—green; Marquis Test—brown → green.

Thin-layer Chromatography. *System TA*—Rf 53; *system TB*—Rf 15; *system TC*—Rf 13. (*Acidified iodoplatinate solution*, strong reaction.)

High Pressure Liquid Chromatography. *System HA*—k' 2.1.

Ultraviolet Spectrum. Aqueous acid—277 nm; aqueous alkali—237 nm, 298 nm.

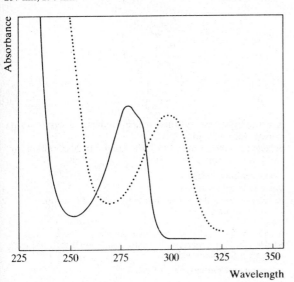

Infra-red Spectrum. Principal peaks at wavenumbers 1570, 1255, 1304, 754, 1227, 1241 (KBr disk).

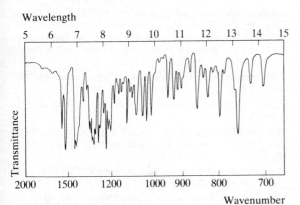

Mass Spectrum. Principal peaks at m/z 230, 271, 55, 256, 164, 270, 71, 124.

Quantification. GAS CHROMATOGRAPHY. In urine: cyclazocine and norcyclazocine, sensitivity 40 ng, FID—R. F. Kaiko and C. E. Inturrisi, *J. Chromat.*, 1974, **100**, 63–72.

GAS CHROMATOGRAPHY-MASS SPECTROMETRY. In plasma: comparison with radioimmunoassay, detection limits 110 pg/ml and 20 pg/ml respectively—J. E. Peterson *et al.*, *J. pharm. Sci.*, 1979, **68**, 1447–1450.

Disposition in the Body. Absorbed after oral administration. About 20% of a dose is excreted in the urine unchanged together with 24% as conjugated cyclazocine, 4% as norcyclazocine, and 11% as conjugated norcyclazocine.

Dose. Cyclazocine has been given in maintenance doses of about 4 mg daily; doses of 10 mg have been given to extend the effect to 48 hours.

Cyclizine   *Antihistamine/Anti-emetic*

1-Benzhydryl-4-methylpiperazine
$C_{18}H_{22}N_2 = 266.4$
CAS—82-92-8

$$C_6H_5 \cdot CH \cdot C_6H_5$$

A white or creamy-white crystalline powder. M.p. 106° to 109°. Practically **insoluble** in water; soluble 1 in 6 of ethanol, 1 in 1 of chloroform, and 1 in 6 of ether.

Cyclizine Hydrochloride
Synonym. Cyclizinium Chloride
Proprietary Names. Marezine (tablets); Marzine; Valoid (tablets). It is an ingredient of Diconal, Migril, and Wellconal.
$C_{18}H_{22}N_2,HCl = 302.8$
CAS—303-25-3
A white crystalline powder, or small colourless crystals. M.p. about 285°, with decomposition.
Soluble 1 in about 125 of water, 1 in about 120 of ethanol, and 1 in 75 of chloroform; practically insoluble in ether.

Cyclizine Lactate
Proprietary Names. Marezine (injection); Valoid (injection).
$C_{18}H_{22}N_2,C_3H_6O_3 = 356.5$
CAS—5897-19-8
Freely **soluble** in water.

Dissociation Constant. pK_a 2.4, 7.8.

Colour Tests. Liebermann's Test—orange; Marquis Test—yellow.

Thin-layer Chromatography. *System TA*—Rf 57; *system TB*—Rf 49; *system TC*—Rf 41. (*Dragendorff spray*, positive; *acidified iodoplatinate solution*, positive; *Marquis reagent*, yellow.)

Gas Chromatography. *System GA*—cyclizine RI 2020, norcyclizine RI 2050; *system GB*—RI 2081; *system GC*—RI 2348; *system GF*—RI 2320.

High Pressure Liquid Chromatography. *System HA*—cyclizine k' 2.9, norcyclizine k' 2.2.

Ultraviolet Spectrum. Aqueous acid—257 nm, 262 nm ($A_1^1 = 28$ a), 268 nm; aqueous alkali—260 nm ($A_1^1 = 16$ b). (See below)

Infra-red Spectrum. Principal peaks at wavenumbers 716, 756, 701, 984, 1125, 1496 (cyclizine hydrochloride, KBr disk). (See below)

Mass Spectrum. Principal peaks at m/z 99, 56, 167, 207, 194, 266, 195, 165.

Quantification. GAS CHROMATOGRAPHY. In plasma or urine: cyclizine and norcyclizine, sensitivity 10 ng/ml for cyclizine, AFID—G. Land *et al.*, *J. Chromat.*, 1981, **222**; *Biomed. Appl.*, **11**, 135–140. In blood or urine: sensitivity 10 ng/ml and 5 ng/ml,

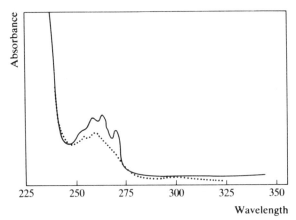

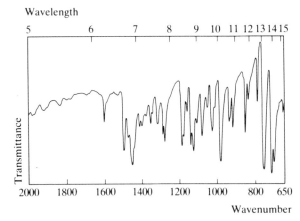

respectively, AFID—D. S. Griffin and R. C. Baselt. *J. analyt. Toxicol.*, 1984, *8*, 97–99.

Disposition in the Body. Cyclizine is extensively metabolised by *N*-demethylation to form norcyclizine, a metabolite which is widely distributed throughout the tissues and especially in lungs, kidneys, liver, and spleen. After a dose of 50 mg of cyclizine thrice daily, 1 to 1.8 mg of norcyclizine is excreted in the urine in 4 days.

THERAPEUTIC CONCENTRATION.
Following a single oral dose of 50 mg of cyclizine hydrochloride to 1 subject, a peak blood concentration of 0.069 µg/ml was attained in 2 hours (D. S. Griffin and R. C. Baselt, *ibid.*).
On the first day after termination of therapy with oral doses of 50 mg thrice daily to 4 subjects, plasma concentrations of norcyclizine were in the range of 0.004 to 0.022 µg/ml (mean 0.014) (R. Kuntzman *et al.*, *J. Pharmac. exp. Ther.*, 1967, *158*, 332–339).

TOXICITY.
In a fatality attributed principally to cyclizine, postmortem concentrations were: blood 15 µg/ml, liver 108 µg/g; doxepin was also detected at concentrations of 0.7 µg/ml and 6 µg/g in the blood and liver, respectively (J. F. Lewin *et al.*, *Bull. int. Ass. forens. Toxicol.*, 1981, *16*(2), 23–24).
For case histories involving the injection of cyclizine with dipipanone, see under Dipipanone.

HALF-LIFE. Plasma half-life, cyclizine about 24 hours.

PROTEIN BINDING. In plasma, norcyclizine about 60%.

Dose. Up to 150 mg of cyclizine hydrochloride daily.

Cyclobarbitone   *Barbiturate*

Synonyms. Cyclobarbital; Ethylhexabital; Hexemalum.
Note. The name ciclobarbital has been applied to hexobarbitone.
5-(Cyclohex-1-enyl)-5-ethylbarbituric acid
$C_{12}H_{16}N_2O_3 = 236.3$
CAS—52-31-3

A white crystalline powder, which gradually decomposes on storage. M.p. 171° to 175°.
Soluble 1 in 800 of water, 1 in 4 of ethanol, 1 in 20 of chloroform, and 1 in 15 of ether.

Cyclobarbitone Calcium
Synonym. Hexemalcalcium
Proprietary Names. Phanodorm. It is an ingredient of Evidorm.
$(C_{12}H_{15}N_2O_3)_2Ca = 510.6$
CAS—143-76-0
A white or slightly yellowish, crystalline powder.
Soluble 1 in 100 of water; very slightly soluble in ethanol; practically insoluble in chloroform and ether.

Dissociation Constant. pK_a 7.6 (20°).

Partition Coefficient. Log *P* (octanol/pH 7.4), 1.8.

Colour Tests. Koppanyi–Zwikker Test—violet; Mercurous Nitrate—black; Vanillin Reagent—brown-red/green.

Thin-layer Chromatography. *System TD*—Rf 50; *system TE*—Rf 35; *system TF*—Rf 64; *system TH*—Rf 59. (*Mercuric chloride-diphenylcarbazone reagent*, positive; *mercurous nitrate spray*, black; *acidified potassium permanganate solution*, yellow-brown; *Zwikker's reagent*, pink.)

Gas Chromatography. *System GA*—cyclobarbitone RI 1963, ketocyclobarbitone RI 2190; *system GF*—RI 2825.

High Pressure Liquid Chromatography. *System HG*—k′ 5.25; *system HH*—k′ 2.61.

Ultraviolet Spectrum. *Borax buffer 0.05M* (pH 9.2)—239 nm $(A_1^1 = 410 \text{ a})$; M sodium hydroxide (pH 13)—256 nm $(A_1^1 = 320 \text{ b})$.

Infra-red Spectrum. Principal peaks at wavenumbers 1693, 1725, 1745, 1300, 1210, 830 (KBr disk).

Mass Spectrum. Principal peaks at *m/z* 207, 141, 81, 79, 67, 80, 41, 77.

Quantification. See under Amylobarbitone.

Disposition in the Body. Rapidly absorbed after oral administration. The main metabolic reaction appears to be oxidation to ketocyclobarbitone [5-(3-oxocyclohex-1-enyl)-5-ethylbarbituric acid]. Less than 10% of a dose is excreted in the urine unchanged.

THERAPEUTIC CONCENTRATION. In plasma, usually in the range 2 to 10 µg/ml.

After a single oral dose of 300 mg of the calcium salt, given to 6 subjects, peak plasma concentrations of 7.4 to 10.3 µg/ml (mean 8.7) were attained

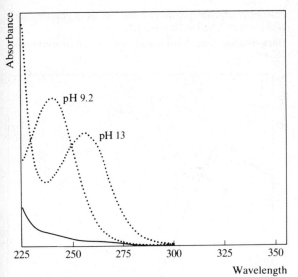

Wavelength

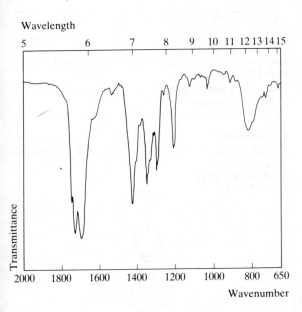

Wavenumber

Cyclobenzaprine

Muscle Relaxant

Synonyms. CBZ; Proheptatriene.

3-(5*H*-Dibenzo[*a,d*]cyclohepten-5-ylidene)-*NN*-dimethylpropylamine

$C_{20}H_{21}N = 275.4$

CAS—303-53-7

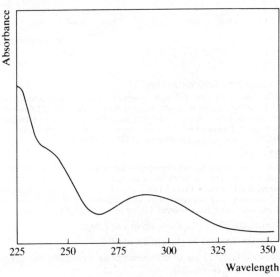

Cyclobenzaprine Hydrochloride

Proprietary Name. Flexeril

$C_{20}H_{21}N,HCl = 311.9$

CAS—6202-23-9

A white crystalline powder. M.p. 215° to 219°.

Freely **soluble** in water and ethanol; slightly soluble in chloroform.

Ultraviolet Spectrum. Aqueous acid—290 nm ($A_1^1 = 407$ b). No alkaline shift.

Infra-red Spectrum. Principal peaks at wavenumbers 764, 778, 800, 968, 988, 880 (KBr disk). (See below)

Mass Spectrum. Principal peaks at *m/z* 58, 59, 42, 215, 202, 57, 189, 43.

Quantification. GAS CHROMATOGRAPHY. In plasma or urine: sensitivity 10 ng/ml, FID—H. B. Hucker and S. C. Stauffer, *J. pharm. Sci.*, 1976, *65*, 1253–1255. In plasma: sensitivity 2 ng/ml, AFID—H. B. Hucker and S. C. Stauffer, *J. Chromat.*, 1976, *124*, 164–168.

Disposition in the Body. Irregularly absorbed after oral administration, and extensively metabolised. The major metabolites are a glucuronide conjugate and 10,11-dihydroxynortriptyline; monodesmethylcyclobenzaprine is a minor metabolite. About 50% of an oral dose is excreted in the urine in 5 days, with less than 1% as unchanged drug. About 14% of a dose is eliminated in the faeces.

in 0.7 to 2.5 hours (D. D. Breimer and A. C. M. Winten, *Eur. J. clin. Pharmac.*, 1976, *9*, 443–450).

TOXICITY. The estimated minimum lethal dose is 2 g. Severe toxic effects are associated with blood concentrations greater than 10 µg/ml.

HALF-LIFE. Plasma half-life, 8 to 17 hours (mean 12), increased in subjects with liver disease.

VOLUME OF DISTRIBUTION. About 0.5 litre/kg.

CLEARANCE. Plasma clearance, about 0.5 ml/min/kg.

PROTEIN BINDING. In plasma, about 70%.

Dose. 100 to 400 mg of cyclobarbitone calcium, as a hypnotic.

Wavelength

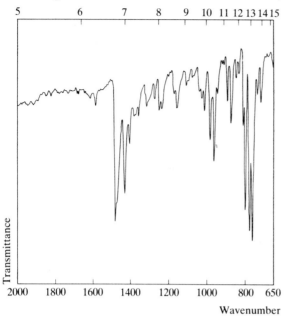

Wavenumber

Practically **insoluble** in water; soluble 1 in 250 of ethanol, 1 in 2 of chloroform, and 1 in 30 of ether.

Ultraviolet Spectrum. Acid ethanol—247 nm; alkaline ethanol—262 nm.

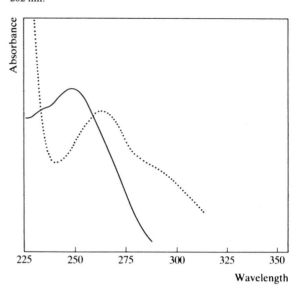

Wavelength

Infra-red Spectrum. Principal peaks at wavenumbers 1204, 1219, 1754, 917, 1162, 1492.

Dose. 200 to 400 mg daily; doses of 800 mg daily have been given in 5-day courses.

THERAPEUTIC CONCENTRATION.

After a single oral dose of 40 mg to 4 subjects, peak plasma concentrations of about 0.027 μg/ml were attained in 4 hours; following oral doses of 20 mg three times a day to 9 subjects, a mean peak plasma concentration of 0.034 μg/ml was reported 6 hours after the first dose on the fourth day (H. B. Hucker *et al.*, *J. clin. Pharmac.*, 1977, *17*, 719–727).

TOXICITY.

In a fatality where cyclobenzaprine was the suspected cause of death, the following postmortem tissue concentrations were reported: blood 0.46 μg/ml, bile 12.0 μg/ml, liver 12.4 μg/g, urine 3.2 μg/ml; low concentrations of morphine and diazepam were also detected (B. K. Beck and T. Lamoreaux, *Bull. int. Ass. forens. Toxicol.*, 1979, *14*(3), 27).

HALF-LIFE. Plasma half-life, about 1 to 3 days.

PROTEIN BINDING. In plasma, about 93%.

Dose. Usually 30 mg of cyclobenzaprine hydrochloride daily; maximum of 60 mg daily.

Cyclofenil
Induction of Ovulation

Proprietary Names. Fertodur; Ondogyne; Ondonid; Rehibin; Sexovid.

4,4′-(Cyclohexylidenemethylene)bis(phenyl acetate)
$C_{23}H_{24}O_4 = 364.4$
CAS—2624-43-3

$CH_3 \cdot CO \cdot O$ — — $O \cdot CO \cdot CH_3$

A white crystalline powder. M.p. 137° to 140°.

Cycloguanil
Antimalarial

1-(4-Chlorophenyl)-1,2-dihydro-2,2-dimethyl-1,3,5-triazine-4,6-diamine
$C_{11}H_{14}ClN_5 = 251.7$
CAS—516-21-2

Cl
NH_2 CH_3
         CH_3
NH_2

Crystals. M.p. 146°.

Cycloguanil Embonate

Synonym. Cycloguanil Pamoate
$C_{11}H_{14}ClN_5, \frac{1}{2}(C_{23}H_{16}O_6) = 445.9$
CAS—609-78-9

A pale greenish-yellow, crystalline powder. M.p. 231° to 234°.
Practically **insoluble** in water; sparingly soluble in dimethylformamide.

Ultraviolet Spectrum. Methanol—237 nm ($A_1^1 = 2250$ b), 278 nm, 289 nm ($A_1^1 = 180$ b), 301 nm.

Infra-red Spectrum. Principal peaks at wavenumbers 1673, 1515, 1628, 1570, 760, 1224 (KBr disk).

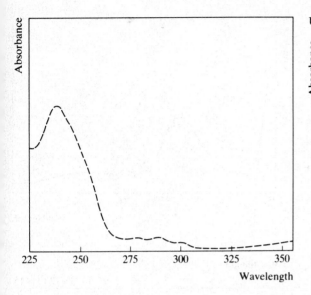

Ultraviolet Spectrum. Aqueous acid—261 nm ($A_1^1 = 508$ a).

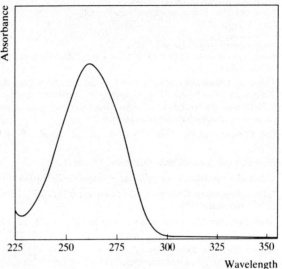

Quantification. See under Proguanil.

Disposition in the Body. Slowly absorbed after intramuscular administration and excreted mainly in the urine.
Cycloguanil is the active metabolite of proguanil.

Dose. The equivalent of 5 to 6 mg/kg of cycloguanil, intramuscularly, every 4 months.

Cyclomethycaine   *Local Anaesthetic*

3-(2-Methylpiperidino)propyl 4-cyclohexyloxybenzoate
$C_{22}H_{33}NO_3 = 359.5$
CAS—139-62-8

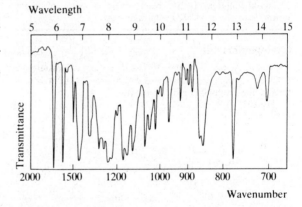

A white crystalline powder.
Sparingly **soluble** in water, ethanol, and ether; very slightly soluble in chloroform.

Cyclomethycaine Sulphate
Proprietary Name. Surfacaine
$C_{22}H_{33}NO_3,H_2SO_4 = 457.6$
CAS—50978-10-4
A white crystalline powder. M.p. 162° to 166°.
Soluble 1 in 50 of water, 1 in 50 of ethanol, and 1 in about 227 of chloroform.

Colour Test. Mandelin's Test—green → brown.

Thin-layer Chromatography. *System TA*—Rf 58; *system TB*—Rf 55; *system TC*—Rf 36; *system TL*—Rf 25. (*Acidified iodoplatinate solution*, positive.)

High Pressure Liquid Chromatography. *System HR*—k' 10.31.

Infra-red Spectrum. Principal peaks at wavenumbers 1704, 1605, 1253, 775, 1170, 1235 (cyclomethycaine sulphate, Nujol mull).

Mass Spectrum. Principal peaks at *m/z* 112, 344, 121, 41, 67, 55, 54, 345.

Use. Cyclomethycaine sulphate has been used in concentrations of 0.5 to 1%.

Cyclopentamine   *Sympathomimetic*

Synonym. Cyclopentadrin
2-Cyclopentyl-1,*N*-dimethylethylamine
$C_9H_{19}N = 141.3$
CAS—102-45-4

Cyclopentamine Hydrochloride

Synonym. Cyclopentaminium Chloride
Proprietary Name. It is an ingredient of Co-Pyronil.
$C_9H_{19}N,HCl = 177.7$
CAS—538-02-3
A white crystalline powder. M.p. 111° to 117°.
Soluble 1 in 1 of water, 1 in 2 of ethanol, and 1 in 1 of chloroform; slightly soluble in ether.

Thin-layer Chromatography. *System TA*—Rf 20; *system TB*—Rf 32; *system TC*—Rf 10. (*Dragendorff spray*, positive; *acidified iodoplatinate solution*, positive; *ninhydrin spray*, positive; *acidified potassium permanganate solution*, positive.)

Gas Chromatography. *System GA*—RI 1087; *system GB*—RI 1095.

High Pressure Liquid Chromatography. *System HA*—k' 1.7.

Ultraviolet Spectrum. No significant absorption, 230 to 360 nm.

Infra-red Spectrum. Principal peaks at wavenumbers 1585, 1020, 1050, 1100, 1082, 1158.

Mass Spectrum. Principal peaks at *m/z* 58, 41, 30, 126, 59, 69, 56, 44.

Disposition in the Body.
TOXICITY. The estimated minimum lethal dose for children up to 2 years is 200 mg when applied to the mucous membranes; the minimum lethal dose for adults may be at least 10 times greater.

Dose. Cyclopentamine hydrochloride has been used as a 0.5 or 1% nasal solution. It has been given in doses of 25 mg intramuscularly, or 5 to 10 mg intravenously.

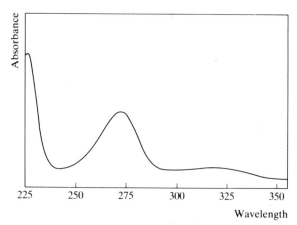

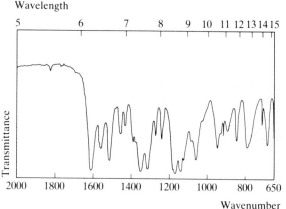

Cyclopenthiazide   *Diuretic*

Proprietary Names. Navidrex. It is an ingredient of Trasidrex.
6-Chloro-3-cyclopentylmethyl-3,4-dihydro-2*H*-1,2,4-benzothiadiazine-7-sulphonamide 1,1-dioxide
$C_{13}H_{18}ClN_3O_4S_2 = 379.9$
CAS—742-20-1

A white powder. M.p. 235°, with decomposition.
Practically **insoluble** in water; soluble 1 in 12 of ethanol and 1 in 600 of chloroform; soluble in ether.

Colour Tests. Koppanyi–Zwikker Test—violet; Liebermann's Test—brown-green; Sulphuric Acid—yellow.

Thin-layer Chromatography. *System TD*—Rf 21; *system TE*—Rf 66; *system TF*—Rf 62.

High Pressure Liquid Chromatography. *System HN*—k' 16.45.

Ultraviolet Spectrum. Aqueous acid—274 nm ($A_1^1 = 556$ a), 319 nm. No alkaline shift.

Infra-red Spectrum. Principal peaks at wavenumbers 1168, 1138, 1605, 1309, 1511, 1060 (KBr disk).

Mass Spectrum. Principal peaks at *m/z* 296, 41, 44, 110, 298, 285, 55, 268.

Dose. 250 to 500 µg daily; maximum of 1.5 mg daily.

Cyclopentobarbitone   *Barbiturate*

Synonyms. Cyclopentenylallyl Barbituric Acid; Cyclopentobarbital.
Proprietary Name. Cyclopal
5-Allyl-5-(cyclopent-2-enyl)barbituric acid
$C_{12}H_{14}N_2O_3 = 234.3$
CAS—76-68-6

Crystals. M.p. 139° to 140°.
Slightly **soluble** in cold water; more soluble in hot water; freely soluble in ethanol.

Colour Test. Vanillin Reagent—brown-red/green.

Thin-layer Chromatography. *System TD*—Rf 50; *system TE*—Rf 37; *system TF*—Rf 64; *system TH*—Rf 62.

Gas Chromatography. *System GA*—RI 1862.

High Pressure Liquid Chromatography. *System HG*—k' 6.00; *system HH*—k' 3.84.

Ultraviolet Spectrum. *Borax buffer 0.05M* (pH 9.2)—241 nm (A_1^1 = 411 a); M sodium hydroxide (pH 13)—254 nm (A_1^1 = 306 b).

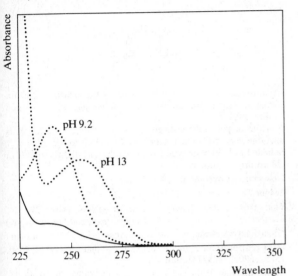

Infra-red Spectrum. Principal peaks at wavenumbers 1700, 1755, 1212, 815, 1319, 848 (KBr disk).

Mass Spectrum. Principal peaks at *m/z* 67, 193, 66, 41, 169, 39, 65, 77.

Dose. Cyclopentobarbitone has been given in a dose of 100 to 200 mg.

Cyclopentolate   *Anticholinergic*

2-Dimethylaminoethyl 2-(1-hydroxycyclopentyl)-2-phenylace-tate
$C_{17}H_{25}NO_3$ = 291.4
CAS—512-15-2

HO CH·CO·O·[CH₂]₂·N(CH₃)₂ with C₆H₅

Cyclopentolate Hydrochloride
Proprietary Names. Cyclogyl; Cyclopen; Mydplegic; Mydrilate; Skiacol P.O.S.; Zyklolat.
$C_{17}H_{25}NO_3,HCl$ = 327.9
CAS—5870-29-1
A white crystalline powder. M.p. 135° to 138°.
Soluble 1 in less than 1 of water and 1 in 5 of ethanol; practically insoluble in ether.

Dissociation Constant. pK_a 7.9.

Colour Test. Mandelin's Test—brown.

Thin-layer Chromatography. *System TA*—Rf 57; *system TB*—Rf 27; *system TC*—Rf 39.

Gas Chromatography. *System GA*—RI 2020.

High Pressure Liquid Chromatography. *System HA*—k' 1.6 (tailing peak).

Ultraviolet Spectrum. Aqueous acid—252 nm (A_1^1 = 5 a), 258 nm (A_1^1 = 6 a), 264 nm (A_1^1 = 5 a). No alkaline shift.

Infra-red Spectrum. Principal peaks at wavenumbers 1148, 1733, 704, 1199, 735, 990 (cyclopentolate hydrochloride, KBr disk).

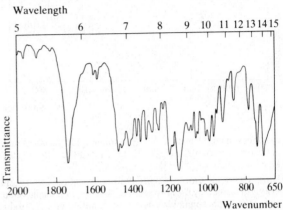

Mass Spectrum. Principal peaks at *m/z* 58, 71, 72, 207, 42, 91, 59, 118.

Use. Cyclopentolate hydrochloride is used as a 0.5 to 1% ophthalmic solution.

Cyclophosphamide   *Antineoplastic*

Proprietary Names. Cytoxan; Endoxan(a); Procytox; Sendoxan.
2-[Bis(2-chloroethyl)amino]perhydro-1,3,2-oxazaphosphorine 2-oxide monohydrate
$C_7H_{15}Cl_2N_2O_2P,H_2O$ = 279.1
CAS—50-18-0 (anhydrous); *6055-19-2* (monohydrate)

A fine, white, crystalline powder which discolours on exposure to light. M.p. 49° to 53°. It liquefies upon loss of its water of crystallisation. In aqueous solutions, at temperatures above 30°, hydrolysis occurs with removal of chlorine.
Soluble 1 in 25 of water and 1 in 1 of ethanol; slightly soluble in ether.

Colour Test. Phosphorus Test—yellow precipitate.

Gas Chromatography. *System GA*—RI 2191.

Ultraviolet Spectrum. No significant absorption, 230 to 360 nm.

Infra-red Spectrum. Principal peaks at wavenumbers 1225, 1044, 975, 1088, 945, 1128 (KBr disk). (See below)

Quantification. GAS CHROMATOGRAPHY. In plasma: sensitivity 10 ng/ml, AFID—N. Van den Bosch and D. De Vos, *J. Chromat.*, 1980, *183*; *Biomed. Appl.*, *9*, 49–56. In plasma or urine: detection limit 10 ng/ml, AFID—T. Facchinetti *et al.*, *J. Chromat.*, 1978, *145*; *Biomed. Appl.*, *2*, 315–318. In plasma:

Wavelength

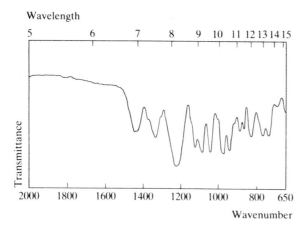

cyclophosphamide metabolites (phosphoramide mustard and nornitrogen mustard), AFID—F. D. Juma *et al.*, *Br. J. clin. Pharmac.*, 1980, *10*, 327–335.

HIGH PRESSURE LIQUID CHROMATOGRAPHY–MASS SPECTROMETRY. In urine: cyclophosphamide, 4-ketocyclophosphamide and carboxyphosphamide, detection limit 10 pg—U. Bahr and H.-R. Schulten, *Biomed. Mass Spectrom.*, 1981, *8*, 553–557.

Disposition in the Body. Well absorbed after oral administration; bioavailability greater than 75%. The parent drug is inactive, but is converted into active metabolites by the liver. The drug and metabolites are widely distributed in the body. It is oxidised to 4-hydroxycyclophosphamide, which is in equilibrium with aldophosphamide, both of which are cytotoxic. 4-Hydroxycyclophosphamide can be oxidised further to 4-ketocyclophosphamide (inactive). Aldophosphamide may be converted to the cytotoxic metabolites phosphoramide mustard and acrolein, or oxidised to inactive carboxyphosphamide. Carboxyphosphamide may be converted to nornitrogen mustard, an active alkylating agent at acid pH. Up to 95% of a dose is excreted in the urine, mostly during the first 48 hours, with up to 25% as unchanged drug and the rest as metabolites. Small amounts are excreted in the bile and faeces.

THERAPEUTIC CONCENTRATION.
After a single intravenous dose of 9.4 mg/kg to a patient, a plasma concentration of about 26 μg/ml of cyclophosphamide was attained immediately after injection, and this fell to about 13 μg/ml after 2 hours. After single intravenous doses of 9 to 12 mg/kg and 40 mg/kg, peak plasma concentrations of unbound alkylating metabolites of about 0.3 to 2 μg/ml (8 studies) and about 2 to 6 μg/ml (7 studies), respectively, were achieved, usually after 2 to 3 hours (C. M. Bagley, jun., *et al.*, *Cancer Res.*, 1973, *33*, 226–233).

HALF-LIFE. Plasma half-life, about 3 to 12 hours (mean 7).

VOLUME OF DISTRIBUTION. About 0.7 litre/kg.

CLEARANCE. Plasma clearance, about 1 ml/min/kg.

SALIVA. Plasma: saliva ratio, about 1.6.

PROTEIN BINDING. In plasma, cyclophosphamide about 12 to 24%, alkylating metabolites about 50 to 60%.

NOTE. For a review of the pharmacokinetics of cyclophosphamide, see L. B. Grochow and M. Colvin, *Clin. Pharmacokinet.*, 1979, *4*, 380–394.

Dose. Regimens usually range from 2 to 6 mg/kg daily, by mouth or intravenously, to 60 to 80 mg/kg as a single intravenous dose every 3 to 4 weeks.

Cycloserine   *Antibiotic/Tuberculostatic*

Synonym. D-Cycloserine
Proprietary Names. Closina; Seromycin.
(*R*)-4-Aminoisoxazolidin-3-one
$C_3H_6N_2O_2 = 102.1$
CAS—68-41-7

An antimicrobial substance produced by the growth of certain strains of *Streptomyces orchidaceus* or *S. garyphalus*, or obtained by synthesis.
A white or pale yellow, hygroscopic, crystalline powder. It is unstable in neutral or acid solutions. M.p. 153° to 155°.
Soluble 1 in 10 of water and 1 in 50 of ethanol; slightly soluble in chloroform and ether.

Dissociation Constant. pK_a 4.5, 7.4 (25°).

Colour Test. Mercurous Nitrate—black.

Thin-layer Chromatography. *System TA*—Rf 44; *system TB*—Rf 01; *system TC*—Rf 01. (*Acidified iodoplatinate solution, positive.*)

Ultraviolet Spectrum. No significant absorption, 230 to 360 nm.

Infra-red Spectrum. Principal peaks at wavenumbers 1577, 1550, 1526, 1620, 934, 877 (KBr disk).

Mass Spectrum. Principal peaks at *m/z* 43, 29, 28, 59, 30, 42, 74, 102.

Disposition in the Body. Readily absorbed after oral administration and widely distributed throughout body fluids and tissues. About 65% of a dose is excreted in the urine unchanged in 72 hours, mostly in the first 24 hours.

THERAPEUTIC CONCENTRATION.
After oral administration of 750 mg, divided into three 6-hourly doses to 11 subjects, followed by a single dose of 500 mg the next morning, peak serum concentrations of 22 to 34 μg/ml (mean 28) were reported 2 to 4 hours after the last dose (M. J. Mattila *et al.*, *Scand. J. resp. Dis.*, 1969, *50*, 291–300).

TOXICITY.
A female subject who ingested a non-fatal overdose of 3 g, had a peak plasma concentration of 91 μg/ml on admission to hospital; following peritoneal dialysis for 20 hours, the plasma concentration declined to 25 μg/ml (R. Atkins *et al.*, *Br. med. J.*, 1965, *1*, 907–908).

HALF-LIFE. Plasma half-life, 4 to 30 hours (mean 10).

PROTEIN BINDING. In plasma, less than 20%.

Dose. 0.25 to 1 g daily.

Cyclothiazide   *Diuretic*

Proprietary Names. Anhydron; Doburil.
6 - Chloro - 3,4 - dihydro - 3 - (norborn - 5 - en - 2 - yl) - 2*H* - 1,2,4 - benzothiadiazine-7-sulphonamide 1,1-dioxide
$C_{14}H_{16}ClN_3O_4S_2 = 389.9$
CAS—2259-96-3

A white powder. M.p. 217° to 225°.

Practically **insoluble** in water; soluble 1 in 70 of ethanol and 1 in 30 of methanol; freely soluble in acetone; practically insoluble in chloroform and ether.

Colour Tests. Koppanyi–Zwikker Test—violet; Liebermann's Test—brown; Sulphuric Acid—orange → red-brown.

Thin-layer Chromatography. *System TA*—Rf 77; *system TD*—Rf 18; *system TE*—Rf 59; *system TF*—Rf 60. (*Acidified potassium permanganate solution*, positive.)

High Pressure Liquid Chromatography. *System HN*—k′ 10.78, 11.91, and 12.81.

Ultraviolet Spectrum. Aqueous acid—272 nm $(A_1^1 = 549 \text{ b})$, 314 nm.

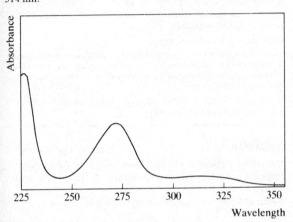

Infra-red Spectrum. Principal peaks at wavenumbers 1596, 1153, 1168, 1307, 1500, 1075 (KBr disk).

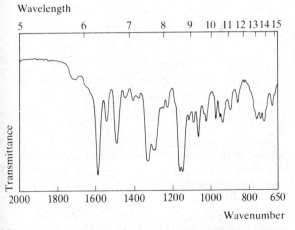

Mass Spectrum. Principal peaks at *m/z* 66, 120, 39, 65, 269, 205, 118, 77.

Dose. 1 to 2 mg daily; up to 6 mg daily may be given.

Cycrimine   *Anticholinergic*

1-Cyclopentyl-1-phenyl-3-piperidinopropan-1-ol

$C_{19}H_{29}NO = 287.4$

CAS—77-39-4

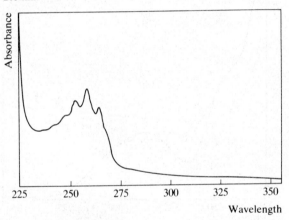

M.p. 90° to 96°.

Cycrimine Hydrochloride

Synonym. Cycriminium Chloride

Proprietary Name. Pagitane Hydrochloride

$C_{19}H_{29}NO,HCl = 323.9$

CAS—126-02-3

A white solid. M.p. about 242°, with decomposition.

Soluble 1 in 175 of water, 1 in 50 of ethanol, and 1 in 35 of chloroform; practically insoluble in ether.

Colour Tests. Liebermann's Test—red-orange; Mandelin's Test—red-brown; Marquis Test—orange → red.

Thin-layer Chromatography. *System TA*—Rf 66; *system TB*—Rf 67; *system TC*—Rf 61. (*Acidified iodoplatinate solution*, positive.)

Gas Chromatography. *System GA*—RI 2114.

Ultraviolet Spectrum. Aqueous acid—251 nm, 256 nm $(A_1^1 = 6 \text{ b})$, 263 nm.

Infra-red Spectrum. Principal peaks at wavenumbers 696, 1117, 755, 751, 1030, 1298 (KBr disk).

Mass Spectrum. Principal peaks at *m/z* 98, 41, 42, 55, 99, 77, 69, 44.

Dose. Usually 3.75 to 20 mg of cycrimine hydrochloride daily.

Cyproheptadine   *Antihistamine*

4-(5*H*-Dibenzo[*a,d*]cyclohepten-5-ylidene)-1-methylpiperidine

$C_{21}H_{21}N = 287.4$

CAS—129-03-3

Crystals. M.p. about 113°.

Cyproheptadine Hydrochloride

Proprietary Names. Antegan; Nuran; Periactin(e); Periactinol; Vimicon.

$C_{21}H_{21}N,HCl,1\frac{1}{2}H_2O = 350.9$

CAS—969-33-5 (anhydrous); *41354-29-4* (sesquihydrate)

A white to slightly yellow, crystalline powder. M.p. 214° to 216°, with decomposition.

Soluble 1 in 275 of water, 1 in 35 of ethanol, 1 in about 16 of chloroform, and 1 in 1.5 of methanol; practically insoluble in ether.

Partition Coefficient. Log *P* (octanol/pH 7.4), 3.2.

Colour Tests. Mandelin's Test—violet-brown; Marquis Test—grey-green; Sulphuric Acid—violet.

Thin-layer Chromatography. *System TA*—Rf 51; *system TB*—Rf 45; *system TC*—Rf 44. (*Acidified iodoplatinate solution*, positive.)

Gas Chromatography. *System GA*—RI 2366; *system GC*—RI 2307; *system GF*—RI 2710.

High Pressure Liquid Chromatography. *System HA*—k' 3.2.

Ultraviolet Spectrum. Aqueous acid—286 nm ($A_1^1 = 433$ a); aqueous alkali—284 nm ($A_1^1 = 377$ b).

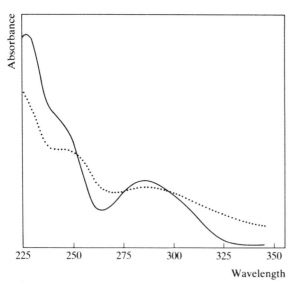

Infra-red Spectrum. Principal peaks at wavenumbers 777, 756, 815, 786, 1640, 960 (cyproheptadine hydrochloride, KBr disk).

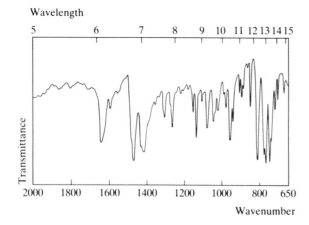

Mass Spectrum. Principal peaks at *m/z* 287, 96, 286, 215, 70, 44, 58, 42.

Quantification. GAS CHROMATOGRAPHY. In plasma or urine: sensitivity 3 ng/ml, AFID—H. B. Hucker and J. E. Hutt, *J. pharm. Sci.*, 1983, *72*, 1069–1070.

Disposition in the Body. Absorbed after oral administration and extensively distributed throughout the tissues. Metabolised by aromatic ring hydroxylation, *N*-demethylation, heterocyclic ring oxidation, and glucuronic acid conjugation; the major metabolite in urine is a quaternary ammonium glucuronide conjugate. About 67 to 77% of a dose is excreted in the urine in 6 days, the remainder being eliminated in the faeces. Of the excreted material, 58 to 65% is conjugated with glucuronic acid, 9 to 11% is conjugated with sulphate, 20 to 26% is excreted as polar material not hydrolysable by glucuronidase or sulphatase, and about 5% is unconjugated.

THERAPEUTIC CONCENTRATION.

After a single oral dose of 5 mg to 2 subjects, peak plasma concentrations of cyproheptadine metabolites of 0.036 and 0.05 µg/ml were attained in 6 to 9 hours; unchanged drug was not detected (K. L. Hintze *et al.*, *Drug Met. Disp.*, 1975, *3*, 1–9).

Dose. 12 to 16 mg of anhydrous cyproheptadine hydrochloride daily; maximum of 32 mg daily.

Cytarabine   *Antineoplastic*

Synonyms. Arabinosylcytosine; Ara-C; Cytosine Arabinoside.

Proprietary Names. Alexan; Aracytin(e); Cytosar; Cytosar-U; Udicil.

4-Amino-1-β-D-arabinofuranosylpyrimidin-2(1*H*)-one

$C_9H_{13}N_3O_5 = 243.2$

CAS—147-94-4

A white crystalline powder. M.p. 212° to 213°.

Soluble 1 in 10 of water, 1 in 1000 of ethanol, and 1 in 1000 of chloroform.

Cytarabine Hydrochloride

$C_9H_{13}N_3O_5,HCl = 279.7$

CAS—69-74-9

A white crystalline powder.

Soluble 1 in 1 of water; less soluble in organic solvents.

Dissociation Constant. pK_a 4.3.

Thin-layer Chromatography. *System TA*—Rf 05; *system TB*—Rf 00; *system TC*—Rf 01. (*Acidified potassium permanganate solution*, positive.)

Ultraviolet Spectrum. Aqueous acid—280 nm ($A_1^1 = 555$ a); aqueous alkali—274 nm.

Infra-red Spectrum. Principal peaks at wavenumbers 1075, 1027, 1145, 1109, 1178, 1002 (KBr disk).

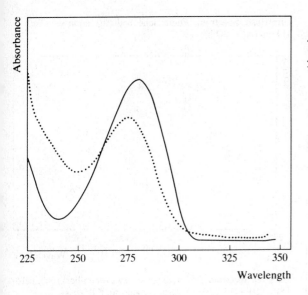

Wavelength

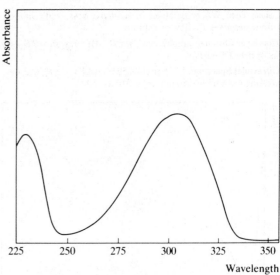

Wavelength

Quantification. GAS CHROMATOGRAPHY. In plasma: detection limit 40 ng/ml, AFID—J. Boutagy and D. J. Harvey, *J. Chromat.*, 1978, *146*; *Biomed. Appl.*, *3*, 283–296.

HIGH PRESSURE LIQUID CHROMATOGRAPHY. In plasma: detection limit 20 ng/ml, UV detection—R. W. Bury and P. J. Keary, *ibid.*, 350–353. In plasma, urine, or cerebrospinal fluid: detection limit 20 ng/ml, UV detection—J. A. Sinkule and W. E. Evans, *J. Chromat.*, 1983, *274*; *Biomed. Appl.*, *25*, 87–93.

Dose. 2 to 4 mg/kg daily, intravenously.

Cytisine   *Alkaloid*

Synonyms. Baptitoxine; Cytiton; Laburnine; Sophorine; Ulexine.

1,2,3,4,5,6 - Hexahydro - 1,5 - methano - 8*H* - pyrido[1,2 - *a*][1,5] diazocin-8-one
$C_{11}H_{14}N_2O = 190.2$
CAS—485-35-8

An alkaloid found in all parts of the laburnum, *Laburnum anagyroides* (Leguminosae), particularly in the pods and seeds, and in some other leguminous plants.
A white or slightly yellowish, crystalline powder. M.p. 154° to 157°.
Soluble 1 in 1.3 of water, 1 in 3.5 of ethanol, and 1 in 2 of chloroform.

Thin-layer Chromatography. *System TA*—Rf 40; *system TB*—Rf 01; *system TC*—Rf 10. (*Acidified iodoplatinate solution*, positive.)

Ultraviolet Spectrum. Aqueous acid—232 nm, 302 nm ($A_1^1 = 344$ b).

Infra-red Spectrum. Principal peaks at wavenumbers 1650, 1540, 1565, 1140, 790, 1311 (KBr disk).

Mass Spectrum. Principal peaks at *m/z* 44, 146, 147, 39, 41, 190, 42, 148.

Quantification. ULTRAVIOLET SPECTROPHOTOMETRY. In blood— H. G. H. Richards and A. Stephens, *Medicine, Sci. Law*, 1970, *10*, 260–266.

Disposition in the Body.

TOXICITY. Cytisine is a highly toxic alkaloid which resembles nicotine in its actions. Fatalities have occurred after the ingestion of laburnum seeds, but recovery is more usual.

In a fatality due to the ingestion of laburnum seeds (estimated amount ingested 50 mg), a blood concentration of 6.8 µg/ml of cytisine was reported; the stomach contained 23 laburnum pods (H. G. H. Richards and A. Stephens, *ibid.*).

NOTE. For reviews of laburnum poisoning in children see R. G. Mitchell, *Lancet*, 1951, *2*, 57–58, and A. Bramley and R. Goulding, *Br. med. J.*, 1981, *283*, 1220–1221.

Danthron   *Purgative*

Synonyms. Antrapurol; Chrysazin; Chryzacin; Dantron; Dianthon; Dioxyanthrachinonum.
Proprietary Names. Dorbane; Duolax; Modane; Roydan. It is an ingredient of Dorbanex, Dorbantyl, Doxidan, Normacol X, and Normax.

1,8-Dihydroxyanthraquinone
$C_{14}H_8O_4 = 240.2$
CAS—117-10-2

An orange crystalline powder. M.p. 190° to 197°.
Practically **insoluble** in water; soluble 1 in 2500 of ethanol, 1 in 30 of chloroform, and 1 in 500 of ether; soluble in solutions of alkali hydroxides.

Colour Test. When dissolved in *sulphuric acid*—red; dilution with water gives a yellow precipitate.

Thin-layer Chromatography. *System TD*—Rf 80; *system TE*—Rf 43; *system TF*—Rf 69.

Ultraviolet Spectrum. Methanol—252 nm ($A_1^1 = 915$ a), 283 nm; alkaline methanol—280 nm ($A_1^1 = 510$ a).

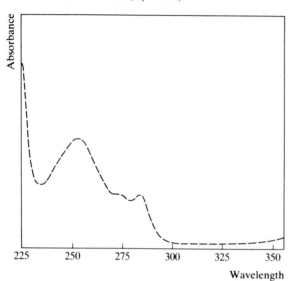

Infra-red Spectrum. Principal peaks at wavenumbers 1264, 740, 1620, 1597, 1152, 1197 (KBr disk).

Mass Spectrum. Principal peaks at *m/z* 240, 212, 241, 184, 138, 92, 128, 63.

Dose. 50 to 150 mg daily.

Dantrolene   *Muscle Relaxant*

1 - [5 - (4 - Nitrophenyl)furfurylideneamino]imidazolidine - 2,4 - dione
$C_{14}H_{10}N_4O_5 = 314.3$
CAS—7261-97-4

NO$_2$ ... CH:N—N ... O ... NH ... O

Crystals. M.p. 279° to 280°.
Practically **insoluble** in water.

Dantrolene Sodium

Proprietary Names. Dantamacrin; Dantrium.
$C_{14}H_9N_4NaO_5,3\frac{1}{2}H_2O = 399.3$
CAS—14663-23-1 (anhydrous); *24868-20-0* (hemiheptahydrate)
An orange powder.
Slightly **soluble** in water; its solubility increases in alkaline solution. Soluble 1 in 40 to 1 in 50 of acetone, and 1 in 25 of propylene glycol.

Dissociation Constant. pK_a 7.5.

Thin-layer Chromatography. *System TD*—Rf 19; *system TE*—Rf 09; *system TF*—Rf 36.

Ultraviolet Spectrum. Dantrolene sodium: aqueous alkali— 314 nm ($A_1^1 = 487$ b).

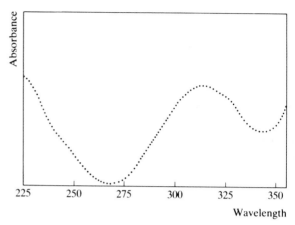

Infra-red Spectrum. Principal peaks at wavenumbers 1600, 1225, 1510, 850, 1713, 1108 (dantrolene sodium, KBr disk).

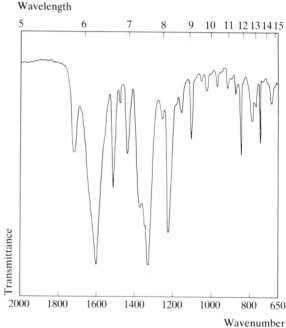

Quantification. SPECTROFLUORIMETRY. In plasma, blood, urine or tissues: sensitivity 100 ng/ml in plasma, blood and urine, 400 ng/ml in bile and tissues—R. D. Hollifield and J. D. Conklin, *J. pharm. Sci.*, 1973, **62**, 271–274.

HIGH PRESSURE LIQUID CHROMATOGRAPHY. In plasma or urine: dantrolene, 5-hydroxydantrolene and *p*-acetamidodantrolene, detection limit 20 ng/ml, UV detection—E. W. Wuis *et al.*, *J. Chromat.*, 1982, *231*; *Biomed. Appl.*, *20*, 401–409.

Disposition in the Body. Slowly and incompletely absorbed after oral administration. Metabolised by oxidation to 5-hydroxydantrolene, which is active, and by reduction followed by acetylation to form the *p*-acetamido derivative. About 20% of an oral dose is excreted in the urine as metabolites, mainly the 5-hydroxy derivative; less than 5% of a dose is excreted in the urine as unchanged drug; up to about 50% of a dose may be excreted in the bile.

THERAPEUTIC CONCENTRATION.

Following a single oral dose of 100 mg to 8 subjects, peak plasma concentrations of 0.7 to 1.7 µg/ml (mean 1.2) of dantrolene and 0.2 to 0.5 µg/ml (mean 0.4) of 5-hydroxydantrolene were attained in about 1 to 8 hours and 1 to 22 hours respectively (W. J. Meyler *et al.*, *Eur. J. clin. Pharmac.*, 1979, *16*, 203–209).

In 4 subjects receiving daily oral doses of 25 to 50 mg 2 to 4 times a day, plasma-dantrolene concentrations were fairly stable and remained between about 0.03 and 0.1 µg/ml; concentrations in an additional 2 subjects fluctuated between about 0.03 and 0.2 µg/ml; plasma concentrations of 5-hydroxydantrolene and *p*-acetamidodantrolene ranged from about 0.1 to 0.3 µg/ml (J. J. Vallner *et al.*, *Curr. ther. Res.*, 1979, *25*, 79–91).

TOXICITY. Fatalities due to liver damage have been reported.

HALF-LIFE. Plasma half-life, dantrolene 4 to 22 hours (mean 9), 5-hydroxydantrolene 8 to 29 hours (mean 16).

NOTE. For a review of the pharmacokinetics of dantrolene see R. M. Pinder *et al.*, *Drugs*, 1977, *13*, 3–23.

Dose. Initially 25 mg of dantrolene sodium daily, increased to a maximum of 400 mg daily.

Dapsone *Antileprotic*

Synonyms. DADPS; DDS; Diaphenylsulfone; Disulone; Sulphonyldianiline.
Proprietary Names. Avlosulfon. It is an ingredient of Maloprim.
Bis(4-aminophenyl) sulphone
$C_{12}H_{12}N_2O_2S = 248.3$
CAS—80-08-0

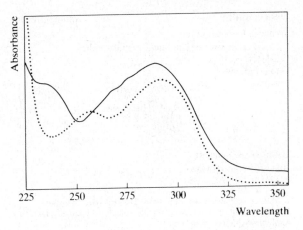

A white or slightly yellowish-white crystalline powder. It discolours on exposure to light but this is not accompanied by significant decomposition. M.p. 175° to 181°.
Soluble 1 in 7000 of water and 1 in about 36 of ethanol; freely soluble in acetone; soluble in dilute mineral acids.

Dissociation Constant. pK_a 1.3, 2.5.

Gas Chromatography. *System GA*—RI 2880.

Ultraviolet Spectrum. Aqueous acid—288 nm ($A_1^1 = 350$ b); aqueous alkali—256 nm, 292 nm.

Infra-red Spectrum. Principal peaks at wavenumbers 1150, 1276, 1592, 1107, 685, 1633 (KBr disk).

Mass Spectrum. Principal peaks at *m/z* 108, 248, 140, 65, 92, 141, 109, 80.

Quantification. GAS CHROMATOGRAPHY. In plasma: dapsone and monoacetyldapsone, ECD—H. P. Burchfield *et al.*, *Analyt. Chem.*, 1973, *45*, 916–920.

HIGH PRESSURE LIQUID CHROMATOGRAPHY. In raw material, dosage forms or biological fluids: detection limit 10 pg using

fluorescence detection and 250 pg using UV detection—C. A. Mannan *et al.*, *J. pharm. Sci.*, 1977, *66*, 1618–1623. In plasma: dapsone and monoacetyldapsone, detection limit 5 ng/ml, UV detection—C. R. Jones and S. M. Ovenell, *J. Chromat.*, 1979, *163*; *Biomed. Appl.*, *5*, 179–185. In serum: dapsone and monoacetyldapsone, sensitivity 200 ng/ml, UV detection—J. Zuidema *et al.*, *J. Chromat.*, 1980, *182*; *Biomed. Appl.*, *8*, 130–135.

THIN-LAYER CHROMATOGRAPHY. In plasma or saliva: detection limit 20 ng/ml—R. A. Ahmad and H. J. Rogers, *Eur. J. clin. Pharmac.*, 1980, *17*, 129–133.

Disposition in the Body. Slowly and almost completely absorbed after oral administration and widely distributed throughout the body. It is acetylated to monoacetyldapsone, the extent of which is genetically determined. It is also metabolised by *N*-oxidation to mono-*N*-hydroxydapsone, together with glucuronic acid and sulphate conjugation of dapsone and the metabolites. Enterohepatic recycling occurs. About 70 to 90% of a dose is excreted in the urine, about 10 to 20% as unchanged drug, about 50% as dapsone conjugates, and about 30% as *N*-oxidation products (mostly conjugated). Small amounts are eliminated in the faeces. About 30 to 50% of a single dose is excreted in the urine within 24 hours and more than 70% in 3 days, but there is wide individual variation.

THERAPEUTIC CONCENTRATION.

After a single oral dose of 50 mg to 6 subjects, plasma concentrations of dapsone were 1.02 to 1.44 µg/ml (mean 1.24) in 3 slow acetylators, and 1.03 to 1.48 µg/ml (mean 1.23) in 3 rapid acetylators, after 4 hours. The concentrations of monoacetyldapsone were 0.15 to 0.38 µg/ml (mean 0.25) in the slow acetylators and 0.63 to 1.66 µg/ml (mean 0.98) in the rapid acetylators, after 4 hours (J. T. Biggs and L. Levy, *Proc. Soc. exp. Biol. Med.*, 1971, *137*, 692–695).

TOXICITY. Toxic effects are likely to occur at serum concentrations above 10 µg/ml.

In 1 case of fatal overdosage, a 22-month-old child died 55 hours after ingesting about 5 g of dapsone. The concentrations in the plasma and cerebrospinal fluid were 150 µg/ml and 33 µg/ml, respectively, 42 hours after ingestion. Postmortem concentrations were: blood 135 µg/ml, brain 90 µg/g, liver 165 µg/g, and urine 400 µg/ml (R. Davies, *Lancet*, 1950, *1*, 905–906).

HALF-LIFE. Plasma half-life, 10 to 50 hours (mean 24).

PROTEIN BINDING. In plasma, dapsone 50 to 80%, monoacetyldapsone 98 to 100%.

Dose. 50 to 100 mg daily.

Debrisoquine

Antihypertensive

Synonym. Isocaramidine

1,2,3,4-Tetrahydroisoquinoline-2-carboxamidine

$C_{10}H_{13}N_3 = 175.2$

CAS—1131-64-2

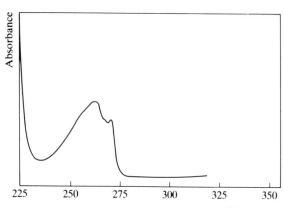

Debrisoquine Sulphate

Proprietary Name. Declinax

$(C_{10}H_{13}N_3)_2,H_2SO_4 = 448.5$

CAS—581-88-4

A white crystalline powder. M.p. about 274°, with decomposition.

Soluble 1 in 40 of water; very slightly soluble in ethanol; practically insoluble in chloroform and ether.

Dissociation Constant. pK_a 11.9.

Colour Tests. Mandelin's Test—green; Marquis Test—red-brown.

Thin-layer Chromatography. *System TA*—Rf 01; *system TB*—Rf 00; *system TC*—Rf 00. (*Acidified iodoplatinate solution*, positive.)

Gas Chromatography. *System GA*—not eluted.

High Pressure Liquid Chromatography. *System HA*—k' 1.2.

Ultraviolet Spectrum. Aqueous acid—262 nm ($A_1^1 = 17.7$ a), 270 nm. No alkaline shift.

Infra-red Spectrum. Principal peaks at wavenumbers 1614, 1090, 1650, 1583, 750, 715 (debrisoquine sulphate, KBr disk).

Mass Spectrum. Principal peaks at m/z 132, 104, 44, 175, 103, 117, 43, 130.

Quantification. GAS CHROMATOGRAPHY. In blood, plasma, saliva or urine: debrisoquine and 4-hydroxydebrisoquine, sensitivity 3 ng/ml, AFID—M. S. Lennard *et al.*, *J. Chromat.*, 1977, *133*, 161–166. In urine: ECD—J. R. Idle *et al.*, *Br. J. clin. Pharmac.*, 1979, *7*, 257–266.

GAS CHROMATOGRAPHY-MASS SPECTROMETRY. In plasma: sensitivity 1 ng/ml for debrisoquine and 5 ng/ml for 4-hydroxy-debrisoquine—S. L. Malcolm and T. R. Marten, *Analyt. Chem.*, 1976, *48*, 807–809.

Disposition in the Body. Rapidly absorbed after oral administration. The main metabolic reaction is 4-hydroxylation; aromatic

hydroxylation at positions 5, 6, 7, and 8 also occurs and acidic ring-opened metabolites are also formed. There is no evidence of glucuronic acid conjugation in man. The extent of 4-hydroxylation of debrisoquine is genetically determined. About 75% of a dose is excreted in the urine in 24 hours. Excretion of unchanged drug ranges from 8 to 80% of a dose. About 90% of the population are extensive metabolisers of debrisoquine, in these subjects, about 10 to 40% of a dose is excreted as 4-hydroxydebrisoquine; the remaining 10% are poor metabolisers and excrete less than 2% as the 4-hydroxy metabolite. Acidic ring-opened metabolites account for up to 15% of a dose and the 5-, 6-, 7-, and 8-hydroxy metabolites for about 7%. About 12% of a dose is eliminated in the faeces.

THERAPEUTIC CONCENTRATION.

Following a single oral dose of 20 mg to 3 subjects, peak plasma concentrations of 0.010, 0.013, and 0.024 µg/ml of debrisoquine were reported at 1.5 to 3.5 hours; peak concentrations of the 4-hydroxy metabolite averaging 0.035 µg/ml were attained in 1.5 to 2.5 hours. The 4-hydroxy metabolite was eliminated more rapidly than debrisoquine and was not detectable after 24 hours (J. H. Silas *et al.*, *Br. J. clin. Pharmac.*, 1978, *5*, 27–34).

Maximum steady-state plasma concentrations of 0.015 to 0.18 µg/ml (mean 0.08), and 0 to 0.05 µg/ml (mean 0.02) for debrisoquine and 4-hydroxydebrisoquine respectively, were reported in 13 patients receiving daily oral doses of 40 mg (J. H. Silas *et al.*, *Br. med. J.*, 1977, *1*, 422–425).

HALF-LIFE. Plasma half-life, debrisoquine about 16 to 30 hours, 4-hydroxydebrisoquine about 10 hours.

DISTRIBUTION IN BLOOD. Plasma: whole blood ratio, 0.45.

PROTEIN BINDING. In plasma, about 25%.

Dose. The equivalent of 10 to 120 mg of debrisoquine daily; up to 300 mg or more daily may be given.

Decamethonium Bromide

Muscle Relaxant

Proprietary Name. Syncurine

NN'-Decamethylenebis(trimethylammonium) dibromide

$C_{16}H_{38}Br_2N_2 = 418.3$

CAS—156-74-1 (decamethonium); *541-22-0* (bromide)

$$[(CH_3)_3\overset{+}{N}\cdot[CH_2]_{10}\cdot\overset{+}{N}(CH_3)_3]\,2Br^-$$

A white, hygroscopic, crystalline powder. M.p. about 265°, with decomposition.

Freely **soluble** in water and ethanol; practically insoluble in ether.

Wavelength

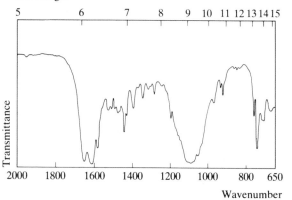

Wavenumber

Thin-layer Chromatography. *System TA*—Rf 00; *system TN*—Rf 56; *system TO*—Rf 16. (*Acidified iodoplatinate solution*, positive.)

Ultraviolet Spectrum. Aqueous acid—227 nm ($A_1^1 = 584$ b).

Infra-red Spectrum. Principal peaks at wavenumbers 1627, 910, 965, 1030, 1136, 1063 (KBr disk).

Dose. Initially 2 to 2.5 mg by intravenous injection.

Decoquinate   *Coccidiostat (Veterinary)*

Proprietary Name. Deccox
Ethyl 6-decyloxy-7-ethoxy-4-hydroxyquinoline-3-carboxylate
$C_{24}H_{35}NO_5 = 417.5$
CAS—18507-89-6

A cream to buff-coloured microcrystalline powder. M.p. about 242°.
Practically **insoluble** in water and ethanol; slightly soluble in chloroform and ether; soluble in acetone.

Colour Tests. Liebermann's Test—orange (slow); Mandelin's Test—red-brown.

Gas Chromatography. *System GA*—not eluted.

Ultraviolet Spectrum. Methanolic acid—265 nm ($A_1^1 = 1000$ b).

Infra-red Spectrum. Principal peaks at wavenumbers 1695, 1613, 1497, 1263, 1205, 1558 (KBr disk).

Dehydroemetine   *Antiprotozoal*

2,3-Didehydro-6′,7′,10,11-tetramethoxyemetan
$C_{29}H_{38}N_2O_4 = 478.6$
CAS—4914-30-1

Dehydroemetine Hydrochloride
Proprietary Name. Dametine
$C_{29}H_{38}N_2O_4,2HCl = 551.6$
CAS—2228-39-9
A white crystalline powder.
Soluble 1 in 30 of water.

Colour Test. Marquis Test—orange.

Thin-layer Chromatography. *System TA*—Rf 43; *system TB*—Rf 06; *system TC*—Rf 21. (*Acidified iodoplatinate solution*, positive.)

Ultraviolet Spectrum. Aqueous acid—230 nm ($A_1^1 = 290$ a), 283 nm.

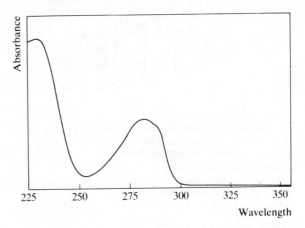

Infra-red Spectrum. Principal peaks at wavenumbers 1121, 1222, 1508, 1252, 1205, 1022 (dehydroemetine hydrochloride, KBr disk).

Mass Spectrum. Principal peaks at *m/z* 192, 193, 287, 176, 191, 286, 270, 285.

Dose. 60 to 180 mg of dehydroemetine hydrochloride daily, intramuscularly.

Demecarium Bromide   *Anticholinesterase*

Proprietary Names. Humorsol; Tosmilen(e).
3,3′-[*NN*′-Decamethylenebis(methylcarbamoyloxy)]bis(*NNN*-trimethylanilinium) dibromide
$C_{32}H_{52}Br_2N_4O_4 = 716.6$
CAS—56-94-0

A white or slightly yellow, slightly hygroscopic, crystalline powder. M.p. 163° to 168°, with decomposition.
Freely **soluble** in water and ethanol; soluble in ether.

Thin-layer Chromatography. *System TA*—Rf 00. (*Acidified iodoplatinate solution*, positive.)

Ultraviolet Spectrum. Aqueous acid—259 nm ($A_1^1 = 14$ b), 265 nm. No alkaline shift.

Infra-red Spectrum. Principal peaks at wavenumbers 1724, 1216, 1149, 1178, 1124, 943 (KBr disk).

Use. As a 0.25 to 0.5% ophthalmic solution.

Demeclocycline   *Antibiotic*

Synonyms. Demethylchlortetracycline; DMCT.
Proprietary Name. Ledermycin (drops and syrup)
7-Chloro-6-demethyltetracycline
$C_{21}H_{21}ClN_2O_8 = 464.9$
CAS—127-33-3

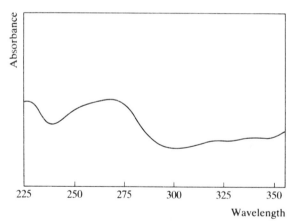

A yellow crystalline powder.

Sparingly **soluble** in water; soluble 1 in 200 of ethanol and 1 in 40 of methanol; soluble in dilute hydrochloric acid and in solutions of alkali hydroxides and carbonates.

Demeclocycline Hydrochloride

Proprietary Names. Declomycin; Ledermycin(e) (capsules and tablets). It is an ingredient of Declostatin and Deteclo.

$C_{21}H_{21}ClN_2O_8,HCl = 501.3$
CAS—64-73-3

A yellow, amphoteric, crystalline powder.

Soluble 1 in 30 to 1 in 60 of water, 1 in 45 to 1 in 200 of ethanol, and 1 in 50 of methanol; practically insoluble in chloroform and ether; soluble in aqueous solutions of alkali hydroxides and carbonates.

Dissociation Constant. pK_a 3.3, 7.2, 9.3 (25°).

Partition Coefficient. Log P (octanol/pH 7.5), −1.3.

Colour Tests. Benedict's Reagent—red; Formaldehyde–Sulphuric Acid—orange → brown-red; Mandelin's Test—violet-brown; Marquis Test—yellow → green; Nessler's Reagent—brown; Sulphuric Acid—brown-blue.

Thin-layer Chromatography. *System TA*—Rf 05, streaking. (Location under ultraviolet light, orange fluorescence; *acidified potassium permanganate solution*, positive.)

Ultraviolet Spectrum. Aqueous acid—268 nm ($A_1^1 = 398$ a); aqueous alkali—241 nm ($A_1^1 = 364$ b), 276 nm ($A_1^1 = 304$ b), 388 nm ($A_1^1 = 385$ b).

Infra-red Spectrum. Principal peaks at wavenumbers 1616, 1573, 1660, 1190, 1298, 1315 (KBr disk).

Disposition in the Body. Readily absorbed after oral administration and slowly excreted in the urine.

HALF-LIFE. Plasma half-life, about 10 to 15 hours.

PROTEIN BINDING. In plasma, 40 to 90%.

Dose. Usually 600 mg of demeclocycline hydrochloride daily; up to 1.2 g daily has been given.

Demeton-S   *Pesticide*

Synonyms. Isosystox; Mercaptofos Teolovy.

OO-Diethyl *S*-2-ethylthioethyl phosphorothioate
$C_8H_{19}O_3PS_2 = 258.3$
CAS—126-75-0

$$(C_2H_5 \cdot O)_2 \cdot \overset{\overset{\displaystyle O}{\|}}{P} - S \cdot [CH_2]_2 \cdot S \cdot CH_2 \cdot CH_3$$

A colourless oil.

Soluble 1 in 500 of water; soluble in most organic solvents.

Demeton-S-methyl

Synonyms. Methyl-mercaptofos Teolovy; Metaisosystox.

Note. The name Demeton-methyl used to be applied to a mixture of demeton-S-methyl and demeton-O-methyl but this mixture has been replaced by demeton-S-methyl.

Proprietary Names. Azotox; Demetox; DSM; Duratox; Metasystox 55.

$C_6H_{15}O_3PS_2 = 230.3$
CAS—919-86-8

A pale yellow oil of low viscosity. In solution or upon storage, demeton-S-methyl is oxidised to the sulphoxide and the sulphone. Refractive index 1.5065.

Soluble 1 in 300 of water; soluble in most organic solvents.

Colour Tests. Palladium Chloride—brown-orange; Phosphorus Test—yellow.

Gas Chromatography. Demeton-S-methyl: *system GA*—RI 1628; *system GK*—retention time 0.70 relative to caffeine.

Infra-red Spectrum. Principal peaks at wavenumbers 1020, 1250, 775, 793, 826, 1190 (demeton-S-methyl).

Mass Spectrum. Principal peaks at *m/z* 88, 60, 109, 142, 79, 47, 111, 61 (demeton-S-methyl).

Disposition in the Body. Demeton-S and demeton-S-methyl are very readily absorbed by all routes and have a particularly high toxicity following percutaneous absorption. They are rapidly hydrolysed in the tissues to the corresponding sulphoxide and sulphone.

TOXICITY. Demeton-S and demeton-S-methyl exert a direct inhibitory action on cholinesterase. The estimated minimum lethal dose is 5 g but exposure to 300 mg daily may be dangerous.

In a fatality due to the ingestion of demeton-S-methyl, the following postmortem tissue concentrations were reported: blood 10 µg/ml, bile 58 µg/ml, kidney 5 µg/g, liver 17 µg/g, urine 121 µg/ml (R. A. Hall and E. D. Carson, *Bull. int. Ass. forens. Toxicol.*, 1970, 7(3), 6).

Demoxepam   *Tranquilliser*

Synonym. Chlordiazepoxide Lactam

7-Chloro-1,3-dihydro-5-phenyl-2*H*-1,4-benzodiazepin-2-one 4-oxide
$C_{15}H_{11}ClN_2O_2 = 286.7$
CAS—963-39-3

A white crystalline powder.
Soluble in chloroform.

Absorbance / Wavelength

225   250   275   300   325   350

Dissociation Constant. pK_a 4.5, 10.6.

Partition Coefficient. Log P (octanol/pH 7.4), 1.5.

Colour Test. Formaldehyde–Sulphuric Acid—orange.

Thin-layer Chromatography. *System TA*—Rf 63; *system TB*—Rf 00; *system TC*—Rf 35; *system TD*—Rf 15; *system TE*—Rf 44; *system TF*—Rf 22. (*Acidified iodoplatinate solution*, positive; *acidified potassium permanganate solution*, positive.)

Gas Chromatography. *System GA*—demoxepam RI 2529, oxazepam RI 2336; *system GG*—demoxepam RI 3043, oxazepam RI 2803.

High Pressure Liquid Chromatography. *System HI*—demoxepam k′ 2.42, oxazepam k′ 4.62; *system HK*—demoxepam k′ 0.03, oxazepam k′ 0.73.

Ultraviolet Spectrum. Aqueous acid—237 nm, 305 nm; aqueous alkali—243 nm, 255 nm, 310 nm; methanol—236 nm ($A_1^1 = 1340$ b), 310 nm.

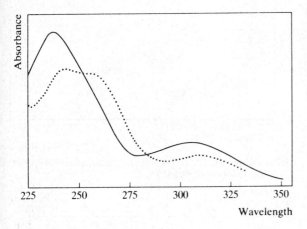

Wavelength

Infra-red Spectrum. Principal peaks at wavenumbers 1678, 690, 1240, 1265, 755, 717.

Mass Spectrum. Principal peaks at m/z 285, 286, 269, 287, 241, 242, 77, 270.

Quantification. SPECTROFLUORIMETRY. In plasma: demoxepam and chlordiazepoxide, sensitivity 250 ng/ml—B. A. Koechlin and L. D'Arconte, *Analyt. Biochem.*, 1963, *5*, 195–207.

GAS CHROMATOGRAPHY. In serum: demoxepam and chlordiazepoxide, ECD—S. R. Sun and D. J. Hoffman, *J. pharm. Sci.*, 1978, *67*, 1647–1648.

Disposition in the Body. Well absorbed after oral administration. About 10% of a dose is excreted in the urine in 24 hours and about 60% in 7 days, including about 27% as unchanged demoxepam and about 5% as conjugated oxazepam. Other urinary metabolites include the 5-(4-hydroxyphenyl) and 9-hydroxy derivatives. Approximately 15% of the dose is eliminated in the faeces in 7 days with about 2% as desmethyldiazepam.

Demoxepam is a metabolite of chlordiazepoxide.

THERAPEUTIC CONCENTRATION.

Following a single oral dose of 20 mg of demoxepam given to 6 subjects, peak plasma concentrations of 0.50 to 0.74 μg/ml (mean 0.6) were attained in 2 to 8 hours (M. A. Schwartz *et al.*, *J. pharm. Sci.*, 1971, *60*, 1500–1503).

HALF-LIFE. Plasma half-life, 14 to 95 hours (mean 40).

Denatonium Benzoate

Alcohol Denaturant

Proprietary Name. Bitrex

Benzyldiethyl(2,6-xylylcarbamoylmethyl)ammonium benzoate
$C_{28}H_{34}N_2O_3 = 446.6$
CAS—3734-33-6

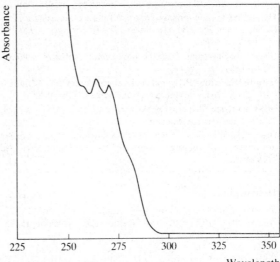

A white crystalline powder. M.p. 166° to 170°.

Soluble in water; soluble 1 in about 2 of ethanol and 1 in about 3 of chloroform; very slightly soluble in ether.

Colour Test. Mandelin's Test—violet.

Thin-layer Chromatography. *System TA*—Rf 10. (*Acidified iodoplatinate solution*, positive.)

Ultraviolet Spectrum. Aqueous acid—263 nm ($A_1^1 = 36$ b), 269 nm.

Wavelength

Infra-red Spectrum. Principal peaks at wavenumbers 1550, 1596, 1680, 719, 704, 757.

Deoxycortone

Corticosteroid

Synonyms. Decortone; Deoxycorticosterone; Desoxycorticosterone; Desoxycortone; 21-Hydroxyprogesterone.

21-Hydroxypregn-4-ene-3,20-dione
$C_{21}H_{30}O_3 = 330.5$
CAS—64-85-7

Crystals. M.p. 141° to 142°.
Freely **soluble** in ethanol and acetone.

Deoxycortone Acetate

Proprietary Names. Cortiron; Doca; Percorten; Syncortyl. It is an ingredient of Plex-Hormone.
$C_{23}H_{32}O_4 = 372.5$
CAS—56-47-3
Colourless crystals or white or creamy-white crystalline powder. M.p. 155° to 161°.
Practically **insoluble** in water; soluble 1 in 50 of ethanol, 1 in 30 of acetone, 1 in 1.5 of chloroform, and 1 in 170 of ether.

Deoxycortone Pivalate

Synonyms. Deoxycortone Trimethylacetate; Desoxycorticosterone Pivalate.
Proprietary Name. Percorten M
$C_{26}H_{38}O_4 = 414.6$
CAS—808-48-0
A white or creamy-white crystalline powder. M.p. 198° to 206°. A solution in dioxan is dextrorotatory.
Practically **insoluble** in water; soluble 1 in 350 to 1 in 500 of ethanol, 1 in 3 of chloroform, and 1 in 60 of dioxan; slightly soluble in ether.

Colour Tests. Antimony Pentachloride—orange; Naphthol–Sulphuric Acid—orange-red/blue-black; Sulphuric Acid—yellow (green-yellow fluorescence under ultraviolet light).

Thin-layer Chromatography. Deoxycortone acetate: *system TP*—Rf 86; *system TQ*—Rf 52; *system TR*—Rf 98; *system TS*—Rf 95. (*DPST solution.*)

Ultraviolet Spectrum. Deoxycortone acetate: ethanol—240 nm ($A_1^1 = 445$ a).

Infra-red Spectrum. Principal peaks at wavenumbers 1242, 1667, 1744, 1718, 1203, 1610 (deoxycortone acetate, KBr disk).

Mass Spectrum. Principal peaks at m/z 43, 55, 299, 91, 147, 79, 253, 271 (deoxycortone acetate).

Dose. Usually 1 to 5 mg of deoxycortone acetate daily, intramuscularly; sublingual doses of 2 to 10 mg daily have also been given.

Deptropine   *Antihistamine*

Synonym. Dibenzheptropine
(1R,3r,5S)-3-(10,11-Dihydro-5H-dibenzo[a,d]cyclohepten-5-yloxy)tropane
$C_{23}H_{27}NO = 333.5$
CAS—604-51-3

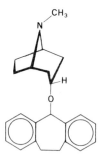

Deptropine Citrate

Proprietary Names. Brontine. It is an ingredient of Brontisol.
$C_{23}H_{27}NO,C_6H_8O_7 = 525.6$
CAS—2169-75-7
A white to off-white microcrystalline powder.
Very slightly **soluble** in water and ethanol; soluble 1 in 100 of methanol; practically insoluble in chloroform and ether.

Colour Tests. Mandelin's Test—yellow; Marquis Test—yellow.

Thin-layer Chromatography. *System TA*—Rf 13; *system TB*—Rf 24; *system TC*—Rf 04. (*Acidified potassium permanganate solution, positive.*)

Gas Chromatography. *System GA*—RI 2615.

High Pressure Liquid Chromatography. *System HA*—k' 5.0 (tailing peak).

Ultraviolet Spectrum. Methanol—266 nm ($A_1^1 = 18.6$ b), 272 nm.

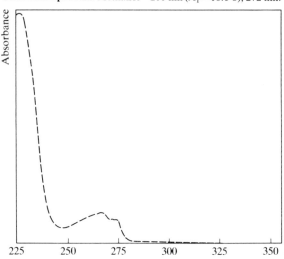

Infra-red Spectrum. Principal peaks at wavenumbers 1059, 1040, 751, 760, 738, 1114 (KBr disk).

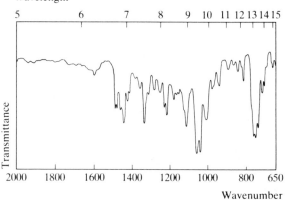

Mass Spectrum. Principal peaks at m/z 83, 140, 82, 124, 43, 96, 97, 42.

Dose. 2 mg of deptropine citrate daily.

Dequalinium Chloride   *Antibacterial/Antifungal*

Synonyms. Decalinium Chloride; Decaminum.
Proprietary Names. Dequadin; Dequavagyn; Labosept; Optipect Halstabletten; Phylletten; Sorot.
1,1'-Decamethylenebis(4-amino-2-methylquinolinium chloride)
$C_{30}H_{40}Cl_2N_4 = 527.6$
CAS—6707-58-0 (dequalinium); *522-51-0* (chloride)

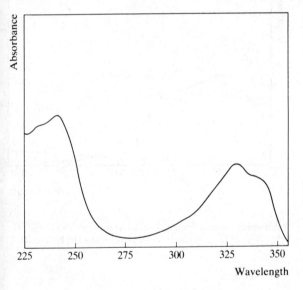

A creamy-white powder. M.p. about 315°, with decomposition. Slightly **soluble** in water; soluble 1 in 30 of boiling water, 1 in 60 of methanol, and 1 in 200 of propylene glycol.

Dequalinium Acetate

$C_{34}H_{46}N_4O_4 = 574.8$
CAS—4028-98-2

A white or pinkish-buff, slightly hygroscopic powder. M.p. about 280°, with decomposition.
Soluble 1 in 2 of water and 1 in 12 of ethanol.

Colour Tests. Aromaticity (Method 2)—red/brown-violet; Liebermann's Test—yellow (→ orange at 100°).

Thin-layer Chromatography. *System TA*—Rf 03. (*Acidified iodoplatinate solution*, positive.)

Ultraviolet Spectrum. Water—240 nm ($A_1^1 = 812$ b), 326 nm ($A_1^1 = 469$ b), 335 nm ($A_1^1 = 406$ b); aqueous acid—241 nm, 330 nm.

Infra-red Spectrum. Principal peaks at wavenumbers 1605, 1660, 765, 1560, 1540, 1307 (KCl disk).

Dose. Lozenges containing 250 μg of dequalinium chloride are available.

Deserpidine   *Antihypertensive*

Synonyms. Canescine; 11-Demethoxyreserpine.
Proprietary Names. Harmonyl. It is an ingredient of Enduronyl.
Methyl 11 - demethoxy - 18 - *O* - (3,4,5 - trimethoxybenzoyl)-reserpate
$C_{32}H_{38}N_2O_8 = 578.7$
CAS—131-01-1

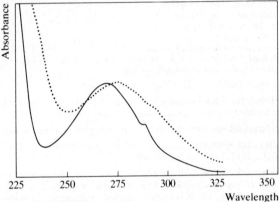

An alkaloid isolated from the root of *Rauwolfia canescens* (Apocynaceae).
Crystals. M.p. 230° to 234°, with decomposition.
Practically **insoluble** in water; soluble in hot ethanol and chloroform.

Colour Tests. Mandelin's Test—blue → green; Marquis Test—grey-green.

Thin-layer Chromatography. *System TA*—Rf 72; *system TB*—Rf 03; *system TC*—Rf 77. (*Acidified iodoplatinate solution*, positive.)

High Pressure Liquid Chromatography. *System HA*—k′ 0.4.

Ultraviolet Spectrum. Aqueous acid—269 nm; aqueous alkali—275 nm.

Infra-red Spectrum. Principal peaks at wavenumbers 1225, 1127, 1715, 1100, 1184, 1590 (KBr disk).

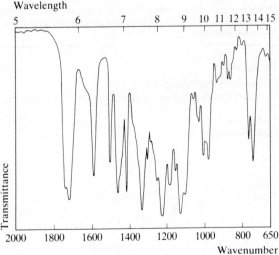

Mass Spectrum. Principal peaks at m/z 578, 195, 577, 367, 351, 579, 366, 365.

Dose. 0.25 to 1 mg daily.

Desferrioxamine
Chelating Agent

Synonyms. Deferoxamine; DFM; DFOM.
30-Amino-3,14,25-trihydroxy-3,9,14,20,25-penta-azatriacontane-2,10,13,21,24-pentaone
$C_{25}H_{48}N_6O_8 = 560.7$
CAS—70-51-9

$$NH_2 \cdot [CH_2]_5 \cdot \underset{HO}{N} \cdot \underset{O}{C} \cdot [CH_2]_2 \cdot \underset{O}{C} \cdot NH \cdot [CH_2]_5 \cdot \underset{HO}{N} \cdot \underset{O}{C} \cdot [CH_2]_2 \cdot \underset{O}{C} \cdot NH \cdot [CH_2]_5 \cdot \underset{HO}{N} \cdot \underset{O}{C} \cdot CH_3$$

Desferrioxamine Mesylate

Synonyms. Deferoxamine Mesylate; Desferrioxamine B Mesylate; Desferrioxamine Methanesulphonate.
Proprietary Name. Desferal
$C_{25}H_{48}N_6O_8,CH_3SO_3H = 656.8$
CAS—138-14-7
A white to cream-coloured powder.
Soluble 1 in 5 of water and 1 in 20 of ethanol; practically insoluble in dehydrated alcohol, chloroform, and ether.

Colour Test. Mandelin's Test—blue → violet.

Thin-layer Chromatography. *System TA*—Rf 08, streaking. (*Acidified potassium permanganate solution*, positive.)

Ultraviolet Spectrum. No significant absorption, 230 to 360 nm.

Infra-red Spectrum. Principal peaks at wavenumbers 1628, 1195, 1562, 1265, 1149, 1041 (KBr disk).

Disposition in the Body. Poorly absorbed after oral administration. It specifically chelates ferric iron to an octahedral complex, ferrioxamine, which is readily excreted in the urine. Theoretically, 100 mg of desferrioxamine can chelate approximately 8.5 mg of iron. About 13 to 65% of a ^{59}Fe-labelled dose is excreted in the urine in 24 hours.

Dose. In acute iron poisoning: 5 g of desferrioxamine mesylate by mouth, with 2 g intramuscularly, and up to 15 mg/kg/hour by intravenous infusion.

Desipramine
Antidepressant

Synonyms. Desmethylimipramine; DMI.
3-(10,11-Dihydro-5*H*-dibenz[*b,f*]azepin-5-yl)-*N*-methylpropylamine
$C_{18}H_{22}N_2 = 266.4$
CAS—50-47-5

$CH_2 \cdot [CH_2]_2 \cdot NH \cdot CH_3$

Desipramine Hydrochloride

Proprietary Names. Norpramin; Pertofran(e).
$C_{18}H_{22}N_2,HCl = 302.8$
CAS—58-28-6
A white crystalline powder. M.p. about 214°.
Soluble 1 in 20 of water, 1 in 20 of ethanol, and 1 in about 4 of chloroform; practically insoluble in ether; freely soluble in methanol.

Dissociation Constant. pK$_a$ 10.2 (24°).

Partition Coefficient. Log P (octanol/pH 7.4), 1.4.

Colour Tests. Forrest Reagent—blue; Mandelin's Test—yellow → blue.

Thin-layer Chromatography. *System TA*—Rf 26; *system TB*—Rf 20; *system TC*—Rf 11. (*Dragendorff spray*, positive; *FPN reagent*, blue; *acidified iodoplatinate solution*, positive; *Marquis reagent*, blue.)

Gas Chromatography. *System GA*—RI 2242.

High Pressure Liquid Chromatography. *System HA*—desipramine k′ 2.1, didesmethylimipramine k′ 1.3, 2-hydroxydesipramine k′ 1.2; *system HF*—desipramine k′ 3.60.

Ultraviolet Spectrum. Aqueous acid—250 nm (A$_1^1$ = 308 a). No alkaline shift.

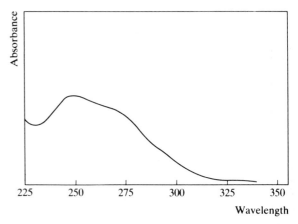

Infra-red Spectrum. Principal peaks at wavenumbers 746, 741, 763, 1230, 1590, 1104 (desipramine hydrochloride, KBr disk).

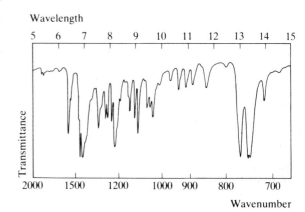

Mass Spectrum. Principal peaks at *m/z* 235, 195, 208, 44, 234, 193, 194, 71; 2-hydroxydesipramine 44, 209, 211, 250, 210, 224, 42, 251.

Quantification. See also under Imipramine.

GAS CHROMATOGRAPHY. In plasma or serum: detection limit 1 ng/ml, AFID—E. Antal *et al.*, *J. Chromat.*, 1980, *183*; *Biomed. Appl.*, *9*, 149–157.

Disposition in the Body. Well absorbed after oral administration. Metabolised by aromatic hydroxylation and possibly hydroxylamine formation; *N*-demethylation to form didesmethylimipramine may occur to a minor extent. 2-Hydroxydesipramine, the major metabolite, is active. Less than 5% of a dose is excreted in urine in 24 hours as unchanged drug; the urinary excretion of unchanged drug is pH-dependent and is increased in acidic urine; the hydroxylated metabolites are excreted mainly as glucuronide conjugates. The extent of 2-hydroxylation is genetically determined.

Desipramine is the major active metabolite of imipramine and lofepramine.

THERAPEUTIC CONCENTRATION. Plasma concentrations vary considerably between individual subjects.

After administration of a single oral dose of 50 mg to 4 subjects, peak plasma-desipramine concentrations of 0.008 to 0.015 µg/ml (mean 0.012) were attained in 3 to 6 hours; peak plasma concentrations of 2-hydroxydesipramine of 0.011 to 0.013 µg/ml were attained in about 2 to 4 hours (C. L. De Vane *et al.*, *Eur. J. clin. Pharmac.*, 1981, *19*, 61–64).

Following daily oral doses of about 2.5 mg/kg to 47 subjects, minimum steady-state plasma concentrations of 0.02 to 0.88 µg/ml (mean 0.17) of desipramine and 0.007 to 0.13 µg/ml (mean 0.04) of 2-hydroxydesipramine were reported (J. L. Bock *et al.*, *Clin. Pharmac. Ther.*, 1983, *33*, 322–328).

TOXICITY. Plasma concentrations greater than 0.4 µg/ml may produce toxic effects. Fatalities are comparatively rare, but may occur with plasma concentrations greater than 10 µg/ml.

Recovery has occurred in 2 subjects after the ingestion of up to 2 g; peak plasma concentrations of 1.56 µg/ml and 1.58 µg/ml were reported (J. T. Biggs, *J. Am. med. Ass.*, 1977, *238*, 135–138).

In 1 fatal case, a blood concentration of 3 µg/ml and a liver concentration of 140 µg/g were reported (R. C. Baselt and R. H. Cravey, *J. analyt. Toxicol.*, 1977, *1*, 81–103).

The following postmortem concentrations were found after the death of a 2-year-old child: blood 8 µg/ml, liver blood 22 µg/ml, bile 67 µg/ml, urine 2 µg/ml (A. E. Robinson *et al.*, *J. analyt. Toxicol.*, 1979, *3*, 3–13).

HALF-LIFE. Plasma half-life, 10 to 35 hours.

PROTEIN BINDING. In plasma, about 70 to 90%.

NOTE. For a review of the pharmacokinetics of tricyclic antidepressants see G. Molnar and R. N. Gupta, *Biopharm. Drug Disp.*, 1980, *1*, 283–305.

Dose. 25 to 200 mg of desipramine hydrochloride daily; up to 300 mg daily has been given.

Deslanoside   *Cardiac Glycoside*

Synonyms. Deacetyl-lanatoside C; Desacetyl-lanatoside C.
Proprietary Names. Cedilanid-D; Cedilanid(e); Desace.
Note. The name Cedilanid(e) is also applied to preparations of lanatoside C.

3β-[(O-β-D-Glucopyranosyl-(1 → 4)-O-2,6-dideoxy-β-D-*ribo*-hexopyranosyl-(1 → 4)-O-2,6-dideoxy-β-D-*ribo*-hexopyranosyl-(1 → 4)-2,6-dideoxy-β-D-*ribo*-hexopyranosyl)oxy]-12β,14-dihydroxy-5β,14β-card-20(22)-enolide
$C_{47}H_{74}O_{19} = 943.1$
CAS—17598-65-1

White hygroscopic crystals or crystalline powder. M.p. about 220°.

Practically **insoluble** in water; soluble 1 in 300 of ethanol and 1 in 200 of methanol; practically insoluble in chloroform and ether.

Colour Test. Dissolve 2 to 3 mg in 5 ml of a solution containing 0.5 ml of a 9% ferric chloride solution and 100 ml of *acetic acid*; underlay with 5 ml of *sulphuric acid*—intense blue in the acetic acid layer and a brown ring free from red at the junction of the two liquids (see also Lanatoside C).

Thin-layer Chromatography. *System TK*—Rf 27. (*Perchloric acid solution*, followed by examination under ultraviolet light, blue fluorescence; p-*anisaldehyde reagent*, blue.)

Disposition in the Body. Incompletely absorbed after oral administration and metabolised to digoxin. After intravenous administration, about 80% of a single dose is excreted in the urine in 72 hours, mostly as unchanged drug, and about 10% of a dose is eliminated in the faeces. During maintenance treatment, about 30% of a daily dose is excreted in the 24-hour urine. After oral administration digoxin accounts for about 50% of the total urinary excretion material.

Deslanoside is a metabolite of lanatoside C.

THERAPEUTIC CONCENTRATION.

After an intravenous dose of 400 µg given to 5 subjects, a mean plasma concentration of 0.03 µg/ml was reported at 15 minutes, declining to 0.001 µg/ml at 48 hours; after an oral dose of 800 µg given to 5 subjects, a mean peak plasma concentration of 0.003 µg/ml was attained in 2 hours (A. Marzo *et al.*, *Farmaco, Edn prat.*, 1982, *37*, 28–37).

HALF-LIFE. Plasma half-life, about 33 hours.

DISTRIBUTION IN BLOOD. Plasma: whole blood ratio, 1.4.

PROTEIN BINDING. In plasma, weakly bound.

Dose. For rapid digitalisation, 0.8 to 1.6 mg intravenously.

Desmetryne   *Herbicide*

Proprietary Name. Semeron 25 WP
2-Isopropylamino-4-methylamino-6-methylthio-1,3,5-triazine
$C_8H_{15}N_5S = 213.3$
CAS—1014-69-3

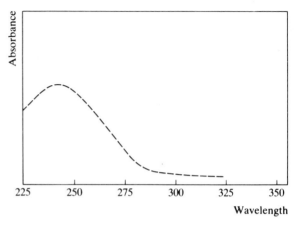

Ultraviolet Spectrum. Methanol—243 nm ($A_1^1 = 450$ b).

Infra-red Spectrum. Principal peaks at wavenumbers 1639, 1052, 1612, 1086, 1265, 1694.

Use. Topically as a 0.05% cream or ointment.

A white crystalline solid. M.p. 84° to 86°.
Very slightly **soluble** in water; readily soluble in organic solvents.

Thin-layer Chromatography. *System TA*—Rf 73. (*Dragendorff spray*, positive.)

Gas Chromatography. *System GA*—RI 1795; *system GK*—retention time 0.95 relative to caffeine.

Ultraviolet Spectrum. Aqueous acid—258 nm ($A_1^1 = 450$ b).

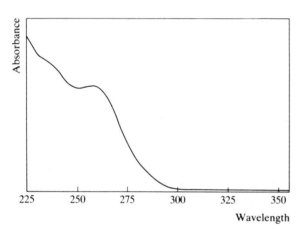

Infra-red Spectrum. Principal peaks at wavenumbers 1531, 1587, 1258, 806, 1292, 1163 (KBr disk).

Mass Spectrum. Principal peaks at *m/z* 213, 57, 58, 198, 82, 171, 43, 99.

Desonide   *Corticosteroid*

Synonyms. Desfluorotriamcinolone Acetonide; 16-Hydroxy-prednisolone 16,17-Acetonide.

Proprietary Names. Apolar; Locapred; Tridesilon; Tridésonit.

11β,21 - Dihydroxy - 16α,17α - isopropylidenedioxypregna - 1,4 - diene-3,20-dione
$C_{24}H_{32}O_6 = 416.5$
CAS—638-94-8

White powder or crystals.

Dexamethasone   *Corticosteroid*

Synonyms. Desamethasone; 9α-Fluoro-16α-methylprednisolone.
Proprietary Names. Aeroseb-Dex; Decaderm; Decadron (elixir and tablets); Decalix; Decaspray; Dexacortisyl; Dexalocal; Dexasone (tablets); Dexone; Dezone (tablets); Fortecortin (tablets); Hexadrol (tablets); Maxidex; Millicorten; Miral; Oradexon (tablets). It is an ingredient of Maxitrol.
9α-Fluoro-11β,17α,21-trihydroxy-16α-methylpregna-1,4-diene-3,20-dione
$C_{22}H_{29}FO_5 = 392.5$
CAS—50-02-2

Dexamethasone is a synthetic glucocorticoid and is an isomer of betamethasone.
A white crystalline powder. M.p. about 250° to 253°, with decomposition. A solution in dioxan is dextrorotatory.
Practically **insoluble** in water; soluble 1 in 42 of ethanol and 1 in 165 of chloroform; sparingly soluble in acetone and methanol; very slightly soluble in ether.

Dexamethasone Acetate
Synonym. Dexamethasone 21-Acetate
Proprietary Names. Decadron-LA; Dexacen-La-8; Dexasone L.A.; Fortecortin (suspension for injection).
$C_{24}H_{31}FO_6 = 434.5$
CAS—1177-87-3 (anhydrous); 55812-90-3 (monohydrate)
A white powder. M.p. about 225°, with decomposition.
Practically **insoluble** in water; soluble 1 in 40 of ethanol, 1 in 25 of dehydrated alcohol, 1 in 33 of chloroform, and 1 in 1000 of ether; freely soluble in acetone and methanol.

Dexamethasone Isonicotinate

Synonym. Dexamethasone 21-Isonicotinate
Proprietary Names. Auxison(e). It is an ingredient of Dexa-Rhinaspray.
$C_{28}H_{32}FNO_6 = 497.6$
CAS—2265-64-7

Dexamethasone Sodium Phosphate

Synonym. Sodium 9α-Fluoro-16α-methylprednisolone 21-Phosphate
Proprietary Names. Dalaron; Decadron (injection); Decasone; Dexacen-4; Dexasone (injection); Dezone (injection); Fortecortin (injection); Hexadrol (injection); Novadex; Oradexon (injection); Savacort-D; Turbinaire Decadron.
$C_{22}H_{28}FNa_2O_8P = 516.4$
CAS—2392-39-4
A white or slightly yellow, very hygroscopic, crystalline powder.
Soluble 1 in 2 of water; sparingly soluble in dehydrated alcohol; practically insoluble in chloroform and ether.

Dexamethasone Tebutate

Synonyms. Dexamethasone Butylacetate; Dexamethasone TBA; Dexamethasone Tertiary Butyl Acetate.
Proprietary Name. Decadron-TBA
$C_{28}H_{39}FO_6 = 490.6$
CAS—24668-75-5
Practically **insoluble** in water; soluble in ethanol and acetone.

Colour Tests. Antimony Pentachloride—green; Naphthol–Sulphuric Acid—yellow-green/yellow; Sulphuric Acid—orange-pink.

Thin-layer Chromatography. *System TP*—Rf 32; *system TQ*—Rf 08; *system TR*—Rf 00; *system TS*—Rf 00. (*DPST solution.*)

Gas Chromatography. *System GA*—RI 2970.

High Pressure Liquid Chromatography. *System HT*—k′ 4.8.

Ultraviolet Spectrum. Methanol—240 nm ($A_1^1 = 385$ a).

Infra-red Spectrum. Principal peaks at wavenumbers 1663, 896, 1622, 1695, 1052, 1603.

Mass Spectrum. Principal peaks at *m/z* 121, 122, 315, 43, 147, 223, 135, 41.

Quantification. HIGH PRESSURE LIQUID CHROMATOGRAPHY. In plasma or tissues: sensitivity 10 ng in plasma, UV detection—B. Cham *et al.*, *Ther. Drug Monit.*, 1980, *2*, 373–377.

RADIOIMMUNOASSAY. In plasma or urine: sensitivity 1 ng/ml—J. English *et al.*, *Eur. J. clin. Pharmac.*, 1975, *9*, 239–244.

Disposition in the Body. Rapidly absorbed after oral administration. Up to 65% of a dose is excreted in the urine in 24 hours, mainly as metabolites.

HALF-LIFE. Plasma half-life, about 2 to 5 hours.

VOLUME OF DISTRIBUTION. About 1 litre/kg.

DISTRIBUTION IN BLOOD. Plasma: whole blood ratio, 1.2.

PROTEIN BINDING. In plasma, about 67%.

REFERENCE. S. E. Tsuei *et al.*, *J. Pharmacokinet. Biopharm.*, 1979, *7*, 249–264.

Dose. 0.5 to 9 mg daily.

Dexamphetamine   *Central Stimulant*

Synonym. Dextroamphetamine
Proprietary Names. It is an ingredient of Biphetamine and Durophet.
(*S*)-α-Methylphenethylamine
$C_9H_{13}N = 135.2$
CAS—51-64-9

$$C_6H_5 \cdot CH_2 \cdot \overset{\overset{\displaystyle H}{|}}{\underset{\underset{\displaystyle CH_3}{|}}{C}} - NH_2$$

Dexamphetamine Phosphate

Synonyms. Dextroamphetamine Phosphate; Monobasic Dextroamphetamine Phosphate.
$C_9H_{13}N,H_3PO_4 = 233.2$
CAS—7528-00-9
A white crystalline powder.
Soluble 1 in 20 of water; slightly soluble in ethanol; practically insoluble in chloroform and ether.

Dexamphetamine Sulphate

Synonym. Dextro Amphetamine Sulphate
Proprietary Names. Dexampex; Dexedrine; Diphylets; Ferndex. It is an ingredient of Dexamyl and Eskatrol.
$(C_9H_{13}N)_2,H_2SO_4 = 368.5$
CAS—51-63-8
A white or almost white crystalline powder. M.p. 295° to 300°.
Soluble 1 in 9 to 1 in 10 of water and 1 in 800 of ethanol; practically insoluble in ether.

For analytical data and Quantification see under Amphetamine.

Disposition in the Body. Well absorbed after oral administration. It is approximately twice as potent as amphetamine. For information on metabolism, excretion, and pharmacokinetics, see under Amphetamine.

Dose. 5 to 60 mg of dexamphetamine sulphate daily.

Dexbrompheniramine   *Antihistamine*

(+)-3-(4-Bromophenyl)-*NN*-dimethyl-3-(2-pyridyl)propylamine
$C_{16}H_{19}BrN_2 = 319.2$
CAS—132-21-8

An oily liquid.

Dexbrompheniramine Maleate

Proprietary Names. It is an ingredient of Disophrol, Drixoral, and Halin.
$C_{16}H_{19}BrN_2,C_4H_4O_4 = 435.3$
CAS—2391-03-9
A white crystalline powder. M.p. 103° to 113°.
Soluble 1 in 1.2 of water, 1 in 2.5 of ethanol, and 1 in 2 of chloroform; very slightly soluble in ether.

For analytical data see under Brompheniramine.

Disposition in the Body. See under Brompheniramine. Dexbrompheniramine is approximately twice as potent as brompheniramine.

TOXICITY.

The following postmortem concentrations of dexbrompheniramine were reported in a fatality involving the ingestion of dexbrompheniramine and 3 other drugs: blood 0.2 μg/ml, liver 4.5 μg/g (R. C. Baselt and E. M. Gross, *J. analyt. Toxicol.*, 1977, *1*, 168–170).

Dose. Usually 8 mg of dexbrompheniramine maleate daily; up to 18 mg daily has been given in sustained-release preparations.

Dexchlorpheniramine   *Antihistamine*

(+) - 3 - (4 - Chlorophenyl) - *NN* - dimethyl - 3 - (2 - pyridyl)pro-pylamine
$C_{16}H_{19}ClN_2 = 274.8$
CAS—25523-97-1

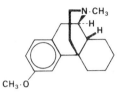

An oily liquid.
Soluble in chloroform.

Dexchlorpheniramine Maleate
Proprietary Names. Destral; Polaramin(e).
$C_{16}H_{19}ClN_2,C_4H_4O_4 = 390.9$
CAS—2438-32-6
A white crystalline powder. M.p. 110° to 115°.
Soluble 1 in 1.1 of water, 1 in 2 of ethanol, and 1 in 1.7 of chloroform; very slightly soluble in ether.

For analytical data see under Chlorpheniramine.

Disposition in the Body. See under Chlorpheniramine. Dexchlorpheniramine is more potent than chlorpheniramine.

Dose. 6 to 8 mg of dexchlorpheniramine maleate daily; up to 18 mg daily has been given in sustained-release preparations.

Dexpanthenol   *Vitamin B Activity*

Synonyms. Dextro-Pantothenyl Alcohol; Pantothenol.
Proprietary Names. Bepanthen(e); Ilopan; Motilyn; Panthoderm.
(*R*) - 2,4 - Dihydroxy - *N* - (3 - hydroxypropyl) - 3,3 - dimethylbutyramide
$C_9H_{19}NO_4 = 205.3$
CAS—81-13-0

$$HOCH_2 \cdot \underset{\underset{CH_3}{|}}{\overset{\overset{CH_3}{|}}{C}} - \underset{\underset{H}{|}}{\overset{\overset{OH}{|}}{C}} - CO \cdot NH \cdot [CH_2]_3 \cdot OH$$

A clear, colourless or slightly yellow, hygroscopic, viscous liquid.
Miscible with water and ethanol; soluble 1 in 70 of chloroform and 1 in 200 of ether.

Thin-layer Chromatography. *System TA*—Rf 70. (*Acidified potassium permanganate solution*, positive, developing slowly.)

Gas Chromatography. *System GA*—RI 1807.

Ultraviolet Spectrum. No significant absorption, 230 to 360 nm.

Infra-red Spectrum. Principal peaks at wavenumbers 1629, 1035, 1064, 1520, 1282, 1250 (thin film).

Dose. Dexpanthenol has been given in doses of 250 to 500 mg intramuscularly.

Dextromethorphan   *Cough Suppressant*

(+)-3-Methoxy-9a-methylmorphinan
$C_{18}H_{25}NO = 271.4$
CAS—125-71-3

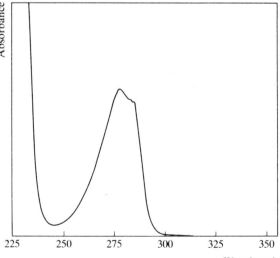

An almost white or slightly yellow crystalline powder. M.p. 109° to 113°.
Practically **insoluble** in water; freely soluble in chloroform.

Dextromethorphan Hydrobromide
Proprietary Names. Balminil D.M.; Broncho-Grippol-DM; Cosylan; DM Syrup; Dormethan; Robidex; Romilar; Sedatuss; Tussorphan. It is an ingredient of Actifed Compound Linctus, Benafed, Benylin (fortified linctus), CoTylenol (liquid), Dexylets, Lotussin, Paranorm, Rondec-DM, Syrtussar, Tancolin, Tusana, Tussils, and Unitussin.
$C_{18}H_{25}NO,HBr,H_2O = 370.3$
CAS—125-69-9 (anhydrous); *6700-34-1* (monohydrate)
A white crystalline powder. M.p. about 125°, with decomposition.
Soluble 1 in 60 to 1 in 65 of water and 1 in 10 of ethanol; freely soluble in chloroform with the separation of water; practically insoluble in ether.

Dissociation Constant. pK_a 8.3.

Colour Tests. Aromaticity (Method 2)—yellow/orange-red; Liebermann's Test—black.

Thin-layer Chromatography. *System TA*—Rf 34; *system TB*—Rf 44; *system TC*—Rf 17. (*Acidified iodoplatinate solution*, positive.)

Gas Chromatography. *System GA*—dextromethorphan RI 2140, dextrorphan RI 2230.

High Pressure Liquid Chromatography. *System HA*—dextromethorphan k' 5.6 (tailing peak), dextrorphan k' 4.7 (tailing peak).

Ultraviolet Spectrum. Aqueous acid—278 nm ($A_1^1 = 70$ a). No alkaline shift.

Infra-red Spectrum. Principal peaks at wavenumbers 1496, 1242, 1040, 1300, 1280, 1070 (dextromethorphan hydrobromide, KBr disk).

Wavelength

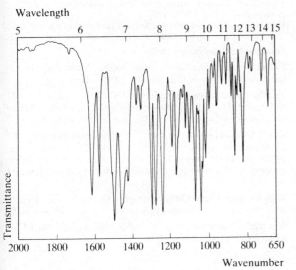

Wavenumber

Mass Spectrum. Principal peaks at m/z 59, 271, 150, 270, 31, 214, 42, 171; dextrorphan 59, 257, 150, 256, 31, 76, 42, 157.

Quantification. SPECTROFLUORIMETRY. In plasma: dextrorphan—G. Ramachander *et al., J. pharm. Sci.,* 1977, *66,* 1047–1048.

GAS CHROMATOGRAPHY. In serum: dextromethorphan, sensitivity 1 ng/ml, ECD—J. W. Barnhart and E. N. Massad, *J. Chromat.,* 1979, *163*; *Biomed. Appl.,* 5, 390–395.

HIGH PRESSURE LIQUID CHROMATOGRAPHY. In plasma: dextrorphan, sensitivity 20 ng/ml, fluorescence detection—R. Gillilan *et al., Analyt. Lett. (Part B),* 1980, *13,* 381–387. In urine: dextromethorphan and metabolites, sensitivity 17 to 90 ng/ml in non-hydrolysed urine and 110 to 210 ng/ml in hydrolysed urine, UV detection—Y. H. Park *et al., J. pharm. Sci.,* 1984, *73,* 24–29.

Disposition in the Body. Well absorbed after oral administration. Metabolised by *N*- and *O*-demethylation followed by sulphate or glucuronic acid conjugation. The major metabolite is dextrorphan, (+)-3-hydroxy-*N*-methylmorphinan; (+)-3-hydroxymorphinan has also been identified. About 50% of a dose is excreted in the urine in 24 hours, mostly as the glucuronide and sulphate conjugates of the metabolites; about 8% of a dose is excreted as unchanged drug in 6 hours.

THERAPEUTIC CONCENTRATION.
Following a single oral dose of 30 mg to 6 subjects, a mean peak plasma concentration of 0.38 µg/ml of conjugated dextrorphan was attained in 2 hours (G. Ramachander *et al., J. pharm. Sci.,* 1977, *66,* 1047–1048).
After an oral dose of 20 mg of dextromethorphan hydrobromide given to 12 subjects, peak serum concentrations of less than 0.001 µg/ml to 0.008 µg/ml (mean 0.0018) of dextromethorphan were attained in about 2.5 hours (J. W. Barnhart and E. N. Massad, *J. Chromat.,* 1979, *163*; *Biomed. Appl.,* 5, 390–395).

TOXICITY. The estimated minimum lethal dose is 0.5 g.

Dose. 15 to 120 mg of dextromethorphan hydrobromide daily.

Dextromoramide

Narcotic Analgesic

Synonyms. Dextrodiphenopyrine; *d*-Moramid; Pyrrolamidol.
(+)-1-(3-Methyl-4-morpholino-2,2-diphenylbutyryl)-pyrrolidine
$C_{25}H_{32}N_2O_2 = 392.5$
CAS—357-56-2

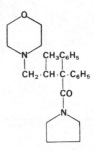

A white amorphous or microcrystalline powder. M.p. 184°. Practically **insoluble** in water; soluble 1 in 50 of ethanol, 1 in 3 of chloroform, 1 in 30 of isopropyl alcohol, and 1 in 45 of methanol; slightly soluble in ether.

Dextromoramide Tartrate

Synonym. Dextromoramide Acid Tartrate
Proprietary Names. Jetrium; Palfium.
$C_{25}H_{32}N_2O_2,C_4H_6O_6 = 542.6$
CAS—2922-44-3
A white amorphous or crystalline powder. M.p. about 190°, with slight decomposition.
Soluble 1 in 25 of water, 1 in 85 of ethanol, and 1 in 40 of methanol; slightly soluble in chloroform and isopropyl alcohol; very slightly soluble in ether.

Colour Test. Liebermann's Test (100°)—green.

Thin-layer Chromatography. *System TA*—Rf 76; *system TB*—Rf 40; *system TC*—Rf 71. (*Dragendorff spray,* positive; *acidified iodoplatinate solution,* positive.)

Gas Chromatography. *System GA*—RI 2940; *system GC*—RI 3625.

High Pressure Liquid Chromatography. *System HA*—k' 0.7; *system HC*—k' 0.09.

Ultraviolet Spectrum. Aqueous acid—254 nm, 259 nm ($A_1^1 = 10.6$ a), 264 nm. No alkaline shift.

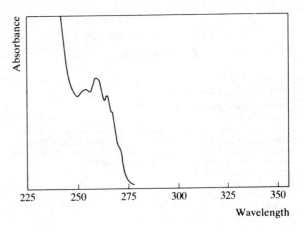

Wavelength

Infra-red Spectrum. Principal peaks at wavenumbers 1623, 703, 1107, 717, 858, 1002 (Nujol mull).

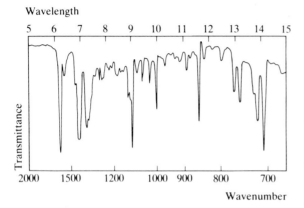

Mass Spectrum. Principal peaks at m/z 100, 265, 128, 266, 44, 98, 56, 101.

Disposition in the Body. Absorbed after oral administration. Metabolic reactions may include *N*-oxidation, hydroxylation, and amide hydrolysis; it is possible that 2-hydroxydextromoramide is a major metabolite. Excreted in the urine, partly as unchanged drug.

TOXICITY. The estimated minimum lethal dose is 500 mg. Fatalities have occurred at blood concentrations greater than 0.04 µg/ml.

The following postmortem disposition was found in a fatal case after the injection of dextromoramide and diazepam: blood, dextromoramide 0.5 µg/ml, diazepam 0.13 µg/ml; liver, dextromoramide 0.9 µg/g, diazepam 0.37 µg/g; urine, dextromoramide not detected, diazepam 0.33 µg/ml (P. Ashton *et al.*, *Bull. int. Ass. forens. Toxicol.*, 1978, *14*(2), 22–24).

Dose. The equivalent of 5 to 20 mg of dextromoramide, repeated as necessary.

Dextropropoxyphene   *Narcotic Analgesic*

Synonym. Propoxyphene
(+)-(1*S*,2*R*)-1-Benzyl-3-dimethylamino-2-methyl-1-phenyl-propyl propionate
$C_{22}H_{29}NO_2 = 339.5$
CAS—469-62-5

$$(CH_3)_2N \cdot CH_2 - \underset{\underset{H}{|}}{\overset{\overset{CH_3}{|}}{C}} - \underset{\underset{C_6H_5}{|}}{\overset{\overset{O \cdot CO \cdot CH_2 \cdot CH_3}{|}}{C}} - CH_2 \cdot C_6H_5$$

Crystals. M.p. 75° to 76°.
Very slightly **soluble** in water.

Dextropropoxyphene Hydrochloride

Synonym. Propoxyphene Hydrochloride
Proprietary Names. Algaphan; Algodex; Antalvic; Daraphen; Darvon; Depronal; Depronal SA; Develin; Dolene; Dolocap; Erantin; Mardon; Novopropoxyn; Pro-65; Proxagesic; SK-65; 642 Tablets. It is an ingredient of Cosalgesic, Dextrogesic, and Distalgesic.
$C_{22}H_{29}NO_2,HCl = 375.9$
CAS—1639-60-7
A white or slightly yellow powder. M.p. 163° to 169°.
Soluble 1 in 0.3 of water, 1 in 1.5 of ethanol, and 1 in 0.6 of chloroform; practically insoluble in ether.

Dextropropoxyphene Napsylate

Synonym. Propoxyphene Napsylate
Proprietary Names. Darvon-N; Doloxene. It is an ingredient of Darvocet-N, Distalgesic Soluble, Dolasan, and Napsalgesic.
$C_{22}H_{29}NO_2,C_{10}H_8O_3S,H_2O = 565.7$
CAS—17140-78-2 (anhydrous); *26570-10-5* (monohydrate)
A white powder. M.p. 158° to 165°.
Practically **insoluble** in water; soluble 1 in 13 to 1 in 15 of ethanol, and 1 in 3 of chloroform; soluble in acetone and methanol.

Dissociation Constant. pK_a 6.3.

Colour Tests. Liebermann's Test—brown; Mandelin's Test—grey-brown; Marquis Test—black-violet → green.

Thin-layer Chromatography. *System TA*—Rf 68; *system TB*—Rf 59; *system TC*—Rf 55. (*Dragendorff spray*, positive; *acidified iodoplatinate solution*, positive; *Marquis reagent*, violet.)

Gas Chromatography. *System GA*—dextropropoxyphene RI 2188, norpropoxyphene RI 2395; *system GB*—dextropropoxyphene RI 1938; *system GC*—dextropropoxyphene RI 2173; *system GF*—dextropropoxyphene RI 2370, norpropoxyphene RI 3025.

High Pressure Liquid Chromatography. *System HA*—dextropropoxyphene k' 1.9, norpropoxyphene k' 1.3; *system HC*—k' 0.19.

Ultraviolet Spectrum. Aqueous acid—252 nm, 257 nm ($A_1^1 = 12$ a), 263 nm. No alkaline shift.

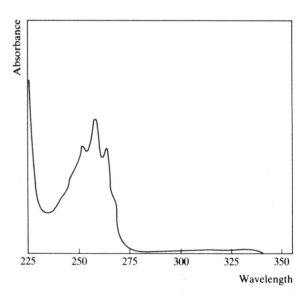

Infra-red Spectrum. Principal peaks at wavenumbers 1730, 1175, 725, 704, 776, 1026 (Nujol mull).

Mass Spectrum. Principal peaks at m/z 58, 117, 208, 115, 193, 91, 179, 130 (no peaks above 210); norpropoxyphene 44, 208, 117, 58, 193, 130, 57, 29.

Quantification. SPECTROFLUORIMETRY. In blood, urine or tissues: limit of detection 10 ng—J. C. Valentour *et al.*, *Clin. Chem.*, 1974, *20*, 275–277.

GAS CHROMATOGRAPHY. In plasma: dextropropoxyphene and norpropoxyphene, FID—M. Cleeman, *J. Chromat.*, 1977, *132*,

Wavelength

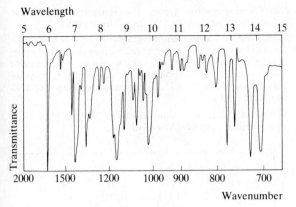

287–294. In plasma: review of thermal decomposition of dextropropoxyphene during gas chromatography—B. J. Millard *et al., J. pharm. Sci.*, 1980, *69*, 1177–1179. In plasma or urine: sensitivity 50 ng/ml for dextropropoxyphene and 100 ng/ml for norpropoxyphene, AFID—P. A. Margot *et al., J. chromatogr. Sci.*, 1983, *21*, 201–204.

HIGH PRESSURE LIQUID CHROMATOGRAPHY. In plasma or breast milk: dextropropoxyphene and norpropoxyphene, sensitivity 20 ng/ml, UV detection—R. L. Kunka *et al., J. pharm. Sci.*, 1985, *74*, 103–104.

Disposition in the Body. Readily and completely absorbed but undergoes considerable first-pass metabolism; bioavailability about 40%. Rapidly distributed and concentrated in the brain, lungs, liver, and kidneys. The main metabolic reaction is *N*-demethylation which produces norpropoxyphene, the major metabolite, and also dinorpropoxyphene which is dehydrated to cyclic dinorpropoxyphene. Norpropoxyphene has less than half the activity of dextropropoxyphene. In 24 hours, about 35% of a dose is excreted in urine with about 13% of the dose as norpropoxyphene and up to 5% as unchanged drug. A total of 60 to 70% of a dose is excreted in urine in about 5 days; about 18% of the dose may be eliminated in the faeces over the same period.

THERAPEUTIC CONCENTRATION. In plasma, usually in the range 0.05 to 0.75 µg/ml.

Peak plasma concentrations of dextropropoxyphene of 0.17 to 0.37 µg/ml (mean 0.23) were attained 2 hours after administration of a single oral dose of 130 mg to 6 subjects; peak norpropoxyphene concentrations of 0.19 to 0.42 µg/ml (mean 0.27) were attained in 4 hours (K. Verebely and C. E. Inturrisi, *Clin. Pharmac. Ther.*, 1974, *15*, 302–309).

Following daily oral dosing of 195 mg to 3 subjects, steady-state plasma concentrations were: dextropropoxyphene 0.24 to 0.75 µg/ml (mean 0.4); norpropoxyphene 0.6 to 3.0 µg/ml (mean 1.5) (K. Verebely and C. E. Inturrisi, *J. Chromat.*, 1973, *75*, 195–205).

TOXICITY. The estimated minimum lethal dose is 0.5 g. Blood concentrations in the region of 1 µg/ml are likely to cause toxic reactions; concentrations of 2 µg/ml or more may be lethal. In fatalities in which dextropropoxyphene is involved, it is common to find much greater concentrations in the liver and lungs than in the blood. Addicts can ingest 10 times the normal dosage before showing toxicity whereas children show toxic symptoms after only one-twentieth of the normal dose.

In a review of a number of fatalities, blood concentrations in 23 cases ranged from 1 to 60 µg/ml (mean 13) and liver concentrations in 73 cases ranged from 5 to 550 µg/g (mean 97) (R. H. Cravey *et al., J. forens. Sci.*, 1974, *19*, 72–80).

In 6 fatalities attributed to dextropropoxyphene overdose, the following postmortem tissue concentrations, µg/ml or µg/g (mean, *n*), were reported:

	Dextropropoxyphene	Norpropoxyphene
Blood	1.1–4.9 (3.5, 6)	1.4–5.9 (3.5, 6)
Brain	2.8–25.2 (14, 4)	4–9.1 (6, 4)
Liver	5.7–229 (117, 6)	24.2–73.2 (50, 6)
Urine	1.5–60.2 (17, 5)	1.6–287 (68, 5)

(A. J. McBay, *Clin. Chem.*, 1976, *22*, 1319–1321).

HALF-LIFE. Plasma half-life, dextropropoxyphene 8 to 24 hours (mean 15), norpropoxyphene 20 to 50 hours (mean 29).

VOLUME OF DISTRIBUTION. About 16 litres/kg.

CLEARANCE. Plasma clearance, about 15 ml/min/kg.

PROTEIN BINDING. In plasma, about 70 to 80%.

NOTE. For a review of dextropropoxyphene pharmacokinetics and overdose, see R. J. Young, *Drugs*, 1983, *26*, 70–79.

Dose. Usually 195 to 260 mg of dextropropoxyphene hydrochloride, or 300 to 400 mg of the napsylate, daily.

Dextrorphan
Cough Suppressant

(+)-9a-Methylmorphinan-3-ol
$C_{17}H_{23}NO = 257.4$
CAS—125-73-5

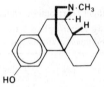

Crystals. M.p. 198° to 199°.

Thin-layer Chromatography. *System TA*—Rf 35; *system TB*—Rf 13; *system TC*—Rf 07. (*Dragendorff spray*, positive; *acidified iodoplatinate solution*, positive.)

Gas Chromatography. *System GA*—RI 2230.

High Pressure Liquid Chromatography. *System HA*—k′ 4.7 (tailing peak).

Ultraviolet Spectrum. Aqueous acid—279 nm ($A_1^1 = 79$ a); aqueous alkali—240 nm ($A_1^1 = 339$ a), 299 nm ($A_1^1 = 119$ a).

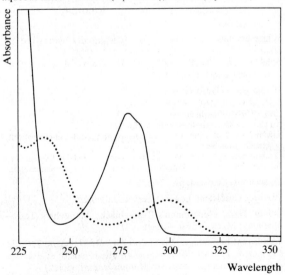

Infra-red Spectrum. Principal peaks at wavenumbers 1240, 1495, 1280, 1580, 756, 1610 (KBr disk).

Wavelength

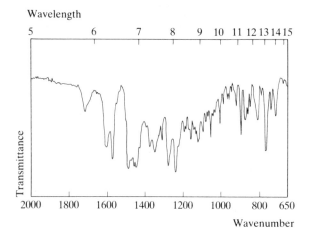

Mass Spectrum. Principal peaks at m/z 59, 257, 150, 256, 31, 76, 42, 157.

Quantification. See under Dextromethorphan.

Disposition in the Body. Dextrorphan is the major metabolite of dextromethorphan but has less antitussive activity.

Diamorphine

Narcotic Analgesic

Synonyms. Acetomorphine; Diacetylmorphine; Heroin.
3,6-*O*-Diacetylmorphine
$C_{21}H_{23}NO_5 = 369.4$
CAS—561-27-3

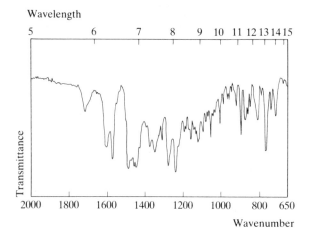

White crystals. M.p. about 170°. It is rapidly hydrolysed by alkalis.
Soluble 1 in 1700 of water, 1 in 31 of ethanol, 1 in 1.5 of chloroform, and 1 in 100 of ether.

Diamorphine Hydrochloride
$C_{21}H_{23}NO_5, HCl, H_2O = 423.9$
CAS—1502-95-0 (anhydrous)
An almost white crystalline powder. M.p. 229° to 233°.
Soluble 1 in 1.6 of water, 1 in 12 of ethanol, and 1 in 1.6 of chloroform; practically insoluble in ether.
Diamorphine hydrolyses in aqueous solution to 3-*O*- and 6-*O*-mono-acetylmorphine and morphine to a significant extent at room temperature.

Dissociation Constant. pK_a 7.6 (23°).

Partition Coefficient. Log P (ether/pH 7.0), 0.2.

Colour Tests. Liebermann's Test—black; Mandelin's Test—blue-grey; Marquis Test—violet.

Thin-layer Chromatography. System *TA*—Rf 47; system *TB*—Rf 15; system *TC*—Rf 38. (*Dragendorff spray*, positive; *acidified iodoplatinate solution*, positive; *Marquis reagent*, violet.)

Gas Chromatography. System *GA*—diamorphine RI 2614, 6-monoacetylmorphine RI 2537, morphine RI 2454.

High Pressure Liquid Chromatography. System *HA*—diamorphine k' 3.0 (tailing peak), 6-monoacetylmorphine k' 3.6 (tailing peak), morphine k' 3.8 (tailing peak); *system HC*—diamorphine k' 0.66, 6-monoacetylmorphine k' 0.80, morphine k' 1.30; *system HS*—diamorphine k' 0.35, 6-monoacetylmorphine k' 1.00, morphine k' 5.16.

Ultraviolet Spectrum. Aqueous acid—279 nm $(A_1^1 = 46 \text{ a})$; aqueous alkali—299 nm $(A_1^1 = 69 \text{ a})$.

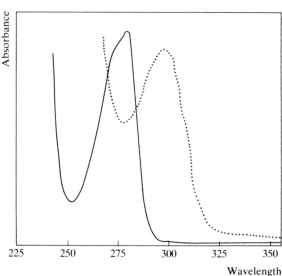

Infra-red Spectrum. Principal peaks at wavenumbers 1245, 1764, 1178, 1215, 911, 1736 (diamorphine hydrochloride, Nujol mull). Two polymorphic forms may occur.

Wavelength

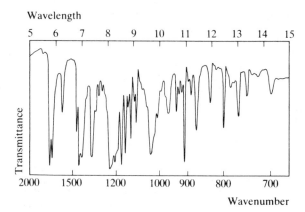

Mass Spectrum. Principal peaks at m/z 327, 43, 369, 268, 310, 42, 215, 204; 6-monoacetylmorphine 327, 268, 42, 43, 215, 44, 328, 269; morphine 285, 162, 42, 215, 286, 124, 44, 284.

Quantification. GAS CHROMATOGRAPHY. In blood: diamorphine and 6-monoacetylmorphine, sensitivity 100 ng/ml, AFID—D. A. Smith and W. J. Cole, *J. Chromat.*, 1975, *105*, 377–381. In illicit heroin samples—G. Machata and W. Vycudlik, *J. analyt. Toxicol.*, 1980, *4*, 318–321.

HIGH PRESSURE LIQUID CHROMATOGRAPHY. In illicit samples, using reversed phase ion-pair chromatography—I. S. Lurie *et al.*, *J. forens. Sci.*, 1982, *27*, 519–526. In blood: diamorphine, 6-monoacetylmorphine, and morphine, sensitivity 12.5 ng/ml, UV detection—J. G. Umans *et al.*, *J. Chromat.*, 1982, *233*; *Biomed. Appl.*, *22*, 213–225.

Disposition in the Body. Readily absorbed after oral administration or by injection. Rapidly hydrolysed to 6-monoacetylmorphine in blood and then more slowly metabolised to morphine which is the major active metabolite; normorphine is also formed to a minor extent; small quantities of codeine are occasionally seen in the urine of addicts, but this is thought to arise from the presence of acetylcodeine as an impurity in illicit heroin samples. All metabolites may be conjugated with glucuronic acid. Up to 80% of a dose is excreted in the urine in 24 hours, mainly as morphine-3-glucuronide with about 5 to 7% of the dose as free morphine, 1% as 6-monoacetylmorphine, 0.1% as unchanged drug, and trace amounts of other metabolites; after inhalation, 14 to 20% of the dose appears in the urine; morphine metabolites are excreted in the bile.

THERAPEUTIC CONCENTRATION. Because of its rapid hydrolysis, diamorphine is difficult to detect in plasma. Morphine plasma concentrations are usually in the range 0.01 to 0.07 µg/ml.

Diamorphine was detected in blood 2 minutes after an intravenous dose of 4 to 5 mg given to 4 subjects, but declined to a blood concentration of less than 0.01 µg/ml within 10 to 15 minutes (C. E. Inturrisi *et al.*, *New Engl. J. Med.*, 1984, *310*, 1213–1217).

TOXICITY. Diamorphine is 2 to 3 times more potent than morphine. The estimated minimum lethal dose is 200 mg, but addicts may be able to tolerate up to 10 times as much; fatalities have occurred after doses of 10 mg.

The following postmortem disposition (total morphine and conjugates) was reported in 2 cases of suicide: blood 0.38 and 0.41 µg/ml, brain 0.25 and 0.35 µg/g, kidney 0.70 and 1.51 µg/g, liver 0.35 and 0.66 µg/g, urine 0.49 and 0.10 µg/ml (D. Reed *et al.*, *Forens. Sci.*, 1977, *9*, 49–52).

In a review of 40 cases of death due to injection of diamorphine by addicts, the following postmortem disposition (total morphine and conjugates) was reported: blood 0.01 to 1.4 µg/ml (mean 0.19, 34 cases), bile 0.02 to 300 µg/ml (mean 22.5, 38 cases), brain 0.02 to 0.60 µg/g (mean 0.20, 21 cases), lung 0.02 to 4.2 µg/g (mean 0.46, 36 cases), urine 0.1 to 120 µg/ml (mean 13.2, 23 cases) (R. G. Richards *et al.*, *J. forens. Sci.*, 1976, *21*, 467–482).

HALF-LIFE. Plasma half-life, diamorphine about 3 minutes, morphine about 2 to 3 hours.

VOLUME OF DISTRIBUTION. Morphine about 3 to 5 litres/kg.

CLEARANCE. Plasma clearance, morphine about 15 to 20 ml/min/kg.

PROTEIN BINDING. In plasma, morphine about 20 to 35%.

NOTE. For a review of the metabolism and excretion of diamorphine see U. Boerner *et al.*, *Drug Met. Rev.*, 1975, *4*, 39–73.

Dose. 5 to 10 mg of diamorphine hydrochloride every 4 hours.

Diamphenethide   *Anthelmintic (Veterinary)*

Synonym. Diamfenetide
Proprietary Name. Coriban
$\beta\beta'$-Oxybis(aceto-*p*-phenetidide)
$C_{20}H_{24}N_2O_5 = 372.4$
CAS—36141-82-9

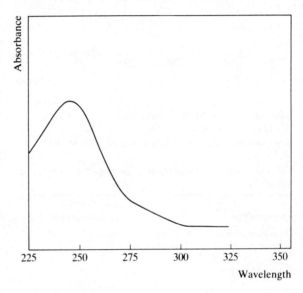

A white to pale buff-coloured powder.

Practically **insoluble** in water; soluble 1 in 160 of ethanol, 1 in 500 of chloroform, and 1 in 150 of methanol; practically insoluble in ether.

Colour Test. Mandelin's Test—grey-green.

Thin-layer Chromatography. *System TA*—Rf 81. (*Acidified iodoplatinate solution*, positive.)

Ultraviolet Spectrum. Aqueous acid—244 nm.

Absorbance / Wavelength

Infra-red Spectrum. Principal peaks at wavenumbers 1653, 1508, 1529, 1238, 1136, 1597 (KBr disk).

Diamthazole   *Antifungal*

Synonyms. Amycazol; Dimazole.
6-(2-Diethylaminoethoxy)-2-dimethylaminobenzothiazole
$C_{15}H_{23}N_3OS = 293.4$
CAS—95-27-2

Diamthazole Hydrochloride
Proprietary Name. Asterol
$C_{15}H_{23}N_3OS,2HCl = 366.3$
CAS—136-96-9

A white, hygroscopic, crystalline powder.

Soluble in water, ethanol, and methanol; very slightly soluble in chloroform and ether.

Colour Test. Liebermann's Test—green.

Thin-layer Chromatography. *System TA*—Rf 52; *system TB*—Rf 30; *system TC*—Rf 30. (*Acidified iodoplatinate solution*, positive.)

Ultraviolet Spectrum. Aqueous acid—270 nm ($A_1^1 = 370$ b), 293 nm.

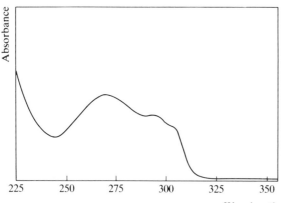

Infra-red Spectrum. Principal peaks at wavenumbers 1015, 1041, 667, 1548, 1602, 1190 (KBr disk).

Mass Spectrum. Principal peaks at m/z 86, 100, 44, 30, 29, 42, 58, 56.

Use. Diamthazole hydrochloride has been used in a concentration of 5%.

Diaveridine   *Coccidiostat (Veterinary)*

Proprietary Name. It is an ingredient of Saquadil.

5-Veratrylpyrimidine-2,4-diyldiamine
$C_{13}H_{16}N_4O_2 = 260.3$
CAS—5355-16-8

A white or creamy-white crystalline powder. M.p. about 233°. Very slightly **soluble** in water and ethanol; soluble 1 in 600 of chloroform.

Colour Tests. Mandelin's Test—green; Marquis Test—grey → violet-brown.

Thin-layer Chromatography. *System TA*—Rf 58. (*Acidified iodoplatinate solution*, positive.)

Ultraviolet Spectrum. Aqueous acid—276 nm ($A_1^1 = 300$ a).

Infra-red Spectrum. Principal peaks at wavenumbers 1630, 1645, 1598, 1250, 1510, 1570 (KBr disk).

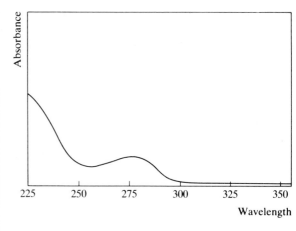

Diazepam   *Tranquilliser*

Proprietary Names. Alupram; Apozepam; Atensine; Dialar; Diazemuls; D-Tran; Ducene; E-Pam; Evacalm; Lorinon; Meval; Neo-Calme; Novodipam; Paxel; Pro-Pam; Serenack; Solis; Stesolid; Stress-Pam; Tensium; Valium; Valrelease; Vivol.

7-Chloro-1,3-dihydro-1-methyl-5-phenyl-2H-1,4-benzodiazepin-2-one
$C_{16}H_{13}ClN_2O = 284.7$
CAS—439-14-5

A white or yellow crystalline powder. M.p. 131° to 135°.
Very slightly **soluble** in water; soluble 1 in 25 of ethanol, 1 in 2 of chloroform, and 1 in 39 of ether.

Dissociation Constant. pK_a 3.3 (20°).

Partition Coefficient. Log P (octanol/pH 7.4), 2.7.

Colour Test. Formaldehyde–Sulphuric Acid—orange.

Thin-layer Chromatography. *System TA*—Rf 75; *system TB*—Rf 23; *system TC*—Rf 73; *system TD*—Rf 58; *system TE*—Rf 77; *system TF*—Rf 48. (*Dragendorff spray*, positive; *FPN reagent*, yellow; *acidified iodoplatinate solution*, positive; *Marquis reagent*, yellow.)

Gas Chromatography. *System GA*—diazepam RI 2425, desmethyldiazepam RI 2496, oxazepam RI 2336, temazepam RI 2633; *system GF*—diazepam RI 3045; *system GG*—diazepam RI 2940, desmethyldiazepam RI 3041, oxazepam RI 2803, temazepam RI 3125.

High Pressure Liquid Chromatography. *System HA*—diazepam k' 0.1, desmethyldiazepam k' 0.2; *system HI*—diazepam k' 9.47, desmethyldiazepam k' 8.00, oxazepam k' 4.62, temazepam k' 5.68; *system HJ*—diazepam k' 2.29; *system HK*—diazepam k' 2.49, desmethyldiazepam k' 1.99, oxazepam k' 0.73, temazepam k' 0.60.

Ultraviolet Spectrum. Aqueous acid—242 nm $(A_1^1 = 1020\ a)$, 284 nm, 366 nm.

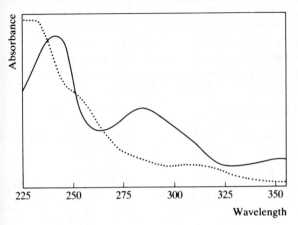

Wavelength

Infra-red Spectrum. Principal peaks at wavenumbers 1681, 1313, 705, 840, 1125, 740 (K Br disk).

Wavelength

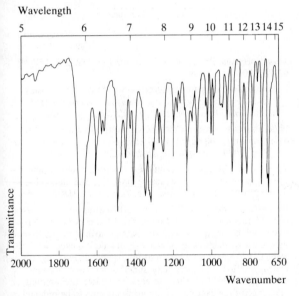

Wavenumber

Mass Spectrum. Principal peaks at m/z 256, 283, 284, 285, 257, 255, 258, 286; desmethyldiazepam 242, 269, 270, 241, 243, 271, 244, 272; oxazepam 257, 77, 268, 239, 205, 267, 233, 259; temazepam 271, 273, 300, 272, 256, 77, 255, 257.

Quantification. GAS CHROMATOGRAPHY. In plasma, saliva, or urine: diazepam and metabolites, sensitivity about 7.5 ng/ml, ECD—J. L. Valentine et al., Analyt. Lett. (Part B), 1982, 15, 1665–1683. In whole blood: diazepam and desmethyldiazepam, limit of detection 10 ng/ml, AFID—H. H. McCurdy et al., J. analyt. Toxicol., 1979, 3, 195–198.

HIGH PRESSURE LIQUID CHROMATOGRAPHY. In blood, plasma or urine: diazepam and metabolites, sensitivity 50 ng/ml in blood or plasma, 200 ng/ml in urine, UV detection—S. Cotler et al., J. Chromat., 1981, 222; Biomed. Appl., 11, 95–106. In plasma: diazepam and desmethyldiazepam, comparison with a gas chromatographic method, UV detection—V. A. Raisys et al., J. Chromat., 1980, 183; Biomed. Appl., 9, 441–448.

RADIOIMMUNOASSAY. In blood, plasma or saliva: sensitivity 30 ng/ml in blood or plasma, 300 pg/ml in saliva—R. Dixon and T. Crews, J. analyt. Toxicol., 1978, 2, 210–213.

Disposition in the Body. Rapidly and completely absorbed after oral administration. The main metabolic reactions are N-demethylation, 3-hydroxylation, and glucuronic acid conjugation. The major active metabolite is desmethyldiazepam (nor-dazepam) which accumulates during chronic dosing; other metabolites include oxazepam and temazepam, both of which are active. Only small traces of unchanged diazepam are excreted in the urine and the relative amounts of metabolites are variable and appear to be dose-dependent. About 70% of a dose is excreted in the urine, mainly as oxazepam glucuronide and conjugated desmethyldiazepam, together with smaller amounts of conjugated temazepam. About 10% of the dose may be eliminated in the faeces.

Diazepam is a metabolite of ketazolam and medazepam.

THERAPEUTIC CONCENTRATION. In plasma, usually in the range 0.1 to 2.5 µg/ml. After discontinuation of chronic therapy, concentrations of desmethyldiazepam may be substantially higher than diazepam and both unchanged drug and metabolite are still detectable 7 days after cessation of dosing.

Following a single oral dose of 10 mg to 4 subjects, peak blood concentrations of 0.14 to 0.19 µg/ml (mean 0.15) were attained in 1 to 1.5 hours; average peak concentrations of 0.03 µg/ml of desmethyldiazepam were attained after 24 hours (S. A. Kaplan et al., J. pharm. Sci., 1973, 62, 1789–1796).

After chronic daily oral dosing of 5 mg twice daily to 15 subjects, steady-state plasma concentrations were: diazepam 0.09 to 0.37 µg/ml (mean 0.23), desmethyldiazepam 0.13 to 0.46 µg/ml (mean 0.29), oxazepam 0.01 to 0.03 µg/ml (mean 0.02), temazepam 0.01 to 0.05 µg/ml (mean 0.03) (I. A. Zingales, J. Chromat., 1973, 75, 55–78).

TOXICITY. Toxic effects may be produced by blood concentrations greater than 1.5 µg/ml; fatalities caused by diazepam alone are rare, but may occur at blood concentrations greater than 5 µg/ml.

In a review of 914 drug-related deaths in which diazepam was involved it was found to be the sole cause of death in only 2 cases; postmortem concentrations of diazepam in the 2 cases were: blood 5 and 19 µg/ml, liver 13 µg/g in the first case (B. S. Finkle et al., J. Am. med. Ass., 1979, 242, 429–434).

In a fatality due to diazepam and alcohol ingestion, postmortem tissue-diazepam concentrations were: blood 1.3 µg/ml, bile 4.5 µg/ml, brain 2.4 µg/g, kidney 11.7 µg/g, liver 11.4 µg/g, urine 6.6 µg/ml (R. K. Simon, Bull. int. Ass. forens. Toxicol., 1976, 12(1), 19–20).

HALF-LIFE. Plasma half-life, diazepam 20 to 100 hours (mean 48), desmethyldiazepam about 40 to 100 hours but there is considerable intersubject variation—see under Nordazepam. The plasma half-life appears to be increased in elderly subjects and neonates, and in subjects with liver disease; sex differences have also been suggested.

VOLUME OF DISTRIBUTION. Diazepam and desmethyldiazepam, 0.5 to 2.5 litres/kg, increased in elderly subjects.

CLEARANCE. Plasma clearance, diazepam about 0.3 to 0.5 ml/min/kg, desmethyldiazepam about 0.1 to 0.3 ml/min/kg.

DISTRIBUTION IN BLOOD. Plasma: whole blood ratio, diazepam 1.8, desmethyldiazepam 1.7.

PROTEIN BINDING. In plasma, diazepam 98 to 99%, desmethyldiazepam about 97%.

NOTE. For a review of the clinical pharmacokinetics of diazepam see M. Mandelli et al., Clin. Pharmacokinet., 1978, 3, 72–91.

Dose. Usually 5 to 30 mg daily.

Diazinon

Pesticide

Synonym. Dimpylate
Proprietary Names. Basudin; Diazitol.
OO-Diethyl *O*-(2-isopropyl-6-methylpyrimidin-4-yl) phosphoro-thioate
$C_{12}H_{21}N_2O_3PS = 304.3$
CAS—333-41-5

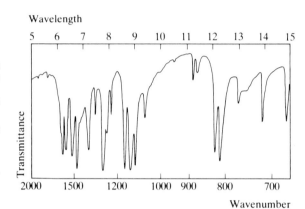

The pure compound is a colourless liquid; the technical grade is a pale to dark brown liquid. It is stable in alkaline solutions but is slowly hydrolysed in water and dilute acids.
Slightly **soluble** in water; miscible with ethanol, ether, and petroleum oils.

Colour Tests. Palladium Chloride—orange-brown; Phosphorus Test—yellow.

Thin-layer Chromatography. *System TW*—Rf 82.

Gas Chromatography. *System GA*—RI 1758; *system GK*—retention time 0.79 relative to caffeine.

Ultraviolet Spectrum. Hexane—248 nm ($A_1^1 = 170$ b).

Infra-red Spectrum. Principal peaks at wavenumbers 1020, 1587, 971, 1562, 823, 1159.

Mass Spectrum. Principal peaks at *m/z* 137, 179, 152, 93, 153, 199, 97, 43.

Quantification. GAS CHROMATOGRAPHY. In postmortem tissues: FID or ECD—A. Poklis *et al.*, *Forens. Sci. Int.*, 1980, *15*, 135–140.

Disposition in the Body. Rapidly absorbed from the lungs and through the skin.

TOXICITY. The estimated minimum lethal dose is 25 g.

In 2 fatalities due to diazinon ingestion, postmortem tissue concentrations were: blood 0.7, 33 µg/ml, brain 12, 62 µg/g, kidney 3, – µg/g, liver 30, 345 µg/g, adipose tissue 37, – µg/g (W. H. Wall, *Bull. int. Ass. forens. Toxicol.*, 1981, *16*(2), 27–28).

In a fatality attributed to diazinon, the following postmortem tissue concentrations were reported: blood 277 µg/ml, bile 200 µg/ml, brain 2 µg/g, kidney 0.1 µg/g, liver 4 µg/g (A. Poklis *et al.*, *Forens. Sci. Int.*, 1980, *15*, 135–140).

Diazoxide

Antihypertensive/Hyperglycaemic

Proprietary Names. Eudemine; Hyperstat; Hypertonalum; Proglicem; Proglycem.
7-Chloro-3-methyl-2*H*-1,2,4-benzothiadiazine 1,1-dioxide
$C_8H_7ClN_2O_2S = 230.7$
CAS—364-98-7

A white or creamy-white crystalline powder. M.p. 330° to 331°. Practically **insoluble** in water, chloroform, and ether; soluble 1 in 250 of ethanol; very soluble in solutions of alkali hydroxides; freely soluble in dimethylformamide.

Dissociation Constant. pK_a 8.5.

Thin-layer Chromatography. *System TA*—Rf 82; *system TB*—Rf 01; *system TC*—Rf 28.

Gas Chromatography. *System GA*—not eluted.

High Pressure Liquid Chromatography. *System HA*—k' 0.1.

Ultraviolet Spectrum. Aqueous alkali—280 nm ($A_1^1 = 585$ a).

Infra-red Spectrum. Principal peaks at wavenumbers 1139, 1294, 1166, 1495, 1112, 812 (KBr disk).

Mass Spectrum. Principal peaks at *m/z* 125, 189, 230, 127, 191, 63, 232, 90.

Quantification. GAS CHROMATOGRAPHY–MASS SPECTROMETRY. In plasma or urine: sensitivity 10 ng/ml—W. Sadee *et al.*, *J. Pharmacokinet. Biopharm.*, 1973, *1*, 295–305.

HIGH PRESSURE LIQUID CHROMATOGRAPHY. In plasma or urine: detection limit 100 ng/ml, UV detection—T. B. Vree *et al.*, *J. Chromat.*, 1979, *164*; *Biomed. Appl.*, 6, 228–234.

THIN-LAYER CHROMATOGRAPHY–ULTRAVIOLET SPECTROPHOTO-METRY. In plasma, urine or faeces: diazoxide and metabolites—A. W. Pruitt *et al.*, *J. Pharmac. exp. Ther.*, 1974, *188*, 248–256.

Disposition in the Body. Readily absorbed after oral administration. Metabolised by oxidation to the 3-hydroxymethyl derivative which is conjugated with sulphate or further metabolised to the 3-carboxy derivative. About 90% of a dose is excreted in the urine in 5 to 6 days, of which 6 to 50% is unchanged drug; the 3-hydroxymethyl and 3-carboxy metabolites each account for about 20 to 30% of the excreted material; the amount of unchanged drug excreted in the urine appears to be reduced in hypertensive patients; about 2% of a dose is eliminated in the faeces.

THERAPEUTIC CONCENTRATION. In plasma, usually in the range 15 to 50 µg/ml.

Following a single oral dose of 300 mg to 2 subjects, peak plasma concentrations of about 15 to 20 µg/ml were attained in 3 to 6 hours (A. W. Pruitt *et al.*, *Clin. Pharmac. Ther.*, 1973, *14*, 73–82).

TOXICITY. Toxic effects may be associated with plasma concentrations greater than 100 µg/ml.

HALF-LIFE. Plasma half-life, adults, about 20 to 70 hours; appears to be lower in children.

VOLUME OF DISTRIBUTION. About 0.2 to 0.3 litre/kg.

CLEARANCE. Plasma clearance, about 0.1 ml/min/kg.

DISTRIBUTION IN BLOOD. Plasma: whole blood ratio, about 1.7.

Wavelength

Transmittance

Wavenumber

PROTEIN BINDING. In plasma, about 90%; decreased in subjects with renal impairment.

NOTE. For a review of the pharmacokinetics of diazoxide see R. M. Pearson, *Clin. Pharmacokinet.*, 1977, *2*, 198–204.

Dose. In the treatment of intractable hypoglycaemia: initially 5 mg/kg daily, by mouth. In hypertensive crises: 300 mg intravenously.

Dibenzepin   *Antidepressant*

10 - (2 - Dimethylaminoethyl) - 5,10 - dihydro - 5 - methyl - 11*H* - dibenzo[*b,e*][1,4]diazepin-11-one
$C_{18}H_{21}N_3O = 295.4$
CAS—4498-32-2

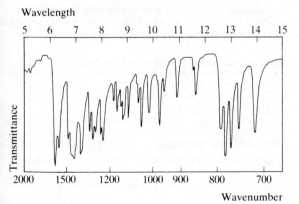

M.p. 116° to 117°.

Dibenzepin Hydrochloride
Proprietary Names. Deprex; Écatril; Noveril.
Note. Deprex is also used as a proprietary name for amitriptyline hydrochloride.
$C_{18}H_{21}N_3O,HCl = 331.8$
CAS—315-80-0
A colourless, fine crystalline powder. M.p. about 237°.
Soluble 1 in 16 of water; soluble in ethanol and chloroform.

Partition Coefficient. Log *P* (octanol/pH 7.4), 1.7.

Colour Test. Mandelin's Test—green.

Thin-layer Chromatography. *System TA*—Rf 54; *system TB*—Rf 20; *system TC*—Rf 35. (*Acidified iodoplatinate solution*, positive.)

Gas Chromatography. *System GA*—RI 2443; *system GF*—RI 2885.

High Pressure Liquid Chromatography. *System HA*—k' 2.8; *system HF*—k' 0.50.

Ultraviolet Spectrum. No significant absorption, 230 to 360 nm.

Infra-red Spectrum. Principal peaks at wavenumbers 1639, 775, 761, 1603, 1250, 1316 (dibenzepin hydrochloride, KBr disk).

Wavelength

Transmittance

Wavenumber

Mass Spectrum. Principal peaks at *m/z* 58, 224, 209, 71, 225, 72, 210, 180.

Quantification. ULTRAVIOLET SPECTROPHOTOMETRY. In blood, urine or tissues: detection limit 500 ng/g for dibenzepin plus desmethyl metabolites—H. Christensen and S. Felby, *Acta pharmac. tox.*, 1975, *37*, 393–401.

GAS CHROMATOGRAPHY. In blood, urine or tissues: dibenzepin and desmethyl metabolites, detection limit 300 ng/g, AFID—H.-J. Schlicht and H.-P. Gelbke, *J. Chromat.*, 1978, *166*, 599–603.

Disposition in the Body. Readily absorbed after oral administration; rapidly and extensively metabolised, mainly by *N*-demethylation. About 20 to 30% of a dose is excreted in the urine as free and conjugated desmethyl metabolites in 24 hours, together with about 1% of the dose as unchanged drug.

THERAPEUTIC CONCENTRATION.
During daily oral treatment with doses of 8 mg/kg of dibenzepin hydrochloride given to 12 patients for 22 days, mean plasma concentrations of 0.18 µg/ml of dibenzepin and 0.28 µg/ml of *N*-monodesmethyldibenzepin (demethylated in the side-chain) were reported, determined 4 hours after a dose. Plasma concentrations declined slightly during therapy (R. Gauch and J. Modestin, *Arzneimittel-Forsch.*, 1973, *23*, 687–690).

TOXICITY. The estimated minimum lethal dose is about 3 g; doses greater than 1.5 g may result in serious poisoning. Patients liable to arrhythmias are particularly susceptible to toxic effects.
The following tissue disposition of total dibenzepin and metabolites was reported in 6 suicides due to the ingestion of dibenzepin: blood 23 to 147 µg/g (mean 73), liver 255 to 566 µg/g (mean 386), urine 63 to 695 µg/g (mean 230, 4 cases) (H. Christensen and S. Felby, *Acta pharmac. tox.*, 1975, *37*, 393–401).
In a fatality due to the ingestion of 3.6 g of dibenzepin, the following postmortem tissue concentrations were reported for dibenzepin and total desmethyl metabolites, respectively: blood 23, – µg/ml; bile 113, 137 µg/ml; brain 42, 12 µg/g; kidney 63, 38 µg/g; liver 130, 134 µg/g; urine 350, 258 µg/ml (H.-J. Schlicht and H.-P. Gelbke, *J. Chromat.*, 1978, *166*, 599–603).

HALF-LIFE. Plasma half-life, about 4 hours (dibenzepin plus desmethyl metabolites).

Dose. 240 to 560 mg of dibenzepin hydrochloride daily.

Dibromopropamidine   *Antibacterial/Antifungal*

4,4'-Trimethylenedioxybis(3-bromobenzamidine)
$C_{17}H_{18}Br_2N_4O_2 = 470.2$
CAS—496-00-4

Dibromopropamidine Isethionate
Proprietary Names. Brolene (eye ointment); Brulidine.
$C_{17}H_{18}Br_2N_4O_2,2C_2H_6O_4S = 722.4$
CAS—614-87-9
A white crystalline powder. M.p. 226°.
Soluble 1 in 2 of water and 1 in 60 of ethanol; practically insoluble in chloroform and ether.

Colour Tests. Aromaticity (Method 2)—yellow/brown; Liebermann's Test—black.

Thin-layer Chromatography. *System TA*—Rf 01. (*Acidified iodoplatinate solution*, positive.)

Ultraviolet Spectrum. Aqueous acid—261 nm ($A_1^1 = 512$ a).

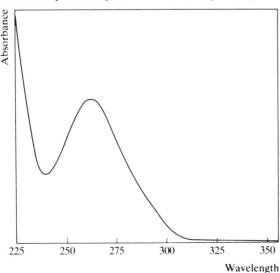

Infra-red Spectrum. Principal peaks at wavenumbers 1190, 1654, 1266, 1047, 1600, 1306 (dibromopropamidine isethionate, KBr disk).

Use. Dibromopropamidine isethionate is used in a concentration of 0.15%.

Dibutyl Phthalate
Insect Repellent

Synonyms. Butyl Phthalate; DBP.
Dibutyl benzene-1,2-dicarboxylate
$C_{16}H_{22}O_4 = 278.3$
CAS—84-74-2

A clear, colourless or faintly yellow, somewhat viscous liquid. Wt per ml about 1.045 g. B.p. about 330°. Refractive index 1.492 to 1.495.
Soluble 1 in 2500 of water; miscible with ethanol, ether, and most other organic solvents.

Gas Chromatography. *System GA*—RI 1913.

Ultraviolet Spectrum. Methanol—274 nm ($A_1^1 = 45$ b).

Mass Spectrum. Principal peaks at m/z 149, 41, 29, 57, 56, 104, 32, 65.

Dichloralphenazone
Hypnotic/Sedative

Synonym. Dichloralantipyrine
Proprietary Names. Bonadorm; Chloralol; Welldorm. It is an ingredient of Midrid and Paedo-Sed.
A complex of chloral hydrate and phenazone.
$C_{15}H_{18}Cl_6N_2O_5 = 519.0$
CAS—480-30-8

$[CCl_3 \cdot CH(OH)_2]_2$

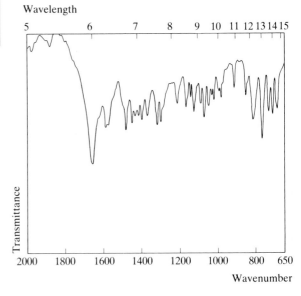

A white microcrystalline powder. M.p. 64° to 67°.
Soluble 1 in 10 of water, 1 in 1 of ethanol, and 1 in 2 of chloroform; soluble in dilute acids.
Note. It is decomposed by dilute alkalis with the liberation of chloroform. In aqueous and ethanolic solutions it dissociates into chloral hydrate and phenazone.

Gas Chromatography. *System GA*—phenazone RI 1848.

Ultraviolet Spectrum. Phenazone: aqueous acid—230 nm ($A_1^1 = 590$ b); aqueous alkali—242 nm ($A_1^1 = 494$ a), 256 nm.

Infra-red Spectrum. Principal peaks at wavenumbers 1656, 767, 1587, 1562, 1315, 1298 (KBr disk).

Mass Spectrum. Principal peaks at m/z 188, 47, 82, 96, 29, 77, 84, 56.

Quantification. See under Chloral Hydrate and Phenazone.

Disposition in the Body. After administration, dichloralphenazone acts as a mixture of chloral hydrate and phenazone and reference should be made to the entries under these substances.

TOXICITY.

Blood concentrations of 20 µg/ml of trichloroethanol and 40 µg/ml of phenazone were reported in a comatose subject following an overdose of dichloralphenazone; the subject eventually recovered (R. J. Armstrong and H. M. Stone, *Bull. int. Ass. forens. Toxicol.*, 1972, *8*(4), 8–9).

Dose. 0.65 to 1.95 g daily.

Dichlorodifluoromethane
Aerosol Propellent/Refrigerant

Synonyms. Difluorodichloromethane; Propellent 12; Refrigerant 12.
Proprietary Names. Arcton 12. It is an ingredient of PR Spray and Skefron.

$CCl_2F_2 = 120.9$
CAS—75-71-8
A colourless non-inflammable gas which, when liquefied by compression, forms a clear colourless liquid. F.p. $-155°$. B.p. about $-29.8°$.

Gas Chromatography. *System GA*—RI 305; *system GI*—retention time 0.9 min.

Mass Spectrum. Principal peaks at m/z 85, 87, 101, 50, 103, 31, 66, 35.

Dichlorophen   *Anthelmintic*

Synonym. Di-phenthane-70
Proprietary Names. Anthiphen; Dicestal (vet.); Ovis; Plath-Lyse; Wespuril.
2,2′-Methylenebis(4-chlorophenol)
$C_{13}H_{10}Cl_2O_2 = 269.1$
CAS—97-23-4

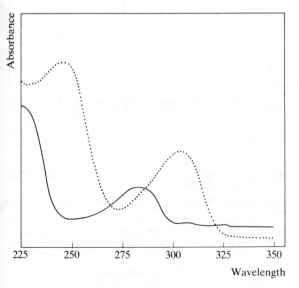

A white or slightly cream-coloured powder. M.p. about 175°. Practically **insoluble** in water; soluble 1 in 1 of ethanol and 1 in less than 1 of ether.

Colour Tests. Aromaticity (Method 2)—yellow/brown; Folin-Ciocalteu Reagent—blue; Liebermann's Test—violet-brown; Millon's Reagent—red.

Thin-layer Chromatography. *System TD*—Rf 58; *system TE*—Rf 34; *system TF*—Rf 67.

Gas Chromatography. *System GA*—RI 2140.

Ultraviolet Spectrum. Aqueous acid—282 nm; aqueous alkali—245 nm ($A_1^1 = 650$ a), 304 nm.

Infra-red Spectrum. Principal peaks at wavenumbers 1226, 817, 1111, 1162, 1245, 1170 (KBr disk).

Mass Spectrum. Principal peaks at m/z 128, 141, 268, 130, 270, 77, 143, 233.

Dose. Usually 6 g daily for 2 or 3 days; a single dose of 9 g has also been given.

Dichlorophenoxyacetic Acid   *Herbicide*

Synonym. 2,4-D
Proprietary Names. Cornox D; Destox; Dicotox; Dioweed; Dormone; Fernimine; For-ester; Iso-planatox; Palormone D; Silvapron D; Syford; Vigon-DC. It is an ingredient of Econal, Nettle Ban, Spontox, and Stancide BWK 75.
2,4-Dichlorophenoxyacetic acid
$C_8H_6Cl_2O_3 = 221.0$
CAS—94-75-7

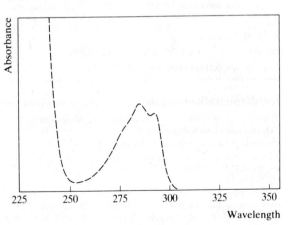

A white powder which is corrosive. M.p. about 140°.
Very slightly **soluble** in water; soluble in aqueous solutions of alkalis and in alcohols.

Thin-layer Chromatography. *System TD*—Rf 04; *system TE*—Rf 04; *system TF*—Rf 06.

Gas Chromatography. Dichlorophenoxyacetic acid methyl ester: *system GA*—RI 1605; *system GK*—retention time 0.65 relative to caffeine. Dichlorophenoxyacetic acid iso-octyl ester: *system GK*—retention times 1.12, 1.18 relative to caffeine.

Ultraviolet Spectrum. Ethanol—284 nm ($A_1^1 = 95$ b), 292 nm.

Infra-red Spectrum. Principal peaks at wavenumbers 1090, 1230, 795, 1264, 1247, 1724 (Nujol mull). (See below)
Mass Spectrum. Principal peaks at m/z 199, 45, 175, 145, 111, 109, 234, 133 (dichlorophenoxyacetic acid methyl ester).

Wavelength

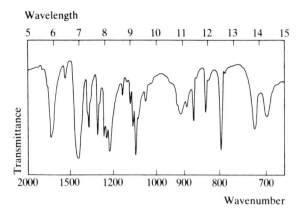

Quantification. GAS CHROMATOGRAPHY. In plasma or urine: FID—J. D. Kohli et al., Xenobiotica, 1974, 4, 97–100. In urine: sensitivity 100 ng/ml, ECD—A. E. Smith and B. J. Hayden, J. Chromat., 1979, 171, 482–485.

Disposition in the Body. Readily absorbed after ingestion but poorly absorbed through the skin. After ingestion, about 80% is excreted in the urine unchanged in 4 days, and about 13% is excreted as conjugates.

BLOOD CONCENTRATION.
After ingestion of 5 mg/kg by 6 subjects, average peak plasma concentrations of about 35 µg/ml were attained in 7 to 24 hours (J. D. Kohli et al., Xenobiotica, 1974, 4, 97–100).

TOXICITY. The estimated minimum lethal dose is 7 g. The maximum permissible atmospheric concentration is 10 mg/m³ and the maximum acceptable daily intake is 300 µg/kg. Dichlorophenoxyacetic acid is very irritating to the eyes, nose, and throat.

The following postmortem tissue concentrations have been reported in 4 fatalities involving ingestion of dichlorophenoxyacetic acid: blood 126 to 826 µg/ml (mean 447, 4 cases), bile 573 µg/ml (1 case), brain 13 and 66 µg/g (2 cases), kidney 62 to 82 µg/g (mean 69, 3 cases), liver 21 to 183 µg/g (mean 134, 4 cases), urine 111 and 264 µg/ml (2 cases) (K. Nielsen et al., Acta pharmac. tox., 1965, 22, 224–234; A. Coutselenis et al., Forens. Sci., 1977, 10, 203–204; J. E. Ryall, Bull. int. Ass. forens. Toxicol., 1978, 14(2), 17–18; M. Watson, ibid., 18).

HALF-LIFE. Plasma half-life, about 12 to 33 hours.

VOLUME OF DISTRIBUTION. About 0.1 litre/kg.

Dichlorotetrafluoroethane   *Aerosol Propellent/Refrigerant*

Synonyms. Cryofluorane; Propellent 114; Refrigerant 114; Tetrafluorodichloroethane.
Proprietary Names. Arcton 33; Arcton 114.
1,2-Dichloro-1,1,2,2-tetrafluoroethane
$CClF_2 \cdot CClF_2 = 170.9$
CAS—76-14-2
A colourless non-inflammable gas which, when liquefied by compression, forms a clear colourless liquid. B.p. about 3.5°.
In the liquid state it is practically **immiscible** with water, but miscible with dehydrated alcohol.

Gas Chromatography. *System GA*—RI 361; *system GI*—retention time 2.0 min.

Mass Spectrum. Principal peaks at m/z 85, 135, 87, 137, 31, 101, 100, 50.

Dichlorphenamide   *Carbonic Anhydrase Inhibitor*

Synonyms. DCPA; Dichlorophenamide; Diclofenamide.
Proprietary Names. Daranide; Oralcon; Oratrol.
4,5-Dichlorobenzene-1,3-disulphonamide
$C_6H_6Cl_2N_2O_4S_2 = 305.2$
CAS—120-97-8

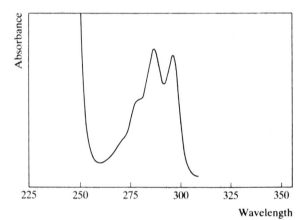

A white crystalline powder. M.p. about 240°.
Practically **insoluble** in water and chloroform; soluble 1 in 30 of ethanol; slightly soluble in ether; freely soluble in pyridine; soluble in solutions of alkali hydroxides and carbonates.

Dissociation Constant. pK_a 7.4, 8.6.

Partition Coefficient. Log P (ether/pH 7.4), 1.0.

Colour Test. Koppanyi–Zwikker Test—violet.

Thin-layer Chromatography. *System TA*—Rf 82; *system TD*—Rf 14; *system TE*—Rf 33; *system TF*—Rf 64. (*Acidified iodoplatinate solution*, positive.)

Ultraviolet Spectrum. Aqueous acid—286 nm ($A_1^1 = 60$ a), 296 nm.

Infra-red Spectrum. Principal peaks at wavenumbers 1162, 1176, 882, 702, 907, 1123 (KBr disk).

Mass Spectrum. Principal peaks at m/z 304, 306, 64, 74, 109, 177, 176, 48.

Quantification. GAS CHROMATOGRAPHY. In rabbit serum: sensitivity 20 ng/ml, ECD—C. Schmitt et al., J. pharm. Sci., 1979, 68, 381–383.

Dose. 100 to 200 mg daily in the treatment of glaucoma.

Wavelength

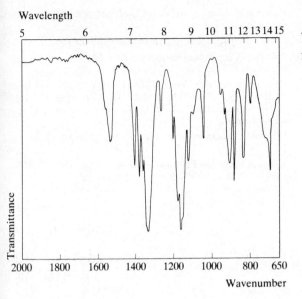

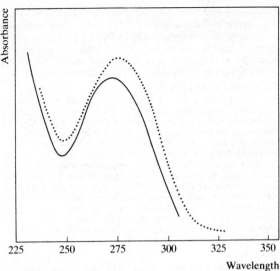

Diclofenac   *Analgesic*

Synonym. Diclophenac

[2-(2,6-Dichloroanilino)phenyl]acetic acid

$C_{14}H_{11}Cl_2NO_2 = 296.2$

CAS—15307-86-5

Crystals. M.p. 156° to 158°.

Diclofenac Sodium

Proprietary Names. Voltaren(e); Voltarol.

$C_{14}H_{10}Cl_2NNaO_2 = 318.1$

CAS—15307-79-6

Crystals. M.p. 283° to 285°.

Colour Tests. Liebermann's Test—red-brown; Mandelin's Test—red-brown; Marquis Test—brown (slow).

Thin-layer Chromatography. *System TD*—Rf 25; *system TE*—Rf 13; *system TF*—Rf 40; *system TG*—Rf 29. (*Chromic acid solution,* red.)

Gas Chromatography. *System GA*—RI 2271; *system GD*—retention time of methyl derivative 1.42 relative to n-$C_{16}H_{34}$.

High Pressure Liquid Chromatography. *System HD*—k' 11.5; *system HV*—retention time 0.85 relative to meclofenamic acid.

Ultraviolet Spectrum. Aqueous acid—273 nm ($A_1^1 = 309$ b); aqueous alkali—275 nm ($A_1^1 = 351$ b).

Infra-red Spectrum. Principal peaks at wavenumbers 1572, 756, 1504, 775, 1286, 1308 (diclofenac sodium, KBr disk).

Mass Spectrum. Principal peaks at m/z 214, 216, 242, 295, 215, 297, 179, 178.

Wavelength

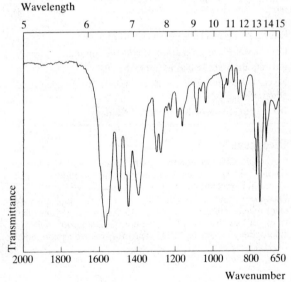

Quantification. GAS CHROMATOGRAPHY. In plasma: detection limit 100 ng/ml, ECD—M. Ikeda *et al., J. Chromat.,* 1980, *183*; *Biomed. Appl., 9,* 41–47.

GAS CHROMATOGRAPHY (CAPILLARY COLUMN). In urine: diclofenac and hydroxy metabolites, ECD—W. Schneider and P. H. Degen, *J. Chromat.,* 1981, *217,* 263–271.

HIGH PRESSURE LIQUID CHROMATOGRAPHY. In plasma: sensitivity 5 ng/ml, UV detection—K. K. H. Chan *et al., Analyt. Lett. (Part B),* 1982, *15,* 1649–1663.

Disposition in the Body. Well absorbed after oral administration but undergoes significant first-pass metabolism; bioavailability about 50 to 60%. Up to about 70% of a dose is excreted in the urine in 3 days, including 20 to 40% as conjugates of the major metabolite 4'-hydroxydiclofenac (active) and up to about 15% as conjugates of unchanged diclofenac. Other metabolites identified in the urine include 5-hydroxydiclofenac (about 12% of the dose), 3'-hydroxydiclofenac, and 4',5-dihydroxydiclofenac. About 10 to 20% of a dose is excreted in the bile as 4'-hydroxydiclofenac and less than 5% as unchanged drug.

THERAPEUTIC CONCENTRATION.

After a single oral dose of 50 mg as an enteric-coated tablet, administered to 12 subjects under fasting conditions, peak plasma concentrations of 0.75 to 2.0 µg/ml (mean 1.3) were attained in about 2 hours. A similar dose administered under non-fasting conditions produced peak plasma concentrations of 0.05 to 1.8 µg/ml (mean 0.8) in about 5 hours (J. V. Willis *et al.*, *Eur. J. clin. Pharmac.*, 1981, *19*, 33–37).

Following oral administration of 50 mg of diclofenac sodium three times a day to 4 subjects, peak plasma concentrations of 0.1 to 2.2 µg/ml (mean 0.8) of diclofenac and 0.3 to 2.0 µg/ml (mean 1.2) of 4'-hydroxydiclofenac were reported 3 hours after a dose; peak concentrations in synovial fluid of 0.1 to 0.6 µg/ml (mean 0.3) of diclofenac and 0.2 to 1.0 µg/ml (mean 0.6) of 4'-hydroxydiclofenac were attained in 3 hours; concentrations in synovial fluid exceeded those in plasma after 4 hours (P. D. Fowler *et al.*, *Eur. J. clin. Pharmac.*, 1983, *25*, 389–394).

TOXICITY.

A 19-year-old man was admitted to hospital following the ingestion of 1.5 g of diclofenac sodium and 4 g of chlormezanone. Plasma-diclofenac concentrations of 60.1 µg/ml and 0.19 µg/ml were reported at 7 and 15 hours, respectively; chlormezanone could not be determined. The subject recovered after about 2 days (P. Netter *et al.*, *Eur. J. clin. Pharmac.*, 1984, *26*, 535–536).

HALF-LIFE. Plasma half-life, about 1 to 2 hours.

CLEARANCE. Plasma clearance, about 4 ml/min/kg.

PROTEIN BINDING. In plasma, more than 99%.

NOTE. For a review of diclofenac see R. W. Brogden *et al.*, *Drugs*, 1980, *20*, 24–48.

Dose. 75 to 150 mg of diclofenac sodium daily.

Dicophane

Pesticide

Synonyms. Chlorophenothane; Chlorphenothanum; Clofenotanum; DDT; Dichlorodiphenyltrichloroethane; Dichophanum; Parachlorocidum; Penticidum.

Dicophane contains about 70% of 1,1,1-trichloro-2,2-bis(4-chlorophenyl)ethane (*pp'*-DDT) together with varying quantities of an isomer, 1,1,1-trichloro-2-(2-chlorophenyl)-2-(4-chlorophenyl)ethane (*op'*-DDT) and other related compounds.
$C_{14}H_9Cl_5 = 354.5$
CAS—50-29-3

White or nearly white crystals, small granules, flakes, or powder. M.p. about 109°. The technical product is a waxy solid of indefinite melting point.

Practically **insoluble** in water; soluble 1 in 50 of ethanol, 1 in 6 of boiling ethanol, 1 in 2.5 of acetone, 1 in 3.5 of chloroform, and 1 in 4 of ether.

Colour Tests. Liebermann's Test—brown; Nitric–Sulphuric Acid—red → orange → green.

Heat a small quantity with a 0.5% solution of hydroquinone in *sulphuric acid*—red.

NOTE. Dicophane does not react to the Fujiwara Test.

Thin-layer Chromatography. *System TD*—Rf 82; *system TE*—Rf 87; *system TF*—Rf 74.

Gas Chromatography. *System GA*—*pp'*-DDT RI 2299, *op'*-DDT RI 2218, *pp'*-DDE RI 2130, *op'*-DDE RI 2070; *system GK*—*pp'*-DDT retention time 1.32, *op'*-DDT retention time 1.24, both relative to caffeine.

Ultraviolet Spectrum. Methanol—236 nm ($A_1^1 = 510$ b), 267 nm ($A_1^1 = 19$ b).

Infra-red Spectrum. Principal peaks at wavenumbers 775, 790, 1500, 1100, 1022, 850 (KBr disk).

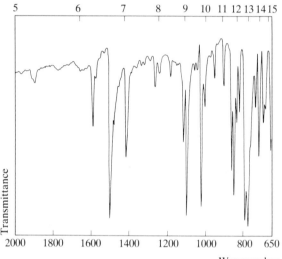

Wavelength

Wavenumber

Mass Spectrum. Principal peaks at *m/z* 235, 237, 165, 236, 75, 239, 82, 199 (*pp'*-DDT).

Quantification. GAS CHROMATOGRAPHY. In serum: dicophane and metabolites, ECD—W. E. Dale *et al.*, *J. Ass. off. analyt. Chem.*, 1970, *53*, 1287–1292. In blood or tissues: dicophane and metabolites, sensitivity, blood <1 ng/ml, tissues <5 ng/g, ECD—J. L. Radomski and A. Rey, *J. chromatogr. Sci.*, 1970, *8*, 108–114. In urine: dichlorodiphenylacetic acid (DDA), detection limit 50 pg, ECD—H. Della Fiorentina *et al.*, *J. Chromat.*, 1978, *157*, 421–426.

Disposition in the Body. Dicophane dry powder is poorly absorbed from the gastro-intestinal tract and is not absorbed through the skin. Solutions of dicophane in oils are rapidly absorbed through intact skin and are also readily absorbed from the gastro-intestinal tract. Dicophane is metabolised to a small extent by dehydrochlorination to dichlorodiphenyldichloroethylene (DDE) which is less toxic; DDE does not appear to be metabolised further and is stored indefinitely in adipose tissues. Most of the DDE present in human fat is thought to be due to preformed DDE taken in the diet rather than being due to ingestion of dicophane. The major metabolic route for dicophane is dechlorination to dichlorodiphenyldichloroethane (DDD) followed by degradation to dichlorodiphenylacetic acid (DDA) which is the major urinary excretion product. Urinary concentrations of DDA are indicative of storage of DDT in adipose tissue.

The following tissue concentrations of total DDT plus metabolites were reported in 35 industrially-exposed subjects: blood 0.11 to 2.2 μg/ml (mean 0.6), fat 38 to 647 μg/g (mean 204), urine 0.05 to 3.4 μg/ml (mean 1.3); DDE accounted for about 40% of the material stored in fat and 6% of the urinary material compared to about 80% and 60%, respectively, reported for members of the general population (E. R. Laws et al., Archs. envir. Hlth, 1967, 15, 766–775).

Fat residues ranging from 0.04 to 17 μg/g (mean 2.6) of total DDT were reported in 236 subjects, without occupational exposure, in the United Kingdom in 1976–77 (D. C. Abbott et al., Br. med. J., 1981, 283, 1425–1428).

TOXICITY. The estimated minimum lethal dose is 30 g but a single oral dose of 10 mg/kg may produce toxic symptoms; the maximum permissible atmospheric concentration is 1 mg/m³ and the maximum acceptable daily intake is 5 μg/kg. The toxicity of some of the organic solvents, such as kerosene, used in the application of dicophane has probably contributed to dicophane fatalities.

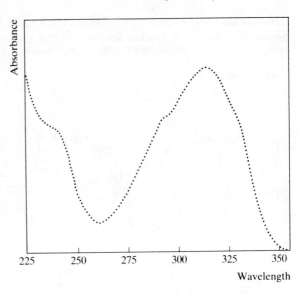

Absorbance / Wavelength

Dicoumarol   *Anticoagulant*

Synonyms. Bishydroxycoumarin; Dicoumarin; Dicumarol; Melitoxin.
Proprietary Name. Dufalone
3,3'-Methylenebis(4-hydroxycoumarin)
$C_{19}H_{12}O_6 = 336.3$
CAS—66-76-2

A white or creamy-white crystalline powder. M.p. about 290°. Practically **insoluble** in water, ethanol, and ether; slightly soluble in chloroform; freely soluble in solutions of alkali hydroxides.

Dissociation Constant. pK_a 4.4, 8.0.

Thin-layer Chromatography. *System TD*—Rf 18; *system TE*—Rf 32; *system TF*—Rf 32. (*Acidified potassium permanganate solution,* positive.)

Ultraviolet Spectrum. Aqueous alkali—314 nm ($A_1^1 = 756$ a).

Mass Spectrum. Principal peaks at m/z 336, 121, 120, 215, 162, 92, 337, 187.

Quantification. ULTRAVIOLET SPECTROPHOTOMETRY. In plasma: sensitivity 2 μg/ml—R. Nagashima et al., J. pharm. Sci., 1968, 57, 58–67.

Disposition in the Body. Slowly and irregularly absorbed after oral administration. It is extensively metabolised with less than 1% of a dose being excreted in the urine as unchanged drug.

THERAPEUTIC CONCENTRATION.

After a single oral dose of 150 mg to 8 subjects, a mean peak plasma concentration of 16.7 μg/ml was attained in 12 hours (H. M. Solomon and J. J. Schrogie, Clin. Pharmac. Ther., 1967, 8, 65–69).
Following daily oral administration of 2 mg/kg to 3 subjects, plasma concentrations of 44 to 59 μg/ml (mean 53) were reported on the 6th day (E. S. Vesell and J. G. Page, J. clin. Invest., 1968, 47, 2657–2663).

TOXICITY. Fatalities, usually due to severe haemorrhage, have been reported following daily oral doses of 100 mg or more.

HALF-LIFE. Plasma half-life, dose-dependent and may range from 7 to 100 hours.

PROTEIN BINDING. In plasma, more than 99%.

Dose. Maintenance, 25 to 150 mg daily.

Dicyclomine   *Anticholinergic*

Synonym. Dicycloverine
2-Diethylaminoethyl bicyclohexyl-1-carboxylate
$C_{19}H_{35}NO_2 = 309.5$
CAS—77-19-0

$CO \cdot O \cdot [CH_2]_2 \cdot N(C_2H_5)_2$

Dicyclomine Hydrochloride

Proprietary Names. Atumin; Benacol; Bentyl; Bentylol; Cyclobec; Formulex; Menospasm; Merbentyl; Or-Tyl; Pasmin; Procyclomin; Spasmoban; Viscerol. It is an ingredient of Diarrest, Kolanticon, Kolantyl, and Ovol.
$C_{19}H_{35}NO_2,HCl = 346.0$
CAS—67-92-5
A white crystalline powder. M.p. 169° to 174°.
Soluble 1 in 20 of water, 1 in 5 of ethanol, and 1 in 2 of chloroform; practically insoluble in ether.

Thin-layer Chromatography. *System TA*—Rf 68; *system TB*—Rf 67; *system TC*—Rf 64. (*Acidified iodoplatinate solution,* positive.)

Gas Chromatography. *System GA*—RI 2097; *system GF*—RI 2265.

High Pressure Liquid Chromatography. *System HA*—k' 1.1.

Ultraviolet Spectrum. No significant absorption, 230 to 360 nm.

Infra-red Spectrum. Principal peaks at wavenumbers 1714, 1214, 1136, 1197, 1184, 1155 (dicyclomine hydrochloride, K Br disk).

Wavelength

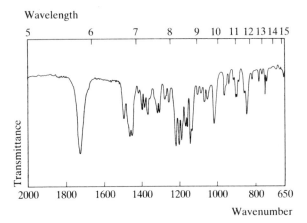

Mass Spectrum. Principal peaks at m/z 86, 71, 99, 58, 55, 56, 100, 87.

Quantification. GAS CHROMATOGRAPHY. In plasma: sensitivity 1 ng/ml, AFID—P. J. Meffin *et al.*, *Analyt. Chem.*, 1973, *45*, 1964–1966.

Disposition in the Body. Rapidly absorbed after oral administration. About 80% of a dose is excreted in the urine and 10% is eliminated in the faeces.

THERAPEUTIC CONCENTRATION.

After a single oral dose of 20 mg to 1 subject, a peak plasma concentration of about 0.02 µg/ml was attained in about 1.5 hours; following administration of 40 mg to the same subject as a sustained-release preparation, a maximum plasma concentration of about 0.08 µg/ml was reported after about 2.5 hours (P. J. Meffin *et al.*, *ibid.*).

TOXICITY. Fatalities have been reported in children after the ingestion of about 0.2 g of a sustained-release preparation.

HALF-LIFE. Plasma half-life, about 5 hours.

Dose. 30 to 80 mg of dicyclomine hydrochloride daily.

Dieldrin
Insecticide

Proprietary Name. Dilstan EC-15

Dieldrin contains about 85% of HEOD, 1,2,3,4,10,10-hexachloro-6,7-epoxy-1,4,4a,5,6,7,8,8a-octahydro-1,4:5,8-dimethanonaphthalene, the remaining 15% being mainly chlorinated organic compounds related to HEOD.

$C_{12}H_8Cl_6O = 380.9$

CAS—60-57-1 (HEOD)

A light-tan, flaky, crystalline solid.

Practically **insoluble** in water; soluble 1 in 4 of ethanol, 1 in 40 of carbon tetrachloride, and 1 in 1 of methanol; moderately soluble in chloroform.

Colour Tests. Nitric–Sulphuric Acid—pink; Sulphuric Acid–Fuming Sulphuric Acid—red.

Gas Chromatography. *System GA*—RI 2110; *system GK*—retention time 1.13, relative to caffeine.

Ultraviolet Spectrum. No significant absorption, 230 to 360 nm.

Infra-red Spectrum. Principal peaks at wavenumbers 848, 811, 1038, 700, 1005, 912 (K Cl disk).

Wavelength

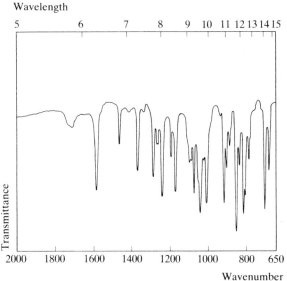

Mass Spectrum. Principal peaks at m/z 79, 82, 81, 263, 77, 108, 265, 80.

Quantification. GAS CHROMATOGRAPHY. In blood or tissues: ECD—A. Steentoft, *Medicine, Sci. Law*, 1979, *19*, 268–269.

Disposition in the Body. Both dieldrin powder and solutions are readily absorbed after oral administration, through the lungs, and through intact skin. Dieldrin is selectively stored in body fat and persists for several weeks after cessation of exposure. It is eliminated in the faeces mainly as unknown hydrophilic metabolites; a small amount is excreted in the urine as metabolites but very little as unchanged dieldrin.

Dieldrin is a metabolite of aldrin.

BLOOD CONCENTRATION. Blood concentrations averaging 0.001 µg/ml have been reported in subjects with no occupational exposure to dieldrin.

Serum concentrations ranging from 0.001 to 0.137 µg/ml (mean 0.02) were reported in 71 industrially-exposed workers and fat concentrations of 0.6 to 32 µg/g (mean 6) were reported in 28 of these subjects (W. T. Hayes and A. Curley, *Archs envir. Hlth*, 1968, *16*, 155–162).

Steady-state blood concentrations of about 0.007 and 0.02 µg/ml were reported in 2 groups of 3 subjects who received doses of 0.05 mg and 0.21 mg daily for 2 years; maximum fat concentrations of 1.3 to 1.6 µg/g and 2.2 to 4.9 µg/g were reported in the same subjects (C. G. Hunter *et al.*, *Archs . envir. Hlth*, 1969, *18*, 12–21).

Fat residues in 236 non-exposed subjects were reported to be in the range <0.01 to 0.5 µg/g (mean 0.1) (D. C. Abbott *et al.*, *Br. med. J.*, 1981, *283*, 1425–1428).

TOXICITY. The estimated minimum lethal dose is 5 g; ingestion of 10 mg/kg may produce toxic effects. The maximum permissible atmospheric concentration is 0.25 mg/m³ and the maximum acceptable daily intake is 0.1 µg/kg. Blood concentrations greater than 0.15 µg/ml are usually toxic. Several fatalities due to accidental or deliberate ingestion of dieldrin have been reported. A serum concentration of 0.27 µg/ml and a fat concentration of 47 µg/g were reported 3 days after ingestion of dieldrin by a 4-year-old boy who survived (L. K. Garrettson and A. Curley, *Archs envir. Hlth*, 1969, **19**, 814–822).

In a fatality due to the ingestion of dieldrin, postmortem blood and liver concentrations of 0.5 µg/ml and 29 µg/g, respectively, were reported (A. Steentoft, *Medicine, Sci. Law*, 1979, **19**, 268–269).

HALF-LIFE. Blood half-life, 50 to 170 days (mean 97).

DISTRIBUTION IN BLOOD. Plasma: whole blood ratio, about 1.5.

PROTEIN BINDING. In plasma, more than 99%.

Dienoestrol   *Oestrogen*

Synonyms. Dehydrostilbestrol; Dienestrol; Oestrodienolum.
Proprietary Names. Cycladiene; DV; Estraguard; Hormofemin.

(*E,E*)-4,4'-[Di(ethylidene)ethylene]diphenol
$C_{18}H_{18}O_2 = 266.3$
CAS—84-17-3; 13029-44-2 (E,E)

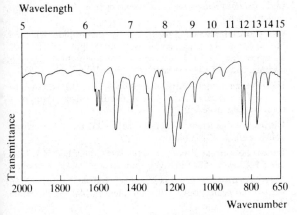

White crystals or crystalline powder. M.p. 227° to 234°.
Practically **insoluble** in water; soluble 1 in 8 of ethanol, 1 in 5 of acetone, and 1 in 15 of ether; slightly soluble in chloroform.
Caution. Dienoestrol is a powerful oestrogen. Contact with the skin or inhalation should be avoided.

Colour Tests. Antimony Pentachloride—red; Naphthol–Sulphuric Acid—orange-brown/yellow; Sulphuric Acid—orange-red.
Dissolve about 0.5 mg in 0.2 ml of *acetic acid*, add 1 ml of *phosphoric acid*, and heat on a water-bath for 3 minutes—violet, becoming slightly more blue on dilution with 3 ml of *acetic acid*. (This test distinguishes dienoestrol from stilboestrol, which produces a yellow colour.)

Thin-layer Chromatography. *System TP*—Rf 72; *system TQ*—Rf 25; *system TR*—Rf 34; *system TS*—Rf 05, streaking may occur.

Infra-red Spectrum. Principal peaks at wavenumbers 1206, 827, 1173, 1510, 1248, 775 (KBr disk).

Wavelength

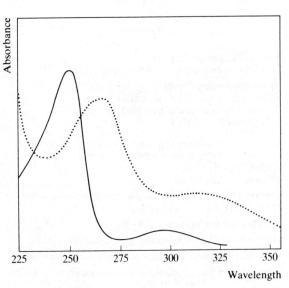

Disposition in the Body. Readily absorbed after oral administration. It is excreted in the urine mainly as a glucuronide conjugate.

Dose. Dienoestrol has been given by mouth in doses of 0.5 to 30 mg daily. It is used as a 0.01 to 0.025% vaginal cream.

Diethazine   *Anticholinergic*

Synonym. Eazamine
10-(2-Diethylaminoethyl)phenothiazine
$C_{18}H_{22}N_2S = 298.4$
CAS—60-91-3

An oily liquid.

Diethazine Hydrochloride
$C_{18}H_{22}N_2S,HCl = 334.9$
CAS—341-70-8
A white or slightly cream-coloured crystalline powder. M.p. 185° to 188°.
Soluble 1 in 2.5 of water, 1 in 5 of ethanol, and 1 in 2 of chloroform; practically insoluble in ether.

Dissociation Constant. pK_a 9.1 (20°).

Colour Tests. Formaldehyde–Sulphuric Acid—red-violet; Forrest Reagent—red; FPN Reagent—orange; Mandelin's Test—green → violet (excess reagent); Marquis Test—violet-brown.

Thin-layer Chromatography. *System TA*—Rf 58; *system TB*—Rf 57; *system TC*—Rf 51. (*Acidified iodoplatinate solution*, positive.)

Gas Chromatography. *System GA*—RI 2377.

High Pressure Liquid Chromatography. *System HA*—k' 3.4.

Ultraviolet Spectrum. Aqueous acid—250 nm ($A_1^1 = 1200$ b), 298 nm; aqueous alkali—265 nm.

Infra-red Spectrum. Principal peaks at wavenumbers 748, 1245, 1587, 1282, 1562, 1219 (KBr disk).

Mass Spectrum. Principal peaks at m/z 86, 298, 87, 30, 58, 299, 212, 180.

Dose. Diethazine hydrochloride has been given in doses of 0.15 to 1.5 g daily.

Diethyl Phthalate

Plasticiser/Solvent

Synonym. Ethyl Phthalate
Diethyl benzene-1,2-dicarboxylate
$C_{12}H_{14}O_4 = 222.2$
CAS—84-66-2

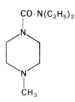

A clear, colourless, somewhat viscous liquid. Wt per ml about 1.117 g. B.p. about 295°. Refractive index 1.500 to 1.505. Practically **insoluble** in water; miscible with ethanol and ether.

Gas Chromatography. *System GA*—RI 1564.

Infra-red Spectrum. Principal peaks at wavenumbers 1733, 1287, 1086, 1132, 744, 1044 (thin film).

Mass Spectrum. Principal peaks at m/z 149, 177, 150, 65, 76, 105, 176, 104.

Diethylcarbamazine

Antifilarial

NN-Diethyl-4-methylpiperazine-1-carboxamide
$C_{10}H_{21}N_3O = 199.3$
CAS—90-89-1

A crystalline powder. M.p. 49°.
Soluble in water, ethanol, chloroform, and ether.

Diethylcarbamazine Citrate

Synonyms. Diethylcarbamazine Acid Citrate; Ditrazini Citras.
Proprietary Names. Banocide; Hetrazan; Notézine.
$C_{10}H_{21}N_3O,C_6H_8O_7 = 391.4$
CAS—1642-54-2
A white, crystalline, slightly hygroscopic powder. M.p. 136° to 141°. Very **soluble** in water; soluble 1 in 35 of ethanol; practically insoluble in chloroform and ether.

Dissociation Constant. pK_a 7.7 (20°).

Thin-layer Chromatography. *System TA*—Rf 52; *system TB*—Rf 17; *system TC*—Rf 26. (*Dragendorff spray*, positive.)

Gas Chromatography. *System GA*—RI 1497.

High Pressure Liquid Chromatography. *System HA*—k' 1.4.

Ultraviolet Spectrum. No significant absorption, 230 to 360 nm.

Infra-red Spectrum. Principal peaks at wavenumbers 1618, 1258, 1217, 1712, 1105, 1149 (KBr disk).

Mass Spectrum. Principal peaks at m/z 71, 72, 58, 100, 83, 56, 70, 44.

Quantification. GAS CHROMATOGRAPHY. In plasma or urine: detection limit 10 ng/ml, AFID—G. D. Allen *et al.*, *J. Chromat.*, 1979, *164*; *Biomed. Appl.*, 6, 521–526.

Disposition in the Body. Readily absorbed after oral administration. About 50% of a dose is excreted in the urine as unchanged drug and 10% as the *N*-oxide metabolite in 48 hours; the excretion of unchanged drug is pH-dependent being increased in acidic urine (pH 5) but decreasing to less than 10% in alkaline urine (pH 8).

THERAPEUTIC CONCENTRATION.
Following a single oral dose of 50 mg to 5 subjects, peak plasma concentrations of 0.08 to 0.20 µg/ml were attained in about 1 to 2 hours; a secondary rise in plasma concentrations was observed at 3 to 9 hours (G. Edwards *et al.*, *Clin. Pharmac. Ther.*, 1981, *30*, 551–557).

HALF-LIFE. Plasma half-life, about 10 hours under alkaline urinary pH conditions or 3 hours if an acidic urinary pH is maintained.

PROTEIN BINDING. In plasma, not significantly bound.

Dose. 1 to 6 mg/kg of diethylcarbamazine citrate daily, by mouth.

Diethylpropion

Anorectic

Synonym. Amfepramone
2-Diethylaminopropiophenone
$C_{13}H_{19}NO = 205.3$
CAS—90-84-6

$$C_6H_5 \cdot CO \cdot \overset{\displaystyle CH_3}{\underset{}{CH}} \cdot N(C_2H_5)_2$$

Diethylpropion Hydrochloride

Proprietary Names. Dietec; D.I.P.; Moderatan Diffucap; Nobensine-75; Prefamone; Regenon; Regibon; Tenuate Dospan; Tepanil. It is an ingredient of Apisate.
Note. The name Tepanil is also applied to phenylpropanolamine hydrochloride.
$C_{13}H_{19}NO,HCl = 241.8$
CAS—134-80-5
A white to off-white, fine, crystalline powder. M.p. about 175°, with decomposition.
Soluble 1 in 0.5 of water, 1 in 3 of ethanol, and 1 in 3 of chloroform; practically insoluble in ether.

Colour Test. Liebermann's Test—yellow.

Thin-layer Chromatography. *System TA*—Rf 76; *system TB*—Rf 62; *system TC*—Rf 63. (*Dragendorff spray*, positive; *FPN reagent*, pink; *acidified iodoplatinate solution*, positive; *Marquis reagent*, violet-brown.)

Gas Chromatography. *System GA*—diethylpropion RI 1486, norephedrine RI 1313; *system GB*—diethylpropion RI 1507, norephedrine RI 1353; *system GC*—diethylpropion RI 1715, norephedrine RI 1383; *system GF*—diethylpropion RI 1655.

High Pressure Liquid Chromatography. *System HA*—diethylpropion k' 1.7, norephedrine k' 0.9; *system HC*—diethylpropion k' 0.16, norephedrine k' 0.70.

Ultraviolet Spectrum. Aqueous acid—253 nm ($A_1^1 = 673$ a); aqueous alkali—246 nm.

Infra-red Spectrum. Principal peaks at wavenumbers 701, 1230, 1682, 1287, 973, 1594 (diethylpropion hydrochloride, KBr disk).

Mass Spectrum. Principal peaks at m/z 100, 44, 72, 101, 77, 56, 42, 105 (no peaks above 110); norephedrine 44, 77, 79, 51, 45, 42, 107, 105.

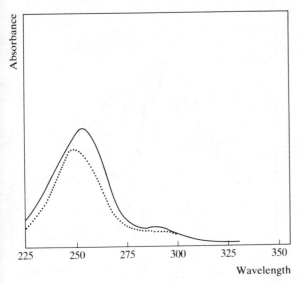

Absorbance

225   250   275   300   325   350

Wavelength

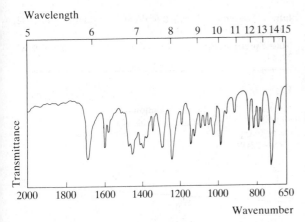

Wavelength

5   6   7   8   9   10   11 12 13 14 15

Transmittance

2000   1800   1600   1400   1200   1000   800   650

Wavenumber

Quantification. GAS CHROMATOGRAPHY. In urine: diethylpropion and metabolites, sensitivity 300 ng/ml, FID—B. Testa and A. H. Beckett, *J. Chromat.*, 1972, *71*, 39–54.

GAS CHROMATOGRAPHY–MASS SPECTROMETRY. In plasma: sensitivity 600 pg/ml—G. J. Wright *et al.*, *Drug Met. Rev.*, 1975, *4*, 267–276.

Disposition in the Body. Readily absorbed after oral administration. Metabolised by *N*-dealkylation, reduction, deamination, and *N*-hydroxylation primarily to active metabolites; keto-reduction is stereoselective resulting in the formation of *threo*-hydroxylated metabolites; glucuronide formation also occurs along with the formation of hippuric and mandelic acids. About 80 to 90% of a dose is excreted in the urine; the amount excreted in the urine is reduced when the urine is alkaline; of the urinary excreted material, *N*-ethylaminopropiophenone, norephedrine (phenylpropanolamine), and hippuric acid are the main metabolites together with small amounts of unchanged drug, aminopropiophenone, *N*-diethylnorephedrine, and *N*-ethylnorephedrine.

THERAPEUTIC CONCENTRATION.
Following a single oral dose of 75 mg to 5 subjects, a mean peak plasma concentration of 0.007 µg/ml was attained in 0.5 hour; total concentrations

of the monodesethyl and didesethyl metabolites reached an average peak of 0.19 µg/ml at 2 hours (G. J. Wright *et al.*, *ibid.*).

TOXICITY. The estimated minimum lethal doses are 200 mg for a child and 2 g for an adult.

The following disposition was reported in a case of fatal overdose resulting from the injection of illicit diethylpropion tablets: blood 5.4 µg/ml, bile 14.4 µg/ml, kidney 0.9 µg/g, liver 0.9 µg/g, injection site 43.2 µg/g (R. R. Fysh and J. F. Taylor, *Bull. int. Ass. forens. Toxicol.*, 1978, *14*(2), 16–17).

HALF-LIFE. Derived from urinary excretion data, 1.5 to 3 hours in subjects whose urines are acidic.

Dose. Usually 75 mg of diethylpropion hydrochloride daily.

Diethylthiambutene   *Narcotic Analgesic (Veterinary)*

NN-Diethyl-1-methyl-3,3-di-(2-thienyl)prop-2-enylamine
$C_{16}H_{21}NS_2 = 291.5$
CAS—86-14-6

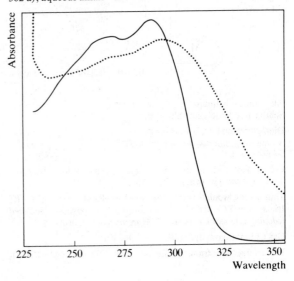

Diethylthiambutene Hydrochloride
$C_{16}H_{21}NS_2,HCl = 327.9$
CAS—132-19-4
A white crystalline powder. M.p. 151° to 154°.
Soluble 1 in 2 of water and 1 in 1 of ethanol; practically insoluble in ether.

Colour Tests. Liebermann's Test (100°)—orange; Mandelin's Test—green→green-blue; Marquis Test—violet; Sulphuric Acid—orange.
Cold *nitric acid* gives a pink-brown colour changing to green.

Thin-layer Chromatography. *System TA*—Rf 70; *system TB*—Rf 61; *system TC*—Rf 43. (*Dragendorff spray*, positive; *acidified iodoplatinate solution*, positive; *Marquis reagent*, red-violet.)

Gas Chromatography. *System GA*—RI 2008.

High Pressure Liquid Chromatography. *System HA*—k' 2.0.

Ultraviolet Spectrum. Aqueous acid—268 nm, 288 nm ($A_1^1 = 362$ a); aqueous alkali—295 nm.

Absorbance

225   250   275   300   325   350

Wavelength

Infra-red Spectrum. Principal peaks at wavenumbers 716, 743, 851, 833, 1244, 1618 (diethylthiambutene hydrochloride, KBr disk).

Mass Spectrum. Principal peaks at m/z 276, 111, 219, 42, 277, 97, 29, 100.

Diethyltoluamide   *Insect Repellent*

Synonym. Deet
Proprietary Name. Autan
NN-Diethyl-*m*-toluamide
$C_{12}H_{17}NO = 191.3$
CAS—134-62-3

A colourless or faintly yellow liquid. Wt per ml 0.997 to 1.000 g. Practically **immiscible** with water; miscible with ethanol, chloroform, and ether.

Thin-layer Chromatography. *System TA*—Rf 73. (*Acidified iodoplatinate solution*, positive.)

Gas Chromatography. *System GA*—RI 1583.

Ultraviolet Spectrum. No significant absorption, 230 to 360 nm.

Infra-red Spectrum. Principal peaks at wavenumbers 1629, 1284, 794, 1305, 1581, 1095 (KBr disk).

Quantification. GAS CHROMATOGRAPHY–MASS SPECTROMETRY. In urine: diethyltoluamide and metabolites—A. Wu *et al.*, *J. High Resolut. Chromat. Chromat. Commun.*, 1979, **2**, 558–562.

Use. As a 50 to 75% solution.

Diethyltryptamine   *Hallucinogen*

Synonyms. D.E.T.; *NN*-Diethyltryptamine.
3-(2-Diethylaminoethyl)indole
$C_{14}H_{20}N_2 = 216.3$
CAS—61-51-8

An orange oily liquid.
Soluble in ethanol and chloroform.

Diethyltryptamine Hydrochloride
A white crystalline powder. M.p. 87° to 89°.
Soluble in water.

Colour Tests. Mandelin's Test—grey-green → yellow; Marquis Test—yellow → brown.

Thin-layer Chromatography. *System TA*—Rf 46; *system TB*—Rf 15; *system TC*—Rf 10. (*Dragendorff spray*, positive; *acidified iodoplatinate solution*, positive; *Marquis reagent*, brown.)

Gas Chromatography. *System GA*—RI 1910.

Ultraviolet Spectrum. Aqueous acid—278 nm $(A_1^1 = 270 \text{ a})$, 287 nm.

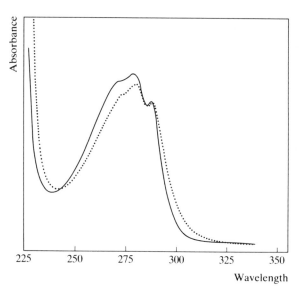

Wavelength

Infra-red Spectrum. Principal peaks at wavenumbers 740, 1111, 1063, 1086, 1234, 724.

Mass Spectrum. Principal peaks at m/z 86, 30, 58, 29, 130, 87, 77, 42.

Diflunisal   *Analgesic*

Proprietary Names. Dolobid; Donobid.
5-(2,4-Difluorophenyl)salicylic acid
$C_{13}H_8F_2O_3 = 250.2$
CAS—22494-42-4

White crystals or crystalline powder. M.p. about 212°.
Practically **insoluble** in water; soluble in ethanol, ether, and in dilute alkalis.

Colour Tests. Ferric Chloride—violet; Folin–Ciocalteu Reagent—blue; McNally's Test—violet.

Thin-layer Chromatography. *System TD*—Rf 08; *system TE*—Rf 16; *system TF*—Rf 10; *system TG*—Rf 37. (*Chromic acid solution*, blue-grey.)

Gas Chromatography. *System GD*—retention time of methyl derivative 1.20 relative to n-$C_{16}H_{34}$.

High Pressure Liquid Chromatography. *System HD*—k' 4.1; *system HV*—retention time 0.77 relative to meclofenamic acid.

Ultraviolet Spectrum. Acid methanol—251 nm $(A_1^1 = 560 \text{ a})$, 315 nm $(A_1^1 = 130 \text{ a})$; aqueous alkali—277 nm.

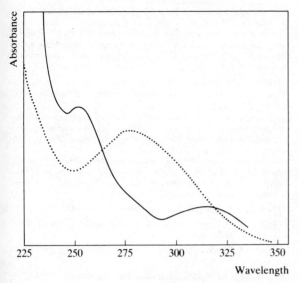

Infra-red Spectrum. Principal peaks at wavenumbers 1683, 1492, 1248, 1220, 1150, 978, (KBr disk). Two polymorphic forms may occur.

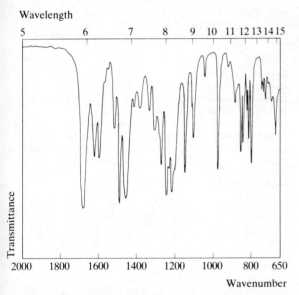

Mass Spectrum. Principal peaks at m/z 232, 250, 175, 204, 176, 233, 102, 78.

Quantification. SPECTROFLUORIMETRY. In plasma: sensitivity 500 ng—D. J. Tocco et al., *Drug Met. Disp.*, 1975, *3*, 453–466.

GAS CHROMATOGRAPHY. In plasma or urine: sensitivity 1 µg/ml, FID—D. J. Tocco et al., *idem*.

HIGH PRESSURE LIQUID CHROMATOGRAPHY. In plasma or urine: sensitivity 50 ng/ml, fluorescence detection—J. E. Ray and R. O. Day, *J. pharm. Sci.*, 1983, *72*, 1403–1405.

Disposition in the Body. Well absorbed after oral administration. Up to about 80% of a dose is excreted in the urine in 24 hours, mostly as the ester and ether glucuronides. Less than 3% of a dose is eliminated in the faeces.

THERAPEUTIC CONCENTRATION.
After a single oral dose of 500 mg given to 5 subjects, peak plasma concentrations of 58 to 92 µg/ml (mean 77) were attained in 2 hours (R. Verbeeck et al., *Br. J. clin. Pharmac.*, 1979, *7*, 273–282).

Following oral administration of 500 mg twice daily to 6 subjects, steady-state plasma concentrations of 66 to 183 µg/ml were reported (E. Wåhlin-Boll et al., *Eur. J. clin. Pharmac.*, 1981, *20*, 375–378).

TOXICITY. Diflunisal appears to be relatively non-toxic.
A 47-year-old woman went into a coma after ingesting 29 g of diflunisal but subsequently recovered uneventfully (H. P. Upadhyay and S. K. Gupta, *Br. med. J.*, 1978, *2*, 640).

HALF-LIFE. Plasma half-life, about 5 to 12 hours (dose-dependent).

VOLUME OF DISTRIBUTION. About 0.1 litre/kg.

CLEARANCE. Plasma clearance, about 0.1 ml/min/kg.

PROTEIN BINDING. In plasma, about 99%.

NOTE. For a review of the pharmacokinetics of diflunisal see R. N. Brogden et al., *Drugs*, 1980, *19*, 84–106.

Dose. 0.5 to 1 g daily.

Digitoxin
Cardiac Glycoside

Synonyms. Digitaline Cristallisée; Digitoxoside.
Proprietary Names. Asthenthilo; Crystodigin; Digimerck; Digitaline Nativelle; Digitox; Digitrin; Ditaven; Purodigin.

3β-[(O-2,6-Dideoxy-β-D-*ribo*-hexopyranosyl-(1→4)-O-2,6-dideoxy-β-D-*ribo*-hexopyranosyl-(1→4)-2,6-dideoxy-β-D-*ribo*-hexopyranosyl)oxy]-14-hydroxy-5β,14β-card-20(22)-enolide
$C_{41}H_{64}O_{13} = 764.9$
CAS—71-63-6

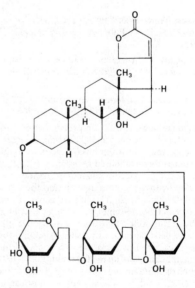

A glycoside obtained from suitable species of *Digitalis* (Scrophulariaceae).

A white or pale buff-coloured, microcrystalline powder. M.p. about 256°.

Practically **insoluble** in water; soluble 1 in 150 of ethanol and 1 in 40 of chloroform; slightly soluble in ether and methanol; freely soluble in a mixture of equal volumes of chloroform and methanol.

Colour Test. Antimony Pentachloride—yellow→brown→ black-violet.

Thin-layer Chromatography. *System TK*—Rf 72. (*Perchloric acid solution,* followed by examination under ultraviolet light, red fluorescence; p-*anisaldehyde reagent,* blue.)

Gas Chromatography. *System GA*—RI 1902.

High Pressure Liquid Chromatography. *System HM*—k′ 5.4. For further information on allied compounds and metabolites, see p. 217.

Infra-red Spectrum. Principal peaks at wavenumbers 1072, 1058, 1010, 1740, 1168, 990 (KBr disk).

Wavelength

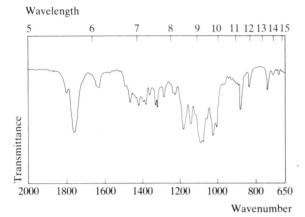

Mass Spectrum. Principal peaks at m/z 43, 29, 39, 41, 45, 57, 68, 58.

Quantification. THIN-LAYER CHROMATOGRAPHY. In serum: sensitivity 1 to 2 ng—D. B. Faber *et al.,* *J. Chromat.,* 1977, *143*; *Biomed. Appl.,* *1,* 95–103.

RADIOIMMUNOASSAY. In serum, urine or cerebrospinal fluid: sensitivity 5 ng/ml—A. K. Nore *et al.,* *Clin. Chem.,* 1980, *26,* 321–323.

FLUOROIMMUNOASSAY. In serum: sensitivity 1 ng/ml—M. H. H. Al-Hakiem *et al.,* *Clin. Chem.,* 1982, *28,* 1364–1366.

Disposition in the Body. Readily absorbed after oral administration; bioavailability greater than 90%. High concentrations are found in the kidney, ventricular myocardium, liver, and skeletal muscle. Extensively metabolised by hydrolysis to digitoxigenin bisdigitoxoside, digitoxigenin monodigitoxoside and digitoxigenin, and by hydroxylation to digoxin and the corresponding digoxigenin derivatives, all of which are active. Epimerisation to the inactive metabolites, epidigitoxigenin and epidigoxigenin, followed by glucuronide conjugation also occurs; dihydrodigitoxin has also been detected in plasma. About 60 to 80% of a single dose is excreted in the urine over a period of 3 weeks, mainly as metabolites, and up to 20% is eliminated in the faeces. The excretion of digitoxin and its active and inactive metabolites is very variable and is independent of dose and route of administration. About 20 to 50% of a dose appears to be excreted as unchanged drug in urine and faeces in variable proportions, and the amount of unchanged drug in the urine has been reported to be greater during maintenance treatment than in single dose studies.

Digitoxin is a metabolite of acetyldigitoxin.

THERAPEUTIC CONCENTRATION. In serum, usually in the range 0.01 to 0.03 µg/ml.

After a single oral dose of 20 µg/kg, given to 6 children, peak serum concentrations of 0.02 to 0.05 µg/ml were attained in 1.5 to 2.5 hours (A. Larsen and L. Storstein, *Clin. Pharmac. Ther.,* 1983, *33,* 717–726).

Following daily oral doses of 0.1 mg to 7 subjects, steady-state serum concentrations of 0.009 to 0.026 µg/ml (mean 0.017) were reported (K. Haustein, *Eur. J. clin. Pharmac.,* 1981, *19,* 45–51).

TOXICITY. The estimated minimum lethal dose is 3 mg. Toxic effects are usually associated with serum concentrations of about 0.03 µg/ml or more.

In a fatality due to the ingestion of 15 mg of digitoxin, a plasma concentration of 0.32 µg/ml was attained 4 hours after ingestion; death occurred after 14 hours (M. Mercier, *Bull. int. Ass. forens. Toxicol.,* 1971, *7*(4), 10–11).

A subject who ingested 10 mg of digitoxin recovered following treatment with activated charcoal; a plasma concentration of 0.26 µg/ml was reported 4 hours after the dose, decreasing to 0.027 µg/ml at 80 hours (S. Pond, *et al., Lancet,* 1981, *2,* 1177–1178).

HALF-LIFE. Plasma half-life, 3 to 16 days (mean 7).

VOLUME OF DISTRIBUTION. 0.4 to 0.8 litre/kg (mean 0.6); increased in children.

CLEARANCE. Plasma clearance, about 0.04 ml/min/kg; increased in children.

DISTRIBUTION IN BLOOD. Plasma: whole blood ratio, about 1.7.

PROTEIN BINDING. In plasma, about 95%.

NOTE. For a review of the clinical pharmacokinetics of digitoxin see D. Perrier *et al., Clin. Pharmacokinet.,* 1977, *2,* 292–311.

Dose. Maximum initial total dose of 1.6 mg over 1 to 2 days; maintenance, 50 to 200 µg daily.

Digoxin
Cardiac Glycoside

Synonym. Digoxosidum

Proprietary Names. Allocor (injection); Cardiox; Coragoxine; Digacin; Digoxin(e) Nativelle; Eudigox; Lanoxin(e); Lenoxin; Natigoxin; Novodigal; Prodigox.

3β-[(O-2,6-Dideoxy-β-D-*ribo*-hexopyranosyl-(1→4)-O-2,6-dideoxy-β-D-*ribo*-hexopyranosyl-(1→4)-2,6-dideoxy-β-D-*ribo*-hexopyranosyl)oxy]-12β,14-dihydroxy-5β,14β-card-20(22)-enolide

$C_{41}H_{64}O_{14} = 780.9$

CAS—20830-75-5

A glycoside obtained from the leaves of *Digitalis lanata* (Scrophulariaceae).

Colourless crystals or a white powder. M.p. about 240°, with decomposition.

Practically **insoluble** in water, dehydrated alcohol, and ether; soluble 1 in 122 of ethanol (80%) and 1 in 4 of pyridine; slightly soluble in chloroform; freely soluble in a mixture of equal volumes of chloroform and methanol.

Colour Test. Antimony Pentachloride—yellow → brown → black-violet.

Thin-layer Chromatography. *System TD*—Rf 01; *system TE*—Rf 33; *system TF*—Rf 05; *system TK*—Rf 62. (*Perchloric acid solution*, followed by examination under ultraviolet light, blue fluorescence; p-*anisaldehyde reagent*, blue.)

High Pressure Liquid Chromatography. *System HM*—k' 11.3. For further information on allied compounds and metabolites, see p. 217.

Infra-red Spectrum. Principal peaks at wavenumbers 1075, 1709, 1055, 1020, 1160, 1110 (KBr disk).

Wavelength

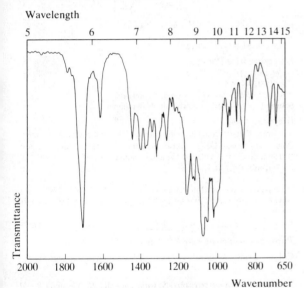

Mass Spectrum. Principal peaks at m/z 73, 58, 57, 43, 41, 39, 29, 45 (no peaks above 360).

Quantification. HIGH PRESSURE LIQUID CHROMATOGRAPHY. In urine: tritiated digoxin and metabolites, sensitivity 8 pg/ml for digoxin—M. H. Gault *et al.*, *J. Chromat.*, 1980, *182*; *Biomed. Appl.*, 8, 465–472.

HIGH PRESSURE LIQUID CHROMATOGRAPHY–RADIOIMMUNO-ASSAY. In plasma: digoxin and metabolites—H. A. Nelson *et al.*, *J. Chromat.*, 1979, *163*; *Biomed. Appl.*, 5, 169–177.

RADIOIMMUNOASSAY. In haemolysed blood—S. M. Fletcher *et al.*, *J. forens. Sci. Soc.*, 1979, *19*, 183–188. In serum or urine: dihydrodigoxin, sensitivity 250 pg/ml—V. P. Butler jun. *et al.*, *J. Pharmac. exp. Ther.*, 1982, *221*, 123–131.

REVIEW. See W. J. F. van der Vijgh—*Pharm. Weekbl.*, 1978, *113*, 585–594.

Disposition in the Body. The absorption of digoxin after oral administration is variable and subject to bioavailability differences; absorption occurs mainly in the small intestine and is delayed in the presence of food. The mean bioavailability is about 67% from tablets, 80% from elixirs, and up to 100% from encapsulated elixirs. Digoxin is rapidly distributed throughout the body and less than 20% of the total digoxin in the body is located in the blood. High concentrations are found in the heart and kidneys, but the skeletal muscles form the largest digoxin store. Digoxin is metabolised by stepwise removal of the sugar moieties to form digoxigenin, which is further metabolised to inactive metabolites which may be excreted in the free or conjugated form. Reduction to dihydrodigoxin, which is relatively inactive, also occurs. Up to 80% of a dose is excreted in the urine in 7 days with 27% of the dose in the first 24 hours; the remainder is eliminated in the faeces via the bile. In most patients, 80 to 90% of the material excreted in the urine is unchanged, up to 10% is in the dihydro form, and a small amount includes digoxigenin and the mono- and bisdigitoxo-sides. In about 10% of patients, however, between 20 and 55% is excreted as metabolites, mainly dihydrodigoxin. Of the material excreted in the bile, about 50% is unchanged, about 25% is digoxin bisdigitoxoside, about 25% is digoxin monodigitoxoside, and about 1% is digoxigenin.

Digoxin is a metabolite of deslanoside, digitoxin, lanatoside C, and medigoxin.

THERAPEUTIC CONCENTRATION. In serum, usually in the range 0.001 to 0.0025 µg/ml. Blood concentrations are significantly lower in hyperthyroidism, but increased in hypothyroidism and in patients with renal failure; children tolerate higher serum concentrations than adults.

Following a single oral dose of 0.25 mg to 6 subjects, a mean peak serum concentration of 0.001 µg/ml was attained in 1 hour (J. C. Panisset *et al.*, *Can. med. Ass. J.*, 1973, *109*, 700–702).

Steady-state plasma concentrations of 0.0004 to 0.0021 µg/ml (mean 0.0011) were reported in 14 patients on an oral daily dosage of 0.125 to 0.25 mg (J. Gayes and D. Greenblatt, *J. clin. Pharmac.*, 1978, *5*, 92–93).

TOXICITY. Toxic effects are usually associated with serum concentrations of 0.0014 to **0.0028** to 0.007 µg/ml and fatalities with concentrations of 0.0015 to **0.010** to 0.03 µg/ml.

In 7 fatalities involving ingestion of digoxin, postmortem 'serum' concentrations of 0.007 to 0.024 µg/ml (mean 0.013) were reported; in a fatality involving intramuscular injection of 1 mg of digoxin in an infant, a postmortem 'serum' concentration of 0.071 µg/ml was reported (A. C. Moffat, *Acta pharmac. tox.*, 1974, *35*, 386–394).

Postmortem blood concentrations vary according to the origin of the sample; serum from the right heart of 10 patients, in whom digoxin was not implicated as the cause of death, was found to contain 0.001 to 0.004 µg/ml of digoxin (mean 0.002), whereas serum from the femoral vein contained 0.0007 to 0.003 µg/ml (mean 0.001) (D. W. Holt and J. G. Benstead, *J. clin. Path.*, 1975, *28*, 483–486).

Serum-digoxin concentrations usually increase after death; average postmortem: antemortem ratios varying from 1.42 for blood from the femoral vein to 1.96 for heart blood have been reported; in contrast, postmortem vitreous humour concentrations were usually lower than antemortem values (T. E. Vorpahl and J. I. Coe, *J. forens. Sci.*, 1978, *23*, 329–334).

The following distribution was observed in a 3-day-old child who received a total of 4 mg of digoxin and died several hours later: blood 0.03 µg/ml, brain 0.0009 µg/g, kidney 0.13 µg/g, liver 0.034 µg/g (M. Selesky *et al.*, *J. forens. Sci.*, 1977, *22*, 409–417).

In a suicide due to digoxin overdose, the following postmortem tissue concentrations were reported: blood 0.022 µg/ml, brain 0.0097 µg/g, heart 0.043 µg/g, kidney 1.4 µg/g, liver 0.081 µg/g, lung 0.053 µg/g (R. Aderjan *et al.*, *Arch. Tox.*, 1979, *42*, 107–114).

HALF-LIFE. Plasma half-life, about 20 to 50 hours, prolonged in subjects with renal impairment.

VOLUME OF DISTRIBUTION. About 5 to 10 litres/kg.

CLEARANCE. Plasma clearance, about 1 to 4 ml/min/kg.

DISTRIBUTION IN BLOOD. Plasma: whole blood ratio, 0.93.

PROTEIN BINDING. In plasma, 20 to 40%.

NOTE. For reviews of the pharmacokinetics of digoxin see E. Iisalo, *Clin. Pharmacokinet.*, 1977, *2*, 1–16 and J. K. Aronson, *ibid.*, 1980, *5*, 137–149.

Dose. 125 to 750 µg daily. For rapid digitalisation, an initial dose of 0.75 to 1.5 mg may be given.

Dihydralazine   *Antihypertensive*

Synonym. Dihydrallazine
1,4-Dihydrazinophthalazine
$C_8H_{10}N_6 = 190.2$
CAS—484-23-1

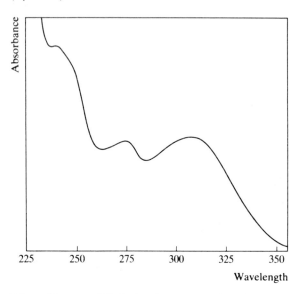

Orange crystalline needles which decompose at about 180°.

Dihydralazine Sulphate
Proprietary Name. Nepresol
$C_8H_{10}N_6,H_2SO_4 = 288.3$
CAS—7327-87-9
A white to slightly yellow crystalline powder. M.p. 245°.
Slightly **soluble** in water; practically insoluble in ethanol, chloroform, and methanol.

Colour Tests. Mandelin's Test—yellow; Nessler's Reagent—black.

Thin-layer Chromatography. *System TA*—Rf 55; *system TB*—Rf 36; *system TC*—Rf 02.

Ultraviolet Spectrum. Aqueous acid—240 nm, 274 nm, 306 nm ($A_1^1 = 323$ a).

(graph: Absorbance versus Wavelength, x-axis 225 to 350)

Infra-red Spectrum. Principal peaks at wavenumbers 1608, 1575, 1537, 1136, 769, 1100 (KBr disk).

Quantification. GAS CHROMATOGRAPHY. In plasma: dihydralazine plus acid-labile hydrazones, sensitivity 5 ng/ml, ECD—P. H. Degen *et al.*, *J. Chromat.*, 1982, *233*; *Biomed. Appl.*, *22*, 375–380.

Dose. Dihydralazine sulphate has been given in doses of 12.5 to 150 mg daily.

Dihydrocodeine   *Narcotic Analgesic*

Synonyms. Drocode; Hydrocodeine.
Proprietary Name. Remedacen
7,8-Dihydro-3-*O*-methylmorphine
$C_{18}H_{23}NO_3 = 301.4$
CAS—125-28-0

Crystals. M.p. 112° to 113°.

Dihydrocodeine Phosphate
$C_{18}H_{23}NO_3,H_3PO_4 = 399.4$
CAS—24204-13-5
A white to yellowish-white crystalline powder.
Soluble 1 in 3 of water; slightly soluble in ethanol.

Dihydrocodeine Tartrate
Synonyms. Dihydrocodeine Acid Tartrate; Dihydrocodeine Bitartrate.
Proprietary Names. DF 118; Fortuss; Paracodin; Rikodeine; Tuscodin. It is an ingredient of Onadox-118 and Paramol.
$C_{18}H_{23}NO_3,C_4H_6O_6 = 451.5$
CAS—5965-13-9
Colourless crystals or white crystalline powder. M.p. 190° to 194°.
Soluble 1 in 5 of water; sparingly soluble in ethanol; practically insoluble in ether.

Dissociation Constant. pK$_a$ 8.8 (25°).

Partition Coefficient. Log *P* (ether/pH 7.0), −1.5.

Colour Tests. Mandelin's Test—grey-green; Marquis Test—violet.

Thin-layer Chromatography. *System TA*—Rf 26; *system TB*—Rf 08; *system TC*—Rf 13. (*Dragendorff spray*, positive; *acidified iodoplatinate solution*, positive; *Marquis reagent*, blue-violet.)

Gas Chromatography. *System GA*—RI 2363; *system GC*—RI 2702; *system GF*—RI 2840.

High Pressure Liquid Chromatography. *System HA*—k′ 7.2 (tailing peak); *system HC*—k′ 2.50.

Ultraviolet Spectrum. Aqueous acid—283 nm ($A_1^1 = 47$ a). No alkaline shift.

Infra-red Spectrum. Principal peaks at wavenumbers 1495, 1271, 1040, 1250, 1055, 1149 (Nujol mull).

Mass Spectrum. Principal peaks at *m/z* 301, 44, 42, 59, 164, 70, 302, 242.

Quantification. GAS CHROMATOGRAPHY. In blood, bile, liver blood or urine: FID—M. A. Peat and A. Sengupta, *Forens. Sci.*, 1977, *9*, 21–32.

Disposition in the Body. Well absorbed after oral administration but appears to undergo extensive first-pass metabolism; bioavailability about 20%. Little is known about the metabolic fate

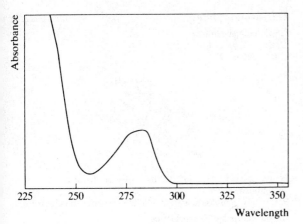

Absorbance

Wavelength

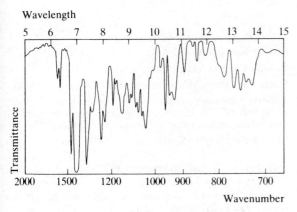

Wavelength

Transmittance

Wavenumber

of dihydrocodeine, but it is likely that *N*-demethylation to form nordihydrocodeine, *O*-demethylation producing dihydromorphine and conjugation occur, similarly to codeine. After an oral dose of 52 mg, 20 to 30% is excreted in the urine in 24 hours; this is increased to about 35% when the urine is acid. After an intramuscular dose of about 43 mg under conditions of controlled acidic urinary pH, 40 to 60% is excreted in the urine in 24 hours. About 30 to 45% of the urinary excreted material is conjugated.

THERAPEUTIC CONCENTRATION.
Following single oral doses of 30 mg and 60 mg to 7 subjects, mean peak plasma concentrations of 0.072 and 0.146 µg/ml were attained in 1.7 hours; the corresponding peak plasma concentrations of acidic metabolites were 0.56 and 1.48 µg/ml (F. J. Rowell *et al.*, *Eur. J. clin. Pharmac.*, 1983, *25*, 419–424).

TOXICITY. The estimated minimum lethal dose is 0.5 g, but addicts may be able to tolerate up to ten times as much, whereas 25 mg may be fatal in children.
In a fatality attributed to an oral overdose of dihydrocodeine, the following postmortem tissue concentrations were reported: blood 12 µg/ml, bile 5340 µg/ml, liver 620 µg/g, urine 570 µg/ml; chlordiazepoxide was also detected. In a second case in which the death of an addict occurred rapidly after an intravenous overdose of dihydrocodeine, the postmortem concentrations were: blood 720 µg/ml, bile 3 µg/ml, liver blood 364 µg/ml, urine 7 µg/ml; pentobarbitone and paracetamol were also detected (M. A. Peat and A. Sengupta, *Forens. Sci.*, 1977, *9*, 21–32).
In four fatalities due to ingestion of dihydrocodeine, postmortem blood concentrations of 7.2 to 12.0 µg/ml (mean 9.0) were reported (S. C. Patterson, *Forens. Sci. Int.*, 1985, *27*, 129–133).

HALF-LIFE. Plasma half-life, about 4 hours.

VOLUME OF DISTRIBUTION. About 1 litre/kg.
CLEARANCE. Plasma clearance, about 4 ml/min/kg.
Dose. 30 to 60 mg of dihydrocodeine tartrate every 4 to 6 hours.

Dihydroergotamine   *Treatment of Migraine*

9,10 - Dihydro - 12' - hydroxy - 2' - methyl - 5'α - benzylergotaman - 3',6',18-trione
$C_{33}H_{37}N_5O_5 = 583.7$
CAS—5111-12-6

White crystals. M.p. 239°.
Practically **insoluble** in water; slightly soluble in ethanol and chloroform.

Dihydroergotamine Mesylate
Synonym. Dihydroergotamine Methanesulphonate
Proprietary Names. DET MS; D.H.E. 45; Dihydergot; Ikaran; Séglor; Tonopres.
$C_{33}H_{37}N_5O_5,CH_3SO_3H = 679.8$
CAS—6190-39-2
A white to slightly yellowish, or an off-white to slightly red, microcrystalline powder.
Soluble 1 in 125 of water, 1 in 90 of ethanol, 1 in 175 of chloroform, and 1 in 2600 of ether; soluble in acetone.

Dihydroergotamine Tartrate
$(C_{33}H_{37}N_5O_5)_2,C_4H_6O_6 = 1318$
CAS—5989-77-5
Colourless crystals or a white crystalline powder. M.p. about 203°, with decomposition.
Very slightly **soluble** in water; sparingly soluble in ethanol; soluble in pyridine.

Dissociation Constant. pK_a 6.9 (24°).

Colour Tests. *p*-Dimethylaminobenzaldehyde—violet; Mandelin's Test—violet-brown; Marquis Test—grey-brown.

Thin-layer Chromatography. *System TA*—Rf 60; *system TB*—Rf 01; *system TC*—Rf 28; *system TL*—Rf 14; *system TM*—Rf 40. (*Van Urk reagent*, blue.)

Gas Chromatography. *System GA*—RI 2315.

High Pressure Liquid Chromatography. *System HA*—k' 0.6; *system HP*—k' 11.4.

Ultraviolet Spectrum. Aqueous acid—280 nm ($A_1^1 = 108$ a). No alkaline shift. (See below)

Infra-red Spectrum. Principal peaks at wavenumbers 1660, 1210, 1712, 1053, 1140, 768 (KBr disk). (See below)

Mass Spectrum. Principal peaks at *m/z* 70, 125, 91, 153, 43, 41, 44, 244 (no peaks above 340).

Quantification. RADIOIMMUNOASSAY. In plasma—J. Rosenthaler and H. Munzer, *Experientia*, 1979, *32*, 234–240.

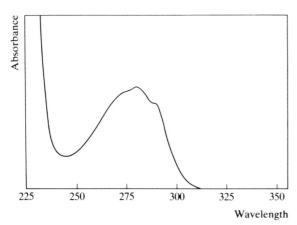

Dihydromorphine

Narcotic Analgesic

7,8-Dihydromorphine
$C_{17}H_{21}NO_3 = 287.4$
CAS—509-60-4

White crystals. M.p. of the hydrated compound, 157°, with decomposition.
Practically **insoluble** in water; soluble in ethanol and chloroform.

Dihydromorphine Hydrochloride
$C_{17}H_{21}NO_3,HCl = 323.8$
CAS—1421-28-9
Crystals.
Very **soluble** in water; slightly soluble in ethanol.

Dissociation Constant. pK_a 8.6.

Partition Coefficient. Log *P* (octanol/pH 7.4), −1.0.

Colour Tests. Mandelin's Test—grey; Marquis Test—red-violet.

Thin-layer Chromatography. *System TA*—Rf 25; *system TB*—Rf 01; *system TC*—Rf 03. (*Dragendorff spray*, positive; *acidified iodoplatinate solution*, positive; *Marquis reagent*, violet.)

Gas Chromatography. *System GA*—RI 2451; *system GC*—RI 2504.

High Pressure Liquid Chromatography. *System HA*—k' 5.7 (tailing peak); *system HC*—k' 2.75.

Ultraviolet Spectrum. Aqueous acid—283 nm ($A_1^1 = 45$ a); aqueous alkali—297 nm ($A_1^1 = 82$ b).

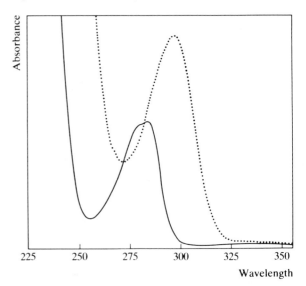

Disposition in the Body. Poorly absorbed after oral administration and undergoes extensive first-pass metabolism with considerable intersubject variation; bioavailability less than 5%. After oral administration less than 5% of a dose is excreted in the urine unchanged in 24 hours, compared to about 11% after intravenous administration. The major metabolite is the 8′-hydroxy derivative, which is active.

THERAPEUTIC CONCENTRATION.

Following single oral doses of 10, 20, and 30 mg to 6 subjects, mean plasma concentrations of about 0.0002, 0.0006, and 0.001 µg/ml, respectively, were attained in about 0.5 to 1 hour (P. J. Little *et al.*, *Br. J. clin. Pharmac.*, 1982, *13*, 785–790).

HALF-LIFE. Plasma half-life, about 2 to 4 hours; a longer terminal elimination half-life of about 20 to 30 hours has also been reported.

VOLUME OF DISTRIBUTION. 6 to 23 litres/kg (mean 14).

CLEARANCE. Plasma clearance, 7 to 22 ml/min/kg (mean 15).

Dose. 1 to 3 mg of dihydroergotamine mesylate, repeated if necessary to a maximum of 10 mg daily.

Infra-red Spectrum. Principal peaks at wavenumbers 1245, 760, 940, 747, 1085, 1145 (KBr disk).

Mass Spectrum. Principal peaks at *m/z* 287, 70, 44, 164, 42, 288, 59, 230.

Dihydrostreptomycin

Antibiotic

4-O-[2-O-(2-Deoxy-2-methylamino-α-L-glucopyranosyl)-5-deoxy-3-C-hydroxymethyl-α-L-lyxofuranosyl]-NN'-diamidino-D-streptamine

$C_{21}H_{41}N_7O_{12} = 583.6$

CAS—128-46-1

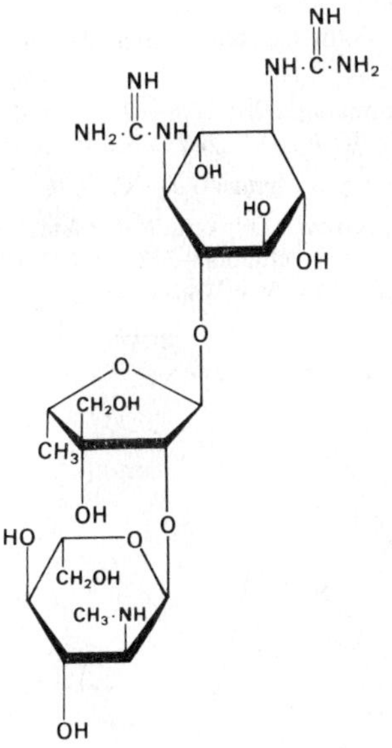

Dihydrostreptomycin Sulphate

Proprietary Names. Abiocine; Enterastrept; Solvo-strept. It is an ingredient of Guanimycin.

$(C_{21}H_{41}N_7O_{12})_2,3H_2SO_4 = 1461$

CAS—5490-27-7

A white hygroscopic solid.
Very **soluble** in water; practically insoluble in ethanol, chloroform, and ether.

Dissociation Constant. pK$_a$ 7.8.

Colour Tests. Nessler's Reagent—yellow → brown; Palladium Chloride—brown (slow).

Thin-layer Chromatography. *System TA*—Rf 01. (*Acidified potassium permanganate solution*, positive.)

Ultraviolet Spectrum. No significant absorption, 230 to 360 nm.

Infra-red Spectrum. Principal peaks at wavenumbers 1111, 1666, 1052, 1724, 1250, 1515.

Dose. The equivalent of 0.5 to 1 g of dihydrostreptomycin has been given daily, intramuscularly.

Dihydrotachysterol

Vitamin D Activity

Synonym. Dichysterol
Proprietary Names. AT 10; Calcamine; Dihydral; Dygratyl; Hytakerol; Tachyrol.

(5E,7E,22E)-10α-9,10-Secoergosta-5,7,22-trien-3β-ol

$C_{28}H_{46}O = 398.7$

CAS—67-96-9

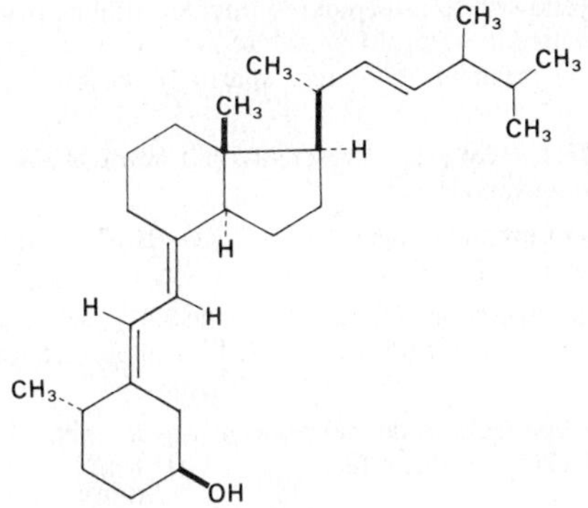

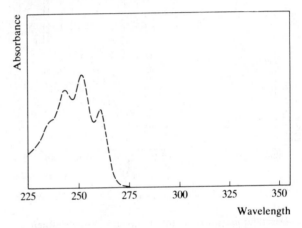

Colourless crystals or white crystalline powder. M.p. 123° to 129°. May also occur in a form melting at about 113°.
Practically **insoluble** in water; soluble 1 in 20 of ethanol, 1 in 0.7 of chloroform, and 1 in 3 of ether.

Ultraviolet Spectrum. Methanol—242 nm, 251 nm (A$_1^1$ = 990 a), 261 nm.

Infra-red Spectrum. Principal peaks at wavenumbers 1056, 967, 1018, 1009, 870, 980 (KBr disk).

Dose. Initially 0.25 to 2.5 mg daily.

Di-iodohydroxyquinoline

Anti-amoebic

Synonyms. Diiodohydroxyquin; Diodoxyquinoléine; Iodo-quinol.
Proprietary Names. Diodoquin; Direxiode; Embequin; Flora-quin; Moebiquin; Yodoxin.

5,7-Di-iodoquinolin-8-ol

$C_9H_5I_2NO = 397.0$

CAS—83-73-8

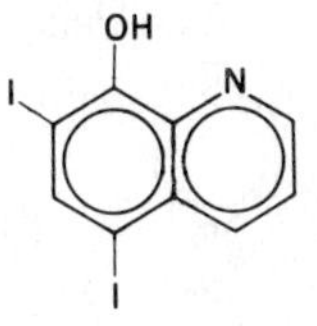

A light yellowish to tan-coloured microcrystalline powder, not readily wetted in water. M.p. 200° to 215°, with decomposition. Practically **insoluble** in water; sparingly soluble in ethanol, acetone, and ether.

Colour Test. Heat a few crystals with 1 ml of *sulphuric acid*—violet iodine vapour.

Thin-layer Chromatography. *System TD*—Rf 17; *system TE*—Rf 28; *system TF*—Rf 19.

Ultraviolet Spectrum. Dilute 5 ml of a 0.01% w/v solution in dioxan to 100 ml with dehydrated alcohol—258 nm ($A_1^1 = 1060$ b).

Infra-red Spectrum. Principal peaks at wavenumbers 1204, 781, 806, 920, 1265, 869 (KBr disk).

Wavelength

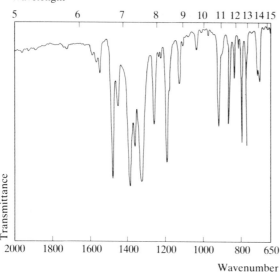

Wavenumber

Mass Spectrum. Principal peaks at *m/z* 397, 115, 242, 398, 88, 143, 271, 62.

Quantification. COLORIMETRY. In urine: sensitivity 10 μg/ml—L. Berggren and O. Hansson, *Clin. Pharmac. Ther.*, 1968, *9*, 67–70.

Disposition in the Body. Incompletely and irregularly absorbed from the small intestine. About 5% of a dose is excreted in the urine as the glucuronide conjugate in 10 hours.

Dose. Usually 1.8 g daily.

Diloxanide   *Anti-amoebic*

Synonym. Diloxan
2,2-Dichloro-4'-hydroxy-*N*-methylacetanilide
$C_9H_9Cl_2NO_2 = 234.1$
CAS—579-38-4

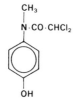

A white crystalline powder. M.p. 175°.
Slightly **soluble** in water; soluble 1 in 8 of ethanol, 1 in 35 of chloroform, and 1 in 66 of ether.

Diloxanide Furoate

Proprietary Names. Furamide. It is an ingredient of Entamizole.
$C_{14}H_{11}Cl_2NO_4 = 328.2$
CAS—3736-81-0
A white crystalline powder. M.p. 114° to 116°.
Very slightly **soluble** in water; soluble 1 in 100 of ethanol, 1 in 2.5 of chloroform, and 1 in 130 of ether.

Colour Tests. Folin–Ciocalteu Reagent—blue; Liebermann's Test—yellow.

Thin-layer Chromatography. *System TA*—Rf 66; *system TB*—Rf 16; *system TC*—Rf 74. (*Acidified iodoplatinate solution*, positive.)

Gas Chromatography. *System GA*—RI 2420.

Ultraviolet Spectrum. Diloxanide furoate: aqueous acid—262 nm ($A_1^1 = 224$ b); ethanol—258 nm ($A_1^1 = 705$ a). Diloxanide: ethanol—278 nm ($A_1^1 = 104$ a).

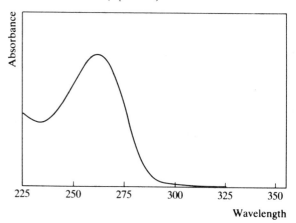

Wavelength

Infra-red Spectrum. Principal peaks at wavenumbers 1678, 1197, 1093, 1290, 1727, 1167 (KBr disk).

Wavelength

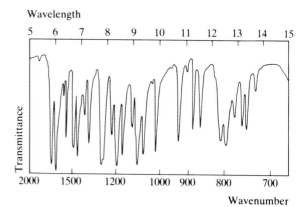

Wavenumber

Mass Spectrum. Principal peaks at *m/z* 95, 327, 39, 329, 96, 122, 244, 67 (diloxanide furoate).

Disposition in the Body. After oral administration diloxanide furoate is hydrolysed to diloxanide and then readily absorbed; it is excreted in the urine and faeces.

Dose. 1.5 g of diloxanide furoate daily.

Dimefline   *Respiratory Stimulant*

8-Dimethylaminomethyl-7-methoxy-3-methyl-2-phenyl-4*H*-chromen-4-one

$C_{20}H_{21}NO_3 = 323.4$

CAS—1165-48-6

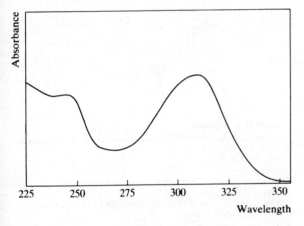

Dimefline Hydrochloride

Proprietary Name. Remeflin(e)

$C_{20}H_{21}NO_3,HCl = 359.9$

CAS—2740-04-7

A white crystalline powder. It decomposes at about 213°.

Soluble in water and ethanol; practically insoluble in chloroform and ether.

Colour Test. Liebermann's Test—orange.

Thin-layer Chromatography. *System TA*—Rf 59; *system TB*—Rf 15; *system TC*—Rf 48. (*Acidified iodoplatinate solution*, positive.)

Gas Chromatography. *System GA*—RI 2555.

Ultraviolet Spectrum. Aqueous acid—309 nm ($A_1^1 = 950$ b).

Infra-red Spectrum. Principal peaks at wavenumbers 1637, 1278, 1602, 1081, 699, 1136 (KBr disk).

Mass Spectrum. Principal peaks at *m/z* 279, 163, 323, 58, 277, 308, 280, 322.

Dose. Dimefline hydrochloride has been given in doses of 16 to 48 mg daily.

Dimenhydrinate   *Antihistamine*

Synonyms. Anautin; Chloranautine; Diphenhydramine Theoclate.

Proprietary Names. Amosyt; Andrumin; Dimate; Dramamine; Dramocen; Epha-retard; Gravol; Nauseatol; Novodimenate; Novomina; Travamine; Vomex A.

The diphenhydramine salt of 8-chlorotheophylline.

$C_{17}H_{21}NO,C_7H_7ClN_4O_2 = 470.0$

CAS—523-87-5

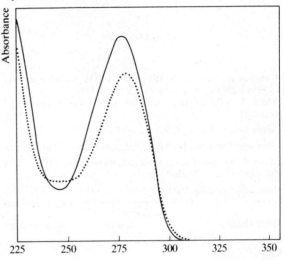

A white crystalline powder. M.p. 102° to 107°.

Soluble 1 in 95 of water, 1 in 2 of ethanol, and 1 in 2 of chloroform; sparingly soluble in ether.

Gas Chromatography. *System GA*—RI 1844; *system GB*—RI 1875.

Ultraviolet Spectrum. Aqueous acid—276 nm ($A_1^1 = 268$ a); aqueous alkali—278 nm.

Infra-red Spectrum. Principal peaks at wavenumbers 1640, 1685, 1118, 755, 712, 1255 (KBr disk).

Mass Spectrum. Principal peaks at m/z 58, 73, 45, 43, 57, 167, 44, 165.

Quantification. HIGH PRESSURE LIQUID CHROMATOGRAPHY. In serum: detection limit 50 ng/ml, UV detection—G. Skofitsch and F. Lembeck, *Arzneimittel-Forsch.*, 1983, *33*, 1674–1676.

Dose. 100 to 300 mg daily.

Dimercaprol   *Chelating Agent*

Synonyms. BAL; British Anti-Lewisite; Dimercaptopropanol.
Proprietary Name. Sulfactin
2,3-Dimercaptopropan-1-ol
$C_3H_8OS_2 = 124.2$
CAS—59-52-9

$$\underset{HS\cdot CH_2\cdot \overset{\displaystyle SH}{CH}\cdot CH_2OH}{}$$

A clear, colourless or slightly yellow liquid. Relative density 1.239 to 1.259. Refractive index 1.568 to 1.574.
Soluble 1 in 20 of water; miscible with ethanol, ether, and methanol.

Colour Test. Palladium Chloride—yellow.

Ultraviolet Spectrum. No significant absorption, 230 to 360 nm.

Infra-red Spectrum. Principal peaks at wavenumbers 1022, 1050, 990, 1270, 1235, 1170 (thin film).

Dose. 2.5 to 4 mg/kg, intramuscularly, up to 6 times daily.

Dimethadione   *Anticonvulsant*

5,5-Dimethyloxazolidine-2,4-dione
$C_5H_7NO_3 = 129.1$
CAS—695-53-4

Crystals. M.p. 76° to 77°.

Dissociation Constant. pK_a 6.1 (37°).

Colour Tests. Koppanyi–Zwikker Test—violet; Mercurous Nitrate—black.

Ultraviolet Spectrum. No significant absorption, 230 to 360 nm.

Infra-red Spectrum. Principal peaks at wavenumbers 1740, 1760, 1815, 1188, 1280, 1007.

Quantification. See under Troxidone.

Disposition in the Body. Dimethadione is the active metabolite of troxidone. It is very slowly excreted in the urine over a period of several days, the rate of excretion being increased in alkaline urine.

TOXICITY. Toxic effects may be associated with plasma concentrations greater than 1000 µg/ml.

HALF-LIFE. Derived from urinary excretion data, 6 to 13 days.

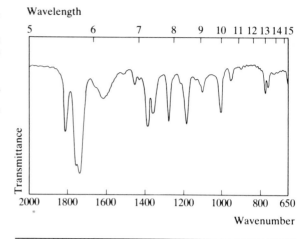

Wavelength

Dimethindene   *Antihistamine*

Synonyms. Dimethpyrindene; Dimethylpyrindene.
NN-Dimethyl-2-{3-[1-(2-pyridyl)ethyl]-1H-inden-2-yl}-ethylamine
$C_{20}H_{24}N_2 = 292.4$
CAS—5636-83-9

Dimethindene Maleate

Proprietary Names. Fenistil; Fenostil; Forhistal; Triten. It is an ingredient of Vibrocil.
$C_{20}H_{24}N_2,C_4H_4O_4 = 408.5$
CAS—3614-69-5
A white to off-white crystalline powder. M.p. about 161°, with decomposition.
Soluble 1 in 63 of water, 1 in 185 of ethanol, and 1 in 10 of chloroform; practically insoluble in ether.

Colour Tests. Cyanogen Bromide—orange-pink; Mandelin's Test—green; Marquis Test—violet→blue.

Thin-layer Chromatography. *System TA*—Rf 42; *system TB*—Rf 36; *system TC*—Rf 13. (*Acidified iodoplatinate solution*, positive.)

Gas Chromatography. *System GA*—RI 2258; *system GC*—RI 2669.

High Pressure Liquid Chromatography. *System HA*—k' 5.1.

Ultraviolet Spectrum. Aqueous acid—260 nm ($A_1^1 = 613$ b).

Infra-red Spectrum. Principal peaks at wavenumbers 763, 1590, 724, 747, 1570, 1050.

Mass Spectrum. Principal peaks at m/z 58, 59, 72, 45, 292, 218, 42, –.

Quantification. GAS CHROMATOGRAPHY. In serum or urine: sensitivity 10 ng/ml, FID—M. M. Wermeille and G. A. Huber, *J. Chromat.*, 1982, *228*; *Biomed. Appl.*, *17*, 187–194.

Dose. Up to 6 mg of dimethindene maleate daily.

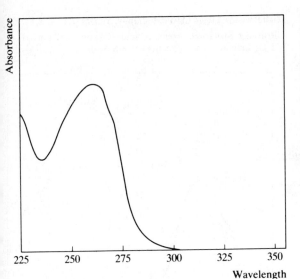

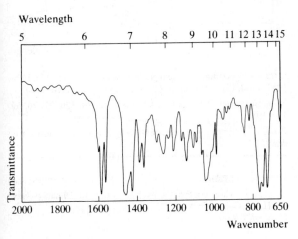

Wavelength

Thin-layer Chromatography. *System TA*—Rf 61; *system TB*—Rf 55; *system TC*—Rf 46; *system TL*—Rf 28. (*Acidified iodoplatinate solution*, positive.)

Gas Chromatography. *System GA*—RI 2030.

High Pressure Liquid Chromatography. *System HA*—k' 2.2; *system HR*—k' 11.24.

Ultraviolet Spectrum. Aqueous acid—261 nm, 269 nm (A_1^1 = 159 a), 331 nm.

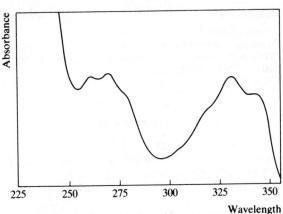

Infra-red Spectrum. Principal peaks at wavenumbers 1576, 1631, 1499, 1155, 1115, 751 (KBr disk).

Mass Spectrum. Principal peaks at *m*/*z* 71, 58, 72, 43, 159, 56, 42, 201.

Use. Dimethisoquin hydrochloride is used in a concentration of 0.5%.

Dimethisoquin
Local Anaesthetic

Synonyms. Chinisocaine; Quinisocaine.

2-(3-Butyl-1-isoquinolyloxy)-*NN*-dimethylethylamine

$C_{17}H_{24}N_2O = 272.4$

CAS—86-80-6

O·[CH₂]₂·N(CH₃)₂ ... CH₂·[CH₂]₂·CH₃

A liquid. B.p. about 156°.

Dimethisoquin Hydrochloride
Proprietary Names. Haenal; Isochinol; Pruralgan; Pruralgin; Quotane.

$C_{17}H_{24}N_2O,HCl = 308.9$

CAS—2773-92-4

A white crystalline powder. M.p. 144° to 148°.

Soluble 1 in 8 of water, 1 in 3 of ethanol, and 1 in 2 of chloroform; very slightly soluble in ether.

Dimethisterone
Progestational Steroid

Synonym. 6α,21-Dimethylethisterone

17β - Hydroxy - 6α,21 - dimethyl - 17α - pregn - 4 - en - 20 - yn - 3 - one monohydrate

$C_{23}H_{32}O_2,H_2O = 358.5$

CAS—79-64-1 (anhydrous); *41354-30-7* (monohydrate)

A white crystalline powder. M.p. about 100°, with decomposition.

Practically **insoluble** in water; soluble 1 in 3 of ethanol, 1 in 0.7 of chloroform, and 1 in 1 of pyridine.

Colour Tests. Antimony Pentachloride—brown; Naphthol-Sulphuric Acid—red-brown/brown-green; Sulphuric Acid—orange-red.

Thin-layer Chromatography. *System TP*—Rf 80; *system TQ*—Rf 42; *system TR*—Rf 91; *system TS*—Rf 95.

Ultraviolet Spectrum. Dimethisterone anhydrous: dehydrated alcohol—240 nm (A_1^1 = 467 a).

Infra-red Spectrum. Principal peaks at wavenumbers 1658, 1605, 1275, 876, 1281, 1241 (KBr disk).

Mass Spectrum. Principal peaks at m/z 67, 137, 91, 138, 55, 79, 41, 95.

Dose. Dimethisterone has been given in doses of 15 mg daily.

Dimethoate   *Pesticide*

Synonym. Fosfamid
Proprietary Names. Rogor E; Roxion.
OO-Dimethyl *S*-methylcarbamoylmethyl phosphorodithioate
$C_5H_{12}NO_3PS_2$ = 229.2
CAS—60-51-5

$$(CH_3 \cdot O)_2 \overset{\overset{\displaystyle S}{\|}}{P} - S \cdot CH_2 \cdot CO \cdot NH \cdot CH_3$$

A white solid. M.p. 51° to 52°.
Soluble 1 in 40 of water; soluble in most organic solvents except saturated hydrocarbons.

Colour Tests. Palladium Chloride—yellow; Phosphorus Test—yellow.

Thin-layer Chromatography. *System TW*—Rf 19.

Gas Chromatography. *System GA*—RI 1725; *system GK*—retention time 0.86 relative to caffeine.

Infra-red Spectrum. Principal peaks at wavenumbers 1010, 1666, 819, 666, 1538, 1176.

Mass Spectrum. Principal peaks at m/z 87, 93, 125, 58, 47, 63, 79, 42.

Dimethothiazine   *Antihistamine*

Synonyms. Dimetiotazine; Fonazine.
10-(2-Dimethylaminopropyl)-*NN*-dimethylphenothiazine-2-sulphonamide
$C_{19}H_{25}N_3O_2S_2$ = 391.5
CAS—7456-24-8

Dimethothiazine Mesylate
Proprietary Names. Banistyl; Migristene; Promaquid.
$C_{19}H_{25}N_3O_2S_2,CH_3SO_3H$ = 487.6
CAS—7455-39-2; 13115-40-7
A white crystalline powder. M.p. about 175°.
Very **soluble** in water; practically insoluble in ether.

Colour Tests. Formaldehyde–Sulphuric Acid—yellow; Forrest Reagent—red; FPN Reagent—red; Mandelin's Test—red-violet; Marquis Test—red.

Thin-layer Chromatography. *System TA*—Rf 56; *system TB*—Rf 13; *system TC*—Rf 48. (*Acidified iodoplatinate solution*, positive.)

Gas Chromatography. *System GA*—RI 3078.

High Pressure Liquid Chromatography. *System HA*—k' 2.1.

Ultraviolet Spectrum. Aqueous acid—235 nm, 262 nm (A_1^1 = 675 a); aqueous alkali—268 nm (A_1^1 = 808 b).

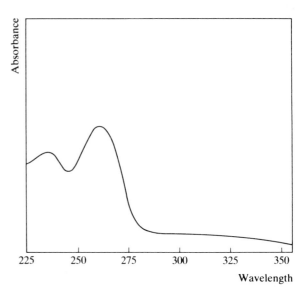

Infra-red Spectrum. Principal peaks at wavenumbers 1205, 1190, 1057, 1160, 1220, 717 (dimethothiazine mesylate, KBr disk).

Mass Spectrum. Principal peaks at m/z 72, 73, 320, 71, 70, 56, 210, 198.

Dose. Usually the equivalent of 60 to 120 mg of dimethothiazine daily.

Dimethoxanate   *Cough Suppressant*

2-(2-Dimethylaminoethoxy)ethyl phenothiazine-10-carboxylate
$C_{19}H_{22}N_2O_3S$ = 358.5
CAS—477-93-0

Dimethoxanate Hydrochloride
Proprietary Name. Cotrane
$C_{19}H_{22}N_2O_3S,HCl$ = 394.9
CAS—518-63-8
Crystals. M.p. 161° to 163°, with decomposition.

Colour Tests. Mandelin's Test—green → brown; Marquis Test—violet.

Thin-layer Chromatography. *System TA*—Rf 39; *system TB*—Rf 18; *system TC*—Rf 24. (*Dragendorff spray*, positive; *FPN reagent*, violet; *acidified iodoplatinate solution*, positive; *Marquis reagent*, brown; *ninhydrin spray*, positive.)

Gas Chromatography. *System GA*—RI 2029.

High Pressure Liquid Chromatography. *System HA*—k' 5.8 (tailing peak).

Ultraviolet Spectrum. Aqueous acid—254 nm $(A_1^1 = 24 \, b)$. No alkaline shift.

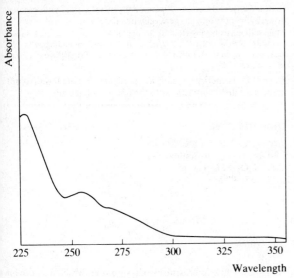

Wavelength

Infra-red Spectrum. Principal peaks at wavenumbers 1718, 1317, 1217, 1250, 763, 1298 (KBr disk).

Mass Spectrum. Principal peaks at m/z 58, 116, 198, 199, 72, 59, 42, 44.

Dose. Dimethoxanate hydrochloride has been given in doses of 75 to 200 mg daily.

Dimethyl Phthalate

Insect Repellent

Synonyms. DMP; Methyl Phthalate.
Proprietary Name. Affel
Dimethyl benzene-1,2-dicarboxylate
$C_{10}H_{10}O_4 = 194.2$
CAS—131-11-3

CO·O·CH₃
CO·O·CH₃

A colourless liquid. Wt per ml 1.186 to 1.192 g. B.p. about 280°, with decomposition. Refractive index 1.515 to 1.517.
Soluble 1 in 250 of water; miscible with ethanol, ether, and most organic solvents.

Gas Chromatography. *System GA*—RI 1406.

Ultraviolet Spectrum. Ethanol—275 nm $(A_1^1 = 75 \, b)$.

Mass Spectrum. Principal peaks at m/z 163, 77, 164, 135, 194, 76, 92, 50.

Use. Topically in concentrations of at least 40%.

Dimethyl Sulphoxide

Solvent

Synonyms. Dimethyl Sulfoxide; Dimexide; DMSO; Methyl Sulphoxide.
Proprietary Names. Deltan; Kemsol; Rimso-50. It is an ingredient of Herpid and Iduridin.

$CH_3 \cdot SO \cdot CH_3 = 78.13$
CAS—67-68-5

A colourless, hygroscopic, viscous liquid. Wt per ml 1.099 to 1.101 g. F.p. not lower than 18.3°. B.p. 189° to 192°. Refractive index 1.478 to 1.479.
Miscible with water with the evolution of heat, with ethanol, acetone, chloroform, ether, and most organic solvents.

Colour Tests. It decolorises a 1% potassium permanganate solution.
Cautiously add 1.5 ml dropwise to 2.5 ml of *hydriodic acid* cooled in ice and filter rapidly—unstable violet residue which is soluble in chloroform giving a red solution.

Ultraviolet Spectrum. No significant absorption, 230 to 360 nm.

Mass Spectrum. Principal peaks at m/z 63, 78, 45, 61, 46, 62, 48, 47.

Quantification. GAS CHROMATOGRAPHY. In serum or urine: dimethyl sulphoxide and sulphone metabolite, FID—H. B. Hucker *et al.*, *J. Pharmac. exp. Ther.*, 1967, *155*, 309–317. In plasma, serum, urine or cerebrospinal fluid: sensitivity 10 µg/ml, FID—S. E. Garretson and J. P. Aitchison, *J. analyt. Toxicol.*, 1982, *6*, 76–81.

Disposition in the Body. Readily absorbed after injection or after oral or percutaneous administration. Widely distributed throughout the body. It is oxidised to dimethyl sulphone. After an oral dose, about 30 to 70% is excreted in the urine unchanged and about 20% as the sulphone; after percutaneous administration, about 13% is excreted unchanged and about 18% as the sulphone; about 3% of a dose is eliminated through the lungs as dimethyl sulphide.

BLOOD CONCENTRATION.
After an oral dose of 1 g/kg to 6 subjects, peak serum concentrations of dimethyl sulphoxide of 1029 to 3380 µg/ml (mean 2200) were attained in 1 to 4 hours, and peak concentrations of the sulphone metabolite of 260 to 600 µg/ml were reported after about 72 hours. After percutaneous administration of 1 g/kg to 2 subjects, peak serum concentrations of about 500 µg/ml of dimethyl sulphoxide and 350 µg/ml of the sulphone metabolite were reported after 4 to 8 hours and 36 to 72 hours respectively (H. B. Hucker *et al.*, *J. Pharmac. exp. Ther.*, 1967, *155*, 309–317).

TOXICITY. Dimethyl sulphoxide has low systemic toxicity, but gives local toxic effects.

HALF-LIFE. Plasma half-life, dimethyl sulphoxide about 10 to 20 hours, sulphone metabolite about 70 hours.

REFERENCE. H. B. Hucker *et al.*, *ibid.*

Dimethylamphetamine

Central Stimulant

N,N,α-Trimethylphenethylamine
$C_{11}H_{17}N = 163.3$
CAS—4075-96-1

N(CH₃)₂
|
C₆H₅·CH₂·CH·CH₃

Dissociation Constant. pK_a 9.8.

Gas Chromatography. *System GA*—RI 1236; *system GB*—RI 1261; *system GC*—RI 1429.

High Pressure Liquid Chromatography. *System HB*—k′ 11.08; *system HC*—k′ 1.89.

Mass Spectrum. Principal peaks at m/z 72, 91, 73, 44, 42, 56, 70, 65.

Dimethyltryptamine

Hallucinogen

Synonyms. NN-Dimethyltryptamine; DMT.
3-(2-Dimethylaminoethyl)indole
$C_{12}H_{16}N_2 = 188.3$
CAS—61-50-7

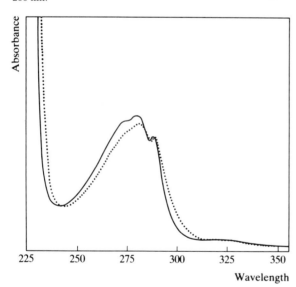

An active principle obtained from the seeds and leaves of *Piptadenia peregrina* (Mimosaceae).
Crystals. M.p. 44° to 47°.
Freely **soluble** in dilute acetic acid and dilute mineral acids.

Dimethyltryptamine Hydrochloride
A white crystalline powder. M.p. 165° to 168°.
Soluble in water.

Colour Test. Marquis Test—orange.

Thin-layer Chromatography. *System TA*—Rf 40; *system TB*—Rf 09; *system TC*—Rf 09. (*Dragendorff spray*, positive; *acidified iodoplatinate solution*, positive; *Marquis reagent*, grey-brown; *Van Urk reagent*, blue.)

Gas Chromatography. *System GA*—RI 1810.

Ultraviolet Spectrum. Aqueous acid—279 nm ($A_1^1 = 327$ a), 288 nm.

Infra-red Spectrum. Principal peaks at wavenumbers 743, 1113, 1235, 1050, 812, 1010 (KBr disk).

Mass Spectrum. Principal peaks at *m/z* 58, 188, 130, 59, 42, 143, 129, 115.

Quantification. GAS CHROMATOGRAPHY–MASS SPECTROMETRY. In blood: sensitivity 10 pg/ml—R. W. Walker *et al., J. Chromat.*, 1979, *162*; *Biomed. Appl.*, *4*, 539–546. In urine: sensitivity 100 pg/ml—M. Räisänen and J. Kärrkkäinen, *ibid.*, 579–584.

Disposition in the Body. It is inactive when taken orally. After intramuscular injection it is rapidly and extensively metabolised, primarily to indol-3-ylacetic acid. About 33% of a dose is excreted in the urine in 6 hours as free and conjugated (glucuronide) indol-3-ylacetic acid; less than 0.1% of a dose is excreted unchanged in the urine in 24 hours.

BLOOD CONCENTRATION. Plasma concentrations of endogenous dimethyltryptamine are generally less than 0.001 µg/ml.
After intramuscular injection of 0.7 mg/kg to 11 subjects, peak blood concentrations averaged 0.1 µg/ml at 0.17 hour, coinciding with the maximum psychoactive effects (J. Kaplan *et al., Psychopharmacologia*, 1974, *28*, 239–245).

TOXICITY. Dimethyltryptamine produces hallucinations and perceptual distortion similar to the effects of lysergide.

Dimetridazole

Antiprotozoal (Veterinary)

Proprietary Name. Emtryl
1,2-Dimethyl-5-nitroimidazole
$C_5H_7N_3O_2 = 141.1$
CAS—551-92-8

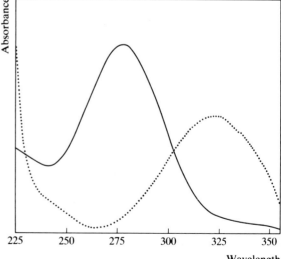

An almost white to brownish-yellow powder, which darkens on exposure to light. M.p. 138° to 141°.
Slightly **soluble** in water; soluble 1 in 30 of ethanol, 1 in 5 of chloroform, and 1 in 170 of ether.

Dimetridazole Hydrochloride
$C_5H_7N_3O_2,HCl = 177.6$
CAS—25332-20-1
Crystals. M.p. 195°.
Freely **soluble** in water and ethanol.

Colour Test. Methanolic Potassium Hydroxide—violet (when boiled).

Thin-layer Chromatography. *System TA*—Rf 63. (*Acidified potassium permanganate solution*, strong reaction.)

Gas Chromatography. *System GA*—RI 1353.

Ultraviolet Spectrum. Aqueous acid—277 nm ($A_1^1 = 405$ b); aqueous alkali—322 nm ($A_1^1 = 500$ b).

Infra-red Spectrum. Principal peaks at wavenumbers 1181, 1258, 1515, 825, 746, 1119 (KBr disk).

Diminazene   *Antiprotozoal/Antibacterial*

1,3-Bis(4-amidinophenyl)triazene
$C_{14}H_{15}N_7 = 281.3$
CAS—536-71-0

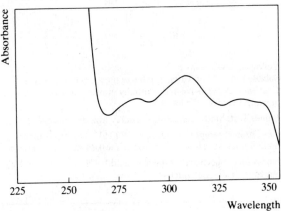

Diminazene Aceturate
Proprietary Name. Berenil
$C_{22}H_{29}N_9O_6,4H_2O = 587.6$
CAS—908-54-3 (anhydrous)
A yellow powder. M.p. 217°, with decomposition.
Soluble 1 in 14 of water; slightly soluble in ethanol; very slightly soluble in chloroform and ether.

Thin-layer Chromatography. *System TA*—Rf 00; *system TB*—Rf 00; *system TC*—Rf 00. (*Acidified iodoplatinate solution*, positive.)

Ultraviolet Spectrum. Diminazene aceturate: aqueous acid—257 nm ($A_1^1 = 305$ a); aqueous alkali—247 nm (broad) ($A_1^1 = 239$ b).

Infra-red Spectrum. Principal peaks at wavenumbers 1610, 1635, 1588, 1171, 1267, 1198 (KBr disk).

Mass Spectrum. Principal peaks at *m/z* 30, 43, 72, 102, 73, 42, 118, 99.

Dimoxyline   *Antispasmodic*

Synonym. Dioxyline
1-(4-Ethoxy-3-methoxybenzyl)-6,7-dimethoxy-3-methyliso-quinoline
$C_{22}H_{25}NO_4 = 367.4$
CAS—147-27-3

Crystals. M.p. 124° to 125°.

Dimoxyline Phosphate
Proprietary Names. Paveril Phosphate; Paverona.
$C_{22}H_{25}NO_4,H_3PO_4 = 465.4$
CAS—5667-46-9
A white crystalline powder. M.p. about 198°, with decomposition.
Soluble 1 in 25 of water and 1 in 320 of ethanol.

Colour Tests. Mandelin's Test—green; Marquis Test—brown.

Thin-layer Chromatography. *System TA*—Rf 68; *system TB*—Rf 16; *system TC*—Rf 75. (*Acidified iodoplatinate solution*, positive.)

Gas Chromatography. *System GA*—RI 2895.

Ultraviolet Spectrum. Aqueous acid—285 nm, 309 nm ($A_1^1 = 179$ b), 335 nm.

Infra-red Spectrum. Principal peaks at wavenumbers 1504, 1247, 1208, 1145, 1225, 865 (KCl disk).

Mass Spectrum. Principal peaks at *m/z* 352, 367, 338, 366, 29, 368, 353, 339.

Disposition in the Body. Absorbed from the gastro-intestinal tract. Metabolised in the liver and excreted in the urine.

Dose. 0.3 to 1.6 g of dimoxyline phosphate daily.

Dinitolmide   *Coccidiostat (Veterinary)*

Synonyms. Dinitrotoluamide; Methyldinitrobenzamide.
Proprietary Name. Salcostat
3,5-Dinitro-*o*-toluamide
$C_8H_7N_3O_5 = 225.2$
CAS—148-01-6

A cream-coloured to light tan-coloured powder. M.p. 177° to 181°.
Practically **insoluble** in water; soluble 1 in 100 of ethanol, 1 in 15 of acetone, 1 in 650 of chloroform, and 1 in 850 of ether.

Colour Tests. Methanolic Potassium Hydroxide—green; Nessler's Reagent—brown-orange.

Thin-layer Chromatography. *System TA*—Rf 75. (*Acidified iodoplatinate solution*, positive, developing slowly.)

Infra-red Spectrum. Principal peaks at wavenumbers 1527, 1672, 1612, 738, 1595, 1289 (KBr disk).

Dinitro-orthocresol   *Insecticide/Herbicide*

Synonyms. Dinitrocresol; Dinitrol; Ditrosol; DN; DNC; DNOC; KIII; KIV.
Proprietary Names. Cresofin; Sandolin A.

2-Methyl-4,6-dinitrophenol
$C_7H_6N_2O_5 = 198.1$
CAS—534-52-1

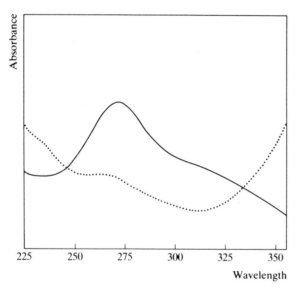

Yellowish crystals. M.p. 86°.
Soluble 1 in 7500 of water; soluble in most organic solvents.
Caution. It is explosive and is usually moistened with up to 10% of water to reduce the hazard.

Colour Test. Methanolic Potassium Hydroxide—orange (100°).

Gas Chromatography. *System GA*—RI 1617. Dinitro-orthocresol methyl ether: *system GK*—retention time 0.74 relative to caffeine.

Ultraviolet Spectrum. Aqueous acid—271 nm ($A_1^1 = 631$ b); aqueous alkali—265 nm ($A_1^1 = 251$ b).

Infra-red Spectrum. Principal peaks at wavenumbers 1605, 1232, 1090, 1218, 1546, 1156 (Nujol mull).

Mass Spectrum. Principal peaks at *m/z* 182, 165, 89, 90, 212, 51, 65, 91 (dinitro-orthocresol methyl ether).

Quantification. COLORIMETRY. In blood or tissues—M. L. Fenwick and V. H. Parker, *Analyst, Lond.*, 1955, *80*, 774–776.

Disposition in the Body. Absorbed through the skin, by inhalation, or by accidental ingestion. It acts as a cumulative poison causing an increase in the metabolic rate, and it is eliminated slowly over a period of weeks. After ingestion, less than 5% is excreted unchanged in the urine.

TOXICITY. The acute toxic dose is about 200 mg and the maximum permissible atmospheric concentration is 0.2 mg/m³. Blood concentrations greater than about 50 µg/ml are associated with severe toxicity.

NOTE. For a review of poisoning by dinitro-orthocresol see P. L. Bidstrup *et al.*, *Lancet*, 1952, *1*, 794–795.

Diperodon   *Local Anaesthetic*

Synonym. Diperocaine
Proprietary Name. Diothane
3-Piperidinopropylene bis(phenylcarbamate) monohydrate
$C_{22}H_{27}N_3O_4,H_2O = 415.5$
CAS—101-08-6 (anhydrous); *51552-99-9* (monohydrate)

A white to cream-coloured powder.
Practically **insoluble** in water; soluble 1 in 3 of ethanol, 1 in 10 of chloroform, 1 in 4 of ether, and 1 in 1 of methanol.

Diperodon Hydrochloride
$C_{22}H_{27}N_3O_4,HCl = 433.9$
CAS—537-12-2
A white crystalline powder. M.p. about 198°.
Soluble 1 in 100 of water; soluble in ethanol; slightly soluble in acetone; practically insoluble in ether.

Colour Tests. Liebermann's Test—brown; Mandelin's Test—red → green.

Thin-layer Chromatography. *System TA*—Rf 70; *system TB*—Rf 15; *system TC*—Rf 58; *system TL*—Rf 66. (*Acidified iodoplatinate solution,* positive.)

Gas Chromatography. *System GA*—RI 2370.

High Pressure Liquid Chromatography. *System HR*—k' 2.48.

Ultraviolet Spectrum. Aqueous acid—232 nm ($A_1^1 = 1320$ b).

Infra-red Spectrum. Principal peaks at wavenumbers 1210, 1705, 1530, 1600, 1305, 1050 (KBr disk).

Mass Spectrum. Principal peaks at *m/z* 98, 119, 91, 99, 124, 64, 41, 55.

Use. Diperodon has been applied topically in a concentration of 1%.

Diphemanil Methylsulphate   *Anticholinergic*

Synonyms. Diphemanil Methylsulfate; Diphenmethanil Methylsulphate; Vagophemanil Methylsulphate.
Proprietary Name. Prantal
4-Benzhydrylidene-1,1-dimethylpiperidinium methylsulphate
$C_{20}H_{24}N,CH_3SO_4 = 389.5$
CAS—62-97-5

A white, hygroscopic, crystalline powder. M.p. 189° to 196°.
Soluble 1 in 33 of water, 1 in 33 of ethanol, and 1 in 33 of chloroform; very slightly soluble in ether.

Colour Tests. Liebermann's Test—brown; Mandelin's Test—brown; Marquis Test—orange-red; Sulphuric Acid—orange.

Thin-layer Chromatography. *System TA*—Rf 02. (*Acidified iodoplatinate solution*, positive.)

Infra-red Spectrum. Principal peaks at wavenumbers 708, 1250, 1230, 1010, 765, 699 (KBr disk).

Dose. 400 to 800 mg daily.

Diphenadione   *Anticoagulant/Rodenticide*

Synonym. Diphacinone
Proprietary Name. Diphacin (rodenticide)
2-(Diphenylacetyl)indan-1,3-dione
$C_{23}H_{16}O_3 = 340.4$
CAS—82-66-6

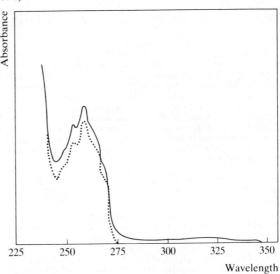

Yellow crystals or crystalline powder. M.p. 144° to 150°. Practically **insoluble** in water; soluble 1 in less than 100 of ethanol and chloroform; soluble in ether and glacial acetic acid.

Colour Tests. Liebermann's Test—orange-brown; Methanolic Potassium Hydroxide—yellow; Sulphuric Acid—yellow.

Thin-layer Chromatography. *System TD*—Rf 11; *system TE*—Rf 46; *system TF*—Rf 33. (*Acidified potassium permanganate solution*, positive.)

Gas Chromatography. *System GA*—RI 2934.

Ultraviolet Spectrum. Aqueous acid—336 nm ($A_1^1 = 675$ b). No alkaline shift.

Mass Spectrum. Principal peaks at *m/z* 173, 340, 168, 167, 165, 341, 174, 322.

Dose. Maintenance, 2.5 to 5 mg daily.

Diphenhydramine   *Antihistamine*

Synonym. Benzhydramine
2-Benzhydryloxy-*NN*-dimethylethylamine
$C_{17}H_{21}NO = 255.4$
CAS—58-73-1

$$CH \cdot O \cdot [CH_2]_2 \cdot N(CH_3)_2$$
with two C_6H_5 groups attached to CH

Note. Diphenhydramine is an isomer of phenyltoloxamine.

Diphenhydramine Di(acefyllinate)
Synonym. Bietanautine
Proprietary Name. Nautamine
$C_{17}H_{21}NO,2C_9H_{10}N_4O_4 = 731.8$
CAS—6888-11-5

Diphenhydramine Hydrochloride
Synonym. Dimedrolum
Proprietary Names. Alergicap; Benadryl; Bidramine; Dolestan; Halbmond; Histergan; Insomnal; Lensen; Pheramin; Somnium; Valdrene; Wehydryl. It is an ingredient of Benafed, Benylin, Caladryl, Globolotion, Guanor, Histalix, Lotussin, Noradran, Pharmidone, Propain, Ticipect, and Uniflu.

$C_{17}H_{21}NO,HCl = 291.8$
CAS—147-24-0
A white crystalline powder which slowly darkens on exposure to light. M.p. 167° to 172°.
Soluble 1 in 1 of water, 1 in 2 of ethanol, and 1 in 2 of chloroform; practically insoluble in ether.

Dissociation Constant. pK_a 9.0 (25°).

Partition Coefficient. Log P (octanol), 3.3.

Colour Tests. Liebermann's Test—brown-orange; Mandelin's Test—yellow; Marquis Test—yellow; Sulphuric Acid—orange.

Thin-layer Chromatography. *System TA*—Rf 55; *system TB*—Rf 45; *system TC*—Rf 33. (*Dragendorff spray*, positive; *FPN reagent*, pink; *acidified iodoplatinate solution*, positive; *Marquis reagent*, yellow; *ninhydrin spray*, positive.)

Gas Chromatography. *System GA*—RI 1873; *system GB*—RI 1872; *system GC*—RI 2378; *system GF*—RI 2105.

High Pressure Liquid Chromatography. *System HA*—k' 3.3.

Ultraviolet Spectrum. Aqueous acid—252 nm, 257 nm ($A_1^1 = 17$ a).

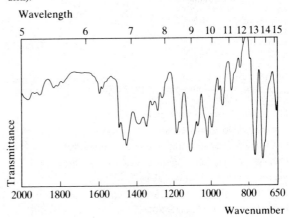

Infra-red Spectrum. Principal peaks at wavenumbers 713, 754, 1103, 1017, 1180, 991 (diphenhydramine hydrochloride, KBr disk).

Mass Spectrum. Principal peaks at m/z 58, 73, 45, 167, 165, 166, 44, 152 (no peaks above 200); didesmethyldiphenhydramine 30, 167, 45, 168, 165, 183, 166, 152; monodesmethyldiphenhydramine 44, 167, 168, 165, 183, 105, 152, 77.

Quantification. GAS CHROMATOGRAPHY. In blood, urine or tissues: FID—R. C. Backer *et al.*, *J. analyt. Toxicol.*, 1977, *1*, 227–228.

GAS CHROMATOGRAPHY (CAPILLARY COLUMN). In serum: sensitivity 2.5 ng/ml, AFID—D. Lutz *et al.*, *J. clin. Chem. clin. Biochem.*, 1983, *21*, 595–597.

Disposition in the Body. Readily absorbed after oral administration, but undergoes extensive first-pass metabolism by *N*-dealkylation and oxidative deamination to form monodesmethyl and didesmethyl metabolites, and diphenylmethoxyacetic acid which may be conjugated with glutamine or glycine; bioavailability about 50%. Up to 65% of a dose is excreted in the urine in 96 hours. The major urinary metabolite appears to be diphenylmethoxyacetic acid in free or conjugated form; very little is excreted as unchanged drug.

THERAPEUTIC CONCENTRATION. In plasma, usually in the range 0.1 to 1.0 μg/ml.

Following a single oral dose of 100 mg of diphenhydramine hydrochloride to 4 subjects, peak plasma concentrations of 0.08 to 0.16 μg/ml (mean 0.11) were obtained 2 to 4 hours after administration; total amine concentrations were approximately 50% higher due to the presence of *N*-dealkylated metabolites. After single oral doses of 100 mg to a further 4 subjects, the concentration of acidic metabolites increased over a period of 24 hours to about 2 μg/ml. After multiple oral doses of 50 mg of diphenhydramine hydrochloride four times daily to 4 subjects, maximum steady-state plasma-diphenhydramine concentrations of 0.10 to 0.27 μg/ml were reported; the maximum steady-state amine concentrations were between 0.17 and 0.37 μg/ml (A. J. Glazko *et al.*, *Clin. Pharmac. Ther.*, 1974, *16*, 1066–1076).

TOXICITY. The estimated minimum lethal dose is 3 g. Toxic effects may be produced by plasma concentrations greater than 1 μg/ml.

In 4 fatalities due to overdosage of diphenhydramine, the following postmortem concentrations were obtained: blood 8 to 31 μg/ml (mean 20), brain 8 and 32 μg/g (2 cases), kidney 13 μg/g (1 case), liver 23 to 47 μg/g (mean 34), urine 40 and 6.4 μg/ml (2 cases) (R. C. Backer *et al.*, *J. analyt. Toxicol.*, 1977, *1*, 227–228; R. C. Baselt and R. H. Cravey, *ibid.*, 81–103; C. Peclet *et al.*, *Bull. int. Ass. forens. Toxicol.*, 1981, *16*(1), 26–27). In 2 fatalities attributed to diphenhydramine, the following postmortem tissue concentrations were reported (μg/ml or μg/g):

	Diphen-hydramine	Diphenylmethoxy-acetic acid
Blood	19.7, 6.9	3.0, 15.3
Heart blood	50, 14.7	3.6, 19
Kidney	114, —	—, —
Liver	260, —	—, —
Lung	460, —	—, —
Urine	34.9, 376	0.3, 20.4

In the first case death occurred within 3 hours whereas the second subject survived for 12 hours after ingestion (R. Aderjan *et al.*, *Z. Rechtsmed.*, 1982, *88*, 263–270).

HALF-LIFE. Plasma half-life, about 9 hours.

VOLUME OF DISTRIBUTION. About 8 litres/kg.

CLEARANCE. Plasma clearance, about 10 ml/min/kg.

DISTRIBUTION IN BLOOD. Plasma: whole blood ratio, about 1.3.

SALIVA. Plasma: saliva ratio, about 3.

PROTEIN BINDING. In plasma, 80 to 98%.

Dose. 75 to 200 mg of diphenhydramine hydrochloride daily.

Diphenidol   *Anti-emetic*

Synonym. Difenidol
1,1-Diphenyl-4-piperidinobutan-1-ol
$C_{21}H_{27}NO = 309.5$
CAS—972-02-1

M.p. 103° to 104°.

Diphenidol Hydrochloride
Proprietary Names. Vontril; Vontrol.
$C_{21}H_{27}NO,HCl = 345.9$
CAS—3254-89-5
A white crystalline powder. M.p. 214° to 221°, with decomposition. Sparingly **soluble** in water and chloroform; soluble in ethanol; practically insoluble in ether.

Colour Tests. Liebermann's Test—brown; Mandelin's Test—yellow; Marquis Test—yellow; Sulphuric Acid—orange.

Thin-layer Chromatography. *System TA*—Rf 61; *system TB*—Rf 56; *system TC*—Rf 45. (*Acidified iodoplatinate solution*, positive.)

Gas Chromatography. *System GA*—RI 2384.

Ultraviolet Spectrum. Aqueous acid—252 nm, 258 nm.

Infra-red Spectrum. Principal peaks at wavenumbers 697, 701, 749, 773, 1123, 1219 (KBr disk).

Mass Spectrum. Principal peaks at m/z 98, 99, 105, 77, 55, 41, 127, 111.

Disposition in the Body. Absorbed from the gastro-intestinal tract; peak blood concentrations are attained in 1.5 to 3 hours. It is excreted in the urine and faeces.

Dose. The equivalent of 25 to 50 mg of diphenidol every 4 hours; maximum of 300 mg daily.

Diphenoxylate   *Narcotic Antidiarrhoeal*

Ethyl 1-(3-cyano-3,3-diphenylpropyl)-4-phenylpiperidine-4-carboxylate
$C_{30}H_{32}N_2O_2 = 452.6$
CAS—915-30-0

Diphenoxylate Hydrochloride
Proprietary Names. It is an ingredient of Diarsed, Lomotil, Reasec, and Retardin.
Preparations of diphenoxylate hydrochloride usually contain subclinical amounts of atropine sulphate in an attempt to prevent abuse by deliberate overdosage.
$C_{30}H_{32}N_2O_2,HCl = 489.1$
CAS—3810-80-8

A white crystalline powder. M.p. 220° to 226°.
Sparingly **soluble** in water; soluble 1 in 50 of ethanol and 1 in 2.5 of chloroform; soluble in methanol; practically insoluble in ether.

Dissociation Constant. pK_a 7.1.

Colour Test. Sodium Picrate—orange.

Thin-layer Chromatography. *System TA*—Rf 74; *system TB*—Rf 42; *system TC*—Rf 81. (*Dragendorff spray*, positive; *acidified iodoplatinate solution*, positive; *Marquis reagent*, orange.)

Gas Chromatography. *System GA*—RI 2443.

High Pressure Liquid Chromatography. *System HA*—diphenoxylate k' 0.2, diphenoxylic acid k' 0.6 (tailing peak).

Ultraviolet Spectrum. Methanol—252 nm, 258 nm ($A_1^1 = 14$ a), 264 nm.

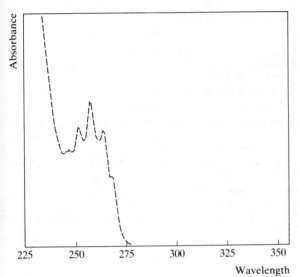

Infra-red Spectrum. Principal peaks at wavenumbers 1728, 697, 1183, 1120, 1215, 1495 (KBr disk).

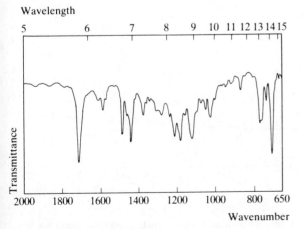

Mass Spectrum. Principal peaks at m/z 246, 42, 247, 91, 103, 165, 115, 56; diphenoxylic acid 218, 42, 219, 91, 165, 155, 193, 115.

Quantification. GAS CHROMATOGRAPHY. In plasma or urine: TCD—S. Abu al Ragheb *et al., Medicine, Sci. Law,* 1982, *22,* 210–214.

GAS CHROMATOGRAPHY–MASS SPECTROMETRY. In plasma: diphenoxylic acid, sensitivity 20 ng/ml—G. C. Ford *et al., Biomed. Mass Spectrom.,* 1976, *3,* 45–47.

Disposition in the Body. Rapidly absorbed after oral administration but it is usually administered together with a small quantity of atropine and this may delay absorption, especially with high doses. It is extensively metabolised by hydrolysis, hydroxylation, and conjugation with glucuronic acid. The major metabolites are diphenoxylic acid (difenoxin), which is active, and hydroxydiphenoxylic acid in both free and conjugated forms. About 14% and 50% of a dose, respectively, is excreted in the urine and faeces in 96 hours; less than 0.1% of a dose is excreted in the urine as unchanged drug in 24 hours.

THERAPEUTIC CONCENTRATION.

After an oral dose of 5 mg, peak plasma concentrations of diphenoxylate of about 0.01 μg/ml were attained in 2 hours and peak concentrations of diphenoxylic acid of about 0.04 μg/ml were attained in the same period (A. Karim *et al., Clin. Pharmac. Ther.,* 1972, *13,* 407–419).

TOXICITY. Diphenoxylate has addiction-producing properties. The estimated minimum lethal dose is 0.2 g although recovery has occurred after the ingestion of 0.75 g.

A postmortem blood concentration of 0.34 μg/ml was reported in a 3½-year-old child who died after ingesting diphenoxylate (S. Abu al Ragheb *et al., Medicine, Sci. Law,* 1982, *22,* 210–214).

HALF-LIFE. Plasma half-life, diphenoxylate about 2.5 hours, diphenoxylic acid about 4 hours.

VOLUME OF DISTRIBUTION. About 4 litres/kg.

Dose. Initially 10 mg of diphenoxylate hydrochloride, followed by 5 mg every 6 hours.

Diphenyl   *Fungistatic*

Synonym. Phenylbenzene
Biphenyl
$C_{12}H_{10} = 154.2$
CAS—92-52-4

A white crystalline powder. M.p. about 69°. B.p. 254° to 255°. Practically **insoluble** in water; soluble in ethanol and ether.

Gas Chromatography. *System GA*—RI 1389.

Infra-red Spectrum. Principal peaks at wavenumbers 740, 710, 1573, 1175, 1018, 918 (KBr disk).

Diphenylpyraline   *Antihistamine*

Synonym. Diphenylpyrilene
4-Benzhydryloxy-1-methylpiperidine
$C_{19}H_{23}NO = 281.4$
CAS—147-20-6

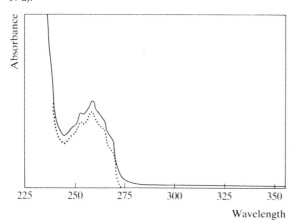

Diphenylpyraline Hydrochloride

Proprietary Names. Allerzine; Anti-Hist; Diafen; Hispril; Histalert; Histryl; Kolton (gel); Lergoban; Lyssipoll. It is an ingredient of Eskornade and Expansyl.

$C_{19}H_{23}NO,HCl = 317.9$

CAS—132-18-3

A white crystalline powder. M.p. 204° to 209°.

Soluble 1 in 1 of water, 1 in 3 of ethanol, and 1 in 2 of chloroform; practically insoluble in ether.

Colour Tests. Liebermann's Test—red-orange; Mandelin's Test—yellow; Marquis Test—yellow.

Thin-layer Chromatography. *System TA*—Rf 46; *system TB*—Rf 37; *system TC*—Rf 28. (*Dragendorff spray*, positive; *FPN reagent*, pink; *acidified iodoplatinate solution*, positive; *Marquis reagent*, brown; *ninhydrin spray*, positive.)

Gas Chromatography. *System GA*—RI 2099; *system GB*—RI 2136; *system GC*—RI 2447; *system GF*—RI 2405.

High Pressure Liquid Chromatography. *System HA*—k' 3.3 (tailing peak).

Ultraviolet Spectrum. Aqueous acid—253 nm, 258 nm ($A_1^1 = 17$ a).

Infra-red Spectrum. Principal peaks at wavenumbers 1070, 709, 1050, 696, 765, 1101 (diphenylpyraline hydrochloride, KCl disk).

Mass Spectrum. Principal peaks at m/z 99, 114, 98, 167, 70, 165, 57, 43.

Quantification. GAS CHROMATOGRAPHY. In urine: FID— G. Graham and A. G. Bolt, *J. Pharmacokinet. Biopharm.*, 1974, 2, 191–195.

Disposition in the Body. Absorbed after oral administration. Less than 10% of a dose is excreted in the urine as unchanged drug. Possible metabolites include the *N*-oxide and *N*-desmethyldiphenylpyraline.

HALF-LIFE. Derived from urinary excretion data, 24 to 40 hours.

Dose. 10 to 20 mg of diphenylpyraline hydrochloride daily.

Dipipanone   *Narcotic Analgesic*

Synonyms. Phenylpiperone; Piperidyl Methadone; Piperidyl-amidone.

(±)-4,4-Diphenyl-6-piperidinoheptan-3-one

$C_{24}H_{31}NO = 349.5$

CAS—467-83-4

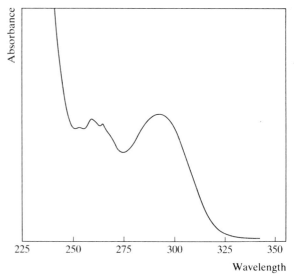

Dipipanone Hydrochloride

Proprietary Names. It is an ingredient of Diconal and Wellconal.

$C_{24}H_{31}NO,HCl,H_2O = 404.0$

A white crystalline powder. M.p. 124° to 127°.

Soluble 1 in 40 of water, 1 in 1.5 of ethanol, and 1 in 6 of acetone; practically insoluble in ether.

Dissociation Constant. pK_a 8.5 (25°).

Colour Test. Mandelin's Test—green → blue.

Thin-layer Chromatography. *System TA*—Rf 66; *system TB*—Rf 66; *system TC*—Rf 33. (*Dragendorff spray*, positive; *acidified iodoplatinate solution*, positive.)

Gas Chromatography. *System GA*—RI 2474; *system GC*—RI 2894; *system GF*—RI 2710.

High Pressure Liquid Chromatography. *System HA*—k' 2.2; *system HC*—k' 1.61.

Ultraviolet Spectrum. Aqueous acid—259 nm, 265 nm, 293 nm ($A_1^1 = 15.6$ a).

Infra-red Spectrum. Principal peaks at wavenumbers 1708, 698, 1491, 1110, 1092, 1030 (KBr disk).

Mass Spectrum. Principal peaks at m/z 112, 264, 113, 91, 179, 110, 178, 115.

Wavelength

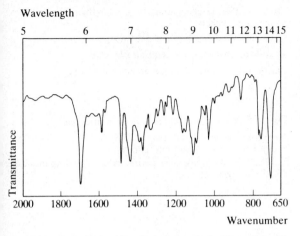

Transmittance

| | | | | | | | | |
| 2000 | 1800 | 1600 | 1400 | 1200 | 1000 | 800 | 650 |

Wavenumber

Disposition in the Body. Absorbed after oral administration with rapid onset of action. It is excreted in the urine and faeces. Prolonged use of dipipanone may produce dependence of the morphine type.

TOXICITY. The estimated minimum lethal dose is 0.1 g.

In two fatalities following intravenous injection of Diconal® (dipipanone with cyclizine), the following postmortem tissue concentrations (µg/ml or µg/g) were reported:

	Cyclizine	Dipipanone
Blood	2.0, 0.5	6.2, 0.5
Bile	20, —	—, —
Liver	3.0, —	5.2, —
Urine	0.5, 9.5	—, 18.5

In 34 addicts, urinary concentrations of free dipipanone ranged from 0 to 5.2 µg/ml (mean 1.6) (T. M. T. Sheehan *et al.*, The Abuse of Preparations Containing Dipipanone and Cyclizine, in *Forensic Toxicology—Proceedings of the European Meeting of the International Association of Forensic Toxicologists*, J. S. Oliver (Ed.), London, Croom Helm, 1979).

Dose. 10 to 30 mg of dipipanone hydrochloride every 6 hours.

Diprenorphine   *Narcotic Antagonist (Veterinary)*

(6*R*,7*R*,14*S*)-17-Cyclopropylmethyl-7,8-dihydro-7-(1-hydroxy-1-methylethyl)-6-*O*-methyl-6,14-ethano-17-normorphine
$C_{26}H_{35}NO_4 = 425.6$
CAS—14357-78-9

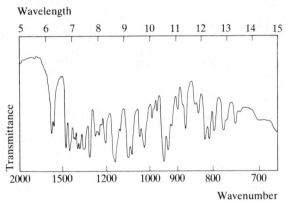

A white microcrystalline powder. M.p. 190° to 192°.

Diprenorphine Hydrochloride

Proprietary Name. Revivon
$C_{26}H_{35}NO_4,HCl = 462.0$
CAS—16808-86-9
A white crystalline powder.
Soluble 1 in 30 of water, 1 in 160 of ethanol, and 1 in 2500 of chloroform; practically insoluble in ether.

Colour Tests. Liebermann's Test—black; Mandelin's Test—grey; Marquis Test—grey-violet.

Thin-layer Chromatography. *System TA*—Rf 70. (*Acidified iodoplatinate solution*, positive.)

High Pressure Liquid Chromatography. *System HA*—k' 0.6.

Ultraviolet Spectrum. Aqueous acid—230 nm ($A_1^1 = 158$ b), 286 nm ($A_1^1 = 36$ a); aqueous alkali—246 nm ($A_1^1 = 184$ b), 299 nm ($A_1^1 = 58$ a).

Infra-red Spectrum. Principal peaks at wavenumbers 1160, 947, 1311, 1092, 1078, 934 (KBr disk).

Wavelength

Transmittance

| | | | | | | |
| 2000 | 1500 | 1200 | 1000 | 900 | 800 | 700 |

Wavenumber

Diprophylline   *Xanthine Bronchodilator*

Synonyms. Dihydroxypropyltheophyllinum; Dyphylline; Glyphyllinum; Hyphylline.

Proprietary Names. Aerophylline; Airet; Asthmolysin; Dilin; Dilor; Droxine; Dyflex; Emfabid; Lufyllin; Neothylline; Neutraphylline; Protophylline; Silbephylline; Zäpfchen. It is an ingredient of Noradran and Tedral Expect.

7-(2,3-Dihydroxypropyl)theophylline
$C_{10}H_{14}N_4O_4 = 254.2$
CAS—479-18-5

A white crystalline powder. M.p. 160° to 165°.

Soluble 1 in 3 of water and 1 in 50 of ethanol; slightly soluble in chloroform; practically insoluble in ether.

Colour Test. Amalic Acid Test—yellow/violet.

Thin-layer Chromatography. *System TA*—Rf 48; *system TB*—Rf 00; *system TC*—Rf 12. (*Acidified potassium permanganate solution*, positive.)

Ultraviolet Spectrum. Aqueous acid—273 nm ($A_1^1 = 380$ a). No alkaline shift. (See below)

Infra-red Spectrum. Principal peaks at wavenumbers 1660, 1700, 1039, 747, 1562, 1234 (KBr disk). (See below)

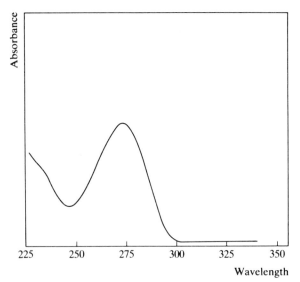

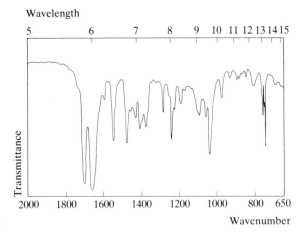

Mass Spectrum. Principal peaks at *m/z* 180, 223, 194, 254, 109, 95, 193, 166.

Quantification. GAS CHROMATOGRAPHY. In serum or saliva: FID—Z. K. Shihabi and R. P. Dave, *Clin. Chem.*, 1977, *23*, 942–943.

HIGH PRESSURE LIQUID CHROMATOGRAPHY. In plasma, saliva or urine: limit of detection 25 ng/ml for plasma and 50 ng/ml for saliva—L. Gisclon *et al.*, *Res. Commun. chem. Path. Pharmac.*, 1979, *23*, 523–531. In serum: sensitivity 1 µg/ml, UV detection—N. Paterson, *J. Chromat.*, 1982, *232*; *Biomed. Appl.*, *21*, 450–455.

Disposition in the Body. Rapidly and almost completely absorbed after oral administration; bioavailability about 90%. About 83% of a dose is excreted in the urine as unchanged drug in 24 hours; less than 1% of a dose is eliminated in the faeces.

THERAPEUTIC CONCENTRATION. In plasma, usually in the range 10 to 20 µg/ml.

After a single oral dose of 1.2 g to 6 subjects, peak plasma concentrations of 18 to 29 µg/ml (mean 22) were attained in about 0.5 hour and peak saliva concentrations of 7 to 17 µg/ml (mean 12) were reported at 0.7 hour (L. G. Gisclon *et al.*, *Am. J. hosp. Pharm.*, 1979, *36*, 1179–1184).

TOXICITY. Plasma concentrations greater than 20 µg/ml may produce toxic effects.

HALF-LIFE. Plasma half-life, about 2 hours.

VOLUME OF DISTRIBUTION. About 0.8 litre/kg.

CLEARANCE. Plasma clearance, about 5 ml/min/kg.

Dose. 0.6 to 1.6 g daily.

Dipyridamole   *Antithrombotic/Anti-anginal Vasodilator*

Proprietary Names. Coronarine; Dipyrida; Functiocardon; Natyl; Péridamol; Persantin(e); Prandiol.
2,2′,2″,2‴ - [(4,8 - Dipiperidinopyrimido[5,4 - *d*]pyrimido - 2,6 - diyl)dinitrilo]tetraethanol
$C_{24}H_{40}N_8O_4 = 504.6$
CAS—58-32-2

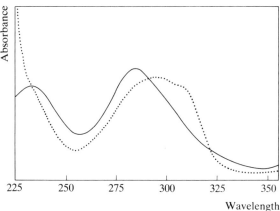

An intensely yellow crystalline powder. Solutions have a yellowish-blue fluorescence. M.p. 164° to 167°.
Practically **insoluble** in water; very soluble in ethanol; soluble in chloroform, methanol, and dilute acids; practically insoluble in ether.

Dissociation Constant. pK$_a$ 6.4.

Colour Tests. Mandelin's Test—violet; Marquis Test—orange.

Thin-layer Chromatography. *System TA*—Rf 68; *system TB*—Rf 00; *system TC*—Rf 37. (*Acidified iodoplatinate solution*, positive.)

Gas Chromatography. *System GA*—RI 1640.

High Pressure Liquid Chromatography. *System HA*—k′ 0.2.

Ultraviolet Spectrum. Acid methanol—230 nm, 285 nm (A$_1^1$ = 650 a); aqueous alkali—295 nm.

Infra-red Spectrum. Principal peaks at wavenumbers 1526, 1214, 1010, 1076, 1041, 1251 (KBr disk).

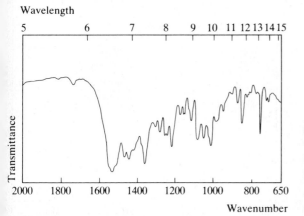

Wavelength

Mass Spectrum. Principal peaks at m/z 504, 473, 429, 505, 221, 474, 84, 430.

Quantification. SPECTROFLUORIMETRY. In serum—J. M. Steyn, *J. Chromat.*, 1979, *164*; Biomed. Appl., 6, 487–494.

HIGH PRESSURE LIQUID CHROMATOGRAPHY. In plasma or whole blood: fluorescence detection—K. M. Wolfram and T. D. Bjornsson, *J. Chromat.*, 1980, *183*; Biomed. Appl., 9, 57–64. In plasma: sensitivity 2 ng/ml, UV detection—J. Rosenfeld *et al.*, *J. Chromat.*, 1982, *231*; Biomed. Appl., 20, 216–221.

Disposition in the Body. Readily absorbed after oral administration. Eliminated mainly in the faeces; excretion may be delayed due to enterohepatic circulation. Small amounts are excreted in the urine as the glucuronide conjugate.

THERAPEUTIC CONCENTRATION.

After a single oral dose of 100 mg given to 6 subjects, peak serum concentrations of about 2 μg/ml were attained in 1 hour (F. Nielsen-Kudsk and A. K. Pederson, *Acta pharmac. tox.*, 1979, *44*, 391–399).

Following oral administration of 50 mg three times a day to 10 subjects, maximum steady-state plasma concentrations of 0.4 to 2.6 μg/ml (mean 1.4) were reported; trough concentrations were 0.1 to 1.5 μg/ml (mean 0.7). In 10 subjects given 75 mg twice daily, the corresponding maximum and minimum steady-state concentrations were 0.5 to 4 μg/ml (mean 1.7) and 0.1 to 2.6 μg/ml (mean 0.9) (C. Mahony *et al.*, *J. clin. Pharmac.*, 1983, *23*, 123–126).

HALF-LIFE. Plasma half-life, about 12 hours.

VOLUME OF DISTRIBUTION. About 2.5 litres/kg.

CLEARANCE. Plasma clearance, about 2 ml/min/kg.

PROTEIN BINDING. In plasma, more than 90%.

Dose. 300 to 600 mg daily (antithrombotic); 150 mg daily (anti-anginal).

Dipyrone   *Analgesic*

Synonyms. Aminopyrine-sulphonate Sodium; Analginum; Metamizol; Methampyrone; Natrium Novaminsulfonicum; Noramidazophenum; Noraminophenazonum; Novamidazofen; Sodium Noramidopyrine Methanesulphonate; Sulpyrine. *Proprietary Names.* Novalgin(e); Novaminsulfon. It is an ingredient of Isaverin (vet.).

Sodium *N*-(2,3-dimethyl-5-oxo-1-phenyl-3-pyrazolin-4-yl)-*N*-methylaminomethanesulphonate monohydrate
$C_{13}H_{16}N_3NaO_4S,H_2O = 351.4$
CAS—68-89-3 (anhydrous); *5907-38-0* (monohydrate)

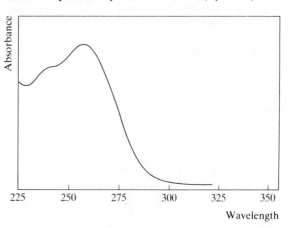

A white or yellowish-white crystalline powder. M.p. 172°.
Soluble 1 in 1.5 of water and 1 in 30 of ethanol; very slightly soluble in chloroform; practically insoluble in ether.

Colour Tests. Ferric Chloride—violet; Folin–Ciocalteu Reagent—blue; Liebermann's Test (100°)—blue; Mandelin's Test—brown; Nitrous Acid—transient blue.

Thin-layer Chromatography. *System TA*—Rf 84; *system TB*—Rf 00; *system TC*—Rf 01. (*Acidified iodoplatinate solution*, white.)

Gas Chromatography. *System GA*—RI 1983.

High Pressure Liquid Chromatography. *System HD*—k' 0.1; *system HW*—k' 0.45.

Ultraviolet Spectrum. Aqueous acid—258 nm $(A_1^1 = 266\ a)$.

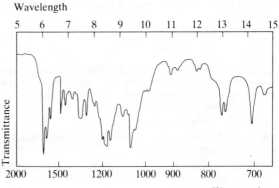

Infra-red Spectrum. Principal peaks at wavenumbers 1672, 1064, 1179, 1163, 1208, 1639 (KBr disk).

Wavelength

Mass Spectrum. Principal peaks at m/z 56, 42, 83, 57, 77, 51, 97, 54.

Quantification. HIGH PRESSURE LIQUID CHROMATOGRAPHY. In plasma or urine: detection limits 1 μg/ml for dipyrone and 250 ng/ml for 4-methylaminophenazone, UV detection—G. Asmardi and F. Jamali, *J. Chromat.*, 1983, *277*; *Biomed. Appl.*, *28*, 183–189.

Disposition in the Body. Rapidly absorbed after oral administration and extensively metabolised. The major metabolites are 4-methylaminophenazone, 4-aminophenazone, 4-formylaminophenazone, and 4-acetylaminophenazone. About 70% of a dose is excreted in the urine in 24 hours as metabolites.

THERAPEUTIC CONCENTRATION.

Following a single oral dose of 1 g given to 12 slow acetylators and 11 rapid acetylators (determined with reference to dapsone), the following mean peak plasma concentrations (μg/ml, time in hours) were reported:

	Slow acetylators	Rapid acetylators
4-Acetylaminophenazone	1.6 (16.1)	4.4 (10.0)
4-Aminophenazone	2.7 (6.7)	1.6 (3.2)
4-Formylaminophenazone	1.8 (7.7)	2.5 (6.6)
4-Methylaminophenazone	10.0 (1.6)	11.0 (1.2)

(M. Levy *et al., Eur. J. clin. Pharmac.*, 1984, *27*, 453–458).

TOXICITY. The estimated minimum lethal dose is 5 g, but fatalities from acute poisoning are rare.

HALF-LIFE. Plasma half-life, 4-acetylaminophenazone about 10.6 hours, 4-aminophenazone about 5 hours, 4-formylaminophenazone about 10 hours, and 4-methylaminophenazone about 3.3 hours.

Dose. 0.5 to 1 g up to 3 times daily.

Diquat   *Herbicide*

Synonym. Deiquat
1,1'-Ethylene-2,2'-bipyridyldiylium ion
$C_{12}H_{12}N_2 = 184.2$
CAS—2764-72-9

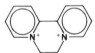

Diquat Dibromide

Proprietary Names. Aquacide; Reglone. It is an ingredient of Pathclear and Weedol.
$C_{12}H_{12}Br_2N_2 = 344.0$
CAS—85-00-7
Yellow crystals. M.p. about 335°.
Soluble in water.
Note. Unless otherwise stated, the analytical information given below refers to diquat dibromide. For information on the monoene and diene reduction products for GC–MS analysis, see under Quaternary Ammonium Herbicides, p. 80.

Colour Test. Sodium Dithionite—green.

Thin-layer Chromatography. *System TA*—Rf 00. (*Acidified iodoplatinate solution*, positive.)

Gas Chromatography. *System GK*—monoene reduction product retention time 0.40, diene reduction product retention time 0.49, both relative to caffeine.

Ultraviolet Spectrum. Aqueous acid—310 nm ($A_1^1 = 518$ b).

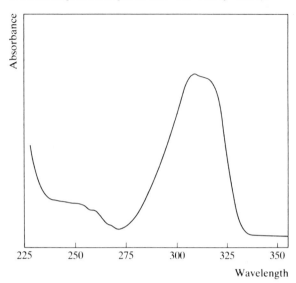

Infra-red Spectrum. Principal peaks at wavenumbers 1522, 1498, 1140, 1166, 1097, 1632 (KBr disk).

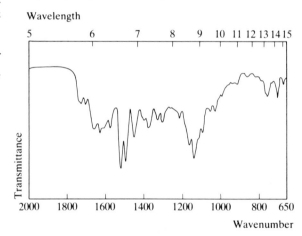

Mass Spectrum. Principal peaks at m/z 83, 108, 96, 54, 111, 192, 84, 55 (monoene reduction product); 54, 108, 81, 190, 111, 135, 83, 80 (diene reduction product).

Quantification. HIGH PRESSURE LIQUID CHROMATOGRAPHY. In urine: diquat and paraquat, detection limit <1 μg/ml, UV detection—R. Gill *et al., J. Chromat.*, 1983, *255*, 483–490.

Disposition in the Body. Absorbed from the gastro-intestinal tract; slightly absorbed through the skin.

TOXICITY. Diquat produces similar adverse effects to those of paraquat except that it does not seem to cause the progressive fibrosis in the lungs. A fatality after ingestion of about 2 g has been reported and the ingestion of about 20 to 50 ml of a 20% concentrate has caused death within 2 to 7 days. The maximum permissible atmospheric concentration is 0.5 mg/m³ (as the dibromide) and the maximum acceptable daily intake (as the dichloride) is 5 μg/kg.

A young man drank several mouthfuls of a 20% concentrate of diquat and died 7 days later. The following postmortem concentrations were reported: blood 0.6 µg/ml, heart 0.11 µg/g, kidney 1.19 µg/g, liver 0.33 µg/g, lung 0.56 µg/g, and spleen 1.04 µg/g (H. Schönborn *et al.*, *Arch. Tox.*, 1971, *27*, 204–216).

A 44-year-old woman ingested an unknown quantity of diquat and died about 16 hours after being found. The following postmortem concentrations were reported: kidney 11.6 µg/g and liver 5.1 µg/g (L. K. Pannell and B. M. Thomson, *Bull. int. Ass. forens. Toxicol.*, 1981, *16*(2), 24–25).

Disopyramide

Anti-arrhythmic

Proprietary Names. Durbis (capsules); Rythmodan (capsules).

4-Di-isopropylamino-2-phenyl-2-(2-pyridyl)butyramide
$C_{21}H_{29}N_{3}O = 339.5$
CAS—3737-09-5

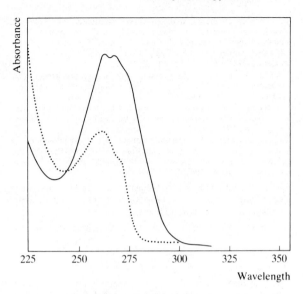

A white powder. M.p. about 95°.
Soluble 1 in 200 of water, 1 in 10 of ethanol, 1 in 5 of chloroform, and 1 in 5 of ether.

Disopyramide Phosphate

Proprietary Names. Dirythmin; Durbis (injection); Norpace; Rythmodan (injection and tablets); Rythmodul.
$C_{21}H_{29}N_{3}O,H_{3}PO_{4} = 437.5$
CAS—22059-60-5
A white powder. M.p. about 205°, with decomposition.
Soluble 1 in 20 of water and 1 in 50 of ethanol; practically insoluble in chloroform and ether.

Dissociation Constant. pK_a 8.4.

Thin-layer Chromatography. *System TA*—Rf 45; *system TB*—Rf 07; *system TC*—Rf 08.

Gas Chromatography. *System GA*—RI 2495; *system GF*—RI 2910.

High Pressure Liquid Chromatography. *System HA*—disopyramide k′ 2.4, *N*-monodesisopropyldisopyramide k′ 1.8.

Ultraviolet Spectrum. Aqueous acid—263 nm, 269 nm ($A_1^1 = 199$ a); aqueous alkali—261 nm.

Infra-red Spectrum. Principal peaks at wavenumbers 1664, 1585, 697, 1163, 1562, 760 (KBr disk).

Mass Spectrum. Principal peaks at *m/z* 195, 212, 114, 30, 194, 72, 44, 43 (no peaks above 240).

Quantification. GAS CHROMATOGRAPHY. In plasma: sensitivity 100 ng/ml, FID—E. N. Foster and P. R. Reid, *J. Chromat.*, 1979, *178*, 571–574. In plasma, urine or postmortem tissues: FID—R. W. Michalek *et al.*, *J. analyt. Toxicol.*, 1982, *6*, 255–257. In serum: sensitivity 100 ng/ml for disopyramide and the desalkyl metabolite, AFID—J. E. Bredesen, *Clin. Chem.*, 1980, *26*, 638–640.

HIGH PRESSURE LIQUID CHROMATOGRAPHY. In plasma or urine: disopyramide and the desalkyl metabolite, detection limit 50 ng/ml, UV detection—C. Charette *et al.*, *J. Chromat.*, 1983, *274*; *Biomed. Appl.*, *25*, 219–230.

REVIEW. For a comparison of GC, HPLC and GC–MS methods, see J. W. Vasiliades *et al.*, *Clin. Chem.*, 1979, *25*, 1900–1904.

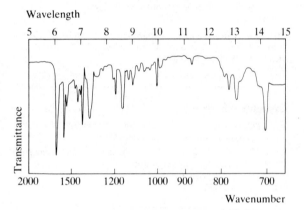

Disposition in the Body. Rapidly and almost completely absorbed after oral administration and widely distributed throughout the body; bioavailability about 80%. The major metabolite, *N*-monodesisopropyldisopyramide, is about one half as active as disopyramide. Up to about 50 to 60% of a dose is excreted in the urine in 5 days as unchanged drug, with about 20 to 30% as the desalkyl metabolite; about 10 to 15% of a dose is eliminated in the faeces.

THERAPEUTIC CONCENTRATION. In plasma, usually in the range 2 to 5 µg/ml.

After a single oral dose of 100 mg of disopyramide phosphate to 6 subjects, peak plasma concentrations of 1.8 to 3.6 µg/ml (mean 2.7) were attained in about 2 hours (R. E. Ranney *et al.*, *Archs int. Pharmacodyn. Thér.*, 1971, *191*, 162–188).

Following oral daily doses averaging 6 mg/kg to 63 subjects, mean steady-state plasma concentrations of 3.3 µg/ml for disopyramide and 0.99 µg/ml for the desalkyl metabolite were reported; plasma concentrations were higher in 17 subjects with renal dysfunction (mean 4.3), but lower in subjects concurrently taking enzyme-inducing drugs (M. Aitio, *Br. J. clin. Pharmac.*, 1981, *11*, 369–376).

TOXICITY. Toxic effects are usually associated with plasma concentrations greater than about 8 µg/ml.

In a fatality attributed to disopyramide overdosage, the following postmortem concentrations were reported for disopyramide and the desalkyl metabolite, respectively: blood 26.6 and 5.9 μg/ml, bile 349 and 145 μg/ml, kidney 147 and 6.7 μg/g, liver 35.8 and 11.2 μg/g (W. H. Anderson *et al.*, *J. forens. Sci.*, 1980, *25*, 33–39).

In 3 fatalities due to disopyramide overdose, postmortem blood concentrations of 8.5, 34, and 114 μg/ml were reported; the dose was estimated to be about 6 to 7 g in 2 of the cases. In a further 2 fatalities, antemortem plasma concentrations, determined 9 hours and 3 hours after ingestion, respectively, were 4.3 and 35 μg/ml (A. M. Hayler *et al.*, *Lancet*, 1978, *1*, 968–969).

In a fatality due to the ingestion of about 15 g of disopyramide, the following postmortem tissue concentrations were reported: blood 57 μg/ml, brain 29 μg/g, liver 115 μg/g, urine 1500 μg/ml (R. W. Michalek *et al.*, *J. analyt. Toxicol.*, 1982, *6*, 255–257).

HALF-LIFE. Plasma half-life, disopyramide 3 to 11 hours (dose-dependent), increased in subjects with renal impairment; desalkyl metabolite about 13 hours.

VOLUME OF DISTRIBUTION. About 0.7 litre/kg (dose-dependent); unbound drug about 2 litres/kg.

CLEARANCE. Plasma clearance, about 0.5 to 2 ml/min/kg (dose-dependent); unbound drug about 6 ml/min/kg.

PROTEIN BINDING. In plasma, disopyramide about 35 to 80% (concentration-dependent), desalkyl metabolite about 30 to 70% (concentration-dependent); considerable intersubject variation occurs.

NOTE. For reviews of disopyramide see R. C. Heel *et al.*, *Drugs*, 1978, *15*, 331–368, and A. Karim *et al.*, *J. Pharmacokinet. Biopharm.*, 1982, *10*, 465–494.

Dose. 300 to 800 mg daily.

Distigmine Bromide   *Anticholinesterase*

Synonyms. Bispyridostigmine Bromide; Hexamarium Bromide.
Proprietary Name. Ubretid
1,1' - Dimethyl - 3,3' - [NN' - hexamethylenebis(methyl-carbamoyloxy)]dipyridinium dibromide
$C_{22}H_{32}Br_2N_4O_4 = 576.3$
CAS—15876-67-2

A crystalline powder. Decomposes at 149°.
Freely **soluble** in water.

Thin-layer Chromatography. *System TA*—Rf 00. (*Acidified iodoplatinate solution*, positive.)

Ultraviolet Spectrum. Aqueous acid—270 nm ($A_1^1 = 160$ a).

Infra-red Spectrum. Principal peaks at wavenumbers 1735, 1255, 1170, 1507, 1135, 1295 (KBr disk).

Disposition in the Body. Poorly absorbed after oral administration. Less than 5% of an oral dose is excreted in the urine in 24 hours, compared to 50% of an intramuscular dose.

Dose. 5 to 20 mg daily, by mouth.

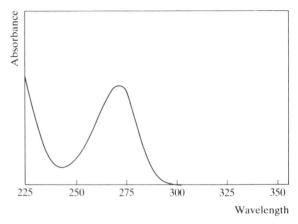

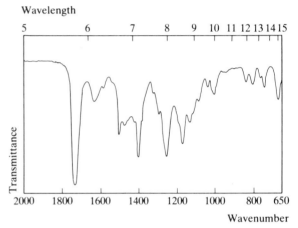

Disulfiram   *Alcohol Deterrent*

Synonyms. Éthyldithiourame; TTD.
Proprietary Names. Antabus(e); Espéral; Ro-Sulfiram-500.
Tetraethylthiuram disulphide
$C_{10}H_{20}N_2S_4 = 296.5$
CAS—97-77-8

$$(C_2H_5)_2N \cdot \overset{\overset{S}{\|}}{C} \cdot S \cdot S \cdot \overset{\overset{S}{\|}}{C} \cdot N(C_2H_5)_2$$

A white powder. M.p. 69° to 73°.
Practically **insoluble** in water; soluble 1 in 65 of ethanol, 1 in 2 of chloroform, and 1 in 20 of ether; soluble in acetone.

Colour Tests. Palladium Chloride—orange.
Dissolve 50 mg in 5 ml of ethanol and add 1 ml of *potassium cyanide solution*—yellow → green → blue-green.

Thin-layer Chromatography. *System TA*—Rf 71; *system TB*—Rf 38; *system TC*—Rf 78.

Gas Chromatography. *System GA*—RI 2141.

Infra-red Spectrum. Principal peaks at wavenumbers 1267, 1193, 1492, 1147, 966, 913 (Nujol mull).

Mass Spectrum. Principal peaks at *m/z* 116, 88, 29, 44, 60, 148, 56, 27.

Wavelength

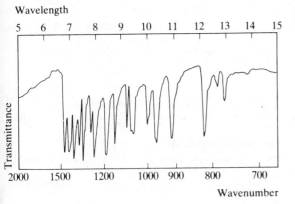

Transmittance

Wavenumber

Plasma half-life, disulfiram about 7 hours, diethyl-dithiocarbamic acid about 15 hours, carbon disulphide about 9 hours.

NOTE. For a review of disulfiram see J. F. Brien *et al.*, *Drug Met. Rev.*, 1983, *14*, 113–126.

Dose. 800 mg on the first day, reducing to a maintenance dose of 100 to 200 mg daily.

Disulphamide   *Diuretic*

Synonym. Disulfamide
Proprietary Names. Diluen; Toluidrin.
5-Chlorotoluene-2,4-disulphonamide
$C_7H_9ClN_2O_4S_2 = 284.7$
CAS—671-88-5

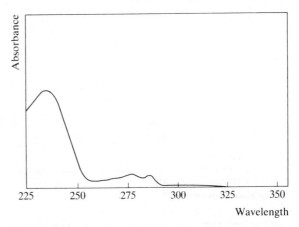

A white or creamy-white crystalline powder. M.p. about 260°.
Soluble 1 in 500 of cold water, 1 in 50 of boiling water, 1 in 50 of ethanol, and 1 in 1000 of ether; slightly soluble in chloroform.

Ultraviolet Spectrum. Aqueous acid—235 nm ($A_1^1 = 336$ b), 276 nm, 285 nm.

Absorbance

Wavelength

Infra-red Spectrum. Principal peaks at wavenumbers 1320, 1172, 1552, 965, 675, 1550 (KBr disk).

Dose. Disulphamide has been given in doses of 100 to 200 mg daily.

Quantification. GAS CHROMATOGRAPHY. In blood: disulfiram and metabolites, sensitivity 10 ng/ml using head-space analysis and FPD—A. M. Sauter and J. P. von Wartburg, *J. Chromat.*, 1977, *133*, 167–172.

HIGH PRESSURE LIQUID CHROMATOGRAPHY. In plasma or urine: disulfiram and metabolites, sensitivity 200 ng/ml, UV detection—J. C. Jensen and M. D. Faiman, *J. Chromat.*, 1980, *181*; *Biomed. Appl.*, 7, 407–416. In plasma: disulfiram and dithiocarbamate metabolites, sensitivity 50 ng/ml, UV detection—P. D. Masso and P. A. Kramer, *J. Chromat.*, 1981, *224*; *Biomed. Appl.*, 13, 457–464.

Disposition in the Body. Disulfiram produces hypersensitivity to alcohol by inhibiting the oxidation of acetaldehyde, the primary metabolite of alcohol; the concentrations of acetaldehyde in the blood and expired air are increased by 5 to 10 times. Disulfiram is incompletely absorbed after oral administration; the maximum effect usually occurs about 12 hours after ingestion, possibly because it is highly lipid soluble and is likely to be initially localised in fat. The metabolites include diethyldithiocarbamic acid, methyl diethyldithiocarbamate, diethylamine, carbon disulphide and inorganic sulphate; glucuronide conjugation may occur. Up to about 20% of a dose is eliminated unchanged in the faeces, up to 50% of a dose may be excreted from the lungs as carbon disulphide, and the remainder is slowly excreted as metabolites in the urine; about 20% of a dose is still present in the body up to 7 days after ingestion.

THERAPEUTIC CONCENTRATION.
Following a single oral dose of 250 mg to 15 subjects, mean peak plasma concentrations of 0.38 μg/ml of disulfiram, 0.77 μg/ml of diethyldithiocarbamic acid, 0.30 μg/ml of methyl diethyldithiocarbamate, and 1.7 μg/ml of diethylamine were attained in about 9 hours; a mean peak plasma concentration of 22 μg/ml of carbon disulphide was reported at 6 hours; there was considerable intersubject variability in the plasma concentrations (M. D. Faiman *et al.*, *Clin. Pharmac. Ther.*, 1984, *36*, 520–526).

TOXICITY. Severe toxic reactions may occur after administration of disulfiram if the blood concentration of acetaldehyde is greater than 5 μg/ml; with very high concentrations of alcohol in the blood the administration of as little as 0.5 to 1 g of disulfiram has proved fatal in some cases. Fatalities due to disulfiram-induced hepatitis have been reported and there have also been reports of severe phenytoin intoxication after simultaneous administration.

In a fatality due to ingestion of disulfiram and alcohol, postmortem blood concentrations of 8 μg/ml of sodium diethyldithiocarbamate and 9600 μg/ml of ethanol were reported (F. Martens and A. Heyndrickx, *Bull. int. Ass. forens. Toxicol.*, 1975, *11*(2), 18–19).

Dithranol   *Dermatological Agent*

Synonyms. Anthralin; Dioxyanthranol.
Proprietary Names. Anthra-Derm; Antraderm; Dithrocream; Lasan. It is an ingredient of Dithrolan, Psoradrate, Psorin, and Stie-Lasan.

1,8-Dihydroxy-9-anthrone
$C_{14}H_{10}O_3 = 226.2$
CAS—1143-38-0

A yellow to yellowish-brown crystalline powder. M.p. 175° to 181°.

Practically **insoluble** in water; slightly soluble in ethanol and ether; soluble in acetone and chloroform.

Caution. Dithranol is a powerful irritant and should be kept away from the eyes and tender parts of the skin.

Dithranol Triacetate

Synonym. Dithranol Acetate
Proprietary Name. Exolan (cream)
$C_{20}H_{16}O_6 = 352.3$
CAS—16203-97-7

Ultraviolet Spectrum. Aqueous alkali—276 nm ($A_1^1 = 490$ b); methanol—256 nm ($A_1^1 = 467$ b), 288 nm ($A_1^1 = 358$ b), 360 nm ($A_1^1 = 418$ b).

Infra-red Spectrum. Principal peaks at wavenumbers 1598, 1278, 1615, 1222, 1168, 1635 (KCl disk).

Use. Topically in concentrations of 0.05 to 1%.

Diuron   *Herbicide*

Proprietary Names. Karmex. It is an ingredient of Dexuron and Krovar.

1-(3,4-Dichlorophenyl)-3,3-dimethylurea
$C_9H_{10}Cl_2N_2O = 233.1$
CAS—330-54-1

Crystals. M.p. 158° to 159°.

Practically **insoluble** in water; soluble in acetone; sparingly soluble in hydrocarbon solvents.

Colour Tests. Liebermann's Test—orange; Marquis Test—pink-orange.

Gas Chromatography. Two decomposition products are formed on-column. *System GA*—3,4-dichloroaniline RI 1323; *system GK*—3,4-dichloroaniline retention time 0.36 and 3,4-dichlorophenyl isocyanate retention time 0.13, both relative to caffeine.

Ultraviolet Spectrum. Ethanol—250 nm ($A_1^1 = 1124$ b), 287 nm.

Mass Spectrum. Principal peaks at m/z 72, 44, 73, 42, 232, 187, 124, 45.

Dixyrazine   *Tranquilliser*

Proprietary Name. Esucos
2-(2-{4-[2-Methyl-3-(phenothiazin-10-yl)propyl]piperazin-1-yl}ethoxy)ethanol
$C_{24}H_{33}N_3O_2S = 427.6$
CAS—2470-73-7

A white to slightly greyish or yellowish powder.

Very slightly **soluble** in water; soluble in ethanol, chloroform, and ether.

Dissociation Constant. pK_a 7.8 (25°).

Ultraviolet Spectrum. Methanol—255 nm ($A_1^1 = 980$ b), 305 nm.

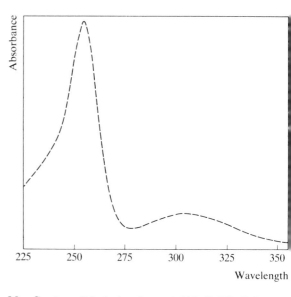

Mass Spectrum. Principal peaks at m/z 212, 42, 187, 45, 70, 180, 56, 98.

Quantification. GAS CHROMATOGRAPHY–MASS SPECTROMETRY. In plasma or serum: sensitivity 400 pg/ml—G. Brante *et al.*, *Eur. J. clin. Pharmac.*, 1981, **20**, 307–310.

Dose. 12.5 to 75 mg daily.

Dobutamine   *Sympathomimetic*

(±)-4-{2-[3-(4-Hydroxyphenyl)-1-methylpropylamino]ethyl}-pyrocatechol
$C_{18}H_{23}NO_3 = 301.4$
CAS—34368-04-2

Dobutamine Hydrochloride

Proprietary Name. Dobutrex
$C_{18}H_{23}NO_3, HCl = 337.8$
CAS—52663-81-7

A white powder. M.p. 189° to 191°.

Sparingly **soluble** in water and ethanol; soluble in methanol and pyridine.

Dissociation Constant. pK_a 9.5.

Colour Tests. Ammoniacal Silver Nitrate—black; *p*-Dimethyl-aminobenzaldehyde—orange/violet; Ferric Chloride—green; Folin–Ciocalteu Reagent—blue; Methanolic Potassium Hydroxide—brown-pink; Millon's Reagent—red; Nessler's Reagent—black; Palladium Chloride—orange → brown; Potassium Dichromate—green-brown.

Thin-layer Chromatography. *System TA*—Rf 52; *system TB*—Rf 00; *system TC*—Rf 01.

Ultraviolet Spectrum. Aqueous acid—279 nm $(A_1^1 = 131 \text{ b})$; aqueous alkali—236 nm, 292 nm.

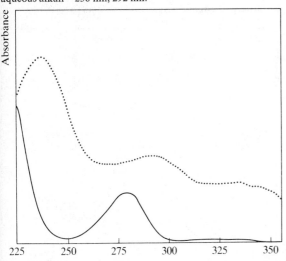

Infra-red Spectrum. Principal peaks at wavenumbers 1520, 1280, 1266, 1190, 1200, 1220 (dobutamine hydrochloride, KBr disk).

Mass Spectrum. Principal peaks at *m/z* 58, 107, 30, 178, 77, 56, 57, 137.

Quantification. HIGH PRESSURE LIQUID CHROMATOGRAPHY. In equine plasma: detection limit 100 pg/ml, electrochemical detection—G. E. Hardee and J. W. Lai, *Analyt. Lett. (Part B)*, 1983, *16*, 69–75.

Disposition in the Body. Inactive after oral administration. After intravenous administration, it is rapidly metabolised by glucuronide conjugation and 3-*O*-methylation to inactive metabolites which are excreted in the urine, mostly in the first 2 hours.

HALF-LIFE. Plasma half-life, about 2 minutes.

Dose. Usually 2.5 to 10 µg/kg/min of dobutamine hydrochloride, by intravenous infusion.

Docusate Sodium
Anionic Surfactant

Synonyms. Dioctyl Sodium Sulphosuccinate; DSS; Sodium Dioctyl Sulphosuccinate.
Proprietary Names. Aerosol OT; Afko-Lube; Audinorm; Bu-Lax; Colace; Comfolax; Constiban; Dilax; Dioctyl; Dio-Medicone; Disonate; Doxinate; Molcer; Regulex; Soliwax; Waxsol. It is an ingredient of Dorbantyl, Dulcodos, Klyx, Migraleve, and Normax.

Sodium 1,4-bis(2-ethylhexyl) sulphosuccinate
$C_{20}H_{37}NaO_7S = 444.6$
CAS—10041-19-7 [1,4-bis(2-ethylhexyl) sulphosuccinate]; *577-11-7* (sodium salt)

White, hygroscopic, waxy masses or flakes.
Slowly **soluble** 1 in 70 of water, higher concentrations forming a thick gel; soluble 1 in 3 of ethanol, 1 in 1 of chloroform, and 1 in 1 of ether.

Docusate Calcium
Synonym. Dioctyl Calcium Sulphosuccinate
Proprietary Names. Surfak. It is an ingredient of Doxidan.
$C_{40}H_{74}CaO_{14}S_2 = 883.2$
CAS—128-49-4
A white amorphous solid.
Soluble 1 in 3300 of water; freely soluble in ethanol, chloroform, and ether.

Docusate Potassium
Synonym. Dioctyl Potassium Sulphosuccinate
Proprietary Names. Dialose; Kasof; Rectalad.
$C_{20}H_{37}KO_7S = 460.7$
CAS—7491-09-0
A white amorphous solid.
Sparingly **soluble** in water; soluble in ethanol; very soluble in light petroleum.

Colour Tests. To 5 ml of a 0.1% solution add 1 ml of *dilute sulphuric acid*, 10 ml of chloroform, and 0.2 ml of *dimethyl yellow solution*, and shake—the chloroform layer is coloured red. Add 50 mg of cetrimide and shake—the colour of the chloroform layer changes to yellow.

Infra-red Spectrum. Principal peaks at wavenumbers 1724, 1250, 1052, 1020, 1612, 1086.

Dose. 50 to 500 mg daily as a laxative.

Dodecyl Gallate
Antoxidant

Synonym. Lauryl Gallate
Proprietary Names. Progallin LA. It is an ingredient of Embanox 7.

Dodecyl 3,4,5-trihydroxybenzoate
$C_{19}H_{30}O_5 = 338.4$
CAS—1166-52-5

A white or creamy-white powder. M.p. 96° to 97.5°.
Practically **insoluble** in water; soluble 1 in 3.5 of ethanol, 1 in 60 of chloroform, and 1 in 4 of ether.

Colour Tests. Ammoniacal Silver Nitrate—black; Ferric Chloride—blue; Folin–Ciocalteu Reagent—blue; Methanolic Potassium Hydroxide—orange; Nessler's Reagent—black.

Ultraviolet Spectrum. Methanol—275 nm $(A_1^1 = 300 \text{ b})$.

Dofamium Chloride   *Cationic Disinfectant*

Synonym. Phenamylium Chloride

Dimethyl [2 - (*N* - methyldodecanamido)ethyl] [(phenyl-carbamoyl)methyl]ammonium chloride

$C_{25}H_{44}ClN_3O_2 = 454.1$

CAS—54063-35-3

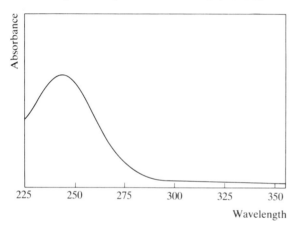

A white crystalline powder.
Soluble in water.

Colour Test. Mandelin's Test—red → brown.

Thin-layer Chromatography. *System TA*—Rf 03. (*Acidified iodoplatinate solution*, positive.)

Gas Chromatography. *System GA*—RI 1676, 1898, and 1974.

Ultraviolet Spectrum. Aqueous acid—244 nm ($A_1^1 = 242$ b).

Infra-red Spectrum. Principal peaks at wavenumbers 1670, 1626, 760, 1538, 1592, 1298.

DOM   *Hallucinogen*

Synonym. 2,5-Dimethoxy-4-methylamphetamine
2,5-Dimethoxy-4,α-dimethylphenethylamine

$C_{12}H_{19}NO_2 = 209.3$

CAS—15588-95-1

DOM is reported to be the active principle of the hallucinogenic preparation known as STP. (STP has also been used as a synonym for DOM.)

Melting-points of 59° and 70° have been reported.
Practically **insoluble** in water; soluble in chloroform.

Colour Test. Marquis Test—yellow.

Thin-layer Chromatography. *System TA*—Rf 51; *system TB*—Rf 16; *system TC*—Rf 17. (*Dragendorff spray*, positive; *FPN reagent*, positive; *acidified iodoplatinate solution*, positive; *Marquis reagent*, yellow; *ninhydrin spray*, positive; *acidified potassium permanganate solution*, positive.)

Gas Chromatography. *System GA*—RI 1616.

High Pressure Liquid Chromatography. *System HC*—k′ 1.13.

Ultraviolet Spectrum. Aqueous acid—289 nm ($A_1^1 = 221$ b).

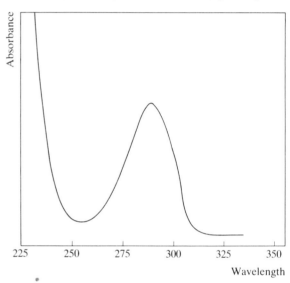

Infra-red Spectrum. Principal peaks at wavenumbers 1208, 1041, 1541, 1515, 1634, 1094.

Mass Spectrum. Principal peaks at *m/z* 44, 166, 151, 57, 43, 91, 135, 209.

Disposition in the Body. About 20% of an ingested dose is excreted in the urine unchanged in 24 hours; peak urinary excretion occurs 3 to 6 hours after ingestion.

REFERENCE. S. H. Snyder *et al.*, *Science*, 1967, *158*, 669–670.

Domiphen Bromide   *Cationic Disinfectant*

Synonym. Phenododecinium Bromide
Proprietary Name. Bradosol

It consists chiefly of dodecyldimethyl(2-phenoxyethyl)-ammonium bromide

$C_{22}H_{40}BrNO = 414.5$

CAS—13900-14-6 (domiphen); *538-71-6* (bromide)

Colourless or faintly yellow crystalline flakes. M.p. 106° to 116°.
Soluble 1 in less than 2 of water and of ethanol, and 1 in 30 of acetone.

Colour Test. Dissolve 10 mg in 10 ml of water, add 0.1 ml of a 0.5% aqueous eosin solution and 100 ml of water—pink.

Thin-layer Chromatography. *System TA*—Rf 05. (*Acidified iodoplatinate solution*, positive.)

Gas Chromatography. *System GA*—RI 2310.

Ultraviolet Spectrum. Methanol—268 nm ($A_1^1 = 30$ a), 277 nm.

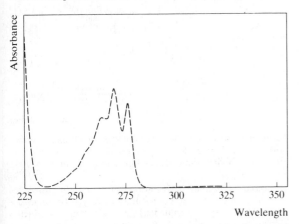

Infra-red Spectrum. Principal peaks at wavenumbers 1228, 752, 1500, 1600, 689, 1080 (KBr disk).

Dose. Lozenges containing 500 µg of domiphen bromide are available.

Dopamine   *Sympathomimetic*

Synonym. 3-Hydroxytyramine
4-(2-Aminoethyl)pyrocatechol
$C_8H_{11}NO_2 = 153.2$
CAS—51-61-6

CH₂·CH₂·NH₂ structure:

CH$_2$·CH$_2$·NH$_2$ benzene ring with OH, OH

Crystals.

Dopamine Hydrochloride

Proprietary Names. Intropin; Revimine; Revivan.

$C_8H_{11}NO_2,HCl = 189.6$
CAS—62-31-7
A white crystalline powder. M.p. about 241°, with decomposition.
Soluble in water and ethanol.

Dissociation Constant. pK_a 8.8, 10.6 (20°).

Colour Tests. Ammoniacal Silver Nitrate—orange-brown/black; *p*-Dimethylaminobenzaldehyde—orange/violet; Ferric Chloride—green; Folin–Ciocalteu Reagent—blue; Marquis Test—brown-violet; Methanolic Potassium Hydroxide—blue → orange → brown; Nessler's Reagent—black; Potassium Dichromate—green → brown (30 s).

Thin-layer Chromatography. *System TA*—Rf 18, streaking. (*Acidified potassium permanganate solution*, positive.)

Gas Chromatography. *System GA*—RI 2175.

High Pressure Liquid Chromatography. *System HA*—k' 2.7 (tailing peak).

Ultraviolet Spectrum. Aqueous acid—280 nm ($A_1^1 = 178$ a).

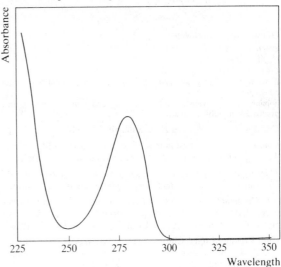

Infra-red Spectrum. Principal peaks at wavenumbers 1503, 1287, 1190, 1174, 813, 1115 (KBr disk).

Quantification. See under Levodopa.

Disposition in the Body. Dopamine is a naturally occurring catecholamine and is considered to be the metabolic precursor of noradrenaline. It is inactivated after oral administration. It is excreted mainly as 3,4-dihydroxyphenylacetic acid (DOPAC) and 3-methoxy-4-hydroxyphenylacetic acid (homovanillic acid); noradrenaline and 3-methoxytyramine are also metabolites. Dopamine is a metabolite of levodopa.

Dose. Initially 2 to 5 µg/kg/min of dopamine hydrochloride, by intravenous infusion.

Dothiepin   *Antidepressant*

Synonym. Dosulepin
3-(Dibenzo[*b,e*]thiepin-11(6*H*)-ylidene)-*NN*-dimethylpropyl-amine
$C_{19}H_{21}NS = 295.4$
CAS—113-53-1

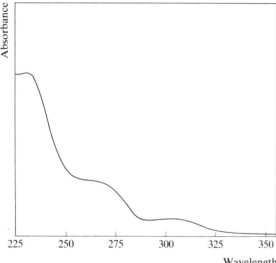

CH·CH₂·CH₂·N(CH₃)₂

Dothiepin Hydrochloride

Proprietary Name. Prothiaden

$C_{19}H_{21}NS,HCl = 331.9$

CAS—897-15-4

A white to faintly yellow crystalline powder. M.p. about 224°, with decomposition.

Soluble 1 in 2 of water, 1 in 8 of ethanol, and 1 in 2 of chloroform; practically insoluble in ether.

Partition Coefficient. Log *P* (octanol/pH 7.4), 2.8.

Colour Tests. Liebermann's Test—red-brown; Mandelin's Test—green; Marquis Test—brown; Sulphuric Acid—violet.

Thin-layer Chromatography. *System TA*—Rf 51; *system TB*—Rf 50; *system TC*—Rf 42. (*Acidified iodoplatinate solution,* positive.)

Gas Chromatography. *System GA*—dothiepin RI 2380, monodesmethyldothiepin RI 2390, dothiepin sulphoxide RI 2450; *system GF*—dothiepin RI 2770, dothiepin sulphoxide RI 2820.

High Pressure Liquid Chromatography. *System HA*—dothiepin k′ 3.2, dothiepin sulphoxide k′ 4.6 (tailing peak), monodesmethyldothiepin k′ 2.2; *system HF*—k′ 3.60.

Ultraviolet Spectrum. Aqueous acid—230 nm ($A^1_1 = 770$ a), 303 nm.

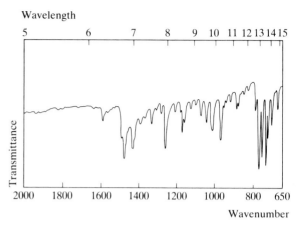

Wavelength

Infra-red Spectrum. Principal peaks at wavenumbers 763, 727, 747, 1252, 963, 717 (dothiepin hydrochloride, KBr disk).

Mass Spectrum. Principal peaks at m/z 58, 236, 40, 202, 235, 203, 42, 44; desmethyldothiepin 44, 204, 203, 202, 41, 221, 57, 55; dothiepin sulphoxide 58, 44, 31, 59, 57, 42, 45, 40.

Quantification. GAS CHROMATOGRAPHY. In plasma: detection limit 4 ng, AFID—L. A. Gifford *et al., J. Chromat.,* 1975, *105,* 107–113.

GAS CHROMATOGRAPHY–MASS SPECTROMETRY. In plasma or whole blood: dothiepin, monodesmethyldothiepin and dothiepin sulphoxide, limit of detection 1 ng/ml—K. P. Maguire *et al., J. Chromat.,* 1981, *222; Biomed. Appl., 11,* 399–408.

HIGH PRESSURE LIQUID CHROMATOGRAPHY. In plasma or serum: dothiepin and monodesmethyldothiepin, limit of detection 10 ng/ml, UV detection—R. R. Brodie *et al., J. int. med. Res.,* 1977, *5,* 387–390.

Disposition in the Body. Well absorbed after oral administration. The main metabolic reactions are demethylation to monodesmethyldothiepin (northiaden) and oxidation to dothiepin sulphoxide. About 50 to 60% of a dose is excreted in the urine in 24 hours, mainly as metabolites, and 15 to 40% of a dose is eliminated in the faeces in the same period. Enterohepatic circulation has been reported.

THERAPEUTIC CONCENTRATION. Plasma concentrations vary considerably between individual subjects.

Following a single oral dose of 75 mg to 7 subjects, peak plasma concentrations of 0.03 to 0.07 μg/ml (mean 0.05) of dothiepin and 0.003 to 0.02 μg/ml (mean 0.01) of monodesmethyldothiepin were attained in about 3 hours and 6 hours respectively. Peak blood concentrations of dothiepin sulphoxide of 0.03 to 0.15 μg/ml (mean 0.08) were reported in 4 subjects at 5 hours (K. P. Maguire *et al., Br. J. clin. Pharmac.,* 1981, *12,* 405–409).

Following oral administration of 25 mg given 3 times a day to 5 subjects for 12 days, minimum steady-state serum concentrations of 0.02 to 0.06 μg/ml (mean 0.04) of dothiepin, and <0.01 to 0.05 μg/ml (mean 0.02) of monodesmethyldothiepin, were reported (B. R. S. Nakra *et al., J. int. med. Res.,* 1977, *5,* 391–397).

TOXICITY. Fatalities have been associated with blood concentrations of 1 to **5** to 19 μg/ml.

In 7 deaths attributed to dothiepin overdose, the following postmortem tissue concentrations were reported: blood 0.3 to 2.5 μg/ml (mean 1.5), bile 12 to 268 μg/ml (mean 117, 4 cases), liver 2 and 14 μg/g (2 cases), liver blood 0.6, 2.9, and 23.5 μg/ml (3 cases), urine 0.4 to 5.1 μg/ml (mean 3.2, 5 cases) (A. E. Robinson *et al., J. analyt. Toxicol.,* 1979, *3,* 3–13 and A. E. Robinson *et al., Z. Rechtsmed.,* 1974, *74,* 261–266).

A 36-year-old female was admitted to hospital 3 hours after the ingestion of 2 to 3 g of dothiepin with alcohol. After 24 hours, following treatment by haemoperfusion, she appeared to be recovering but toxic symptoms reappeared after 48 hours followed by death 56 hours after ingestion. The following plasma concentrations were reported (μg/ml):

Hours after ingestion	Dothiepin	Monodesmethyl-dothiepin
4.5	2.51	0
6.0	1.88	0.13
17.5	1.07	0.32
57.5*	4.54	1.28

*postmortem

(L. Bloodworth *et al., Postgrad. med. J.,* 1984, *60,* 442–444).

HALF-LIFE. Plasma half-life, dothiepin 11 to 40 hours (mean 22), monodesmethyldothiepin 22 to 60 hours (mean 33), dothiepin sulphoxide 13 to 35 hours (mean 20).

DISTRIBUTION IN BLOOD. Plasma: whole blood ratio, about 1.4.

NOTE. For a review of the pharmacokinetics of tricyclic antidepressants see G. Molnar and R. N. Gupta, *Biopharm. Drug Disp.*, 1980, *1*, 283–305.

Dose. 75 to 150 mg of dothiepin hydrochloride daily; up to 225 mg daily has been given.

Doxapram
Respiratory Stimulant

1-Ethyl-4-(2-morpholinoethyl)-3,3-diphenylpyrrolidin-2-one
$C_{24}H_{30}N_2O_2 = 378.5$
CAS—309-29-5

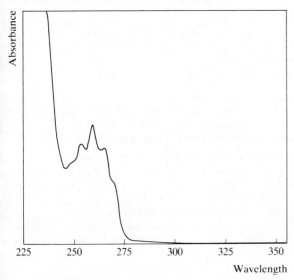

Doxapram Hydrochloride

Proprietary Names. Dopram; Doxapril.

$C_{24}H_{30}N_2O_2, HCl, H_2O = 433.0$
CAS—113-07-5 (anhydrous); *7081-53-0* (monohydrate)
A white crystalline powder. M.p. about 220°.

Soluble 1 in 50 of water; sparingly soluble in ethanol; soluble in chloroform; practically insoluble in ether.

Colour Tests. Liebermann's Test—orange; Mandelin's Test—blue.

Thin-layer Chromatography. *System TA*—Rf 64; *system TB*—Rf 20; *system TC*—Rf 70. (*Acidified iodoplatinate solution, positive.*)

Gas Chromatography. *System GA*—RI 2906; *system GC*—RI 2230.

High Pressure Liquid Chromatography. *System HA*—k' 0.4.

Ultraviolet Spectrum. Aqueous acid—253 nm, 259 nm ($A_1^1 = 12$ c), 265 nm.

Infra-red Spectrum. Principal peaks at wavenumbers 1683, 753, 710, 1253, 696, 764 (doxapram hydrochloride, KBr disk).

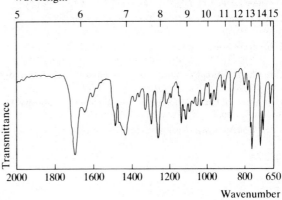

Wavelength

Mass Spectrum. Principal peaks at *m/z* 100, 113, 56, 101, 87, 378, 194, 91.

Quantification. GAS CHROMATOGRAPHY. In plasma: detection limit 10 ng/ml, AFID—R. H. Robson and L. F. Prescott, *J. Chromat.*, 1977, *143*; *Biomed. Appl.*, 1, 527–529.

Disposition in the Body. Readily absorbed after oral administration; bioavailability about 60%. The major metabolite is the 2-ketomorpholino derivative.

THERAPEUTIC CONCENTRATION.

Following an intravenous injection of 1.5 mg/kg to 6 subjects, plasma concentrations of 1.6 to 4.3 µg/ml (mean 2.6) were reported after 2 minutes declining to 0.6 to 1.5 µg/ml (mean 0.9) at 2 hours. Following intravenous infusion of 6.5 mg/kg to 6 subjects, peak plasma concentrations of 3.3 to 5.2 µg/ml (mean 4.1) were reported at the end of the infusion; peak concentrations of the 2-ketomorpholino metabolite of 1.1 to 2.0 µg/ml (mean 1.6) were attained 0.2 to 2 hours after the end of the infusion (J. A. Clements *et al.*, *Eur. J. clin. Pharmac.*, 1979, *16*, 411–416).

HALF-LIFE. Plasma half-life, about 7 hours.

VOLUME OF DISTRIBUTION. About 3 litres/kg.

CLEARANCE. Plasma clearance, about 5 ml/min/kg.

Dose. 1 to 1.5 mg/kg of doxapram hydrochloride by intravenous injection.

Doxepin
Antidepressant

A mixture of the *cis-* and *trans-*isomers of 3-(dibenz[*b,e*]oxepin-11(6*H*)-ylidene)-*NN*-dimethylpropylamine.
$C_{19}H_{21}NO = 279.4$
CAS—1668-19-5

An oily liquid.

Doxepin Hydrochloride

Proprietary Names. Adapin; Aponal; Quitaxon; Sinequan; Sinquan.

$C_{19}H_{21}NO, HCl = 315.8$
CAS—1229-29-4
A white crystalline powder. M.p. 185° to 191°.

Absorbance

225   250   275   300   325   350
Wavelength

Soluble 1 in 1.5 of water, 1 in 1 of ethanol, and 1 in 2 of chloroform; very slightly soluble in ether.

Dissociation Constant. pK_a 9.0 (25°).

Partition Coefficient. Log P (octanol/pH 7.4), 2.4.

Colour Tests. Liebermann's Test—black; Mandelin's Test—brown; Marquis Test—brown; Sulphuric Acid—orange.

Thin-layer Chromatography. *System TA*—Rf 51; *system TB*—Rf 52; *system TC*—Rf 37. (*Acidified iodoplatinate solution*, positive.)

Gas Chromatography. *System GA*—doxepin RI 2217, monodesmethyldoxepin RI 2235; *system GF*—RI 2570.

High Pressure Liquid Chromatography. *System HA*—doxepin k' 3.7, monodesmethyldoxepin k' 2.2; *system HF*—k' 2.27.

Ultraviolet Spectrum. Aqueous acid—292 nm (A_1^1 = 231 a).

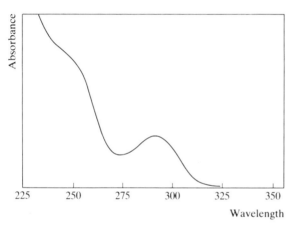

Infra-red Spectrum. Principal peaks at wavenumbers 750, 1006, 768, 1198, 1290, 1219 (doxepin hydrochloride, KBr disk).

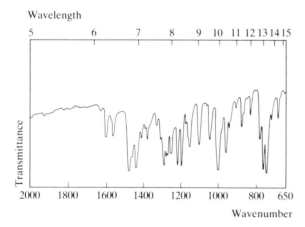

Mass Spectrum. Principal peaks at m/z 58, 220, 219, 59, 191, 189, 42, 205.

Quantification. GAS CHROMATOGRAPHY. In plasma: sensitivity 10 ng/ml, FID—J. E. O'Brien and O. N. Hinsvark, *J. pharm. Sci.*, 1976, *65*, 1068–1069. In plasma: sensitivity 2 ng/ml for doxepin and 1 ng/ml for monodesmethyldoxepin, AFID—

M. T. Rosseel *et al.*, *J. pharm. Sci.*, 1978, *67*, 802–805. In plasma: sensitivity 2.5 ng/ml, ECD—J. E. Wallace *et al.*, *J. analyt. Toxicol.*, 1978, *2*, 44–49.

GAS CHROMATOGRAPHY–MASS SPECTROMETRY. In blood, urine or tissues: doxepin and monodesmethyldoxepin—G. de Groot *et al.*, *J. analyt. Toxicol.*, 1978, *2*, 13–17.

HIGH PRESSURE LIQUID CHROMATOGRAPHY. In plasma: detection limit 5 ng/ml for doxepin and monodesmethyldoxepin, UV detection—R. D. Faulkner and C. Lee, *J. pharm. Sci.*, 1983, *72*, 1165–1167.

RADIOIMMUNOASSAY. In serum or plasma: doxepin and monodesmethyldoxepin, sensitivity 2.5 ng/ml—R. Virtanen *et al.*, *Acta pharmac. tox.*, 1980, *47*, 274–278.

Disposition in the Body. Well absorbed after oral administration, but undergoes extensive first-pass demethylation; bioavailability 15 to 45%. Other metabolic reactions include N-oxidation, aromatic hydroxylation, and glucuronic acid conjugation. Monodesmethyldoxepin is an active metabolite. Less than 1% of a dose is excreted in the urine as unchanged drug in 24 hours.

THERAPEUTIC CONCENTRATION. In plasma, usually in the range 0.02 to 0.15 μg/ml.

After a single oral dose of 75 mg given to 7 subjects, peak plasma concentrations of 0.01 to 0.05 μg/ml (mean 0.03) of doxepin were attained in 2 to 4 hours and peak plasma concentrations of 0.005 to 0.014 μg/ml (mean 0.01) of monodesmethyldoxepin were reported at 2 to 10 hours (V. E. Ziegler *et al.*, *Clin. Pharmac. Ther.*, 1978, *23*, 573–579).

Daily oral doses of 75 to 200 mg given to 5 subjects, produced steady-state plasma concentrations of 0.05 to 0.15 μg/ml of doxepin; in two of these subjects plasma concentrations for monodesmethyldoxepin of 0.09 and 0.10 μg/ml were reported (J. E. O'Brien and O. N. Hinsvark, *J. pharm. Sci.*, 1976, *65*, 1068–1069).

TOXICITY. Doses in excess of 500 mg are likely to produce severe toxic effects and the estimated minimum lethal dose is 1 g. Blood concentrations greater than 0.1 μg/ml may be associated with toxic reactions and fatalities have been associated with blood concentrations of 1 to **8** to 18 μg/ml.

In 5 deaths due to overdosage of doxepin, the postmortem blood concentrations ranged from 9 to 19 μg/ml (mean 13) and in 3 of these cases, liver concentrations of 71, 75, and 500 μg/g were reported (J. S. Oliver and A. A. Watson, *Medicine, Sci. Law*, 1974, *14*, 280–283).

In a report of 4 fatalities attributed to overdose of doxepin, the following postmortem blood and tissue concentrations, μg/ml or μg/g (mean), were found:

	Doxepin	Monodesmethyldoxepin
Blood	0.7–29 (9.3)	0.1–6.2 (1.7)
Bile	38–195 (95)	1.0–19 (7.1)
Brain	9–21 (14)	1.5–22 (7.2)
Kidney	3.3–19 (12)	0.5–9.0 (3.0)
Liver	22–38 (32)	1.2–20 (7.5)
Urine	2.1–12 (7.5)	0.7–6.4 (2.8)

(G. de Groot *et al.*, *J. analyt. Toxicol.*, 1978, *2*, 18–20).

HALF-LIFE. Plasma half-life, doxepin 8 to 25 hours (mean 17), monodesmethyldoxepin 33 to 80 hours (mean 51).

VOLUME OF DISTRIBUTION. About 20 litres/kg.

CLEARANCE. Plasma clearance, about 15 ml/min/kg.

DISTRIBUTION IN BLOOD. Plasma: whole blood ratio, doxepin about 0.8 but there is considerable intersubject variation; monodesmethyldoxepin about 0.6.

PROTEIN BINDING. In plasma, about 80%.

NOTE. For a review of the pharmacokinetics of tricyclic antidepressants see G. Molnar and R. N. Gupta, *Biopharm. Drug Disp.*, 1980, *1*, 283–305.

Dose. The equivalent of 30 to 300 mg of doxepin daily.

Doxorubicin

Antineoplastic

Synonyms. Adriamycin; 14-Hydroxydaunorubicin.

(1*S*,3*S*)-3-Glycoloyl-1,2,3,4,6,11-hexahydro-3,5,12-trihydroxy-10-methoxy-6,11-dioxonaphthacen-1-yl 3-amino-2,3,6-trideoxy-α-L-lyxopyranoside
$C_{27}H_{29}NO_{11} = 543.5$
CAS—23214-92-8

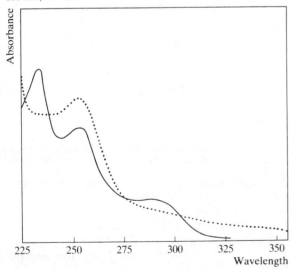

An antibiotic isolated from *Streptomyces peucetius* var. *caesius.*

Doxorubicin Hydrochloride

Proprietary Names. Adriamycin; Adriblastin(a); Adriblastine.
$C_{27}H_{29}NO_{11},HCl = 580.0$
CAS—25316-40-9
An orange-red, hygroscopic, crystalline powder. M.p. 204° to 205°, with decomposition.
Soluble in water and methanol; soluble 1 in 75 of ethanol; practically insoluble in chloroform, ether, and other organic solvents.
Caution. Doxorubicin hydrochloride is irritant; avoid contact with skin and mucous membranes.

Dissociation Constant. pK_a 8.2, 10.2.

Colour Tests. Mandelin's Test—green; Marquis Test—violet.

Thin-layer Chromatography. *System TA*—Rf 12. (Visible red streak).

Ultraviolet Spectrum. Aqueous acid—233 nm, 253 nm, 290 nm; aqueous alkali—253 nm; methanol—233 nm ($A_1^1 = 702$ b), 253 nm, 290 nm.

Infra-red Spectrum. Principal peaks at wavenumbers 1282, 990, 1010, 1587, 1612, 1204 (doxorubicin hydrochloride).

Dose. 1.2 to 2.4 mg/kg, intravenously, as a single dose every 3 weeks.

Doxycycline

Antibiotic

Synonym. Doxycycline Monohydrate .
Proprietary Names. Doxin; Doxitard; Doxychel; Vibramycin-D; Vibravenös.
6-Deoxy-5β-hydroxytetracycline monohydrate
$C_{22}H_{24}N_2O_8,H_2O = 462.5$
CAS—564-25-0 (anhydrous); *17086-28-1* (monohydrate)

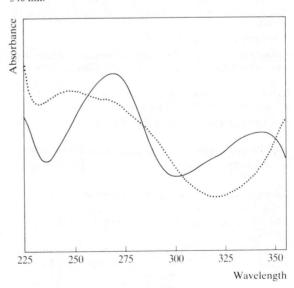

A yellow crystalline powder.
Very slightly **soluble** in water; sparingly soluble in ethanol; practically insoluble in chloroform and ether; freely soluble in dilute acids and alkali hydroxides.

Doxycycline Hydrochloride

Synonyms. Doxycycline Hyclate; Doxycyclini Chloridum.
Proprietary Names. Doxatet; Doxychel; Doxylar; Dumoxin; Idocyklin; Nordox; Vibramycin(e); Vibra-Tabs; Vibraveineuse.
$C_{22}H_{24}N_2O_8,HCl,\frac{1}{2}C_2H_5OH,\frac{1}{2}H_2O = 512.9$
CAS—10592-13-9 ($C_{22}H_{24}N_2O_8,HCl$); *24390-14-5* ($C_{22}H_{24}N_2O_8,HCl$, $\frac{1}{2}C_2H_5OH,\frac{1}{2}H_2O$)
A yellow crystalline powder. M.p. about 200°, with decomposition.
Soluble 1 in 3 of water, 1 in 60 of ethanol, and 1 in 4 of methanol; practically insoluble in chloroform and ether.

Dissociation Constant. pK_a 3.5, 7.7, 9.5 (20°).

Partition Coefficient. Log *P* (octanol/pH 7.5), −0.2.

Colour Tests. Benedict's Reagent—red; Formaldehyde–Sulphuric Acid—yellow; Mandelin's Test—green → yellow; Marquis Test—yellow; Sulphuric Acid—yellow.

Thin-layer Chromatography. *System TA*—Rf 12, streaking. (*Acidified iodoplatinate solution*, positive.)

Ultraviolet Spectrum. Aqueous acid—269 nm ($A_1^1 = 412$ b), 346 nm.

Infra-red Spectrum. Principal peaks at wavenumbers 1580, 1613, 1660, 1244, 1220, 1040 (doxycycline hydrochloride, KBr disk).

Quantification. HIGH PRESSURE LIQUID CHROMATOGRAPHY. In serum or urine: detection limit 50 ng/ml in serum, UV detection—A. P. De Leenheer and H. J. C. Nelis, *J. pharm. Sci.,* 1979, *68,* 999–1002.

Disposition in the Body. Readily and almost completely absorbed after oral administration; peak plasma concentrations are attained in about 2 hours. It does not appear to be significantly metabolised. About 40% of a dose is excreted in the urine unchanged in 72 hours (about 24% in the first 24 hours).

HALF-LIFE. Plasma half-life, about 22 hours.

PROTEIN BINDING. In plasma, about 82 to 90%.

NOTE. For a review of doxycycline see B. A. Cunha *et al., Ther. Drug Monit.,* 1982, *4,* 115–135.

Dose. The equivalent of 100 to 200 mg of doxycycline daily; a one-day course of 300 to 600 mg has also been given.

Doxylamine   *Antihistamine*

Synonym. Histadoxylamine
NN-Dimethyl-2-[α-methyl-α-(2-pyridyl)benzyloxy]ethylamine
$C_{17}H_{22}N_2O = 270.4$
CAS—469-21-6

A liquid. B.p. about 140°.

Doxylamine Succinate

Proprietary Names. Decapryn; Hoggar N; Mereprine; Unisom. It is an ingredient of Bendectin, Debendox, Nethaprin, and Syndol.
$C_{17}H_{22}N_2O,C_4H_6O_4 = 388.5$
CAS—562-10-7
A white or creamy-white powder. M.p. 103° to 108°.

Soluble 1 in 1 of water, 1 in 2 of ethanol, 1 in 2 of chloroform, and 1 in 370 of ether.

Dissociation Constant. pK_a 4.4, 9.2.

Colour Tests. Cyanogen Bromide—orange-pink; Liebermann's Test—red-orange; Marquis Test—violet; Sulphuric Acid—pink.

Thin-layer Chromatography. *System TA*—Rf 48; *system TB*—Rf 41; *system TC*—Rf 10. (*Acidified iodoplatinate solution,* positive.)

Gas Chromatography. *System GA*—RI 1906; *system GF*—RI 2170.

High Pressure Liquid Chromatography. *System HA*—k' 4.4.

Ultraviolet Spectrum. Aqueous acid—261 nm (A_1^1 = 335 a). No alkaline shift.

Infra-red Spectrum. Principal peaks at wavenumbers 700, 1590, 1123, 1086, 1041, 751 (KBr disk).

Mass Spectrum. Principal peaks at *m/z* 58, 71, 72, 167, 182, 42, 180, 59.

Quantification. GAS CHROMATOGRAPHY-MASS SPECTROMETRY. In plasma: sensitivity 100 ng/ml—A. Cailleux *et al., J. chromatogr. Sci.,* 1981, *19,* 163–176.

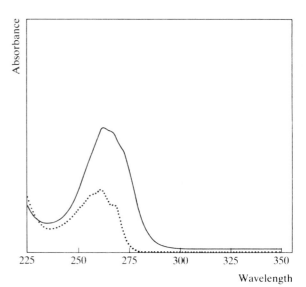

HIGH PRESSURE LIQUID CHROMATOGRAPHY. In plasma: detection limit 5 ng/ml, UV detection—K. J. Kohlhof *et al., J. pharm. Sci.,* 1983, *72,* 961–962.

Dose. Usually up to 100 mg of doxylamine succinate daily.

Droperidol   *Tranquilliser*

Proprietary Names. Dehydrobenzperidol; Dridol; Droleptan; Inapsine. It is an ingredient of Innovar and Thalamonal.
1-{1-[3-(4-Fluorobenzoyl)propyl]-1,2,3,6-tetrahydro-4-pyridyl}benzimidazolin-2-one
$C_{22}H_{22}FN_3O_2 = 379.4$
CAS—548-73-2

A white to light tan-coloured, amorphous or microcrystalline powder, which gradually darkens on exposure to light. M.p. 144° to 148°.

Practically **insoluble** in water; soluble 1 in 140 of ethanol, 1 in 4 of chloroform, and 1 in 500 of ether.

Dissociation Constant. pK_a 7.6.

Colour Test. Mandelin's Test—blue → green.

Thin-layer Chromatography. *System TA*—Rf 67; *system TB*—Rf 02; *system TC*—Rf 48. (*Acidified iodoplatinate solution,* positive.)

Gas Chromatography. *System GA*—RI 3430.

High Pressure Liquid Chromatography. *System HA*—k' 0.6.

Ultraviolet Spectrum. Aqueous acid—248 nm (A_1^1 = 443 a), 276 nm; aqueous alkali—246 nm, 288 nm.

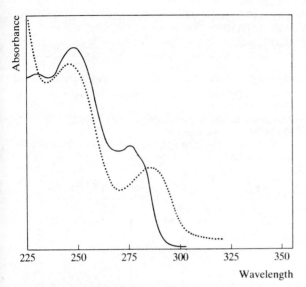

Infra-red Spectrum. Principal peaks at wavenumbers 1685, 1705, 1595, 1230, 752, 1156 (KBr disk).

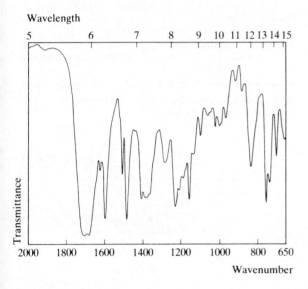

Mass Spectrum. Principal peaks at m/z 246, 165, 42, 123, 199, 247, 214, 108.

Quantification. GAS CHROMATOGRAPHY. In plasma: sensitivity 30 ng/ml, FID—M. P. Quaglio *et al.*, *Boll. chim.-farm.*, 1982, *121*, 276–284.

Disposition in the Body. Absorbed after oral administration. About 75% of a dose is excreted in the urine with less than 10% as unchanged drug; about 22% of a dose is eliminated in the faeces.

HALF-LIFE. Plasma half-life, about 2 to 3 hours.

PROTEIN BINDING. In plasma, about 85 to 90%.

Dose. 5 to 20 mg every 4 to 8 hours.

Dropropizine   *Cough Suppressant*

Proprietary Name. Ribex
3-(4-Phenylpiperazin-1-yl)propane-1,2-diol
$C_{13}H_{20}N_2O_2 = 236.3$
CAS—17692-31-8

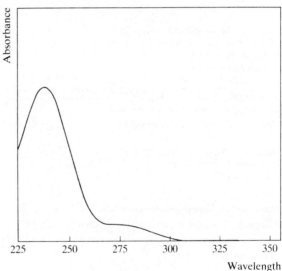

A white crystalline powder. M.p. 108° to 109°.
Soluble in chloroform and in dilute acetic acid.

Colour Tests. Liebermann's Test—red-orange; Mandelin's Test—orange (slow).
Cold *nitric acid* gives a red colour.

Thin-layer Chromatography. *System TA*—Rf 65. (*Acidified iodoplatinate solution*, strong reaction.)

Gas Chromatography. *System GA*—RI 2112.

Ultraviolet Spectrum. Aqueous acid—238 nm ($A_1^1 = 330$ a).

Infra-red Spectrum. Principal peaks at wavenumbers 1595, 1238, 1500, 760, 1060, 925 (KBr disk).

Dose. Dropropizine has been given in doses of 90 to 120 mg daily.

Drostanolone Propionate   *Anabolic Steroid*

Synonym. Dromostanolone Propionate
Proprietary Names. Drolban; Masterid; Masteril; Masteron; Permastril.
2α-Methyl-3-oxo-5α-androstan-17β-yl propionate
$C_{23}H_{36}O_3 = 360.5$
CAS—58-19-5 (drostanolone); *521-12-0* (propionate)

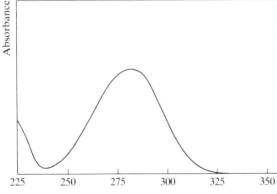

A white to creamy-white crystalline powder. M.p. 127° to 133°. Practically **insoluble** in water; soluble 1 in 30 of ethanol, 1 in 2 of chloroform, and 1 in 20 of ether.

Infra-red Spectrum. Principal peaks at wavenumbers 1715, 1200, 1735, 1035, 1087, 1265 (KBr disk).

Dose. Usually 100 mg thrice weekly, by intramuscular injection.

Dyclonine
Local Anaesthetic

4'-Butoxy-3-piperidinopropiophenone
$C_{18}H_{27}NO_2 = 289.4$
CAS—586-60-7

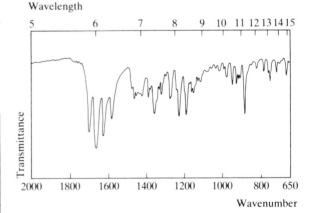

Dyclonine Hydrochloride
Synonym. Dyclocaine Chloride
Proprietary Name. Dyclone
$C_{18}H_{27}NO_2,HCl = 325.9$
CAS—536-43-6
White crystals or white crystalline powder. M.p. 173° to 178°.
Soluble 1 in 60 of water, 1 in 24 of ethanol, and 1 in 2.3 of chloroform; soluble in acetone; practically insoluble in ether.

Colour Tests. Aromaticity (Method 2)—yellow/orange; Liebermann's Test (100°)—orange.

Thin-layer Chromatography. *System TA*—Rf 60; *system TB*—Rf 49; *system TC*—Rf 40; *system TL*—Rf 25. (*Acidified iodoplatinate solution*, positive.)

Gas Chromatography. *System GA*—RI 1678.

High Pressure Liquid Chromatography. *System HR*—k' 2.78.

Ultraviolet Spectrum. Aqueous acid—282 nm ($A_1^1 = 580$ b).

Infra-red Spectrum. Principal peaks at wavenumbers 1178, 1605, 1229, 1672, 1575, 965 (dyclonine hydrochloride, KBr disk).

Use. Dyclonine hydrochloride is applied as a 0.5 or 1% solution.

Dydrogesterone
Progestational Steroid

Synonyms. Dehydroprogesterone; Didrogesteron; Isopregnenone.
Proprietary Names. Duphaston; Gynorest; Terolut.
9β,10α-Pregna-4,6-diene-3,20-dione
$C_{21}H_{28}O_2 = 312.5$
CAS—152-62-5

A white to pale yellow crystalline powder. M.p. 167° to 171°. Practically **insoluble** in water; soluble 1 in 40 to 1 in 52 of ethanol, 1 in 17 of acetone, 1 in 2 of chloroform, and 1 in 140 of ether.

Colour Tests. Antimony Pentachloride—orange; Naphthol–Sulphuric Acid—orange-red; Sulphuric Acid—orange (green–yellow fluorescence under ultraviolet light).

Thin-layer Chromatography. *System TP*—Rf 86; *system TQ*—Rf 53; *system TR*—Rf 96; *system TS*—Rf 98. (p-*Toluenesulphonic acid solution*, positive.)

Ultraviolet Spectrum. Dehydrated alcohol—286 nm ($A_1^1 = 838$ a).

Infra-red Spectrum. Principal peaks at wavenumbers 1660, 1622, 1697, 1581, 1232, 1197 (KBr disk).

Wavelength

Mass Spectrum. Principal peaks at *m/z* 43, 91, 227, 268, 312, 79, 55, 77.

Disposition in the Body. Rapidly absorbed after oral administration. The major metabolites are 20α-hydroxydydrogesterone and 21-hydroxydydrogesterone. About 50% of a dose is excreted in the urine in 24 hours, as metabolites.

Dose. Usually 20 to 30 mg daily.

Ecgonine
Alkaloid

Synonym. Laevo-ecgonine
(1*R*,2*R*,3*s*,5*S*)-3-Hydroxytropane-2-carboxylic acid
$C_9H_{15}NO_3 = 185.2$
CAS—481-37-8

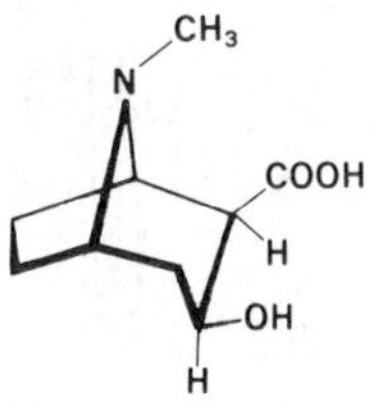

M.p. 198°, with decomposition; the dry substance melts at 205°.
Soluble in water; slightly soluble in ethanol; practically insoluble in ether.

Dissociation Constant. pK_a 2.8, 11.1.

Thin-layer Chromatography. *System TA*—Rf 17. (*Acidified iodoplatinate solution*, positive.)

Gas Chromatography. *System GA*—not eluted.

High Pressure Liquid Chromatography. *System HA*—k′ 1.1.

Ultraviolet Spectrum. Ethanol—275 nm.

Infra-red Spectrum. Principal peaks at wavenumbers 1688, 1210, 1200, 1223, 1134, 1179 (ecgonine hydrochloride, KBr disk).

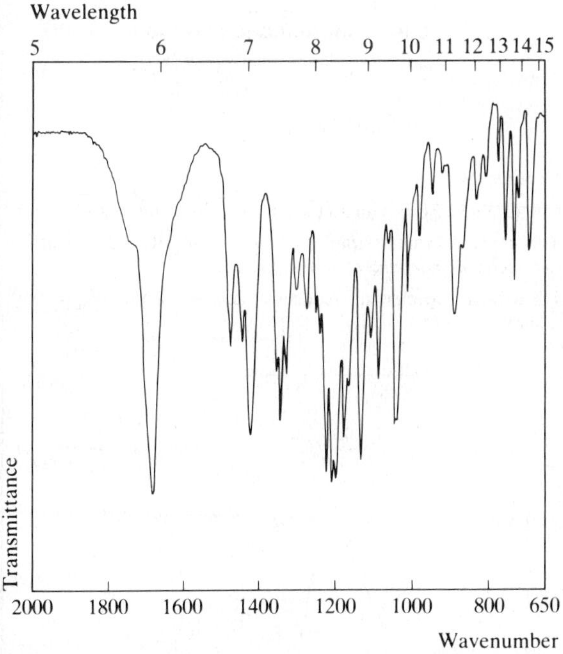

Mass Spectrum. Principal peaks at *m/z* 82, 97, 42, 83, 96, 57, 94, 55.

Disposition in the Body. Ecgonine and its methyl ester are metabolites of cocaine.

Econazole
Antifungal

1-[2,4-Dichloro-β-(4-chlorobenzyloxy)phenethyl]imidazole
$C_{18}H_{15}Cl_3N_2O = 381.7$
CAS—27220-47-9

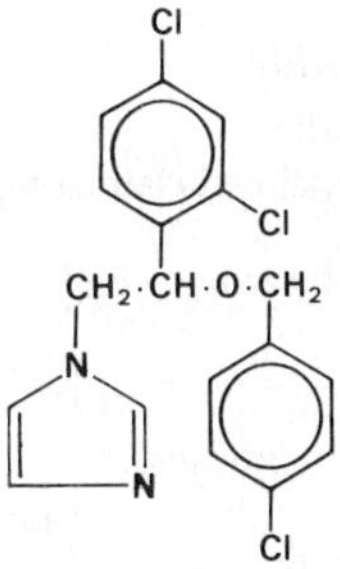

M.p. 87°.

Econazole Nitrate

Proprietary Names. Ecostatin; Epi-Pevaryl; Gyno-Pevaryl; Pevaryl. It is an ingredient of Econacort.
$C_{18}H_{15}Cl_3N_2O,HNO_3 = 444.7$
CAS—24169-02-6; 68797-31-9
A white crystalline powder. M.p. about 164°, with decomposition.
Very slightly **soluble** in water and ether; soluble 1 in 125 of ethanol, 1 in 60 of chloroform, and 1 in 25 of methanol.

Ultraviolet Spectrum. Methanolic acid—265 nm ($A_1^1 = 12$ b), 271 nm ($A_1^1 = 12.5$ a), 280 nm ($A_1^1 = 7.6$ a).

Infra-red Spectrum. Principal peaks at wavenumbers 1090, 1310, 805, 825, 1010, 1040 (econazole nitrate, KBr disk).

Quantification. HIGH PRESSURE LIQUID CHROMATOGRAPHY. In plasma: sensitivity 200 ng/ml, UV detection—R. R. Brodie *et al.*, *J. Chromat.*, 1978, *155*, 209–213.

Disposition in the Body. About 10% of a topical dose is absorbed and after vaginal application about 5% of the dose is absorbed. Following oral administration, about 40% of the dose is excreted in the urine and 30% is eliminated in the faeces, in 5 days.

BLOOD CONCENTRATION.
A mean peak plasma concentration of 2.6 µg/ml has been reported 2.5 hours after oral administration of 250 mg of econazole to 8 subjects (R. C. Heel *et al.*, *Drugs*, 1978, *16*, 177–201).

Uses. Econazole nitrate is applied topically in a concentration of 1%, or as pessaries.

Ecothiopate Iodide
Anticholinesterase

Synonyms. Diethoxyphosphinylthiocholine Iodide; Echothiopate Iodide; Echothiophate Iodide; Ecostigmine Iodide.
Proprietary Names. Echodide; Phospholine Iodide; Phospholinjod.
(2-Diethoxyphosphinylthioethyl)trimethylammonium iodide
$C_9H_{23}INO_3PS = 383.2$
CAS—6736-03-4 (ecothiopate); *513-10-0* (iodide)

A white, hygroscopic, crystalline powder. M.p. about 119°, with decomposition.
Soluble 1 in 1 of water, 1 in 25 of ethanol, and 1 in 3 of methanol; practically insoluble in chloroform and ether.

Colour Test. Palladium Chloride—orange.

Thin-layer Chromatography. *System TA*—Rf 02. (*Acidified iodoplatinate solution*, positive.)

Use. As a 0.03 to 0.25% ophthalmic solution.

Edrophonium Chloride

Anticholinesterase

Proprietary Name. Tensilon

Ethyl(3-hydroxyphenyl)dimethylammonium chloride
$C_{10}H_{16}ClNO = 201.7$
CAS—312-48-1 (edrophonium); *116-38-1* (chloride)

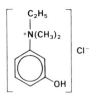

A white crystalline powder. M.p. 165° to 170°, with decomposition.

Soluble 1 in 0.5 of water and 1 in 5 of ethanol; practically insoluble in chloroform and ether.

Colour Test. Mandelin's Test—blue-green.

Thin-layer Chromatography. *System TA*—Rf .07. (*Acidified iodoplatinate solution*, positive.)

Ultraviolet Spectrum. Aqueous acid—273 nm ($A_1^1 = 110$ a); aqueous alkali—240 nm ($A_1^1 = 550$ b), 294 nm ($A_1^1 = 170$ b).

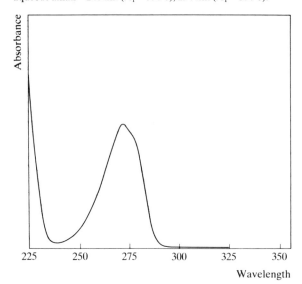

Infra-red Spectrum. Principal peaks at wavenumbers 1609, 690, 1217, 1495, 934, 1280 (KBr disk).

Disposition in the Body.

THERAPEUTIC CONCENTRATION.

Following intravenous injections of 100 µg/kg to 5 subjects, plasma concentrations of 0.8 to 3.9 µg/ml (mean 1.6) were reported at 2 minutes, declining to 0.038 to 0.056 µg/ml (mean 0.048) at 1 hour (T. N. Calvey et al., *Clin. Pharmac. Ther.*, 1976, **19**, 813–820).

TOXICITY. The estimated minimum lethal dose is 100 mg.

Wavelength

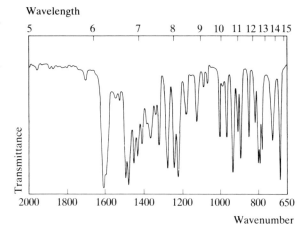

Wavenumber

HALF-LIFE. Plasma half-life, about 0.5 hour.

Dose. 2 to 10 mg intravenously, in the diagnosis of myasthenia gravis.

Embutramide

Narcotic Analgesic

Proprietary Name. It is an ingredient of Tanax (vet.).

N-(β,β-Diethyl-*m*-methoxyphenethyl)-4-hydroxybutyramide
$C_{17}H_{27}NO_3 = 293.4$
CAS—15687-14-6

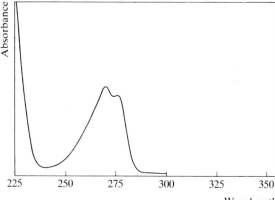

Crystals. M.p. 70°.

Colour Tests. Mandelin's Test—brown; Marquis Test—blue.

Thin-layer Chromatography. *System TA*—Rf 72. (*Acidified potassium permanganate solution*, positive.)

Ultraviolet Spectrum. Aqueous acid—271 nm ($A_1^1 = 50$ b), 276 nm.

Wavelength

Infra-red Spectrum. Principal peaks at wavenumbers 1652, 1248, 1037, 1595, 1562, 1063 (KBr disk).

Quantification. ULTRAVIOLET SPECTROPHOTOMETRY. In blood or urine—E. Bertol *et al.*, *J. pharm. biomed. Analysis*, 1983, *1*, 373–377.

Disposition in the Body.

TOXICITY.

In 3 fatalities due to the injection of a preparation containing embutramide and mebezonium iodide, the following postmortem concentrations (µg/ml) were reported:

	Embutramide	Mebezonium iodide
Blood	3.0, 15.5, 12.1	4.5, 6.0, 7.5
Urine	2.0, 6.3, 4.5	0.8, 2.0, 1.8

(E. Bertol *et al.*, *idem.*).

Emepronium Bromide   *Anticholinergic*

Proprietary Names. Cetiprin; Uro-Ripirin.

Ethyldimethyl(1-methyl-3,3-diphenylpropyl)ammonium bromide

$C_{20}H_{28}BrN = 362.4$

CAS—27892-33-7 (emepronium); *3614-30-0* (bromide)

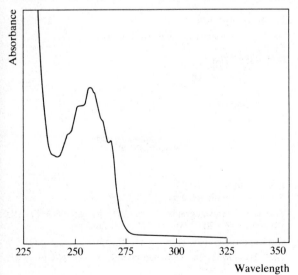

A white crystalline powder. M.p. 201° to 206°.
Soluble in water, ethanol, and chloroform.

Colour Test. Liebermann's Test—brown.

Thin-layer Chromatography. *System TA*—Rf 05. (*Acidified iodoplatinate solution*, strong reaction.)

Gas Chromatography. *System GA*—RI 1973.

High Pressure Liquid Chromatography. *System HA*—k' 5.2.

Ultraviolet Spectrum. Aqueous acid—253 nm, 258 nm ($A_1^1 = 13$ a), 268 nm.

Infra-red Spectrum. Principal peaks at wavenumbers 708, 699, 752, 1102, 742, 1134 (KBr disk).

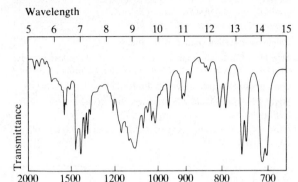

Quantification. GAS CHROMATOGRAPHY. In serum: sensitivity 200 pg/ml, ECD—P. Hartvig *et al.*, *J. pharm. Sci.*, 1976, *65*, 1707–1709.

Disposition in the Body. Poorly absorbed after oral administration; less than 5% of a dose is excreted in the urine in 24 hours, partly as metabolites. After intramuscular administration, about 30% of a dose is excreted in the urine in 3 days and 45% is eliminated in the faeces in the same period.

THERAPEUTIC CONCENTRATION.

Following a single oral dose of 150 mg to 5 subjects, peak serum concentrations of 0.017 to 0.10 µg/ml were attained in about 2 hours (J. Vessman *et al.*, *Acta pharm. suec.*, 1970, *7*, 363–372).

HALF-LIFE. Plasma half-life, about 7 to 11 hours.

Dose. 200 to 600 mg daily.

Emetine   *Anti-amoebic*

Synonyms. Ipecine; Methylcephaëline.

6′,7′,10,11-Tetramethoxyemetan

$C_{29}H_{40}N_2O_4 = 480.6$

CAS—483-18-1

An alkaloid present in ipecacuanha, the dried root, or rhizome and roots, of *Cephaëlis ipecacuanha* (= *Uragoga ipecacuanha*) (Rubiaceae) or *C. acuminata*.
A white amorphous powder. M.p. 74°.
Slightly **soluble** in water; soluble in ethanol, chloroform, and ether.

Emetine Hydrochloride

Synonym. Emetine Dihydrochloride
$C_{29}H_{40}N_2O_4, 2HCl, 7H_2O = 679.7$
CAS—316-42-7 (anhydrous); *7083-71-8* (hydrate)

A white or very slightly yellow, crystalline powder. M.p. 235° to 255°, after drying.
Soluble 1 in 8 of water, 1 in 12 of ethanol (90%), and 1 in 4 of chloroform; practically insoluble in ether.

Dissociation Constant. pK_a 7.4, 8.3 (25°).

Colour Test. Liebermann's Test—black.

Thin-layer Chromatography. *System TA*—Rf 54; *system TB*—Rf 09; *system TC*—Rf 34. (*Acidified iodoplatinate solution*, positive.)

Gas Chromatography. *System GA*—RI 2505.

High Pressure Liquid Chromatography. *System HA*—k′ 7.1 (tailing peak).

Ultraviolet Spectrum. Aqueous acid—230 nm ($A_1^1 = 341$ a), 282 nm ($A_1^1 = 158$ a).

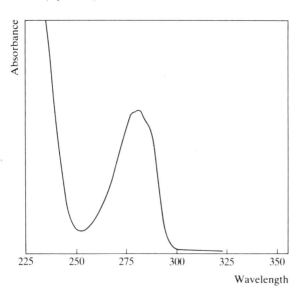

Infra-red Spectrum. Principal peaks at wavenumbers 1514, 1256, 1228, 1110, 1200, 1150 (KBr disk).

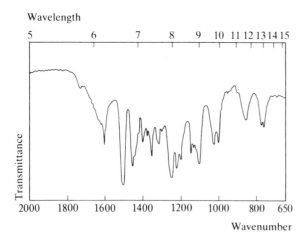

Mass Spectrum. Principal peaks at m/z 192, 206, 272, 480, 288, 246, 205, 191.

Quantification. HIGH PRESSURE LIQUID CHROMATOGRAPHY. In plasma: sensitivity 10 ng/ml, fluorescence detection—S. J. Bannister *et al.*, *J. Chromat.*, 1979, *176*, 381–390. In blood or urine: sensitivity 5 ng/ml, fluorescence detection—D. J. Crouch *et al.*, *J. analyt. Toxicol.*, 1984, *8*, 63–65.

Disposition in the Body. Rapidly absorbed after oral administration and after injection; concentrated in the liver, kidneys, lungs, and spleen. It is excreted only very slowly in the urine and detectable concentrations are found up to 60 days after treatment.

TOXICITY. The minimum lethal dose is 150 mg.
In a fatality which occurred after chronic ingestion of about 70 mg of emetine daily for 3 months, the following postmortem tissue concentrations were reported: blood 2.4 µg/g, bile 1.9 µg/g, kidney 7.4 µg/g, liver 14 µg/g (A. G. Adler *et al.*, *J. Am. med. Ass.*, 1980, *243*, 1927–1928).

Dose. Up to 60 mg of emetine hydrochloride daily, subcutaneously or intramuscularly, for no longer than 10 days.

Emylcamate   *Tranquilliser/Muscle Relaxant*

1-Ethyl-1-methylpropyl carbamate
$C_7H_{15}NO_2 = 145.2$
CAS—78-28-4

$$NH_2 \cdot CO \cdot O \cdot \underset{\underset{CH_3}{|}}{\overset{\overset{C_2H_5}{|}}{C}} \cdot CH_2 \cdot CH_3$$

A white crystalline powder. M.p. 56° to 58°.
Soluble 1 in 250 of water; freely soluble in ethanol and ether.

Gas Chromatography. *System GA*—RI 1105.

Ultraviolet Spectrum. No significant absorption, 230 to 360 nm.

Infra-red Spectrum. Principal peaks at wavenumbers 1690, 1610, 1041, 1170, 1150, 1010 (KCl disk).

Mass Spectrum. Principal peaks at m/z 73, 43, 84, 55, 69, 41, 44, 85.

Dose. Emylcamate was formerly given in doses of 600 to 800 mg daily.

Enallylpropymal   *Barbiturate*

5-Allyl-5-isopropyl-1-methylbarbituric acid
$C_{11}H_{16}N_2O_3 = 224.3$
CAS—1861-21-8

Crystals. M.p. 56° to 57°.
Soluble in organic solvents.

Thin-layer Chromatography. *System TD*—Rf 71; *system TE*—Rf 58; *system TF*—Rf 71; *system TH*—Rf 87.

Gas Chromatography. *System GA*—RI 1561.

High Pressure Liquid Chromatography. *System HG*—k′ 8.65; *system HH*—k′ 6.96.

Ultraviolet Spectrum. *Borax buffer 0.05M* (pH 9.2)—245 nm ($A_1^1 = 329$ b); M sodium hydroxide (pH 13)—244 nm ($A_1^1 = 362$ b).

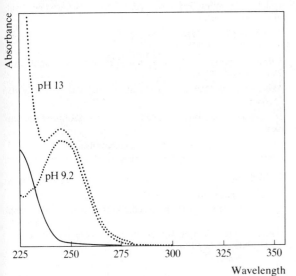

Infra-red Spectrum. Principal peaks at wavenumbers 1689, 1718, 1550, 1640, 1285, 672.

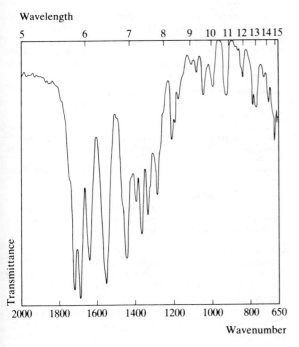

Mass Spectrum. Principal peaks at *m/z* 181, 41, 182, 39, 124, 53, 138, 97.

Endosulfan   *Pesticide*

Synonym. Benzoepin
Proprietary Name. Thiodan
1,4,5,6,7,7 - Hexachloro - 8,9,10 - trinorborn - 5 - en - 2,3 - ylenedimethyl sulphite
$C_9H_6Cl_6O_3S = 406.9$
CAS—115-29-7; 959-98-8 (α); 33213-65-9 (β)

Endosulfan is a mixture of 2 stereoisomers: the α-isomer, m.p. 109°, accounts for about 70% of the technical grade and the β-isomer, m.p. 213°, for about 30%.
The technical grade is a brownish crystalline solid. M.p. 70° to 100°.
Practically **insoluble** in water; moderately soluble in most organic solvents.

Gas Chromatography. *System GA*—RI 2085; *system GK*—retention time 1.10 relative to caffeine.

Mass Spectrum. Principal peaks at *m/z* 195, 36, 237, 41, 241, 75, 239, 170.

Quantification. GAS CHROMATOGRAPHY. In blood or tissues: ECD or FID—A. Coutselinis *et al., Forens. Sci.*, 1976, *8*, 251–254.

GAS CHROMATOGRAPHY–MASS SPECTROMETRY. In serum, urine or tissues: detection limit 2 ng for α-endosulfan—J. Demeter *et al., Quant. Mass Spectrom. Life Sci.*, 1978, *2*, 471–481.

Disposition in the Body.

TOXICITY.
In 3 fatalities attributed to the ingestion of endosulfan, the following postmortem tissue concentrations were reported: blood 4, 7, and 8 µg/ml; brain 0.25, 0.28, and 0.3 µg/g; kidney 2.4, 2.8, and 3.2 µg/g; liver 0.8, 1.4, and 1 µg/g (A. Coutselinis *et al., Forens. Sci.*, 1978, *11*, 75).

Endrin   *Insecticide*

1,2,3,4,10,10 - Hexachloro - 6,7 - epoxy - 1,4,4a,5,6,7,8,8a - octahydro-1,4:5,8-dimethanonaphthalene
$C_{12}H_8Cl_6O = 380.9$
CAS—72-20-8

A white crystalline solid. M.p. about 230°, with decomposition. Practically **insoluble** in water; sparingly soluble in ethanol.

Colour Tests. Nitric–Sulphuric Acid—pink; Sulphuric Acid–Fuming Sulphuric Acid—pink-orange.

Gas Chromatography. *System GA*—RI 2183; *system GK*—retention time 1.19 relative to caffeine.

Infra-red Spectrum. Principal peaks at wavenumbers 851, 750, 724, 1049, 889, 1010 (Nujol mull).

Mass Spectrum. Principal peaks at m/z 67, 81, 263, 36, 79, 82, 261, 265.

Quantification. COLORIMETRY. In blood, urine or tissues: sensitivity 4 µg/ml—R. T. Sane and S. S. Kamat, *Forens. Sci. Int.*, 1981, *18*, 63–66.

Enflurane
General Anaesthetic

Synonym. Methylflurether
Proprietary Names. Alyrane; Efrane; Ethrane.
2-Chloro-1,1,2-trifluoroethyl difluoromethyl ether
$C_3H_2ClF_5O = 184.5$
CAS—13838-16-9

$$CHF_2 \cdot O \cdot CF_2 \cdot CHClF$$

A colourless volatile liquid. B.p. 55.5° to 57.5°. Relative density 1.516 to 1.519.

Gas Chromatography. *System GA*—RI 462; *system GI*—retention time 8.3 min.

Quantification. GAS CHROMATOGRAPHY. In blood: detection limit 1.5 µg/ml, TCD—M. S. Miller and A. J. Gandolfi, *Anesthesiology*, 1979, *51*, 542–544.

Disposition in the Body. Readily absorbed on inhalation. About 50% of a dose is exhaled unchanged in 18 hours and more than 80% is exhaled in 5 days. Less than 5% of a dose is excreted in the urine as non-volatile metabolites. Difluoromethoxydifluoroacetic acid has been identified as a urinary metabolite.

THERAPEUTIC CONCENTRATION.

In 10 subjects receiving anaesthesia with 0.5 to 2.5% v/v of enflurane, a mean peak venous blood concentration of 95 µg/ml was attained in 30 minutes, declining to 0.5 µg/ml at 90 minutes after discontinuation of anaesthesia (I. M. Corall *et al.*, *Br. J. Anaesth.*, 1977, *49*, 881–885).
A mean peak serum-fluoride concentration of 0.2 µg/ml was attained 3 hours after induction in 18 subjects receiving 0.6 to 2% v/v of enflurane (P. Duvaldestin *et al.*, *Clin. Pharmac. Ther.*, 1981, *29*, 61–64).

HALF-LIFE. About 36 hours.

Dose. For induction of anaesthesia, up to 4% of the vapour by inhalation; maintenance, 0.5 to 3%.

Enoxolone
Dermatological Agent

Synonyms. Glycyrrhetic Acid; Glycyrrhetinic Acid.
Proprietary Names. PO 12. It is an ingredient of Biosone GA.
3β-Hydroxy-11-oxo-olean-12-en-30-oic acid
$C_{30}H_{46}O_4 = 470.7$
CAS—471-53-4

A white or faintly cream-coloured powder. M.p. 296°.
Very sparingly **soluble** in water; soluble in ethanol and ether; freely soluble in chloroform.

Colour Tests. Antimony Pentachloride—orange-brown → violet; Naphthol–Sulphuric Acid—red-brown/orange; Sulphuric Acid—yellow.

Thin-layer Chromatography. *System TD*—Rf 21; *system TE*—Rf 07; *system TF*—Rf 46.

Ultraviolet Spectrum. Aqueous acid—254 nm; aqueous alkali—260 nm ($A_1^1 = 338$ b).

Mass Spectrum. Principal peaks at m/z 303, 262, 135, 175, 41, 55, 43, 95.

Disposition in the Body. Enoxolone is a metabolite of carbenoxolone.

Use. Has been used topically in a concentration of 2%.

Ephedrine
Sympathomimetic

Synonym. Hydrated Ephedrine
Proprietary Names. It is an ingredient of Asmapax and Franol Expect.
(1R,2S)-2-Methylamino-1-phenylpropan-1-ol hemihydrate
$C_{10}H_{15}NO,\frac{1}{2}H_2O = 174.2$
CAS—50906-05-3

An alkaloid obtained from species of *Ephedra*, or prepared synthetically.
Colourless crystals or white crystalline powder or granules which decompose on exposure to light. M.p. 40° to 43° without previous drying; in warm weather it slowly volatilises.
Soluble 1 in 20 of water and 1 in less than 1 of ethanol; soluble in chloroform with turbidity due to separation of water; soluble in ether.

Anhydrous Ephedrine
Synonym. Ephedrine
$C_{10}H_{15}NO = 165.2$
CAS—299-42-3
Unctuous deliquescent colourless crystals, or white crystalline powder. It rapidly absorbs carbon dioxide and decomposes on exposure to light. M.p. about 38°.
Soluble 1 in 20 of water; very soluble in ethanol; soluble in chloroform; freely soluble in ether.

Ephedrine Hydrochloride
Synonyms. Ephedrinium Chloratum; *l*-Ephedrinum Hydrochloricum.
Proprietary Names. It is an ingredient of many proprietary preparations—see *Martindale, The Extra Pharmacopoeia*, 28th Edn.
$C_{10}H_{15}NO,HCl = 201.7$
CAS—50-98-6
Colourless crystals or white crystalline powder. M.p. 217° to 220°.
Soluble 1 in 3 to 1 in 4 of water and 1 in 14 to 1 in 17 of ethanol; very slightly soluble in chloroform; practically insoluble in ether.

Ephedrine Sulphate
Proprietary Names. Ectasule Minus. It is an ingredient of Enuretrol, Expansyl, and Franol Plus.
$(C_{10}H_{15}NO)_2,H_2SO_4 = 428.5$
CAS—134-72-5
Fine white crystals or powder which darken on exposure to light. M.p. 258°, with decomposition.
Soluble 1 in 1.3 of water and 1 in 90 of ethanol.

Dissociation Constant. pK_a 9.6 (25°).

Partition Coefficient. Log P (octanol), 1.0.

Colour Test. Liebermann's Test—red-orange.

Thin-layer Chromatography. *System TA*—Rf 30; *system TB*—Rf 05; *system TC*—Rf 05. (*Dragendorff spray*, positive; *acidified iodoplatinate solution*, positive; *Marquis reagent*, brown; *ninhydrin spray*, positive; *acidified potassium permanganate solution*, positive.)

Gas Chromatography. *System GA*—ephedrine RI 1363, norephedrine RI 1313; *system GB*—ephedrine RI 1386, norephedrine RI 1353; *system GC*—ephedrine RI 1467, norephedrine RI 1383.

High Pressure Liquid Chromatography. *System HA*—ephedrine k' 1.0, norephedrine k' 0.9; *system HB*—ephedrine k' 5.68, norephedrine k' 3.87; *system HC*—ephedrine k' 1.79, norephedrine k' 0.70.

Ultraviolet Spectrum. Aqueous acid—251 nm, 257 nm ($A_1^1 = 12$ a), 263 nm. No alkaline shift.

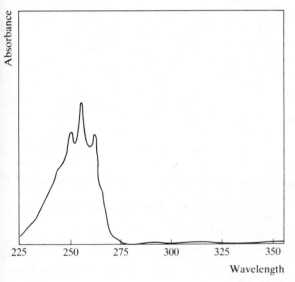

Absorbance / Wavelength

Infra-red Spectrum. Principal peaks at wavenumbers 994, 699, 754, 1049, 1242, 670 (ephedrine hydrochloride, KBr disk).

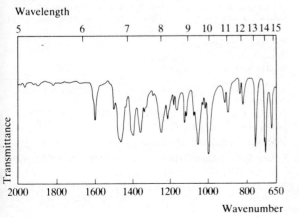

Wavelength / Transmittance / Wavenumber

Mass Spectrum. Principal peaks at m/z 58, 146, 56, 105, 77, 42, 106, 40; norephedrine 44, 77, 79, 51, 45, 42, 107, 105.

Quantification. GAS CHROMATOGRAPHY. In plasma or urine: sensitivity 2 ng/ml in plasma, ECD—K. K. Midha *et al.*, *J. pharm. Sci.*, 1979, *68*, 557–560.

Disposition in the Body. Readily absorbed after oral or percutaneous administration. Metabolised by *N*-demethylation to norephedrine (phenylpropanolamine) and by oxidative deamination followed by conjugation. Accumulates in the liver, lungs, kidneys, spleen, and brain. About 90% of a dose is excreted in the urine in 24 hours, with about 55 to 75% of the dose as unchanged drug, 8 to 20% as norephedrine, and 4 to 13% as deaminated metabolites such as benzoic acid, hippuric acid, and 1-phenylpropane-1,2-diol. In acidic urine, excretion of unchanged drug is increased slightly, whereas in alkaline urine, about 20 to 35% of the dose is excreted unchanged and the proportion of norephedrine is increased.
Ephedrine is a metabolite of methylephedrine.

THERAPEUTIC CONCENTRATION. In plasma, usually in the range 0.035 to 0.08 µg/ml.

After a single oral dose of 22 mg of the hydrochloride to 10 subjects, peak plasma concentrations of 0.04 to 0.14 µg/ml (mean 0.08) were attained; after daily oral doses of 33 mg of the hydrochloride to 10 subjects, peak plasma concentrations of 0.07 to 0.12 µg/ml (mean 0.08) were obtained (J. F. Costello *et al.*, *Br. J. clin. Pharmac.*, 1975, *2*, 180P–181P).

TOXICITY. The estimated minimum lethal dose in children up to 2 years of age is 200 mg and for adults 2 g but fatalities are rare. Single doses of up to 400 mg have been given without causing serious toxic effects.

HALF-LIFE. Plasma half-life, 3 to 11 hours but may be increased when the urine is alkaline and decreased when it is acid.

Dose. 45 to 240 mg of ephedrine hydrochloride or sulphate daily.

Epithiazide

Diuretic

Synonym. Epitizide
Proprietary Name. It is an ingredient of Thiaver.
6-Chloro-3,4-dihydro-3-(2,2,2-trifluoroethylthiomethyl)-2*H*-1,2,4-benzothiadiazine-7-sulphonamide 1,1-dioxide
$C_{10}H_{11}ClF_3N_3O_4S_3 = 425.8$
CAS—1764-85-8

A white crystalline powder. M.p. 206° to 207°.
Practically **insoluble** in water; soluble in alkaline solutions.

Ultraviolet Spectrum. Aqueous acid—272 nm, 315 nm. (See below)

Infra-red Spectrum. Principal peaks at wavenumbers 1176, 1314, 1167, 1126, 1603, 1269 (Nujol mull).

Dose. 8 to 12 mg daily.

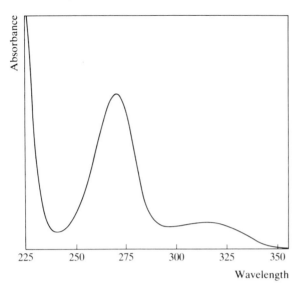

function, and extensive enterohepatic circulation occurs. Metabolised by 25-hydroxylation in the liver followed by 1α- or 24-hydroxylation in the kidney; possibly conjugated with glucuronic acid or sulphate. Excreted mainly in the bile together with small amounts of metabolites in the urine; unchanged ergocalciferol does not appear to be excreted in the urine.

BLOOD CONCENTRATION. Normal serum concentrations of 25-hydroxyergocalciferol are about 0.01 to 0.04 μg/ml but there are considerable intersubject and seasonal variations.

HALF-LIFE. About 40 days.

PROTEIN BINDING. In blood, bound to α- and β-lipoproteins.

Dose. 0.025 to 5 mg daily.

Ergometrine   *Ergot Alkaloid*

Synonyms. Ergobasine; Ergonovine.
N-[(S)-2-Hydroxy-1-methylethyl]-D-lysergamide
$C_{19}H_{23}N_3O_2 = 325.4$
CAS—60-79-7

Colourless crystals. Solutions in water give a blue fluorescence. M.p. 162°.
Slightly **soluble** in water; more soluble in ethanol; sparingly soluble in chloroform.

Ergometrine Maleate

Synonyms. Ergometrinhydrogenmaleat; Ergonovine Bimaleate; Ergonovine Maleate.
Proprietary Names. Ergomine; Ergotrate; Ermalate; Ermetrine. It is an ingredient of Syntometrine.
$C_{19}H_{23}N_3O_2,C_4H_4O_4 = 441.5$
CAS—129-51-1
A white or yellowish, slightly hygroscopic, microcrystalline powder. It darkens with age and on exposure to light. Solutions in water and ethanol give a blue fluorescence. M.p. about 185°, with decomposition.
Soluble 1 in 40 of water and 1 in 100 of ethanol; practically insoluble in chloroform and ether.

Ergometrine Tartrate

Synonym. Ergonovinum Tartaricum
$(C_{19}H_{23}N_3O_2)_2,C_4H_6O_6 = 800.9$
CAS—129-50-0
White or slightly reddish-yellow, very light, matted masses of acicular crystals.
Soluble in water and ethanol; slightly soluble in chloroform and ether.

Dissociation Constant. pK$_a$ 6.8 (20°).

Partition Coefficient. Log P (ether), −0.9.

Colour Tests. p-Dimethylaminobenzaldehyde—violet; Marquis Test—brown.

Thin-layer Chromatography. *System TA*—Rf 57; *system TB*—Rf 00; *system TC*—Rf 12; *system TL*—Rf 08; *system TM*—Rf 26. (*Van Urk reagent*, blue.)

Ergocalciferol   *Vitamin*

Synonyms. Calciferol; Irradiated Ergosterol; Viosterol; Vitamin D$_2$.
Proprietary Names. Deltar; Drisdol; Endo D; Farmobion D$_2$; Ostelin; Radiostol; Sterogyl-15; Vidue; Vigantolo.
Note. Ergocalciferol is also used as a rodenticide. It is an ingredient of Sorexa C.R.
(5Z,7E,22E)-9,10-Secoergosta-5,7,10(19),22-tetraen-3β-ol
$C_{28}H_{44}O = 396.7$
CAS—50-14-6

Colourless or slightly yellow crystals, or white or slightly yellow crystalline powder. M.p. 113° to 119°.
Practically **insoluble** in water; soluble 1 in 2 of ethanol, 1 in 10 of acetone, 1 in 0.7 of chloroform, and 1 in 2 of ether.

Ultraviolet Spectrum. Ethanol—265 nm (A$_1^1$ = 475 b).

Infra-red Spectrum. Principal peaks at wavenumbers 973, 1059, 1079, 1712, 893, 1000 (KBr disk).

Quantification. See under Cholecalciferol.

Disposition in the Body. Well absorbed after oral administration; absorption may be decreased with impaired liver and biliary

High Pressure Liquid Chromatography. *System HA*—k' 0.4; *system HP*—k' 0.50.

Ultraviolet Spectrum. Aqueous acid—313 nm ($A_1^1 = 240$ a); aqueous alkali—310 nm.

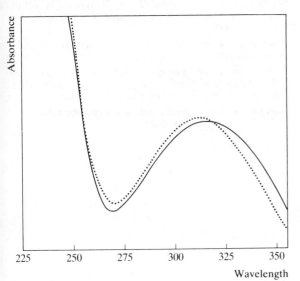

Infra-red Spectrum. Principal peaks at wavenumbers 1634, 754, 748, 1044, 1212, 1541.

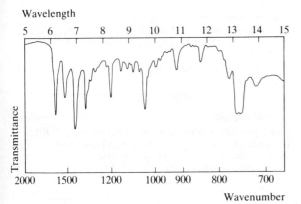

Mass Spectrum. Principal peaks at *m/z* 221, 72, 325, 54, 196, 55, 207, 181.

Disposition in the Body. More rapidly absorbed from the gastrointestinal tract than ergotamine. Metabolised by hydroxylation and glucuronic acid conjugation and possibly *N*-demethylation. Peak plasma concentrations are attained within 60 to 90 minutes and are more than tenfold those achieved with an equivalent dose of ergotamine. It is less toxic than ergotamine. Ergometrine has been reported to be detected unchanged in urine up to 8 hours after injection, the maximum concentration usually occurring 2 to 3 hours after an injection. It is mainly excreted in the bile as 12-hydroxyergometrine glucuronide.

Dose. 0.4 to 1.5 mg of ergometrine maleate daily, by mouth; doses of 200 to 500 μg are given intramuscularly.

Ergotamine   *Ergot Alkaloid*

12′-Hydroxy-2′-methyl-5′α-benzylergotaman-3′,6′,18-trione
$C_{33}H_{35}N_5O_5 = 581.7$
CAS—113-15-5

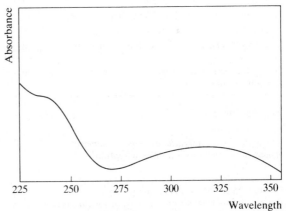

Hygroscopic crystals which darken and decompose on exposure to air, heat, and light. M.p. 212° to 214°, with decomposition. Practically **insoluble** in water; slightly soluble in ethanol; freely soluble in chloroform.

Ergotamine Tartrate
Proprietary Names. Ergomar; Ergostat; Gynergen(e); Lingraine. It is an ingredient of Cafergot, Effergot, and Migril.
$(C_{33}H_{35}N_5O_5)_2, C_4H_6O_6 = 1313$
CAS—379-79-3
Colourless crystals or white or yellowish-white crystalline powder. M.p. about 180°, with decomposition.
Soluble 1 in about 500 of water and 1 in 500 of ethanol; practically insoluble in chloroform and ether.

Dissociation Constant. pK$_a$ 6.4 (24°).

Colour Tests. *p*-Dimethylaminobenzaldehyde—violet; Mandelin's Test—violet-brown; Marquis Test—brown.

Thin-layer Chromatography. *System TA*—Rf 63; *system TB*—Rf 01; *system TC*—Rf 34; *system TL*—Rf 23; *system TM*—Rf 48. (*Van Urk reagent*, blue.)

Gas Chromatography. *System GA*—RI 2366.

High Pressure Liquid Chromatography. *System HA*—k' 0.4; *system HP*—k' 9.58.

Ultraviolet Spectrum. Aqueous acid—316 nm ($A_1^1 = 133$ a); aqueous alkali—310 nm ($A_1^1 = 148$ b).

Infra-red Spectrum. Principal peaks at wavenumbers 1631, 1712, 750, 1208, 1136, 1160 (KBr disk). (See below)

Mass Spectrum. Principal peaks at *m/z* 125, 44, 70, 91, 41, 40, 244, 153 (no peaks above 250).

Wavelength

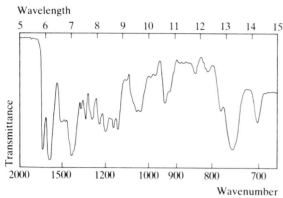

Quantification. HIGH PRESSURE LIQUID CHROMATOGRAPHY. In plasma or serum: ergotamine and methylergometrine, detection limit 100 pg/ml, fluorescence detection—P. O. Edlund, *J. Chromat.*, 1981, *226*; *Biomed. Appl.*, *15*, 107–115.

RADIOIMMUNOASSAY. In plasma—H. F. Schran *et al.*, *Clin. Chem.*, 1979, *25*, 1928–1933.

Disposition in the Body. Poorly absorbed after oral administration; the extent and rate of absorption is increased if caffeine is administered concurrently. Ergotamine is rapidly metabolised in the liver and is excreted mainly in the bile as metabolites; only traces of unchanged drug are excreted in the urine or faeces.

THERAPEUTIC CONCENTRATION.

After a single oral dose of 2 mg of ergotamine tartrate administered to 11 subjects, peak plasma concentrations of 0.0001 to 0.0009 µg/ml (mean 0.0006) were attained in 0.5 to 3 hours; following an intramuscular dose of 0.5 mg given to 10 subjects, peak plasma concentrations of 0.0009 to 0.004 µg/ml (mean 0.002) were attained in about 0.5 hour (V. Ala-Hurula *et al.*, *Eur. J. clin. Pharmac.*, 1979, *15*, 51–55).

TOXICITY. Ergotamine is highly toxic; in large repeated doses it can produce all the symptoms of ergot poisoning. Fatal poisoning has occurred after the oral administration of 26 mg of ergotamine over a period of several days, and also following single injections of only 0.5 to 1.5 mg.

In 12 cases of non-fatal ergotamine overdose, plasma concentrations of 0 to 0.003 µg/ml (mean 0.0008) were reported 1.7 to 5 hours after ingestion (D. Lamb *et al.*, *Human Toxicol.*, 1983, *2*, 424).

HALF-LIFE. Plasma half-life, about 2 hours.

VOLUME OF DISTRIBUTION. About 2 litres/kg.

CLEARANCE. Plasma clearance, about 5 to 18 ml/min/kg (mean 11).

Dose. Not more than 8 mg of ergotamine tartrate in a day or 12 mg in any one week.

Ergotoxine

Ergot Derivative

Synonym. Ecboline

Ergotoxine is a mixture of the 3 isomorphous alkaloids ergocornine, ergocristine, and ergocryptine.
$C_{31}H_{39}N_5O_5 = 561.7$
CAS—8006-25-5

Crystals. M.p. 190°, with decomposition.
Practically **insoluble** in water; soluble in ethanol; very soluble in chloroform; slightly soluble in ether.

Ergotoxine Esylate

Synonym. Ergotoxine Ethanesulphonate
$C_{31}H_{39}N_5O_5,C_2H_5SO_3H = 671.8$
CAS—8047-28-7

Colourless crystals which decompose at 209°.
Sparingly **soluble** in water; more soluble in ethanol.

Colour Test. *p*-Dimethylaminobenzaldehyde—violet.

Thin-layer Chromatography. *System TA*—Rf 66; *system TB*—Rf 01; *system TC*—Rf 62; *system TL*—Rf 48; *system TM*—Rf 67. (*Acidified potassium permanganate solution*, strong reaction; *Van Urk reagent*, blue.)

Gas Chromatography. *System GA*—ergocristine RI 2495, ergocryptine RI 2184.

High Pressure Liquid Chromatography. *System HA*—ergocornine k' 0.4, ergocristine k' 0.3, ergocryptine k' 0.4; *system HP*—ergocornine k' 10.2, ergocristine k' 17.3, ergocryptine k' 15.2.

Infra-red Spectrum. Principal peaks at wavenumbers 1639, 1721, 758, 1534, 1212, 1294 (KBr disk).

Wavelength

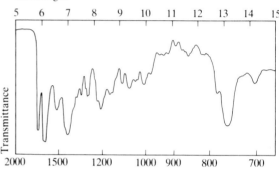

Mass Spectrum. Principal peaks at *m/z* 43, 70, 29, 71, 27, 154, 41, 267; ergocornine 43, 70, 71, 54, 44, 154, 267, 55; ergocristine 70, 125, 71, 91, 153, 267, 154, 221; ergocryptine 43, 70, 71, 154, 41, 209, 69, 267.

Dose. Ergotoxine esylate was formerly given parenterally in doses of 0.5 to 1 mg.

Erythromycin

Antibiotic

Proprietary Names. Abboticine; Bram-mycin; Emu-V; E-Mycin (tablets); Eratrex; Eryc; Erycen; Erycinum (tablets); Erythromid; Ilocap; Ilotycin; Retcin; Robimycin.
$C_{37}H_{67}NO_{13} = 733.9$
CAS—114-07-8 (erythromycin A)

An antimicrobial substance produced by the growth of certain strains of *Streptomyces erythreus*. It is a mixture consisting largely of erythromycin A with lesser amounts of erythromycins B and C.

White or slightly yellow, slightly hygroscopic, crystals or powder. M.p. about 135°.

Soluble 1 in 1000 of water, less soluble at higher temperatures; soluble 1 in 5 of ethanol, 1 in 6 of chloroform, and 1 in 5 of ether.

Erythromycin Estolate

Synonyms. Erythromycin Propionate Lauryl Sulphate; Propionyl Erythromycin Lauryl Sulphate.

Proprietary Names. Eromycin; Ilosone; Neo-Erycinum; Novorythro; Propiocine; Togiren.

$C_{40}H_{71}NO_{14},C_{12}H_{26}O_4S = 1056$
CAS—3521-62-8

A white crystalline powder. M.p. 135° to 138°.

Practically **insoluble** in water; soluble 1 in 2 of ethanol, 1 in 15 of acetone, and 1 in 10 of chloroform.

Erythromycin Ethylsuccinate

Proprietary Names. Abboticin(e); Anamycin; Arpimycin; EES; E-Mycin E; Eromerzin; Erythrocin IM; Erythrocine; Erythroped; Pediamycin; Wyamycin E.

$C_{43}H_{75}NO_{16} = 862.1$
CAS—1264-62-6

A white or slightly yellow crystalline powder.
Very slightly **soluble** in water; freely soluble in ethanol and chloroform.

Erythromycin Gluceptate

Synonym. Erythromycin Glucoheptonate
Proprietary Names. Erycinum; Ilotycin Gluceptate.

$C_{37}H_{67}NO_{13},C_7H_{14}O_8 = 960.1$
CAS—23067-13-2

A white, slightly hygroscopic powder.
Freely **soluble** in water, ethanol, and methanol; slightly soluble in chloroform; practically insoluble in ether.

Erythromycin Lactobionate

Proprietary Names. Abboticin; Erythrocin I.V. Lactobionate; Erythrocine Lactobionate.

$C_{37}H_{67}NO_{13},C_{12}H_{22}O_{12} = 1092$
CAS—3847-29-8

White or slightly yellow crystals or powder.
Freely **soluble** in water, ethanol, and methanol; slightly soluble in chloroform; practically insoluble in ether.

Erythromycin Propionate

Proprietary Names. Éry 500; Propiocine.

$C_{40}H_{71}NO_{14} = 790.0$
CAS—134-36-1

A white powder.
Slightly **soluble** in water; freely soluble in ethanol and chloroform.

Erythromycin Stearate

Proprietary Names. Abboticin(e); Bristamycin; Dowmycin-E; E-Mycin (capsules); Erostin; Erypar; Erythrocin(e); Ethril; Ethryn; Novorythro; Pfizer-E.

$C_{37}H_{67}NO_{13},C_{18}H_{36}O_2 = 1018$
CAS—643-22-1

White or slightly yellow crystals or powder.
Practically **insoluble** in water; partly soluble in ethanol, chloroform, and ether.

Dissociation Constant. pK_a 8.9.

Colour Test. Marquis Test—brown.

Infra-red Spectrum. Principal peaks at wavenumbers 1050, 1168, 1074, 1010, 1108, 1734 (KBr disk).

Quantification. HIGH PRESSURE LIQUID CHROMATOGRAPHY. In serum: erythromycin and erythromycin ethylsuccinate, detection limits < 10 ng/ml, derivatisation and fluorescence detection—K. Tsuji, *J. Chromat.*, 1978, *158*, 337–348.

Disposition in the Body. Erythromycin base is destroyed by gastric acid; erythromycin stearate is hydrolysed in the intestine and absorbed as free erythromycin; the estolate is absorbed as the ester and then hydrolysed. About 5 to 10% of a dose is excreted in the urine unchanged and large amounts of unchanged drug are excreted in the bile.

THERAPEUTIC CONCENTRATION.

Following single oral doses of 250 mg, 500 mg, and 1 g of a preparation containing enteric-coated pellets of erythromycin base to 23 subjects, mean peak serum concentrations of 1.9, 3.8, and 6.5 µg/ml, respectively, were attained in about 2 hours. After a single oral dose of 500 mg of erythromycin stearate to the same subjects, a mean peak serum concentration of 2.9 µg/ml was attained in about 2 hours (K. Josefsson *et al., Br. J. clin. Pharmac.*, 1982, *13*, 685–691).

Following oral administration of 250 mg of erythromycin four times a day to 16 subjects, maximum and minimum steady-state plasma concentrations of 1.7 and 0.45 µg/ml were reported on the third day, compared to 1.34 and 0.58 µg/ml respectively, following repeated oral administration of erythromycin estolate (A. R. DiSanto *et al., J. clin. Pharmac.*, 1980, *20*, 437–443).

HALF-LIFE. Plasma half-life, about 1 to 3 hours (dose-dependent).

VOLUME OF DISTRIBUTION. About 0.7 litre/kg.

CLEARANCE. Plasma clearance, about 7 ml/min/kg.

DISTRIBUTION IN BLOOD. Plasma: whole blood ratio, 0.43.

PROTEIN BINDING. In plasma, erythromycin about 70 to 80%, erythromycin propionate about 90 to 99%, erythromycin stearate about 90%.

Dose. 1 to 4 g daily.

Etafedrine   *Sympathomimetic*

Synonym. Ethylephedrine
(−)-2-(Ethylmethylamino)-1-phenylpropan-1-ol
$C_{12}H_{19}NO = 193.3$
CAS—48141-64-6

Etafedrine Hydrochloride

Proprietary Name. It is an ingredient of Nethaprin and Nethaprin Dospan.

$C_{12}H_{19}NO,HCl = 229.7$
CAS—5591-29-7

Crystals. M.p. 183° to 184°.
Soluble 1 in 1.5 of water and 1 in 8 of ethanol.

Thin-layer Chromatography. *System TA*—Rf 44; *system TB*—Rf 35; *system TC*—Rf 09. (*Acidified potassium permanganate solution,* positive.)

Gas Chromatography. *System GA*—RI 1519; *system GB*—RI 1510; *system GC*—RI 1737.

High Pressure Liquid Chromatography. *System HA*—k' 1.9.

Ultraviolet Spectrum. Aqueous acid—251 nm, 257 nm ($A_1^1 = 10$ a), 263 nm. (See below)

Infra-red Spectrum. Principal peaks at wavenumbers 697, 1051, 1020, 1000, 740, 1115 (KBr disk).

Mass Spectrum. Principal peaks at *m/z* 86, 58, 87, 42, 56, 77, 44, 43.

Dose. 80 to 200 mg of etafedrine hydrochloride daily.

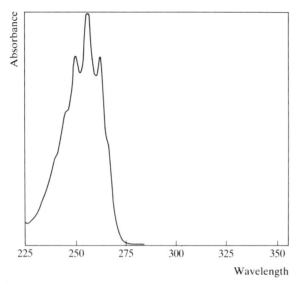

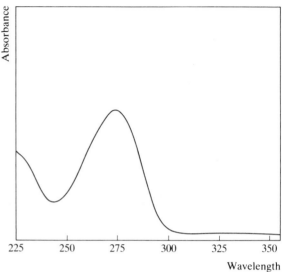

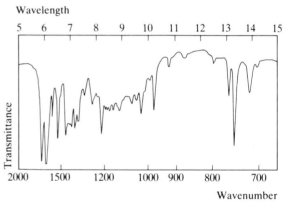

Etamiphylline

Xanthine Bronchodilator

Synonym. Etamphyllin
7-(2-Diethylaminoethyl)theophylline
$C_{13}H_{21}N_5O_2 = 279.3$
CAS—314-35-2

A waxy solid. M.p. 75°.
Very **soluble** in water; slightly soluble in ethanol and ether.

Etamiphylline Camsylate

Synonym. Diétamiphylline Camphosulfonate
Proprietary Names. Camphophyline; Millophylline.
$C_{23}H_{37}N_5O_6S = 511.6$
CAS—19326-29-5
A white crystalline powder. M.p. 198° to 202°.
Very **soluble** in water; soluble in ethanol and chloroform; very slightly soluble in ether.

Colour Test. Amalic Acid Test—yellow/pink.

Thin-layer Chromatography. *System TA*—Rf 54; *system TB*—Rf 12; *system TC*—Rf 39. (*Acidified iodoplatinate solution*, positive.)

High Pressure Liquid Chromatography. *System HA*—k' 1.2.

Ultraviolet Spectrum. Water—274 nm ($A_1^1 = 320$ b).

Infra-red Spectrum. Principal peaks at wavenumbers 1656, 1706, 748, 1543, 1220, 1600.

Mass Spectrum. Principal peaks at *m/z* 86, 109, 30, 151, 87, 81, 99, 58.

Dose. 0.3 to 1.2 g of etamiphylline camsylate daily.

Etenzamide

Analgesic

Synonyms. Aethoxybenzamidum; Ethbenzamide; Ethenzamide; Ethylsalicylamide; Salicylamide o-Ethyl Ether.
Proprietary Name. Trancalgyl
2-Ethoxybenzamide
$C_9H_{11}NO_2 = 165.2$
CAS—938-73-8

A white crystalline powder. M.p. 131° to 134°.
Practically **insoluble** in cold water; slightly soluble in boiling water and in ether; soluble in ethanol and acetone; freely soluble in chloroform.

Colour Tests. Liebermann's Test—brown; Mandelin's Test—green-brown; Marquis Test—red; Nessler's Reagent—brown-orange (weak).

Thin-layer Chromatography. *System TA*—Rf 64; *system TB*—Rf 03; *system TC*—Rf 59. (*Acidified iodoplatinate solution*, positive.)

Gas Chromatography. *System GA*—RI 1542.

High Pressure Liquid Chromatography. *System HD*—k' 0.55; *system HW*—k' 4.6.

Ultraviolet Spectrum. Aqueous acid—234 nm $(A_1^1 = 540 \text{ c})$, 293 nm.

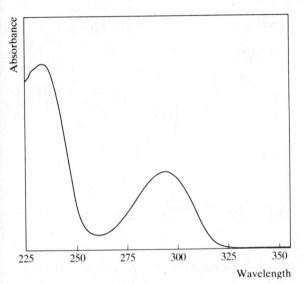

Infra-red Spectrum. Principal peaks at wavenumbers 1634, 1233, 753, 1276, 1114, 1587 (KBr disk).

Mass Spectrum. Principal peaks at *m/z* 120, 92, 105, 148, 150, 121, 133, 65.

Dose. Etenzamide has been given in doses of up to 4 g daily.

Ethacridine   *Disinfectant*

6,9-Diamino-2-ethoxyacridine
$C_{15}H_{15}N_3O = 253.3$
CAS—442-16-0

NH₂

O·C₂H₅

NH₂   **N**

Orange crystals. M.p. 226°.

Ethacridine Lactate

Synonyms. Acrinol; Acrinol Lactate; Aethacridinium Lacticum; Lacto-acridine.

Proprietary Names. Metifex; Rivanol.

$C_{15}H_{15}N_3O,C_3H_6O_3 = 343.4$
CAS—1837-57-6

A yellow crystalline powder. It forms yellow fluorescent solutions. M.p. about 245°, with decomposition.

Slowly **soluble** 1 in 15 of water, 1 in 9 of boiling water, and 1 in about 150 of ethanol.

Colour Test. Marquis Test—orange → red.

Thin-layer Chromatography. *System TA*—Rf 60. (*Van Urk reagent*, yellow.)

Ultraviolet Spectrum. Aqueous acid—268 nm $(A_1^1 = 2062 \text{ a})$.

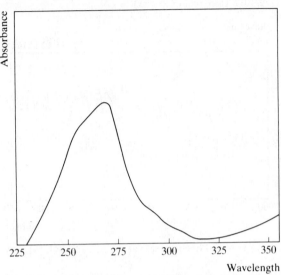

Infra-red Spectrum. Principal peaks at wavenumbers 1113, 1630, 1495, 1226, 1591, 1034 (KBr disk).

Dose. Ethacridine lactate has been given, by mouth, in doses of 200 to 600 mg daily.

Ethacrynic Acid   *Diuretic*

Synonyms. Etacrynic Acid; Etacrynsäure.

Proprietary Names. Edecril; Edecrin(e) (tablets); Hydromedin (tablets).

[2,3-Dichloro-4-(2-ethylacryloyl)phenoxy]acetic acid
$C_{13}H_{12}Cl_2O_4 = 303.1$
CAS—58-54-8

O·CH₂·COOH

Cl

Cl

CH₂:C·CO
|
C₂H₅

A white crystalline powder. M.p. about 123°.

Very slightly **soluble** in water; soluble 1 in 1.6 of ethanol, 1 in 6 of chloroform, and 1 in 3.5 of ether.

Caution. Ethacrynic acid, especially in the form of dust, is irritating to the skin, eyes, and mucous membranes.

Ethacrynate Sodium

Synonyms. Etacrynate Sodium; Sodium Etacrynate; Sodium Ethacrynate.

Proprietary Names. Edecrin(e) (injection); Hydromedin (injection).

$C_{13}H_{11}Cl_2NaO_4 = 325.1$
CAS—6500-81-8

Dissociation Constant. pK_a 3.5 (20°).

Thin-layer Chromatography. *System TD*—Rf 03; *system TE*—Rf 04; *system TF*—Rf 06.

Gas Chromatography. *System GA*—not eluted.

Ultraviolet Spectrum. Acid methanol—270 nm ($A_1^1 = 115$ a).

Infra-red Spectrum. Principal peaks at wavenumbers 1726, 1249, 1279, 1077, 1586, 1661 (KBr disk).

Wavelength

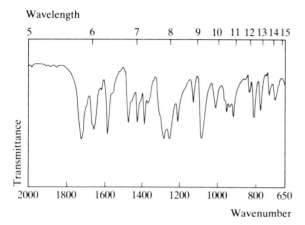

Mass Spectrum. Principal peaks at *m/z* 247, 189, 249, 191, 243, 55, 29, 245.

Quantification. GAS CHROMATOGRAPHY–MASS SPECTROMETRY. In plasma: detection limit 10 to 20 ng/ml—W. Stuber *et al.*, *J. Chromat.*, 1982, *227*; *Biomed. Appl.*, *16*, 193–198.

Disposition in the Body. Readily absorbed after oral administration and distributed to the liver and kidneys. After intravenous administration, 60% is excreted in the urine and 30% in the bile in 24 hours; urinary excretion is pH-dependent and the material excreted in the urine consists of unchanged drug, a cysteine conjugate, and a third unstable metabolite, in approximately equal proportions.

TOXICITY. Thrombocytopenia and fatal agranulocytosis have been reported during chronic treatment.

HALF-LIFE. Plasma half-life, 0.5 to 1 hour.

PROTEIN BINDING. In plasma, significantly bound.

Dose. Usually 50 to 150 mg daily; maximum of 400 mg daily.

Ethambutol   *Antituberculous Agent*

Synonym. EMB

$(+)$-(R,R)-*NN'*-Ethylenebis(2-aminobutan-1-ol)

$C_{10}H_{24}N_2O_2 = 204.3$

CAS—74-55-5

$$C_2H_5{-}\underset{\underset{CH_2OH}{|}}{\overset{\overset{H}{|}}{C}}{-}NH{\cdot}CH_2{\cdot}CH_2{\cdot}NH{-}\underset{\underset{H}{|}}{\overset{\overset{CH_2OH}{|}}{C}}{-}C_2H_5$$

M.p. 88°.

Ethambutol Hydrochloride

Proprietary Names. Dexambutol; EMB-Fatol; Etibi; Myambutol. It is an ingredient of Mynah.

$C_{10}H_{24}N_2O_2,2HCl = 277.2$

CAS—1070-11-7

A white, crystalline, hygroscopic powder. M.p. 199° to 204°.

Soluble 1 in 1 of water, 1 in 4 of ethanol, 1 in 850 of chloroform, and 1 in 9 of methanol; very slightly soluble in ether.

Dissociation Constant. pK_a 6.3, 9.5 (20°).

Thin-layer Chromatography. *System TA*—Rf 30; *system TB*—Rf 03; *system TC*—Rf 02. (*Acidified potassium permanganate solution, positive.*)

Ultraviolet Spectrum. No significant absorption, 230 to 360 nm.

Infra-red Spectrum. Principal peaks at wavenumbers 1090, 1061, 1142, 987, 1050, 1009 (KBr disk).

Wavelength

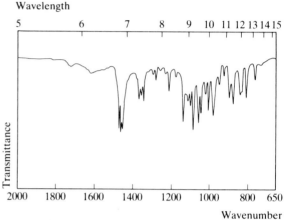

Mass Spectrum. Principal peaks at *m/z* 102, 30, 72, 44, 116, 55, 173, 71.

Quantification. GAS CHROMATOGRAPHY. In plasma: sensitivity 10 ng/ml, ECD—C. S. Lee and L. H. Wang, *J. pharm. Sci.*, 1980, *69*, 362–363.

GAS CHROMATOGRAPHY–MASS SPECTROMETRY. In plasma: detection limit 36 ng/ml—M. R. Holdiness *et al.*, *J. Chromat.*, 1981, *224*, 415–422.

Disposition in the Body. Readily absorbed after oral administration. About 50 to 70% of a dose is excreted in the urine as unchanged drug in 24 hours, and up to 15% may be excreted as inactive aldehyde and carboxylic acid metabolites; up to 20% of an oral dose may be eliminated in the faeces.

THERAPEUTIC CONCENTRATION. In plasma, usually in the range 2.5 to 6.5 μg/ml.

After a single oral dose of 15 mg/kg to 6 subjects, peak plasma concentrations of 3.2 to 5.6 μg/ml (mean 4) were attained in 2 to 4 hours (C. S. Lee *et al.*, *Clin. Pharmac. Ther.*, 1977, *22*, 615–621).

TOXICITY. Toxic effects are usually associated with plasma concentrations greater than 6 μg/ml.

In a fatality due to the ingestion of ethambutol and rifampicin, the following postmortem concentrations were reported for ethambutol and rifampicin, respectively: blood 84 and 182 μg/ml, urine 6800 and 3300 μg/ml; low concentrations of ethanol were also detected (D. B. Jack *et al.*, *Lancet*, 1978, *2*, 1107–1108).

HALF-LIFE. Plasma half-life, about 10 to 15 hours.

CLEARANCE. Plasma clearance, about 9 ml/min/kg.

DISTRIBUTION IN BLOOD. Plasma: whole blood ratio, 0.6 to 0.9.

PROTEIN BINDING. In plasma, about 10 to 40% (concentration-dependent).

Dose. 15 to 25 mg/kg of ethambutol hydrochloride daily; 50 mg/kg has been given twice weekly.

Ethamivan

Respiratory Stimulant

Synonyms. Etamivan; Vanillic Acid Diethylamide; Vanillic Diethylamide.

Proprietary Names. Clairvan; Vandid.

NN-Diethylvanillamide
$C_{12}H_{17}NO_3 = 223.3$
CAS—304-84-7

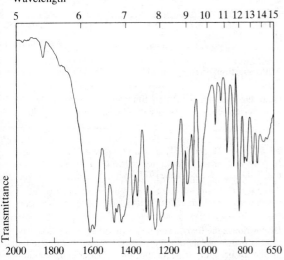

A white crystalline powder. M.p. 94° to 99°.

Soluble 1 in 100 of water, 1 in 2 of ethanol, 1 in 1.5 of chloroform, and 1 in 50 of ether.

Colour Tests. Ferric Chloride—green; Folin–Ciocalteu Reagent—blue; Liebermann's Test—black.

Thin-layer Chromatography. *System TD*—Rf 38; *system TE*—Rf 40; *system TF*—Rf 35.

Gas Chromatography. *System GC*—RI 2409.

Ultraviolet Spectrum. Aqueous acid—280 nm ($A_1^1 = 153$ a).

Infra-red Spectrum. Principal peaks at wavenumbers 1608, 1270, 1585, 1240, 1300, 1543 (KBr disk).

Wavelength

Mass Spectrum. Principal peaks at *m/z* 151, 72, 223, 123, 222, 152, 52, 29.

Dose. Ethamivan has been given intravenously in doses of up to 10 ml of a 5% solution; doses of 40 to 240 mg daily have been given by mouth.

Ethanol

Central Depressant

Synonyms. Alcohol; Ethyl Alcohol.
$CH_3 \cdot CH_2OH = 46.07$
CAS—64-17-5

Ethanol of the *British Pharmacopoeia* is Dehydrated Alcohol (Absolute Alcohol) which contains 99.4 to 100% v/v of C_2H_6O, sp. gr. 0.7904 to 0.7935 (20°/20°). Ethanol (96%) of the *B.P.* contains 96.0 to 96.6% v/v of C_2H_6O, sp. gr. 0.8062 to 0.8087 (20°/20°). Rectified Spirit is ethanol (90%). In the *United States Pharmacopeia*, Alcohol contains 94.9 to 96.0% v/v of C_2H_6O, sp. gr. 0.812 to 0.816 (15.56°).

A clear, colourless, mobile, volatile, readily inflammable, hygroscopic liquid. Ethanol (96%) boils at about 78°.

Miscible with water, chloroform, and ether.

Industrial Methylated Spirit

Synonym. IMS

A mixture of ethanol, of an appropriate strength, 95 parts by volume with wood naphtha 5 parts by volume.

Note. Two other classes of methylated spirits are recognised in the United Kingdom: mineralised methylated spirits and denatured ethanol. Mineralised methylated spirits is ethanol of an appropriate strength, 90 parts by volume mixed with wood naphtha 9.5 parts by volume and crude pyridine 0.5 parts by volume, and to every 2000 litres of this mixture is added 7.5 litres of mineral naphtha (petroleum oil) and 3.0 g of methyl violet. Denatured ethanol is ethanol, of a strength not less than 85% v/v, 98 parts by volume mixed with propanol 2 parts by volume, and to the resulting mixture is added denatonium benzoate 10 µg/ml, or solid quassin 120 µg/ml, or sucrose octa-acetate 4000 µg/ml.

Surgical Spirit (*B.P.*) is a mixture of castor oil 2.5 ml, diethyl phthalate 2 ml, and methyl salicylate 0.5 ml, diluted to 100 ml with industrial methylated spirit.

Rubbing Alcohol (*U.S.P.*) is a mixture of acetone 8 volumes, methyl isobutyl ketone 1.5 volumes, and Alcohol 100 volumes; the mixture contains not less than 3550 µg/ml of sucrose octa-acetate, or 14 µg/ml of denatonium benzoate.

Colour Test. Potassium Dichromate (Method 2)—green.

Gas Chromatography. *System GA*—RI 421; *system GI*—retention time 1.9 min.

Mass Spectrum. Principal peaks at *m/z* 31, 45, 29, 27, 46, 43, 30, 42.

Quantification. ALCOHOL DEHYDROGENASE METHOD. In blood: sensitivity 500 µg/ml—A. Poklis and M. A. Mackell, *Clin. Chem.*, 1982, *28*, 2125–2127.

GAS CHROMATOGRAPHY. In blood or urine: direct injection, FID—B. R. Manno and J. E. Manno, *J. analyt. Toxicol.*, 1978, *2*, 257–261. In biological materials: head-space analysis, sensitivity ethanol 125 µg, acetaldehyde 1 µg, FID—C. L. Mendenhall *et al.*, *J. Chromat.*, 1980, *190*, 197–200.

GAS CHROMATOGRAPHY—MASS SPECTROMETRY. In plasma: sensitivity 5 ng—W. E. Pereira *et al.*, *Clinica chim. Acta*, 1974, *51*, 109–112.

REVIEWS. In breath—M. F. Mason and K. M. Dubowski, *J. forens. Sci.*, 1976, *21*, 9–41. In blood—R. H. Cravey and N. C. Jain, *J. chromatogr. Sci.*, 1974, *12*, 209–213, and P. Fabiani, *Pharm. Biol.*, 1979, *13*, 39–40.

Disposition in the Body. Readily absorbed from the stomach and small intestine after oral administration but absorption may be delayed by the presence of food; rapidly distributed throughout the body fluids. Metabolised in the liver by alcohol dehydrogenase to acetaldehyde and then further oxidised to acetate and carbon dioxide. More than 90% is metabolised and is excreted by the lungs and in the urine, saliva, sweat, and other secretions together with unchanged alcohol. The body can metabolise about 10 to 15 ml per hour. The rate of metabolism may be accelerated following repeated excessive use.

BLOOD CONCENTRATION.

After administration of 15, 30, 45, and 60 ml of 95% ethanol to 8 fasting subjects, peak blood concentrations of 25 to 290 µg/ml (mean 199), 180 to

620 µg/ml (mean 440), 410 to 860 µg/ml (mean 680) and 630 to 1120 µg/ml (mean 860) respectively were attained in 0.3, 0.5, 0.8 and 1 hour (P. K. Wilkinson *et al.*, *J. Pharmacokinet. Biopharm.*, 1977, *5*, 207–224).

After administration of 0.5 g/kg of ethanol to 4 subjects, blood-acetaldehyde concentrations of 0.02 to 0.06 µg/ml were reported after 40 to 80 minutes (J. M. Christensen *et al.*, *Clinica chim. Acta*, 1981, *116*, 389–395).

TOXICITY. The minimum lethal dose is about 500 ml of 50% v/v spirit ingested in about 1 hour. In the United Kingdom it is illegal to be in charge of a motor vehicle with a concentration greater than 800 µg/ml in the blood or 1070 µg/ml in the urine or 35 µg/ml in the breath. Toxic effects are associated with blood concentrations of 840 to **2400** to 4500 µg/ml, and subjects with concentrations of 3000 µg/ml or more are considered to be clinically drunk. Blood concentrations of 2250 to **4000** to 6030 µg/ml have been associated with fatalities. The maximum permissible atmospheric concentration is 1000 ppm.

In 10 fatalities due to the ingestion of ethanol, the following postmortem tissue concentrations were reported: blood 4230 to 17660 µg/ml (mean 7410), bile 1250 to 27950 µg/ml (mean 7860), brain 3100 to 9120 µg/g (mean 4430), kidney 2850 to 10430 µg/g (mean 4830), liver 2450 to 11610 µg/g (mean 4470), urine 4850 to 9400 µg/ml (mean 6190) (G. Christopoulos *et al.*, *J. Chromat.*, 1973, *87*, 455–472).

HALF-LIFE. Plasma half-life, dose-dependent.

VOLUME OF DISTRIBUTION. About 0.6 litre/kg.

DISTRIBUTION IN BLOOD. Plasma: whole blood ratio, 1.2.

SALIVA. Plasma: saliva ratio, about 0.93.

PROTEIN BINDING. In plasma, not significantly bound.

Ethanolamine   *Sclerosing Agent*

Synonyms. Aethanolaminum; Hydroxyethylamine; Monoethanolamine; Olamine.
Proprietary Name. Ethamolin (oleate)
2-Aminoethanol
$NH_2 \cdot CH_2 \cdot CH_2OH = 61.08$
CAS—141-43-5

A clear, colourless or pale yellow, viscous liquid. Wt per ml 1.014 to 1.023 g. B.p. about 170°.

Miscible with water, ethanol, and chloroform; slightly soluble in ether.

Dissociation Constant. pK_a 9.4 (25°).

Gas Chromatography. *System GA*—RI 780.

Mass Spectrum. Principal peaks at *m/z* 42, 31, 61, 43, 29, 27, 44, 41.

Dose. Ethanolamine Oleate Injection (*B.P.*) is administered intravenously in a dose of 2 to 5 ml.

Ethchlorvynol   *Hypnotic*

Synonym. β-Chlorovinyl Ethyl Ethynyl Carbinol
Proprietary Name. Placidyl
1-Chloro-3-ethylpent-1-en-4-yn-3-ol
$C_7H_9ClO = 144.6$
CAS—113-18-8

$$CH\vdots C \cdot \overset{\overset{\displaystyle OH}{|}}{C} \cdot CH\vdots CHCl$$
$$\underset{\displaystyle C_2H_5}{|}$$

A colourless to yellow, slightly viscous liquid which darkens on exposure to air and light. Wt per ml about 1.072 g. Refractive index, at 20°, 1.4770 to 1.4805.

Practically **immiscible** with water; miscible with ethanol, chloroform, ether, and most other organic solvents.

Colour Test. Ammoniacal Silver Nitrate—white precipitate/yellow.

Gas Chromatography. *System GA*—RI 1030; *system GI*—retention time 35.2 min.

Infra-red Spectrum. Principal peaks at wavenumbers 935, 950, 830, 1010, 1063, 980.

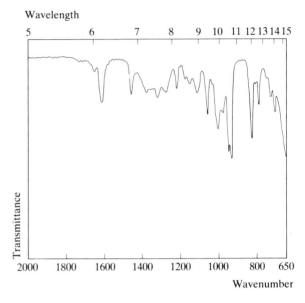

Mass Spectrum. Principal peaks at *m/z* 115, 117, 89, 53, 109, 51, 91, 39.

Quantification. ULTRAVIOLET SPECTROPHOTOMETRY. In blood, serum or urine—J. E. Wallace *et al.*, *Clin. Chem.*, 1974, *20*, 159–162.

GAS CHROMATOGRAPHY. In blood or urine: detection limit 1 µg/ml, FID—H. H. McCurdy, *J. analyt. Toxicol.*, 1977, *1*, 164–165. In plasma or urine: sensitivity 2 µg/ml, FID—R. J. Flanagan and T. D. Lee, *J. Chromat.*, 1977, *137*, 119–126.

REVIEW. For an evaluation of gas chromatographic and colorimetric methods see R. R. Bridges and T. A. Jennison, *J. analyt. Toxicol.*, 1984, *8*, 263–268.

Disposition in the Body. Rapidly absorbed after oral administration. It is extensively metabolised; the major metabolite found in the blood and urine of poisoned patients is 1-chloro-3-ethynylpent-1-ene-3,4-diol; other metabolites include 1-chloro-3-ethynylpent-1-ene-3,5-diol and 1-chloro-3-ethylpent-1-ene-3,4-diol. Ethchlorvynol is highly localised in the tissues, particularly in adipose tissue, and is released very slowly. Less than 0.1% of a dose is excreted in the urine in 24 hours as unchanged drug or its glucuronide conjugate.

THERAPEUTIC CONCENTRATION. In plasma, usually in the range 5 to 20 µg/ml.

Following a single oral dose of 500 mg to 8 subjects, a mean peak plasma concentration of 6.5 µg/ml was attained in 1 hour (L. M. Cummins *et al.*, *J. pharm. Sci.*, 1971, *60*, 261–263).

TOXICITY. The estimated minimum lethal dose is 15 g, although death has occurred after the acute ingestion of 2.5 g. Plasma concentrations greater than about 20 µg/ml are associated with toxic effects. Prolonged use of ethchlorvynol may lead to dependence of the barbiturate–alcohol type.

In a review of 13 fatalities due to overdosage with ethchlorvynol, postmortem blood concentrations were in the range 14 to 400 µg/ml (mean 119) (C. J. Rehling, Poison Residues in Human Tissues, in *Progress in Chemical Toxicology*, Vol. 3, A. Stolman (Ed.), New York, Academic Press, 1967, pp. 363–386).

In 3 fatalities due to ethchlorvynol, the following postmortem tissue concentrations were reported: blood 85, 22 and 66 µg/ml; brain 57, –, 285 µg/g; kidney 54, 63, and 860 µg/g; liver 70, 60, and 507 µg/g; adipose tissue 1040 and 142 µg/g (2 cases) (R. H. Cravey and R. C. Baselt, *J. forens. Sci.*, 1968, *13*, 532–536 and C. L. Winek, *Forens. Sci. Int.*, 1981, *17*, 219–224).

HALF-LIFE. Plasma half-life, 19 to 32 hours (mean 23), increased in overdose cases.

VOLUME OF DISTRIBUTION. About 2 to 3 litres/kg.

DISTRIBUTION IN BLOOD. Plasma: whole blood ratio, about 1.1.

PROTEIN BINDING. In plasma, about 60%.

Dose. 0.2 to 1 g, as a hypnotic.

Ethebenecid   *Uricosuric*

Synonym. Etebenecid
4-Diethylsulphamoylbenzoic acid
$C_{11}H_{15}NO_4S = 257.3$
CAS—1213-06-5

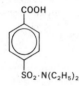

Crystals. M.p. 192° to 194°.

Dissociation Constant. pK_a 3.3 (25°).

Ultraviolet Spectrum. Methanol—246 nm ($A_1^1 = 460$ b).

Infra-red Spectrum. Principal peaks at wavenumbers 1694, 729, 1162, 1282, 1298, 934.

Dose. Ethebenecid has been given in doses of 1 to 3 g daily.

Ether   *General Anaesthetic*

Synonyms. Diethyl Oxide; Ethyl Ether; Ethyl Oxide.

Diethyl ether
$(C_2H_5)_2O = 74.12$
CAS—60-29-7

A clear, colourless, volatile, inflammable, very mobile liquid. B.p. 34° to 36°.

Soluble 1 in 10 to 1 in 12 of water; miscible with ethanol and chloroform.

Anaesthetic Ether (*B.P.*) is highly purified ether containing not more than 0.002% w/v of a stabiliser such as propyl gallate or hydroquinone.

Solvent Ether (*B.P.*) is not so highly purified and is without a stabiliser.

Caution. Ether is very volatile and inflammable, and mixtures of its vapour with oxygen, nitrous oxide, or air at certain concentrations are explosive. It should not be used in the presence of an open flame or any electrical apparatus liable to produce a spark; precautions should be taken against the production of static electrical discharge. Explosive peroxides are generated by the atmospheric oxidation of solvent ether and it is dangerous to distil a sample which contains peroxides.

Gas Chromatography. *System GA*—RI 515; *system GI*—retention time 5.9 min.

Mass Spectrum. Principal peaks at *m/z* 31, 59, 29, 45, 74, 27, 41, 43.

Disposition in the Body. Absorbed into the circulation after inhalation; the blood:gas partition coefficient is high (about 12). About 90% of a dose is slowly exhaled unchanged and very little is metabolised; a small amount may be excreted unchanged in the urine. Acetaldehyde is believed to be a minor metabolite.

THERAPEUTIC CONCENTRATION. In plasma, during anaesthesia, usually in the range 500 to 1500 µg/ml.

TOXICITY. The estimated minimum lethal oral dose is 30 ml; the maximum permissible atmospheric concentration is 400 ppm. Atmospheric concentrations of 2000 ppm may cause dizziness and 100 000 ppm may be rapidly fatal.

In four elderly persons who died after being given ether with other medication, ether concentrations (µg/ml or µg/g) immediately after operation were: blood 600, 3750, 2880, 190; brain 700, 610, 2720, 310; liver 400, 1280, 260, 230; lung 200, 1580, 210, –; in the second case the urine contained 340 µg/ml (J. E. Campbell, *J. forens. Sci.*, 1960, *5*, 501–549).

Dose. For induction of anaesthesia, 10 to 20% of the vapour by inhalation; maintenance, 3 to 10%.

Ethiazide   *Diuretic*

6-Chloro-3-ethyl-3,4-dihydro-2*H*-1,2,4-benzothiadiazine-7-sulphonamide 1,1-dioxide
$C_9H_{12}ClN_3O_4S_2 = 325.8$
CAS—1824-58-4

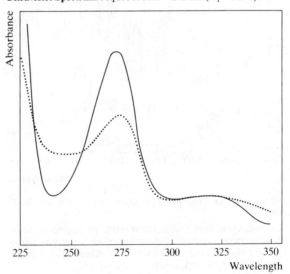

Crystals. M.p. 269° to 270°.

Thin-layer Chromatography. *System TD*—Rf 11; *system TE*—Rf 50; *system TF*—Rf 50.

Ultraviolet Spectrum. Aqueous acid—272 nm ($A_1^1 = 345$ b).

Infra-red Spectrum. Principal peaks at wavenumbers 1163, 1172, 1603, 1312, 781, 1510 (Nujol mull).

Mass Spectrum. Principal peaks at m/z 296, 298, 205, 221, 64, 63, 41, 125.

Dose. Usually 5 to 10 mg daily.

Ethinamate   *Hypnotic*

Proprietary Names. Valamin; Valmid.
1-Ethynylcyclohexyl carbamate
$C_9H_{13}NO_2 = 167.2$
CAS—126-52-3

A white powder. M.p. 94° to 98°.
Soluble 1 in 400 of water and 1 in about 3 of ethanol; freely soluble in chloroform and ether.

Colour Test. Ammoniacal Silver Nitrate—yellow/brown.

Thin-layer Chromatography. *System TA*—Rf 76; *system TD*—Rf 49; *system TE*—Rf 74; *system TF*—Rf 59. (*Furfuraldehyde reagent*, positive; *acidified potassium permanganate solution*, positive.)

Gas Chromatography. *System GA*—RI 1363.

Ultraviolet Spectrum. No significant absorption, 230 to 360 nm.

Infra-red Spectrum. Principal peaks at wavenumbers 1713, 1041, 1694, 1030, 1052, 1250 (KBr disk).

Wavelength

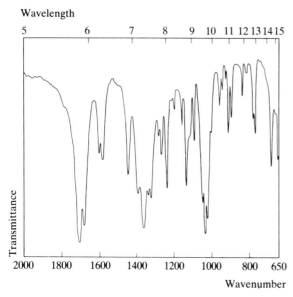

Mass Spectrum. Principal peaks at m/z 91, 81, 106, 78, 39, 95, 68, 43.

Quantification. GAS CHROMATOGRAPHY. In plasma or urine: ethinamate and *trans*-4-hydroxyethinamate, sensitivity 500 ng/ml for ethinamate in plasma, FID—J. W. Kleber *et al.*, *J. pharm. Sci.*, 1977, *66*, 992–994.

Disposition in the Body. Rapidly absorbed after oral administration. Metabolised by hydroxylation to 4-hydroxyethinamate, which exists as stereoisomers, and conjugated with glucuronic acid. About 40% of a dose is excreted in the urine in 24 hours as *trans*-4-hydroxyethinamate or its glucuronide conjugate; only a small amount is excreted unchanged in the urine; 3- and 2-hydroxyethinamate have also been detected in urine.

THERAPEUTIC CONCENTRATION. In plasma, usually in the range 5 to 10 µg/ml.

After a single oral dose of 1 g to 8 subjects, peak blood concentrations of 3.8 to 11.7 µg/ml (mean 6.5) were attained in 1 to 2 hours (J. M. Clifford *et al.*, *Clin. Pharmac. Ther.*, 1974, *16*, 376–389).

TOXICITY. The estimated minimum lethal dose is 15 g but recovery has occurred after ingestion of as much as 28 g. Prolonged use of ethinamate may lead to dependence of the barbiturate–alcohol type. Blood concentrations greater than 100 µg/ml have been associated with fatalities.

HALF-LIFE. Plasma half-life, about 2 hours.

Dose. 0.5 to 1 g, as a hypnotic.

Ethinyloestradiol   *Oestrogen*

Synonyms. Ethinyl Estradiol; Etinilestradiol.
Proprietary Names. Edrol; Estigyn; Estinyl; Farmacyrol; Feminone; Gynolett; Lynoral; Primogyn C; Progynon C.
Ethinyloestradiol is an ingredient of many oral contraceptives—see *Martindale, The Extra Pharmacopoeia*, 28th Edn.
19-Nor-17α-pregna-1,3,5(10)-trien-20-yne-3,17β-diol
$C_{20}H_{24}O_2 = 296.4$
CAS—57-63-6

A fine, white to slightly yellowish-white, crystalline powder. There are two forms, one melts at 141° to 146° and the other at 180° to 186°.
Practically **insoluble** in water; soluble 1 in 6 of ethanol, 1 in 20 of chloroform, and 1 in 4 of ether.
Caution. Ethinyloestradiol is a powerful oestrogen. Contact with the skin or inhalation should be avoided.

Colour Tests. Ammoniacal Silver Nitrate—white precipitate/yellow; Antimony Pentachloride—brown→black; Liebermann's Test—black; Naphthol–Sulphuric Acid—brown-red/pink; Sulphuric Acid—red-orange.

Thin-layer Chromatography. *System TP*—Rf 72; *system TQ*—Rf 30; *system TR*—Rf 40; *system TS*—Rf 40, streaking may occur.

Gas Chromatography. *System GA*—RI 2719.

Ultraviolet Spectrum. Ethanol—281 nm ($A_1^1 = 70$ a).

Infra-red Spectrum. Principal peaks at wavenumbers 1252, 1505, 1298, 1285, 1020, 1060 (KBr disk).

Mass Spectrum. Principal peaks at m/z 213, 160, 159, 296, 133, 145, 212, 157.

Dose. 10 to 150 µg daily; up to 2 mg daily may be given.

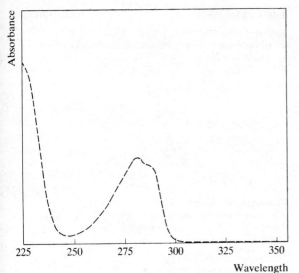

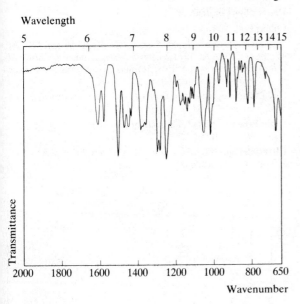

Practically **insoluble** in water; soluble 1 in 30 of ethanol, 1 in 45 of acetone, 1 in 350 of chloroform, and 1 in 600 of ether; soluble in methanol.

Colour Tests. Nessler's Reagent—brown-orange; Palladium Chloride—brown.

Thin-layer Chromatography. *System TA*—Rf 65; *system TB*—Rf 00; *system TC*—Rf 36. (*Acidified iodoplatinate solution*, positive.)

Gas Chromatography. *System GA*—RI 1756.

Ultraviolet Spectrum. Aqueous acid—230 nm ($A_1^1 = 635$ a), 275 nm; aqueous alkali—277 nm.

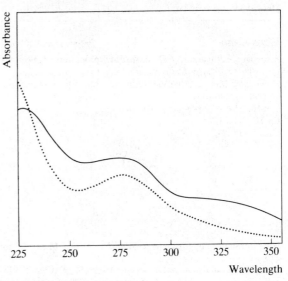

Infra-red Spectrum. Principal peaks at wavenumbers 1588, 808, 865, 1275, 1140, 880 (KBr disk).

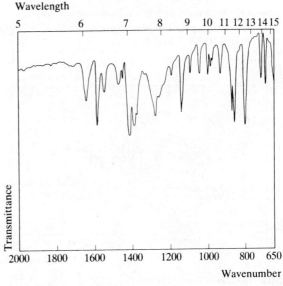

Ethionamide   *Antituberculous Agent*

Synonym. Etionamida
Proprietary Names. Trecator; Trescatyl.
2-Ethylpyridine-4-carbothioamide
$C_8H_{10}N_2S = 166.2$
CAS—536-33-4

A bright yellow crystalline powder, darkening on exposure to light. M.p. 158° to 165°.

Mass Spectrum. Principal peaks at *m/z* 166, 165, 167, 138, 133, 105, 60, 106.

Quantification. HIGH PRESSURE LIQUID CHROMATOGRAPHY. In plasma, serum or urine: detection limit 10 ng/ml, UV detection—P. J. Jenner and G. A. Ellard, *J. Chromat.*, 1981, *225*; *Biomed. Appl.*, *14*, 245–251.

Disposition in the Body. Readily absorbed after oral administration and widely distributed throughout the body. Peak plasma concentrations are attained 2 to 3 hours after a dose. It is extensively metabolised and is excreted in the urine mainly as metabolites with little unchanged drug. The metabolites include ethionamide sulphoxide, 2-ethylisonicotinic acid, and 2-ethyl-isonicotinamide.

Dose. 0.5 to 1 g daily.

Ethisterone   *Progestational Steroid*

Synonyms. Aethisteron; Anhydrohydroxyprogesterone; Ethinyl-testosterone; Praegnin; Pregneninolone; Pregnin.
Proprietary Names. Etherone; Gestone-Oral. It is an ingredient of Trimone Sublets.

17β-Hydroxy-17α-pregn-4-en-20-yn-3-one
$C_{21}H_{28}O_2 = 312.5$
CAS—434-03-7

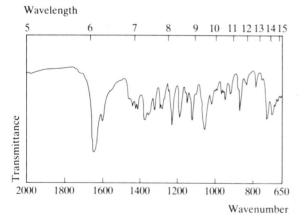

A white, slightly hygroscopic, crystalline powder. M.p. 272° to 276°.
Practically **insoluble** in water; soluble 1 in 1000 of ethanol, 1 in 750 of acetone, 1 in 110 of chloroform, 1 in 3000 of ether, and 1 in 35 of pyridine.

Thin-layer Chromatography. *System TP*—Rf 78; *system TQ*—Rf 39; *system TR*—Rf 80; *system TS*—Rf 00.

Ultraviolet Spectrum. Dehydrated alcohol—240 nm ($A_1^1 = 520$ a).

Infra-red Spectrum. Principal peaks at wavenumbers 1660, 1060, 1235, 1612, 1127, 723 (KBr disk).

Wavelength

Mass Spectrum. Principal peaks at *m/z* 122, 121, 91, 147, 161, 43, 107, 120.

Dose. 25 to 100 mg daily.

Ethoheptazine   *Narcotic Analgesic*

Synonym. Heptacyclazine
Ethyl 1-methyl-4-phenylperhydroazepine-4-carboxylate
$C_{16}H_{23}NO_2 = 261.4$
CAS—77-15-6

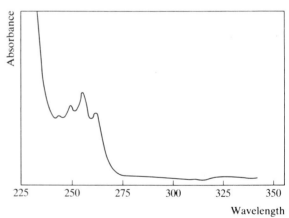

A liquid.

Ethoheptazine Citrate
Proprietary Names. Zactane. It is an ingredient of Ecuagesico, Equagesic, Zactipar, Zactirin, Zactrin, and Zamintol.
$C_{16}H_{23}NO_2,C_6H_8O_7 = 453.5$
CAS—6700-56-7
A white powder. M.p. about 140°.
Soluble in water and ethanol; practically insoluble in ether.

Dissociation Constant. pK_a 8.5.

Colour Test. Marquis Test—orange.

Thin-layer Chromatography. *System TA*—Rf 40; *system TB*—Rf 45; *system TC*—Rf 19. (*Dragendorff* spray, positive; *acidified iodoplatinate solution*, positive; *Marquis reagent*, orange; *acidified potassium permanganate solution*, positive.)

Gas Chromatography. *System GA*—RI 1857; *system GB*—RI 1882; *system GC*—RI 1630; *system GF*—RI 2110.

High Pressure Liquid Chromatography. *System HA*—k′ 3.3; *system HC*—k′ 1.55.

Ultraviolet Spectrum. Aqueous acid—251 nm, 257 nm ($A_1^1 = 8$ c), 263 nm. No alkaline shift.

Infra-red Spectrum. Principal peaks at wavenumbers 1727, 1193, 1094, 695, 1248, 1030 (KBr disk).

Mass Spectrum. Principal peaks at *m/z* 57, 58, 70, 42, 44, 188, 84, 43.

Quantification. GAS CHROMATOGRAPHY. In plasma or postmortem tissues: sensitivity 1 μg/ml, AFID—R. H. Drost *et al.*, *J. Chromat.*, 1983, *277*; *Biomed. Appl.*, *28*, 352–355.

Disposition in the Body. Readily absorbed after oral administration; peak blood concentrations are attained within 1 hour of a dose. It is extensively metabolised and is excreted in the urine.

TOXICITY. The estimated minimum lethal dose is 1 g.

In a fatality due to the ingestion of an unknown amount of ethoheptazine, the following postmortem concentrations were reported: blood 15 µg/g, brain 4.5 µg/g, kidney 2.4 µg/g, liver 10.0 µg/g, spleen 3.1 µg/g (R. H. Drost *et al.*, *ibid.*).

Dose. 225 to 600 mg of ethoheptazine citrate daily.

Ethomoxane   *Tranquilliser*

N-Butyl-8-ethoxy-1,4-benzodioxan-2-ylmethylamine
$C_{15}H_{23}NO_3 = 265.4$
CAS—3570-46-5

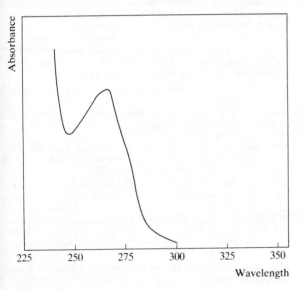

A liquid.

Ethomoxane Hydrochloride
$C_{15}H_{23}NO_3,HCl = 301.8$
CAS—6038-78-4
Crystals. M.p. 196° to 197°.

Colour Tests. Mandelin's Test—red-brown; Marquis Test—red-violet.

Thin-layer Chromatography. *System TA*—Rf 60; *system TB*—Rf 34; *system TC*—Rf 47. (*Acidified iodoplatinate solution*, positive.)

Gas Chromatography. *System GA*—RI 1975.

Ultraviolet Spectrum. Aqueous acid—267 nm ($A_1^1 = 23.5$ a).

Infra-red Spectrum. Principal peaks at wavenumbers 1120, 1279, 1594, 1493, 1097, 1252 (K Br disk).

Mass Spectrum. Principal peaks at *m/z* 86, 44, 30, 265, 41, 180, 29, 87.

Ethopropazine   *Anticholinergic*

Synonyms. Isothazine; Phenopropazine; Profenamine.
10-(2-Diethylaminopropyl)phenothiazine
$C_{19}H_{24}N_2S = 312.5$
CAS—522-00-9

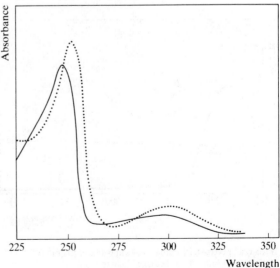

Crystals. M.p. 53° to 55°.

Ethopropazine Hybenzate
Synonym. Profenamine Hibenzate
$C_{19}H_{24}N_2S,C_{14}H_{10}O_4 = 554.7$
A white crystalline powder. M.p. about 188°, with decomposition. Practically **insoluble** in water; slightly soluble in methanol.

Ethopropazine Hydrochloride
Proprietary Names. Lysivane; Parsidol; Parsitan.
$C_{19}H_{24}N_2S,HCl = 348.9$
CAS—1094-08-2
A white crystalline powder, which darkens in colour on exposure to light. M.p. about 210°, with decomposition.
Soluble 1 in 225 of water, 1 in 35 of ethanol, and 1 in 7 of chloroform; practically insoluble in ether.

Dissociation Constant. pK_a 9.6 (20°).

Partition Coefficient. Log *P* (octanol), 4.8.

Colour Tests. Formaldehyde–Sulphuric Acid—red-violet; Forrest Reagent—pink; FPN Reagent—orange→yellow; Liebermann's Test—red-brown; Mandelin's Test—green→violet; Marquis Test—violet.

Thin-layer Chromatography. *System TA*—Rf 67; *system TB*—Rf 64; *system TC*—Rf 47. (*Dragendorff spray*, positive; *FPN reagent*, pink; *acidified iodoplatinate solution*, positive; *Marquis reagent*, orange; *ninhydrin spray*, positive.)

Gas Chromatography. *System GA*—RI 2357; *system GF*—RI 2775.

High Pressure Liquid Chromatography. *System HA*—k' 2.4.

Ultraviolet Spectrum. Aqueous acid—250 nm ($A_1^1 = 881$ a), 299 nm; aqueous alkali—253 nm, 302 nm.

Infra-red Spectrum. Principal peaks at wavenumbers 748, 1248, 1590, 1282, 1568, 1125 (KBr disk).

Mass Spectrum. Principal peaks at *m/z* 100, 101, 44, 72, 198, 180, 42, 29.

Dose. 50 to 500 mg of ethopropazine hydrochloride daily.

Ethosuximide

Anticonvulsant

Synonym. Ethosuccimide
Proprietary Names. Emeside; Ethymal; Petnidan; Pyknolepsinum; Suxinutin; Zarondan; Zarontin.
2-Ethyl-2-methylsuccinimide
$C_7H_{11}NO_2 = 141.2$
CAS—77-67-8

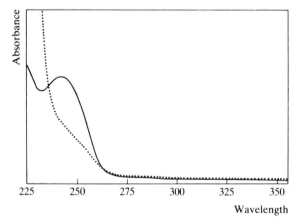

A white powder or waxy solid. M.p. 46° to 52°.
Soluble 1 in 4.5 of water and 1 in less than 1 of ethanol, chloroform, and ether.

Dissociation Constant. pK_a 9.5 (20°).

Colour Test. Koppanyi–Zwikker Test—violet.

Thin-layer Chromatography. *System TA*—Rf 70; *system TD*—Rf 50; *system TE*—Rf 57; *system TF*—Rf 56.

Gas Chromatography. *System GA*—ethosuximide RI 1206, 3-hydroxyethosuximide RI 1320, 1-hydroxyethylethosuximide RI 1370; *system GE*—ethosuximide retention time 0.18 relative to phenytoin.

High Pressure Liquid Chromatography. *System HE*—k' 0.91.

Ultraviolet Spectrum. Aqueous acid—244 nm ($A_1^1 = 9.9$ b).

Infra-red Spectrum. Principal peaks at wavenumbers 1700, 1777, 1208, 1130, 1303, 730 (KBr disk).

Wavelength

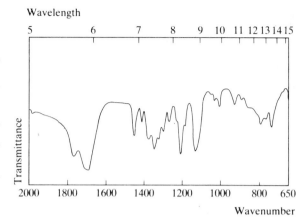

Mass Spectrum. Principal peaks at *m/z* 113, 70, 55, 42, 41, 39, 85, 69.

Quantification. GAS CHROMATOGRAPHY. In plasma or serum: sensitivity 500 ng/ml, ECD—J. E. Wallace *et al.*, *Clin. Chem.*, 1979, *25*, 252–255. In plasma or urine: ethosuximide and phensuximide, sensitivity 2.5 µg/ml, FID—E. van der Kleijn *et al.*, *J. Pharm. Pharmac.*, 1973, *25*, 324–327.

HIGH PRESSURE LIQUID CHROMATOGRAPHY. In plasma or serum: ethosuximide and other anticonvulsants, sensitivity about 2 µg/ml, UV detection—J. A. Christofides and D. E. Fry, *Clin. Chem.*, 1980, *26*, 499–501. In serum: ethosuximide and other anticonvulsants, sensitivity 1 µg/ml, UV detection—P. M. Kabra *et al.*, *J. analyt. Toxicol.*, 1978, *2*, 127–133.

Disposition in the Body. Readily absorbed after oral administration. Metabolised by hydroxylation to 3-hydroxyethosuximide and 1-hydroxyethylethosuximide; the latter is further oxidised to produce 2-acetyl-2-methylsuccinimide; an additional metabolite, 2-carboxymethyl-2-methylsuccinimide has also been reported. None of the metabolites are pharmacologically active. About 25% of a dose is excreted in the urine in 24 hours as 1-hydroxyethylethosuximide glucuronide and about 14% as the unconjugated metabolite. Up to about 20% of a dose is excreted as unchanged drug in the urine over a 9-day period.

THERAPEUTIC CONCENTRATION. In plasma, usually in the range 40 to 100 µg/ml.
After a single oral dose of 500 mg to 5 children, peak plasma concentrations of 28 to 51 µg/ml (mean 39) were attained in 3 to 7 hours (R. A. Buchanan *et al.*, *J. clin. Pharmac.*, 1969, *9*, 393–398).
Steady-state serum concentrations of 31 to 68 µg/ml (mean 49) were reported in 5 young adults receiving daily oral doses of 1 g (E. B. Solow and J. B. Green, *Clinica chim. Acta*, 1971, *33*, 87–90).

TOXICITY. The estimated minimum lethal dose is 5 g. Toxic effects may be observed at plasma concentrations greater than about 100 µg/ml.
In a fatality involving ethosuximide, the following postmortem tissue concentrations were reported: blood 250 µg/ml, liver 280 µg/g, urine 120 µg/ml; phenobarbitone was also detected (M. Rousseau *et al.*, *Bull. int. Ass. forens. Toxicol.*, 1980, *15*(2), 5–6).

HALF-LIFE. Plasma half-life, 40 to 60 hours in adults and about 30 hours in children.

VOLUME OF DISTRIBUTION. About 0.7 litre/kg.

SALIVA. Plasma:saliva ratio, about 1.1.

PROTEIN BINDING. In plasma, not significantly bound.

Dose. 0.5 to 2 g daily.

Ethotoin
Anticonvulsant

Proprietary Name. Peganone
3-Ethyl-5-phenylhydantoin
$C_{11}H_{12}N_2O_2 = 204.2$
CAS—86-35-1

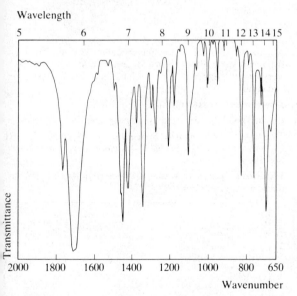

A white crystalline powder. M.p. about 90°.
Practically **insoluble** in water; soluble 1 in 4 of dehydrated alcohol, 1 in 1.5 of chloroform, and 1 in 25 of ether.

Dissociation Constant. pK_a 8.5.

Thin-layer Chromatography. *System TD*—Rf 53.

Gas Chromatography. *System GA*—RI 1800; *system GE*—retention time 0.57 relative to phenytoin.

High Pressure Liquid Chromatography. *System HE*—k' 2.81.

Ultraviolet Spectrum. Dehydrated alcohol—259 nm ($A_1^1 = 11$ b), 265 nm ($A_1^1 = 8$ b).

Infra-red Spectrum. Principal peaks at wavenumbers 1716, 700, 760, 820, 1780, 1100 (KBr disk).

Wavelength

Mass Spectrum. Principal peaks at m/z 104, 105, 204, 77, 78, 133, 51, 132.

Quantification. GAS CHROMATOGRAPHY. In serum: detection limit 1 µg/ml, FID—N.-E. Larsen and J. Naestoft, *J. Chromat.*, 1974, *92*, 157–161.

GAS CHROMATOGRAPHY–MASS SPECTROMETRY. In urine: ethotoin and some metabolites, sensitivity 5 µg/ml—J. Naestoft and N.-E. Larsen, *J. Chromat.*, 1977, *143*; *Biomed. Appl.*, *1*, 161–169.

Disposition in the Body. Readily absorbed after oral administration. Extensively metabolised by *N*-de-ethylation and ring cleavage, 5-hydroxylation, and *p*-hydroxylation of the phenyl ring. During chronic therapy, less than 5% of the dose is excreted in the urine in 24 hours as unchanged drug, together with 5 to 14% of the dose as desethylethotoin, 17 to 35% as 5-hydroxy-ethotoin, 14 to 32% as conjugated *p*-hydroxyethotoin, and small amounts of other phenyl-substituted oxidation products. 2-Phenylhydantoic acid may account for about 10% of the dose.

THERAPEUTIC CONCENTRATION. In plasma, usually in the range 6 to 20 µg/ml.
Following single oral doses of 500, 1500 and 2500 mg to 5 subjects, peak plasma concentrations of 9 to 15 µg/ml (mean 12), 30 to 59 µg/ml (mean 42) and 37 to 75 µg/ml (mean 54), respectively, were attained in about 1.5, 3.5 and 3.5 hours (M. C. Meyer *et al.*, *Clin. Pharmac. Ther.*, 1983, *33*, 329–334).
During daily oral dosing with 30 mg/kg to 7 subjects, minimum steady-state plasma concentrations of 4.5 to 14 µg/ml (mean 10) were reported; following daily oral treatment with 60 mg/kg to 6 subjects, minimum steady-state plasma concentrations of 14 to 50 µg/ml (mean 30) were reported (O. Sjö *et al.*, *Clin. exp. Pharmac. Physiol.*, 1975, *2*, 185–192).

TOXICITY. The estimated minimum lethal dose is 5 g.

HALF-LIFE. Plasma half-life, 3 to 11 hours (dose-dependent).

Dose. Initially 1 g daily, increasing to 2 to 3 g daily.

Ethoxazene
Analgesic

Synonyms. *p*-Ethoxychrysoidine; Etoxazene.
4-(4-Ethoxyphenylazo)benzene-1,3-diyldiamine
$C_{14}H_{16}N_4O = 256.3$
CAS—94-10-0

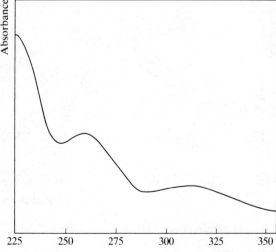

M.p. 117° to 120°.

Ethoxazene Hydrochloride
Proprietary Name. Serenium
$C_{14}H_{16}N_4O,HCl = 292.8$
CAS—2313-87-3
A reddish powder.
Practically **insoluble** in water; soluble in boiling water and in ethanol.

Colour Test. Marquis Test—violet.

Thin-layer Chromatography. *System TA*—Rf 65; *system TB*—Rf 00; *system TC*—Rf 56. (*Dragendorff spray*, positive.)

Gas Chromatography. *System GA*—not eluted.

Ultraviolet Spectrum. Aqueous acid—261 nm ($A_1^1 = 308$ b), 310 nm.

Infra-red Spectrum. Principal peaks at wavenumbers 1245, 1624, 1635, 1600, 1185, 1501 (KBr disk).

Dose. Ethoxazene hydrochloride has been given in doses of 300 mg daily.

Ethoxzolamide
Carbonic Anhydrase Inhibitor

Synonym. Ethoxyzolamide
Proprietary Names. Cardrase; Ethamide; Glaucotensil; Redupresin.
6-Ethoxybenzothiazole-2-sulphonamide
$C_9H_{10}N_2O_3S_2 = 258.3$
CAS—452-35-7

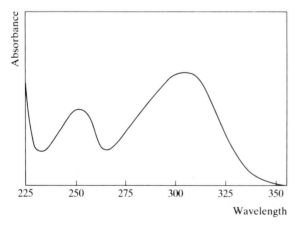

A white or slightly yellow crystalline powder. M.p. 189° to 195°. Practically **insoluble** in water; slightly soluble in ethanol, chloroform, and ether.

Dissociation Constant. pK$_a$ 8.1.

Partition Coefficient. Log P (octanol/pH 7.4), 2.2.

Colour Tests. Koppanyi–Zwikker Test—violet; Liebermann's Test—yellow; Marquis Test—yellow.

Thin-layer Chromatography. *System TA*—Rf 76; *system TD*—Rf 43; *system TE*—Rf 43; *system TF*—Rf 65. (*Marquis reagent*, positive.)

Gas Chromatography. *System GA*—RI 2578.

Ultraviolet Spectrum. Aqueous acid—253 nm, 304 nm ($A_1^1 = 96$ a).

Infra-red Spectrum. Principal peaks at wavenumbers 1170, 1490, 1263, 824, 1224, 1036 (KBr disk).

Dose. In the treatment of glaucoma, 250 to 500 mg daily.

Ethyl Acetate
Flavouring Agent/Solvent

Synonym. Acetic Ether
$CH_3 \cdot CO \cdot O \cdot C_2H_5 = 88.11$
CAS—141-78-6
A colourless inflammable liquid. Sp. gr. 0.894 to 0.898. B.p. 77°. **Soluble** 1 in 15 of water; miscible with ethanol, chloroform, and ether.

Gas Chromatography. *System GA*—RI 596; *system GI*—retention time 9.4 min.

Mass Spectrum. Principal peaks at *m/z* 43, 61, 45, 70, 29, 27, 73, 42.

Ethyl Biscoumacetate
Anticoagulant

Synonyms. Aethylis Biscoumacetas; BOEA; Ethyldicoumarol; Neodicumarinum.
Proprietary Names. Stabilène; Tromexan(e).
Ethyl bis(4-hydroxycoumarin-3-yl)acetate
$C_{22}H_{16}O_8 = 408.4$
CAS—548-00-5

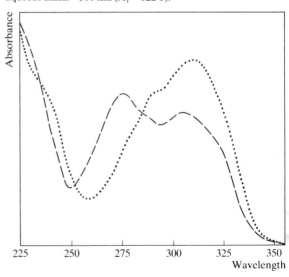

A white to yellowish-white, fine crystalline powder. There are two forms, one melts at about 155° and the other at about 180°. Very slightly **soluble** in water; soluble in ethanol, chloroform, and ether.

Dissociation Constant. pK$_a$ 3.1.

Colour Test. Sulphuric Acid—orange-yellow.

Thin-layer Chromatography. *System TD*—Rf 04; *system TE*—Rf 24; *system TF*—Rf 32. (*Acidified potassium permanganate solution*, positive.)

Ultraviolet Spectrum. Water—275 nm ($A_1^1 = 449$ b), 303 nm; aqueous alkali—311 nm ($A_1^1 = 622$ b).

Infra-red Spectrum. Principal peaks at wavenumbers 1653, 1600, 768, 1560, 754, 1730.

Mass Spectrum. Principal peaks at m/z 121, 318, 317, 173, 120, 362, 44, 31.

Quantification. HIGH PRESSURE LIQUID CHROMATOGRAPHY. In plasma: sensitivity 100 ng/ml, UV detection—M. Arman and F. Jamali, *J. Chromat.*, 1983, *272*; *Biomed. Appl.*, *23*, 406–410.

Disposition in the Body. Readily absorbed after oral administration and extensively metabolised. About 5 to 15% of a dose is excreted in the urine as hydroxyethyl biscoumacetate and only traces are excreted unchanged.

THERAPEUTIC CONCENTRATION.
Following a single oral dose of 300 mg to 4 subjects, peak plasma concentrations of 10.2 to 12.4 µg/ml (mean 11.2) were attained in 1 to 1.5 hours (M. Arman and F. Jamali, *ibid.*).

HALF-LIFE. Plasma half-life, about 1 to 2 hours.

PROTEIN BINDING. In plasma, about 90%.

Dose. Maintenance, 300 to 600 mg daily.

Ethyl Gallate　*Antoxidant*

Proprietary Name. Progallin A
Ethyl 3,4,5-trihydroxybenzoate
$C_9H_{10}O_5 = 198.2$
CAS—831-61-8

A white to creamy-white crystalline powder. M.p. 151° to 154°.
Soluble 1 in 500 of water, 1 in 3 of ethanol, 1 in 3 of ether, and 1 in 3 of propylene glycol.

Colour Test. Ferric Chloride—violet-black → blue-black.

Ultraviolet Spectrum. Methanol—275 nm ($A_1^1 = 540$ b).

Ethyl Hydroxybenzoate　*Preservative*

Synonyms. Aethylum Hydroxybenzoicum; Ethylis Paraoxybenzoas; Ethylparaben.
Proprietary Names. Nipagin A. It is an ingredient of Nipasept and Nipastat.
Ethyl *p*-hydroxybenzoate
$C_9H_{10}O_3 = 166.2$
CAS—120-47-8

Colourless crystals or white crystalline powder. M.p. 115° to 118°.

Soluble 1 in 1500 of water, 1 in 2 of ethanol, 1 in 1.2 of acetone, 1 in 10 of chloroform, and 1 in 3.5 of ether.

Sodium Ethyl Hydroxybenzoate

Proprietary Name. Nipagin A Sodium
$C_9H_9NaO_3 = 188.2$
CAS—35285-68-8
A white hygroscopic crystalline powder.
Soluble 1 in 2 of water and 1 in 3 of ethanol (50%).

Colour Test. Millon's Reagent—red.

Ultraviolet Spectrum. Aqueous acid—254 nm ($A_1^1 = 956$ b); aqueous alkali—295 nm ($A_1^1 = 1390$ b).

Infra-red Spectrum. Principal peaks at wavenumbers 1290, 1673, 1170, 1240, 1610, 1590 (KBr disk).

Ethyl Nicotinate　*Topical Vasodilator*

Proprietary Names. It is an ingredient of Cremathurm and Transvasin.
$C_8H_9NO_2 = 151.2$
CAS—614-18-6

A liquid. M.p. 8° to 9°. B.p. 225°.
Very **soluble** in water, ethanol, and ether.

Thin-layer Chromatography. *System TA*—Rf 00. (*Acidified potassium permanganate solution*, positive.)

Ultraviolet Spectrum. Aqueous acid—261 nm ($A_1^1 = 341$ a).

Infra-red Spectrum. Principal peaks at wavenumbers 1286, 1724, 1110, 740, 1591, 1025 (KBr disk).

Use. Topically in concentrations of 1 to 2%.

Ethylene Glycol　*Antifreeze/Solvent*

Synonyms. Ethylene Alcohol; Glycol.
Ethane-1,2-diol
$HOCH_2 \cdot CH_2OH = 62.07$
CAS—107-21-1
A colourless, hygroscopic, syrupy liquid. Wt per ml about 1.114 g. F.p. about $-13°$. B.p. about 197°.
Miscible with water, ethanol, and acetone.

Gas Chromatography. *System GA*—RI 798; *system GI*—retention time 17.0 min (tailing peak).

Mass Spectrum. Principal peaks at m/z 31, 33, 29, 32, 43, 28, 27, 42.

Quantification. SPECTROFLUORIMETRY. In serum: sensitivity 50 µg/ml—J. M. Meola *et al.*, *Clin. Chem.*, 1980, *26*, 1709.

GAS CHROMATOGRAPHY. In plasma: sensitivity 50 µg/ml, FID—D. W. Robinson and D. S. Reive, *J. analyt. Toxicol.*, 1981, *5*, 69–72.

REVIEW. For a review of assay methods see D. J. Doedens, *Vet. Hum. Toxicol.*, 1983, *25*, 96–101.

Disposition in the Body. Ethylene glycol is metabolised initially to glycoaldehyde and subsequently to lactic acid and oxalic acid. Calcium oxalate crystals are deposited in the kidneys and some oxalate may be excreted in the urine together with unchanged ethylene glycol.

TOXICITY. Ethylene glycol itself is probably non-toxic and the serious toxic effects are due to the metabolites. In adults the minimum lethal dose is about 100 ml although survival has been reported after ingestion of 250 ml. Toxic effects are usually associated with plasma concentrations greater than 500 µg/ml. The maximum permissible atmospheric concentration of ethylene glycol vapour is 100 ppm.

In a fatal case of ethylene glycol poisoning the serum concentration 12 hours after ingestion was 1000 µg/ml and the urine concentration was 2700 µg/ml; in a second fatal case a serum concentration of 7100 µg/ml was found 6 hours after ingestion of 500 ml (D. A. L. Bowen et al., *Medicine, Sci. Law*, 1978, *18*, 102–107).

In 4 fatalities due to drinking varying amounts of antifreeze mixture, the volumes of ethylene glycol ingested and the postmortem blood concentrations were as follows: 150 ml, 80 µg/ml after 36 hours; 300 ml, 560 µg/ml after 18 hours; 500 ml, 600 µg/ml after 24 hours; 1500 ml, 4100 µg/ml after 28 hours (E. W. Walton, *Medicine, Sci. Law*, 1978, *18*, 231–237).

A 51-year-old man ingested 600 ml of antifreeze solution but recovered after treatment. A blood concentration of 6500 µg/ml of ethylene glycol was reported 2½ hours after ingestion; pharmacokinetic studies indicated that the volume of distribution of ethylene glycol was about 0.8 litre/kg and the plasma half-life was about 3 hours (C. D. Peterson et al., *New Engl. J. Med.*, 1981, *304*, 21–23).

A 36-year-old man was admitted to hospital 6 hours after ingesting 500 ml of an antifreeze mixture containing ethylene glycol and methanol; initial serum concentrations were 1900 µg/ml for ethylene glycol and 1130 µg/ml for methanol; the subject recovered after treatment with ethanol and haemodialysis (N. P. Vites et al., *Lancet*, 1984, *1*, 562).

Ethylenediamine Hydrate   *Pharmaceutical Adjuvant*

$NH_2 \cdot CH_2 \cdot CH_2 \cdot NH_2, H_2O = 78.11$
CAS—107-15-3 (anhydrous); *6780-13-8* (monohydrate)
A clear, colourless or slightly yellow, strongly alkaline liquid. It is hygroscopic and absorbs carbon dioxide from the air. It solidifies on cooling to a crystalline mass (m.p. 10°). Wt per ml about 0.96 g. B.p. about 120°.
Miscible with water and ethanol; soluble 1 in 130 of chloroform; slightly soluble in ether.
Caution. It is irritant to the skin and mucous membranes.

Dissociation Constant. pK_a 7.2, 10.0 (20°).

Colour Test. Dissolve 1 ml in 5 ml of water and to 3 drops of this solution add 2 ml of a 1% solution of copper sulphate and shake—violet-blue.

Mass Spectrum. Principal peaks at m/z 30, 42, 43, 27, 44, 29, 31, 41.

Quantification. HIGH PRESSURE LIQUID CHROMATOGRAPHY. In plasma or urine: detection limit 50 ng/ml in plasma, UV detection—I. A. Cotgreave and J. Caldwell, *Biopharm. Drug Disp.*, 1983, *4*, 53–62.

Disposition in the Body. Absorbed after oral administration and rapidly metabolised.

TOXICITY. The maximum permissible atmospheric concentration is 10 ppm.

HALF-LIFE. Plasma half-life, about 0.5 to 1 hour.

REFERENCE. I. A. Cotgreave and J. Caldwell, *J. Pharm. Pharmac.*, 1983, *35*, 378–382.

Use. Ethylenediamine hydrate is used in the manufacture of aminophylline and in the preparation of aminophylline injections.

Ethylmorphine   *Narcotic Analgesic*

3-*O*-Ethylmorphine
$C_{19}H_{23}NO_3 = 313.4$
CAS—76-58-4

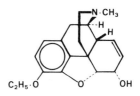

Crystals. M.p. 199° to 201°.

Ethylmorphine Hydrochloride
Synonym. Chlorhydrate de Codéthyline
Proprietary Name. It is an ingredient of Natirose.
$C_{19}H_{23}NO_3, HCl, 2H_2O = 385.9$
CAS—125-30-4 (anhydrous)
A white crystalline powder. M.p. about 123°, with decomposition.
Soluble 1 in 12 of water, 1 in 25 of ethanol, 1 in 1 of warm ethanol, and 1 in 250 of chloroform; practically insoluble in ether.

Dissociation Constant. pK_a 8.2 (20°).

Colour Test. Marquis Test—yellow → violet → black.

Thin-layer Chromatography. *System TA*—Rf 40; *system TB*—Rf 07; *system TC*—Rf 22. (*Dragendorff spray*, positive; *acidified iodoplatinate solution*, positive; *Marquis reagent*, blue-violet.)

Gas Chromatography. *System GA*—RI 2411.

High Pressure Liquid Chromatography. *System HA*—k' 3.7 (tailing peak); *system HC*—k' 1.06; *system HS*—k' 1.45.

Ultraviolet Spectrum. Aqueous acid—284 nm ($A_1^1 = 48$ a); aqueous alkali—281 nm.

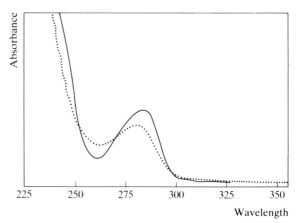

Infra-red Spectrum. Principal peaks at wavenumbers 1064, 1045, 1129, 1499, 1185, 1264 (ethylmorphine hydrochloride, Nujol mull).

Mass Spectrum. Principal peaks at m/z 313, 162, 314, 124, 284, 59, 42, 243.

Quantification. GAS CHROMATOGRAPHY (CAPILLARY COLUMN). In blood, urine or postmortem tissues: AFID—P. Demedts et al., *J. analyt. Toxicol.*, 1983, *7*, 113–115.

Disposition in the Body. Absorbed after oral administration.

TOXICITY. The estimated minimum lethal dose is 500 mg.

Wavelength

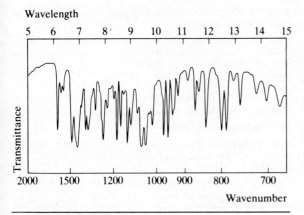

2000   1500   1200   1000   900   800   700

Wavenumber

Ethylnoradrenaline
Sympathomimetic

Synonym. Ethylnorepinephrine
2-Amino-1-(3,4-dihydroxyphenyl)butan-1-ol
$C_{10}H_{15}NO_3 = 197.2$
CAS—536-24-3

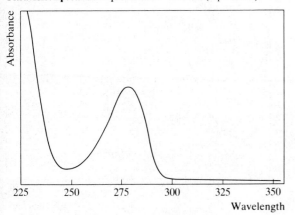

Ethylnoradrenaline Hydrochloride
Proprietary Name. Bronkephrine
$C_{10}H_{15}NO_3,HCl = 233.7$
CAS—3198-07-0
A crystalline solid. M.p. 189° to 194°.
Soluble in water.

Dissociation Constant. pK_a 8.4 (25°).

Colour Tests. Ferric Chloride—green; Mandelin's Test—orange; Marquis Test—orange→brown; Nessler's Reagent—black.

Thin-layer Chromatography. *System TA*—Rf 42; *system TB*—Rf 01; *system TC*—Rf 02. (*Acidified potassium permanganate solution, positive.*)

Ultraviolet Spectrum. Aqueous acid—278 nm ($A_1^1 = 154$ b).

225   250   275   300   325   350

Wavelength

Infra-red Spectrum. Principal peaks at wavenumbers 1500, 1529, 1280, 1265, 1052, 1600 (KBr disk).

Mass Spectrum. Principal peaks at *m/z* 58, 41, 56, 30, 124, 65, 59, 93.

Dose. 1 to 2 mg of ethylnoradrenaline hydrochloride, subcutaneously or intramuscularly.

Ethyloestrenol
Anabolic Steroid

Synonym. Ethylestrenol
Proprietary Names. Maxibolin; Orabolin; Orgabolin.
19-Nor-17α-pregn-4-en-17β-ol
$C_{20}H_{32}O = 288.5$
CAS—965-90-2

A white crystalline powder. M.p. about 89°.
Practically **insoluble** in water; soluble 1 in 9 of ethanol, 1 in 2 of chloroform, and 1 in 6 of ether.

Thin-layer Chromatography. *System TP*—Rf 79; *system TQ*—Rf 50; *system TR*—Rf 94; *system TS*—Rf 99.

Ultraviolet Spectrum. No significant absorption, 230 to 360 nm.

Infra-red Spectrum. Principal peaks at wavenumbers 975, 994, 964, 1299, 1142, 1165 (Nujol mull).

Dose. Usually 2 to 4 mg daily.

Ethynodiol Diacetate
Progestational Steroid

Proprietary Names. Femulen; Lutométrodiol. It is an ingredient of AlfamesE, Anoryol, Conova 30, Demulen, Metrulen, and Ovulen.
19-Nor-17α-pregn-4-en-20-yne-3β,17β-diol diacetate
$C_{24}H_{32}O_4 = 384.5$
CAS—1231-93-2 (ethynodiol); *297-76-7* (diacetate)

A white crystalline powder. M.p. 126° to 131°.
Very slightly **soluble** in water; soluble 1 in 15 of ethanol, 1 in 1 of chloroform, and 1 in 3.5 of ether.

Thin-layer Chromatography. *System TP*—Rf 83; *system TQ*—Rf 61; *system TR*—Rf 95; *system TS*—Rf 99.

Gas Chromatography. *System GA*—RI 2445 and 2779.

Infra-red Spectrum. Principal peaks at wavenumbers 1252, 1226, 1746, 1737, 1012, 1028 (KBr disk).

Dose. 0.5 to 6 mg daily.

Etidocaine
Local Anaesthetic

(±)-2-(*N*-Ethylpropylamino)butyro-2′,6′-xylidide
$C_{17}H_{28}N_2O = 276.4$
CAS—36637-18-0

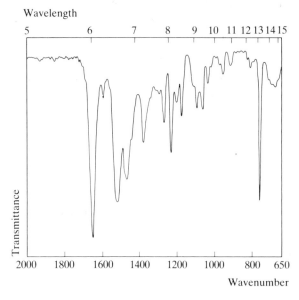

A white crystalline powder. M.p. 87° to 91°.
Soluble 1 in about 7000 of water; freely soluble in organic solvents.

Etidocaine Hydrochloride
Proprietary Name. Duranest
$C_{17}H_{28}N_2O,HCl = 312.9$
CAS—36637-19-1
A white crystalline powder. M.p. 202° to 205°, with decomposition.
Soluble 1 in 10 of water and 1 in 5 of chloroform; practically insoluble in ether.

Dissociation Constant. pK_a 7.9.

Ultraviolet Spectrum. Aqueous acid—262 nm $(A_1^1 = 17 a)$, 271 nm $(A_1^1 = 14 a)$.

Infra-red Spectrum. Principal peaks at wavenumbers 1650, 1520, 765, 1235, 1272, 1180 (KBr disk).

Quantification. Gas Chromatography. In plasma or urine: etidocaine and *N*-desalkyl metabolites, sensitivity 20 ng/ml, FID—D. J. Morgan *et al.*, *Eur. J. clin. Pharmac.*, 1977, *12*, 359–365.

Disposition in the Body. Rapidly absorbed into the circulation after epidural administration. Extensively metabolised by *N*-dealkylation, hydrolysis, and ring hydroxylation. Desethyletidocaine and despropyletidocaine are detectable in plasma. Less than 1% of a dose is excreted in the urine unchanged in 48 hours.

TOXICITY. Plasma concentrations greater than 2 µg/ml may be associated with toxic effects.

HALF-LIFE. Plasma half-life, after intravenous administration, about 2.5 hours, increased to about 6 hours after epidural administration.

VOLUME OF DISTRIBUTION. About 2 litres/kg.

CLEARANCE. Plasma clearance, about 15 ml/min/kg.

DISTRIBUTION IN BLOOD. Plasma: whole blood ratio, 1.7.

PROTEIN BINDING. In plasma, about 94%.

NOTE. For a review of the pharmacokinetics of local anaesthetics see G. T. Tucker and L. E. Mather, *Clin. Pharmacokinet.*, 1979, *4*, 241–278.

Dose. Etidocaine hydrochloride is administered by injection as 0.5 to 1.5% solutions; maximum dose, 300 mg.

Etilefrine
Sympathomimetic

Synonyms. Ethyladrianol; Ethylnorphenylephrine.
2-Ethylamino-1-(3-hydroxyphenyl)ethanol
$C_{10}H_{15}NO_2 = 181.2$
CAS—709-55-7

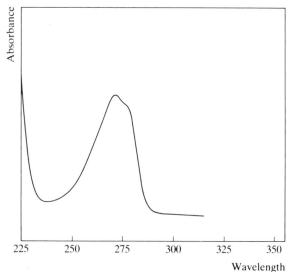

A white crystalline powder. M.p. 147° to 148°.
Soluble 1 in 25 of water and 1 in 15 of ethanol.

Etilefrine Hydrochloride
Proprietary Names. Circupon RR; Effortil; Tonus-forte-Tablinen; Tri-Effortil.
$C_{10}H_{15}NO_2,HCl = 217.7$
CAS—943-17-9
A white crystalline powder. M.p. 121°.
Freely **soluble** in water; soluble in ethanol; practically insoluble in chloroform.

Dissociation Constant. pK_a 9.0, 10.2 (25°).

Colour Tests. Folin–Ciocalteu Reagent—blue; Liebermann's Test—black; Mandelin's Test—grey → green → brown; Marquis Test—red.

Thin-layer Chromatography. *System TA*—Rf 41; *system TB*—Rf 03; *system TC*—Rf 02. (*Acidified potassium permanganate solution, positive.*)

Gas Chromatography. *System GA*—RI 1685.

Ultraviolet Spectrum. Aqueous acid—272 nm ($A_1^1 = 102$ a); aqueous alkali—237 nm ($A_1^1 = 491$ b), 290 nm ($A_1^1 = 167$ a).

Infra-red Spectrum. Principal peaks at wavenumbers 1597, 1068, 797, 1305, 1279, 1222 (etilefrine hydrochloride, KBr disk).

Mass Spectrum. Principal peaks at m/z 58, 30, 59, 77, 29, 95, 65, 57.

Dose. Etilefrine hydrochloride has been given in doses of 15 to 50 mg daily.

Etisazole
Antifungal (Veterinary)

N-Ethyl-1,2-benzisothiazol-3-ylamine
$C_9H_{10}N_2S = 178.3$
CAS—7716-60-1

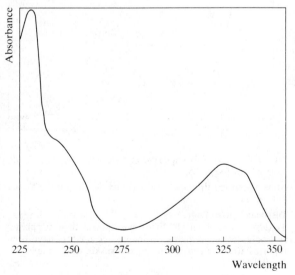

A white to slightly brown crystalline powder. M.p. 78°.

Etisazole Hydrochloride
Proprietary Name. Netrosylla
$C_9H_{10}N_2S,HCl = 214.7$
CAS—7716-59-8
A crystalline powder. M.p. 182° to 186°.
Sparingly **soluble** in water; freely soluble in ethanol and methanol; slightly soluble in chloroform and ether.

Colour Test. Liebermann's Test—red-brown.

Thin-layer Chromatography. *System TA*—Rf 74. (*Acidified iodoplatinate solution, positive.*)

Gas Chromatography. *System GA*—RI 1668.

Ultraviolet Spectrum. Aqueous acid—232 nm ($A_1^1 = 1200$ b), 323 nm.

Infra-red Spectrum. Principal peaks at wavenumbers 1608, 1314, 1292, 772, 706, 1111 (KBr disk).

Etofenamate
Analgesic

Proprietary Name. Rheumon
2-(2-Hydroxyethoxy)ethyl *N*-(ααα-trifluoro-*m*-tolyl)anthranilate
$C_{18}H_{18}F_3NO_4 = 369.3$
CAS—30544-47-9

A pale yellow viscous liquid.
Practically **insoluble** in water; soluble in organic solvents.

Ultraviolet Spectrum. Aqueous acid—284 nm ($A_1^1 = 287$ b), 349 nm ($A_1^1 = 165$ b).

Quantification. GAS CHROMATOGRAPHY. In plasma, tissues or urine: FID—H.-D. Dell *et al.*, *Arzneimittel-Forsch.*, 1981, *31*, 17–21.

Disposition in the Body. Well absorbed from the gastro-intestinal tract and through the skin. The unchanged drug is found in small amounts in urine, together with hydroxylated derivatives of etofenamate and flufenamic acid.

THERAPEUTIC CONCENTRATION.
Following a single oral dose of 300 mg to 6 subjects, a mean peak plasma concentration of 10.0 µg/ml was attained in 1 hour; following topical administration of 6 g to 6 subjects, a mean peak plasma concentration of 0.15 µg/ml was attained in 2 hours (H.-D. Dell *et al.*, *Arzneimittel-Forsch.*, 1977, *27*, 1322–1325).

HALF-LIFE. Plasma half-life, about 1.6 hours after ingestion and about 3.3 hours after topical administration.

Use. Topically in a concentration of 5%.

Etofylline
Xanthine Bronchodilator

Synonyms. Aethophyllinum; Hydroxyaethyltheophyllinum; Oxyetophylline.
Proprietary Names. Bio-Phyllin; Oxyphylline.
7-(2-Hydroxyethyl)theophylline
$C_9H_{12}N_4O_3 = 224.2$
CAS—519-37-9

A white crystalline powder. M.p. 161° to 166°.
Soluble in water; slightly soluble in ethanol; sparingly soluble in chloroform; practically insoluble in ether.

Gas Chromatography. *System GA*—RI 2090.

Ultraviolet Spectrum. Aqueous acid—270 nm ($A_1^1 = 416$ b).

Dose. Up to 1.5 g daily.

Etomidate
General Anaesthetic

Proprietary Name. Hypnomidat(e)
(+)-Ethyl 1-(α-methylbenzyl)imidazole-5-carboxylate
$C_{14}H_{16}N_2O_2 = 244.3$
CAS—33125-97-2

A white or yellowish crystalline or amorphous powder. M.p. about 67°.

Dissociation Constant. pK_a 4.2.

Thin-layer Chromatography. *System TA*—Rf 67; *system TB*—Rf 26; *system TC*—Rf 71.

Gas Chromatography. *System GA*—RI 2008.

Ultraviolet Spectrum. Water—242 nm ($A_1^1 = 450$ b).

Infra-red Spectrum. Principal peaks at wavenumbers 1212, 1708, 712, 1112, 1132, 664 (KBr disk).

Mass Spectrum. Principal peaks at m/z 105, 104, 77, 79, 244, 106, 108, 27.

Quantification. GAS CHROMATOGRAPHY (CAPILLARY COLUMN). In plasma: detection limit 5 ng/ml, AFID—A. G. de Boer *et al.*, *J. Chromat.*, 1979, *162*; *Biomed. Appl.*, *4*, 591–595.

GAS CHROMATOGRAPHY-MASS SPECTROMETRY. In plasma: sensitivity 1 ng/ml—M. J. Van Hamme *et al.*, *J. pharm. Sci.*, 1977, *66*, 1344–1346.

HIGH PRESSURE LIQUID CHROMATOGRAPHY. In plasma: detection limit 2 ng/ml, UV detection—E. O. Ellis and P. R. Beck, *J. Chromat.*, 1982, *232*; *Biomed. Appl.*, *21*, 207–211.

Disposition in the Body. Rapidly distributed after intravenous injection. It is metabolised in the liver by hydrolysis and N-dealkylation to inactive metabolites. About 90% of a dose is excreted in the urine as the carboxylic acid derivative, together with mandelic acid and benzoic acid; less than 5% is excreted as unchanged drug.

THERAPEUTIC CONCENTRATION.
After intravenous injection of 0.3 mg/kg to 8 subjects, plasma concentrations of 0.22 to 0.41 µg/ml (mean 0.32) were reported at 4 minutes (M. J. Van Hamme *et al.*, *Anesthesiology*, 1978, *49*, 274–277).

HALF-LIFE. Plasma half-life, 2 to 11 hours (mean 5).

VOLUME OF DISTRIBUTION. About 4 to 5 litres/kg.

CLEARANCE. Plasma clearance, 9 to 18 ml/min/kg.

DISTRIBUTION IN BLOOD. Plasma: whole blood ratio, 0.62.

PROTEIN BINDING. In plasma, about 75%.

REFERENCE. M. J. Van Hamme *et al.*, *ibid.*

Dose. 300 µg/kg intravenously, with supplementary doses of 100 to 200 µg/kg, as required.

Etorphine
Narcotic Analgesic (Veterinary)

Synonym. 19-Propylorvinol
$(6R,7R,14R)$-7,8-Dihydro-7-(1-hydroxy-1-methylbutyl)-6-O-methyl-6,14-ethenomorphine
$C_{25}H_{33}NO_4 = 411.5$
CAS—14521-96-1

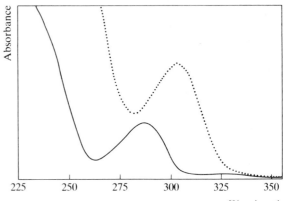

M.p. 214° to 215°.
Soluble 1 in 30 000 of water; freely soluble in ethanol, chloroform, and ether.
Caution. It is dangerous to smell or taste this material.

Etorphine Hydrochloride

Proprietary Name. It is an ingredient of Immobilon.
$C_{25}H_{33}NO_4,HCl = 448.0$
CAS—13764-49-3
A white microcrystalline powder. M.p. 266° to 267°.
Soluble 1 in 40 of water, 1 in 30 of ethanol, and 1 in 2200 of chloroform; practically insoluble in ether.

Partition Coefficient. Log P (octanol/pH 7.4), 1.9.

Colour Test. Marquis Test—blue-grey → yellow-brown.

Thin-layer Chromatography. *System TA*—Rf 73; *system TB*—Rf 07; *system TC*—Rf 61. (*Acidified iodoplatinate solution*, positive; *Marquis reagent*, grey; *acidified potassium permanganate solution*, positive.)

High Pressure Liquid Chromatography. *System HA*—k′ 0.6; *system HC*—k′ 1.11.

Ultraviolet Spectrum. Aqueous acid—289 nm ($A_1^1 = 37$ a); aqueous alkali—302 nm ($A_1^1 = 65$ a).

Infra-red Spectrum. Principal peaks at wavenumbers 1113, 1195, 1205, 1155, 1088, 1005.

Mass Spectrum. Principal peaks at m/z 44, 215, 411, 324, 45, 164, 42, 216.

Disposition in the Body.
TOXICITY. It is about 400 times more potent than morphine; several cases of poisoning, including one fatality, have been reported after accidental pricking of the skin with an injection needle.

Wavelength

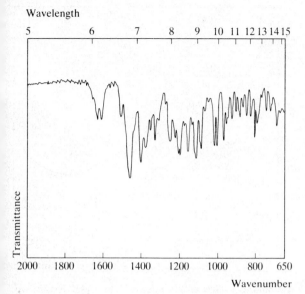

Wavenumber

Use. With acepromazine as a sedative for the control of large animals, and with methotrimeprazine as a neuroleptanalgesic in small animals.

Eucatropine   *Anticholinergic*

1,2,2,6-Tetramethyl-4-piperidyl mandelate
$C_{17}H_{25}NO_3 = 291.4$
CAS—100-91-4

Eucatropine Hydrochloride
$C_{17}H_{25}NO_3,HCl = 327.9$
CAS—536-93-6
A white granular powder. M.p. 183° to 186°.
Very **soluble** in water; freely soluble in ethanol and chloroform; practically insoluble in ether.

Thin-layer Chromatography. *System TA*—Rf 46; *system TB*—Rf 18; *system TC*—Rf 13. (*Acidified iodoplatinate solution*, positive.)

Gas Chromatography. *System GA*—RI 2026.

Ultraviolet Spectrum. Aqueous acid—252 nm, 258 nm ($A_1^1 = 6.8$ a), 264 nm.

Infra-red Spectrum. Principal peaks at wavenumbers 1720, 1235, 1740, 1295, 1145, 1262 (KBr disk).

Mass Spectrum. Principal peaks at m/z 124, 276, 58, 140, 56, 72, 125, 41.

Use. Eucatropine hydrochloride is used as a 2 to 10% ophthalmic solution.

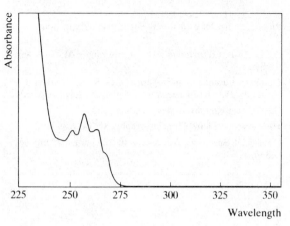

Eugenol   *Essential Oil*

Synonyms. 4-Allylguaiacol; Caryophyllic Acid; Eugenic Acid.
4-Allyl-2-methoxyphenol
$C_{10}H_{12}O_2 = 164.2$
CAS—97-53-0

Eugenol is the principal constituent of clove oil.
A colourless or pale yellow liquid with an odour of clove. It darkens in colour with age or on exposure to air. Wt per ml 1.064 to 1.068 g. B.p. about 254°. Refractive index, at 20°, 1.540 to 1.542.
Practically **insoluble** in water; soluble 1 in 2 of ethanol (70%); miscible with ethanol, chloroform, and ether.

Dissociation Constant. pK_a 9.8 (20°).

Gas Chromatography. *System GA*—RI 1368.

Ultraviolet Spectrum. Aqueous alkali—246 nm ($A_1^1 = 552$ b), 296 nm ($A_1^1 = 262$ b); ethanol—232 nm ($A_1^1 = 406$ b), 282 nm ($A_1^1 = 193$ b).

Mass Spectrum. Principal peaks at m/z 164, 149, 131, 137, 103, 77, 133, 165.

Famprofazone   *Analgesic*

4 - Isopropyl - 1 - methyl - 5 - [N - methyl - N - (α - methylphenethyl)aminomethyl]-2-phenyl-4-pyrazolin-3-one
$C_{24}H_{31}N_3O = 377.5$
CAS—22881-35-2

A white crystalline powder. M.p. 132° to 133°.
Practically **insoluble** in water; slightly soluble in dilute acetic acid.

Colour Tests. Liebermann's Test—red-orange; Marquis Test—orange.

Thin-layer Chromatography. *System TA*—Rf 72; *system TB*—Rf 37; *system TC*—Rf 74. (*Acidified iodoplatinate solution*, positive.)

Gas Chromatography. *System GA*—RI 3059.

High Pressure Liquid Chromatography. *System HD*—k′ 2.5.

Ultraviolet Spectrum. Aqueous acid—243 nm, 279 nm ($A_1^1 = 248$ a).

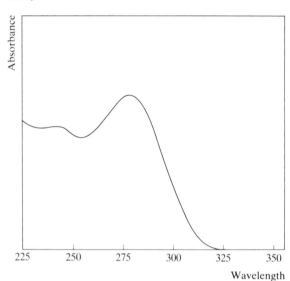

Mass Spectrum. Principal peaks at *m/z* 286, 229, 91, 81, 287, 41, 77, 228.

Dose. Famprofazone has been given in doses of up to 150 mg daily.

Fazadinium Bromide   *Muscle Relaxant*

Proprietary Name. Fazadon
1,1′-Azobis(3-methyl-2-phenyl-1*H*-imidazo[1,2-*a*]pyridinium) dibromide
$C_{28}H_{24}Br_2N_6 = 604.3$
CAS—36653-54-0 (fazadinium); *49564-56-9* (bromide)

A yellow solid. M.p. 215°.
Soluble in water.

Ultraviolet Spectrum. Aqueous acid—283 nm ($A_1^1 = 188$ a).

Infra-red Spectrum. Principal peaks at wavenumbers 1280, 1220, 1160, 1250, 760, 780 (Nujol mull).

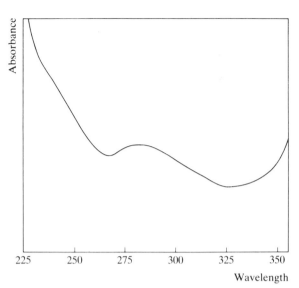

Quantification. SPECTROFLUORIMETRY. In plasma: sensitivity 50 ng/ml—A. M. Pastorino, *Arzneimittel-Forsch.*, 1978, *28*, 1728–1730.

Disposition in the Body. About 50% of a dose is excreted in the urine in 24 hours, mainly unchanged. Extensive biliary excretion has been reported.

THERAPEUTIC CONCENTRATION.
Following an intravenous dose of 70 mg to 5 subjects, the mean plasma concentration was > 10 µg/ml at 2 minutes and 2.2 µg/ml at 1 hour (J. D'Souza *et al.*, *J. Pharm. Pharmac.*, 1979, *31*, 416–418).

HALF-LIFE. Plasma half-life, about 1 hour.

VOLUME OF DISTRIBUTION. About 0.3 litre/kg.

CLEARANCE. Plasma clearance, about 3 ml/min/kg.

PROTEIN BINDING. In plasma, about 17%.

Dose. Initially, the equivalent of 0.75 to 1 mg/kg of fazadinium, intravenously.

Fenbendazole   *Anthelmintic*

Proprietary Name. Panacur (vet.)
Methyl 5-phenylthio-1*H*-benzimidazol-2-ylcarbamate
$C_{15}H_{13}N_3O_2S = 299.3$
CAS—43210-67-9

A light brownish-grey crystalline powder. M.p. 233°, with decomposition.
Practically **insoluble** in water; freely soluble in dimethyl sulphoxide.

Ultraviolet Spectrum. Aqueous acid—289 nm, 302 nm; aqueous alkali—238 nm, 312 nm; ethanol—296 nm ($A_1^1 = 416$ b).

Mass Spectrum. Principal peaks at *m/z* 267, 299, 266, 31, 51, 268, 29, 77.

Dose. Fenbendazole has been given in doses of 1 to 1.5 g.

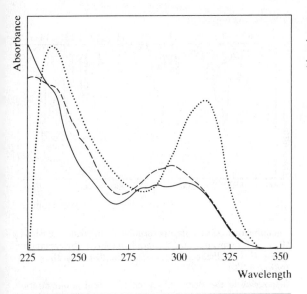

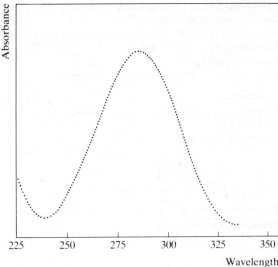

Fenbufen   *Analgesic*

Proprietary Names. Cinopal; Lederfen.

4-(Biphenyl-4-yl)-4-oxobutyric acid

$C_{16}H_{14}O_3 = 254.3$

CAS—36330-85-5

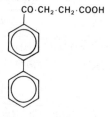

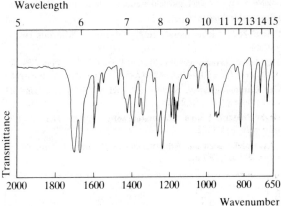

Crystals. M.p. about 180°.

Colour Tests. Liebermann's Test—red-brown; Marquis Test—orange→brown; Sulphuric Acid—yellow.

Thin-layer Chromatography. *System TD*—Rf 18; *system TE*—Rf 04; *system TF*—Rf 30; *system TG*—Rf 09.

Gas Chromatography. *System GD*—retention time of methyl derivative 1.79 relative to n-$C_{16}H_{34}$.

High Pressure Liquid Chromatography. *System HD*—k' 4.0; *system HV*—retention time 0.81 relative to meclofenamic acid.

Ultraviolet Spectrum. Aqueous alkali—285 nm ($A_1^1 = 835$ a).

Infra-red Spectrum. Principal peaks at wavenumbers 764, 1674, 1708, 1242, 1268, 829 (KBr disk).

Mass Spectrum. Principal peaks at m/z 181, 152, 153, 254, 182, 151, 76, 127.

Quantification. GAS CHROMATOGRAPHY. In plasma: limit of detection, fenbufen 50 ng/ml, metabolites (i) and (ii) (see under Disposition) 100 ng/ml, FID—G. Cuisinaud *et al., J. Chromat.*, 1978, *148*, 509–513.

HIGH PRESSURE LIQUID CHROMATOGRAPHY. In serum or urine: fenbufen and metabolites, sensitivity 500 ng/ml in serum, 1 μg/ml in urine, UV detection—G. E. Van Lear *et al., J. pharm. Sci.*,

1978, *67*, 1662–1664. In serum: fenbufen and metabolites (i) and (ii), detection limit 500 ng/ml, UV detection—J. S. Fleitman *et al., J. Chromat.*, 1982, *228*; *Biomed. Appl.*, *17*, 372–376.

Disposition in the Body. Readily absorbed after oral administration, and extensively metabolised to active metabolites. A number of metabolites have been identified including (i) 4-(biphenyl-4-yl)-4-hydroxybutyric acid, (ii) biphenyl-4-ylacetic acid, (iii) (4′-hydroxybiphenyl-4-yl)acetic acid, and (iv) 4-hydroxy-(4′-hydroxybiphenyl-4-yl)butyric acid. About 40% of a dose is excreted in the urine in 24 hours. The major urinary metabolites are metabolite (iii), about 11% of the dose, and metabolite (iv), about 17% of the dose; metabolites (i) and (ii) are excreted in amounts less than about 3% of the dose. Very little unchanged drug is excreted in the urine. Less than 2% of the dose is eliminated in the faeces in 24 hours.

THERAPEUTIC CONCENTRATION.

After a single oral dose of 600 mg administered to 3 subjects, mean peak serum concentrations of 8.1 μg/ml of fenbufen and 64.9 μg/ml of metabolite (i) were attained in about 2 hours. A mean peak serum concentration of 13.2 μg/ml of metabolite (ii) was attained in about 8 hours (F. S. Chiccarelli *et al., Arzneimittel-Forsch.*, 1980, *30*, 728–735).

HALF-LIFE. Plasma half-life, fenbufen and metabolites (i) and (ii), about 10 hours.

PROTEIN BINDING. In plasma, fenbufen and metabolite (ii), more than 99%; metabolite (i), about 98%.

NOTE. For a review of the pharmacokinetics of fenbufen see R. N. Brogden *et al.*, *Drugs*, 1981, *21*, 1–22.

Dose. 600 to 900 mg daily.

Fencamfamin   *Central Stimulant*

N-Ethyl-3-phenyl-8,9,10-trinorbornan-2-ylamine
$C_{15}H_{21}N = 215.3$
CAS—1209-98-9

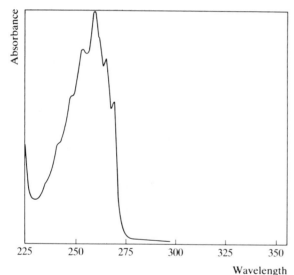

Practically **insoluble** in water; soluble in chloroform.

Fencamfamin Hydrochloride

Proprietary Name. It is an ingredient of Reactivan.
$C_{15}H_{21}N,HCl = 251.8$
CAS—2240-14-4
A white crystalline solid. M.p. 192°.
Soluble in water, ethanol, and chloroform; practically insoluble in ether.

Dissociation Constant. pK_a 8.7 (25°).

Colour Tests. Liebermann's Test—red-orange; Marquis Test—orange.

Thin-layer Chromatography. *System TA*—Rf 54; *system TB*—Rf 62; *system TC*—Rf 34. (*Acidified iodoplatinate solution*, positive.)

Gas Chromatography. *System GA*—RI 1677; *system GB*—RI 1745; *system GC*—RI 2180.

High Pressure Liquid Chromatography. *System HA*—k′ 1.3; *system HC*—k′ 0.72.

Ultraviolet Spectrum. Aqueous acid—253 nm, 259 nm ($A_1^1 = 10$ a), 265 nm, 269 nm.

Infra-red Spectrum. Principal peaks at wavenumbers 708, 756, 1042, 797, 738, 1492 (fencamfamin hydrochloride, Nujol mull).

Mass Spectrum. Principal peaks at *m/z* 98, 215, 58, 84, 91, 56, 71, 186.

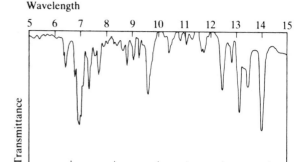

Quantification. GAS CHROMATOGRAPHY. In urine: sensitivity 40 ng/ml for fencamfamin, 50 ng/ml for the desethyl metabolite, ECD—F. T. Delbeke and M. Debackere, *Biopharm. Drug Disp.*, 1981, *2*, 17–30.

Disposition in the Body. Absorbed after oral administration. Metabolised by de-ethylation. About 10 to 30% of a dose is excreted in the urine as unchanged drug and desethylfencamfamin in 3 days. The extent and rate of excretion is dependent on the urinary pH.

HALF-LIFE. Derived from urinary excretion data, about 16 hours.

REFERENCE. F. T. Delbeke and M. Debackere, *ibid.*

Dose. Usually 30 mg of fencamfamin hydrochloride daily.

Fenclofenac   *Analgesic*

Proprietary Names. Feclan; Flenac; Gidalon.
[2-(2,4-Dichlorophenoxy)phenyl]acetic acid
$C_{14}H_{10}Cl_2O_3 = 297.1$
CAS—34645-84-6

A white powder. M.p. about 136°.
Slightly **soluble** in water, but less soluble in acid solutions; freely soluble in most organic solvents.

Dissociation Constant. pK_a 5.5.

Colour Tests. Liebermann's Test—orange (slow), (→ brown at 100°); Marquis Test—red (slow).

Thin-layer Chromatography. *System TG*—Rf 20.

Gas Chromatography. *System GD*—retention times of methyl derivative 1.55 and 1.26 relative to *n*-$C_{16}H_{34}$.

High Pressure Liquid Chromatography. *System HV*—retention time 0.91 relative to meclofenamic acid.

Ultraviolet Spectrum. Methanol—270 nm ($A_1^1 = 72$ b), 276 nm.

Infra-red Spectrum. Principal peaks at wavenumbers 1242, 1258, 1707, 1215, 1100, 772 (KBr disk).

Mass Spectrum. Principal peaks at *m/z* 296, 215, 217, 298, 216, 152, 181, 251.

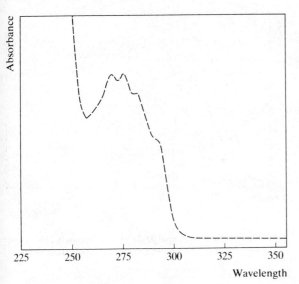

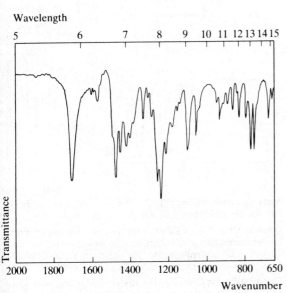

Quantification. GAS CHROMATOGRAPHY. In plasma: sensitivity 300 ng/ml, ECD—R. Henson *et al., Eur. J. drug Met. Pharmacokinet.,* 1980, *5,* 217–223.

Disposition in the Body. Well absorbed after oral administration. More than 90% of a dose is excreted in the urine in the form of conjugates of the drug and hydroxylated metabolites.

THERAPEUTIC CONCENTRATION.

A single oral dose of 600 mg to 9 subjects produced a mean peak plasma concentration of 63 µg/ml in 3 to 4 hours. Daily oral doses of 1200 mg to 5 subjects produced a mean steady-state plasma concentration of 87 µg/ml (R. Henson *et al., ibid.*).

Following daily oral doses of 10 to 25 mg/kg to 18 children for 3 weeks, maximum steady-state plasma concentrations of 52 to 372 µg/ml (mean 120) were reported 2 to 8 hours after a dose (A.-L. Makela *et al., Eur. J. clin. Pharmac.,* 1983, *25,* 381–388).

HALF-LIFE. Plasma half-life, 15 to 40 hours (mean 26).

VOLUME OF DISTRIBUTION. About 0.2 litre/kg.

DISTRIBUTION IN BLOOD. Plasma: whole blood ratio, about 1.7.

PROTEIN BINDING. In plasma, about 99%.

Dose. 0.6 to 1.2 g daily.

Fendosal
Analgesic

Proprietary Name. Alnovin

5-(4,5-Dihydro-2-phenyl-3*H*-benz[*e*]indol-3-yl)salicylic acid

$C_{25}H_{19}NO_3 = 381.4$

CAS—53597-27-6

A yellow powder. M.p. 239° to 241°.

Practically **insoluble** in water; soluble 1 in 50 of ethanol; slightly soluble in alkaline solutions, and in propylene glycol.

Dissociation Constant. pK_a 3.1.

Ultraviolet Spectrum. Aqueous alkali—292 nm ($A_1^1 = 564$ b).

Infra-red Spectrum. Principal peaks at wavenumbers 1675, 1242, 1500, 1615, 1298, 765 (KBr disk).

Dose. Fendosal has been given in doses of 200 to 400 mg.

Fenethylline
Xanthine Stimulant

Synonyms. Amfetyline; 7-Ethyltheophylline Amphetamine.

7-[2-(α-Methylphenethylamino)ethyl]theophylline

$C_{18}H_{23}N_5O_2 = 341.4$

CAS—3736-08-1

Practically **insoluble** in water; soluble in chloroform.

Fenethylline Hydrochloride

Proprietary Name. Captagon

$C_{18}H_{23}N_5O_2,HCl = 377.9$

CAS—1892-80-4

A white crystalline powder.

Soluble in water.

Colour Tests. Amalic Acid Test—pink-orange/violet; Marquis Test—orange.

Thin-layer Chromatography. *System TA*—Rf 55; *system TB*—Rf 03; *system TC*—Rf 45. (*Acidified iodoplatinate solution,* positive.)

Gas Chromatography. *System GA*—RI 2830.

High Pressure Liquid Chromatography. *System HC*—k' 0.27.

Ultraviolet Spectrum. Aqueous acid—275 nm ($A_1^1 = 242$ a). No alkaline shift. (See below)

Infra-red Spectrum. Principal peaks at wavenumbers 1664, 1705, 1600, 1546, 746, 1219 (KBr disk).

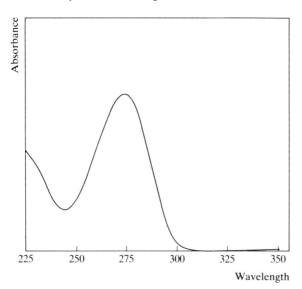

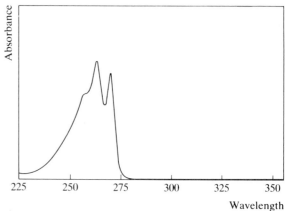

Infra-red Spectrum. Principal peaks at wavenumbers 1165, 1116, 1070, 698, 793, 1202 (fenfluramine hydrochloride, KBr disk).

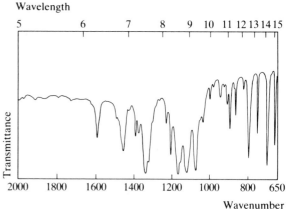

Mass Spectrum. Principal peaks at m/z 250, 70, 207, 91, 251, 119, 148, 56.

Dose. Fenethylline hydrochloride has been given in doses of 25 to 100 mg daily.

Fenfluramine   *Anorectic*

N-Ethyl-α-methyl-3-trifluoromethylphenethylamine
$C_{12}H_{16}F_3N = 231.3$
CAS—458-24-2

CH₃ group structure:

$CH_2 \cdot CH \cdot NH \cdot C_2H_5$ with CH_3 and CF_3 substituents on phenyl ring.

Practically **insoluble** in water; soluble in chloroform.

Fenfluramine Hydrochloride
Proprietary Names. Ponderal; Ponderax; Pondimin.
$C_{12}H_{16}F_3N,HCl = 267.7$
CAS—404-82-0
A white crystalline powder. M.p. 168° to 172°.
Soluble 1 in 20 of water, 1 in 10 of ethanol, and 1 in 10 of chloroform; practically insoluble in ether.

Dissociation Constant. pK_a 9.1 (25°).

Colour Test. Liebermann's Test (at 100°)—yellow.

Thin-layer Chromatography. *System TA*—Rf 48; *system TB*—Rf 41; *system TC*—Rf 16. (*Acidified iodoplatinate solution*, positive.)

Gas Chromatography. *System GA*—fenfluramine RI 1222, norfenfluramine RI 1133; *system GB*—fenfluramine RI 1158, norfenfluramine RI 1066; *system GC*—fenfluramine RI 1621, norfenfluramine RI 1470.

High Pressure Liquid Chromatography. *System HA*—fenfluramine k' 1.3, norfenfluramine k' 1.0; *system HC*—k' 0.88.

Ultraviolet Spectrum. Aqueous acid—264 nm ($A_1^1 = 22$ a), 271 nm.

Mass Spectrum. Principal peaks at m/z 72, 44, 159, 73, 58, 42, 109, 56; norfenfluramine 44, 42, 159, 43, 45, 184, 41, 109.

Quantification. GAS CHROMATOGRAPHY. In plasma or urine; fenfluramine and norfenfluramine, detection limits fenfluramine 5 ng/ml and norfenfluramine 100 pg/ml in plasma, ECD—K. K. Midha *et al.*, *Can. J. pharm. Sci.*, 1979, *14*, 18–21.

Disposition in the Body. Readily absorbed after oral administration and accumulates in the tissues. The major metabolite in the blood is the *N*-desethyl derivative, norfenfluramine, which is active. It is also metabolised by oxidation to *m*-trifluoromethyl-benzoic acid which is conjugated with glycine to form *m*-trifluoromethylhippuric acid. The rate of elimination is influenced by urinary pH and urinary flow. In acidic urine about 23% of a dose is excreted unchanged, and about 17% as norfenfluramine in 48 hours; the remainder consists of *m*-trifluoromethylhippuric acid; in alkaline urine about 2% is excreted as unchanged drug and norfenfluramine; when the urinary pH is not controlled, 3 to 10% may be excreted as unchanged drug and 3 to 14% as norfenfluramine. Up to 5% of a dose is eliminated in the faeces as fenfluramine and norfenfluramine.

THERAPEUTIC CONCENTRATION. In plasma, usually in the range 0.05 to 0.15 μg/ml.

There is considerable intersubject variation in plasma concentrations and it has been reported that the therapeutic effect (weight loss) is greater in those patients who can tolerate higher plasma concentrations (more than 0.2 µg/ml) (J. A. Innes *et al.*, *Br. med. J.*, 1977, *2*, 1322–1325).

A single oral dose of 60 mg administered to 5 subjects, resulted in a mean plasma concentration of 0.06 µg/ml of fenfluramine in 2 to 4 hours and 0.016 µg/ml of norfenfluramine in 4 to 6 hours. Steady-state plasma concentrations of 0.04 to 0.12 µg/ml of fenfluramine were attained in 3 to 4 days after daily administration of 60 mg, in divided doses, to 6 subjects; concentrations of norfenfluramine were similar (D. B. Campbell, *Br. J. Pharmac.*, 1971, *43*, 465P–466P).

TOXICITY. In adults the minimum lethal dose is probably in excess of 2 g but for young children as little as 200 mg may cause death. Toxic effects may be produced when the plasma concentration is greater than about 0.5 µg/ml, and death has occurred at concentrations above 6 µg/ml.

Three children aged 6 years, 3 years, and 1 year 9 months ingested between them about 4 g of fenfluramine hydrochloride. The youngest and the oldest child died; postmortem blood concentrations were 6.5 and 16 µg/ml respectively and liver concentrations were 48 and 136 µg/g; a urine concentration of 60 µg/ml was found in the younger child (R. G. Gold *et al.*, *Lancet*, 1969, *2*, 1306).

A 13-year-old boy died after ingesting 2 g of fenfluramine hydrochloride; postmortem concentrations, µg/ml or µg/g, were:

	Fenfluramine	Norfenfluramine
Blood	6.5	0.75
Bile	64.5	10.2
Brain	42	5.3
Kidney	27.1	1.5
Liver	49	8.5
Urine	89	10

(M. R. Fleisher and D. B. Campbell, *Lancet*, 1969, *2*, 1306–1307).

HALF-LIFE. Plasma half-life, 11 to 30 hours (mean 20).

DISTRIBUTION IN BLOOD. Plasma:whole blood ratio, about 0.74.

PROTEIN BINDING. In plasma, about 30%.

NOTE. For a review of fenfluramine see R. M. Pinder *et al.*, *Drugs*, 1975, *10*, 241–323. For a review of fenfluramine poisoning see K. E. von Muhlendahl and E. G. Krienke, *Clin. Toxicol.*, 1979, *14*, 97–106.

Dose. Initially 40 mg of fenfluramine hydrochloride daily, increasing to 60 to 120 mg daily.

Fenoprofen   *Analgesic*

(±)-2-(3-Phenoxyphenyl)propionic acid
$C_{15}H_{14}O_3 = 242.3$
CAS—31879-05-7

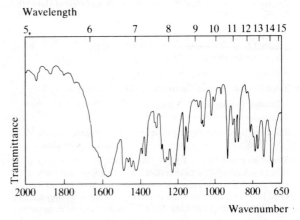

Fenoprofen Calcium

Proprietary Names. Fenopron; Fepron; Nalfon; Nalgésic; Progesic.
$(C_{15}H_{13}O_3)_2Ca,2H_2O = 558.6$
CAS—34597-40-5 (anhydrous); *53746-45-5* (dihydrate)
A white crystalline powder. M.p. 105° to 110°.
Soluble 1 in 400 to 1 in 500 of water, 1 in 15 of ethanol, and 1 in 300 of chloroform.

Dissociation Constant. pK_a 4.5 (25°).

Partition Coefficient. Log *P* (octanol/pH 7.4), 0.8.

Colour Tests. Liebermann's Test—red-brown; Marquis Test—pink.

Thin-layer Chromatography. *System TD*—Rf 42; *system TE*—Rf 09; *system TF*—Rf 53; *system TG*—Rf 16. (*Ludy Tenger reagent*, orange.)

Gas Chromatography. *System GA*—RI 2021; *system GD*—retention time of methyl derivative 1.31 relative to *n*-$C_{16}H_{34}$.

High Pressure Liquid Chromatography. *System HD*—k' 7.9.

Ultraviolet Spectrum. Aqueous acid—272 nm ($A_1^1 = 72$ a); methanol—273 nm ($A_1^1 = 72$ a), 280 nm.

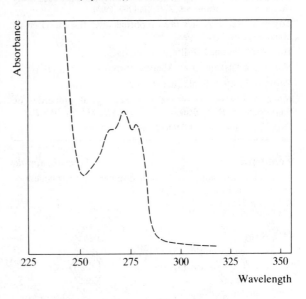

Infra-red Spectrum. Principal peaks at wavenumbers 1562, 1225, 696, 1211, 1268, 1248 (fenoprofen calcium, KBr disk).

Mass Spectrum. Principal peaks at *m/z* 197, 241, 198, 77, 242, 104, 91, 103.

Quantification. GAS CHROMATOGRAPHY. In plasma: sensitivity 250 ng/ml, FID—J. F. Nash *et al.*, *J. pharm. Sci.*, 1971, *60*, 1062–1064.

HIGH PRESSURE LIQUID CHROMATOGRAPHY. In plasma: sensitivity 500 ng/ml, UV detection—R. J. Bopp *et al.*, *J. pharm. Sci.*, 1981, *70*, 507–509.

Disposition in the Body. Readily absorbed after oral administration. About 90% of a dose is excreted in the urine in 24 hours, about 3% of the excreted material being unchanged drug, about 45% fenoprofen glucuronide, about 42% 4-hydroxyfenoprofen glucuronide, and about 2% free 4-hydroxyfenoprofen. About 2% of a dose is eliminated in the faeces in 24 hours.

THERAPEUTIC CONCENTRATION.

After a single oral dose of 250 mg administered to 4 subjects, peak plasma concentrations of 23 to 31 µg/ml (mean 27) were attained in 0.5 to 2 hours (A. Rubin *et al.*, *J. pharm. Sci.*, 1971, *60*, 1797–1801).

TOXICITY. Recovery has been reported after the ingestion of about 60 g.

HALF-LIFE. Plasma half-life, 2 to 3 hours.

VOLUME OF DISTRIBUTION. About 0.1 litre/kg.

PROTEIN BINDING. In plasma, about 99%.

NOTE. For a review of the pharmacological properties of fenoprofen see R. N. Brogden *et al.*, *Drugs*, 1977, *13*, 241–265.

Dose. The equivalent of 0.9 to 2.4 g of fenoprofen daily.

Fenoterol   *Sympathomimetic*

1 - (3,5 - Dihydroxyphenyl) - 2 - (4 - hydroxy - α - methylphenethyl-amino)ethanol
$C_{17}H_{21}NO_4 = 303.4$
CAS—13392-18-2

Fenoterol Hydrobromide
Proprietary Names. Berotec; Partusisten. It is an ingredient of Duovent.
$C_{17}H_{21}NO_4,HBr = 384.3$
CAS—1944-12-3
A white crystalline powder. M.p. about 230°, with decomposition.
Soluble 1 in 10 of water and 1 in 11 of ethanol; practically insoluble in chloroform and ether.

Dissociation Constant. pK_a 8.5, 10.0.

High Pressure Liquid Chromatography. *System HA*—k′ 0.7.

Ultraviolet Spectrum. Aqueous acid—275 nm ($A_1^1 = 107$ a); aqueous alkali—295 nm ($A_1^1 = 190$ b).

Infra-red Spectrum. Principal peaks at wavenumbers 1605, 1510, 700, 1160, 1575, 1200 (fenoterol hydrobromide, KBr disk).

Disposition in the Body. Rapidly but incompletely absorbed after inhalation or oral administration. It undergoes extensive first-pass metabolism by sulphate conjugation. About 35% of an oral dose is excreted in the urine in 24 hours, mainly as the inactive sulphate conjugate, and less than 2% as unchanged drug; about 40% of an oral dose is eliminated in the faeces.

THERAPEUTIC CONCENTRATION.

After oral administration of 5 mg of tritiated fenoterol to 8 subjects, peak plasma radioactivity equivalent to about 0.04 µg/ml of fenoterol was attained in 2 hours; most of the radioactivity was due to metabolites. Following inhalation of a 200-µg or 500-µg metered-dose by 3 subjects, peak plasma radioactivity equivalent to about 0.0003 to 0.0004 µg/ml of fenoterol was reported (L. Buchelt and K. L. Rominger, *Med. Proc.*, 1972, *18*, 15–20).

HALF-LIFE. Plasma half-life, about 6 to 7 hours.

NOTE. For a review of the pharmacokinetics of fenoterol see R. C. Heel *et al.*, *Drugs*, 1978, *15*, 3–32.

Dose. Up to 360 µg of fenoterol hydrobromide every 4 hours, by aerosol inhalation; 15 to 20 mg daily has been given by mouth.

Fenpipramide   *Antispasmodic (Veterinary)*

2,2-Diphenyl-4-piperidinobutyramide
$C_{21}H_{26}N_2O = 322.4$
CAS—77-01-0

White crystals. M.p. 188°.
Practically **insoluble** in water; soluble in chloroform.

Fenpipramide Hydrochloride
Proprietary Name. It is an ingredient of Efosin.
$C_{21}H_{26}N_2O,HCl,H_2O = 376.9$
CAS—14007-53-5 (anhydrous)
A white crystalline powder.
Soluble in water, ethanol, and chloroform.

Colour Test. Liebermann's Test—orange.

Thin-layer Chromatography. *System TA*—Rf 54; *system TB*—Rf 05; *system TC*—Rf 16. (*Acidified iodoplatinate solution*, positive.)

Ultraviolet Spectrum. Aqueous acid—253 nm, 259 nm ($A_1^1 = 12$ a), 265 nm.

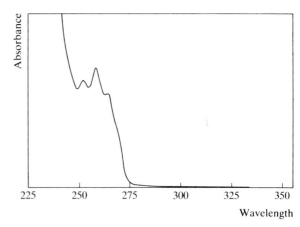

Infra-red Spectrum. Principal peaks at wavenumbers 1618, 1684, 695, 712, 702, 764 (KBr disk).

Mass Spectrum. Principal peaks at *m/z* 98, 112, 99, 55, 42, 41, 211, 84.

Fenpiprane   *Antispasmodic (Veterinary)*

1-(3,3-Diphenylpropyl)piperidine
$C_{20}H_{25}N = 279.4$
CAS—3540-95-2

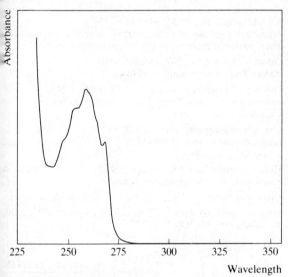

Crystals. M.p. 41° to 43°.
Practically **insoluble** in water; soluble in chloroform.

Fenpiprane Hydrochloride
Proprietary Name. It is an ingredient of Efosin.
$C_{20}H_{25}N,HCl = 315.9$
CAS—3329-14-4
A white crystalline powder. M.p. 211° to 213°.
Soluble in water and chloroform.

Colour Tests. Liebermann's Test—brown; Mandelin's Test—green; Marquis Test—red.

Thin-layer Chromatography. *System TA*—Rf 61. (*Acidified iodoplatinate solution*, positive.)

Ultraviolet Spectrum. Aqueous acid—259 nm ($A_1^1 = 16.7$ a), 268 nm.

Infra-red Spectrum. Principal peaks at wavenumbers 1492, 1631, 1092, 698, 1010, 1600 (KBr disk).

Fenproporex   *Anorectic*

Synonym. N-2-Cyanoethylamphetamine
Proprietary Names. Appetitzügler (hydrochloride); Perphoxen(e) (hydrochloride).
(±)-3-(α-Methylphenethylamino)propionitrile
$C_{12}H_{16}N_2 = 188.3$
CAS—15686-61-0; 18305-29-8 (hydrochloride)

$$CH_3$$
$$C_6H_5 \cdot CH_2 \cdot CH \cdot NH \cdot [CH_2]_2 \cdot CN$$

Gas Chromatography. *System GA*—RI 1619.

Ultraviolet Spectrum. Aqueous acid—252 nm, 257 nm, 263 nm.

Infra-red Spectrum. Principal peaks at wavenumbers 745, 1583, 697, 1019, 707, 1139 (fenproporex hydrochloride, KBr disk).

Dose. Fenproporex has been given as the hydrochloride in usual doses equivalent to 20 mg of the base daily.

Fentanyl   *Narcotic Analgesic*

Synonym. Phentanyl
N-(1-Phenethyl-4-piperidyl)propionanilide
$C_{22}H_{28}N_2O = 336.5$
CAS—437-38-7

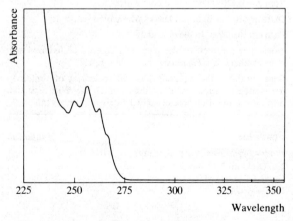

Crystals. M.p. 83° to 84°.
Sparingly **soluble** in water.

Fentanyl Citrate
Proprietary Names. Fentanest; Leptanal; Sublimaze. It is an ingredient of Hypnorm (vet.), Innovar, and Thalamonal.
$C_{22}H_{28}N_2O,C_6H_8O_7 = 528.6$
CAS—990-73-8
White granules or a white glistening crystalline powder. M.p. 147° to 152°.
Soluble 1 in 40 of water, 1 in 140 of ethanol, 1 in 350 of chloroform, and 1 in 10 of methanol; slightly soluble in ether.
Caution. Avoid contact with skin and the inhalation of particles of fentanyl citrate.

Partition Coefficient. Log *P* (octanol/pH 7.4), 2.3.

Colour Test. Marquis Test—orange.

Thin-layer Chromatography. *System TA*—Rf 70; *system TB*—Rf 45; *system TC*—Rf 74. (*Acidified iodoplatinate solution*, positive.)

Gas Chromatography. *System GA*—RI 2650.

High Pressure Liquid Chromatography. *System HA*—k' 0.8; *system HC*—k' 1.11.

Ultraviolet Spectrum. Aqueous acid—251 nm, 257 nm ($A_1^1 = 13$ a), 263 nm.

Infra-red Spectrum. Principal peaks at wavenumbers 1660, 701, 1493, 1263, 1273, 1236 (KBr disk). (See below)

Mass Spectrum. Principal peaks at *m/z* 245, 146, 42, 189, 44, 105, 29, 43.

Wavelength

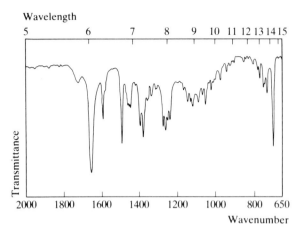

Transmittance

Wavenumber

Quantification. GAS CHROMATOGRAPHY. In plasma: sensitivity 20 pg/ml, AFID—J. A. Phipps *et al.*, *J. Chromat.*, 1983, *272*; *Biomed. Appl.*, *23*, 392–395.

RADIOIMMUNOASSAY. In plasma: sensitivity 60 pg/ml—M. Michiels *et al.*, *Eur. J. clin. Pharmac.*, 1977, *12*, 153–158.

Disposition in the Body. Rapidly metabolised in the liver. Two metabolites, norfentanyl and despropionylfentanyl, have been detected in plasma at concentrations similar to those of fentanyl. About 70% of a dose is excreted in the urine in 72 hours, mostly as metabolites, with about 10 to 20% of a dose being excreted as unchanged drug in 48 hours. About 9% of a dose is eliminated in the faeces.

THERAPEUTIC CONCENTRATION.

Following intravenous injection of 0.2 mg to 6 subjects, plasma concentrations of about 0.002 μg/ml were reported after 2 minutes (M. Michiels *et al.*, *ibid.*).

Following a single intravenous dose of 60 μg/kg to 5 subjects, plasma concentrations of 0.03 to 0.2 μg/ml (mean 0.1) were reported at 1 minute, decreasing to 0.01 μg/ml at 1 hour (J. G. Bovill and P. S. Sebel, *Br. J. Anaesth.*, 1980, *52*, 795–801).

TOXICITY. The estimated minimum lethal dose is 2 mg.

HALF-LIFE. Plasma half-life, about 1 to 6 hours (dose-dependent).

VOLUME OF DISTRIBUTION. About 3 litres/kg.

DISTRIBUTION IN BLOOD. Plasma:whole blood ratio, 1.0.

PROTEIN BINDING. In plasma, about 80%.

NOTE. For a review of the pharmacokinetics of fentanyl see L. E. Mather, *Clin. Pharmacokinet.*, 1983, *8*, 422–446.

Dose. Initially, the equivalent of 50 to 200 μg of fentanyl, intravenously; supplementary doses of 50 μg. With assisted respiration, an initial dose of up to 3500 μg may be given.

Fenticlor   *Antifungal*

Proprietary Names. ADT; Antimyk.
4,4′-Dichloro-2,2′-thiodiphenol
$C_{12}H_8Cl_2O_2S = 287.2$
CAS—97-24-5

A white crystalline powder. M.p. 176°.
Practically **insoluble** in water; freely soluble in ethanol.

Infra-red Spectrum. Principal peaks at wavenumbers 1269, 825, 1209, 818, 889, 1104.

Use. Fenticlor has been applied topically in concentrations of up to 2%.

Feprazone   *Analgesic*

Synonyms. Phenylprenazone; Prenazone.
Proprietary Names. Methrazone; Zepelin.
4-(3-Methylbut-2-enyl)-1,2-diphenylpyrazolidine-3,5-dione
$C_{20}H_{20}N_2O_2 = 320.4$
CAS—30748-29-9

A white crystalline powder. M.p. about 157°.
Practically **insoluble** in water; slightly soluble in ethanol and ether; soluble in acetone; readily soluble in chloroform.

Colour Tests. *p*-Dimethylaminobenzaldehyde—red/-; Liebermann's Test—brown-orange (→ brown at 100°).

Thin-layer Chromatography. *System TG*—Rf 45. (*Chromic acid* solution, yellow; *Ludy Tenger reagent*, orange; *mercurous nitrate* spray, positive.)

Gas Chromatography. *System GA*—RI 2380; *system GD*—retention time of methyl derivative 1.81 relative to *n*-$C_{16}H_{34}$; *system GF*—RI 2800.

High Pressure Liquid Chromatography. *System HV*—retention time 0.92 relative to meclofenamic acid.

Ultraviolet Spectrum. Methanolic alkali—266 nm ($A_1^1 = 700$ b).

Infra-red Spectrum. Principal peaks at wavenumbers 1715, 1300, 767, 1745, 715, 703 (KBr disk).

Wavelength

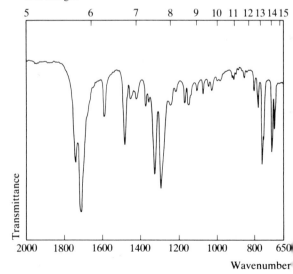

Transmittance

Wavenumber

Mass Spectrum. Principal peaks at *m/z* 183, 77, 252, 320, 184, 41, 69, 51.

Quantification. HIGH PRESSURE LIQUID CHROMATOGRAPHY. In plasma: detection limit, feprazone 100 ng/ml, 4-(3-hydroxy-methyl)feprazone 200 ng/ml, UV detection—H. Spahn and E. Mutschler, *J. Chromat.*, 1982, *232*; *Biomed. Appl.*, *21*, 145–153.

Disposition in the Body. Absorbed after oral administration. Metabolised by hydroxylation to 4-(3-hydroxymethyl)feprazone. Less than 1% of a dose is excreted unchanged in the urine.

THERAPEUTIC CONCENTRATION.

Following a single oral dose of 400 mg to 8 subjects, peak plasma concentrations of 30.2 to 54.7 µg/ml (mean 40.6) were attained in 4 to 8 hours; peak plasma concentrations of 1.09 to 3.60 µg/ml (mean 1.9) of the 4-(3-hydroxymethyl) metabolite were reported at about 27 hours (H. Spahn and E. Mutschler, *Arzneimittel-Forsch.*, 1985, *35*, 167–169).

HALF-LIFE. Plasma half-life, 6 to 30 hours (mean 20).

PROTEIN BINDING. In plasma, 90 to 99%.

Dose. 200 to 600 mg daily.

Flavoxate   *Antispasmodic*

2-Piperidinoethyl 3-methyl-4-oxo-2-phenyl-4*H*-chromene-8-carboxylate

$C_{24}H_{25}NO_4 = 391.5$

CAS—15301-69-6

Soluble in chloroform.

Flavoxate Hydrochloride

Proprietary Names. Genurin; Spasuret; Urispas.

$C_{24}H_{25}NO_4,HCl = 427.9$

CAS—3717-88-2

A creamy-white crystalline powder. M.p. 230° to 236°.

Soluble 1 in 150 of water, 1 in 500 of ethanol, 1 in 40 of chloroform, and 1 in 120 of methanol; practically insoluble in ether.

Colour Test. Liebermann's Test—yellow.

Thin-layer Chromatography. *System TA*—Rf 62; *system TB*—Rf 36; *system TC*—Rf 67. (*Acidified iodoplatinate solution*, strong reaction.)

Gas Chromatography. *System GA*—not eluted.

High Pressure Liquid Chromatography. *System HA*—k' 2.2.

Ultraviolet Spectrum. Aqueous acid—241 nm ($A_1^1 = 360$ b), 293 nm, 320 nm.

Infra-red Spectrum. Principal peaks at wavenumbers 1633, 1121, 1718, 1255, 759, 1272 (KBr disk).

Mass Spectrum. Principal peaks at *m/z* 98, 111, 99, 147, 55, 41, 42, 96.

Dose. 300 to 800 mg of flavoxate hydrochloride daily.

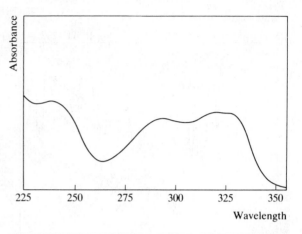

Floctafenine   *Analgesic*

Proprietary Name. Idarac

2,3 - Dihydroxypropyl *N* - (8 - trifluoromethyl - 4 - quinolyl)-anthranilate

$C_{20}H_{17}F_3N_2O_4 = 406.4$

CAS—23779-99-9

A yellowish-white powder. M.p. 175° to 179°.

Slightly **soluble** in water; soluble in ethanol; very slightly soluble in chloroform and ether; freely soluble in dimethylformamide and pyridine.

Ultraviolet Spectrum. Aqueous acid—233 nm ($A_1^1 = 547$ a), 348 nm ($A_1^1 = 450$ a); aqueous alkali—249 nm ($A_1^1 = 392$ b), 359 nm ($A_1^1 = 390$ b).

Infra-red Spectrum. Principal peaks at wavenumbers 1585, 1305, 1252, 1131, 1605, 1070 (KBr disk). (See below)

Quantification. THIN-LAYER CHROMATOGRAPHY–SPECTRO-PHOTOMETRY. In blood or urine: floctafenic acid and hydroxy-floctafenic acid—R. K. Lynn *et al.*, *J. clin. Pharmac.*, 1979, *19*, 20–30.

Disposition in the Body. Absorbed after oral administration. It is rapidly metabolised to floctafenic acid which is thought to be responsible for most of the analgesic activity. About 25% of a dose is excreted in the urine as floctafenic acid and hydroxyfloc-tafenic acid in 48 hours.

THERAPEUTIC CONCENTRATION.

A single oral dose of 400 mg administered to 7 subjects, produced peak blood concentrations of floctafenic acid of 0.9 to 3.8 µg/ml (mean 2.0) in 0.5 to 2.5 hours (R. K. Lynn *et al.*, *ibid.*).

PROTEIN BINDING. In plasma, floctafenic acid, extensively bound.

Dose. 0.8 to 1.6 g daily.

Wavelength

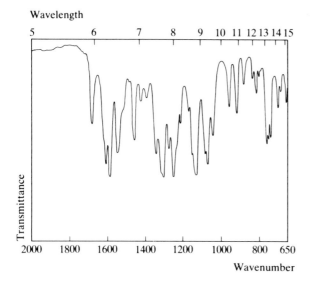

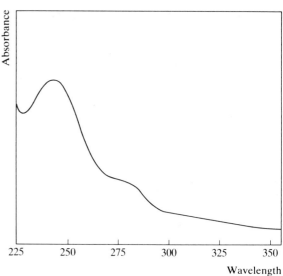

Wavelength

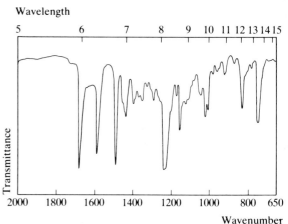

Fluanisone   *Tranquilliser*

Synonym. Haloanisone

Proprietary Names. Sedalande. It is an ingredient of Hypnorm (vet.).

4'-Fluoro-4-[4-(2-methoxyphenyl)piperazin-1-yl]butyrophenone
$C_{21}H_{25}FN_2O_2 = 356.4$
CAS—1480-19-9

An almost white to buff-coloured crystalline powder. M.p. 72° to 76°.

Practically **insoluble** in water; soluble 1 in 12 of ethanol, 1 in 1 of chloroform, and 1 in 22 of ether.

Colour Test. Mandelin's Test—brown.

Thin-layer Chromatography. *System TA*—Rf 73. (*Acidified potassium permanganate solution*, positive.)

Gas Chromatography. *System GA*—RI 2732.

Ultraviolet Spectrum. Acid isopropyl alcohol—243 nm ($A_1^1 = 550$ a).

Infra-red Spectrum. Principal peaks at wavenumbers 1690, 1235, 1497, 1598, 1155, 750 (KBr disk).

Mass Spectrum. Principal peaks at m/z 205, 218, 123, 356, 219, 162, 95, 190.

Dose. Fluanisone has been given in doses of 5 to 7.5 mg daily.

Fluclorolone Acetonide   *Corticosteroid*

Synonym. Flucloronide
Proprietary Name. Topilar

9α,11β - Dichloro - 6α - fluoro - 21 - hydroxy - 16α,17α - isopropyl-idenedioxypregna-1,4-diene-3,20-dione
$C_{24}H_{29}Cl_2FO_5 = 487.4$
CAS—3693-39-8

A white crystalline powder. M.p. about 245°, with decomposition.

Practically **insoluble** in water; soluble in ethanol, chloroform, and methanol.

Ultraviolet Spectrum. Methanol—236 nm ($A_1^1 = 242$ b).

Infra-red Spectrum. Principal peaks at wavenumbers 1666, 1086, 1052, 1063, 1724, 1639.

Use. Topically as a 0.025% cream or ointment.

Flucloxacillin
Antibiotic

Synonym. Floxacillin

(6R)-6-[3-(2-Chloro-6-fluorophenyl)-5-methylisoxazole-4-carboxamido]penicillanic acid
$C_{19}H_{17}ClFN_3O_5S = 453.9$
CAS—5250-39-5

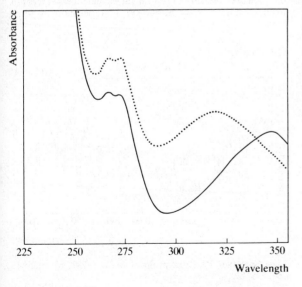

Flucloxacillin Sodium

Proprietary Names. Flopen; Floxapen (also as the magnesium salt); Heracillin; Ladropen; Stafoxil; Staphylex. It is an ingredient of Magnapen.

$C_{19}H_{16}ClFN_3NaO_5S,H_2O = 493.9$
CAS—1847-24-1 (anhydrous); *34214-51-2* (monohydrate)
A white, hygroscopic, crystalline powder.
Soluble 1 in 1 of water, 1 in 8 of ethanol, 1 in 8 of acetone, and 1 in 2 of methanol.

Dissociation Constant. pK$_a$ 2.7.

Ultraviolet Spectrum. Aqueous acid—268 nm, 274 nm, 344 nm; aqueous alkali—268 nm, 274 nm, 318 nm.

Infra-red Spectrum. Principal peaks at wavenumbers 1603, 1767, 1622, 1495, 1660, 794 (flucloxacillin sodium, KBr disk).

Dose. The equivalent of 1 to 2 g of flucloxacillin daily.

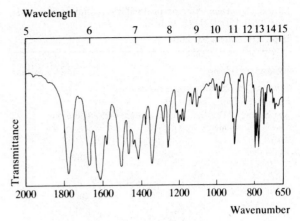

Flucytosine
Antifungal

Synonym. 5-Fluorocytosine
Proprietary Names. Alcobon; Ancobon; Ancotil.
4-Amino-5-fluoropyrimidin-2(1H)-one
$C_4H_4FN_3O = 129.1$
CAS—2022-85-7

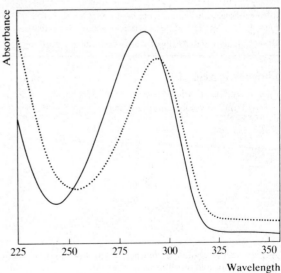

A white crystalline powder. M.p. about 295°, with decomposition.
Soluble 1 in 67 of water; slightly soluble in ethanol; practically insoluble in chloroform and ether.

Dissociation Constant. pK$_a$ 2.9, 10.7.

Ultraviolet Spectrum. Aqueous acid—286 nm ($A_1^1 = 709$ a); aqueous alkali—293 nm.

Infra-red Spectrum. Principal peaks at wavenumbers 1676, 1638, 1548, 1230, 1516, 1211 (KBr disk).

Dose. 50 to 200 mg/kg daily.

Fludrocortisone
Corticosteroid

Synonym. 9α-Fluorohydrocortisone
Proprietary Name. Astonin-H
9α-Fluoro-11β,17α,21-trihydroxypregn-4-ene-3,20-dione
$C_{21}H_{29}FO_5 = 380.5$
CAS—127-31-1

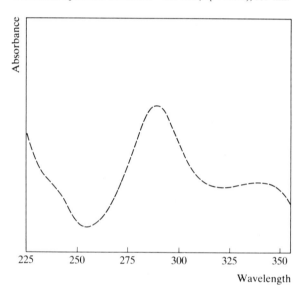

Crystals which decompose between 260° and 262°.
Very **soluble** in water.

Fludrocortisone Acetate
Synonym. 9α-Fluorohydrocortisone 21-acetate
Proprietary Names. Florinef; Scherofluron.
$C_{23}H_{31}FO_6 = 422.5$
CAS—514-36-3
A white to pale yellow, hygroscopic, crystalline powder. There are two forms one of which melts at about 209° and the other at about 225°. A solution in dioxan is dextrorotatory.
Practically **insoluble** in water; soluble 1 in 50 of ethanol, 1 in 50 of chloroform, and 1 in 250 of ether.

Colour Tests. Antimony Pentachloride—orange; Naphthol–Sulphuric Acid—violet/brown; Sulphuric Acid—orange (green fluorescence under ultraviolet light.)

Thin-layer Chromatography. Fludrocortisone acetate: *system TP*—Rf 58; *system TQ*—Rf 12; *system TR*—Rf 30; *system TS*—Rf 00. (*DPST solution.*)

Ultraviolet Spectrum. Fludrocortisone acetate: dehydrated alcohol—240 nm ($A_1^1 = 405$ a).

Infra-red Spectrum. Principal peaks at wavenumbers 1651, 1271, 1714, 1736, 1246, 1041 (fludrocortisone acetate, KBr disk).

Dose. Usually 100 to 300 μg of fludrocortisone acetate daily.

Flufenamic Acid
Analgesic

Proprietary Names. Arlef; Meralen; Sastridex; Surika.
N-(ααα-Trifluoro-*m*-tolyl)anthranilic acid
$C_{14}H_{10}F_3NO_2 = 281.2$
CAS—530-78-9

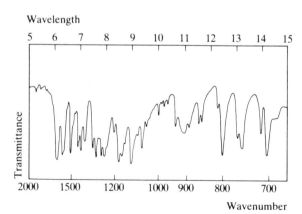

A pale yellow crystalline powder. M.p. 124° to 125°, with resolidification and remelting at 134° to 136°.

Practically **insoluble** in water; soluble 1 in 4 of ethanol, 1 in 7 of chloroform, and 1 in 3 of ether.

Dissociation Constant. pK_a 3.9.

Thin-layer Chromatography. *System TG*—Rf 37. (*Chromic acid solution*, blue.)

Gas Chromatography. *System GA*—RI 1950; *system GD*—retention time of methyl derivative 1.26 relative to $n\text{-}C_{16}H_{34}$.

High Pressure Liquid Chromatography. *System HD*—k′ 19.7; *system HV*—retention time 1.00 relative to meclofenamic acid.

Ultraviolet Spectrum. Methanol—288 nm ($A_1^1 = 593$ a), 339 nm.

Infra-red Spectrum. Principal peaks at wavenumbers 1115, 1176, 1653, 1284, 1265, 1600 (KBr disk). Five polymorphic forms occur.

Mass Spectrum. Principal peaks at *m/z* 263, 281, 166, 92, 145, 167, 235, 139.

Quantification. HIGH PRESSURE LIQUID CHROMATOGRAPHY. In plasma: flufenamic acid and mefenamic acid, detection limit 1 μg/ml, UV detection—C. K. Lin *et al.*, *J. pharm. Sci.*, 1980, **69**, 95–97.

Disposition in the Body. Readily absorbed after oral administration. Metabolised by hydroxylation and glucuronic acid conjugation. About 50% of a dose is excreted in the urine in 72 hours and about 36% is eliminated in the faeces. The material excreted in the urine consists mainly of conjugated flufenamic acid and free and conjugated 4'-hydroxyflufenamic acid with smaller amounts of the 5'-hydroxy and dihydroxy derivatives.

THERAPEUTIC CONCENTRATION.
Following oral administration of 200 mg three times daily for 4 days to 10 subjects, plasma concentrations of 0.3 to 17 µg/ml (mean 6.4) were reported 2 hours after the morning dose (R. A. Buchanan *et al.*, *Curr. ther. Res.*, 1969, *11*, 533–538).

HALF-LIFE. Plasma half-life, about 3 hours.

PROTEIN BINDING. In plasma, extensively bound.

Dose. 400 to 600 mg daily.

Flugestone   *Progestational Steroid (Veterinary)*

Synonym. Flurogestone
9α-Fluoro-11β,17α-dihydroxypregn-4-ene-3,20-dione
$C_{21}H_{29}FO_4 = 364.5$
CAS—337-03-1

Flugestone Acetate
Proprietary Name. Chronogest
$C_{23}H_{31}FO_5 = 406.5$
CAS—2529-45-5
A white or creamy-white powder. M.p. 266° to 269°.
Very slightly **soluble** in water; soluble 1 in 23 of ethanol, 1 in 2.5 of chloroform, and 1 in 100 of methanol.

Ultraviolet Spectrum. Flugestone acetate: methanol—238 nm $(A_1^1 = 425 \text{ b})$.

Flumethasone   *Corticosteroid*

Proprietary Name. Fluvet (vet.)
6α,9α-Difluoro-11β,17α,21-trihydroxy-16α-methylpregna-1,4-diene-3,20-dione
$C_{22}H_{28}F_2O_5 = 410.5$
CAS—2135-17-3

Flumethasone Pivalate
Synonym. Flumethasone Trimethylacetate
Proprietary Names. Locacorten; Locorten.
$C_{27}H_{36}F_2O_6 = 494.6$
CAS—2002-29-1
A white crystalline powder.
Practically **insoluble** in water; soluble 1 in 89 of ethanol, 1 in 350 of chloroform, and 1 in 2800 of ether.

Ultraviolet Spectrum. Methanol—238 nm $(A_1^1 = 438 \text{ a})$.

Infra-red Spectrum. Principal peaks at wavenumbers 1664, 1623, 901, 1733, 1139, 1160 (flumethasone pivalate, KBr disk).

Use. Flumethasone pivalate is used topically in a concentration of 0.02%.

Flunitrazepam   *Hypnotic*

Proprietary Names. Narcozep; Rohypnol; Roipnol.
5-(2-Fluorophenyl)-1,3-dihydro-1-methyl-7-nitro-2H-1,4-benzodiazepin-2-one
$C_{16}H_{12}FN_3O_3 = 313.3$
CAS—1622-62-4

An almost white to pale yellow crystalline solid. M.p. about 170°.
Sparingly **soluble** in water; soluble 1 in 172 of ethanol, 1 in 3 of chloroform, 1 in 300 of ether, and 1 in 100 of methanol.

Dissociation Constant. pK_a 1.8.

Colour Test. Formaldehyde–Sulphuric Acid—orange.

Thin-layer Chromatography. System *TA*—Rf 63; *system TB*—Rf 10; *system TC*—Rf 72; *system TD*—Rf 54; *system TE*—Rf 77; *system TF*—Rf 48.

Gas Chromatography. System *GA*—flunitrazepam RI 2645, 7-amino-1-desmethylflunitrazepam RI 2825, 7-aminoflunitrazepam RI 2723, desmethylflunitrazepam RI 2740; *system GG*—flunitrazepam RI 3190.

High Pressure Liquid Chromatography. System *HI*—k' 3.15; *system HK*—k' 0.47.

Ultraviolet Spectrum. Methanol—252 nm $(A_1^1 = 516 \text{ a})$, 308 nm $(A_1^1 = 332 \text{ a})$.

Infra-red Spectrum. Principal peaks at wavenumbers 1697, 1620, 1490, 1528, 1107, 783 (KBr disk). (See below)

Mass Spectrum. Principal peaks at *m/z* 285, 312, 313, 286, 266, 238, 294, 284; 7-amino-1-desmethylflunitrazepam 269, 240, 241, 268, 270, 107, 121, 213; 7-aminoflunitrazepam 283, 44, 255, 282, 254, 284, 264, 256; desmethylflunitrazepam 298, 271, 299, 224, 272, 270, 252, 280.

Quantification. GAS CHROMATOGRAPHY. In plasma: sensitivity 500 pg/ml, ECD—Y. C. Sumirtapura *et al.*, *Arzneimittel-Forsch.*, 1982, *32*, 252–257.

Wavelength

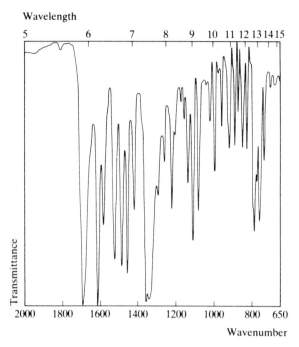

HIGH PRESSURE LIQUID CHROMATOGRAPHY. In plasma: sensitivity 1 ng/ml, UV detection—T. B. Vree *et al.*, *J. Chromat.*, 1977, *143*; *Biomed. Appl.*, *1*, 530–534.

RADIOIMMUNOASSAY. In plasma or whole blood: sensitivity 150 pg/ml—R. Dixon *et al.*, *J. pharm. Sci.*, 1981, *70*, 230–231.

Disposition in the Body. Readily absorbed after oral administration; bioavailability 80 to 90%. The major metabolites are desmethylflunitrazepam and 7-aminoflunitrazepam which are active; other metabolites include 3-hydroxyflunitrazepam, 3-hydroxy-7-acetamidoflunitrazepam, and 7-amino-1-desmethyl-flunitrazepam. Flunitrazepam is excreted in the urine almost entirely as metabolites with less than 1% as unchanged drug. About 10% of a dose is eliminated in the faeces.

THERAPEUTIC CONCENTRATION.
After single oral doses of 1 mg and 2 mg given to 11 and 5 subjects, mean peak plasma concentrations of 0.0025 and 0.015 μg/ml, respectively, were attained in about 1 hour (R. S. J. Clarke *et al.*, *Br. J. Anaesth.*, 1980, *52*, 437–445).

Following oral doses of 2 mg daily for 28 days given to 7 subjects, a mean peak plasma concentration of about 0.02 μg/ml was reported 3 hours after the last dose (E. Wickstrom *et al.*, *Eur. J. clin. Pharmac.*, 1980, *17*, 189–196).

HALF-LIFE. Plasma half-life, 10 to 70 hours (mean 25).

VOLUME OF DISTRIBUTION. About 4 litres/kg.

CLEARANCE. Plasma clearance, about 2 ml/min/kg.

DISTRIBUTION IN BLOOD. Plasma: whole blood ratio, about 0.75.

PROTEIN BINDING. In plasma, about 78%.

NOTE. For a review of flunitrazepam see M. A. K. Mattila and H. M. Larni, *Drugs*, 1980, *20*, 353–374.

Dose. 1 to 2 mg, as a hypnotic.

Flunixin   *Analgesic*

2-(2-Methyl-3-trifluoromethylanilino)nicotinic acid
$C_{14}H_{11}F_3N_2O_2 = 296.2$
CAS—38677-85-9

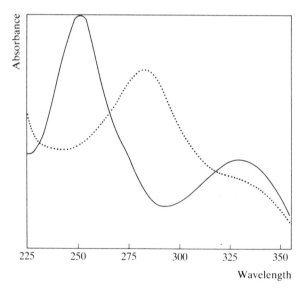

Crystals. M.p. 226° to 228°.

Flunixin Meglumine
$C_{14}H_{11}F_3N_2O_2, C_7H_{17}NO_5 = 491.5$
CAS—42461-84-7
Colourless crystals. M.p. 135° to 137°.

Thin-layer Chromatography. *System TG*—Rf 33. (*Ludy Tenger reagent*, orange.)

Gas Chromatography. *System GD*—retention time of methyl derivative 1.39 relative to *n*-$C_{16}H_{34}$.

High Pressure Liquid Chromatography. *System HV*—retention time 0.99 relative to meclofenamic acid.

Ultraviolet Spectrum. Aqueous acid—252 nm, 327 nm; aqueous alkali—281 nm ($A_1^1 = 490$ b).

Infra-red Spectrum. Principal peaks at wavenumbers 1122, 1315, 1572, 1237, 1142, 1165.

Quantification. HIGH PRESSURE LIQUID CHROMATOGRAPHY. In equine plasma: detection limit 50 ng/ml, UV detection—G. E. Hardee *et al.*, *J. liq. Chromat.*, 1982, *5*, 1991–2003.

Wavelength

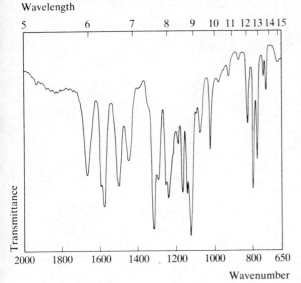

Wavenumber

Fluocinolone Acetonide *Corticosteroid*

Synonym. 6α,9α-Difluoro-16α-hydroxyprednisolone Acetonide

Proprietary Names. Dermalar; Fluoderm; Fluonid; Jellin; Synalar; Synamol; Synandone; Synemol.

6α,9α-Difluoro-11β,21-dihydroxy-16α,17α-isopropylidenedioxy-pregna-1,4-diene-3,20-dione

$C_{24}H_{30}F_2O_6 = 452.5$

CAS—67-73-2

A white crystalline powder. M.p. about 270°, with decomposition. A solution in dioxan is dextrorotatory.

Practically **insoluble** in water; soluble 1 in 26 of dehydrated alcohol, 1 in 10 of acetone, 1 in 15 to 1 in 25 of chloroform, and 1 in 350 of ether; soluble in methanol.

Colour Tests. Naphthol–Sulphuric Acid—green/yellow; Sulphuric Acid—yellow (green fluorescence under ultraviolet light).

Thin-layer Chromatography. *System TP*—Rf 42; *system TQ*—Rf 08; *system TR*—Rf 10; *system TS*—Rf 01. (*DPST solution.*)

Ultraviolet Spectrum. Ethanol—240 nm ($A_1^1 = 360$ a).

Infra-red Spectrum. Principal peaks at wavenumbers 1669, 1074, 1629, 910, 1056, 1615 (KBr disk).

Use. Topically in concentrations of 0.01 to 0.2%.

Fluocinonide *Corticosteroid*

Synonym. Fluocinolone Acetonide 21-Acetate

Proprietary Names. Lidemol; Lidex; Metosyn; Topsymin; Topsyn(e).

6α,9α-Difluoro-11β,21-dihydroxy-16α,17α-isopropylidenedioxy-pregna-1,4-diene-3,20-dione 21-acetate

$C_{26}H_{32}F_2O_7 = 494.5$

CAS—356-12-7

A white to cream-coloured crystalline powder. M.p. about 300°, with decomposition.

Practically **insoluble** in water; soluble 1 in 70 of ethanol, 1 in 10 of acetone, and 1 in 10 of chloroform; very slightly soluble in ether.

Ultraviolet Spectrum. Methanol—240 nm ($A_1^1 = 360$ a).

Infra-red Spectrum. Principal peaks at wavenumbers 1670, 1240, 1730, 1750, 1070, 1635 (KBr disk).

Use. Topically in a concentration of 0.05%.

Fluocortolone *Corticosteroid*

Synonym. 6α-Fluoro-16α-methyldehydrocorticosterone

Proprietary Names. Ultralan (tablets). It is an ingredient of Ultralanum.

6α-Fluoro-11β,21-dihydroxy-16α-methylpregna-1,4-diene-3,20-dione

$C_{22}H_{29}FO_4 = 376.5$

CAS—152-97-6

A white crystalline powder. M.p. 188° to 191°.

Practically **insoluble** in water; soluble 1 in 120 of ethanol; soluble in chloroform and ether.

Fluocortolone Hexanoate

Synonym. Fluocortolone Caproate

Proprietary Names. It is an ingredient of Ultradil Plain, Ultralan (cream and lotion), and Ultralanum.

$C_{28}H_{39}FO_5 = 474.6$

CAS—303-40-2

A white to creamy-white crystalline powder. M.p. about 244°.

Practically **insoluble** in water and ether; very slightly soluble in ethanol and methanol; soluble 1 in 18 of chloroform.

Fluocortolone Pivalate

Synonym. Fluocortolone Trimethylacetate

Proprietary Names. It is an ingredient of Ultradil Plain, Ultralan (cream and lotion), and Ultralanum Plain (cream).

$C_{27}H_{37}FO_5 = 460.6$

CAS—29205-06-9

A white to creamy-white crystalline powder. M.p. about 187°.

Practically **insoluble** in water; soluble 1 in 36 of ethanol and 1 in 3 of chloroform; freely soluble in dioxan; slightly soluble in ether.

Colour Tests. Antimony Pentachloride—green-yellow; Naphthol–Sulphuric Acid—red-brown/red-brown; Sulphuric Acid—orange-yellow.

Thin-layer Chromatography. Fluocortolone hexanoate: *system TP*—Rf 79; *system TQ*—Rf 39; *system TR*—Rf 88; *system TS*—Rf 00. (p-*Toluenesulphonic acid solution*, positive.) Fluocortolone pivalate: *system TP*—Rf 78; *system TQ*—Rf 35; *system TR*—Rf 89; *system TS*—Rf 58.

Ultraviolet Spectrum. Methanol—242 nm ($A_1^1 = 429$ a).

Infra-red Spectrum. Principal peaks at wavenumbers 1658, 1163, 1622, 1722, 1176, 1747 (fluocortolone hexanoate, KBr disk); 1662, 1159, 1725, 1619, 1605, 1285 (fluocortolone pivalate, KBr disk).

Dose. Fluocortolone has been given by mouth in doses of 5 to 60 mg daily.

Fluopromazine
Tranquilliser

Synonym. Triflupromazine
Proprietary Name. Vesprin (suspension)
NN - Dimethyl - 3 - (2 - trifluoromethylphenothiazin - 10 - yl)-propylamine
$C_{18}H_{19}F_3N_2S = 352.4$
CAS—146-54-3

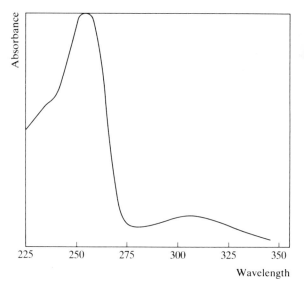

CH₂·[CH₂]₂·N(CH₃)₂ / CF₃ (structural formula)

A pale amber viscous oily liquid, which forms into large irregular crystals during prolonged storage.
Practically **insoluble** in water.

Fluopromazine Hydrochloride

Proprietary Names. Psyquil; Siquil; Vesprin (injection and tablets).
$C_{18}H_{19}F_3N_2S,HCl = 388.9$
CAS—1098-60-8
A white to pale tan crystalline powder. M.p. 170° to 178°.
Soluble 1 in less than 1 of water and of ethanol, and 1 in 1.7 of chloroform; practically insoluble in ether.

Dissociation Constant. pK$_a$ 9.2 (24°).

Colour Tests. Formaldehyde–Sulphuric Acid—red; Forrest Reagent—orange; FPN Reagent—orange; Mandelin's Test—red-brown; Marquis Test—red-violet.

Thin-layer Chromatography. System TA—Rf 54; system TB—Rf 49; system TC—Rf 35. (*Acidified iodoplatinate solution*, positive.)

Gas Chromatography. System GA—RI 2211; system GF—RI 2550.

High Pressure Liquid Chromatography. System HA—k' 2.7.

Ultraviolet Spectrum. Aqueous acid—256 nm ($A_1^1 = 874$ a), 305 nm.

Infra-red Spectrum. Principal peaks at wavenumbers 1117, 1316, 1159, 1237, 1075, 1030 (KBr disk).

Mass Spectrum. Principal peaks at m/z 58, 352, 86, 353, 85, 306, 42, 266.

Dose. 20 to 150 mg of fluopromazine hydrochloride daily.

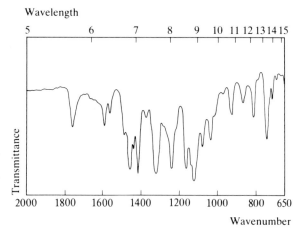

Fluoroacetamide
Rodenticide

Synonym. Compound 1081
$FCH_2·CO·NH_2 = 77.06$
CAS—640-19-7
A fine fluffy white powder which decomposes if heated appreciably above 100°.
Very **soluble** in water; relatively insoluble in organic solvents.

Colour Test. Nessler's Reagent—brown-orange.

Infra-red Spectrum. Principal peaks at wavenumbers 1667, 1036, 1117, 1020, 810, 1239 (Nujol mull).

Quantification. See under Fluoroacetic Acid.

Disposition in the Body. Rapidly absorbed after ingestion or through cuts and abrasions. It is converted to fluoroacetic acid and then to fluorocitric acid.

TOXICITY. Fluoroacetamide is extremely toxic to animals and man but its lethal action is slower than sodium fluoroacetate.

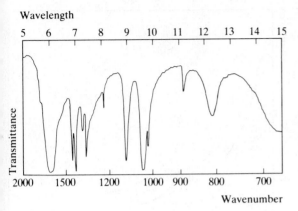

Wavelength

Transmittance

Wavenumber

A white to yellowish-white crystalline powder. M.p. about 280°, with decomposition.

Practically **insoluble** in water; soluble 1 in 200 of ethanol and 1 in 2200 of chloroform; very slightly soluble in ether.

Ultraviolet Spectrum. Methanol—241 nm ($A_1^1 = 375$ a).

Use. Usually applied as a 0.025% cream or ointment and is also available as a 0.1% ophthalmic suspension.

Fluoroacetic Acid   *Rodenticide*

Synonyms. Fluoroethanoic Acid; Gifblaar Poison; Monofluoro-acetic Acid.

$FCH_2 \cdot COOH = 78.04$

CAS—144-49-0

Fluoroacetic acid is the toxic principle of the South African plant gifblaar, *Dichapetalum cymosum* (= *Chailletia cymosa*) (Dichapetalaceae). Crystals. M.p. 33° to 35°. B.p. 165° to 168°. **Soluble** in water and ethanol; practically insoluble in most common organic solvents.

Sodium Fluoroacetate

Synonyms. Compound 1080; Sodium Monofluoroacetate.

$FCH_2 \cdot CO \cdot ONa = 100.0$

CAS—62-74-8

A white hygroscopic powder which decomposes at about 200°.
Very **soluble** in water; relatively insoluble in organic solvents.

Quantification. GAS CHROMATOGRAPHY. In tissues: detection limit 100 ng/g, ECD—I. Okuno *et al.*, *J. Ass. off. analyt. Chem.*, 1982, *65*, 1102–1105.

GAS CHROMATOGRAPHY–MASS SPECTROMETRY. In tissues: detection limits 700 ng/g for fluoroacetamide, 100 ng/g for fluoroacetic acid—H. M. Stevens *et al.*, *Forens. Sci.*, 1976, *8*, 131–137.

Disposition in the Body. Fluoroacetic acid and sodium fluoro-acetate are absorbed rapidly through cuts and abrasions but less rapidly from intact skin. Sodium fluoroacetate is converted to fluorocitric acid which inhibits the citric acid cycle and leads to accumulation of citrate.

TOXICITY. Fluoroacetic acid and sodium fluoroacetate are extremely toxic to animals and man; the minimum lethal dose is about 5 mg/kg. Toxic effects are delayed for several hours following ingestion or absorption through the skin. The maximum permissible atmospheric concentration is 50 µg/m³.

Fluorometholone   *Corticosteroid*

Proprietary Names. Delmeson; Efflumidex; FML; Oxylone.

9α-Fluoro-11β,17α-dihydroxy-6α-methylpregna-1,4-diene-3,20-dione

$C_{22}H_{29}FO_4 = 376.5$

CAS—426-13-1

Fluorouracil   *Antineoplastic*

Synonyms. 5-Fluorouracil; 5-FU.

Proprietary Names. Adrucil; Effluderm; Efudex; Efudix; Fluoroplex.

5-Fluoropyrimidine-2,4(1*H*,3*H*)-dione

$C_4H_3FN_2O_2 = 130.1$

CAS—51-21-8

A white crystalline powder which decomposes at about 282°. Sparingly **soluble** in water; slightly soluble in ethanol; practically insoluble in chloroform and ether. Solutions discolour on storage. *Caution.* Fluorouracil is irritant; avoid contact with skin and mucous membranes.

Dissociation Constant. pK$_a$ 8.0, 13.0.

Partition Coefficient. Log *P* (octanol/pH 7.4), −1.0.

Ultraviolet Spectrum. Aqueous acid—266 nm ($A_1^1 = 552$ a).

Infra-red Spectrum. Principal peaks at wavenumbers 1653, 1242, 1718, 816, 1220, 1495 (KBr disk).

Dose. Initially 12 mg/kg daily intravenously, to a maximum of 1 g daily, for 3 or 4 days.

Fluoxymesterone   *Androgen*

Synonym. Fluorohydroxymethyltestosterone

Proprietary Names. Halotestin; Oratestin; Ora-Testryl; Testoral; Ultandren.

Note. Testoral is also used as a proprietary name for testosterone.

9α-Fluoro-11β,17β-dihydroxy-17α-methylandrost-4-en-3-one

$C_{20}H_{29}FO_3 = 336.4$

CAS—76-43-7

A white or creamy-white crystalline powder. M.p. about 278°. Practically **insoluble** in water; soluble 1 in 70 of ethanol and 1 in 200 of chloroform.

Colour Tests. Antimony Pentachloride—brown; Naphthol–Sulphuric Acid—green-yellow/yellow; Sulphuric Acid—yellow (green fluorescence under ultraviolet light).

Thin-layer Chromatography. *System TP*—Rf 51; *system TQ*—Rf 09; *system TR*—Rf 38; *system TS*—Rf 16, streaking may occur.

Ultraviolet Spectrum. Dehydrated alcohol—240 nm ($A_1^1 = 495$ a).

Infra-red Spectrum. Principal peaks at wavenumbers 1654, 867, 1036, 1247, 926, 1282 (KBr disk).

Mass Spectrum. Principal peaks at m/z 43, 71, 55, 79, 91, 109, 123, 336.

Dose. 2 to 10 mg daily; up to 30 mg daily may be given.

Flupenthixol   *Tranquilliser*

2 - {4 - [3 - (2 - Trifluoromethylthioxanthen - 9 - ylidene)propyl]-piperazin-1-yl}ethanol
$C_{23}H_{25}F_3N_2OS = 434.5$
CAS—2709-56-0

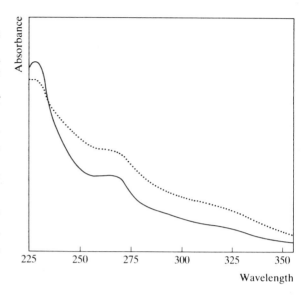

Flupenthixol Decanoate
Proprietary Names. Depixol (injection); Fluanxol Depot.
$C_{33}H_{43}F_3N_2O_2S = 588.8$
CAS—30909-51-4
A yellow oil.
Very slightly **soluble** in water; soluble in ethanol; freely soluble in chloroform and ether.

Flupenthixol Hydrochloride
Proprietary Names. Depixol (tablets); Émergil; Fluanxol (tablets).
$C_{23}H_{25}F_3N_2OS,2HCl = 507.4$
CAS—2413-38-9
A white or yellowish-white powder. M.p. 230° to 240°.
Soluble in water and ethanol; very slightly soluble in chloroform; practically insoluble in ether.

Partition Coefficient. Log *P* (octanol/pH 7.0), 3.0.

Colour Tests. Formaldehyde–Sulphuric Acid—red (orange fluorescence under ultraviolet light); Liebermann's Test—red; Mandelin's Test—red; Marquis Test—orange-red; Sulphuric Acid—orange (fluoresces under ultraviolet light).

Thin-layer Chromatography. *System TA*—Rf 62; *system TB*—Rf 05; *system TC*—Rf 33. (*Acidified iodoplatinate solution*, strong reaction.)

Gas Chromatography. *System GA*—not eluted.

High Pressure Liquid Chromatography. *System HA*—flupenthixol k' 1.2, flupenthixol sulphoxide k' 1.3.

Ultraviolet Spectrum. Aqueous acid—230 nm.

Infra-red Spectrum. Principal peaks at wavenumbers 1119, 1320, 1160, 1081, 1253, 1287 (KBr disk).

Mass Spectrum. Principal peaks at m/z 143, 70, 100, 144, 42, 98, 58, 56.

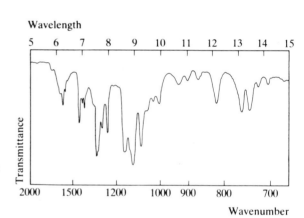

Quantification. RADIOIMMUNOASSAY. In serum: *cis*-flupenthixol, sensitivity 300 pg/ml—A. Jørgensen, *Life Sci.*, 1978, *23*, 1533–1542.

Disposition in the Body. Readily absorbed after oral administration; bioavailability about 55%. Flupenthixol decanoate is very slowly absorbed from the site of intramuscular injection. Peak plasma concentrations are attained about 3 to 6 hours after oral administration and 3 to 7 days after intramuscular injection. The main metabolic reactions are sulphoxidation, side-chain N-dealkylation and glucuronic acid conjugation. N-Desalkylflupenthixol and flupenthixol sulphoxide are the major metabolites found in plasma (both are inactive). Numerous metabolites are excreted in the urine and faeces and there is evidence of enterohepatic circulation.

NOTE. For information on the pharmacokinetics of flupenthixol see A. Jørgensen, *Eur. J. clin. Pharmac.*, 1980, *18*, 355–360.

Dose. For psychoses, the equivalent of 6 to 18 mg of flupenthixol daily, by mouth.

Fluphenazine
Tranquilliser

Synonym. Triflumethazine

2-{4-[3-(2-Trifluoromethylphenothiazin-10-yl)propyl]piper-azin-1-yl}ethanol

$C_{22}H_{26}F_3N_3OS = 437.5$

CAS—69-23-8

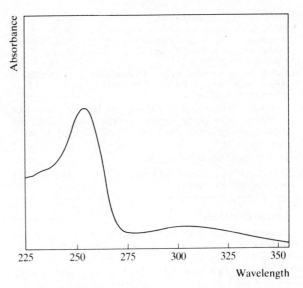

Fluphenazine Decanoate

Proprietary Names. Anatensol Decanoate; Dapotum D; Lyogen-Depot; Modecate; Prolixin Decanoate; Siqualone Decanoate.

$C_{32}H_{44}F_3N_3O_2S = 591.8$

CAS—5002-47-1

A pale yellow viscous liquid or a yellow crystalline oily solid. Practically **insoluble** in water; miscible with dehydrated alcohol, chloroform, and ether.

Fluphenazine Enanthate

Synonym. Fluphenazine Heptanoate

Proprietary Names. Moditen (injection); Prolixin Enanthate; Siqualone Enanthate.

$C_{29}H_{38}F_3N_3O_2S = 549.7$

CAS—2746-81-8

A pale yellow to yellow-orange, clear to slightly turbid, viscous liquid or a yellow crystalline oily solid. Practically **insoluble** in water; soluble 1 in less than 1 of ethanol and of chloroform, and 1 in 2 of ether.

Fluphenazine Hydrochloride

Proprietary Names. Anatensol; Dapotum; Lyogen; Moditen (tablets); Omca; Pacinol; Permitil; Prolixin; Siqualone. It is an ingredient of Motipress and Motival.

$C_{22}H_{26}F_3N_3OS,2HCl = 510.4$

CAS—146-56-5

A white crystalline powder. M.p. about 230°.

Soluble 1 in 10 or less of water; slightly soluble in ethanol, acetone, and chloroform; practically insoluble in ether.

Dissociation Constant. pK_a 3.9, 8.1.

Partition Coefficient. Log *P* (octanol/pH 7.0), 3.5.

Colour Tests. Formaldehyde–Sulphuric Acid—red; Forrest Reagent—orange; FPN Reagent—orange; Mandelin's Test—brown; Marquis Test—red.

Thin-layer Chromatography. *System TA*—Rf 63; *system TB*—Rf 06; *system TC*—Rf 23. (*Dragendorff spray*, positive; *FPN reagent*, pink; *acidified iodoplatinate solution*, positive; *Marquis reagent*, brown; *ninhydrin spray*, positive.)

Gas Chromatography. *System GA*—RI 3065.

High Pressure Liquid Chromatography. *System HA*—k' 1.2.

Ultraviolet Spectrum. Aqueous acid—256 nm ($A_1^1 = 690$ a), 306 nm.

Infra-red Spectrum. Principal peaks at wavenumbers 1116, 767, 1245, 1144, 1084, 836 (fluphenazine hydrochloride, KBr disk).

Mass Spectrum. Principal peaks at *m/z* 280, 143, 42, 70, 437, 406, 113, 56.

Quantification. GAS CHROMATOGRAPHY. In plasma: sensitivity 500 pg/ml, AFID—J. I. Javaid *et al.*, *J. chromatogr. Sci.*, 1981,

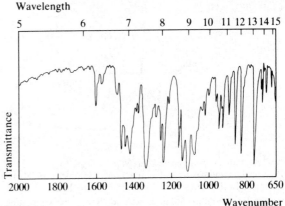

19, 439–443. In urine: free and conjugated fluphenazine, sensitivity 2 ng/ml, AFID—R. Whelpton and S. H. Curry, *J. Pharm. Pharmac.*, 1976, *28*, 869–873.

GAS CHROMATOGRAPHY–MASS SPECTROMETRY. In plasma: sensitivity 80 pg/ml—G. McKay *et al.*, *Biomed. Mass Spectrom.*, 1983, *10*, 550–555.

HIGH PRESSURE LIQUID CHROMATOGRAPHY–RADIOIMMUNO-ASSAY. In plasma: fluphenazine, related phenothiazines and metabolites, detection limit 160 pg for fluphenazine—S. A. Goldstein and H. Van Vunakis, *J. Pharmac. exp. Ther.*, 1981, *217*, 36–43.

Disposition in the Body. The hydrochloride is well absorbed after oral administration; the decanoate and enanthate are slowly absorbed from sites of injection. Fluphenazine is metabolised by sulphoxidation, hydroxylation, and conjugation with glucuronic acid or sulphate. Fluphenazine sulphoxide and 7-hydroxy-fluphenazine have been detected in urine and faeces. After an oral dose of the hydrochloride, 20% is excreted in the urine and 60% is eliminated in the faeces in 7 days; after an intramuscular dose of the enanthate, 26% is eliminated in the faeces and 14% excreted in the urine in 14 days; after an intramuscular dose of the decanoate, 17% is eliminated in the faeces and 6% excreted in the urine in 30 days.

THERAPEUTIC CONCENTRATION.
Following a single oral dose of 5 mg of fluphenazine hydrochloride to 6 subjects, peak plasma concentrations of 0.0003 to 0.001 µg/ml (mean 0.0006) were attained in 2.8 hours (K. K. Midha *et al.*, *Eur. J. clin. Pharmac.*, 1983, *25*, 709–711).

Following daily oral doses of 20 mg of fluphenazine hydrochloride to 18 subjects, steady-state plasma concentrations of 0.0002 to 0.004 µg/ml were reported (J. I. Javaid *et al.*, *J. chromatogr. Sci.*, 1981, *19*, 439–443).

HALF-LIFE. Plasma half-life, fluphenazine hydrochloride about 33 hours; fluphenazine decanoate about 5 to 12 days and fluphenazine enanthate about 3 to 4 days, following intramuscular injection.

PROTEIN BINDING. In plasma, about 99%.

Dose. Usually 1 to 5 mg of fluphenazine hydrochloride daily; up to 20 mg daily has been given.

Flurandrenolone   *Corticosteroid*

Synonyms. Fludroxycortide; Fluorandrenolone; 6α-Fluoro-16α-hydroxyhydrocortisone 16,17-Acetonide; Flurandrenolide.
Proprietary Names. Cordran; Drenison; Haelan; Sermaka.
6α - Fluoro - 11β,21 - dihydroxy - 16α,17α - isopropylidenedioxy-pregn-4-ene-3,20-dione
$C_{24}H_{33}FO_6 = 436.5$
CAS—1524-88-5

A white, fluffy, crystalline powder. M.p. 247° to 255°.
Practically **insoluble** in water and ether; soluble 1 in 72 of ethanol, 1 in 10 of chloroform, and 1 in 25 of methanol.

Colour Tests. Naphthol–Sulphuric Acid—green, brown dichroism/yellow; Sulphuric Acid—yellow (green fluorescence under ultraviolet light).

Ultraviolet Spectrum. Methanol—235 nm ($A_1^1 = 324$ a).

Infra-red Spectrum. Principal peaks at wavenumbers 1675, 1701, 1059, 1045, 1095, 1079 (KBr disk).

Use. Topically in concentrations of 0.0125 to 0.05%.

Flurazepam   *Hypnotic*

7-Chloro-1-(2-diethylaminoethyl)-5-(2-fluorophenyl)-1,3-di-hydro-2*H*-1,4-benzodiazepin-2-one
$C_{21}H_{23}ClFN_3O = 387.9$
CAS—17617-23-1

White crystals. M.p. 77° to 82°.
Soluble in chloroform.

Flurazepam Hydrochloride
Synonym. Flurazepam Dihydrochloride
Proprietary Names of Flurazepam Hydrochloride and Monohydrochloride. Dalmadorm; Dalmane; Felmane; Flunox; Remdue.
$C_{21}H_{23}ClFN_3O,2HCl = 460.8$
CAS—1172-18-5
An off-white to yellow crystalline powder. M.p. about 212°, with decomposition.
Soluble 1 in 2 of water, 1 in 4 of ethanol, 1 in 90 of chloroform, and 1 in 3 of methanol; very slightly soluble in ether.

Flurazepam Monohydrochloride
Proprietary Names. See above under flurazepam hydrochloride.
$C_{21}H_{23}ClFN_3O,HCl = 424.3$
CAS—36105-20-1
A white crystalline powder.
Very **soluble** in water; freely soluble in ethanol; practically insoluble in ether.

Dissociation Constant. pK$_a$ 1.9, 8.2.

Partition Coefficient. Log *P* (octanol/pH 7.4), 2.3.

Colour Test. Formaldehyde–Sulphuric Acid—pink.

Thin-layer Chromatography. *System TA*—Rf 62; *system TB*—Rf 30; *system TC*—Rf 48; *system TD*—Rf 03; *system TE*—Rf 74; *system TF*—Rf 03. (*Acidified iodoplatinate solution*, positive.)

Gas Chromatography. *System GA*—flurazepam RI 2785, N^1-desalkylflurazepam RI 2471, N^1-desalkyl-3-hydroxyflurazepam RI 2240, N^1-(2-hydroxyethyl)flurazepam RI 2688; *system GF*—flurazepam RI 3210; *system GG*—flurazepam RI 3220.

High Pressure Liquid Chromatography. *System HA*—flurazepam k' 1.3, N^1-desalkylflurazepam k' 0.1; *system HI*—N^1-desalkylflurazepam k' 5.19, N^1-(2-hydroxyethyl)flurazepam k' 4.27; *system HJ*—flurazepam k' 3.19; *system HK*—flurazepam k' 6.50, N^1-desalkylflurazepam k' 1.52, N^1-(2-hydroxyethyl)flurazepam k' 1.43.

Ultraviolet Spectrum. Aqueous acid—236 nm ($A_1^1 = 620$ b), 284 nm; aqueous alkali—231 nm ($A_1^1 = 856$ b), 312 nm ($A_1^1 = 53$ b).

Infra-red Spectrum. Principal peaks at wavenumbers 1672, 1613, 1316, 1211, 1171, 1100 (KBr disk).

Mass Spectrum. Principal peaks at *m/z* 86, 87, 99, 58, 84, 387, 315, 56; N^1-desalkylflurazepam 260, 259, 288, 287, 261, 289, 262, 290; didesethylflurazepam 30, 313, 246, 211, 273, 274, 302, 183; N^1-(2-hydroxyethyl)flurazepam 288, 273, 331, 287, 304, 290, 289, 275.

Quantification. SPECTROFLUORIMETRY. In blood or urine: flurazepam and metabolites, sensitivity 10 ng/ml—J. A. F. de Silva and N. Strojny, *J. pharm. Sci.*, 1971, *60*, 1303–1314.

GAS CHROMATOGRAPHY. In blood or urine: limits of detection, N^1-(2-hydroxyethyl)flurazepam and flurazepam-N^1-ylacetic acid 300 pg/ml, flurazepam 500 pg/ml, N^1-desalkylflurazepam and N^1-desalkyl-3-hydroxyflurazepam 2 ng/ml, ECD—M. Hasegawa *et al.*, *Chem. pharm. Bull.*, 1975, *23*, 1826–1833. In plasma: sensitivity, flurazepam 3 ng/ml, N^1-(2-hydroxyethyl)flurazepam 1 ng/ml, N^1-desalkylflurazepam 600 pg/ml, ECD—S. F. Cooper and D. Drolet, *J. Chromat.*, 1982, *231*; *Biomed. Appl.*, *20*, 321–331.

HIGH PRESSURE LIQUID CHROMATOGRAPHY. In urine: N^1-(2-hydroxyethyl)flurazepam, sensitivity 500 ng/ml, UV detection—R. E. Weinfeld and K. F. Miller, *J. Chromat.*, 1981, *223*; *Biomed. Appl.*, *12*, 123–130.

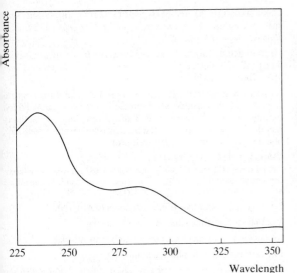

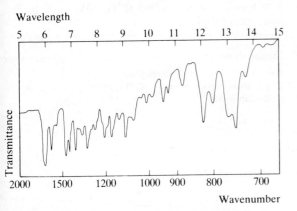

Wavenumber

RADIOIMMUNOASSAY. In plasma: sensitivity 100 pg/ml—W. Glover *et al.*, *J. pharm. Sci.*, 1980, *69*, 601–602.

Disposition in the Body. Readily absorbed after oral administration; about 70% of a dose is metabolised during the first pass through the liver. The major metabolites in blood are N^1-desalkylflurazepam and N^1-(2-hydroxyethyl)flurazepam which are both pharmacologically active and accumulate on daily administration; 7-chloro-5-(2-fluorophenyl) - 1,3 - dihydro - 2 - oxo - $2H$ - 1,4 - benzodiazepin - 1 - acetaldehyde has also been detected in plasma. Other active metabolites found in urine include monodesethyl- and didesethylflurazepam and N^1-desalkyl-3-hydroxyflurazepam, but these are not detectable in blood. Up to 60% of a dose may be excreted in the urine in 48 hours, with about 40% of the dose as a glucuronide/sulphate conjugate of N^1-(2-hydroxyethyl)flurazepam and about 4% as conjugated N^1-desalkyl-3-hydroxyflurazepam and conjugated flurazepam-N^1-ylacetic acid; only trace amounts of unchanged flurazepam and the unconjugated metabolites are present. N^1-(Hydroxyethyl)-3-hydroxyflurazepam has also been detected. About 9% of a dose is eliminated in the faeces.

THERAPEUTIC CONCENTRATION. Flurazepam is rapidly metabolised and hence blood concentrations of the unchanged drug are low and quickly decrease; for normal doses the peak concentration is usually in the range 0.0005 to 0.03 µg/ml. The blood

concentration of N^1-desalkylflurazepam is usually in the range 0.04 to 0.06 µg/ml.

Following a single oral dose of 30 mg of flurazepam hydrochloride to 2 subjects, peak blood concentrations were attained as follows: flurazepam, 0.001 and 0.005 µg/ml at 3 hours; N^1-(2-hydroxyethyl)flurazepam 0.005 and 0.01 µg/ml at 3 hours; N^1-desalkylflurazepam, 0.010 and 0.012 µg/ml at 24 hours (J. A. F. de Silva *et al.*, *J. pharm. Sci.*, 1974, *63*, 1837–1841).

Following daily oral doses of 15 mg to 18 subjects, steady-state plasma concentrations of N^1-desalkylflurazepam of 0.03 to 0.15 µg/ml (mean 0.08) were reported (D. J. Greenblatt *et al.*, *Clin. Pharmac. Ther.*, 1981, *30*, 475–486).

TOXICITY. Blood concentrations greater than 0.2 µg/ml of flurazepam or 0.5 µg/ml of N^1-desalkylflurazepam may be toxic, and blood concentrations greater than 0.5 µg/ml of flurazepam may be fatal.

In a fatality attributed to flurazepam overdose, the following postmortem concentrations (µg/ml or µg/g) were reported for flurazepam, N^1-desalkylflurazepam, and N^1-(2-hydroxyethyl)flurazepam, respectively: blood 0.51, 0.14, 9; urine 7, 3.9, 98. The amount ingested was estimated to be more than 2.4 g (R. Aderjan and R. Mattern, *Arch. Tox.*, 1979, *43*, 69–75).

In a 5-year-old child who died following the ingestion of flurazepam and phenobarbitone, the following postmortem tissue concentrations were reported for flurazepam, N^1-desalkylflurazepam and N^1-(2-hydroxyethyl)flurazepam, respectively: blood 3.2, 1.8 and 2.5 µg/ml; brain 0.8, 0.7 and 0.7 µg/g, kidney 0.9, 0.6 and 1.1 µg/g, liver 2.7, 3.1 and 3.5 µg/g. Phenobarbitone concentrations were consistent with a therapeutic dose and low concentrations of phenytoin were also detected (S. D. Ferrara *et al.*, *J. forens. Sci.*, 1979, *24*, 61–69).

HALF-LIFE. Plasma half-life, flurazepam 2 to 3 hours, N^1-desalkylflurazepam 2 to 5 days, N^1-(2-hydroxyethyl)flurazepam 10 to 20 hours.

PROTEIN BINDING. In plasma, flurazepam about 97%, N^1-desalkylflurazepam about 98% and N^1-(2-hydroxyethyl)flurazepam about 90%.

NOTE. For a review of the pharmacokinetics of flurazepam see D. J. Greenblatt *et al.*, *Clin. Pharmac. Ther.*, 1975, *17*, 1–14.

Dose. The equivalent of 15 to 30 mg of flurazepam, as a hypnotic.

Flurbiprofen   *Analgesic*

Proprietary Names. Cebutid; Froben.

2-(2-Fluorobiphenyl-4-yl)propionic acid
$C_{15}H_{13}FO_2 = 244.3$
CAS—5104-49-4

A colourless crystalline solid. M.p. about 110°.

Slightly **soluble** in water; freely soluble in most organic solvents.

Colour Tests. Liebermann's Test—brown; Marquis Test—red.

Thin-layer Chromatography. *System TD*—Rf 30; *system TE*—Rf 07; *system TF*—Rf 41; *system TG*—Rf 16. (*Ludy Tenger reagent*, orange.)

Gas Chromatography. *System GA*—RI 2032; *system GD*—retention time of methyl derivative 1.30 relative to *n*-$C_{16}H_{34}$.

High Pressure Liquid Chromatography. *System HV*—retention time 0.89 relative to meclofenamic acid.

Ultraviolet Spectrum. Aqueous acid—247 nm ($A_1^1 = 787$ b). No alkaline shift.

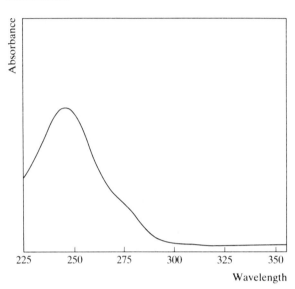

Infra-red Spectrum. Principal peaks at wavenumbers 1695, 1220, 707, 930, 773, 960 (KBr disk).

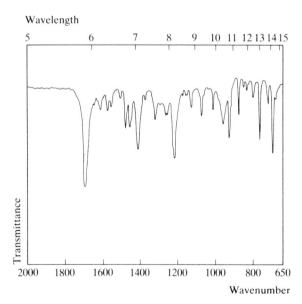

Mass Spectrum. Principal peaks at *m/z* 199, 244, 200, 178, 179, 184, 183, 245.

Quantification. Gas Chromatography. In plasma: sensitivity 50 ng/ml, ECD—D. G. Kaiser *et al.*, *J. pharm. Sci.*, 1974, *63*, 567–570.

Gas Chromatography–Mass Spectrometry. In plasma: sensitivity 1 ng/ml—K. Kawahara *et al.*, *J. Chromat.*, 1981, *223*; *Biomed. Appl.*, *12*, 202–207.

High Pressure Liquid Chromatography. In serum: sensitivity 40 ng/ml, UV detection—B. G. Snider *et al.*, *J. pharm. Sci.*, 1981, *70*, 1347–1349.

Disposition in the Body. Readily absorbed after oral administration. About 95% of a dose is excreted in the urine in 24 hours, mainly as the 4'-hydroxy, 3',4'-dihydroxy, and 4'-methoxy metabolites, which are excreted partly as conjugates; about 25% of a dose is excreted as unchanged drug.

Therapeutic Concentration.

After a single oral dose of 100 mg, administered to 6 subjects, peak serum concentrations of 9.1 to 16.6 µg/ml (mean 12) were attained in about 1.5 hours (N. Cardoe *et al.*, *Curr. med. Res. Opinion*, 1977, *5*, 21–25).

Half-life. Plasma half-life, 2 to 6 hours (mean 3.5).

Volume of Distribution. About 0.1 litre/kg.

Clearance. Plasma clearance, about 0.3 ml/min/kg.

Protein Binding. In plasma, about 99%.

Note. For a review of the pharmacokinetics of flurbiprofen see R. N. Brogden *et al.*, *Drugs*, 1979, *18*, 417–438.

Dose. 150 to 300 mg daily.

Fluspirilene   *Tranquilliser*

Proprietary Names. Imap; Redeptin.

8-[4,4-Bis(4-fluorophenyl)butyl]-1-phenyl-1,3,8-triazaspiro-[4.5]decan-4-one
$C_{29}H_{31}F_2N_3O = 475.6$
CAS—1841-19-6

A white to yellowish, amorphous or crystalline powder. M.p. about 190°.

Practically **insoluble** in water; slightly soluble in ethanol and ether; sparingly soluble in acetone; freely soluble in chloroform.

Thin-layer Chromatography. *System TA*—Rf 69; *system TB*—Rf 04; *system TC*—Rf 59.

Gas Chromatography. *System GA*—RI 1017.

Ultraviolet Spectrum. Methanol—252 nm ($A_1^1 = 295$ a), 273 nm, 293 nm.

Infra-red Spectrum. Principal peaks at wavenumbers 1710, 1505, 1596, 1220, 743, 1230 (KBr disk). Polymorphism may occur.

Mass Spectrum. Principal peaks at *m/z* 244, 42, 72, 475, 109, 245, 85, 476.

Dose. Usually 2 to 8 mg weekly, by deep intramuscular injection; maximum of 20 mg weekly.

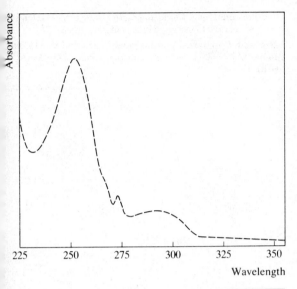

Absorbance

225   250   275   300   325   350

Wavelength

Folic Acid

Vitamin

Synonyms. Folacin; Folinsyre; Pteroylglutamic Acid; Pteroyl-monoglutamic Acid.
Proprietary Names. Folasic; Foldine; Folettes; Folsan; Folvite; Novofolacid. It is an ingredient of Co-Ferol, Fefol, Folex-350, Folvron, Hepanorm, Kelfolate, Pregaday, and Pregfol.

N-[4-(2-Amino-4-hydroxypteridin-6-ylmethylamino)benzoyl]-L(+)-glutamic acid
$C_{19}H_{19}N_7O_6 = 441.4$
CAS—59-30-3

A yellow to orange microcrystalline powder.
Practically **insoluble** in water, ethanol, chloroform, and ether. Soluble in dilute solutions of alkali hydroxides and carbonates, yielding a clear orange-brown solution; soluble in hydrochloric acid and in sulphuric acid, yielding very pale yellow solutions. Solutions are inactivated by ultraviolet light; alkaline solutions are sensitive to oxidation and acid solutions are sensitive to heat.

Dissociation Constant. pK_a 4.7, 6.8, 9.0 (30°).

Ultraviolet Spectrum. Aqueous alkali—256 nm ($A_1^1 = 549$ a), 283 nm ($A_1^1 = 539$ a).

Infra-red Spectrum. Principal peaks at wavenumbers 1686, 1602, 1636, 1191, 1567, 1225 (KBr disk).

Dose. 2.5 to 20 mg daily.

Formaldehyde

Disinfectant

Synonyms. Formic Aldehyde; Methanal; Methylene Oxide; Oxomethane.
HCHO = 30.03
A colourless inflammable gas.
Very **soluble** in water; slightly soluble in ethanol and ether.

Formaldehyde Solution

Synonyms. Formalin; Formol.
Proprietary Names. Emoform; Formitrol; Lysoform; Veracur.
CAS—50-00-0
An aqueous solution containing 34 to 38% w/w of CH_2O, with methanol as a stabilising agent.
A colourless liquid. Wt per ml about 1.08 g.
Miscible with water and ethanol; immiscible with chloroform and ether.

Colour Tests. Chromotropic Acid—red.
Add a little resorcinol to a solution containing formaldehyde, shake, then carefully add *sulphuric acid* to form a layer under the solution—red-violet ring at the junction of the two layers.

Mass Spectrum. Principal peaks at m/z 29, 30, 28, 31, 32, –, –, –.

Disposition in the Body. Rapidly metabolised in the body tissues to formic acid and methanol, especially in the liver and erythrocytes; the formic acid may then be excreted in the urine as formates, or metabolised to labile methyl groups.
Formaldehyde is a metabolite of methanol.

TOXICITY. Formaldehyde is very irritant to mucous membranes and inhalation of the vapour causes intense irritation of the respiratory tract which may lead to bronchitis and pneumonia. Atmospheric concentrations of 2 to 3 ppm may cause mild irritation of the mucous membranes and exposure to concentrations of 10 to 20 ppm for only a few minutes may cause moderate to severe irritation. Adverse effects have been reported as a result of release of formaldehyde fumes from synthetic foam insulation. Few fatalities have been recorded but 30 ml of Formaldehyde Solution may be fatal in an adult. The maximum permissible atmospheric concentration is 2 ppm or 3 mg/m³.
In a fatality due to the ingestion of about 125 ml of Formaldehyde Solution, the following postmortem concentrations were reported: blood, methanol 0.4 µg/ml, formaldehyde, a trace; stomach contents, methanol 0.9 g, formaldehyde 4.5 g (B. Finkle, *Bull. int. Ass. forens. Toxicol.*, 1975, *11*(2), 26).
In a fatality due to the ingestion of 120 ml of Formaldehyde Solution, the following blood concentrations were reported 0.5 hour after ingestion: formic acid 500 µg/ml, formaldehyde 4.8 µg/ml, methanol 420 µg/ml; after 17 hours they had declined to 300, 2 and 70 µg/ml respectively; death occurred approximately 28 hours after ingestion (J. T. Eells *et al.*, *J. Am. med. Ass.*, 1981, *246*, 1237–1238).

Formic Acid

Synonym. Aminic Acid
HCOOH = 46.03
CAS—64-18-6
A colourless liquid containing about 25% w/w of CH_2O_2. Wt per ml about 1.05 g. B.p. about 101°.
Miscible with water, ethanol, and ether.

Dissociation Constant. pK_a 3.8 (25°).

Colour Test. When warmed with *sulphuric acid* in a tube, carbon monoxide is evolved; the gas can be ignited at the mouth of the tube and burns with a blue flame.

Mass Spectrum. Principal peaks at m/z 29, 46, 45, 28, 44, 30, 47, –.

Quantification. ULTRAVIOLET SPECTROPHOTOMETRY. In urine: determination at 340 nm before and after treatment with formate dehydrogenase, sensitivity 500 ng/ml—G. Triebig and K. H. Schaller, *Clinica chim. Acta*, 1980, *108*, 355–360.

GAS CHROMATOGRAPHY. In blood or urine: head-space analysis, sensitivity 5 μg/ml, FID—C. Abolin *et al.*, *Biochem. Med.*, 1980, *15*, 209–218.

Disposition in the Body. Formic acid is an intermediate in normal metabolism; when administered it probably takes part in the metabolism of 1-carbon compounds to produce methyl groups; it is excreted in the urine and also undergoes oxidation to carbon dioxide. Together with formaldehyde, it is a metabolite of methanol and the two are probably mainly responsible for the effect of methanol on vision.

Formic acid concentrations of 2 to 30 μg/ml (mean 13) were reported in the urine of normal subjects (G. Triebig and K. H. Schaller, *Clinica chim. Acta*, 1980, *108*, 355–360).

TOXICITY. The minimum lethal dose is about 30 ml. Formic acid is dangerously caustic to the skin. The maximum permissible atmospheric concentration is 5 ppm or 9 mg/m^3; the estimated acceptable daily intake is up to 3 mg/kg.

Ingestion of more than 45 g was fatal in 14 out of 16 subjects (D. B. Jefferys and H. M. Wiseman, *Human Toxicol.*, 1983, *2*, 423).

Three subjects who intentionally swallowed between 1 mouthful and 100 ml of descaling agents containing 40 to 55% v/v of formic acid, died 5 to 14 days after ingestion (R. B. Naik *et al.*, *Postgrad. med. J.*, 1980, *56*, 451–456).

NOTE. Formic acid is the principal ingredient (about 60%) of several proprietary preparations used for descaling kettles.

Frusemide   *Diuretic*

Synonyms. Furosemide; Fursemide.

Proprietary Names. Aluzine; Diural; Diuresal; Dryptal; Frusetic; Frusid; Fur-O-Ims; Furoside; Impugan; Lasilix; Lasix; Neo-Renal; Novosemide; Uritol. It is an ingredient of Diumide-K, Frumil, Frusene, Lasikal, Lasilactone, and Lasipressin.

4-Chloro-*N*-furfuryl-5-sulphamoylanthranilic acid
$C_{12}H_{11}ClN_2O_5S = 330.7$
CAS—54-31-9

A white or slightly yellow crystalline powder. M.p. about 206°, with decomposition.

Practically **insoluble** in water and chloroform; soluble 1 in 75 of ethanol, 1 in 15 of acetone, and 1 in 850 of ether; freely soluble in dimethylformamide and solutions of alkali hydroxides.

Dissociation Constant. pK$_a$ 3.9 (20°).

Colour Tests. Koppanyi–Zwikker Test—violet; Liebermann's Test—black; Sulphuric Acid—yellow.

Thin-layer Chromatography. *System TD*—Rf 01; *system TE*—Rf 07; *system TF*—Rf 12; *system TG*—Rf 19. (*Mercurous nitrate spray*, positive; *acidified potassium permanganate solution*, positive; *Van Urk reagent*, pink-brown.)

Gas Chromatography. *System GD*—retention time of methyl derivative 2.64 relative to *n*-C$_{16}$H$_{34}$.

High Pressure Liquid Chromatography. *System HV*—retention time 0.45 relative to meclofenamic acid.

Ultraviolet Spectrum. Aqueous acid—235 nm (A$_1^1$ = 1333 a), 274 nm (A$_1^1$ = 600 a), 342 nm; aqueous alkali—271 nm (A$_1^1$ = 580 a), 333 nm.

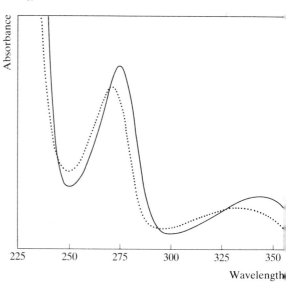

Infra-red Spectrum. Principal peaks at wavenumbers 1143, 1668, 1565, 1240, 1590, 1260 (KBr disk).

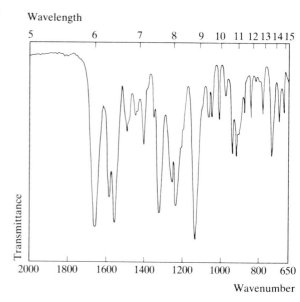

Mass Spectrum. Principal peaks at *m/z* 81, 53, 330, 96, 82, 332, 64, 63.

Quantification. GAS CHROMATOGRAPHY. In plasma or urine: sensitivity 20 ng/ml, ECD—E. Keller *et al.*, *Eur. J. clin. Pharmac.*, 1981, *20*, 27–33.

HIGH PRESSURE LIQUID CHROMATOGRAPHY. In plasma or urine: detection limits 100 ng/ml in plasma and 500 ng/ml in urine, fluorescence detection—A. L. M. Kerremans *et al.*, *J. Chromat.*, 1982, *229*; *Biomed. Appl.*, *18*, 129–139. In plasma or urine: frusemide and its glucuronide metabolite, sensitivity 8 ng/ml for frusemide in plasma, fluorescence detection—D. E. Smith *et al.*, *Drug Met. Disp.*, 1980, *8*, 337–342.

Disposition in the Body. Rapidly but incompletely absorbed after oral administration; bioavailability about 65%. Up to 90% of an intravenous dose is excreted in the urine, mainly as unchanged drug with up to 14% of the dose as a glucuronide conjugate. 2-Amino-4-chloro-5-sulphamoylanthranilic acid has been reported as a metabolite in several studies, but in other cases it has not been detected and it has been suggested that it is an analytical artefact produced during acid extraction procedures. In normal subjects, about 6 to 18% of a dose is eliminated in the faeces after intravenous administration; this may be increased to about 60% in renal failure.

THERAPEUTIC CONCENTRATION.
Following a single oral dose of 80 mg to 8 fasting subjects, peak serum concentrations of 1.8 to 4.9 µg/ml (mean 2.3) were attained in 60 to 70 minutes (M. R. Kelly *et al.*, *Clin. Pharmac. Ther.*, 1974, *15*, 178–186). Plasma concentrations averaging 7.5 µg/ml were reported 10 minutes after an intravenous dose of 40 mg to 9 subjects (D. E. Smith *et al.*, *Drug Met. Disp.*, 1980, *8*, 337–342).

HALF-LIFE. Plasma half-life, about 1 to 3 hours, increased in subjects with renal failure, congestive heart failure, liver disease, and in neonates (up to about 20 hours).

VOLUME OF DISTRIBUTION. About 0.1 to 0.2 litre/kg, increased in subjects with liver disease, nephrotic syndrome, and in neonates.

CLEARANCE. Plasma clearance, about 1 to 3 ml/min/kg, decreased in uraemia, heart failure, and neonates.

PROTEIN BINDING. In plasma, about 97%, decreased in patients with cirrhosis and uraemia.

NOTE. For reviews of frusemide pharmacokinetics see L. Z. Benet, *J. Pharmacokinet. Biopharm.*, 1979, *7*, 1–27 and R. E. Cutler and A. D. Blair, *Clin. Pharmacokinet.*, 1979, *4*, 279–296.

Dose. Usually 20 to 80 mg daily; in oliguria, maximum single dose of 2 g.

Furaltadone   *Antibacterial (Veterinary)*

Synonyms. Furmethonol; Nitrofurmethonum.
(±)-5-Morpholinomethyl-3-(5-nitrofurfurylideneamino)-2-oxazolidone
$C_{13}H_{16}N_4O_6 = 324.3$
CAS—139-91-3; 59302-14-6 (±)

A yellow crystalline powder. M.p. about 205°.
Soluble 1 in 2000 of water, 1 in 1000 of ethanol, and 1 in 300 of chloroform; practically insoluble in ether.

Colour Test. Marquis Test—yellow.

Thin-layer Chromatography. *System TA*—Rf 43; *system TB*—Rf 00; *system TC*—Rf 40. (*Acidified iodoplatinate solution*, positive.)

Ultraviolet Spectrum. Aqueous acid—255 nm, 362 nm.

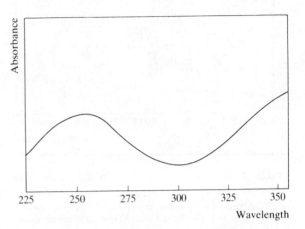

Infra-red Spectrum. Principal peaks at wavenumbers 1755, 1226, 1250, 1110, 1020, 1315 (KBr disk).

Mass Spectrum. Principal peaks at *m/z* 100, 56, 101, 42, 185, 184, 41, 128.

Furazolidone   *Antimicrobial*

Synonym. Nifurazolidonum
Proprietary Names. Coryzium (vet.); Furoxane; Furoxone; Neftin (vet.); Tricofuron.
3-(5-Nitrofurfurylideneamino)-2-oxazolidone
$C_8H_7N_3O_5 = 225.2$
CAS—67-45-8

A yellow crystalline powder. M.p. about 259°, with decomposition.
Very slightly **soluble** in water and ethanol; slightly soluble in chloroform; practically insoluble in ether.

Colour Test. Dissolve 1 mg in 1 ml of dimethylformamide with 0.05 ml of M ethanolic potassium hydroxide—deep blue.

Thin-layer Chromatography. *System TA*—Rf 44; *system TB*—Rf 00; *system TC*—Rf 47.

Ultraviolet Spectrum. After solution in dimethylformamide and dilution with water—259 nm, 367 nm ($A_1^1 = 754$ a).

Infra-red Spectrum. Principal peaks at wavenumbers 1227, 1739, 1015, 1250, 1101, 738 (Nujol mull). (See below)

Mass Spectrum. Principal peaks at *m/z* 87, 79, 51, 225, 42, 50, 86, 80.

Dose. 400 mg daily.

Wavelength

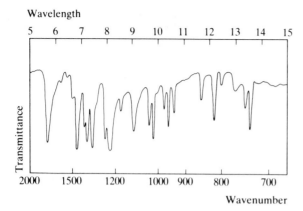

Fusidic Acid *Antibiotic*

Proprietary Name. Fucidin (suspension)

ent-16α-Acetoxy-3β,11β-dihydroxy-4β,8β,14α-trimethyl-18-nor-5β,10α-cholesta-(17Z)-17(20),24-dien-21-oic acid hemihydrate
$C_{31}H_{48}O_6, \frac{1}{2}H_2O = 525.7$
CAS—6990-06-3 (anhydrous)

A white crystalline powder. M.p. about 193°.
Practically **insoluble** in water; soluble 1 in 5 of ethanol, 1 in 4 of chloroform, and 1 in 60 of ether.

Sodium Fusidate

Synonym. Fusidate Sodium
Proprietary Name. Fucidin(e) (tablets)
$C_{31}H_{47}NaO_6 = 538.7$
CAS—751-94-0
A white, slightly hygroscopic, crystalline powder.
Soluble 1 in 1 of water, 1 in 1 of ethanol, and 1 in 350 of chloroform; practically insoluble in ether.

Dissociation Constant. pK_a 5.4.

Infra-red Spectrum. Principal peaks at wavenumbers 1267, 1547, 1706, 1238, 1020, 966 (sodium fusidate, KBr disk).

Quantification. HIGH PRESSURE LIQUID CHROMATOGRAPHY. In plasma: sensitivity 500 ng/ml, UV detection—A. H. Hikal, *Int. J. Pharmaceut.*, 1983, *13*, 297–301.

Dose. 1.5 to 3 g of sodium fusidate daily.

Gallamine Triethiodide *Muscle Relaxant*

Synonym. Bencurine Iodide
Proprietary Name. Flaxedil
2,2′,2″-(Benzene-1,2,3-triyltrioxy)tris(tetraethylammonium) tri-iodide
$C_{30}H_{60}I_3N_3O_3 = 891.5$
CAS—153-76-4 (gallamine); *65-29-2* (triethiodide)

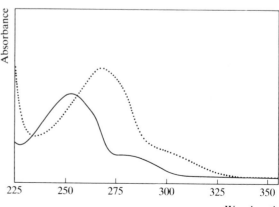

A white, or faintly cream-coloured, hygroscopic powder. M.p. about 235°, with decomposition.

Soluble 1 in 0.6 of water, 1 in 115 of ethanol, and 1 in 1500 of chloroform; slightly soluble in acetone; practically insoluble in ether.

Thin-layer Chromatography. *System TA*—Rf 00; *system TN*—Rf 34; *system TO*—Rf 05. (*Acidified iodoplatinate solution*, positive.)

Gas Chromatography. *System GA*—RI 2625.

Ultraviolet Spectrum. Aqueous acid—225 nm $(A_1^1 = 525 a)$, 266 nm $(A_1^1 = 9 a)$.

Infra-red Spectrum. Principal peaks at wavenumbers 1100, 1120, 1260, 1000, 780, 1600 (KBr disk).

Quantification. SPECTROFLUORIMETRY. In plasma: sensitivity 50 ng—M. I. Ramzan *et al.*, *Eur. J. clin. Pharmac.*, 1980, *17*, 135–143.

Disposition in the Body. Slowly and incompletely absorbed after oral administration; absorbed after intramuscular administration but is generally given by the intravenous route. Small amounts enter the cerebrospinal fluid. Almost 100% of a dose is excreted unchanged in the urine in 24 to 30 hours. Negligible amounts are excreted in the bile.

HALF-LIFE. Plasma half-life, 2 to 3 hours; greatly increased in renal failure.

VOLUME OF DISTRIBUTION. About 0.3 litre/kg.

CLEARANCE. Plasma clearance, about 1.4 ml/min/kg.

Dose. 40 to 120 mg intravenously.

Gelsemine *Central Depressant*

$C_{20}H_{22}N_2O_2 = 322.4$
CAS—509-15-9
An alkaloid present in gelsemium, the dried rhizome and roots of *Gelsemium sempervirens* (Loganiaceae).
Crystals. M.p. 178°.
Slightly **soluble** in water; soluble in ethanol, chloroform, and ether.

Colour Test. Mandelin's Test—red → green.

Thin-layer Chromatography. *System TA*—Rf 49. (*Acidified iodoplatinate solution*, positive.)

Gas Chromatography. *System GA*—RI 2850.

Ultraviolet Spectrum. Aqueous acid—252 nm $(A_1^1 = 220 \text{ b})$; aqueous alkali—268 nm.

Infra-red Spectrum. Principal peaks at wavenumbers 1715, 1620, 1100, 747, 759, 1237.

Disposition in the Body.
TOXICITY. Death has been caused by the ingestion of 4 ml of a 1:1 fluid extract.

Gentamicin   *Antibiotic*

CAS—1403-66-3
A mixture of isomeric aminoglycoside antibiotics (gentamicin C_1, gentamicin C_{1A}, and gentamicin C_2) produced by *Micromonospora purpurea*.
A white amorphous powder. M.p. 102° to 108°.
Freely **soluble** in water; sparingly soluble in ethanol and chloroform.

Gentamicin Sulphate

Proprietary Names. Alcomicin; Cidomycin; Garamycin; Genoptic; Gentalline; Genticin; Gentigan; Lugacin; Refobacin; Sulmycin.
CAS—1405-41-0
A white to buff-coloured powder.
Soluble in water; practically insoluble in ethanol, chloroform, and ether.

Colour Tests. Nessler's Reagent (100°)—black; Ninhydrin (heat for 4 min)—violet.

Ultraviolet Spectrum. Aqueous acid—247 nm; aqueous alkali—251 nm.

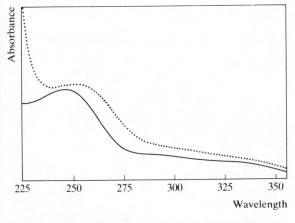

Infra-red Spectrum. Principal peaks at wavenumbers 1120, 1060, 1625, 1525, 1290, 880 (KBr disk).

Quantification. See also under Amikacin.

HIGH PRESSURE LIQUID CHROMATOGRAPHY. In plasma or urine: gentamicin components C_1, C_{1A} and C_2, sensitivity 500 ng/ml, fluorescence detection—J. D'Souza and R. I. Ogilvie, *J. Chromat.*, 1982, *232*; *Biomed. Appl.*, *21*, 212–218.

IMMUNOASSAY. In serum: enzyme immunoassay, detection limit 100 ng/ml—P. J. Wills and R. Wise, *Antimicrob. Ag. Chemother.*, 1979, *16*, 40–42. In serum: fluoroimmunoassay—A. J. Munro *et al., J. antimicrob. Chemother.*, 1982, *9*, 47–51.

REVIEW. For a review of methods for the determination of gentamicin in serum, see W. Hospes *et al., Pharm. Weekbl., Sci. Edn*, 1982, *4*, 32–37.

Disposition in the Body. Poorly absorbed after oral administration but rapidly absorbed after intramuscular injection; it is also absorbed systemically following topical application to wounds. In normal subjects it is rapidly excreted in the urine as unchanged drug, up to 80% of a dose being excreted in 24 hours. It accumulates in the tissues and there may be considerable intersubject variation in the pharmacokinetics. Gentamicin may be detected in serum and urine for several days after cessation of treatment.

THERAPEUTIC CONCENTRATION. During treatment the serum concentration should be in the range 4 to 12 µg/ml and should be monitored regularly, especially in patients who have renal insufficiency. During multiple dosing, the trough concentration immediately preceding a dose should not exceed 2 µg/ml.
A single intramuscular dose of 1 mg/kg given to 10 subjects, produced a mean peak serum concentration of 5.8 µg/ml in 0.5 to 1 hour (M. Chung *et al., Antimicrob. Ag. Chemother.*, 1980, *17*, 184–187).

TOXICITY. Toxic effects may be produced at serum concentrations of 12 µg/ml or more, or during chronic treatment, if the trough serum concentration exceeds 2 µg/ml.

HALF-LIFE. Plasma half-life, about 2 to 4 hours, increased in renal failure; a very long terminal elimination phase of several days has also been reported.

VOLUME OF DISTRIBUTION. About 0.2 litre/kg.

CLEARANCE. Plasma clearance, about 1 ml/min/kg.

PROTEIN BINDING. In plasma, less than 30%.

Dose. The equivalent of 3 to 5 mg/kg of gentamicin daily, given parenterally.

Gestronol Hexanoate   *Progestational Steroid*

Synonym. Gestonorone Caproate
Proprietary Name. Depostat
3,20-Dioxo-19-norpregn-4-en-17α-yl hexanoate
$C_{26}H_{38}O_4 = 414.6$
CAS—1253-28-7

A white to creamy-white crystalline powder. M.p. 124° to 130°; a polymorph melting at 119° to 123° may also occur.
Soluble in ethanol and methanol; freely soluble in acetone and chloroform; sparingly soluble in ether.

Ultraviolet Spectrum. Methanol—240 nm $(A_1^1 = 415 \text{ b})$.

Infra-red Spectrum. Principal peaks at wavenumbers 1733, 1667, 1715, 1266, 1250, 1618 (KBr disk).

Dose. 200 to 400 mg intramuscularly every 5 to 7 days.

Glafenine
Analgesic

Synonym. Glaphenine
Proprietary Names. Glifan; Glifanan.
2,3-Dihydroxypropyl *N*-(7-chloro-4-quinolyl)anthranilate
$C_{19}H_{17}ClN_2O_4 = 372.8$
CAS—3820-67-5

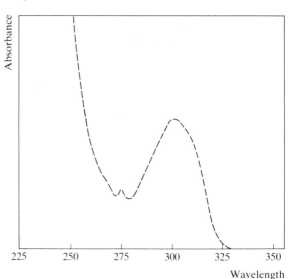

A white or slightly yellow crystalline powder. M.p. about 165°.
Practically **insoluble** in water; slightly soluble in acetone and
chloroform; soluble in dilute acids.

Ultraviolet Spectrum. Aqueous acid—345 nm ($A_1^1 = 467$ b).

Quantification. HIGH PRESSURE LIQUID CHROMATOGRAPHY. In
plasma: glafenine and metabolites, detection limits 500 ng/ml
for glafenine and hydroxyglafenic acid, 200 ng/ml for glafenic
acid, UV detection—M. C. Tournet *et al., J. Chromat.*, 1981,
224; *Biomed. Appl.*, *13*, 348–352.

Disposition in the Body. Absorbed after oral administration with
peak plasma concentrations occurring about 1 to 2 hours after
ingestion. It is hydrolysed to glafenic acid which is excreted in
the urine as an acylglucuronide conjugate; glafenic acid is found
in plasma at concentrations greater than those of unchanged
drug. Small amounts of unconjugated *N*-oxide of glafenic acid,
and hydroxyglafenic acid which is mainly conjugated, have also
been found in urine.

TOXICITY. Plasma concentrations greater than 75 µg/ml may be
associated with toxic effects.

HALF-LIFE. About 1 to 2 hours.

Dose. Up to 1.2 g daily.

Glibenclamide
Antidiabetic

Synonyms. Glybenclamide; Glyburide; Glycbenzcyclamide.
Proprietary Names. Daonil; Diaβeta; Euglucon; Libanil; Malix;
Miglucan.
1 - {4 - [2 - (5 - Chloro - 2 - methoxybenzamido)ethyl]benzenesul-
phonyl}-3-cyclohexylurea
$C_{23}H_{28}ClN_3O_5S = 494.0$
CAS—10238-21-8

A white crystalline powder. M.p. 172° to 174°.
Practically **insoluble** in water and ether; soluble 1 in 330 of
ethanol, 1 in 36 of chloroform, and 1 in 250 of methanol.

Dissociation Constant. pK_a 5.3.

Colour Tests. Aromaticity (Method 2)—yellow/orange; Liebermann's Test (100°)—orange (15 s).

Thin-layer Chromatography. *System TA*—Rf 80. (*Acidified
iodoplatinate solution*, positive.)

Ultraviolet Spectrum. Methanol—275 nm, 300 nm ($A_1^1 =$
63 a).

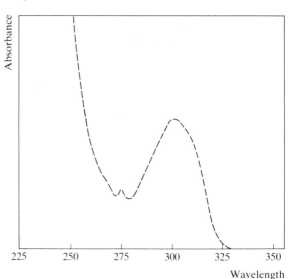

Infra-red Spectrum. Principal peaks at wavenumbers 1524, 1160,
1623, 1718, 1276, 823 (KBr disk).

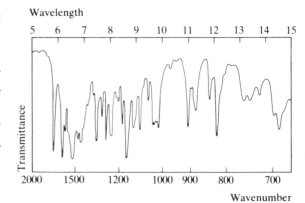

Quantification. GAS CHROMATOGRAPHY. In plasma: sensitivity
5 ng/ml, ECD—D. Castoldi and O. Tofanetti, *Clinica chim.
Acta*, 1979, *93*, 195–198.

HIGH PRESSURE LIQUID CHROMATOGRAPHY. In serum: sensitivity
10 ng/ml, fluorescence detection—W. J. Adams *et al., Analyt.
Chem.*, 1982, *54*, 1287–1291.

Disposition in the Body. Readily absorbed after oral administration; widely distributed throughout the body and metabolised
mainly by 4-*trans*- and 3-*cis*-hydroxylation of the cyclohexyl ring.
About 20 to 50% of a dose is excreted in the urine in 24 hours,
mainly as metabolites; about 45 to 75% of a dose is eliminated
in the faeces over a period of 5 days.

After a single oral dose of 5 mg to 2 subjects, peak plasma concentrations of 0.17 to 0.36 μg/ml were attained in 3 hours (L. Balant *et al.*, *Eur. J. clin. Pharmac.*, 1975, *8*, 63-69).

TOXICITY.
In a suicide attempt, a concentration of 0.6 μg/ml was found in the serum initially. After 84 hours the concentration had declined to <0.1 μg/ml (M. Berger *et al.*, *Dt. med. Wschr.*, 1977, *102*, 586–587).

HALF-LIFE. Plasma half-life, 5 to 16 hours.

VOLUME OF DISTRIBUTION. About 0.3 litre/kg.

DISTRIBUTION IN BLOOD. Plasma: whole blood ratio, 2.

PROTEIN BINDING. In plasma, about 99%.

NOTE. For reviews of the pharmacokinetics of hypoglycaemic drugs see L. Balant, *Clin. Pharmacokinet.*, 1981, *6*, 215–241 and J. E. Jackson and R. Bressler, *Drugs*, 1981, *22*, 211–245.

Dose. 5 to 15 mg daily.

Glibornuride
Antidiabetic

Proprietary Names. Gluborid; Glutril.

1-[(2S,3R)-2-Hydroxyborn-3-yl]-3-tosylurea

$C_{18}H_{26}N_2O_4S = 366.5$

CAS—26944-48-9

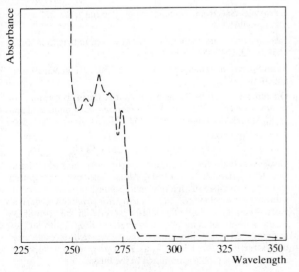

Crystals. M.p. 186° to 189°.

Colour Tests. Koppanyi–Zwikker Test—violet; Mercurous Nitrate—black.

Thin-layer Chromatography. *System TD*—Rf 40; *system TE*—Rf 05; *system TF*—Rf 60.

Gas Chromatography. *System GA*—RI 1520, 1690, and 1780.

Ultraviolet Spectrum. Ethanol—257 nm, 264 nm $(A_1^1 = 17 \text{ a})$, 275 nm.

Infra-red Spectrum. Principal peaks at wavenumbers 1170, 1682, 1520, 1710, 1050, 1100 (KBr disk).

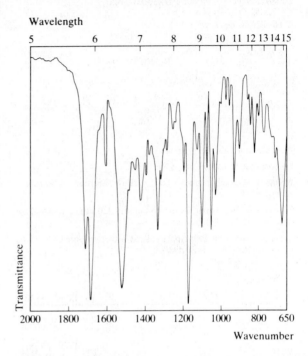

Mass Spectrum. Principal peaks at *m/z* 91, 155, 197, 65, 84, 39, 95, 41.

Quantification. SPECTROFLUORIMETRY. In plasma or serum: detection limit 40 ng/ml—R. Becker, *Arzneimittel-Forsch.*, 1977, *27*, 102-104.

HIGH PRESSURE LIQUID CHROMATOGRAPHY. In serum: sensitivity 500 ng/ml, UV detection—K. Harzer, *J. Chromat.*, 1980, *183*; *Biomed. Appl.*, *9*, 115–117.

Disposition in the Body. Readily absorbed after oral administration. Extensively metabolised by hydroxylation to a series of inactive or almost inactive compounds and by oxidation to a *p*-carboxy derivative. About 60 to 70% of a dose is excreted in the urine as metabolites; four hydroxylated derivatives account for about 75% of the urinary material, *p*-hydroxyglibornuride accounts for about 6%, and *p*-carboxyglibornuride for about 7%; the remainder of a dose is eliminated in the faeces.

THERAPEUTIC CONCENTRATION.
After an oral dose of 50 mg to 7 subjects, peak plasma concentrations of 1.6 to 3.4 μg/ml were attained in about 3 to 4 hours (G. Rentsch *et al.*, *Arzneimittel-Forsch.*, 1972, *22*, 2209–2212).

HALF-LIFE. Plasma half-life, 5 to 11 hours (mean 8).

VOLUME OF DISTRIBUTION. 0.15 to 0.35 litre/kg.

PROTEIN BINDING. In plasma, about 95%.

NOTE. For reviews of the pharmacokinetics of sulphonylurea hypoglycaemic drugs, see L. Balant, *Clin. Pharmacokinet.*, 1981, *6*, 215–241, and J. E. Jackson and R. Bressler, *Drugs*, 1981, *22*, 211–245.

Dose. 12.5 to 75 mg daily.

Gliclazide

Antidiabetic

Proprietary Names. Diamicron; Dramion.
1-(3-Azabicyclo[3.3.0]oct-3-yl)-3-tosylurea
$C_{15}H_{21}N_3O_3S = 323.4$
CAS—21187-98-4

A crystalline solid. M.p. about 181°.

Dissociation Constant. pK_a 5.8.

Colour Tests. Liebermann's Test—yellow; Mercurous Nitrate—black.

Ultraviolet Spectrum. Aqueous acid—230 nm ($A_1^1 = 440$ b); aqueous alkali—263 nm ($A_1^1 = 20$ b).

Infra-red Spectrum. Principal peaks at wavenumbers 1707, 1162, 920, 667, 1089, 997 (KBr disk).

Quantification. HIGH PRESSURE LIQUID CHROMATOGRAPHY. In serum: detection limit 200 ng/ml, UV detection—M. Kimura *et al.*, *J. Chromat.*, 1980, *183*; *Biomed. Appl.*, *9*, 467–473. In plasma: sensitivity 300 ng/ml, UV detection—M. Kimura *et al.*, *Chem. pharm. Bull.*, 1980, *28*, 344–346.

Disposition in the Body. Absorbed after oral administration. It is extensively metabolised by hydroxylation, *N*-oxidation, and oxidation to several inactive metabolites; the *p*-carboxy metabolite, which accounts for about 1% of the plasma concentration, has no hypoglycaemic activity but has some antithrombotic activity. About 60 to 70% of a dose is excreted in the urine with less than 5% as unchanged drug. The *p*-carboxy and *N*-oxide metabolites account for about 40% of the dose. About 10 to 20% of the dose is eliminated in the faeces as metabolites.

THERAPEUTIC CONCENTRATION.

After a single oral dose of 80 mg to 23 subjects, peak plasma concentrations of 0.7 to 4.9 μg/ml were attained in about 4 hours. Following daily oral administration of 80 mg to 144 subjects, steady-state plasma concentrations of 0.3 to 8.2 μg/ml (mean 2.5) were reported (D. B. Campbell *et al.*, Pharmacokinetics and Metabolism of Gliclazide, in *Gliclazide and the Treatment of Diabetes*, H. Keen *et al.* (Ed.), London, Royal Society of Medicine, 1980, pp. 71–82).

HALF-LIFE. Plasma half-life, 6 to 14 hours (mean 10).

PROTEIN BINDING. In plasma, 85 to 95%.

REFERENCE. D. B. Campbell *et al.*, *ibid*. See also B. Holmes *et al.*, *Drugs*, 1984, *27*, 301–327.

Dose. 40 to 320 mg daily.

Glipizide

Antidiabetic

Synonym. Glydiazinamide
Proprietary Names. Glibenese; Minidiab; Minodiab.
1 - Cyclohexyl - 3 - {4 - [2 - (5 - methylpyrazine - 2 - carboxamido)-ethyl]benzenesulphonyl}urea
$C_{21}H_{27}N_5O_4S = 445.5$
CAS—29094-61-9

A white powder. M.p. about 205°.
Practically **insoluble** in water and ethanol; soluble in chloroform, dimethylformamide, and in dilute solutions of alkali hydroxides; sparingly soluble in acetone.

Colour Test. Mercurous Nitrate—black.

Thin-layer Chromatography. *System TA*—Rf 87; *system TB*—Rf 00; *system TC*—Rf 41.

Ultraviolet Spectrum. Aqueous acid—276 nm ($A_1^1 = 231$ a). No alkaline shift.

Infra-red Spectrum. Principal peaks at wavenumbers 1528, 1690, 1650, 1159, 1032, 900 (KBr disk).

Mass Spectrum. Principal peaks at *m/z* 150, 121, 56, 93, 39, 151, 66, 94.

Quantification. HIGH PRESSURE LIQUID CHROMATOGRAPHY. In serum: sensitivity 20 ng/ml, UV detection—E. Wåhlin-Boll and A. Melander, *J. Chromat.*, 1979, *164*; *Biomed. Appl.*, *6*, 541–546.

RADIOIMMUNOASSAY. In plasma: sensitivity 1 ng/ml—E. Maggi *et al.*, *Eur. J. clin. Pharmac.*, 1981, *21*, 251–255.

Disposition in the Body. Readily absorbed after oral administration; bioavailability almost 100%. Metabolised by hydroxylation to form a number of inactive metabolites, principally the 4-*trans*-hydroxycyclohexyl and 3-*cis*-hydroxycyclohexyl derivatives. About 65 to 85% of a dose is excreted in the urine in 24 hours, with about 3 to 10% as unchanged drug, up to 80% as hydroxylated metabolites, mainly the 4-*trans*-hydroxycyclohexyl derivative, and about 1 to 2% as an *N*-acetamido metabolite; about 11% of a dose is eliminated in the faeces.

Wavelength

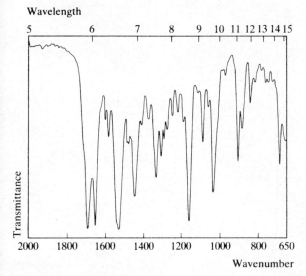

THERAPEUTIC CONCENTRATION.
After a single oral dose of 5 mg given to 6 subjects, peak serum concentrations of 0.11 to 0.49 µg/ml (mean 0.33) were attained in about 1.6 hours (E. Wåhlin-Boll *et al.*, *Clin. Pharmacokinet.*, 1982, *7*, 363–372).

HALF-LIFE. Plasma half-life, 2 to 6 hours.

VOLUME OF DISTRIBUTION. About 0.2 litre/kg.

CLEARANCE. Plasma clearance, about 0.6 ml/min/kg.

PROTEIN BINDING. In plasma, about 98%.

NOTE. For a review of the pharmacokinetics of glipizide see R. N. Brogden *et al.*, *Drugs*, 1979, *18*, 329–353.

Dose. 2.5 to 30 mg daily.

Gliquidone   *Antidiabetic*

Proprietary Name. Glurenorm
1-Cyclohexyl-3-{4-[2-(3,4-dihydro-7-methoxy-4,4-dimethyl-1,3-dioxo-2(1*H*)-isoquinolyl)ethyl]benzenesulphonyl}urea
$C_{27}H_{33}N_3O_6S = 527.6$
CAS—33342-05-1

A white or slightly yellow crystalline substance. M.p. about 178°. Practically **insoluble** in water; slightly soluble in ethanol and methanol; soluble in acetone and chloroform.

Colour Test. Koppanyi–Zwikker Test—violet.

Ultraviolet Spectrum. Methanol—311 nm ($A_1^1 = 50$ a); aqueous alkali—276 nm.

Infra-red Spectrum. Principal peaks at wavenumbers 1700, 1652, 1160, 1285, 1295, 1530 (KBr disk).

Quantification. RADIOIMMUNOASSAY. In plasma: sensitivity 1 ng/ml—Z. Kopitar and H. E. Kompa, *Arzneimittel-Forsch.*, 1975, *25*, 1469–1472.

Wavelength

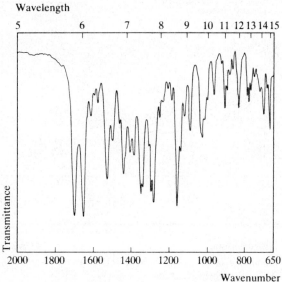

Disposition in the Body. Readily absorbed after oral administration. Extensively metabolised by hydroxylation and demethylation to inactive metabolites. Less than 5% of a dose is excreted in the urine and about 95% is eliminated in the faeces, via the bile.

THERAPEUTIC CONCENTRATION.
After a single oral dose of 15 mg to 10 subjects, peak plasma concentrations of about 0.7 µg/ml, and peak blood concentrations of about 0.37 µg/ml were reported (Z. Kopitar, *Arzneimittel-Forsch.*, 1975, *25*, 1455–1460).

HALF-LIFE. Plasma half-life, about 1.5 hours.

DISTRIBUTION IN BLOOD. Plasma: whole blood ratio, about 1.9.

PROTEIN BINDING. In plasma, about 99%.

Dose. 15 to 180 mg daily.

Gloxazone   *Anaplasmodastat (Veterinary)*

3-Ethoxy-2-oxobutyraldehyde bis(thiosemicarbazone)
$C_8H_{16}N_6OS_2 = 276.4$
CAS—2507-91-7

A yellow powder.
Practically **insoluble** in water and ether; slightly soluble in chloroform.

Colour Test. Palladium Chloride—red.

Thin-layer Chromatography. *System TA*—Rf 77. (*Acidified iodoplatinate solution*, positive.)

Ultraviolet Spectrum. Aqueous acid—329 nm; aqueous alkali—303 nm. (See below)

Infra-red Spectrum. Principal peaks at wavenumbers 1587, 1079, 1228, 1259, 1575, 1022 (KBr disk).

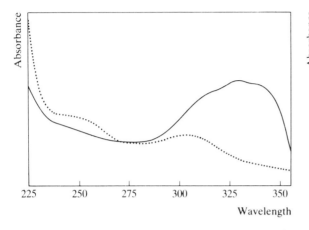

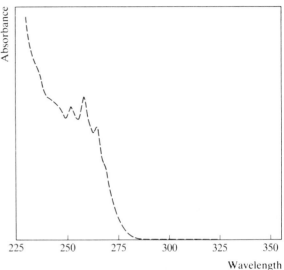

Glutethimide

Hypnotic

Proprietary Names. Doriden(e); Dorimide.
2-Ethyl-2-phenylglutarimide
$C_{13}H_{15}NO_2 = 217.3$
CAS—77-21-4

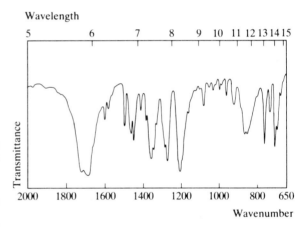

Colourless crystals or white crystalline powder. M.p. 85° to 89°. Practically **insoluble** in water; soluble 1 in 5 of ethanol, 1 in less than 1 of chloroform, and 1 in 12 of ether; freely soluble in acetone.

Dissociation Constant. pK_a 9.2.

Colour Tests. Koppanyi-Zwikker Test—violet; Liebermann's Test—red-orange; Mercurous Nitrate—black.

Thin-layer Chromatography. *System TA*—Rf 75; *system TD*—Rf 63; *system TE*—Rf 78; *system TF*—Rf 62. (*Dragendorff spray*, weak reaction; *acidified iodoplatinate solution*, positive; *mercuric chloride-diphenylcarbazone reagent*, positive; *mercurous nitrate spray*, black.)

Gas Chromatography. *System GA*—glutethimide RI 1836, 4-hydroxyglutethimide RI 1875, 2-phenylglutarimide RI 1778; *system GF*—RI 2315.

High Pressure Liquid Chromatography. *System HE*—k' 7.97.

Ultraviolet Spectrum. Ethanol—252 nm, 258 nm ($A_1^1 = 18$ a), 264 nm.

Infra-red Spectrum. Principal peaks at wavenumbers 1686, 1710, 1200, 1270, 1281, 704 (KBr disk).

Mass Spectrum. Principal peaks at m/z 189, 132, 117, 160, 91, 115, 103, 77; 4-hydroxyglutethimide 146, 233, 103, 133, 91, 117, 115, 77; 2-phenylglutarimide 104, 189, 103, 117, 78, 91, 51, 146.

Quantification. GAS CHROMATOGRAPHY. In plasma, tissues or urine: glutethimide and 4-hydroxyglutethimide, sensitivity 200 ng/ml for glutethimide and 500 ng/ml for 4-hydroxyglutethimide in plasma, FID—A. R. Hansen and L. J. Fischer, *Clin. Chem.*, 1974, *20*, 236–242. In serum: sensitivity 250 ng/ml, FID—D. Kadar and W. Kalow, *J. Chromat.*, 1972, *72*, 21–27.

GAS CHROMATOGRAPHY-MASS SPECTROMETRY. In plasma or urine: glutethimide and six metabolites, sensitivity 50 ng/ml—K. A. Kennedy *et al.*, *Biomed. Mass Spectrom.*, 1978, *5*, 679–685.

Disposition in the Body. Irregularly absorbed from the gastro-intestinal tract; absorption is enhanced if alcohol is taken concomitantly. Widely distributed in body tissues and fat. Glutethimide is a racemate; the (+)-isomer is metabolised in the liver to 4-hydroxyglutethimide and the (−)-isomer to 2-(1-hydroxyethyl)-2-phenylglutarimide. 4-Hydroxyglutethimide is twice as active as glutethimide in animals but does not appear to contribute to the effects of single therapeutic doses in man; however it tends to accumulate in the plasma during intoxication and may contribute to the central nervous depression in overdose cases. Both hydroxylated metabolites are converted to glucuronides and undergo enterohepatic circulation; they are still being excreted in the urine after more than 48 hours. 2-Ethyl-2-(4-hydroxyphenyl)glutarimide is a major metabolite during chronic administration. Other metabolites include 2-phenylglutarimide, α-phenyl-γ-butyrolactone, and 2-ethyl-2-phenylglutaconimide which are pharmacologically active; numerous other mono- and dihydroxyphenyl metabolites have been isolated from human urine. Less than 2% of a dose is excreted unchanged in the urine in 24 hours. 2-Phenylglutarimide and 2-ethyl-2-phenylglutaconimide each account for about 2 to 4% of the dose as urinary excretion products and the remainder consists largely of glucuronide conjugates of the hydroxylated metabolites.

THERAPEUTIC CONCENTRATION.
Following single oral doses of 500 mg to 6 subjects, peak plasma concentrations of 2.8 to 7.1 µg/ml (mean 4.3) were attained in 1 to 6 hours (mean 2) (S. Curry *et al.*, *Clin. Pharmac. Ther.*, 1971, *12*, 849–857).

TOXICITY. The estimated minimum lethal dose is 5 g although recoveries have occurred after the ingestion of up to 10 g. Blood concentrations of 3.4 to **27** to 48 µg/ml of glutethimide have been associated with toxic effects and concentrations of 25 to **48** to 90 µg/ml have been associated with fatalities. Postmortem blood concentrations of about 10 µg/ml may be indicative of poisoning if the survival time has been prolonged.

In a review of 11 fatalities, blood concentrations of glutethimide were reported to range from 10 to 97 µg/ml (mean 45) and liver concentrations from 63 to 141 µg/g (mean 89) (R. C. Baselt and R. H. Cravey, *J. analyt. Toxicol.*, 1977, *1*, 81–103).

HALF-LIFE. Plasma half-life, 5 to 22 hours (mean 12); in acute intoxication the plasma half-life has an average value of about 40 hours but may exceed 100 hours.

VOLUME OF DISTRIBUTION. About 3 litres/kg.

PROTEIN BINDING. In plasma, about 54%.

Dose. Usually 250 to 500 mg, as a hypnotic.

Glyceryl Trinitrate   *Anti-anginal Vasodilator*

Synonyms. Glonoin; Nitroglycerin; Nitroglycerol; Trinitrin; Trinitroglycerin.
Proprietary Names. Cardabid; Coro-Nitro; Lénitral; Nitora; Nitro-Bid; Nitrocine; Nitrocontin; Nitroglyn; Nitrol; Nitrolingual; Nitrong; Nitro-SA; Nitrospan; Nitrostabilin; Nitrostat; Nitrovas; Percutol; Suscard Buccal; Sustac; Transiderm-Nitro; Trates; Tridil. It is an ingredient of Cardiac Dellipsoids D 18 and Natirose.
Propane-1,2,3-triol trinitrate
$C_3H_5N_3O_9 = 227.1$
CAS—55-63-0

$$O \cdot NO_2$$
$$|$$
$$NO_2 \cdot O \cdot CH_2 \cdot CH \cdot CH_2 \cdot O \cdot NO_2$$

A colourless, slightly volatile, oily liquid. It explodes on rapid heating or on percussion. Wt per ml about 1.6 g.
Soluble 1 in 800 of water and 1 in 4 of ethanol; miscible with chloroform and ether.
Caution. In fatty or oily solution it is safe and stable but in alcoholic solution the substance must be handled with the utmost caution.

Colour Test. Ferrous Sulphate—red.

Thin-layer Chromatography. *System TD*—Rf 71; *system TE*—Rf 86; *system TF*—Rf 72.

Infra-red Spectrum. Principal peaks at wavenumbers 1647, 1279, 843, 1013, 903, 754.

Quantification. GAS CHROMATOGRAPHY (CAPILLARY COLUMN). In plasma: sensitivity 25 pg/ml, ECD—P. K. Noonan *et al.*, *J. pharm. Sci.*, 1984, *73*, 923–927.

HIGH PRESSURE LIQUID CHROMATOGRAPHY. In plasma: limit of detection 500 pg/ml—R. J. Spanggord and R. G. Keck, *J. pharm. Sci.*, 1980, *69*, 444–446.

Disposition in the Body. Readily absorbed from the skin and mucous membranes; less readily absorbed after oral administration. It is rapidly metabolised in the body to dinitrates, which are active, and to inactive mononitrates. About 20% of a sublingual dose is excreted in the urine in 24 hours, mainly as the mononitrate.

THERAPEUTIC CONCENTRATION.
After sublingual administration of 0.3 mg to 1 subject, a blood concentration of about 0.001 µg/ml was attained in 3 minutes; following an oral dose of 6.5 mg or application of an ointment containing 16 mg of glyceryl trinitrate to the same subject, peak blood concentrations of about 0.0002 to 0.0003 µg/ml were reported, 20 to 60 minutes after the dose (H. P. Blumenthal *et al.*, *Br. J. clin. Pharmac.*, 1977, *4*, 241–242).

Following sublingual administration of 0.5 mg to 6 subjects, a mean peak plasma concentration of 0.0014 µg/ml was attained in 3 minutes; after oral administration of 6.4 mg, a peak plasma concentration of 0.0026 µg/ml was reported at 2 to 4 hours, and after topical administration of 35 mg, a mean peak plasma concentration of 0.0025 µg/ml was attained in 1 hour. Plasma nitrate and nitrite concentrations were undetectable after sublingual administration; after oral administration peak plasma concentrations of about 0.5 µg/ml of nitrate and nitrite were attained in 5 and 2 hours respectively, and following topical administration, peak concentrations of about 0.7 µg/ml were reported at 5 hours and 1 hour respectively (A. Bashir *et al.*, *Br. J. clin. Pharmac.*, 1982, *14*, 779–784).

TOXICITY. The estimated minimum oral lethal dose is 2 g and the maximum permissible atmospheric concentration is 0.2 ppm.

HALF-LIFE. Plasma half-life, after intravenous administration about 2 to 5 minutes; after sublingual administration about 5 minutes.

VOLUME OF DISTRIBUTION. About 3 litres/kg.

NOTE. For a review of the pharmacokinetics of organic nitrates, see M. G. Bogaert, *Clin. Pharmacokinet.*, 1983, *8*, 410–421. For a review of intravenous glyceryl trinitrate see E. M. Sorkin *et al.*, *Drugs*, 1984, *27*, 45–80.

Dose. Usually the equivalent of 0.5 to 1 mg of glyceryl trinitrate sublingually, repeated as required; doses of 5.2 to 38.4 mg daily are given by mouth as sustained-release tablets.

Glycopyrronium Bromide   *Anticholinergic*

Synonym. Glycopyrrolate
Proprietary Names. Asécryl; Robinul.
3 - (α - Cyclopentylmandeloyloxy) - 1,1 - dimethylpyrrolidinium bromide
$C_{19}H_{28}BrNO_3 = 398.3$
CAS—596-51-0

A white crystalline powder. M.p. 193° to 198°.
Soluble 1 in about 5 of water and 1 in 10 of ethanol; practically insoluble in chloroform and ether.

Colour Test. The following test is performed on glycopyrronium nitrate (see page 128): Liebermann's Test—black.

Thin-layer Chromatography. *System TA*—Rf 03. (*Acidified iodoplatinate solution*, positive.)

Gas Chromatography. *System GA*—RI 2120.

High Pressure Liquid Chromatography. *System HA*—k' 3.2 (tailing peak).

Ultraviolet Spectrum. Aqueous acid—252 nm, 258 nm ($A_1^1 =$ 7.1 a), 264 nm.

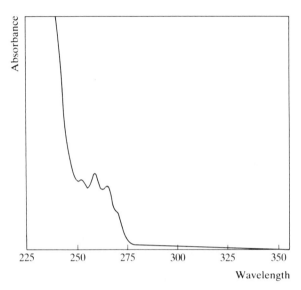

Infra-red Spectrum. Principal peaks at wavenumbers 1738, 1225, 1164, 1178, 1115, 1192.

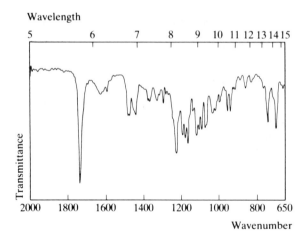

Dose. 2 to 12 mg daily.

Glymidine   *Antidiabetic*

Synonyms. Glidiazine Sodique; Glycodiazine; Sodium Glymidine.

Proprietary Names. Gondafon; Lycanol; Redul.

The sodium salt of N-[5-(2-methoxyethoxy)pyrimidin-2-yl]-benzenesulphonamide.

$C_{13}H_{14}N_3NaO_4S = 331.3$

CAS—3459-20-9

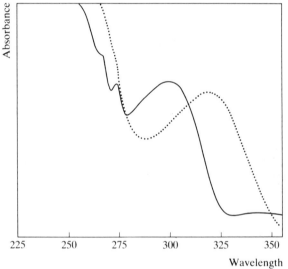

A white crystalline powder. M.p. about 223°.

Soluble in water; slightly soluble in ethanol.

Colour Tests. Koppanyi–Zwikker Test—pink-violet; Mercurous Nitrate—black.

Thin-layer Chromatography. *System TA*—Rf 76; *system TB*—Rf 00; *system TC*—Rf 65.

Gas Chromatography. *System GJ*—retention time of methyl derivative 0.53 relative to griseofulvin.

Ultraviolet Spectrum. Aqueous acid—273 nm, 299 nm; aqueous alkali—243 nm, 317 nm.

Infra-red Spectrum. Principal peaks at wavenumbers 1130, 1092, 1267, 1247, 691, 1220 (KBr disk).

Mass Spectrum. Principal peaks at *m/z* 244, 59, 77, 29, 43, 31, 45, 55.

Quantification. SPECTROFLUORIMETRY. In plasma (glymidine) or urine (desmethyl and carboxy metabolites): detection limit, 1 μg/ml for glymidine in plasma—H. Held *et al.*, *Arzneimittel-Forsch.*, 1970, *20*, 1927–1929.

GAS CHROMATOGRAPHY. In blood: sensitivity 1.5 μg/ml, ECD—H. J. Schlicht *et al.*, *J. Chromat.*, 1978, *155*, 178–181.

THIN-LAYER CHROMATOGRAPHY–SPECTROPHOTOMETRY. In plasma: glymidine and metabolites, sensitivity 2.5 μg/ml—J. C. Soyfer *et al.*, *Chim. Ther.*, 1969, *4*, 131–135.

Disposition in the Body. Almost completely absorbed after oral administration. Metabolised by demethylation to an active metabolite and oxidation to an inactive carboxy derivative. About 85 to 95% of a dose is excreted in the urine in 48 hours, with less than 1% of the urinary material as unchanged drug, 20 to 40% as the desmethyl metabolite, and 60 to 80% as the carboxy metabolite; about 6% of a dose is eliminated in the faeces.

HALF-LIFE. Plasma half-life, about 2 to 6 hours, increased in subjects with hepatic disease.

PROTEIN BINDING. In plasma, about 80%.

REFERENCE. E. Gerhards *et al.*, *Arzneimittel-Forsch.*, 1964, *14*, 394–402.

Dose. 0.5 to 2 g daily.

Griseofulvin
Antifungal

Synonym. Curling Factor

Proprietary Names. Fulcin; Fulvicin; Grifulvin V; Grisactin; Grisaltin; Grisefuline; Griseostatin; Grisovin; Gris-PEG; Lamoryl; Likuden M; Neo-Fulcin.

(2*S*,6′*R*)-7-Chloro-2′,4,6-trimethoxy-6′-methylbenzofuran-2-spiro-1′-cyclohex-2′-ene-3,4′-dione
$C_{17}H_{17}ClO_6 = 352.8$
CAS—126-07-8

A white to pale cream-coloured powder. M.p. 217° to 224°.
Very slightly **soluble** in water; soluble 1 in 300 of dehydrated alcohol, 1 in 20 of acetone, and 1 in 25 of chloroform; soluble in dimethylformamide.

Colour Test. Dissolve 5 mg in 1 ml of *sulphuric acid* and add 5 mg of powdered potassium dichromate—red.

Gas Chromatography. *System GA*—RI 2700.

Ultraviolet Spectrum. Dehydrated alcohol—236 nm, 291 nm ($A_1^1 = 686$ a).

Infra-red Spectrum. Principal peaks at wavenumbers 1220, 1611, 1210, 1583, 1135, 800 (KBr disk).

Mass Spectrum. Principal peaks at *m/z* 138, 352, 215, 310, 214, 69, 321, 354.

Dose. 0.5 to 1 g daily.

Guaiphenesin
Expectorant

Synonyms. Glyceryl Guaiacolate; Glycerylguayacolum; Guaiacol Glycerol Ether; Guaiacyl Glyceryl Ether; Guaifenesin; Guajacolum Glycerolatum.

Proprietary Names. Balminil (expectorant); Broncho-Grippex; Corutol (expectorant); 2/G (expectorant); Gaiapect; Glycotuss; Glytuss; Guiatuss; Hytuss; Motussin; Myoscain 'E'; Reorganin; Resyl; Robitussin; Sedatuss (expectorant); S-T Expect; Tussanca.

It is an ingredient of many proprietary preparations—see *Martindale, The Extra Pharmacopoeia*, 28th Edn.

3-(2-Methoxyphenoxy)propane-1,2-diol
$C_{10}H_{14}O_4 = 198.2$
CAS—93-14-1

White or slightly grey crystals or crystalline aggregates. M.p. 78° to 82°.

Soluble 1 in 33 of water, 1 in 11 of ethanol, 1 in 11 of chloroform, and 1 in 100 of ether.

Colour Tests. Liebermann's Test—black; Mandelin's Test—grey-green; Marquis Test—violet.

Thin-layer Chromatography. *System TD*—Rf 11; *system TE*—Rf 37; *system TF*—Rf 17.

Gas Chromatography. *System GA*—RI 1650.

Ultraviolet Spectrum. Aqueous acid—273 nm ($A_1^1 = 125$ a). No alkaline shift.

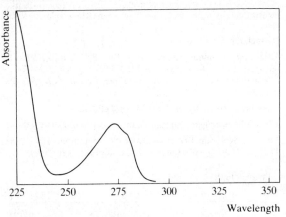

Infra-red Spectrum. Principal peaks at wavenumbers 1255, 1510, 740, 1230, 1125, 1020 (KBr disk).

Mass Spectrum. Principal peaks at *m/z* 124, 109, 198, 81, 77, 125, 52, 31.

Quantification. GAS CHROMATOGRAPHY. In plasma: detection limit 15 ng/ml, ECD—S. Singhawangcha *et al.*, *J. Chromat.*, 1980, *183*; *Biomed. Appl.*, 9, 433–439. In blood: ECD—W. R. Maynard, jun., and R. B. Bruce, *J. pharm. Sci.*, 1970, *59*, 1346–1348.

Disposition in the Body. Readily absorbed after oral administration. It is rapidly metabolised by oxidation to β-(2-methoxyphenoxy)lactic acid; about 40% of a dose is excreted as this metabolite in the urine in 3 hours.

THERAPEUTIC CONCENTRATION.

After a single oral dose of 600 mg given to 3 subjects, a mean peak blood concentration of about 1.4 µg/ml was attained in 15 minutes (W. R. Maynard, jun., and R. B. Bruce, *ibid.*).

TOXICITY.

In a fatality due to ingestion of cough syrup containing guaiphenesin and hydrocodone, postmortem blood concentrations of 14 and 3 µg/ml respectively were reported (R. H. Cravey per R. C. Baselt, *Disposition of Toxic Drugs and Chemicals in Man*, 2nd Edn, Davis, California, Biomedical Publications, 1982, pp. 357–358).

HALF-LIFE. Blood half-life, about 1 hour.

VOLUME OF DISTRIBUTION. About 1 litre/kg.

Dose. 100 to 200 mg every 2 to 4 hours.

Guanethidine
Antihypertensive

1-[2-(Perhydroazocin-1-yl)ethyl]guanidine
$C_{10}H_{22}N_4 = 198.3$
CAS—55-65-2

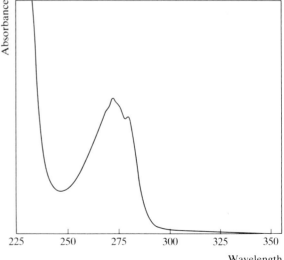

Guanethidine Monosulphate

Synonym. Guanethidine Sulphate

Proprietary Names. Antipres; Ismelin. It is an ingredient of Esimil and Ganda.

$C_{10}H_{22}N_4,H_2SO_4 = 296.4$

CAS—645-43-2

A colourless crystalline powder. M.p. about 250°, with decomposition.

Soluble 1 in 1.5 of water; practically insoluble in ethanol, chloroform, and ether.

Dissociation Constant. pK_a 8.3, 11.4 (20°).

Thin-layer Chromatography. *System TA*—Rf 01; *system TB*—Rf 00; *system TC*—Rf 02; *system TN*—Rf 56; *system TO*—Rf 50. (*Dragendorff* spray, positive; *acidified iodoplatinate solution,* positive.)

Gas Chromatography. *System GA*—not eluted.

Ultraviolet Spectrum. No significant absorption, 230 to 360 nm.

Infra-red Spectrum. Principal peaks at wavenumbers 1030, 1143, 1127, 1070, 1050, 1630 (guanethidine sulphate, KBr disk).

Wavelength

Mass Spectrum. Principal peaks at *m/z* 126, 44, 30, 42, 41, 55, 43, 58.

Quantification. GAS CHROMATOGRAPHY–MASS SPECTROMETRY. In plasma or urine: guanethidine and other guanido-containing drugs, sensitivity 100 ng/ml using FID and 1 ng/ml using MID— J. H. Hengstmann *et al., Analyt. Chem.,* 1974, *46,* 34–39.

RADIOIMMUNOASSAY. In plasma: sensitivity 4 ng/ml—L. J. Loeffler and A. W. Pittman, *J. pharm. Sci.,* 1979, *68,* 1419–1423.

Disposition in the Body. Incompletely absorbed after oral administration; bioavailability about 20%. Up to about 25% of an oral dose is excreted in the urine in 24 hours as unchanged drug and two metabolites, guanethidine N-oxide and 2-(6-carboxyhexylamino)ethylguanidine; the proportion of metabolites to unchanged drug is variable. A total of about 40% of an oral dose is excreted in the urine in 9 days and about 40 to 47% is eliminated in the faeces as unchanged drug in 6 days.

THERAPEUTIC CONCENTRATION. In plasma, usually in the range 0.008 to 0.017 µg/ml.

After a single oral ^{3}H-labelled dose of 50 mg to 1 subject, a peak plasma-guanethidine concentration of 0.009 µg/ml was attained in 3 hours and was almost constant over the period 1 to 12 hours, declining slowly to about 0.003 µg/ml at 24 hours; a peak total metabolite concentration of about 0.04 µg/ml was reported at 2 to 4 hours (C. McMartin *et al., Clin. Pharmac. Ther.,* 1970, *11,* 423–431).

Following daily oral doses of 25 mg to 8 subjects, steady-state plasma-guanethidine concentrations of 0.003 to 0.016 µg/ml (mean 0.009) were reported; after oral doses of 37.5 mg daily to 8 subjects, the steady-state plasma-guanethidine concentrations ranged from 0.008 to 0.015 µg/ml (mean 0.011) (I. E. Walter *et al., Clin. Pharmac. Ther.,* 1975, *18,* 571–580).

HALF-LIFE. Plasma half-life, about 4 to 8 days.

PROTEIN BINDING. In plasma, not significantly bound.

NOTE. For a review of guanethidine disposition, see G. Lukas, *Drug Met. Rev.,* 1973, *2,* 101–116.

Dose. Usually 10 to 100 mg of guanethidine monosulphate daily; up to 300 mg daily may be given.

Guanoclor   *Antihypertensive*

1-[2-(2,6-Dichlorophenoxy)ethylamino]guanidine

$C_9H_{12}Cl_2N_4O = 263.1$

CAS—5001-32-1

Guanoclor Sulphate

Proprietary Name. Vatensol

$(C_9H_{12}Cl_2N_4O)_2,H_2SO_4 = 624.3$

CAS—551-48-4

A white crystalline powder. M.p. about 208°.

Soluble 1 in about 400 of water.

Colour Test. Mandelin's Test—violet→ orange→ brown-yellow.

Thin-layer Chromatography. *System TA*—Rf 03; *system TB*—Rf 00; *system TC*—Rf 00. (*Acidified iodoplatinate solution*, positive.)

Ultraviolet Spectrum. Aqueous acid—272 nm ($A_1^1 = 14$ b), 278 nm.

Infra-red Spectrum. Principal peaks at wavenumbers 1672, 1134, 1652, 1050, 765, 1243 (KBr disk).

Mass Spectrum. Principal peaks at m/z 162, 43, 63, 164, 30, 44, 98, 42.

Dose. 10 to 120 mg of guanoclor sulphate daily; doses of 200 mg or more daily have been given.

Guanoxan   *Antihypertensive*

1-(1,4-Benzodioxan-2-ylmethyl)guanidine
$C_{10}H_{13}N_3O_2 = 207.2$
CAS—2165-19-7

Crystals. M.p. 164° to 165°.

Guanoxan Sulphate
$(C_{10}H_{13}N_3O_2)_2,H_2SO_4 = 512.5$
CAS—5714-04-5
A white crystalline powder. M.p. about 206°.
Soluble 1 in 50 of water.

Dissociation Constant. pK_a 12.3.

Colour Tests. Mandelin's Test—green, sometimes violet, depending on relative proportions of test material and reagent; Marquis Test—violet.

Thin-layer Chromatography. *System TA*—Rf 01; *system TB*—Rf 00; *system TC*—Rf 00. (*Acidified potassium permanganate solution*, positive.)

Ultraviolet Spectrum. Aqueous acid—275 nm ($A_1^1 = 104$ b).

Infra-red Spectrum. Principal peaks at wavenumbers 1115, 1495, 1264, 1665, 1592, 748 (KBr disk).

Mass Spectrum. Principal peaks at m/z 30, 72, 43, 135, 121, 148, 52, 56.

Dose. 10 to 50 mg of guanoxan sulphate daily; doses of 120 mg or more daily have been given.

Halazone   *Disinfectant*

Synonym. Pantocide
4-(Dichlorosulphamoyl)benzoic acid
$C_7H_5Cl_2NO_4S = 270.1$
CAS—80-13-7

A white crystalline powder containing about 52% of 'available chlorine'. M.p. about 194°, with decomposition.

Very slightly **soluble** in water, chloroform, and ether; soluble 1 in 140 of ethanol; soluble in glacial acetic acid, and in aqueous solutions of alkali hydroxides and carbonates.

Ultraviolet Spectrum. Aqueous acid—237 nm; aqueous alkali—229 nm ($A_1^1 = 382$ b).

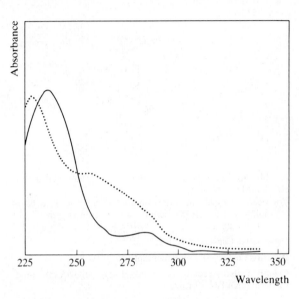

Mass Spectrum. Principal peaks at m/z 121, 65, 36, 185, 50, 38, 76, 39.

Halcinonide   *Corticosteroid*

Proprietary Names. Halciderm; Halcimat; Halog.
21 - Chloro - 9α - fluoro - 11β - hydroxy - 16α,17α - isopropylidenedi-oxypregn-4-ene-3,20-dione
$C_{24}H_{32}ClFO_5 = 455.0$
CAS—3093-35-4

Crystals. M.p. 264° to 265°, with decomposition.

Ultraviolet Spectrum. Methanolic acid—238 nm ($A_1^1 = 370$ b). No alkaline shift.

Infra-red Spectrum. Principal peaks at wavenumbers 1660, 1060, 1730, 1080, 1250, 1175 (KBr disk).

Mass Spectrum. Principal peaks at m/z 377, 43, 55, 246, 278, 59, 378, 41.

Use. Topically in concentrations of 0.025 to 0.1%.

Haloperidol

Tranquilliser

Proprietary Names. Dozic; Fortunan; Haldol; Serenace; Serenase; Sigaperidol.

4-[4-(4-Chlorophenyl)-4-hydroxypiperidino]-4'-fluorobutyrophenone

$C_{21}H_{23}ClFNO_2 = 375.9$

CAS—52-86-8

A white to faintly yellowish, amorphous or microcrystalline powder. M.p. 147° to 152°.

Practically **insoluble** in water; soluble 1 in 50 to 1 in 60 of ethanol, 1 in 15 to 1 in 20 of chloroform, 1 in 200 of ether, and 1 in 55 of methanol.

Dissociation Constant. pK_a 8.3.

Partition Coefficient. Log P (octanol/pH 7.4), 4.3.

Colour Tests. Aromaticity (Method 2)—yellow/orange-red; Liebermann's Test—brown.

Thin-layer Chromatography. *System TA*—Rf 67; *system TB*—Rf 10; *system TC*—Rf 27. (*Acidified iodoplatinate solution,* positive.)

Gas Chromatography. *System GA*—RI 2942.

High Pressure Liquid Chromatography. *System HA*—k' 1.2.

Ultraviolet Spectrum. Methanolic acid—245 nm ($A_1^1 = 340$ a). No alkaline shift.

Infra-red Spectrum. Principal peaks at wavenumbers 832, 1151, 1673, 1217, 1136, 1598 (KBr disk).

Wavelength

Transmittance

Wavenumber

Mass Spectrum. Principal peaks at m/z 224, 42, 237, 226, 123, 206, 239, 56 (no peaks above 240).

Quantification. GAS CHROMATOGRAPHY. In serum or cerebrospinal fluid: sensitivity 500 pg/ml, AFID—D. R. Abernethy *et al., J. Chromat.,* 1984, *307*; *Biomed. Appl., 32,* 194–199.

GAS CHROMATOGRAPHY–MASS SPECTROMETRY. In serum: detection limit 100 pg—M. A. Moulin *et al., J. Chromat.,* 1979, *178*, 324–329.

HIGH PRESSURE LIQUID CHROMATOGRAPHY. In plasma or serum: haloperidol and reduced metabolite, sensitivity 1 ng/ml, electrochemical detection—E. R. Korpi *et al., Clin. Chem.,* 1983, *29*, 624–628.

RADIOIMMUNOASSAY. In plasma: sensitivity 400 pg/ml—F. J. Rowell *et al., Clin. Chem.,* 1981, *27*, 1249–1254.

Disposition in the Body. Readily absorbed after oral administration; bioavailability about 65%. Haloperidol is localised in the tissues and rapidly taken up by the brain. It is slowly excreted in the urine, about 40% of a dose being eliminated in 5 days with only about 1% of the dose as unchanged drug; about 15% of a dose is excreted in the bile. Metabolites which have been identified in urine are 4-fluorobenzoylpropionic acid and 4-fluorophenylaceturic acid (the glycine conjugate of 4-fluorophenylacetic acid), both of which are inactive. Haloperidol is also metabolised by reduction of the ketone group to a secondary alcohol.

THERAPEUTIC CONCENTRATION. There is considerable intersubject variation in steady-state blood concentrations. However, for normal doses (up to 15 mg per day), the serum concentration is usually below 0.05 µg/ml.

Steady-state serum concentrations of 0.0008 to 0.033 µg/ml (mean 0.0065) were attained after daily oral administration of 1 to 14 mg (mean 6) to 34 patients (A. O. Forsman and R. Öhman, *Curr. ther. Res.,* 1977, *21*, 396–411).

TOXICITY. The minimum lethal dose is probably in excess of 3 g. Toxic effects may appear with blood concentrations greater than about 0.05 µg/ml but there is considerable intersubject variation.

HALF-LIFE. Plasma half-life, 10 to 40 hours (mean 20).

VOLUME OF DISTRIBUTION. 10 to 30 litres/kg (mean 18).

CLEARANCE. Plasma clearance, 8 to 17 ml/min/kg (mean 12).

DISTRIBUTION IN BLOOD. Plasma: whole blood ratio, about 0.93.

PROTEIN BINDING. In plasma, about 90%.

Dose. 1 to 15 mg daily; up to 200 mg daily has been given.

Halopyramine

Antihistamine

Synonyms. Chloropyramine; Chlortripelennamine.

N-(4-Chlorobenzyl)-$N'N'$-dimethyl-N-(2-pyridyl)ethylenediamine

$C_{16}H_{20}ClN_3 = 289.8$

CAS—59-32-5

A yellow oil.

Halopyramine Hydrochloride

Proprietary Names. Synopen; Synpen.

$C_{16}H_{20}ClN_3, HCl = 326.3$

CAS—6170-42-9

A white powder. M.p. 172°.

Freely **soluble** in water, ethanol, and chloroform; practically insoluble in ether.

Colour Test. Cyanogen Bromide—yellow.

Thin-layer Chromatography. *System TA*—Rf 52; *system TB*—Rf 41; *system TC*—Rf 28. (*Acidified iodoplatinate solution*, positive.)

Gas Chromatography. *System GA*—RI 2234.

High Pressure Liquid Chromatography. *System HA*—k' 4.2.

Ultraviolet Spectrum. Aqueous acid—239 nm ($A_1^1 = 515$ a), 315 nm; aqueous alkali—248 nm, 313 nm.

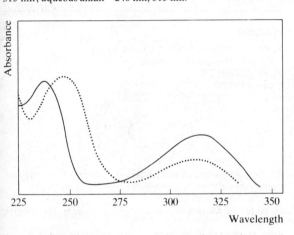

Infra-red Spectrum. Principal peaks at wavenumbers 1494, 1598, 769, 1562, 1010, 1098 (KBr disk).

Mass Spectrum. Principal peaks at *m/z* 58, 125, 71, 72, 36, 127, 79, 219.

Dose. Halopyramine hydrochloride has been given in doses of up to 150 mg daily.

Halothane
General Anaesthetic

Synonyms. Alotano; Phthorothanum.

Proprietary Names. Fluothane; Rhodialothan; Somnothane.

2-Bromo-2-chloro-1,1,1-trifluoroethane

$CF_3 \cdot CHBrCl = 197.4$

CAS—151-67-7

A colourless, mobile, heavy, non-inflammable liquid. B.p. 49° to 51°. Refractive index, at 20°, 1.3695 to 1.3705.

Halothane contains thymol 0.01% w/w as a preservative.

Soluble 1 in 400 of water; miscible with dehydrated alcohol, chloroform, and ether.

Gas Chromatography. *System GA*—RI 533; *system GI*—retention time 8.5 min.

Mass Spectrum. Principal peaks at *m/z* 117, 198, 196, 119, 129, 67, 127, 98.

Quantification. GAS CHROMATOGRAPHY. In whole blood: direct injection, FID—W. J. Cole *et al., Br. J. Anaesth.,* 1975, *47,* 1043–1047. In blood: FID—M. K. Tham *et al., Anesthesiology,* 1972, *37,* 647–649. In plasma, serum or urine: trifluoroacetic acid (TFA) and bromide, detection limit, TFA 300 ng/ml in

plasma, 1 µg/ml in urine, FID—R. M. Maiorino *et al., J. analyt. Toxicol.,* 1980, *4,* 250–254. In blood or tissues: 2-chloro-1,1-difluoroethylene and 2-chloro-1,1,1-trifluoroethane, limit of detection 200 and 300 pg/ml, respectively, in blood, FID—R. M. Maiorino *et al., J. Chromat.,* 1979, *164;* *Biomed. Appl., 6,* 63–72.

Disposition in the Body. Rapidly absorbed upon inhalation; blood:gas partition coefficient about 2.4. It accumulates in adipose tissue. About 60 to 80% of an absorbed dose is exhaled unchanged from the lungs in 24 hours and smaller amounts continue to be exhaled for several days or weeks. A variable amount is metabolised in the liver by debromination and dechlorination; replacement of a fluorine atom by a methoxy group followed by glucuronic acid conjugation occurs to a limited extent. Other metabolites which have been detected in expired air and in blood are 2-chloro-1,1,1-trifluoroethane and 2-chloro-1,1-difluoroethylene. Up to about 20% of a dose may be excreted in the urine as trifluoroacetic acid and its salts. Bromide ion is slowly excreted in the urine.

THERAPEUTIC CONCENTRATION. During surgical anaesthesia, concentrations in blood are usually in the range 22 to 84 µg/ml. Venous blood concentrations lag behind arterial concentrations during induction and decline less rapidly during recovery.

Blood concentrations ranging from 50.5 to 106.5 µg/ml were reported in 8 patients following anaesthesia with 1.5% halothane for 20 minutes. At recovery 10 minutes later the range was 22 to 30 µg/ml; traces were still detectable after 44 hours; bromide concentrations increased during the post-anaesthetic period (M. M. Atallah and I. C. Geddes, *Br. J. Anaesth.,* 1973, *45,* 464–470).

Peak plasma-bromide concentrations occurred in surgical patients 2 to 3 days after anaesthesia and ranged from 52 to 180 µg/ml (J. H. Tinker *et al., Anesthesiology,* 1976, *44,* 194–196).

TOXICITY. The minimum lethal dose by ingestion or inhalation is about 10 ml although one case of recovery after the ingestion of 250 ml has been reported. Blood concentrations of 7 to **40** to 310 µg/ml have been associated with fatalities.

In one fatality involving the ingestion of 35 ml of halothane, the following postmortem tissue concentrations were reported: blood 650 µg/ml, brain 1560 µg/g, lung 500 µg/g, liver 880 µg/g, spleen 230 µg/g, urine 20 µg/ml; salicylate and an unidentified barbiturate were also present (J. A. E. Spencer and N. M. Green, *J. Am. med. Ass.,* 1968, *205,* 702–703).

Dose. For induction of anaesthesia, 2 to 3% of the vapour by inhalation; maintenance, 0.5 to 1.5%.

Haloxon
Anthelmintic (Veterinary)

Proprietary Name. Equilox

Bis(2-chloroethyl) 3-chloro-4-methylcoumarin-7-yl phosphate

$C_{14}H_{14}Cl_3O_6P = 415.6$

CAS—321-55-1

$(ClCH_2 \cdot CH_2 \cdot O)_2 \overset{\overset{\displaystyle O}{\|}}{P} - O$

CH_3

A white powder. M.p. 88° to 93°.

Practically **insoluble** in water; soluble 1 in 9 of ethanol, 1 in 4 of acetone, and 1 in 2 of chloroform.

Ultraviolet Spectrum. After solution in dioxan and dilution with acid methanol—290 nm, 312 nm.

Infra-red Spectrum. Principal peaks at wavenumbers 1738, 1010, 1070, 1036, 1277, 1605 (KBr disk).

Halquinol

Antimicrobial

Synonyms. Chlorhydroxyquinoline; Chlorquinol.

Proprietary Names. Capitrol (chloroxine); Quixalin(e); Quixalud (vet.).

A mixture of the chlorinated products of quinolin-8-ol containing 57 to 74% of 5,7-dichloroquinolin-8-ol (chloroxine), 23 to 40% of 5-chloroquinolin-8-ol, and not more than 4% of 7-chloroquinolin-8-ol.

CAS—8067-69-4

A yellowish-white to yellowish-grey, voluminous powder.

Practically **insoluble** in water; soluble 1 in 250 of ethanol, 1 in 50 of chloroform, and 1 in 130 of ether; soluble in acids.

Colour Tests. Mandelin's Test—yellow; Marquis Test—yellow; Sulphuric Acid—yellow.

Thin-layer Chromatography. *System TA*—Rf 19, streaking. (*Acidified iodoplatinate solution*, positive.)

Gas Chromatography. *System GA*—RI 1743.

Ultraviolet Spectrum. Aqueous acid—258 nm ($A_1^1 = 2187$ a); aqueous alkali—259 nm, 343 nm; methanol—248 nm, 263 nm, 334 nm.

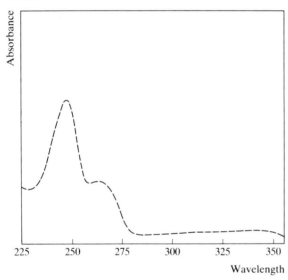

Infra-red Spectrum. Principal peaks at wavenumbers 1512, 1282, 812, 1200, 950, 785 (KBr disk).

Dose. 3 to 4 g daily for 5 days.

Harmaline

Hallucinogen

3,4-Dihydroharmine
$C_{13}H_{14}N_2O = 214.3$
CAS—304-21-2

An alkaloid obtained from peganum, the dried seeds of *Peganum harmala* (Zygophyllaceae). It is also found, together with harmine, in the South American hallucinogenic drink 'caapi', also known as 'Yagé' and 'ayahuasca'.

M.p. 249° to 250°, with decomposition.

Slightly **soluble** in water, ethanol, and ether.

Colour Tests. Mandelin's Test—green-brown; Marquis Test—brown-green.

Thin-layer Chromatography. *System TA*—Rf 38. (*Acidified iodoplatinate solution*, positive.)

Ultraviolet Spectrum. Aqueous acid—256 nm; aqueous alkali—330 nm; methanol—260 nm ($A_1^1 = 288$ b), 344 nm ($A_1^1 = 468$ b).

Mass Spectrum. Principal peaks at m/z 213, 214, 170, 198, 169, 115, 63, 143.

Harman

Alkaloid

Synonyms. Aribine; Harmane; Loturine.

1-Methyl-9*H*-pyrido[3,4-*b*]indole
$C_{12}H_{10}N_2 = 182.2$
CAS—486-84-0

An alkaloid present in passion flower, the dried flowering and fruiting tops of *Passiflora incarnata* (Passifloraceae).

Crystals. M.p. about 238°.

Sparingly **soluble** in hot water; soluble in ethanol, chloroform, and ether.

Note. Harman may be found in tobacco smoke and in home-made wine. It may also be found as a putrefactive base, particularly in cases where embalming has taken place. It is a condensation product of tryptophan and acetaldehyde.

Colour Tests. Mandelin's Test—green; Marquis Test—green.

Thin-layer Chromatography. *System TA*—Rf 70. (*Acidified iodoplatinate solution*, positive.)

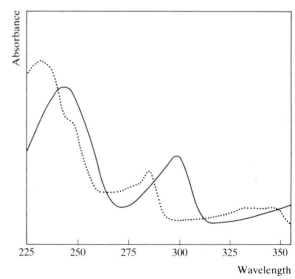

Gas Chromatography. *System GA*—RI 1952.

Ultraviolet Spectrum. Aqueous acid—245 nm ($A_1^1 = 1987$ a), 300 nm; aqueous alkali—232 nm, 284 nm.

Infra-red Spectrum. Principal peaks at wavenumbers 751, 1317, 1235, 1504, 1245, 1567.

Mass Spectrum. Principal peaks at m/z 182, 57, 43, 55, 40, 69, 41, 181.

Harmine   *Hallucinogen*

7-Methoxy-1-methyl-9H-pyrido[3,4-b]indole
$C_{13}H_{12}N_2O = 212.3$
CAS—442-51-3

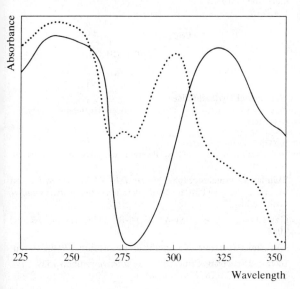

An alkaloid obtained from peganum, the dried seeds of *Peganum harmala* (Zygophyllaceae). Harmine is identical with an alkaloid known as banisterine or telepathine obtained from *Banisteria caapi* (Malpighiaceae) and with the alkaloid, yageine, from *Haemadictyon amazonicum* (Apocynaceae). It is also found, together with harmaline, in the South American hallucinogenic drink 'caapi', also known as 'Yagé' and 'ayahuasca'.
Crystals. M.p. 261°, with decomposition or sublimation.
Slightly **soluble** in water, ethanol, chloroform, and ether.

Dissociation Constant. pK$_a$ 7.6 (20°).

Colour Tests. *p*-Dimethylaminobenzaldehyde—red; Mandelin's Test—blue→green; Marquis Test—orange.

Thin-layer Chromatography. *System TA*—Rf 63; *system TB*—Rf 00; *system TC*—Rf 22. (*Acidified iodoplatinate solution*, positive.)

Gas Chromatography. *System GA*—RI 2291.

High Pressure Liquid Chromatography. *System HA*—k′ 0.8.

Ultraviolet Spectrum. Aqueous acid—247 nm ($A_1^1 = 1927$ a), 319 nm; aqueous alkali—243 nm, 275 nm, 300 nm.

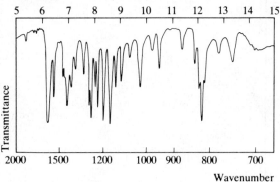

Infra-red Spectrum. Principal peaks at wavenumbers 1165, 817, 1629, 1200, 1282, 1239 (KBr disk).

Mass Spectrum. Principal peaks at m/z 212, 169, 197, 213, 106, 211, 170, 168.

Heptabarbitone   *Barbiturate*

Synonym. Heptabarbital (distinguish from Heptobarbitalum)
Proprietary Name. Medomin(e)
5-(Cyclohept-1-enyl)-5-ethylbarbituric acid
$C_{13}H_{18}N_2O_3 = 250.3$
CAS—509-86-4

A white crystalline powder. M.p. 167° to 171°.
Very slightly **soluble** in water; soluble 1 in 30 of ethanol, 1 in 20 of acetone, and 1 in 75 of chloroform; soluble in solutions of alkali hydroxides.

Dissociation Constant. pK$_a$ 7.5 (20°).

Partition Coefficient. Log P (octanol/pH 7.4), 2.2.

Colour Tests. Koppanyi–Zwikker Test—violet; Mercurous Nitrate—black; Vanillin Reagent—violet-red/colourless.

Thin-layer Chromatography. *System TD*—Rf 50; *system TE*—Rf 30; *system TF*—Rf 65; *system TH*—Rf 62. (*Mercuric chloride-diphenylcarbazone reagent*, positive; *mercurous nitrate spray*, black; *acidified potassium permanganate solution*, yellow-brown; *Zwikker's reagent*, pink.)

Gas Chromatography. *System GA*—heptabarbitone RI 2058, 3′-hydroxyheptabarbitone RI 2275, 3′-oxoheptabarbitone RI 2320; *system GF*—RI 2940.

High Pressure Liquid Chromatography. *System HG*—k′ 9.90; *system HH*—k′ 4.93.

Ultraviolet Spectrum. *Borax buffer 0.05M* (pH 9.2)—239 nm ($A_1^1 = 413$ a); M sodium hydroxide (pH 13)—255 nm ($A_1^1 = 326$ b). (See below)

Infra-red Spectrum. Principal peaks at wavenumbers 1673, 1761, 1718, 1237, 1292, 1303 (KBr disk). (See below)

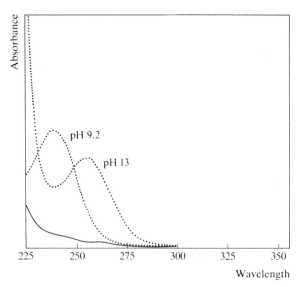

Wavelength

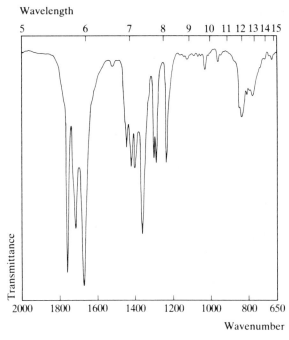

Wavenumber

Mass Spectrum. Principal peaks at m/z 221, 43, 78, 93, 80, 41, 141, 39.

Quantification. See under Amylobarbitone.

Disposition in the Body. Readily absorbed after oral administration. Less than 1% of a dose is excreted unchanged in the urine. Major metabolites which have been identified in the urine are 3′-oxoheptabarbitone and 3′-hydroxyheptabarbitone.

THERAPEUTIC CONCENTRATION. In plasma, usually in the range 1 to 4 µg/ml.

After a single oral dose of 200 mg administered to 7 subjects, peak plasma concentrations of 1.3 to 2.4 µg/ml (mean 1.9) were attained in 1.5 to 4 hours (D. D. Breimer *et al.*, *Eur. J. clin. Pharmac.*, 1975, *9*, 169–178).

TOXICITY. The estimated minimum lethal dose is 2 g. Plasma concentrations greater than about 8 µg/ml may produce toxic effects.

HALF-LIFE. Plasma half-life, 6 to 11 hours.

VOLUME OF DISTRIBUTION. About 1 litre/kg.

NOTE. For a review of the clinical pharmacokinetics of barbiturates, see D. D. Breimer, *Clin. Pharmacokinet.*, 1977, *2*, 93–109.

Dose. 150 to 400 mg daily.

Heptachlor   *Insecticide*

1,4,5,6,7,8,8-Heptachloro-3a,4,7,7a-tetrahydro-4,7-methano-indene
$C_{10}H_5Cl_7 = 373.3$
CAS—76-44-8

The pure substance is a white crystalline solid and the technical grade is a soft, waxy solid which contains about 72% of heptachlor and 28% of related compounds. Heptachlor may be found as an impurity in chlordane. M.p. 95° to 96° (pure substance), 46° to 74° (technical grade).
Practically **insoluble** in water; soluble 1 in 22 of ethanol.

Gas Chromatography. *System GA*—RI 1880; *system GK*—retention time 0.85 relative to caffeine.

Mass Spectrum. Principal peaks at m/z 100, 272, 274, 270, 237, 102, 65, 276.

Heptaminol   *Cardiac Stimulant/Vasodilator*

6-Amino-2-methylheptan-2-ol
$C_8H_{19}NO = 145.2$
CAS—372-66-7

Heptaminol Hydrochloride
Proprietary Names. Coreptil; Cortensor; Eoden; Hept-a-myl; Heptylon.
$C_8H_{19}NO,HCl = 181.7$
CAS—543-15-7
A white crystalline powder.
Very **soluble** in water; soluble in ethanol; practically insoluble in acetone and ether.

Thin-layer Chromatography. *System TA*—Rf 23; *system TB*—Rf 01; *system TC*—Rf 02. (*Acidified potassium permanganate solution*, positive.)

Gas Chromatography. *System GA*—RI 1118; *system GB*—RI 1084.

Ultraviolet Spectrum. No significant absorption, 230 to 360 nm.

Infra-red Spectrum. Principal peaks at wavenumbers 1529, 1537, 896, 1622, 1153, 1614 (KBr disk).

Mass Spectrum. Principal peaks at m/z 44, 43, 59, 56, 69, 55, 41, 113.

Quantification. HIGH PRESSURE LIQUID CHROMATOGRAPHY. In plasma or urine: sensitivity 100 ng/ml in plasma, fluorescence detection—R. R. Brodie *et al.*, *J. Chromat.*, 1983, *274*; *Biomed. Appl.*, *25*, 179–186.

Dose. Heptaminol hydrochloride has been given in doses of 0.3 to 1.6 g daily.

Heteronium Bromide   *Anticholinergic*

1,1-Dimethyl-3-(α-2-thienylmandeloyloxy)pyrrolidinium bromide
$C_{18}H_{22}BrNO_3S = 412.3$
CAS—7247-57-6

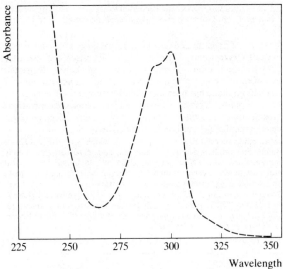

A white crystalline powder. M.p. 182° to 184°.
Very **soluble** in water and ethanol.

Thin-layer Chromatography. *System TA*—Rf 03. (*Acidified iodoplatinate solution*, positive.)

Ultraviolet Spectrum. Aqueous acid—234 nm ($A_1^1 = 235$ b).

Infra-red Spectrum. Principal peaks at wavenumbers 1735, 1219, 1085, 1234, 1063, 700.

Hexachlorophane   *Disinfectant*

Synonym. Hexachlorophene
Proprietary Names. Hexaphenyl; Phaisohex; Phisoscrub; Ster-Zac. It is an ingredient of Anacal.
2,2′-Methylenebis(3,4,6-trichlorophenol)
$C_{13}H_6Cl_6O_2 = 406.9$
CAS—70-30-4

A white or pale buff, crystalline powder. M.p. 161° to 167°.
Practically **insoluble** in water; soluble 1 in 3.5 of ethanol, 1 in less than 1 of acetone, and 1 in less than 1 of ether; soluble in chloroform, possibly with turbidity.

Dissociation Constant. pK_a 5.7.

Colour Tests. Ferric Chloride—violet (transient); Fuming Nitric Acid—orange-red/orange/orange-brown.

Gas Chromatography. *System GA*—RI 2807.

Ultraviolet Spectrum. Ethanol—299 nm ($A_1^1 = 155$ a); aqueous alkali—249 nm ($A_1^1 = 400$ b), 320 nm ($A_1^1 = 312$ a).

Infra-red Spectrum. Principal peaks at wavenumbers 1276, 1182, 737, 1139, 960, 1213 (KBr disk).

Quantification. GAS CHROMATOGRAPHY. In blood: ECD—W. Dodson *et al.*, *Clin. Chem.*, 1977, *23*, 944–947. In blood or urine: ECD—R. S. Browning *et al.*, *J. pharm. Sci.*, 1968, *57*, 2165–2166.

Disposition in the Body. Absorbed after oral administration and through the skin. Percutaneous absorption may be significant in premature infants and through damaged skin. After topical application, up to about 10% may be excreted in the urine over a period of 4 to 5 days.

BLOOD CONCENTRATION.
Cord-blood concentrations of 0.003 to 0.18 μg/ml (mean 0.02) were reported in 50 neonates at birth. After washing once daily for 1 to 11 days with a 3% solution of hexachlorophane diluted with 50 to 100 ml of water, whole blood concentrations of 0.009 to 0.65 μg/ml (mean 0.11) were attained (A. Curley *et al.*, *Lancet*, 1971, *2*, 296–297).
After whole-body washing with 30 ml of a 3% skin-cleansing product once daily, blood concentrations in 36 adults reached a plateau of about

0.6 µg/ml after 3 to 5 weeks and decreased to about 0.3 to 0.4 µg/ml after 7 to 8 weeks (B. Calesnick *et al.*, *Toxic. appl. Pharmac.*, 1975, *32*, 204–211).

TOXICITY. The estimated minimum lethal dose is 5 g. A number of deaths have occurred after accidental ingestion and also after chronic application for the treatment of burns. Repeated exposure of neonates and infants to high concentrations of hexachlorophane has been associated with spongy lesions of the brain. Fatalities have been associated with blood concentrations greater than 2 µg/ml although recovery has occurred after development of plasma concentrations up to 90 µg/ml.

In an epidemic of percutaneous poisoning which occurred in 1972 in infants and children due to exposure to a talcum powder accidentally contaminated with 6% of hexachlorophane, 36 children died. An antemortem serum concentration of 1.15 µg/ml was reported in 1 child and the following postmortem tissue concentrations were reported: brain 1 to 149 µg/g (mean 21, 23 cases), kidney 17 to 43 µg/g (mean 26, 4 cases), liver 12.5 to 1080 µg/g (mean 133, 25 cases), lung 10 to 67 µg/g (mean 30, 17 cases), and skin 1 to 392 µg/g (mean 52, 30 cases) (G. Martin-Bouyer *et al.*, *Lancet*, 1982, *1*, 91–95).

Use. In soaps and creams at a concentration of 0.25 to 3%.

Hexamethonium Bromide   *Antihypertensive*

Synonyms. Hexamethone Bromide; Hexonium Bromide.
NN'-Hexamethylenebis(trimethylammonium) dibromide
$C_{12}H_{30}Br_2N_2 = 362.2$
CAS—60-26-4 (hexamethonium); *55-97-0* (dibromide)

$$[(CH_3)_3N^+ \cdot [CH_2]_6 \cdot N^+ (CH_3)_3]2Br^-$$

A white or creamy-white hygroscopic powder. M.p. about 280°, with decomposition.
Soluble 1 in less than 1 of water and 1 in 60 of ethanol; practically insoluble in chloroform and ether.

Hexamethonium Iodide

Synonym. Hexonium Iodide
Proprietary Name. Gastrometonio
$C_{12}H_{30}I_2N_2 = 456.2$
CAS—870-62-2
A white, slightly hygroscopic, crystalline powder.
Soluble 1 in 2 of water; practically insoluble in ethanol.

Thin-layer Chromatography. *System TA*—Rf 00; *system TN*—Rf 36; *system TO*—Rf 10. (*Acidified iodoplatinate solution*, positive.)

Ultraviolet Spectrum. No significant absorption, 230 to 360 nm.

Infra-red Spectrum. Principal peaks at wavenumbers 913, 970, 1630, 945, 1063, 1000 (KBr disk).

Dose. Hexamethonium bromide has been given parenterally in doses of up to 500 mg daily.

Hexamine   *Antibacterial (Urinary)*

Synonyms. Aminoform; Esammina; Formine; Hexamethylenamine; Hexamethylenetetramine; Methenamine; Urotropine.
Proprietary Names. Antihydral; Urotropina.
1,3,5,7-Tetra-azatricyclo[3.3.1.1^3,7]decane
$C_6H_{12}N_4 = 140.2$
CAS—100-97-0

Colourless lustrous crystals or white crystalline powder. It sublimes at about 260° without melting.
Soluble 1 in 1.5 of water, 1 in 8 of ethanol (90%), 1 in 12 of chloroform, and 1 in 320 of ether.

Hexamine Hippurate

Synonym. Methenamine Hippurate
Proprietary Names. Hiprex; Urex.
$C_6H_{12}N_4, C_9H_9NO_3 = 319.4$
CAS—5714-73-8
A white crystalline powder. M.p. 105° to 110°.
Soluble in water and ethanol.

Hexamine Mandelate

Synonym. Methenamine Mandelate
Proprietary Names. Mandaze; Mandelamine; Methandine; Renelate; Sterine. It is an ingredient of G-500.
$C_6H_{12}N_4, C_8H_8O_3 = 292.3$
CAS—587-23-5
A white crystalline powder. M.p. about 127°, with decomposition.
Very soluble in water; soluble 1 in 10 of ethanol, 1 in 20 of chloroform, and 1 in 350 of ether.

Colour Test. Mix 100 mg with an equal amount of salicylic acid and heat with 1 ml of *sulphuric acid*—a red colour is produced.

Thin-layer Chromatography. *System TA*—Rf 30; *system TB*—Rf 04; *system TC*—Rf 13. (*Acidified iodoplatinate solution*, positive.)

Gas Chromatography. *System GA*—RI 1210.

Ultraviolet Spectrum. Aqueous acid—251 nm, 257 nm ($A_1^1 = 15.5$ b), 263 nm.

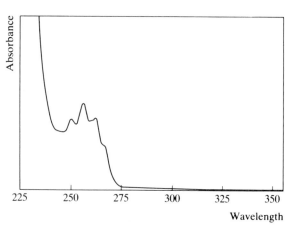

Wavelength

Infra-red Spectrum. Principal peaks at wavenumbers 1232, 812, 671, 1010, 1044, 724 (Nujol mull).

Mass Spectrum. Principal peaks at *m/z* 42, 140, 112, 41, 85, 43, 71, 141.

Quantification. COLORIMETRY. In urine: hexamine and formaldehyde, sensitivity 25 µg/ml for hexamine, 5 µg/ml for formaldehyde—R. Gollamudi *et al.*, *Biopharm. Drug Disp.*, 1979, *1*, 27–36.

GAS CHROMATOGRAPHY. In serum or urine: sensitivity <5 µg/ml in serum—A.-L. Nieminen *et al.*, *J. Chromat.*, 1980, *181*; *Biomed. Appl.*, 7, 11–16.

Disposition in the Body. Readily absorbed after oral administration and rapidly excreted unchanged in the urine. In acidic urine it is slowly hydrolysed, with the liberation of formaldehyde; this may also occur in the acid gastric secretions and 10 to 30% of a dose may be hydrolysed in the stomach.

Dose. Usually 2 g of hexamine hippurate or 4 g of hexamine mandelate daily.

Hexethal   *Barbiturate*

5-Ethyl-5-hexylbarbituric acid
$C_{12}H_{20}N_2O_3 = 240.3$
CAS—77-30-5

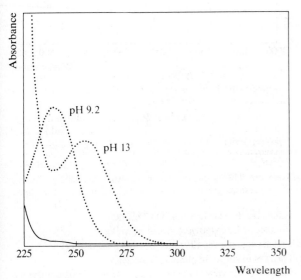

Hexethal Sodium

$C_{12}H_{19}N_2NaO_3 = 262.3$
CAS—144-00-3
A white or slightly yellowish powder.
Very **soluble** in water; soluble in ethanol; practically insoluble in ether.
Aqueous solutions are unstable and decompose on standing.

Thin-layer Chromatography. *System TD*—Rf 53; *system TE*—Rf 44; *system TF*—Rf 67; *system TH*—Rf 74.

Gas Chromatography. *System GA*—RI 1858.

High Pressure Liquid Chromatography. *System HG*—k′ 34.28; *system HH*—k′ 20.39.

Ultraviolet Spectrum. *Borax buffer 0.05M* (pH 9.2)—238 nm ($A_1^1 = 423$ b); M sodium hydroxide (pH 13)—253 nm ($A_1^1 = 323$ b).

Infra-red Spectrum. Principal peaks at wavenumbers 1698, 1720, 1757, 1316, 1230, 850 (hexethal sodium).

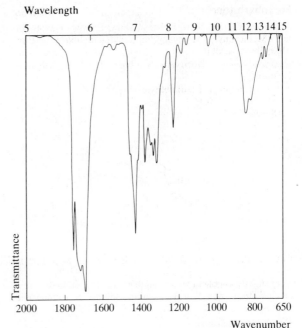

Mass Spectrum. Principal peaks at *m/z* 156, 141, 55, 41, 157, 43, 98, 39.

Hexetidine   *Antimicrobial*

Proprietary Names. Collu-Hextril; Glypesin; Hexoral; Hextril; Oraldene; Steri/Sol.

5-Amino-1,3-bis(2-ethylhexyl)perhydro-5-methylpyrimidine
$C_{21}H_{45}N_3 = 339.6$
CAS—141-94-6

A viscous oil. Wt per ml about 0.87 g. Refractive index 1.466. Practically **insoluble** in water; miscible with ethanol, acetone, and chloroform.

Dissociation Constant. pK_a 8.3.

Thin-layer Chromatography. *System TA*—Rf 70. (*Acidified iodoplatinate solution*, positive.)

Gas Chromatography. *System GA*—RI 2093.

Ultraviolet Spectrum. No significant absorption, 230 to 360 nm.

Infra-red Spectrum. Principal peaks at wavenumbers 1093, 854, 1300, 910, 1176, 1234 (thin film).

Mass Spectrum. Principal peaks at *m/z* 142, 57, 42, 197, 185, 339, 240, 226.

Use. As a 0.1% solution.

Hexobarbitone   *Barbiturate*

Synonyms. Ciclobarbital; Enhexymalum; Enimal; Hexobarbital; Methexenyl; Methyl-cyclohexenylmethyl-barbitursäure; Methylhexabarbital.

Proprietary Names. Noctivane; Sombulex. It is an ingredient of Evidorm.

5-(Cyclohex-1-enyl)-1,5-dimethylbarbituric acid
$C_{12}H_{16}N_2O_3 = 236.3$
CAS—56-29-1

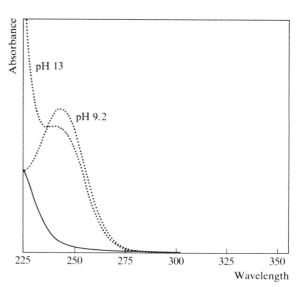

Colourless crystals or a white crystalline powder. M.p. 144° to 148°.

Very slightly **soluble** in water; soluble 1 in 45 of ethanol, 1 in 4 of chloroform, and 1 in 80 of ether; soluble in acetone and methanol.

Hexobarbitone Sodium

Synonyms. Enhexymalnatrium; Hexenalum; Narcosanum Solubile; Sodium Hexobarbital; Soluble Hexobarbitone.

Proprietary Name. Evipan-Natrium

$C_{12}H_{15}N_2NaO_3 = 258.3$
CAS—50-09-9

A white, very hygroscopic powder. It discolours on exposure to air.

Very **soluble** in water, ethanol, acetone, and methanol; soluble in chloroform; very slightly soluble in ether. A solution in water slowly decomposes.

Dissociation Constant. pK_a 8.2 (20°).

Colour Tests. Koppanyi–Zwikker Test—violet; Mercurous Nitrate—black; Vanillin Reagent—brown/violet.

Thin-layer Chromatography. *System TD*—Rf 65; *system TE*—Rf 48; *system TF*—Rf 65; *system TH*—Rf 85. (*Mercuric chloride-diphenylcarbazone reagent*, positive; *mercurous nitrate spray*, black; *acidified potassium permanganate solution*, yellow-brown on violet.)

Gas Chromatography. *System GA*—RI 1857; *system GF*—RI 2380.

High Pressure Liquid Chromatography. *System HG*—k′ 7.37; *system HH*—k′ 5.67.

Ultraviolet Spectrum. *Borax buffer 0.05M* (pH 9.2)—243 nm ($A_1^1 = 331$ a); *M sodium hydroxide* (pH 13)—243 nm ($A_1^1 = 301$ b).

Infra-red Spectrum. Principal peaks at wavenumbers 1720, 1665, 1748, 1200, 1275, 1045 (KBr disk).

Mass Spectrum. Principal peaks at m/z 221, 81, 157, 80, 79, 155, 41, 77; 3′-oxohexobarbitone 250, 95, 39, 235, 66, 207, 41, 193.

Quantification. See under Amylobarbitone.

Disposition in the Body. Readily absorbed after oral administration. The sodium salt has a very short duration of action and is usually administered intravenously. Hexobarbitone is inactivated in the liver by *N*-demethylation and oxidation. About 32% of a dose is excreted in the urine in 24 hours as 3′-oxohexobarbitone, 5% as 3′-hydroxyhexobarbitone, and 18% as

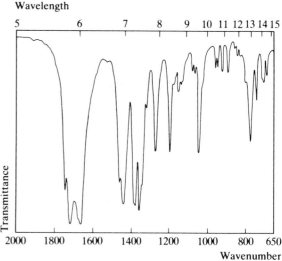

1,5-dimethylbarbituric acid; less than 1% of a dose is excreted unchanged in the urine in 24 hours.

THERAPEUTIC CONCENTRATION. In plasma, usually in the range 1 to 5 µg/ml.

Following a single oral dose of 500 mg to 6 subjects, peak plasma concentrations of 4.9 to 10.9 µg/ml (mean 7) were attained in about 1 hour (N. P. E. Vermeulen *et al.*, *Br. J. clin. Pharmac.*, 1983, *15*, 459–464).

TOXICITY. The estimated minimum lethal dose is 2 g. Plasma concentrations greater than about 8 µg/ml may produce toxic effects.

HALF-LIFE. Plasma half-life, 3 to 7 hours.

VOLUME OF DISTRIBUTION. About 1 litre/kg.

CLEARANCE. Plasma clearance, about 3.5 ml/min/kg.

PROTEIN BINDING. In plasma, 42 to 52%.

NOTE. For a review of the pharmacokinetics of barbiturates see D. D. Breimer, *Clin. Pharmacokinet.*, 1977, *2*, 93–109.

Dose. 250 to 500 mg, as a hypnotic; up to 750 mg daily, as a sedative.

Hexobendine
Anti-anginal Vasodilator

NN'-Ethylenebis(3-methylaminopropyl 3,4,5-trimethoxybenz-oate)
$C_{30}H_{44}N_2O_{10} = 592.7$
CAS—54-03-5

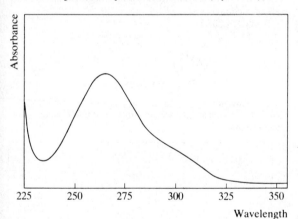

M.p. 75° to 77°.

Hexobendine Hydrochloride
Proprietary Names. Reoxyl; Ustimon.
$C_{30}H_{44}N_2O_{10},2HCl = 665.6$
CAS—50-62-4
A white crystalline powder. M.p. 170° to 174°.
Soluble in water and chloroform; slightly soluble in ethanol; practically insoluble in ether.

Colour Tests. Liebermann's Test—black; Mandelin's Test—violet.

Thin-layer Chromatography. *System TA*—Rf 47; *system TB*—Rf 10; *system TC*—Rf 44. (*Acidified iodoplatinate solution*, positive.)

Gas Chromatography. *System GA*—not eluted.

Ultraviolet Spectrum. Aqueous acid—265 nm ($A_1^1 = 311$ a).

Infra-red Spectrum. Principal peaks at wavenumbers 1123, 1219, 1703, 1585, 1497, 1171 (KBr disk).

Mass Spectrum. Principal peaks at m/z 296, 195, 58, 297, 253, 196, 212, 84.

Dose. Hexobendine hydrochloride has been given in doses of 60 to 180 mg daily.

Hexocyclium Methylsulphate
Anticholinergic

Proprietary Names. Tral; Traline.
4-(β-Cyclohexyl-β-hydroxyphenethyl)-1,1-dimethylpiperazinium methylsulphate
$C_{20}H_{33}N_2O,CH_3SO_4 = 428.6$
CAS—6004-98-4 (hexocyclium); *115-63-9* (methylsulphate)

A white powder. M.p. 200° to 210°.
Soluble 1 in 2 of water; slightly soluble in chloroform; practically insoluble in ether.

Colour Tests. Mandelin's Test—blue-violet; Marquis Test—violet.

Thin-layer Chromatography. *System TA*—Rf 02. (*Acidified iodoplatinate solution*, positive.)

Ultraviolet Spectrum. Aqueous acid—252 nm, 257 nm ($A_1^1 = 5.3$ b), 264 nm.

Infra-red Spectrum. Principal peaks at wavenumbers 1224, 1005, 748, 1052, 700, 770 (KBr disk).

Dose. Initially, 100 mg daily.

Hexoestrol
Oestrogen

Synonyms. Dihydrostilboestrol; Hexanoestrol; Hexestrol; Synestrol; Synoestrol.
Proprietary Names. Cycloestrol; Hormoestrol (tablets).
meso-4,4'-(1,2-Diethylethylene)diphenol
$C_{18}H_{22}O_2 = 270.4$
CAS—5635-50-7; 84-16-2 (meso)

Colourless crystals or white crystalline powder. M.p. 185° to 188°.
Very slightly **soluble** in water; soluble in ethanol, acetone, and ether; slightly soluble in chloroform.

Hexoestrol Dipropionate
Proprietary Names. Hormoestrol (injection); Neoestrolo.
$C_{24}H_{30}O_4 = 382.5$
CAS—4825-53-0
A white crystalline powder. M.p. 127° to 128°.
Sparingly **soluble** in water; soluble in warm ethanol and ether.

Gas Chromatography. *System GA*—RI 2402.

Ultraviolet Spectrum. Ethanol—230 nm ($A_1^1 = 775$ b), 280 nm ($A_1^1 = 135$ a); aqueous alkali—242 nm ($A_1^1 = 965$ b), 297 nm ($A_1^1 = 175$ b). (See below)

Infra-red Spectrum. Principal peaks at wavenumbers 1175, 1523, 1220, 840, 857, 1615 (KBr disk).

Dose. Hexoestrol has been given in doses of 1 to 5 mg daily.

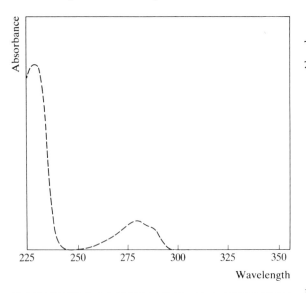

Wavelength

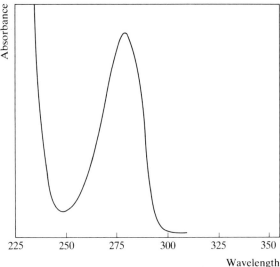

Wavelength

Hexoprenaline

Sympathomimetic

NN' - Hexamethylenebis[4 - (2 - amino - 1 - hydroxyethyl)-pyrocatechol]
$C_{22}H_{32}N_2O_6 = 420.5$
CAS—3215-70-1

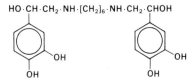

Hexoprenaline Hydrochloride
Proprietary Name. Ipradol
$C_{22}H_{32}N_2O_6,2HCl = 493.4$
CAS—4323-43-7
Crystals. M.p. 197° to 198°.

Hexoprenaline Sulphate
Proprietary Names. Etoscol; Ipradol.
$C_{22}H_{32}N_2O_6,H_2SO_4 = 518.6$
CAS—32266-10-7
A white crystalline powder. M.p. 214°, with decomposition.
Soluble in water and dilute hydrochloric acid; practically insoluble in ethanol.

Colour   Tests.   Ammoniacal   Silver   Nitrate—red → brown → black/—; Ferric Chloride—orange; Folin–Ciocalteu Reagent—blue; Mandelin's Test—orange-yellow; Marquis Test—red;   Methanolic   Potassium   Hydroxide—orange → brown; Nessler's Reagent—black; Potassium Dichromate (Method 1)—green → brown (30 s); Sulphuric Acid—orange-yellow.

Thin-layer Chromatography. *System TA*—Rf 03; *system TB*—Rf 01; *system TC*—Rf 00. (*Acidified iodoplatinate solution*, positive.)

Ultraviolet Spectrum. Aqueous acid—280 nm ($A_1^1 = 129$ a).

Infra-red Spectrum. Principal peaks at wavenumbers 1102, 1242, 1190, 1605, 1517, 1280 (hexoprenaline sulphate, KBr disk).

Mass Spectrum. Principal peaks at *m/z* 30, 27, 124, 56, 123, 87, 78, 41.

Dose. Hexoprenaline sulphate has been given in doses of 0.75 to 1.5 mg daily.

Hexyl Nicotinate

Topical Vasodilator

Proprietary Name. It is an ingredient of Transvasin.

n-Hexyl nicotinate
$C_{12}H_{17}NO_2 = 207.3$
CAS—23597-82-2

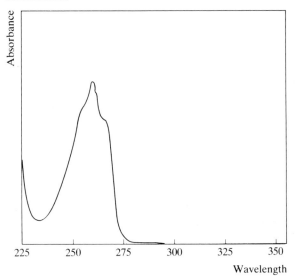

A pale yellow liquid.
Practically **insoluble** in water; soluble in ethanol, chloroform, and methanol.

Wavelength

Thin-layer Chromatography. *System TA*—Rf 70. (*Acidified iodoplatinate solution*, positive.)

Ultraviolet Spectrum. Aqueous acid—260 nm ($A_1^1 = 268$ b).

Infra-red Spectrum. Principal peaks at wavenumbers 1724, 1276, 1111, 741, 1022, 1590 (KBr disk).

Use. Topically in a concentration of 2%.

Hexylcaine   *Local Anaesthetic*

2-Cyclohexylamino-1-methylethyl benzoate
$C_{16}H_{23}NO_2 = 261.4$
CAS—532-77-4

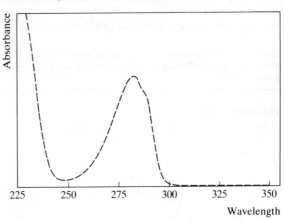

Hexylcaine Hydrochloride
Proprietary Name. Cyclaine
$C_{16}H_{23}NO_2,HCl = 297.8$
CAS—532-76-3
A white powder. M.p. 182° to 184°.
Soluble 1 in 17 of water; freely soluble in ethanol and chloroform; practically insoluble in ether.

Dissociation Constant. pK_a 9.1.

Thin-layer Chromatography. *System TA*—Rf 01. (*Acidified iodoplatinate solution*, positive.)

Gas Chromatography. *System GA*—RI 1965.

Ultraviolet Spectrum. Aqueous acid—232 nm ($A_1^1 = 485$ a), 275 nm ($A_1^1 = 43$ a).

Infra-red Spectrum. Principal peaks at wavenumbers 1270, 1718, 1105, 710, 1068, 1022 (KBr disk).

Mass Spectrum. Principal peaks at m/z 112, 77, 105, 139, 55, 41, 96, 56.

Use. Hexylcaine hydrochloride has been used in concentrations of up to 5%.

Hexylresorcinol   *Anthelmintic*

Proprietary Name. Oxana
4-Hexylbenzene-1,3-diol
$C_{12}H_{18}O_2 = 194.3$
CAS—136-77-6

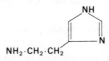

White or yellowish-white acicular crystals, crystalline plates or crystalline powder. It acquires a brownish-pink tint on exposure to light and air. M.p. 62° to 68°.
Soluble 1 in 2000 of water; freely soluble in ethanol, chloroform, and ether.

Caution. Hexylresorcinol is irritating to the oral mucosa, to the respiratory tract, and to the skin; ethanolic solutions have vesicant properties.

Colour Test. Ferric Chloride—green.

Gas Chromatography. *System GA*—RI 1777.

Ultraviolet Spectrum. Methanol—282 nm ($A_1^1 = 160$ c).

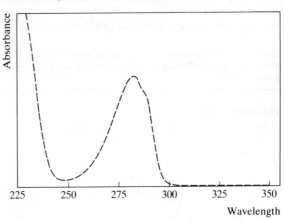

Wavelength

Infra-red Spectrum. Principal peaks at wavenumbers 970, 980, 1185, 1616, 1150, 1205 (KBr disk).

Disposition in the Body. Partly absorbed after oral administration. About 20 to 30% of a dose is rapidly excreted unchanged in the urine and the remainder is eliminated in the faeces.

Dose. 1 g as a single dose.

Histamine   *Diagnostic Agent (Gastric Secretion)*

Synonym. Ergotidine
2-(Imidazol-4-yl)ethylamine
$C_5H_9N_3 = 111.1$
CAS—51-45-6

Deliquescent acicular crystals. M.p. 83° to 84°.
Freely **soluble** in water, ethanol, and hot chloroform; sparingly soluble in ether.

Histamine Acid Phosphate
Synonyms. Histamine Diphosphate; Histamine Phosphate.
Proprietary Names. It is an ingredient of Akrotherm and Cremathurm.
$C_5H_9N_3,2H_3PO_4 = 307.1$
CAS—51-74-1
Colourless crystals. M.p. 130° to 133°.
Soluble 1 in 4 of water; slightly soluble in ethanol; practically insoluble in ether.

Histamine Hydrochloride
Synonym. Histamine Dihydrochloride
$C_5H_9N_3,2HCl = 184.1$
CAS—56-92-8
Hygroscopic colourless crystals or white crystalline powder. M.p. about 245°, with decomposition.
Very **soluble** in water; soluble in ethanol and acetone; practically insoluble in chloroform and ether.

Dissociation Constant. pK$_a$ 5.9, 9.7 (25°).

Thin-layer Chromatography. *System TA*—Rf 13. (*Acidified iodoplatinate solution*, positive.)

Gas Chromatography. *System GA*—RI 1497.

Ultraviolet Spectrum. No significant absorption, 230 to 360 nm.

Infra-red Spectrum. Principal peaks at wavenumbers 840, 1622, 1522, 1084, 802, 1577 (histamine hydrochloride, KBr disk).

Mass Spectrum. Principal peaks at *m/z* 82, 30, 81, 54, 28, 55, 83, 41.

Dose. Histamine acid phosphate is given subcutaneously, in a dose of 40 µg/kg, following administration of a large dose of an antihistamine.

Histapyrrodine   *Antihistamine*

N-Benzyl-*N*-phenyl-2-(pyrrolidin-1-yl)ethylamine
C$_{19}$H$_{24}$N$_2$ = 280.4
CAS—493-80-1

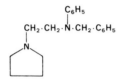

An oil.

Histapyrrodine Hydrochloride
Proprietary Name. Domistan
C$_{19}$H$_{24}$N$_2$,HCl = 316.9
CAS—6113-17-3
A white powder. M.p. 196°.

Colour Test. Mandelin's Test—red-violet.

Thin-layer Chromatography. *System TA*—Rf 60. (*Acidified iodoplatinate solution*, positive.)

High Pressure Liquid Chromatography. *System HA*—k′ 3.0.

Ultraviolet Spectrum. Aqueous acid—250 nm (A$_1^1$ = 141 a), 295 nm.

Infra-red Spectrum. Principal peaks at wavenumbers 1513, 1604, 750, 698, 1500, 732.

Dose. Histapyrrodine hydrochloride has been given in doses of 50 to 150 mg daily.

Homatropine   *Anticholinergic*

(1*R*,3*r*,5*S*)-Tropan-3-yl (±)-mandelate
C$_{16}$H$_{21}$NO$_3$ = 275.3
CAS—87-00-3

Small white prismatic crystals or coarse crystalline powder. M.p. 99° to 100°.
Practically **insoluble** in water; soluble in ethanol, chloroform, and ether.

Homatropine Hydrobromide
Synonym. Tropyl Mandelate Hydrobromide
Proprietary Name. Homat
C$_{16}$H$_{21}$NO$_3$,HBr = 356.3
CAS—51-56-9
Colourless crystals or a white crystalline powder. M.p. 214° to 217°, with decomposition.
Soluble 1 in 6 of water, 1 in 60 of ethanol, and 1 in 420 of chloroform; practically insoluble in ether.

Dissociation Constant. pK$_a$ 9.9 (20°).

Thin-layer Chromatography. *System TA*—Rf 01; *system TB*—Rf 01; *system TC*—Rf 01. (*Acidified iodoplatinate solution*, positive.)

Gas Chromatography. *System GA*—RI 2072.

High Pressure Liquid Chromatography. *System HA*—k′ 4.2 (tailing peak).

Ultraviolet Spectrum. Aqueous acid—252 nm, 258 nm (A$_1^1$ = 7.3 a), 264 nm. No alkaline shift.

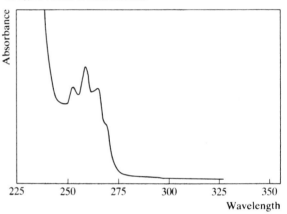

Infra-red Spectrum. Principal peaks at wavenumbers 1730, 1172, 1030, 735, 1063, 1125 (KBr disk).

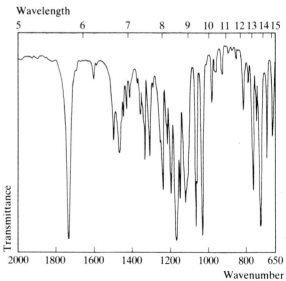

Mass Spectrum. Principal peaks at m/z 124, 107, 82, 83, 42, 77, 79, 94.

Use. Homatropine hydrobromide is used as a 2% ophthalmic solution.

Homatropine Methobromide   *Anticholinergic*

Synonyms. Homatropine Methylbromide; Methylhomatropinium Bromide.
Proprietary Names. Homapin; Mesopin; Novatrin.
(1*R*,3*r*,5*S*)-3-[(±)-Mandeloyloxy]-8-methyltropanium bromide
$C_{16}H_{21}NO_3,CH_3Br = 370.3$
CAS—80-49-9
A white powder. M.p. about 190°.
Very **soluble** in water; freely soluble in ethanol; practically insoluble in acetone and ether.

Thin-layer Chromatography. *System TA*—Rf 02. (*Acidified iodoplatinate solution*, positive.)

Ultraviolet Spectrum. Aqueous acid—252 nm, 258 nm ($A_1^1 = 5.8$ b), 264 nm.

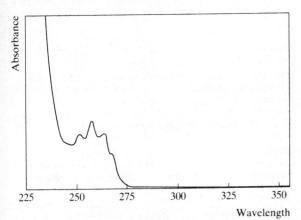

Infra-red Spectrum. Principal peaks at wavenumbers 1724, 1179, 1160, 1195, 1044, 935 (KBr disk).

Dose. Usually 12 to 40 mg daily.

Homidium Bromide   *Trypanocide (Veterinary)*

Synonym. Ethidium Bromide
3,8-Diamino-5-ethyl-6-phenylphenanthridinium bromide
$C_{21}H_{20}BrN_3 = 394.3$
CAS—1239-45-8

A dark purple crystalline or amorphous powder. M.p. 245°, with decomposition.
Soluble 1 in 20 of water and 1 in 750 of chloroform.

Colour Test. The following test is performed on homidium nitrate (see page 128): Mandelin's Test—yellow.

Thin-layer Chromatography. *System TA*—Rf 55. (*Acidified potassium permanganate solution*, positive.)

Ultraviolet Spectrum. Aqueous acid—242 nm, 283 nm ($A_1^1 = 785$ a).

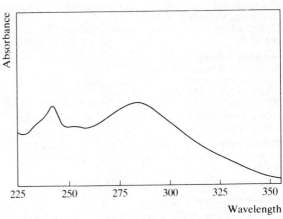

Infra-red Spectrum. Principal peaks at wavenumbers 1628, 1492, 1260, 1312, 836, 1077 (KBr disk).

Homochlorcyclizine   *Antihistamine*

1-(4-Chlorobenzhydryl)perhydro-4-methyl-1,4-diazepine
$C_{19}H_{23}ClN_2 = 314.9$
CAS—848-53-3

A white crystalline powder.
Soluble in dilute acetic acid.

Thin-layer Chromatography. *System TA*—Rf 28. (*Acidified iodoplatinate solution*, positive.)

Ultraviolet Spectrum. Aqueous acid—233 nm ($A_1^1 = 457$ b), 258 nm, 263 nm, 270 nm.
Infra-red Spectrum. Principal peaks at wavenumbers 1135, 1010, 1600, 1618, 1630, 720 (KBr disk).

Dose. Homochlorcyclizine has been given in doses of 30 to 60 mg daily.

Hordenine   *Sympathomimetic*

4-(2-Dimethylaminoethyl)phenol
$C_{10}H_{15}NO = 165.2$
CAS—539-15-1

CH₂·CH₂·N(CH₃)₂ — $CH_2 \cdot CH_2 \cdot N(CH_3)_2$

OH

Hordenine occurs naturally in germinating barley and other Gramineae. Crystals. M.p. 117° to 118°.
Slightly **soluble** in water; very soluble in ethanol, chloroform, and ether.

Hordenine Sulphate

$(C_{10}H_{15}NO)_2,H_2SO_4,2H_2O = 464.6$
CAS—622-64-0 (anhydrous); *6202-17-1* (dihydrate)
Crystals. M.p. 197°, and 210° after drying at 100°.
Soluble in water; slightly soluble in ethanol; practically insoluble in ether.

Colour Tests. Mandelin's Test—grey-green; Marquis Test—brown → green.

Thin-layer Chromatography. *System TA*—Rf 40; *system TB*—Rf 05; *system TC*—Rf 06. (*Acidified potassium permanganate solution, positive.*)

High Pressure Liquid Chromatography. *System HB*—k′ 2.00.

Ultraviolet Spectrum. Aqueous acid—274 nm.

Infra-red Spectrum. Principal peaks at wavenumbers 1252, 1512, 820, 1612, 1270, 869 (KBr disk).

Mass Spectrum. Principal peaks at *m/z* 58, 42, 59, 30, 77, 107, 57, 51.

Hydralazine

Antihypertensive

Synonym. Hydrallazine
1-Hydrazinophthalazine
$C_8H_8N_4 = 160.2$
CAS—86-54-4

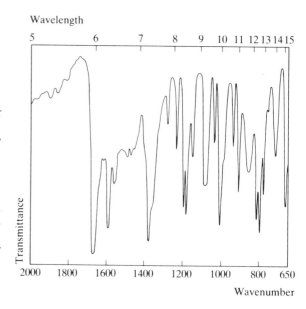

NH·NH₂

Yellow crystals. M.p. 172° to 173°.

Hydralazine Hydrochloride

Synonym. Apressinum
Proprietary Names. Apresolin(e); Dralzine.
$C_8H_8N_4,HCl = 196.6$
CAS—304-20-1
A white crystalline powder. M.p. about 275°, with decomposition.
Soluble 1 in 25 of water and 1 in 500 of ethanol; practically insoluble in chloroform and ether.

Dissociation Constant. pK_a 0.5, 7.1.

Colour Test. Nessler's Reagent—black.

Thin-layer Chromatography. *System TA*—Rf 51; *system TB*—Rf 38; *system TC*—Rf 11. (*Acidified iodoplatinate solution*, positive.)

Gas Chromatography. *System GA*—RI 1528.

Ultraviolet Spectrum. Water—240 nm ($A_1^1 = 675$ a), 260 nm ($A_1^1 = 675$ a), 304 nm, 315 nm.

Infra-red Spectrum. Principal peaks at wavenumbers 1665, 790, 1582, 1000, 810, 1175 (hydralazine hydrochloride, KBr disk).

Wavelength

[Infra-red spectrum: Transmittance vs Wavenumber, axis from 2000 to 650; wavelength scale 5 to 15]

Transmittance

2000   1800   1600   1400   1200   1000   800   650

Wavenumber

Mass Spectrum. Principal peaks at *m/z* 160, 103, 89, 131, 115, 76, 161, 104.

Quantification. HIGH PRESSURE LIQUID CHROMATOGRAPHY. In plasma: limit of detection 1 ng/ml for hydralazine and 200 pg/ml for hydralazine pyruvic acid hydrazone, fluorescence detection—P. A. Reece *et al.*, *J. Chromat.*, 1980, *181*; *Biomed. Appl.*, 7, 427–440. In blood: sensitivity 1 ng/ml, UV detection—T. M. Ludden *et al.*, *J. pharm. Sci.*, 1983, *72*, 693–695.

NOTE. Spectrophotometric and gas chromatographic assays have been shown to be non-selective due to interference from acid-labile hydrazones—see P. A. Reece *et al.*, *J. pharm. Sci.*, 1978, *67*, 1150–1153 and T. M. Ludden *et al.*, *Clin. Pharmacokinet.*, 1982, *7*, 185–205.

Disposition in the Body. Readily absorbed after oral administration. It undergoes first-pass acetylation, the extent of which is genetically determined; bioavailability 30 to 35% in slow acetylators, 10 to 16% in rapid acetylators. The major metabolites are: 3-methyl-1,2,4-triazolo[3,4-*a*]phthalazine (MTP—the acetylation product); hydralazine pyruvic acid hydrazone (HPH) which is the major plasma metabolite; 4-(2-acetylhydrazino)phthalazin-1-one (*N*-AcHPZ) which is the major urinary metabolite; 3-hydroxymethyl-1,2,4-triazolo[3,4-*a*]phthalazine (3-OHMTP). About 65% of a dose is excreted in the urine in 24 hours. In rapid acetylators, about 30% is excreted as *N*-AcHPZ and 10 to 30% as conjugated 3-OHMTP; in slow acetylators, about 15 to 20% is excreted as *N*-AcHPZ and up to 10% as conjugated 3-OHMTP. Other metabolites include phthalazin-1-one (PZ), 1,2,4-triazolo[3,4-*a*]phthalazine (TP), 9-hydroxy-MTP, phthalazine, tetrazolo[5,1-*a*]phthalazine, and hydrazones of hydralazine formed with acetone and α-ketoglutaric acid. About 10% of a dose is eliminated in the faeces.

THERAPEUTIC CONCENTRATION.
Following a single oral dose of 1 mg/kg to 4 rapid acetylators, a mean peak plasma-hydralazine concentration of 0.05 µg/ml was attained in 0.4 hour and a mean peak plasma-HPH concentration of 0.26 µg/ml was attained in 0.6 hour; after the same dose was given to 4 slow acetylators the corresponding peak plasma concentrations were 0.17 µg/ml of hydralazine and 0.54 µg/ml of HPH in 0.3 hour and 1 hour respectively (A. Shepherd *et al.*, *Clin. Pharmac. Ther.*, 1980, *28*, 804–811).

HALF-LIFE. Plasma half-life, hydralazine 0.4 to 2 hours, HPH about 4 hours, MTP about 1.5 to 2 hours.

VOLUME OF DISTRIBUTION. About 3 to 8 litres/kg.

NOTE. For a review of the pharmacokinetics of hydralazine see T. M. Ludden *et al.*, *Clin. Pharmacokinet.*, 1982, *7*, 185–205.

Dose. 50 to 200 mg of hydralazine hydrochloride daily.

Hydrastine   *Alkaloid*

6,7 - Dimethoxy - 3 - (5,6,7,8 - tetrahydro - 6 - methyl - 1,3 - dioxolo-[4,5-*g*]isoquinolin-5-yl)isobenzofuran-1(3*H*)-one
$C_{21}H_{21}NO_6 = 383.4$
CAS—118-08-1

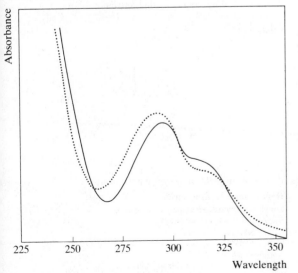

An alkaloid obtained from hydrastis, the dried rhizome and roots of golden seal, *Hydrastis canadensis* (Ranunculaceae). Crystals. M.p. 132°.
Practically **insoluble** in water; soluble 1 in 210 of ethanol, 1 in 1 of chloroform, and 1 in 245 of ether.

Hydrastine Hydrochloride
$C_{21}H_{21}NO_6,HCl = 419.9$
CAS—5936-28-7
A white or creamy-white hygroscopic powder. M.p. about 116°.
Soluble in water and ethanol; slightly soluble in chloroform.

Dissociation Constant. pK_a 6.2 (25°).

Colour Tests. Liebermann's Test—green; Mandelin's Test—red-brown → red.

Thin-layer Chromatography. *System TA*—Rf 61. (*Acidified iodoplatinate solution, positive.*)

Absorbance

225   250   275   300   325   350

Wavelength

Gas Chromatography. *System GA*—RI 2988.

Ultraviolet Spectrum. Aqueous acid—294 nm ($A_1^1 = 195$ b); aqueous alkali—292 nm.

Infra-red Spectrum. Principal peaks at wavenumbers 1760, 1501, 1037, 1260, 1020, 1111 (KBr disk).

Dose. Hydrastine hydrochloride was formerly given in doses of 15 to 60 mg.

Hydrastinine   *Alkaloid*

5,6,7,8-Tetrahydro-6-methyl-1,3-dioxolo[4,5-*g*]isoquinolin-5-ol
$C_{11}H_{13}NO_3 = 207.2$
CAS—6592-85-4

An alkaloid produced by oxidation of hydrastine.
A white crystalline substance. M.p. 117°.
Slightly **soluble** in hot water; soluble in ethanol, chloroform, and ether.

Hydrastinine Hydrochloride
$C_{11}H_{11}NO_2,HCl = 225.7$
CAS—4884-68-8
Pale yellow crystals or crystalline powder. M.p. 212°, with decomposition. Very **soluble** in water and ethanol; sparingly soluble in chloroform and ether. Solutions in water show a blue fluorescence.

Colour Test. Mandelin's Test—orange → green.

Thin-layer Chromatography. *System TA*—Rf 00. (*Acidified iodoplatinate solution, positive.*)

Gas Chromatography. *System GA*—RI 1590.

Ultraviolet Spectrum. Aqueous acid—249 nm, 306 nm, 363 nm.
Infra-red Spectrum. Principal peaks at wavenumbers 1235, 1032, 1499, 925, 1075, 934 (KBr disk).

Dose. Hydrastinine hydrochloride was formerly given in doses of 15 to 60 mg.

Hydrochlorothiazide   *Diuretic*

Synonym. Chlorosulthiadil
Proprietary Names. Chlorzide; Delco-Retic; Dichlotride; Direma; Diucen-H; Diuchlor H; Esidrex; Esidrix; Hydro-Aquil; HydroDIURIL; HydroSaluric; Hydro-Z; Hydrozide; Jen-Diril; Lexor; Loqua; Mictrin; Natrimax; Neo-Codema; Novohydrazide; Oretic; Ro-Hydrazide; Thiuretic; Urozide. It is an ingredient of Aldoril, Amilco, Co-Betaloc, Dyazide, Dytenzide, Esimil, Hydromet, Hydropres, Moducren, Moduretic, Secadrex, Sotazide, and Tolerzide.

6 - Chloro - 3,4 - dihydro - 2*H* - 1,2,4 - benzothiadiazine - 7 - sulphon-amide 1,1-dioxide
$C_7H_8ClN_3O_4S_2 = 297.7$
CAS—58-93-5

A white crystalline powder. M.p. about 268°, with decomposition.

Practically **insoluble** in water, chloroform, and ether; soluble 1 in 200 of ethanol and 1 in 20 of acetone; freely soluble in dimethylformamide and solutions of alkali hydroxides.

Dissociation Constant. pK$_a$ 7.0, 9.2.

Colour Tests. Chromotropic Acid—violet, after dilution; Koppanyi–Zwikker Test—violet; Liebermann's Test—blue-green.

Thin-layer Chromatography. *System TD*—Rf 04; *system TE*—Rf 34; *system TF*—Rf 39. (*Mercuric chloride–diphenylcarbazone reagent*, positive.)

Gas Chromatography. *System GA*—not eluted.

High Pressure Liquid Chromatography. *System HN*—k′ 0.70.

Ultraviolet Spectrum. Aqueous acid—272 nm (A$_1^1$ = 644 a), 318 nm; aqueous alkali—274 nm (A$_1^1$ = 520 a), 324 nm.

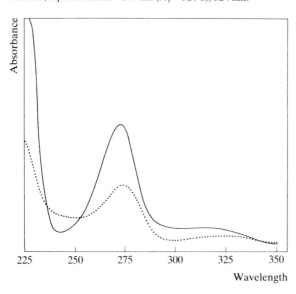

Wavelength

Infra-red Spectrum. Principal peaks at wavenumbers 1318, 1180, 1150, 1168, 1602, 1060 (KBr disk).

Mass Spectrum. Principal peaks at *m/z* 269, 205, 221, 297, 271, 62, 285, 124.

Quantification. GAS CHROMATOGRAPHY. In blood or plasma: sensitivity 5 ng/ml, ECD—E. Redalieu *et al.*, *J. pharm. Sci.*, 1978, *67*, 726–728. In plasma, erythrocytes or urine: detection limit 10 ng/ml in plasma, ECD and FID—B. Lindström *et al.*, *J. Chromat.*, 1975, *114*, 459–462.

HIGH PRESSURE LIQUID CHROMATOGRAPHY. In plasma or urine: hydrochlorothiazide and chlorothiazide, sensitivity 10 ng/ml in plasma and 2 µg/ml in urine, UV detection—R. H. Barbhaiya *et al.*, *J. pharm. Sci.*, 1981, *70*, 291–295.

Disposition in the Body. Rapidly but incompletely absorbed after oral administration; bioavailability about 70%. More than 95% of an intravenous dose is excreted unchanged in the urine. About 65% of an oral dose is excreted in the urine unchanged in 24 hours.

THERAPEUTIC CONCENTRATION.

Peak plasma concentrations of 0.18 to 0.43 µg/ml (mean 0.26) were attained in 2 to 4 hours, following a single oral dose of 50 mg given to 8 subjects (B. Beerman *et al.*, *Eur. J. clin. Pharmac.*, 1977, *12*, 297–303).

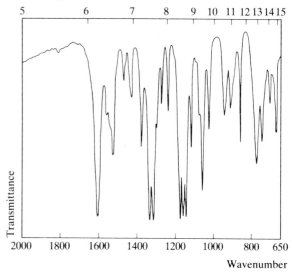

Wavenumber

Steady-state plasma concentrations of 0.05 to 0.16 µg/ml (mean 0.1) were achieved after daily oral doses of 75 mg to 8 subjects (B. Beerman and M. Groschinsky-Grind, *Eur. J. clin. Pharmac.*, 1978, *13*, 195–201).

HALF-LIFE. Plasma half-life, 6 to 15 hours.

VOLUME OF DISTRIBUTION. About 3 litres/kg.

DISTRIBUTION IN BLOOD. Plasma : whole blood ratio, 0.41.

PROTEIN BINDING. In plasma, about 40%.

NOTE. For a review of the pharmacokinetics of diuretics, see B. Beerman and M. Groschinsky-Grind, *Clin. Pharmacokinet.*, 1980, *5*, 221–245.

Dose. 25 to 200 mg daily.

Hydrocodone   *Narcotic Analgesic/Antitussive*

Synonym. Dihydrocodeinone
6-Deoxy-7,8-dihydro-3-*O*-methyl-6-oxomorphine
C$_{18}$H$_{21}$NO$_3$ = 299.4
CAS—125-29-1

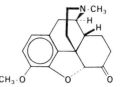

M.p. 198°.
Practically **insoluble** in water; soluble in ethanol.

Hydrocodone Hydrochloride
Synonym. Dihydrocodeinone Hydrochloride
Proprietary Name. Dicodid (injection)
C$_{18}$H$_{21}$NO$_3$,HCl,2½H$_2$O = 380.9
CAS—25968-91-6 (anhydrous)
A white crystalline powder.
Soluble 1 in 2 of water; soluble in ethanol.

Hydrocodone Phosphate
$C_{18}H_{21}NO_3,1\frac{1}{2}H_3PO_4 = 446.4$
CAS—34366-67-1
A white or yellowish-white crystalline powder.
Soluble in water; practically insoluble in ethanol, chloroform, and ether.

Hydrocodone Tartrate
Synonyms. Dihydrocodeinone Acid Tartrate; Hydrocodone Acid Tartrate; Hydrocodone Bitartrate; Hydrocone Bitartrate.
Proprietary Names. Codone; Corutol DH; Dicodid (tablets); Hycodan; Hycon; Robidone. It is an ingredient of Hycomine.
$C_{18}H_{21}NO_3,C_4H_6O_6,2\frac{1}{2}H_2O = 494.5$
CAS—143-71-5 (anhydrous); *34195-34-1* (hemipentahydrate).
White crystals or crystalline powder.
Soluble 1 in 10 of water and 1 in 150 of ethanol; practically insoluble in chloroform and ether.

Dissociation Constant. pK_a 8.3 (20°).

Colour Test. Marquis Test—yellow → brown → violet.

Thin-layer Chromatography. *System TA*—Rf 25; *system TB*—Rf 04; *system TC*—Rf 20. (*Dragendorff spray*, positive; *acidified iodoplatinate solution*, positive; *Marquis reagent*, violet.)

Gas Chromatography. *System GA*—RI 2440; *system GC*—RI 3028; *system GF*—RI 2930.

High Pressure Liquid Chromatography. *System HA*—k' 7.1 (tailing peak); *system HC*—k' 2.17.

Ultraviolet Spectrum. Aqueous acid—280 nm ($A_1^1 = 41$ a). No alkaline shift.

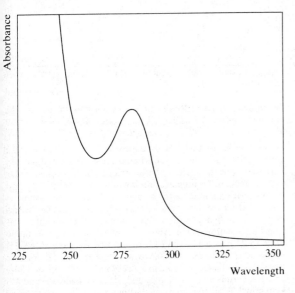

Infra-red Spectrum. Principal peaks at wavenumbers 1720, 1270, 1500, 959, 1055, 800 (KBr disk).

Mass Spectrum. Principal peaks at *m/z* 299, 242, 59, 243, 42, 96, 70, 214.

Quantification. GAS CHROMATOGRAPHY. In serum: sensitivity 1 ng/ml, ECD—J. W. Barnhart and W. J. Caldwell, *J. Chromat.*, 1977, *130*, 243–249. In postmortem blood: detection limit 100 ng/ml, AFID—G. Cimbura and E. Koves, *J. analyt. Toxicol.*, 1981, *5*, 296–299.

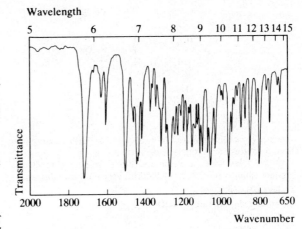

GAS CHROMATOGRAPHY–MASS SPECTROMETRY. In urine: hydrocodone and metabolites, sensitivity 10 ng/ml—E. J. Cone and W. D. Darwin, *Biomed. Mass Spectrom.*, 1978, *5*, 291–295.

RADIOIMMUNOASSAY. In plasma: sensitivity 10 ng/ml—I. L. Honigberg and J. T. Stewart, *J. pharm. Sci.*, 1980, *69*, 1171–1173.

Disposition in the Body. Absorbed after oral administration. Metabolised by demethylation and reduction of the 6-keto group. About 26% of a dose is excreted in the urine in 72 hours, with 12% of the dose as unchanged drug, 5% as norhydrocodone, 4% as conjugated hydromorphone, 3% as 6-hydrocodol, and 0.1% as conjugated 6-hydromorphol. Hydrocodol and hydromorphol exist as stereoisomers. The unconjugated metabolites are thought to be active.
Hydrocodone is a metabolite of codeine.

THERAPEUTIC CONCENTRATION.
After a single oral dose of 10 mg of hydrocodone tartrate to 5 subjects, peak serum concentrations of 0.018 to 0.032 µg/ml (mean 0.023) were attained in 1.5 hours (J. W. Barnhart and W. J. Caldwell, *J. Chromat.* 1977, *130*, 243–249).

TOXICITY. The estimated lethal dose is 200 mg. Fatalities have occurred at blood concentrations greater than 0.1 µg/ml.
In 2 fatalities due to the ingestion of hydrocodone and phenyltolamine, the following postmortem concentrations were reported: blood, hydrocodone 0.3 µg/ml (both cases), bile, hydrocodone 14.3, – µg/ml, hydromorphone 98, 48 µg/ml; in the first case phenyltolamine was present in bile at a concentration of 0.4 µg/ml (J. I. Park *et al.*, *J. forens. Sci.*, 1982, *27*, 223–224).

HALF-LIFE. Plasma half-life, about 4 hours.

Dose. 15 to 40 mg of hydrocodone tartrate daily.

Hydrocortisone   *Corticosteroid*

Synonyms. Compound F; Cortisol; 17-Hydroxycorticosterone.
Note. Cortisol is also used as a proprietary name for cortisone acetate.
Proprietary Names. Cobadex; Cortenema; Cortril; Dioderm; Efcortelan; Hydrocortistab; Hydrocortisyl; Hydrocortone.
Hydrocortisone and its esters are ingredients of many proprietary preparations—see *Martindale, The Extra Pharmacopoeia*, 28th Edn.

11β,17α,21-Trihydroxypregn-4-ene-3,20-dione
$C_{21}H_{30}O_5 = 362.5$
CAS—50-23-7

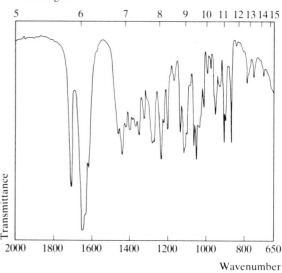

A white crystalline powder. M.p. about 214°, with decomposition. A solution in dioxan is dextrorotatory.
Practically **insoluble** in water and ether; soluble 1 in 40 of ethanol; slightly soluble in chloroform; very soluble in dioxan.

Hydrocortisone Acetate

Synonym. Hydrocortisone 21-Acetate
$C_{23}H_{32}O_6 = 404.5$
CAS—50-03-3
A white crystalline powder. M.p. about 220°, with decomposition.
Practically **insoluble** in water and ether; soluble 1 in 230 of ethanol; slightly soluble in chloroform.

Hydrocortisone Butyrate

Synonym. Hydrocortisone 17-Butyrate
$C_{25}H_{36}O_6 = 432.6$
CAS—13609-67-1

Hydrocortisone Cypionate

Synonyms. Hydrocortisone Cipionate; Hydrocortisone Cyclopentylpropionate.
$C_{29}H_{42}O_6 = 486.6$
CAS—508-99-6
A white crystalline powder.
Practically **insoluble** in water; soluble in ethanol; very soluble in chloroform; slightly soluble in ether.

Hydrocortisone Hydrogen Succinate

Synonyms. Cortisol Hemisuccinate; Hydrocortisone Hemisuccinate.
$C_{25}H_{34}O_8 = 462.5$
CAS—2203-97-6
A white crystalline powder. M.p. 170° to 173° or 210° to 214°.
Practically **insoluble** in water; soluble 1 in 40 of ethanol and 1 in 7 of dehydrated alcohol.

Hydrocortisone Sodium Phosphate

$C_{21}H_{29}Na_2O_8P = 486.4$
CAS—6000-74-4
A white or light yellow hygroscopic powder.
Soluble 1 in 4 of water; slightly soluble in ethanol; practically insoluble in chloroform and ether.

Hydrocortisone Sodium Succinate

Synonym. Hydrocortisone 21-Sodium Succinate
$C_{25}H_{35}NaO_8 = 484.5$
CAS—125-04-2
A white, hygroscopic, crystalline powder or amorphous solid. M.p. 169° to 171°.
Soluble 1 in 3 of water and 1 in 34 of ethanol; practically insoluble in chloroform and ether. It is unstable in aqueous solution.

Hydrocortisone Valerate

Synonym. Hydrocortisone 17-Valerate
$C_{26}H_{38}O_6 = 446.6$
CAS—57524-89-7

Dissociation Constant. Hydrocortisone sodium succinate, pK_a 5.1.

Colour Tests. Antimony Pentachloride—orange; Naphthol–Sulphuric Acid—yellow-brown/yellow-brown; Sulphuric Acid—green, orange dichroism (green fluorescence under ultraviolet light).

Thin-layer Chromatography. Hydrocortisone: *system TP*—Rf 27; *system TQ*—Rf 02; *system TR*—Rf 08; *system TS*—Rf 00. Hydrocortisone acetate: *system TP*—Rf 51; *system TQ*—Rf 11; *system TR*—Rf 38; *system TS*—Rf 00. Hydrocortisone hydrogen succinate: *system TP*—Rf 08; *system TQ*—Rf 00; *system TR*—Rf 00; *system TS*—Rf 00. Hydrocortisone sodium phosphate: *system TP*—Rf 00; *system TQ*—Rf 00; *system TR*—Rf 00; *system TS*—Rf 00. (*DPST solution.*)

High Pressure Liquid Chromatography. System *HT*—k' 5.8.

Ultraviolet Spectrum. Ethanol—240 nm ($A_1^1 = 435$ a).

Infra-red Spectrum. Principal peaks at wavenumbers 1640, 1702, 1610, 1232, 1042, 1115 (KBr disk).

Wavelength

Quantification. HIGH PRESSURE LIQUID CHROMATOGRAPHY. In plasma: sensitivity 5 ng/ml, UV detection—R. D. Toothaker *et al.*, *J. pharm. Sci.*, 1982, **71**, 573–576.

Disposition in the Body. Hydrocortisone (cortisol) is the main glucocorticoid secreted by the adrenal cortex. It is administered parenterally as the sodium phosphate or sodium succinate ester in emergencies. Hydrocortisone is readily absorbed after oral administration and through the skin; hydrocortisone acetate is less well absorbed. It is metabolised in the liver and other tissues by reduction, hydroxylation, side-chain cleavage, and conjugation with glucuronic acid. About 90% of a dose is excreted in the urine in 24 hours; less than 1% is excreted unchanged, 40% is the 5α- and 5β- forms of tetrahydrocortisol and the 5β- form of tetrahydrocortisone, 17% is a mixture of the 5α- and 5β- and 20α- and 20β-cortols and cortolones, and 6% is 11-hydroxy- and 11-keto-etiocholanolone; most of the metabolites are excreted as glucuronide conjugates; at plasma concentrations of greater than 0.2 µg/ml, the amount of unchanged hydrocortisone excreted in the urine is increased.

BLOOD CONCENTRATION. Endogenous hydrocortisone exhibits a diurnal variation in plasma concentrations; in the morning, concentrations are in the approximate range 0.08 to 0.20 µg/ml and in the evening, in the range 0.04 to 0.10 µg/ml.

Following a single intravenous injection of 40 mg to 6 subjects, a mean plasma concentration of 1.85 µg/ml was reported at 10 minutes (R. D. Toothaker and P. G. Welling, *J. Pharmacokinet. Biopharm.*, 1982, **10**, 147–156).

HALF-LIFE. Plasma half-life, about 1.5 hours.

VOLUME OF DISTRIBUTION. About 0.3 litre/kg.

PROTEIN BINDING. In plasma, more than 90%.

Dose. 10 to 30 mg daily, by mouth. In the treatment of certain medical emergencies, the equivalent of 100 to 500 mg of hydrocortisone by intravenous injection, 3 or 4 times daily.

Hydroflumethiazide   *Diuretic*

Synonym. Trifluoromethylhydrothiazide

Proprietary Names. Di-Ademil; Diucardin; Hydrenox; Leodrine; Rontyl; Saluron. It is an ingredient of Aldactide, Rautrax, and Salutensin.

3,4-Dihydro-6-trifluoromethyl-2H-1,2,4-benzothiadiazine-7-sulphonamide 1,1-dioxide

$C_8H_8F_3N_3O_4S_2 = 331.3$

CAS—135-09-1

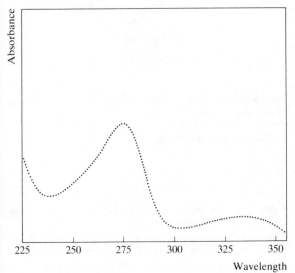

White or cream-coloured glistening crystals or crystalline powder. M.p. 270° to 275°.

Soluble 1 in 3000 of water, 1 in about 50 of ethanol, and 1 in 4 of acetone; practically insoluble in chloroform and ether.

Dissociation Constant. pK_a 8.5, 10.0 (20°).

Colour Tests. Chromotropic Acid—violet, after dilution; Koppanyi-Zwikker Test—violet; Liebermann's Test—blue-green.

Thin-layer Chromatography. *System TD*—Rf 07; *system TE*—Rf 40; *system TF*—Rf 47. (Location under ultraviolet light, violet fluorescence; *acidified potassium permanganate solution*, faint reaction.)

High Pressure Liquid Chromatography. *System HN*—k' 1.30.

Ultraviolet Spectrum. Aqueous acid—273 nm ($A_1^1 = 578$ a), 325 nm; aqueous alkali—274 nm, 333 nm.

Infra-red Spectrum. Principal peaks at wavenumbers 1151, 1180, 1125, 1052, 1300, 1525 (KBr disk).

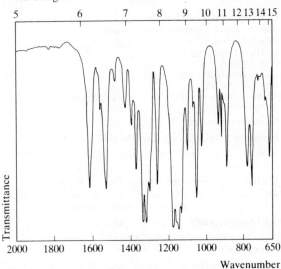

Mass Spectrum. Principal peaks at m/z 303, 331, 239, 255, 30, 158, 64, 159.

Quantification. SPECTROFLUORIMETRY. In plasma or urine: detection limit 10 ng/ml in plasma and 100 ng/ml in urine—O. Brørs *et al.*, *Eur. J. clin. Pharmac.*, 1977, *11*, 149–154.

THIN-LAYER CHROMATOGRAPHY–SPECTROFLUORIMETRY. In plasma or urine: detection limit 10 ng/ml in plasma and 500 ng/ml in urine—Y. Garceau *et al.*, *J. pharm. Sci.*, 1974, *63*, 1793–1795.

Disposition in the Body. Incompletely but fairly rapidly absorbed after oral administration. During daily dosing, 50 to 70% of a dose is excreted in the 24-hour urine as unchanged drug and about 2% as 2,4-disulphamyl-5-trifluoromethylaniline (DTA).

THERAPEUTIC CONCENTRATION.

Following single oral doses of 100 mg to 12 subjects, peak plasma concentrations of 0.17 to 0.6 µg/ml (mean 0.4) were attained in 2 to 4 hours (G. Yakatan *et al.*, *J. clin. Pharmac.*, 1977, *17*, 37–47).

HALF-LIFE. Derived from urinary excretion data, 5 to 18 hours (dose-dependent).

DISTRIBUTION IN BLOOD. Plasma:whole blood ratio, about 0.7.

PROTEIN BINDING. In plasma, about 75%.

Dose. 25 to 200 mg daily.

Hydromorphone   *Narcotic Analgesic*

Synonyms. 7,8-Dihydromorphinone; Dimorphone.

6-Deoxy-7,8-dihydro-6-oxomorphine

$C_{17}H_{19}NO_3 = 285.3$

CAS—466-99-9

A fine, white, crystalline powder. M.p. about 260°, with decomposition.

Slightly **soluble** in water; freely soluble in ethanol; very soluble in chloroform.

Hydromorphone Hydrochloride

Synonym. Dihydromorphinone Hydrochloride
Proprietary Name. Dilaudid
$C_{17}H_{19}NO_3,HCl = 321.8$
CAS—71-68-1
A white crystalline powder, which is affected by light. M.p. 305° to 315°, with decomposition.
Soluble 1 in 3 of water and 1 in 100 of ethanol (90%); practically insoluble in chloroform and ether.

Dissociation Constant. pK_a 8.2 (20°).

Partition Coefficient. Log P (heptane/pH 7.4), −4.0.

Colour Tests. Mandelin's Test—violet → orange; Marquis Test—yellow → red → violet.

Thin-layer Chromatography. *System TA*—Rf 23; *system TB*—Rf 03; *system TC*—Rf 09. (*Dragendorff spray*, positive; *acidified iodoplatinate solution*, positive; *Marquis reagent*, violet.)

Gas Chromatography. *System GA*—RI 2467.

High Pressure Liquid Chromatography. *System HA*—k' 7.9 (tailing peak).

Ultraviolet Spectrum. Aqueous acid—280 nm $(A_1^1 = 50\,a)$; aqueous alkali—290 nm.

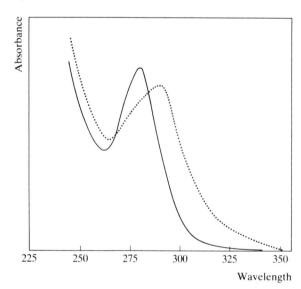

Infra-red Spectrum. Principal peaks at wavenumbers 1727, 1247, 1279, 1034, 757, 1500 (KBr disk).

Mass Spectrum. Principal peaks at *m/z* 285, 96, 229, 228, 70, 214, 115, 200.

Quantification. GAS CHROMATOGRAPHY. In urine: hydromorphone and metabolites, FID—E. J. Cone *et al.*, *J. pharm. Sci.*, 1977, *66*, 1709–1713. In postmortem blood: limit of detection 100 ng/ml, AFID—G. Cimbura and E. Koves, *J. analyt. Toxicol.*, 1981, *5*, 296–299.

GAS CHROMATOGRAPHY–MASS SPECTROMETRY. In blood, serum or tissue homogenates: sensitivity 80 ng/ml—J. J. Saady *et al.*, *J. analyt. Toxicol.*, 1982, *6*, 235–237.

RADIOIMMUNOASSAY. In plasma: sensitivity 2.5 ng/ml—I. L. Honigberg and J. T. Stewart, *J. pharm. Sci.*, 1980, *69*, 1171–1173.

Disposition in the Body. Rapidly but incompletely absorbed after oral administration; bioavailability about 60% but there is considerable intersubject variation. About 6% of a dose is excreted in the urine in 24 hours as free hydromorphone with about 30% as conjugated hydromorphone and only traces of the active 6α- and 6β-hydroxy metabolites.
Hydromorphone is a metabolite of hydrocodone.

THERAPEUTIC CONCENTRATION.

Following a single oral dose of 4 mg to 6 subjects, peak plasma concentrations of 0.018 to 0.027 µg/ml (mean 0.022) were attained in about 1 hour (J. J. Vallner *et al.*, *J. clin. Pharmac.*, 1981, *21*, 152–156).

TOXICITY. The estimated minimum lethal dose is 200 mg. Plasma concentrations greater than 0.1 µg/ml may be toxic.

In a fatality attributed to hydromorphone overdose, the following tissue concentrations were reported: blood 1.2 µg/ml, brain a trace, kidney 1.2 µg/g, liver 0.4 µg/g, urine 1.1 µg/ml; diazepam was also detected (R. C. Baselt, *Bull. int. Ass. forens. Toxicol.*, 1978, *14*(2), 20).

The following postmortem tissue concentrations were reported in a fatality due to an injected overdose of hydromorphone: blood 0.17 µg/ml, bile 8.6 µg/ml, kidney 0.13 µg/g, liver 0.07 µg/g (H. C. Walls, *Bull. int. Ass. forens. Toxicol.*, 1976, *12*(3), 7–8).

HALF-LIFE. Plasma half-life, 1.5 to 4 hours.

VOLUME OF DISTRIBUTION. About 1 litre/kg.

Dose. 2 to 4 mg of hydromorphone hydrochloride every 4 to 6 hours.

Hydroquinidine   *Anti-arrhythmic*

Synonyms. Dihydrochinidin; Dihydroquinidine; Hydroconchinine.
(8R,9S)-10,11-Dihydro-6′-methoxycinchonan-9-ol
$C_{20}H_{26}N_2O_2 = 326.4$
CAS—1435-55-8

An alkaloid present in the bark of species of *Cinchona* (Rubiaceae). Crystals. M.p. about 169°.
Soluble in ethanol and ether.

Hydroquinidine Hydrochloride

$C_{20}H_{26}N_2O_2,HCl = 362.9$
CAS—1476-98-8
Colourless crystals. M.p. 273° to 274°.
Freely **soluble** in chloroform and methanol; less readily soluble in water and ethanol.

Colour Tests. Sulphuric Acid—yellow (fluoresces under ultraviolet light); Thalleioquin Test—green.

Thin-layer Chromatography. *System TA*—Rf 45; *system TB*—Rf 03; *system TC*—Rf 08. (*Acidified iodoplatinate solution*, positive.)

Gas Chromatography. *System GA*—RI 2810.

Ultraviolet Spectrum. Aqueous acid—250 nm ($A_1^1 = 1240$ b), 316 nm, 345 nm ($A_1^1 = 180$ b).

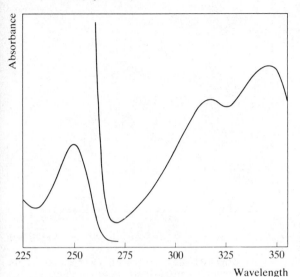

Infra-red Spectrum. Principal peaks at wavenumbers 1509, 1261, 1620, 1234, 854, 1030.

Mass Spectrum. Principal peaks at m/z 138, 326, 55, 110, 189, 82, 160, 139.

Dose. Usually 450 to 600 mg of hydroquinidine hydrochloride daily.

Hydroquinine   *Alkaloid*

Synonym. Dihydroquinine
(8S,9R)-10,11-Dihydro-6'-methoxycinchonan-9-ol
$C_{20}H_{26}N_2O_2 = 326.4$
CAS—522-66-7

An alkaloid present in the bark of species of *Cinchona* (Rubiaceae). Crystals. M.p. 173°.
Practically **insoluble** in water; soluble in ethanol, chloroform, and ether.

Colour Tests. Sulphuric Acid—yellow (fluoresces under ultraviolet light); Thalleioquin Test—green.

Thin-layer Chromatography. *System TA*—Rf 44; *system TB*—Rf 02; *system TC*—Rf 07. (*Acidified iodoplatinate solution*, positive.)

Gas Chromatography. *System GA*—RI 1450.

Ultraviolet Spectrum. Aqueous acid—250 nm ($A_1^1 = 915$ b), 316 nm, 345 nm ($A_1^1 = 167$ b).

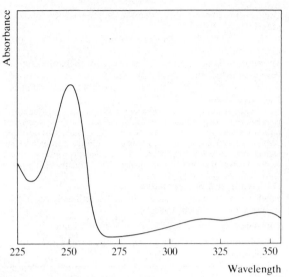

Infra-red Spectrum. Principal peaks at wavenumbers 1240, 1225, 1507, 1623, 1026, 1132 (KBr disk).

Mass Spectrum. Principal peaks at m/z 138, 55, 189, 82, 41, 110, 326, 42.

Hydroquinone   *Depigmenting Agent/Antoxidant*

Synonyms. Hydroquinol; Quinol.
Proprietary Names. Eldopaque; Eldoquin; Phiaquin.
Benzene-1,4-diol
$C_6H_6O_2 = 110.1$
CAS—123-31-9

Fine white crystals, or white crystalline powder, which darken on exposure to light and air. M.p. 172° to 174°.
Soluble 1 in 17 of water, 1 in 4 of ethanol, 1 in 51 of chloroform, and 1 in 16 of ether.

Partition Coefficient. Log P (octanol/pH 7.4), 0.6.

Colour Tests. Ammoniacal Silver Nitrate—grey-yellow/brown; Benedict's Reagent—red; Ferric Chloride—green.

Gas Chromatography. *System GA*—RI 1220.

Ultraviolet Spectrum. Ethanol—295 nm ($A_1^1 = 282$ b).

Infra-red Spectrum. Principal peaks at wavenumbers 1210, 1192, 1520, 760, 1240, 813 (KBr disk).

Use. As a 2 to 5% ointment for depigmentation of the skin.

Hydroxocobalamin   *Haemopoietic Vitamin*

Synonyms. Vitamin B_{12a}; Vitamin B_{12b}.
Proprietary Names. Alpha Redisol; Alpha-Ruvite; Cobalin-H; Hydroxo B_{12}; Neo-Betalin 12; Neo-Cytamen; Novobedouze; Rubesol-LA; Sytobex-H.

Coα-[α-(5,6-Dimethylbenzimidazol-1-yl)]-*Coβ*-hydroxocobamide
$C_{62}H_{89}CoN_{13}O_{15}P = 1346$
CAS—13422-51-0

Hydroxocobalamin occurs either as aquocobalamin chloride [α-(5,6-dimethylbenzimidazol-1-yl)aquocobamide chloride], $C_{62}H_{90}ClCoN_{13}O_{15}P$, or as aquocobalamin sulphate, $C_{124}H_{180}Co_2N_{26}O_{34}P_2S$.

Note. In acid solutions, hydroxocobalamin takes up a hydrogen ion which converts the hydroxyl group to a co-ordinated water molecule, and in this form it is known as aquocobalamin, which is basic and forms salts with acids. In solution, aquocobalamin exists in equilibrium with hydroxocobalamin and, since it is more stable in acid solution, it usually occurs commercially in the form of aquocobalamin (E. L. Smith *et al.*, *Analyst, Lond.*, 1962, *87*, 183–186).

Dark red crystals or crystalline powder.

Soluble 1 in 50 of water and 1 in 100 of ethanol; practically insoluble in chloroform and ether.

Ultraviolet Spectrum. Acetic acid—274 nm, 351 nm.

Dose. Initially 0.25 to 1 mg, by intramuscular injection, daily or on alternate days.

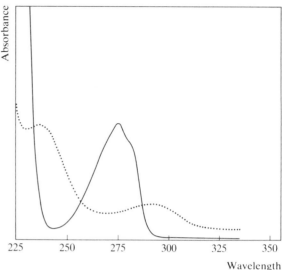

Wavelength

Hydroxyamphetamine
Sympathomimetic

Synonym. Oxamphetamine
(±)-4-(2-Aminopropyl)phenol
$C_9H_{13}NO = 151.2$
CAS—103-86-6; 1518-86-1 (±)

Crystals. M.p. 125° to 126°.
Soluble in water, ethanol, and chloroform.

Hydroxyamphetamine Hydrobromide
Proprietary Name. Paredrine
$C_9H_{13}NO,HBr = 232.1$
CAS—306-21-8; 140-36-3 (±)
A white crystalline powder. M.p. 189° to 192°.
Soluble 1 in 1 of water and 1 in 2.5 of ethanol; slightly soluble in chloroform; practically insoluble in ether.

Dissociation Constant. pK_a 9.3 (25°).

Thin-layer Chromatography. *System TA*—Rf 35; *system TB*—Rf 02; *system TC*—Rf 02. (*Acidified potassium permanganate solution*, positive.)

Gas Chromatography. *System GA*—RI 1320.

High Pressure Liquid Chromatography. *System HB*—k' 2.24; *system HC*—k' 1.11.

Ultraviolet Spectrum. Aqueous acid—275 nm ($A_1^1 = 103$ a); aqueous alkali—238 nm ($A_1^1 = 672$ b), 294 nm.

Infra-red Spectrum. Principal peaks at wavenumbers 1259, 1517, 1599, 1102, 813, 1111 (KBr disk).

Mass Spectrum. Principal peaks at *m/z* 44, 82, 80, 107, 77, 108, 81, 79.

Disposition in the Body. Readily absorbed after oral administration. About 90% of a dose is excreted in the urine in 24 hours as free and conjugated hydroxyamphetamine, with about 4% of the dose as free and conjugated 4'-hydroxynorephedrine.

TOXICITY. The estimated minimum lethal dose, intranasally, in children up to 2 years of age is 200 mg, and in adults about 2 g.

Dose. Hydroxyamphetamine hydrobromide has been given in doses of 60 to 240 mg daily.

Hydroxychloroquine
Antimalarial

Synonym. Oxichlorochin
2-{*N*-[4-(7-Chloro-4-quinolylamino)pentyl]-*N*-ethylamino}-ethanol
$C_{18}H_{26}ClN_3O = 335.9$
CAS—118-42-3

Crystals. M.p. 89° to 91°.

Hydroxychloroquine Sulphate
Proprietary Names. Ercoquin; Plaquenil; Quensyl.
$C_{18}H_{26}ClN_3O,H_2SO_4 = 433.9$
CAS—747-36-4
A white crystalline powder. There are 2 forms, one melting at about 198° and the other at about 240°.
Soluble 1 in 5 of water; practically insoluble in ethanol, chloroform, and ether.

Thin-layer Chromatography. *System TA*—Rf 45; *system TB*—Rf 00; *system TC*—Rf 02. (*Acidified iodoplatinate solution*, positive.)

Gas Chromatography. *System GA*—RI 2872.

Ultraviolet Spectrum. Aqueous acid—235 nm ($A_1^1 = 560$ a), 256 nm, 329 nm, 343 nm; aqueous alkali—253 nm, 330 nm.

Infra-red Spectrum. Principal peaks at wavenumbers 1579, 1608, 1530, 1050, 1150, 810 (KBr disk).

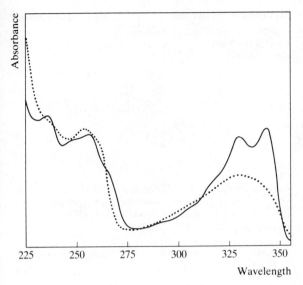

Wavelength

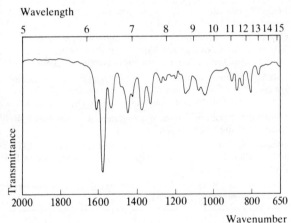

Wavenumber

Mass Spectrum. Principal peaks at *m/z* 102, 245, 247, 304, 305, 306, 58, 126.

Quantification. ULTRAVIOLET SPECTROPHOTOMETRY. In blood or urine—R. A. Dalley and D. Hainsworth, *J. forens. Sci. Soc.*, 1965, 5, 99–101.

SPECTROFLUORIMETRY. In plasma—E. W. McChesney *et al.*, *Antibiotics Chemother.*, 1962, *12*, 583–594.

Disposition in the Body. Rapidly and almost completely absorbed after oral administration. It is metabolised by de-ethylation. About 6% of a single dose is excreted in the urine over a period of 10 days and about 25% of a dose is eliminated in the faeces in 3 days as unchanged drug plus the de-ethylated metabolites. During daily therapy, less than 13% of a dose is excreted in the 24-hour urine with 8% of the dose as unchanged drug, 2% as desethylchloroquine, 2% as desethylhydroxychloroquine, and 0.5% as didesethylchloroquine.

THERAPEUTIC CONCENTRATION.

After an oral dose of hydroxychloroquine sulphate equivalent to 310 mg of the base to 6 subjects, peak plasma concentrations of 0.003 to 0.20 µg/ml (mean 0.08) were attained in 3 hours. Following oral administration of hydroxychloroquine diphosphate equivalent to 1264 mg of the base to

3 subjects, peak plasma concentrations of 0.29 to 1.0 µg/ml (mean 0.64) were attained in 3 hours and therapeutic concentrations greater than 0.01 µg/ml were maintained for 240 hours (E. W. McChesney *et al.*, *ibid.*).

TOXICITY.

In a fatality due to the ingestion of at least 12 g, the following postmortem tissue concentrations were reported: blood 48 µg/ml, heart blood 61 µg/ml, liver 71 µg/g, urine 970 µg/ml (R. A. Dalley and D. Hainsworth, *J. forens. Sci. Soc.*, 1965, *5*, 99–101).

HALF-LIFE. Plasma half-life, about 3 days.

Dose. For an acute attack of malaria, 2 g of hydroxychloroquine sulphate given over three days (1.2 g on the first day). In rheumatoid arthritis, initially 400 to 800 mg daily.

Hydroxyephedrine   *Sympathomimetic*

Synonyms. p-Hydroxyephedrine; Methylsynephrine; Oxyephedrine.

1-(4-Hydroxyphenyl)-2-methylaminopropan-1-ol
$C_{10}H_{15}NO_2 = 181.2$
CAS—365-26-4

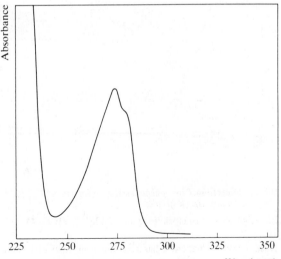

A crystalline powder. M.p. 152° to 154°.
Sparingly **soluble** in water, ethanol, and ether; freely soluble in dilute acids and sodium hydroxide solution.

Hydroxyephedrine Hydrochloride

$C_{10}H_{15}NO_2,HCl = 217.7$
CAS—942-51-8
A crystalline powder. M.p. 209° to 211°.
Soluble 1 in 3 of water and 1 in 10 of ethanol; sparingly soluble in acetone.

Colour Tests. Liebermann's Test—black; Mandelin's Test—green; Marquis Test—yellow.

Wavelength

Thin-layer Chromatography. *System TA*—Rf 35, streaking. (*Acidified potassium permanganate solution*, positive.)

Gas Chromatography. *System GA*—RI 1682.

High Pressure Liquid Chromatography. *System HB*—k' 0.73.

Ultraviolet Spectrum. Aqueous acid—273 nm ($A_1^1 = 75$ b); aqueous alkali—242 nm ($A_1^1 = 760$ b), 290 nm ($A_1^1 = 131$ b).

Infra-red Spectrum. Principal peaks at wavenumbers 980, 1238, 835, 1157, 1129, 792 (KBr disk).

Mass Spectrum. Principal peaks at *m/z* 58, 30, 59, 56, 77, –, –, –.

Dose. Hydroxyephedrine hydrochloride has been given in doses of 10 mg daily.

Hydroxyphenamate   *Tranquilliser*

Synonym. Oxyfenamate
Proprietary Name. Listica
2-Hydroxy-2-phenylbutyl carbamate
$C_{11}H_{15}NO_3 = 209.2$
CAS—50-19-1

$$C_6H_5 \cdot \underset{\underset{C_2H_5}{|}}{\overset{\overset{OH}{|}}{C}} \cdot CH_2 \cdot O \cdot CO \cdot NH_2$$

A white crystalline powder. M.p. 55° to 57°.
Soluble 1 in 40 of water; soluble in ethanol and chloroform.

Thin-layer Chromatography. *System TA*—Rf 74. (*Van Urk reagent*, positive.)

Gas Chromatography. *System GA*—RI 1724.

Ultraviolet Spectrum. Aqueous acid—251 nm, 257 nm ($A_1^1 = 9.0$ a), 263 nm.

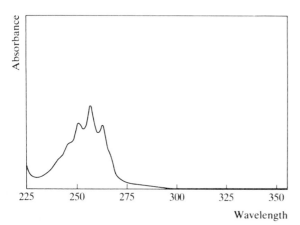

Infra-red Spectrum. Principal peaks at wavenumbers 1715, 1072, 700, 1603, 1110, 760 (KBr disk).

Mass Spectrum. Principal peaks at *m/z* 135, 57, 91, 77, 43, 119, 105, 180.

Dose. Hydroxyphenamate has been given in doses of 600 mg daily.

Hydroxyprogesterone   *Progestational Steroid*

17α-Hydroxypregn-4-ene-3,20-dione
$C_{21}H_{30}O_3 = 330.5$
CAS—68-96-2

A crystalline powder. M.p. 222° to 223° with rapid heating; with slow heating it undergoes molecular rearrangement accompanied by partial resolidification and melts at 276°.

Hydroxyprogesterone Hexanoate

Synonyms. 17 AHPC; Hydroxyprogesterone Caproate.
Proprietary Names. Delalutin; Hyproval PA; Proluton Depot; Relutin.
$C_{27}H_{40}O_4 = 428.6$
CAS—630-56-8
A white or creamy-white crystalline powder. M.p. 120° to 124°.
Practically **insoluble** in water; soluble 1 in 10 of ethanol, 1 in 0.4 of chloroform, and 1 in 10 of ether.

Colour Tests. Antimony Pentachloride—orange; Naphthol–Sulphuric Acid—orange-red/blue, violet dichroism; Sulphuric Acid—yellow (green fluorescence under ultraviolet light).

Thin-layer Chromatography. Hydroxyprogesterone hexanoate: *system TP*—Rf 81; *system TQ*—Rf 55; *system TR*—Rf 99; *system TS*—Rf 90. (*p-Toluenesulphonic acid solution*, positive.)

Ultraviolet Spectrum. Hydroxyprogesterone hexanoate: dehydrated alcohol—240 nm ($A_1^1 = 395$ a).

Infra-red Spectrum. Principal peaks at wavenumbers 1728, 1670, 1177, 1188, 1716, 1224 (hydroxyprogesterone hexanoate, KBr disk).

Dose. Usually 250 to 500 mg of hydroxyprogesterone hexanoate weekly, by intramuscular injection.

Hydroxyquinoline   *Antibacterial/Antifungal*

Synonyms. Oxine; Oxyquinoline; 8-Quinolinol.
Quinolin-8-ol
$C_9H_7NO = 145.2$
CAS—148-24-3

A white or faintly yellow crystalline powder. M.p. 76°.
Soluble 1 in 1500 of water; soluble in ethanol, acetone, and chloroform.

Hydroxyquinoline Sulphate

Synonyms. Chinosolum; Oxyquinol; Oxyquinoline Sulphate.
Proprietary Name. Sérorhinol
$(C_9H_7NO)_2,H_2SO_4 = 388.4$
CAS—134-31-6
A light yellow powder. M.p. about 178°.
Soluble 1 in 1 of water and 1 in 100 of ethanol; practically insoluble in chloroform and ether.

Potassium Hydroxyquinoline Sulphate

Synonyms. Oxyquinol Potassium; Potassium Oxyquinoline Sulphate.

Proprietary Names. It is an ingredient of Auralgicin, Quinoderm, and Quinoped.

An equimolecular mixture of potassium sulphate and quinolin-8-ol sulphate, containing the equivalent of 50% of quinolin-8-ol.

A pale yellow microcrystalline powder. It partly liquefies at 172° to 184°.

Soluble 1 in 2 of water; partly soluble in ethanol; practically insoluble in ether.

Dissociation Constant. pK_a 5.0, 9.9 (20°).

Colour Test. Ferric Chloride—green.

Thin-layer Chromatography. *System TA*—Rf 32, streaking. (*Acidified iodoplatinate solution*, positive.)

Ultraviolet Spectrum. Aqueous acid—251 nm ($A_1^1 = 3930$ a), 308 nm ($A_1^1 = 105$ a), 318 nm, 356 nm.

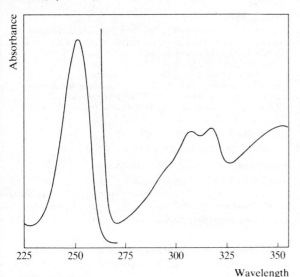

Infra-red Spectrum. Principal peaks at wavenumbers 1509, 779, 709, 1282, 1219, 1190.

Mass Spectrum. Principal peaks at m/z 145, 117, 122, 89, 105, 90, 63, 146.

Use. Potassium hydroxyquinoline sulphate is used topically in concentrations of 0.05 to 0.5%.

Hydroxystilbamidine   *Antifungal/Antiprotozoal*

Synonym. Oxistilbamidine

2-Hydroxystilbene-4,4'-dicarboxamidine

$C_{16}H_{16}N_4O = 280.3$

CAS—495-99-8

Yellow crystals. M.p. 235°.

Hydroxystilbamidine Isethionate

$C_{16}H_{16}N_4O,2C_2H_6O_4S = 532.6$

CAS—533-22-2

A fine, yellow, crystalline powder, which decomposes on exposure to light. M.p. about 280°.

Soluble in water; slightly soluble in ethanol; practically insoluble in ether.

Colour Tests. Folin–Ciocalteu Reagent—blue; Liebermann's Test—black; Mandelin's Test—blue-green.

Thin-layer Chromatography. *System TA*—Rf 01; *system TB*—Rf 00; *system TC*—Rf 00. (*Acidified iodoplatinate solution*, positive.)

Ultraviolet Spectrum. Aqueous acid—344 nm ($A_1^1 = 1093$ a); aqueous alkali—310 nm ($A_1^1 = 811$ b).

Infra-red Spectrum. Principal peaks at wavenumbers 1196, 1028, 1667, 1597, 742, 1053 (hydroxystilbamidine isethionate, KBr disk).

Mass Spectrum. Principal peaks at m/z 96, 44, 43, 31, 45, 27, 78, 264.

Dose. 225 or 250 mg of hydroxystilbamidine isethionate daily or on alternate days, by intravenous infusion.

Hydroxyurea   *Antineoplastic*

Synonym. Hydroxycarbamide

Proprietary Names. Hydrea; Litalir.

$HO \cdot NH \cdot CO \cdot NH_2 = 76.05$

CAS—127-07-1

A white crystalline powder. It is hygroscopic and decomposes in the presence of moisture. M.p. above 133°, with decomposition. Freely **soluble** in water and hot ethanol; slightly soluble in ethanol.

Ultraviolet Spectrum. No significant absorption, 230 to 360 nm.

Infra-red Spectrum. Principal peaks at wavenumbers 1639, 1592, 1111, 1492, 812, 758 (KBr disk).

Dose. 20 to 30 mg/kg daily or 80 mg/kg every third day, by mouth.

Hydroxyzine   *Antihistamine/Tranquilliser*

2-{2-[4-(4-Chlorobenzhydryl)piperazin-1-yl]ethoxy}ethanol

$C_{21}H_{27}ClN_2O_2 = 374.9$

CAS—68-88-2

Hydroxyzine Embonate

Synonym. Hydroxyzine Pamoate

Proprietary Names. Masmoran; Vistaril (capsules and oral suspension).

$C_{21}H_{27}ClN_2O_2,C_{23}H_{16}O_6 = 763.3$

CAS—10246-75-0

A pale yellow powder.

Practically **insoluble** in water, chloroform, ether, and methanol; soluble 1 in 700 of ethanol and 1 in 10 of dimethylformamide.

Hydroxyzine Hydrochloride

Proprietary Names. Atarax; Atazina; Sedaril; Vistaril (injection). It is an ingredient of Cartrax, Enarax, and Vistrax.

$C_{21}H_{27}ClN_2O_2,2HCl = 447.8$
CAS—2192-20-3
A white crystalline powder. M.p. about 200°, with decomposition.
Soluble 1 in 1 of water, 1 in 4.5 of ethanol, and 1 in 13 of chloroform; practically insoluble in ether.

Dissociation Constant. pK_a 2.1, 7.1.

Thin-layer Chromatography. *System TA*—Rf 68; *system TB*—Rf 09; *system TC*—Rf 54. (*Dragendorff spray*, positive; *acidified iodoplatinate solution*, positive; *Marquis reagent*, green.)

Gas Chromatography. *System GA*—RI 2849.

High Pressure Liquid Chromatography. *System HA*—k' 1.4.

Ultraviolet Spectrum. Aqueous acid—232 nm ($A_1^1 = 416$ a), 258 nm, 263 nm, 270 nm. No alkaline shift.

Infra-red Spectrum. Principal peaks at wavenumbers 1082, 1130, 1005, 1149, 1063, 800 (KBr disk).

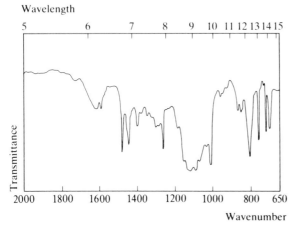

Mass Spectrum. Principal peaks at *m/z* 201, 203, 165, 45, 299, 166, 202, 56.

Quantification. GAS CHROMATOGRAPHY–MASS SPECTROMETRY. In plasma: sensitivity 2 ng/ml—H. G. Fouda *et al.*, *J. pharm. Sci.*, 1979, *68*, 1456–1458.

Disposition in the Body.

THERAPEUTIC CONCENTRATION.

Following a single oral dose of 100 mg of the hydrochloride given to 4 subjects, peak plasma concentrations of 0.074 to 0.089 µg/ml (mean 0.083) were attained in 2 to 4 hours (H. G. Fouda *et al.*, *ibid.*).

TOXICITY.

A plasma concentration of 102.7 µg/ml was reported 8.5 hours after the ingestion of about 500 mg of hydroxyzine by a 13-month-old child; the child recovered within 72 hours (B. E. Magera, *Pediatrics*, 1981, *67*, 280–283).

In a fatality due to hydroxyzine, the following postmortem tissue concentrations were reported: blood 39 µg/ml, brain 163 µg/g, bile 122 µg/ml, liver 414 µg/g, urine 19 µg/ml (G. R. Johnson, *J. analyt. Toxicol.*, 1982, *6*, 69–70).

HALF-LIFE. Plasma half-life, about 3 hours.

Dose. 75 to 400 mg of hydroxyzine hydrochloride daily.

Hyoscine   *Anticholinergic*

Synonym. Scopolamine
(−)-(1*S*,3*s*,5*R*,6*R*,7*S*)-6,7-Epoxytropan-3-yl (*S*)-tropate
$C_{17}H_{21}NO_4 = 303.4$
CAS—51-34-3

An alkaloid found in various solanaceous plants, particularly species of *Datura*, *Scopolia*, and *Duboisia*.
A viscous liquid which forms a crystalline monohydrate with a m.p. of 59°.
Soluble 1 in 10 of water; freely soluble in ethanol, chloroform, and ether.

Hyoscine Hydrobromide

Synonyms. Scopolamine Bromhydrate; Scopolamine Hydrobromide.
Proprietary Names. Joy-rides; Quick Kwells; Scopos; Sereen. It is an ingredient of Omnopon-Scopolamine.
$C_{17}H_{21}NO_4,HBr,3H_2O = 438.3$
CAS—114-49-8 (anhydrous); *6533-68-2* (trihydrate)
Colourless transparent crystals or white crystalline powder; slightly efflorescent in dry air. M.p. about 197°, with decomposition.
Soluble 1 in 3.5 of water and 1 in 30 of ethanol; practically insoluble in chloroform and ether.

Dissociation Constant. pK_a 7.6 (23°).

Partition Coefficient. Log *P* (octanol/pH 7.4), 1.2.

Colour Test. Liebermann's Test—red-orange.

Thin-layer Chromatography. *System TA*—Rf 01; *system TB*—Rf 06; *system TC*—Rf 39. (*Dragendorff spray*, positive; *acidified iodoplatinate solution*, positive; *Marquis reagent*, pink.)

Gas Chromatography. *System GA*—RI 2303; *system GF*—RI 2885.

High Pressure Liquid Chromatography. *System HA*—k' 1.1.

Ultraviolet Spectrum. Aqueous acid—251 nm, 257 nm ($A_1^1 = 6.3$ a), 263 nm.

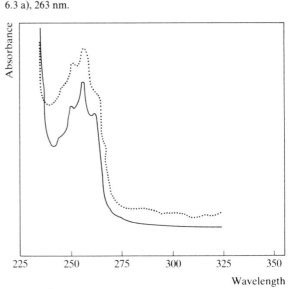

Infra-red Spectrum. Principal peaks at wavenumbers 1730, 853, 1166, 736, 705, 1047 (hyoscine hydrobromide, KBr disk).

Wavelength

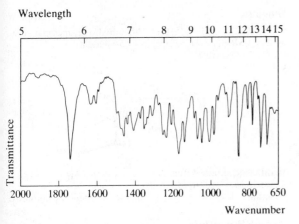

Wavelength

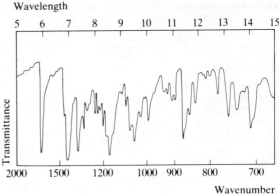

Mass Spectrum. Principal peaks at m/z 94, 138, 42, 108, 136, 41, 96, 97.

Quantification. GAS CHROMATOGRAPHY–MASS SPECTROMETRY. In plasma or urine: sensitivity 50 pg/ml—W. F. Bayne *et al.*, *J. pharm. Sci.*, 1975, **64**, 288–291.

Disposition in the Body. Readily absorbed after oral administration and extensively metabolised. About 5% of an oral dose is excreted in the urine as unchanged drug.

THERAPEUTIC CONCENTRATION.

Following a single oral dose equivalent to 415 μg of hyoscine to 10 subjects, a mean peak plasma concentration of 0.0003 μg/ml was attained in 0.5 to 1 hour, decreasing to 50% of the peak concentration in 2 to 4 hours (C. Muir and R. Metcalfe, *J. pharm. biomed. Analysis*, 1983, **1**, 363–367).

TOXICITY. The lethal dose in children may be as low as 10 mg but fatalities after hyoscine poisoning are rare.

PROTEIN BINDING. Bound to plasma proteins.

Dose. 0.6 to 2.4 mg of hyoscine hydrobromide daily.

Hyoscine Butylbromide   *Anticholinergic*

Synonyms. Butylscopolamonii Bromidum; Hyoscine-*N*-Butyl Bromide; Scopolamine Butylbromide.

Proprietary Name. Buscopan

(−) - (1*S*,3*s*,5*R*,6*R*,7*S*) - 8 - Butyl - 6,7 - epoxy - 3 - [(*S*) - tropoyl-oxy]tropanium bromide

$C_{21}H_{30}BrNO_4 = 440.4$

CAS—149-64-4

A white crystalline powder. M.p. 140° to 144°.

Soluble 1 in 1 of water, 1 in 50 of ethanol, and 1 in 5 of chloroform; practically insoluble in ether.

Colour Tests. Aromaticity (Method 2)—colourless/yellow; Liebermann's Test—orange.

Thin-layer Chromatography. *System TA*—Rf 08. (*Acidified iodoplatinate solution*, positive.)

Ultraviolet Spectrum. Aqueous acid—252 nm ($A_1^1 = 3.7$ a), 258 nm ($A_1^1 = 4.6$ a), 264 nm ($A_1^1 = 3.6$ a).

Infra-red Spectrum. Principal peaks at wavenumbers 1175, 1721, 1052, 874, 1072, 709 (Nujol mull).

Disposition in the Body. Poorly absorbed after oral administration. About 90% of an oral dose is eliminated in the faeces and less than 10% is excreted in the urine. After intravenous administration, about 40% of a dose is excreted in the urine.

HALF-LIFE. Plasma half-life, about 8 hours.

PROTEIN BINDING. In plasma, about 10%.

Dose. 20 mg given parenterally, repeated if necessary; 80 mg daily, by mouth.

Hyoscine Methobromide   *Anticholinergic*

Synonyms. Epoxymethamine Bromide; Hyoscine Methylbromide; Methoscopolamine Bromide; Scopolamine Methylbromide.

Proprietary Names. Holopon; Pamine.

(−) - (1*S*,3*s*,5*R*,6*R*,7*S*) - 6,7 - Epoxy - 8 - methyl - 3 - [(*S*) - tropoyl-oxy]tropanium bromide

$C_{18}H_{24}BrNO_4 = 398.3$

CAS—155-41-9

White crystals or crystalline powder. M.p. about 225°, with decomposition.

Soluble 1 in 3 of water, 1 in 100 of ethanol, and 1 in 40 of methanol; practically insoluble in chloroform.

Colour Test. Aromaticity (Method 2)—colourless/yellow.

Ultraviolet Spectrum. Aqueous acid—253 nm ($A_1^1 = 3.7$ b), 258 nm ($A_1^1 = 4.4$ a), 264 nm ($A_1^1 = 3.4$ b).

Infra-red Spectrum. Principal peaks at wavenumbers 1718, 1180, 1174, 1042, 923, 858 (KBr disk).

Dose. 10 to 12.5 mg daily.

Hyoscine Methonitrate   *Anticholinergic*

Synonyms. Hyoscine Methylnitrate; Methscopolamine Nitrate; Methylhyoscini Nitras; Methylscopolamini Nitras; Scopolamine Methylnitrate.

Proprietary Name. Skopyl

(−) - (1*S*,3*s*,5*R*,6*R*,7*S*) - 6,7 - Epoxy - 8 - methyl - 3 - [(*S*) - tropoyloxy]tropanium nitrate

$C_{18}H_{24}N_2O_7 = 380.4$

CAS—6106-46-3

Colourless hygroscopic crystals or a white crystalline powder. M.p. 194° to 199°.

Soluble 1 in 1.5 of water and 1 in 40 of ethanol; practically insoluble in chloroform and ether.

Colour Tests. Aromaticity (Method 2)—colourless/violet (transient); Liebermann's Test—orange.

Thin-layer Chromatography. *System TA*—Rf 02. (*Acidified iodoplatinate solution*, positive.)

Ultraviolet Spectrum. Aqueous acid—251 nm ($A_1^1 = 4.3$ a), 257 nm ($A_1^1 = 5.1$ a), 263 nm ($A_1^1 = 3.8$ a).

Infra-red Spectrum. Principal peaks at wavenumbers 1735, 1175, 1185, 1317, 860, 923 (KBr disk).

Dose. Up to 12 mg daily.

Hyoscyamine   *Anticholinergic*

Synonym. l-Hyoscyamine
Proprietary Name. Cystospaz
$(-)-(1R,3r,5S)$-Tropan-3-yl (S)-tropate
$C_{17}H_{23}NO_3 = 289.4$
CAS—101-31-5

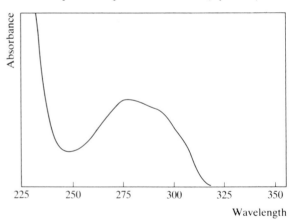

An alkaloid obtained from various solanaceous plants, *Hyoscyamus muticus* and *Duboisia myoporoides* being the best sources. It is the laevo-isomer of atropine.
A white crystalline powder. M.p. 106° to 109°.
Soluble 1 in 280 of water, 1 in 1 of chloroform, and 1 in 48 of ether; freely soluble in ethanol.

Hyoscyamine Hydrobromide
Synonym. Hyoscyamine Bromhydrate
Proprietary Name. It is an ingredient of Natirose.
$C_{17}H_{23}NO_3,HBr = 370.3$
CAS—306-03-6
White prismatic crystals or crystalline powder. M.p. about 149°.
Freely **soluble** in water; soluble 1 in 2.5 of ethanol and 1 in 1.7 of chloroform; very slightly soluble in ether.

Hyoscyamine Sulphate
Proprietary Names. Anaspaz; Cystospaz-M; Egacen(e); Egazil; Levsin; Levsinex; Peptard.
$(C_{17}H_{23}NO_3)_2,H_2SO_4,2H_2O = 712.9$
CAS—620-61-1 (anhydrous); *6835-16-1* (dihydrate)
Colourless needles or a white deliquescent crystalline powder. M.p. about 203°, with decomposition.
Soluble 1 in 0.5 of water and 1 in 5 of ethanol; sparingly soluble in dehydrated alcohol; practically insoluble in chloroform and ether.

Dissociation Constant. pK_a 9.7 (21°).

Colour Test. Liebermann's Test—red-orange.

Thin-layer Chromatography. *System TA*—Rf 18. (*Acidified iodoplatinate solution*, positive.)

Gas Chromatography. *System GA*—RI 2192.

High Pressure Liquid Chromatography. *System HA*—k' 3.7 (tailing peak).

Ultraviolet Spectrum. Aqueous acid—252 nm $(A_1^1 = 6.2$ a), 258 nm $(A_1^1 = 8.2$ a), 264 nm $(A_1^1 = 6.2$ a).

Infra-red Spectrum. Principal peaks at wavenumbers 1738, 1160, 1025, 1145, 1225, 1050 (hyoscyamine hydrobromide, KBr disk).

Quantification. See under Atropine.

Dose. 0.6 to 1.2 mg daily.

Ibogaine   *Alkaloid*

$(-)$-7-Ethyl-6,6a,7,8,9,10,12,13-octahydro-2-methoxy-6,9-methano-5H-pyrido[1,2-a]azepino[4,5-b]indole
$C_{20}H_{26}N_2O = 310.4$
CAS—83-74-9

An alkaloid obtained from *Tabernanthe iboga* (Apocynaceae).
Crystals. M.p. 152° to 153°.
Practically **insoluble** in water; soluble in ethanol, chloroform, and ether.

Ibogaine Hydrochloride
$C_{20}H_{26}N_2O,HCl = 346.9$
CAS—5934-55-4
Crystals. M.p. 299° to 300°, with decomposition.
Soluble in water, ethanol, and methanol; slightly soluble in chloroform; practically insoluble in ether.

Colour Tests. Liebermann's Test—black; Mandelin's Test—grey → violet; Marquis Test—grey → orange.

Thin-layer Chromatography. *System TA*—Rf 65; *system TB*—Rf 28; *system TC*—Rf 50. (*Acidified iodoplatinate solution*, positive.)

Gas Chromatography. *System GA*—RI 2872.

High Pressure Liquid Chromatography. *System HA*—k' 2.1.

Ultraviolet Spectrum. Aqueous acid—278 nm $(A_1^1 = 212$ c).

Infra-red Spectrum. Principal peaks at wavenumbers 1490, 1210, 1140, 810, 1020, 835 (ibogaine hydrochloride, KBr disk).

Mass Spectrum. Principal peaks at *m/z* 136, 310, 135, 225, 149, 122, 155, 311.

Quantification. GAS CHROMATOGRAPHY. In urine: detection limit 5 ng, AFID—G. P. Cartoni and A. Giarusso, *J. Chromat.*, 1972, *71*, 154–158.

Ibomal   *Barbiturate*

Synonyms. Bromoaprobarbitone; Isopropyl-bromallyl-barbitursäure; Propallylonal.
Proprietary Name. Noctal

5-(2-Bromoallyl)-5-isopropylbarbituric acid
$C_{10}H_{13}BrN_2O_3 = 289.1$
CAS—545-93-7

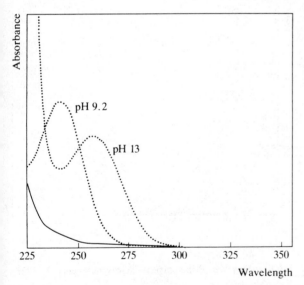

A white crystalline powder. M.p. 179° to 182°.
Very slightly **soluble** in water; soluble in ethanol; slightly soluble in ether.

Dissociation Constant. pK_a 7.7 (20°).

Colour Test. Koppanyi–Zwikker Test—violet.

Thin-layer Chromatography. *System TD*—Rf 50; *system TE*—Rf 31; *system TF*—Rf 67; *system TH*—Rf 61.

Gas Chromatography. *System GA*—ibomal RI 1883, 5-(2-acetonyl)-5-isopropylbarbituric acid RI 1770.

High Pressure Liquid Chromatography. *System HG*—k' 4.01; *system HH*—k' 2.58.

Ultraviolet Spectrum. *Borax buffer 0.05M* (pH 9.2)—240 nm ($A_1^1 = 307$ a); M sodium hydroxide (pH 13)—257 nm ($A_1^1 = 240$ b).

Infra-red Spectrum. Principal peaks at wavenumbers 1700, 1722, 1210, 1300, 830, 1622.

Mass Spectrum. Principal peaks at *m/z* 167, 209, 43, 124, 39, 41, 53, 140.

Disposition in the Body. Metabolised by side-chain oxidation to 5-(2-acetonyl)-5-isopropylbarbituric acid. About 6 to 16% of a dose is slowly excreted in the urine as the metabolite with about 1 to 3% as unchanged drug; the metabolite is still detectable in urine 9 days after a single dose.

THERAPEUTIC CONCENTRATION. In plasma, usually in the range 0.3 to 10 µg/ml.

TOXICITY. Blood concentrations greater than about 10 µg/ml may be toxic or lethal.

PROTEIN BINDING. In plasma, about 34%.

Dose. 100 to 400 mg, as a hypnotic.

Ibuprofen

Analgesic

Proprietary Names. Amersol; Apsifen; Brufen; Ebufac; Fenbid; Inabrin; Inflam; Librofem; Motrin; Nurofen; Paxofen; Proflex; Relcofen; Seclodin; Uniprofen.
2-(4-Isobutylphenyl)propionic acid
$C_{13}H_{18}O_2 = 206.3$
CAS—15687-27-1

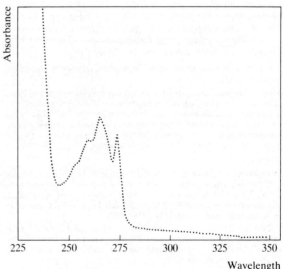

A white powder or crystals. M.p. 75° to 78°.
Practically **insoluble** in water; soluble 1 in 1.5 of ethanol, 1 in 1 of chloroform, and 1 in 2 of ether.

Dissociation Constant. pK_a 4.4, 5.2.

Colour Tests. Liebermann's Test—brown-orange; Marquis Test—brown (→ orange at 100°).

Thin-layer Chromatography. *System TD*—Rf 46; *system TE*—Rf 07; *system TF*—Rf 54; *system TG*—Rf 18.

Gas Chromatography. *System GA*—RI 1631; *system GD*—retention time of methyl derivative 0.89 relative to n-$C_{16}H_{34}$.

High Pressure Liquid Chromatography. *System HD*—k' 15.1.

Ultraviolet Spectrum. Aqueous alkali—265 nm ($A_1^1 = 18.5$ a), 273 nm.

Infra-red Spectrum. Principal peaks at wavenumbers 1721, 1232, 779, 1185, 1273, 870 (KBr disk). (See below)

Mass Spectrum. Principal peaks at *m/z* 163, 161, 119, 91, 206, 117, 107, 164.

Wavelength

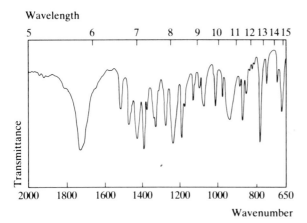

Transmittance

Wavenumber

Quantification. GAS CHROMATOGRAPHY. In serum: sensitivity 500 ng/ml, FID—D. J. Hoffman, *J. pharm. Sci.*, 1977, *66*, 749–750. In serum: sensitivity 100 ng/ml, ECD—D. G. Kaiser and R. S. Martin, *J. pharm. Sci.*, 1978, *67*, 627–630.

GAS CHROMATOGRAPHY–MASS SPECTROMETRY. In biological fluids: sensitivity 1 ng—J. B. Whitlam and J. H. Vine, *J. Chromat.*, 1980, *181*; *Biomed. Appl.*, *7*, 463–468.

HIGH PRESSURE LIQUID CHROMATOGRAPHY. In biological fluids: sensitivity, 1 µg/ml for ibuprofen in plasma, 5 µg/ml for ibuprofen or the hydroxy or carboxy metabolites in urine, UV detection—G. F. Lockwood and J. G. Wagner, *J. Chromat.*, 1982, *232*; *Biomed. Appl.*, *21*, 335–343.

Disposition in the Body. Readily and almost completely absorbed after oral administration. More than 60% of a dose is excreted in the urine in 24 hours, including about 9% of the dose as the 2-hydroxy metabolite, 2-[4-(2-hydroxy-2-methylpropyl)phenyl]-propionic acid, about 17% as the conjugated hydroxy metabolite, about 16% as the 2-carboxy metabolite, 2-[4-(carboxypropyl)phenyl]propionic acid, and about 19% as the conjugated carboxy metabolite (both metabolites are inactive); less than 10% of a dose is excreted unchanged. The remainder of the dose is probably eliminated in the faeces after excretion in the bile; excretion is virtually complete within 24 hours.

THERAPEUTIC CONCENTRATION. In plasma, usually in the range 20 to 30 µg/ml.

After a single oral dose of 200 mg to 2 subjects, peak plasma concentrations of 18 and 24 µg/ml of ibuprofen were attained in 1.5 hours; peak plasma concentrations of the hydroxy and carboxy metabolites of 0.6 and 1 µg/ml, and 1.7 and 2.1 µg/ml, respectively, were attained in 3 hours; plasma concentrations after oral doses of 200 mg three times daily for 14 days were of the same order (R. Mills *et al.*, *Xenobiotica*, 1973, *3*, 589–598).

TOXICITY.

In an attempted suicide involving the ingestion of 12 g of ibuprofen, an initial serum concentration of 840 µg/ml was reported; this declined to 220 µg/ml at 3 hours; chlorpheniramine was also detected in the urine. The subject was comatose but recovered within 24 hours (D. P. Hunt and R. J. Leigh, *Br. med. J.*, 1980, *281*, 1458–1459).

In 2 overdoses due to ibuprofen, plasma concentrations of 400 and 711 µg/ml were reported about 1.5 hours after ingestion. In the first case, the estimated dose was 14 to 16 g; both subjects recovered (H. Court *et al.*, *Br. med. J.*, 1981, *282*, 1073).

HALF-LIFE. Plasma half-life, about 2 hours.

VOLUME OF DISTRIBUTION. About 0.1 litre/kg.

PROTEIN BINDING. In plasma, about 99%.

Dose. 0.6 to 2.4 g daily.

Idobutal
Barbiturate

Synonym. n-Butylallylbarbituric Acid
5-Allyl-5-butylbarbituric acid
$C_{11}H_{16}N_2O_3 = 224.3$
CAS—3146-66-5

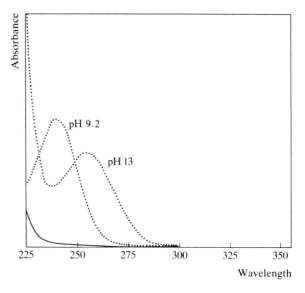

$CH_3 \cdot [CH_2]_2 \cdot CH_2$
$CH_2:CH \cdot CH_2$

Crystals. M.p. 128°.
Slightly **soluble** in water; freely soluble in ethanol and ether.

Thin-layer Chromatography. *System TD*—Rf 55; *system TE*—Rf 41; *system TF*—Rf 69; *system TH*—Rf 71.

Gas Chromatography. *System GA*—RI 1698.

High Pressure Liquid Chromatography. *System HG*—k′ 8.12; *system HH*—k′ 4.77.

Ultraviolet Spectrum. *Borax buffer 0.05M* (pH 9.2)—239 nm ($A_1^1 = 434$ b); M sodium hydroxide (pH 13)—254 nm ($A_1^1 = 328$ b).

pH 9.2

pH 13

Wavelength

Infra-red Spectrum. Principal peaks at wavenumbers 1696, 1728, 1755, 835, 1290, 1207.

Mass Spectrum. Principal peaks at *m/z* 167, 41, 168, 124, 39, 97, 141, 67.

Idoxuridine
Antiviral

Synonyms. IDU; 5 IDUR.
Proprietary Names. Herplex; Idoxene; Iduviran; Kerecid; Ophthalmadine; Stoxil. It is an ingredient of Herpid and Iduridin.
2′-Deoxy-5-iodouridine
$C_9H_{11}IN_2O_5 = 354.1$
CAS—54-42-2

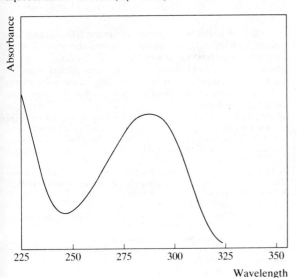

Colourless crystals or a white crystalline powder. It decomposes on heating with the liberation of iodine vapour.

Soluble 1 in 500 of water, 1 in 400 of ethanol, and 1 in 230 of methanol; practically insoluble in chloroform and ether.

Dissociation Constant. pK$_a$ 8.3.

Colour Test. Iodine Test—positive.

Ultraviolet Spectrum. Aqueous acid—288 nm (A$_1^1$ = 220 a); aqueous alkali—279 nm (A$_1^1$ = 162 a).

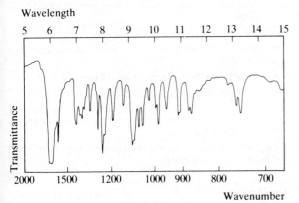

Infra-red Spectrum. Principal peaks at wavenumbers 1667, 1259, 1096, 1605, 1289, 1070 (KBr disk).

Use. Solutions of idoxuridine in dimethyl sulphoxide are used topically in concentrations of 5 to 40%.

Imipramine

Antidepressant

3-(10,11-Dihydro-5H-dibenz[b,f]azepin-5-yl)-NN-dimethyl-propylamine
C$_{19}$H$_{24}$N$_2$ = 280.4
CAS—50-49-7

Imipramine structure with CH$_2$·[CH$_2$]$_2$·N(CH$_3$)$_2$

Imipramine Embonate

Synonym. Imipramine Pamoate
Proprietary Name. Tofranil-PM
(C$_{19}$H$_{24}$N$_2$)$_2$,C$_{23}$H$_{16}$O$_6$ = 949.2
CAS—10075-24-8
A yellow powder.
Practically **insoluble** in water; soluble in ethanol, chloroform, and ether.

Imipramine Hydrochloride

Synonym. Imizine
Proprietary Names. Antipress; Berkomine; Imavate; Impril; Iramil; Janimine; Praminil; Presamine; Tofranil; W.D.D.
C$_{19}$H$_{24}$N$_2$,HCl = 316.9
CAS—113-52-0
A white or slightly yellow crystalline powder. M.p. 170° to 174°.
Soluble 1 in 2 of water, 1 in 1.5 of ethanol, and 1 in 1.5 of chloroform; practically insoluble in ether.

Dissociation Constant. pK$_a$ 9.5 (24°).

Partition Coefficient. Log *P* (octanol/pH 7.4), 2.5.

Colour Tests. Forrest Reagent—blue; FPN Reagent—blue; Liebermann's Test—blue; Mandelin's Test—blue (add water).

Thin-layer Chromatography. *System TA*—Rf 48; *system TB*—Rf 49; *system TC*—Rf 23. (*Dragendorff spray*, positive; *FPN reagent*, blue; *acidified iodoplatinate solution*, positive; *Marquis reagent*, blue.)

Gas Chromatography. *System GA*—imipramine RI 2223, desipramine RI 2242, 2-hydroxyimipramine RI 2540; *system GF*—RI 2540.

High Pressure Liquid Chromatography. *System HA*—imipramine k' 4.2, desipramine k' 2.1, 2-hydroxydesipramine k' 1.2, 2-hydroxyimipramine k' 3.1; *system HF*—imipramine k' 4.17, desipramine k' 3.60.

Ultraviolet Spectrum. Aqueous acid—251 nm (A$_1^1$ = 298 a); aqueous alkali—252 nm. (See below)

Infra-red Spectrum. Principal peaks at wavenumbers 740, 747, 765, 1230, 1110, 756 (imipramine hydrochloride, KBr disk). (See below)

Mass Spectrum. Principal peaks at *m/z* 58, 235, 85, 234, 236, 195, 193, 208; desipramine 235, 195, 208, 44, 234, 193, 194, 71; 2-hydroxyimipramine 58, 251, 250, 211, 85, 42, 209, 296; 2-hydroxydesipramine 44, 209, 211, 250, 210, 224, 42, 251.

Quantification. GAS CHROMATOGRAPHY. In plasma: imipramine and desipramine, detection limit 10 ng/ml, AFID—S. Dawling and R. A. Braithwaite, *J. Chromat.*, 1978, *146*; *Biomed. Appl.*, 3, 449–456.

GAS CHROMATOGRAPHY-MASS SPECTROMETRY. In serum or plasma: imipramine and desipramine, sensitivity 4 ng/ml—D. Alkalay *et al.*, *Biomed. Mass Spectrom.*, 1979, 6, 200–204.

HIGH PRESSURE LIQUID CHROMATOGRAPHY. In plasma: imipramine, desipramine and the 2-hydroxy metabolites, sensitivity

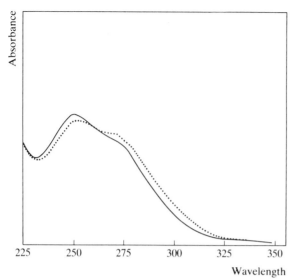

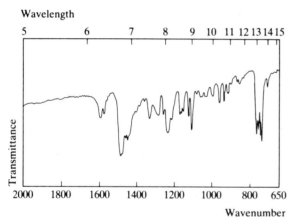

small amounts of didesmethylimipramine, free iminodibenzyl, and 10-hydroxydesipramine are also found. The excretion of unchanged drug and unconjugated metabolites is pH-dependent and is increased in acid urine. About 20% of a dose is eliminated in the faeces.

THERAPEUTIC CONCENTRATION. Plasma concentrations vary considerably between individual subjects; therapeutic effect has been correlated with plasma concentrations of imipramine plus desipramine greater than 0.1 μg/ml.

Following a single oral dose of 50 mg to 8 subjects, peak plasma concentrations of 0.010 to 0.083 μg/ml (mean 0.03) of imipramine and 0.004 to 0.014 μg/ml (mean 0.008) of desipramine were attained in about 3.4 hours, and 4.8 hours respectively (N. Sistovaris *et al., J. Chromat.,* 1983, *277*; *Biomed. Appl., 28,* 273–281).

After daily oral doses of 50 to 300 mg (mean 100) to 24 subjects, the following steady-state plasma concentrations were reported: imipramine 0.01 to 0.11 μg/ml (mean 0.05), desipramine 0.02 to 0.33 μg/ml (mean 0.09), 2-hydroxyimipramine 0 to 0.02 μg/ml (mean 0.01), 2-hydroxydesipramine 0 to 0.06 μg/ml (mean 0.03), didesmethylimipramine 0 to 0.04 μg/ml (mean 0.007) (L. F. Gram *et al., Clin. Pharmac. Ther.,* 1983, *33,* 335–342).

TOXICITY. In adults the estimated minimum lethal dose is 1 g, although fatalities have occurred with less and patients have survived the ingestion of as much as 5 g. In children, as little as 350 mg may be fatal. Blood concentrations greater than 0.5 μg/ml (imipramine and desipramine) may cause toxic effects and imipramine concentrations of 0.8 to **4.5** to 13 μg/ml have been associated with fatalities.

In 5 fatalities attributed to overdosage with imipramine, the following postmortem concentrations were found: blood 0.3 to 4.1 μg/ml (mean 2.7), bile 19.2 to 71.7 μg/ml (mean 46, 4 cases), liver blood 0.2 to 9.6 μg/ml (mean 4.6), urine 0.8 to 12.7 μg/ml (mean 5.3, 3 cases) (A. E. Robinson *et al., J. analyt. Toxicol.,* 1979, *3,* 3–13).

A 49-year-old female was found dead after having ingested 33 tablets equivalent to 925 mg of imipramine; blood and tissue concentrations were as follows: blood 14 μg/ml, bile 88 μg/ml, brain 25 μg/g, liver 75 μg/g (K. D. Singh *et al., Bull. int. Ass. forens. Toxicol.,* 1978, *14*(2), 21).

In 2 fatalities due to imipramine overdose, the following postmortem tissue concentrations were reported (μg/ml or μg/g):

	Imipramine	Desipramine
Blood	10, 3	3, trace
Kidney	9, —	6, —
Liver	16, 46	10, 13
Urine	—, 64	—, 13

(A. E. Hodda, *Bull. int. Ass. forens. Toxicol.,* 1974, *10*(3), 8–9).

HALF-LIFE. Plasma half-life, imipramine 8 to 20 hours, increased in children, elderly subjects, and after overdose; desipramine 10 to 35 hours.

VOLUME OF DISTRIBUTION. 10 to 20 litres/kg.

CLEARANCE. Plasma clearance, about 15 ml/min/kg, decreased in elderly subjects.

DISTRIBUTION IN BLOOD. Plasma: whole blood ratio, 0.98.

PROTEIN BINDING. In plasma, 85 to 95%.

NOTE. For a review of the pharmacokinetics of tricyclic antidepressants see G. Molnar and R. N. Gupta, *Biopharm. Drug Disp.,* 1980, *1,* 283–305.

Dose. 30 to 200 mg of imipramine hydrochloride daily; up to 300 mg daily has been given.

5 ng/ml, electrochemical detection—R. F. Suckow and T. B. Cooper, *J. pharm. Sci.,* 1981, *70,* 257–261. In plasma or serum: imipramine and desipramine, sensitivity 5 ng/ml, UV detection—P. M. Kabra *et al., Clinica chim. Acta,* 1981, *111,* 123–132.

REVIEW. Comparison of GC, GC–MS and RIA methods— K. K. Midha *et al., J. analyt. Toxicol.,* 1980, *4,* 237–243.

Disposition in the Body. Readily absorbed after oral administration and widely distributed throughout the tissues; bioavailability about 50%, but there is considerable intersubject variation. Imipramine undergoes considerable first-pass metabolism, mainly by demethylation to the primary active metabolite desipramine. Other major metabolic reactions include hydroxylation at the 2- or 10-positions followed by conjugation. The extent of 2-hydroxylation appears to be genetically determined. 2-Hydroxyimipramine and 2-hydroxydesipramine appear to be active. A large number of metabolites have been identified in the urine and less than 10% of a dose is excreted unchanged. A total of about 40% of a dose is excreted in the urine in 24 hours and about 70% in 72 hours. Of the urinary material, up to 40% consists of free and conjugated 2-hydroxydesipramine, up to about 25% is free and conjugated 2-hydroxyimipramine, and about 15% is free and conjugated 2-hydroxyiminodibenzyl;

Imolamine   *Anti-anginal Vasodilator*

2-(5-Imino-3-phenyl-1,2,4-oxadiazolin-4-yl)triethylamine
$C_{14}H_{20}N_4O = 260.3$
CAS—318-23-0

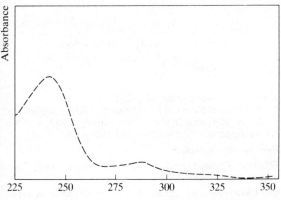

Imolamine Hydrochloride

Proprietary Name. Irrigor
$C_{14}H_{20}N_4O,HCl = 296.8$
CAS—15823-89-9
A white powder. M.p. 154° to 155°.
Soluble 1 in 1 of water and 1 in 500 of ethanol; slightly soluble in chloroform.

Thin-layer Chromatography. *System TA*—Rf 56. (*Acidified iodoplatinate solution*, positive.)

Gas Chromatography. *System GA*—RI 2177.

Infra-red Spectrum. Principal peaks at wavenumbers 1638, 698, 752, 1610, 1500, 1070 (KBr disk).

Dose. Imolamine hydrochloride has been given in doses of 30 to 90 mg daily.

Indapamide   *Diuretic*

Proprietary Names. Fludex; Lozol; Natrilix.
4-Chloro-*N*-(2-methylindolin-1-yl)-3-sulphamoylbenzamide hemihydrate
$C_{16}H_{16}ClN_3O_3S,\frac{1}{2}H_2O = 374.8$
CAS—26807-65-8 (anhydrous)

Colour Tests. Koppanyi–Zwikker Test—violet; Liebermann's Test—violet-red; Mandelin's Test—red; Marquis Test—orange → violet; Mercurous Nitrate—black; Sulphuric Acid—pink (slow).

Thin-layer Chromatography. *System TD*—Rf 38; *system TE*—Rf 67; *system TF*—Rf 61.

High Pressure Liquid Chromatography. *System HA*—k' 0.1.

Ultraviolet Spectrum. Ethanol—242 nm ($A_1^1 = 627$ b), 288 nm.

Mass Spectrum. Principal peaks at m/z 147, 131, 130, 132, 119, 148, 365, 218.

Quantification. HIGH PRESSURE LIQUID CHROMATOGRAPHY. In blood, plasma or urine: sensitivity 25 ng/ml in plasma, 50 ng/ml in blood and urine, UV detection—R. L. Choi *et al.*, *J. Chromat.*, 1982, *230*; *Biomed. Appl.*, *19*, 181–187. In urine: indapamide and 4-chloro-3-sulphamoylbenzoic acid, sensitivity 25 ng/ml, UV detection—P. Pietta *et al.*, *J. Chromat.*, 1982, *228*; *Biomed. Appl.*, *17*, 377–381.

Disposition in the Body. Rapidly absorbed after oral administration. It is extensively metabolised and about 60% of a dose is slowly excreted in the urine over a period of 8 days with less than 5% as unchanged drug. About 20% of a dose is slowly eliminated in the faeces.

THERAPEUTIC CONCENTRATION.

Following a single oral dose of 5 mg to 22 subjects, a mean peak plasma concentration of 0.26 µg/ml was attained in about 2 to 3 hours (P. E. Grebow *et al.*, *Eur. J. clin. Pharmac.*, 1982, *22*, 295–299).

Following daily oral doses of 2.5 mg to 6 subjects, steady-state plasma concentrations of 0.02 to 0.05 µg/ml (mean 0.03) were attained in 3 days (D. B. Campbell *et al.*, *Curr. med. Res. Opinion*, 1977, *5*, Suppl. 1, 13–24).

HALF-LIFE. Plasma half-life, about 15 hours.

PROTEIN BINDING. In plasma, about 80%.

NOTE. For a review of indapamide see M. Chaffman *et al.*, *Drugs*, 1984, *28*, 189–235.

Dose. 2.5 to 5 mg daily.

Indomethacin   *Analgesic*

Proprietary Names. Amuno; Artracin; Confortid; Imbrilon; Indocid; Indocin; Indoflex; Indolar; Mobilan; Rheumacin.
[1-(4-Chlorobenzoyl)-5-methoxy-2-methylindol-3-yl]acetic acid
$C_{19}H_{16}ClNO_4 = 357.8$
CAS—53-86-1

A white to yellow-tan, crystalline powder. M.p. about 158° to 162°. It exhibits **polymorphism**.
Practically **insoluble** in water; soluble 1 in 50 of ethanol, 1 in 30 of chloroform, and 1 in about 40 of ether; soluble in acetone.

Dissociation Constant. pK_a 4.5.

Partition Coefficient. Log P (octanol/pH 7.4), -1.0.

Colour Tests. Liebermann's Test—black; Mandelin's Test—grey; Marquis Test—orange; Sulphuric Acid—orange.

Thin-layer Chromatography. *System TD*—Rf 16; *system TE*—Rf 06; *system TF*—Rf 20; *system TG*—Rf 20. (*Chromic acid solution*, grey-brown; *acidified potassium permanganate solution*, positive.)

Gas Chromatography. *System GA*—RI 2685; *system GD*—retention times of methyl derivative 1.55 and 0.49 relative to n-$C_{16}H_{34}$.

High Pressure Liquid Chromatography. *System HD*—k' 6.95; *system HV*—retention time 0.87 relative to meclofenamic acid.

Ultraviolet Spectrum. Methanolic acid—318 nm ($A_1^1 = 180$ a); aqueous alkali—230 nm, 279 nm ($A_1^1 = 213$ a). (See below)

Absorbance

225   250   275   300   325   350

Wavelength

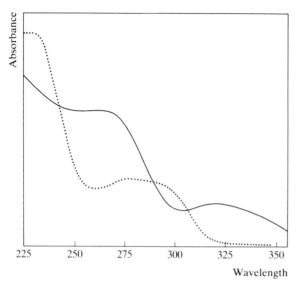

Infra-red Spectrum. Principal peaks at wavenumbers 1681, 1228, 1218, 1706, 1299, 1065 (KBr disk).

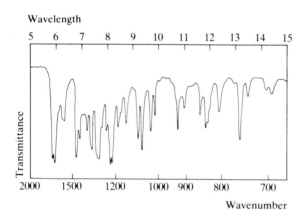

Mass Spectrum. Principal peaks at m/z 139, 141, 357, 111, 359, 140, 113, 75.

Quantification. GAS CHROMATOGRAPHY. In plasma or urine: indomethacin and desmethylindomethacin, sensitivity 10 ng/ml, ECD—P. Guissou et al., J. Chromat., 1983, 277; Biomed. Appl., 28, 368–373.

HIGH PRESSURE LIQUID CHROMATOGRAPHY. In plasma or urine: indomethacin and desmethylindomethacin, sensitivity 25 ng/ml for indomethacin in plasma, fluorescence detection—M. S. Bernstein and M. A. Evans, J. Chromat., 1982, 229; Biomed. Appl., 18, 179–187.

THIN-LAYER CHROMATOGRAPHY. In plasma or urine: sensitivity 30 ng/ml—I. Soendergaard and E. Steiness, J. Chromat., 1979, 162; Biomed. Appl., 4, 485–488.

RADIOIMMUNOASSAY. In plasma or urine: sensitivity 50 ng/ml— L. E. Hare et al., J. pharm. Sci., 1977, 66, 486–489.

Disposition in the Body. Readily and almost completely absorbed after oral administration. Indomethacin is subject to considerable enterohepatic circulation. Metabolic reactions include O-demethylation, N-deacetylation, and glucuronic acid conjugation, the major metabolites being desmethylindomethacin (DMI), deschlorobenzoylindomethacin (DBI), and desmethyl-deschlorobenzoylindomethacin (DMBI) and their glucuronides. These substances, together with unchanged indomethacin and its glucuronide, are excreted in both the urine (up to about 60% of the dose in 48 hours) and in the faeces (up to about 30% of the dose in 96 hours) in variable amounts. Expressed as a percentage of the dose, the average amounts excreted in the urine in 48 hours are: unchanged indomethacin 5 to 20% (dependent on urinary pH), indomethacin glucuronide 6 to 26%, DMI and its glucuronide 8 to 23%, DBI and its glucuronide 4 to 20%, DMBI and its glucuronide less than 3%; in the faeces the major metabolites found are DMBI (up to about 16%) and DMI (up to about 12%), with only small amounts of unchanged indomethacin and DBI.

THERAPEUTIC CONCENTRATION. In plasma, usually in the range 0.5 to 3 µg/ml.

After a single oral dose of 50 mg given to 20 subjects, peak plasma concentrations of 1.0 to 3.0 µg/ml (mean 1.9) were attained in 1 to 4 hours (K. C. Kwan et al., J. Pharmacokinet. Biopharm., 1976, 4, 255–280). Steady-state plasma concentrations of 0.31 to 0.63 µg/ml (mean 0.49) were attained in about 6 days after oral doses of 25 mg three times a day to 5 subjects (G. Alván et al., Clin. Pharmac. Ther., 1975, 18, 364–373).

TOXICITY. Toxic effects may be produced by plasma concentrations greater than 5 µg/ml.

HALF-LIFE. Plasma half-life, 3 to 15 hours.

VOLUME OF DISTRIBUTION. About 1 litre/kg.

CLEARANCE. Plasma clearance, 1 to 2 ml/min/kg.

DISTRIBUTION IN BLOOD. Plasma: whole blood ratio, 1.9.

PROTEIN BINDING. In plasma, 90 to 99%.

NOTE. For a review of the pharmacokinetics of indomethacin see L. Helleberg, Clin. Pharmacokinet., 1981, 6, 245–258.

Dose. 50 to 200 mg daily.

Indoprofen   *Analgesic*

Synonym. Isindone
Proprietary Name. Flosint
2-[4-(1-Oxoisoindolin-2-yl)phenyl]propionic acid
$C_{17}H_{15}NO_3 = 281.3$
CAS—31842-01-0

A white crystalline powder. M.p. 212°.
Practically **insoluble** in water; very slightly soluble in chloroform; freely soluble in dimethylformamide; slightly soluble in methanol; sparingly soluble in 0.1M sodium hydroxide.

Dissociation Constant. pK_a 5.8.

Thin-layer Chromatography. *System TG*—Rf 08. (*Ludy Tenger reagent*, brown-black.)

Gas Chromatography. *System GD*—retention times of methyl derivative 2.27 and 2.07 relative to n-$C_{16}H_{34}$.

High Pressure Liquid Chromatography. *System HD*—k' 1.2; *system HV*—retention time 0.52 relative to meclofenamic acid.

Ultraviolet Spectrum. Methanol—282 nm ($A_1^1 = 505$ a).

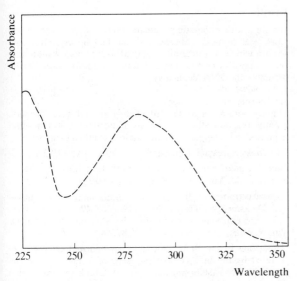

Infra-red Spectrum. Principal peaks at wavenumbers 1680, 1510, 730, 1300, 1220, 1605 (KBr disk).

Quantification. GAS CHROMATOGRAPHY. In plasma: sensitivity 400 ng/ml, FID—R. V. Smith *et al.*, *J. pharm. Sci.*, 1977, *66*, 132–134.

HIGH PRESSURE LIQUID CHROMATOGRAPHY. In plasma or urine: sensitivity 500 ng/ml, UV detection—K. Lanbeck *et al.*, *J. Chromat.*, 1980, *182*; *Biomed. Appl.*, 8, 262–266.

Disposition in the Body. Rapidly and almost completely absorbed after oral administration. About 80 to 90% of a dose is excreted in the urine in 24 hours as the glucuronide conjugate together with small amounts of unchanged drug and metabolites.

THERAPEUTIC CONCENTRATION.
After a single oral dose of 100 mg given to 4 subjects, peak plasma concentrations of 6.9 to 14.3 μg/ml were attained in 1 to 1.5 hours; following a single oral dose of 200 mg, peak plasma concentrations of 14.2 to 26.1 μg/ml were reported at 0.5 to 2 hours (V. Tamassia *et al.*, *Eur. J. clin. Pharmac.*, 1976, *10*, 257–262).

TOXICITY. Indoprofen was suspended from use in the United Kingdom in December 1983 because of reports of side-effects and fatalities.

HALF-LIFE. Plasma half-life, about 2 hours.

VOLUME OF DISTRIBUTION. About 0.1 litre/kg.

CLEARANCE. Plasma clearance, about 0.7 ml/min/kg.

PROTEIN BINDING. In plasma, about 99%.

Dose. Indoprofen has been given in doses of 200 to 800 mg daily.

Indoramin   *Antihypertensive*

N-[1-(2-Indol-3-ylethyl)-4-piperidyl]benzamide
$C_{22}H_{25}N_3O = 347.5$
CAS—26844-12-2

Indoramin Hydrochloride
Proprietary Name. Baratol
$C_{22}H_{25}N_3O,HCl = 383.9$
CAS—33124-53-7 (*x*HCl)
Crystals. M.p. 250° to 253°.
Slightly **soluble** in water and chloroform; sparingly soluble in ethanol; soluble in methanol.

Dissociation Constant. pK$_a$ 7.7.

Ultraviolet Spectrum. Ethanol—273 nm ($A_1^1 = 187$ b), 279 nm ($A_1^1 = 190$ b), 289 nm ($A_1^1 = 159$ b).

Infra-red Spectrum. Two major polymorphic forms exist. Principal peaks at wavenumbers 1640, 1535, 1316, 745, 1575, 715 (indoramin hydrochloride form I, Nujol mull); 1620, 1630, 1540, 1560, 740, 1317 (indoramin hydrochloride form II, Nujol mull).

Quantification. HIGH PRESSURE LIQUID CHROMATOGRAPHY. In plasma: sensitivity 1 ng/ml, fluorescence detection—A. J. Swaisland, *Analyst, Lond.*, 1981, *106*, 717–719.

Disposition in the Body. Readily absorbed after oral administration, but undergoes extensive first-pass metabolism to active metabolites. About 35% of a dose is excreted in the urine in 5 days, mainly as metabolites; less than 10% of a dose is excreted in the urine as unchanged drug; about 47% of a dose is eliminated in the faeces, mainly as metabolites. 6-hydroxyindoramin has been identified as a major metabolite. Other metabolites include acid-labile conjugates of indoramin and 6-hydroxyindoramin.

THERAPEUTIC CONCENTRATION.
Following a single oral dose of 50 mg to 6 middle-aged female subjects, peak plasma concentrations of 0.004 to 0.090 μg/ml (mean 0.02) were attained in about 3 hours. After the same dose given to 5 elderly female subjects, peak plasma concentrations of 0.011 to 0.090 μg/ml (mean 0.04) were attained after about 4 hours (H. M. Norbury *et al.*, *Eur. J. clin. Pharmac.*, 1984, *27*, 247–249).
Following daily oral doses of 150 mg given to 5 subjects, steady-state plasma concentrations of 0.08 to 0.22 μg/ml (mean 0.13) were reported (G. H. Draffan *et al.*, *Br. J. clin. Pharmac.*, 1976, *3*, 489–495).

TOXICITY.
In a fatality attributed to indoramin overdose, an antemortem plasma concentration of 6.4 μg/ml was reported together with an alcohol concentration of 2250 μg/ml (R. Hunter, *Br. med. J.*, 1982, *285*, 1011).

HALF-LIFE. Plasma half-life, 2 to 8 hours (mean 5), increased in elderly subjects.

VOLUME OF DISTRIBUTION. About 7 litres/kg.

CLEARANCE. Plasma clearance, about 20 ml/min/kg.

PROTEIN BINDING. In plasma, about 70 to 90% (concentration-dependent).

Dose. The equivalent of 50 to 200 mg of indoramin daily.

Inositol Nicotinate   *Vasodilator*

Synonyms. Hexanicotinoyl Inositol; Inositol Niacinate.
Proprietary Names. Dilcit; Dilexpal; Hexanicit; Hexopal; Linodil; Palohex; Vasodil.
meso-Inositol hexanicotinate
$C_{42}H_{30}N_6O_{12} = 810.7$
CAS—6556-11-2

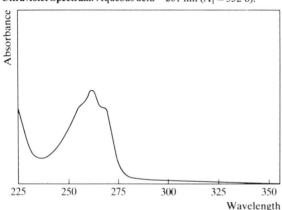

A white crystalline powder. M.p. about 255°.

Practically **insoluble** in water and most organic solvents; soluble 1 in 100 of chloroform; soluble in dilute acids.

Thin-layer Chromatography. *System TA*—Rf 57; *system TB*—Rf 01; *system TC*—Rf 43. (*Acidified iodoplatinate solution*, positive.)

Ultraviolet Spectrum. Aqueous acid—261 nm ($A_1^1 = 352$ b).

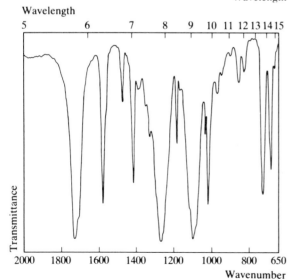

Infra-red Spectrum. Principal peaks at wavenumbers 1272, 1734, 1102, 1593, 1025, 718 (KBr disk).

Dose. 1.5 to 4 g daily.

Insulin   *Antidiabetic*

Insulin is an amphoteric pancreatic protein which is extracted from beef or pork pancreas and purified by crystallisation. Insulin which is structurally identical with human insulin may be produced by chemical manipulation of animal insulin or by recombinant DNA technology.

CAS—9004-10-8

A white crystalline powder.

Slightly **soluble** in water; practically insoluble in ethanol, chloroform, and ether; soluble in dilute solutions of mineral acids and, with degradation, in solutions of alkali hydroxides.

Ultraviolet Spectrum. Aqueous acid—276 nm ($A_1^1 = 10.3$ a).

Quantification. ENZYME IMMUNOASSAY. In serum: sensitivity 5 μU/ml—M. Yoshioka *et al.*, *Clin. Chem.*, 1979, *25*, 35–38.

RADIOIMMUNOASSAY. In serum, subcutaneous fat, or tissues— S. J. Dickson *et al.*, *Forens. Sci.*, 1977, *9*, 37–42. In serum: free, total, and antibody-bound insulin—W. D. Gennaro and J. D. Van Norman, *Clin. Chem.*, 1975, *21*, 873–879.

Disposition in the Body. Insulin is an endogenous hormone secreted by the beta cells of the islets of Langerhans in the pancreas; it consists of two linked polypeptide chains. Ineffective after oral administration due to rapid inactivation by proteolytic enzymes, but well absorbed after subcutaneous or intramuscular injection. It circulates in the blood as a polymer with a molecular weight of 17 000 to 43 000 and is rapidly taken up by the tissues. About 50% of endogenous insulin in the portal vein is metabolised in a single passage through the liver. It is reduced to two separate chains by glutathione insulin transhydrogenase. The intact molecule or reduced chains may be metabolised by insulin-specific protease to peptides and amino acids. Insulin is filtered at the glomeruli but is reabsorbed and metabolised in the renal tubules, and only small amounts are excreted unchanged in the urine. It is also excreted in the bile.

THERAPEUTIC CONCENTRATION. In normal subjects, endogenous blood-insulin concentrations vary throughout the day. The fasting or basal concentration in the plasma is usually in the range of 5 to 40 μU/ml (mean 17), with 50 to 100 μU/ml in the portal vein. During absorption of food the peripheral blood concentration may increase by 10 to 15 times.

Serum-insulin concentrations were measured in 21 diabetics; the daily dose varied from 3 to 80 units (mean 36) and the treatment period from one month to 35 years. The concentration of free insulin in the serum was in the range 10 to 440 μU/ml (mean 47) and total insulin (free and antibody-bound) varied from 67 to 17 020 μU/ml (mean 2676) (W. D. Gennaro and J. D. Van Norman, *ibid.*).

TOXICITY.

A non-diabetic male, aged 32 years, was found unconscious after a self-administered injection of at least 980 units of lente and soluble insulins. On admission, the serum-insulin concentration was 1830 to 2010 μU/ml. He died 9 days later and the following postmortem concentrations were reported: serum 42.5 μU/ml and bile 768 μU/ml (W. Q. Sturner and R. S. Putman, *J. forens. Sci.*, 1972, *17*, 514–521).

PROTEIN BINDING. In plasma, about 5% in normal subjects, but in diabetics the binding capacity may be extremely high due to formation of insulin-binding antibodies.

NOTE. For a review of the biochemistry and forensic aspects of insulin see S. M. Fletcher, *J. forens. Sci. Soc.*, 1983, *23*, 5–17.

Dose. Usually 10 to 100 units or more, a day, subcutaneously.

Iprindole
Antidepressant

Synonym. Pramindole
3-(6,7,8,9,10,11-Hexahydro-5*H*-cyclo-oct[*b*]indol-5-yl)-*NN*-dimethylpropylamine
$C_{19}H_{28}N_2 = 284.4$
CAS—5560-72-5

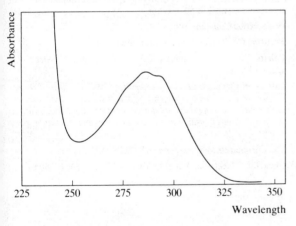

Iprindole Hydrochloride
Proprietary Name. Prondol
$C_{19}H_{28}N_2,HCl = 320.9$
CAS—20432-64-8
A white powder. M.p. about 144°.
Soluble in water, ethanol, and chloroform.

Dissociation Constant. pK_a 8.2.

Thin-layer Chromatography. *System TA*—Rf 47; *system TB*—Rf 49; *system TC*—Rf 34. (*Acidified iodoplatinate solution*, positive.)

Gas Chromatography. *System GA*—RI 2335.

High Pressure Liquid Chromatography. *System HA*—k′ 4.1; *system HF*—k′ 10.83.

Ultraviolet Spectrum. Aqueous acid—287 nm ($A_1^1 = 248$ a), 293 nm; aqueous alkali—302 nm.

[Graph: Absorbance vs Wavelength, 225–350 nm]

Infra-red Spectrum. Principal peaks at wavenumbers 738, 1650, 1612, 1145, 1173, 1040 (KBr disk).

Mass Spectrum. Principal peaks at *m/z* 58, 170, 284, 213, 145, 212, 159, 144.

Quantification. GAS CHROMATOGRAPHY. In plasma: sensitivity 5 ng/ml, AFID—G. Caillé *et al.*, *Biopharm. Drug Disp.*, 1982, *3*, 11–17.

Disposition in the Body. Well absorbed after oral administration. It is slowly excreted in the urine, about 50% of a dose being eliminated in 3 days and it is still detectable one week after administration; only about 5% of a dose is excreted in the urine as unchanged drug.

THERAPEUTIC CONCENTRATION.
After a single oral dose of 60 mg given to 5 subjects, peak plasma concentrations of 0.05 to 0.09 µg/ml (mean 0.07) were attained in 2 to 4 hours. Following oral administration of 30 mg three times daily to 4 subjects, plasma concentrations of 0.03 to 0.08 µg/ml (mean 0.06) were reported 10 hours after the final daily dose on day 21 (G. Caillé *et al.*, *ibid.*).

HALF-LIFE. Plasma half-life, about 35 to 70 hours (mean 52).

Dose. The equivalent of 45 to 180 mg of iprindole daily.

Iproniazid
Antidepressant (Monoamine Oxidase Inhibitor)

2′-Isopropylisonicotinohydrazide
$C_9H_{13}N_3O = 179.2$
CAS—54-92-2

Crystals. M.p. 113°.
Soluble in water and ethanol.

Iproniazid Phosphate
Proprietary Name. Marsilid
$C_9H_{13}N_3O,H_3PO_4 = 277.2$
CAS—305-33-9
A white crystalline powder.
Soluble 1 in 5 of water and 1 in 90 of ethanol; practically insoluble in chloroform and ether.

Partition Coefficient. Log *P* (chloroform/pH 7.4), 0.

Colour Tests. Cyanogen Bromide—orange-pink; Nessler's Reagent—black.

Thin-layer Chromatography. *System TA*—Rf 69; *system TB*—Rf 01; *system TC*—Rf 23. (*Dragendorff spray*, positive; *acidified iodoplatinate solution*, positive; *acidified potassium permanganate solution*, positive.)

Gas Chromatography. *System GA*—RI 1593.

Ultraviolet Spectrum. Aqueous acid—266 nm ($A_1^1 = 235$ c); aqueous alkali—242 nm, 307 nm.

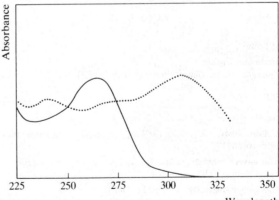

Infra-red Spectrum. Principal peaks at wavenumbers 975, 1090, 1672, 1110, 1065, 1025 (KBr disk). (See below)

Mass Spectrum. Principal peaks at *m/z* 123, 31, 58, 106, 79, 43, 78, 51; isonicotinic acid 123, 51, 78, 106, 50, 52, 105, 39.

Wavelength

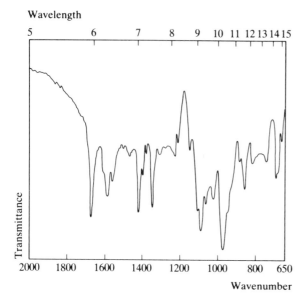

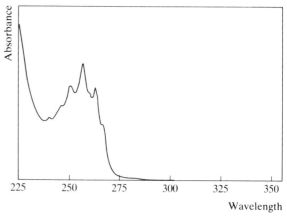

Quantification. GAS CHROMATOGRAPHY. In urine: FID—R. M. de Sagher *et al.*, *J. pharm. Sci.*, 1976, *65*, 878–882.

Disposition in the Body. Readily absorbed after oral administration. It is excreted in the urine mainly as metabolites, principally isonicotinic acid, with up to 15% as unchanged drug.

HALF-LIFE. Plasma half-life, about 10 hours.

Dose. The equivalent of 25 to 150 mg of iproniazid daily.

Isoaminile   *Cough Suppressant*

4-Dimethylamino-2-isopropyl-2-phenylvaleronitrile
$C_{16}H_{24}N_2 = 244.4$
CAS—77-51-0

$$CH_3 \cdot CH \cdot CH_2 \cdot \underset{\underset{N(CH_3)_2}{|}}{\overset{\overset{CH(CH_3)_2}{|}}{C}} \cdot CN \quad C_6H_5$$

A liquid.

Isoaminile Citrate

Proprietary Names. Dimyril; Peracon (citrate or cyclamate).
$C_{16}H_{24}N_2, C_6H_8O_7 = 436.5$
CAS—28416-66-2
Crystals. M.p. 63° to 64°.
Soluble in water.

Colour Tests. Liebermann's Test—red-orange; Sodium Picrate—orange.

Thin-layer Chromatography. *System TA*—Rf 68; *system TB*—Rf 58; *system TC*—Rf 54.

Gas Chromatography. *System GA*—RI 1830.

Ultraviolet Spectrum. Aqueous acid—252 nm, 258 nm ($A_1^1 = 7.3$ a), 264 nm.

Mass Spectrum. Principal peaks at *m/z* 72, 58, 71, 42, 73, 70, 56, 44.

Dose. 40 mg of isoaminile citrate 3 to 5 times daily.

Isocarboxazid *Antidepressant (Monoamine Oxidase Inhibitor)*

Proprietary Name. Marplan
2′-Benzyl-5-methylisoxazole-3-carbohydrazide
$C_{12}H_{13}N_3O_2 = 231.3$
CAS—59-63-2

$$CH_3 - \text{(isoxazole ring)} - CO \cdot NH \cdot NH \cdot CH_2 \cdot C_6H_5$$

A white or creamy-white crystalline powder. M.p. 105° to 108°. Slightly **soluble** in water; soluble 1 in 150 of ethanol, 1 in 3 of chloroform, and 1 in 50 of ether.

Dissociation Constant. pK_a 10.4.

Partition Coefficient. Log *P* (octanol/pH 7.4), 1.5.

Colour Tests. Liebermann's Test—red-orange; Nessler's Reagent—black.

Thin-layer Chromatography. *System TA*—Rf 71; *system TB*—Rf 17; *system TC*—Rf 74. (*Dragendorff spray*, positive; *FPN reagent*, pink-yellow; *acidified iodoplatinate solution*, positive; *Marquis reagent*, brown; *acidified potassium permanganate solution*, positive.)

Gas Chromatography. *System GA*—RI 1949.

Ultraviolet Spectrum. Aqueous alkali—274 nm ($A_1^1 = 240$ b).

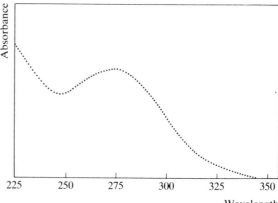

Infra-red Spectrum. Principal peaks at wavenumbers 1670, 750, 705, 870, 815, 1595 (KBr disk).

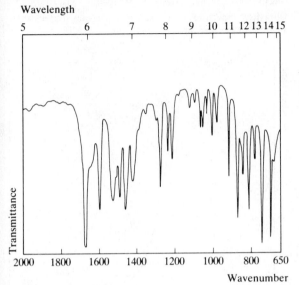

Wavelength

Mass Spectrum. Principal peaks at *m/z* 91, 127, 106, 110, 43, 92, 65, 120; hippuric acid 105, 135, 51, 134, 77, 106, 50, 78.

Disposition in the Body. Rapidly absorbed after oral administration. Metabolised by oxidation to benzoic acid followed by glycine conjugation to form hippuric acid; an active metabolite, benzhydrazine, has been detected in animal studies but its formation in man has not been confirmed. About 60% of a dose is excreted in the urine in 24 hours and about 70% in 8 days; 90% of the excreted material is hippuric acid and about 2% is unchanged drug.

THERAPEUTIC CONCENTRATION. Peak plasma concentrations are attained about 4 hours after oral administration. Maximal therapeutic effects are attained within 5 to 10 days after beginning treatment.

TOXICITY. Toxic reactions from overdosage may occur in a matter of hours despite the long delay in onset of a therapeutic response. A fatality has been reported 24 hours after ingestion of 400 mg.

HALF-LIFE. Plasma half-life, about 36 hours.

Dose. 10 to 30 mg daily.

Isoetharine   *Sympathomimetic*

Synonym. N-Isopropylethylnoradrenaline
1-(3,4-Dihydroxyphenyl)-2-isopropylaminobutan-1-ol
$C_{13}H_{21}NO_3 = 239.3$
CAS—530-08-5

$$(CH_3)_2CH \cdot NH \cdot \underset{\underset{C_2H_5}{|}}{CH} \cdot CHOH$$

Isoetharine Hydrochloride

Synonym. Etyprenalinum Hydrochloridum
Proprietary Names. Asthmalitan Depot; Bronkosol; Numotac.
$C_{13}H_{21}NO_3,HCl = 275.8$
CAS—50-96-4
A white crystalline solid. M.p. 196° to 208°, with decomposition.
Soluble in water; sparingly soluble in ethanol; practically insoluble in ether.

Isoetharine Mesylate

Synonym. Isoetharine Methanesulphonate
Proprietary Names. Bronkometer. It is an ingredient of Bronchilator.
$C_{13}H_{21}NO_3,CH_4O_3S = 335.4$
CAS—7279-75-6
White crystals. M.p. 162° to 168°.
Freely **soluble** in water; soluble in ethanol; practically insoluble in acetone and ether.

Colour Tests. Ammoniacal Silver Nitrate—red/brown-orange; Ferric Chloride—green; Folin–Ciocalteu Reagent—blue; Mandelin's Test—brown; Marquis Test—yellow → orange; Methanolic Potassium Hydroxide—red → orange → yellow; Nessler's Reagent—black; Palladium Chloride—orange → brown; Potassium Dichromate (Method 1)—green → brown (30 s).

Thin-layer Chromatography. *System TA*—Rf 59; *system TB*—Rf 00; *system TC*—Rf 00. (*Acidified potassium permanganate solution*, positive.)

Ultraviolet Spectrum. Aqueous acid—278 nm ($A_1^1 = 132$ a).

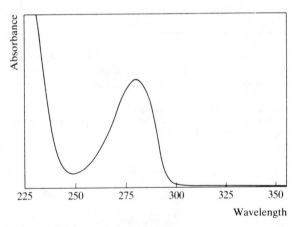

Wavelength

Infra-red Spectrum. Principal peaks at wavenumbers 1200, 1287, 1075, 1114, 1518, 1160 (KBr disk).

Mass Spectrum. Principal peaks at *m/z* 100, 58, 41, 101, 43, 56, 65, 30.

Quantification. HIGH PRESSURE LIQUID CHROMATOGRAPHY. In plasma: sensitivity 500 pg/ml, electrochemical detection—G. B. Park *et al.*, *J. pharm. Sci.*, 1982, **71**, 932–934.

Dose. 30 to 80 mg of isoetharine hydrochloride daily.

Isometheptene   *Sympathomimetic*

1,5,N-Trimethylhex-4-enylamine
$C_9H_{19}N = 141.3$
CAS—503-01-5

$$CH_3 \cdot NH \cdot \underset{\underset{CH_3}{|}}{CH} \cdot [CH_2]_2 \cdot CH:C(CH_3)_2$$

A colourless or slightly yellow oily liquid. B.p. 176° to 178°. Practically **insoluble** in water; soluble in ethanol, chloroform, and ether.

Isometheptene Hydrochloride

Proprietary Name. Octinum (injection)
$C_9H_{19}N,HCl = 177.7$
CAS—6168-86-1
An almost white, very hygroscopic, crystalline powder. M.p. about 68°.
Soluble in water and ethanol.

Isometheptene Mucate

Synonym. Isometheptene Galactarate
Proprietary Names. Octinum (tablets). It is an ingredient of Midrid.
$(C_9H_{19}N)_2,C_6H_{10}O_8 = 492.7$
CAS—7492-31-1
A white crystalline powder. M.p. about 148°, with decomposition.
Freely **soluble** in water; soluble in ethanol; practically insoluble in chloroform and ether.

Colour Test. Mandelin's Test—brown.

Thin-layer Chromatography. *System TA*—Rf 24. (*Acidified potassium permanganate solution*, positive.)

Gas Chromatography. *System GA*—RI 1052; *system GB*—RI 994.

Ultraviolet Spectrum. No significant absorption, 230 to 360 nm.

Mass Spectrum. Principal peaks at m/z 58, 55, 41, 44, 43, 128, 59, 56.

Dose. Isometheptene mucate has been given in doses of up to 520 mg daily.

Isoniazid
Antituberculous Agent

Synonyms. INAH; INH; Isonicotinic Acid Hydrazide; Isonicotinoylhydrazine; Isonicotinylhydrazide; Isonicotinylhydrazine; Tubazid.
Proprietary Names. Isotamine; Isotinyl; Neoteben; Niconyl; Nydrazid; Panazid; Rimifon; Teebaconin. It is an ingredient of Mynah, Rifinah, and Rimactazid.
Isonicotinohydrazide
$C_6H_7N_3O = 137.1$
CAS—54-85-3

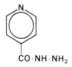

Colourless crystals or white crystalline powder. M.p. 170° to 174°.
Soluble 1 in 8 of water, 1 in about 45 of ethanol, and 1 in 1000 of chloroform; very slightly soluble in ether.

Isoniazid Aminosalicylate

Synonym. Pasiniazid
Proprietary Names. Dipasic; Paraniazide.
$C_6H_7N_3O,C_7H_7NO_3 = 290.3$
CAS—2066-89-9
Yellow crystals. M.p. 140° to 142°.
Soluble in water and methanol.

Dissociation Constant. pK_a 1.8, 3.5, 10.8 (20°).

Partition Coefficient. Log P (octanol/pH 7.4), −1.1.

Colour Tests. Cyanogen Bromide—orange; Nessler's Reagent—black.

Thin-layer Chromatography. *System TA*—Rf 47; *system TB*—Rf 01; *system TC*—Rf 11. (*Acidified iodoplatinate solution*, positive.)

Gas Chromatography. *System GA*—RI 1670.

Ultraviolet Spectrum. Aqueous acid—266 nm $(A_1^1 = 390 \, a)$; aqueous alkali—298 nm.

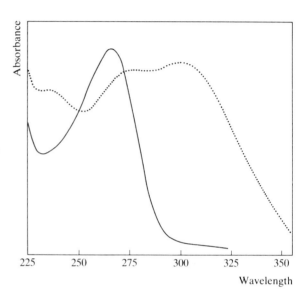

Infra-red Spectrum. Principal peaks at wavenumbers 1653, 1541, 1621, 676, 992, 845 (KBr disk).

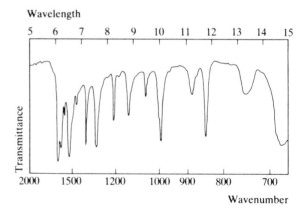

Mass Spectrum. Principal peaks at m/z 106, 78, 51, 137, 50, 79, 107, 31; isonicotinic acid 123, 51, 78, 106, 50, 52, 105, 39.

Quantification. SPECTROFLUORIMETRY. In plasma: isoniazid and acetylisoniazid—W. A. Olson *et al.*, *Clin. Chem.*, 1977, *23*, 745–748.

GAS CHROMATOGRAPHY. In urine: sensitivity 2 µg/ml for isoniazid and acetylisoniazid, 400 ng/ml for hydrazine, monoacetylhydrazine and diacetylhydrazine, AFID—J. A. Timbrell *et al.*, *J. Chromat.*, 1977, *138*, 165–172.

GAS CHROMATOGRAPHY-MASS SPECTROMETRY. In plasma: detection limit-100 ng/ml for isoniazid and acetylisoniazid, 50 ng/ml for hydrazine metabolites—B. H. Lauterburg et al., J. Chromat., 1981, 224; Biomed. Appl., 13, 431–438.

HIGH PRESSURE LIQUID CHROMATOGRAPHY. In plasma: isoniazid and acetylisoniazid, limit of detection 100 ng/ml, UV detection—M. R. Holdiness, J. liq. Chromat., 1982, 5, 707–714.

Disposition in the Body. Readily absorbed after oral administration; bioavailability about 80%. The main metabolic reaction is acetylation and the rate at which this occurs shows genetic variation, approximately 40% of the population being rapid acetylators and the remainder slow acetylators. Other metabolic reactions which occur are hydrolysis, glycine conjugation, hydrazone formation, and N-methylation. Metabolites include acetylisoniazid, isonicotinic acid, isonicotinylglycine, and mono- and diacetylhydrazine. All the metabolites are inactive with the exception of monoacetylhydrazine which is a reactive metabolite and is hepatotoxic. Up to about 70% of a dose is excreted in the urine in 24 hours, most being excreted in the first 12 hours. In slow acetylators, about 30% of the dose is excreted in the urine as unchanged drug, up to about 25% as acetylisoniazid, about 10% as isonicotinic acid, and about 8% as diacetylhydrazine. In rapid acetylators, about 10% of a dose is excreted as unchanged drug, up to 45% as acetylisoniazid, about 20% as isonicotinic acid, and about 25% as diacetylhydrazine. Small amounts of monoacetylhydrazine are also excreted in the urine. Less than 10% of a dose is eliminated in the faeces.

THERAPEUTIC CONCENTRATION. In plasma, usually in the range 3 to 10 µg/ml.

Following a single oral dose of 300 mg to 6 fasting subjects classified as slow acetylators, mean peak serum concentrations of 7.2 µg/ml of isoniazid and 1.7 µg/ml of acetylisoniazid were attained in 0.6 and 3.7 hour respectively. Following a single oral dose of 300 mg given to 4 rapid acetylators, mean peak serum concentrations of 7.2 µg/ml of isoniazid and 4.5 µg/ml of acetylisoniazid were attained in 0.4 hours and 2.6 hours, respectively (P. Männistö et al., J. antimicrob. Chemother., 1982, 10, 427–434).

TOXICITY. Serious toxic symptoms may occur with doses of 3 g or more. In children, toxic effects have occurred after ingestion of 0.9 g or more but a child has recovered after taking as much as 20 g. Toxic effects have been associated with plasma concentrations greater than 20 µg/ml.

A 16-year-old girl who had ingested an unknown quantity of isoniazid had a serum concentration of 127 µg/ml on admission to hospital and died 7 hours later. Two children aged 1½ and 2½ years had serum concentrations of 103 µg/ml and 35 µg/ml, respectively, on admission to hospital following ingestion of isoniazid and subsequently recovered (J. Miller et al., Am. J. Dis. Child., 1980, 134, 290–292).

A postmortem blood concentration of 150 µg/ml was reported in a fatality due to isoniazid overdose (A. C. McBay, Bull. int. Ass. forens. Toxicol., 1968, 5(3), 2).

HALF-LIFE. Plasma half-life, about 1 hour in rapid acetylators and 3 to 5 hours in slow acetylators.

VOLUME OF DISTRIBUTION. About 0.8 litre/kg.

CLEARANCE. Plasma clearance, about 2.5 and about 7 ml/min/kg in slow and rapid acetylators, respectively.

PROTEIN BINDING. In plasma, not significantly bound.

NOTE. For a review of the pharmacokinetics of isoniazid see W. W. Weber and D. W. Hein, Clin. Pharmacokinet., 1979, 4, 401–422.

Dose. Usually 4 to 5 mg/kg daily, by mouth, to a maximum of 300 mg daily.

Isoprenaline   *Sympathomimetic*

Synonyms. Isopropylarterenol; Isopropylnoradrenaline; Isoproterenol.

1-(3,4-Dihydroxyphenyl)-2-isopropylaminoethanol
$C_{11}H_{17}NO_3 = 211.3$
CAS—7683-59-2

$$(CH_3)_2CH \cdot NH \cdot CH_2 \cdot CHOH$$

Crystals. M.p. 155°.

Isoprenaline Hydrochloride

Synonym. Isoproterenol Hydrochloride
Proprietary Names. Aerolone; Isuprel; Norisodrine; Proternol; Saventrine. It is an ingredient of Brontisol, Duo-Autohaler, Medihaler-duo, and PIB.
$C_{11}H_{17}NO_3,HCl = 247.7$
CAS—51-30-9
A white crystalline powder. It gradually darkens on exposure to air and light. M.p. 165° to 170°, with decomposition.
Soluble 1 in less than 1 of water and 1 in about 50 of ethanol; practically insoluble in chloroform and ether. Aqueous solutions become pink to brownish-pink on standing exposed to air, and almost immediately so when made alkaline.

Isoprenaline Sulphate

Synonym. Isoproterenol Sulfate
Proprietary Names. Aleudrin(e); Ingelan; Iso-Autohaler; Medihaler Iso; Norisodrine. It is an ingredient of Intal Compound.
$(C_{11}H_{17}NO_3)_2,H_2SO_4,2H_2O = 556.6$
CAS—299-95-6 (anhydrous); 6700-39-6 (dihydrate)
A white crystalline powder. It gradually darkens on exposure to light and air. M.p. about 128°, with decomposition.
Soluble 1 in 4 of water; slightly soluble in ethanol; practically insoluble in chloroform and ether. Aqueous solutions become pink to brownish-pink on standing exposed to air, and almost immediately so when made alkaline.

Dissociation Constant. pK_a 8.6, 10.1, 12.0 (20°).

Colour Tests. Ammoniacal Silver Nitrate—red → red-brown/brown; Ferric Chloride—green; Folin–Ciocalteu Reagent—blue; Mandelin's Test—brown; Marquis Test—brown → violet; Methanolic Potassium Hydroxide—orange → yellow; Nessler's Reagent—black; Potassium Dichromate—green → brown (30 s).

Thin-layer Chromatography. System TA—Rf 40; system TB—Rf 00; system TC—Rf 01. (Acidified potassium permanganate solution, positive.)

Gas Chromatography. System GA—RI 1730.

Ultraviolet Spectrum. Aqueous acid—279 nm ($A_1^1 = 134$ a); aqueous alkali—297 nm. (See below)

Infra-red Spectrum. Principal peaks at wavenumbers 1246, 1293, 1535, 1230, 1040, 1607 (isoprenaline hydrochloride, KCl disk). (See below)

Mass Spectrum. Principal peaks at m/z 72, 44, 43, 124, 123, 30, 42, 41.

Quantification. HIGH PRESSURE LIQUID CHROMATOGRAPHY. In plasma or urine: detection limit 40 pg, fluorescence detection—Y. Kishimoto et al., J. Chromat., 1982, 231; Biomed. Appl., 20, 121–127. In plasma or urine: sensitivity 1 ng/ml, electrochemical detection—R. C. Causon et al., J. Chromat., 1984, 306; Biomed. Appl., 31, 257–268.

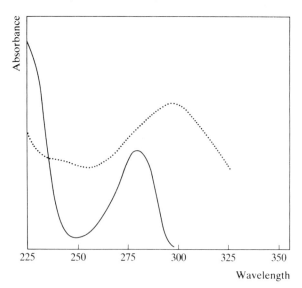

Wavelength

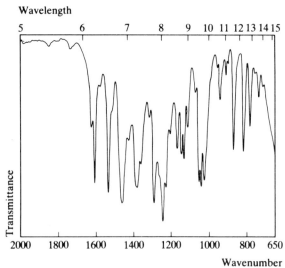

Wavenumber

µg/ml of isoprenaline plus metabolites were attained within 90 minutes; in blood the major component was the sulphate ester together with small amounts of the methylated metabolite (M. E. Conolly *et al.*, *Br. J. Pharmac.*, 1972, *46*, 458–472).

TOXICITY. Estimated minimum lethal dose for children, applied to mucous membranes, 100 mg.

HALF-LIFE. Plasma half-life, 3 to 7 hours.

VOLUME OF DISTRIBUTION. About 0.5 litre/kg.

PROTEIN BINDING. In plasma, about 68%.

Dose. 90 to 840 mg of isoprenaline hydrochloride daily, by mouth, as sustained-release tablets.

Isopropamide Iodide   *Anticholinergic*

Proprietary Names. Darbid; Priamide; Tyrimide. It is an ingredient of Combid, Eskornade, and Stelabid.

(3-Carbamoyl-3,3-diphenylpropyl)di-isopropylmethylammonium iodide

$C_{23}H_{33}IN_2O = 480.4$

CAS—7492-32-2 (isopropamide); *71-81-8* (iodide)

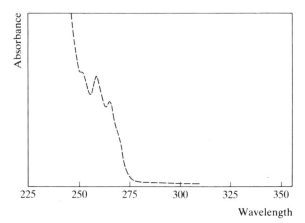

A white to pale yellow crystalline powder. M.p. about 181°.

Soluble 1 in 50 of water, 1 in 10 of ethanol, and 1 in 5 of chloroform; very slightly soluble in ether.

Colour Tests. Aromaticity (Method 2)—colourless/brown; Liebermann's Test—grey.

Thin-layer Chromatography. *System TA*—Rf 05. (*Acidified iodoplatinate solution*, positive.)

High Pressure Liquid Chromatography. *System HA*—k' 2.4 (tailing peak).

Ultraviolet Spectrum. Methanol—259 nm ($A_1^1 = 9.1$ a), 265 nm.

Disposition in the Body. Irregularly absorbed after oral or sublingual administration with extensive metabolism and conjugation occurring in the gut. Only about 10% of an inhaled dose reaches the lungs. Rapidly metabolised by 3-*O*-methylation and sulphate conjugation; 3-*O*-methylisoprenaline exhibits weak activity. After intravenous administration, about 90% of a dose is excreted in the urine in 24 hours, mostly as the conjugated 3-*O*-methyl metabolite, with up to about 15% of the dose as unchanged drug; after inhalation or oral administration, 68 to 94% of a dose is excreted as conjugated isoprenaline, with about 2 to 8% of a dose as the 3-*O*-methyl conjugate and less than 5% as unchanged drug or free 3-*O*-methylisoprenaline; small amounts of a dose are excreted in the bile, mainly as metabolites.

THERAPEUTIC CONCENTRATION.

After a dose of 500 µg administered by aerosol inhalation, plasma concentrations of about 0.0003 µg/ml were attained in 5 minutes in 2 subjects (E. W. Blackwell *et al.*, *Br. J. Pharmac.*, 1970, *39*, 194P–195P).

After an oral dose of 0.2 mg/kg, plasma concentrations of about 0.5

Wavelength

Infra-red Spectrum. Principal peaks at wavenumbers 1650, 1576, 705, 769, 757, 1500 (KBr disk).

Mass Spectrum. Principal peaks at m/z 86, 114, 100, 44, 238, 115, 56, 72.

Dose. The equivalent of 5 to 10 mg of isopropamide every 12 hours.

Isopropyl Alcohol   *Solvent*

Synonyms. Alcohol Isopropylicus; Dimethyl Carbinol; Isopropanol; 2-Propanol; Secondary Propyl Alcohol.
Proprietary Names. Alcojel; Avantine; IPS.1; IPS/C; Sterets. It is an ingredient of Manusept.
Propan-2-ol
$(CH_3)_2 \cdot CHOH = 60.10$
CAS—67-63-0
A clear, colourless, mobile, volatile, inflammable liquid. Wt per ml 0.784 to 0.786 g. B.p. 81° to 83°. Refractive index, at 20°, 1.377 to 1.380.

Miscible with water, ethanol, chloroform, and ether.

Colour Test. Potassium Dichromate (Method 2)—green.

Gas Chromatography. *System GA*—RI 530; *system GI*—retention time 4 min.

Infra-red Spectrum. Principal peaks at wavenumbers 952, 1123, 1162, 819, 1111, 1298.

Mass Spectrum. Principal peaks at m/z 45, 43, 27, 41, 39, 29, 59, 44; acetone 43, 58, 59, 27, 42, 26, 39, 29.

Quantification. GAS CHROMATOGRAPHY. In blood—D. R. Daniel *et al.*, *J. analyt. Toxicol.*, 1981, *5*, 110–112.

Disposition in the Body. Readily absorbed after oral administration and slowly absorbed through intact skin. Isopropyl alcohol is metabolised more slowly than ethanol; it is largely converted to acetone which is slowly excreted from the lungs and in the urine; acetone may be further metabolised to acetate, formate, and carbon dioxide; some unchanged isopropyl alcohol may be excreted in the urine together with its glucuronide conjugate, particularly after large doses.

TOXICITY. The estimated minimum lethal dose is 240 ml. Isopropyl alcohol is about twice as toxic as ethanol and the symptoms of intoxication are similar. Fatalities have been associated with blood concentrations greater than 1000 µg/ml. The maximum permissible atmospheric concentration is 400 ppm. A dose of 16 ml has been ingested daily for 3 days without discomfort but marked depression has been observed following a dose of 23 ml. Recovery has followed treatment by haemodialysis in subjects with initial blood concentrations of up to 4400 µg/ml of isopropyl alcohol.

In a review of 31 fatalities attributed solely to isopropyl alcohol poisoning, postmortem blood concentrations ranged from 100 to 2500 µg/ml (mean 1400) for isopropyl alcohol and 400 to 3000 µg/ml (mean 1700) for acetone (C. B. Alexander *et al.*, *J. forens. Sci.*, 1982, *27*, 541–548).

A woman who died about 3 hours after ingesting isopropyl alcohol was reported to have the following postmortem tissue concentrations: isopropyl alcohol, blood 3300 µg/ml, brain 1800 µg/g, urine 2000 µg/ml; acetone, blood 1200 µg/ml, brain 600 µg/g, urine 700 µg/ml (R. H. Cravey, per R. C. Baselt, *Disposition of Toxic Drugs and Chemicals in Man*, 2nd Edn, Davis, California, Biomedical Publications, 1982, pp. 407–409).

In 4 fatalities due to the ingestion of isopropyl alcohol, the following antemortem or postmortem tissue concentrations were reported: blood 200 to 2000 µg/ml (mean 1300, 4 cases), brain 1000 µg/g (1 case), liver 1000 µg/g (1 case), spleen 1300 µg/g (1 case), urine 1500 and 1800 µg/ml (2 cases) (L. Adelson, *Am. J. clin. Path.*, 1962, *38*, 144–151).

HALF-LIFE. Blood half-life, about 3 hours in subjects with acute intoxication.

Isopropylaminophenazone   *Analgesic (Veterinary)*

Synonym. Isopyrin
Note. The name Isopyrin has also been applied to isoniazid.
4-Isopropylamino-1,5-dimethyl-2-phenyl-4-pyrazolin-3-one
$C_{14}H_{19}N_3O = 245.3$
CAS—3615-24-5

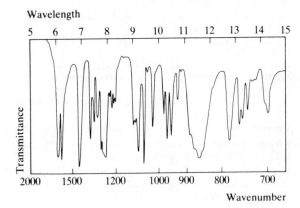

Crystals. M.p. 80°.

Ultraviolet Spectrum. Aqueous acid—260 nm $(A_1^1 = 377$ b); aqueous alkali—271 nm $(A_1^1 = 334$ b); methanol—243 nm $(A_1^1 = 310$ b), 269 nm $(A_1^1 = 381$ b).

Isosorbide Dinitrate   *Anti-anginal Vasodilator*

Synonym. Sorbide Nitrate
Proprietary Names. Carvasin; Cedocard; Coronex; Dilatrate-SR; Iso-Bid; Iso D; Isoket; Isordil; Isotrate; Risordan; Soni-Slo; Sorbichew; Sorbid SA; Sorbidilat; Sorbitrate; Sorquad; Vascardin; Vasotrate.
1,4:3,6-Dianhydro-D-glucitol 2,5-dinitrate
$C_6H_8N_2O_8 = 236.1$
CAS—87-33-2

A white crystalline powder. M.p. about 70°.
Very slightly **soluble** in water; sparingly soluble in ethanol; very soluble in acetone; freely soluble in chloroform; soluble in methanol.
Caution. Isosorbide dinitrate may explode if subjected to percussion or excessive heat.

Ultraviolet Spectrum. No significant absorption, 230 to 360 nm.

Infra-red Spectrum. Principal peaks at wavenumbers 1062, 1618, 862, 1266, 1653, 1089 (isosorbide, Nujol mull).

Wavelength

| 5 | 6 | 7 | 8 | 9 | 10 | 11 | 12 | 13 | 14 | 15 |

Transmittance

| 2000 | 1500 | 1200 | 1000 | 900 | 800 | 700 |

Wavenumber

Mass Spectrum. Principal peaks at *m/z* 43, 31, 29, 61, 60, 85, 73, 44.

Quantification. GAS CHROMATOGRAPHY. In plasma or urine: limit of detection 500 pg/ml, ECD—A. Sioufi and F. Pommier, *J. Chromat.*, 1982, *229*; *Biomed. Appl.*, *18*, 347–353.

GAS CHROMATOGRAPHY (CAPILLARY COLUMN). In plasma: detection limits 500 pg/ml for isosorbide dinitrate, 2 ng/ml for isosorbide 2-mononitrate and 10 ng/ml for isosorbide 5-mononitrate, ECD—Y. Santoni *et al.*, *J. Chromat.*, 1984, *306*; *Biomed Appl.*, *31*, 165–172.

HIGH PRESSURE LIQUID CHROMATOGRAPHY. In plasma: limit of detection 200 pg—W. C. Yu and E. U. Goff, *Analyt. Chem.*, 1983, *55*, 29–32.

Disposition in the Body. Readily absorbed after sublingual or oral administration; bioavailability about 60% after sublingual administration and about 20% orally, but there is considerable intersubject variation. Metabolised by enzymatic denitration followed by glucuronide conjugation. Isosorbide 2-mononitrate and isosorbide 5-mononitrate have some pharmacological activity. About 80% of a dose is excreted in the urine in 24 hours, of which about 50% is isosorbide glucuronide, up to 15% is free and conjugated isosorbide 5-mononitrate, about 1% is free isosorbide 2-mononitrate, and less than 1% is unchanged drug.

THERAPEUTIC CONCENTRATION. Isosorbide 5-mononitrate accumulates in the plasma during chronic treatment.

Following a single oral dose of 20 mg of isosorbide dinitrate to 8 subjects, peak plasma concentrations of 0.02 to 0.09 µg/ml (mean 0.05) of isosorbide dinitrate, 0.02 to 0.06 µg/ml (mean 0.04) of isosorbide 2-mononitrate, and 0.10 to 0.22 µg/ml (mean 0.14) of isosorbide 5-mononitrate, were attained in 0.25, 0.7, and 1 hour respectively (H. Laufen *et al.*, *Arzneimittel-Forsch.*, 1983, *33*, 980–984).

After a single sublingual dose of 5 mg to 6 subjects, peak plasma concentrations of 0.007 to 0.015 µg/ml (mean 0.009) were attained in 10 to 15 minutes (D. F. Assinder *et al.*, *J. pharm. Sci.*, 1977, *66*, 775–778).

HALF-LIFE. Plasma half-life, isosorbide dinitrate about 0.5 to 1.5 hours, isosorbide 2-mononitrate about 2 hours, isosorbide 5-mononitrate 3 to 7 hours. A longer terminal elimination half-life of about 8 hours has been reported for isosorbide dinitrate.

SALIVA. Plasma: saliva ratio, about 1.5.

PROTEIN BINDING. In plasma, about 30%.

NOTE. For a review of the pharmacokinetics of organic nitrates, see M. G. Bogaert, *Clin. Pharmacokinet.*, 1983, *8*, 410–421.

Dose. 10 to 240 mg daily, by mouth.

Isosorbide Mononitrate   *Anti-anginal Vasodilator*

Synonym. Isosorbide 5-Mononitrate
Proprietary Names. Elantan; Ismo; Monit; Mono-Cedocard.
1,4:3,6-Dianhydro-D-glucitol 5-nitrate
$C_6H_9NO_6 = 191.1$
CAS—16051-77-7
Colourless prismatic crystals. M.p. 89° to 91°.
Soluble in water, ethanol, acetone, and methanol; slightly soluble in chloroform and ether.
Caution. Isosorbide mononitrate may explode if subjected to percussion or excessive heat.

Ultraviolet Spectrum. No significant absorption, 230 to 360 nm.

Infra-red Spectrum. Principal peaks at wavenumbers 1280, 1650, 1635, 852, 1090, 968 (KBr disk).

Quantification. GAS CHROMATOGRAPHY (CAPILLARY COLUMN). In plasma: sensitivity 1 ng/ml, ECD—P. Straehl and R. L. Galeazzi, *J. pharm. Sci.*, 1984, *73*, 1317–1319.

Disposition in the Body. Rapidly and almost completely absorbed after oral or sublingual administration; bioavailability almost 100%. Metabolised by enzymatic denitration and by glucuronide conjugation. About 80% of a dose is excreted in the urine in 24 hours.

THERAPEUTIC CONCENTRATION.
Following a single dose of 20 mg given to 19 subjects, peak plasma concentrations of 0.34 to 0.68 µg/ml (mean 0.48) were attained in 1 hour (U. Abshagen *et al.*, *ibid.*).

HALF-LIFE. Plasma half-life, 3 to 7 hours.

VOLUME OF DISTRIBUTION. About 0.6 litre/kg.

CLEARANCE. Plasma clearance, about 1 to 2 ml/min/kg.

SALIVA. Plasma: saliva ratio, about 0.8.

PROTEIN BINDING. In plasma, less than 5%.

Dose. 20 to 120 mg daily.

Isothipendyl   *Antihistamine*

NN - Dimethyl - 1 - (pyrido[3,2 - *b*][1,4]benzothiazin - 10 - yl-methyl)ethylamine
$C_{16}H_{19}N_3S = 285.4$
CAS—482-15-5

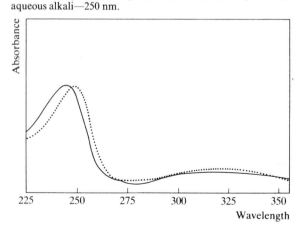

Isothipendyl Hydrochloride

Proprietary Names. Andantol; Nilergex.
$C_{16}H_{19}N_3S,HCl = 321.9$
CAS—1225-60-1
A fine white crystalline powder. M.p. about 212°, with decomposition.
Soluble 1 in 5 of water, 1 in 60 of ethanol, and 1 in 10 of chloroform; practically insoluble in ether.

Colour Test. Marquis Test—orange.

Thin-layer Chromatography. *System TA*—Rf 52; *system TB*—Rf 41; *system TC*—Rf 30. (*Dragendorff spray*, positive; *FPN reagent*, yellow-pink; *acidified iodoplatinate solution*, positive; *Marquis reagent*, pink; *ninhydrin spray*, positive.)

Gas Chromatography. *System GA*—RI 2267.

High Pressure Liquid Chromatography. *System HA*—k' 3.8.

Ultraviolet Spectrum. Aqueous acid—245 nm ($A_1^1 = 860$ a); aqueous alkali—250 nm.

Infra-red Spectrum. Principal peaks at wavenumbers 1017, 1030, 1070, 987, 1090, 1080 (KBr disk).

Mass Spectrum. Principal peaks at m/z 72, 73, 214, 200, 44, 285, 86, 56.

Dose. 12 to 32 mg of isothipendyl hydrochloride daily.

Isoxsuprine   *Vasodilator*

Proprietary Name. Defencin CP (resinate)

1 - (4 - Hydroxyphenyl) - 2 - (1 - methyl - 2 - phenoxyethyl-amino)propan-1-ol

$C_{18}H_{23}NO_3 = 301.4$

CAS—395-28-8

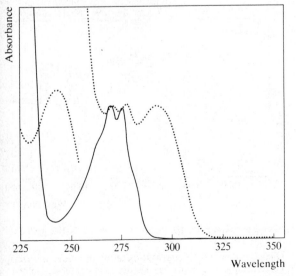

Crystals. M.p. 103°.

Isoxsuprine Hydrochloride

Synonym. Phenoxyisopropylnorsuprifen

Proprietary Names. Duvadilan; Isolait; Vasodilan; Vasoplex.

$C_{18}H_{23}NO_3,HCl = 337.8$

CAS—579-56-6

A white crystalline powder. M.p. about 200°, with decomposition.

Soluble 1 in 500 of water, 1 in 100 of ethanol and dilute sodium hydroxide solution, and 1 in 2500 of dilute hydrochloric acid; practically insoluble in chloroform and ether.

Dissociation Constant. pK_a 8.0, 9.8.

Colour Tests. Mandelin's Test—green; Marquis Test—red-violet.

Thin-layer Chromatography. *System TA*—Rf 78; *system TB*—Rf 02; *system TC*—Rf 32. (*Acidified potassium permanganate solution, positive.*)

Gas Chromatography. *System GA*—RI 2300.

High Pressure Liquid Chromatography. *System HA*—k' 0.8.

Ultraviolet Spectrum. Aqueous acid—269 nm, 274 nm ($A_1^1 = 82$ a); aqueous alkali—243 nm ($A_1^1 = 450$ a), 270 nm, 277 nm, 292 nm ($A_1^1 = 78$ b).

Infra-red Spectrum. Principal peaks at wavenumbers 1514, 1240, 745, 1220, 1043, 1500.

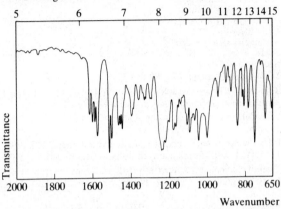

Mass Spectrum. Principal peaks at m/z 178, 44, 135, 179, 77, 84, 107, 41.

Disposition in the Body. Absorbed after oral administration; peak blood concentrations are attained within 1 hour of a dose. It is excreted in the urine partly unchanged and partly as a conjugate.

Dose. Up to 80 mg of isoxsuprine hydrochloride daily.

Kanamycin   *Antibiotic*

Synonym. Kanamycin A

6-*O*-(3-Amino-3-deoxy-α-D-glucopyranosyl)-4-*O*-(6-amino-6-deoxy-α-D-glucopyranosyl)-2-deoxy-D-streptamine

$C_{18}H_{36}N_4O_{11} = 484.5$

CAS—59-01-8

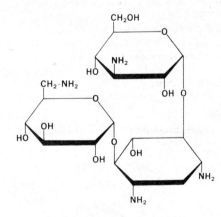

An antimicrobial substance produced by the growth of *Streptomyces kanamyceticus*.

A whitish powder.

Kanamycin Acid Sulphate

Proprietary Name. Kannasyn (powder)

$C_{18}H_{36}N_4O_{11},1.7H_2SO_4 = 651.2$

A white hygroscopic powder.

Soluble 1 in 1 of water; practically insoluble in ethanol, acetone, chloroform, and ether.

Kanamycin Sulphate

Synonym. Kanamycin A Sulphate

Proprietary Names. Kamycine; Kanamytrex; Kanasig; Kannasyn (solution); Kantrex; Klebcil.

$C_{18}H_{36}N_4O_{11},H_2SO_4 = 582.6$

CAS—25389-94-0

A white crystalline powder.

Soluble 1 in 8 of water; practically insoluble in ethanol, acetone, chloroform, and ether.

Dissociation Constant. pK_a 7.2.

Thin-layer Chromatography. *System TA*—Rf 01. (*Acidified potassium permanganate solution*, positive.)

Ultraviolet Spectrum. Aqueous acid—249 nm (A_1^1 = about 3 b), 306 nm.

Infra-red Spectrum. Principal peaks at wavenumbers 1033, 1068, 1143, 1123, 980, 1516 (kanamycin sulphate, KBr disk).

Quantification. SPECTROFLUORIMETRY. In serum or urine: sensitivity 50 ng/ml—A. Csiba, *J. Pharm. Pharmac.*, 1979, *31*, 115–116.

BIOASSAY. Aminoglycoside antibiotics in biological fluids—J. M. Broughall, Aminoglycosides, in *Laboratory Methods in Antimicrobial Chemotherapy*, D. S. Reeves *et al.* (Ed.), Edinburgh, Churchill Livingstone, 1978, pp. 194–207.

Disposition in the Body. Poorly absorbed after oral administration, but rapidly and completely absorbed after intramuscular injection. Up to 95% of a dose is excreted unchanged in the urine in 24 hours, most being excreted within the first 6 hours. A small amount is excreted in the bile.

THERAPEUTIC CONCENTRATION. During treatment, the serum concentration should be in the range 20 to 25 µg/ml and should be monitored regularly, especially in patients who have renal insufficiency. During multiple dosing, the trough concentration immediately preceding a dose should not exceed 10 µg/ml.

TOXICITY. Toxic effects may be produced at serum concentrations of 30 µg/ml or more or, during chronic treatment, if the trough serum concentration exceeds 10 µg/ml.

HALF-LIFE. Plasma half-life, about 2 to 4 hours; increased to 4 to 5 days in renal failure.

VOLUME OF DISTRIBUTION. About 0.3 litre/kg.

CLEARANCE. Plasma clearance, about 1.4 ml/min/kg.

PROTEIN BINDING. In plasma, not significantly bound.

Dose. The equivalent of up to 1.5 g of kanamycin daily, by intramuscular injection.

Ketamine

General Anaesthetic

(±)-2-(2-Chlorophenyl)-2-methylaminocyclohexanone

$C_{13}H_{16}ClNO = 237.7$

CAS—6740-88-1

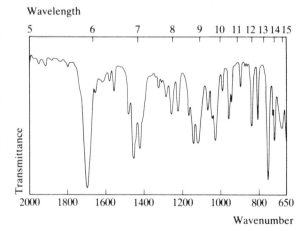

Crystals. M.p. 92° to 93°.

Ketamine Hydrochloride

Proprietary Names. Ketaject; Ketalar; Ketanest.

$C_{13}H_{16}ClNO,HCl = 274.2$

CAS—1867-66-9

A white crystalline powder. M.p. 258° to 261°.

Soluble 1 in 4 of water, 1 in 14 of ethanol, and 1 in 6 of methanol; sparingly soluble in chloroform; practically insoluble in ether.

Dissociation Constant. pK_a 7.5.

Thin-layer Chromatography. *System TA*—Rf 63; *system TB*—Rf 37; *system TC*—Rf 63. (*Acidified iodoplatinate solution*, positive.)

Gas Chromatography. *System GA*—RI 1843.

Ultraviolet Spectrum. Aqueous acid—269 nm (A_1^1 = 25 a), 276 nm.

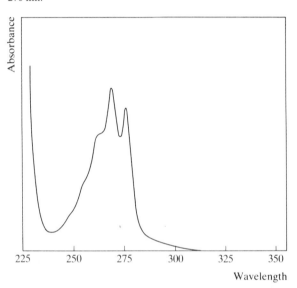

Infra-red Spectrum. Principal peaks at wavenumbers 1696, 747, 1142, 1120, 712, 1027 (KBr disk).

Mass Spectrum. Principal peaks at *m/z* 180, 209, 182, 152, 181, 30, 211, 138.

Quantification. GAS CHROMATOGRAPHY. In serum or urine: ketamine and metabolites, sensitivity 25 ng/ml for ketamine in erum, FID—J. Wieber *et al.*, *Anaesthesist*, 1975, *24*, 260–263.

n plasma or urine: ketamine and norketamine, sensitivity
0 ng/ml, AFID—R. L. Stiller *et al.*, *J. Chromat.*, 1982, *232*;
iomed. Appl., *21*, 305–314.

Disposition in the Body. Rapidly distributed in the tissues
ollowing parenteral administration. About 90% of a dose is
xcreted in the urine in 72 hours, with about 2% of the dose as
nchanged drug, 2% as norketamine, 16% as dehydronorke-
amine, and 80% as conjugates of hydroxylated metabolites.
Norketamine (which has about one-sixth of the potency of
ketamine) and dehydronorketamine are found in the serum in
oncentrations similar to those of ketamine. It has been suggested
that dehydronorketamine may be an analytical artefact rather
than a metabolite.

THERAPEUTIC CONCENTRATION.
Following single intravenous injections of 2.5 mg/kg to 5 subjects, serum
oncentrations of about 1 µg/ml were reported after 15 minutes (J. Wieber
t al., *Anaesthesist*, 1975, *24*, 260–263).

During continuous intravenous infusion at an average rate of 41 µg/kg/
minute to 31 subjects, a mean steady-state plasma concentration of 2.2 µg/
ml was reported; norketamine and dehydronorketamine attained mean
peak plasma concentrations of 1.1 µg/ml and 0.7 µg/ml, respectively, in
about 3 hours; the subjects awoke at an average plasma concentration of
.64 µg/ml (J. Idvall *et al.*, *Br. J. Anaesth.*, 1979, *51*, 1167–1173).

Following an intramuscular injection of 0.5 mg/kg to 6 subjects, peak
plasma concentrations of 0.10 to 0.43 µg/ml (mean 0.24) were attained in
about 0.3 hour; norketamine attained a mean peak plasma concentration
of 0.09 µg/ml at about 1 hour (J. A. Clements *et al.*, *J. pharm. Sci.*, 1982,
71, 539–542).

TOXICITY. Ketamine produces hallucinogenic effects similar to
those of phencyclidine and may be subject to abuse.

HALF-LIFE. Plasma half-life, about 2 to 4 hours.

VOLUME OF DISTRIBUTION. About 4 litres/kg.

CLEARANCE. Plasma clearance, about 17 ml/min/kg.

DISTRIBUTION IN BLOOD. Plasma: whole blood ratio, about 0.6.

PROTEIN BINDING. In plasma, about 20 to 50%.

Dose. The equivalent of 1 to 4.5 mg/kg of ketamine, by slow
intravenous injection or 6.5 to 13 mg/kg, intramuscularly.

Ketazolam   *Tranquilliser*

Proprietary Names. Anxon; Contamex; Loftran; Solatran.

11 - Chloro - 8,12b - dihydro - 2,8 - dimethyl - 12b - phenyl - 4*H* -
[1,3]oxazino[3,2-*d*][1,4]benzodiazepine-4,7(6*H*)-dione
$C_{20}H_{17}ClN_2O_3 = 368.8$
CAS—27223-35-4

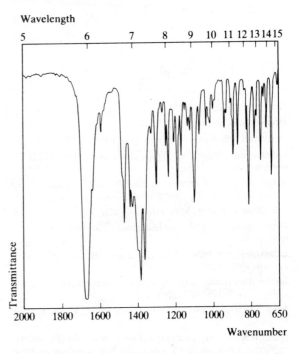

A white crystalline powder. M.p. 183°.
Slightly **soluble** in water.

Colour Test. Formaldehyde–Sulphuric Acid—orange.

Thin-layer Chromatography. *System TA*—Rf 66; *system TB*—Rf
08; *system TC*—Rf 64; *system TD*—Rf 45; *system TE*—Rf 73;

system *TF*—Rf 45. (*Dragendorff spray*, positive; *furfuraldehyde
reagent*, dark grey; *acidified iodoplatinate solution*, positive;
mercuric chloride–diphenylcarbazone reagent, pale blue; *ninhydrin
spray*, pale yellow; *acidified potassium permanganate solution*,
positive.)

Gas Chromatography. Rearrangement to form diazepam occurs
on-column: *system GA*—diazepam RI 2425, oxazepam RI 2336;
system GG—diazepam RI 2940, oxazepam RI 2803.

High Pressure Liquid Chromatography. *System HI*—k′ 12.81;
system HJ—k′ 2.45; *system HK*—k′ 0.04.

Ultraviolet Spectrum. Ethanol—242 nm ($A_1^1 = 492$ a).

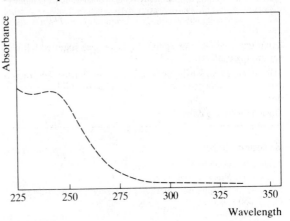

Infra-red Spectrum. Principal peaks at wavenumbers 1675, 820,
1105, 1195, 1308, 1242 (KBr disk).

Mass Spectrum. Principal peaks at *m/z* 256, 284, 283, 285, 84,
257, 258, 255; oxazepam 257, 77, 268, 239, 205, 267, 233, 259.

Disposition in the Body. Readily absorbed after oral administration. Rapidly metabolised by *N*-demethylation to desmethylketazolam and desmethyldiazepam (nordazepam). About 80% of a dose is excreted in the urine as metabolites with only traces of unchanged drug. Of the material excreted in the urine, about 56% is oxazepam and the remainder is a mixture of minor metabolites including diazepam, desmethyldiazepam, temazepam, and other unidentified metabolites. About 20% of a dose is eliminated in the faeces, mainly as metabolites.

THERAPEUTIC CONCENTRATION.
Following a single oral dose of 30 mg of ^{14}C-labelled ketazolam, peak plasma concentrations of about 0.004 μg/ml of ketazolam, 0.017 μg/ml of diazepam, and 0.127 μg/ml of *N*-demethylated metabolites were attained in 2, 10, and 14 hours respectively (F. S. Eberts jun. *et al.*, *Pharmacologist*, 1977, *19*, 165).

TOXICITY. Overdoses of up to 0.5 g have been ingested without serious toxic effects.

HALF-LIFE. Plasma half-life, ketazolam about 1.5 hours, oxazepam 4 to 25 hours (mean 8), diazepam 20 to 100 hours (mean 48).

Dose. 15 to 60 mg daily.

Ketobemidone

Narcotic Analgesic

Synonym. Cetobemidone
Proprietary Name. Cliradon
1-(4-*m*-Hydroxyphenyl-1-methyl-4-piperidyl)propan-1-one
$C_{15}H_{21}NO_2 = 247.3$
CAS—469-79-4

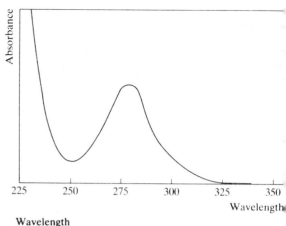

Crystals. M.p. 156° to 157°.

Dissociation Constant. pK$_a$ 8.7 (20°).

Partition Coefficient. Log *P* (heptane/pH 7.4), −3.0.

Colour Tests. Mandelin's Test—blue-green; Marquis Test—orange.

Thin-layer Chromatography. *System TA*—Rf 47; *system TB*—Rf 02; *system TC*—Rf 09. (*Acidified iodoplatinate solution*, positive.)

Gas Chromatography. *System GA*—RI 2035.

High Pressure Liquid Chromatography. *System HA*—k' 2.8 (tailing peak).

Ultraviolet Spectrum. Aqueous acid—280 nm (A$_1^1$ = 81 a); aqueous alkali—300 nm (A$_1^1$ = 126 b).

Infra-red Spectrum. Principal peaks at wavenumbers 1705, 1597, 1248, 777, 699, 1285 (KBr disk).

Mass Spectrum. Principal peaks at *m/z* 70, 71, 42, 44, 57, 190, 29, 247.

Quantification. GAS CHROMATOGRAPHY–MASS SPECTROMETRY. In plasma: ketobemidone and desmethylketobemidone, sensitivity 5 ng/ml—U. Bondesson *et al.*, *Biomed. Mass Spectrom.*, 1983, *10*, 283–286.

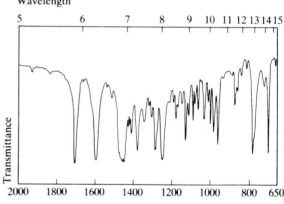

Disposition in the Body. Poorly absorbed after oral or rectal administration; bioavailability about 40%. Metabolised by *N*-demethylation.

HALF-LIFE. Plasma half-life, about 2 hours.

VOLUME OF DISTRIBUTION. About 2 to 3 litres/kg.

CLEARANCE. Plasma clearance, about 10 ml/min/kg.

REFERENCE. P. Anderson *et al.*, *Eur. J. clin. Pharmac.*, 1981, *19*, 217–223.

Dose. Ketobemidone has been given in doses of 5 to 10 mg.

Ketoconazole

Antifungal

Proprietary Name. Nizoral
cis - 1 - Acetyl - 4 - {4 - [2 - (2,4 - dichlorophenyl) - 2 - imidazol - 1 - ylmethyl-1,3-dioxolan-4-ylmethoxy]phenyl}piperazine
$C_{26}H_{28}Cl_2N_4O_4 = 531.4$
CAS—65277-42-1

Crystals. M.p. 146°.

Practically **insoluble** in water; soluble 1 in 54 of ethanol, 1 in about 2 of chloroform, and 1 in 9 of methanol; very slightly soluble in ether.

Ultraviolet Spectrum. Aqueous acid—269 nm ($A_1^1 = 26$ a); aqueous alkali—287 nm ($A_1^1 = 29$ b); methanol—244 nm ($A_1^1 = 280$ b), 296 nm ($A_1^1 = 32$ b).

Infra-red Spectrum. Principal peaks at wavenumbers 1507, 1640, 1240, 1258, 1200, 1221 (KBr disk).

Wavelength

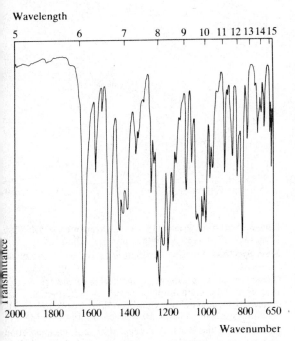

Wavenumber

Quantification. HIGH PRESSURE LIQUID CHROMATOGRAPHY. In plasma: sensitivity < 100 ng/ml, UV detection—K. B. Alton, *J. Chromat.*, 1980, *221*; *Biomed. Appl.*, *10*, 337–344. In serum, plasma, cerebrospinal fluid, or synovial fluid: sensitivity 40 ng/ml, fluorescence detection—V. L. Pascucci *et al.*, *J. pharm. Sci.*, 1983, *72*, 1467–1469.

Disposition in the Body. Readily but incompletely absorbed after oral administration and extensively metabolised to inactive metabolites. About 13% of a dose is excreted in the urine in 4 days and 57% is eliminated in the faeces in the same period.

THERAPEUTIC CONCENTRATION.
Following single oral doses of 200 and 400 mg to 6 subjects, mean peak serum concentrations of 3.6 and 6.5 µg/ml were attained in 2 and 3 hours, respectively (T. K. Daneshmend *et al.*, *J. antimicrob. Chemother.*, 1981, *8*, 299–304).

HALF-LIFE. Plasma half-life, about 6 to 10 hours.

DISTRIBUTION IN BLOOD. Plasma: whole blood ratio, 1.6.

PROTEIN BINDING. In plasma, about 99%.

NOTE. For a review of the pharmacokinetics of systemic antifungal drugs see T. K. Daneshmend and D. W. Warnock, *Clin. Pharmacokinet.*, 1983, *8*, 17–42.

Dose. 200 to 400 mg daily.

Ketoprofen   *Analgesic*

Proprietary Names. Alrheumat; Orudis; Oruvail; Profénid.
2-(3-Benzoylphenyl)propionic acid
$C_{16}H_{14}O_3 = 254.3$
CAS—22071-15-4

CH₃·CH·COOH

CO·C₆H₅

A white crystalline powder. M.p. 93° to 96°.
Practically **insoluble** in water; freely soluble in ethanol, chloroform, and ether.

Partition Coefficient. Log *P* (octanol/pH 7.4), 0.

Colour Tests. Aromaticity (Method 2)—colourless/yellow; Koppanyi–Zwikker Test—violet.

Thin-layer Chromatography. *System TD*—Rf 27; *system TE*—Rf 07; *system TF*—Rf 40; *system TG*—Rf 14. (*Ludy Tenger reagent*, orange.)

Gas Chromatography. *System GD*—retention time of methyl derivative 1.45 relative to *n*-C₁₆H₃₄.

High Pressure Liquid Chromatography. *System HD*—k' 2.4; *system HV*—retention time 0.66 relative to meclofenamic acid.

Ultraviolet Spectrum. Aqueous acid—260 nm ($A_1^1 = 665$ a); aqueous alkali—262 nm ($A_1^1 = 647$ a).

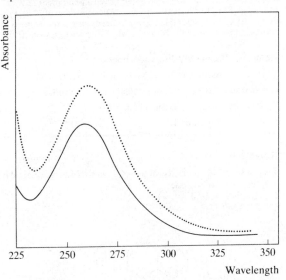

Wavelength

Infra-red Spectrum. Principal peaks at wavenumbers 1656, 1693, 1284, 714, 690, 1226 (KBr disk). Two polymorphic forms may occur. (See below)

Mass Spectrum. Principal peaks at *m/z* 105, 177, 77, 209, 254, 210, 103, 181.

Quantification. GAS CHROMATOGRAPHY. In plasma: detection limit 130 ng/ml, ECD—P. Stenberg *et al.*, *J. Chromat.*, 1979, *177*, 145–148.

HIGH PRESSURE LIQUID CHROMATOGRAPHY. In plasma or urine: limit of detection 50 ng/ml, UV detection—C. M. Kaye *et al.*, *Br. J. clin. Pharmac.*, 1981, *11*, 395–398.

Wavelength

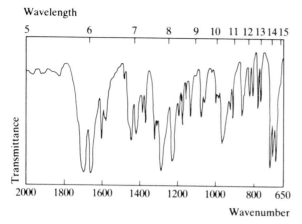

Disposition in the Body. Readily absorbed after oral, rectal, or intramuscular administration. About 75% of a single oral dose is excreted in the urine in 24 hours, mostly in the first 6 hours, about 90% of which is the glucuronide conjugate; hydroxylation may also occur.

THERAPEUTIC CONCENTRATION.

After oral administration of 100 mg as capsules, to 7 subjects, peak plasma concentrations of 6.0 to 14.3 μg/ml (mean 10) were attained in 0.45 to 2.5 hours; a single rectal dose of 100 mg, produced peak plasma concentrations of 4.7 to 10.5 μg/ml (mean 7.5) in 0.75 to 1.5 hours, and an intramuscular dose of 100 mg produced peak concentrations of 8.3 to 13.2 μg/ml (mean 10.4) in 0.33 to 0.5 hour. After oral doses of 50 mg four times a day to 7 subjects, mean maximum steady-state concentrations of 5.6 μg/ml were reported (T. Ishizaki *et al.*, *Eur. J. clin. Pharmac.*, 1980, *18*, 407–414).

HALF-LIFE. Plasma half-life, 1 to 4 hours.

VOLUME OF DISTRIBUTION. About 0.1 to 0.2 litre/kg.

CLEARANCE. Plasma clearance, about 1 to 2 ml/min/kg.

PROTEIN BINDING. In plasma, about 95%.

Dose. 100 to 200 mg daily.

Ketotifen

Anti-allergic

4 - (1 - Methyl - 4 - piperidylidene) - 4H - benzo[4,5]cyclohepta[1, 2-*b*]thiophen-10(9H)-one
$C_{19}H_{19}NOS = 309.4$
CAS—34580-13-7

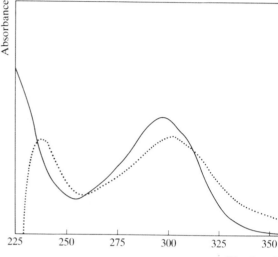

Crystals. M.p. 151° to 153°.

Ketotifen Fumarate
Proprietary Name. Zaditen
$C_{19}H_{19}NOS,C_4H_4O_4 = 425.5$
CAS—34580-14-8
A white crystalline powder. M.p. 190° to 196°, with decomposition.

Slightly **soluble** in water; soluble in ethanol; sparingly soluble in chloroform.

Gas Chromatography. *System GA*—RI 2607.

Ultraviolet Spectrum. Aqueous acid—297 nm ($A_1^1 = 475$ a) aqueous alkali—237 nm, 302 nm.

Infra-red Spectrum. Principal peaks at wavenumbers 1650, 1280, 1255, 1302, 1720, 1180 (ketotifen fumarate, KBr disk).

Mass Spectrum. Principal peaks at m/z 309, 96, 42, 58, 98, 70, 57, 44.

Quantification. GAS CHROMATOGRAPHY–MASS SPECTROMETRY. In plasma: detection limit 50 pg/ml for ketotifen and the desmethyl metabolite, 300 pg/ml for 10-hydroxyketotifen—C. Julien-Larose *et al.*, *Biomed. Mass Spectrom.*, 1983, *10*, 136–142.

Disposition in the Body. Absorbed after oral administration. Metabolised by 10-hydroxylation, N-demethylation, and glucuronic acid conjugation. It is excreted in the urine and faeces as unchanged drug and metabolites.

THERAPEUTIC CONCENTRATION.

Following a single oral dose of 2 mg to 3 subjects, a peak plasma concentration of about 0.0006 μg/ml was attained in 2 hours; a peak plasma concentration of about 0.015 μg/ml of ketotifen glucuronide was attained in about 4 hours (C. Julien-Larose *et al.*, *ibid.*).

TOXICITY.

In 8 cases of overdose involving ingestion of up to 120 mg, drowsiness and other toxic effects were reported but in each case full recovery occurred within 12 hours. In 3 cases involving the ingestion of 10, 50, and 120 mg, plasma concentrations were 0.016, 0.054, and 0.122 μg/ml, respectively, at 5, 3, and 20 hours after ingestion (D. B. Jefferys and G. N. Volans, *Br. med. J.*, 1981, *282*, 1755–1756 and 2014).

In a fatality involving ketotifen, a postmortem blood concentration of 1.2 μg/ml was reported (A. H. Stead and A. C. Moffat, personal communication).

Dose. The equivalent of 2 to 4 mg of ketotifen daily.

Labetalol

Antihypertensive

Synonym. Ibidomide
5 - [1 - Hydroxy - 2 - (1 - methyl - 3 - phenylpropylamino) ethyl]salicylamide
$C_{19}H_{24}N_2O_3 = 328.4$
CAS—36894-69-6

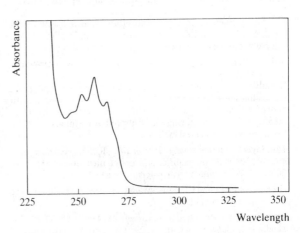

OH

CO·NH₂

CH₃

C₆H₅·CH₂·CH₂·CH·NH·CH₂·CHOH

Labetalol Hydrochloride

Proprietary Names. Trandate; Vescal.
$C_{19}H_{24}N_2O_3,HCl = 364.9$
CAS—32780-64-6
A white crystalline solid. M.p. about 180°.
Soluble in water and ethanol; practically insoluble in chloroform and ether.

Dissociation Constant. pK_a 7.4 (phenol), 8.7 ($-NH_2$).

Colour Tests. Ferric Chloride—violet; Folin–Ciocalteu Reagent—blue; Liebermann's Test—brown-orange; Mandelin's Test—green-blue; Marquis Test—red → brown-red; Nessler's Reagent (100°)—black.

Gas Chromatography. *System GA*—RI 1280.

High Pressure Liquid Chromatography. *System HA*—k' 1.7 (tailing peak).

Ultraviolet Spectrum. Aqueous acid—302 nm ($A_1^1 = 95$ a); aqueous alkali—246 nm ($A_1^1 = 267$ a), 333 nm ($A_1^1 = 161$ a).

Infra-red Spectrum. Principal peaks at wavenumbers 1680, 1643, 1502, 1270, 820, 1250 (labetalol hydrochloride, Nujol mull).

Quantification. HIGH PRESSURE LIQUID CHROMATOGRAPHY. In plasma, serum, or whole blood: detection limit 10 ng/ml, UV detection—I. J. Hidalgo and K. T. Muir, *J. Chromat.*, 1984, *305*; *Biomed. Appl.*, *30*, 222–227. In postmortem tissues: UV detection—L. K. Panell *et al.*, *J. analyt. Toxicol.*, 1982, *6*, 193–195.

RADIORECEPTOR ASSAY. In plasma: sensitivity 5 ng/ml—J. G. Kelly *et al.*, *Br. J. clin. Pharmac.*, 1981, *12*, 258–260.

Disposition in the Body. Well absorbed after oral administration but undergoes extensive first-pass metabolism; bioavailability 10 to 80% (mean 30). The major metabolites are glucuronides of labetalol. Up to about 60% of a dose is excreted in the urine in 24 hours as conjugates, one of which has been identified as the *O*-phenylglucuronide; about 5% of a dose is excreted as unchanged drug.

THERAPEUTIC CONCENTRATION.
After a single oral dose of 100 mg given to 6 subjects, peak plasma concentrations of 0.09 to 0.25 µg/ml (mean 0.16) were attained in about 0.5 hour; following a single oral dose of 200 mg to the same subjects, peak plasma concentrations of 0.09 to 0.27 µg/ml (mean 0.19) were reported at about 1 hour (J. J. McNeil *et al.*, *Br. J. clin. Pharmac.*, 1979, *8*, Suppl. 2, 157S–161S).
Following oral administration of 200 mg twice daily to 9 subjects, average steady-state plasma concentrations of 0.04 to 0.18 µg/ml (mean 0.09) were reported (J. J. McNeil *et al.*, *Br. J. clin. Pharmac.*, 1982, *13*, Suppl. 1, 75S–80S).

TOXICITY.
A 68-year-old subject suffering from chronic respiratory disease died about 1 hour after inadvertently being given 200 mg of labetalol. Postmortem kidney and liver concentrations of 10.6 and 20.5 µg/g respectively, were reported and were considered to be consistent with a therapeutic dose; death was attributed to respiratory disease (L. K. Panell *et al.*, *J. analyt. Toxicol.*, 1982, *6*, 193–195).

HALF-LIFE. Plasma half-life, 3 to 6 hours.

VOLUME OF DISTRIBUTION. About 3 to 10 litres/kg (mean 7).

CLEARANCE. Plasma clearance, 10 to 40 ml/min/kg (mean 25).

PROTEIN BINDING. In plasma, about 50%.

NOTE. For a review of the pharmacokinetics of labetalol see J. J. McNeil and W. J. Louis, *Clin. Pharmacokinet.*, 1984, *9*, 157–167.

Dose. 200 to 800 mg of labetalol hydrochloride daily; doses of 2.4 g daily have been given.

Lachesine Chloride   *Anticholinergic*

(2-Benziloyloxyethyl)ethyldimethylammonium chloride
$C_{20}H_{26}ClNO_3 = 363.9$
CAS—1164-38-1

$$\left[\begin{array}{c} C_6H_5 \\ HO\cdot\overset{|}{C}\cdot CO\cdot O\cdot [CH_2]_2\cdot \overset{+}{N}\cdot C_2H_5 \\ C_6H_5 \end{array} \begin{array}{c} CH_3 \\ \\ CH_3 \end{array} \right] Cl^-$$

A white amorphous powder. M.p. 212° to 214°.
Soluble 1 in 3 of water and 1 in 10 of ethanol (90%); very slightly soluble in chloroform and ether.

Colour Tests. Mandelin's Test—orange → green; Marquis Test—orange → green → blue.

Thin-layer Chromatography. *System TA*—Rf 02. (*Acidified iodoplatinate solution*, positive.)

Gas Chromatography. *System GA*—RI 1852.

Ultraviolet Spectrum. Aqueous acid—252 nm, 258 nm ($A_1^1 = 12$ b), 264 nm. No alkaline shift.

[Graph: vertical axis labelled "Absorbance", horizontal axis labelled "Wavelength", with marks at 225, 250, 275, 300, 325, 350]

Infra-red Spectrum. Principal peaks at wavenumbers 1739, 1241, 699, 743, 1176, 1191 (KBr disk).

Use. As a 1% ophthalmic solution.

Lanatoside C   *Cardiac Glycoside*

Synonym. Celanide
Proprietary Names. Cedilanid(e); Celadigal; Lanimerck; Lanocide.
Note. The name Cedilanid(e) is also applied to a preparation of deslanoside.

3β-[(*O*-β-D-Glucopyranosyl-(1 → 4)-*O*-3-acetyl-2,6-dideoxy-β-D - *ribo* - hexopyranosyl - (1 → 4) - *O* - 2,6 - dideoxy - β - D - *ribo* - hexopyranosyl - (1 → 4) - 2,6 - dideoxy - β - D - *ribo* - hexopyranosyl)oxy]-12β,14-dihydroxy-5β,14β-card-20(22)-enolide
$C_{49}H_{76}O_{20} = 985.1$
CAS—17575-22-3

A glycoside obtained from the leaves of the woolly foxglove, *Digitalis lanata* (Scrophulariaceae).

Colourless or white hygroscopic crystals or white crystalline powder. It melts above 240°, indistinctly and with decomposition.

Practically **insoluble** in water and ether; sparingly soluble in ethanol; soluble 1 in 2000 of chloroform and 1 in 20 of methanol; soluble in dioxan and pyridine.

Colour Tests. Antimony Pentachloride—yellow → brown → black-violet.

Dissolve 2 to 3 mg in 5 ml of a solution containing 0.5 ml of 9% ferric chloride solution and 100 ml of *acetic acid*; underlay with 5 ml of *sulphuric acid*—an intense blue colour forms in the acetic acid layer and a brown ring free from red at the junction of the two liquids (see also Deslanoside).

Thin-layer Chromatography. *System TK*—Rf 36. (*Perchloric acid solution*, followed by examination under ultraviolet light, blue fluorescence; p-*anisaldehyde reagent*, blue.)

High Pressure Liquid Chromatography. *System HM*—lanatoside C k′ 39.5, digoxin k′ 11.3.

Mass Spectrum. Principal peaks at *m/z* 41, 43, 29, 55, 39, 57, 73, 81; digoxin 73, 58, 57, 43, 41, 39, 29, 45 (no peaks above 360).

Quantification. RADIOIMMUNOASSAY. In serum—A. C. Moffat, *Acta pharmac. tox.*, 1974, *35*, 386–394.

Disposition in the Body. Poorly absorbed after oral administration; it is converted to digoxin in the gastro-intestinal tract and very little unchanged drug is found in the plasma or urine after oral administration. Hydrolysis to derivatives of digoxigenin and deacetylation to deslanoside also occur. After an oral dose, about 18% is excreted in the urine in 24 hours, mostly as digoxin and metabolites of digoxigenin; after intravenous administration, about 30% of a dose is excreted in the urine in 24 hours with about 70% of the urinary material consisting of unchanged drug and the remainder being digoxin and deslanoside. A total of about 60% of an intravenous dose is excreted in the urine in 5 days.

THERAPEUTIC CONCENTRATION. In serum, usually in the range 0.0004 to 0.001 μg/ml.

Following a single oral dose of 0.5 mg of ³H-lanatoside C to 9 subjects, peak plasma concentrations of unchanged drug plus metabolites of about 0.002 μg/ml were attained after about 1 hour and a second peak of approximately the same concentration was reported in each subject after 5 to 8 hours (S. Aldous *et al.*, *Aust. J. pharm. Sci.*, 1972, *1*, 35–41).

TOXICITY.

A postmortem blood concentration of 0.047 μg/ml was reported in a fatality involving an overdose of lanatoside C; death occurred 48 hours after ingestion (A. C. Moffat, *Acta pharmac. tox.*, 1974, *35*, 386–394).

DISTRIBUTION IN BLOOD. Plasma: whole blood ratio, 1.2.

PROTEIN BINDING. In plasma, about 25%.

Dose. For slow digitalisation, 1.5 to 2 mg daily for 3 to 5 days; maintenance, 0.25 to 1.5 mg daily.

Levallorphan   *Narcotic Antagonist*

(−)-9a-Allylmorphinan-3-ol
$C_{19}H_{25}NO = 283.4$
CAS—152-02-3

White crystals. M.p. 180° to 182°.

Levallorphan Tartrate

Proprietary Names. Lorfan. It is an ingredient of Pethilorfan.
$C_{19}H_{25}NO,C_4H_6O_6 = 433.5$
CAS—71-82-9
A white crystalline powder. M.p. 174° to 177°.

Soluble 1 in about 20 of water, 1 in 100 of ethanol, 1 in 3300 of chloroform, 1 in 5000 of ether, and 1 in 13 of methanol.

Dissociation Constant. pK_a 4.5, 6.9.

Partition Coefficient. Log *P* (octanol/pH 7.4), 2.3.

Colour Tests. Aromaticity (Method 2)—yellow/orange; Liebermann's Test—black.

Thin-layer Chromatography. *System TA*—Rf 67; *system TB*—Rf 19; *system TC*—Rf 24. (*Dragendorff spray*, positive; *FPN reagent*, yellow; *acidified iodoplatinate solution*, positive; *Marquis reagent*, grey.)

Gas Chromatography. *System GA*—RI 2359.

High Pressure Liquid Chromatography. *System HA*—k′ 1.9 (tailing peak); *system HC*—k′ 1.46.

Ultraviolet Spectrum. Aqueous acid—279 nm ($A_1^1 = 71$ a); aqueous alkali—240 nm ($A_1^1 = 312$ a), 299 nm.

Infra-red Spectrum. Principal peaks at wavenumbers 759, 1271, 747, 1575, 1242, 932 (Nujol mull).

Mass Spectrum. Principal peaks at *m/z* 283, 282, 256, 176, 157, 43, 41, 57.

Disposition in the Body. Levallorphan is effective within 1 minute of intravenous injection and the effects may last up to 4 hours. It is metabolised by *N*-dealkylation and glucuronic acid conjugation.

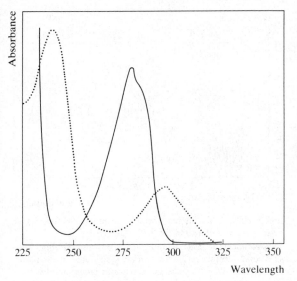

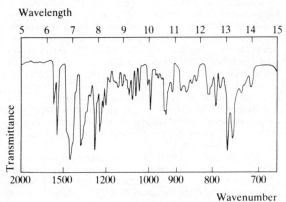

TOXICITY. The estimated minimum lethal dose is 0.2 g or 2 g for an addict.

Dose. 0.5 to 1 mg of levallorphan tartrate intravenously, repeated if necessary.

Levamisole   *Anthelmintic*

Synonym. *l*-Tetramisole
(*S*)-2,3,5,6-Tetrahydro-6-phenylimidazo[2,1-*b*]thiazole
$C_{11}H_{12}N_2S = 204.3$
CAS—14769-73-4

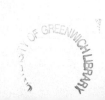

A white crystalline powder. M.p. 60° to 62°.
Soluble in dilute acetic acid and in chloroform.

Levamisole Hydrochloride

Proprietary Names. Cyverm (vet.); Ergamisol; Ketrax; Nemicide (vet.); Nilverm (vet.); Solaskil.

$C_{11}H_{12}N_2S,HCl = 240.8$
CAS—16595-80-5
A white to pale cream-coloured crystalline powder. M.p. 227° to 229°.
Soluble 1 in 2 of water and 1 in 5 of methanol; practically insoluble in ether.

Dissociation Constant. pK_a 8.0.

Colour Tests. Liebermann's Test—red-orange; Mandelin's Test —orange → grey-green.

Thin-layer Chromatography. *System TA*—Rf 62; *system TB*—Rf 18; *system TC*—Rf 48. (*Acidified iodoplatinate solution*, positive.)

Gas Chromatography. *System GA*—RI 1928.

Infra-red Spectrum. Principal peaks at wavenumbers 1587, 1575, 1197, 699, 1150, 1248 (KBr disk).

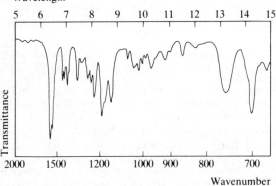

Mass Spectrum. Principal peaks at *m/z* 204, 148, 73, 101, 203, 127, 104, 205.

Quantification. GAS CHROMATOGRAPHY. In plasma: sensitivity 4 ng/ml, AFID—F. Rousseau *et al.*, *Eur. J. drug Met. Pharmacokinet.*, 1981, *6*, 281–288.

HIGH PRESSURE LIQUID CHROMATOGRAPHY. In sheep or cattle plasma: detection limit 20 ng/ml, UV detection—S. Marriner *et al.*, *Analyst, Lond.*, 1980, *105*, 993–996.

Disposition in the Body. Readily absorbed after oral administration, but extensively metabolised. It is almost completely excreted in the urine and faeces within 48 hours.

THERAPEUTIC CONCENTRATION.

Following single oral doses of 2.5 mg/kg and 5 mg/kg to 11 subjects, mean peak plasma concentrations of 0.7 and 1.5 µg/ml, respectively, were attained within 2 hours (M. Luyckx *et al.*, *Eur. J. drug Met. Pharmacokinet.*, 1982, *7*, 247–254).

HALF-LIFE. Plasma half-life, about 4 hours.

Dose. The equivalent of 2.5 to 5 mg/kg of levamisole daily, for 2 or 3 days.

Levamphetamine   *Central Stimulant*

Synonyms. (−)-Amphetamine; Laevo-amphetamine.
(−)-α-Methylphenethylamine
$C_9H_{13}N = 135.2$
CAS—156-34-3

$$C_6H_5 \cdot CH_2 \cdot \overset{\overset{\displaystyle NH_2}{|}}{CH} \cdot CH_3$$

For analytical data see under Amphetamine.

Levodopa
Dopaminergic Agent

Synonyms. Dihydroxyphenylalanine; Dopa; L-Dopa; Laevo-dopa.

Proprietary Names. Bendopa; Berkdopa; Brocadopa; Dopar; Eldopal; Larodopa; Levopa; Syndopa. It is an ingredient of Madopar, Prolopa, and Sinemet.

(−)-3-(3,4-Dihydroxyphenyl)-L-alanine
$C_9H_{11}NO_4 = 197.2$
CAS—59-92-7

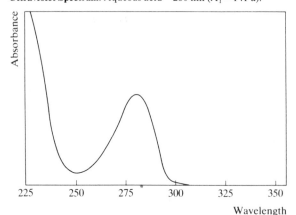

A white or slightly cream-coloured crystalline powder, which darkens on exposure to air and light. M.p. about 275°, with decomposition.

Soluble 1 in 300 of water; practically insoluble in ethanol, chloroform, and ether; soluble in aqueous solutions of mineral acids and alkali carbonates.

Dissociation Constant. pK_a 2.3, 8.7, 9.7, 13.4 (25°).

Colour Tests. Ammoniacal Silver Nitrate—yellow → brown/black; Ferric Chloride—green; Folin–Ciocalteu Reagent—blue; Methanolic Potassium Hydroxide—pink → red-brown; Millon's Reagent (cold)—brown-red; Nessler's Reagent—black; Palladium Chloride—orange (→ brown); Potassium Dichromate (Method 1)—green → brown.

Ultraviolet Spectrum. Aqueous acid—280 nm ($A_1^1 = 141$ a).

Infra-red Spectrum. Principal peaks at wavenumbers 1647, 1562, 1117, 1241, 1274, 1520 (KBr disk).

Mass Spectrum. Principal peaks at m/z 123, 124, 77, 44, 51, 74, 53, 39.

Quantification. GAS CHROMATOGRAPHY. In plasma: levodopa and dopamine, ECD—Y. Mizuno, *Clinica chim. Acta*, 1977, *74*, 11–19.

HIGH PRESSURE LIQUID CHROMATOGRAPHY. In plasma: levodopa and 3,4-dihydroxyphenylacetic acid, sensitivity 1 ng/ml, electrochemical detection—E. Nissinen and J. Taskinen, *J. Chromat.*, 1982, *231*; *Biomed. Appl.*, *20*, 459–462. In urine: levodopa and

Wavelength

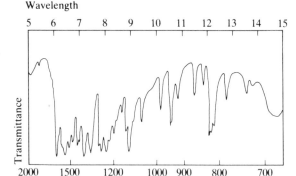

Wavenumber

metabolites, UV and fluorescence detection—J. Seki *et al.*, *Chem. pharm. Bull.*, 1981, *29*, 789–795.

Disposition in the Body. Rapidly absorbed from the small bowel after oral administration and widely distributed in the tissues; less than 1% of a dose reaches the brain; bioavailability about 33%. Extensively metabolised mainly by decarboxylation to dopamine, which is further metabolised, and also by methylation to 3-O-methyldopa which accumulates in the central nervous system; most of a dose is decarboxylated by the gastric mucosa before entering the systemic circulation; the decarboxylase activity is inhibited by carbidopa and benserazide. Dopamine is further metabolised to noradrenaline, 3-methoxytyramine, and to the two major excretory metabolites, 3,4-dihydroxyphenylacetic acid (DOPAC) and 3-methoxy-4-hydroxyphenylacetic acid (homovanillic acid, HVA). During prolonged therapy, the rate of levodopa metabolism appears to increase, possibly due to enzyme induction. About 70 to 80% of a dose is excreted in the urine in 24 hours. Of the material excreted in the urine, about 50% is DOPAC and HVA, 10% is dopamine, up to 30% is 3-O-methyldopa, and less than 1% is unchanged drug. Less than 1% of a dose is eliminated in the faeces. During prolonged therapy the ratio of the amount of DOPAC produced to that of HVA may be increased.

THERAPEUTIC CONCENTRATION. There is considerable intersubject variation in plasma concentrations and there appears to be no significant correlation between plasma concentrations of levodopa or its metabolites and therapeutic effect.

Following single oral doses of 1.5 g to 42 subjects, peak plasma-levodopa concentrations averaged about 1 μg/ml at 1 to 2 hours but there was a tenfold variation in peak concentrations. Peak plasma concentrations of 3-O-methyldopa of about 1.5 μg/ml were attained in about 4 hours and concentrations of HVA in the cerebrospinal fluid reached a maximum of about 0.15 μg/ml in 8 hours (S. Bergmann *et al.*, *Br. J. clin. Pharmac.*, 1974, *1*, 417–424).

HALF-LIFE. Plasma half-life, about 1 hour which may be increased by concomitant administration of peripheral decarboxylase inhibitors; 3-O-methyldopa about 13 hours.

CLEARANCE. Plasma clearance, about 23 ml/min/kg.

Dose. Initially, 0.25 to 1 g daily; maintenance, up to 8 g daily.

Levomethadyl Acetate
Narcotic Analgesic

Synonyms. *l*-Acetylmethadol; LAAM; LAM; Levacetylmethadol.

(−)-4-Dimethylamino-1-ethyl-2,2-diphenylpentyl acetate
$C_{23}H_{31}NO_2 = 353.5$
CAS—1477-40-3 (levomethadyl); *34433-66-4* (acetate)

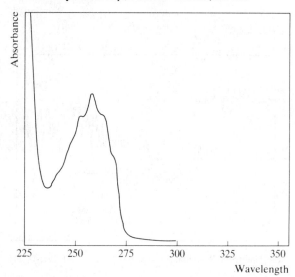

CH₃·CH₂ C₆H₅   CH₃

CH₃·CO·O·CH·C·CH₂·CH·N(CH₃)₂

C₆H₅

M.p. about 70°.

Levomethadyl Acetate Hydrochloride
$C_{23}H_{31}NO_2,HCl = 390.0$
CAS—38821-43-1
Crystals. M.p. 215°.
Soluble in water.

Dissociation Constant. pK_a 8.3.

Colour Tests. Mandelin's Test—grey-green; Marquis Test—violet-brown → grey-green.

Thin-layer Chromatography. *System TA*—Rf 57; *system TB*—Rf 62; *system TC*—Rf 39. (*Acidified iodoplatinate solution*, positive.)

Gas Chromatography. *System GA*—RI 2187.

High Pressure Liquid Chromatography. *System HA*—k′ 1.7.

Ultraviolet Spectrum. Aqueous acid—253 nm, 258 nm.

Infra-red Spectrum. Principal peaks at wavenumbers 1240, 1735, 702, 1496, 1015, 1031.

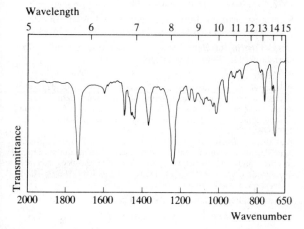

Mass Spectrum. Principal peaks at *m/z* 72, 73, 43, 91, 224, 56, 71, 129.

Quantification. GAS CHROMATOGRAPHY. In plasma: sensitivity 10 ng/ml for levomethadyl acetate using FID, 5 ng/ml and 25 ng/ml for L-α-noracetylmethadol and L-α-dinoracetylmethadol, respectively, using ECD—F. L. S. Tse and P. G. Welling, *Biopharm. Drug Disp.*, 1980, *1*, 203–209.

GAS CHROMATOGRAPHY–MASS SPECTROMETRY. In plasma, whole blood or tissues: levomethadyl acetate and demethylated metabolites, sensitivity 5 ng/ml—T. A. Jennison *et al.*, *J. chromatogr. Sci.*, 1979, *17*, 64–74.

HIGH PRESSURE LIQUID CHROMATOGRAPHY. In plasma or urine: levomethadyl acetate and metabolites, sensitivity 6 ng/ml for levomethadyl acetate, L-α-noracetylmethadol and methadol, 10 ng/ml for L-α-dinoracetylmethadol, normethadol, and dinormethadol—C.- H. Kiang *et al.*, *J. Chromat.*, 1981, *222*; *Biomed. Appl.*, *11*, 81–93.

RADIOIMMUNOASSAY. In biological fluids: sensitivity 50 pg—K. L. McGilliard and G. D. Olsen, *J. Pharmac. exp. Ther.*, 1980, *215*, 205–212.

Disposition in the Body. Absorbed after oral administration. It is metabolised principally by *N*-demethylation to L-α-noracetylmethadol and L-α-dinoracetylmethadol which are active narcotics, and also by deacetylation to methadol which is also active; further demethylation to normethadol and dinormethadol also occurs. L-α-Noracetylmethadol, L-α-dinoracetylmethadol and, in some subjects, unchanged drug accumulate during chronic oral administration, but there is considerable intersubject variation. About 20 to 25% of a dose is excreted in the urine as unchanged drug and demethylated metabolites, and about 2% as methadol and normethadol.

THERAPEUTIC CONCENTRATION.

After a single oral dose of 60 mg given to 5 subjects, peak plasma concentrations of 0.09 to 0.16 μg/ml (mean 0.13) of levomethadyl acetate and 0.04 to 0.05 μg/ml of L-α-noracetylmethadol were attained in about 2 to 4 hours and 2 to 6 hours, respectively; following chronic oral treatment with 85 mg three times a week for three months to 3 subjects, peak plasma concentrations were: levomethadyl acetate 0.16 to 0.23 μg/ml (mean 0.20), L-α-noracetylmethadol 0.15 to 0.30 μg/ml (mean 0.24), and L-α-dinoracetylmethadol, mean 0.27 μg/ml (G. L. Henderson *et al.*, *Clin. Pharmac. Ther.*, 1977, *21*, 16–25).

TOXICITY.

The following postmortem tissue concentrations, μg/ml (mean, *n*), were reported in 9 heroin addicts who died unexpectedly during treatment with levomethadyl acetate:

	Levomethadyl Acetate	L-α-Noracetyl-methadol	L-α-Dinoracetyl-methadol
Blood	0.01–0.12 (0.05, 7)	0.01–0.22 (0.08, 7)	0.01–0.17 (0.05,7)
Brain	0.04, 0.24 (2)	0.07, 0.42 (2)	0.14, 0.34 (2)
Kidney	0.01–0.69 (0.28, 6)	0.01–1.2 (0.5, 6)	0.04–1.1 (0.66, 6)
Liver	0.01–0.7 (0.31, 7)	0.01–1.43 (0.70, 7)	0.03–2.08 (1.0, 7)
Lung	0.03–2.49 (0.95, 3)	0.04–6.0 (2.3, 3)	0.21–8.52 (3.8, 3)
Urine	0.05–1.76 (0.72, 4)	0.22–3.04 (1.1, 4)	0.46–2.0 (1.0, 4)

Other drugs (mainly diazepam, methadone or morphine) were detected in all subjects except one in which the cause of death was multiple stab wounds (D. M. Chinn *et al.*, *J. analyt. Toxicol.*, 1979, *3*, 143–149).

HALF-LIFE. Plasma half-life, levomethadyl acetate about 50 hours, L-α-noracetylmethadol 30 to 65 hours, L-α-dinoracetylmethadol about 170 hours.

Dose. Usually up to 80 mg three times a week.

Levopropoxyphene   *Cough Suppressant*

(−)-1-Benzyl-3-dimethylamino-2-methyl-1-phenylpropyl propionate
$C_{22}H_{29}NO_2 = 339.5$
CAS—2338-37-6

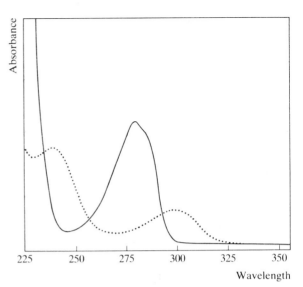

Crystals. M.p. 75° to 76°.

Levopropoxyphene Napsylate

Synonym. Levopropoxyphene Naphthalene-2-sulphonate
Proprietary Name. Novrad
$C_{22}H_{29}NO_2,C_{10}H_8O_3S,H_2O = 565.7$
CAS—5714-90-9 (anhydrous); *55557-30-7* (monohydrate)
A white powder. M.p. 158° to 165°.
Very slightly **soluble** in water; soluble 1 in 17 of ethanol and 1 in 2 of
chloroform; soluble in acetone and methanol.
For analytical data see under Dextropropoxyphene.

Dose. The equivalent of 50 to 100 mg of levopropoxyphene every
4 hours.

Levorphanol   *Narcotic Analgesic*

Synonyms. Levorphan; Methorphinan.
(−)-9a-Methylmorphinan-3-ol
$C_{17}H_{23}NO = 257.4$
CAS—77-07-6

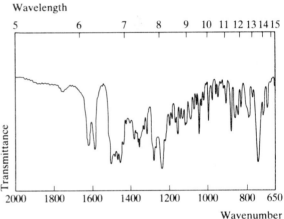

Crystals. M.p. 198° to 199°.

Levorphanol Tartrate

Synonym. Levorphanol Bitartrate
Proprietary Names. Dalmadorm; Dalmate; Dormador; Dromoran; Levo-
Dromoran.
$C_{17}H_{23}NO,C_4H_6O_6,2H_2O = 443.5$
CAS—125-72-4 (anhydrous); *5985-38-6* (dihydrate)
A white crystalline powder. M.p. 114° to 117°.
Soluble 1 in about 45 of water and 1 in about 110 of ethanol; practically
insoluble in chloroform.

Dissociation Constant. pK_a 8.2 (20°).

Partition Coefficient. Log *P* (octanol/pH 7.4), 1.1.

Thin-layer Chromatography. *System TA*—Rf 35; *system TB*—Rf
13; *system TC*—Rf 07. (*Dragendorff spray*, positive; *acidified
iodoplatinate solution*, positive.)

Gas Chromatography. *System GA*—RI 2230; *system GC*—RI
2230.

High Pressure Liquid Chromatography. *System HA*—k' 4.4
(tailing peak); *system HC*—k' 3.20.

Ultraviolet Spectrum. Aqueous acid—279 nm $(A_1^1 = 79 \text{ a})$;
aqueous alkali—240 nm $(A_1^1 = 339 \text{ a})$, 299 nm $(A_1^1 = 119 \text{ a})$.

Infra-red Spectrum. Principal peaks at wavenumbers 1238, 1495,
753, 1278, 1578, 1608 (KBr disk).

Mass Spectrum. Principal peaks at *m/z* 59, 257, 150, 256, 44, 31,
200, 157.

Quantification. GAS CHROMATOGRAPHY–MASS SPECTROMETRY.
In plasma: sensitivity 1 ng/ml—B. H. Min *et al.*, *J. Chromat.*,
1982, *231*; *Biomed. Appl.*, *20*, 194–199.

RADIOIMMUNOASSAY. In plasma: sensitivity 1 ng/ml—R. Dixon
et al., *Res. Commun. chem. Path. Pharmac.*, 1981, *32*, 545–548.

Disposition in the Body. Absorbed after oral administration.
Metabolised by 3-glucuronidation.

TOXICITY.

Postmortem concentrations in a 41-year-old female found dead after
having ingested an unknown quantity of levorphanol were: blood 2.7
µg/ml, bile 24 µg/ml, brain 1.8 µg/g, kidney 3.4 µg/g, liver 5.4 µg/g, lung
17 µg/g, urine 2.3 µg/ml (J. E. Turner *et al.*, *J. analyt. Toxicol.*, 1977, *1*,
103–104).

A 61-year-old man ingested 30 mg of levorphanol and died about 18 hours
later. The antemortem blood concentration was 0.8 µg/ml. Concentrations
in other fluids and tissues (samples taken after the body had been
embalmed) were: bile 15 µg/ml, kidney 1 µg/g, liver 11 µg/g (L. R.
Bednarczyk, *J. analyt. Toxicol.*, 1979, *3*, 217–219).

HALF-LIFE. Plasma half-life, about 13 hours.

Dose. 1.5 to 9 mg of levorphanol tartrate daily.

Lidoflazine

Anti-anginal

Synonym. Ordiflazine

Proprietary Names. Clinium; Corflazine.

4 - [3 - (4,4' - Difluorobenzhydryl)propyl]piperazin - 1 - ylaceto - 2',
6'-xylidide

$C_{30}H_{35}F_2N_3O = 491.6$

CAS—3416-26-0

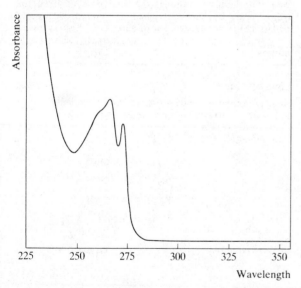

A white or slightly yellow amorphous powder. M.p. 158° to 161°.
Practically **insoluble** in water; soluble 1 in 90 of ethanol and 1 in
220 of ether; very soluble in chloroform.

Colour Tests. Mandelin's Test—yellow; Marquis Test—yellow.

Thin-layer Chromatography. *System TA*—Rf 70; *system TB*—Rf
11; *system TC*—Rf 63. (*Acidified iodoplatinate solution*, positive.)

Gas Chromatography. *System GA*—not eluted.

High Pressure Liquid Chromatography. *System HA*—k' 0.6.

Ultraviolet Spectrum. Acid isopropyl alcohol—266 nm ($A_1^1 =$
47 b), 272 nm.

Infra-red Spectrum. Principal peaks at wavenumbers 1505, 1645,
1220, 1155, 835, 775 (KBr disk).

Mass Spectrum. Principal peaks at *m/z* 343, 70, 344, 109, 42,
113, 491, 56.

Disposition in the Body. Well absorbed after oral administration.
It is excreted mainly as metabolites, the major metabolites being
bis(4-fluorophenyl)butyric acid and the glucuronide conjugate
of bis(4-fluorophenyl)butan-1-ol. In 7 days, about 40% of an oral
dose is excreted in the urine and about 40% is eliminated in the
faeces.

THERAPEUTIC CONCENTRATION.

After a single oral dose of 120 mg given with food, peak plasma
concentrations of about 0.06 μg/ml were attained in about 1 hour.
Following repeated oral administration of 120 mg three times a day, a
mean steady-state plasma concentration of 0.12 μg/ml was reported
(P. M. Vanhoutte and J. M. Van Nueten, Lidoflazine, in *New Drugs
Annual: Cardiovascular Drugs*, A. Scriabine (Ed.), New York, Raven
Press, 1973, pp. 203–226).

HALF-LIFE. Plasma half-life, about 1 day.

REFERENCE. P. M. Vanhoutte and J. M. Van Nueten, *ibid*.

Dose. 120 to 360 mg daily.

Lignocaine

Local Anaesthetic/Anti-arrhythmic

Synonym. Lidocaine

2-Diethylaminoaceto-2',6'-xylidide

$C_{14}H_{22}N_2O = 234.3$

CAS—137-58-6

A white to slightly yellow crystalline powder. M.p. 66° to 69°.
Practically **insoluble** in water; very soluble in ethanol and
chloroform; freely soluble in ether.

Lignocaine Hydrochloride

Synonym. Lidocaine Hydrochloride

Proprietary Names. Anestacon; Laryng-O-Jet; Lidocaton; Lignostab;
Ultracaine; Uro-Jet; Xylocaine; Xylocard.

$C_{14}H_{22}N_2O,HCl,H_2O = 288.8$

CAS—73-78-9 (anhydrous); *6108-05-0* (monohydrate)

A white crystalline powder. M.p. 74° to 79°.

Soluble 1 in 0.7 of water, 1 in 1.5 of ethanol, and 1 in 40 of chloroform;
practically insoluble in ether.

Dissociation Constant. pK_a 7.9 (25°).

Colour Test. To a 2% solution in water, add 1 ml of dilute nitric
acid and 3 ml of *mercuric nitrate solution* and heat to boiling—
yellow or yellow-green.

Thin-layer Chromatography. *System TA*—Rf 70; *system TB*—Rf
35; *system TC*—Rf 73; *system TL*—Rf 63. (*Dragendorff spray*,
positive; *acidified iodoplatinate solution*, positive; *Marquis reagent*, pink.)

Gas Chromatography. *System GA*—RI 1870; *system GF*—RI
2240.

High Pressure Liquid Chromatography. *System HA*—lignocaine
k' 0.6, monoethylglycinexylidide k' 1.2; *system HQ*—k' 0.79.

Ultraviolet Spectrum. Aqueous acid—263 nm ($A_1^1 = 19$ a),
272 nm. (See below)

Infra-red Spectrum. Principal peaks at wavenumbers 1662, 1495,
762, 1204, 1290, 1086 (KBr disk). (See below)

Mass Spectrum. Principal peaks at *m/z* 86, 87, 58, 44, 72, 42,
120, 85.

Quantification. GAS CHROMATOGRAPHY. In blood, serum or
tissues: sensitivity 100 ng/ml, AFID—B. Levine *et al., J. analyt.
Toxicol.*, 1983, **7**, 123–124. In plasma: lignocaine and monoethylglycinexylidide, sensitivity 300 ng/ml, AFID—J. D. Hawkins *et al., Ther. Drug Monit.*, 1982, **4**, 103–106.

Absorbance (y-axis)

Wavelength (x-axis: 225, 250, 275, 300, 325, 350)

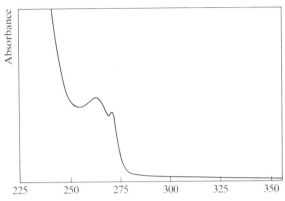

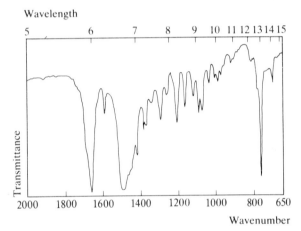

HIGH PRESSURE LIQUID CHROMATOGRAPHY. In serum: sensitivity 100 ng/ml for lignocaine, 50 ng/ml for monoethylglycinexylidide and glycinexylidide, UV detection—R. Lindberg *et al.*, *Clin. Chem.*, 1983, *29*, 1572–1573.

Disposition in the Body. Readily absorbed from the gastro-intestinal tract, mucous membranes, and after intramuscular injection; oral bioavailability is low due to first-pass metabolism. Metabolic reactions include *N*-de-ethylation, hydrolysis, and ring hydroxylation. About 3% of a dose is excreted in the urine as unchanged drug in 24 hours, 40 to 70% as 4-hydroxy-2,6-xylidine, and about 4% as the active monoethylglycinexylidide; excretion of unchanged drug is increased if the urine is acid. Other metabolites include glycinexylidide (active), 2,6-xylidine, 3′-hydroxylignocaine, and 3′-hydroxymonoethylglycinexylidide. Glycinexylidide and the hydroxy metabolites are excreted as acid-hydrolysable conjugates. Glycinexylidide has also been detected in plasma after prolonged intravenous infusion.

THERAPEUTIC CONCENTRATION. In plasma, usually in the range 2 to 5 μg/ml.

Intravenous infusions at rates varying between 16 and 143 μg/min/kg were given to 31 patients; after about 10 hours, blood concentrations, normalised to an infusion rate of 10 μg/min/kg, were 0.1 to 3.2 μg/ml (mean 1.1) for lignocaine and 0.02 to 2.27 μg/ml (mean 0.25) for monoethylglycinexylidide (H. Halkin *et al.*, *Clin. Pharmac. Ther.*, 1975, *17*, 669–675).

Following intravenous infusions at rates varying between 20 and 50 μg/min/kg to 24 subjects, the following steady-state serum concentrations

were reported: lignocaine 1.7 to 11.4 μg/ml (mean 5.7), monoethylglycinexylidide 0.2 to 5.2 μg/ml (mean 2.0), glycinexylidide 0 to 1.4 μg/ml (mean 0.5) (D. E. Drayer *et al.*, *Clin. Pharmac. Ther.*, 1983, *34*, 14–22).

TOXICITY. Toxic effects are associated with plasma concentrations greater than 6 μg/ml, and fatalities with blood concentrations greater than 14 μg/ml.

In a fatality due to accidental intravenous injection of 2 g of lignocaine, the following postmortem tissue concentrations were reported: blood 30 μg/ml, brain 135 μg/g, heart 106 μg/g, kidney 204 μg/g, lung 87 μg/g, skeletal muscle 20 μg/g (A. Poklis *et al.*, *J. forens. Sci.*, 1984, *29*, 1229–1236).

In 3 fatalities involving accidental ingestion of 25 g, the following postmortem tissue concentrations were reported: blood 44, 92, 11 μg/ml, brain 17, 32, 7 μg/g, kidney 66, –, 68 μg/g, liver 70, 96, 20 μg/g, lung 94, 130, 49 μg/g, urine 59, –, – μg/ml; in the first 2 cases death occurred within a few minutes of ingestion whereas the third subject survived for 24 hours (T. Borkowski and A. Dluzneiwska, *ibid.*, 1976, *12*(3), 17–18).

HALF-LIFE. Plasma half-life, lignocaine 1 to 2 hours, increased in subjects with liver disease or after acute myocardial infarction; monoethylglycinexylidide about 1 to 2 hours, glycinexylidide about 10 hours.

VOLUME OF DISTRIBUTION. About 1 to 2 litres/kg.

CLEARANCE. Plasma clearance, about 5 to 20 ml/min/kg.

PROTEIN BINDING. In plasma, about 70% at therapeutic concentrations but there is considerable intersubject variation and binding appears to be concentration-dependent.

NOTE. For a review of the pharmacokinetics of lignocaine see N. L. Benowitz and W. Meister, *Clin. Pharmacokinet.*, 1978, *3*, 177–201.

Dose. For local anaesthesia, the total dose of lignocaine hydrochloride by injection should not exceed 300 mg (4.5 mg/kg), unless administered with adrenaline. For ventricular arrhythmias, initally 50 to 100 mg intravenously, followed by an infusion.

Lincomycin   *Antibiotic*

Methyl 6-amino-6,8-dideoxy-*N*-[(2*S*,4*R*)-1-methyl-4-propyl-prolyl]-1-thio-α-D-*erythro*-D-*galacto*-octopyranoside
$C_{18}H_{34}N_2O_6S = 406.5$
CAS—154-21-2

Soluble in water, and most organic solvents.

Lincomycin Hydrochloride
Proprietary Names. Albiotic; Cillimycin; Lincocin(e); Mycivin.
$C_{18}H_{34}N_2O_6S,HCl,H_2O = 461.0$
CAS—859-18-2 (anhydrous); *7179-49-9* (monohydrate)
A white crystalline powder.
Soluble 1 in 1 of water, 1 in 40 of ethanol, and 1 in 20 of dimethylformamide; soluble in methanol; practically insoluble in chloroform and ether.

Dissociation Constant. pK$_a$ 7.5.

Colour Test. Sodium Nitroprusside (Method 3)—violet.

Thin-layer Chromatography. *System TA*—Rf 67. (*Acidified potassium permanganate solution*, positive.)

Ultraviolet Spectrum. No significant absorption, 230 to 360 nm.

Infra-red Spectrum. Principal peaks at wavenumbers 1655, 1104, 1075, 1564, 1040, 1262 (lincomycin hydrochloride, KBr disk).

Dose. The equivalent of 1.5 to 2 g of lincomycin daily.

Lindane   *Pesticide*

Synonyms. 666; Benhexachlor; Gamma Benzene Hexachloride; Gamma-BHC; Gamma-HCH; HCH; Hexicide.

Proprietary Names. Aphtiria; Élentol; Esoderm; Gamene; GBH; Hexicid; Jacutin; Kwell; Kwellada; Lorexane; Quellada; Scabene.

1α,2α,3β,4α,5α,6β-Hexachlorocyclohexane
$C_6H_6Cl_6 = 290.8$
CAS—58-89-9

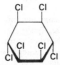

A white crystalline powder. M.p. about 112°.
Practically **insoluble** in water; soluble 1 in 19 of dehydrated alcohol, 1 in 2 of acetone, 1 in 3.5 of chloroform, and 1 in 5.5 of ether.

Partition Coefficient. Log *P* (octanol), 3.7.

Gas Chromatography. *System GA*—RI 1745; *system GK*—retention time 0.76 relative to caffeine.

Infra-red Spectrum. Principal peaks at wavenumbers 680, 665, 695, 778, 840, 950 (KBr disk).

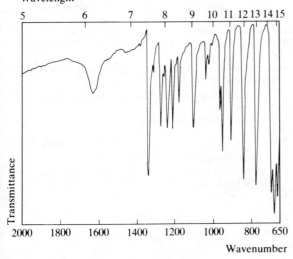

Wavelength

Mass Spectrum. Principal peaks at *m/z* 181, 183, 109, 219, 111, 217, 51, 221.

Quantification. GAS CHROMATOGRAPHY. In blood: ECD—N. Jain *et al.*, *J. Pharm. Pharmac.*, 1965, *17*, 362–367. In blood or tissues: sensitivity 1 ng/ml, ECD—J. L. Radomski and A. Ray, *J. chromatogr. Sci.*, 1970, *8*, 108–114.

Disposition in the Body. Readily absorbed after ingestion, inhalation, or through the skin. It is stored in the body fat and adrenal glands. Metabolised by oxidation and dehydrohalogenation to a series of chlorinated phenols which are excreted mainly in the urine in free and conjugated form.

After intravenous administration, about 25% of the dose is excreted in the urine; after topical administration about 10% of the dose is recovered in the urine (R. J. Feldmann and H. J. Maibach, *Toxic. appl. Pharmac.*, 1974, *28*, 126–132).

BLOOD CONCENTRATION.

Blood-lindane concentrations in subjects with low occupational exposure ranged from 0.001 to 0.009 µg/ml (mean 0.004), and concentrations in subjects with high dermal occupational exposure ranged from 0.006 to 0.093 µg/ml (mean 0.031) (T. H. Milby *et al.*, *J. occup. Med.*, 1968, *10*, 584–587).

Average serum concentrations of 0.07, 0.19 and 0.04 µg/ml of α-benzene hexachloride (α-BHC), β-BHC and γ-BHC, respectively, were reported in 57 subjects who worked in a factory manufacturing lindane; β-BHC was the only isomer observed to accumulate on chronic exposure. A mean fat concentration of 45.6 µg/g of β-BHC was reported in 8 subjects (K. Baumann *et al.*, *Int. Archs occup. envir. Hlth*, 1980, *47*, 119–127).

TOXICITY. Lindane is not highly toxic when applied externally in the concentrations usually employed (0.1 to 1%), but when ingested it may cause convulsions; dusts may irritate the nose and throat when used in a confined space. Blood concentrations greater than 0.02 µg/ml have been associated with toxic effects. The estimated minimum oral lethal dose is 200 mg/kg and the maximum permissible atmospheric concentration is 0.5 mg/m³. Toxic doses or long term exposure may cause liver necrosis. The maximum acceptable daily intake is 10 µg/kg.

A young girl who ingested about 1.6 g of lindane was found to have a serum concentration of 0.84 µg/ml after 2 hours, following convulsions; the concentration decreased to 0.49 µg/ml after 4 hours; urinary concentrations of individual free phenolic metabolites determined 5.5 hours after ingestion ranged from 0.04 to 0.74 µg/ml (H. G. Starr and N. J. Clifford, *Archs envir. Hlth*, 1972, *25*, 374–375).

A fat concentration of 343 µg/g was reported in a fatality due to lindane (W. J. Hayes and W. K. Vaughn, *Toxic. appl. Pharmac.*, 1977, *42*, 235–252).

HALF-LIFE. Derived from urinary excretion data, about 26 hours.

Use. Topically in concentrations of 0.1 to 1%.

Liothyronine   *Thyroid Agent*

Synonyms. L-Tri-iodothyronine. The abbreviation T_3 is often used for tri-iodothyronine.

4-*O*-(4-Hydroxy-3-iodophenyl)-3,5-di-iodo-L-tyrosine
$C_{15}H_{12}I_3NO_4 = 651.0$
CAS—6893-02-3

Crystals. M.p. 236°, with decomposition.

Liothyronine Sodium

Synonym. Sodium Liothyronine

Proprietary Names. Cynomel; Cytomel; Ro-Thyronine; Tertroxin; Ti-Tre. It is an ingredient of Euthroid and Thyrolar.

$C_{15}H_{11}I_3NNaO_4 = 673.0$
CAS—55-06-1
A white to buff-coloured solid or crystalline powder.

Practically **insoluble** in water, chloroform, ether, and most other organic solvents; soluble 1 in 500 of ethanol; soluble in solutions of alkali hydroxides.

Dissociation Constant. pK_a 8.5.

Ultraviolet Spectrum. Liothyronine sodium: aqueous alkali—319 nm ($A_1^1 = 65$ a).

Infra-red Spectrum. Principal peaks at wavenumbers 1608, 1180, 1493, 1250, 1535, 1320 (KBr disk).

Quantification. See under Thyroxine.

Disposition in the Body. Absorbed after oral or intramuscular administration. It is metabolised by conjugation with glucuronic acid or sulphate, de-iodination, oxidative deamination, and decarboxylation. It is excreted mainly in the bile and faeces, and is subject to enterohepatic circulation; some iodide is excreted in the urine.

Endogenous serum concentrations range from 0.0010 to 0.0016 µg/ml, in normal subjects.

HALF-LIFE. Plasma half-life, about 2 days.

PROTEIN BINDING. In plasma, more than 99%.

Dose. Up to 100 µg of liothyronine sodium daily.

Lithium Carbonate   *Tranquilliser*

Proprietary Names. Camcolit; Carbolith; Eskalith; Hypnorex; Liskonum; Lithane; Lithizine; Lithobid; Lithonate; Lithotabs; Manialith; Phasal; Priadel; Quilonum retard; Téralithe.

$Li_2CO_3 = 73.89$

CAS—554-13-2

A white granular powder. M.p. about 618°.

Soluble 1 in 100 of water and 1 in 140 of boiling water; very slightly soluble in ethanol; soluble, with effervescence, in dilute mineral acids.

Lithium Citrate

Proprietary Names. Arthri-Sel; Cibalith-S; Litarex; Lithonate-S.

$C_6H_5Li_3O_7,4H_2O = 282.0$

CAS—919-16-4 (anhydrous); *6080-58-6* (tetrahydrate)

A white, somewhat deliquescent, crystalline powder.

Soluble 1 in 2 of water; practically insoluble in ethanol and ether.

Quantification. ATOMIC ABSORPTION SPECTROPHOTOMETRY. In postmortem blood: sensitivity 145 nmol/litre—I. M. B. Scott, *J. forens. Sci. Soc.*, 1982, *22*, 41–42.

EMISSION FLAME PHOTOMETRY. In blood or urine: sensitivity 2 nmol/litre in blood, 30 nmol/litre in urine—R. Robertson *et al.*, *Clinica chim. Acta.*, 1973, *45*, 25–31. In serum: sensitivity 50 nmol/litre (comparison with atomic absorption spectrophotometry)—A. L. Levi and E. M. Katz, *Clin. Chem.*, 1970, *16*, 840–842.

Disposition in the Body. Readily absorbed after oral administration. About 97% of a dose is excreted unchanged in the urine in 10 days with 50 to 60% in the first 24 hours. The urinary excretion of lithium appears to be slower in the elderly than the young and also appears to occur more slowly at night, resulting in a diurnal rhythm in excretion rate; its excretion is also markedly influenced by sodium and, possibly, potassium status; in subjects where the sodium intake is reduced, lithium is reabsorbed by the renal tubules and in subjects who have a high sodium intake the excretion of lithium is increased. Lithium is widely distributed throughout the body and concentrations in the cerebrospinal fluid may reach 50% of those in plasma.

THERAPEUTIC CONCENTRATION. Lithium plasma concentrations should be monitored 12 hours after a dose to ensure that they are within the range 0.5 to 1.2 mmol/litre.

Following a single oral dose of 600 mg to 10 subjects, peak plasma concentrations of 0.45 to 0.80 mmol/litre (mean 0.64) were attained in about 2 hours (J. M. Meinhold *et al.*, *J. clin. Pharmac.*, 1979, *19*, 701–703). After daily oral doses of 1.5 to 1.7 g to 16 subjects, steady-state serum concentrations were in the range 0.7 to 0.9 mmol/litre (J. L. Marini and M. H. Sheard, *J. clin. Pharmac.*, 1976, *16*, 276–283).

TOXICITY. Toxic effects may be produced by serum concentrations greater than 2 mmol/litre. Blood concentrations of about 5 mmol/litre or more are usually fatal, although in one instance of survival which occurred after the ingestion of 22.5 g of lithium carbonate, the maximum serum concentration was 8.2 mmol/litre; a fatality due to the acute ingestion of lithium carbonate in which the serum concentration was 2.43 mmol/litre on admission to hospital and 1.93 mmol/litre at the time of death has also been reported.

In 3 fatalities due to lithium intoxication, the following postmortem tissue concentrations were reported: blood 1.9, 3.0, and 4.6 mmol/litre, brain 1.4, 5.2, and 4.2 mmol/kg, kidney 1.9, 5.9, and 9.6 mmol/kg, liver 1.9, 2.9, and 6.7 mmol/kg, urine 4.9, –, and 6.7 mmol/litre (Z. Kosa and A. Benko, *Bull. int. Ass. forens. Toxicol.*, 1981, *16*(2), 19–20 and A. Alha *et al.*, *ibid.*, 20–21).

In one subject who ingested an unknown amount, the serum concentration at 48 hours was 6.8 mmol/litre; death occurred after 21 days and the following postmortem tissue distribution was reported: serum 0.4 mmol/litre, brain 0.35 to 0.85 mmol/kg, kidney 0.60 mmol/kg, liver 0.22 mmol/kg, lung 0.51 mmol/kg (A. Amidsen *et al.*, *Acta psychiat. scand.*, 1974, *255*, *Suppl.* 4, 25–33).

HALF-LIFE. Plasma half-life, about 20 hours after a single dose but appears to be dependent on the duration of treatment. In patients on their first course of treatment a plasma half-life averaging 31 hours has been reported; this increased to 40 hours in subjects receiving lithium for less than one year and 58 hours in those taking the drug for longer than one year.

VOLUME OF DISTRIBUTION. About 0.8 litre/kg.

CLEARANCE. Apparent plasma clearance after a single dose, about 0.4 ml/min/kg, decreased in uraemia and in the elderly.

DISTRIBUTION IN BLOOD. Lithium is taken up by erythrocytes to a variable extent which appears to be partly genetically determined.

The erythrocyte:plasma ratio was reported to range from 0.19 to 1.0 (mean 0.5), in 42 subjects (J. A. Smith *et al.*, *Med. J. Aust.*, 1979, *1*, 631–632).

SALIVA. Plasma : saliva ratio, about 0.4 but there is considerable intersubject variation.

Dose. Usually 0.6 to 1.2 g daily; up to 2 g daily may be given for the first 5 to 7 days.

Lobeline   *Respiratory Stimulant*

Synonym. Alpha-lobeline

2-[6-(β-Hydroxyphenethyl)-1-methyl-2-piperidyl]acetophenone

$C_{22}H_{27}NO_2 = 337.5$

CAS—90-69-7

An alkaloid obtained from *Lobelia inflata* (Lobeliaceae).

Crystals. M.p. 130° to 131°.

Sparingly **soluble** in water; soluble in hot ethanol, chloroform, and ether.

Lobeline Hydrochloride
$C_{22}H_{27}NO_2,HCl = 373.9$
CAS—134-63-4
A white crystalline or granular powder. M.p. not lower than 180°.
Soluble 1 in 40 of water and 1 in 12 of ethanol; very soluble in chloroform; very slightly soluble in ether.

Lobeline Sulphate
Proprietary Names. Lobatox; Nikoban; Unilobin.
$(C_{22}H_{27}NO_2)_2,H_2SO_4 = 773.0$
CAS—134-64-5

Colour Tests. Mandelin's Test—grey; Marquis Test—red-violet.

Thin-layer Chromatography. *System TA*—Rf 61; *system TB*—Rf 17; *system TC*—Rf 35. (*Acidified iodoplatinate solution*, positive.)

Gas Chromatography. *System GA*—RI 1780.

Ultraviolet Spectrum. Aqueous acid—248 nm ($A_1^1 = 416$ a).

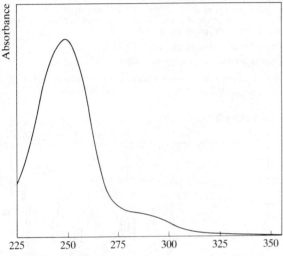

Infra-red Spectrum. Principal peaks at wavenumbers 1687, 700, 1211, 1115, 1052, 769 (KBr disk).

Mass Spectrum. Principal peaks at *m/z* 96, 105, 77, 97, 216, 42, 218, 51.

Dose. Lobeline hydrochloride was formerly given intramuscularly in doses of 3 to 10 mg.

Lofepramine   *Antidepressant*
Synonym. Lopramine
4'-Chloro-2-[3-(10,11-dihydro-5*H*-dibenz[*b*,*f*]azepin-5-yl)-*N*-methylpropylamino]acetophenone
$C_{26}H_{27}ClN_2O = 419.0$
CAS—23047-25-8

Colourless crystals, which become discoloured in air. M.p. 106°. Practically **insoluble** in water; slightly soluble in ethanol; soluble in chloroform.

Lofepramine Hydrochloride
Proprietary Names. Gamanil; Gamonil; Tymelyt.
$C_{26}H_{27}ClN_2O,HCl = 455.4$
CAS—26786-32-3
Colourless crystals or yellowish-white microcrystalline powder. M.p. 152° to 154°.
Slightly **soluble** in water; freely soluble in ethanol and chloroform.

High Pressure Liquid Chromatography. *System HA*—lofepramine k' 0.6, desipramine k' 2.1, 2-hydroxydesipramine k' 1.2.

Ultraviolet Spectrum. Methanol—255 nm ($A_1^1 = 596$ a).

Infra-red Spectrum. Principal peaks at wavenumbers 1700, 1235, 1495, 1590, 1100, 763 (lofepramine hydrochloride, KBr disk).

Mass Spectrum. Principal peaks at *m/z* 58, 234, 193, 192, 42, 235, 194, 59; desipramine 235, 195, 208, 44, 234, 193, 194, 71; 2-hydroxydesipramine 44, 209, 211, 250, 210, 224, 42, 251.

Quantification. GAS CHROMATOGRAPHY. In plasma: limit of detection, lofepramine 1 ng/ml, desipramine 2 ng/ml, FID—R. Lundgren *et al.*, *Acta pharm. suec.*, 1977, *14*, 81–94.

GAS CHROMATOGRAPHY–MASS SPECTROMETRY. In plasma or urine: sensitivity 2 ng/ml for lofepramine and desipramine, and 20 ng/ml for 2-hydroxydesipramine—K. Matsubayashi *et al.*, *J. Chromat.*, 1977, *143*; *Biomed. Appl.*, *1*, 571–580.

Disposition in the Body. Readily absorbed after oral administration but undergoes extensive first-pass demethylation to desipramine which is the principal active metabolite. It is also metabolised by *N*-oxidation, hydroxylation, and conjugation and is excreted in the urine mainly as metabolites; a second active metabolite, 2-hydroxydesipramine, has been reported to be the major unconjugated urinary metabolite.

THERAPEUTIC CONCENTRATION.
After a single oral dose of 2 mg/kg given to 6 subjects, peak plasma-lofepramine concentrations of 0.04 to 0.14 µg/ml (mean 0.09) were attained in about 1 hour; peak plasma-desipramine concentrations of 0.01 to 0.02 µg/ml were attained in 3 to 8 hours in 4 subjects. When a similar dose was given to the same subjects on a second occasion some weeks later, peak plasma-lofepramine concentrations of 0.05 to 0.27 µg/ml (mean 0.13) were reported. Following oral doses of 70 mg three times a day for 10 days to 3 subjects, plasma concentrations of about 0.003 µg/ml of lofepramine and 0.01 to 0.05 µg/ml (mean 0.025) of desipramine were reported, determined immediately prior to a dose (G. P. Forshell *et al.*, *Eur. J. clin. Pharmac.*, 1976, *9*, 291–298).

PROTEIN BINDING. In plasma, about 99%.

Dose. 70 to 210 mg daily.

Loperamide   *Antidiarrhoeal*
4-(4-*p*-Chlorophenyl-4-hydroxypiperidino)-*NN*-dimethyl-2,2-diphenylbutyramide
$C_{29}H_{33}ClN_2O_2 = 477.0$
CAS—53179-11-6

Loperamide Hydrochloride
Proprietary Names. Arret; Blox; Imodium; Lopemid.
$C_{29}H_{33}ClN_2O_2,HCl = 513.5$
CAS—34552-83-5

A white or yellowish-white, amorphous or microcrystalline powder. M.p. about 225°, with some decomposition.
Slightly **soluble** in water; freely soluble in chloroform and methanol.

Thin-layer Chromatography. *System TA*—Rf 70; *system TB*—Rf 09; *system TC*—Rf 32. (*Dragendorff spray*.)

Ultraviolet Spectrum. Acid isopropyl alcohol—254 nm, 260 nm ($A_1^1 = 14$ b), 266 nm.

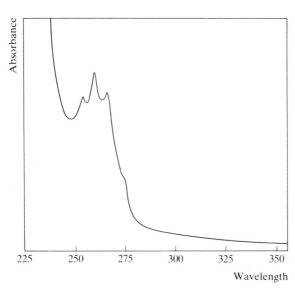

Infra-red Spectrum. Principal peaks at wavenumbers 1600, 700, 830, 765, 964, 986 (loperamide hydrochloride, KBr disk).

Mass Spectrum. Principal peaks at *m/z* 238, 42, 239, 224, 240, 56, 72, 226.

Quantification. RADIOIMMUNOASSAY. In serum or urine—H. S. Weintraub *et al.*, *Curr. ther. Res.*, 1977, *21*, 867–876.

Disposition in the Body. Poorly absorbed after oral administration. About 1 to 2% of a dose is excreted in the urine as free or conjugated loperamide in 48 hours. Up to 10% of a dose may be excreted in the urine in 8 days and about 40% is eliminated in the faeces over the same period.

THERAPEUTIC CONCENTRATION.
Following oral administration of capsules containing 8 mg of loperamide hydrochloride to 6 subjects, peak serum concentrations of about 0.002 µg/ml were attained in about 4 to 5 hours (J. M. Killinger *et al.*, *J. clin. Pharmac.*, 1979, *19*, 211–218).

HALF-LIFE. Plasma half-life, 7 to 15 hours (mean 11).

PROTEIN BINDING. In plasma, about 97%.

NOTE. For a review of the pharmacokinetics of loperamide see R. C. Heel *et al.*, *Drugs*, 1978, *15*, 33–52.

Dose. Up to 16 mg of loperamide hydrochloride daily.

Loprazolam   *Hypnotic*

6-(2-Chlorophenyl)-2,4-dihydro-2-(4-methylpiperazin-1-yl-methylene)-8-nitro-1*H*-imidazo[1,2-*a*][1,4]benzodiazepin-1-one
$C_{23}H_{21}ClN_6O_3 = 464.9$
CAS—*61197-73-7*

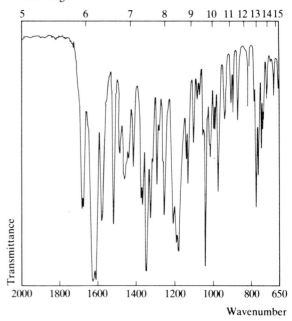

Crystals. M.p. 214° to 215°.

Loprazolam Mesylate
Proprietary Name. Dormonoct
$C_{23}H_{21}ClN_6O_3,CH_4SO_3,H_2O = 579.0$
A yellow powder. M.p. 242° to 245°, with decomposition.
Soluble 1 in about 100 of water, 1 in about 200 of ethanol, and 1 in about 500 of chloroform; practically insoluble in ether.

Dissociation Constant. pK$_a$ 6.0 (24°).

Ultraviolet Spectrum. Ethanol—330 nm ($A_1^1 = 884$ b).

Infra-red Spectrum. Principal peaks at wavenumbers 1628, 1610, 1045, 1182, 1192, 1518 (loprazolam mesylate, KBr disk).

Disposition in the Body. Readily absorbed after oral administration.

THERAPEUTIC CONCENTRATION.
Following a single oral dose of 2 mg to 8 subjects, a mean peak serum concentration of 0.0097 µg/ml was attained in 2.4 hours. Following repeated oral doses of 2 mg daily for 8 days, a mean peak serum concentration of 0.012 µg/ml was reported 2.2 hours after the last dose (L. A. Stevens *et al.*, *Eur. J. clin. Pharmac.*, 1983, *25*, 651–655).

HALF-LIFE. Plasma half-life, 4 to 11 hours (mean 7).

Dose. The equivalent of 1 to 2 mg of loprazolam, as a hypnotic.

Lorazepam
Tranquilliser

Proprietary Names. Almazine; Ativan; Tavor; Temesta.

7-Chloro-5-(2-chlorophenyl)-1,3-dihydro-3-hydroxy-2H-1,4-benzodiazepin-2-one

$C_{15}H_{10}Cl_2N_2O_2 = 321.2$

CAS—846-49-1

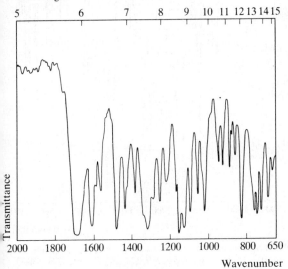

A white powder. M.p. 166° to 168°.

Practically **insoluble** in water; soluble in ethanol, acetone, and glacial acetic acid; slightly soluble in chloroform and ether.

Dissociation Constant. pK_a 1.3, 11.5 (20°).

Partition Coefficient. Log P (octanol/pH 7.4), 2.4.

Colour Tests. Formaldehyde–Sulphuric Acid—orange; Marquis Test—yellow; Sulphuric Acid—yellow.

Thin-layer Chromatography. *System TA*—Rf 52; *system TB*—Rf 01; *system TC*—Rf 36; *system TD*—Rf 23; *system TE*—Rf 45; *system TF*—Rf 39. (*Acidified iodoplatinate solution*, positive; *acidified potassium permanganate solution*, positive.)

Gas Chromatography. *System GA*—RI 2402; *system GG*—RI 2910.

High Pressure Liquid Chromatography. *System HA*—k' 0.1; *system HI*—k' 4.60; *system HK*—k' 0.14.

Ultraviolet Spectrum. Ethanol—230 nm ($A_1^1 = 1100$ b), 316 nm.

Infra-red Spectrum. Principal peaks at wavenumbers 1685, 1149, 1317, 1120, 1605, 826 (KBr disk).

Wavelength

[Infra-red spectrum chart: x-axis Wavenumber from 2000 to 650, y-axis Transmittance; wavelength scale 5 to 15]

Mass Spectrum. Principal peaks at m/z 291, 239, 274, 293, 75, 302, 276, 138.

Quantification. GAS CHROMATOGRAPHY. In plasma or urine: lorazepam and lorazepam glucuronide, limit of detection 1 ng/ml, ECD—D. J. Greenblatt *et al.*, *J. Chromat.*, 1978, *146*; *Biomed. Appl.*, *3*, 311–320.

GAS CHROMATOGRAPHY–MASS SPECTROMETRY. In plasma or urine: lorazepam and lorazepam glucuronide, limit of detection 2 ng/ml—S. Higuchi *et al.*, *J. Chromat.*, 1979, *164*; *Biomed. Appl.*, *6*, 55–61.

Disposition in the Body. Readily absorbed after oral administration; bioavailability about 95%. About 75% of a dose is excreted in the urine as the inactive glucuronide conjugate within 5 days (up to about 50% in the first 24 hours) and 14% is excreted as conjugates of minor metabolites which include ring-hydroxylation products and quinazoline derivatives; only negligible amounts are excreted as free lorazepam; about 7% of a dose is eliminated in the faeces.

Lorazepam is a metabolite of lormetazepam.

THERAPEUTIC CONCENTRATION. In plasma, usually in the range 0.05 to 0.24 µg/ml. Lorazepam glucuronide accumulates in plasma achieving concentrations greater than those of unchanged drug.

After a single oral dose of 0.05 mg/kg given to 9 subjects, peak plasma concentrations of 0.04 to 0.06 µg/ml (mean 0.05) were attained in about 0.5 to 1.5 hours; the maximum therapeutic effect was associated with plasma concentrations of 0.03 to 0.05 µg/ml and concentrations below 0.01 µg/ml were ineffective (E. G. Bradshaw *et al.*, *Br. J. Anaesth.*, 1981, *53*, 517–522).

Following daily oral doses of 6 mg to 8 subjects, mean steady-state plasma concentrations of 0.09 µg/ml of lorazepam and 0.17 µg/ml of lorazepam glucuronide were reported; in 7 subjects receiving 10 mg daily, the mean steady-state plasma concentrations were 0.16 and 0.27 µg/ml respectively (D. J. Greenblatt *et al.*, *J. clin. Pharmac.*, 1977, *17*, 495–500).

TOXICITY.

Plasma concentrations of 0.3 to 0.6 µg/ml were reported in 3 subjects suffering toxic effects after the ingestion of overdoses of lorazepam; the estimated amounts ingested were 100 and 120 mg in 2 of the cases. The subjects recovered within 24 to 30 hours (M. D. Allen *et al.*, *Am. J. Psychiat.*, 1980, *137*, 1414–1415).

HALF-LIFE. Plasma half-life, lorazepam 9 to 24 hours (mean 14), lorazepam glucuronide about 16 hours.

VOLUME OF DISTRIBUTION. About 1 to 2 litres/kg.

CLEARANCE. Plasma clearance, about 1 ml/min/kg.

PROTEIN BINDING. In plasma, about 90%; decreased in patients with cirrhosis.

NOTE. For reviews of the clinical pharmacokinetics of lorazepam see A. A. Kyriakopoulos *et al.*, *J. clin. Psychiat.*, 1978, *39*, 16–23, and D. J. Greenblatt, *Clin. Pharmacokinet.*, 1981, *6*, 89–105.

Dose. 1 to 10 mg daily.

Lorcainide
Anti-arrhythmic

Synonyms. Isocainide; Socainide.

4'-Chloro-N-(1-isopropyl-4-piperidyl)-2-phenylacetanilide

$C_{22}H_{27}ClN_2O = 370.9$

CAS—59729-31-6

[Chemical structure: $C_6H_5 \cdot CH_2 \cdot CO-N$ attached to a chlorophenyl ring with Cl, and a piperidyl ring with $CH(CH_3)_2$]

Lorcainide Hydrochloride

Proprietary Name. Remivox
$C_{22}H_{27}ClN_2O,HCl = 407.4$
CAS—58934-46-6
Crystals. M.p. 263°.
Freely **soluble** in water, ethanol, chloroform, and methanol.

High Pressure Liquid Chromatography. *System HA*—k' 1.8.

Ultraviolet Spectrum. Water—257 nm ($A_1^1 = 14.3$ b), 263 nm ($A_1^1 = 12.1$ b).

Infra-red Spectrum. Principal peaks at wavenumbers 1649, 716, 1094, 1298, 1153, 1016 (lorcainide hydrochloride, KBr disk).

Quantification. GAS CHROMATOGRAPHY. In plasma or urine: sensitivity 10 ng/ml for lorcainide and norlorcainide, ECD—U. Klotz *et al., Clin. Pharmacokinet.*, 1978, *3*, 407–418. In plasma, urine or tissues: sensitivity 5 ng/ml for lorcainide, 10 ng/ml for norlorcainide, 10 to 15 ng/ml for hydroxylated metabolites, ECD—R. Woestenborghs *et al., J. Chromat.*, 1979, *164*; *Biomed. Appl.*, 6, 169–176.

HIGH PRESSURE LIQUID CHROMATOGRAPHY. In plasma: sensitivity 5 ng/ml for lorcainide and norlorcainide, UV detection—Y. G. Yee and R. E. Kates, *J. Chromat.*, 1981, *223*; *Biomed. Appl.*, *12*, 453–459.

Disposition in the Body. Well absorbed after oral administration but undergoes extensive, saturable, first-pass metabolism; bioavailability about 30% after a single dose of 150 mg but almost 100% during chronic oral dosing. The principal active metabolite, norlorcainide, is found in high concentrations in plasma during chronic oral dosing. Other major metabolites include a 4-hydroxyphenyl derivative and a 4-hydroxy-3-methoxyphenyl compound. After intravenous administration, less than 2% of a dose is excreted in the urine as unchanged drug in 48 hours; a total of about 60% of a dose is excreted in the urine as metabolites in 4 days and 35% is eliminated in the faeces.

THERAPEUTIC CONCENTRATION.
Following oral doses of 100 mg twice a day to 8 subjects for 2 weeks, mean steady-state plasma concentrations of 0.05 to 0.50 µg/ml (mean 0.19) of lorcainide and 0.16 to 0.68 µg/ml (mean 0.32) of norlorcainide, were reported (R. E. Kates *et al., Clin. Pharmac. Ther.*, 1983, *33*, 28–34).

HALF-LIFE. Plasma half-life, lorcainide 3 to 15 hours (mean 8), increased in subjects with cirrhosis of the liver and during chronic oral dosing; norlorcainide 20 to 40 hours (mean 27).

VOLUME OF DISTRIBUTION. About 8 litres/kg but there is considerable intersubject variation.

CLEARANCE. Plasma clearance, 10 to 25 ml/min/kg.

DISTRIBUTION IN BLOOD. Plasma: whole blood ratio, about 1.3.

PROTEIN BINDING. In plasma, 80 to 85%.

NOTE. For a review of lorcainide see C. E. Eiriksson and R. N. Brogden, *Drugs*, 1984, *27*, 279–300.

Dose. The equivalent of 200 to 300 mg of lorcainide daily.

Lormetazepam   *Hypnotic*

Proprietary Names. Loramet; Noctamid.
7-Chloro-5-(2-chlorophenyl)-1,3-dihydro-3-hydroxy-1-methyl-2*H*-1,4-benzodiazepin-2-one
$C_{16}H_{12}Cl_2N_2O_2 = 335.2$
CAS—848-75-9

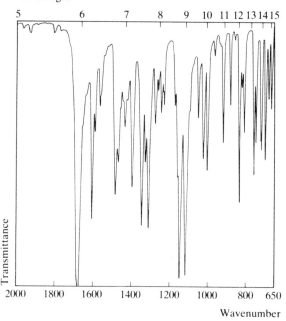

A white crystalline powder. M.p. 209° to 211°, with decomposition.
Practically **insoluble** in water; slightly soluble in ethanol and methanol; freely soluble in chloroform.

Colour Test. Formaldehyde–Sulphuric Acid—orange.

Thin-layer Chromatography. *System TA*—Rf 52; *system TB*—Rf 07; *system TC*—Rf 62; *system TD*—Rf 43; *system TE*—Rf 61; *system TF*—Rf 47. (*Dragendorff spray*, positive; *FPN reagent*, pale yellow; *Marquis reagent*, very weak pale yellow; *mercuric chloride–diphenylcarbazone reagent*, blue, on heating turns pale pink; *acidified potassium permanganate solution*, positive.)

Gas Chromatography. *System GA*—lormetazepam RI 2674, lorazepam RI 2402, decomposition product RI 2727.

High Pressure Liquid Chromatography. *System HI*—k' 6.32; *system HK*—k' 0.08.

Ultraviolet Spectrum. Aqueous acid—231 nm ($A_1^1 = 1030$ b), 311 nm ($A_1^1 = 59$ b).

Infra-red Spectrum. Principal peaks at wavenumbers 1682, 1153, 1121, 1315, 1610, 843 (KBr disk).

Wavelength

Transmittance vs Wavenumber

Mass Spectrum. Principal peaks at *m/z* 305, 307, 306, 309, 308, 334, 102, 75; lorazepam 291, 239, 274, 293, 75, 302, 276, 138.

Quantification. GAS CHROMATOGRAPHY. In plasma: sensitivity 200 pg/ml, ECD—D. M. Pierce *et al., Br. J. clin. Pharmac.*, 1984, *18*, 31–35.

RADIOIMMUNOASSAY. In plasma: detection limit 30 pg/ml—M. Hümpel *et al.*, *Clin. Pharmac. Ther.*, 1980, *28*, 673–679.

Disposition in the Body. Well absorbed after oral administration; bioavailability about 80%. Metabolised to some extent by *N*-demethylation to lorazepam. About 80% of a dose is excreted in the urine as lormetazepam glucuronide in 72 hours, and about 6% as lorazepam glucuronide.

THERAPEUTIC CONCENTRATION.

Single oral doses of 1 mg and 3 mg given to 6 subjects, produced mean peak plasma concentrations of 0.006 and 0.016 µg/ml, respectively, in 2 to 3 hours (M. Hümpel *et al.*, *ibid.*).

HALF-LIFE. Plasma half-life, lormetazepam about 10 hours, appears to be increased in elderly subjects; lormetazepam glucuronide about 13 hours.

VOLUME OF DISTRIBUTION. About 5 litres/kg.

CLEARANCE. Plasma clearance, about 4 ml/min/kg.

PROTEIN BINDING. In plasma, about 90%.

Dose. 0.5 to 2 mg, as a hypnotic.

Loxapine   *Tranquilliser*

Synonym. Oxilapine

Proprietary Name. Loxapac (solution)

2 - Chloro - 11 - (4 - methylpiperazin - 1 - yl)dibenz[*b*,*f*][1,4]-oxazepine

$C_{18}H_{18}ClN_3O = 327.8$

CAS—1977-10-2

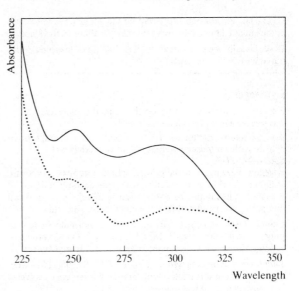

Pale yellowish crystals. M.p. 109° to 110°.

Loxapine Succinate

Proprietary Names. Loxapac (tablets); Loxitane (capsules).

$C_{18}H_{18}ClN_3O,C_4H_6O_4 = 445.9$

CAS—27833-64-3

A white crystalline solid.

Dissociation Constant. pK_a 6.6.

Colour Tests. Liebermann's Test (50–60°)—orange.

Heat with *nitric acid* for 3 minutes at 100° and then dilute tenfold with water—yellow precipitate.

Gas Chromatography. *System GA*—loxapine RI 2530, amoxapine RI 2659.

High Pressure Liquid Chromatography. *System HA*—k′ 1.1.

Ultraviolet Spectrum. Aqueous acid—251 nm ($A_1^1 = 346$ b), 292 nm; aqueous alkali—248 nm ($A_1^1 = 374$ b), 298 nm.

Infra-red Spectrum. Principal peaks at wavenumbers 1590, 1603, 1564, 1109, 1188, 1248.

Mass Spectrum. Principal peaks at *m/z* 70, 83, 42, 257, 193, 56, 228, 164; amoxapine 245, 257, 247, 193, 56, 246, 228, 259.

Quantification. GAS CHROMATOGRAPHY. In serum: sensitivity 2 ng/ml, AFID—J. Vasiliades *et al.*, *J. Chromat.*, 1979, *164*; *Biomed. Appl.*, *6*, 457–470. In plasma or urine: detection limit

140 pg/ml, ECD—S. F. Cooper *et al.*, *Xenobiotica*, 1979, *9*, 405–414. In serum or urine: loxapine and metabolites, ECD (serum) or FID (urine)—T. B. Cooper and R. G. Kelly, *J. pharm. Sci.*, 1979, *68*, 216–219.

Disposition in the Body. Readily absorbed after oral administration. The major urinary metabolite appears to be 8-hydroxyloxapine; other metabolites which have been identified include 7-hydroxyloxapine, desmethyl-loxapine (amoxapine) and its 7-hydroxy and 8-hydroxy derivatives, loxapine *N*-oxide, and 8-methoxyloxapine. Some unchanged drug is also excreted in the urine.

THERAPEUTIC CONCENTRATION. There is considerable intersubject variation in plasma concentrations.

After a single oral dose of 25 mg to 25 subjects, mean peak serum concentrations of 0.02 µg/ml of loxapine, 0.05 µg/ml of 8-hydroxyloxapine and 0.006 µg/ml of 8-hydroxyamoxapine were attained in 1 to 2 hours (M. A. Khan *et al.*, *Curr. ther. Res.*, 1980, *28*, 277–283).

Two subjects receiving 100 mg daily were found to have serum concentrations, respectively, of 0.031 µg/ml and 0.006 µg/ml of loxapine, 0.072 µg/ml and 0.041 µg/ml of 8-hydroxyloxapine and 0.064 µg/ml and 0.031 µg/ml of 8-hydroxyamoxapine immediately prior to a morning dose (T. B. Cooper and R. G. Kelly, *J. pharm. Sci.*, 1979, *68*, 216–219).

TOXICITY.

In a fatality attributed to loxapine overdose, the following postmortem tissue concentrations, µg/ml or µg/g, were reported:

	Blood	Brain	Liver	Lung	Spleen
Loxapine	1.22	4.46	11.88	4.98	3.96
8-Hydroxyloxapine (conjugated)	1.51	—	7.98	1.59	0.93
8-Hydroxyloxapine (unconjugated)	0.76	3.80	4.38	3.28	3.26
Amoxapine	1.01	4.84	10.00	3.80	6.30
8-Hydroxyamoxapine (conjugated)	1.92	—	1.89	1.32	—
8-Hydroxyamoxapine (unconjugated)	1.98	3.71	25.47	9.44	14.17

(T. B Cooper *et al.*, *J. analyt. Toxicol.*, 1981, *5*, 99–100).

A 22-year-old female ingested about 2.5 g of loxapine and died after 12 days in coma. Concentrations on admission to hospital were: blood 1.9 µg/ml, urine 0.4 µg/ml; 24 hours later the urine concentration was 8 µg/ml; in a second fatality, postmortem blood and liver concentrations of 7.7 µg/ml and 150 µg/g were reported (P. Reynolds *et al.*, *Clin. Toxicol.*, 1979, *14*, 181–185).

Absorbance

225   250   275   300   325   350

Wavelength

HALF-LIFE. Plasma half-life, loxapine 1 to 4 hours, 8-hydroxyloxapine about 8 hours, 8-hydroxyamoxapine about 36 to 48 hours.

Dose. Usually the equivalent of 20 to 100 mg of loxapine daily; maximum of 250 mg daily.

Lymecycline   *Antibiotic*

Synonyms. Limeciclina; Tetracycline-L-methylenelysine.
Proprietary Name. Tetralysal
A water-soluble combination of tetracycline, lysine, and formaldehyde with a molecular weight of approximately 603.
CAS—992-21-2
A yellow, very hygroscopic powder which darkens on exposure to light and air. M.p. above 200°, with slow decomposition.
Soluble 1 in less than 1 of water; slightly soluble in ethanol and methanol; practically insoluble in chloroform and ether.

Colour Tests. Benedict's Reagent—red; Formaldehyde–Sulphuric Acid—brown-red; Mandelin's Test—violet-brown → yellow; Marquis Test—orange; Sulphuric Acid—red-brown.

Thin-layer Chromatography. *System TA*—Rf 05, streaking. (Location under ultraviolet light, orange fluorescence; *acidified potassium permanganate solution*, positive.)

Ultraviolet Spectrum. Aqueous acid—269 nm $(A_1^1 = 292\ a)$, 356 nm; aqueous alkali—239 nm, 267 nm.

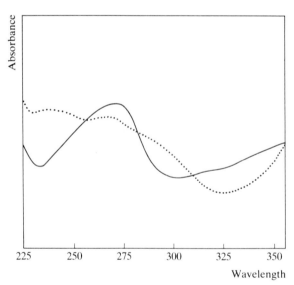

Dose. Usually 816 mg (the equivalent of 600 mg of tetracycline) daily.

Lynoestrenol   *Progestational Steroid*

Synonyms. Lynenol; Lynestrenol.
Proprietary Names. Exluton(a); Orgametril.
It is an ingredient of many oral contraceptives, see *Martindale, The Extra Pharmacopoeia*, 28th Edn.
19-Nor-17α-pregn-4-en-20-yn-17β-ol
$C_{20}H_{28}O = 284.4$
CAS—52-76-6

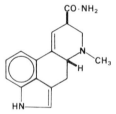

A white crystalline powder. M.p. 160° to 164°.
Practically **insoluble** in water; soluble 1 in 15 of ethanol, 1 in 8 of chloroform, and 1 in 12 of ether.

Thin-layer Chromatography. *System TP*—Rf 77; *system TQ*—Rf 55; *system TR*—Rf 99; *system TS*—Rf 97.

Ultraviolet Spectrum. No significant absorption, 230 to 360 nm.

Infra-red Spectrum. Principal peaks at wavenumbers 683, 1040, 1014, 1053, 813, 1266 (KBr disk).

Mass Spectrum. Principal peaks at *m/z* 91, 79, 67, 201, 77, 105, 93, 120.

Dose. 2.5 mg daily, for courses of 22 days.

Lysergamide   *Hallucinogen*

Synonyms. Ergine; Lysergic Acid Amide.
9,10-Didehydro-6-methylergoline-8β-carboxamide
$C_{16}H_{17}N_3O = 267.3$
CAS—478-94-4

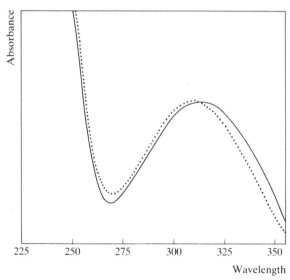

Lysergamide is found in *Rivea corymbosa*, *Ipomoea* spp. (Convolvulaceae), and ergot.
Crystals. It decomposes at 242°.

Colour Test. Marquis Test—brown.

Thin-layer Chromatography. *System TA*—Rf 60; *system TL*—Rf 06; *system TM*—Rf 27. (*Van Urk reagent*, blue.)

High Pressure Liquid Chromatography. *System HA*—k′ 0.5; *system HP*—k′ 0.33.

Ultraviolet Spectrum. Aqueous acid—313 nm; aqueous alkali—309 nm.

Infra-red Spectrum. Principal peaks at wavenumbers 1670, 760, 783, 1618, 1158, 1270 (KBr disk).

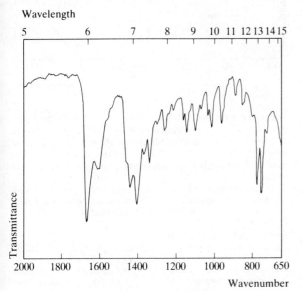

Mass Spectrum. Principal peaks at *m/z* 267, 221, 207, 180, 223, 154, 196, 268.

Lysergic Acid   *Hallucinogen*

9,10-Didehydro-6-methylergoline-8β-carboxylic acid
$C_{16}H_{16}N_2O_2 = 268.3$
CAS—82-58-6

A white crystalline powder. M.p. 240°, with decomposition. Slightly **soluble** in water; soluble in dilute acids and alkalis.

Dissociation Constant. pK_a 3.4, 6.3.

Colour Tests. Mandelin's Test—green-brown; Marquis Test—brown.

Thin-layer Chromatography. *System TA*—Rf 58; *system TD*—Rf 00; *system TE*—Rf 00; *system TF*—Rf 00; *system TL*—Rf 00; *system TM*—Rf 00. (Location under ultraviolet light, violet fluorescence; *mercuric chloride–diphenylcarbazone reagent*, blue; *acidified potassium permanganate solution*, positive; *Van Urk reagent*, blue.)

High Pressure Liquid Chromatography. *System HA*—k′ 0.8 (tailing peak); *system HP*—k′ 0.00.

Ultraviolet Spectrum. Aqueous acid—305 nm; aqueous alkali—308 nm.

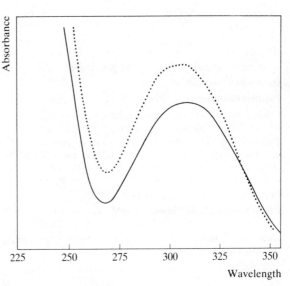

Infra-red Spectrum. Principal peaks at wavenumbers 1592, 787, 758, 1308, 691, 1015.

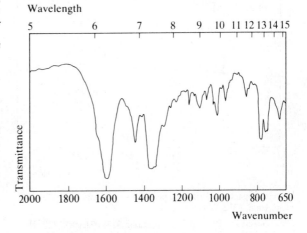

Mass Spectrum. Principal peaks at *m/z* 268, 224, 154, 180, 207, 223, 192, 179.

Lysergide   *Hallucinogen*

Synonyms. LSD; LSD 25; Lysergic Acid Diethylamide.
(+)-*NN*-Diethyl-D-lysergamide
$C_{20}H_{25}N_3O = 323.4$
CAS—50-37-3

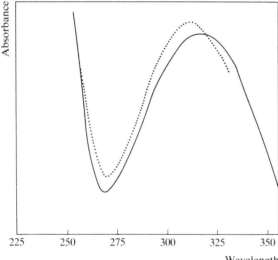

A colourless crystalline substance. M.p. 80° to 85°.

Dissociation Constant. pK$_a$ 7.5.

Partition Coefficient. Log P (octanol), 3.0.

Colour Tests. *p*-Dimethylaminobenzaldehyde—violet; Mandelin's Test—grey; Marquis Test—grey.

Thin-layer Chromatography. *System TA*—Rf 60; *system TB*—Rf 03; *system TC*—Rf 39; *system TL*—Rf 24; *system TM*—Rf 70. (*Dragendorff* spray, positive; *acidified iodoplatinate solution*, positive; *Marquis reagent*, grey; *Van Urk reagent*, blue.)

Gas Chromatography. *System GA*—RI 3445.

High Pressure Liquid Chromatography. *System HA*—lysergide k' 0.7; *system HP*—lysergide k' 1.83, 2-oxylysergide k' 0.92.

Ultraviolet Spectrum. Aqueous acid—315 nm (A$_1^1$ = 225 a); aqueous alkali—310 nm.

Infra-red Spectrum. Principal peaks at wavenumbers 1626, 1307, 1136, 1066, 1212, 749 (KBr disk).

Mass Spectrum. Principal peaks at *m/z* 323, 221, 181, 222, 207, 72, 223, 324.

Quantification. HIGH PRESSURE LIQUID CHROMATOGRAPHY–RADIOIMMUNOASSAY. In biological fluids: sensitivity 1 ng/ml, fluorescence detection—P. W. Twitchett *et al.*, *J. Chromat.*, 1978, *150*, 73–84.

THIN-LAYER CHROMATOGRAPHY (HIGH PERFORMANCE). In illicit dosage forms: limit of detection 2 ng—L. Kraus *et al.*, *Bull. Narcot.*, 1980, *32*, 67–71.

FLUOROIMMUNOASSAY. In biological fluids: sensitivity 4 ng/ml—A. R. Hubbard *et al.*, *Analyt. Proc.*, 1983, *20*, 606–608.

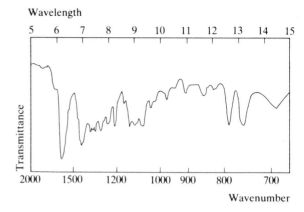

Disposition in the Body. Readily absorbed after oral administration; it is believed to undergo extensive biotransformation in the liver to inactive metabolites. About 1% of a dose is excreted unchanged in the urine in 24 hours. 2-Oxylysergide is a major metabolite although 13-hydroxy- and 14-hydroxylysergide also appear.

Single doses of 200 to 400 μg were administered to 8 subjects; the urinary concentration of lysergide or a closely related metabolite ranged from 0.001 to 0.055 μg/ml in the 24 hours after ingestion (A. Taunton-Rigby *et al.*, *Science*, 1973, *181*, 165–166).

BLOOD CONCENTRATION.

A single oral dose of 160 μg was administered to 13 subjects; plasma concentrations measured at intervals over a period of 2½ hours varied considerably but were in the range 0 to 0.009 μg/ml (D. G. Upshall and D. G. Wailling, *Clinica chim. Acta*, 1972, *36*, 67–73).

TOXICITY. Hallucinatory effects are produced with doses of 200 to 400 μg but recovery has occurred after much larger doses (up to 10 mg). Plasma concentrations greater than 0.001 μg/ml have been associated with toxic effects.

HALF-LIFE. Plasma half-life, about 3 hours.

VOLUME OF DISTRIBUTION. About 0.3 litre/kg.

PROTEIN BINDING. In plasma, about 90%, decreasing to about 65% in overdose subjects.

Dose. In psychotherapy, doses of 100 to 750 μg have been given.

Mafenide   *Sulphonamide*

Synonyms. Bensulfamide; Benzamsulfonamide; 4-Homosulphanilamide; Sulfabenzamine.

α-Aminotoluene-*p*-sulphonamide
C$_7$H$_{10}$N$_2$O$_2$S = 186.2
CAS—138-39-6

A white powder. M.p. 151° to 154°.
Sparingly **soluble** in water; soluble in methanol and in dilute acids and alkalis.

Mafenide Acetate

Proprietary Names. Napaltan; Sulfamylon.

$C_7H_{10}N_2O_2S,C_2H_4O_2 = 246.3$

CAS—13009-99-9

A white crystalline powder. M.p. 162° to 171°.

Freely **soluble** in water; sparingly soluble in ethanol.

Mafenide Hydrochloride

Synonyms. Homosulfaminum; Maphenide.

$C_7H_{10}N_2O_2S,HCl = 222.7$

CAS—138-37-4

A colourless or white crystalline powder. M.p. about 260°.

Soluble 1 in 1.7 of water and 1 in 100 of ethanol; practically insoluble in chloroform and ether.

Mafenide Propionate

Proprietary Name. Sulfomyl

$C_7H_{10}N_2O_2S,C_3H_6O_2 = 260.3$

Colourless crystals. M.p. 158°.

Soluble in water.

Colour Test. Koppanyi–Zwikker Test—violet.

Thin-layer Chromatography. *System TA*—Rf 49; *system TD*—Rf 01; *system TE*—Rf 27; *system TF*—Rf 01. (*Acidified iodoplatinate solution,* positive.)

Gas Chromatography. *System GA*—not eluted.

Ultraviolet Spectrum. Aqueous acid—267 nm $(A_1^1 = 41 a)$, 274 nm.

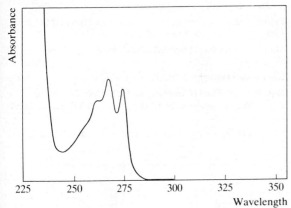

Infra-red Spectrum. Principal peaks at wavenumbers 1151, 1316, 1299, 897, 1089, 1592 (KBr disk).

Mass Spectrum. Principal peaks at m/z 106, 30, 77, 185, 105, 104, 89, 141.

Quantification. THIN-LAYER CHROMATOGRAPHY. In serum: detection limit 1 µg/ml—J. M. Steyn, *J. Chromat.,* 1977, *143*; *Biomed. Appl.,* *1*, 210–213.

Disposition in the Body. Absorbed from wounds into the circulation and metabolised to *p*-carboxybenzenesulphonamide which is excreted in the urine.

Use. Topically as a cream containing 8.5% mafenide (as the acetate).

Malathion   *Pesticide*

Synonyms. Carbofos; Compound 4047; OMS-1.

Proprietary Names. Derbac (liquid); Prioderm; Suleo-M.

Diethyl 2-(dimethoxyphosphinothioylthio)succinate

$C_{10}H_{19}O_6PS_2 = 330.4$

CAS—121-75-5

$$(CH_3 \cdot O)_2 \overset{\overset{\text{S}}{\|}}{P} - S \cdot CH \cdot CO \cdot O \cdot C_2H_5$$
$$CH_2 \cdot CO \cdot O \cdot C_2H_5$$

A colourless to light amber liquid which decomposes in strong acid or high humidity. Although stable in light, it decomposes at high temperatures. F.p. 2.85°. Refractive index 1.4985.

Very slightly **soluble** in water; miscible with many organic solvents.

Colour Tests. Palladium Chloride—brown; Phosphorus Test—yellow; Sodium Nitroprusside (Method 2)—violet.

Thin-layer Chromatography. *System TW*—Rf 74.

Gas Chromatography. *System GA*—RI 1917; *system GK*—retention time 1.03 relative to caffeine.

Infra-red Spectrum. Principal peaks at wavenumbers 1018, 1748, 1174, 1209, 824, 1250 (thin film).

Mass Spectrum. Principal peaks at m/z 125, 93, 127, 173, 158, 99, 55, 79.

Quantification. COLORIMETRY. In blood or tissues—A. Faragó, *Arch. Tox.,* 1967, *23*, 11–16.

GAS CHROMATOGRAPHY. In urine: dialkyl phosphate residues, detection limits 40 ng/ml to 130 ng/ml, FID—S. J. Reid and R. R. Watts, *J. analyt. Toxicol.,* 1981, *5*, 126–132. In urine: malathion α-mono- and dicarboxylic acid and alkyl phosphate metabolites, detection limit 2 ng/ml for the dicarboxylic acid and 5 ng/ml for the α-monocarboxylic acid, FID—D. E. Bradway and T. M. Shafik, *J. agric. Fd Chem.,* 1977, *25*, 1342–1344.

Disposition in the Body. Absorbed after oral ingestion but absorbed only slowly and to a small extent through intact skin. It is metabolised by conversion to malaoxon, the toxic keto analogue, and by hydrolysis to malathion α-mono- and dicarboxylic acids which are the major metabolites. Other hydrolysis products include dimethylthiophosphoric acid (DMTP) and dimethyldithiophosphoric acid (DMDTP) which have been detected in the urine of subjects exposed to malathion. After ingestion, up to 25% is excreted in the 24-hour urine as ether-extractable phosphates, mostly in the first 8 hours.

TOXICITY. Malathion is less toxic than most other organophosphorus pesticides; the estimated minimum lethal dose is 25 g; the maximum permissible atmospheric concentration is 10 mg/m^3 and the maximum acceptable daily intake is 20 µg/kg.

In 4 fatalities due to the ingestion of 25 to 70 g of malathion, the following postmortem concentrations were reported: blood 100 to 1880 µg/ml (mean 815), kidney 190 to 1880 µg/g (mean 1308), liver 200 to 1700 µg/g (mean 1215) (A. Faragó, *Arch. Tox.,* 1967, *23*, 11–16).

In a poisoning case due to the ingestion of 200 ml of a 50% malathion preparation, the following concentrations were reported in the urine collected over the period 24 to 48 hours after ingestion: malathion α-monocarboxylic acid 223 µg/ml, dicarboxylic acid metabolite 12 µg/ml, dimethylthiophosphoric acid 96 µg/ml, dimethyldithiophosphoric acid 20 µg/ml, dimethylphosphoric acid 50 µg/ml, monomethyl phosphate 8 µg/ml (D. E. Bradway and T. M. Shafik, *J. agric. Fd Chem.,* 1977, *25*, 1342–1344).

HALF-LIFE. Derived from urinary excretion data, about 3 hours.

Use. Topically in concentrations of 0.5 or 1% in the treatment of pediculosis.

Mandelic Acid   *Antibacterial (Urinary)*

Synonyms. Amygdalic Acid; Phenylglycollic Acid; Racemic Mandelic Acid.

2-Hydroxy-2-phenylacetic acid

$C_8H_8O_3 = 152.1$

CAS—90-64-2; 611-72-3 ($\pm$)

OH
|
CH$_2$·COOH

White crystals, which turn yellow on exposure to light. M.p. 119° to 121°.

Soluble 1 in 6 of water, 1 in 1 of ethanol, 1 in 45 of chloroform, and 1 in 6 of ether.

Ammonium Mandelate

C$_8$H$_7$O$_3$NH$_4$ = 169.2
CAS—530-31-4
A white, very hygroscopic, crystalline powder, which discolours on exposure to light.
Very **soluble** in water; sparingly soluble in ethanol.

Calcium Mandelate

Synonym. Calcium Amygdalate
(C$_8$H$_7$O$_3$)$_2$Ca = 342.4
CAS—134-95-2
A white crystalline powder.
Soluble 1 in 100 of water and 1 in 4500 of ethanol (90%).

Dissociation Constant. pK$_a$ 3.4 (25°).

Gas Chromatography. *System GA*—RI 1487.

Ultraviolet Spectrum. Aqueous acid—251 nm (A$_1^1$ = 10.9 b), 257 nm (A$_1^1$ = 13.7 b), 262 nm (A$_1^1$ = 11.2 b). No alkaline shift.

Infra-red Spectrum. Principal peaks at wavenumbers 1710, 1060, 1245, 1185, 690, 720 (KBr disk).

Mass Spectrum. Principal peaks at *m/z* 107, 79, 77, 51, 152, 105, 50, 78.

Disposition in the Body. Mandelic acid is a urinary metabolite of several drugs and toxic chemicals and is also found endogenously in normal urine at concentrations of up to 5 µg/ml.

Dose. Mandelic acid has been given in doses of 12 g daily, usually as the calcium or ammonium salt.

Mannomustine   *Antineoplastic*

Synonyms. BCM; Mannitol Mustard.
1,6-Bis(2-chloroethylamino)-1,6-dideoxy-D-mannitol
C$_{10}$H$_{22}$Cl$_2$N$_2$O$_4$ = 305.2
CAS—576-68-1

CH$_2$·NH·CH$_2$·CH$_2$Cl
|
HO—C—H
|
HO—C—H
|
H—C—OH
|
H—C—OH
|
CH$_2$·NH·CH$_2$·CH$_2$Cl

M.p. 278°, with decomposition.
Soluble in water.

Mannomustine Hydrochloride

C$_{10}$H$_{22}$Cl$_2$N$_2$O$_4$,2HCl = 378.1
CAS—551-74-6
A white crystalline powder. M.p. 241°, with decomposition.
Soluble 1 in 2 of water; slightly soluble in ethanol; practically insoluble in chloroform and ether.

Ultraviolet Spectrum. No significant absorption, 230 to 360 nm.

Infra-red Spectrum. Principal peaks at wavenumbers 1065, 1013, 1298, 1284, 1102, 1581 (mannomustine hydrochloride, KBr disk).

Dose. Mannomustine hydrochloride has been given in doses of 50 to 100 mg daily, by intravenous injection.

Maprotiline   *Antidepressant*

3-(9,10-Dihydro-9,10-ethanoanthracen-9-yl)-*N*-methylpropyl-amine
C$_{20}$H$_{23}$N = 277.4
CAS—10262-69-8

CH$_2$·CH$_2$·CH$_2$·NH·CH$_3$

M.p. 92° to 94°.

Maprotiline Hydrochloride

Proprietary Name. Ludiomil
C$_{20}$H$_{23}$N,HCl = 313.9
CAS—10347-81-6
A white crystalline powder. M.p. 230° to 232°.
Soluble in water and some organic solvents.

Colour Tests. Liebermann's Test—orange-brown; Mandelin's Test—blue; Marquis Test—red.

Thin-layer Chromatography. *System TA*—Rf 15; *system TB*—Rf 17; *system TC*—Rf 05.

Gas Chromatography. *System GA*—RI 2356.

High Pressure Liquid Chromatography. *System HA*—maprotiline k' 2.2, desmethylmaprotiline k' 1.1; *system HF*—maprotiline k' 4.92.

Ultraviolet Spectrum. Aqueous acid—265 nm, 272 nm (A$_1^1$ = 52 b).

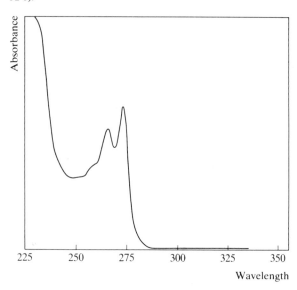

Infra-red Spectrum. Principal peaks at wavenumbers 759, 1140, 1592, 1032, 1308, 935 (maprotiline hydrochloride, KBr disk).

Wavelength

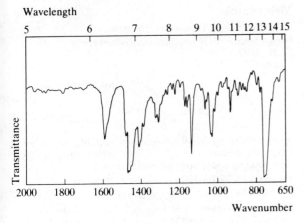

Mass Spectrum. Principal peaks at m/z 44, 70, 59, 277, 71, 191, 278, 203.

Quantification. GAS CHROMATOGRAPHY. In blood: sensitivity 20 ng/ml for maprotiline and 50 ng/ml for desmethylmaprotiline, AFID—A. Sioufi and A. Richard, *J. Chromat.*, 1980, *221*; *Biomed. Appl.*, *10*, 393–398. In blood: sensitivity 10 ng/ml, ECD—D. Alkalay *et al.*, *Analyt. Lett. (Part B)*, 1982, *15*, 1493–1503.

GAS CHROMATOGRAPHY–MASS SPECTROMETRY. In plasma: maprotiline and desmethylmaprotiline, sensitivity 2 ng/ml—S. P. Jindal *et al.*, *J. pharm. Sci.*, 1980, *69*, 684–687.

HIGH PRESSURE LIQUID CHROMATOGRAPHY. In plasma: maprotiline and desmethylmaprotiline, detection limit 2 ng/ml, UV detection—H. J. Kuss and E. Festenauer, *J. Chromat.*, 1981, *204*, 349–353.

Disposition in the Body. Slowly but completely absorbed following oral administration. It appears to undergo significant first-pass metabolism; bioavailability about 70%. After intravenous administration, about 57% of a dose is excreted in the urine and 30% in the faeces over a period of 21 days; less than 10% of the dose is excreted as unchanged drug. The principal metabolite is the desmethyl derivative, which has been shown to be active in animals, but hydroxylation also occurs to form phenolic derivatives which may be further converted to aromatic methoxy ethers or excreted as glucuronide conjugates; N-oxidation also occurs and maprotiline N-oxide has been reported to be active; numerous minor metabolites have been identified in urine.

THERAPEUTIC CONCENTRATION. Blood concentrations vary considerably between subjects and there appears to be no clear correlation between clinical response, dose, side-effects, and blood or plasma concentrations. Peak blood concentrations are usually attained 3 to 8 hours after a single dose.

After a single oral dose of 75 mg to 6 subjects, peak blood concentrations of 0.012 to 0.037 µg/ml (mean 0.023) and peak plasma concentrations of 0.016 to 0.031 µg/ml (mean 0.024) were attained in 4 to 8 hours (K. P. Maguire *et al.*, *Eur. J. clin. Pharmac.*, 1980, *18*, 249–254).

After daily oral doses of 50, 100, and 150 mg to 7 subjects, steady-state blood concentrations were: 0.02 to 0.15 µg/ml (mean 0.07), 0.07 to 0.25 µg/ml (mean 0.14), and 0.14 to 0.32 µg/ml (mean 0.22) (W. Riess *et al.*, *J. int. med. Res.*, 1975, *3*, Suppl. 2, 16–41).

Following daily oral doses of 150 mg to 4 subjects for 22 days, steady-state serum concentrations of 0.05 to 0.24 µg/ml of maprotiline and 0.02 to 0.13 µg/ml of desmethylmaprotiline were reported (R. N. Gupta *et al.*, *Clin. Chem.*, 1977, *23*, 1849–1852).

TOXICITY.
The following postmortem tissue distribution was reported in a suicide case: axillary blood 6.2 µg/ml, cardiac blood 2.0 µg/ml, bile 161 µg/ml, kidney 34.0 µg/g, liver 82.0 µg/g (A. E. Robinson *et al.*, *J. analyt. Toxicol.*, 1979, *3*, 3–13).

In a fatality due to the ingestion of 4.5 to 6 g of maprotiline, the following postmortem tissue concentrations were reported: blood 44.5 µg/ml, brain 158 µg/g, liver 605 µg/g, urine 12.6 µg/ml (T. A. Rejent and R. E. Doyle, *ibid.*, 1982, *6*, 199–201).

HALF-LIFE. Plasma half-life, 20 to 70 hours (mean 45).

VOLUME OF DISTRIBUTION. 23 to 70 litres/kg (mean 52).

CLEARANCE. Plasma clearance, 6 to 20 ml/min/kg (mean 15).

DISTRIBUTION IN BLOOD. The plasma:whole blood ratio has been reported to vary between individuals and may also vary between single and multiple dosing (see K. P. Maguire *et al.*, *Eur. J. clin. Pharmac.*, 1980, *18*, 249–254).

PROTEIN BINDING. In plasma, about 90%.

NOTE. For a review of the pharmacokinetics of maprotiline see R. M. Pinder *et al.*, *Drugs*, 1977, *13*, 321–352.

Dose. 30 to 150 mg of maprotiline hydrochloride daily.

Mazindol
Anorectic

Proprietary Names. Mazanor; Mazildene; Sanorex; Teronac.

5-(4-Chlorophenyl)-2,5-dihydro-3H-imidazo[2,1-a]isoindol-5-ol
$C_{16}H_{13}ClN_2O = 284.7$
CAS—22232-71-9

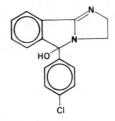

Crystals. M.p. 198° to 199°.

Dissociation Constant. pK_a 8.6.

Colour Test. Sulphuric Acid—orange.

Thin-layer Chromatography. *System TA*—Rf 63; *system TB*—Rf 06; *system TC*—Rf 13.

Gas Chromatography. *System GA*—RI 2355.

High Pressure Liquid Chromatography. *System HA*—k' 1.8; *system HC*—k' 0.20.

Ultraviolet Spectrum. Aqueous acid—271 nm ($A_1^1 = 509$ a); aqueous alkali—269 nm ($A_1^1 = 170$ b), 275 nm ($A_1^1 = 173$ b). (See below)

Infra-red Spectrum. Principal peaks at wavenumbers 763, 1656, 1063, 1175, 674, 1093 (KBr disk). (See below)

Mass Spectrum. Principal peaks at m/z 266, 268, 267, 255, 231, 102, 88, 176.

Disposition in the Body. Absorbed after oral administration and slowly excreted in the urine, partly unchanged and partly as metabolites.

HALF-LIFE. About 12 to 24 hours.

Dose. 2 to 3 mg daily.

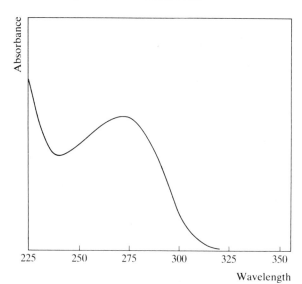

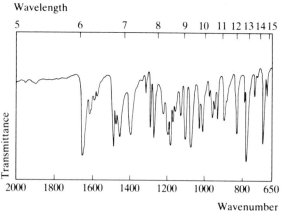

Mebanazine   *Antidepressant (Monoamine Oxidase Inhibitor)*

α-Methylbenzylhydrazine
$C_8H_{12}N_2 = 136.2$
CAS—65-64-5

$$C_6H_5 \cdot \overset{\displaystyle CH_3}{\underset{}{CH}} \cdot NH \cdot NH_2$$

Practically **insoluble** in water, ethanol, and ether; soluble in chloroform.

Colour Tests. Nessler's Reagent—black; Palladium Chloride—black; Sulphuric Acid—orange.

Thin-layer Chromatography. *System TA*—Rf 70; *system TB*—Rf 48; *system TC*—Rf 69.

Gas Chromatography. *System GA*—RI 1240.

High Pressure Liquid Chromatography. *System HA*—k' 0.2.

Ultraviolet Spectrum. Aqueous acid—251 nm, 257 nm, 261 nm, 267 nm.

Infra-red Spectrum. Principal peaks at wavenumbers 699, 1175, 760, 1199, 1292, 1070 (Nujol mull).

Dose. Mebanazine has been given in doses of 5 to 30 mg daily.

Mebendazole   *Anthelmintic*

Proprietary Names. Telmin (vet.); Vermox.
Methyl 5-benzoyl-1*H*-benzimidazol-2-ylcarbamate
$C_{16}H_{13}N_3O_3 = 295.3$
CAS—31431-39-7

A white to slightly yellow amorphous powder. M.p. about 290°. Practically **insoluble** in water, ethanol, chloroform, ether, and dilute mineral acids; freely soluble in formic acid.

Thin-layer Chromatography. *System TA*—Rf 65; *system TB*—Rf 00; *system TC*—Rf 59. (*Dragendorff spray*.)

Ultraviolet Spectrum. Acid isopropyl alcohol—234 nm ($A_1^1 = 1000$ b), 288 nm ($A_1^1 = 524$ b); alkaline isopropyl alcohol—270 nm ($A_1^1 = 802$ b), 355 nm ($A_1^1 = 653$ b).

Infra-red Spectrum. Principal peaks at wavenumbers 1635, 1260, 1590, 1730, 1230, 705 (KBr disk).

Mass Spectrum. Principal peaks at *m/z* 186, 218, 77, 295, 263, 105, 51, 158.

Quantification. HIGH PRESSURE LIQUID CHROMATOGRAPHY. In plasma: detection limit 10 ng/ml for mebendazole, 60 ng/ml for the 5-(α-hydroxy) metabolite and 30 ng/ml for the 2-amino metabolite, UV detection—R. J. Allan *et al.*, *J. Chromat.*, 1980, *183*; *Biomed. Appl.*, *9*, 311–319.

Disposition in the Body. Poorly absorbed after oral administration. Metabolised to the 5-(α-hydroxy) derivative and by decarboxylation to the 2-amino metabolite, both of which are detectable in plasma at concentrations higher than those of unchanged mebendazole. Less than 10% of a dose is excreted in the urine; the major urinary metabolite is the 2-amino-5-(α-hydroxy) derivative. Biliary excretion and enterohepatic circulation have been reported.

THERAPEUTIC CONCENTRATION.

Following single oral doses of 10 mg/kg to 5 subjects, peak plasma concentrations of 0.018 to 0.116 µg/ml (mean 0.07) were attained in 2.5 to 7 hours (mean 5) (P. A. Braithwaite *et al.*, *Eur. J. clin. Pharmac.*, 1982, *22*, 161–169).

HALF-LIFE. Plasma half-life, 1.5 to 9 hours.

VOLUME OF DISTRIBUTION. About 2 litres/kg.

DISTRIBUTION IN BLOOD. Plasma: whole blood ratio, about 1.2.

PROTEIN BINDING. In plasma, about 95%.

REFERENCE. P. A. Braithwaite *et al.*, *ibid.*

Dose. Usually 200 mg daily for 3 days.

Mebeverine   *Antispasmodic*

4-[Ethyl(4-methoxy-α-methylphenethyl)amino]butyl veratrate
$C_{25}H_{35}NO_5 = 429.6$
CAS—3625-06-7

Soluble in chloroform.

Mebeverine Hydrochloride

Synonym. CSAG 144

Proprietary Names. Colofac; Duspatal; Duspatalin.

$C_{25}H_{35}NO_5,HCl = 466.0$

CAS—2753-45-9

A white crystalline powder. M.p. 131° to 136°.

Soluble in water and ethanol; sparingly soluble in ether.

Colour Test. Liebermann's Test—black.

Thin-layer Chromatography. *System TA*—Rf 63; *system TB*—Rf 40; *system TC*—Rf 53. (*Acidified iodoplatinate solution*, positive.)

Gas Chromatography. *System GA*—not eluted.

High Pressure Liquid Chromatography. *System HA*—k' 1.9.

Ultraviolet Spectrum. Aqueous acid—262 nm ($A_1^1 = 307$ b); aqueous alkali—269 nm, 290 nm.

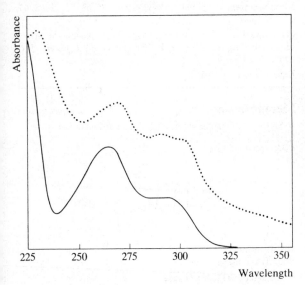

Infra-red Spectrum. Principal peaks at wavenumbers 1216, 1266, 1132, 1510, 1715, 1174 (mebeverine hydrochloride, KBr disk).

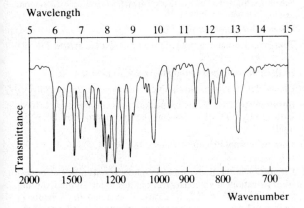

Mass Spectrum. Principal peaks at *m/z* 308, 165, 309, 121, 55, 154, 98, 56.

Disposition in the Body.

TOXICITY.

In a fatality attributed to the ingestion of mebeverine and thioridazine, the following postmortem concentrations were reported: mebeverine, blood 36 µg/ml, liver 15 µg/g, urine 24 µg/ml; thioridazine, not detected in blood and urine, liver 2 µg/g (G. del Villar, *Bull. int. Ass. forens. Toxicol.*, 1977, *13*(1&2), 23–24).

Dose. 405 mg of mebeverine hydrochloride daily.

Mebezonium Iodide   *Muscle Relaxant*

Proprietary Name. It is an ingredient of Tanax (vet.).

4,4'-Methylenebis(cyclohexyltrimethylammonium) di-iodide

$C_{19}H_{40}I_2N_2 = 550.3$

CAS—7681-78-9

A white crystalline powder. M.p. 260°, with decomposition.

Soluble in water.

Thin-layer Chromatography. *System TA*—Rf 00. (*Acidified iodoplatinate solution*, positive.)

Infra-red Spectrum. Principal peaks at wavenumbers 961, 888, 831, 1621, 985, 1020 (KBr disk).

Quantification. THIN-LAYER CHROMATOGRAPHY–ULTRAVIOLET SPECTROPHOTOMETRY. In blood or urine—E. Bertol *et al.*, *J. pharm. biomed. Analysis*, 1983, *1*, 373–377.

Disposition in the Body.

TOXICITY.

In 3 fatalities due to the injection of a preparation containing mebezonium iodide and embutramide, the following postmortem concentrations (µg/ml) were reported:

	Mebezonium iodide	Embutramide
Blood	4.5, 6.0, 7.5	3.0, 15.5, 12.1
Urine	0.8, 2.0, 1.8	2.0, 6.3, 4.5

(E. Bertol *et al.*, *ibid.*).

Mebhydrolin   *Antihistamine*

Proprietary Name. Fabahistin (tablets)

5-Benzyl-1,2,3,4-tetrahydro-2-methyl-γ-carboline

$C_{19}H_{20}N_2 = 276.4$

CAS—524-81-2

A white crystalline powder. M.p. 95°.

Practically **insoluble** in water; soluble in ethanol, chloroform, and ether.

Mebhydrolin Napadisylate

Synonyms. Diazolinum; Mebhydrolin Naphthalenedisulphonate.

Proprietary Names. Fabahistin (suspension); Incidal; Omeril.

$(C_{19}H_{20}N_2)_2,C_{10}H_8O_6S_2 = 841.1$

CAS—6153-33-9

A white powder.

Very slightly **soluble** in water, ethanol, chloroform, and ether.

Dissociation Constant. pK$_a$ 6.7.

Colour Tests. Mandelin's Test—blue; Marquis Test—grey-blue.

Thin-layer Chromatography. *System TA*—Rf 57; *system TB*—Rf 28; *system TC*—Rf 45. (*Acidified iodoplatinate solution*, positive.)

Gas Chromatography. *System GA*—RI 2465; *system GC*—RI 2739; *system GF*—RI 2920.

High Pressure Liquid Chromatography. *System HA*—k' 3.0 (tailing peak).

Ultraviolet Spectrum. Aqueous acid—286 nm (A$_1^1$ = 409 b), 320 nm.

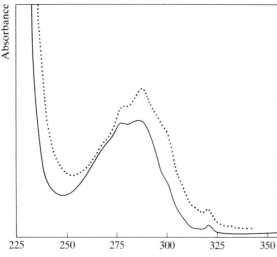

Infra-red Spectrum. Principal peaks at wavenumbers 737, 1134, 1316, 695, 1122, 1212 (thin film).

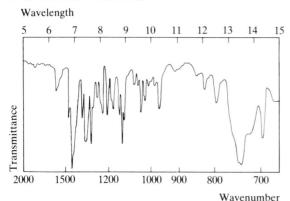

Mass Spectrum. Principal peaks at *m/z* 91, 233, 30, 232, 31, 276, 275, 65.

Dose. 150 to 300 mg daily.

Mebutamate   *Tranquilliser*

Proprietary Names. Axiten; Mebutina; No-Press; Sigmafon.

2-*sec*-Butyl-2-methyltrimethylene dicarbamate
C$_{10}$H$_{20}$N$_2$O$_4$ = 232.3
CAS—64-55-1

$$NH_2 \cdot CO \cdot O \cdot CH_2 \cdot \underset{\underset{CH_3 \cdot CH \cdot CH_2 \cdot CH_3}{|}}{\overset{\overset{CH_3}{|}}{C}} \cdot CH_2 \cdot O \cdot CO \cdot NH_2$$

A white crystalline powder. M.p. 77° to 79°.
Slightly **soluble** in water.

Colour Tests. Furfuraldehyde—black; Nessler's Reagent—brown (slow):

Thin-layer Chromatography. *System TD*—Rf 10; *system TE*—Rf 59; *system TF*—Rf 35.

Gas Chromatography. *System GA*—RI 1889.

Ultraviolet Spectrum. No significant absorption, 230 to 360 nm.

Infra-red Spectrum. Principal peaks at wavenumbers 1682, 1070, 1710, 1601, 1140, 788 (KBr disk).

Mass Spectrum. Principal peaks at *m/z* 97, 55, 69, 72, 71, 98, 43, 62.

Quantification. GAS CHROMATOGRAPHY. In plasma or urine: sensitivity 1 µg/ml, FID—J. F. Douglas *et al.*, *J. pharm. Sci.*, 1969, *58*, 145–146.

Dose. 0.9 to 1.2 g daily.

Mecamylamine   *Antihypertensive*

N-Methyl-2,3,3-trimethylbicyclo[2.2.1]hept-2-ylamine
C$_{11}$H$_{21}$N = 167.3
CAS—60-40-2

An oily liquid.
Slightly **soluble** in water.

Mecamylamine Hydrochloride
Proprietary Names. Inversine; Mevasine.
C$_{11}$H$_{21}$N,HCl = 203.8
CAS—826-39-1
A white crystalline powder. M.p. about 245°, with decomposition.
Soluble 1 in 5 of water and 1 in 12 of ethanol; freely soluble in chloroform; practically insoluble in ether.

Dissociation Constant. pK$_a$ 11.3.

Thin-layer Chromatography. *System TA*—Rf 16; *system TB*—Rf 51; *system TC*—Rf 02.

High Pressure Liquid Chromatography. *System HA*—k' 1.7.

Ultraviolet Spectrum. No significant absorption, 230 to 360 nm.

Infra-red Spectrum. Principal peaks at wavenumbers 1111, 1068, 1078, 1592, 1098, 890 (mecamylamine hydrochloride, Nujol mull).

Mass Spectrum. Principal peaks at *m/z* 98, 84, 71, 56, 41, 42, 99, 124.

Disposition in the Body. Almost completely absorbed after oral administration; high concentrations are found in the liver and kidney. More than 50% of a dose is excreted in 24 hours as unchanged drug in acid urine; the excretion is reduced if the urine is alkaline.

Dose. 5 to 30 mg of mecamylamine hydrochloride daily.

Wavelength

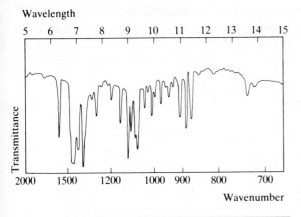

O·CH₂·CO·O·[CH₂]₂·N(CH₃)₂

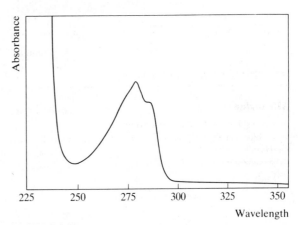

Meclofenamic Acid   *Analgesic*

Proprietary Name. Arquel (vet.)
N-(2,6-Dichloro-*m*-tolyl)anthranilic acid
$C_{14}H_{11}Cl_2NO_2 = 296.2$
CAS—644-62-2

White crystals.
Practically **insoluble** in water.

Meclofenamate Sodium

Proprietary Name. Meclomen
$C_{14}H_{10}Cl_2NNaO_2 = 318.1$
CAS—6385-02-0
M.p. 289° to 291°.
Sparingly **soluble** in water.

Thin-layer Chromatography. *System TG*—Rf 38. (*Chromic acid solution*, violet.)

Gas Chromatography. *System GA*—RI 2420; *system GD*—retention time of methyl derivative 1.62 relative to n-$C_{16}H_{34}$.

High Pressure Liquid Chromatography. Meclofenamic acid is used as a reference substance in *System HV*.

Ultraviolet Spectrum. Aqueous alkali—275 nm ($A_1^1 = 240$ b), 319 nm ($A_1^1 = 180$ b); methanol—242 nm ($A_1^1 = 342$ b), 282 nm ($A_1^1 = 235$ b), 331 nm ($A_1^1 = 235$ b).

Dose. The equivalent of 200 to 400 mg of meclofenamic acid daily.

Meclofenoxate   *Central Stimulant*

Synonyms. Centrophenoxine; Clofenoxine; Clophenoxate; Deanol 4-Chlorophenoxyacetate; Meclofenoxane.
2-Dimethylaminoethyl 4-chlorophenoxyacetate
$C_{12}H_{16}ClNO_3 = 257.7$
CAS—51-68-3

Meclofenoxate Hydrochloride

Proprietary Names. Helfergin; Lucidril.
$C_{12}H_{16}ClNO_3,HCl = 294.2$
CAS—3685-84-5
A white powder. M.p. 136°.
Soluble in water. It rapidly hydrolyses in aqueous solution.

Thin-layer Chromatography. *System TA*—Rf 77; *system TB*—Rf 26; *system TC*—Rf 42. (*Acidified potassium permanganate solution*, positive.)

Gas Chromatography. *System GA*—RI 1770; *system GB*—RI 1804; *system GC*—RI 2200.

High Pressure Liquid Chromatography. *System HA*—k' 1.7.

Ultraviolet Spectrum. Aqueous acid—277 nm ($A_1^1 = 44$ a).

Infra-red Spectrum. Principal peaks at wavenumbers 1167, 1183, 1742, 1080, 833, 1768 (KBr disk).

Mass Spectrum. Principal peaks at m/z 58, 111, 71, 42, 75, 59, 141, 113.

Dose. 0.9 to 1.5 g of meclofenoxate hydrochloride daily.

Mecloqualone   *Hypnotic*

Proprietary Name. Nubarène
3-(2-Chlorophenyl)-2-methylquinazolin-4(3H)-one
$C_{15}H_{11}ClN_2O = 270.7$
CAS—340-57-8

Crystals. M.p. 125° to 128°.

Gas Chromatography. *System GA*—RI 2255.

Infra-red Spectrum. Principal peaks at wavenumbers 1682, 1605, 768, 782, 1282, 1583.

Wavelength

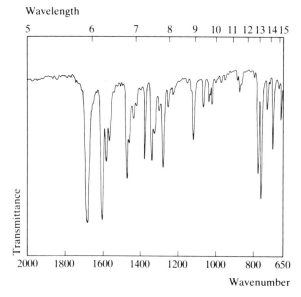

Dose. 150 to 300 mg, as a hypnotic.

Meclozine
Antihistamine

Synonyms. Histamethizine; Meclizine.
1-(4-Chlorobenzhydryl)-4-(3-methylbenzyl)piperazine
$C_{25}H_{27}ClN_2 = 391.0$
CAS—569-65-3

Meclozine Hydrochloride
Synonym. Meclizinium Chloride
Proprietary Names. Ancolan; Antivert; Bonamine; Bonine; Calmonal; Peremesin; Postafen(e); Sea-legs. It is an ingredient of Ancoloxin.
$C_{25}H_{27}ClN_2,2HCl = 463.9$
CAS—1104-22-9 (anhydrous); *31884-77-2* (monohydrate)
A white or slightly yellowish crystalline powder. M.p. 217° to 224°, with decomposition.
Soluble 1 in 1000 of water, 1 in 25 of ethanol, and 1 in 5 of chloroform; practically insoluble in ether; freely soluble in pyridine.

Dissociation Constant. pK_a 3.1, 6.2 (25°).

Colour Test. Liebermann's Test—red-orange.

Thin-layer Chromatography. *System TA*—Rf 76; *system TB*—Rf 58; *system TC*—Rf 79; *system TL*—Rf 70. (*Dragendorff spray*, positive; *acidified iodoplatinate solution*, positive; *Marquis reagent*, brown-yellow; *ninhydrin spray*, positive.)

Gas Chromatography. *System GA*—RI 3033.

High Pressure Liquid Chromatography. *System HA*—k′ 0.7.

Ultraviolet Spectrum. Ethanol—230 nm $(A_1^1 = 391 \text{ a})$, 266 nm $(A_1^1 = 27 \text{ b})$, 273 nm.

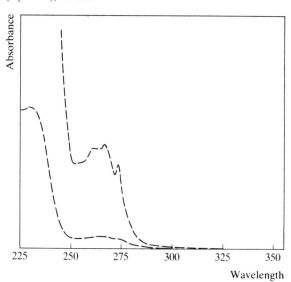

Infra-red Spectrum. Principal peaks at wavenumbers 700, 720, 760, 940, 805, 1491 (meclozine hydrochloride, KBr disk).

Wavelength

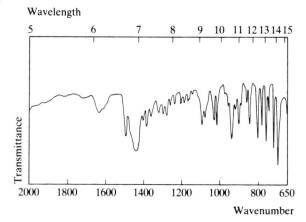

Mass Spectrum. Principal peaks at *m/z* 189, 105, 201, 285, 165, 166, 190, 134.

Quantification. GAS CHROMATOGRAPHY–MASS SPECTROMETRY. In plasma: detection limit 5 ng/ml—H. G. Fouda *et al.*, *Biomed. Mass Spectrom.*, 1978, *5*, 491–494.

Dose. Usually 50 to 150 mg of meclozine hydrochloride daily.

Medazepam
Tranquilliser

Proprietary Names. Nobrium; Raporan.
7-Chloro-2,3-dihydro-1-methyl-5-phenyl-1*H*-1,4-benzodiazepine
$C_{16}H_{15}ClN_2 = 270.8$
CAS—2898-12-6

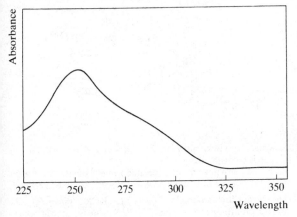

A white to greenish-yellow crystalline powder. M.p. 100° to 103°.

Practically **insoluble** in water; soluble 1 in 8 of ethanol, 1 in 1 of chloroform, and 1 in 5 of ether.

Dissociation Constant. pK_a 6.2 (37°).

Partition Coefficient. Log P (octanol/pH 7.4), 4.0.

Colour Tests. Formaldehyde–Sulphuric Acid—orange (add water).
Cold *nitric acid* gives a red colour.

Thin-layer Chromatography. *System TA*—Rf 67; *system TB*—Rf 40; *system TC*—Rf 74; *system TD*—Rf 56; *system TE*—Rf 79; *system TF*—Rf 40. (*Acidified iodoplatinate solution*, positive.)

Gas Chromatography. *System GA*—medazepam RI 2226, desmethyldiazepam RI 2496, diazepam RI 2425; *system GF*—medazepam RI 2640, diazepam RI 3045; *system GG*—medazepam RI 2620, desmethyldiazepam RI 3041, diazepam RI 2940.

High Pressure Liquid Chromatography. *System HA*—medazepam k′ 0.2, desmethyldiazepam k′ 0.2, diazepam k′ 0.1; *system HJ*—k′ 7.05; *system HK*—k′ 4.44.

Ultraviolet Spectrum. Aqueous acid—253 nm ($A_1^1 = 860$ a).

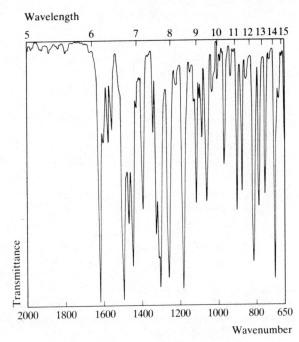

Infra-red Spectrum. Principal peaks at wavenumbers 1610, 1178, 1298, 700, 1255, 815 (KBr disk).

Mass Spectrum. Principal peaks at m/z 242, 207, 244, 270, 243, 271, 269, 165; desmethyldiazepam 242, 269, 270, 241, 243, 271, 244, 272; desmethylmedazepam 193, 255, 228, 256, 257, 165, 230, 258; diazepam 256, 283, 284, 285, 257, 255, 258, 286.

Quantification. GAS CHROMATOGRAPHY. In plasma or urine: sensitivity 40 ng/ml, ECD—J. A. F. de Silva and C. V. Puglisi, *Analyt. Chem.*, 1970, *42*, 1725–1736. In whole blood: detection limit 80 ng/ml, FID—M. S. Greaves, *Clin. Chem.*, 1974, *20*, 141–147.

Disposition in the Body. Readily absorbed after oral administration. The active metabolites desmethyldiazepam (nordazepam)

and diazepam may be detected in the blood shortly after dosing; desmethyldiazepam accumulates during chronic treatment. Desmethylmedazepam has also been detected in plasma. A total of up to about 75% of a dose is excreted in the urine and about 20% is eliminated in the faeces. The major urinary metabolite is oxazepam glucuronide, 2 to 3% of a dose being excreted in this form in 72 hours; other urinary metabolites include desmethyldiazepam and temazepam.

THERAPEUTIC CONCENTRATION.
Following single oral doses of 10 mg given to 4 subjects, peak plasma concentrations of 0.14 to 0.26 µg/ml (mean 0.21) of medazepam were attained in about 1 hour (D. M. Hailey and E. S. Baird, *Br. J. Anaesth.*, 1979, *51*, 493–496).

Doses of 10 to 50 mg given daily to 20 subjects, resulted in the following steady-state plasma concentrations: medazepam 0.01 to 0.16 µg/ml (mean 0.06), diazepam 0 to 0.12 µg/ml (mean 0.03), desmethyldiazepam 0.2 to 1.7 µg/ml (mean 0.7) (A. J. Bond *et al.*, *Br. J. clin. Pharmac.*, 1977, *4*, 51–56).

HALF-LIFE. Plasma half-life, medazepam 1 to 2 hours, desmethyldiazepam about 40 to 100 hours, but there is considerable intersubject variation—see under Nordazepam.

DISTRIBUTION IN BLOOD. Plasma: whole blood ratio, 1.9.

PROTEIN BINDING. In plasma, almost completely bound.

Dose. 10 to 40 mg daily.

Medigoxin
Cardiac Glycoside

Synonyms. β-Methyl Digoxin; β-Methyldigoxin; Metildigoxin.
Proprietary Names. Lanitop; Metidi.

3β-[(O-2,6-Dideoxy-4-O-methyl-β-D-*ribo*-hexopyranosyl-(1 → 4)-O-2,6-dideoxy-β-D-*ribo*-hexopyranosyl-(1 → 4)-2,6-dideoxy-β-D-*ribo*-hexopyranosyl)oxy]-12β,14-dihydroxy-5β,14β-card-20(22)-enolide
$C_{42}H_{66}O_{14} = 795.0$
CAS—30685-43-9

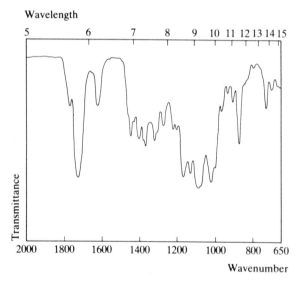

A white crystalline powder. M.p. 162° to 168°.
Very slightly **soluble** in water; soluble in ethanol and chloroform.

Infra-red Spectrum. Principal peaks at wavenumbers 1085, 1014, 1730, 1163, 1130, 864 (KBr disk).

Wavelength

[Infra-red spectrum: x-axis Wavenumber from 2000 to 650 (labelled 2000, 1800, 1600, 1400, 1200, 1000, 800, 650); top axis Wavelength labelled 5, 6, 7, 8, 9, 10, 11, 12, 13, 14, 15; y-axis Transmittance]

Quantification. RADIOIMMUNOASSAY. In plasma: sensitivity 200 pg/ml (comparison with methods using radiolabelled drug)— E. R. Garrett and P. H. Hinderling, *J. pharm. Sci.*, 1977, *66*, 806–810.

Disposition in the Body. Rapidly and almost completely absorbed after oral administration. Metabolised by demethylation to digoxin and by hydrolysis to the bis- and mono-glycosides. About 75% of a dose is excreted in the urine over a period of several days with about 25 to 30% being excreted in the first 24 hours. Of the material excreted in the urine, about 30 to 50% is unchanged drug, 15% consists of conjugated bis- and mono-glycosides, and the remainder is digoxin. About 15 to 30% of a dose is eliminated in the faeces over a period of 7 days.

THERAPEUTIC CONCENTRATION.
Following a single oral dose of 0.4 mg to 17 subjects, a mean peak plasma concentration of 0.003 µg/ml was attained in about 1 hour. Following daily oral doses of 0.15 to 0.2 mg to 18 subjects, steady-state plasma concentrations of 0.0006 to 0.002 µg/ml (mean 0.001) were reported (D. Boerner *et al.*, *Eur. J. clin. Pharmac.*, 1976, *9*, 307–314).

TOXICITY.
In a fatality in which death occurred about 1 hour after ingestion of a medigoxin overdose, the following postmortem tissue concentrations of glycosides were reported: blood 0.075 µg/ml, bile 2.4 µg/ml, kidney 0.237 µg/g, liver 0.047 µg/g, left ventricular myocardium 0.14 µg/g, right ventricular myocardium 0.16 µg/g, urine 0.91 µg/ml (N. Rietbrock *et al.*, *Dtsch. med. Wschr.*, 1978, *103*, 1841–1844).

HALF-LIFE. Plasma half-life, 40 to 70 hours.

VOLUME OF DISTRIBUTION. About 6 to 10 litres/kg.

CLEARANCE. Plasma clearance, about 2 ml/min/kg.

DISTRIBUTION IN BLOOD. Plasma: whole blood ratio, 1.1.

PROTEIN BINDING. In plasma, about 10 to 30%.

Dose. For rapid digitalisation, 600 µg daily for 2 to 4 days; maintenance, 200 to 300 µg daily.

Medroxyprogesterone Acetate   *Progestational Steroid*

Synonyms. Methylacetoxyprogesterone; Metipregnone.
Proprietary Names. Amen; Clinovir; Curretab; Depo-Provera; Farlutal; Luteodione; Lutoral; Metilgestene; Prodasone; Provera.

6α-Methyl-3,20-dioxopregn-4-en-17α-yl acetate
$C_{24}H_{34}O_4 = 386.5$
CAS—520-85-4 (medroxyprogesterone); *71-58-9* (acetate)

A white crystalline powder. M.p. about 204°. A solution in dioxan is dextrorotatory.
Practically **insoluble** in water; soluble 1 in 800 of ethanol, 1 in 50 of acetone, and 1 in 10 of chloroform; slightly soluble in ether.

Thin-layer Chromatography. *System TP*—Rf 80; *system TQ*—Rf 50; *system TR*—Rf 98; *system TS*—Rf 85, streaking may occur.

Ultraviolet Spectrum. Ethanol—241 nm ($A_1^1 = 426$ a).

Infra-red Spectrum. Principal peaks at wavenumbers 1727, 1669, 1258, 1608, 967, 1188 (medroxyprogesterone, KBr disk).

Quantification. GAS CHROMATOGRAPHY. In plasma: detection limit 5 ng/ml, ECD—E. Rossi *et al.*, *J. Chromat.*, 1979, *169*, 416–421.

GAS CHROMATOGRAPHY–MASS SPECTROMETRY. In plasma: detection limit 1 ng—G. Phillipou and R. G. Frith, *Clinica chim. Acta*, 1980, *103*, 129–133.

HIGH PRESSURE LIQUID CHROMATOGRAPHY. In plasma: sensitivity 4 ng/ml, UV detection—G. Milano *et al.*, *J. Chromat.*, 1982, *232*; *Biomed. Appl.*, *21*, 413–417.

Dose. 2.5 to 10 mg daily, by mouth; up to 1 g daily may be given.

Mefenamic Acid

Analgesic

Proprietary Names. Parkemed; Ponstan; Ponstel; Ponstyl.

N-(2,3-Xylyl)anthranilic acid

$C_{15}H_{15}NO_2 = 241.3$

CAS—61-68-7

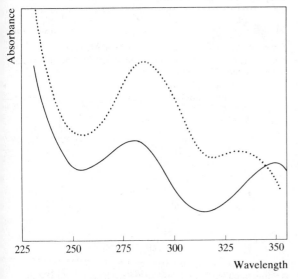

A white to greyish-white microcrystalline powder. M.p. about 230°, with effervescence.

Practically **insoluble** in water; soluble 1 in 185 of ethanol, 1 in 150 of chloroform, and 1 in 80 of ether; soluble in solutions of alkali hydroxides.

Dissociation Constant. pK_a 4.2.

Colour Test. Liebermann's Test—blue.

Thin-layer Chromatography. *System TD*—Rf 41; *system TE*—Rf 14; *system TF*—Rf 54; *system TG*—Rf 32. (*Chromic acid solution, green.*)

Gas Chromatography. *System GA*—RI 2201; *system GD*—retention time of methyl derivative 1.45 relative to $n\text{-}C_{16}H_{34}$.

High Pressure Liquid Chromatography. *System HD*—k′ 21.1; *system HV*—retention time 0.95 relative to meclofenamic acid.

Ultraviolet Spectrum. Acid methanol—279 nm ($A_1^1 = 357$ a), 350 nm; aqueous alkali—285 nm ($A_1^1 = 420$ a, 322 nm).

Infra-red Spectrum. Principal peaks at wavenumbers 1255, 1647, 1572, 1504, 757, 1163 (KBr disk).

Mass Spectrum. Principal peaks at *m/z* 223, 241, 208, 222, 194, 180, 77, 224; 3′-carboxymefenamic acid 44, 180, 209, 227, 223, 77, 208, 179; 3′-hydroxymethylmefenamic acid 209, 257, 180, 208, 210, 77, 44, 194.

Quantification. GAS CHROMATOGRAPHY. In serum: sensitivity 1 µg/ml, FID—L. J. Dusci and L. P. Hackett, *J. Chromat.*, 1978, *161*, 340–342.

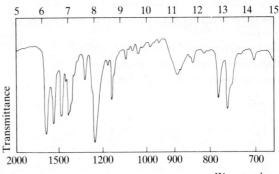

HIGH PRESSURE LIQUID CHROMATOGRAPHY. In plasma: mefenamic acid and flufenamic acid, UV detection—C. K. Lin *et al.*, *J. pharm. Sci.*, 1980, *69*, 95–97.

Disposition in the Body. Readily absorbed after oral administration. Metabolised by hydroxylation of the 3′-methyl group followed by oxidation to produce the 3′-carboxy metabolite; glucuronide conjugation also occurs. About 50% of a dose is excreted in the urine in 48 hours, mainly as conjugated metabolites; about 20% of a dose is eliminated in the faeces, mostly as unconjugated 3′-carboxymefenamic acid.

THERAPEUTIC CONCENTRATION.

Following a single oral dose of 1 g to 6 subjects, a mean peak plasma concentration of 10 µg/ml was attained in about 2 hours; the free and conjugated 3′-hydroxymethyl and 3′-carboxy metabolites attained similar concentrations after about 3 hours, and 6 to 8 hours respectively (A. J. Glazko, *Ann. phys. Med.*, 1966, *9*, *Suppl.*, 23–26).

After oral administration of 250 mg 3 times a day for four days to 10 subjects, peak plasma concentrations of 0.3 to 2.4 µg/ml (mean 0.9) were reported 2 hours after the morning dose (R. A. Buchanan *et al.*, *Curr. ther. Res.*, 1968, *10*, 592–596).

TOXICITY. Toxic effects are usually associated with plasma concentrations greater than 10 µg/ml.

In a survey of 29 cases of mefenamic acid overdose, plasma concentrations were in the range 11 to 148 µg/ml; in 11 of the cases convulsions occurred (mean plasma concentration 73 µg/ml). All the patients recovered (M. Balali-Mood *et al.*, *Lancet*, 1981, *1*, 1354–1356).

HALF-LIFE. Plasma half-life, about 3 to 4 hours.

PROTEIN BINDING. In plasma, about 99%.

Dose. Up to 1.5 g daily.

Mefruside

Diuretic

Proprietary Names. Baycaron; Mefrusal.

4-Chloro-N^1-methyl-N^1-(tetrahydro-2-methylfurfuryl)benzene-1,3-disulphonamide

$C_{13}H_{19}ClN_2O_5S_2 = 382.9$

CAS—7195-27-9

A white powder. M.p. 148° to 149°.

Practically **insoluble** in water; soluble in dilute solutions of sodium hydroxide.

Colour Tests. Koppanyi–Zwikker Test—violet; Liebermann's Test—blue; Mercurous Nitrate—black.

Thin-layer Chromatography. *System TD*—Rf 45; *system TE*—Rf 65; *system TF*—Rf 58.

Gas Chromatography. *System GA*—RI 2950.

High Pressure Liquid Chromatography. *System HN*—k' 8.67.

Ultraviolet Spectrum. Methanol—276 nm ($A_1^1 = 44$ a), 284 nm.

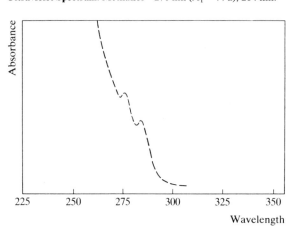

Wavelength

Infra-red Spectrum. Principal peaks at wavenumbers 1162, 1176, 819, 1041, 746, 909.

Mass Spectrum. Principal peaks at m/z 85, 43, 42, 86, 44, 41, 75, 110.

Quantification. GAS CHROMATOGRAPHY. In blood, plasma, erythrocytes or urine: sensitivity 5 ng/ml in plasma, AFID—H. L. J. Fleuren *et al.*, *Arzneimittel-Forsch.*, 1979, *29*, 1041–1047. In plasma, erythrocytes or urine: 5-oxomefruside and its hydroxycarboxylic acid analogue, sensitivity 25 ng, AFID—H. L. J. Fleuren *et al.*, *J. Chromat.*, 1980, *182*; *Biomed. Appl.*, 8, 179–190.

HIGH PRESSURE LIQUID CHROMATOGRAPHY. In urine: mefruside and its metabolites, UV detection—C. J. Little *et al.*, *Analyt. Chem.*, 1977, *49*, 1311–1313.

Disposition in the Body. Readily absorbed after oral administration. About 13% of a dose is excreted in the urine as 5-oxomefruside, about 35 to 55% as the hydroxycarboxylic acid analogue of 5-oxomefruside, and up to about 15% as a conjugate of this acid analogue. Both of these metabolites appear to be active. Less than 1% of the dose is excreted as unchanged drug.

THERAPEUTIC CONCENTRATION. There is considerable intersubject variation in plasma concentrations after therapeutic doses. Peak plasma concentrations of 0.07 to 0.13 µg/ml were attained 2 to 5 hours after a single oral dose of 50 mg to 6 subjects (H. L. J. Fleuren *et al.*, *Eur. J. clin. Pharmac.*, 1980, *17*, 59–69).

HALF-LIFE. Plasma half-life, mefruside 3 to 12 hours (mean 7), 5-oxomefruside 10 to 14 hours, hydroxycarboxylic acid analogue 8 to 12 hours.

VOLUME OF DISTRIBUTION. About 6 litres/kg.

CLEARANCE. Plasma clearance, 5 to 30 ml/min/kg (mean 13).

DISTRIBUTION IN BLOOD. Plasma: whole blood ratio, about 0.03.

REFERENCE. H. L. J. Fleuren *et al.*, *Eur. J. clin. Pharmac.*, 1980, *17*, 59–69.

Dose. 25 to 100 mg daily.

Megestrol Acetate

Progestational Steroid

Proprietary Names. Megace; Niagestin; Pallace.
6-Methyl-3,20-dioxopregna-4,6-dien-17α-yl acetate
$C_{24}H_{32}O_4 = 384.5$
CAS—3562-63-8 (megestrol); *595-33-5* (acetate)

A white to creamy-white crystalline powder. M.p. about 217°. A solution in chloroform is dextrorotatory.
Practically **insoluble** in water; soluble 1 in 55 of ethanol, 1 in 0.8 of chloroform, and 1 in 130 of ether; soluble in acetone.

Thin-layer Chromatography. *System TP*—Rf 80; *system TQ*—Rf 50; *system TR*—Rf 98; *system TS*—Rf 85, streaking may occur.

Ultraviolet Spectrum. Dehydrated alcohol—287 nm ($A_1^1 = 630$ a).

Infra-red Spectrum. Principal peaks at wavenumbers 1263, 1249, 1733, 1662, 1712, 1630 (KBr disk).

Mass Spectrum. Principal peaks at m/z 281, 43, 282, 187, 107, 91, 55, 105.

Dose. 40 to 320 mg daily.

Melphalan

Antineoplastic

Synonyms. PAM; Phenylalanine Nitrogen Mustard.
Note. Merphalan is the racemic form of melphalan; medphalan is the D-isomer of melphalan.
Proprietary Name. Alkeran
4-Bis(2-chloroethyl)amino-L-phenylalanine
$C_{13}H_{18}Cl_2N_2O_2 = 305.2$
CAS—148-82-3

A white to buff-coloured powder. M.p. about 177° to 180°, with decomposition.
Practically **insoluble** in water, chloroform, and ether; slightly soluble in ethanol; soluble in dilute mineral acids.

Ultraviolet Spectrum. Methanol—260 nm ($A_1^1 = 707$ a), 301 nm.

Infra-red Spectrum. Principal peaks at wavenumbers 1621, 1513, 1186, 1160, 1250, 1205 (KBr disk).

Quantification. HIGH PRESSURE LIQUID CHROMATOGRAPHY. In plasma: sensitivity 10 ng/ml, fluorescence detection—K. W. Woodhouse and D. B. Henderson, *Br. J. clin. Pharmac.*, 1982,

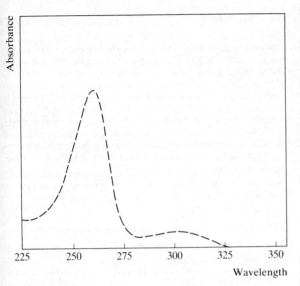

Absorbance

225   250   275   300   325   350

Wavelength

13, 605P. In plasma: sensitivity 50 ng/ml, UV detection—S. Y. Chang *et al.*, *J. pharm. Sci.*, 1978, *67*, 679–682.

Dose. 200 to 300 μg/kg daily, by mouth, for 4 to 6 days.

Menadione   *Vitamin K Analogue*

Synonyms. Menaphthene; Menaphthone; Methylnaphthochinonum; Vitamin K_3.
Proprietary Name. Bilkaby
2-Methyl-1,4-naphthoquinone
$C_{11}H_8O_2 = 172.2$
CAS—58-27-5

A bright yellow crystalline powder. On exposure to light it decomposes and darkens to light brown. M.p. 105° to 107°.
Practically **insoluble** in water; soluble 1 in 60 of ethanol; freely soluble in chloroform; soluble in ether.
Caution. The powder is irritating to the respiratory tract and to the skin. The ethanolic solution has vesicant properties.

Menadione Sodium Bisulphite
Synonyms. Kavitanum; Vikasolum.
Proprietary Name. K Thrombin
$C_{11}H_8O_2NaHSO_3,3H_2O = 330.3$
CAS—130-37-0 (anhydrous); *6147-37-1* (trihydrate)
A white, hygroscopic, crystalline powder.
Soluble 1 in 3 of water; very slightly soluble in ethanol, chloroform, and ether.

Colour Test. Dissolve about 0.5 mg in 5 ml of ethanol and add 2 ml of *strong ammonia solution* and a few drops of ethyl cyanoacetate—violet; add 5 ml of *sodium hydroxide solution*—brown-yellow. The violet colour is destroyed on the addition of acid or on exposure to sunlight.

Ultraviolet Spectrum. Aqueous acid—244 nm ($A_1^1 = 1052$ b), 249 nm ($A_1^1 = 1133$ b), 261 nm ($A_1^1 = 990$ b), 340 nm ($A_1^1 = 159$ b).

Dose. Menadione is usually administered by intramuscular injection as a 0.5% solution in oil.

Menthol   *Decongestant/Antipruritic*

Synonym. Mentol
p-Menthan-3-ol
$C_{10}H_{20}O = 156.3$
CAS—89-78-1; 1490-04-6; 2216-51-5 (−); 15356-70-4 (±)

Menthol is natural laevo-menthol, obtained from the volatile oils of various species of *Mentha* (Labiatae), or synthetic laevo-menthol, or racemic menthol.
Colourless crystals or crystalline powder. M.p. of natural or synthetic (−)-menthol, 41° to 44° and of (±)-menthol, 27° to 28° (rising on prolonged stirring to 30° to 32°).
Very slightly **soluble** in water; soluble 1 in 0.2 of ethanol, 1 in 0.25 of chloroform, and 1 in 0.4 of ether.

Ultraviolet Spectrum. No significant absorption, 230 to 360 nm.

Infra-red Spectrum. Principal peaks at wavenumbers 1046, 1026, 995, 1102, 1078, 979 (Nujol mull).

Mass Spectrum. Principal peaks at *m/z* 81, 95, 71, 41, 67, 55, 138, 123.

Disposition in the Body. Menthol is excreted in the bile and urine as a glucuronide conjugate; the various stereoisomers differ quantitatively in the extent to which they conjugate with glucuronic acid. Menthol may occur in the conjugated form as a metabolite of pulagone which is a constituent of pulegium oil.

TOXICITY. The minimum lethal dose has been estimated to be about 2 g. The application of drops or ointments containing menthol to the nostrils of infants is dangerous and may cause instant collapse. Ingestion of excess menthol may cause severe abdominal pain and coma.

Mepacrine   *Antimalarial/Antiprotozoal*

Synonyms. Acrichinum; Acrinamine; Atebrine; Chinacrina; Quinacrine.
6-Chloro-9-(4-diethylamino-1-methylbutylamino)-2-methoxy-acridine
$C_{23}H_{30}ClN_3O = 400.0$
CAS—83-89-6

Mepacrine Hydrochloride
Synonyms. Antimalarinae Chlorhydras; Erion; Quinacrine Hydrochloride.

Proprietary Name. Atabrine
$C_{23}H_{30}ClN_3O,2HCl,2H_2O = 508.9$
CAS—69-05-6 (anhydrous); *6151-30-0* (dihydrate)
A bright yellow crystalline powder. M.p. about 250°, with decomposition.
Soluble 1 in about 35 of water; soluble in ethanol; very slightly soluble in chloroform; practically insoluble in ether.

Mepacrine Mesylate

Synonym. Mepacrine Methanesulphonate
$C_{23}H_{30}ClN_3O,2CH_3SO_3H,H_2O = 610.2$
CAS—316-05-2 (anhydrous)
Bright yellow crystals.
Soluble 1 in 3 of water and 1 in 36 of ethanol.

Dissociation Constant. pK_a 7.7, 10.3 (20°).

Colour Tests. Mandelin's Test—violet → yellow; Marquis Test—yellow.

Thin-layer Chromatography. *System TA*—Rf 43; *system TB*—Rf 15; *system TC*—Rf 05. (*Acidified iodoplatinate solution*, positive.)

Ultraviolet Spectrum. Aqueous acid—279 nm ($A_1^1 = 1706$ a), 343 nm; aqueous alkali—270 nm, 345 nm.

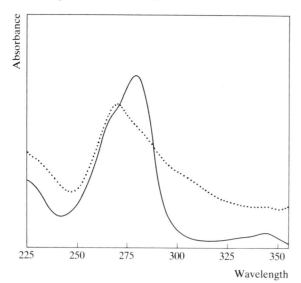

Infra-red Spectrum. Principal peaks at wavenumbers 1245, 1627, 1587, 1500, 1560, 1522 (mepacrine hydrochloride, KBr disk).

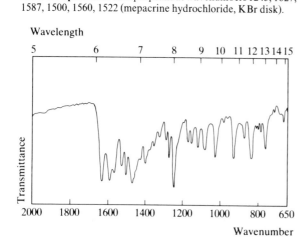

Mass Spectrum. Principal peaks at *m/z* 86, 36, 126, 30, 58, 38, 112, 99.

Disposition in the Body. Readily absorbed after oral administration; it appears in the blood within 2 hours, peak concentrations being attained in 8 hours. Mepacrine accumulates in the body during chronic administration and is widely distributed, high concentrations being found in the liver, lungs, and spleen; it also persists in the skin and finger-nails. The urine and skin may become yellow. It is excreted very slowly in the urine and bile with significant amounts detectable in the urine for at least 2 months after the discontinuation of therapy. Several metabolites are excreted but these account for not more than 5% of the dose.

TOXICITY. Large doses may give rise to nausea and vomiting and occasionally to transient mental disturbances. Attempts at suicide with massive doses have not been successful.

HALF-LIFE. About 5 days.

DISTRIBUTION IN BLOOD. Concentrated in the erythrocytes.

PROTEIN BINDING. In plasma, about 90%.

Dose. 300 to 900 mg daily.

Mepenzolate Bromide   *Anticholinergic*

Proprietary Names. Cantil; Colibantil; Gastropidil.
3-Benziloyloxy-1,1-dimethylpiperidinium bromide
$C_{21}H_{26}BrNO_3 = 420.3$
CAS—25990-43-6 (mepenzolate); *76-90-4* (bromide)

A white or light cream-coloured powder. M.p. about 230°, with decomposition.
Soluble 1 in 110 of water, 1 in 120 of dehydrated alcohol, 1 in about 630 of chloroform, and 1 in about 8 of methanol; practically insoluble in ether.

Colour Tests. The following tests are performed on mepenzolate nitrate (see page 128): Liebermann's Test—brown; Marquis Test—orange (transient).

Thin-layer Chromatography. *System TA*—Rf 01. (*Acidified iodoplatinate solution*, positive.)

Gas Chromatography. *System GA*—RI 2327.

High Pressure Liquid Chromatography. *System HA*—k' 4.1 (tailing peak).

Ultraviolet Spectrum. Aqueous acid—252 nm, 258 nm ($A_1^1 = 11$ b), 261 nm, 263 nm.

Infra-red Spectrum. Principal peaks at wavenumbers 1220, 1727, 1163, 763, 1062, 1093 (KBr disk).

Mass Spectrum. Principal peaks at *m/z* 97, 105, 77, 96, 42, 183, 98, 82.

Dose. 75 to 200 mg daily.

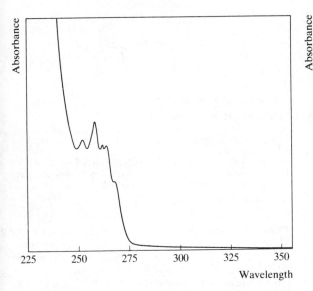

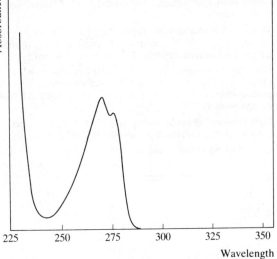

Mephenesin *Muscle Relaxant*

Synonyms. Cresoxydiol; Glykresin.
Proprietary Names. Decontractyl; Rhex.
3-(*o*-Tolyloxy)propane-1,2-diol
$C_{10}H_{14}O_3 = 182.2$
CAS—59-47-2

White crystals or crystalline aggregates. M.p. 70° to 73°.

Soluble 1 in 100 of water, 1 in 8 of ethanol, and 1 in 12 of chloroform; soluble in ether.

Mephenesin Carbamate
$C_{11}H_{15}NO_4 = 225.2$
CAS—533-06-2
White crystals. M.p. 93°.
Slightly **soluble** in water; very soluble in ethanol; soluble 1 in 50 of chloroform.

Colour Tests. Mephenesin carbamate: Mandelin's Test—grey-brown; Marquis Test—red.

Thin-layer Chromatography. *System TA*—Rf 64; *system TB*—Rf 02; *system TC*—Rf 43. (*Marquis reagent*, positive.)
Mephenesin carbamate: *system TD*—Rf 14; *system TE*—Rf 55; *system TF*—Rf 36. (*Furfuraldehyde reagent*, positive.)

Gas Chromatography. *System GA*—RI 1568.

High Pressure Liquid Chromatography. *System HA*—k' 0.2.

Ultraviolet Spectrum. Aqueous acid—270 nm ($A_1^1 = 87$ a), 276 nm. No alkaline shift.

Infra-red Spectrum. Principal peaks at wavenumbers 1047, 1248, 1124, 1493, 756, 748 (Nujol mull).

Mass Spectrum. Principal peaks at *m/z* 108, 107, 91, 182, 109, 77, 79, 31; mephenesin carbamate 118, 108, 182, 91, 225, 107, 57, 75.

Disposition in the Body. Readily absorbed after oral administration and widely distributed throughout the tissues. It is rapidly metabolised to the inactive metabolites, β-(*o*-tolyloxy)lactic acid and β-(2-methyl-4-hydroxyphenoxy)lactic acid. Less than 2% of a dose is excreted in the urine as unchanged drug.

THERAPEUTIC CONCENTRATION.
Following a single oral dose of 3 g to 4 subjects, a mean peak plasma concentration of about 10 μg/ml was attained in 0.5 hour (I. London and R. B. Poet, *Proc. Soc. exp. Biol. Med.*, 1957, *94*, 191).

TOXICITY.
A 43-year-old woman, who ingested between 5.5 and 11 g of mephenesin recovered within about 10 hours following treatment (D. W. Barron and T. G. Milliken, *Lancet*, 1960, *1*, 262).

Dose. 0.5 to 6 g of mephenesin daily.

Mephentermine *Sympathomimetic*

Synonyms. Mephenterdrine; Mephetedrine.
N,α,α-Trimethylphenethylamine
$C_{11}H_{17}N = 163.3$
CAS—100-92-5

A clear, colourless to pale yellow liquid.
Practically **insoluble** in water; very soluble in ethanol.

Mephentermine Sulphate
Proprietary Name. Wyamine Sulfate
$(C_{11}H_{17}N)_2,H_2SO_4,2H_2O = 460.6$
CAS—1212-72-2 (anhydrous); *6190-60-9* (dihydrate)
Colourless crystals or white crystalline powder.
Soluble 1 in about 18 of water and 1 in 150 of ethanol; practically insoluble in chloroform and ether.

Dissociation Constant. pK_a 10.4.

Colour Tests. Liebermann's Test—red-orange; Marquis Test—orange → brown.

Thin-layer Chromatography. *System TA*—Rf 25; *system TB*—Rf 34; *system TC*—Rf 08. (*Dragendorff spray*, positive; *acidified iodoplatinate solution*, positive; *Marquis reagent*, brown.)

Gas Chromatography. *System GA*—mephentermine RI 1239, phentermine RI 1147; *system GB*—mephentermine RI 1278, phentermine RI 1182; *system GC*—mephentermine RI 1668, phentermine RI 1450.

High Pressure Liquid Chromatography. *System HA*—mephentermine k' 1.5, phentermine k' 0.6; *system HC*—k' 2.48.

Ultraviolet Spectrum. Aqueous acid—251 nm, 257 nm ($A_1^1 = $ 10 c), 263 nm.

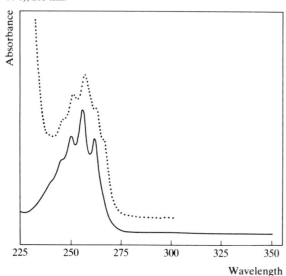

Infra-red Spectrum. Principal peaks at wavenumbers 1111, 711, 1162, 696, 763, 1587.

Mass Spectrum. Principal peaks at *m/z* 72, 91, 73, 56, 148, 65, 57, 42; phentermine 58, 91, 42, 41, 134, 65, 59, 40.

Quantification. GAS CHROMATOGRAPHY. In urine: mephentermine, chlorphentermine and phentermine, FID—A. H. Beckett and L. G. Brookes, *J. Pharm. Pharmac.*, 1971, **23**, 288–294.

Disposition in the Body. Readily absorbed after oral or parenteral administration and rapidly metabolised by demethylation and hydroxylation. About 50 to 85% of a dose is excreted in the urine unchanged, together with 15 to 20% as phentermine. Conjugated *N*-hydroxymephentermine has also been detected in the urine in small quantities.

TOXICITY. The estimated minimum lethal dose in children up to 2 years of age is 200 mg, and in adults is 2 g.

HALF-LIFE. Derived from urinary excretion data, about 6 to 20 hours.

Dose. The equivalent of 15 to 80 mg of mephentermine has been given parenterally.

Mepivacaine   *Local Anaesthetic*

(1-Methyl-2-piperidyl)formo-2',6'-xylidide
$C_{15}H_{22}N_2O = 246.4$
CAS—96-88-8

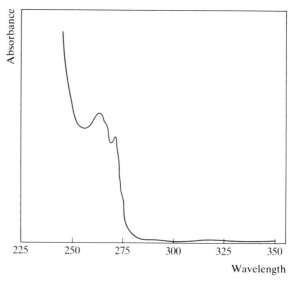

Yellow-white crystals. M.p. 149° to 153°.

Mepivacaine Hydrochloride

Proprietary Names. Carbocain(e); Chlorocain; Meaverin; Scandicain(e).
$C_{15}H_{22}N_2O,HCl = 282.8$
CAS—1722-62-9
A white crystalline powder. M.p. 255° to 262°, with decomposition. Freely **soluble** in water and methanol; soluble 1 in 10 of ethanol; very slightly soluble in chloroform; practically insoluble in ether.

Dissociation Constant. pK_a 7.7 (20°).

Colour Test. Liebermann's Test—brown-orange.

Thin-layer Chromatography. *System TA*—Rf 65; *system TB*—Rf 27; *system TC*—Rf 62; *system TL*—Rf 48. (*Dragendorff spray*, positive; *acidified iodoplatinate solution*, positive; *Marquis reagent*, brown; *ninhydrin spray*, positive.)

Gas Chromatography. *System GA*—RI 2071; *system GF*—RI 2345.

High Pressure Liquid Chromatography. *System HA*—k' 0.9; *system HQ*—k' 1.09.

Ultraviolet Spectrum. Aqueous acid—263 nm ($A_1^1 = 18$ a), 271 nm.

Infra-red Spectrum. Principal peaks at wavenumbers 1650, 1523, 760, 1220, 1123, 1265 (KBr disk).

Mass Spectrum. Principal peaks at *m/z* 98, 99, 70, 42, 96, 55, 41, 40 (no peaks above 100).

Quantification. GAS CHROMATOGRAPHY. In blood: sensitivity 40 ng, FID—J. H. Asling *et al.*, *Anesthesiology*, 1969, **31**, 458–461. In urine: mepivacaine and 3 metabolites, FID—J. Thomas and P. Meffin, *J. med. Chem.*, 1972, **15**, 1046–1049.

Disposition in the Body. Rapidly absorbed into the circulation following epidural and paracervical injection. Rapidly metabolised by hydroxylation to the 3'- and 4'-hydroxy metabolites and

Wavelength

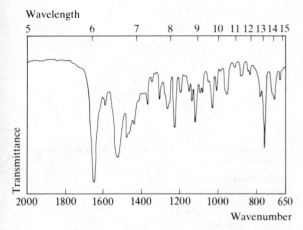

by *N*-demethylation to 2′,6′-pipecoloxylidide (PPX). Less than 10% of a dose is excreted in the urine as unchanged drug in 24 hours; about 16% of a dose is excreted in the 24-hour urine as 3′-hydroxymepivacaine, 12% as 4′-hydroxymepivacaine, and 2% as 2′,6′-pipecoloxylidide; the excretion of unchanged drug is increased in acid urine and in neonates.

THERAPEUTIC CONCENTRATION. In plasma, usually in the range 2 to 5 µg/ml.

Following epidural administration of 250 to 580 mg to 8 subjects, plasma concentrations at delivery were 3.7 to 5.5 µg/ml (mean 4.7) for mepivacaine and <0.1 to 0.38 µg/ml for 2′,6′-pipecoloxylidide (P. Meffin *et al.*, *Clin. Pharmac. Ther.*, 1973, *14*, 218–225).

Following paracervical injection of 200 mg to 5 subjects, peak plasma concentrations of 1.4 to 4.0 µg/ml (mean 2.3) were attained in about 30 minutes (K. Teramo and A. Rajamaki, *Br. J. Anaesth.*, 1971, *43*, 300–312).

TOXICITY.

Mepivacaine had been given as a local anaesthetic (between 75 and 150 ml of a 2% solution) to a young woman who died while undergoing cosmetic surgery. Postmortem concentrations were: blood 50 µg/ml, bile 50 µg/ml, brain 51 µg/g, kidney 51 µg/g, liver 75 µg/g, spleen 72 µg/g. Salicylate and glutethimide were also found in the blood and urine (I. Sunshine and W. W. Fike, *New Engl. J. Med.*, 1964, *271*, 487–490).

HALF-LIFE. Plasma half-life, about 2 to 3 hours.

VOLUME OF DISTRIBUTION. About 1 litre/kg.

CLEARANCE. Plasma clearance, about 5 ml/min/kg.

DISTRIBUTION IN BLOOD. Plasma: whole blood ratio, 1.1.

PROTEIN BINDING. In plasma, about 77%.

NOTE. For a review of the pharmacokinetics of local anaesthetics see G. T. Tucker and L. E. Mather, *Clin. Pharmacokinet.*, 1979, *4*, 241–278.

Dose. Mepivacaine hydrochloride is given by injection in doses of up to 400 mg; maximum of 1 g in 24 hours.

Meprobamate   *Tranquilliser*

Synonym. Meprotanum
Proprietary Names. Equanil; Lan-Dol; Meditran; Mep-E; Meprate; Mepriam; Mepron; Meprospan; Milonorm; Miltown; Neo-Tran; Novomepro; Oasil; Procalmadiol; Quietal; Restenil; SK-Bamate. It is an ingredient of Deprol, Ecuagesico, Equagesic, Milpath, Miltrate, and Tenavoid.

2-Methyl-2-propyltrimethylene dicarbamate
$C_9H_{18}N_2O_4 = 218.3$
CAS—57-53-4

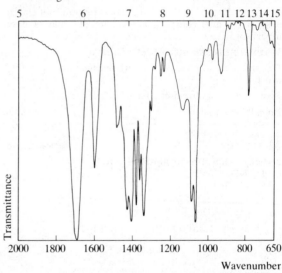

Colourless crystals or white crystalline powder. M.p. 103° to 107°.

Soluble 1 in 240 of water, 1 in 7 of ethanol, 1 in 80 of chloroform, and 1 in 70 of ether; freely soluble in acetone.

Partition Coefficient. Log *P* (octanol), 0.7.

Colour Tests. Furfuraldehyde—black; Nessler's Reagent (100°)—grey-black.

Thin-layer Chromatography. *System TD*—Rf 09; *system TE*—Rf 60; *system TF*—Rf 34. (*Furfuraldehyde reagent*, positive; *Van Urk reagent*, yellow.)

Gas Chromatography. *System GA*—RI 1796; *system GF*—RI 2460.

Ultraviolet Spectrum. No significant absorption, 230 to 360 nm.

Infra-red Spectrum. Principal peaks at wavenumbers 1688, 1069, 1090, 1590, 1310, 1140 (KBr disk).

Wavelength

Mass Spectrum. Principal peaks at *m/z* 83, 84, 55, 56, 43, 71, 41, 62 (no peaks above 160).

Quantification. GAS CHROMATOGRAPHY. In plasma or urine: FID—L. Martis and R. H. Levy, *J. pharm. Sci.*, 1974, *63*, 834–837.

HIGH PRESSURE LIQUID CHROMATOGRAPHY. In plasma: UV detection, comparison with a GC method—R. N. Gupta and F. Eng, *J. High Resolut. Chromat. Chromat. Commun.*, 1980, *3*, 419–420.

Disposition in the Body. Readily absorbed after oral administration. About 90% of a dose is excreted in the urine in 24 hours, with about 10 to 20% of the dose as unchanged drug and the remainder as metabolites, mainly 2-hydroxypropylmeprobamate and meprobamate *N*-glucuronide. About 10% of the dose is eliminated in the faeces.

Meprobamate is a minor metabolite of tybamate and is a metabolite of carisoprodol.

THERAPEUTIC CONCENTRATION. In plasma, usually in the range 5 to 20 µg/ml.

Following two oral doses of 800 mg, given to 5 subjects over a period of 1.5 hours, peak blood concentrations of 18.6 to 26.6 µg/ml (mean 23.8) were attained in about 3.5 hours (K. D. Parker et al., Clin. Toxicol., 1970, 3, 131–145).

TOXICITY. The estimated minimum lethal dose is 12 g, although recovery has occurred after much larger doses. Blood concentrations greater than about 50 µg/ml may cause coma and fatalities have usually been associated with blood concentrations greater than about 70 µg/ml.

In a review of 12 deaths attributed to meprobamate overdose, the blood concentrations were in the range 142 to 346 µg/ml (mean 226); in 9 of these cases, concentrations in the liver were 147 to 412 µg/g (mean 238) (S. Felby, Acta pharmac. tox., 1970, 28, 334–337).

The following postmortem tissue concentrations were reported in 16 fatalities due solely to meprobamate ingestion: blood 35 to 240 µg/ml (mean 95), liver 58 to 360 µg/g (mean 148) (R. C. Baselt and R. H. Cravey, J. analyt. Toxicol., 1977, 1, 81–103).

A man ingested about 200 g of meprobamate and, when admitted to hospital, was comatose and had a serum concentration of 111 µg/ml. After treatment by haemoperfusion he recovered consciousness, but 19 hours later relapsed into profound coma; the serum concentration was 260 µg/ml. Recovery occurred after further treatment (W. E. Hoy et al., Ann. intern. Med., 1980, 93, 455–459).

HALF-LIFE. Plasma half-life, 6 to 17 hours (mean 11); it may be much longer after chronic administration and may be dose-dependent.

VOLUME OF DISTRIBUTION. About 0.7 litre/kg.

DISTRIBUTION IN BLOOD. Plasma: whole blood ratio, about 0.2 to 0.3.

PROTEIN BINDING. In plasma, about 20%.

Dose. 1.2 to 2.4 g daily.

Meprylcaine   Local Anaesthetic

2-Methyl-2-propylaminopropyl benzoate
$C_{14}H_{21}NO_2 = 235.3$
CAS—495-70-5

$$C_6H_5 \cdot CO \cdot O \cdot CH_2 \cdot \underset{\underset{CH_3}{|}}{\overset{\overset{CH_3}{|}}{C}} \cdot NH \cdot [CH_2]_2 \cdot CH_3$$

An oil.
Practically **insoluble** in water; soluble in ethanol and ether.

Meprylcaine Hydrochloride
$C_{14}H_{21}NO_2,HCl = 271.8$
CAS—956-03-6
A white crystalline powder. M.p. 150° to 153°.
Soluble 1 in 6 of water, 1 in 5 of ethanol, 1 in 3 of chloroform, and 1 in 12 of ether.

Ultraviolet Spectrum. Aqueous acid—232 nm ($A_1^1 = 422$ b).

Mass Spectrum. Principal peaks at m/z 100, 58, 105, 77, 56, 101, 41, 70.

Meptazinol   Narcotic Analgesic

Proprietary Name. Meptid (tablets)
3-(3-Ethyl-1-methylperhydroazepin-3-yl)phenol
$C_{15}H_{23}NO = 233.4$
CAS—54340-58-8

Crystals. M.p. 127° to 133°.
Very slightly **soluble** in water; soluble in ethanol; sparingly soluble in chloroform and ether.

Meptazinol Hydrochloride
Proprietary Name. Meptid (injection)
$C_{15}H_{23}NO,HCl = 269.8$
CAS—59263-76-2; 34154-59-1 ($\pm$)
A white crystalline powder. M.p. 183° to 187°.
Soluble 1 in about 4 of water and 1 in 12 of ethanol; very slightly soluble in chloroform; practically insoluble in ether.

Dissociation Constant. pK_a 8.7 ($-NH_2$), 11.9 (phenol).

High Pressure Liquid Chromatography. System HA—k' 3.1.

Ultraviolet Spectrum. Ethanol—277 nm ($A_1^1 = 91$ b).

Infra-red Spectrum. Principal peaks at wavenumbers 1580, 708, 795, 1225, 1205, 1300 (meptazinol hydrochloride, KBr disk).

Quantification. HIGH PRESSURE LIQUID CHROMATOGRAPHY. In plasma: detection limit 3 ng/ml, fluorescence detection—T. Frost, Analyst, Lond., 1981, 106, 999–1001.

Disposition in the Body. Readily and almost completely absorbed after oral administration; bioavailability 2 to 19% (mean 9) due to extensive first-pass metabolism. Rapidly absorbed after intramuscular or rectal administration. It is excreted rapidly in the urine, mainly as the glucuronide conjugate, with less than 5% of a dose as unchanged drug, and about 5 to 10% as 7-oxomeptazinol. Both metabolites are inactive. Over 50% of a dose is excreted in the urine in 9 hours and over 60% in 24 hours. Less than 10% of an oral dose is eliminated in the faeces.

THERAPEUTIC CONCENTRATION.

Following a single oral dose of 200 mg to 9 subjects, peak plasma concentrations of 0.01 to 0.11 µg/ml (mean 0.06) were attained in 0.25 to 2 hours; accumulation in plasma did not occur after repeated oral administration (H. M. Norbury et al., Eur. J. clin. Pharmac., 1983, 25, 77–80).

After a single intramuscular dose of 50 mg to 4 subjects, peak plasma concentrations of 0.19 to 0.26 µg/ml (mean 0.22) were attained in 10 minutes (G. Davies et al., Eur. J. clin. Pharmac., 1982, 23, 535–538).

HALF-LIFE. Plasma half-life, about 2 hours.

VOLUME OF DISTRIBUTION. About 5 litres/kg.

CLEARANCE. Plasma clearance, about 30 ml/min/kg.

PROTEIN BINDING. In plasma, about 27%.

Dose. 200 mg, by mouth, every 4 hours; the equivalent of 50 to 100 mg of meptazinol parenterally.

Mepyramine   Antihistamine

Synonyms. Pyranisamine; Pyrilamine.
N-p-Anisyl-N'N'-dimethyl-N-(2-pyridyl)ethylenediamine
$C_{17}H_{23}N_3O = 285.4$
CAS—91-84-9

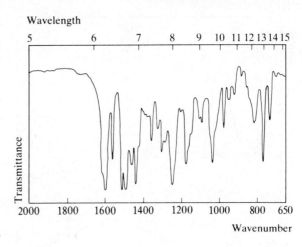

An oily liquid.

Mepyramine Maleate

Proprietary Names. Anthisan. It is an ingredient of Flavelix and Triotussic.
$C_{17}H_{23}N_3O, C_4H_4O_4 = 401.5$
CAS—59-33-6
A white or creamy-white crystalline powder. M.p. 99° to 103°.
Soluble 1 in 0.5 of water, 1 in 2.5 of ethanol, and 1 in 1.5 of chloroform; slightly soluble in ether.

Dissociation Constant. pK_a 4.0, 8.9 (25°).

Partition Coefficient. Log P (octanol), 2.8.

Colour Tests. Cyanogen Bromide—yellow; Mandelin's Test—violet; Marquis Test—violet.

Thin-layer Chromatography. *System TA*—Rf 51; *system TB*—Rf 39; *system TC*—Rf 25. (*Dragendorff spray*, positive; *acidified iodoplatinate solution*, positive; *Marquis reagent*, red.)

Gas Chromatography. *System GA*—RI 2220; *system GF*—RI 2560.

High Pressure Liquid Chromatography. *System HA*—k′ 3.9.

Ultraviolet Spectrum. Aqueous acid—239 nm ($A_1^1 = 633$ a), 316 nm; aqueous alkali—248 nm, 312 nm.

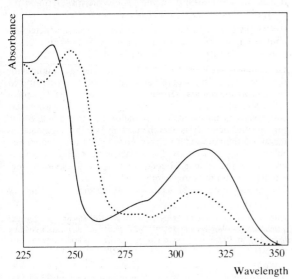

Infra-red Spectrum. Principal peaks at wavenumbers 1492, 1512, 1598, 1247, 1175, 1035 (KBr disk).

Mass Spectrum. Principal peaks at m/z 121, 58, 72, 71, 214, 122, 215, 78.

Quantification. GAS CHROMATOGRAPHY. In postmortem tissues: FID—G. R. Johnson, *Clin. Toxicol.*, 1981, *18*, 907–909.

Disposition in the Body. Absorbed after oral administration.

TOXICITY.
In a fatality due to mepyramine ingestion, the following postmortem tissue concentrations were reported: blood 11 μg/ml, brain 71 μg/g, liver 18 μg/g (G. R. Johnson, *ibid.*).

Dose. 0.3 to 1 g of mepyramine maleate daily.

Mequitazine   *Antihistamine*

Proprietary Names. Metaplexan; Mircol; Primalan.
10-(Quinuclidin-3-ylmethyl)phenothiazine
$C_{20}H_{22}N_2S = 322.5$
CAS—29216-28-2

M.p. about 143°.
Practically **insoluble** in water; soluble in ethanol and chloroform.

Colour Tests. Formaldehyde–Sulphuric Acid—red-violet; Forrest Reagent—red; FPN Reagent—orange-red; Liebermann's Test—green; Mandelin's Test—red; Marquis Test—red (slow); Sulphuric Acid (100°)—red (slow).

Thin-layer Chromatography. *System TA*—Rf 10; *system TB*—Rf 06; *system TC*—Rf 06.

Gas Chromatography. *System GA*—RI 2760.

High Pressure Liquid Chromatography. *System HA*—k′ 8.3 (tailing peak).

Ultraviolet Spectrum. Aqueous acid—256 nm ($A_1^1 = 1060$ a), 307 nm. No alkaline shift. (See below)

Infra-red Spectrum. Principal peaks at wavenumbers 751, 1250, 742, 1220, 729, 1042 (KBr disk). (See below)

Dose. 10 mg daily.

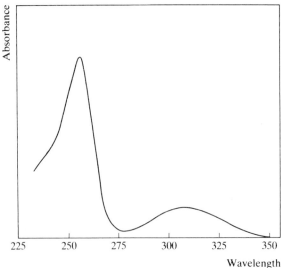

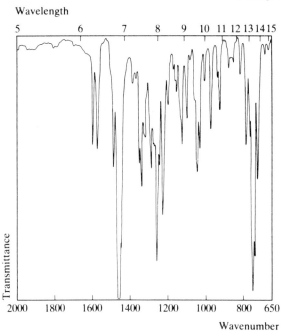

A yellow crystalline powder which darkens on exposure to air and light. M.p. above 308°, with decomposition.

Practically **insoluble** in water, chloroform, and ether; soluble 1 in 950 of ethanol; soluble in solutions of alkali hydroxides.

Dissociation Constant. pK$_a$ 7.7, 11.0 (20°).

Gas Chromatography. *System GA*—RI 1517.

Ultraviolet Spectrum. Mercaptopurine monohydrate: aqueous acid—325 nm (A$_1^1$ = 1165 a); aqueous alkali—231 nm (A$_1^1$ = 831 a), 310 nm (A$_1^1$ = 1160 a).

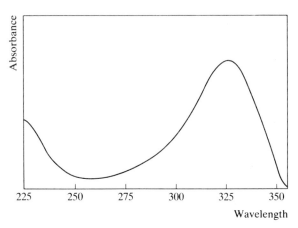

Infra-red Spectrum. Principal peaks at wavenumbers 1610, 1220, 1570, 1010, 865, 780 (KBr disk).

Quantification. GAS CHROMATOGRAPHY–MASS SPECTROMETRY. In plasma: detection limit 2 ng/ml—S. Floberg *et al.*, *J. Chromat.*, 1981, *225*; *Biomed. Appl.*, *14*, 73–81.

HIGH PRESSURE LIQUID CHROMATOGRAPHY. In plasma: detection limit <2 ng/ml, fluorescence detection—R. E. Jonkers *et al.*, *J. Chromat.*, 1982, *233*; *Biomed. Appl.*, *22*, 249–255.

Disposition in the Body. Readily absorbed after oral administration; bioavailability about 16% and very variable. It is distributed throughout the body water and diffuses into the cerebrospinal fluid. Mercaptopurine is activated in the body by intracellular conversion to nucleotide forms including the ribonucleotide thioinosinic acid. It is metabolised by xanthine oxidase to inactive 6-thiouric acid which is excreted in the urine; inorganic sulphate may also be present. About 50% of an oral dose is excreted in the urine in 24 hours, up to 8% as unchanged drug. Small amounts are excreted for up to 17 days.

Mercaptopurine is a metabolite of azathioprine.

THERAPEUTIC CONCENTRATION.

After a single oral dose of 75 mg/m^2 to 14 children (mean age 13 years) with acute lymphoblastic leukaemia, peak plasma concentrations of 0.04 to 0.28 µg/ml (mean 0.14) were attained in 0.5 to 4 hours (mean 2) (S. Zimm *et al.*, *New Engl. J. Med.*, 1983, *308*, 1005–1009).

TOXICITY.

A 64-year-old woman took 200 mg of mercaptopurine every 8 hours for about 2 weeks, because of an error in dispensing. She died 3 days later and the following postmortem concentrations were reported: blood 110 µg/ml, bile 16 µg/ml, brain 10 µg/g, kidney 33 µg/g (R.-L. Lin *et al.*, *J. forens. Sci.*, 1982, *27*, 454–460).

HALF-LIFE. Plasma half-life, about 0.5 to 1.5 hours.

PROTEIN BINDING. In plasma, about 20%.

Dose. Initially 2.5 mg/kg daily, by mouth.

Mercaptopurine   *Antineoplastic*

Synonym. 6MP

Proprietary Name. Puri-Nethol

Purine-6-thiol monohydrate

C$_5$H$_4$N$_4$S,H$_2$O = 170.2

CAS—50-44-2 (anhydrous); *6112-76-1* (monohydrate)

Mersalyl Acid   *Diuretic*

A mixture of {3-[2-(carboxymethoxy)benzamido]-2-methoxypropyl}hydroxymercury ($C_{13}H_{17}HgNO_6 = 483.9$) and its anhydrides.
CAS—486-67-9 ($C_{13}H_{17}HgNO_6$)

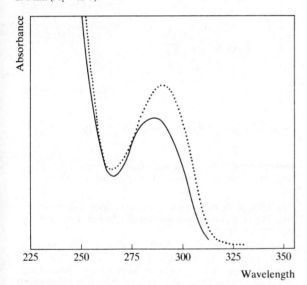

A white, slightly hygroscopic powder.
Sparingly **soluble** in water and dilute mineral acids; readily soluble in solutions of alkali hydroxides.

Mersalyl Sodium

Synonym. Mersalyl
$C_{13}H_{16}HgNNaO_6 = 505.9$
CAS—492-18-2
A white deliquescent powder.
Soluble 1 in 1 of water, 1 in 3 of ethanol, and 1 in 2 of methanol; practically insoluble in chloroform and ether.

Thin-layer Chromatography. *System TA—Rf 24.*

Ultraviolet Spectrum. Aqueous acid—286 nm; aqueous alkali—290 nm ($A_1^1 = 63$ b).

Dose. 50 to 200 mg of mersalyl sodium, intramuscularly.

Mescaline   *Hallucinogen*

3,4,5-Trimethoxyphenethylamine
$C_{11}H_{17}NO_3 = 211.3$
CAS—54-04-6

An alkaloid obtained from the cactus *Lophophora williamsii* (= *Anhalonium williamsii* = *A. lewinii*) (Cactaceae), which grows in the northern regions of Mexico. The cactus is also known by the names 'peyote' or 'peyotl' and dried slices of the cactus are called 'mescal buttons'.
Crystals which take up carbon dioxide from the air. M.p. 35° to 36°.
Soluble in water, ethanol, and chloroform; practically insoluble in ether.

Colour Tests. Liebermann's Test—black; Marquis Test—orange.

Thin-layer Chromatography. *System TA*—Rf 20; *system TB*—Rf 04; *system TC*—Rf 10. (*Dragendorff spray*, positive; *FPN reagent*, positive; *acidified iodoplatinate solution*, positive; *Marquis reagent*, yellow; *ninhydrin spray*, positive.)

Gas Chromatography. *System GA*—RI 1688.

High Pressure Liquid Chromatography. *System HA*—k' 1.3; *system HB*—k' 16.82; *system HC*—k' 2.17.

Ultraviolet Spectrum. Aqueous acid—268 nm ($A_1^1 = 34$ c). No alkaline shift.

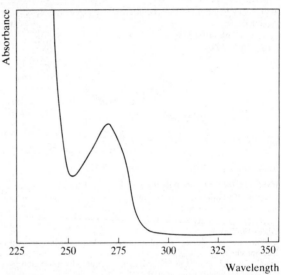

Infra-red Spectrum. Principal peaks at wavenumbers 1127, 1242, 1592, 996, 1513, 834 (mescaline hydrochloride, KBr disk).

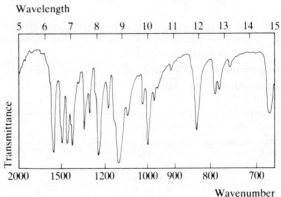

Mass Spectrum. Principal peaks at m/z 182, 30, 181, 167, 211, 183, 151, 148.

Quantification. GAS CHROMATOGRAPHY–MASS SPECTROMETRY. In plasma—C. Van Peteghem *et al.*, *J. pharm. Sci.*, 1980, *69*, 118–120.

Disposition in the Body. Readily absorbed after oral administration. It is concentrated in the kidneys, liver, and spleen. About 90% of a dose is excreted in the urine in 24 hours with about 30% as 3,4,5-trimethoxyphenylacetic acid, which is inactive; the remainder is mostly unchanged drug, together with 3,4-dihydroxy-5-methoxyphenylacetic acid which is excreted as a glutamine conjugate. Other metabolites include *N*-acetylmescaline and *N*-acetyl-3,4-dimethoxy-5-hydroxyphenethylamine.

TOXICITY. Mescaline induces psychotic changes similar to those produced by lysergide, but it is less potent. The effects of a single dose may persist for about 12 hours.

PROTEIN BINDING. In plasma, partly bound.

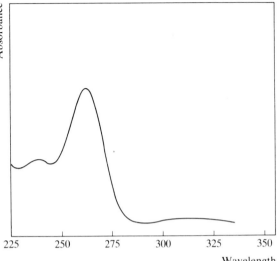
Absorbance — Wavelength

Mesoridazine   *Tranquilliser*

Synonym. Mesuridazine

10 - [2 - (1 - Methyl - 2 - piperidyl)ethyl] - 2 - (methylsulphinyl)-phenothiazine

$C_{21}H_{26}N_2OS_2 = 386.6$

CAS—5588-33-0

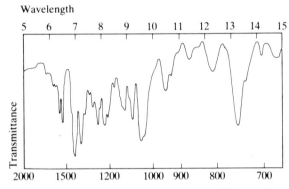
Transmittance — Wavenumber

Soluble in chloroform.

Mesoridazine Benzenesulphonate

Synonym. Mesoridazine Besylate

Proprietary Name. Serentil

$C_{21}H_{26}N_2OS_2,C_6H_6O_3S = 544.7$

CAS—32672-69-8

A white to pale yellow, crystalline powder. M.p. about 178°, with decomposition.

Soluble 1 in 1 of water, 1 in 11 of ethanol, 1 in 3 of chloroform, and 1 in 6300 of ether; freely soluble in methanol.

Colour Tests. Formaldehyde–Sulphuric Acid—violet; Forrest Reagent—red; FPN Reagent—red; Mandelin's Test—green-brown; Marquis Test—red → violet; Sulphuric Acid—violet → blue.

Thin-layer Chromatography. *System TA*—Rf 38; *system TB*—Rf 03; *system TC*—Rf 06. (*Acidified iodoplatinate solution*, positive.)

Gas Chromatography. *System GA*—not eluted.

High Pressure Liquid Chromatography. *System HA*—k′ 5.0.

Ultraviolet Spectrum. Aqueous acid—238 nm, 262 nm ($A_1^1 = 773$ b), 310 nm.

Infra-red Spectrum. Principal peaks at wavenumbers 1050, 752, 1239, 1282, 1562, 1091 (KBr disk).

Mass Spectrum. Principal peaks at m/z 98, 70, 99, 42, 386, 126, 55, 41.

Quantification. GAS CHROMATOGRAPHY. In plasma: limit of detection 50 ng/ml, FID—E. C. Dinovo *et al.*, *J. pharm. Sci.*, 1976, *65*, 667–669.

HIGH PRESSURE LIQUID CHROMATOGRAPHY. In whole blood: UV detection—J. R. McCutcheon, *J. analyt. Toxicol.*, 1979, *3*, 105–107.

Disposition in the Body. Readily absorbed after oral administration. The major metabolite is sulforidazine which is pharmacologically active.

Mesoridazine is a major metabolite of thioridazine.

THERAPEUTIC CONCENTRATION.

Following a single intramuscular injection of 2 mg/kg to 6 subjects, peak plasma concentrations of 0.1 to 1.1 µg/ml (mean 0.5) for mesoridazine, and 0.1 to 0.6 µg/ml (mean 0.3) for sulforidazine, were attained in about 4 hours (L. A. Gottschalk *et al.*, Plasma Levels of Mesoridazine and its Metabolites, in *Pharmacokinetics of Psychoactive Drugs*, L. A. Gottschalk and S. Merlis (Ed.), New York, Spectrum Publications, 1976, pp. 171–189).

TOXICITY.

In a fatality attributed to the ingestion of 2.5 g, the following postmortem tissue concentrations were reported: blood 3 µg/ml, kidney 17 µg/g, liver 114 µg/g; in a second case in which 8 g had been ingested, the postmortem blood concentration was 4 µg/ml (P. T. Donlon and J. P. Tupin, *Archs gen. Psychiat.*, 1977, *34*, 955–957).

HALF-LIFE. Plasma half-life, mesoridazine 2 to 9 hours (mean 5), sulforidazine 6 to 25 hours (mean 13).

Dose. The equivalent of 150 mg of mesoridazine daily; up to 400 mg daily has been given.

Mesterolone

Androgen

Proprietary Names. Mestoranum; Pro-viron.
17β-Hydroxy-1α-methyl-5α-androstan-3-one
$C_{20}H_{32}O_2 = 304.5$
CAS—1424-00-6

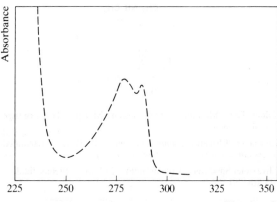

A white crystalline powder. M.p. about 210°.
Practically **insoluble** in water; soluble 1 in 50 of ethanol, 1 in 6 of chloroform, and 1 in 150 of ether.

Ultraviolet Spectrum. No significant absorption, 230 to 360 nm.

Infra-red Spectrum. Principal peaks at wavenumbers 1706, 1068, 1055, 1252, 1238, 1032 (KBr disk).

Dose. 50 to 100 mg daily.

Mestranol

Oestrogen

Synonyms. EE3ME; Ethinyloestradiol-3-methyl Ether.
Proprietary Names. It is an ingredient of Metrulen, Norinyl, Ortho-Novin, and Syntex Menophase.
3-Methoxy-19-nor-17α-pregna-1,3,5(10)-trien-20-yn-17β-ol
$C_{21}H_{26}O_2 = 310.4$
CAS—72-33-3

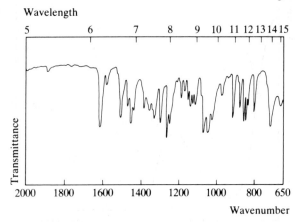

A white to creamy-white, crystalline powder. M.p. 146° to 154°.
Practically **insoluble** in water; soluble 1 in 44 of ethanol, 1 in 4.5 of chloroform, and 1 in 23 of ether.
Caution. Mestranol is a powerful oestrogen. Contact with the skin or inhalation should be avoided.

Colour Tests. Antimony Pentachloride—green; Liebermann's Test—red; Naphthol–Sulphuric Acid—red/red; Sulphuric Acid—orange-red (yellow fluorescence under ultraviolet light).

Thin-layer Chromatography. *System TP*—Rf 86; *system TQ*—Rf 52; *system TR*—Rf 90; *system TS*—Rf 90.

Gas Chromatography. *System GA*—RI 2612.

Ultraviolet Spectrum. Methanol—278 nm ($A_1^1 = 61$ a), 287 nm.

Infra-red Spectrum. Principal peaks at wavenumbers 1255, 1060, 1035, 1612, 1291, 1241 (KBr disk).

Mass Spectrum. Principal peaks at *m/z* 227, 310, 174, 284, 147, 160, 173, 199.

Dose. Up to 100 µg daily.

Metaldehyde

Molluscicide

Proprietary Names. It is an ingredient of many proprietary preparations used for the destruction of slugs. As a compressed fuel, it is known as 'Meta'.
A polymer of acetaldehyde.
$(C_2H_4O)_x$
CAS—9002-91-9
A white crystalline solid which burns readily with a non-luminous carbon-free flame and sublimes at 100°. In the presence of acids it decomposes slowly to acetaldehyde.
Practically **insoluble** in water.

Colour Test. Add 1 drop of *sulphuric acid* to a small amount of solid, then add a trace of pyrocatechol—violet-red.

Infra-red Spectrum. Principal peaks at wavenumbers 1094, 1113, 1163, 1074, 975, 1205 (KBr disk).

Disposition in the Body.
TOXICITY. Metaldehyde probably decomposes slowly in the body to acetaldehyde which is further oxidised. Fatalities have occurred after the ingestion of about 3 g.

Metanephrine

Synonym. Metadrenaline
(*R*)-1-(4-Hydroxy-3-methoxyphenyl)-2-methylaminoethanol
$C_{10}H_{15}NO_3 = 197.2$
CAS—5001-33-2

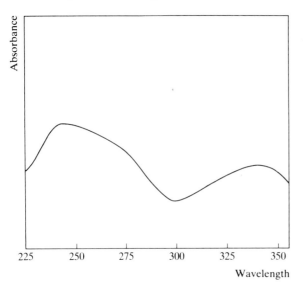

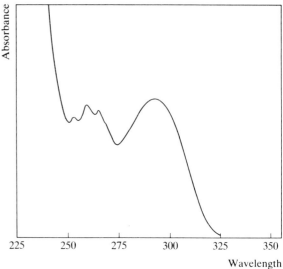

Methadone

Narcotic Analgesic

Synonyms. Amidone; Phenadone.
(±)-6-Dimethylamino-4,4-diphenylheptan-3-one
$C_{21}H_{27}NO = 309.5$
CAS—76-99-3; 297-88-1 (±)

$$CH_3 \cdot CH_2 \cdot CO \cdot \underset{\underset{C_6H_5}{|}}{\overset{\overset{C_6H_5}{|}}{C}} \cdot CH_2 \cdot \underset{}{\overset{\overset{CH_3}{|}}{CH}} \cdot N(CH_3)_2$$

Methadone Hydrochloride

Proprietary Names. Dolophine Hydrochloride; Eptadone; Mephenon; Physeptone.
$C_{21}H_{27}NO,HCl = 345.9$
CAS—1095-90-5; 125-56-4 (±)
Colourless crystals or white crystalline powder. M.p. 233° to 236°.
Soluble 1 in 12 of water, 1 in 7 of ethanol, and 1 in 3 of chloroform; practically insoluble in ether.

Dissociation Constant. pK_a 8.3 (20°).

Partition Coefficient. Log P (octanol/pH 7.4), 2.1.

Colour Tests. Liebermann's Test—brown-orange; Mandelin's Test—green → blue.

Thin-layer Chromatography. *System TA*—Rf 48; *system TB*—Rf 61; *system TC*—Rf 20. (*Dragendorff spray*, positive; *acidified iodoplatinate solution*, positive.)

Gas Chromatography. *System GA*—methadone RI 2148, 2-ethylidene-1,5-dimethyl-3,3-diphenylpyrrolidine (EDDP) RI 2030, 2-ethyl-5-methyl-3,3-diphenyl-1-pyrroline (EMDP) RI 1950; *system GB*—RI 2124; *system GC*—RI 2470; *system GF*—methadone RI 2370, EDDP RI 2280, EMDP RI 2190.

High Pressure Liquid Chromatography. *System HA*—methadone k′ 2.2, 2-ethylidene-1,5-dimethyl-3,3-diphenylpyrrolidine k′ 2.8, 2-ethyl-5-methyl-3,3-diphenyl-1-pyrroline k′ 0.2; *system HC*—k′ 1.03.

Ultraviolet Spectrum. Aqueous acid—253 nm, 259 nm, 264 nm, 292 nm ($A_1^1 = 18$ a).

Infra-red Spectrum. Principal peaks at wavenumbers 710, 1709, 769, 1107, 943, 1133 (methadone hydrochloride, Nujol mull).

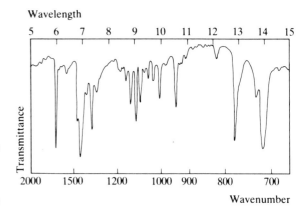

Mass Spectrum. Principal peaks at m/z 72, 73, 91, 293, 223, 165, 85, 71; EMDP 208, 193, 130, 115, 91, 165, 179, 207.

Quantification. SPECTROFLUORIMETRY. In plasma or tissues— C. H. Chi and B. N. Dixit, *J. pharm. Sci.*, 1979, *68*, 1097–1099.

GAS CHROMATOGRAPHY. In blood, plasma or urine: methadone and EDDP, sensitivity < 5 ng/ml, AFID—P. Jacob *et al.*, *J. analyt. Toxicol.*, 1981, *5*, 292–295. In blood, urine or tissues: methadone and metabolites, detection limit 20 ng/ml for methadone, FID—B. C. Thompson and Y. H. Caplan, *J. analyt. Toxicol.*, 1977, *1*, 66–69.

GAS CHROMATOGRAPHY-MASS SPECTROMETRY. In plasma, saliva or urine: methadone and metabolites, sensitivity 20 ng/ml for methadone in plasma or saliva—G. I. Kang and F. S. Abbott, *J. Chromat.*, 1982, *231*; *Biomed. Appl.*, *20*, 311–319.

HIGH PRESSURE LIQUID CHROMATOGRAPHY. In plasma: sensitivity 200 ng/ml, UV detection—R. G. Buice *et al.*, *Res. Commun. Subst. Abuse*, 1982, *3*, 97–107.

REVIEW. N. Jain *et al.*, *J. analyt. Toxicol.*, 1977, *1*, 6–9.

Disposition in the Body. Rapidly absorbed after oral administration, and widely distributed in the tissues, with higher concentrations in the liver, lungs, and kidneys than in the blood. The main metabolic reaction is *N*-demethylation resulting in a substance which spontaneously cyclises to form the major metabolites, 2-ethylidene-1,5-dimethyl-3,3-diphenylpyrrolidine (EDDP) and 2-ethyl-5-methyl-3,3-diphenyl-1-pyrroline (EMDP), neither of which are active. Hydroxylation to methadol followed by *N*-demethylation to normethadol also occurs to some extent. Other metabolic reactions occur and there are at least eight known metabolites. In subjects on methadone maintenance, about 20 to 60% of a dose is excreted in the urine in 24 hours, with up to about 33% of the dose as unchanged drug and up to about 43% as EDDP; EMDP accounts for about 5 to 10% of the dose. The ratio of EDDP to unchanged methadone is usually very much higher in the urine of patients on methadone maintenance treatment than in simple overdose cases. Urinary excretion of unchanged drug is pH-dependent, being increased in acid urine. Up to 30% of a dose may be eliminated in the faeces, but this appears to decrease with increasing dosage. About 75% of the total excreted material is unconjugated.

THERAPEUTIC CONCENTRATION. In plasma, usually in the range 0.05 to 1.0 μg/ml. During methadone maintenance treatment there are often considerable fluctuations in plasma concentrations from day to day, and there appears to be a decrease in concentration as dispositional tolerance develops.

A single oral dose of 15 mg given to 5 subjects, resulted in a mean peak plasma concentration of 0.07 μg/ml at about 4 hours (C. E. Inturrisi and K. Verebely, *Clin. Pharmac. Ther.*, 1972, *13*, 923–930).

Steady-state plasma concentrations of 0.14 to 0.22 μg/ml (mean 0.18) were attained with daily oral doses of 0.46 to 0.58 mg/kg given to 6 subjects; with oral doses of 0.85 to 1.33 mg/kg, the steady-state plasma concentrations were 0.34 to 0.58 μg/ml (mean 0.42) (K. Verebely *et al.*, *Clin. Pharmac. Ther.*, 1975, *18*, 180–190).

TOXICITY. The estimated minimum lethal dose is 50 mg but addicts on maintenance treatment may tolerate doses of 200 mg or more. In non-addicted subjects, toxic reactions are associated with plasma concentrations in the region of 1 to 2 μg/ml and concentrations above 2 μg/ml may be lethal.

In 3 cases in which death was attributed to methadone overdose, liver concentrations of 1.9, 1.3, and 0.7 μg/g and urine concentrations of 13, 25, and 4 μg/ml, respectively, were reported (P. E. Nelson and R. C. Selkirk, *Forens. Sci.*, 1975, *6*, 175–186).

In 23 fatalities in which methadone was involved, the following postmortem tissue concentrations, μg/ml or μg/g (mean, *n*), were reported:

	Methadone	EDDP
Blood	0–3 (1.2, *21*)	0–0.4 (0.1, *10*)
Bile	1.1–75 (13, *18*)	0.2–315 (41, *18*)
Brain	0.23–2.2 (0.9, 7)	—
Kidney	0.51–18.3 (3.5, *19*)	0.5–3.1 (1.2, *14*)
Liver	0.05–49.5 (6, *23*)	0.02–2.7 (0.6, *16*)
Lung	1.6–110 (16, *17*)	0.01–0.98 (0.2, *10*)
Spleen	1.6–20.9 (5.3, 7)	0–0.98 (0.7, *4*)
Urine	0.52–76.2 (21, *22*)	0.4–46.2 (11, *17*)

(J. C. Garriott *et al.*, *Clin. Toxicol.*, 1973, *6*, 163–173; A. E. Robinson and F. M. Williams, *J. Pharm. Pharmac.*, 1971, *23*, 353–358; A. E. Robinson and A. T. Holder, *J. chromatogr. Sci.*, 1974, *12*, 281–284; A. E. Robinson and A. T. Holder, *Z. Rechtsmed.*, 1973, *72*, 306–311; G. Norheim, *Z. Rechtsmed.*, 1973, *73*, 219–224).

HALF-LIFE. Plasma half-life, after a single dose, 10 to 25 hours (mean 15); increased during long-term maintenance therapy to 13 to 55 hours (mean 30).

VOLUME OF DISTRIBUTION. About 5 litres/kg.

CLEARANCE. Plasma clearance, about 2 ml/min/kg.

DISTRIBUTION IN BLOOD. Plasma:whole blood ratio, about 1.3.

PROTEIN BINDING. In plasma, up to 90%, but there is considerable intersubject variation.

Dose. Initially 5 to 10 mg of methadone hydrochloride every 6 hours; doses of 30 mg have been given.

Methallenoestril   *Oestrogen*

Synonym. Methallenoestrol
Proprietary Name. Vallestril
3-(6-Methoxy-2-naphthyl)-2,2-dimethylvaleric acid
$C_{18}H_{22}O_3 = 286.4$
CAS—517-18-0

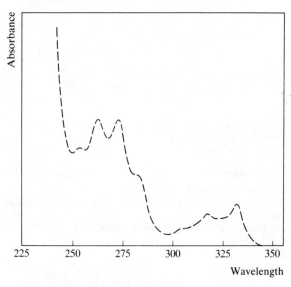

A white crystalline powder. M.p. about 138°.
Very slightly **soluble** in water; soluble 1 in 10 of ethanol, 1 in 2 of chloroform, and 1 in 8 of ether.

Thin-layer Chromatography. *System TP*—Rf 79; *system TQ*—Rf 18; *system TR*—Rf 70; *system TS*—Rf 54, streaking may occur.

Ultraviolet Spectrum. Methanol—253 nm, 264 nm ($A_1^1 = 180$ a), 273 nm ($A_1^1 = 180$ a), 317 nm, 332 nm.

Infra-red Spectrum. Principal peaks at wavenumbers 1689, 1232, 1270, 857, 1606, 1149 (KBr disk).

Dose. 3 to 9 mg daily.

Methallibure   *Hypothalamus and Pituitary Suppressant*

1-Methyl-6-(1-methylallyl)-2,5-dithiobiurea
$C_7H_{14}N_4S_2 = 218.3$
CAS—926-93-2

$$CH_2{:}CH{\cdot}CH{\cdot}NH{\cdot}C{\cdot}NH{\cdot}NH{\cdot}C{\cdot}NH{\cdot}CH_3$$
$$\underset{CH_3}{|} \quad \underset{S}{\|} \quad \underset{S}{\|}$$

A white powder. M.p. about 187°.

Practically **insoluble** in water and chloroform; soluble 1 in 100 of acetone and 1 in 200 of methanol; soluble in pyridine.

Caution. Protective gloves should be worn when handling methallibure.

Colour Tests. Nessler's Reagent (100°)—black; Palladium Chloride—orange.

Thin-layer Chromatography. *System TA*—Rf 79. (*Acidified iodoplatinate solution*, positive.)

Gas Chromatography. *System GA*—not eluted.

Ultraviolet Spectrum. Aqueous acid—243 nm $(A_1^1 = 1340 \text{ b})$; aqueous alkali—293 nm.

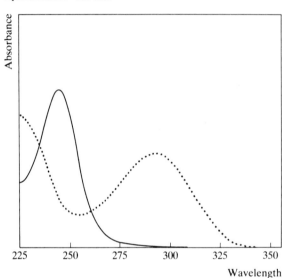

Wavelength

Infra-red Spectrum. Principal peaks at wavenumbers 1524, 1577, 1209, 1025, 1147, 1258 (KBr disk).

Methandienone
Anabolic Steroid

Synonym. Methandrostenolone

Proprietary Names. Danabol; Dianabol; Metastenol; Vetanabol (vet.).

17β-Hydroxy-17α-methylandrosta-1,4-dien-3-one
$C_{20}H_{28}O_2 = 300.4$
CAS—72-63-9

A white or faintly yellowish-white, crystalline powder. M.p. 163° to 167°.

Practically **insoluble** in water; soluble 1 in 2 of ethanol, 1 in less than 1 of chloroform, and 1 in 70 of ether.

Thin-layer Chromatography. *System TP*—Rf 65; *system TQ*—Rf 10; *system TR*—Rf 87; *system TS*—Rf 61.

Gas Chromatography. *System GA*—RI 2672.

Ultraviolet Spectrum. Dehydrated alcohol—245 nm $(A_1^1 = 516 \text{ a})$.

Infra-red Spectrum. Principal peaks at wavenumbers 1660, 1620, 886, 1601, 1160, 1240 (KBr disk).

Wavelength

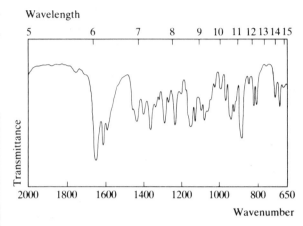

Wavenumber

Quantification. GAS CHROMATOGRAPHY. In urine: sensitivity 30 ng for methandienone, 10 ng for 17-epimethandienone and 6β-hydroxy-17-epimethandienone—H. H. Dürbeck *et al.*, *J. Chromat.*, 1978, *167*, 117–124.

HIGH PRESSURE LIQUID CHROMATOGRAPHY. In urine: sensitivity 5 ng, UV detection—C. G. B. Frischkorn and H. E. Frischkorn, *J. Chromat.*, 1978, *151*, 331–338.

Dose. Initially 2.5 to 5 mg daily.

Methanol
Solvent

Synonym. Methyl Alcohol

$CH_3OH = 32.04$
CAS—67-56-1

A clear, colourless, highly inflammable liquid. B.p. 63.5° to 65.7°. Refractive index 1.328 to 1.329.

Miscible with water, ethanol, chloroform, and ether.

Note. The commercial substance known as 'wood naphtha', 'pyroxylic spirit' or 'wood spirit' contains 60 to 90% of methanol, together with acetone and other empyreumatic impurities. The variety used for denaturing ethanol (see under Ethanol) contains not less than 72% v/v of methanol.

Colour Test. Potassium Dichromate (Method 2)—green.

Gas Chromatography. *System GA*—RI 491; *system GI*—retention time 0.7 min.

Mass Spectrum. Principal peaks at *m/z* 31, 32, 29, 30, 28, 33, 34, 27; formic acid 29, 46, 45, 28, 44, 30, 47, –.

Quantification. GAS CHROMATOGRAPHY. In blood or urine: direct injection, FID—B. R. Manno and J. E. Manno, *J. analyt. Toxicol.*, 1978, *2*, 257–261.

Disposition in the Body. Readily absorbed after oral administration and distributed in the body according to the water content of the tissues; it may also be absorbed by inhalation or through intact skin. It is metabolised, much more slowly than ethanol, by oxidation to formaldehyde, formic acid, and possibly other products. Oxidation to formaldehyde is probably accomplished by alcohol dehydrogenase since the metabolism is inhibited by ethanol. Maximum concentrations of formic acid in the blood and urine occur 2 to 3 days after ingestion. Small amounts of methanol are excreted unchanged in the urine and expired air and about 10% of a dose is excreted in the urine as formic acid. Endogenous blood-methanol concentrations are approximately 1.5 µg/ml, and urinary formic acid concentrations are usually about 12 to 17 µg/ml.

TOXICITY. The initial effects of methanol are much milder than those of ethanol and toxic effects are not usually seen until after a latent period of 8 to 36 hours; the symptoms may include severe upper abdominal pain, visual disturbance often proceeding to incurable blindness, severe metabolic acidosis, and prolonged coma which may terminate in death from respiratory failure. The fatal dose varies greatly but is usually between 100 and 200 ml in adults, although ingestion of 30 ml is potentially lethal; permanent blindness has been caused by as little as 10 ml. Toxic effects are usually associated with blood concentrations greater than 100 µg/ml and blood concentrations greater than 200 µg/ml are indicative of severe poisoning and may be lethal. The maximum permissible atmospheric concentration is 200 ppm.

In an incident involving the consumption of contraband 'vodka' subsequently found to be a mixture of methanol and water, 57 people were poisoned; 17 of the 57 died and 2 became blind. Postmortem heart-blood concentrations of 230 to 2680 µg/ml (mean 1205) were reported in 15 subjects (S. E. H. Tonkabony, *Forens. Sci.*, 1975, *6*, 1–3).

The following postmortem tissue concentrations were reported in 3 fatalities due to methanol ingestion: blood 2100, 2600, and 3200 µg/ml; brain 2700, 2500, and 3100 (brain blood) µg/g; kidney –, 2600, and 3300 (kidney blood) µg/g; liver 2200, 2200, and 2400 (liver blood) µg/g; urine 3000, 1200, – µg/ml (H. Bremer and D. Tiess, *Bull. int. Ass. forens. Toxicol.*, 1976, *12*(1), 21; L. R. Bednarczyk and M. Commiskey, *ibid.*, 1978, *14*(2), 14; H. Bremer and D. Tiess, *ibid.*, 1978, *13*(3), 21–22).

A 44-year-old man suffering from methanol intoxication was found comatose and had a serum concentration of 5830 µg/ml on admission. The subject died 40 hours later and the following postmortem concentrations were found (µg/ml or µg/g): blood 1420, bile 1750, brain 1590, heart 930, kidney 1300, liver 1070, lung 1270, vitreous humour 1730 (N. B. Wu Chen *et al.*, *J. forens. Sci.*, 1985, *30*, 213–216).

VOLUME OF DISTRIBUTION. About 0.6 litre/kg.

PROTEIN BINDING. In plasma, not significantly bound.

Methanthelinium Bromide   *Anticholinergic*

Synonyms. Bromuro de Metantelina; Dixamonum Bromidum; Methantheline Bromide; Methanthine Bromide.
Proprietary Names. Banthine; Bronerg; Evogal; Vagantin; Xantenol.

Diethylmethyl[2 - (xanthen - 9 - ylcarbonyloxy)ethyl]ammonium bromide
$C_{21}H_{26}BrNO_3 = 420.3$
CAS—5818-17-7 (methanthelinium); *53-46-3* (bromide)

A white crystalline powder. M.p. 171° to 177°.
Soluble 1 in less than 5 of water, ethanol, and chloroform; practically insoluble in ether. Aqueous solutions decompose on standing.

Colour Tests. Mandelin's Test—orange; Marquis Test—orange.

Thin-layer Chromatography. *System TA*—Rf 02. (*Acidified iodoplatinate solution*, positive.)

Ultraviolet Spectrum. Aqueous acid—282 nm ($A_1^1 = 65$ a).

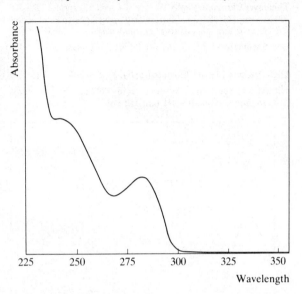

Infra-red Spectrum. Principal peaks at wavenumbers 1155, 1248, 1724, 761, 1200, 755 (KBr disk).

Mass Spectrum. Principal peaks at m/z 72, 181, 85, 152, 42, 44, 58, 43.

Dose. Methanthelinium bromide has been given in doses of 200 to 400 mg daily.

Methapyrilene   *Antihistamine*

Synonym. Thenylpyramine
NN-Dimethyl-N'-(2-pyridyl)-N'-(2-thenyl)ethylenediamine
$C_{14}H_{19}N_3S = 261.4$
CAS—91-80-5

A liquid.

Methapyrilene Fumarate
$(C_{14}H_{19}N_3S)_2,3C_4H_4O_4 = 871.0$
CAS—33032-12-1
A white crystalline powder. M.p. 133° to 137°.
Soluble 1 in 20 of water and 1 in 30 of ethanol.

Methapyrilene Hydrochloride
Synonym. Methapyrilenium Chloride
$C_{14}H_{19}N_3S,HCl = 297.8$
CAS—135-23-9
A white crystalline powder. M.p. 161° to 165°.
Soluble 1 in 0.5 of water, 1 in 5 of ethanol, and 1 in 3 of chloroform; practically insoluble in ether.

Dissociation Constant. pK_a 3.7, 8.9 (25°).

Colour Tests. Liebermann's Test—red-brown; Mandelin's Test—black-violet; Marquis Test—black-violet; Sulphuric Acid—orange.

Thin-layer Chromatography. *System TA*—Rf 52; *system TB*—Rf 43; *system TC*—Rf 26. (*Dragendorff spray*, positive; *acidified iodoplatinate solution*, positive; *Marquis reagent*, violet.)

Gas Chromatography. *System GA*—RI 1981; *system GF*—RI 2305.

High Pressure Liquid Chromatography. *System HA*—k' 4.1.

Ultraviolet Spectrum. Aqueous acid—237 nm ($A_1^1 = 720$ a), 314 nm; aqueous alkali—241 nm, 312 nm.

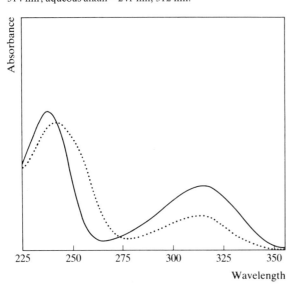

Infra-red Spectrum. Principal peaks at wavenumbers 1592, 765, 1558, 1250, 1158, 1316 (KBr disk).

Mass Spectrum. Principal peaks at m/z 58, 97, 72, 71, 42, 191, 79, 78.

Quantification. GAS CHROMATOGRAPHY. In plasma or urine: sensitivity 10 ng/ml in plasma, 50 ng/ml in urine, AFID—R. C. Baselt and S. Franch, *J. Chromat.*, 1980, *183*; *Biomed. Appl.*, *9*, 234–238. In blood, urine or tissues: FID—C. L. Winek *et al.*, *Clin. Toxicol.*, 1977, *11*, 287–294.

Disposition in the Body. Variably and incompletely absorbed after oral administration. Less than 2% of a dose is excreted in the urine as unchanged drug in 24 hours.

THERAPEUTIC CONCENTRATION.
After a single oral dose of 50 mg to 8 subjects, peak plasma concentrations of 0.006 to 0.05 µg/ml (mean 0.024) were attained in about 1.5 hours (E. P. Calandre *et al.*, *Clin. Pharmac. Ther.*, 1981, *29*, 527–532).

TOXICITY. Methapyrilene has been shown to be carcinogenic in rats and is little used. Fatalities have occurred after ingestion of 7 g or more and toxic effects have been associated with plasma concentrations greater than 30 µg/ml. In 13 fatalities attributed to methapyrilene overdose, reported blood concentrations ranged from 2 to 380 µg/ml (mean 50) (salicylamide and ethanol were also detected in several cases).

The following postmortem tissue concentrations were reported in one fatality: blood 9 µg/ml, kidney 52 µg/g, liver 82 µg/g, lung 119 µg/g, urine 200 µg/ml (C. A. Ainsworth and J. D. Biggs, *Clin. Toxicol.*, 1977, *11*, 281–286).

HALF-LIFE. Plasma half-life, about 1 to 2 hours.

VOLUME OF DISTRIBUTION. About 4 litres/kg.

CLEARANCE. Plasma clearance, about 30 ml/min/kg.

DISTRIBUTION IN BLOOD. Plasma: whole blood ratio, about 1.0.

Dose. Methapyrilene hydrochloride has been given in doses of up to 200 mg daily.

Methaqualone   *Hypnotic/Sedative*

Synonym. Methachalonum
Proprietary Names. Mequin; Normi-Nox; Quäälude.
A preparation containing methaqualone and diphenhydramine hydrochloride was formerly marketed under the proprietary name Mandrax.
2-Methyl-3-*o*-tolylquinazolin-4(3*H*)-one
$C_{16}H_{14}N_2O = 250.3$
CAS—72-44-6

A white crystalline powder. M.p. 114° to 117°.
Practically **insoluble** in water; soluble 1 in 12 of ethanol, 1 in 1 of chloroform, and 1 in 50 of ether.

Methaqualone Hydrochloride
Proprietary Names. Parest; Rouqualone; Sleepinal; Tualone.
$C_{16}H_{14}N_2O,HCl = 286.8$
CAS—340-56-7
A white crystalline powder. M.p. about 250°, with decomposition.
Soluble 1 in 65 of water, 1 in 31 of ethanol, and 1 in 13 of chloroform; soluble in acetone; practically insoluble in ether.

Dissociation Constant. pK_a 2.5.

Thin-layer Chromatography. *System TA*—Rf 70; *system TB*—Rf 37; *system TC*—Rf 80; *system TD*—Rf 63. (*Dragendorff spray*, positive; *acidified iodoplatinate solution*, positive.)

Gas Chromatography. *System GA*—methaqualone RI 2125, 2-hydroxymethylmethaqualone RI 2360, 2'-hydroxymethylmethaqualone RI 2410, 3'-hydroxymethylmethaqualone RI 2490, 4'-hydroxymethylmethaqualone RI 2520, 6-hydroxymethylmethaqualone RI 2525; *system GF*—methaqualone RI 2580.

High Pressure Liquid Chromatography. *System HA*—k' 0.2.

Ultraviolet Spectrum. Aqueous acid—234 nm ($A_1^1 = 1320$ a), 269 nm; aqueous alkali—265 nm ($A_1^1 = 347$ b), 306 nm.

Infra-red Spectrum. Principal peaks at wavenumbers 1682, 1599, 1565, 770, 1265, 697 (KBr disk).

Mass Spectrum. Principal peaks at m/z 235, 250, 91, 233, 236, 65, 76, 132; 4'-hydroxymethaqualone 251, 266, 249, 77, 143, 76, 252, 39.

Quantification. GAS CHROMATOGRAPHY. In plasma or saliva: methaqualone and the 2'-hydroxymethyl metabolite, sensitivity 20 ng/ml, AFID—M. A. Peat and B. S. Finkle, *J. analyt. Toxicol.*, 1980, *4*, 114–118.

GAS CHROMATOGRAPHY (CAPILLARY COLUMN)–MASS SPECTROMETRY. In urine: methaqualone and metabolites—L. Kazyak *et al.*, *Clin. Chem.*, 1977, *23*, 2001–2006.

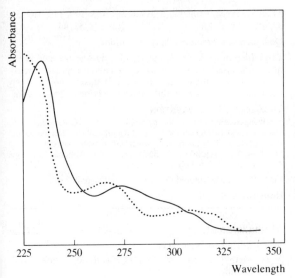

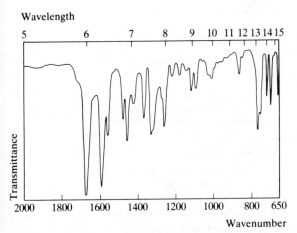

HIGH PRESSURE LIQUID CHROMATOGRAPHY. In plasma: detection limit 1 ng/ml, UV detection—R. A. Hux *et al.*, *Analyt. Chem.*, 1982, *54*, 113–117.

RADIOIMMUNOASSAY–THIN-LAYER CHROMATOGRAPHY. In urine: methaqualone and metabolites, sensitivity 1 μg/ml—R. D. Budd *et al.*, *J. Chromat.*, 1980, *190*, 129–132.

REVIEW. S. S. Brown, *Methodol. Dev. Biochem.*, 1976, *5*, 179–184.

Disposition in the Body. Readily absorbed after oral administration and widely distributed throughout the body. The major metabolites are 4'-hydroxymethaqualone, 2'-hydroxymethyl-methaqualone and their *O*-glucuronides or *O*-methyl ethers, and methaqualone *N*-oxide. A large number of metabolites are known and there is considerable intersubject variation in the relative amounts produced. About 40 to 50% of a dose is excreted in the urine in 72 hours, mostly as conjugated metabolites, with less than 2% of a dose as unchanged drug. In 24 hours, about 10% of a dose is excreted in the urine as the conjugated 4'-hydroxy metabolite, 7% as the *N*-oxide, 5% as the conjugated 2'-hydroxymethyl derivative, and about 3% each as the conjugated

2-hydroxymethyl, 3'-hydroxy, and 6-hydroxy metabolites. Up to 4% of a dose may be eliminated unchanged in the faeces.

THERAPEUTIC CONCENTRATION. In plasma, usually in the range 0.4 to 5 μg/ml.

After a single oral dose of 250 mg of the base to 7 subjects, peak plasma concentrations of 1.0 to 4.0 μg/ml (mean 2.2) were attained in 2 hours; following an equivalent dose of the hydrochloride, peak plasma concentrations of 2.0 to 4.9 μg/ml (mean 3.7) were attained in 1 hour (S. Goenechea *et al.*, *Arch. Tox.*, 1973, *31*, 25–30).

After daily oral doses of 300 mg to 8 subjects, a mean maximum steady-state plasma concentration of 3.7 μg/ml was reported (R. K. Nayak *et al.*, *J. Pharmacokinet. Biopharm.*, 1974, *2*, 107–121).

TOXICITY. The estimated minimum lethal dose is 5 g in non-tolerant subjects. Drug accumulation is likely in chronic dosing because of the long half-life. Toxic effects may be associated with plasma concentrations greater than 2 μg/ml, and plasma concentrations greater than about 8 μg/ml are likely to produce coma and may be lethal. The 2'-hydroxymethyl metabolite, which has been found unconjugated in both blood and urine in overdose cases, may contribute to the degree of intoxication. Abuse of methaqualone, particularly when taken in conjunction with diphenhydramine, has been reported.

In 6 fatal cases, postmortem blood concentrations of 5 to 42 μg/ml (mean 22) and liver concentrations of 26 to 89 μg/g (mean 55) were reported (R. C. Baselt and R. H. Cravey, *J. analyt. Toxicol.*, 1977, *1*, 81–102).

In 19 mildly poisoned patients the plasma concentration on admission to hospital ranged from 2 to 20 μg/ml (mean 9). In 9 more severe cases, a mean peak concentration of 27 μg/ml was reached within 12 hours of admission to hospital (A. A. H. Lawson and S. S. Brown, *Br. med. J.*, 1966, *2*, 1455–1456).

HALF-LIFE. Plasma half-life, about 20 to 60 hours (mean 35); a slower terminal elimination half-life of up to about 72 hours has also been reported.

VOLUME OF DISTRIBUTION. About 6 litres/kg.

DISTRIBUTION IN BLOOD. Plasma: whole blood ratio about 1.1 at therapeutic concentrations decreasing to about 0.5 at concentrations of 20 μg/ml.

SALIVA. Plasma: saliva ratio, about 9.

PROTEIN BINDING. In plasma, about 75 to 95% (concentration-dependent).

NOTE. For a review of the pharmacokinetics of hypnotic drugs see D. D. Breimer, *Clin. Pharmacokinet.*, 1977, *2*, 93–109.

Dose. Usually up to 300 mg daily.

Metharbitone   *Barbiturate*

Synonyms. Endiemal; Metharbital.
Proprietary Name. Gemonil
5,5-Diethyl-1-methylbarbituric acid
$C_9H_{14}N_2O_3 = 198.2$
CAS—50-11-3

A white crystalline powder. M.p. 151° to 155°.

Soluble 1 in 830 of water, 1 in 23 of ethanol, and 1 in 40 of ether.

Dissociation Constant. pK_a 8.3 (20°).

Colour Tests. Koppanyi–Zwikker Test—violet; Mercurous Nitrate—black.

Thin-layer Chromatography. *System TD*—Rf 66; *system TE*—Rf 53; *system TF*—Rf 67; *system TH*—Rf 86. (*Mercurous nitrate spray*, black; *Zwikker's reagent*, faint pink.)

Gas Chromatography. *System GA*—metharbitone RI 1472, barbitone RI 1497.

High Pressure Liquid Chromatography. *System HG*—metharbitone k′ 2.69, barbitone k′ 1.11; *system HH*—metharbitone k′ 1.99, barbitone k′ 0.63.

Ultraviolet Spectrum. *Borax buffer 0.05M* (pH 9.2)—244 nm ($A_1^1 = 433$ a); M sodium hydroxide (pH 13)—244 nm ($A_1^1 = 458$ b).

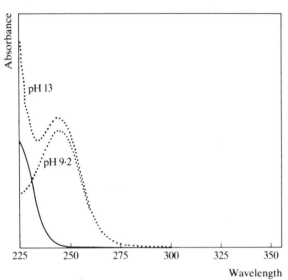

Infra-red Spectrum. Principal peaks at wavenumbers 1655, 1699, 1755, 1275, 1205, 815 (KBr disk).

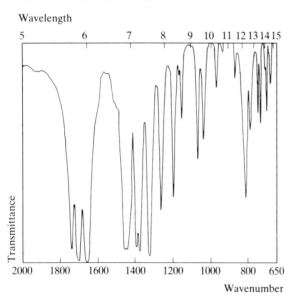

Mass Spectrum. Principal peaks at *m/z* 155, 170, 112, 169, 55, 82, 41, 39; barbitone 156, 141, 55, 155, 98, 39, 82, 43.

Quantification. See under Amylobarbitone.

Disposition in the Body. About 1% of a dose is excreted in the urine in 48 hours as unchanged drug and about 10% as the active metabolite, barbitone; the remainder is thought to be slowly excreted in the urine as barbitone over a period of 2 to 3 weeks.

THERAPEUTIC CONCENTRATION.

Following daily oral doses of 300 mg for 14 days to 1 subject, metharbitone reached a peak plasma concentration of 5 μg/ml shortly after a dose, but was undetectable 8 hours later when the plasma concentration of barbitone was 26 μg/ml (T. C. Butler and W. J. Waddell, *Neurology, Minneap.*, 1958, *8*, 106–112).

TOXICITY. The estimated minimum lethal dose is 2 g.

Dose. 100 to 300 mg daily.

Methazolamide   *Carbonic Anhydrase Inhibitor*

Proprietary Name. Neptazane

N - (4 - Methyl - 2 - sulphamoyl - Δ^2 - 1,3,4 - thiadiazolin - 5 - ylidene)acetamide

$C_5H_8N_4O_3S_2 = 236.3$

CAS—554-57-4

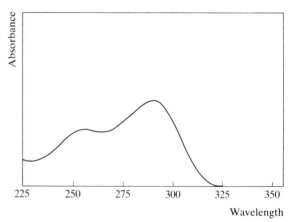

A white or faintly yellow, crystalline powder. M.p. about 213°. Very slightly **soluble** in water and ethanol; slightly soluble in acetone; soluble in dimethylformamide.

Dissociation Constant. pK$_a$ 7.3.

Partition Coefficient. Log *P* (ether/pH 7.4), −0.2.

Colour Test. Koppanyi–Zwikker Test—violet.

Thin-layer Chromatography. *System TA*—Rf 72. (*Acidified iodoplatinate solution*, positive.)

Gas Chromatography. *System GA*—RI 2187.

Ultraviolet Spectrum. Aqueous acid—255 nm, 290 nm ($A_1^1 = 396$ a); aqueous alkali—288 nm ($A_1^1 = 568$ a).

Mass Spectrum. Principal peaks at *m/z* 43, 221, 83, 236, 56, 223, 222, 55.

Quantification. GAS CHROMATOGRAPHY–MASS SPECTROMETRY. In blood, plasma or urine: sensitivity <1 ng/ml in plasma— W. F. Bayne *et al.*, *J. pharm. Sci.*, 1981, *70*, 75–81.

Disposition in the Body. Well absorbed after oral administration. About 15 to 20% of a dose may be excreted in the urine in 24 hours, of which about half is unchanged drug.

THERAPEUTIC CONCENTRATION.
After a single oral dose of 50 mg to 1 subject, peak concentrations of 19.1 and 0.08 µg/ml in blood and plasma respectively were reported at 3 hours; the corresponding concentrations, 3 hours after a dose of 150 mg to a different subject were 36.1 and 1.4 µg/ml. Following oral doses of 100 mg three times a day to 1 subject, steady-state concentrations of about 40 µg/ml and about 9.5 µg/ml were reported for blood and plasma respectively (W. F. Bayne *et al.*, *ibid.*).

DISTRIBUTION IN BLOOD. Plasma : erythrocyte ratio appears to be concentration-dependent, saturation of the carbonic anhydrase in the erythrocytes occurring at about 40 µg/ml.

PROTEIN BINDING. In plasma, about 55%.

Dose. In the treatment of glaucoma, 100 to 300 mg daily.

Methdilazine   *Antihistamine*

Proprietary Name. Tacaryl (chewable tablets)
10-(1-Methylpyrrolidin-3-ylmethyl)phenothiazine
$C_{18}H_{20}N_2S = 296.4$
CAS—1982-37-2

A light tan, crystalline powder. M.p. 83° to 88°.
Practically **insoluble** in water; soluble 1 in 2 of ethanol, 1 in 1 of chloroform, and 1 in 8 of ether.

Methdilazine Hydrochloride
Proprietary Names. Dilosyn; Tacaryl (syrup and tablets).
$C_{18}H_{20}N_2S,HCl = 332.9$
CAS—1229-35-2
A light tan, crystalline powder, which darkens on exposure to light. M.p. 184° to 190°.
Soluble 1 in 2 of water, 1 in 2 of ethanol, and 1 in 6 of chloroform; practically insoluble in ether.

Dissociation Constant. pK_a 7.5.

Colour Tests. Formaldehyde–Sulphuric Acid—red-violet; Forrest Reagent—red-orange; FPN Reagent—red; Liebermann's Test—green-brown; Mandelin's Test—green → violet; Marquis Test—red-violet.

Thin-layer Chromatography. *System TA*—Rf 29; *system TB*—Rf 32; *system TC*—Rf 15. (*Acidified iodoplatinate solution*, positive.)

Gas Chromatography. *System GA*—RI 2467; *system GF*—RI 2920.

High Pressure Liquid Chromatography. *System HA*—k′ 6.0.

Ultraviolet Spectrum. Aqueous acid—253 nm $(A_1^1 = 982 a)$, 302 nm; aqueous alkali—255 nm, 308 nm.

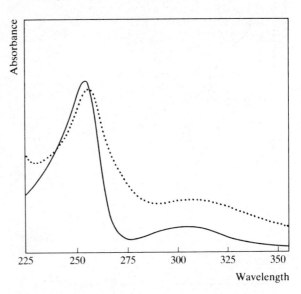

Infra-red Spectrum. Principal peaks at wavenumbers 753, 1242, 1319, 1222, 1277, 1031 (methdilazine hydrochloride, KBr disk).

Mass Spectrum. Principal peaks at *m/z* 97, 98, 296, 199, 55, 212, 96, 198.

Dose. Usually 14.4 to 28.8 mg daily.

Methicillin   *Antibiotic*

Synonyms. Dimethoxyphenecillin; Dimethoxyphenyl Penicillin.
(6R)-6-(2,6-Dimethoxybenzamido)penicillanic acid
$C_{17}H_{20}N_2O_6S = 380.4$
CAS—61-32-5

Methicillin Sodium
Synonym. Meticillinum Natricum
Proprietary Names. Azapen; Celbenin; Flabelline; Metin; Pénistaph; Staphcillin.
$C_{17}H_{19}N_2NaO_6S,H_2O = 420.4$
CAS—132-92-3 (anhydrous); *7246-14-2* (monohydrate)
A fine white crystalline powder. M.p. 196° to 197°, with decomposition.
Soluble 1 in 0.6 of water and 1 in 35 of ethanol; slightly soluble in chloroform; practically insoluble in ether; freely soluble in methanol.

Dissociation Constant. pK_a 2.8 (25°).

Ultraviolet Spectrum. Water—280 nm $(A_1^1 = 61 a)$. (See below)

Infra-red Spectrum. Principal peaks at wavenumbers 1607, 1766, 1673, 1500, 1093, 1260 (methicillin sodium, KBr disk). (See below)

Dose. Up to 12 g of methicillin sodium daily, by slow intravenous injection.

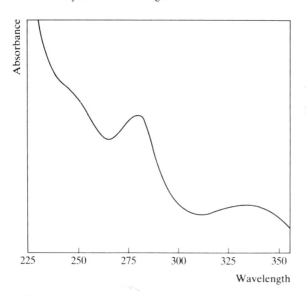

Wavelength

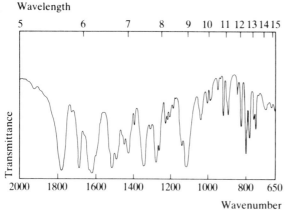

Wavenumber

Methimazole
Antithyroid Agent

Synonyms. Mercazolylum; Thiamazole; Tiamazol.
Proprietary Names. Antitiroide GW; Favistan; Strumazol; Tapazole.
1-Methylimidazole-2-thiol
$C_4H_6N_2S = 114.2$
CAS—60-56-0

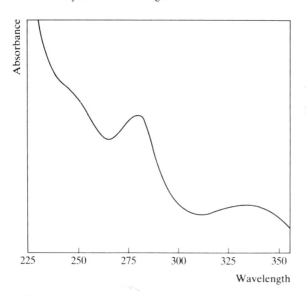

A white to pale buff, crystalline powder. M.p. 144° to 147°.
Soluble 1 in 5 of water, 1 in 5 of ethanol, and 1 in about 5 of chloroform; freely soluble in acetone; slightly soluble in ether.

Colour Test. Palladium Chloride—orange.

Thin-layer Chromatography. *System TA*—Rf 62; *system TB*—Rf 01; *system TC*—Rf 52. (*Acidified iodoplatinate solution*, positive.)

Gas Chromatography. *System GA*—RI 1550.

Ultraviolet Spectrum. Aqueous acid—252 nm ($A_1^1 = 1505$ a).

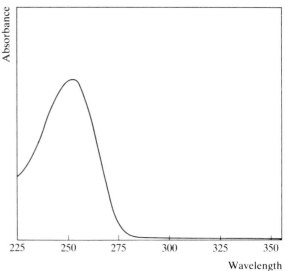

Wavelength

Infra-red Spectrum. Principal peaks at wavenumbers 1570, 1271, 740, 1250, 765, 675 (KBr disk).

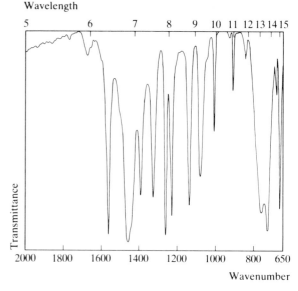

Wavenumber

Mass Spectrum. Principal peaks at *m/z* 114, 42, 72, 113, 69, 81, 54, 115.

Quantification. See under Carbimazole.

Disposition in the Body. Absorbed after oral administration and widely distributed throughout the body. About 10% of a dose is excreted in the urine as unchanged drug. 3-Methyl-2-thiohydantoin has been identified in plasma and urine as a minor metabolite.
Methimazole is the active metabolite of carbimazole.

THERAPEUTIC CONCENTRATION.
Following a single oral dose of 60 mg given to 11 subjects, peak serum concentrations of 0.5 to 2.5 µg/ml (mean 1.3) were attained in about 1 to 3 hours (A. Melander *et al.*, *Eur. J. clin. Pharmac.*, 1980, *17*, 295–299).

HALF-LIFE. Plasma half-life, about 3 to 5 hours.

VOLUME OF DISTRIBUTION. About 0.5 litre/kg.

PROTEIN BINDING. In plasma, not significantly bound.

NOTE. For a review of the pharmacokinetics of antithyroid agents see J. P. Kampmann and J. M. Hansen, *Clin. Pharmacokinet.*, 1981, *6*, 401–428.

Dose. Initially, 15 to 60 mg daily; maintenance, 5 to 15 mg daily.

Methindizate   *Antispasmodic (Veterinary)*

2-(1-Methylperhydroindol-3-yl)ethyl benzilate
$C_{25}H_{31}NO_3 = 393.5$
CAS—15687-33-9

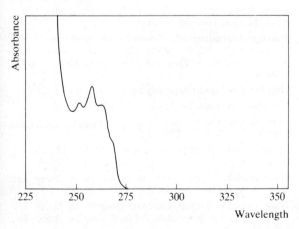

Methindizate Hydrochloride
Proprietary Name. It is an ingredient of Isaverin.
$C_{25}H_{31}NO_3,HCl = 430.0$
A fine, white, crystalline powder. M.p. 159° to 160°.
Freely **soluble** in water and ethanol; practically insoluble in chloroform and ether.

Colour Tests. Liebermann's Test—orange → brown; Mandelin's Test—brown; Marquis Test—orange → green; Sulphuric Acid—orange.

Thin-layer Chromatography. *System TA*—Rf 36. (*Acidified iodoplatinate solution*, positive.)

Ultraviolet Spectrum. Aqueous acid—251 nm, 257 nm ($A_1^1 = 10.3$ b).

Infra-red Spectrum. Principal peaks at wavenumbers 1739, 1238, 1227, 702, 1058, 1093 (KBr disk).

Methisazone   *Antiviral*

Synonyms. N-Methylisatin β-Thiosemicarbazone; Metisazone.
Proprietary Name. Marboran
1-Methylindoline-2,3-dione 3-thiosemicarbazone
$C_{10}H_{10}N_4OS = 234.3$
CAS—1910-68-5

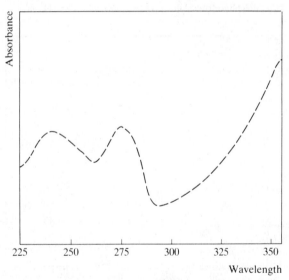

A very fine, orange-yellow powder. M.p. about 248°, with decomposition.
Practically **insoluble** in water; soluble 1 in 25 of acetone and 1 in 800 of chloroform; soluble in warm dilute solutions of alkali hydroxides.

Colour Tests. Mandelin's Test—violet → yellow; Palladium Chloride—yellow → orange → brown.

Thin-layer Chromatography. *System TA*—Rf 65; *system TB*—Rf 03; *system TC*—Rf 68. (*Acidified iodoplatinate solution*, positive.)

Ultraviolet Spectrum. Ethanol—241 nm, 274 nm ($A_1^1 = 588$ b).

Infra-red Spectrum. Principal peaks at wavenumbers 1605, 1493, 1097, 1673, 1040, 826 (KBr disk).

Mass Spectrum. Principal peaks at *m/z* 234, 146, 179, 206, 131, 91, 117, 118.

Dose. Usually 6 g daily (prophylactic dose).

Methixene   *Anticholinergic*

9-(1-Methyl-3-piperidylmethyl)thioxanthene
$C_{20}H_{23}NS = 309.5$
CAS—4969-02-2

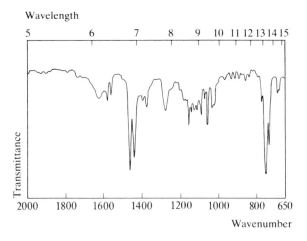

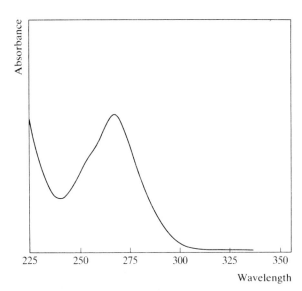

A slightly yellow viscous liquid.

Methixene Hydrochloride

Proprietary Names. Tremaril; Tremonil; Trest.
$C_{20}H_{23}NS,HCl = 345.9$
CAS—1553-34-0
A white crystalline powder. M.p. about 216°.
Soluble in water, ethanol, and chloroform.

Colour Tests. Formaldehyde–Sulphuric Acid—orange; Liebermann's Test—red-orange; Mandelin's Test—orange; Sulphuric Acid—orange (fluoresces under ultraviolet light).

Thin-layer Chromatography. *System TA*—Rf 50; *system TB*—Rf 48; *system TC*—Rf 25. (*Acidified iodoplatinate solution*, positive.)

Gas Chromatography. *System GA*—RI 2461; *system GF*—RI 2895.

High Pressure Liquid Chromatography. *System HA*—k' 3.6.

Ultraviolet Spectrum. Aqueous acid—268 nm ($A_1^1 = 324$ a).

Infra-red Spectrum. Principal peaks at wavenumbers 750, 729, 1052, 1162, 1086, 1280 (KBr disk).

Mass Spectrum. Principal peaks at m/z 99, 197, 44, 58, 112, 309, 41, 42.

Disposition in the Body. Absorbed after oral administration. It is excreted in the urine, partly unchanged, partly as its two isomeric sulphoxides, and partly as the stereoisomeric sulphoxides of *N*-demethylated methixene.

Dose. 7.5 to 60 mg of methixene hydrochloride daily.

Methocarbamol   *Muscle Relaxant*

Synonym. Guaiphenesin Carbamate
Proprietary Names. Delaxin; Lumirelax; Miowas; Robamol; Robaxin; Traumacut. It is an ingredient of Robaxisal Forte.
2-Hydroxy-3-(2-methoxyphenoxy)propyl carbamate
$C_{11}H_{15}NO_5 = 241.2$
CAS—532-03-6

A white powder. M.p. about 94° or, if previously ground to a fine powder, about 90°.
Soluble 1 in 40 of water; soluble in ethanol only with heating; sparingly soluble in chloroform; soluble in propylene glycol.

Colour Tests. Liebermann's Test—violet; Mandelin's Test—green; Marquis Test—blue-violet.

Thin-layer Chromatography. *System TA*—Rf 70; *system TD*—Rf 07; *system TE*—Rf 49; *system TF*—Rf 23. (*Furfuraldehyde reagent*, positive; *acidified potassium permanganate solution*, positive.)

High Pressure Liquid Chromatography. *System HA*—k' 0.1.

Ultraviolet Spectrum. Methanol—275 nm ($A_1^1 = 101$ a).

Infra-red Spectrum. Principal peaks at wavenumbers 1667, 1248, 1119, 1215, 1010, 1080 (KBr disk).

Mass Spectrum. Principal peaks at m/z 124, 118, 198, 109, 43, 57, 125, 77.

Quantification. COLORIMETRY. In serum—A. A. Forist and R. W. Judy, *J. pharm. Sci.*, 1971, *60*, 1686–1688.

HIGH PRESSURE LIQUID CHROMATOGRAPHY. In blood: UV detection—K. Sprague and A. Poklis, *J. Can. Soc. forens. Sci.*, 1980, *13*, 31–36.

Disposition in the Body. Absorbed after oral administration. Metabolised by demethylation and *p*-hydroxylation followed by

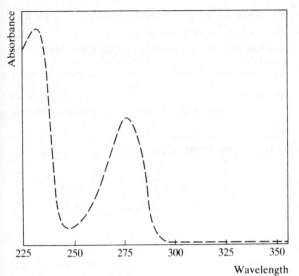

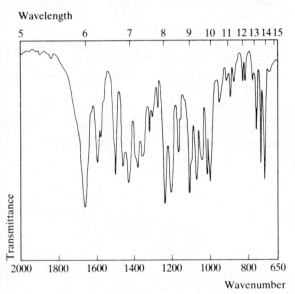

conjugation with glucuronic acid or sulphate. About 98% of a dose is excreted in the urine in 72 hours, with less than 1% as unchanged drug and the remainder as free and conjugated metabolites; most of the excretion occurs in the first 8 hours.

THERAPEUTIC CONCENTRATION.
Following a single oral dose of 2 g to 1 subject, a peak serum concentration of 25.8 µg/ml was attained in 1 hour (A. A. Forist and R. W. Judy, *J. pharm. Sci.*, 1971, *60*, 1686–1688).

TOXICITY.
In a fatality due to ingestion of methocarbamol and alcohol, the following postmortem tissue concentrations were reported: blood, methocarbamol 525 µg/ml, alcohol 1400 µg/ml, salicylate 20 µg/ml; urine, methocarbamol 575 µg/ml (M. Kemal *et al.*, *J. forens. Sci.*, 1982, *27*, 217–222).

HALF-LIFE. Plasma half-life, about 1 to 2 hours.

Dose. 4 to 6 g daily.

Methohexitone   *Barbiturate*

Synonym. Methohexital
α-(±)-5-Allyl-1-methyl-5-(1-methylpent-2-ynyl)barbituric acid
$C_{14}H_{18}N_2O_3 = 262.3$
CAS—151-83-7; 18652-93-2

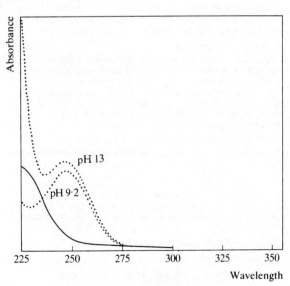

A white to faintly yellowish-white, crystalline powder. M.p. 92° to 96°.
Very slightly **soluble** in water; slightly soluble in ethanol and chloroform.

Methohexitone Sodium
Synonyms. Enallynymalnatrium; Sodium Methohexital.
Proprietary Names. Brevital Sodium; Brietal Sodium.
$C_{14}H_{17}N_2NaO_3 = 284.3$
CAS—309-36-4
A white crystalline substance.
Soluble in water.

Dissociation Constant. pK_a 8.3.

Colour Tests. Koppanyi–Zwikker Test—violet; Mercurous Nitrate—black; Vanillin Reagent—violet-brown/colourless.

Thin-layer Chromatography. *System TD*—Rf 73; *system TE*—Rf 58; *system TF*—Rf 72; *system TH*—Rf 93. (*Mercuric chloride-diphenylcarbazone reagent*, positive; *mercurous nitrate spray*, black; *acidified potassium permanganate solution*, yellow-brown; *Zwikker's reagent*, faint pink.)

Gas Chromatography. *System GA*—RI 1766.

High Pressure Liquid Chromatography. *System HG*—k' 27.61; *system HH*—k' 20.48.

Ultraviolet Spectrum. *Borax buffer 0.05M* (pH 9.2)—246 nm ($A_1^1 = 276$ a); M sodium hydroxide (pH 13)—246 nm ($A_1^1 = 308$ b).

Infra-red Spectrum. Principal peaks at wavenumbers 1680, 1709, 1316, 1193, 1253, 1040 (methohexitone sodium).

Wavelength

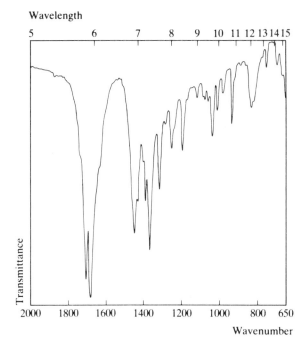

Mass Spectrum. Principal peaks at m/z 41, 81, 53, 221, 79, 39, 178, 233.

Quantification. See also under Amylobarbitone.

GAS CHROMATOGRAPHY. In blood or plasma: methohexitone and 4′-hydroxymethohexitone, sensitivity 50 ng/ml in plasma and 100 ng/ml in blood, AFID—H. Heusler et al., J. Chromat., 1981, 226; Biomed. Appl., 15, 403–412.

Disposition in the Body. Methohexitone has a very short duration of action. It rapidly enters the brain and upon redistribution is localised in body fat but to a lesser extent than thiopentone. Less than 1% of a dose is excreted unchanged in the urine in 24 hours; the major metabolite is 4′-hydroxymethohexitone.

THERAPEUTIC CONCENTRATION.

Following an intravenous dose of 2 mg/kg of methohexitone to 6 subjects, venous blood concentrations of 3.9 to 8.6 μg/ml were reported at 1 to 3 minutes (I. Sunshine et al., Br. J. Anaesth., 1966, 38, 23–28).

After a slow intravenous infusion of 3 mg/kg of methohexitone sodium over a period of 60 minutes to 1 subject, a peak plasma concentration of about 3 μg/ml was reported (D. D. Breimer, Br. J. Anaesth., 1976, 48, 643–649).

TOXICITY. The estimated minimum lethal dose is 1 g.

The following postmortem tissue concentrations were reported in a fatal case involving the intravenous self-administration of methohexitone: blood 103 μg/ml, kidney 45 μg/g, liver 41 μg/g, spleen 41 μg/g; alcohol was also found in the blood (B. Finkle, 1967—personal communication).

In a fatality due to the injection of about 300 mg of methohexitone, postmortem blood and liver concentrations of 2 μg/ml and 17 μg/g, respectively, were reported (J. E. Ryall, Bull. int. Ass. forens. Toxicol., 1981, 16(2), 36–37).

HALF-LIFE. Plasma half-life, about 1 to 2 hours.

VOLUME OF DISTRIBUTION. About 1 litre/kg.

CLEARANCE. Plasma clearance, about 12 ml/min/kg.

DISTRIBUTION IN BLOOD. Plasma:whole blood ratio, about 1.5.

PROTEIN BINDING. In plasma, about 73%.

Dose. For induction of anaesthesia, 50 to 120 mg of methohexitone sodium, by slow intravenous injection.

Methoin   *Anticonvulsant*

Synonyms. Mephenetoin; Mephenytoin; Methantoin; Phenantoin.

Proprietary Name. Mesantoin

5-Ethyl-3-methyl-5-phenylhydantoin

$C_{12}H_{14}N_2O_2 = 218.3$

CAS—50-12-4

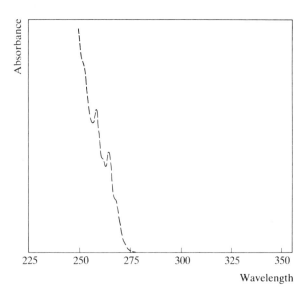

Colourless lustrous crystals or white crystalline powder. M.p. 136° to 140°.

Soluble 1 in 1400 of water, 1 in 15 of ethanol, 1 in 3 of chloroform, and 1 in 90 of ether.

Dissociation Constant. pK_a 8.1.

Colour Tests. Koppanyi–Zwikker Test—violet; Liebermann's Test—red-orange; Mercurous Nitrate—black.

Thin-layer Chromatography. *System TD*—Rf 62; *system TE*—Rf 76; *system TF*—Rf 58.

Gas Chromatography. *System GA*—RI 1791; *system GE*—retention time 0.55 for methoin and 0.73 for 5-ethyl-5-phenylhydantoin, both relative to phenytoin.

Ultraviolet Spectrum. Ethanol—257 nm ($A_1^1 = 11$ a), 264 nm.

Infra-red Spectrum. Principal peaks at wavenumbers 1704, 1754, 733, 1052, 1302, 702 (KBr disk).

Mass Spectrum. Principal peaks at m/z 189, 104, 190, 77, 44, 105, 132, 103.

Wavelength

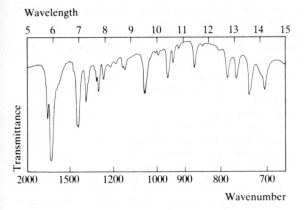

Quantification. GAS CHROMATOGRAPHY. In serum: sensitivity 5 µg/ml for methoin and 10 µg/ml for 5-ethyl-5-phenylhydantoin, FID—V. A. Raisys et al., Clin. Chem., 1979, 25, 172–175.

GAS CHROMATOGRAPHY–MASS SPECTROMETRY. In plasma: sensitivity 10 ng/ml for methoin and 50 ng/ml for 5-ethyl-5-phenylhydantoin—W. Yonekawa and H. J. Kupferberg, J. Chromat., 1979, 163; Biomed. Appl., 5, 161–167.

HIGH PRESSURE LIQUID CHROMATOGRAPHY. In serum: methoin and 5-ethyl-5-phenylhydantoin, sensitivity 1 µg/ml, UV detection—P. M. Kabra et al., J. analyt. Toxicol., 1978, 2, 127–133. In urine: methoin and metabolites, UV detection—A. Küpfer et al., J. Chromat., 1982, 232; Biomed. Appl., 21, 93–100.

Disposition in the Body. Rapidly absorbed after oral administration. During chronic administration, the major metabolite is 5-ethyl-5-phenylhydantoin (nirvanol) which is a more active anticonvulsant than methoin and accounts for at least 22% of the daily dose in the 24-hour urine. After a single dose, the major metabolite is 4′-hydroxymethoin which is excreted in the urine as a glucuronide conjugate and accounts for 43% of a dose in 24 hours; only about 1% of a single dose is excreted in the urine as 5-ethyl-5-phenylhydantoin; 5-ethyl-5-(4-hydroxyphenyl)hydantoin has also been detected in the urine in both free and conjugated forms, together with minor amounts of other conjugated hydroxy metabolites; very little unchanged drug is excreted in the urine.

THERAPEUTIC CONCENTRATION. In plasma, methoin plus metabolites, usually in the range 15 to 40 µg/ml.

Following a single oral dose of 7 mg/kg to 5 subjects, peak serum concentrations of about 3 µg/ml each of methoin and 5-ethyl-5-phenylhydantoin were attained in about 1 hour and 27 hours respectively (A. S. Troupin, Ann. Neurol., 1979, 6, 410–414).

A mean steady-state serum concentration of 26 µg/ml of total hydantoin was reported for 173 subjects receiving daily oral doses averaging 6.8 mg/kg; methoin concentrations averaged 8% of the total hydantoin concentration (A. S. Troupin et al., Epilepsia, 1976, 17, 403–414).

TOXICITY. The estimated minimum lethal dose is 5 g. Methoin gives rise to toxic symptoms more frequently than phenytoin and cases of fatal aplastic anaemia have been reported; the toxicity of the drug is attributed to the proven toxicity of 5-ethyl-5-phenylhydantoin. Acute overdosage may result in coma.

HALF-LIFE. Plasma half-life, after a single dose, methoin about 7 hours, 5-ethyl-5-phenylhydantoin about 95 hours; the half-life of the metabolite decreases to about 72 hours during chronic treatment.

SALIVA. Plasma:saliva ratio, about 1.6.

PROTEIN BINDING. In plasma, about 40%.

Dose. Initially, 50 to 100 mg daily; maintenance, 200 to 600 mg daily.

Methoprotryne   *Herbicide*

2-Isopropylamino-4-(3-methoxypropylamino)-6-methylthio-1,3,5-triazine
$C_{11}H_{21}N_5OS = 271.4$
CAS—841-06-5

A crystalline solid. M.p. 68° to 70°.

Soluble 1 in 3000 of water; soluble in most organic solvents.

Thin-layer Chromatography. System TA—Rf 74. (Dragendorff spray, positive.)

Gas Chromatography. System GA—RI 2098.

Infra-red Spectrum. Principal peaks at wavenumbers 1538, 811, 1304, 1121, 1272, 1175 (KBr disk).

Methoserpidine   *Antihypertensive*

Synonym. 10-Methoxydeserpidine
Proprietary Name. Decaserpyl
Methyl 11-demethoxy-10-methoxy-18-O-(3,4,5-trimethoxybenzoyl)reserpate
$C_{33}H_{40}N_2O_9 = 608.7$
CAS—865-04-3

A cream-coloured, hygroscopic, microcrystalline powder, which darkens on exposure to light. M.p. about 171°, with decomposition.

Practically **insoluble** in water; soluble 1 in 60 of ethanol, 1 in 5 of chloroform, and 1 in 8 of dioxan.

Colour Tests. Mandelin's Test—grey-violet; Marquis Test—grey.

Thin-layer Chromatography. System TA—Rf 72; system TB—Rf 04; system TC—Rf 77. (Acidified iodoplatinate solution, positive.)

High Pressure Liquid Chromatography. System HA—k′ 0.5.

Ultraviolet Spectrum. Dehydrated alcohol—273 nm ($A_1^1 = 300$ a). (See below)

Infra-red Spectrum. Principal peaks at wavenumbers 1120, 1220, 1710, 1088, 1180, 1740 (KBr disk). (See below)

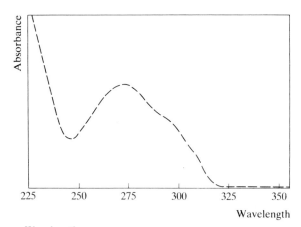

Wavelength

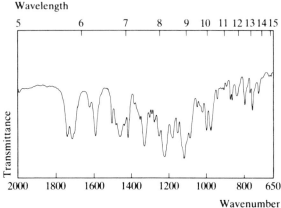

Wavenumber

Mass Spectrum. Principal peaks at m/z 608, 195, 607, 397, 609, 395, 381, 396.

Dose. 15 to 50 mg daily.

Methotrexate

Antineoplastic

Synonyms. Amethopterin; 4-Amino-10-methylfolic Acid; α-Methopterin.

Proprietary Names of Methotrexate and Methotrexate Sodium. Emtexate; Ledertrexate; Mexate.

A mixture of 4-amino-10-methylpteroyl-L-glutamic acid and related substances.

$C_{20}H_{22}N_8O_5 = 454.4$
CAS—59-05-2

A yellow to orange-brown, crystalline powder. M.p. 182° to 189°.

Practically **insoluble** in water, ethanol, chloroform, and ether; very soluble in dilute solutions of alkali hydroxides and carbonates.

Caution. Methotrexate is irritant; avoid contact with skin and mucous membranes.

Dissociation Constant. pK_a 3.8, 4.8, 5.6.

Colour Tests. Mandelin's Test—red; Mercurous Nitrate—black; Nessler's Reagent—orange.

Ultraviolet Spectrum. Aqueous acid—243 nm ($A_1^1 = 372$ a), 307 nm ($A_1^1 = 430$ a); aqueous alkali—258 nm ($A_1^1 = 500$ a), 303 nm ($A_1^1 = 500$ a).

Infra-red Spectrum. Principal peaks at wavenumbers 1600, 1511, 1634, 1305, 1200, 1538 (Nujol mull).

Quantification. HIGH PRESSURE LIQUID CHROMATOGRAPHY. In serum or urine: methotrexate and 3 metabolites, detection limit 12.5 ng/ml for methotrexate in serum, UV detection—Y. Y. Z. Farid *et al.*, *J. pharm. biomed. Analysis*, 1983, *1*, 55–63. In plasma, urine or cerebrospinal fluid: methotrexate and 2 metabolites, sensitivity 50 ng/ml, UV detection—H. Breithaupt *et al.*, *Analyt. Biochem.*, 1982, *121*, 103–113. In serum: methotrexate and 7-hydroxymethotrexate, sensitivity 100 ng/ml for methotrexate, UV detection—G. J. Lawson *et al.*, *J. Chromat.*, 1981, *223*; *Biomed. Appl.*, *12*, 225–231.

RADIOIMMUNOASSAY. In serum, urine or cerebrospinal fluid: sensitivity 450 pg/ml—G. W. Aherne *et al.*, *Br. J. Cancer*, 1977, *36*, 608–617.

Disposition in the Body. When given in low doses, it is rapidly absorbed after oral administration to give plasma concentrations equivalent to those obtained by intravenous administration; higher doses may be less well absorbed. It is distributed mainly in the extracellular spaces but a proportion penetrates cell membranes and is strongly bound to dihydrofolate reductase. Small amounts of methotrexate diffuse into the cerebrospinal fluid, higher concentrations being achieved with high doses. The major metabolite appears to be 4-amino-10-methylpteroic acid; 7-hydroxymethotrexate has been detected after high doses; 7-hydroxy-4-amino-10-methylpteroic acid has also been reported to be a metabolite. About 50 to 95% of a dose is excreted unchanged in the urine in 24 hours (dose-dependent); after oral administration, about 30% of a dose may be excreted as metabolites as a result of the action of intestinal bacteria prior to absorption; after intravenous administration, up to about 10% of a dose is excreted in the urine as metabolites and up to about 15% of a dose may be excreted in the bile.

THERAPEUTIC CONCENTRATION.

After single oral doses of 15 mg/m² to 10 fasting subjects (children), peak serum concentrations of 0.18 to 0.73 µg/ml (mean 0.41) were attained in 1 to 2 hours (C. R. Pinkerton *et al.*, *Lancet*, 1980, *2*, 944–946).

Following intravenous infusion of 50 to 250 mg/kg over 6 hours to 14 subjects, peak plasma concentrations of 45 to 450 µg/ml were attained (R. G. Stoller *et al.*, *New Engl. J. Med.*, 1977, *297*, 630–634).

TOXICITY. Toxic effects are usually associated with plasma concentrations greater than 4.5 µg/ml, 24 hours after a dose, or 0.45 µg/ml, 48 hours after a dose.

HALF-LIFE. Plasma half-life, about 4 to 10 hours; a longer terminal elimination phase of 10 to 70 hours (mean 27) has also been reported.

VOLUME OF DISTRIBUTION. About 0.8 litre/kg.

DISTRIBUTION IN BLOOD. Plasma: whole blood ratio, 0.9.

PROTEIN BINDING. In plasma, variously reported as 50 to 95%.

NOTE. For reviews of the clinical pharmacokinetics of methotrexate see D. D. Shen and D. L. Azarnoff, *Clin. Pharmacokinet.*, 1978, *3*, 1–13, F. M. Balis *et al.*, *ibid.*, 1983, *8*, 202–232, and Y.-M. Wang and T. Fujimoto, *ibid.*, 1984, *9*, 335–348.

Dose. 10 to 25 mg weekly, by mouth.

Methotrimeprazine

Tranquilliser

Synonym. Levomepromazine

Proprietary Names of Methotrimeprazine and its Salts. Levoprome; Minozinan; Neurocil; Nozinan. Methotrimeprazine is an ingredient of Immobilon (for small animals).

(−) - *NN* - Dimethyl - 3 - (2 - methoxyphenothiazin - 10 - yl) - 2 - methylpropylamine
$C_{19}H_{24}N_2OS = 328.5$
CAS—60-99-1

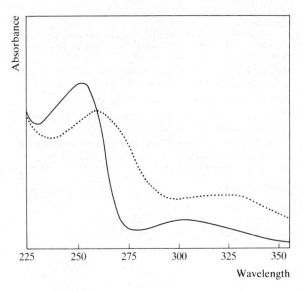

A fine, white, crystalline powder. M.p. about 126°.
Practically **insoluble** in water; sparingly soluble in ethanol; soluble 1 in 2 of chloroform and 1 in 10 of methanol; freely soluble in ether.

Methotrimeprazine Hydrochloride

$C_{19}H_{24}N_2OS,HCl = 364.9$
CAS—4185-80-2
Very **soluble** in water and ethanol.

Methotrimeprazine Maleate

Synonym. Methotrimeprazine Hydrogen Maleate
$C_{19}H_{24}N_2OS,C_4H_4O_4 = 444.5$
CAS—7104-38-3; 17086-29-2
A white crystalline powder. M.p. about 187°, with decomposition.
Very slightly **soluble** in water; slightly soluble in ethanol; soluble in chloroform; practically insoluble in ether.

Dissociation Constant. pK$_a$ 9.2.

Partition Coefficient. Log *P* (octanol), 4.7.

Colour Tests. Formaldehyde–Sulphuric Acid—blue; Forrest Reagent—violet; FPN Reagent—violet; Mandelin's Test—blue-violet; Marquis Test—blue-violet.

Thin-layer Chromatography. System *TA*—Rf 57; *system TB*—Rf 49; *system TC*—Rf 38. (*Dragendorff spray*, positive; *FPN reagent*, violet; *acidified iodoplatinate solution*, positive; *Marquis reagent*, violet.)

Gas Chromatography. System *GA*—RI 2514; *system GF*—RI 2965.

High Pressure Liquid Chromatography. System *HA*—k′ 3.2.

Ultraviolet Spectrum. Aqueous acid—250 nm (A$_1^1$ = 783 a), 302 nm; aqueous alkali—259 nm, 323 nm.

Infra-red Spectrum. Principal peaks at wavenumbers 1580, 1270, 1175, 1030, 1205, 752 (KBr disk).

Mass Spectrum. Principal peaks at m/z 58, 328, 100, 228, 185, 329, 242, 229.

Quantification. GAS CHROMATOGRAPHY. In plasma or erythrocytes: methotrimeprazine and metabolites, AFID—S. G. Dahl *et al., Ther. Drug Monit.,* 1982, *4,* 81–87.

GAS CHROMATOGRAPHY–MASS SPECTROMETRY. In plasma or urine: methotrimeprazine and metabolites—S. G. Dahl and M. Garle, *J. pharm. Sci.,* 1977, *66,* 190–193.

HIGH PRESSURE LIQUID CHROMATOGRAPHY. In plasma: limit of detection 2 ng/ml, UV detection—J. E. Holt *et al., Br. J. clin. Pharmac.,* 1982, *13,* 282P.

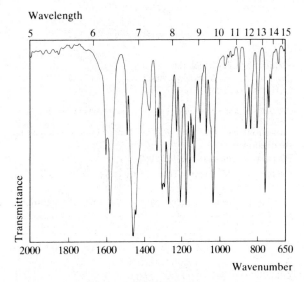

Disposition in the Body. Readily absorbed after oral administration and widely distributed throughout the body. The major metabolites are the sulphoxide and *N*-monodesmethyl derivative (active); hydroxylation also occurs. Less than 1% of a dose is excreted in the urine as unchanged drug in 24 hours. About 10% of a dose is excreted in the urine as the sulphoxide.

THERAPEUTIC CONCENTRATION.

After a single oral dose of 50 mg to 5 subjects, peak plasma concentrations of 0.016 to 0.04 µg/ml were attained in 1 to 4 hours; concentrations of the sulphoxide metabolite exceeded those of unchanged drug in each case (S. G. Dahl, *Clin. Pharmac. Ther.,* 1976, *19,* 435–442).

Following daily oral doses of 300 to 400 mg to 4 subjects, steady-state plasma concentrations of 0.05 to 0.14 µg/ml (mean 0.08) were reported; steady-state plasma concentrations of the sulphoxide metabolite ranged from 0.26 to 0.39 µg/ml (mean 0.33); the *N*-monodesmethyl metabolite was also detected (S. G. Dahl and M. Garle, *J. pharm. Sci.,* 1977, *66,* 190–193).

TOXICITY.
The following postmortem concentrations were reported in a fatality attributed to methotrimeprazine overdose: blood 8 μg/ml, liver 160 μg/g (R. Bonnichsen *et al.*, *Z. Rechtsmed.*, 1970, *67*, 158–169).

HALF-LIFE. Plasma half-life, methotrimeprazine 15 to 77 hours (mean 27), sulphoxide metabolite 10 to 30 hours (mean 20).

VOLUME OF DISTRIBUTION. About 30 litres/kg.

DISTRIBUTION IN BLOOD. Plasma:whole blood ratio, about 1.2 but there is considerable intersubject variation.

Dose. Usually 25 to 50 mg of methotrimeprazine maleate daily; up to 1 g daily has been given.

Methoxamine   *Sympathomimetic*

Synonym. Methoxamedrine
2-Amino-1-(2,5-dimethoxyphenyl)propan-1-ol
$C_{11}H_{17}NO_3 = 211.3$
CAS—390-28-3

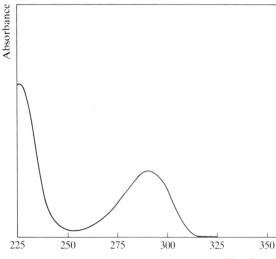

Methoxamine Hydrochloride
Proprietary Names. Vasoxine; Vasoxyl.
$C_{11}H_{17}NO_3,HCl = 247.7$
CAS—61-16-5
Colourless or white plate-like crystals or white crystalline powder. M.p. 214° to 219°.
Soluble 1 in 2.5 of water and 1 in 12 of ethanol; very slightly soluble in chloroform and ether.

Dissociation Constant. pK_a 9.2 (25°).

Colour Tests. Mandelin's Test—green-yellow; Marquis Test—violet-brown→green.

Thin-layer Chromatography. *System TA*—Rf 55. (*Acidified potassium permanganate solution*, positive.)

Gas Chromatography. *System GA*—RI 1726; *system GB*—RI 1735.

High Pressure Liquid Chromatography. *System HA*—k' 0.9.

Ultraviolet Spectrum. Aqueous acid—290 nm; water—290 nm $(A_1^1 = 161 \text{ a})$. No alkaline shift.

Infra-red Spectrum. Principal peaks at wavenumbers 1496, 1219, 1022, 1276, 1179, 1050 (methoxamine hydrochloride, KBr disk).

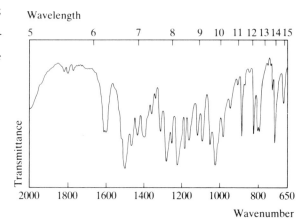

Mass Spectrum. Principal peaks at *m/z* 168, 137, 44, 139, 43, 152, 124, 167.

Dose. 5 to 20 mg of methoxamine hydrochloride intramuscularly.

Methoxsalen   *Pigmenting Agent*

Synonyms. Ammoidin; 8-Methoxypsoralen; Metoxaleno; Xanthotoxin.
Proprietary Names. Deltasoralen; Meladinine; Oxsoralen.
9-Methoxy-7*H*-furo[3,2-*g*]chromen-7-one
$C_{12}H_8O_4 = 216.2$
CAS—298-81-7

A constituent of the fruits of *Ammi majus*.
White to cream-coloured fluffy crystals. M.p. 143° to 148°.
Practically **insoluble** in water; soluble in boiling ethanol and in acetone; freely soluble in chloroform; sparingly soluble in ether.

Gas Chromatography. *System GA*—RI 1980.

Ultraviolet Spectrum. Aqueous acid—247 nm, 304 nm.

Infra-red Spectrum. Principal peaks at wavenumbers 1705, 1150, 1100, 1580, 1020, 1000 (Nujol mull).

Dose. 20 mg daily; doses of up to 50 mg have been given.

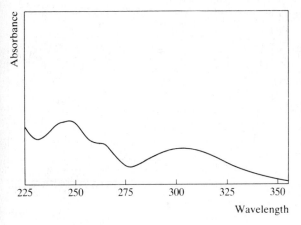

Absorbance

225   250   275   300   325   350

Wavelength

Methoxyamphetamine   *Hallucinogen*

Synonym. p-Methoxyamphetamine
α-Methyl-4-methoxyphenethylamine
$C_{10}H_{15}NO = 165.2$
CAS—23239-32-9

A colourless oil.
Practically **insoluble** in water; soluble in chloroform and dilute acids.

Methoxyamphetamine Hydrochloride
$C_{10}H_{15}NO,HCl = 201.7$
CAS—3706-26-1
White crystals.
Soluble in water.

Colour Test. Mandelin's Test—green.

Thin-layer Chromatography. *System TA*—Rf 73; *system TB*—Rf 36; *system TC*—Rf 77. (*Acidified iodoplatinate solution*, positive.)

Gas Chromatography. *System GA*—RI 1385.

High Pressure Liquid Chromatography. *System HB*—k′ 14.95.

Ultraviolet Spectrum. Aqueous acid—274 nm ($A_1^1 = 80$ b). No alkaline shift.

Infra-red Spectrum. Principal peaks at wavenumbers 1512, 1259, 1033, 808, 1190, 1623 (methoxyamphetamine hydrochloride).

Mass Spectrum. Principal peaks at m/z 44, 122, 121, 78, 77, 42, 51, 52.

Quantification. GAS CHROMATOGRAPHY. In urine: sensitivity 70 ng/ml—B. M. Angrist *et al.*, *Nature*, 1970, *225*, 651–652.

Disposition in the Body. Absorbed after oral administration. About 80% of a dose is excreted in the urine in 24 hours with up to 15% of the dose as unchanged drug, about 25% as free 4-hydroxyamphetamine, 50% as conjugated 4-hydroxyamphetamine, and 5% each as 4-hydroxynorephedrine and a conjugated

N-oxidation product. The extent of O-demethylation appears to be genetically determined being decreased in poor metabolisers.

TOXICITY. Methoxyamphetamine is about 3 times as potent as methylenedioxyamphetamine and appears to be more toxic.

In 9 fatalities due to the ingestion or intravenous administration of methoxyamphetamine, the following postmortem tissue concentrations were reported: blood 0.3 to 1.9 µg/ml, bile 0.4 to 3 µg/ml, liver 0.5 to 10.3 µg/g, urine 6 to 175 µg/ml; alcohol was also detected in 4 cases (G. Cimbura, *Can. med. Ass. J.*, 1974, *110*, 1263–1264).

Methoxychlor   *Pesticide*

Synonyms. Dimethoxy-DT; DMDT; Methoxy-DDT.
1,1,1-Trichloro-2,2-bis(4-methoxyphenyl)ethane
$C_{16}H_{15}Cl_3O_2 = 345.7$
CAS—72-43-5

The technical product contains about 88% of methoxychlor and about 12% of related isomers.
The pure pp′-isomer occurs as colourless crystals; the technical product is a grey powder. M.p. pure isomer, about 89°; technical product, 77°.
Practically **insoluble** in water; soluble in ethanol and aromatic solvents; very soluble in ether.

Colour Test. Liebermann's Test—black-violet.

Gas Chromatography. *System GA*—op′-methoxychlor RI 2417; *system GK*—pp′-methoxychlor retention time 1.46, op′-methoxychlor retention time 1.40, both relative to caffeine.

Ultraviolet Spectrum. Hexane—276 nm ($A_1^1 = 100$ b), shoulder at 283 nm.

Mass Spectrum. Principal peaks at m/z 121, 227, 228, 114, 152, 122, 63, 165 (op′-methoxychlor); 227, 228, 114, 152, 212, 63, 169, 115 (pp′-methoxychlor).

Disposition in the Body. Methoxychlor is less persistent than dicophane. It is stored in the fat to a limited extent and disappears in 2 to 4 weeks after cessation of exposure. It is eliminated mainly in the faeces; small amounts are excreted in the urine.

TOXICITY. Methoxychlor is the least toxic of the chlorinated hydrocarbon insecticides. The maximum permissible atmospheric concentration is 10 mg/m³ and the maximum permissible concentration in food is 14 µg/g.

Methoxyflurane   *General Anaesthetic*

Proprietary Name. Penthrane
2,2-Dichloro-1,1-difluoroethyl methyl ether
$CHCl_2 \cdot CF_2 \cdot O \cdot CH_3 = 165.0$
CAS—76-38-0

A clear, almost colourless, non-inflammable mobile liquid. Wt per ml 1.423 to 1.427 g. B.p. 103° to 108°.
Methoxyflurane (*B.P.*) contains butylated hydroxytoluene 0.01% w/w.

Soluble 1 in 500 of water; miscible with ethanol, chloroform, and ether.

Gas Chromatography. *System GA*—RI 701; *system GI*—retention time 17.6 min.

Ultraviolet Spectrum. No significant absorption, 230 to 360 nm.

Infra-red Spectrum. Principal peaks at wavenumbers 1315, 1063, 1136, 833, 1204, 1234.

Quantification. GAS CHROMATOGRAPHY. In blood: FID—W. J. Cole *et al.*, *Br. J. Anaesth.*, 1975, *47*, 1043–1047. In blood: sensitivity 10 μg/ml, FID—P. L. Jones *et al.*, *Br. J. Anaesth.*, 1972, *44*, 124–130.

Dose. For maintenance of anaesthesia, 0.2 to 0.5% of the vapour by inhalation.

Methoxyphenamine   *Sympathomimetic*

Synonyms. Methoxiphenadrin; Mexyphamine.
2-Methoxy-*N*,α-dimethylphenethylamine
$C_{11}H_{17}NO = 179.3$
CAS—93-30-1

An oil.

Methoxyphenamine Hydrochloride
Proprietary Names. Orthoxine. It is an ingredient of Orthoxicol.
$C_{11}H_{17}NO,HCl = 215.7$
CAS—5588-10-3
White crystals or powder. M.p. about 130°.
Freely **soluble** in water, ethanol, and chloroform; slightly soluble in ether.

Dissociation Constant. pK_a 10.1.

Partition Coefficient. Log *P* (chloroform/pH 7.4), 0.0.

Colour Tests. Mandelin's Test—blue-green; Marquis Test—red.

Thin-layer Chromatography. *System TA*—Rf 23; *system TB*—Rf 24; *system TC*—Rf 04. (*Acidified iodoplatinate solution*, positive.)

Gas Chromatography. *System GA*—RI 1361; *system GB*—RI 1370; *system GC*—RI 1670.

High Pressure Liquid Chromatography. *System HA*—k' 1.7; *system HB*—k' 32.17.

Ultraviolet Spectrum. Aqueous acid—271 nm ($A_1^1 = 92$ a). No alkaline shift.

Infra-red Spectrum. Principal peaks at wavenumbers 1236, 749, 1047, 1125, 1026, 1175 (Nujol mull).

Mass Spectrum. Principal peaks at *m/z* 58, 91, 59, 56, 30, 42, 121, 78.

Disposition in the Body. Readily absorbed after oral administration. Metabolites identified in urine include the *N*-desmethyl, *O*-desmethyl, and 5-hydroxy derivatives and their glucuronide and/or sulphate conjugates. Unchanged drug is also excreted in the urine.

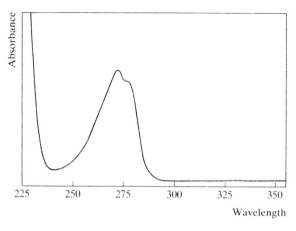

TOXICITY. The estimated minimum lethal dose for children up to 2 years of age is 200 mg and for adults is 2 g.

Dose. 50 to 100 mg of methoxyphenamine hydrochloride every 4 hours.

Methsuximide   *Anticonvulsant*

Synonym. Mesuximide
Proprietary Names. Celontin; Petinutin.
N,2-Dimethyl-2-phenylsuccinimide
$C_{12}H_{13}NO_2 = 203.2$
CAS—77-41-8

A white to greyish-white crystalline powder. M.p. 50° to 56°.
Soluble 1 in 350 of water, 1 in 3 of ethanol, 1 in less than 1 of chloroform, and 1 in 2 of ether.

Thin-layer Chromatography. *System TA*—Rf 76.

Gas Chromatography. *System GA*—RI 1622; *system GE*—retention time 0.35 for methsuximide and 0.50 for *N*-desmethylmethsuximide, relative to phenytoin.

High Pressure Liquid Chromatography. *System HE*—k' 6.02.

Ultraviolet Spectrum. Methanol—247 nm ($A_1^1 = 21$ a), 252 nm, 258 nm, 264 nm.

Infra-red Spectrum. Principal peaks at wavenumbers 1705, 1282, 1030, 699, 1775, 1086 (KBr disk).

Mass Spectrum. Principal peaks at *m/z* 118, 117, 203, 103, 77, 78, 119, 91.

Quantification. GAS CHROMATOGRAPHY. In serum: sensitivity 1 μg/ml, FID—J. Bonitati, *Clin. Chem.*, 1976, *22*, 341–345. In plasma or serum: *N*-desmethylmethsuximide, sensitivity 500 ng/ml, ECD—J. E. Wallace *et al.*, *Clin. Chem.*, 1979, *25*, 252–255.

HIGH PRESSURE LIQUID CHROMATOGRAPHY. In serum: sensitivity 1 μg/ml, UV detection—P. M. Kabra *et al.*, *J. analyt. Toxicol.*, 1978, *2*, 127–133.

Disposition in the Body. Rapidly absorbed after oral administration and metabolised to the active *N*-desmethyl derivative.

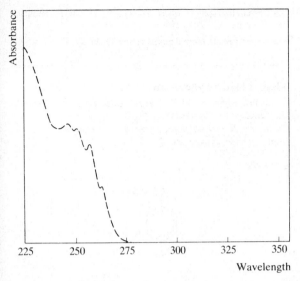

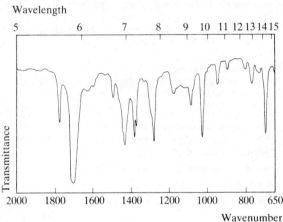

Less than 1% of a dose is excreted in the urine as unchanged drug. The major urinary metabolites are conjugated 4-hydroxyphenyl derivatives; minor metabolites include the 3-hydroxy, 2-hydroxymethyl, and 2-dihydrodihydroxyphenyl derivatives. Methsuximide increases its own rate of metabolism on chronic dosing.

THERAPEUTIC CONCENTRATION. In plasma, N-desmethylmethsuximide, usually in the range 10 to 40 µg/ml.

Following daily oral doses of 600 to 1200 mg to 8 subjects experiencing good seizure control, steady-state plasma concentrations of 0.01 to 0.11 µg/ml (mean 0.04) and 16 to 37 µg/ml (mean 25) for methsuximide and the N-desmethyl metabolite, respectively, were reported (J. M. Strong *et al.*, *Neurology, Minneap.*, 1974, *24*, 250–255).

TOXICITY. The estimated minimum lethal dose is 5 g. Toxic effects are usually associated with plasma N-desmethylmethsuximide concentrations of more than 40 µg/ml.

In a case of severe coma, which began several hours after the ingestion of nearly 10 g in a suicide attempt, blood concentrations of 18 µg/ml of methsuximide and 44 µg/ml of the N-desmethyl metabolite were reported 14 hours after ingestion; the coma persisted for about 80 hours and correlated with the presence of the N-desmethyl metabolite in the blood (S. B. Karch, *J. Am. med. Ass.*, 1973, *223*, 1463–1465).

HALF-LIFE. Plasma half-life, methsuximide about 3 hours, but may reduce to one quarter of this value on chronic dosing; N-desmethylmethsuximide about 30 to 40 hours.

PROTEIN BINDING. In plasma, not significantly bound.

Dose. 0.3 to 1.2 g daily; up to 3.6 g daily has been given.

Methyclothiazide   *Diuretic*

Proprietary Names. Aquatensen; Duretic; Enduron; Thiazidil. It is an ingredient of Enduronyl.

6 - Chloro - 3 - chloromethyl - 3,4 - dihydro - 2 - methyl - 2H - 1,2,4 - benzothiadiazine-7-sulphonamide 1,1-dioxide

$C_9H_{11}Cl_2N_3O_4S_2 = 360.2$

CAS—135-07-9

A white crystalline powder. M.p. 216°.

Very slightly **soluble** in water and chloroform; soluble 1 in about 90 of ethanol; freely soluble in acetone and pyridine; soluble in solutions of alkali hydroxides and carbonates.

Dissociation Constant. pK$_a$ 9.4.

Colour Tests. Koppanyi–Zwikker Test—violet; Sulphuric Acid—orange.

Thin-layer Chromatography. *System TD*—Rf 19; *system TE*—Rf 53; *system TF*—Rf 50.

Gas Chromatography. *System GA*—not eluted.

High Pressure Liquid Chromatography. *System HN*—k' 3.82.

Ultraviolet Spectrum. Aqueous acid—270 nm (A$_1^1$ = 525 b), 314 nm; aqueous alkali—264 nm, 300 nm.

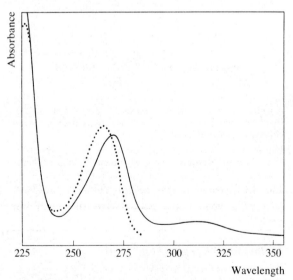

Infra-red Spectrum. Principal peaks at wavenumbers 1158, 1595, 715, 1063, 1515, 1300 (KBr disk). (See below)

Mass Spectrum. Principal peaks at m/z 310, 64, 36, 312, 42, 43, 62, 63.

Wavelength

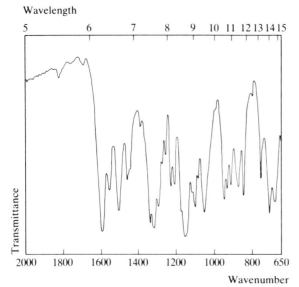

Transmittance

Wavenumber

Quantification. HIGH PRESSURE LIQUID CHROMATOGRAPHY. In plasma: detection limit 1.5 ng/ml, UV detection—C. A. Hartman *et al.*, *J. Chromat.*, 1981, *226*; *Biomed. Appl.*, *15*, 510–513.

Dose. 2.5 to 10 mg daily.

Methyl Benzoquate   *Coccidiostat (Veterinary)*

Synonym. Nequinate
Methyl 7-benzyloxy-6-butyl-1,4-dihydro-4-oxoquinoline-3-carboxylate
$C_{22}H_{23}NO_4 = 365.4$
CAS—13997-19-8

A white or creamy-white, amorphous powder. M.p. about 208°. Practically **insoluble** in water; very slightly soluble in ethanol, chloroform, and methanol.

Colour Tests. Liebermann's Test—red-orange; Mandelin's Test—brown; Marquis Test—red-brown; Sulphuric Acid—yellow.

Ultraviolet Spectrum. Methanolic acid—261 nm ($A_1^1 = 1955$ a).

Infra-red Spectrum. Principal peaks at wavenumbers 1621, 1689, 1250, 1089, 1211, 1550 (KBr disk).

Methyl Ethyl Ketone   *Solvent*

Synonym. Ethyl Methyl Ketone
Butan-2-one
$CH_3 \cdot CO \cdot CH_2 \cdot CH_3 = 72.11$
CAS—78-93-3
An inflammable liquid. B.p. 80°.
Soluble 1 in about 4 of water; miscible with ethanol and ether.

Gas Chromatography. *System GA*—RI 579; *system GI*—retention time 7.3 min.

Mass Spectrum. Principal peaks at *m/z* 43, 29, 27, 72, 57, 42, 44, 41.

Methyl Hydroxybenzoate   *Preservative*

Synonyms. Metagin; Methyl Parahydroxybenzoate; Methylis Oxybenzoas; Methylparaben.
Proprietary Names. Methyl Chemosept; Nipagin M.
Methyl *p*-hydroxybenzoate
$C_8H_8O_3 = 152.1$
CAS—99-76-3

Colourless crystals or a fine, white, crystalline powder. M.p. 125° to 128°.
Soluble 1 in 400 to 1 in 500 of water, 1 in 20 of boiling water, 1 in 3 to 1 in 3.5 of ethanol, 1 in 40 of chloroform, and 1 in 10 of ether.

Sodium Methyl Hydroxybenzoate

Synonyms. Sodium Methylparaben; Soluble Methyl Hydroxybenzoate.
Proprietary Name. Nipagin M Sodium
$C_8H_7NaO_3 = 174.1$
CAS—5026-62-0
A white, hygroscopic, crystalline powder.
Soluble 1 in 2 of water and 1 in 50 of ethanol.

Dissociation Constant. pK_a 8.4 (22°).

Gas Chromatography. *System GA*—RI 1419.

Ultraviolet Spectrum. Ethanol—257 nm ($A_1^1 = 1075$ a).

Mass Spectrum. Principal peaks at *m/z* 121, 152, 40, 93, 65, –, –, –.

Methyl Nicotinate   *Topical Vasodilator*

Proprietary Names. It is an ingredient of Algipan, Cremalgex, and Cremalgin.
$C_7H_7NO_2 = 137.1$
CAS—93-60-7

White crystals or crystalline powder; it darkens to a reddish colour on storage. M.p. 40° to 42°.
Soluble 1 in 0.7 of water and ethanol, 1 in 0.4 of chloroform, and 1 in 1 of ether.

Dissociation Constant. pK_a 3.1 (22°).

Thin-layer Chromatography. *System TA*—Rf 61; *system TB*—Rf 37; *system TC*—Rf 66.

Gas Chromatography. *System GA*—RI 1100.

Ultraviolet Spectrum. Water—264 nm ($A_1^1 = 230$ b).

Infra-red Spectrum. Principal peaks at wavenumbers 1282, 1718, 1111, 741, 1022, 703 (KBr disk).

Mass Spectrum. Principal peaks at m/z 78, 106, 51, 137, 50, 136, 107, 79.

Use. Topically in a concentration of 1%.

Methyl Salicylate   *Analgesic*

Synonym. Wintergreen Oil
Methyl 2-hydroxybenzoate
$C_8H_8O_3 = 152.1$
CAS—119-36-8

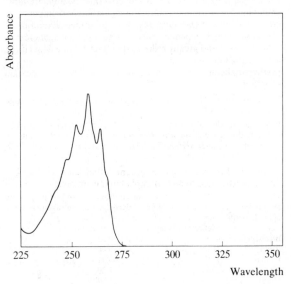

A colourless or pale yellow liquid. Relative density 1.182 to 1.187. B.p. about 221°, with some decomposition. Refractive index 1.535 to 1.538.
Very slightly **soluble** in water; miscible with ethanol (90%) and with most organic solvents.

Gas Chromatography. *System GA*—methyl salicylate RI 1193, salicylic acid RI 1308.

High Pressure Liquid Chromatography. *System HD*—methyl salicylate k′ 3.9, salicylic acid k′ 0.7.

Ultraviolet Spectrum. Ethanol—238 nm $(A_1^1 = 581$ a), 306 nm $(A_1^1 = 280$ a).

Infra-red Spectrum. Principal peaks at wavenumbers 1680, 705, 1310, 1220, 760, 1255 (thin film).

Mass Spectrum. Principal peaks at m/z 120, 92, 152, 121, 65, 64, 93, 63; salicylic acid 120, 92, 138, 64, 39, 63, 121, 65.

Disposition in the Body. Poorly absorbed through intact skin; absorbed after oral ingestion. It is incompletely hydrolysed to salicylic acid.

TOXICITY. Methyl salicylate is more toxic than salicylic acid. Deaths have occurred in children after ingestion of as little as 4 ml and doses of 30 ml are usually fatal in adults.

In a fatality due to the ingestion of about 120 ml of methyl salicylate, postmortem salicylic acid concentrations were, blood 615 μg/ml and liver 455 μg/g (J. Ryall, *Bull. int. Ass. forens. Toxicol.*, 1974, *10*(1), 10).

Use. Topically in liniments and ointments or in undiluted form.

Methylamphetamine   *Central Stimulant*

Synonyms. d-Deoxyephedrine; Desoxyephedrine; Methamphetamine; Phenylmethylaminopropane.
(+)-N,α-Dimethylphenethylamine
$C_{10}H_{15}N = 149.2$
CAS—537-46-2

$$C_6H_5 \cdot CH_2 \cdot \underset{\underset{CH_3}{|}}{CH} \cdot NH \cdot CH_3$$

A clear, colourless, slowly volatile, mobile liquid. Wt per ml 0.921 to 0.922 g. B.p. about 214°.
Slightly **soluble** in water; miscible with ethanol, chloroform, and ether.

Methylamphetamine Hydrochloride

Proprietary Names. Desoxyn; Methampex; Pervitin.
$C_{10}H_{15}N,HCl = 185.7$
CAS—51-57-0
White crystals or crystalline powder. M.p. 172° to 174°.
Soluble 1 in 2 of water, 1 in 4 of ethanol, and 1 in 5 of chloroform; practically insoluble in ether.

Dissociation Constant. pK_a 10.1.

Colour Test. Marquis Test—orange.

Thin-layer Chromatography. *System TA*—Rf 31; *system TB*—Rf 28; *system TC*—Rf 13. (*Dragendorff spray*, positive; *acidified iodoplatinate solution*, positive; *Marquis reagent*, brown; *ninhydrin spray*, positive; *acidified potassium permanganate solution*, positive.)

Gas Chromatography. *System GA*—methylamphetamine RI 1176, amphetamine RI 1123; *system GB*—methylamphetamine RI 1200, amphetamine RI 1134; *system GC*—methylamphetamine RI 1722, amphetamine RI 1536; *system GF*—methylamphetamine RI 1335, amphetamine RI 1315.

High Pressure Liquid Chromatography. *System HA*—methylamphetamine k′ 2.0, amphetamine k′ 0.9; *system HB*—methylamphetamine k′ 10.52, amphetamine k′ 8.48; *system HC*—methylamphetamine k′ 2.07, amphetamine k′ 0.98.

Ultraviolet Spectrum. Aqueous acid—252 nm, 257 nm $(A_1^1 = 12.1$ a), 263 nm.

Infra-red Spectrum. Principal peaks at wavenumbers 747, 698, 1060, 1491, 1590, 1085 (methylamphetamine hydrochloride, KBr disk). (See below)

Mass Spectrum. Principal peaks at m/z 58, 91, 59, 134, 65, 56, 42, 57; amphetamine 44, 91, 40, 42, 65, 45, 39, 43.

Quantification. GAS CHROMATOGRAPHY. In urine: methylamphetamine and amphetamine, detection limit 10 ng/ml, ECD—M. Terada *et al.*, *J. Chromat.*, 1982, *237*, 285–292.

RADIOIMMUNOASSAY. In urine: sensitivity 1 ng—S. Inayama *et al.*, *Chem. pharm. Bull.*, 1980, *28*, 2779–2782.

Disposition in the Body. Readily absorbed after oral administration. About 70% of a dose is excreted in the urine in 24 hours. Under normal conditions, up to 43% of a dose is excreted as

Wavelength

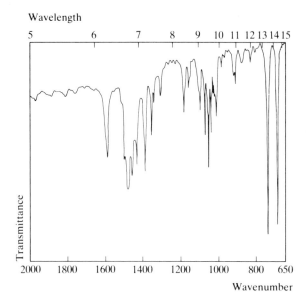

unchanged drug, up to 15% as 4-hydroxymethylamphetamine, and about 5% as amphetamine, the major active metabolite. A number of other metabolites have been identified. Excretion of unchanged drug is dependent on the urinary pH, being increased in acidic urine and greatly reduced (to about 2% of a dose) if the urine is alkaline.

Methylamphetamine is a metabolite of benzphetamine and selegiline.

THERAPEUTIC CONCENTRATION. In plasma, usually in the range 0.01 to 0.05 µg/ml.

Following a single oral dose of 12.5 mg of methylamphetamine hydrochloride to 10 subjects, a mean peak blood concentration of about 0.02 µg/ml was attained in about 2 hours (R. C. Driscoll et al., J. pharm. Sci., 1971, 60, 1492–1495).

TOXICITY. The estimated minimum lethal dose is 1 g, but fatalities attributed to methylamphetamine are rare.

The following postmortem tissue concentrations, µg/ml or µg/g, were reported in a 25-year-old female found dead after the intravenous abuse of methylamphetamine followed by ingestion of about 1.5 g:

	Methylamphetamine	Amphetamine
Blood	43	0.35
Brain	101.8	0.86
Kidney	75.5	0.72
Liver	174.6	1.30
Urine	277.5	10.0

(T. Kojima et al., Forens. Sci. Int., 1984, 24, 87–93).

In 3 fatalities caused by the intravenous self-administration of methylamphetamine, the following postmortem tissue concentrations, µg/ml or µg/g, were reported:

	Methylamphetamine	Amphetamine
Blood	0, 0.1, 0.6	0.1, 0, 0.5
Brain	0.2, 0.3, 0.8	0.2, 0, 0.8
Kidney	1.0, –, 0.2	0.8, –, 0.2
Liver	0.6, 0.7, 0.4	0.2, 0, 0.3
Urine	1.0, –, –	4.0, –, –

(R. H. Cravey and D. Reed, J. forens. Sci. Soc., 1970, 10, 109–112).

HALF-LIFE. Plasma half-life, about 9 hours.

Dose. 2.5 to 25 mg of methylamphetamine hydrochloride daily, by mouth; 15 to 20 mg intramuscularly, or 10 to 15 mg intravenously.

Methylchlorophenoxyacetic Acid   *Herbicide*

Synonym. MCPA

4-Chloro-2-methylphenoxyacetic acid

$C_9H_9ClO_3 = 200.6$

CAS—4841-22-9

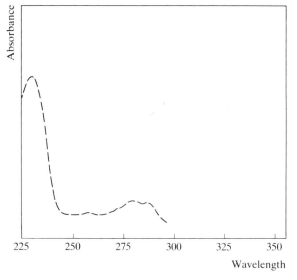

A white crystalline solid. M.p. pure compound, 118° to 119°; technical product, 100° to 115°.

Very slightly **soluble** in water; soluble 1 in 160 of ethanol and 1 in 80 of ether.

Colour Test. Liebermann's Test—black.

Thin-layer Chromatography. *System TD*—Rf 09; *system TE*—Rf 05; *system TF*—Rf 11.

Gas Chromatography. Methylchlorophenoxyacetic acid methyl ester: *system GK*—retention time 0.54 relative to caffeine.

Ultraviolet Spectrum. Methanol—280 nm ($A_1^1 = 80$ a), 287 nm.

Infra-red Spectrum. Principal peaks at wavenumbers 1247, 1198, 1748, 1499, 1143, 806 (Nujol mull).

Mass Spectrum. Principal peaks at m/z 141, 214, 125, 155, 46, 77, 89, 143 (methylchlorophenoxyacetic acid methyl ester).

Methyldopa   *Antihypertensive*

Synonyms. Alpha-methyldopa; Methyldopum Hydratum; Metildopa.

Proprietary Names. Aldomet (tablets); Dopamet; Medimet-250; Medomet; Novomedopa; Presinol; Sembrina. It is an ingredient of Aldoclor, Aldoril, and Hydromet.

(−)-3-(3,4-Dihydroxyphenyl)-2-methyl-L-alanine sesquihydrate

$C_{10}H_{13}NO_4, 1\frac{1}{2}H_2O = 238.2$

CAS—555-30-6 (anhydrous); *41372-08-1* (sesquihydrate)

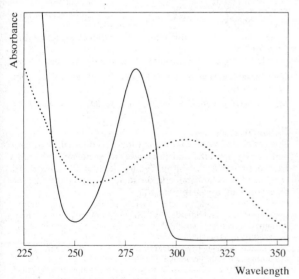

Colourless crystals or a white to yellowish-white, fine powder. M.p. about 310°.

Soluble 1 in 100 of water, 1 in 400 of ethanol, and 1 in 0.5 of dilute hydrochloric acid; practically insoluble in chloroform and ether.

Dissociation Constant. pK_a 2.2 (—COOH), 9.2 (—OH), 10.6 (—NH_2), 12.0 (—OH), (25°).

Colour Tests. Ammoniacal Silver Nitrate—red-brown/black; Ferric Chloride—green; Folin–Ciocalteu Reagent—blue; Mandelin's Test—orange; Marquis Test—yellow→violet; Methanolic Potassium Hydroxide—yellow→orange; Nessler's Reagent—black; Potassium Dichromate (Method 1)—green→brown (30s).

Thin-layer Chromatography. *System TA*—Rf 49; *system TB*—Rf 01; *system TC*—Rf 01. (*Mercuric chloride-diphenylcarbazone reagent*, white-blue; *acidified potassium permanganate solution*, positive; *Van Urk reagent*, violet.)

Ultraviolet Spectrum. Aqueous acid—279 nm ($A_1^1 = 130$ a); aqueous alkali—302 nm.

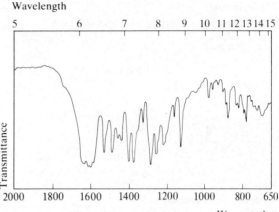

Infra-red Spectrum. Principal peaks at wavenumbers 1600, 1288, 1261, 1530, 1123, 1219 (KBr disk).

Mass Spectrum. Principal peaks at m/z 88, 42, 123, 124, 89, 77, 51, 44.

Quantification. SPECTROFLUORIMETRY. In plasma or urine: sensitivity 100 ng/ml—B. K. Kim and R. T. Koda, *J. pharm. Sci.*, 1977, *66*, 1632–1634.

HIGH PRESSURE LIQUID CHROMATOGRAPHY. In plasma or breast milk: electrochemical detection—J. A. Hoskins and S. B. Holliday, *J. Chromat.*, 1982, *230*; *Biomed. Appl.*, *19*, 162–167. In urine: sensitivity 5 μg/ml, electrochemical detection—G. M. Kochak and W. D. Mason, *Analyt. Lett. (Part B)*, 1981, *14*, 439–449.

Disposition in the Body. Poorly absorbed after oral administration. It is mainly excreted as unchanged drug and as the mono-*O*-sulphate conjugate. After oral dosage, about 40% of the dose is excreted in the urine in 48 hours, of which about 40% is the conjugate. A considerable amount of unchanged drug is eliminated in the faeces. After intravenous administration, the amount of conjugate excreted is much less than after oral dosage; a total of 52 to 82% of an intravenous dose is excreted in the urine in 36 hours, only about 2% of which is the conjugate. Other metabolites and their conjugates which have been identified in the urine in small amounts (each less than 5% of the dose) include 3-*O*-methyl-α-methyldopa, α-methyldopamine, 3-*O*-methyl-α-methyldopamine, and 3,4-dihydroxyphenylacetone. Methyldopa is a metabolite of methyldopate.

THERAPEUTIC CONCENTRATION. In plasma, usually in the range 1 to 5 μg/ml.

After a single oral dose of 750 mg administered to 12 subjects, mean peak plasma concentrations of 2.6 μg/ml of unchanged drug and 1.3 μg/ml of the conjugate were attained in 3 hours. An intravenous infusion of 250 mg given over 90 minutes to 12 subjects produced, at the end of the infusion period, a mean peak plasma concentration of 7.5 μg/ml; no conjugate was found in the plasma (K. C. Kwan *et al.*, *J. Pharmac. exp. Ther.*, 1976, *198*, 264–277).

TOXICITY.

In a fatality involving the ingestion of methyldopa, postmortem blood and urine concentrations of 9 and 1400 μg/ml, respectively, were reported (V. Tamminen and A. Alha, *Bull. int. Ass. forens. Toxicol.*, 1970, *7*(2), 2–3).

HALF-LIFE. Plasma half-life, about 2 hours; a longer terminal elimination half-life has also been reported.

VOLUME OF DISTRIBUTION. About 0.6 litre/kg.

CLEARANCE. Plasma clearance, about 3 ml/min/kg.

PROTEIN BINDING. In plasma, less than 20%.

NOTE. For a review of the pharmacokinetics of methyldopa see E. Myhre *et al.*, *Clin. Pharmacokinet.*, 1982, *7*, 221–233.

Dose. The equivalent of 0.5 to 3 g of anhydrous methyldopa daily.

Methyldopate   *Antihypertensive*

Ethyl 3-(3,4-dihydroxyphenyl)-2-methyl-L-alaninate
$C_{12}H_{17}NO_4 = 239.3$
CAS—2544-09-4

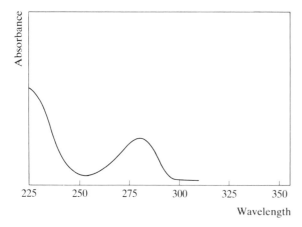

Methyldopate Hydrochloride

Proprietary Name. Aldomet (injection)
$C_{12}H_{17}NO_4,HCl = 275.7$
CAS—2508-79-4
A white crystalline powder.
Soluble 1 in 1 of water, 1 in 3 of ethanol, and 1 in 2 of methanol; slightly soluble in chloroform; practically insoluble in ether.

Colour Tests. Ammoniacal Silver Nitrate—orange-brown/ orange-brown; Ferric Chloride—green; Folin–Ciocalteu Reagent—blue; Mandelin's Test—orange; Marquis Test— yellow → violet; Methanolic Potassium Hydroxide— blue → orange; Nessler's Reagent—black; Potassium Dichromate (Method 1)—green → brown (30s).

Thin-layer Chromatography. *System TA*—Rf 65. (*Acidified potassium permanganate solution*, positive.)

Ultraviolet Spectrum. Aqueous acid—280 nm ($A_1^1 = 115$ a).

Infra-red Spectrum. Principal peaks at wavenumbers 1527, 1726, 1516, 1290, 1240, 1215 (KBr disk).

Quantification. HIGH PRESSURE LIQUID CHROMATOGRAPHY. In plasma or breast milk: electrochemical detection—J. A. Hoskins and S. B. Holliday, *J. Chromat.*, 1982, *230*; *Biomed. Appl.*, *19*, 162–167.

Disposition in the Body. Metabolised by de-esterification to methyldopa; a small amount of sulphate conjugation also occurs.

THERAPEUTIC CONCENTRATION.
After an intravenous dose of 250 mg to 5 subjects, peak plasma concentrations of 0.8 to 2.2 µg/ml (mean 1.6) of free and esterified methyldopa, and 1.0 to 2.2 µg/ml (mean 1.5) of conjugated methyldopa

Wavelength

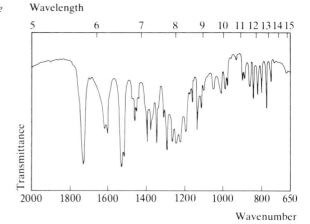

were attained in about 1 hour (J. A. Saavedra *et al.*, *Eur. J. clin. Pharmac.*, 1975, *8*, 381–386).

HALF-LIFE. Plasma half-life, about 4 hours.

VOLUME OF DISTRIBUTION. About 2 litres/kg.

Dose. Usually 250 to 500 mg of methyldopate hydrochloride, by intravenous infusion, every 6 hours.

Methylene Chloride   *Solvent*

Dichloromethane
$CH_2Cl_2 = 84.93$
CAS—75-09-2
A clear, colourless, volatile liquid. Wt per ml about 1.32 g. B.p. 39° to 41°.
Soluble 1 in 50 of water; miscible with ethanol and ether.

Gas Chromatography. *System GA*—RI 515; *system GI*—retention time 1.9 min.

Mass Spectrum. Principal peaks at *m/z* 49, 84, 86, 51, 47, 35, 88, 41.

Disposition in the Body.

TOXICITY. Methylene chloride is widely used in paint strippers and several non-fatal and fatal cases of accidental inhalation have been reported. The maximum permissible atmospheric concentration is 200 ppm and the temporary estimated acceptable daily intake is up to 500 µg/kg.
In a fatality involving the accidental inhalation of a paint stripper containing methylene chloride, the following postmortem tissue concentrations were reported: blood 510 µg/ml, brain 248 µg/g, liver 144 µg/g (J. Bonventre *et al.*, *J. analyt. Toxicol.*, 1977, *1*, 158–160).
In a fatality following the intentional inhalation of a paint stripper containing methylene chloride, the following postmortem tissue concentrations were reported: blood 252 µg/ml, brain 125 µg/g, liver 130 µg/g, lungs 67 µg/g, urine 10 µg/ml (A. Franc, *Bull. Int. Ass. forens. Toxicol.*, 1983, *17*(2), 22–25).

Methylenedioxyamphetamine   *Hallucinogen*

Synonym. MDA
α-Methyl-3,4-methylenedioxyphenethylamine
$C_{10}H_{13}NO_2 = 179.2$
CAS—4764-17-4

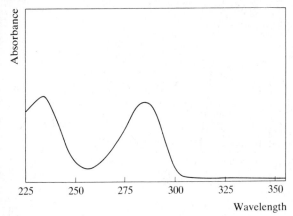

A white powder.
Soluble in chloroform and dilute acetic acid.

Colour Tests. Liebermann's Test—black; Mandelin's Test—green→blue; Marquis Test—blue-black; Sulphuric Acid—violet.

Thin-layer Chromatography. *System TA*—Rf 39; *system TB*—Rf 17; *system TC*—Rf 12. (*Acidified potassium permanganate solution*, positive.)

Gas Chromatography. *System GA*—RI 1472.

High Pressure Liquid Chromatography. *System HC*—k' 0.98.

Ultraviolet Spectrum. Aqueous acid—233 nm ($A_1^1 = 216$ b), 285 nm.

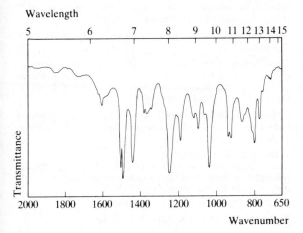

Infra-red Spectrum. Principal peaks at wavenumbers 1490, 1257, 1038, 1504, 799, 1188 (KBr disk).

Mass Spectrum. Principal peaks at m/z 44, 136, 51, 135, 77, 42, 78, 45.

Quantification. COLORIMETRY. In plasma or urine—M. M. DeMayo *et al.*, *J. forens. Sci.*, 1972, *17*, 444–446.

GAS CHROMATOGRAPHY. In biological tissues: FID—G. Cimbura, *J. forens. Sci.*, 1972, *17*, 329–333. In plasma or urine: sensitivity 125 ng/ml, FID—K. K. Midha *et al.*, *J. pharm. Sci.*, 1976, *65*, 188–197.

Disposition in the Body.
TOXICITY. The estimated lethal dose is 0.5 g.

In 5 fatalities due to the ingestion of methylenedioxyamphetamine, the following postmortem tissue concentrations were reported: blood 6 to 26 µg/ml (mean 14, 5 cases), bile 5 to 9 µg/ml (mean 6, 3 cases), liver 8 to 17 µg/g (mean 11, 3 cases), urine 46 to 160 µg/ml (mean 102, 3 cases) (G. Cimbura, *J. forens. Sci.*, 1972, *17*, 329–333).

In a fatality in which death occurred shortly after the ingestion of methylenedioxyamphetamine, the following postmortem concentrations were reported: blood 2.3 µg/ml, bile 7 µg/ml, liver 11 µg/g, urine 175 µg/ml (T. Lukabzewski, *Clin. Toxicol.*, 1979, *15*, 405–409).

Methylephedrine   *Sympathomimetic*

Synonyms. l-Methylephedrine; *l-N*-Methylephedrine.
(−)-2-Dimethylamino-1-phenylpropan-1-ol
$C_{11}H_{17}NO = 179.3$
CAS—552-79-4

$$\underset{C_6H_5 \cdot CH \cdot CH \cdot N(CH_3)_2}{\overset{OH\ \ \ CH_3}{|\ \ \ \ \ |}}$$

Soluble in chloroform and ether.

Methylephedrine Hydrochloride
Proprietary Name. It is an ingredient of Pholcomed (expectorant).
$C_{11}H_{17}NO,HCl = 215.7$
CAS—38455-90-2
A white crystalline powder. M.p. 190° to 195°.
Freely **soluble** in water; soluble in ethanol; practically insoluble in ether.

Dissociation Constant. pK_a 9.3 (25°).

Thin-layer Chromatography. *System TA*—Rf 32. (*Acidified iodoplatinate solution*, positive.)

Gas Chromatography. *System GA*—methylephedrine RI 1400, ephedrine RI 1363; *system GB*—methylephedrine RI 1440, ephedrine RI 1386; *system GC*—methylephedrine RI 1480, ephedrine RI 1467.

High Pressure Liquid Chromatography. *System HA*—methylephedrine k' 2.3, ephedrine k' 1.0; *system HC*—methylephedrine k' 1.83, ephedrine k' 1.79.

Ultraviolet Spectrum. Aqueous acid—251 nm, 257 nm ($A_1^1 = 11$ a), 263 nm. (See below)

Infra-red Spectrum. Principal peaks at wavenumbers 742, 1039, 702, 1052, 990, 1162 (KBr disk). (See below)

Mass Spectrum. Principal peaks at m/z 58, 72, 30, 77, 56, 44, 42, 73; ephedrine 58, 146, 56, 105, 77, 42, 106, 40.

Disposition in the Body. Absorbed after oral administration. About 32% of a dose is excreted in the urine unchanged and 8% is excreted as the demethylated metabolite, ephedrine; the rate of excretion is dependent on the urinary pH.

Dose. Methylephedrine hydrochloride has been given in doses of 160 to 200 mg daily.

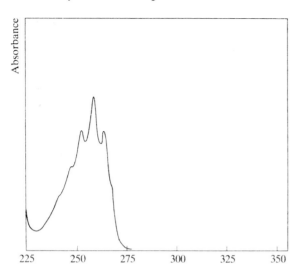

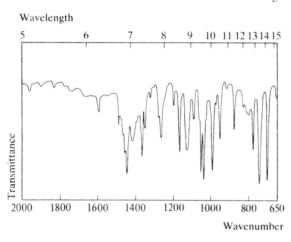

Methylergometrine Maleate

Proprietary Name. Methergin(e)
$C_{20}H_{25}N_3O_2, C_4H_4O_4 = 455.5$
CAS—57432-61-8
A white or pinkish-tan, crystalline powder, which darkens on exposure to light. M.p. 185° to 195°, with decomposition.
Soluble 1 in 200 of water and 1 in 140 of ethanol giving a blue fluorescence; practically insoluble in chloroform and ether.

Dissociation Constant. pK_a 6.7 (24°).

Colour Tests. Mandelin's Test—violet-brown; Marquis Test—grey-brown.

Thin-layer Chromatography. *System TA*—Rf 62; *system TB*—Rf 00; *system TC*—Rf 14; *system TL*—Rf 12; *system TM*—Rf 31. (*Van Urk reagent*, blue.)

Gas Chromatography. *System GA*—not eluted.

High Pressure Liquid Chromatography. *System HA*—k' 0.4; *system HP*—k' 0.83.

Ultraviolet Spectrum. Aqueous acid—313 nm ($A_1^1 = 255$ a); aqueous alkali—310 nm.

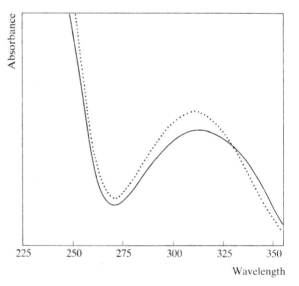

Infra-red Spectrum. Principal peaks at wavenumbers 1580, 1490, 1650, 1620, 1065, 1103 (KBr disk).

Mass Spectrum. Principal peaks at *m/z* 339, 221, 196, 181, 207, 223, 222, 72.

Quantification. HIGH PRESSURE LIQUID CHROMATOGRAPHY. In plasma or serum: methylergometrine and ergotamine, detection limit 100 pg/ml, fluorescence detection—P. O. Edlund, *J. Chromat.*, 1981, *226*; *Biomed. Appl.*, *15*, 107–115.

Disposition in the Body. Rapidly absorbed after oral administration. About 2 to 3% of a dose is excreted in the urine as unchanged drug in 24 hours.

THERAPEUTIC CONCENTRATION.

After a single oral dose of 0.25 mg to 6 subjects, peak plasma concentrations of about 0.003 µg/ml were attained in 0.5 hour (R. Mantyla *et al.*, *Int. J. clin. Pharmac. Biopharm.*, 1978, *16*, 254–257).

HALF-LIFE. Plasma half-life, about 2 hours.

VOLUME OF DISTRIBUTION. About 0.5 litre/kg.

Methylergometrine   *Uterine Stimulant*

Synonyms. Methylergobasine; Methylergonovine.
N-[(S)-1-(Hydroxymethyl)propyl]-D-lysergamide
$C_{20}H_{25}N_3O_2 = 339.4$
CAS—113-42-8

Crystals. M.p. 172°, with decomposition.
Slightly **soluble** in water; very soluble in ethanol.

Wavelength

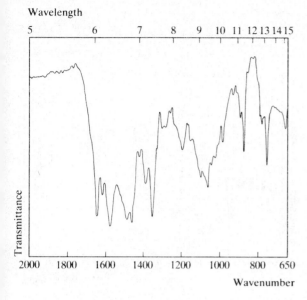

PROTEIN BINDING. In plasma, about 35%.

Dose. 0.375 to 1 mg of methylergometrine maleate daily, for up to 7 days.

Methylpentynol

Hypnotic/Sedative

Synonyms. Meparfynol; Methylparafynol.
Proprietary Name. Allotropal
3-Methylpent-1-yn-3-ol
$C_6H_{10}O = 98.14$
CAS—77-75-8

$$CH{:}C{\cdot}\underset{\underset{CH_3}{|}}{\overset{\overset{OH}{|}}{C}}{\cdot}CH_2{\cdot}CH_3$$

A colourless or pale yellow liquid. Wt per ml 0.865 to 0.873 g. B.p. about 120°. Refractive index, at 20°, 1.430 to 1.432.
Soluble 1 in 10 of water; miscible with organic solvents.

Methylpentynol Carbamate
Synonym. Mepentamate
Proprietary Name. N-Oblivon
$C_7H_{11}NO_2 = 141.2$
CAS—302-66-9
A white powder. M.p. 53° to 56°.
Soluble 1 in less than 200 of water, 1 in 1 of ethanol, and 1 in 2 of chloroform.

Thin-layer Chromatography. Methylpentynol carbamate: *system TD*—Rf 49; *system TE*—Rf 74; *system TF*—Rf 62. (*Furfuraldehyde reagent*, positive; *acidified potassium permanganate solution*, positive.)

Gas Chromatography. *System GA*—RI 715; *system GI*—retention time 20.1 min.

Infra-red Spectrum. Principal peaks at wavenumbers 917, 1126, 1156, 995, 1030, 1050 (thin film).

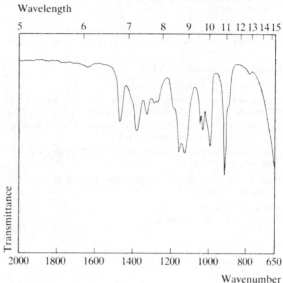

Mass Spectrum. Principal peaks at *m/z* 69, 83, 43, 79, 41, 81, 53, 80 (methylpentynol carbamate).

Quantification. GAS CHROMATOGRAPHY. In serum (methylpentynol) or urine (4-hydroxymethylpentynol): FID—J. Grove and B. K. Martin, *J. Chromat.*, 1977, *133*, 267–272.

Disposition in the Body. Absorbed after oral administration. It is almost completely metabolised with less than 1% being excreted in the urine as unchanged drug in 7 days; higher amounts of unchanged drug may be excreted after large doses. The major metabolite is the *N*-glucuronide which accounts for about 80% of the dose; the 4-hydroxy metabolite accounts for about 13% of a dose.

TOXICITY. A fatality has been reported after a dose of 5 g although recoveries have occurred after ingestion of up to 10 g. Repeated medication may cause toxic reactions in the liver and skin.

A liver concentration of 1100 µg/g and a urine concentration of 410 µg/ ml were reported in one fatal poisoning case (J. V. Jackson, 1967— personal communication).

Dose. 0.5 to 1 g daily.

Methylphenidate

Central Stimulant

Synonyms. Methyl Phenidate; Methyl Phenidylacetate.
Methyl α-phenyl-α-(2-piperidyl)acetate
$C_{14}H_{19}NO_2 = 233.3$
CAS—113-45-1

Crystals. M.p. 74° to 75°.
Practically **insoluble** in water; soluble in ethanol and ether.

Methylphenidate Hydrochloride

Proprietary Names. Methidate; Ritalin.
$C_{14}H_{19}NO_2,HCl = 269.8$
CAS—298-59-9
Fine, white, crystalline powder or acicular crystals.
Freely **soluble** in water and methanol; soluble in ethanol; slightly soluble in acetone and chloroform.

Dissociation Constant. pK_a 8.8.

Colour Test. Liebermann's Test—orange.

Thin-layer Chromatography. *System TA*—Rf 57; *system TB*—Rf 34; *system TC*—Rf 34. (*Dragendorff spray*, positive; *acidified iodoplatinate solution*, positive; *ninhydrin spray*, positive; *acidified potassium permanganate solution*, positive.)

Gas Chromatography. *System GA*—RI 1737; *system GC*—RI 2200; *system GF*—RI 1935.

High Pressure Liquid Chromatography. *System HA*—k' 1.7; *system HC*—k' 0.36.

Ultraviolet Spectrum. Aqueous acid—251 nm, 257 nm ($A_1^1 = 9.0$ a), 264 nm. No alkaline shift.

Wavelength

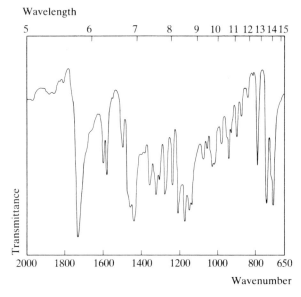

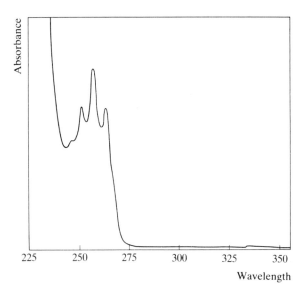

Infra-red Spectrum. Principal peaks at wavenumbers 1735, 1175, 1210, 1150, 705, 740 (methylphenidate hydrochloride, KCl disk).

Mass Spectrum. Principal peaks at *m/z* 84, 91, 85, 56, 55, 150, 41, 118 (no peaks above 150).

Quantification. GAS CHROMATOGRAPHY. In urine: sensitivity 30 ng/ml, AFID—R. Dugal *et al., J. analyt. Toxicol.*, 1978, *2*, 101–106. In urine: ritalinic acid, sensitivity about 1 µg/ml, FID—H. W. Allen and B. Sedgwick, *J. analyt. Toxicol.*, 1984, *8*, 61–62.

GAS CHROMATOGRAPHY–MASS SPECTROMETRY. In blood or urine: methylphenidate and ritalinic acid, sensitivity about 2 ng/ml and 60 ng/ml respectively—R. M. Milberg *et al., Biomed. Mass Spectrom.*, 1975, *2*, 2–8.

HIGH PRESSURE LIQUID CHROMATOGRAPHY. In serum: methylphenidate and ritalinic acid, sensitivity 20 ng/ml, UV detection—S. J. Soldin *et al., Clin. Chem.*, 1979, *25*, 401–404.

Disposition in the Body. Readily absorbed after oral administration. About 80% of a dose is excreted in the urine in 24 hours, of which 60 to 80% is ritalinic acid and 5 to 12% is 6-oxo-α-phenylpiperidine-2-acetic acid; only a small amount is excreted as unchanged drug.

THERAPEUTIC CONCENTRATION.

Following a single oral dose of 20 mg to 2 subjects, peak plasma concentrations of 0.013 and 0.058 µg/ml were attained in 3 hours; ritalinic acid concentrations averaged 0.22 µg/ml at the same time (R. M. Milberg *et al., Biomed. Mass Spectrom.*, 1975, *2*, 2–8).

Following oral doses of 10 to 30 mg daily, administered to 4 hyperkinetic children, peak plasma concentrations of 0.008 to 0.023 µg/ml (mean 0.018) were reported (B. L. Hungund *et al., Br. J. clin. Pharmac.*, 1979, *8*, 571–576).

TOXICITY. The estimated minimum lethal dose for adults is 2 g but few instances of serious toxicity due to overdosage have been reported. Abuse and dependence of the amphetamine type is not uncommon.

Urine concentrations of 0.8 to 40 µg/ml (mean 16) were reported in six arrested drivers who showed signs of drowsiness or hyperactivity (B. Schubert, *Acta chem. scand.*, 1970, *24*, 433–438).

HALF-LIFE. Plasma half-life, about 2 hours, ritalinic acid about 8 hours.

PROTEIN BINDING. In plasma, about 15%.

Dose. Usually up to 60 mg of methylphenidate hydrochloride daily.

Methylphenobarbitone   *Barbiturate*

Synonyms. Enphenemalum; Mephobarbital; Phemitone.
Proprietary Names. Mebaral; Prominal.
5-Ethyl-1-methyl-5-phenylbarbituric acid
$C_{13}H_{14}N_2O_3 = 246.3$
CAS—115-38-8

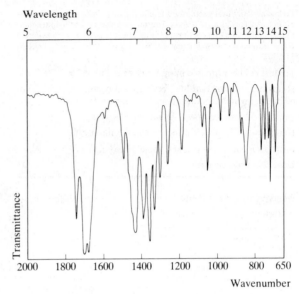

Wavelength

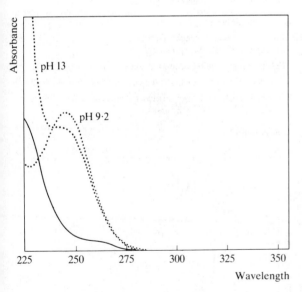

Colourless crystals or white crystalline powder. M.p. 176° to 181°.

Practically **insoluble** in water; soluble 1 in 240 of ethanol, 1 in 40 of chloroform, and 1 in 200 of ether; soluble in solutions of ammonia, alkali hydroxides, and carbonates.

Dissociation Constant. pK_a 7.8 (20°).

Colour Tests. Koppanyi–Zwikker Test—violet; Liebermann's Test—red-orange; Mercurous Nitrate—black.

Thin-layer Chromatography. *System TD*—Rf 70; *system TE*—Rf 43; *system TF*—Rf 69; *system TH*—Rf 72. (*Mercurous nitrate spray*, black; *Zwikker's reagent*, faint pink.)

Gas Chromatography. *System GA*—methylphenobarbitone RI 1891, phenobarbitone RI 1957.

High Pressure Liquid Chromatography. *System HG*—k' 7.27; *system HH*—k' 3.84.

Ultraviolet Spectrum. *Borax buffer 0.05M* (pH 9.2)—244 nm ($A_1^1 = 355$ c); M sodium hydroxide (pH 13)—243 nm ($A_1^1 = 329$ b).

Infra-red Spectrum. Principal peaks at wavenumbers 1707, 1684, 1754, 720, 1298, 1050 (KBr disk).

Mass Spectrum. Principal peaks at m/z 218, 117, 118, 146, 103, 77, 91, 115; phenobarbitone 204, 117, 146, 161, 77, 103, 115, 118.

Quantification. See also under Amylobarbitone.

GAS CHROMATOGRAPHY. In plasma or serum: methylphenobarbitone and phenobarbitone, FID—W. D. Hooper *et al.*, *J. Chromat.*, 1975, *110*, 206–209.

GAS CHROMATOGRAPHY–MASS SPECTROMETRY. In plasma: methylphenobarbitone and phenobarbitone, detection limit 20 ng/ml for both compounds—W. D. Hooper *et al.*, *J. Chromat.*, 1981, *223*; *Biomed. Appl.*, *12*, 426–431.

HIGH PRESSURE LIQUID CHROMATOGRAPHY. In serum: methylphenobarbitone, phenobarbitone and other anticonvulsants, sensitivity 500 ng/ml, UV detection—P. M. Kabra *et al.*, *J. analyt. Toxicol.*, 1978, *2*, 127–133. In urine: the metabolites phenobarbitone, p-hydroxyphenobarbitone and p-hydroxymethylphenobarbitone, detection limit 500 ng/ml for each compound, UV detection—H. E. Kunze *et al.*, *Ther. Drug Monit.*, 1981, *3*, 45–49.

Disposition in the Body. Incompletely absorbed after oral administration; bioavailability about 70%. Metabolised by N-demethylation to the active metabolite, phenobarbitone, and by p-hydroxylation. Over a period of 10 days, less than 2% of a dose is excreted in the urine as unchanged drug, about 30 to 35% is excreted as p-hydroxymethylphenobarbitone both free and conjugated, and up to 10% may be excreted as phenobarbitone. Small amounts of p-hydroxyphenobarbitone, 5-ethyl-5-(4-hydroxy-3-methoxyphenyl)barbituric acid, and 5-ethyl-5-(4-hydroxy-3-methoxyphenyl)-1-methylbarbituric acid have also been detected in the urine.

THERAPEUTIC CONCENTRATION.

Following a single oral dose of 800 mg to 2 subjects, peak plasma concentrations of about 3 µg/ml were attained in 3 to 6 hours; peak phenobarbitone plasma concentrations of 2 to 3 µg/ml were attained in 4 to 6 days (W. D. Hooper *et al.*, *Ther. Drug Monit.*, 1981, *3*, 39–44).

Following daily oral doses of 60 to 600 mg to 11 subjects, steady-state plasma concentrations of 0.2 to 1.7 μg/ml (mean 0.9) of methylphenobarbitone and 4 to 32 μg/ml (mean 15) of phenobarbitone were reported (H. J. Kupferberg and J. Longacre-Shaw, *Ther. Drug Monit.*, 1979, *1*, 117–122).

TOXICITY. The estimated minimum lethal dose is 2 g.

HALF-LIFE. Plasma half-life, methylphenobarbitone about 50 to 60 hours, phenobarbitone about 100 hours.

VOLUME OF DISTRIBUTION. About 2 to 3 litres/kg.

CLEARANCE. Plasma clearance, about 0.5 ml/min/kg.

PROTEIN BINDING. In plasma, about 40 to 60%.

Dose. 90 to 600 mg daily.

Methylpiperidyl Benzilate   *Hallucinogen*

1-Methyl-3-piperidyl benzilate
$C_{20}H_{23}NO_3 = 325.4$
CAS—3321-80-0

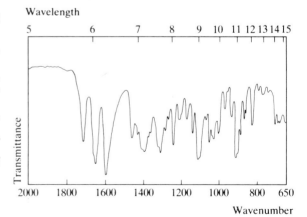

A clear liquid.
Practically **insoluble** in water; soluble in chloroform and most organic solvents.

Methylpiperidyl Benzilate Hydrochloride

A white powder. M.p. 212° to 218°, with decomposition.
Soluble in water; practically insoluble in chloroform.

Colour Tests. Liebermann's Test—brown; Mandelin's Test—orange → brown → green; Marquis Test—orange → green → blue; Sulphuric Acid—orange.

Thin-layer Chromatography. *System TA*—Rf 60. (*Acidified iodoplatinate solution*, positive.)

Ultraviolet Spectrum. Aqueous acid—251 nm ($A_1^1 = 18$ b), 257 nm ($A_1^1 = 20$ b).

Infra-red Spectrum. Principal peaks at wavenumbers 1734, 1195, 965, 685, 1160, 720 (methylpiperidyl benzilate hydrochloride, KBr disk).

Mass Spectrum. Principal peaks at *m/z* 97, 105, 77, 183, 84, 36, 42, 51.

Methylprednisolone   *Corticosteroid*

Synonym. 6α-Methylprednisolone
Proprietary Names. Medrol; Medrone; Urbason.
11β,17α,21-Trihydroxy-6α-methylpregna-1,4-diene-3,20-dione
$C_{22}H_{30}O_5 = 374.5$
CAS—83-43-2

A white crystalline powder. M.p. about 240° to 243°, with decomposition. A solution in dioxan is dextrorotatory.
Practically **insoluble** in water; soluble 1 in 100 of dehydrated alcohol; slightly soluble in chloroform and ether; sparingly soluble in dioxan and methanol.

Methylprednisolone Acetate

Synonym. 6α-Methylprednisolone 21-Acetate
Proprietary Names. Depo-Medrone; Medrone (cream).
$C_{24}H_{32}O_6 = 416.5$
CAS—53-36-1
A white crystalline powder. M.p. about 225°, with decomposition.
Practically **insoluble** in water; slightly soluble in ethanol; soluble 1 in 250 of chloroform and 1 in 1500 of ether; soluble in dioxan.

Methylprednisolone Hemisuccinate

Synonym. Methylprednisolone Hydrogen Succinate
$C_{26}H_{34}O_8 = 474.5$
CAS—2921-57-5
A white hygroscopic solid.
Very slightly **soluble** in water; freely soluble in ethanol; soluble in acetone.

Methylprednisolone Sodium Succinate

Synonym. Sodium 6α-Methylprednisolone 21-Succinate
Proprietary Name. Solu-Medrone
$C_{26}H_{33}NaO_8 = 496.5$
CAS—2375-03-3
A white, hygroscopic, amorphous powder.
Soluble 1 in 1.5 of water and 1 in 12 of ethanol; practically insoluble in chloroform and ether.

Thin-layer Chromatography. *System TP*—Rf 23; *system TQ*—Rf 80; *system TR*—Rf 03; *system TS*—Rf 00.

High Pressure Liquid Chromatography. *System HT*—k' 7.5.

Ultraviolet Spectrum. Dehydrated alcohol—240 nm ($A_1^1 = 400$ a).

Infra-red Spectrum. Principal peaks at wavenumbers 1595, 1650, 1114, 914, 1313, 1248 (KBr disk).

Wavelength

Dose. Usually 4 to 48 mg daily.

Methyltestosterone   *Androgen*

Proprietary Names. Android; Glosso-Stérandryl; Metandren; Neohombreol M; Oreton Methyl; Testoviron (tablets); Testred; Virilon; Virormone-Oral. It is an ingredient of Menolet, Mixogen (tablets), Plex-Hormone (tablets), and Trimone Sublets.

17β-Hydroxy-17α-methylandrost-4-en-3-one
$C_{20}H_{30}O_2 = 302.5$
CAS—58-18-4

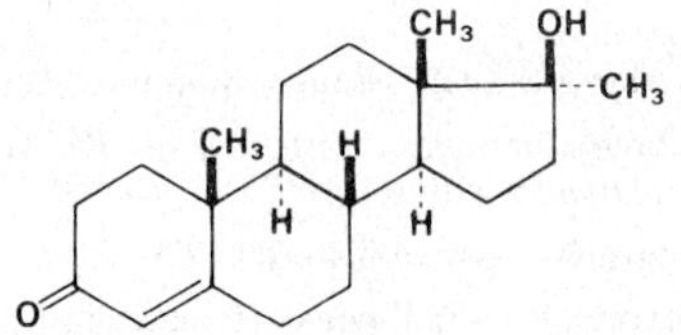

A white or slightly yellowish-white, slightly hygroscopic, crystalline powder. M.p. 162° to 168°. A solution in ethanol is dextrorotatory.

Practically **insoluble** in water; soluble 1 in 5 of ethanol; freely soluble in chloroform; slightly soluble in ether.

Thin-layer Chromatography. *System TP*—Rf 70; *system TQ*—Rf 16; *system TR*—Rf 91; *system TS*—Rf 71.

Gas Chromatography. *System GA*—RI 2643.

Ultraviolet Spectrum. Ethanol—241 nm $(A_1^1 = 540 \text{ a})$.

Infra-red Spectrum. Principal peaks at wavenumbers 1660, 1160, 1239, 950, 1612, 1090 (KBr disk).

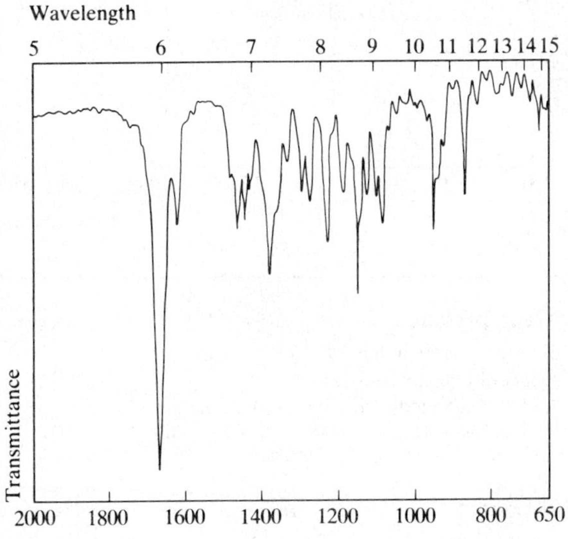

Wavelength

Wavenumber

Mass Spectrum. Principal peaks at m/z 302, 124, 43, 91, 79, 121, 105, 122.

Quantification. SPECTROFLUORIMETRY. In plasma or serum: sensitivity 1 ng/ml—D. Alkalay *et al.*, *J. pharm. Sci.*, 1972, *61*, 1746–1749.

Dose. 5 to 80 mg daily, by mouth; up to 200 mg daily has been given.

Methylthiouracil   *Antithyroid Agent*

Proprietary Name. Thyreostat
2,3-Dihydro-2-thioxo-6-methylpyrimidin-4(1*H*)-one
$C_5H_6N_2OS = 142.2$
CAS—56-04-2

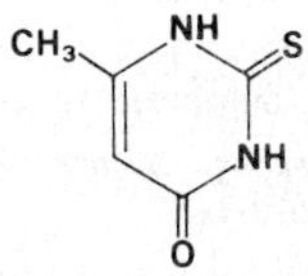

A white crystalline powder. M.p. about 330°, with decomposition.

Soluble 1 in 2000 of water, 1 in 150 of boiling water, and 1 in 800 of ethanol; slightly soluble in chloroform and ether; freely soluble in solutions of ammonium hydroxide and sodium hydroxide.

Dissociation Constant. pK_a 8.2 (20°).

Ultraviolet Spectrum. Aqueous acid—276 nm $(A_1^1 = 1190 \text{ b})$; aqueous alkali—256 nm $(A_1^1 = 850 \text{ b})$.

Infra-red Spectrum. Principal peaks at wavenumbers 1645, 1170, 1564, 1198, 850, 1240.

Dose. Initially, 200 to 400 mg daily; maintenance, 50 to 150 mg daily.

5-Methyltryptamine   *Hallucinogen*

3-(2-Aminoethyl)-5-methylindole
$C_{11}H_{14}N_2 = 174.2$
CAS—1821-47-2

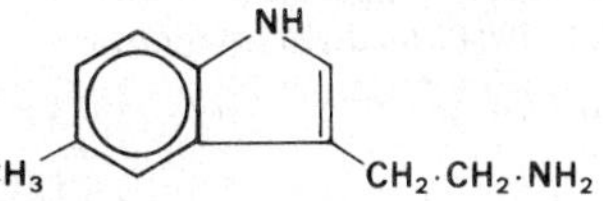

5-Methyltryptamine Hydrochloride
$C_{11}H_{14}N_2,HCl = 210.7$
CAS—1010-95-3
M.p. 289° to 292°.

Colour Tests. Mandelin's Test—green-orange; Marquis Test—orange → brown; Sulphuric Acid—yellow.

Thin-layer Chromatography. *System TA*—Rf 56. (*Acidified iodoplatinate solution*, positive.)

Gas Chromatography. *System GA*—RI 1795.

Infra-red Spectrum. Principal peaks at wavenumbers 800, 1515, 1612, 1587, 1234, 1315 (5-methyltryptamine hydrochloride).

α-Methyltryptamine   *Hallucinogen*

3-(2-Aminopropyl)indole
$C_{11}H_{14}N_2 = 174.2$
CAS—299-26-3

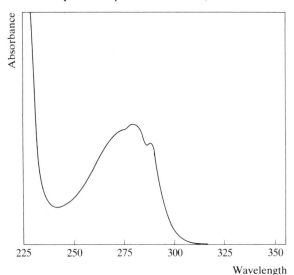

A white crystalline powder. M.p. 98° to 108°.
Soluble in chloroform and dilute acetic acid.

Colour Tests. Mandelin's Test—green → orange; Marquis Test—orange → brown; Sulphuric Acid—yellow.

Thin-layer Chromatography. *System TA*—Rf 58. (*Acidified iodoplatinate solution*, positive.)

Gas Chromatography. *System GA*—RI 1740.

Ultraviolet Spectrum. Aqueous acid—279 nm, 288 nm.

Infra-red Spectrum. Principal peaks at wavenumbers 1215, 1170, 1050, 750, 1520, 790 (α-methyltryptamine esylate, KBr disk).

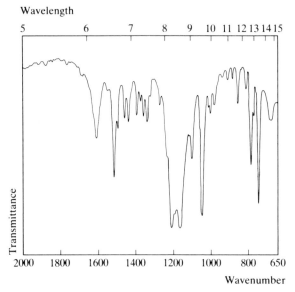

N-Methyltryptamine

Hallucinogen

3-(2-Methylaminoethyl)indole
$C_{11}H_{14}N_2 = 174.2$
CAS—61-49-4

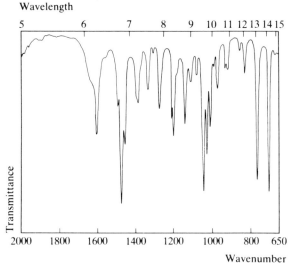

Colour Tests. Marquis Test—orange; Sulphuric Acid—yellow.

Thin-layer Chromatography. *System TA*—Rf 18. (*Acidified iodoplatinate solution*, positive.)

Gas Chromatography. *System GA*—RI 1770.

Infra-red Spectrum. Principal peaks at wavenumbers 700, 1040, 762, 1025, 1605, 1200 (KBr disk).

Methyprylone

Hypnotic

Synonym. Methyprylon
Proprietary Name. Noludar
3,3-Diethyl-5-methylpiperidine-2,4-dione
$C_{10}H_{17}NO_2 = 183.2$
CAS—125-64-4

A white crystalline powder. M.p. 74° to 78°.
Soluble 1 in 14 of water, 1 in 0.7 of ethanol, 1 in 0.6 of chloroform, and 1 in 3.5 of ether.

Dissociation Constant. pKa 12.0.

Thin-layer Chromatography. *System TA*—Rf 58; *system TD*—Rf 31; *system TE*—Rf 61; *system TF*—Rf 25. (*Acidified potassium permanganate solution*, positive.)

Gas Chromatography. *System GA*—RI 1529; *system GF*—RI 2090.

Infra-red Spectrum. Principal peaks at wavenumbers 1660, 1693, 1085, 1310, 750, 869 (KBr disk).

Wavelength

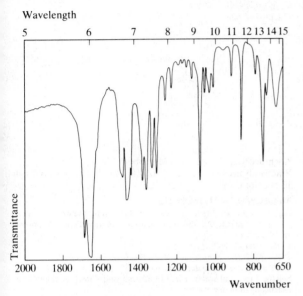

Mass Spectrum. Principal peaks at *m/z* 155, 140, 83, 98, 55, 41, 84, 69.

Quantification. Gas Chromatography. In blood, plasma or urine: methyprylone and methylpersedon, sensitivity 1 μg/ml, FID—R. R. Bridges and M. A. Peat, *J. analyt. Toxicol.*, 1979, *3*, 21–25.

Gas Chromatography (Capillary Column). In blood, urine or tissues: methyprylone and metabolites, FID—M. Van Boven and I. Sunshine, *J. analyt. Toxicol.*, 1979, *3*, 174–176.

Disposition in the Body. Absorbed after oral administration. The principal metabolites are 2,4-dioxo-3,3-diethyl-5-methyltetrahydropyridine (methylpersedon) which is active, 6-oxomethyprylone, 5-hydroxymethyprylone, and 5-carboxymethyprylone. About 60% of a dose is excreted in the urine in 24 hours as free and conjugated metabolites together with 3% of the dose as unchanged drug.

Therapeutic Concentration. In plasma, usually in the range 10 to 20 μg/ml.

Following a single oral dose of 650 mg to 6 subjects, peak plasma concentrations averaging 10.2 μg/ml were attained in 2 hours (L. O. Randell *et al.*, *Archs int. Pharmacodyn. Thér.*, 1956, *106*, 388–394).

Toxicity. Prolonged use of methyprylone may lead to dependence of the barbiturate–alcohol type. Numerous cases of overdose have been reported but there have been few fatalities; death has occurred after the ingestion of 6 g but at least two recoveries following doses of 30 g have been reported. Plasma concentrations of 12 to **75** to 128 μg/ml have been associated with toxic effects and concentrations greater than 50 μg/ml may be lethal.

In one fatality attributed to methyprylone overdose, the following postmortem tissue concentrations, μg/ml or μg/g, were reported:

	Blood	Brain	Kidney	Liver	Spleen	Urine
Methyprylone	158	176	87	90	121	61
Methylpersedon	36	73	21	40	29	123
5-Hydroxymethyprylone	—	—	—	—	—	16
5-Carboxymethyprylone	2	—	10	7	16	80
6-Oxomethyprylone	16	18	9	8	3	68

(M. Van Boven and I. Sunshine, *J. analyt. Toxicol.*, 1979, *3*, 174–176).
In 4 cases of fatal overdose, the following tissue disposition was reported: blood 53 to 66 μg/ml (mean 59), kidney 10 to 108 μg/g (mean 62), liver 62 to 260 μg/g (mean 118), urine 17 to 166 μg/ml (mean 86) (R. C. Baselt, *Disposition of Toxic Drugs and Chemicals in Man*, 2nd Edn, Davis, California, Biomedical Publications, 1982, pp. 527–529).

Half-life. Plasma half-life following a single oral dose, about 4 hours, increased to about 50 hours in acute intoxication.

Dose. 200 to 400 mg, as a hypnotic.

Methysergide
Migraine Prophylactic

N-[1-(Hydroxymethyl)propyl]-1-methyl-D-lysergamide
$C_{21}H_{27}N_3O_2 = 353.5$
CAS—361-37-5

Crystals. M.p. 194° to 196°.

Methysergide Maleate

Synonym. 1-Methyl-D-lysergic Acid Butanolamide Maleate
Proprietary Names. Deseril; Désernil; Sansert.
$C_{21}H_{27}N_3O_2,C_4H_4O_4 = 469.5$
CAS—129-49-7
A white to yellowish-white or reddish-white, crystalline powder.
Soluble 1 in 500 of water, 1 in 165 of ethanol, and 1 in 125 of methanol; practically insoluble in chloroform and ether.

Dissociation Constant. pK_a 6.6 (24°).

Colour Tests. *p*-Dimethylaminobenzaldehyde—violet; Mandelin's Test—brown; Marquis Test—grey.

Thin-layer Chromatography. *System TA*—Rf 65; *system TB*—Rf 01; *system TC*—Rf 21; *system TL*—Rf 12; *system TM*—Rf 33. (*Van Urk reagent*, blue.)

Gas Chromatography. *System GA*—RI 3089.

High Pressure Liquid Chromatography. *System HA*—k′ 0.4; *system HP*—k′ 2.33.

Ultraviolet Spectrum. Aqueous acid—230 nm, 322 nm ($A_1^1 =$ 223 a); aqueous alkali—243 nm, 320 nm.

Infra-red Spectrum. Principal peaks at wavenumbers 1566, 1650, 863, 1615, 1190, 740 (methysergide maleate, KBr disk). (See below)

Wavelength

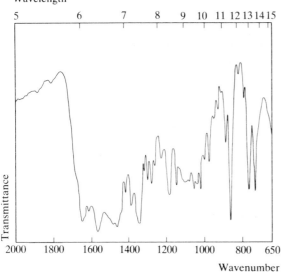

Wavenumber

Mass Spectrum. Principal peaks at m/z 353, 210, 235, 336, 72, 54, 236, 195.

Dose. The equivalent of 2 to 6 mg of methysergide daily.

Metipranolol
Beta-adrenoceptor Blocking Agent

Synonyms. Methypranolum; Trimepranol.

Proprietary Name. Disorat

4-(2-Hydroxy-3-isopropylaminopropoxy)-2,3,6-trimethylphenyl acetate

$C_{17}H_{27}NO_4 = 309.4$

CAS—22664-55-7

A white crystalline powder. M.p. 105° to 109°.

Practically **insoluble** in water; soluble in ethanol; sparingly soluble in ether.

Ultraviolet Spectrum. Aqueous acid—278 nm ($A_1^1 = 44$ b).

Disposition in the Body. Readily absorbed after oral administration and rapidly metabolised to the active metabolite, desacetylmetipranolol. About 20% of a dose is excreted in the urine as unchanged drug.

THERAPEUTIC CONCENTRATION.

After a single oral dose of 40 mg to 13 subjects, peak plasma concentrations of the desacetyl metabolite of 0.034 to 0.214 μg/ml (mean 0.14) were attained in about 1 hour. Oral administration of 20 mg twice daily to 6 subjects, produced mean steady-state plasma concentrations (desacetyl derivative) of 0.06 to 0.08 μg/ml determined on the 6th to 8th day; considerable intersubject variation was reported (O. Mayer, *Int. J. clin. Pharmac. Ther. Toxicol.*, 1980, *18*, 113–120).

HALF-LIFE. Plasma half-life, desacetylmetipranolol about 2 to 4 hours but there is considerable intersubject variation.

Dose. Metipranolol has been given in doses of 10 to 120 mg daily.

Metoclopramide
Anti-emetic

4-Amino-5-chloro-N-(2-diethylaminoethyl)-2-methoxybenzamide

$C_{14}H_{22}ClN_3O_2 = 299.8$

CAS—364-62-5

A white crystalline powder. M.p. about 148°.

Practically **insoluble** in water; soluble 1 in 45 of ethanol and 1 in 15 of chloroform.

Metoclopramide Hydrochloride

Proprietary Names. Maxeran; Maxolon; Metamide; Metox; Mygdalon; Parmid; Paspertin; Primperan; Reglan. It is an ingredient of Migravess and Paramax.

$C_{14}H_{22}ClN_3O_2,HCl,H_2O = 354.3$

CAS—7232-21-5 (anhydrous); *54143-57-6* (monohydrate)

A white crystalline powder. M.p. about 185°.

Soluble 1 in 0.7 of water, 1 in 3 of ethanol, and 1 in 55 of chloroform; practically insoluble in ether.

Dissociation Constant. pK_a 9.0.

Colour Tests. Coniferyl Alcohol—orange; Liebermann's Test—yellow; Mandelin's Test—brown.

Thin-layer Chromatography. *System TA*—Rf 47; *system TB*—Rf 01; *system TC*—Rf 07. (*Acidified iodoplatinate solution*, positive.)

Gas Chromatography. *System GA*—RI 2630.

High Pressure Liquid Chromatography. *System HA*—k′ 5.0.

Ultraviolet Spectrum. Aqueous acid—273 nm ($A_1^1 = 467$ b), 309 nm.

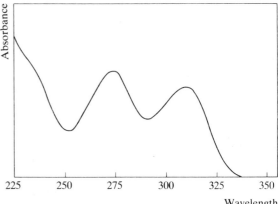

Wavelength

Infra-red Spectrum. Principal peaks at wavenumbers 1590, 1614, 1530, 1496, 1254, 1311 (metoclopramide hydrochloride, KBr disk).

Wavelength

[IR spectrum chart with Wavelength axis top: 5 6 7 8 9 10 11 12 13 14 15; Transmittance on vertical axis; Wavenumber bottom axis: 2000 1800 1600 1400 1200 1000 800 650]

Wavenumber

Mass Spectrum. Principal peaks at m/z 86, 99, 184, 58, 30, 87, 201, 186.

Quantification. GAS CHROMATOGRAPHY. In plasma: sensitivity 5 ng/ml, ECD—L. M. Ross-Lee *et al.*, *J. Chromat.*, 1980, *183*; *Biomed. Appl.*, *9*, 175–184.

HIGH PRESSURE LIQUID CHROMATOGRAPHY. In plasma: sensitivity 10 ng/ml, UV detection—G. Bishop-Freudling and H. Vergin, *J. Chromat.*, 1983, *273*; *Biomed. Appl.*, *24*, 453–457. In serum, saliva or urine: sensitivity 4.5 ng/ml for serum and saliva, 900 ng/ml for urine, UV detection—J. Popović, *Ther. Drug Monit.*, 1984, *6*, 77–82.

Disposition in the Body. Rapidly absorbed after oral administration. Up to about 60% of an oral dose undergoes first-pass metabolism but there is considerable intersubject variation. Up to about 80% of a dose is excreted in the urine in 24 hours with about 10 to 20% as unchanged drug, up to 50% as conjugated metoclopramide (mainly the N-4-sulphate), and a small amount as 2-(4-amino-5-chloro-2-methoxybenzamido)acetic acid.

THERAPEUTIC CONCENTRATION.
After a single oral dose of 10 mg given to 6 subjects, peak plasma concentrations of 0.04 to 0.06 µg/ml (mean 0.05) were attained in 0.5 to 2 hours; following intravenous administration of 10 mg to 6 subjects, plasma concentrations of 0.07 to 0.13 µg/ml were reported after 5 minutes (L. M. Ross-Lee *et al.*, *Eur. J. clin. Pharmac.*, 1981, *20*, 465–471).

TOXICITY. Ingestion by adults of up to 0.8 g without serious adverse effects has been reported.

HALF-LIFE. Plasma half-life, 3 to 6 hours, increased in renal impairment.

VOLUME OF DISTRIBUTION. About 3 litres/kg but there is considerable intersubject variation.

CLEARANCE. Plasma clearance, 7 to 17 ml/min/kg (mean 11).

DISTRIBUTION IN BLOOD. Plasma: whole blood ratio, 0.93.

PROTEIN BINDING. In plasma, about 60 to 70%.

NOTE. For reviews of metoclopramide, see R. A. Harrington *et al.*, *Drugs*, 1983, *25*, 451–494, and D. N. Bateman, *Clin. Pharmacokinet.*, 1983, *8*, 523–529.

Dose. The equivalent of 30 mg of anhydrous metoclopramide hydrochloride daily.

Metocurine Iodide   *Muscle Relaxant*

Synonyms. Dimethyl Tubocurarine Iodide; Dimethyltubocurarine Iodide.
Note. The name dimethyltubocurarine iodide was based on the old empirical formula for Tubocurarine.
Proprietary Name. Metubine Iodide
(+)-6,6',7',12'-Tetramethoxy-2,2,2',2'-tetramethyltubocuraranium di-iodide
$C_{40}H_{48}I_2N_2O_6 = 906.6$
CAS—5152-30-7 (metocurine); *7601-55-0* (iodide)

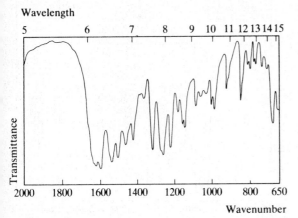

A white to pale yellow, crystalline powder. When heated to 257°, it decomposes with the evolution of gas.
Soluble 1 in 400 of water; very slightly soluble in ethanol; practically insoluble in chloroform and ether; slightly soluble in dilute acids and alkalis.

Colour Tests. Aromaticity (Method 2)—yellow/orange.
Cold *nitric acid* gives a brown colour.

Ultraviolet Spectrum. Aqueous acid—280 nm ($A_1^1 = 74$ b).

Infra-red Spectrum. Principal peaks at wavenumbers 1510, 1220, 1265, 1280, 1125, 1240 (KBr disk).

Disposition in the Body. About 50% of a dose is excreted in the urine unchanged in 48 hours, and about 2% of the dose is excreted in the bile in the same period.

HALF-LIFE. Plasma half-life, about 3 to 4 hours.

VOLUME OF DISTRIBUTION. About 0.4 litre/kg.

CLEARANCE. Plasma clearance, about 1.3 ml/min/kg.

PROTEIN BINDING. In plasma, about 35%.

REFERENCE. D. K. F. Meijer *et al.*, *Anesthesiology*, 1979, *51*, 402–407.

Dose. Initially, 1.5 to 8 mg intravenously.

Metolazone   *Diuretic*

Proprietary Names. Diulo; Metenix; Zaroxolyn.
7-Chloro-1,2,3,4-tetrahydro-2-methyl-4-oxo-3-o-tolylquinazoline-6-sulphonamide
$C_{16}H_{16}ClN_3O_3S = 365.8$
CAS—17560-51-9

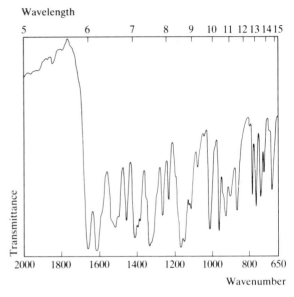

Wavelength

Wavenumber

Colourless crystals. It may occur in two polymorphic forms which melt at 227° and 270°.

Sparingly **soluble** in water; more soluble in alkalis and organic solvents.

Dissociation Constant. pK$_a$ 9.7.

Colour Tests. Koppanyi–Zwikker Test—violet; Liebermann's Test—orange → green-brown; Methanolic Potassium Hydroxide—yellow; Sulphuric Acid—yellow.

Thin-layer Chromatography. *System TD*—Rf 23; *system TE*—Rf 57; *system TF*—Rf 51.

High Pressure Liquid Chromatography. *System HN*—k′ 4.89.

Ultraviolet Spectrum. Aqueous acid—237 nm (A$_1^1$ = 1470 b), 271 nm, 344 nm.

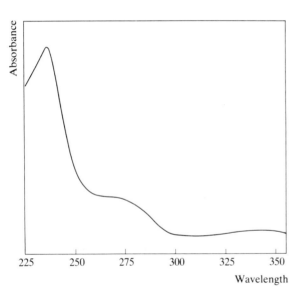

Wavelength

Infra-red Spectrum. Principal peaks at wavenumbers 1610, 1660, 1165, 1145, 962, 1012.

Mass Spectrum. Principal peaks at *m/z* 350, 91, 259, 352, 348, 65, 351, 107.

Quantification. HIGH PRESSURE LIQUID CHROMATOGRAPHY. In plasma: detection limit 2 ng/ml, UV detection—R. R. Brodie *et al.*, *J. Chromat.*, 1981, *226*; *Biomed. Appl.*, *15*, 526–532. In plasma or urine: detection limit 1 ng/ml in plasma and 5 ng/ml in urine, fluorescence detection—C. W. Vose *et al.*, *J. Chromat.*, 1981, *222*; *Biomed. Appl.*, *11*, 311–315.

Disposition in the Body. Incompletely but fairly readily absorbed after oral administration. About 80% of a dose is excreted in the urine as unchanged drug in 48 hours; about 10% is excreted in the bile.

THERAPEUTIC CONCENTRATION.

After a single oral dose of 2.5 mg given to 3 subjects, a mean peak plasma concentration of about 0.01 µg/ml was attained in 5 hours (W. J. Tilstone *et al.*, *Clin. Pharmac. Ther.*, 1974, *16*, 322–329).

HALF-LIFE. Plasma half-life, about 18 hours.

VOLUME OF DISTRIBUTION. About 1.6 litres/kg.

CLEARANCE. Plasma clearance, about 1.4 ml/min/kg.

DISTRIBUTION IN BLOOD. Plasma: whole blood ratio, 0.84.

PROTEIN BINDING. In plasma, 95%.

REFERENCE. W. J. Tilstone *et al.*, *ibid*.

Dose. Usually 2.5 to 10 mg daily; maximum of 80 mg daily.

Metomidate   *Sedative (Veterinary)*

Methyl 1-(α-methylbenzyl)imidazole-5-carboxylate
C$_{13}$H$_{14}$N$_2$O$_2$ = 230.3
CAS—5377-20-8

Metomidate Hydrochloride
Proprietary Name. Hypnodil
C$_{13}$H$_{14}$N$_2$O$_2$,HCl = 266.7
CAS—35944-74-2
An off-white crystalline powder. M.p. about 172°.
Very **soluble** in water.

Colour Test. Liebermann's Test—red-orange.

Thin-layer Chromatography. *System TA*—Rf 73. (*Acidified iodoplatinate solution*, positive.)

Ultraviolet Spectrum. Water—240 nm ($A_1^1 = 408$ b).

Infra-red Spectrum. Principal peaks at wavenumbers 1730, 1230, 725, 770, 1288, 1200 (metomidate hydrochloride, KBr disk).

Metopimazine
Anti-emetic

Proprietary Name. Vogalene
1-[3-(2-Methylsulphonylphenothiazin-10-yl)propyl]piperidine-4-carboxamide
$C_{22}H_{27}N_3O_3S_2 = 445.6$
CAS—14008-44-7

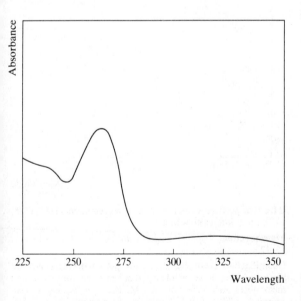

A white crystalline powder. M.p. 170° to 171°.
Soluble in chloroform and dilute acetic acid.

Colour Tests. Formaldehyde–Sulphuric Acid—red; Forrest Reagent—brown; FPN Reagent—orange; Mandelin's Test—green; Marquis Test—red; Sulphuric Acid—red.

Thin-layer Chromatography. *System TA*—Rf 56; *system TB*—Rf 00; *system TC*—Rf 11. (*Acidified iodoplatinate solution*, positive.)

High Pressure Liquid Chromatography. *System HA*—k' 1.4.

Ultraviolet Spectrum. Aqueous acid—264 nm ($A_1^1 = 922$ b), 310 nm.

Infra-red Spectrum. Principal peaks at wavenumbers 1150, 1310, 750, 1665, 1102, 1248 (KBr disk).

Mass Spectrum. Principal peaks at *m/z* 141, 445, 169, 123, 155, 96, 42, 317.

Dose. 5 to 15 mg daily.

Metoprolol
Beta-adrenoceptor Blocking Agent

($\pm$)-1-Isopropylamino-3-[4-(2-methoxyethyl)phenoxy]propan-2-ol
$C_{15}H_{25}NO_3 = 267.4$
CAS—37350-58-6

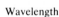

Metoprolol Tartrate

Proprietary Names. Beloc; Betaloc; Lopresor; Lopressor; Seloken. It is an ingredient of Co-Betaloc and Lopresoretic.
$(C_{15}H_{25}NO_3)_2, C_4H_6O_6 = 684.8$
CAS—56392-17-7
A white crystalline powder. M.p. about 120°.
Very **soluble** in water; soluble in ethanol and chloroform; practically insoluble in ether.

Dissociation Constant. pK_a 9.7.

Colour Tests. Liebermann's Test—pink-brown; Mandelin's Test—pink-brown; Marquis Test—pink.

Thin-layer Chromatography. *System TA*—Rf 49; *system TB*—Rf 08; *system TC*—Rf 08.

Gas Chromatography. *System GA*—RI 2010.

High Pressure Liquid Chromatography. *System HA*—k' 1.3.

Ultraviolet Spectrum. Aqueous acid—274 nm ($A_1^1 = 52$ a), 280 nm (inflexion).

Infra-red Spectrum. Principal peaks at wavenumbers 1510, 1245, 1108, 1028, 1175, 810 (KBr disk).

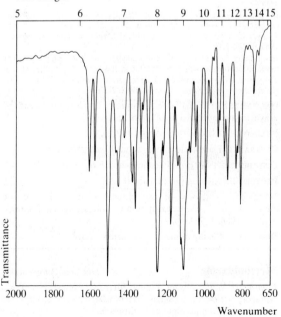

Mass Spectrum. Principal peaks at m/z 72, 30, 107, 56, 45, 41, 44, 43.

Quantification. GAS CHROMATOGRAPHY. In plasma or urine: sensitivity 3 ng/ml, ECD—C. D. Kinney, *J. Chromat.*, 1981, *225*; *Biomed. Appl.*, *14*, 213–218. In plasma or urine: metoprolol metabolites, sensitivity 6 ng/ml, ECD—C. P. Quarterman *et al.*, *J. Chromat.*, 1980, *183*; *Biomed. Appl.*, *9*, 92–98.

GAS CHROMATOGRAPHY-MASS SPECTROMETRY. In plasma or urine: metoprolol and metabolites, sensitivity 300 pg/ml—M. Ervik *et al.*, *Biomed. Mass Spectrom.*, 1981, *8*, 322–326.

HIGH PRESSURE LIQUID CHROMATOGRAPHY. In plasma: sensitivity 3 ng/ml for metoprolol and 12.5 ng/ml for α-hydroxymetoprolol, fluorescence detection—D. B. Pautler and W. J. Jusko, *J. Chromat.*, 1982, *228*; *Biomed. Appl.*, 17, 215–222.

Disposition in the Body. Well absorbed after oral administration; bioavailability about 50% due to extensive first-pass metabolism. About 95% of a dose is excreted in the urine within 48 hours, with about 65% of the dose as the inactive metabolite, 4-(2-hydroxy-3-isopropylaminopropoxy)phenylacetic acid, and about 10% as a further inactive metabolite, 2-hydroxy-3-[4-(2-methoxyethyl)phenoxy]propionic acid. Two active metabolites, α-hydroxymetoprolol and O-desmethylmetoprolol are also excreted in the urine in amounts equivalent to about 10% and less than 1% of the dose, respectively. Up to about 10% of a dose is excreted as unchanged drug.

THERAPEUTIC CONCENTRATION.
Following a single oral dose of 100 mg, given to 6 subjects, peak plasma concentrations of 0.03 to 0.28 µg/ml (mean 0.13) were attained in about 2.5 hours (W. Kirch *et al.*, *Biopharm. Drug Disp.*, 1983, *4*, 73–81).
Following a single oral dose of 100 mg to 8 subjects, a mean peak plasma concentration of metoprolol of 0.12 µg/ml was attained in 2 to 3 hours; the α-hydroxy metabolite reached a mean peak of 0.07 µg/ml in about 3 hours. After repeated administration of 100 mg every 12 hours, the mean peak plasma concentrations on the 8th day were 0.19 µg/ml for metoprolol and 0.07 µg/ml for the α-hydroxy metabolite. The concentration of the metabolite appears to be increased in elderly subjects (C. P. Quarterman *et al.*, *Br. J. clin. Pharmac.*, 1981, *11*, 287–294).

TOXICITY.
In a fatality due to metoprolol, the following postmortem tissue concentrations were reported: blood 4.7 µg/ml, bile 254 µg/ml, kidney 7.1 µg/g, liver 6.3 µg/g, urine 194 µg/ml (M. Stajić *et al.*, *J. analyt. Toxicol.*, 1984, *8*, 228–230).
In a fatality due to metoprolol and salicylate, the following postmortem tissue concentrations were reported: blood, metoprolol 56 µg/ml, salicylate 220 µg/ml; bile, metoprolol 276 µg/ml; liver, metoprolol 230 µg/g (M. Holzbecher *et al.*, *J. forens. Sci. Soc.*, 1982, *27*, 715–717).

HALF-LIFE. Plasma half-life, metoprolol 2 to 7 hours (mean 3), α-hydroxymetoprolol 4 to 12 hours (mean 6).

VOLUME OF DISTRIBUTION. About 4 litres/kg.

CLEARANCE. Plasma clearance, about 13 ml/min/kg.

DISTRIBUTION IN BLOOD. Plasma: whole blood ratio, 0.77.

PROTEIN BINDING. In plasma, about 12%.

NOTE. For a review of the clinical pharmacokinetics of metoprolol see C.-G. Regardh and G. Johnsson, *Clin. Pharmacokinet.*, 1980, *5*, 557–569.

Dose. 100 to 400 mg of metoprolol tartrate daily.

Metronidazole   *Antiprotozoal/Antibacterial*

Proprietary Names. Elyzol; Flagyl; Metrolyl; Metryl; Neo-Tric; Nidazol; Novonidazol; Sãtric; Trichozole; Trikacide; Vaginyl; Zadstat. It is an ingredient of Entamizole.

2-(2-Methyl-5-nitroimidazol-1-yl)ethanol
$C_6H_9N_3O_3 = 171.2$
CAS—443-48-1

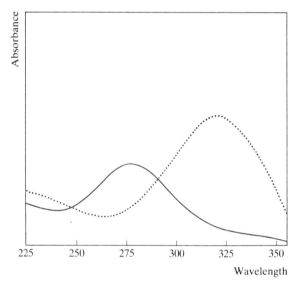

A white to pale yellow crystalline powder or crystals. It darkens on exposure to light. M.p. 159° to 163°.

Soluble 1 in 100 of water, 1 in 200 of ethanol, and 1 in 250 of chloroform; slightly soluble in ether.

Dissociation Constant. pK_a 2.5.

Partition Coefficient. Log P (octanol/pH 7.4), -0.1.

Colour Test. Methanolic Potassium Hydroxide—red.

Thin-layer Chromatography. *System TA*—Rf 58; *system TB*—Rf 02; *system TC*—Rf 36. (*Acidified potassium permanganate solution, positive.*)

Gas Chromatography. *System GA*—RI 1592.

Ultraviolet Spectrum. Aqueous acid—277 nm ($A_1^1 = 377$ a); aqueous alkali—319 nm ($A_1^1 = 520$ b).

Infra-red Spectrum. Principal peaks at wavenumbers 1187, 1535, 1070, 1265, 745, 1160 (KBr disk).

Mass Spectrum. Principal peaks at m/z 81, 124, 54, 53, 125, 171, 45, 42.

Quantification. HIGH PRESSURE LIQUID CHROMATOGRAPHY. In plasma, serum, saliva, whole blood or urine: metronidazole and metabolites, UV detection—C. M. Kaye *et al.*, *Br. J. clin. Pharmac.*, 1980, *9*, 528–529. In plasma: sensitivity 25 ng/ml, UV detection—R. A. Gibson *et al.*, *Clin. Chem.*, 1984, *30*, 784–787.

Disposition in the Body. Readily and almost completely absorbed after oral administration and widely distributed in the body. Metabolised by oxidation to 2-hydroxymethylmetronidazole and 2-methyl-5-nitroimidazol-1-acetic acid, and by conjugation with

Wavelength

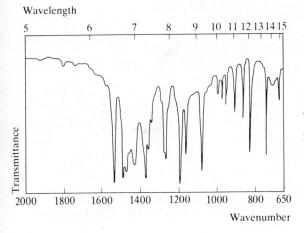

Thin-layer Chromatography. *System TA*—Rf 58; *system TB*—Rf 16; *system TC*—Rf 58. (*Acidified iodoplatinate solution*, positive.)

Gas Chromatography. *System GA*—RI 1860.

Ultraviolet Spectrum. Aqueous acid—260 nm ($A_1^1 = 500$ a).

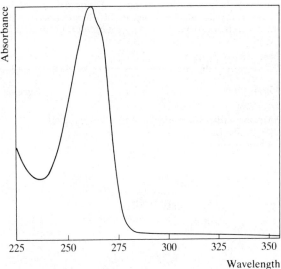

glucuronic acid. About 70 to 80% of a dose is excreted in the urine in 48 hours with less than 10% of the dose as unchanged drug, up to 10% as conjugated metronidazole, about 27% as 2-hydroxymethylmetronidazole, 10% as the conjugated 2-hydroxy methyl metabolite, and 20% as the acid metabolite.

THERAPEUTIC CONCENTRATION.
Following a single oral dose of 400 mg to 7 subjects, peak plasma concentrations of 4.5 to 11.6 µg/ml (mean 6.9) were attained in about 2 hours; a mean peak plasma concentration of 1.6 µg/ml of 2-hydroxy-methylmetronidazole was attained in about 8 hours (J. C. Jensen and R. Gugler, *Clin. Pharmac. Ther.*, 1983, *34*, 481–487).

HALF-LIFE. Plasma half-life, about 8 hours.

VOLUME OF DISTRIBUTION. About 0.5 to 1 litre/kg.

CLEARANCE. Plasma clearance, about 1 ml/min/kg.

PROTEIN BINDING. In plasma, less than 20%.

NOTE. For a review of the pharmacokinetics of metronidazole see E. D. Ralph, *Clin. Pharmacokinet.*, 1983, *8*, 43–62.

Dose. Up to 2.4 g daily for 10 days.

Metyrapone   *Diagnostic Agent (Pituitary Function)*

Synonym. Methopyrapone
Proprietary Name. Metopiron(e)
2-Methyl-1,2-di(3-pyridyl)propan-1-one
$C_{14}H_{14}N_2O = 226.3$
CAS—54-36-4

A white to light amber, fine, crystalline powder which darkens on exposure to light. M.p. 50° to 53°.
Soluble 1 in 100 of water, 1 in 3 of ethanol and chloroform; soluble in methanol.

Colour Test. Cyanogen Bromide—orange.

Infra-red Spectrum. Principal peaks at wavenumbers 1672, 1578, 1255, 714, 699, 970 (KBr disk).

Wavelength

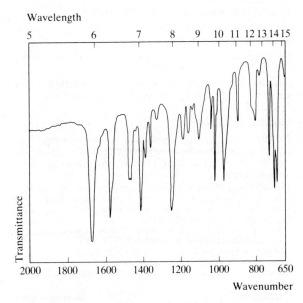

Mass Spectrum. Principal peaks at *m/z* 120, 106, 78, 92, 51, 226, 41, 39.

Quantification. COLORIMETRY. In plasma or tissues: sensitivity 5 µg/ml for metyrapone, 2 µg/ml for 1-hydroxymetyrapone—S. Szeberenyi *et al.*, *J. Chromat.*, 1969, *40*, 417–421.

SPECTROFLUORIMETRY. In plasma—A. W. Meikle *et al.*, *J. Lab. clin. Med.*, 1969, *74*, 515–520.

GAS CHROMATOGRAPHY. In urine: metyrapone and 1-hydroxy-metyrapone, FID—D. M. Hannah and J. G. Sprunt, *J. Pharm. Pharmac.*, 1969, *21*, 877–878.

Disposition in the Body. Metabolised by reduction to the 1-hydroxy derivative which is active. Excreted in the urine mainly as the glucuronide conjugates of 1-hydroxymetyrapone and metyrapone. About 50% of a dose is excreted in the urine in 3 days.

Dose. Up to 4.5 g daily.

Mevinphos   *Pesticide*

Proprietary Name. Phosdrin
2-Methoxycarbonyl-1-methylvinyl dimethyl phosphate
$C_7H_{13}O_6P = 224.1$
CAS—7786-34-7

$$(CH_3 \cdot O)_2 \overset{\overset{O}{\|}}{P} - O \cdot \overset{\overset{CH_3}{|}}{C} : CH \cdot CO \cdot O \cdot CH_3$$

The technical product is a pale yellow to orange liquid.
Miscible with water, ethanol, acetone, carbon tetrachloride, and chloroform.

Colour Test. Phosphorus Test—yellow.

Thin-layer Chromatography. *System TW*—Rf 23.

Gas Chromatography. *System GA*—RI 1450; *system GK*—retention time 0.50 relative to caffeine.

Mass Spectrum. Principal peaks at *m/z* 127, 192, 109, 67, 43, 193, 39, 79.

Quantification. GAS CHROMATOGRAPHY. In postmortem tissues and fluids: AFID—J. F. Lewin and J. L. Love, *Forens. Sci.*, 1974, *4*, 253–255.

Disposition in the Body.

TOXICITY. Mevinphos is extremely toxic by inhalation, ingestion, or percutaneous absorption and the estimated lethal dose is less than 500 mg. The maximum permissible atmospheric concentration is 0.1 mg/m^3.

The following postmortem tissue concentrations were reported in a fatality due to the ingestion of mevinphos: blood 360 μg/ml, brain 3 μg/g, kidney 20 μg/g, liver 240 μg/g, skeletal muscle 86 μg/g, urine 8 μg/ml; alcohol was detected in blood and urine at concentrations of 1250 μg/ml and 1550 μg/ml, respectively; death occurred within 45 minutes of ingestion (J. F. Lewin and J. L. Love, *ibid.*).

A 66-year-old man died about 1 minute after ingesting 28 g of mevinphos (R. Lokan and R. James, *Forens. Sci. Int.*, 1983, *22*, 179–182).

Mexenone   *Sunscreen Agent*

Synonym. Benzophenone-10
Proprietary Names. Uvicone; Uvistat.
2-Hydroxy-4-methoxy-4'-methylbenzophenone
$C_{15}H_{14}O_3 = 242.3$
CAS—1641-17-4

A pale yellow crystalline powder. M.p. 99° to 102°.
Practically **insoluble** in water; soluble 1 in 70 of ethanol and 1 in 7 of acetone.

Ultraviolet Spectrum. Methanol—243 nm ($A_1^1 = 353$ b), 287 nm ($A_1^1 = 640$ a), 325 nm ($A_1^1 = 440$ b).

Infra-red Spectrum. Principal peaks at wavenumbers 1260, 1598, 1637, 1211, 1613, 920 (KBr disk).

Use. Topically in a concentration of 4% in a cream or a solid basis.

Mexiletine   *Anti-arrhythmic*

1-Methyl-2-(2,6-xylyloxy)ethylamine
$C_{11}H_{17}NO = 179.3$
CAS—31828-71-4

Mexiletine Hydrochloride
Proprietary Name. Mexitil
$C_{11}H_{17}NO,HCl = 215.7$
CAS—5370-01-4
A white crystalline powder. M.p. 198° to 204°.
Soluble 1 in 2 of water, 1 in 3 of ethanol, and 1 in 30 of chloroform; practically insoluble in ether.

Dissociation Constant. pK$_a$ 9.0.

Colour Tests. Liebermann's Test—brown; Mandelin's Test—brown-orange; Marquis Test—red.

Thin-layer Chromatography. *System TA*—Rf 40; *system TB*—Rf 04; *system TC*—Rf 04.

Gas Chromatography. *System GA*—RI 1340.

High Pressure Liquid Chromatography. *System HA*—k' 1.2.

Ultraviolet Spectrum. Aqueous acid—260 nm ($A_1^1 = 14$ a).

Infra-red Spectrum. Principal peaks at wavenumbers 1200, 1040, 770, 760, 1595, 1090 (mexiletine hydrochloride, KBr disk).

Wavelength

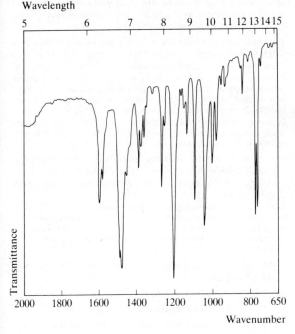

Transmittance

Wavenumber

Mass Spectrum. Principal peaks at m/z 58, 44, 41, 83, 77, 69, 85, 43.

Quantification. GAS CHROMATOGRAPHY. In plasma or urine: sensitivity 50 ng/ml, FID—K. Chan *et al.*, *J. Pharm. Pharmac.*, 1980, *32*, *Suppl.*, 98P. In plasma: detection limits 20 ng/ml for mexiletine and 7 ng/ml for the 2′-hydroxymethyl metabolite; ECD—A. Pachecus *et al.*, *Arzneimittel-Forsch.*, 1982, *32*, 688–693. In blood or plasma: sensitivity 5 ng/ml, AFID—K. J. Smith and P. J. Meffin, *J. Chromat.*, 1980, *181*; *Biomed. Appl.*, *7*, 469–472.

HIGH PRESSURE LIQUID CHROMATOGRAPHY. In plasma, urine or cerebrospinal fluid: detection limit 10 ng/ml, UV detection—H. Breithaupt and M. Wilfling, *J. Chromat.*, 1982, *230*; *Biomed. Appl.*, *19*, 97–105.

Disposition in the Body. Readily absorbed after oral administration; bioavailability 80 to 90%. It is extensively metabolised; the major metabolites are the 4′-hydroxy and 2′-hydroxymethyl derivatives, which may be further metabolised by deamination to the corresponding alcohols. The rate and extent of renal excretion is dependent on the urinary pH. Under normal conditions, up to about 20% of a dose may be excreted in the urine as unchanged drug in 24 hours, but this may be increased to about 50% if the urinary pH is maintained at about 5.

THERAPEUTIC CONCENTRATION. In plasma, usually in the range 0.5 to 2 µg/ml.

Following a single oral dose of 400 mg to 6 subjects, peak plasma concentrations of 0.65 to 0.94 µg/ml (mean 0.77) were attained in about 2 hours (V. Häselbarth *et al.*, *Clin. Pharmac. Ther.*, 1981, *29*, 729–736).

Following daily oral doses of 450 mg to 10 subjects, steady-state plasma concentrations of 0.75 to 2.18 µg/ml (mean 1.6) were reported (K. Ohashi *et al.*, *Arzneimittel-Forsch.*, 1984, *34*, 503–507).

TOXICITY. Serious toxic effects are usually associated with plasma concentrations of about 2 µg/ml or more, although toxicity may occur throughout the therapeutic range.

In a fatality due to the ingestion of 4.4 g, a postmortem blood concentration of about 35 µg/ml was reported (P. Jequier *et al.*, *Lancet*, 1976, *1*, 429).

In a fatality due to a mexiletine overdose, postmortem blood and liver concentrations of 44.3 µg/ml and 636 µg/g, respectively, were reported (R. C. Blackmore and M. D. Ossleton, *Bull. int. Ass. forens. Toxicol.*, 1983, *16*(3), 7–8).

HALF-LIFE. There is considerable intersubject variation and the plasma half-life appears to vary with the urinary pH; it is usually in the range 7 to 25 hours (mean 11 hours in normal subjects, increased in subjects with arrhythmias).

VOLUME OF DISTRIBUTION. About 8 litres/kg but there is considerable intersubject variation.

CLEARANCE. Plasma clearance, about 7 ml/min/kg with considerable intersubject variation.

PROTEIN BINDING. In plasma, about 70%.

NOTE. For a review of mexiletine see C. Y. C. Chew *et al.*, *Drugs*, 1979, *17*, 161–181, and B. G. Wulf, *Clin. Pharm.*, 1983, *2*, 340–346.

Dose. 0.6 to 1 g of mexiletine hydrochloride daily.

Mianserin   *Antidepressant*

1,2,3,4,10, 14b - Hexahydro - 2 - methyldibenzo[*c*, *f*] - pyrazino[1, 2-*a*]azepine
$C_{18}H_{20}N_2 = 264.4$
CAS—24219-97-4

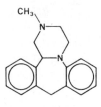

Mianserin Hydrochloride

Proprietary Names. Bolvidon; Norval; Tolvon.
Note. The name Norval was formerly applied to a preparation containing docusate sodium.
$C_{18}H_{20}N_2,HCl = 300.8$
CAS—21535-47-7
White crystals or crystalline powder. M.p. 282° to 284°.
Soluble 1 in 50 of water, 1 in 100 of ethanol, and 1 in 20 of chloroform.

Colour Tests. Liebermann's Test—violet; Mandelin's Test—violet.

Thin-layer Chromatography. *System TA*—Rf 58; *system TB*—Rf 39; *system TC*—Rf 58. (*Acidified iodoplatinate solution*, blue; *Mandelins reagent*, violet.)

Gas Chromatography. *System GA*—RI 2211; *system GF*—RI 2595.

High Pressure Liquid Chromatography. *System HA*—mianserin k′ 1.8, N-desmethylmianserin k′ 2.4.

Ultraviolet Spectrum. Aqueous acid—279 nm ($A_1^1 = 75$ a). (See below)

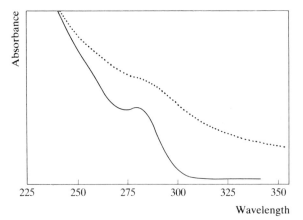

Wavelength

Infra-red Spectrum. Principal peaks at wavenumbers 787, 772, 1138, 1254, 1314, 742 (mianserin hydrochloride, KBr disk).

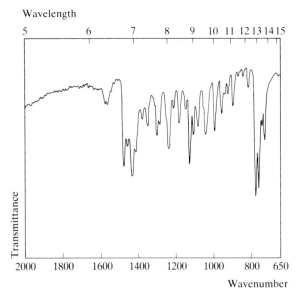

Wavenumber

Mass Spectrum. Principal peaks at m/z 193, 264, 43, 72, 71, 220, 192, 194; *N*-desmethylmianserin 193, 208, 194, 250, 178, 192, 29, 179.

Quantification. GAS CHROMATOGRAPHY. In plasma: detection limit 1 ng/ml, AFID—G. F. Lachâtre *et al.*, *Ther. Drug Monit.*, 1982, *4*, 359–364.

GAS CHROMATOGRAPHY–MASS SPECTROMETRY. In plasma: sensitivity 5 ng/ml—S. P. Jindal *et al.*, *J. analyt. Toxicol.*, 1982, *6*, 34–37.

HIGH PRESSURE LIQUID CHROMATOGRAPHY. In plasma: sensitivity 5 ng/ml, electrochemical detection—R. F. Suckow *et al.*, *J. pharm. Sci.*, 1982, *71*, 889–893.

Disposition in the Body. Readily absorbed after oral administration. The major metabolites are *N*-desmethylmianserin and 8-hydroxymianserin, which are both active, and mianserin *N*-oxide. About 30 to 40% of a dose is excreted in the urine in 24

hours, and a total of about 70% is excreted over a period of several days, mainly as conjugated metabolites. About 5% of a dose is excreted in the urine unchanged.

THERAPEUTIC CONCENTRATION. In plasma, usually in the range 0.015 to 0.07 μg/ml. *N*-Desmethylmianserin is detectable in plasma at concentrations about one-third of those of mianserin.

Following a single oral dose of 60 mg given to 8 subjects, peak plasma concentrations of 0.05 to 0.14 μg/ml (mean 0.10) and peak blood concentrations of 0.04 to 0.09 μg/ml (mean 0.06) were attained in about 3 hours (K. P. Maguire *et al.*, *Eur. J. clin. Pharmac.*, 1982, *21*, 517–520).

Following oral doses of 20 mg three times a day to 10 subjects, minimum steady-state plasma concentrations of 0.03 to 0.09 μg/ml (mean 0.06) were reported (G. F. Lachâtre *et al.*, *Ther. Drug Monit.*, 1982, *4*, 359–364).

TOXICITY. Overdosage does not appear to cause the complications associated with overdose of tricyclic antidepressants. Toxic effects have been associated with plasma concentrations greater than 0.5 μg/ml.

Plasma concentrations of 0.11 μg/ml of mianserin and 0.5 μg/ml of lorazepam were reported on admission to hospital in a comatose subject who had ingested 600 mg of mianserin plus an unknown amount of lorazepam; the patient died the following day (P. Crome and B. Newman, *Br. med. J.*, 1977, *2*, 260).

HALF-LIFE. Plasma half-life, 6 to 39 hours (mean 16), increased in elderly subjects.

VOLUME OF DISTRIBUTION. About 13 litres/kg.

PROTEIN BINDING. In plasma, about 90%.

NOTE. For a review of mianserin see R. Brogden *et al.*, *Drugs*, 1978, *16*, 273–301.

Dose. 30 to 90 mg of mianserin hydrochloride daily; maximum of 200 mg daily.

Miconazole   *Antifungal*

Proprietary Name. Daktarin
1-[2,4-Dichloro-β-(2,4-dichlorobenzyloxy)phenethyl]imidazole
$C_{18}H_{14}Cl_4N_2O = 416.1$
CAS—22916-47-8

A white crystalline powder.
Very slightly **soluble** in water; very soluble in chloroform; soluble in most other organic solvents.

Miconazole Nitrate

Proprietary Names. Albistat; Daktarin (cream); Dermonistat; Gyno-Daktarin; Micatin; Monistat.
$C_{18}H_{14}Cl_4N_2O,HNO_3 = 479.1$
CAS—22832-87-7
A white crystalline powder. M.p. about 182°.
Very slightly **soluble** in water and ether; soluble 1 in 140 of ethanol; slightly soluble in chloroform.

Dissociation Constant. pK$_a$ 6.7.

Thin-layer Chromatography. *System TA*—Rf 73; *system TB*—Rf 11; *system TC*—Rf 67. (*Dragendorff spray.*)

Gas Chromatography. *System GA*—RI 2980.

Ultraviolet Spectrum. Methanol—264 nm, 272 nm (A$_1^1$ = 17 a), 280 nm.

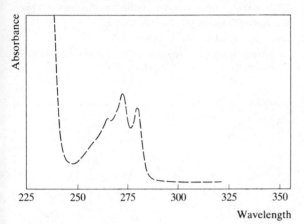

Infra-red Spectrum. Principal peaks at wavenumbers 1085, 1319, 827, 1302, 1038, 812 (miconazole nitrate, KBr disk).

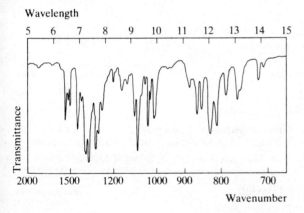

Mass Spectrum. Principal peaks at *m/z* 159, 161, 81, 335, 333, 163, 337, 205.

Quantification. GAS CHROMATOGRAPHY (CAPILLARY COLUMN). In serum: sensitivity 1 ng/ml, ECD—P. T. Männistö *et al.*, *Antimicrob. Ag. Chemother.*, 1982, *21*, 730–733.

HIGH PRESSURE LIQUID CHROMATOGRAPHY. In saliva: sensitivity 500 ng/ml, UV detection—A. Turner and D. W. Warnock, *J. Chromat.*, 1982, *227*; *Biomed. Appl.*, *16*, 229–232.

BIOASSAY. In serum—A. Espinel-Ingroff *et al.*, *Antimicrob. Ag. Chemother.*, 1977, *11*, 365–368.

Disposition in the Body. Incompletely absorbed after oral administration and poorly absorbed after topical administration. Metabolised by oxidation to 2,4-dichloromandelic acid and 2-(2,4-dichlorobenzyloxy)-2-(2,4-dichlorophenyl)acetic acid which are both inactive. About 10 to 20% of an oral or

intravenous dose is excreted in the urine in 6 days, with only about 1% of the dose as unchanged drug. About 50% of an oral dose is eliminated in the faeces, mostly unchanged.

THERAPEUTIC CONCENTRATION.

Following an intravenous infusion of 522 mg to 4 subjects, plasma concentrations of 2.0 to 9.1 μg/ml (mean 6.2) were reported at the end of the infusion (P. J. Lewi *et al.*, *Eur. J. clin. Pharmac.*, 1976, *10*, 49–54).

HALF-LIFE. Plasma half-life, about 24 hours.

VOLUME OF DISTRIBUTION. About 20 litres/kg.

PROTEIN BINDING. In plasma, about 92%.

NOTE. For a review of the pharmacokinetics of systemic antifungal drugs see T. K. Daneshmend and D. W. Warnock, *Clin. Pharmacokinet.*, 1983, *8*, 17–42.

Dose. 0.6 to 3.6 g daily by intravenous infusion; 1 g daily by mouth.

Midazolam   *Hypnotic*

Proprietary Name. Hypnovel (as the hydrochloride)
8 - Chloro - 6 - (2 - fluorophenyl) - 1 - methyl - 4H - imidazo[1,5 - a][1,4]benzodiazepine
C$_{18}$H$_{13}$ClFN$_3$ = 325.8
CAS—59467-70-8

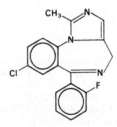

Colourless crystals. M.p. 158° to 160°.
Soluble in water.

Dissociation Constant. pK$_a$ 6.2.

High Pressure Liquid Chromatography. *System HI*—k′ 9.75; *system HJ*—k′ 2.10; *system HK*—k′ 5.90.

Infra-red Spectrum. Principal peaks at wavenumbers 1608, 820, 767, 1310, 1210, 995 (KBr disk). (See below)

Mass Spectrum. Principal peaks at *m/z* 310, 312, 311, 163, 325, 75, 39, 297.

Quantification. GAS CHROMATOGRAPHY. In plasma: limit of detection 500 pg/ml, ECD—M. T. Smith *et al.*, *Eur. J. clin. Pharmac.*, 1981, *19*, 271–278.

HIGH PRESSURE LIQUID CHROMATOGRAPHY. In plasma: midazolam and 1-hydroxymethylmidazolam, sensitivity 15 ng/ml, UV detection—J. Vasiliades and T. H. Sahawneh, *J. Chromat.*, 1981, *225*; *Biomed. Appl.*, *14*, 266–271.

POLAROGRAPHY. In urine: 1-hydroxymethylmidazolam, sensitivity 50 ng/ml—C. V. Puglisi *et al.*, *J. Chromat.*, 1978, *145*; *Biomed. Appl.*, *2*, 81–96.

NOTE. For a comparison of various chromatographic methods see J. Vasiliades and T. H. Sahawneh, *J. Chromat.*, 1982, *228*; *Biomed. Appl.*, *17*, 195–203.

Disposition in the Body. Rapidly absorbed after oral administration; bioavailability 30 to 70%. Metabolised by hydroxylation to 1-hydroxymethylmidazolam (which is active), 4-hydroxymida-

Wavelength

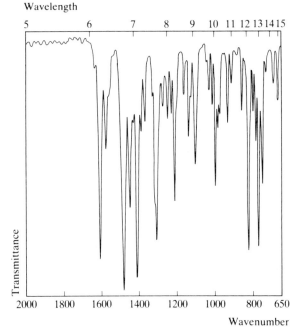

zolam, and 4-hydroxy-1-hydroxymethylmidazolam; the hydroxy metabolites are then conjugated with glucuronic acid. Up to 90% of a dose is excreted in the urine in 24 hours as the conjugated metabolites, mainly as conjugated 1-hydroxymethyl-midazolam (60 to 80% of a dose). Less than 1% of a dose is excreted in the urine as unchanged drug.

THERAPEUTIC CONCENTRATION.
Following a single oral dose of 20 mg to 6 subjects, peak plasma concentrations of 0.13 to 0.37 µg/ml (mean 0.26) of midazolam and 0.07 to 0.25 µg/ml (mean 0.14) of 1-hydroxymethylmidazolam were attained in 0.25 to 0.5 hour (P. Heizmann et al., Br. J. clin. Pharmac., 1983, 16, Suppl., 43S–49S).

HALF-LIFE. Plasma half-life, about 2 hours, increased in elderly subjects.

VOLUME OF DISTRIBUTION. 0.5 to 2 litres/kg.

CLEARANCE. Plasma clearance, 3 to 8 ml/min/kg (mean 5).

PROTEIN BINDING. In plasma, about 95%.

Dose. The equivalent of 70 µg/kg of midazolam by slow intravenous injection; usual dose range 2.5 to 7.5 mg.

Minocycline   *Antibiotic*

6-Desmethyl-6-deoxy-7-dimethylaminotetracycline
$C_{23}H_{27}N_3O_7 = 457.5$
CAS—10118-90-8

A bright yellow-orange amorphous solid.

Minocycline Hydrochloride
Proprietary Names. Klinomycin; Minocin; Minomycin; Mynocine; Ultramycin; Vectrin.
$C_{23}H_{27}N_3O_7,HCl = 493.9$
CAS—13614-98-7
A yellow crystalline powder.
Soluble in water and in solutions of alkali hydroxides and carbonates; slightly soluble in ethanol; practically insoluble in chloroform and ether.

Dissociation Constant. pK_a 2.8, 5.0, 7.8, 9.5.

Colour Test. Sulphuric Acid—yellow.

Ultraviolet Spectrum. Aqueous acid—265 nm ($A_1^1 = 400$ b), 354 nm; aqueous alkali—243 nm ($A_1^1 = 414$ b).

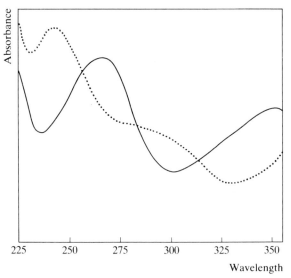

Infra-red Spectrum. Principal peaks at wavenumbers 1600, 1645, 1525, 1225, 1310, 1050 (minocycline hydrochloride, K Br disk).

Dose. The equivalent of 100 to 200 mg of minocycline daily.

Minoxidil   *Antihypertensive*

Proprietary Name. Loniten
2,6-Diamino-4-piperidinopyrimidine 1-oxide
$C_9H_{15}N_5O = 209.3$
CAS—38304-91-5

A white crystalline solid. M.p. about 225°, with decomposition.
Soluble 1 in about 500 of water; readily soluble in ethanol and propylene glycol; practically insoluble in chloroform.

Thin-layer Chromatography. *System TA*—Rf 51; *system TB*—Rf 00; *system TC*—Rf 03.

Ultraviolet Spectrum. Aqueous acid—230 nm, 281 nm ($A_1^1 = 547$ b); aqueous alkali—262 nm, 288 nm.

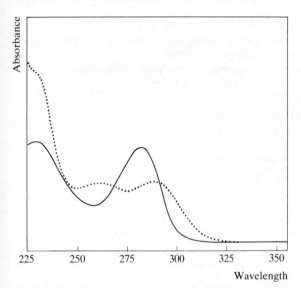

Absorbance

225   250   275   300   325   350
Wavelength

Infra-red Spectrum. Principal peaks at wavenumbers 1640, 1610, 1550, 1231, 1210, 758 (KBr disk).

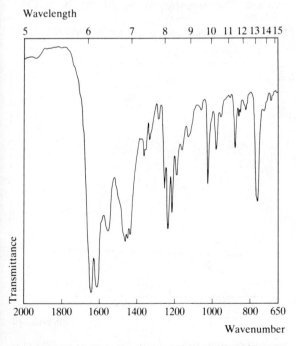

Wavelength

5   6   7   8   9   10 11 12 13 14 15

2000   1800   1600   1400   1200   1000   800   650
Wavenumber

Transmittance

Mass Spectrum. Principal peaks at m/z 84, 209, 67, 43, 110, 41, 192, 164.

Quantification. RADIOIMMUNOASSAY. In serum: limit of detection 3 ng/ml—M. E. Royer *et al.*, *J. pharm. Sci.*, 1977, *66*, 1266–1269.

Disposition in the Body. Readily absorbed after oral administration. More than 80% of a dose is excreted in the urine in 24 hours, mainly as glucuronide conjugates with less than 10% as unchanged drug; about 3% of a dose is eliminated in the faeces.

THERAPEUTIC CONCENTRATION.

Following daily oral administration of 27 to 30 mg to 6 subjects, serum concentrations of 0.04 to 0.25 µg/ml (mean 0.10) were reported 1 to 2 hours after a dose (D. T. Lowenthal *et al.*, *J. clin. Pharmac.*, 1978, *18*, 500–508).

HALF-LIFE. Plasma half-life, about 3 to 4 hours.

PROTEIN BINDING. In plasma, not significantly bound.

NOTE. For a review of minoxidil see V. M. Campese, *Drugs*, 1981, *22*, 257–278.

Dose. 5 to 50 mg daily; up to 100 mg daily has been given.

Molindone   *Tranquilliser*

3 - Ethyl - 6,7 - dihydro - 2 - methyl - 5 - (morpholinomethyl)indol - 4(5*H*)-one
$C_{16}H_{24}N_2O_2 = 276.4$
CAS—7416-34-4

Crystals. M.p. 180° to 181°.

Molindone Hydrochloride
Proprietary Names. Lidone; Moban.
$C_{16}H_{24}N_2O_2,HCl = 312.8$
CAS—15622-65-8
A white crystalline powder.
Freely **soluble** in water and ethanol.

Dissociation Constant. pK_a 6.9 (25°).

Gas Chromatography. *System GA*—RI 2465.

Ultraviolet Spectrum. Aqueous acid—255 nm ($A_1^1 = 41$ b), 299 nm.

Mass Spectrum. Principal peaks at m/z 100, 56, 42, 176, 98, 120, 70, 189.

Disposition in the Body. Readily absorbed after oral administration; peak plasma concentrations of unchanged drug are attained in 1 to 2 hours. It is extensively metabolised and excreted in the urine and faeces almost entirely as metabolites.

Dose. 15 to 225 mg of molindone hydrochloride daily.

6-Monoacetylmorphine

6-*O*-Acetylmorphine
$C_{19}H_{21}NO_4 = 327.4$
CAS—2784-73-8

6-Monoacetylmorphine Hydrochloride

$C_{19}H_{21}NO_4$,HCl = 363.8
CAS—36418-22-1
Crystals.
Soluble in water.

Colour Test. Marquis Test—violet.

Thin-layer Chromatography. *System TA*—Rf 46; *system TB*—Rf 06; *system TC*—Rf 19. (*Acidified iodoplatinate solution*, positive.)

Gas Chromatography. *System GA*—RI 2537.

High Pressure Liquid Chromatography. *System HA*—k′ 3.6 (tailing peak); *system HC*—k′ 0.80; *system HS*—k′ 1.00.

Ultraviolet Spectrum. Aqueous acid—287 nm ($A_1^1 = 45$ b).

Infra-red Spectrum. Principal peaks at wavenumbers 1238, 1730, 1213, 1050, 1030, 1131 (KBr disk).

Wavelength

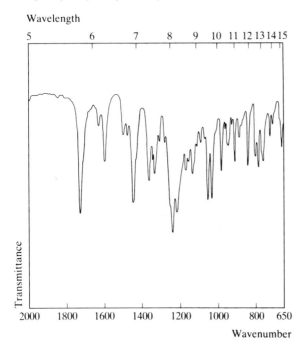

Mass Spectrum. Principal peaks at *m/z* 327, 268, 46, 43, 215, 44, 328, 269.

Disposition in the Body. 6-Monoacetylmorphine is the first hydrolysis product of diamorphine. It is further metabolised to morphine.

Monocrotaline   *Alkaloid*

Synonym. Crotaline
$C_{16}H_{23}NO_6 = 325.4$
CAS—315-22-0

An alkaloid obtained from *Crotalaria spectabilis* and other species of *Crotalaria* (Leguminosae).
A white crystalline powder. M.p. 197° to 198°, with decomposition.
Soluble 1 in 80 of water; soluble in chloroform and dilute acetic acid.

Colour Test. Mandelin's Test—green.

Thin-layer Chromatography. *System TA*—Rf 36. (*Acidified iodoplatinate solution*, positive.)

Infra-red Spectrum. Principal peaks at wavenumbers 1736, 1064, 1110, 1183, 1242, 1174 (KBr disk).

Monosulfiram   *Parasiticide*

Synonym. Sulfiram
Proprietary Name. Tetmosol
Tetraethylthiuram monosulphide
$C_{10}H_{20}N_2S_3 = 264.5$
CAS—95-05-6

$$(C_2H_5)_2N \cdot \overset{\overset{S}{\|}}{C} \cdot S \cdot \overset{\overset{S}{\|}}{C} \cdot N(C_2H_5)_2$$

A yellow or yellowish-brown, soft crystalline powder. M.p. 28.5° to 32°.
Practically **insoluble** in water; soluble 1 in 3 of ethanol; freely soluble in chloroform, ether, and most other organic solvents.

Colour Test. Sodium Nitroprusside (Method 3)—violet.

Thin-layer Chromatography. *System TA*—Rf 75. (*Acidified iodoplatinate solution*, positive.)

Ultraviolet Spectrum. Methanol—281 nm ($A_1^1 = 650$ a).

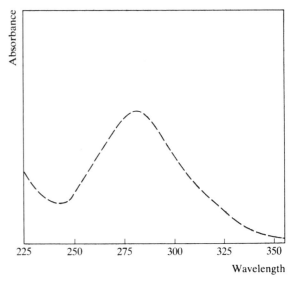

Infra-red Spectrum. Principal peaks at wavenumbers 1270, 1490, 1198, 1142, 968, 915 (KBr disk).

Use. As a 25% alcoholic solution, diluted with 2 or 3 parts of water immediately before use.

Morantel

Anthelmintic (Veterinary)

(*E*) - 1,4,5,6 - Tetrahydro - 1 - methyl - 2 - [2 - (3 - methyl - 2 - thienyl)vinyl]pyrimidine
$C_{12}H_{16}N_2S = 220.3$
CAS—20574-50-9

Crystals. M.p. 239° to 241°.

Morantel Tartrate

$C_{12}H_{16}N_2S,C_4H_6O_6 = 370.4$
CAS—26155-31-7
Pale yellow to greenish-yellow crystals. M.p. 167° to 170°.
Readily **soluble** in water.

Colour Tests. Liebermann's Test—black; Mandelin's Test—violet; Marquis Test—blue-violet; Sulphuric Acid—violet-red.

Thin-layer Chromatography. *System TA*—Rf 60. (*Acidified iodoplatinate solution*, positive.)

Gas Chromatography. *System GA*—not eluted.

Ultraviolet Spectrum. Methanol—322 nm (A$_1^1$ = 864 b).

Infra-red Spectrum. Principal peaks at wavenumbers 1626, 1577, 1319, 1305, 1148, 955 (KBr disk).

Morazone

Analgesic

1,5 - Dimethyl - 4 - (3 - methyl - 2 - phenylmorpholinomethyl) - 2 - phenyl-4-pyrazolin-3-one
$C_{23}H_{27}N_3O_2 = 377.5$
CAS—6536-18-1

A white crystalline powder. M.p. 131° to 134°.
Very **soluble** in ethanol, acetone, chloroform, and methanol.

Morazone Hydrochloride

Proprietary Names. Rosimon-Neu. It is an ingredient of Delimon.
$C_{23}H_{27}N_3O_2,HCl = 413.9$
CAS—50321-35-2
Crystals. M.p. 171° to 172°, with decomposition.
Soluble in water.

Colour Test. Liebermann's Test—red-orange.

Thin-layer Chromatography. *System TA*—Rf 58; *system TB*—Rf 08; *system TC*—Rf 46. (*Acidified iodoplatinate solution*, positive.)

Gas Chromatography. *System GA*—RI 1718.

High Pressure Liquid Chromatography. *System HA*—k' 0.7; *system HD*—k' 0.4; *system HW*—k' 2.05.

Ultraviolet Spectrum. Aqueous acid—258 nm (A$_1^1$ = 212 a); aqueous alkali—244 nm, 263 nm (A$_1^1$ = 201 b).

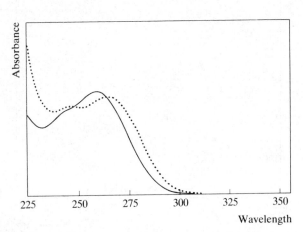

Infra-red Spectrum. Principal peaks at wavenumbers 754, 1656, 700, 1492, 1590, 1117 (thin film).

Mass Spectrum. Principal peaks at *m/z* 201, 176, 202, 56, 258, 70, 71, 42.

Dose. Morazone hydrochloride has been given in doses of 75 to 150 mg.

Morinamide

Antituberculous Agent

Synonym. Morphazinamide
N-Morpholinomethylpyrazine-2-carboxamide
$C_{10}H_{14}N_4O_2 = 222.2$
CAS—952-54-5

Crystals. M.p. 118° to 120°.
Soluble 1 in 3 of water, 1 in 30 of ethanol, and 1 in 2.5 of chloroform.

Morinamide Hydrochloride

Proprietary Name. Piazofolina
$C_{10}H_{14}N_4O_2,HCl = 258.7$
CAS—1473-73-0
A white crystalline powder. M.p. 196°.
Soluble 1 in 2 of water, 1 in 350 of ethanol, and 1 in 2000 of chloroform.

Thin-layer Chromatography. *System TA*—Rf 54; *system TB*—Rf 08; *system TC*—Rf 49. (*Acidified iodoplatinate solution*, weak reaction; *acidified potassium permanganate solution*, positive.)

Gas Chromatography. *System GA*—RI 1906.

Ultraviolet Spectrum. Aqueous acid—269 nm (A$_1^1$ = 340 b), 314 nm. (See below)

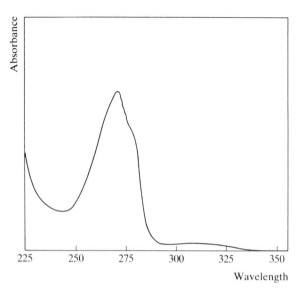

Infra-red Spectrum. Principal peaks at wavenumbers 1667, 1101, 1499, 1125, 1002, 1019 (K Br disk).

Mass Spectrum. Principal peaks at m/z 115, 86, 79, 57, 56, 107, 100, 52.

Dose. Morinamide has been given in doses of 3 g daily.

Morphine

Narcotic Analgesic

Synonym. Morphia
Proprietary Names. Duromorph; Nepenthe.
(4a*R*,5*S*,7a*R*,8*R*,9c*S*) - 4a,5,7a,8,9,9c - Hexahydro - 12 - methyl - 8,9c - iminoethanophenanthro[4,5 - *bcd*]furan - 3,5 - diol monohydrate
$C_{17}H_{19}NO_3,H_2O = 303.4$
CAS—57-27-2 (anhydrous); *6009-81-0* (monohydrate)

The principal alkaloid of opium. A white crystalline powder or colourless or white acicular crystals. M.p. 254° to 256°, with decomposition.
Soluble 1 in 5000 of water, 1 in 250 of ethanol, 1 in 1500 of chloroform, and 1 in 125 of glycerol; practically insoluble in ether.
Note. The solubility can vary according to the method of preparation and the crystalline state.

Morphine Acetate

$C_{17}H_{19}NO_3,C_2H_4O_2,3H_2O = 399.4$
CAS—596-15-6 (anhydrous); *5974-11-8* (trihydrate)
A white amorphous or crystalline powder.
Soluble 1 in 2.5 of water, 1 in 100 of ethanol, and 1 in 5 of glycerol; practically insoluble in ether.

Morphine Hydrochloride

$C_{17}H_{19}NO_3,HCl,3H_2O = 375.8$
CAS—52-26-6 (anhydrous); *6055-06-7* (trihydrate)
Colourless silky crystals or crystalline powder, or cubical white masses. A solution in water is laevorotatory.
Soluble 1 in 24 of water, 1 in 100 of ethanol, and 1 in 10 of glycerol; practically insoluble in chloroform and ether.

Morphine Sulphate

Proprietary Name. MST-Continus
$(C_{17}H_{19}NO_3)_2,H_2SO_4,5H_2O = 758.8$
CAS—64-31-3 (anhydrous); *6211-15-0* (pentahydrate)
White, acicular crystals, cubical masses, or crystalline powder. When exposed to air it gradually loses water of crystallisation. It darkens on prolonged exposure to light. M.p. 250°, with decomposition. A solution in water is laevorotatory.
Soluble 1 in 21 of water and 1 in 1000 of ethanol; practically insoluble in chloroform and ether.

Morphine Tartrate

Proprietary Name. It is an ingredient of Cyclimorph.
$(C_{17}H_{19}NO_3)_2,C_4H_6O_6,3H_2O = 774.8$
CAS—302-31-8 (anhydrous); *6032-59-3* (trihydrate)
Minute, colourless, acicular, efflorescent crystals.
Soluble 1 in 10 of water and 1 in 1000 of ethanol; practically insoluble in chloroform and ether.

Dissociation Constant. pK_a 8.0, 9.9 (20°).

Partition Coefficient. Log *P* (octanol/pH 7.4), −0.1.

Colour Tests. Ferric Chloride—blue; Liebermann's Test—black; Mandelin's Test—blue-grey; Marquis Test—violet.

Thin-layer Chromatography. *System TA*—Rf 37; *system TB*—Rf 00; *system TC*—Rf 09. (*Dragendorff spray*, positive; *acidified iodoplatinate solution*, positive; *Marquis reagent*, violet.)

Gas Chromatography. *System GA*—morphine RI 2454, codeine RI 2376, norcodeine RI 2388; *system GC*—morphine RI 2542, codeine RI 2681.

High Pressure Liquid Chromatography. *System HA*—morphine k' 3.8 (tailing peak), codeine k' 4.8 (tailing peak), morphine *N*-oxide k' 3.2 (tailing peak), norcodeine k' 3.1 (tailing peak), normorphine k' 2.9 (tailing peak); *system HC*—morphine k' 1.30, codeine k' 1.21, morphine-3-glucuronide k' 1.56, norcodeine k' 3.51, normorphine k' 3.92; *system HS*—k' 5.16.

Ultraviolet Spectrum. Aqueous acid—285 nm ($A_1^1 = 52$ a); aqueous alkali—298 nm ($A_1^1 = 92$ a).

Infra-red Spectrum. Principal peaks at wavenumbers 805, 1243, 1118, 945, 1086, 833 (K Br disk).

Mass Spectrum. Principal peaks at m/z 285, 162, 42, 215, 286, 124, 44, 284; codeine 299, 42, 162, 124, 229, 59, 300, 69; norcodeine 285, 81, 215, 148, 286, 164, 110, 115; normorphine 271, 81, 150, 201, 148, 110, 272, 82.

Quantification. GAS CHROMATOGRAPHY. In postmortem tissues: sensitivity 50 ng/ml in blood, 300 ng/g in kidney and liver, 500 ng/ml in urine, FID—G. R. Nakamura and E. L. Way, *Analyt. Chem.*, 1975, *47*, 775–778. In whole blood: sensitivity 1 ng/ml, ECD—S. Felby, *Forens. Sci. Int.*, 1979, *13*, 145–150. In raw opium and opium preparations—D. C. Garratt *et al.*, *Analyst, Lond.*, 1978, *103*, 268–283.

GAS CHROMATOGRAPHY-MASS SPECTROMETRY. In blood, urine or tissues: sensitivity 20 ng/ml—J. J. Saady *et al.*, *J. analyt. Toxicol.*, 1982, *6*, 235–237.

HIGH PRESSURE LIQUID CHROMATOGRAPHY. In plasma or cerebrospinal fluid: sensitivity 1 ng/ml, electrochemical detection—R. D. Todd *et al.*, *J. Chromat.*, 1982, *232*; *Biomed. Appl.*, *21*, 101–110. In plasma or urine: morphine and morphine-3-

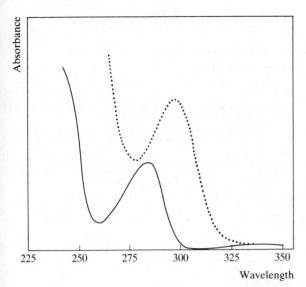

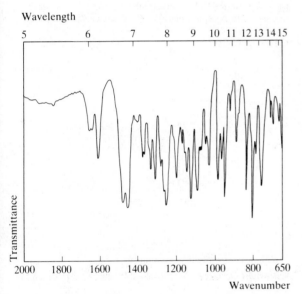

pass metabolism; bioavailability about 20 to 30%. It is widely distributed, mainly in kidneys, liver, lungs, and spleen with lower concentrations in the brain and muscles, but does not accumulate in the tissues. The major metabolic reaction is conjugation to form morphine-3- and 6-glucuronides; other reactions include N-demethylation, O-methylation, and N-oxide formation. After a parenteral dose, up to 90% is excreted in the urine in 24 hours, including about 10% of the dose as free morphine, 65 to 70% as conjugated morphine, up to 10% as morphine-3-ethereal sulphate, 1% as normorphine, and 3% as normorphine glucuronide. After an oral dose, about 60% is excreted in the urine in 24 hours, and about 3% of the dose is excreted as free morphine in 48 hours. The urinary excretion of morphine appears to be pH-dependent to some extent; as the urine becomes more acid, excretion of free morphine rises, and as the urine becomes more alkaline, excretion of the glucuronide conjugate rises. Up to about 10% of a dose may be excreted in the bile.

Morphine is the major active metabolite of diamorphine, and is also a metabolite of codeine.

NOTE. Morphine may be slowly converted to pseudomorphine in cadavers and can be found as such on exhumation.

THERAPEUTIC CONCENTRATION. In plasma, usually in the range 0.01 to 0.07 µg/ml.

A single intramuscular dose of 10 mg of morphine sulphate administered to 5 subjects, produced peak average serum concentrations of 0.051 to 0.062 µg/ml (mean 0.056) within 20 minutes (D. R. Stanski *et al.*, *Clin. Pharmac. Ther.*, 1978, *24*, 52–59).

Following a single intravenous dose of 10 mg of morphine sulphate administered to 12 subjects, a mean serum concentration of free morphine of about 0.05 µg/ml was reported at 15 minutes, and serum concentrations of conjugated morphine of 0.13 to 0.16 µg/ml were reported at 1 hour (S. F. Brunk *et al.*, *J. clin. Pharmac.*, 1974, *14*, 581–587).

Following repeated oral administration of 5 mg every 4 hours to 8 patients, a mean minimum steady-state plasma concentration of 0.011 µg/ml was reported; in 8 patients receiving 30 mg every 4 hours, a mean minimum steady-state plasma concentration of 0.044 µg/ml was reported (T. D. Walsh and B. V. Kadam, *Br. J. clin. Pharmac.*, 1984, *17*, 232P).

TOXICITY. The estimated minimum lethal dose for adults is 200 mg but addicts may be able to tolerate up to ten times as much. Morphine is initially eliminated from the blood fairly quickly and blood concentrations are difficult to interpret, especially as toxic effects depend on the degree of tolerance which has been acquired.

In a survey of 10 fatalities due to morphine overdose in addicts, the following tissue concentrations of total morphine were found: blood 0.2 to 2.3 µg/g (mean 0.7, 7 cases), liver 0.4 to 18.0 µg/g (mean 3.0, 10 cases), muscle 0.1 to 2.0 µg/g (mean 0.8, 6 cases), urine 14 to 81 µg/g (mean 52, 7 cases) (S. Felby *et al.*, *Forens. Sci.*, 1974, *3*, 77–81).

HALF-LIFE. Plasma half-life, about 2 to 3 hours.

VOLUME OF DISTRIBUTION. About 3 to 5 litres/kg.

CLEARANCE. Plasma clearance, about 15 to 20 ml/min/kg.

PROTEIN BINDING. In plasma, 20 to 35%.

NOTE. For a review of the metabolism of morphine see U. Boerner *et al.*, *Drug Met. Rev.*, 1975, *4*, 39–73.

Dose. 5 to 20 mg of morphine hydrochloride, sulphate, or tartrate, by mouth or parenterally, every 4 hours.

---

glucuronide, sensitivities 20 ng/ml and 200 ng/ml respectively, using ion-pair chromatography and UV detection—J. O. Svensson *et al.*, *J. Chromat.*, 1982, *230*; *Biomed. Appl.*, *19*, 427–432.

HIGH PRESSURE LIQUID CHROMATOGRAPHY–IMMUNOASSAY. In blood or urine—P. E. Nelson *et al.*, *J. forens. Sci. Soc.*, 1980, *20*, 195–202.

RADIOIMMUNOASSAY. In serum: detection limit 100 pg—S. Spector, *J. Pharmac. exp. Ther.*, 1971, *178*, 253–258. Comparison with GC—D. R. Stanski *et al.*, *J. pharm. Sci.*, 1982, *71*, 314–317.

Disposition in the Body. Rapidly absorbed after subcutaneous, intravenous, or intramuscular administration. Absorption after oral administration is variable and there is considerable first-

Muzolimine   *Diuretic*

3-Amino-1-[1-(3,4-dichlorophenyl)ethyl]-2-pyrazolin-5-one
$C_{11}H_{11}Cl_2N_3O = 272.1$
CAS—55294-15-0

Crystals.

M.p. 134° to 137°.

Practically **insoluble** in water; soluble 1 in 4 of ethanol, 1 in 9 of acetone, and 1 in 3 of chloroform.

Dissociation Constant. pK_a 9.3.

Ultraviolet Spectrum. Methanolic acid—240 nm ($A_1^1 = 489$ b).

Infra-red Spectrum. Principal peaks at wavenumbers 1690, 1640, 1602, 835, 665, 880 (KBr disk).

Quantification. THIN-LAYER CHROMATOGRAPHY. In plasma or urine: detection limit 2 ng/ml—W. Ritter, *J. Chromat.*, 1977, *142*, 431–440.

Disposition in the Body. Readily absorbed following oral administration. About 5% of a dose is excreted unchanged in the urine in 10 hours.

THERAPEUTIC CONCENTRATION.

After a single oral dose of 30 mg given to 6 subjects, peak plasma concentrations of 0.29 to 0.51 µg/ml (mean 0.44) were attained in 1 to 3 hours (D. Loew *et al.*, *Eur. J. clin. Pharmac.*, 1977, *12*, 341–344).

HALF-LIFE. Plasma half-life, 10 to 17 hours.

Dose. 40 to 80 mg daily.

Myristicin

5-Allyl-1-methoxy-2,3-methylenedioxybenzene
$C_{11}H_{12}O_3 = 192.2$
CAS—607-91-0

The most toxic principle of nutmeg and nutmeg oil. M.p. below −20°. B.p. 276° to 277°. Refractive index 1.5403.
Slightly **soluble** in ethanol; soluble in ether.

Nutmeg

Synonyms. Muscade; Myristica; Nux Moschata.
The dried kernels of the seeds of *Myristica fragrans* (Myristicaceae), containing not less than 5% v/w of volatile oil.

Nutmeg Oil

Synonyms. Essence de Muscade; Myristica Oil; Oleum Myristicae.
CAS—8008-45-5
A volatile oil obtained by distillation from nutmeg. East Indian oil contains about 15% of myristicin and West Indian about 2%.

A colourless, pale yellow, or pale green liquid. Wt per ml, East Indian oil 0.885 to 0.915 g, West Indian oil 0.86 to 0.88 g. Refractive index 1.472 to 1.488.
Freely **soluble** in ethanol (90%); soluble in glacial acetic acid.

Disposition in the Body.

TOXICITY. Severe symptoms of poisoning have been caused by the ingestion of 1 to 1½ nutmegs, and doses of 5 g or more of nutmeg or nutmeg powder will produce a marked depressive action on the central nervous system.

A 28-year-old woman ingested 18.3 g of powdered nutmeg. Following a period of disorientation, delirium and excitement, the patient became semi-stuporous for 12 hours. For some days she complained of numbness, dizziness and nausea and there were further periods of excitement. No specific therapy was given and she was discharged after 7 days (R. C. Green, *J. Am. med. Ass.*, 1959, *171*, 1342–1344).

Two young women consumed 15 and 25 g respectively of ground nutmeg in order to experience its hallucinogenic action. Both became intoxicated but recovered (H. O. Akesson and J. Walinder, *Lancet*, 1965, *1*, 1271–1272).

For a review of the toxic effects and uses of nutmeg see A. T. Weil, *Bull. Narcot.*, 1966, *18* (4), 15–23.

Nabilone   *Anti-emetic*

Proprietary Name. Cesamet

(±)-(6aR,10aR)-3-(1,1-Dimethylheptyl)-6,6a,7,8,10,10a-hexa-hydro-1-hydroxy-6,6-dimethyl-9H-dibenzo[b,d]pyran-9-one
$C_{24}H_{36}O_3 = 372.5$
CAS—51022-71-0

Nabilone is a synthetic cannabinoid.

Ultraviolet Spectrum. Methanol—275 nm ($A_1^1 = 35$ b), 282 nm ($A_1^1 = 35$ b).

Infra-red Spectrum. Principal peaks at wavenumbers 1696, 1619, 1574, 1260, 1100, 1038 (KBr disk).

Mass Spectrum. Principal peaks at m/z 288, 69, 178, 41, 287, 43, 289, 55.

Disposition in the Body. Readily absorbed after oral administration; rapidly distributed into the tissues and metabolised by reduction of the 9-keto group forming a mixture of isomeric alcohols (carbinols) together with several other unidentified metabolites. About 65% of a dose is eliminated in the faeces, and about 20% is excreted in the urine as polar acidic metabolites.

HALF-LIFE. Plasma half-life, about 2 hours.

REFERENCE. A. Rubin *et al.*, *Clin. Pharmac. Ther.*, 1977, *22*, 85–91.

Dose. 2 to 4 mg daily; maximum of 6 mg daily.

Nadolol

Beta-adrenoceptor Blocking Agent

Proprietary Names. Corgard; Solgol. It is an ingredient of Corgaretic.

(2*R*,3*S*) - 5 - (3 - *tert* - Butylamino - 2 - hydroxypropoxy) - 1,2,3,4 - tetrahydronaphthalene-2,3-diol

$C_{17}H_{27}NO_4 = 309.4$

CAS—42200-33-9

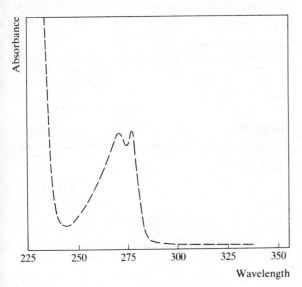

A white crystalline powder. M.p. 124° to 136°.

Soluble in water; freely soluble in ethanol; slightly soluble in chloroform; practically insoluble in ether.

Colour Tests. Liebermann's Test—brown; Mandelin's Test—brown-red; Marquis Test—red; Nessler's Reagent—brown.

Thin-layer Chromatography. *System TA*—Rf 42; *system TB*—Rf 01; *system TC*—Rf 01.

Gas Chromatography. *System GA*—RI 2550.

High Pressure Liquid Chromatography. *System HA*—k' 1.2.

Ultraviolet Spectrum. Aqueous acid—269 nm, 276 nm; methanol—270 nm, 278 nm ($A_1^1 = 38$ a). No alkaline shift.

Wavelength

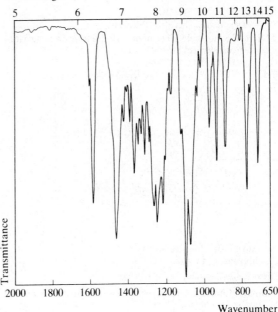

Infra-red Spectrum. Principal peaks at wavenumbers 1092, 1070, 1248, 1262, 1582, 1217 (KBr disk).

Mass Spectrum. Principal peaks at *m/z* 30, 86, 57, 294, 71, 310, 70, 87.

Quantification. SPECTROFLUORIMETRY. In serum or urine: sensitivity <10 ng/ml—E. Ivashkiv, *J. pharm. Sci.*, 1977, *66*, 1168–1172.

GAS CHROMATOGRAPHY–MASS SPECTROMETRY. In serum: detection limit 7 ng/ml—P. T. Funke *et al.*, *J. pharm. Sci.*, 1978, *67*, 653–657.

HIGH PRESSURE LIQUID CHROMATOGRAPHY. In serum: electrochemical detection—P. Surmann, *Arch. Pharm. Berl.*, 1980, *313*, 1052–1054.

Disposition in the Body. Absorbed after oral administration; bioavailability about 30%. It is excreted almost entirely as unchanged drug; about 15 to 21% of the dose is excreted in the urine and 68 to 85% is eliminated in the faeces in 4 days, after oral administration. After intravenous administration, about 75% of a dose is excreted in the urine unchanged.

THERAPEUTIC CONCENTRATION.

Following single oral doses of 60 and 120 mg to 7 subjects, peak plasma concentrations of 0.02 to 0.14 µg/ml (mean 0.07) and 0.05 to 0.25 µg/ml (mean 0.13) were attained in 1 to 4 hours (M. Schäfer-Korting *et al.*, *Eur. J. clin. Pharmac.*, 1984, *26*, 125–127).

Single oral doses of 80 mg to 4 subjects, resulted in peak plasma concentrations of 0.04 to 0.21 µg/ml (mean 0.14) in 1 to 4 hours. During daily oral dosing of 4 subjects with 80 mg a day, peak plasma concentrations of 0.11 to 0.24 µg/ml (mean 0.22) were observed 2 to 4 hours after a morning dose (J. Dreyfuss *et al.*, *J. clin. Pharmac.*, 1979, *19*, 712–720).

HALF-LIFE. Plasma half-life, 6 to 24 hours.

VOLUME OF DISTRIBUTION. About 2 litres/kg.

CLEARANCE. Plasma clearance, about 3 ml/min/kg.

PROTEIN BINDING. In plasma, about 4 to 30% (mean 14).

NOTE. For a review of the pharmacokinetics of nadolol see R. C. Heel *et al.*, *Drugs*, 1980, *20*, 1–23.

Dose. 40 to 240 mg daily.

Naftidrofuryl Oxalate

Vasodilator

Synonym. Nafronyl Oxalate
Proprietary Names. Dusodril; Praxilene.
2-Diethylaminoethyl   3-(1-naphthyl)-2-tetrahydrofurfurylpropionate hydrogen oxalate
$C_{24}H_{33}NO_3, C_2H_2O_4 = 473.6$
CAS—31329-57-4 (naftidrofuryl); *3200-06-4* (oxalate)

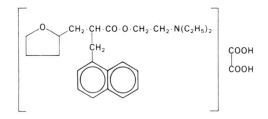

A white powder. M.p. about 108°.
Readily **soluble** in water.

Dissociation Constant. pK_a 8.2 (30°).

Thin-layer Chromatography. *System TA*—Rf 64; *system TB*—Rf 52; *system TC*—Rf 41.

Gas Chromatography. *System GA*—RI 2748.

Ultraviolet Spectrum. Aqueous acid—273 nm, 283 nm (A_1^1 = 141 a). No alkaline shift.

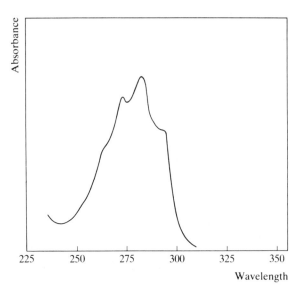

Infra-red Spectrum. Principal peaks at wavenumbers 1730, 1165, 722, 1280, 1620, 1070 (KBr disk).

Mass Spectrum. Principal peaks at *m/z* 86, 99, 100, 141, 87, 71, 44, 58 (naftidrofuryl).

Quantification. HIGH PRESSURE LIQUID CHROMATOGRAPHY. In plasma: sensitivity 20 ng/ml, UV detection—R. R. Brodie *et al.*, *J. Chromat.*, 1979, *164*; *Biomed. Appl.*, *6*, 534–540.

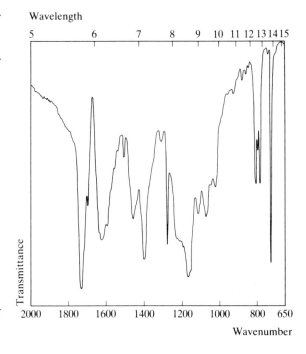

Disposition in the Body. Absorbed after oral administration. It is metabolised by hydrolysis to the free acid, 3-(1-naphthyl)-2-tetrahydrofurfurylpropionic acid. Less than 1% of a dose is excreted in the urine in 48 hours as free or conjugated naftidrofuryl. Most of a dose appears to be excreted in the bile.

THERAPEUTIC CONCENTRATION.
After oral administration of 100 mg to 2 subjects, peak plasma concentrations averaging 0.21 µg/ml were attained in 0.5 to 0.75 hour (R. R. Brodie *et al.*, *ibid.*).

Dose. 300 to 600 mg daily.

Nalbuphine

Narcotic Analgesic

17-Cyclobutylmethyl-7,8-dihydro-14-hydroxy-17-normorphine
$C_{21}H_{27}NO_4 = 357.4$
CAS—20594-83-6

Crystals. M.p. about 231°.

Nalbuphine Hydrochloride
Proprietary Name. Nubain
$C_{21}H_{27}NO_4, HCl = 393.9$
CAS—23277-43-2

Ultraviolet Spectrum. Aqueous acid—284 nm ($A_1^1 = 46$ b); aqueous alkali—297 nm.

Infra-red Spectrum. Principal peaks at wavenumbers 970, 1080, 1033, 1060, 1115, 1495.

Quantification. GAS CHROMATOGRAPHY. In plasma: sensitivity 500 pg/ml, ECD—S. H. Weinstein et al., J. pharm. Sci., 1978, 67, 547–548.

HIGH PRESSURE LIQUID CHROMATOGRAPHY. In plasma: sensitivity 1 ng, electrochemical detection—C. L. Lake et al., J. Chromat., 1982, 233; Biomed. Appl., 22, 410–416.

Disposition in the Body. Absorbed after oral administration, but there is thought to be considerable first-pass metabolism; rapidly absorbed after intramuscular or subcutaneous injection. The major metabolic reaction is conjugation to form nalbuphine glucuronide (inactive); oxidation to 6-oxonalbuphine occurs, and the desalkyl derivative, 7,8-dihydro-14-hydroxynormorphine, has also been identified as a metabolite. Unchanged nalbuphine, its conjugates, and the two metabolites have been detected in the urine.

THERAPEUTIC CONCENTRATION.
Following a single oral dose of 30 mg to 3 subjects, a peak plasma concentration of about 0.015 µg/ml was attained in 1 hour. Following a single intramuscular dose of 10 mg to 6 subjects, peak plasma concentrations of 0.038 to 0.059 µg/ml (mean 0.052) were attained in 15 to 30 minutes (R. E. S. Bullingham, Pharmacokinetics of Nalbuphine, in Opioid Agonist/Antagonist Drugs in Clinical Practice, W. S. Nimmo and G. Smith (Ed.), Oxford, Excerpta Medica, 1984, pp. 115–122).

HALF-LIFE. Plasma half-life, about 5 hours.

NOTE. For a review of nalbuphine see J. K. Errick and R. C. Heel, Drugs, 1983, 26, 191–211.

Dose. 10 to 20 mg of nalbuphine hydrochloride parenterally, every 3 to 6 hours.

Nalidixic Acid

Antibacterial (Urinary)

Synonym. Nalidixinic Acid
Proprietary Names. NegGram; Negram; Uriben. It is an ingredient of Mictral.
1-Ethyl-1,4-dihydro-7-methyl-4-oxo-1,8-naphthyridine-3-carboxylic acid
$C_{12}H_{12}N_2O_3 = 232.2$
CAS—389-08-2

An almost white or very pale yellow crystalline powder. M.p. 225° to 231°.
Practically **insoluble** in water; soluble 1 in 910 of ethanol and 1 in 35 of chloroform; very slightly soluble in ether; soluble in solutions of alkali hydroxides and carbonates.

Dissociation Constant. pK_a 6.0.

Thin-layer Chromatography. *System TD*—Rf 39; *system TE*—Rf 02; *system TF*—Rf 31.

Ultraviolet Spectrum. Aqueous acid—257 nm ($A_1^1 = 1233$ b), 315 nm; aqueous alkali—258 nm ($A_1^1 = 1120$ a), 334 nm.

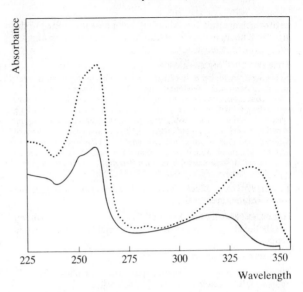

Infra-red Spectrum. Principal peaks at wavenumbers 1613, 1704, 809, 1250, 1225, 1515 (KBr disk).

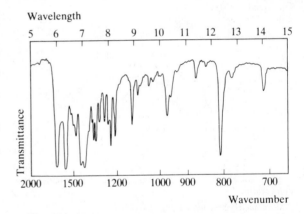

Mass Spectrum. Principal peaks at m/z 188, 189, 159, 132, 53, 173, 131, 145.

Quantification. GAS CHROMATOGRAPHY. In plasma: sensitivity 5 µg/ml, FID—H. Roseboom et al., J. Chromat., 1979, 163; Biomed. Appl., 5, 92–95.

HIGH PRESSURE LIQUID CHROMATOGRAPHY. In plasma or urine: nalidixic acid, 7-hydroxynalidixic acid and 7-carboxynalidixic acid, sensitivity 500 ng/ml, UV detection—G. Cuisinaud et al., J. Chromat., 1980, 181; Biomed. Appl., 7, 399–406.

THIN-LAYER CHROMATOGRAPHY. In plasma: sensitivity 200 ng/ml, fluorescence detection—H. K. L. Hundt and E. C. Barlow, J. Chromat., 1981, 223; Biomed. Appl., 12, 165–172.

Disposition in the Body. Readily absorbed after oral administration. The major metabolite, 7-hydroxynalidixic acid, is active; other metabolites include glucuronide conjugates of nalidixic acid and 7-hydroxynalidixic acid, and a 7-carboxy metabolite, all of which are inactive. About 80% of a dose is excreted in the urine in 8 hours mainly as glucuronide conjugates with about 2 to 3% as unchanged drug.

THERAPEUTIC CONCENTRATION.

Following a single oral dose of 1 g to 11 female subjects, a mean peak plasma concentration of nalidixic acid of 27.3 µg/ml was attained in 1.5 hours; concentrations of 7-hydroxynalidixic acid reached a maximum of about 10 µg/ml within 1 hour. After repeated oral administration of 1 g twice daily to the same subjects, a peak plasma concentration of 33 µg/ml of nalidixic acid was reported on the 7th day. Urinary concentrations of nalidixic acid plus 7-hydroxynalidixic acid following single or multiple dose administration were in excess of about 200 µg/ml for 8 hours in all subjects, and in some cases greater than 50 µg/ml for 12 hours (N. Ferry et al., Clin. Pharmac. Ther., 1981, 29, 695–698).

TOXICITY. Toxic effects have been associated with plasma concentrations greater than 40 µg/ml.

HALF-LIFE. Plasma half-life, nalidixic acid and the 7-hydroxy metabolite about 7 hours; increased in renal failure to about 20 hours.

VOLUME OF DISTRIBUTION. About 0.4 litre/kg.

PROTEIN BINDING. In plasma, nalidixic acid about 93%, 7-hydroxynalidixic acid about 60%.

Dose. 2 to 4 g daily.

Nalorphine

Narcotic Antagonist

17-Allyl-17-normorphine
$C_{19}H_{21}NO_3 = 311.4$
CAS—62-67-9

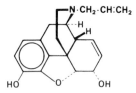

Crystals. M.p. 208°.
Slightly **soluble** in water and ether; soluble in ethanol and chloroform.

Nalorphine Hydrobromide

Proprietary Names. Lethidrone; Norfin.
$C_{19}H_{21}NO_3,HBr = 392.3$
CAS—1041-90-3
A white to creamy-white crystalline powder. M.p. about 206°, with decomposition.
Soluble 1 in 24 of water and 1 in 35 of ethanol. Aqueous solutions may deposit crystals of the dihydrate; the dihydrate is readily soluble in dehydrated alcohol but the solution rapidly yields a deposit of the anhydrous salt.

Nalorphine Hydrochloride

$C_{19}H_{21}NO_3,HCl = 347.8$
CAS—57-29-4
A white crystalline powder which slowly darkens on exposure to air and light. M.p. 260° to 263°.
Soluble 1 in 8 of water and 1 in 35 of ethanol; practically insoluble in chloroform and ether; soluble in dilute solutions of alkali hydroxides.

Dissociation Constant. pK_a 7.8 (20°).

Partition Coefficient. Log P (octanol/pH 7.4), 1.5.

Colour Test. Marquis Test—violet.

Thin-layer Chromatography. *System TA*—Rf 59; *system TB*—Rf 01; *system TC*—Rf 23. (*Acidified iodoplatinate solution,* positive.)

Gas Chromatography. *System GA*—RI 2577.

High Pressure Liquid Chromatography. *System HA*—k' 1.0; *system HC*—k' 0.29.

Ultraviolet Spectrum. Aqueous acid—285 nm ($A_1^1 = 49$ a); aqueous alkali—251 nm ($A_1^1 = 190$ a), 298 nm ($A_1^1 = 81$ a).

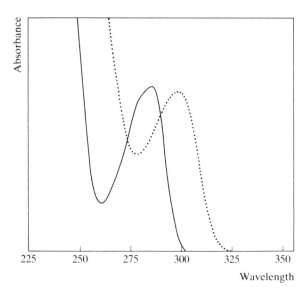

Infra-red Spectrum. Principal peaks at wavenumbers 1505, 1121, 1155, 1304, 805, 945 (nalorphine hydrobromide, KBr disk).

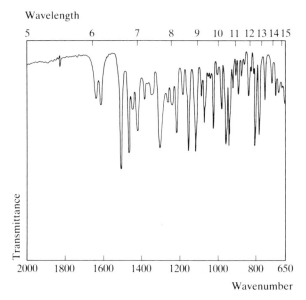

Mass Spectrum. Principal peaks at m/z 311, 312, 41, 188, 80, 82, 81, 241.

Disposition in the Body. Absorbed after oral administration but undergoes extensive first-pass metabolism. It is excreted in the urine mainly as metabolites and glucuronide conjugates with about 2 to 6% of a dose as unchanged drug.

TOXICITY. The estimated minimum lethal dose is 200 mg. The administration of nalorphine to morphine addicts may be followed by a typical withdrawal syndrome.

Dose. 5 to 10 mg of nalorphine hydrobromide intravenously, repeated if necessary.

Naloxone
Narcotic Antagonist

Synonym. Allylnoroxymorphone
17-Allyl-6-deoxy-7,8-dihydro-14-hydroxy-6-oxo-17-normorphine
$C_{19}H_{21}NO_4 = 327.4$
CAS—465-65-6

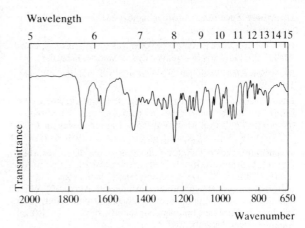

Crystals. M.p. 177° to 180°.
Soluble in chloroform; practically insoluble in ether.

Naloxone Hydrochloride
Proprietary Names. Nalonee; Narcan.
$C_{19}H_{21}NO_4,HCl = 363.8$
CAS—357-08-4 (anhydrous); *51481-60-8* (dihydrate)
A white powder. M.p. 200° to 205°.
Soluble in water; slightly soluble in ethanol; practically insoluble in chloroform and ether.

Dissociation Constant. pK_a 7.9.

Partition Coefficient. Log P (octanol/pH 7.4), 1.5.

Colour Tests. Folin–Ciocalteu Reagent—blue; Liebermann's Test—black; Mandelin's Test—violet → brown; Marquis Test—brown → violet.

Thin-layer Chromatography. *System TA*—Rf 65; *system TB*—Rf 09; *system TC*—Rf 66. (*Acidified iodoplatinate solution,* positive.)

Gas Chromatography. *System GA*—RI 2640.

High Pressure Liquid Chromatography. *System HA*—k′ 1.4; *system HC*—k′ 0.17.

Ultraviolet Spectrum. Aqueous acid—281 nm.

Infra-red Spectrum. Principal peaks at wavenumbers 1244, 1728, 940, 1230, 922, 1050 (KBr disk).

Mass Spectrum. Principal peaks at *m/z* 327, 328, 41, 242, 286, 96, 229, 70.

Quantification. GAS CHROMATOGRAPHY. In biological fluids: sensitivity 5 ng, ECD—P. J. Meffin and K. J. Smith, *J. Chromat.,* 1980, *183*; *Biomed. Appl.,* 9, 352–356.

HIGH PRESSURE LIQUID CHROMATOGRAPHY. In plasma or urine: naloxone and naltrexone, sensitivity 2 to 5 ng/ml for plasma, 10 ng/ml for urine, electrochemical detection—H. Derendorf *et al., J. pharm. Sci.,* 1984, *73*, 621–624.

RADIOIMMUNOASSAY. In plasma: sensitivity <500 pg/ml—E. F. Hahn *et al., J. Pharm. Pharmac.,* 1983, *35*, 833–836.

Wavelength

(Infra-red spectrum figure: Transmittance vs Wavenumber, Wavelength axis marked 5, 6, 7, 8, 9, 10, 11, 12, 13, 14, 15; Wavenumber axis marked 2000, 1800, 1600, 1400, 1200, 1000, 800, 650)

Disposition in the Body. Rapidly absorbed after oral administration but undergoes extensive first-pass metabolism. It is rapidly but incompletely excreted in the urine, mainly as conjugated metabolites, with about 30% of a dose being excreted in 6 hours but only 60% being excreted in 72 hours. Metabolites which have been identified include naloxone-3-glucuronide and the *N*-desalkyl, and 6-hydroxy derivatives together with their glucuronide conjugates.

THERAPEUTIC CONCENTRATION.
Following intravenous administration of 0.4 mg to 9 subjects, mean serum concentrations of 0.01 μg/ml were reported after 2 minutes (S. H. Ngai *et al., Anesthesiology,* 1976, *44*, 398–401).
During constant intravenous infusion of 0.02 mg/min to 3 subjects, steady-state plasma concentrations of 0.014, 0.015 and 0.030 μg/ml were reported (E. F. Hahn *et al., J. Pharm. Pharmac.,* 1983, *35*, 833–836.)

HALF-LIFE. Plasma half-life, about 1 to 2 hours.

VOLUME OF DISTRIBUTION. About 3 litres/kg.

CLEARANCE. Plasma clearance, about 20 to 30 ml/min/kg.

PROTEIN BINDING. In plasma, about 40%.

Dose. 0.4 to 2 mg of naloxone hydrochloride parenterally, repeated as necessary.

Naltrexone
Narcotic Antagonist

17-Cyclopropylmethyl-6-deoxy-7,8-dihydro-14-hydroxy-6-oxo-17-normorphine
$C_{20}H_{23}NO_4 = 341.4$
CAS—16590-41-3

Crystals. M.p. 167° to 174°.

Naltrexone Hydrochloride
$C_{20}H_{23}NO_4,HCl = 377.9$
CAS—16676-29-2
A white powder. M.p. 274° to 276°.
Soluble in water, dilute acids, and alkali.

Ultraviolet Spectrum. Aqueous acid—281 nm ($A_1^1 = 34$ b); aqueous alkali—293 nm.

Infra-red Spectrum. Principal peaks at wavenumbers 1716, 1505, 1280, 1639, 1115, 909 (naltrexone hydrochloride, KBr disk).

Mass Spectrum. Principal peaks at m/z 341, 55, 36, 300, 342, 110, 243, 256.

Quantification. GAS CHROMATOGRAPHY. In plasma, erythrocytes, saliva, or urine: naltrexone, 6β-naltrexol and 2-hydroxy-3-methoxy-6β-naltrexol, sensitivity 0.5 to 1 ng/ml in plasma, ECD and FID—K. Verebey et al., J. analyt. Toxicol., 1980, 4, 33–37.

Disposition in the Body. Rapidly and almost completely absorbed after oral administration. It is metabolised by reduction to 6β-naltrexol which has weak activity; both naltrexone and 6β-naltrexol are conjugated with glucuronic acid. About 40% of an oral dose is excreted in the urine in 24 hours, with about 8% of the dose as naltrexone (mainly conjugated), 26% as 6β-naltrexol (mainly unconjugated), and about 4% as free 2-hydroxy-3-methoxy-6β-naltrexol. About 2% of a dose is eliminated in the faeces in 24 hours, mainly as 6β-naltrexol.

THERAPEUTIC CONCENTRATION.

After a single oral dose of 100 mg to 4 subjects, peak plasma concentrations of 0.01 to 0.06 μg/ml (mean 0.04) of naltrexone and 0.08 to 0.13 μg/ml (mean 0.10) of 6β-naltrexol were attained in 1 to 2 hours and 1 to 4 hours, respectively (K. Verebey et al., Clin. Pharmac. Ther., 1976, 20, 315–328).

HALF-LIFE. Plasma half-life, after oral administration, about 10 hours for naltrexone and about 12 hours for 6β-naltrexol; after intravenous administration, naltrexone about 3 hours.

VOLUME OF DISTRIBUTION. About 20 litres/kg.

CLEARANCE. Plasma clearance, about 70 ml/min/kg.

PROTEIN BINDING. In plasma, about 20%.

NOTE. For a review of the pharmacokinetics of naltrexone see B. L. Crabtree, Clin. Pharm., 1984, 3, 273–280.

Dose. Usually 50 mg of naltrexone hydrochloride daily.

Nandrolone   Anabolic Steroid

Synonym. Nortestosterone
17β-Hydroxyestr-4-en-3-one
$C_{18}H_{26}O_2 = 274.4$
CAS—434-22-0

Crystals. Two polymorphic forms occur; m.p. 111° to 112°, and 124°.

Soluble in ethanol, chloroform, and ether.

Nandrolone Decanoate

Synonym. Nortestosterone Decylate
Proprietary Names. Anabolin LA-100; Androlone-D; Deca-Durabolin; Hybolin Decanoate.
$C_{28}H_{44}O_3 = 428.7$
CAS—360-70-3
A white to creamy-white crystalline powder. M.p. 33° to 37°.
Practically **insoluble** in water; soluble 1 in 1 of ethanol; freely soluble in chloroform and ether.

Nandrolone Phenylpropionate

Synonyms. Nandrolone Phenpropionate; 19-Norandrostenolone Phenylpropionate; Nortestosteronum Phenylpropionicum.
Proprietary Names. Androlone; Durabolin; Hybolin Improved; Nandrolin.
$C_{27}H_{34}O_3 = 406.6$
CAS—62-90-8
A white crystalline powder. M.p. 95° to 99°.
Practically **insoluble** in water; soluble 1 in 20 of ethanol; soluble in chloroform.

Thin-layer Chromatography. Nandrolone decanoate: system TP—Rf 88; system TQ—Rf 49; system TR—Rf 97; system TS—Rf 95. Nandrolone phenylpropionate: system TP—Rf 87; system TQ—Rf 48; system TR—Rf 97; system TS—Rf 95.

Ultraviolet Spectrum. Nandrolone decanoate: dehydrated alcohol—240 nm ($A_1^1 = 407$ a). Nandrolone phenylpropionate: dehydrated alcohol—240 nm ($A_1^1 = 430$ a).

Infra-red Spectrum. Principal peaks at wavenumbers 1679, 1733, 1205, 1178, 1255, 692 (nandrolone phenylpropionate).

Disposition in the Body. In man, nandrolone is excreted in the urine mainly as the two metabolites, 19-norandrosterone and 19-noretiocholanolone. In the horse, the major metabolites are 5α-estrane-3β,17α-diol, excreted mainly as the glucuronide conjugate, and its 17β-epimer which is excreted as the sulphate conjugate.

Dose. By intramuscular injection: 25 to 100 mg of nandrolone decanoate every 3 weeks; 25 to 50 mg of nandrolone phenylpropionate weekly.

Naphazoline   Sympathomimetic

2-(1-Naphthylmethyl)-2-imidazoline
$C_{14}H_{14}N_2 = 210.3$
CAS—835-31-4

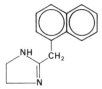

M.p. about 120°.

Naphazoline Hydrochloride

Proprietary Names. Albalon; Clear Eyes; Clera; Naphcon Forte; Privine; Rhino-Mex-N; Vasocon.
$C_{14}H_{14}N_2,HCl = 246.7$
CAS—550-99-2
A white crystalline powder. M.p. about 255°, with decomposition.
Soluble 1 in 6 of water and 1 in 15 of ethanol; very slightly soluble in chloroform; practically insoluble in ether.

Naphazoline Nitrate

Proprietary Names. Imidazyl; Privine; Rinazina. It is an ingredient of Antistin-Privine.
$C_{14}H_{14}N_2,HNO_3 = 273.3$
CAS—5144-52-5
A white crystalline powder. M.p. about 168°.
Soluble 1 in 36 of water and 1 in 16 of ethanol; very slightly soluble in chloroform; practically insoluble in ether.

Dissociation Constant. pK_a 10.9 (20°).

Partition Coefficient. Log P (chloroform/pH 7.4), −0.3.

Colour Tests. Mandelin's Test—brown-violet; Marquis Test—grey-green.

Thin-layer Chromatography. *System TA*—Rf 14; *system TB*—Rf 03; *system TC*—Rf 06. (*Dragendorff spray*, positive; *acidified iodoplatinate solution*, positive; *Marquis reagent*, green.)

Gas Chromatography. *System GA*—RI 2057; *system GB*—RI 2122; *system GC*—RI 2457.

High Pressure Liquid Chromatography. *System HA*—k' 2.4.

Ultraviolet Spectrum. Aqueous acid—271 nm, 281 nm (A_1^1 = 321 a), 288 nm, 291 nm. No alkaline shift.

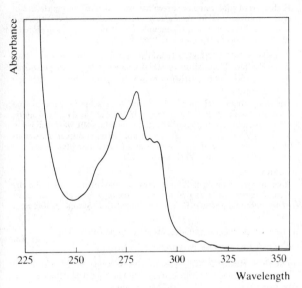

Infra-red Spectrum. Principal peaks at wavenumbers 1615, 780, 1499, 791, 1211, 800 (KBr disk).

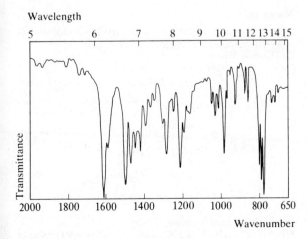

Mass Spectrum. Principal peaks at m/z 209, 210, 141, 115, 153, 208, 46, 181.

Disposition in the Body. Systemic absorption has been reported following topical application of solutions of naphazoline. It is not used systemically but is readily absorbed from the gastro-intestinal tract.

TOXICITY. The estimated minimum lethal dose is 10 mg, intranasally.

Use. Naphazoline hydrochloride and nitrate are used as 0.05 to 0.1% aqueous solutions.

Naphthalene

Synonym. Naphthalin
$C_{10}H_8 = 128.2$
CAS—91-20-3

Colourless transparent scales. M.p. 80°. B.p. 218°.
Practically **insoluble** in water; soluble 1 in 8 of ethanol and 1 in 1.5 of chloroform; very soluble in ether.

Gas Chromatography. *System GA*—RI 1186.

Ultraviolet Spectrum. Ethanol—266 nm (A_1^1 = 411 b), 275 nm (A_1^1 = 454 b), 286 nm (A_1^1 = 307 b).

Naproxen   *Analgesic*

Proprietary Names. Equiproxen (vet.); Floginax; Laser; Naprosyn(e); Proxen; Xenar.
(+)-2-(6-Methoxy-2-naphthyl)propionic acid
$C_{14}H_{14}O_3 = 230.3$
CAS—22204-53-1

A white crystalline powder. M.p. about 156°.
Practically **insoluble** in water; soluble 1 in 25 of ethanol, 1 in 15 of chloroform, and 1 in 40 of ether.

Naproxen Sodium
Proprietary Names. Anaprox; Synflex.
$C_{14}H_{13}NaO_3 = 252.2$
CAS—26159-34-2

Dissociation Constant. pK_a 4.2 (25°).

Colour Tests. Liebermann's Test—black-green; Marquis Test—brown; Sulphuric Acid—orange.

Thin-layer Chromatography. *System TD*—Rf 33; *system TE*—Rf 07; *system TF*—Rf 45; *system TG*—Rf 14. (*Ludy Tenger reagent*, orange.)

Gas Chromatography. *System GA*—RI 2130; *system GD*—retention times of methyl derivative 1.37 and 1.18, relative to *n*-$C_{16}H_{34}$.

High Pressure Liquid Chromatography. *System HD*—k' 3.3; *system HV*—retention time 0.67 relative to meclofenamic acid.

Ultraviolet Spectrum. Aqueous acid—262 nm ($A_1^1 = 208$ b), 272 nm ($A_1^1 = 215$ b), 315 nm ($A_1^1 = 52$ b), 328 nm ($A_1^1 = 63$ b); aqueous alkali—261 nm ($A_1^1 = 218$ b), 271 nm ($A_1^1 = 218$ b), 316 nm, 330 nm.

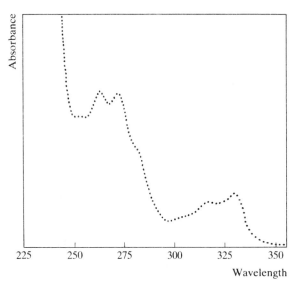

Infra-red Spectrum. Principal peaks at wavenumbers 1724, 1174, 1155, 1223, 1190, 1681 (KBr disk).

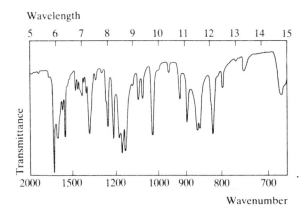

Mass Spectrum. Principal peaks at *m/z* 185, 230, 141, 186, 184, 115, 170, 153.

Quantification. ULTRAVIOLET SPECTROPHOTOMETRY. In serum—M. Holzbecher *et al.*, *Clin. Biochem.*, 1979, *12*, 66–67.

SPECTROFLUORIMETRY. In serum: detection limit 500 ng/ml—M. Anttila, *J. pharm. Sci.*, 1977, *66*, 433–434.

GAS CHROMATOGRAPHY. In serum: sensitivity 2 µg/ml, FID—S. S. Weber *et al.*, *Ther. Drug Monit.*, 1981, *3*, 75–83. In urine: naproxen and metabolites, FID—S. H. Wan and S. B. Matin, *J. Chromat.*, 1979, *170*, 473–478.

HIGH PRESSURE LIQUID CHROMATOGRAPHY. In plasma or urine: naproxen and 6-O-desmethylnaproxen, sensitivity 100 ng/ml, fluorescence detection—J. W. A. van Loenhout *et al.*, *J. liq. Chromat.*, 1982, *5*, 549–561.

Disposition in the Body. Readily and almost completely absorbed after oral or rectal administration. About 50% of a dose is excreted in the urine in 24 hours and about 94% in 5 days together with about 1 to 2% in the faeces. Of the material excreted in the urine, approximately 60% is conjugated naproxen, 5% is 6-O-desmethylnaproxen, and 20% is conjugated desmethylnaproxen. Less than 10% of the excreted material is unchanged drug.

Hydrolysis of conjugated naproxen has been reported during storage of urine samples, and assays carried out immediately after collection suggested that only very small amounts of unchanged drug were excreted (R. A. Upton *et al.*, *J. pharm. Sci.*, 1980, *69*, 1254–1257).

THERAPEUTIC CONCENTRATION. Plasma concentrations are dose-dependent at doses of up to 500 mg twice daily; at larger doses the increase in concentration is non-linear and renal clearance is accelerated.

Following single oral doses of 250 mg to 6 subjects, peak plasma concentrations of 26 to 51 µg/ml (mean 38) were attained in 2 to 4 hours; peak plasma concentrations of 49 to 69 µg/ml (mean 60), were attained in 3 subjects, 2 hours after a single oral dose of 500 mg; peak concentrations of the desmethyl metabolite were about 0.1 to 0.2 µg/ml (G. Tomson *et al.*, *Clin. Pharmac. Ther.*, 1981, *29*, 168–173).

TOXICITY.

A serum concentration of 414 µg/ml was reported in one subject 15 hours after the ingestion of 25 g of naproxen; the only toxic effect was mild gastro-intestinal distress (E. W. Fredell and L. J. Strand, *J. Am. med. Ass.*, 1977, *238*, 938).

HALF-LIFE. Plasma half-life, 10 to 20 hours (mean 14).

VOLUME OF DISTRIBUTION. About 0.1 litre/kg.

PROTEIN BINDING. In plasma, more than 99% at normal therapeutic concentrations; decreased at higher plasma concentrations and in subjects with liver disease.

NOTE. For a review of naproxen see R. N. Brogden *et al.*, *Drugs*, 1979, *18*, 241–277.

Dose. Usually 0.5 to 1 g daily.

Narceine   *Alkaloid*

6-{[6-(2-Dimethylaminoethyl)-4-methoxy-1,3-benzodioxol-5-yl]acetyl}-2,3-dimethoxybenzoic acid
$C_{23}H_{27}NO_8,3H_2O = 499.5$
CAS—131-28-2 (anhydrous)

An alkaloid present in opium.

White silky crystals. M.p. 170° to 171°. The anhydrous substance melts at about 138° and is very hygroscopic.

Slightly **soluble** in water; soluble in ethanol; practically insoluble in chloroform and ether.

Narceine Hydrochloride

$C_{23}H_{27}NO_8,HCl = 481.9$
CAS—4901-03-5
Prismatic crystals. M.p. 192° to 193°.
Slightly **soluble** in hot water and ether; soluble in hot ethanol.

Dissociation Constant. pK_a 3.8 (20°).

Colour Tests. Liebermann's Test—black; Mandelin's Test—green-brown; Marquis Test—brown → green.

Thin-layer Chromatography. *System TA*—Rf 52; *system TB*—Rf 00; *system TC*—Rf 03. (*Acidified iodoplatinate solution,* positive.)

High Pressure Liquid Chromatography. *System HA*—k' 0.7.

Ultraviolet Spectrum. Aqueous acid—277 nm ($A_1^1 = 306$ a). No alkaline shift.

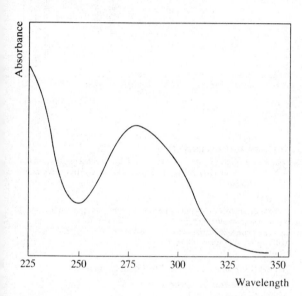

Infra-red Spectrum. Principal peaks at wavenumbers 1253, 1582, 1060, 1090, 1000, 1047 (KCl disk).

Mass Spectrum. Principal peaks at *m/z* 58, 427, 234, 59, 50, 42, 428, 91.

Natamycin

Antifungal

Synonym. Pimaricin
Proprietary Names. Natafucin; Pimafucin(e).
$C_{33}H_{47}NO_{13} = 665.7$
CAS—7681-93-8
An antibiotic produced by the growth of *Streptomyces natalensis.*
A white crystalline powder, which may discolour slightly on storage.
Very slightly **soluble** in water and ethanol; practically insoluble in chloroform; readily soluble in dilute acids and alkalis, forming salts.

Ultraviolet Spectrum. Acid methanol—290 nm ($A_1^1 = 795$ b), 303 nm ($A_1^1 = 1250$ b), 318 nm ($A_1^1 = 1145$ b).

Infra-red Spectrum. Principal peaks at wavenumbers 1062, 1002, 1563, 1709, 1101, 1258 (KBr disk).

Uses. Topically in concentrations of 2 to 5%; by inhalation in a dose of 7.5 mg daily.

Nealbarbitone

Barbiturate

Synonyms. Alneobarbital; Nealbarbital; Neallymalum.
5-Allyl-5-neopentylbarbituric acid
$C_{12}H_{18}N_2O_3 = 238.3$
CAS—561-83-1

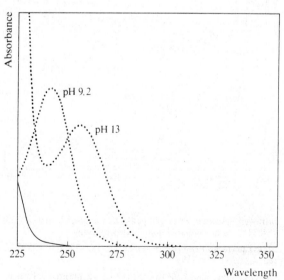

A white or slightly cream-coloured powder. M.p. 155° to 157°.
Soluble 1 in 5000 of water, 1 in 4 of ethanol, 1 in 80 of chloroform, and 1 in 5 of ether; soluble in aqueous solutions of alkalis.

Dissociation Constant. pK_a 7.2 (20°).

Thin-layer Chromatography. *System TD*—Rf 58; *system TE*—Rf 39; *system TF*—Rf 69; *system TH*—Rf 78. (*Mercurous nitrate spray,* black; *acidified potassium permanganate solution,* yellow-brown; *Zwikker's reagent,* pink.)

Gas Chromatography. *System GA*—RI 1720; *system GF*—RI 2460.

High Pressure Liquid Chromatography. *System HG*—k' 10.22; *system HH*—k' 6.19.

Ultraviolet Spectrum. *Borax buffer 0.05M* (pH 9.2)—240 nm ($A_1^1 = 396$ b); M sodium hydroxide (pH 13)—255 nm ($A_1^1 = 303$ b).

Infra-red Spectrum. Principal peaks at wavenumbers 1695, 1752, 1265, 833, 1205, 775 (KBr disk).

Mass Spectrum. Principal peaks at *m/z* 57, 41, 141, 167, 39, 83, 55, 182.

Dose. Nealbarbitone has been given in doses of up to 200 mg as a hypnotic.

Nefopam   *Analgesic*

3,4,5,6-Tetrahydro-5-methyl-1-phenyl-1*H*-2,5-benzoxazocine
$C_{17}H_{19}NO = 253.3$
CAS—13669-70-0

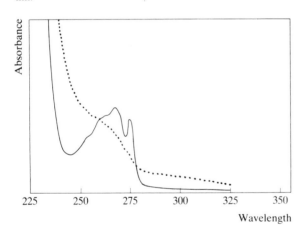

Nefopam Hydrochloride

Proprietary Names. Acupan; Ajan.
$C_{17}H_{19}NO,HCl = 289.8$
CAS—23327-57-3
A white crystalline powder. M.p. about 252°, with decomposition.
Soluble in water, chloroform, and methanol.

Dissociation Constant. pK_a 9.2.

Colour Tests. Liebermann's Test—brown-orange → brown; Marquis Test—orange → brown; Sulphuric Acid—orange.

Thin-layer Chromatography. *System TA*—Rf 50; *system TB*—Rf 33; *system TC*—Rf 32.

Gas Chromatography. *System GA*—RI 2000; *system GF*—RI 2380.

High Pressure Liquid Chromatography. *System HA*—k′ 3.0.

Ultraviolet Spectrum. Aqueous acid—267 nm ($A_1^1 = 29$ b), 275 nm.

Infra-red Spectrum. Principal peaks at wavenumbers 720, 760, 775, 1112, 1130, 1038 (nefopam hydrochloride).

Mass Spectrum. Principal peaks at *m/z* 58, 179, 180, 225, 178, 165, 42, 210.

Quantification. GAS CHROMATOGRAPHY. In plasma, saliva, or cerebrospinal fluid: sensitivity 5 ng/ml, AFID—S. F. Chang *et al.*, *J. Chromat.*, 1981, *226*; *Biomed. Appl.*, *15*, 79–89.

Disposition in the Body. Rapidly absorbed after oral administration. It is extensively metabolised, less than 5% of a dose being excreted unchanged in the urine; metabolites include desmethylnefopam and its *N*-glucuronide, and nefopam *N*-oxide. About 87% of a dose is excreted in the urine and about 8% in the faeces in 5 days.

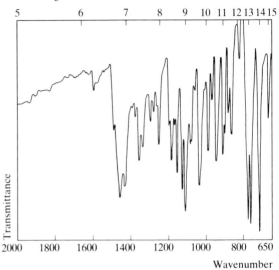

THERAPEUTIC CONCENTRATION.

Following a single oral dose of 90 mg, peak blood concentrations of 0.07 to 0.15 µg/ml were reported at 1 to 3 hours (per R. C. Heel *et al.*, *Drugs*, 1980, *19*, 249–267).

TOXICITY.

A postmortem blood concentration of 11.9 µg/ml was reported in a suicide due to nefopam overdose; in a second non-fatal overdose case, a plasma concentration of 3.8 µg/ml was reported 3 hours after ingestion, declining to 0.9 µg/ml at 19 hours (D. M. Piercy *et al.*, *Br. med. J.*, 1981, *283*, 1508–1509).

HALF-LIFE. Plasma half-life, 3 to 8 hours (mean 4).

PROTEIN BINDING. In plasma, about 75%.

NOTE. For a review of nefopam see R. C. Heel *et al.*, *Drugs*, 1980, *19*, 249–267.

Dose. 90 to 270 mg of nefopam hydrochloride daily.

Neomycin   *Antibiotic*

A mixture of the 2 isomers, neomycins B and C, with neomycin A (neamine), an inactive component and degradation product of neomycins B and C.
$C_{23}H_{46}N_6O_{13} = 614.6$ (neomycin B)
CAS—1404-04-2 (neomycin); 3947-65-7 (neomycin A); 119-04-0 (neomycin B); 66-86-4 (neomycin C)
Neomycin is obtained from certain selected strains of *Streptomyces fradiae*.

Neomycin Sulphate

Synonyms. Fradiomycin Sulphate; Neomycin.
Proprietary Names. It is an ingredient of many proprietary preparations—see *Martindale, The Extra Pharmacopoeia*, 28th Edn.
CAS—1405-10-3
A white to yellowish-white hygroscopic powder.
Slowly **soluble** 1 in 1 of water; very slightly soluble in ethanol; practically insoluble in chloroform and ether.

Neomycin Undecenoate

Synonym. Neomycin Undecylenate
Proprietary Names. It is an ingredient of Audicort.

CAS—1406-04-8
A yellowish-white to pale yellow, waxy, unctuous powder.
Practically **insoluble** in water; very soluble in ethanol; soluble in chloroform.

Thin-layer Chromatography. *System TA*—Rf 00. (*Acidified potassium permanganate solution*, positive.)

Ultraviolet Spectrum. No significant absorption, 230 to 360 nm.

Dose. As an intestinal antiseptic, up to 12 g of neomycin sulphate daily, by mouth; it is also applied topically.

Neopine   *Alkaloid*

Synonym. β-Codeine. It has been incorrectly called hydroxy-codeine.

4,5-Epoxy-3-methoxy-9a-methylmorphin-8-en-6-ol
$C_{18}H_{21}NO_3 = 299.4$
CAS—467-14-1

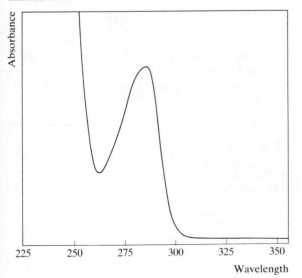

An alkaloid obtained from opium.
Crystals. M.p. about 127°.
Slightly **soluble** in water; soluble in chloroform.

Neopine Hydrobromide

$C_{18}H_{21}NO_3,HBr = 380.3$
Crystals which darken at about 240° and decompose at about 283°.
Practically **insoluble** in water hence ease of separation from other opium alkaloids.

Colour Test. Marquis Test—blue-violet.

Thin-layer Chromatography. *System TA*—Rf 35; *system TB*—Rf 05; *system TC*—Rf 12. (*Acidified iodoplatinate solution*, positive.)

Gas Chromatography. *System GA*—RI 2395.

Ultraviolet Spectrum. Aqueous acid—285 nm ($A_1^1 = 39$ b). No alkaline shift.

Infra-red Spectrum. Principal peaks at wavenumbers 1275, 1500, 1118, 1050, 1250, 782 (KBr disk).

Mass Spectrum. Principal peaks at *m/z* 299, 162, 229, 123, 59, 42, 44, 300.

Neostigmine Bromide   *Anticholinesterase*

Synonym. Synstigmine Bromide
Proprietary Name. Prostigmin(e) (tablets)
3-(Dimethylcarbamoyloxy)-*NNN*-trimethylanilinium bromide
$C_{12}H_{19}BrN_2O_2 = 303.2$
CAS—59-99-4 (neostigmine); *114-80-7* (bromide)

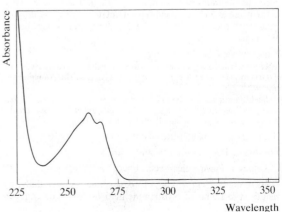

Colourless crystals or a white crystalline, slightly hygroscopic powder. M.p. 171° to 176°, with decomposition.
Soluble 1 in 0.5 of water, 1 in 8 of ethanol, and 1 in 5 of chloroform; practically insoluble in ether.

Neostigmine Methylsulphate

Synonym. Proserinum
Proprietary Name. Prostigmin(e) (injection)
$C_{13}H_{22}N_2O_6S = 334.4$
CAS—51-60-5
Colourless crystals or a white crystalline powder. M.p. 144° to 149°.
Soluble 1 in 0.5 of water and 1 in 6 of ethanol.

Dissociation Constant. pK_a 12.0.

Thin-layer Chromatography. *System TA*—Rf 02. (*Acidified iodoplatinate solution*, positive.)

Gas Chromatography. *System GA*—RI 1770.

High Pressure Liquid Chromatography. *System HA*—k' 4.7 (tailing peak).

Ultraviolet Spectrum. Aqueous acid—260 nm ($A_1^1 = 16$ a), 266 nm. No alkaline shift.

Infra-red Spectrum. Principal peaks at wavenumbers 1711, 1215, 1154, 1176, 948, 690 (KBr disk).

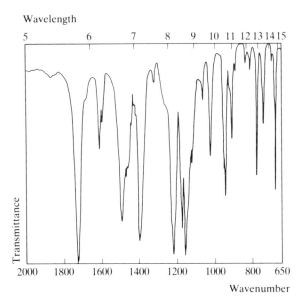

Wavelength

Mass Spectrum. Principal peaks at m/z 72, 42, 208, 108, 65, 73, 66, 39.

Quantification. GAS CHROMATOGRAPHY. In plasma: sensitivity 50 ng/ml, AFID—K. Chan *et al.*, *J. Chromat.*, 1976, *120*, 349–358.

GAS CHROMATOGRAPHY-MASS SPECTROMETRY. In plasma: sensitivity 1 ng/ml—S.- M. Aquilonius *et al.*, *Eur. J. clin. Pharmac.*, 1979, *15*, 367–371.

Disposition in the Body. Poorly absorbed after oral administration. Metabolised by ester hydrolysis to form 3-hydroxytrimethylanilinium bromide, which is active. About 20% of an oral dose is excreted in the urine with less than 5% as unchanged drug; about 50% of an oral dose is eliminated in the faeces. After intramuscular administration, about 80% of a dose is excreted in the urine in 24 hours, with approximately 50% consisting of unchanged drug and 15% as the 3-hydroxytrimethylanilinium metabolite.

THERAPEUTIC CONCENTRATION.
After a single oral dose of 30 mg to 3 subjects, peak plasma concentrations of 0.004 to 0.009 µg/ml were attained in 1 to 2 hours (S.- M. Aquilonius *et al.*, *ibid.*).
Following intravenous administration of 5 mg to 5 subjects, plasma concentrations of 0.84 to 6.25 µg/ml were reported at 2 minutes (N. E. Williams *et al.*, *Br. J. Anaesth.*, 1978, *50*, 1065–1067).

HALF-LIFE. Plasma half-life, about 1 hour.

VOLUME OF DISTRIBUTION. About 1 litre/kg.

CLEARANCE. Plasma clearance, about 11 ml/min/kg.

Dose. Usually 75 to 300 mg of neostigmine bromide daily, by mouth; 1 to 2.5 mg of neostigmine methylsulphate daily, given parenterally.

Nialamide   *Antidepressant (Monoamine Oxidase Inhibitor)*

Proprietary Name. Niamid(e)
2′-(2-Benzylcarbamoylethyl)isonicotinohydrazide
$C_{16}H_{18}N_4O_2 = 298.3$
CAS—51-12-7

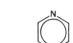

A white crystalline powder. M.p. 151° to 153°.
Soluble 1 in 400 of water, 1 in 40 of ethanol, 1 in 150 of chloroform, and 1 in 10 of methanol.

Partition Coefficient. Log P (octanol/pH 7.4), 0.9.

Colour Tests. Liebermann's Test—red-orange; Mandelin's Test—red; Nessler's Reagent—black.

Thin-layer Chromatography. *System TA*—Rf 70; *system TB*—Rf 02; *system TC*—Rf 25. (*Dragendorff spray*, positive; *acidified iodoplatinate solution*, positive; *Marquis reagent*, brown.)

High Pressure Liquid Chromatography. *System HA*—k′ 1.2 (tailing peak).

Ultraviolet Spectrum. Aqueous acid—266 nm ($A_1^1 = 193$ a); aqueous alkali—307 nm.

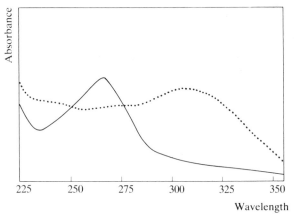

Infra-red Spectrum. Principal peaks at wavenumbers 1625, 1520, 1547, 698, 670, 1600 (KBr disk).

Mass Spectrum. Principal peaks at m/z 91, 177, 44, 106, 45, 78, 123, 51.

Dose. 75 to 150 mg daily.

Nicametate   *Vasodilator*

2-Diethylaminoethyl nicotinate
$C_{12}H_{18}N_2O_2 = 222.3$
CAS—3099-52-3

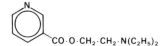

A liquid.

Nicametate Citrate

Proprietary Name. Euclidan
$C_{12}H_{18}N_2O_2, C_6H_8O_7 = 414.4$
CAS—1641-74-3
A white crystalline powder.

Colour Test. Cyanogen Bromide—orange.

Thin-layer Chromatography. *System TA*—Rf 56; *system TB*—Rf 41; *system TC*—Rf 35. (*Acidified iodoplatinate solution*, positive.)

Gas Chromatography. *System GA*—nicametate RI 1608, nicotinic acid RI 1335.

Ultraviolet Spectrum. Aqueous acid—261 nm ($A_1^1 = 120$ b).

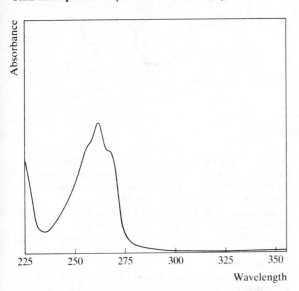

Infra-red Spectrum. Principal peaks at wavenumbers 1729, 1283, 1594, 1130, 1116, 743 (KBr disk).

Mass Spectrum. Principal peaks at *m/z* 86, 30, 58, 123, 78, 51, 29, 42; nicotinic acid 123, 105, 78, 51, 106, 77, 124, 50.

Disposition in the Body. Slowly hydrolysed to nicotinic acid and diethylaminoethanol.

Dose. 300 mg of nicametate citrate daily.

Nicergoline   *Vasodilator*

Synonyms. Nicotergoline; Nimergoline.

Proprietary Name. Sermion
10α-Methoxy-1,6-dimethylergolin-8β-ylmethyl   5-bromonicotinate
$C_{24}H_{26}BrN_3O_3 = 484.4$
CAS—27848-84-6

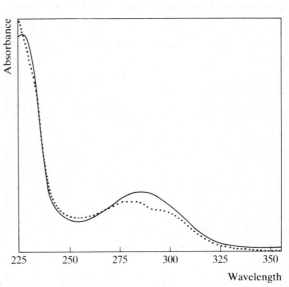

A yellowish-white crystalline powder. M.p. 136° to 138°. Practically **insoluble** in water; soluble in ethanol and chloroform; slightly soluble in ether.

Colour Tests. Liebermann's Test—black; Mandelin's Test—violet-brown → brown; Marquis Test—blue → grey; Sulphuric Acid—violet.

Thin-layer Chromatography. *System TA*—Rf 64. (*Acidified iodoplatinate solution*, positive.)

Gas Chromatography. *System GA*—not eluted.

Ultraviolet Spectrum. Aqueous acid—286 nm; aqueous alkali—280 nm; ethanol—287 nm ($A_1^1 = 200$ b).

Infra-red Spectrum. Principal peaks at wavenumbers 1281, 751, 1718, 1306, 1075, 1103 (KBr disk).

Quantification. RADIOIMMUNOASSAY. In plasma or urine: sensitivity <60 pg/ml—C. A. Bizollon *et al.*, *Eur. J. nucl. Med.*, 1982, 7, 318–321.

Disposition in the Body. Extensively metabolised mainly by hydrolysis and N^1-demethylation and excreted in the urine as free and conjugated (glucuronide) metabolites.

REFERENCE. F. Arcamone *et al.*, *Biochem. Pharmac.*, 1972, *21*, 2205–2213.

Dose. Usually 15 mg daily.

Niclosamide   *Anthelmintic*

Synonym. Phenasale
Proprietary Names. Mansonil (vet.); Niclocide; Trédémine; Yomesan.

2′,5-Dichloro-4′-nitrosalicylanilide
$C_{13}H_8Cl_2N_2O_4 = 327.1$
CAS—50-65-7

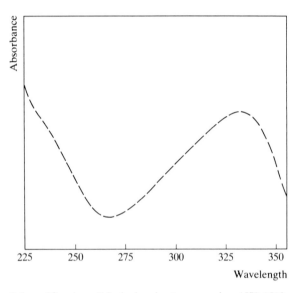

A cream-coloured powder. M.p. about 228°.

Practically **insoluble** in water; soluble 1 in 150 of ethanol, 1 in 400 of chloroform, and 1 in 350 of ether; soluble in acetone.

Colour Tests. Mandelin's Test—green; Methanolic Potassium Hydroxide—yellow.

Thin-layer Chromatography. *System TA*—Rf 91. (*Acidified iodoplatinate solution*, positive.)

Ultraviolet Spectrum. Aqueous alkali—334 nm, 377 nm; methanol—333 nm ($A_1^1 = 527$ b).

Infra-red Spectrum. Principal peaks at wavenumbers 1572, 1515, 1613, 1285, 1650, 1218 (KBr disk).

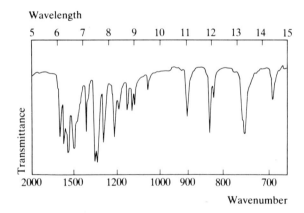

Dose. Usually 2 g as a single dose.

Nicofuranose

Vasodilator

Synonyms. Tetranicotinoylfructofuranose; Tetranicotinoylfructose.

Proprietary Name. Bradilan

β-D-Fructofuranose 1,3,4,6-tetranicotinate
$C_{30}H_{24}N_4O_{10} = 600.5$
CAS—15351-13-0

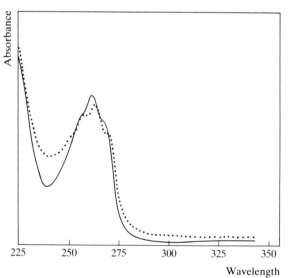

A creamy-white crystalline powder. M.p. 132° to 143°.

Practically **insoluble** in water; soluble 1 in 4 of chloroform and 1 in 70 of methanol; sparingly soluble in dilute solutions of hydrochloric acid and sodium hydroxide.

Colour Tests. Add 50 mg to 5 ml of *potassium cupri-tartrate solution* and heat to boiling for 1 minute—red precipitate.

Fuse 50 mg with 10 mg of 2,4-dinitrochlorobenzene, cool, add about 3 ml of ethanol and 1 ml of M sodium hydroxide—intense red-violet colour.

Thin-layer Chromatography. *System TA*—Rf 61; *system TB*—Rf 42; *system TC*—Rf 70. (*Acidified iodoplatinate solution*, positive.)

Ultraviolet Spectrum. Aqueous acid—262 nm ($A_1^1 = 380$ b); aqueous alkali—263 nm.

Infra-red Spectrum. Principal peaks at wavenumbers 1721, 1271, 1107, 737, 1587, 1022 (KBr disk).

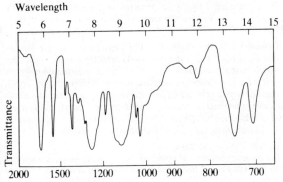

Wavelength

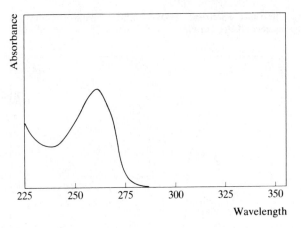

Wavelength

Infra-red Spectrum. Principal peaks at wavenumbers 1680, 1698, 703, 1618, 1594, 1026 (KBr disk).

Mass Spectrum. Principal peaks at m/z 123, 106, 78, 51, 105, 50, 77, 52; nicotinic acid 123, 105, 78, 51, 106, 77, 124, 50.

Mass Spectrum. Principal peaks at m/z 122, 78, 106, 51, 50, 52, 44, 123; nicotinic acid 123, 105, 78, 51, 106, 77, 124, 50.

Disposition in the Body. Slowly hydrolysed in the small intestine to nicotinic acid which is readily absorbed.

Disposition in the Body. It is excreted in the urine as unchanged drug, nicotinic acid, N-methylnicotinamide, and nicotinuric acid.

Nicotinamide is a metabolite of nikethamide.

THERAPEUTIC CONCENTRATION.

Following a single oral dose of 500 mg to 27 subjects, a mean peak plasma concentration of 0.72 µg/ml was attained in 3 hours (H. A. Salmi and H. Frey, *Curr. ther. Res.*, 1974, *16*, 669–674).

Dose. Up to 250 mg daily.

Dose. 1.5 to 3 g daily.

Nicotine   *Insecticide*

Proprietary Name. Nicorette (anti-smoking preparation)

3-(1-Methylpyrrolidin-2-yl)pyridine
$C_{10}H_{14}N_2 = 162.2$
CAS—54-11-5

Nicotinamide   *Vitamin*

Synonyms. Niacinamide; Nicotinic Acid Amide; Nicotylamide; Vitamin PP.
Proprietary Names. Nicobion. It is an ingredient of Apisate and Effico.

Pyridine-3-carboxamide
$C_6H_6N_2O = 122.1$
CAS—98-92-0

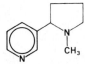

An alkaloid obtained from the dried leaves of the tobacco plant, *Nicotiana tabacum* (Solanaceae).

A colourless to pale yellow, very hygroscopic, oily liquid with an unpleasant pungent odour. It gradually becomes brown on exposure to air or light. Wt per ml about 1.01 g. B.p. 247°, with decomposition. Refractive index 1.5280.

Soluble in water, ethanol, chloroform, and ether.

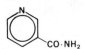

A white crystalline powder or colourless crystals. M.p. 128° to 131°.
Soluble 1 in 1 of water and 1 in 1.5 of ethanol; slightly soluble in chloroform and ether.

Dissociation Constant. pK_a 3.3 (20°).

Partition Coefficient. Log P (octanol), −0.4.

Colour Tests. Cyanogen Bromide—orange; Nessler's Reagent—brown-orange.

Thin-layer Chromatography. *System TA*—Rf 54, streaking.

Gas Chromatography. *System GA*—nicotinamide RI 1436, nicotinic acid RI 1335.

Ultraviolet Spectrum. Aqueous acid—261 nm ($A_1^1 = 451$ a).

Dissociation Constant. pK_a 3.2, 7.9 (25°).

Colour Test. Cyanogen Bromide—orange.

Thin-layer Chromatography. *System TA*—Rf 54; *system TB*—Rf 39; *system TC*—Rf 35. (*Dragendorff spray*, positive; *acidified iodoplatinate solution*, positive.)

Gas Chromatography. *System GA*—nicotine RI 1348, cotinine RI 1678; *system GB*—nicotine RI 1375, cotinine RI 1736; *system GC*—nicotine RI 1573, cotinine RI 2111; *system GF*—nicotine RI 1525, cotinine RI 2195.

High Pressure Liquid Chromatography. *System HA*—nicotine k′ 1.1, cotinine k′ 0.2.

Ultraviolet Spectrum. Aqueous acid—259 nm ($A_1^1 = 338$ a); aqueous alkali—261 nm.

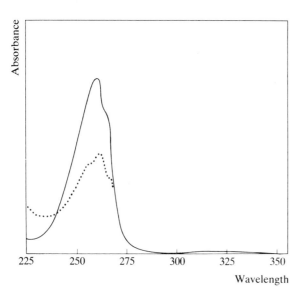

Wavelength

Infra-red Spectrum. Principal peaks at wavenumbers 712, 1022, 810, 1575, 1310, 1040 (thin film).

Wavelength

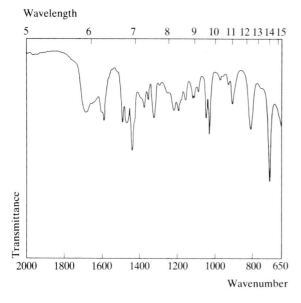

Wavenumber

Mass Spectrum. Principal peaks at m/z 84, 133, 42, 162, 161, 105, 77, 119; cotinine 98, 176, 42, 118, 41, 119, 51, 175; nicotine-1'-N-oxide 84, 178, 161, 133, 118, –, –, –.

Quantification. GAS CHROMATOGRAPHY. In plasma or urine: detection limits in plasma, 5 ng/ml for nicotine and cotinine and 15 ng/ml for the N-oxide; detection limits in urine, 30 ng/ml for nicotine and cotinine and 100 ng/ml for the N-oxide, FID—G. Stehlich et al., J. Chromat., 1982, 232; Biomed. Appl., 21, 295–303.

GAS CHROMATOGRAPHY (CAPILLARY COLUMN). In plasma: sensitivity 1 ng/ml for nicotine, 5 ng/ml for cotinine, AFID—K. G. Verebey et al., J. analyt. Toxicol., 1982, 6, 294–296.

HIGH PRESSURE LIQUID CHROMATOGRAPHY. In plasma or urine: detection limit 2 ng/ml for nicotine or cotinine in urine, UV detection—M. P. Maskarinec et al., J. analyt. Toxicol., 1978, 2, 124–126.

Disposition in the Body. Readily absorbed from the gastro-intestinal tract, the respiratory tract, and from intact skin, and widely distributed throughout the tissues. It is metabolised by oxidation to cotinine and nicotine-1'-N-oxide followed by further degradation to produce hydroxycotinine, norcotinine, and a ring cleavage product. About 5% is excreted unchanged in the urine in 24 hours and about 10% as cotinine; the excretion of unchanged drug is decreased if the urine is alkaline.

BLOOD CONCENTRATION.

In a group of 150 habitual smokers, nicotine concentrations in samples of plasma withdrawn 2 minutes after smoking were in the range 0.003 to 0.063 µg/ml (mean 0.019); corresponding cotinine concentrations ranged from 0.02 to 0.26 µg/ml (mean 0.22) (M. J. Kogan et al., J. forens. Sci., 1981, 26, 6–11).

TOXICITY. Nicotine is highly toxic and, in acute poisoning, death may occur within a few minutes due to respiratory failure arising from paralysis of the respiratory muscles. The lethal dose for an adult is between 40 and 60 mg. Blood concentrations greater than 5 µg/ml may be fatal. The maximum permissible atmospheric concentration is 0.5 mg/m³.

In 5 adults who ingested 20 to 25 g of nicotine and died within 1 hour, postmortem blood concentrations were between 11 and 63 µg/ml (mean 29) (R. C. Baselt and R. H. Cravey, J. analyt. Toxicol., 1977, 1, 81–103).

HALF-LIFE. After inhalation or parenteral administration, plasma half-life, nicotine 0.5 to 2 hours, cotinine 6 to 16 hours (mean 11).

VOLUME OF DISTRIBUTION. About 1 to 3 litres/kg.

CLEARANCE. Plasma clearance, 10 to 30 ml/min/kg.

Nicotinic Acid   *Vitamin/Vasodilator*

Synonym. Niacin
Proprietary Names. Nico-400; Nicobid; Nicolar; Niconacid; Nico-Span; Nicotinex; Nicyl; Vasotherm. It is an ingredient of Equivert and Pernivit.
Pyridine-3-carboxylic acid
$C_6H_5NO_2 = 123.1$
CAS—59-67-6

White or creamy-white crystals or crystalline powder. M.p. 234° to 237°.

Soluble 1 in 55 to 1 in 60 of water and 1 in 100 of ethanol; very slightly soluble in chloroform; practically insoluble in ether; soluble in solutions of alkali hydroxides and carbonates.

Dissociation Constant. pK_a 2.0 (—N=), 4.8 (—COOH), (25°).

Colour Test. Cyanogen Bromide—orange.

Thin-layer Chromatography. System TA—Rf 58; system TD—Rf 01; system TE—Rf 00; system TF—Rf 00.

Gas Chromatography. *System GA*—RI 1335.

Ultraviolet Spectrum. Methanol—263 nm ($A_1^1 = 229$ a).

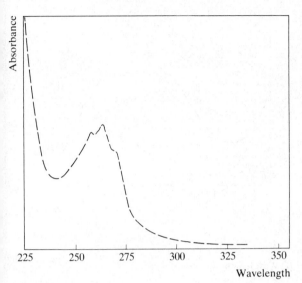

Infra-red Spectrum. Principal peaks at wavenumbers 1300, 744, 1710, 1042, 694, 1180 (KBr disk).

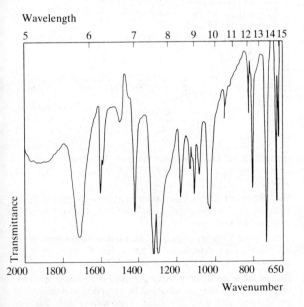

Mass Spectrum. Principal peaks at *m/z* 123, 105, 78, 51, 106, 77, 124, 50; *N*-methylnicotinamide 78, 106, 135, 136, 51, 50, 79, 52.

Quantification. HIGH PRESSURE LIQUID CHROMATOGRAPHY. In plasma or urine: nicotinic acid and nicotinuric acid, sensitivity 500 ng/ml, UV detection—N. Hengen *et al.*, *Clin. Chem.*, 1978,

24, 1740–1743. In plasma: nicotinic acid, nicotinuric acid and nicotinamide, sensitivity 100 ng/ml, 500 ng/ml and 1 µg/ml, respectively—K. Takikawa *et al.*, *J. Chromat.*, 1982, *233*; *Biomed. Appl.*, *22*, 343–348.

Disposition in the Body. Readily absorbed after oral administration. Metabolised to *N*-methylnicotinamide, *N*-methyl-6-oxo-pyridine-3-carboxamide, *N*-methyl-4-oxopyridine-3-carboxamide, and by glycine conjugation to nicotinuric acid. It is rapidly excreted in the urine, and after administration of therapeutic doses about 34% is excreted unchanged in 6 hours. Nicotinic acid is a metabolite of nicergoline, nicotinamide, and nicotinyl tartrate.

THERAPEUTIC CONCENTRATION.

After a single oral dose of 300 mg to 5 subjects, peak plasma concentrations of 3.5 to 18.4 µg/ml (mean 9.3) were attained in about 40 minutes (M. Lesne *et al.*, *Pharm. Acta Helv.*, 1976, *51*, 367–370).

HALF-LIFE. Plasma half-life, about 0.3 to 0.8 hour.

DISTRIBUTION IN BLOOD. Plasma: whole blood ratio, 0.01.

NOTE. For a review of the pharmacokinetics of nicotinic acid see R. Gugler, *Clin. Pharmacokinet.*, 1978, *3*, 425–439.

Dose. Up to 500 mg daily.

Nicotinyl Alcohol   *Vasodilator*

Synonyms. 3-Hydroxymethylpyridine; Nicotinic Alcohol; 3-Pyridinemethanol; *β*-Pyridylcarbinol.

3-Pyridylmethanol

$C_6H_7NO = 109.1$

CAS—100-55-0

A very hygroscopic liquid. Refractive index 1.5425.
Very **soluble** in water and ether.

Nicotinyl Tartrate

Proprietary Names. Roniacol; Ronicol; Tebarcon.

$C_6H_7NO,C_4H_6O_6 = 259.2$

CAS—6164-87-0

A white crystalline powder. M.p. 146° to 149°.

Soluble in water, ethanol, and ether.

Thin-layer Chromatography. *System TA*—Rf 56; *system TB*—Rf 04; *system TC*—Rf 17. (*Dragendorff spray*, positive; *acidified iodoplatinate solution*, positive.)

Gas Chromatography. *System GA*—nicotinyl alcohol RI 1215, nicotinic acid RI 1335.

Ultraviolet Spectrum. Aqueous acid—260 nm. No alkaline shift. (See below)

Infra-red Spectrum. Principal peaks at wavenumbers 675, 1262, 1305, 1556, 1215, 788 (KBr disk).

Mass Spectrum. Principal peaks at *m/z* 109, 108, 80, 53, 51, 39, 91, 27; nicotinic acid 123, 105, 78, 51, 106, 77, 124, 50.

Disposition in the Body. Nicotinyl tartrate is absorbed after oral administration and partly metabolised to nicotinic acid. It is excreted in the urine.

Dose. The equivalent of 100 to 200 mg of nicotinyl alcohol daily; up to 600 mg daily given as a sustained-release preparation.

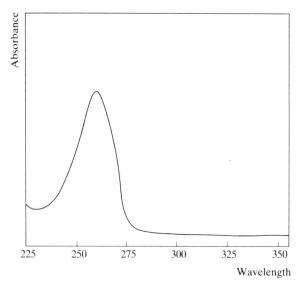

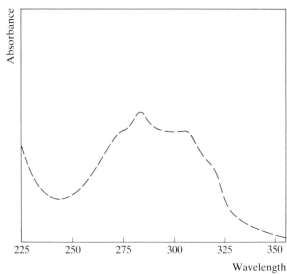

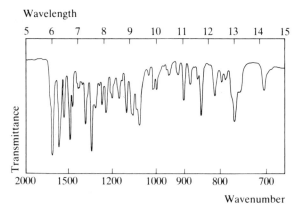

Nicoumalone
Anticoagulant

Synonyms. Acenocoumarol; Acenocumarin.
Proprietary Names. Sinthrome; Sintrom.
4-Hydroxy-3-[1-(4-nitrophenyl)-3-oxobutyl]coumarin
$C_{19}H_{15}NO_6 = 353.3$
CAS—152-72-7

An almost white to buff-coloured powder. M.p. about 198°.
Practically **insoluble** in water and ether; soluble 1 in 400 of ethanol and 1 in 200 of chloroform; soluble in solutions of alkali hydroxides.

Dissociation Constant. pK_a 4.7.

Thin-layer Chromatography. *System TD*—Rf 52; *system TE*—Rf 15; *system TF*—Rf 51. (*Acidified iodoplatinate solution*, positive; *acidified potassium permanganate solution*, positive.)

Gas Chromatography. *System GA*—RI 1779.

Ultraviolet Spectrum. Methanol—283 nm ($A_1^1 = 640$ a), 306 nm.

Infra-red Spectrum. Principal peaks at wavenumbers 1686, 1616, 1508, 1070, 762, 1570 (K Br disk).

Mass Spectrum. Principal peaks at *m/z* 310, 121, 353, 311, 43, 120, 92, 296.

Quantification. GAS CHROMATOGRAPHY. In plasma: detection limit 500 pg, ECD—G. Bianchetti *et al.*, *J. Chromat.*, 1976, *124*, 331–335.

HIGH PRESSURE LIQUID CHROMATOGRAPHY. In serum: sensitivity 15 ng/ml, UV detection—F. A. de Wolff *et al.*, *J. analyt. Toxicol.*, 1980, *4*, 156–159.

THIN-LAYER CHROMATOGRAPHY. In plasma: sensitivity 10 ng/ml, fluorescence detection—G. M. J. van Kempen *et al.*, *J. Chromat.*, 1978, *145*; *Biomed. Appl.*, *2*, 332–335.

Disposition in the Body. Readily absorbed after oral administration. It is extensively metabolised by reduction to a number of metabolites including the amino derivative, and the two diastereoisomers of 4-hydroxy-3-[1-(4-nitrophenyl)-3-hydroxy-butyl]coumarin. Two further inactive metabolites, the 6-hydroxy- and 7-hydroxycoumarin derivatives have been identified in urine. About 50 to 60% of a dose is excreted in the urine in 48 hours, mostly as metabolites, with less than 1% as unchanged drug; about 30% of a dose is eliminated in the faeces.

THERAPEUTIC CONCENTRATION.

After a single oral dose of 12 mg to 2 subjects, peak plasma-nicoumalone concentrations of 0.17 and 0.41 µg/ml were attained in 3 hours; peak concentrations of the amino metabolite of 0.28 and 0.16 µg/ml were reported after 6 to 10 hours (W. Dieterle *et al.*, *Eur. J. clin. Pharmac.*, 1977, *11*, 367–375).

Following a single oral dose of 10 mg to 3 subjects, peak plasma concentrations of about 0.3 µg/ml were attained in 2 to 3 hours; the amino metabolite was not detected in plasma (H. H. W. Thijssen and L. G. Baars, *Br. J. clin. Pharmac.*, 1983, *16*, 491–496).

Following oral administration of 2.5 mg twice daily to 2 subjects, steady-state plasma concentrations of 0.02 to 0.07 µg/ml were reported (G. Bianchetti *et al.*, *J. Chromat.*, 1976, *124*, 331–335).

HALF-LIFE. Plasma half-life, about 8 hours.

VOLUME OF DISTRIBUTION. About 0.3 litre/kg.

CLEARANCE. Plasma clearance, about 0.5 ml/min/kg.

PROTEIN BINDING. In plasma, about 98%.

Dose. Maintenance, 1 to 8 mg daily.

Nifedipine   *Anti-anginal Vasodilator*

Proprietary Names. Adalat(e); Procardia.

Dimethyl 1,4-dihydro-2,6-dimethyl-4-(2-nitrophenyl)pyridine-3,5-dicarboxylate
$C_{17}H_{18}N_2O_6 = 346.3$
CAS—21829-25-4

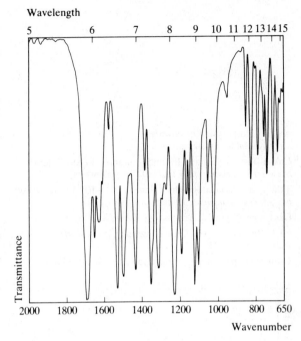

A yellow crystalline powder. M.p. 171° to 175°.
Practically **insoluble** in water; slightly soluble in ethanol; soluble in acetone and chloroform.

Colour Tests. Methanolic Potassium Hydroxide—orange; Sulphuric Acid—orange.

Thin-layer Chromatography. *System TA*—Rf 68; *system TB*—Rf 01; *system TC*—Rf 65.

Gas Chromatography. *System GA*—RI 2170.

High Pressure Liquid Chromatography. *System HA*—k′ 0.2.

Ultraviolet Spectrum. Aqueous acid—238 nm ($A_1^1 = 595$ b), 338 nm ($A_1^1 = 165$ b). No alkaline shift.

Infra-red Spectrum. Principal peaks at wavenumbers 1690, 1225, 1527, 1120, 1496, 1310 (KBr disk).

Mass Spectrum. Principal peaks at *m/z* 329, 284, 224, 268, 330, 285, 225, 270.

Quantification. GAS CHROMATOGRAPHY. In plasma: nifedipine and dimethyl 2,6-dimethyl-4-(2-nitrophenyl)pyridine-3,5-dicarboxylate, detection limit 1 ng/ml, ECD—J. Dokladalova *et al.*, *J. Chromat.*, 1982, *231*; *Biomed. Appl.*, *20*, 451–458.

HIGH PRESSURE LIQUID CHROMATOGRAPHY. In plasma: UV detection—T. Sadanaga *et al.*, *Chem. pharm. Bull.*, 1982, *30*, 3807–3809.

Wavelength

Transmittance

2000   1800   1600   1400   1200   1000   800   650

Wavenumber

Disposition in the Body. Rapidly and almost completely absorbed after oral or sublingual administration. It is completely metabolised. About 70% of a dose is excreted in the urine in 24 hours as metabolites including 5-methoxycarbonyl-2,6-dimethyl-4-(2-nitrophenyl)pyridine-3-carboxylic acid, dimethyl 2,6-dimethyl-4-(2-nitrophenyl)pyridine-3,5-dicarboxylate, and 2-hydroxymethyl-5-methoxycarbonyl-6-methyl-4-(2-nitrophenyl)pyridine-3-carboxylic acid, and its lactone derivative. Up to 15% of a dose is eliminated in the faeces as metabolites in 4 days.

THERAPEUTIC CONCENTRATION.

Following a single oral dose of 10 mg to 9 subjects, a mean peak plasma concentration of 0.07 µg/ml was attained in about 0.6 hour; in a further 3 subjects, absorption was much slower with peak plasma concentrations reported at 2 to 6 hours (T. S. Foster *et al.*, *J. clin. Pharmac.*, 1983, *23*, 161–170).

Following single oral doses of 20, 40, and 60 mg to 8 hypertensive subjects, mean peak plasma concentrations of 0.06, 0.11, and 0.17 µg/ml were reported at 1.6, 2.1, and 1.8 hours, respectively (O. Banzet, *Eur. J. clin. Pharmac.*, 1983, *24*, 145–150).

HALF-LIFE. Plasma half-life, about 2 to 6 hours.

VOLUME OF DISTRIBUTION. About 1 litre/kg.

CLEARANCE. Plasma clearance, about 10 ml/min/kg.

PROTEIN BINDING. In plasma, more than 90%.

Dose. 15 to 60 mg daily.

Nifenazone   *Analgesic*

Synonym. Nicotinylamidoantipyrine

Proprietary Names. Neopiran; Nicopyron; Nicoreumal; Reumatosil.

N-(2,3-Dimethyl-5-oxo-1-phenyl-3-pyrazolin-4-yl)nicotinamide
$C_{17}H_{16}N_4O_2 = 308.3$
CAS—2139-47-1

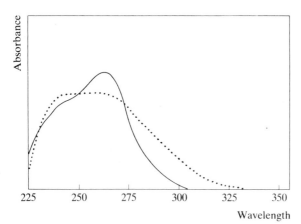

A pale yellow crystalline powder.
Slightly **soluble** in water and ether.

Colour Tests. Cyanogen Bromide—orange; Ferric Chloride—brown-red; Liebermann's Test (100°)—yellow.

Thin-layer Chromatography. System TA—Rf 57. (Acidified potassium permanganate solution, positive.)

Gas Chromatography. System GA—RI 1608.

High Pressure Liquid Chromatography. System HD—k' 0.1; system HW—k' 0.45.

Ultraviolet Spectrum. Aqueous acid—262 nm ($A_1^1 = 502$ a).

Infra-red Spectrum. Principal peaks at wavenumbers 1648, 1670, 1588, 1511, 1302, 1495 (KBr disk).

Dose. 0.5 to 1.5 g daily.

Niflumic Acid
Analgesic

Proprietary Names. Actol; Flaminon; Inflaryl; Nifluril.
2-(ααα-Trifluoro-*m*-toluidino)nicotinic acid
$C_{13}H_9F_3N_2O_2 = 282.2$
CAS—4394-00-7

Crystals. M.p. 204°.

Thin-layer Chromatography. System TG—Rf 28. (*Ludy Tenger reagent*, orange-brown.)

Gas Chromatography. System GD—retention time of methyl derivative 1.38 relative to *n*-$C_{16}H_{34}$.

High Pressure Liquid Chromatography. System HV—retention time 0.93 relative to meclofenamic acid.

Ultraviolet Spectrum. Aqueous acid—255 nm ($A_1^1 = 471$ b), 329 nm ($A_1^1 = 202$ b); aqueous alkali—288 nm ($A_1^1 = 788$ b).

Mass Spectrum. Principal peaks at *m/z* 282, 236, 237, 281, 263, 145, 44, 93.

Dose. 0.5 to 1 g daily.

Nifuratel
Antimicrobial

Synonyms. Methylmercadone; Thiodinone.
Proprietary Names. Inimur; Macmiror; Omnes; Polmiror.
5-Methylthiomethyl-3-(5-nitrofurfurylideneamino)-2-oxazolidone
$C_{10}H_{11}N_3O_5S = 285.3$
CAS—4936-47-4

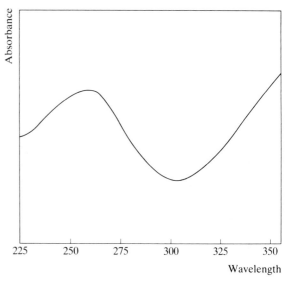

A yellow crystalline powder. M.p. 186° to 188°.
Practically **insoluble** in water; soluble 1 in 400 of chloroform; sparingly soluble in acetone; soluble in dimethylformamide.

Colour Tests. Methanolic Potassium Hydroxide—orange; Palladium Chloride—black.

Thin-layer Chromatography. System TA—Rf 73. (*Acidified iodoplatinate solution*, positive.)

Gas Chromatography. System GA—RI 2590.

Ultraviolet Spectrum. Aqueous acid—259 nm ($A_1^1 = 452$ a), 367 nm.

Infra-red Spectrum. Principal peaks at wavenumbers 1748, 1253, 1232, 1520, 1027, 1126 (KBr disk).

Dose. 600 mg daily.

Nifursol

Antiprotozoal (Veterinary)

Proprietary Name. Salfuride

3,5-Dinitro-2'-(5-nitrofurfurylidene)salicylohydrazide

$C_{12}H_7N_5O_9 = 365.2$

CAS—16915-70-1

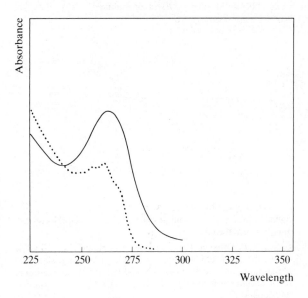

A bright yellow crystalline powder. M.p. 214° to 225°, with decomposition.

Very slightly **soluble** in water, ethanol, and chloroform; soluble 1 in 350 of acetone; practically insoluble in ether; slightly soluble in methanol.

Colour Test. Methanolic Potassium Hydroxide—orange.

Thin-layer Chromatography. *System TA*—Rf 86. (Visible yellow spot; *acidified potassium permanganate solution*, positive.)

Gas Chromatography. *System GA*—not eluted.

Infra-red Spectrum. Principal peaks at wavenumbers 1251, 1281, 1606, 1176, 1674, 1566 (KBr disk).

Nikethamide

Respiratory Stimulant

Synonyms. Cardiamide; Diethylamide Nicotinic Acid; Nicethamidum; Nicorine; Nicotinoyldiethylamidum; Nikethylamide.

Proprietary Names. Coramin(e); Cormed; Juvacor; Kardonyl.

NN-Diethylnicotinamide

$C_{10}H_{14}N_2O = 178.2$

CAS—59-26-7

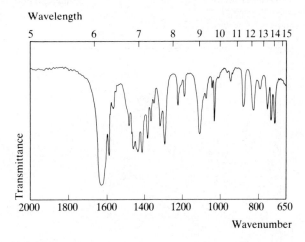

A colourless or slightly yellow, oily liquid or crystalline solid. Relative density 1.060 to 1.066. F.p. 23° to 25°. B.p. 280°. Refractive index 1.524 to 1.526.

Miscible with water, ethanol, chloroform, and ether.

Dissociation Constant. pK_a 3.5 (20°).

Partition Coefficient. Log *P* (octanol), 0.3.

Colour Test. Cyanogen Bromide—orange.

Thin-layer Chromatography. *System TA*—Rf 59; *system TB*—Rf 15; *system TC*—Rf 56. (*Dragendorff spray*, positive; *acidified iodoplatinate solution*, positive.)

Gas Chromatography. *System GA*—nikethamide RI 1525, nicotinamide RI 1436; *system GB*—RI 1513; *system GC*—RI 1852; *system GF*—RI 1895.

Ultraviolet Spectrum. Aqueous acid—264 nm ($A_1^1 = 280$ a); aqueous alkali—256 nm, 261 nm.

Infra-red Spectrum. Principal peaks at wavenumbers 1635, 1590, 1291, 1103, 1316, 712 (KBr disk).

Mass Spectrum. Principal peaks at *m/z* 106, 78, 177, 51, 178, 107, 149, 40; nicotinamide 122, 78, 106, 51, 50, 52, 44, 123.

Quantification. GAS CHROMATOGRAPHY. In canine blood or urine: FID—J. H. Lewis, *J. Chromat.*, 1979, *172*, 295–302.

Disposition in the Body. Rapidly absorbed after oral or parenteral administration and metabolised by *N*-dealkylation to *N*-ethylnicotinamide and nicotinamide; rapidly excreted in the urine; the major urinary metabolite is *N*-ethylnicotinamide.

Dose. 0.5 to 2 g intravenously, repeated if necessary.

Nimorazole

Antiprotozoal

Synonym. Nitrimidazine
Proprietary Names. Acterol Forte; Esclama; Naxogin.
4-[2-(5-Nitroimidazol-1-yl)ethyl]morpholine
$C_9H_{14}N_4O_3 = 226.2$
CAS—6506-37-2

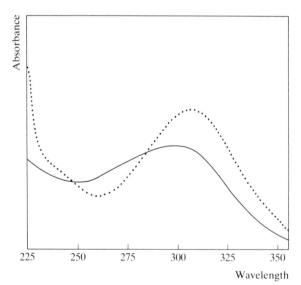

A whitish crystalline powder. M.p. about 110°.

Soluble 1 in 33 of water; soluble in acetone, alcohols, chloroform, and dilute acetic acid.

Colour Test. Dissolve 10 mg in 1 ml of methanol, add 10 ml of water, 10 ml of 6M sodium hydroxide containing 20 mg of alpha-naphthol, and 10 ml of 12M sodium hydroxide, and heat for 30 minutes on a boiling water-bath—an intense brown colour develops.

Thin-layer Chromatography. *System TA*—Rf 57; *system TB*—Rf 03; *system TC*—Rf 44. (*Acidified iodoplatinate solution*, positive.)

Gas Chromatography. *System GA*—RI 1803.

Ultraviolet Spectrum. Aqueous acid—297 nm; aqueous alkali—305 nm.

Mass Spectrum. Principal peaks at *m/z* 100, 56, 42, 101, 55, 54, 41, 30.

Dose. Usually 2 g as a single dose.

Niridazole

Schistosomicide

Proprietary Name. Ambilhar
1-(5-Nitrothiazol-2-yl)imidazolidin-2-one
$C_6H_6N_4O_3S = 214.2$
CAS—61-57-4

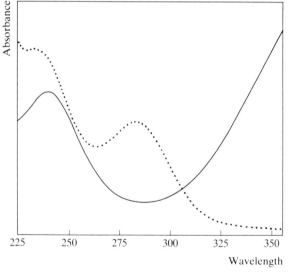

A yellow crystalline powder. M.p. 260° to 264°.

Practically **insoluble** in water, ethanol, acetone, chloroform, and ether; soluble in dimethyl sulphoxide, dimethylformamide, and pyridine.

Colour Test. Methanolic Potassium Hydroxide—yellow.

Thin-layer Chromatography. *System TA*—Rf 54; *system TB*—Rf 01; *system TC*—Rf 44. (Visible yellow spot.)

Ultraviolet Spectrum. Aqueous acid—239 nm; aqueous alkali—233 nm, 282 nm.

Mass Spectrum. Principal peaks at *m/z* 158, 214, 57, 145, 124, 45, 70, 96.

Quantification. GAS CHROMATOGRAPHY. In serum or urine: sensitivity 250 ng/ml, FID—J. J. Miller and R. J. Oake, *J. Chromat.*, 1977, *131*, 442–443.

HIGH PRESSURE LIQUID CHROMATOGRAPHY. In plasma or urine: sensitivity 50 ng/ml, UV detection—J. J. Miller *et al.*, *J. Chromat.*, 1978, *147*, 507–508.

Disposition in the Body. Slowly absorbed after oral administration. It undergoes extensive first-pass metabolism in the liver to inactive metabolites. About 50% of a dose is excreted in the urine as metabolites in 48 hours; niridazole is also excreted as metabolites in bile.

THERAPEUTIC CONCENTRATION.
After a single oral dose of 25 mg/kg, peak blood concentrations of unchanged drug of about 0.2 µg/ml were attained in about 3 hours, and peak blood concentrations of metabolites of about 5 to 10 µg/ml were reported after 6 to 9 hours (J. W. Faigle, *Acta pharmac. tox.*, 1971, *29*, *Suppl.* 3, 233–239).

HALF-LIFE. Plasma half-life, 12 to 15 hours.

PROTEIN BINDING. In plasma, niridazole metabolites extensively bound.

Dose. 25 mg/kg daily, by mouth, up to a maximum of 1.5 g daily.

Nitrazepam   *Hypnotic*

Proprietary Names. Apodorm; Dormicum; Dumolid; Mogadon; Nitrados; Noctesed; Remnos; Somnite; Surem; Unisomnia.
1,3-Dihydro-7-nitro-5-phenyl-2*H*-1,4-benzodiazepin-2-one
$C_{15}H_{11}N_3O_3 = 281.3$
CAS—146-22-5

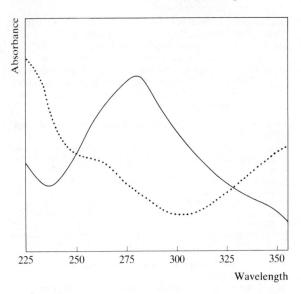

A yellow crystalline powder. M.p. 226° to 230°.
Practically **insoluble** in water; soluble 1 in 120 of ethanol, 1 in 45 of chloroform, and 1 in 900 of ether.

Dissociation Constant. pK_a 3.2, 10.8 (20°).

Partition Coefficient. Log P (octanol/pH 7.4), 2.1.

Colour Test. Formaldehyde–Sulphuric Acid—orange.

Thin-layer Chromatography. *System TA*—Rf 68; *system TB*—Rf 00; *system TC*—Rf 36; *system TD*—Rf 35; *system TE*—Rf 59; *system TF*—Rf 45. (*Dragendorff spray*, positive; *acidified iodoplatinate solution*, positive.)

Gas Chromatography. *System GA*—nitrazepam RI 2750, 7-acetamidonitrazepam RI 3205, 7-aminonitrazepam RI 2828, 2-amino-5-nitrobenzophenone RI 2388; *system GG*—RI 3450.

High Pressure Liquid Chromatography. *System HA*—k′ 0.1; *system HI*—nitrazepam k′ 2.96, 7-acetamidonitrazepam k′ 0.68, 7-aminonitrazepam k′ 0.46; *system HK*—nitrazepam k′ 1.49, 7-acetamidonitrazepam k′ 1.93, 7-aminonitrazepam k′ 0.00.

Ultraviolet Spectrum. Methanolic acid—280 nm ($A_1^1 = 910$ a).

Infra-red Spectrum. Principal peaks at wavenumbers 1690, 1610, 698, 1536, 745, 784 (KBr disk).

Mass Spectrum. Principal peaks at m/z 280, 253, 281, 206, 234, 252, 254, 264; 7-acetamidonitrazepam 293, 265, 264, 292, 43, 222, 223, 294; 7-aminonitrazepam 251, 222, 223, 250, 252, 195, 110, 97; 2-amino-5-nitrobenzophenone 241, 77, 242, 105, 44, 43, 195, 57.

Quantification. SPECTROFLUORIMETRY. In plasma or urine: nitrazepam and metabolites, sensitivity about 10 ng/ml for nitrazepam, 25 ng/ml for the sum of the 7-amino and 7-acetamido metabolites—J. Rieder, *Arzneimittel-Forsch.*, 1973, *23*, 207–211.

GAS CHROMATOGRAPHY. In urine: detection limits 200 pg/ml for nitrazepam using ECD, and 50 ng/ml for metabolites using AFID—L. Kangas, *J. Chromat.*, 1979, *172*, 273–278. In plasma:

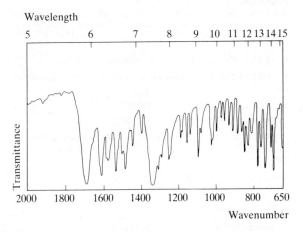

comparison of two procedures using the hydrolysis product and intact drug, sensitivity 200 pg/ml and 1 ng/ml respectively, ECD—L. Kangas, *J. Chromat.*, 1977, *136*, 259–270.

HIGH PRESSURE LIQUID CHROMATOGRAPHY. In plasma, serum or whole blood: limits of detection 5 ng/ml for nitrazepam and 7-acetamidonitrazepam, 50 ng/ml for 7-aminonitrazepam, UV detection—H. Kelly *et al.*, *Clin. Chem.*, 1982, *28*, 1478–1481.

RADIOIMMUNOASSAY. In plasma: sensitivity 4 ng/ml—R. Dixon *et al.*, *Life Sci.*, 1979, *25*, 311–316.

Disposition in the Body. Readily absorbed after oral administration. The major metabolites, 7-aminonitrazepam and the 7-acetamido derivative accumulate to some extent in plasma. Other metabolites include 2-amino-5-nitrobenzophenone and 2-amino-3-hydroxy-5-nitrobenzophenone; all the metabolites are inactive. After oral administration, about 50 to 70% of a dose is excreted in the urine in 120 hours and up to 20% is eliminated in the faeces. Up to about 37% of a dose may be excreted in the first 24 hours with about 5 to 10% of the dose as free 7-acetamidonitrazepam, 5% as 7-aminonitrazepam, 5% as conjugated 2-amino-3-hydroxy-5-nitrobenzophenone, and 20% as unknown acidic compounds. After intravenous administration, about 90% is excreted in the urine in 120 hours and up to about 10% is eliminated in the faeces. Only a small amount (less than 4%) is excreted as unchanged nitrazepam after oral or intravenous administration.

THERAPEUTIC CONCENTRATION. In plasma, usually in the range 0.03 to 0.07 µg/ml.

Following a single oral dose of 5 mg to 9 subjects, peak plasma concentrations of 0.028 to 0.045 µg/ml (mean 0.04) were attained in 0.5 to 4 hours (D. D. Breimer *et al.*, *Br. J. clin. Pharmac.*, 1977, *4*, 709–711).

Following daily oral doses of 5 mg to 4 subjects, steady-state plasma-nitrazepam concentrations of 0.035 to 0.044 µg/ml (mean 0.04) were reported; combined steady-state concentrations of the 7-amino and 7-acetamido metabolites were in the range 0.018 to 0.053 µg/ml (mean 0.03) (J. Rieder and G. Wendt, Pharmacokinetics and Metabolism of the Hypnotic Nitrazepam, in *The Benzodiazepines*, S. Garattini, E. Mussini and L. O. Randall (Ed.), New York, Raven Press, 1973, pp. 99–127).

TOXICITY. Blood concentrations greater than 0.2 µg/ml may produce toxic effects.

In 2 fatalities due to overdoses of nitrazepam, postmortem urine concentrations of 5.9 and 6.0 µg/ml were reported; in the first case alcohol was also present at a blood concentration of 2100 µg/ml (J. S. Oliver and H. Smith, *Forens. Sci.*, 1974, *4*, 183–186).

In a fatality due to ingestion of up to 250 mg of nitrazepam, postmortem blood and liver concentrations of 9 µg/ml and 4 µg/g, respectively, were reported (M. R. Loveland, *Bull. int. Ass. forens. Toxicol.*, 1974, *10* (1), 16–18).

HALF-LIFE. Plasma half-life, 18 to 38 hours (mean 28).

VOLUME OF DISTRIBUTION. About 2 to 3 litres/kg, increased in elderly subjects.

CLEARANCE. Plasma clearance, about 1 ml/min/kg.

PROTEIN BINDING. In plasma, 85 to 88%.

NOTE. For a review of the pharmacokinetics of nitrazepam see L. Kangas and D. D. Breimer, *Clin. Pharmacokinet.*, 1981, *6*, 346–366.

Dose. Usually 5 to 10 mg.

Nitrobenzene

Synonyms. Nitrobenzol; Oil of Mirbane.

$C_6H_5NO_2 = 123.1$

CAS—98-95-3

A pale yellow, oily liquid. Wt per ml about 1.203 g. B.p. 210° to 212°.

Practically **insoluble** in water; miscible with ethanol and ether.

Ultraviolet Spectrum. Ethanol—258 nm ($A_1^1 = 697$ b).

Mass Spectrum. Principal peaks at m/z 77, 51, 123, 50, 65, 93, 30, 78.

Nitrofurantoin   *Antibacterial (Urinary)*

Synonym. Furadonium

Proprietary Names. Berkfurin; Cyantin; Furadantin(e); Furadöine; Furan; Furatine; Ituran; Macrodantin; Nephronex; Nifuran; Nitrex; Novofuran; Trantoin; Urantoin; Urolong. It is an ingredient of Ceduran.

1-(5-Nitrofurfurylideneamino)hydantoin

$C_8H_6N_4O_5 = 238.2$

CAS—67-20-9 (anhydrous); *17140-81-7* (monohydrate)

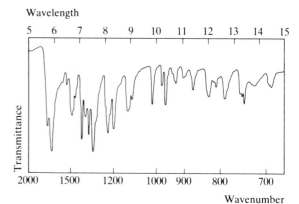

Yellow crystals or fine powder. It is discoloured by alkalis and by exposure to light. M.p. about 271°.

Soluble 1 in 5000 of water, 1 in 2000 of ethanol, 1 in 200 of acetone, and 1 in 16 of dimethylformamide.

Nitrofurantoin Sodium

Proprietary Name. Ivadantin

$C_8H_5N_4NaO_5 = 260.1$

CAS—54-87-5

A yellow to orange-coloured powder.

Dissociation Constant. pK$_a$ 7.2 (25°).

Colour Test. Methanolic Potassium Hydroxide—yellow-orange.

Ultraviolet Spectrum. After solution in dimethylformamide and dilution with water—266 nm, 367 nm ($A_1^1 = 765$ a).

Infra-red Spectrum. Principal peaks at wavenumbers 1718, 1237, 1205, 1770, 1513, 1126 (KBr disk).

Wavelength

Transmittance / Wavenumber

Quantification. SPECTROFLUORIMETRY. In plasma or urine—N. Watari *et al.*, *J. pharm. Sci.*, 1980, *69*, 106–107.

HIGH PRESSURE LIQUID CHROMATOGRAPHY. In plasma or urine: sensitivity 20 ng/ml, UV detection—T. B. Vree *et al.*, *J. Chromat.*, 1979, *162*; *Biomed. Appl.*, *4*, 110–116. In plasma or urine: aminofurantoin and cyanofurantoin, sensitivity 4 µg/ml in plasma, UV detection—B.-A. Hoener and J. L. Wolff, *J. Chromat.*, 1980, *182*; *Biomed. Appl.*, *8*, 246–251.

Disposition in the Body. Readily and almost completely absorbed after oral administration. About 40% of a dose is excreted in the urine unchanged in 24 hours together with small amounts of the reduced metabolite, aminofurantoin.

THERAPEUTIC CONCENTRATION.

Following a single oral dose of 50 mg to 6 fasting subjects, peak plasma concentrations of 0.29 to 0.66 µg/ml (mean 0.43) were attained in 1 to 4 hours (B.-A. Hoener and S. E. Patterson, *Clin. Pharmac. Ther.*, 1981, *29*, 808–816).

HALF-LIFE. Plasma half-life, about 0.5 to 1 hour.

VOLUME OF DISTRIBUTION. About 0.6 litre/kg.

CLEARANCE. Plasma clearance, about 10 ml/min/kg.

DISTRIBUTION IN BLOOD. Plasma: whole blood ratio, 1.3.

PROTEIN BINDING. In plasma, about 60%.

Dose. Usually 400 mg daily.

Nitrofurazone   *Antibacterial*

Synonyms. Furacilinum; Nitrofural.
Proprietary Name. Furacin(e)
5-Nitro-2-furaldehyde semicarbazone
$C_6H_6N_4O_4 = 198.1$
CAS—59-87-0

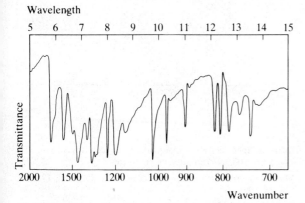

A lemon to brownish-yellow crystalline powder which slowly
darkens on exposure to light and discolours in contact with
alkalis. M.p. about 236°, with decomposition.

Soluble 1 in 4200 of water and 1 in 600 of ethanol; soluble in
dimethylformamide; practically insoluble in chloroform and
ether.

Dissociation Constant. pK_a 10.0.

Colour Test. Methanolic Potassium Hydroxide—red.

Ultraviolet Spectrum. Aqueous acid—261 nm ($A_1^1 = 610$ b);
aqueous alkali—284 nm ($A_1^1 = 475$ b).

Infra-red Spectrum. Principal peaks at wavenumbers 1023, 1250,
1200, 970, 1718, 1585 (Nujol mull).

Wavelength

Transmittance / Wavenumber

Uses. Topically in a concentration of 0.2%; doses of 0.4 to 2 g
daily have been given orally.

Nitroxoline   *Antibacterial (Urinary)*

Proprietary Names. Nibiol; Uro-Coli.
5-Nitroquinolin-8-ol
$C_9H_6N_2O_3 = 190.2$
CAS—4008-48-4

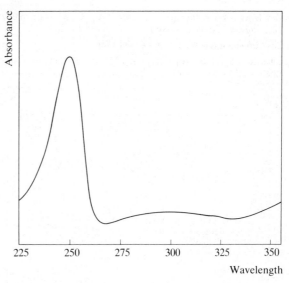

A yellow crystalline powder. M.p. 179° to 182°.
Sparingly **soluble** in ethanol and ether; freely soluble in alkalis
and hot hydrochloric acid.

Colour Tests. Mandelin's Test—green; Methanolic Potassium
Hydroxide—yellow.

Thin-layer Chromatography. *System TA*—Rf 13, streaking.
(Visible yellow spot; *acidified iodoplatinate solution*, positive.)

Ultraviolet Spectrum. Aqueous acid—249 nm ($A_1^1 = 1914$ a),
293 nm.

Absorbance / Wavelength

Infra-red Spectrum. Principal peaks at wavenumbers 1504, 1277,
1307, 1189, 1149, 1565 (KBr disk).

Quantification. HIGH PRESSURE LIQUID CHROMATOGRAPHY. In
plasma or urine: absorbance detection (436 nm)—R. H. A. Sorel
et al., J. Chromat., 1981, *222*; *Biomed. Appl.*, *11*, 241–248.

Disposition in the Body. Readily and almost completely absorbed
after oral administration. About 60% of a dose is excreted in the
urine in 24 hours, mainly as conjugated nitroxoline.

REFERENCE. A. Mrhar *et al., Int. J. clin. Pharmac. Biopharm.*,
1979, *17*, 476–481.

Dose. 300 to 500 mg daily.

Nitroxynil

Anthelmintic (Veterinary)

Synonym. Nitroxinil
4-Hydroxy-3-iodo-5-nitrobenzonitrile
$C_7H_3IN_2O_3 = 290.0$
CAS—1689-89-0

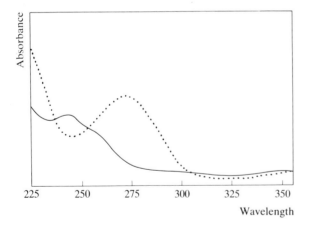

A yellow powder. M.p. 136° to 139°.
Practically **insoluble** in water; soluble 1 in 120 of ethanol and 1 in 60 of ether; soluble in solutions of alkali hydroxides.

Nitroxynil (Eglumine Salt)

Proprietary Name. Trodax
$C_7H_3IN_2O_3,C_8H_19NO_5 = 499.3$
CAS—27917-82-4
Readily **soluble** in water.

Colour Tests. Iodine Test—positive; Methanolic Potassium Hydroxide—yellow.

Thin-layer Chromatography. *System TA*—Rf 83. (*Acidified iodoplatinate solution,* positive.)

Gas Chromatography. *System GA*—RI 1754.

Ultraviolet Spectrum. Aqueous acid—243 nm, 350 nm; aqueous alkali—271 nm $(A_1^1 = 660 \text{ a})$.

Infra-red Spectrum. Principal peaks at wavenumbers 1529, 1245, 1123, 730, 1309, 1600 (KBr disk).

Nomifensine

Antidepressant

8-Amino-1,2,3,4-tetrahydro-2-methyl-4-phenylisoquinoline
$C_{16}H_{18}N_2 = 238.3$
CAS—24526-64-5

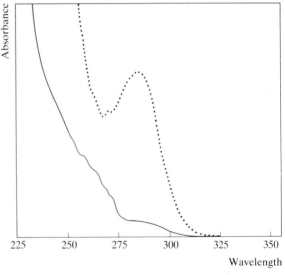

M.p. 179° to 181°.

Nomifensine Maleate

Proprietary Names. Alival; Merital; Psicronizer.
$C_{16}H_{18}N_2,C_4H_4O_4 = 354.4$
CAS—32795-47-4
A white or slightly yellowish powder. M.p. about 195°.
Soluble in dimethylformamide and methanol.

Colour Tests. Coniferyl Alcohol—yellow; Diazotisation—red; Liebermann's Test—orange; Marquis Test—orange (slow).

Thin-layer Chromatography. *System TA*—Rf 56; *system TB*—Rf 08; *system TC*—Rf 29.

Gas Chromatography. *System GA*—RI 2122; *system GF*—RI 2670.

High Pressure Liquid Chromatography. *System HA*—k′ 0.9; *system HF*—k′ 0.42.

Ultraviolet Spectrum. Aqueous alkali—284 nm $(A_1^1 = 75 \text{ b})$; methanol—241 nm $(A_1^1 = 461 \text{ b})$, 292 nm $(A_1^1 = 124 \text{ a})$.

Infra-red Spectrum. Principal peaks at wavenumbers 1580, 877, 741, 1000, 708, 775 (nomifensine maleate).

Mass Spectrum. Principal peaks at m/z 194, 195, 238, 193, 72, 178, 45, 196.

Quantification. GAS CHROMATOGRAPHY. In plasma: detection limit 5 ng/ml, AFID—I. M. McIntyre *et al., Br. J. clin. Pharmac.,* 1981, *12,* 691–694.

RADIOIMMUNOASSAY. In plasma: detection limit 1 ng/ml—I. M. McIntyre *et al., ibid.*

Wavelength

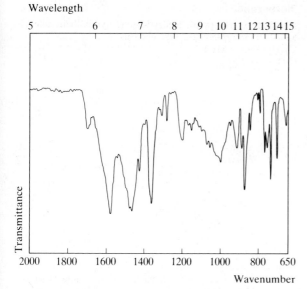

In 26 cases of suspected overdose where the estimated mean dose was 1.15 g, there were few serious toxic reactions; of the subjects who had ingested only nomifensine, only one became comatose and all eventually recovered (S. Dawling *et al.*, *Lancet*, 1979, *1*, 56).

In a fatality involving the ingestion of alcohol and nomifensine, the following postmortem concentrations of nomifensine were reported: blood 17 μg/ml, kidney 141 μg/g, liver 32 μg/g, urine 400 μg/ml; a blood-alcohol concentration of 5000 μg/ml was also reported (A. F. Reyfer *et al.*, *Beitr. Gerichtl. Med.*, 1979, *37*, 313–318).

HALF-LIFE. Plasma half-life, 1.5 to 4 hours, prolonged in severe renal impairment.

PROTEIN BINDING. In plasma, 60 to 75%.

NOTE. For a review of nomifensine see R. N. Brogden *et al.*, *Drugs*, 1979, *18*, 1–24.

Dose. 75 to 200 mg of nomifensine maleate daily.

Noradrenaline   *Sympathomimetic*

Synonyms. l-Arterenol; Levarterenol; Norepinephrine.
(*R*)-2-Amino-1-(3,4-dihydroxyphenyl)ethanol
$C_8H_{11}NO_3 = 169.2$
CAS—51-41-2

Disposition in the Body. Readily absorbed after oral administration. More than 99% of the dose is excreted within 48 hours, about 96% in the urine and about 3% in the faeces. Of the material excreted in the urine, about 60% is the glucuronide conjugate of nomifensine; the metabolites found in urine include 4′-hydroxynomifensine, which is active, 4′-hydroxy-3′-methoxy-nomifensine, and 3′-hydroxy-4′-methoxynomifensine, each of which account for about 7% of the dose. A further four metabolites, accounting for less than 1% of the dose, have also been identified and the remaining material is present as unidentified stable conjugates. After a single dose, less than 5% is usually excreted as unchanged drug. The proportion of free nomifensine found in the urine is dependent on the urinary pH, the time and temperature of storage of the sample, and the extraction procedure, because the glucuronide is readily hydrolysed if the pH is below 7.1 and the sample is not frozen.

THERAPEUTIC CONCENTRATION. A relationship between plasma concentration and clinical effect has not been established. Nomifensine is present in plasma mainly as the glucuronide conjugate; when both free and conjugated nomifensine concentrations are required to be measured, plasma samples must be deep-frozen immediately after collection to prevent hydrolysis. Steady-state concentrations are usually achieved within 5 days.

Following a single oral dose of 100 mg to 6 male subjects, peak plasma concentrations of 0.09 to 0.18 μg/ml (mean 0.13) of free nomifensine and 2.65 to 3.68 μg/ml (mean 3.1) of total nomifensine were attained in 1 to 2 hours; after a single oral dose of 100 mg to 6 female subjects, the corresponding peak plasma concentrations were 0.03 to 0.05 μg/ml (mean 0.04), and 1.95 to 3.32 μg/ml (mean 2.6), for free and total nomifensine respectively (I. M. McIntyre *et al.*, *Br. J. clin. Pharmac.*, 1982, *13*, 740–743).

Following oral administration of 25 mg three times a day to 9 subjects for 6 days, plasma concentrations of 0.005 to 0.017 μg/ml (mean 0.011) were reported 6 hours after a dose (E. Bailey *et al.*, *J. Chromat.*, 1977, *131*, 347–355).

TOXICITY. Ingestion of 3.5 g has been reported without serious toxic effects.

Microcrystals. M.p. 217°, with decomposition.
Slightly **soluble** in water, ethanol, and ether.

Noradrenaline Acid Tartrate
Synonyms. Noradrenaline Tartrate; Norepinephrine Bitartrate.
Proprietary Names. Levophed; Noradrec.
$C_8H_{11}NO_3, C_4H_6O_6, H_2O = 337.3$
CAS—51-40-1 (anhydrous); *69815-49-2* (monohydrate)
A white or faintly grey, crystalline powder which darkens on exposure to air and light. M.p. 98° to 104°, with decomposition.
Soluble 1 in 2.5 of water and 1 in 300 of ethanol; practically insoluble in chloroform and ether.

Noradrenaline Hydrochloride
Proprietary Name. Arterenol
$C_8H_{11}NO_3, HCl = 205.6$
CAS—329-56-6
Crystals. M.p. about 145° to 146°.
Freely **soluble** in water.

Dissociation Constant. pK_a 8.6, 9.8, 12.0 (20°).

Colour Tests. Ammoniacal Silver Nitrate (room temperature)—black; Ferric Chloride—green; Folin–Ciocalteau Reagent—blue; Mandelin's Test—orange; Marquis Test—brown; Methanolic Potassium Hydroxide—blue → orange; Nessler's Reagent—black; Potassium Dichromate (Method 1)—green → brown (30s).

Thin-layer Chromatography. *System TA*—Rf 00; *system TB*—Rf 00; *system TC*—Rf 00. (*Acidified potassium permanganate solution, positive.*)

High Pressure Liquid Chromatography. *System HB*—k′ 0.10.

Ultraviolet Spectrum. Aqueous acid—279 nm ($A_1^1 = 160$ a); aqueous alkali—296 nm.

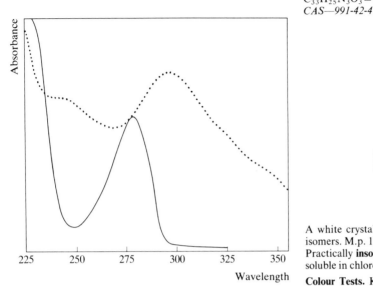

Infra-red Spectrum. Principal peaks at wavenumbers 1265, 1293, 1216, 1200, 1066, 1137 (noradrenaline acid tartrate, KBr disk).

Mass Spectrum. Principal peaks at m/z 44, 45, 58, 76, 60, 43, 42, 46 (no peaks above 90); normetanephrine 153, 93, 30, 65, 152, 154, 125, 110.

Quantification. GAS CHROMATOGRAPHY. In plasma, erythrocytes, serum or urine: FID—H. G. Lovelady and L. L. Foster, *J. Chromat.*, 1975, *108*, 43–52.

RADIOENZYMATIC ASSAY. In plasma: sensitivity 30 pg/ml—H. Hörtnagl *et al.*, *Br. J. clin. Pharmac.*, 1977, *4*, 553–558.

Disposition in the Body. Rapidly metabolised before reaching the systemic circulation and therefore ineffective after oral administration; poorly absorbed after subcutaneous injection; widely distributed throughout the body. The principal metabolic reaction is *O*-methylation catalysed by catechol-*O*-methyltransferase to form normetanephrine; this is followed by oxidative deamination catalysed by monoamine oxidase, to form 4-hydroxy-3-methoxymandelic aldehyde which is converted to 4-hydroxy-3-methoxymandelic acid (vanillylmandelic acid) and to 4-hydroxy-3-methoxyphenyl glycol; the reaction sequence also occurs in reverse, producing 3,4-dihydroxymandelic acid which is methylated to 4-hydroxy-3-methoxymandelic acid; the metabolites are conjugated with glucuronic acid or sulphate or further metabolised. Up to about 16% of an intravenous dose is excreted unchanged in the urine together with methylated and deaminated metabolites in free and conjugated forms; negligible amounts of endogenous noradrenaline are excreted in the urine in normal subjects.

Noradrenaline is a metabolite of dopamine and levodopa.

Endogenous plasma concentrations are approximately in the range 0.0001 to 0.0003 μg/ml.

Dose. Initially, the equivalent of 8 to 12 μg/min of noradrenaline by intravenous infusion.

Norbormide

Rodenticide

5-[α-Hydroxy-α-(2-pyridyl)benzyl]-7-[α-(2-pyridyl)benzylidene]-8,9,10-trinorborn-5-ene-2,3-dicarboximide
$C_{33}H_{25}N_3O_3 = 511.6$
CAS—991-42-4

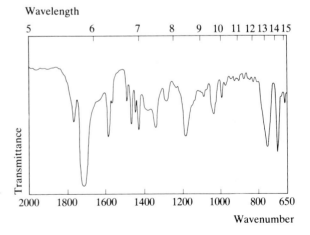

A white crystalline powder consisting of a mixture of stereo-isomers. M.p. 190° to 198°.

Practically **insoluble** in water, ethanol, and ether; very slightly soluble in chloroform.

Colour Tests. Koppanyi–Zwikker Test—violet; Liebermann's Test—green-brown.

Thin-layer Chromatography. *System TA*—Rf 70; *system TB*—Rf 00; *system TC*—Rf 62. (*Acidified iodoplatinate solution*, positive.)

Gas Chromatography. *System GA*—RI 2050.

Ultraviolet Spectrum. Methanolic acid—238 nm, 300 nm ($A_1^1 = 136$ b).

Infra-red Spectrum. Principal peaks at wavenumbers 1708, 701, 751, 1590, 1190, 1754 (KBr disk).

Mass Spectrum. Principal peaks at m/z 91, 58, 86, 106, 231, 45, 77, 230.

Norcodeine

Narcotic Analgesic

Synonyms. *N*-Demethylcodeine; Normorphine 3-Methyl Ether.
3-*O*-Methyl-17-normorphine
$C_{17}H_{19}NO_3 = 285.3$
CAS—467-15-2

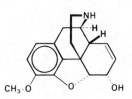

Crystals. M.p. 185°.
Slightly **soluble** in water and ether; soluble in ethanol.

Norcodeine Hydrochloride

$C_{17}H_{19}NO_3,HCl,3H_2O = 375.8$
CAS—14648-14-7 (anhydrous)
Crystals. The anhydrous form decomposes at 309°.
Sparingly **soluble** in water; freely soluble in ethanol.

Dissociation Constant. pK_a 5.7.

Colour Test. Marquis Test—yellow → violet.

Thin-layer Chromatography. *System TA*—Rf 13; *system TB*—Rf
00; *system TC*—Rf 05. (*Dragendorff spray*, positive; *acidified
iodoplatinate solution*, positive; *Marquis reagent*, blue-violet;
ninhydrin spray, positive.)

Gas Chromatography. *System GA*—RI 2388.

High Pressure Liquid Chromatography. *System HA*—k' 3.1
(tailing peak); *system HC*—k' 3.51.

Ultraviolet Spectrum. Aqueous acid—284 nm. No alkaline shift.

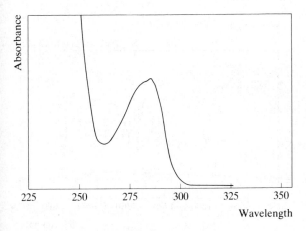

Infra-red Spectrum. Principal peaks at wavenumbers 800, 1515,
1065, 1130, 1290, 1205 (KBr disk). Polymorphism may occur.

Mass Spectrum. Principal peaks at m/z 285, 81, 215, 148, 286,
164, 110, 115.

Disposition in the Body. Norcodeine is a metabolite of codeine.

Wavelength

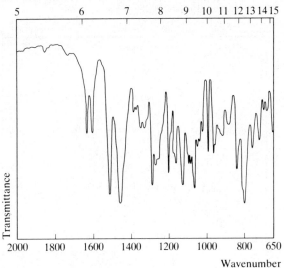

Wavenumber

Nordazepam

Tranquilliser

Synonyms. Demethyldiazepam; Desmethyldiazepam; *N*-Des-
methyldiazepam; Nordiazepam.
Proprietary Name. Madar
7-Chloro-1,3-dihydro-5-phenyl-2*H*-1,4-benzodiazepin-2-one
$C_{15}H_{11}ClN_2O = 270.7$
CAS—1088-11-5

A white or pale yellow crystalline powder. M.p. about 216°.
Practically **insoluble** in water; slightly soluble in ethanol and
chloroform.

Dissociation Constant. pK_a 3.5, 12.0.

Colour Test. Formaldehyde–Sulphuric Acid—orange.

Thin-layer Chromatography. *System TA*—Rf 62; *system TB*—Rf
04; *system TC*—Rf 55; *system TD*—Rf 34; *system TE*—Rf 67;
system TF—Rf 45. (*Dragendorff spray*, positive; *acidified iodoplatinate solution*, positive.)

Gas Chromatography. *System GA*—nordazepam RI 2496, oxazepam RI 2336; *system GG*—nordazepam RI 3041, oxazepam
RI 2803.

High Pressure Liquid Chromatography. *System HA*—k' 0.2;
system HI—nordazepam k' 8.00, oxazepam k' 4.62; *system HK*—
nordazepam k' 1.99, oxazepam k' 0.73.

Ultraviolet Spectrum. Aqueous acid—238 nm ($A_1^1 = 1140$ b), 283 nm, 361 nm; aqueous alkali—240 nm, 340 nm.

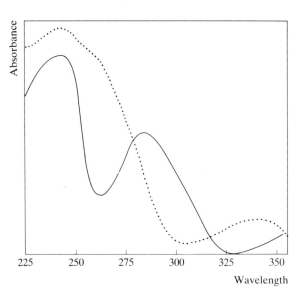

Wavelength

Infra-red Spectrum. Principal peaks at wavenumbers 1680, 700, 1602, 820, 738, 790 (KBr disk).

Mass Spectrum. Principal peaks at m/z 242, 269, 270, 241, 243, 271, 244, 272; oxazepam 257, 77, 268, 239, 205, 267, 233, 259.

Quantification. See also under Diazepam.

GAS CHROMATOGRAPHY. In plasma: sensitivity 1 ng/ml, ECD— A. Viala *et al.*, *J. Chromat.*, 1978, *147*, 349–357.

RADIOIMMUNOASSAY. In serum: sensitivity 3 ng/ml—R. Dixon *et al.*, *J. pharm. Sci.*, 1979, *68*, 1471.

Disposition in the Body. Absorbed after oral administration, maximum blood concentrations being attained in 2 to 4 hours; bioavailability about 50%. It is metabolised to oxazepam and then to oxazepam glucuronide.
Nordazepam is a metabolite of several benzodiazepines including chlordiazepoxide, clorazepate, diazepam, medazepam, and prazepam.

THERAPEUTIC CONCENTRATION.
Following a single oral dose of 10 mg to 2 subjects, a mean peak plasma concentration of 0.17 μg/ml was reported (G. M. Pacifici *et al.*, *Eur. J. drug Met. Pharmacokinet.*, 1982, *7*, 69–72).
Following daily oral doses of 20 to 30 mg to 9 subjects for 10 days, plasma concentrations of 0.63 to 1.84 μg/ml (mean 1.1) were reported 10 hours after a dose (G. Tognoni *et al.*, *Br. J. clin. Pharmac.*, 1975, *2*, 227–232).

HALF-LIFE. The plasma half-life is very variable and values ranging from 25 to over 200 hours have been reported. Mean values which have been reported are usually in the range 40 to 100 hours in normal subjects. The plasma half-life is prolonged in elderly subjects and in subjects with liver disease.

VOLUME OF DISTRIBUTION. 0.5 to 2.5 litres/kg, increased in elderly subjects.

CLEARANCE. Plasma clearance, about 0.1 to 0.3 ml/min/kg.

DISTRIBUTION IN BLOOD. Plasma: whole blood ratio, 1.7.

PROTEIN BINDING. In plasma, about 97%.

Dose. Nordazepam has been given in doses of 10 mg daily.

Norethandrolone
Anabolic Steroid

Synonym. 17α-Ethyl-19-nortestosterone
Proprietary Name. Nilevar
17β-Hydroxy-19-nor-17α-pregn-4-en-3-one
$C_{20}H_{30}O_2 = 302.5$
CAS—52-78-8

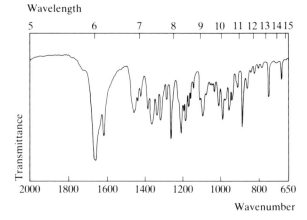

A white crystalline powder. M.p. about 135°.
Practically **insoluble** in water; soluble 1 in 8 of ethanol, 1 in 5 of chloroform, and 1 in 3 of methanol; very soluble in acetone; soluble in ether.

Colour Tests. Antimony Pentachloride—brown; Naphthol–Sulphuric Acid—orange, green dichroism/red-orange; Sulphuric Acid—orange (green-yellow fluorescence under ultraviolet light).

Thin-layer Chromatography. *System TP*—Rf 71; *system TQ*—Rf 20; *system TR*—Rf 95; *system TS*—Rf 78. (p-*Toluenesulphonic acid solution*, positive.)

Ultraviolet Spectrum. Methanol—240 nm ($A_1^1 = 565$ a).

Infra-red Spectrum. Principal peaks at wavenumbers 1650, 1263, 1612, 1210, 894, 1185 (KBr disk).

Wavelength

Mass Spectrum. Principal peaks at m/z 302, 57, 85, 231, 91, 110, 79, 215.

Dose. 10 to 30 mg daily.

Norethisterone

Progestational Steroid

Synonyms. Ethinylnortestosterone; Norethindrone; Norpregneninolone.

Proprietary Names. Micronor; Micronovum; Norfor; Noriday; Norlutin; Nor-QD; Primolut N; Utovlan.

Norethisterone is an ingredient of many proprietary preparations—see *Martindale, The Extra Pharmacopoeia, 28th Edn.*

17β-Hydroxy-19-nor-17α-pregn-4-en-20-yn-3-one

$C_{20}H_{26}O_2 = 298.4$

CAS—68-22-4

A white or creamy-white crystalline powder. M.p. 201° to 208°. Practically **insoluble** in water; soluble 1 in 150 of ethanol, 1 in 30 of chloroform, and 1 in 5 of pyridine; slightly soluble in ether.

Norethisterone Acetate

Synonym. Norethindrone Acetate

Proprietary Names. Milligynon; Norlutate; Primolut Nor; SH 420.
Norethisterone acetate is an ingredient of many proprietary preparations—see *Martindale, The Extra Pharmacopoeia, 28th Edn.*

$C_{22}H_{28}O_3 = 340.5$

CAS—51-98-9

A white or creamy-white crystalline powder. M.p. about 163°. Practically **insoluble** in water; soluble 1 in about 12 of ethanol, 1 in 4 of acetone, 1 in less than 1 of chloroform, 1 in 2 of dioxan, and 1 in 18 of ether.

Colour Tests. Antimony Pentachloride—brown; Naphthol–Sulphuric Acid—orange/orange-brown; Sulphuric Acid—orange (orange fluorescence under ultraviolet light).

Thin-layer Chromatography. Norethisterone: *system TP*—Rf 71; *system TQ*—Rf 22; *system TR*—Rf 87; *system TS*—Rf 63, streaking may occur. Norethisterone acetate: *system TP*—Rf 87; *system TQ*—Rf 39; *system TR*—Rf 98; *system TS*—Rf 90.

Gas Chromatography. *System GA*—RI 2625.

Ultraviolet Spectrum. Ethanol—240 nm ($A_1^1 = 570$ a).

Infra-red Spectrum. Principal peaks at wavenumbers 1649, 1068, 1617, 689, 1272, 660 (KBr disk).

Wavelength

Mass Spectrum. Principal peaks at *m/z* 43, 340, 298, 325, 91, 41, 231, 280 (norethisterone acetate).

Dose. 5 to 25 mg of norethisterone or 2.5 to 15 mg of norethisterone acetate daily; doses of up to 60 mg daily have been given.

Norethynodrel

Progestational Steroid

17β-Hydroxy-19-nor-17α-pregn-5(10)-en-20-yn-3-one

$C_{20}H_{26}O_2 = 298.4$

CAS—68-23-5

A white crystalline powder. M.p. about 174° to 184°. Practically **insoluble** in water; soluble 1 in 30 of ethanol, 1 in 7 of chloroform, and 1 in 60 of ether; soluble in acetone.

Colour Tests. Antimony Pentachloride—green-brown; Naphthol–Sulphuric Acid—orange-red/brown-red; Sulphuric Acid—orange (orange fluorescence under ultraviolet light).
Dissolve 2 mg in 0.3 ml of a 0.5% solution of dinitrobenzene in ethanol and add 2 drops of *benzalkonium chloride solution*. Mix, and add 2 ml of *dilute ammonia solution*—intense violet immediately, changing to red-brown in about 5 minutes.

Thin-layer Chromatography. *System TP*—Rf 79; *system TQ*—Rf 32; *system TR*—Rf 91; *system TS*—Rf 71.

Gas Chromatography. *System GA*—RI 2551.

Ultraviolet Spectrum. No significant absorption, 230 to 360 nm.

Infra-red Spectrum. Principal peaks at wavenumbers 1066, 1690, 1729, 1140, 1008, 1242 (KBr disk).

Wavelength

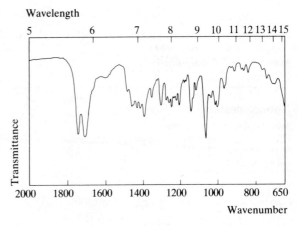

Mass Spectrum. Principal peaks at *m/z* 91, 215, 79, 105, 77, 55, 41, 298.

Dose. 5 to 40 mg daily.

Norharman

Putrefactive Base

Synonym. β-Carboline
9*H*-Pyrido[3,4-*b*]indole
$C_{11}H_8N_2 = 168.2$
CAS—244-63-3

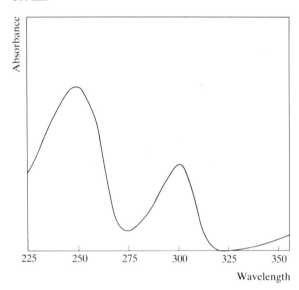

Colourless crystals. M.p. 199°.
Soluble in hot water, ethanol, and ether.

Colour Tests. Mandelin's Test—green → yellow; Marquis Test—green.

Thin-layer Chromatography. *System TA*—Rf 64; *system TB*—Rf 00; *system TC*—Rf 30. (*Acidified iodoplatinate solution*, positive.)

Ultraviolet Spectrum. Aqueous acid—247 nm ($A_1^1 = 1723$ a), 300 nm.

Infra-red Spectrum. Principal peaks at wavenumbers 1247, 731, 747, 1630, 813, 1280 (KBr disk).

Mass Spectrum. Principal peaks at *m/z* 168, 140, 169, 114, 141, 167, 113, 63.

Normetanephrine

Synonym. Normetadrenaline
(*R*)-2-Amino-1-(4-hydroxy-3-methoxyphenyl)ethanol
$C_9H_{13}NO_3 = 183.2$
CAS—97-31-4

Colour Tests. Liebermann's Test—black; Mandelin's Test—green; Marquis Test—orange → violet-brown.

Thin-layer Chromatography. *System TA*—Rf 33. (*Acidified potassium permanganate solution*, positive.)

High Pressure Liquid Chromatography. *System HC*—k' 1.08.

Ultraviolet Spectrum. Aqueous acid—278 nm ($A_1^1 = 85$ b).

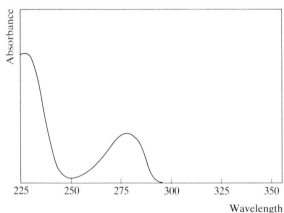

Infra-red Spectrum. Principal peaks at wavenumbers 1529, 1162, 1250, 1037, 1290, 1123 (normetanephrine hydrochloride, KBr disk).

Mass Spectrum. Principal peaks at *m/z* 153, 93, 30, 65, 152, 154, 125, 110.

Disposition in the Body. Normetanephrine is a metabolite of noradrenaline.

Normethadone

Narcotic Analgesic

Synonyms. Desmethylmethadone; Phenyldimazone.
6-Dimethylamino-4,4-diphenylhexan-3-one
$C_{20}H_{25}NO = 295.4$
CAS—467-85-6

$$CH_3 \cdot CH_2 \cdot CO \cdot \underset{\underset{C_6H_5}{|}}{\overset{\overset{C_6H_5}{|}}{C}} \cdot [CH_2]_2 \cdot N(CH_3)_2$$

An oily liquid.

Normethadone Hydrochloride
$C_{20}H_{25}NO, HCl = 331.9$
CAS—847-84-7
Crystals. M.p. 174° to 177°.
Soluble in water and ethanol.

Dissociation Constant. pK_a 9.2.

Colour Test. Mandelin's Test—yellow-green.

Thin-layer Chromatography. *System TA*—Rf 56; *system TB*—Rf 40; *system TC*—Rf 34. (*Acidified iodoplatinate solution*, positive.)

Gas Chromatography. *System GA*—RI 2091.

High Pressure Liquid Chromatography. *System HC*—k' 0.53.

Ultraviolet Spectrum. Aqueous acid—253 nm, 259 nm, 265 nm, 292 nm ($A_1^1 = 19$ a).

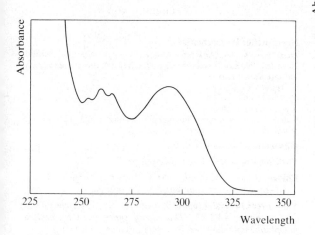

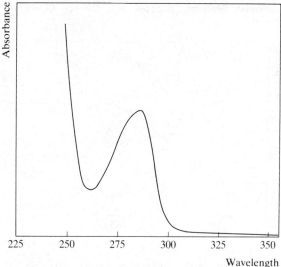

Infra-red Spectrum. Principal peaks at wavenumbers 1711, 701, 1495, 1122, 1032, 760 (KBr disk).

Mass Spectrum. Principal peaks at m/z 58, 72, 29, 42, 71, 57, 59, 224.

Normorphine   *Narcotic Analgesic*

Synonym. Desmethylmorphine
$(-)$-$(5R,6S)$-4,5-Epoxymorphin-7-en-3,6-diol
$C_{16}H_{17}NO_3 = 271.3$
CAS—466-97-7

Infra-red Spectrum. Principal peaks at wavenumbers 1312, 790, 1258, 1066, 1275, 1030 (KBr disk).

Mass Spectrum. Principal peaks at m/z 271, 81, 150, 201, 148, 110, 272, 82.

Disposition in the Body. Normorphine is a metabolite of codeine, diamorphine, and morphine.

Norpipanone   *Narcotic Analgesic*

4,4-Diphenyl-6-piperidinohexan-3-one
$C_{23}H_{29}NO = 335.5$
CAS—561-48-8

Crystals. M.p. 273° to 277°.
Slightly **soluble** in water and ethanol; practically insoluble in chloroform and ether.

Dissociation Constant. pK_a 9.8.

Partition Coefficient. Log P (ether/pH 7.0), -2.8.

Colour Tests. Mandelin's Test—grey-green; Marquis Test—violet.

Thin-layer Chromatography. *System TA*—Rf 17. (*Acidified iodoplatinate solution,* positive.)

Gas Chromatography. *System GA*—RI 2438.

High Pressure Liquid Chromatography. *System HA*—k′ 2.9 (tailing peak); *system HC*—k′ 3.92.

Ultraviolet Spectrum. Aqueous acid—285 nm ($A_1^1 = 57$ b).

Norpipanone Hydrochloride
$C_{23}H_{29}NO,HCl = 371.9$
Crystals. M.p. 181° to 182°.
Soluble in water and ethanol.

Colour Test. Mandelin's Test—brown → blue.

Thin-layer Chromatography. *System TA*—Rf 68; *system TB*—Rf 59; *system TC*—Rf 50. (*Dragendorff spray,* positive; *acidified iodoplatinate solution,* positive; *Marquis reagent,* dull orange.)

Gas Chromatography. *System GA*—RI 2488.

High Pressure Liquid Chromatography. *System HC*—k′ 0.35.

Ultraviolet Spectrum. Aqueous acid—260 nm ($A_1^1 = 17$ b), 294 nm.

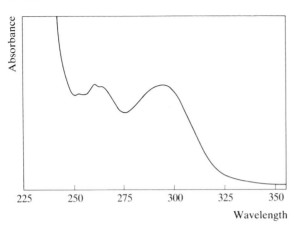

Infra-red Spectrum. Principal peaks at wavenumbers 1705, 700, 1115, 1492, 1600, 1157 (KBr disk).

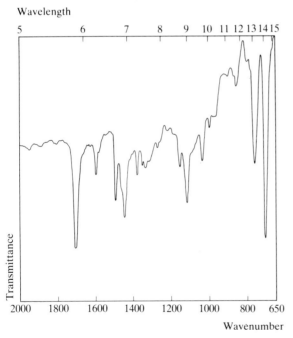

Mass Spectrum. Principal peaks at m/z 98, 111, 99, 42, 55, 41, 29, 112.

Dose. Norpipanone hydrochloride has been given in doses of 18 mg daily.

Nortriptyline
Antidepressant

3-(10,11-Dihydro-5H-dibenzo[a,d]cyclohepten-5-ylidene)-N-methylpropylamine
$C_{19}H_{21}N = 263.4$
CAS—72-69-5

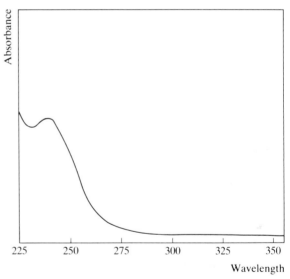

Nortriptyline Hydrochloride
Proprietary Names. Allegron; Altilev; Aventyl; Noritren; Nortab; Nortrilen; Pamelor; Psychostyl; Sensival; Vividyl. It is an ingredient of Motipress and Motival.
$C_{19}H_{21}N,HCl = 299.8$
CAS—894-71-3
A white powder. M.p. 215° to 220°.
Soluble 1 in 50 of water, 1 in 10 of ethanol, and 1 in 5 of chloroform; practically insoluble in ether.

Dissociation Constant. pK_a 9.7.

Partition Coefficient. Log P (octanol/pH 7.4), 1.7.

Colour Tests. Mandelin's Test—brown → green; Marquis Test—orange-brown; Sulphuric Acid—orange.

Thin-layer Chromatography. *System TA*—Rf 34; *system TB*—Rf 27; *system TC*—Rf 16. (*Dragendorff spray*, positive; *acidified iodoplatinate solution*, positive; *Marquis reagent*, brown.)

Gas Chromatography. *System GA*—nortriptyline RI 2210, 10-hydroxynortriptyline RI 2385.

High Pressure Liquid Chromatography. *System HA*—nortriptyline k′ 2.0, 10-hydroxynortriptyline k′ 1.8; *system HF*—k′ 4.58.

Ultraviolet Spectrum. Aqueous acid—239 nm ($A_1^1 = 517$ a). No alkaline shift.

Infra-red Spectrum. Principal peaks at wavenumbers 756, 742, 768, 720, 775, 1590 (nortriptyline hydrochloride, KBr disk).

Mass Spectrum. Principal peaks at m/z 44, 202, 45, 220, 218, 215, 91, –; 10-hydroxynortriptyline 44, 45, 26, 218, 215, 203, 202, 42.

Quantification. See under Amitriptyline.

Disposition in the Body. Readily absorbed after oral administration; bioavailability about 50 to 60% due to first-pass metabolism.

Wavelength

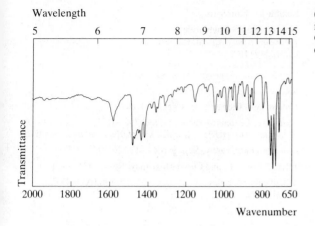

The main metabolic reactions are *N*-demethylation and 10-hydroxylation; glucuronide conjugation of nortriptyline and its metabolites also occurs. Up to 60% of the daily dose is excreted in the urine within 24 hours, with less than 5% as unchanged drug, 30 to 50% as free or conjugated 10-hydroxynortriptyline, 6 to 15% as free and conjugated 10-hydroxydinortriptyline, and about 1% as dinortriptyline.
Nortriptyline is a metabolite of amitriptyline.

THERAPEUTIC CONCENTRATION. In plasma, usually in the range 0.05 to 0.15 µg/ml. Plasma concentrations vary considerably between individuals and are influenced by exposure to other drugs.

Following a single oral dose of 100 mg to 10 subjects, peak plasma concentrations of 0.015 to 0.050 µg/ml (mean 0.03) of nortriptyline and 0.039 to 0.172 µg/ml (mean 0.10) of 10-hydroxynortriptyline were attained in 3 to 24 hours (S. Nakano and L. E. Hollister, *Clin. Pharmac. Ther.*, 1978, *23*, 199–203).

Following average daily oral doses of 82 mg to 62 subjects, the following steady-state plasma concentrations were reported: nortriptyline 0.03 to 0.34 µg/ml (mean 0.12), 10-hydroxynortriptyline 0.04 to 0.42 µg/ml (mean 0.16), conjugated 10-hydroxynortriptyline 0.075 to 1.07 µg/ml (mean 0.37) (S. Dawling *et al.*, *Clin. Pharmac. Ther.*, 1982, *32*, 322–329).

TOXICITY. Relatively few cases of serious intoxication have been attributed to nortriptyline in comparison to the tertiary amine tricyclic antidepressants. Toxic effects are usually associated with blood concentrations greater than 0.25 µg/ml and concentrations above 1 µg/ml may produce coma. Recovery has occurred after the ingestion of 2.5 g.

The following distribution was reported in 9 fatal cases: blood 0 to 26 µg/ml (mean 11, 3 cases), kidney 7 to 94 µg/g (mean 43, 5 cases), liver 8 to 220 µg/g (mean 90, 9 cases), urine 25 to 120 µg/ml (mean 76, 4 cases) (R. Bonnichsen *et al.*, *Z. Rechtsmed.*, 1970, *67*, 190–200).

HALF-LIFE. Plasma half-life, 15 to 90 hours (mean 30).

VOLUME OF DISTRIBUTION. 14 to 40 litres/kg (mean 23).

PROTEIN BINDING. In plasma, 90 to 95%.

NOTE. For a review of tricyclic antidepressants see G. Molnar and R. N. Gupta, *Biopharm. Drug Disp.*, 1980, *1*, 283–305.

Dose. The equivalent of 30 to 100 mg of nortriptyline daily.

Noscapine   *Cough Suppressant*

Synonyms. Narcotine; L-α-Narcotine.
Proprietary Names. Longatin; Noscatuss; Tusscapine. It is an ingredient of Extil.

(3*S*)-6,7-Dimethoxy-3-[(5*R*)-5,6,7,8-tetrahydro-4-methoxy-6-methyl-1,3-dioxolo[4,5-*g*]isoquinolin-5-yl]phthalide
$C_{22}H_{23}NO_7 = 413.4$
CAS—128-62-1

An alkaloid obtained from opium.
Colourless crystals or a fine white crystalline powder. M.p. 174° to 176°, with decomposition.
Practically **insoluble** in water; slightly soluble in ethanol and ether; soluble in acetone and chloroform.

Noscapine Hydrochloride
Proprietary Names. Narcotussin; Noscapect. It is an ingredient of Triotussic.
$C_{22}H_{23}NO_7,HCl,H_2O = 467.9$
CAS—912-60-7 (anhydrous)
Hygroscopic, colourless crystals or a fine white crystalline powder. M.p. about 200°, with decomposition.
Soluble 1 in 4 of water and 1 in 8 of ethanol; freely soluble in chloroform; practically insoluble in ether. Aqueous solutions may deposit the base on standing.

Dissociation Constant. pK_a 6.2 (20°).

Colour Tests. Liebermann's Test—black; Marquis Test—blue-violet (fades).

Thin-layer Chromatography. *System TA*—Rf 64; *system TB*—Rf 22; *system TC*—Rf 74. (*Acidified iodoplatinate solution*, positive.)

Gas Chromatography. *System GA*—RI 3120.

High Pressure Liquid Chromatography. *System HA*—k' 0.3; *system HC*—k' 0.15; *system HS*—k' 0.01.

Ultraviolet Spectrum. Aqueous acid—290 nm, 312 nm ($A_1^1 = 84$ a); aqueous alkali—281 nm, 315 nm.

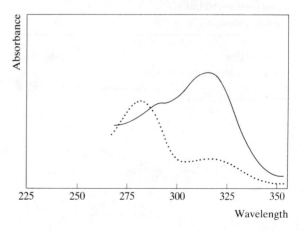

Infra-red Spectrum. Principal peaks at wavenumbers 1745, 1276, 1038, 1010, 1498, 1080 (KBr disk).

Wavelength

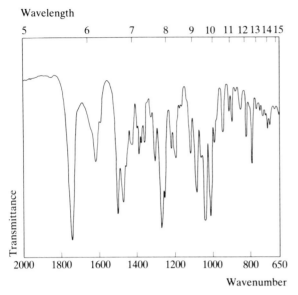

Mass Spectrum. Principal peaks at m/z 220, 221, 205, 147, 42, 193, 77, 118.

Quantification. SPECTROFLUORIMETRY. In plasma or urine: sensitivity 50 ng/ml—S. Vedso, *Acta pharmac. tox.*, 1961, *18*, 119–128.

Disposition in the Body. Rapidly absorbed after oral administration; bioavailability about 30%. About 1% of a dose is excreted in the urine in 6 hours as free and conjugated noscapine.

THERAPEUTIC CONCENTRATION.

Following a single oral dose of 150 mg to 5 subjects, peak plasma concentrations of 0.20 to 0.35 µg/ml (mean 0.27) were attained in 0.5 to 2.5 hours (B. Dahlström *et al.*, *Eur. J. clin. Pharmac.*, 1982, *22*, 535–539).

HALF-LIFE. Plasma half-life, 1.5 to 4 hours (mean 2.5).

VOLUME OF DISTRIBUTION. 3 to 7 litres/kg (mean 5).

CLEARANCE. Plasma clearance, about 20 ml/min/kg.

REFERENCE. B. Dahlström *et al.*, *ibid.*

Dose. Usually 45 to 120 mg daily.

Noxiptyline   *Antidepressant*

Synonyms. Dibenzoxine; Noxiptiline.

10,11 - Dihydro - 5*H* - dibenzo[*a,d*]cyclohepten - 5 - one *O*-(2-dimethylaminoethyl)oxime
$C_{19}H_{22}N_2O = 294.4$
CAS—3362-45-6

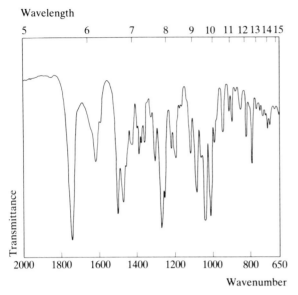

N·O·CH₂·CH₂·N(CH₃)₂

Soluble in chloroform.

Noxiptyline Hydrochloride

Proprietary Names. Agedal; Nogédal.
$C_{19}H_{22}N_2O,HCl = 330.9$
CAS—4985-15-3
A white crystalline powder. M.p. 189° to 191°.

Soluble in water.

Colour Test. Liebermann's Test—black.

Thin-layer Chromatography. *System TA*—Rf 53; *system TB*—Rf 43; *system TC*—Rf 35. (*Acidified iodoplatinate solution*, positive.)

Gas Chromatography. *System GA*—RI 2267.

High Pressure Liquid Chromatography. *System HF*—k' 1.63.

Ultraviolet Spectrum. Aqueous acid—250 nm ($A_1^1 = 477$ a). No alkaline shift.

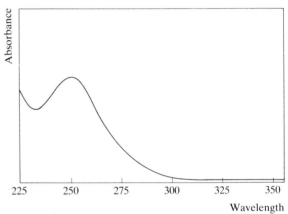

Mass Spectrum. Principal peaks at m/z 58, 71, 208, 72, 59, 42, 89, 57.

Quantification. GAS CHROMATOGRAPHY. In plasma, urine or tablets: detection limit 100 ng/ml, AFID—E. Szyszko and W. Wejman, *J. Chromat.*, 1981, *219*, 291–296.

Dose. The equivalent of 10 to 200 mg of noxiptyline daily.

Noxythiolin   *Antibacterial/Antifungal*

Synonym. Noxytiolin
Proprietary Name. Noxyflex 'S'
1-Hydroxymethyl-3-methyl-2-thiourea
$C_3H_8N_2OS = 120.2$
CAS—15599-39-0

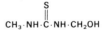

A white crystalline powder. Decomposes between 88° and 90°.
Soluble 1 in 10 of water; soluble in chloroform.

Colour Test. Palladium Chloride—brown.

Thin-layer Chromatography. *System TA*—Rf 74. (*Acidified iodoplatinate solution*, positive.)

Gas Chromatography. *System GA*—RI 2370.

Ultraviolet Spectrum. Methanol—244 nm ($A_1^1 = 1180$ a).

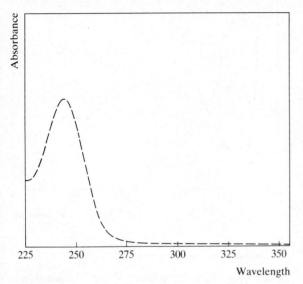

Wavelength

Infra-red Spectrum. Principal peaks at wavenumbers 1558, 1042, 1230, 987, 1026, 1517 (KBr disk).

Use. In concentrations of 1 to 2.5%.

Nystatin   *Antifungal*

Synonyms. Fungicidin; Nistatina.

Proprietary Names. Nyspes; Nystan; Nystavescent.
Nystatin is an ingredient of many proprietary preparations—see *Martindale, The Extra Pharmacopoeia*, 28th Edn.

CAS—1400-61-9

A mixture of antifungal polyenes produced by the growth of certain strains of *Streptomyces noursei*, or by any other means. It consists largely of nystatin A_1. Approximate molecular formula: $C_{47}H_{75}NO_{17} = 926.1$.

A yellow to light brown, hygroscopic powder.
Very slightly **soluble** in water; sparingly soluble in ethanol; practically insoluble in chloroform and ether; freely soluble in dimethylformamide and formamide.

Gas Chromatography. *System GA*—RI 1945.

Ultraviolet Spectrum. Aqueous alkali—291 nm ($A_1^1 = 405$ b), 305 nm ($A_1^1 = 600$ b), 319 nm ($A_1^1 = 530$ b).

Infra-red Spectrum. Principal peaks at wavenumbers 1067, 1000, 1570, 1175, 1316, 847 (Nujol mull).

Uses. Topically in preparations containing 100 000 units per g; orally in doses of 1 500 000 to 4 000 000 units daily.

Obidoxime Chloride   *Cholinesterase Reactivator*

Proprietary Name. Toxogonin

1,1' - (Oxydimethylene)bis(4 - hydroxyiminomethylpyridinium) dichloride
$C_{14}H_{16}Cl_2N_4O_3 = 359.2$
CAS—7683-36-5 (obidoxime); *114-90-9* (chloride)

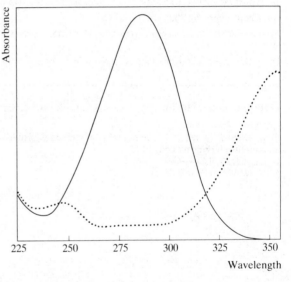

White crystals, occurring in two interchangeable isomeric forms. M.p. 225°, with decomposition.
Freely **soluble** in water; slightly soluble in ethanol and methanol; practically insoluble in chloroform and ether.

Dissociation Constant. pK_a 7.6, 8.3 (25°).

Colour Tests. Mandelin's Test—green → blue; Methanolic Potassium Hydroxide—orange.

Thin-layer Chromatography. *System TA*—Rf 01. (*Acidified iodoplatinate solution*, positive.)

Ultraviolet Spectrum. Aqueous acid—285 nm ($A_1^1 = 947$ a); aqueous alkali—353 nm ($A_1^1 = 1440$ b).

Wavelength

Infra-red Spectrum. Principal peaks at wavenumbers 996, 1090, 1637, 1600, 1282, 847 (KBr disk).

Quantification. POLAROGRAPHY. In serum or urine: sensitivity 4 µg/ml—Z. Koriċanac *et al., Acta pharm. jugosl.*, 1982, *32*, 297–302.

Disposition in the Body. Poorly absorbed after oral administration. After intramuscular administration, more than 80% of a dose is excreted unchanged in the urine in 24 hours.

THERAPEUTIC CONCENTRATION.

Following intramuscular doses of 2.5 to 10 mg/kg to 10 subjects, peak plasma concentrations of 6.3 to 26.5 µg/ml were attained in about 20 minutes (F. R. Sidell and W. A. Groff, *J. pharm. Sci.*, 1970, *59*, 793–797).

HALF-LIFE. Plasma half-life, about 1.4 hours.

DISTRIBUTION IN BLOOD. Plasma: whole blood ratio, 1.9.

Dose. Obidoxime chloride has been given parenterally in doses of 250 mg.

Octamylamine
Antispasmodic

Synonym. Octisamyl
N-Isopentyl-1,5-dimethylhexylamine
$C_{13}H_{29}N = 199.4$
CAS—502-59-0

$$CH_3 \cdot CH \cdot [CH_2]_2 \cdot CH_2 \cdot CH \cdot CH_3$$
$$|\qquad\qquad\qquad\qquad |$$
$$CH_3 \qquad\qquad NH \cdot [CH_2]_2 \cdot CH(CH_3)_2$$

An oily liquid.

Octamylamine Hydrochloride
Proprietary Name. Octometine
$C_{13}H_{29}N,HCl = 235.8$
CAS—5964-56-7
White crystals. M.p. 121°.
Soluble in water, ethanol, and ether.

Thin-layer Chromatography. *System TA*—Rf 22; *system TB*—Rf 28; *system TC*—Rf 11. (*Acidified iodoplatinate solution*, positive.)

Gas Chromatography. *System GA*—RI 1303.

Mass Spectrum. Principal peaks at *m/z* 30, 44, 41, 45, 86, 55, 43, 69.

Dose. Octamylamine hydrochloride is given in doses of 100 to 200 mg.

Octaphonium Chloride
Cationic Disinfectant

Synonym. Phenoctide
Benzyldiethyl{2 - [4 - (1,1,3,3 - tetramethylbutyl)phenoxy]ethyl}-
ammonium chloride monohydrate
$C_{27}H_{42}ClNO,H_2O = 450.1$
CAS—15687-40-8 (anhydrous)

$$(CH_3)_3C \cdot CH_2 \cdot C(CH_3)_2$$
$$Cl^-, H_2O$$
$$C_2H_5$$
$$O \cdot CH_2 \cdot CH_2 \cdot \overset{+}{N} \cdot CH_2 \cdot C_6H_5$$
$$C_2H_5$$

A white crystalline powder.
Soluble 1 in 5 of water; soluble in ethanol and chloroform.

Colour Tests. Liebermann's Test—black; Mandelin's Test—violet-brown; Marquis Test—grey-brown; Sulphuric Acid—grey-brown.

Thin-layer Chromatography. *System TA*—Rf 15, streaking. (*Dragendorff spray*, positive.)

Gas Chromatography. *System GA*—RI 2013.

Ultraviolet Spectrum. Aqueous acid—269 nm ($A_1^1 = 32$ a), 274 nm, 281 nm; ethanol—263 nm ($A_1^1 = 25$ b), 269 nm ($A_1^1 = 30$ b), 274 nm ($A_1^1 = 29$ b), 282 nm ($A_1^1 = 25$ b).

Infra-red Spectrum. Principal peaks at wavenumbers 1240, 840, 760, 1515, 708, 1185 (Nujol mull).

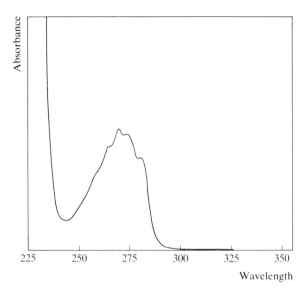

Absorbance

Wavelength

Octatropine Methylbromide
Anticholinergic

Synonyms. Anisotropine Methobromide; Anisotropine Methyl-bromide.
Proprietary Name. Valpin
(1*R*,3*r*,5*S*)-8-Methyl-3-(2-propylvaleryloxy)tropanium bromide
$C_{17}H_{32}BrNO_2 = 362.3$
CAS—80-50-2

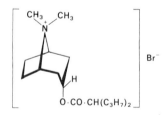

A white, glistening, hygroscopic powder. M.p. 329°.
Soluble in water; freely soluble in ethanol and chloroform; practically insoluble in ether.

Thin-layer Chromatography. *System TA*—Rf 02. (*Acidified iodoplatinate solution*, positive.)

Infra-red Spectrum. Principal peaks at wavenumbers 1735, 1155, 1178, 1040, 1237, 1203 (KBr disk).

Dose. 30 to 150 mg daily.

Oestradiol
Oestrogen

Synonyms. Beta-oestradiol; Dihydrofolliculine; Dihydrotheelin; Dihydroxyoestrin; Estradiol.
Proprietary Names. Estrace; Farmacyrol; Gynoestryl; Oestrogel; Progynon. It is an ingredient of Hormonin and Trisequens.

Estra-1,3,5(10)-triene-3,17β-diol
$C_{18}H_{24}O_2 = 272.4$
CAS—50-28-2

White or creamy-white, hygroscopic crystals or crystalline powder. M.p. 173° to 179°.

Practically **insoluble** in water; soluble 1 in 28 of ethanol, 1 in 17 of acetone, 1 in 435 of chloroform, and 1 in 150 of ether; soluble in dioxan and solutions of alkali hydroxides.

Oestradiol Benzoate

Synonyms. Estradiol Benzoate; Oestradiol Monobenzoate.

Proprietary Names. Benzo-Gynoestryl 5; Benztrone; Gynécormone; Oestramine; Ovocyclin M; Progynon B. It is an ingredient of Mixogen (injection) and Plex-Hormone (injection).

$C_{25}H_{28}O_3 = 376.5$
CAS—50-50-0

Colourless crystals or white or creamy-white crystalline powder. M.p. 190° to 198°.

Practically **insoluble** in water; slightly soluble in ethanol; soluble 1 in 5 of chloroform and 1 in 150 of ether; soluble in dioxan.

Oestradiol Cypionate

Synonyms. Estradiol Cypionate; Oestradiol Cyclopentylpropionate.

Proprietary Names. Depo-Estradiol Cypionate; Neoginon Depositum.

$C_{26}H_{36}O_3 = 396.6$
CAS—313-06-4

A white crystalline powder. M.p. 149° to 153°.

Practically **insoluble** in water; soluble 1 in 40 of ethanol and 1 in 7 of chloroform; soluble in acetone and dioxan; very slightly soluble in ether.

Oestradiol Undecanoate

Synonym. Estradiol Undecylate

Proprietary Names. Progynon Depot; Progynon-Retard.

$C_{29}H_{44}O_3 = 440.7$

CAS—33613-02-4

Oestradiol Valerate

Synonym. Estradiol Valerate

Proprietary Names. Delestrogen; Femogex; Östrogynol sine; Primogyn Depot; Progynon Depot; Progynova. It is an ingredient of Cyclacur and Cyclo-Progynova.

$C_{23}H_{32}O_3 = 356.5$
CAS—979-32-8

A white crystalline powder. M.p. 143° to 150°.

Practically **insoluble** in water; soluble in dioxan and methanol.

Colour Tests. Antimony Pentachloride—brown; Liebermann's Test—black; Naphthol–Sulphuric Acid—blue-green, yellow dichroism/orange; Sulphuric Acid—yellow (green fluorescence under ultraviolet light).

Thin-layer Chromatography. Oestradiol benzoate: *system TP*—Rf 79; *system TQ*—Rf 32; *system TR*—Rf 96; *system TS*—Rf 79.

Gas Chromatography. *System GA*—RI 2659.

Ultraviolet Spectrum. Oestradiol benzoate: ethanol—231 nm $(A_1^1 = 490 \text{ b})$.

Infra-red Spectrum. Principal peaks at wavenumbers 1245, 1054, 1227, 1493, 1276, 821 (KBr disk).

Dose. Up to 2 mg daily, by mouth.

Oestriol   *Oestrogen*

Synonyms. Estriol; Theelol.

Proprietary Names. Hormomed; Ovestin. It is an ingredient of Hormonin and Trisequens.

Estra-1,3,5(10)-triene-3,16α,17β-triol
$C_{18}H_{24}O_3 = 288.4$
CAS—50-27-1

A white crystalline powder. M.p. about 280°.

Practically **insoluble** in water; soluble 1 in about 500 of ethanol; soluble in acetone, chloroform, dioxan, and ether.

Dissociation Constant. pK_a 10.4.

Colour Tests. Antimony Pentachloride—brown; Liebermann's Test—black; Naphthol–Sulphuric Acid—green, yellow dichroism/orange; Sulphuric Acid—no initial colour (yellow-green fluorescence under ultraviolet light).

Gas Chromatography. *System GA*—RI 2970.

Ultraviolet Spectrum. Ethanol—280 nm.

Infra-red Spectrum. Principal peaks at wavenumbers 1228, 1067, 917, 1147, 1250, 1605 (Nujol mull).

Dose. 0.25 to 1 mg daily.

Oestrone   *Oestrogen*

Synonyms. Estrone; Folliculin; Ketohydroxyoestrin.

Proprietary Names. Cristallovar; Femogen; Kolpon; Oestrilin (vaginal preparations). It is an ingredient of Hormonin.

3-Hydroxyestra-1,3,5(10)-trien-17-one
$C_{18}H_{22}O_2 = 270.4$
CAS—53-16-7

Colourless crystals or white to creamy-white crystalline powder. M.p. about 260°, with decomposition.

Practically **insoluble** in water; soluble 1 in 250 of ethanol and 1 in 110 of chloroform; soluble in dioxan; slightly soluble in ether.

Colour Tests. Antimony Pentachloride—brown; Liebermann's Test—black; Naphthol–Sulphuric Acid—green, yellow dichroism/orange; Sulphuric Acid—green-yellow (green fluorescence under ultraviolet light).

Gas Chromatography. *System GA*—RI 2612.

Ultraviolet Spectrum. Methanol—280 nm $(A_1^1 = 78 \text{ a})$.

Infra-red Spectrum. Principal peaks at wavenumbers 1282, 820, 1709, 1244, 921, 1493.

Dose. Oestrone has been given in doses of 0.1 to 5 mg daily by intramuscular injection.

Oleandomycin

Antibiotic

Proprietary Name. Triolmicina
$C_{35}H_{61}NO_{12} = 687.9$
CAS—3922-90-5
An antimicrobial substance produced by the growth of *Streptomyces antibioticus.*
A white amorphous powder.
Moderately **soluble** in water; freely soluble in ethanol, acetone, and methanol.

Oleandomycin Phosphate

$C_{35}H_{61}NO_{12},H_3PO_4 = 785.9$
CAS—7060-74-4
A white crystalline powder.
Soluble 1 in 2.5 of water and 1 in 3 of ethanol; slightly soluble in ether.

Colour Tests. Mandelin's Test—green; Marquis Test—green.

Thin-layer Chromatography. *System TA—Rf 45. (Acidified potassium permanganate solution, positive.)*

Ultraviolet Spectrum. Aqueous acid—242 nm ($A_1^1 = 7$ b).

Infra-red Spectrum. Principal peaks at wavenumbers 1111, 1052, 1075, 1010, 1162, 1190 (oleandomycin phosphate).

Dose. Oleandomycin phosphate has been given in doses of 1 to 2 g daily.

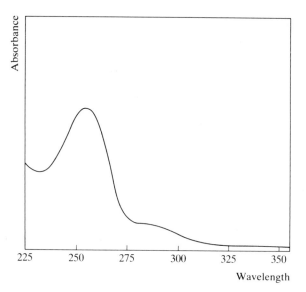

Opipramol

Antidepressant

2-{4-[3-(5*H*-Dibenz[*b,f*]azepin-5-yl)propyl]piperazin-1-yl}-ethanol
$C_{23}H_{29}N_3O = 363.5$
CAS—315-72-0

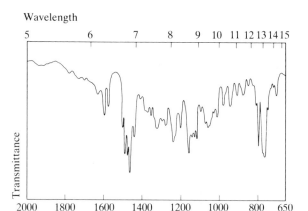

Crystals. M.p. 100° to 101°.

Opipramol Hydrochloride

Proprietary Name. Insidon
$C_{23}H_{29}N_3O,2HCl = 436.4$
CAS—909-39-7
A light yellow, crystalline powder which develops a reddish tinge on prolonged exposure to light. M.p. about 210°, with decomposition.
Very **soluble** in water; soluble in ethanol.

Dissociation Constant. pK_a 3.8.

Colour Tests. Forrest Reagent—blue; Mandelin's Test—yellow-green.

Thin-layer Chromatography. *System TA—Rf 54; system TB—Rf 06; system TC—Rf 22. (Acidified iodoplatinate solution, positive.)*

High Pressure Liquid Chromatography. *System HA—k' 2.2; system HF—k' 1.63.*

Ultraviolet Spectrum. Aqueous acid—253 nm ($A_1^1 = 870$ a). No alkaline shift.

Infra-red Spectrum. Principal peaks at wavenumbers 755, 1155, 790, 1237, 1115, 1126 (KBr disk).

Mass Spectrum. Principal peaks at *m/z* 363, 206, 143, 42, 70, 207, 218, 113.

Quantification. DOUBLE RADIOISOTOPE TECHNIQUE. In biological samples—W. Riess, *Analytica chim. Acta,* 1977, *88,* 109–115.

Disposition in the Body. Readily absorbed after oral administration.

TOXICITY.

Somnolence was reported in a 27-year-old subject following an overdose of opipramol; a maximum serum concentration of 0.115 μg/ml was determined; ethanol was also detected (O. L. Pedersen *et al., Eur. J. clin. Pharmac.,* 1982, *23,* 513–521).

Dose. 150 to 300 mg of opipramol hydrochloride daily.

Orciprenaline
Sympathomimetic

Synonym. Metaproterenol
(±)-1-(3,5-Dihydroxyphenyl)-2-isopropylaminoethanol
$C_{11}H_{17}NO_3 = 211.3$
CAS—586-06-1

$$(CH_3)_2CH \cdot NH \cdot CH_2 \cdot CH \cdot OH$$

HO   OH

Crystals. M.p. 100°.

Orciprenaline Sulphate
Proprietary Names. Alupent; Dosalupent; Metaprel.
$(C_{11}H_{17}NO_3)_2,H_2SO_4 = 520.6$
CAS—5874-97-5
A white crystalline powder. M.p. about 205°.
Soluble 1 in 2 of water and 1 in 1 of ethanol; practically insoluble in chloroform and ether.

Dissociation Constant. pK_a 9.0 (—OH), 10.1 (—NH—), 11.4 (—OH), (25°).

Colour Tests. *p*-Dimethylaminobenzaldehyde—orange/violet; Folin–Ciocalteu Reagent—blue; Marquis Test—yellow; Potassium Dichromate (Method 1)—brown (slow).

Thin-layer Chromatography. *System TA*—Rf 48; *system TB*—Rf 01; *system TC*—Rf 03. (*Acidified potassium permanganate solution*, positive.)

Gas Chromatography. *System GA*—not eluted.

Ultraviolet Spectrum. Aqueous acid—276 nm ($A_1^1 = 89$ a); aqueous alkali—297 nm ($A_1^1 = 155$ a).

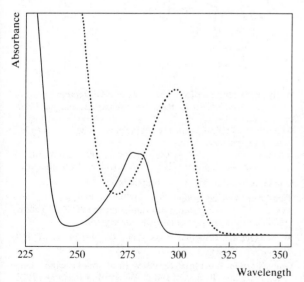

Infra-red Spectrum. Principal peaks at wavenumbers 1086, 1173, 1605, 1010, 1305, 995 (orciprenaline sulphate, KBr disk).

Mass Spectrum. Principal peaks at *m/z* 72, 43, 73, 41, 70, 65, 40, 39.

Dose. 80 mg of orciprenaline sulphate daily.

Orphenadrine
Anticholinergic

Synonyms. Mephenamine; Orphenadin.
NN-Dimethyl-2-(2-methylbenzhydryloxy)ethylamine
$C_{18}H_{23}NO = 269.4$
CAS—83-98-7

CH₃
$$C_6H_5 \cdot CH \cdot O \cdot CH_2 \cdot CH_2 \cdot N(CH_3)_2$$

A liquid.

Orphenadrine Citrate
Proprietary Names. Norflex; Tega-Flex; X-Otag. It is an ingredient of Norgesic.
$C_{18}H_{23}NO,C_6H_8O_7 = 461.5$
CAS—4682-36-4
A white crystalline powder. M.p. 134° to 138°.
Soluble 1 in 70 of water; slightly soluble in ethanol; practically insoluble in chloroform and ether.

Orphenadrine Hydrochloride
Proprietary Names. Biorphen; Disipal.
$C_{18}H_{23}NO,HCl = 305.8$
CAS—341-69-5
A white crystalline powder. M.p. 159° to 162°.
Soluble 1 in 1 of water, 1 in 1 of ethanol, and 1 in 2 of chloroform; practically insoluble in ether.

Dissociation Constant. pK_a 8.4.

Partition Coefficient. Log *P* (heptane), 1.5.

Colour Tests. Mandelin's Test—orange; Marquis Test—yellow-orange; Sulphuric Acid—orange.

Thin-layer Chromatography. *System TA*—Rf 55; *system TB*—Rf 48; *system TC*—Rf 33. (*Dragendorff spray*, positive; *acidified iodoplatinate solution*, positive; *Marquis reagent*, yellow.)

Gas Chromatography. *System GA*—orphenadrine RI 1936, *N*-monodesmethylorphenadrine RI 1920; *system GF*—RI 2185.

High Pressure Liquid Chromatography. *System HA*—orphenadrine k' 3.0, *N*-monodesmethylorphenadrine k' 1.7, orphenadrine *N*-oxide k' 1.1 (tailing peak).

Ultraviolet Spectrum. Aqueous acid—258 nm, 264 nm ($A_1^1 = 24$ a). No alkaline shift. (See below)

Infra-red Spectrum. Principal peaks at wavenumbers 1718, 1216, 1108, 1285, 1585, 1265 (orphenadrine citrate, KBr disk). (See below)

Mass Spectrum. Principal peaks at *m/z* 58, 73, 44, 45, 165, 42, 40, 181 (no peaks above 200); *N*-monodesmethylorphenadrine 44, 59, 165, 166, 181, 179, 178, 43; orphenadrine *N*-oxide 58, 181, 43, 45, 60, 44, 165, 73.

Quantification. GAS CHROMATOGRAPHY. In plasma or urine: orphenadrine and metabolites, sensitivity 10 ng/ml, AFID—J. J. M. Labout *et al.*, *J. Chromat.*, 1977, *144*, 201–208. In postmortem tissues: FID—L. F. Wilkinson *et al.*, *J. analyt. Toxicol.*, 1983, *7*, 72–75.

Disposition in the Body. Readily absorbed after oral administration and rapidly distributed. Up to about 60% of an oral dose is excreted in the urine in 3 days. During 24 hours after dosage, under uncontrolled conditions, about 4% of a dose is excreted as unchanged drug, about 5% as *N*-monodesmethylorphenadrine (tofenacin), about 3% as *NN*-didesmethylorphenadrine, about

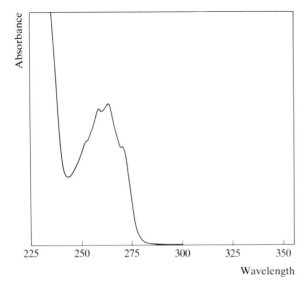

Absorbance

225   250   275   300   325   350

Wavelength

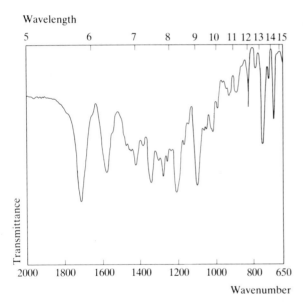

Wavelength

5   6   7   8   9   10   11 12 13 14 15

Transmittance

2000   1800   1600   1400   1200   1000   800   650

Wavenumber

3% as orphenadrine *N*-oxide, about 8% as a conjugate of 2-methylbenzhydryloxyacetic acid, and about 6% as a conjugate of 2-methylbenzhydrol. The urinary excretion appears to be dependent on urinary pH.

THERAPEUTIC CONCENTRATION. In plasma, usually in the range 0.1 to 0.2 µg/ml.

TOXICITY. The lethal dose is estimated to be in excess of about 2 g. Blood concentrations greater than about 0.5 µg/ml may cause toxic reactions and concentrations greater than 5 µg/ml may be lethal.

In a survey of 9 fatalities attributed to orphenadrine overdose, blood concentrations ranged from 1.1 to 37 µg/ml (mean 15); in 5 cases the bile

concentration was 85 to 234 µg/ml (mean 150), and in 7 cases the urine concentration was 3 to 122 µg/ml (mean 53). In one case in which a more complete analysis was reported, the concentrations were: blood 33 µg/ml, bile 202 µg/ml, brain 3.3 µg/g, kidney 15 µg/g, liver 23 µg/g, lung 19.5 µg/g, spleen 26.5 µg/g (A. E. Robinson *et al.*, *Forens. Sci.*, 1977, *9*, 53–62). In a fatality due to an orphenadrine overdose in which death occurred within 2.5 hours of ingestion, the following postmortem concentrations were reported: blood 18.1 µg/ml, liver 242 µg/g, urine 7 µg/ml (L. F. Wilkinson *et al.*, *J. analyt. Toxicol.*, 1983, *7*, 72–75).

HALF-LIFE. Plasma half-life, about 14 hours.

PROTEIN BINDING. In plasma, about 20%.

Dose. 150 to 400 mg of orphenadrine hydrochloride daily.

Ouabain   *Cardiac Glycoside*

Synonyms. G-Strophanthin; Strophanthin-G; Strophanthinum; Strophanthoside-G; Uabaina; Ubaína.

Proprietary Names. Ouabaine Arnaud; Purostrophan; Strodival; Strophoperm.

3β-(α-L-Rhamnopyranosyloxy)-$1\beta,5,11\alpha,14,19$-pentahydroxy-$5\beta,14\beta$-card-20(22)-enolide octahydrate
$C_{29}H_{44}O_{12},8H_2O = 728.8$
CAS—630-60-4 (anhydrous); *11018-89-6* (octahydrate)

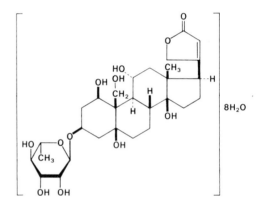

A glycoside obtained from the seeds of *Strophanthus gratus* or from the wood of *Acokanthera schimperi* or *A. ouabaio* (Apocynaceae).

Colourless crystals or white crystalline powder. M.p. about 190°, with decomposition.

Slowly **soluble** 1 in 75 of water; soluble 1 in 100 of ethanol and 1 in 30 of methanol; practically insoluble in chloroform and ether.

Colour Test. Sulphuric Acid—orange-brown (slow).

Thin-layer Chromatography. *SystemTK*—Rf 09. (*Perchloric acid solution*, followed by examination under ultraviolet light, yellow-green fluorescence; p-*anisaldehyde reagent*, yellow.)

Mass Spectrum. Principal peaks at *m/z* 183, 43, 29, 60, 41, 129, 91, 73.

Quantification. RADIOIMMUNOASSAY. In plasma or urine: sensitivity 50 pg/ml—R. Selden and T. W. Smith, *Circulation*, 1972, *45*, 1176–1182.

Disposition in the Body. Irregularly absorbed after oral administration. About 30 to 60% of a dose is excreted in the urine in 24 hours and about 25% is eliminated in the faeces in 3 days. Under steady-state conditions about 40% of the daily dose is excreted in the 24-hour urine.

THERAPEUTIC CONCENTRATION.

After a single intravenous dose of 0.5 mg to 3 subjects, a plasma concentration of about 0.012 µg/ml was reported in 5 minutes; following daily intravenous administration of 0.25 mg to 3 subjects, steady-state plasma concentrations of about 0.0005 µg/ml were attained on the 4th or 5th day (R. Selden and T. W. Smith, *ibid.*).

HALF-LIFE. Plasma half-life, about 10 to 20 hours.

PROTEIN BINDING. In plasma, about 5 to 10%.

Dose. 250 to 500 µg intravenously; further injections of 100 µg may be given up to a total dose of 1 mg in 24 hours.

Oxalic Acid

$HOOC \cdot COOH, 2H_2O = 126.1$
CAS—144-62-7 (anhydrous); *6153-56-6* (dihydrate)
Colourless, transparent, efflorescent crystals.
Soluble 1 in 12 of water, 1 in 3 of ethanol, and 1 in 100 of ether; practically insoluble in chloroform.

Dissociation Constant. pK_a 1.2, 4.2 (25°).

Colour Test. Add a few drops of a strong solution of ferrous sulphate to the acid or to a slightly acid solution of an oxalate—yellow.

Infra-red Spectrum. Principal peaks at wavenumbers 1666, 1250, 1123, 724.

Quantification. COLORIMETRY. In urine—H. Baadenhuijsen and A. P. Jansen, *Clinica chim. Acta*, 1975, *62*, 315–324.

GAS CHROMATOGRAPHY. In blood or serum: FID—P. Nuret and M. Offner, *Clinica chim. Acta*, 1978, *82*, 9–12. In postmortem blood or urine: sensitivity 13 µg/ml, AFID—G. Gauthier *et al.*, *J. Can. Soc. forens. Sci.*, 1980, *13*(4), 1–9.

HIGH PRESSURE LIQUID CHROMATOGRAPHY. In urine: sensitivity 1 µg/ml, electrochemical detection—W. J. Mayer *et al.*, *J. chromatogr. Sci.*, 1979, *17*, 656–660.

Disposition in the Body. Less than 5% of ingested oxalic acid is absorbed in healthy adults. About 8 to 40 mg of oxalic acid is normally excreted in the urine daily; this is derived mainly from the metabolism of dietary ascorbic acid and glycine with small amounts from dietary oxalic acid and other minor metabolic sources. Calcium oxalate is a major constituent of kidney stones and is frequently found as crystals in freshly-voided urine. In normal subjects concentrations of oxalic acid in blood range from about 1 to 3 µg/ml. Small amounts of oxalate are produced as a metabolite of ethylene glycol.

After intravenous administration of oxalic acid to normal subjects, more than 90% of the dose was excreted in the urine in 36 hours (T. D. Elder and J. B. Wyngaarden, *J. clin. Invest.*, 1960, *39*, 1337–1344).

TOXICITY. In dilute solution, oxalic acid and its salts are toxic owing to withdrawal of ionisable calcium from the blood and tissues with resulting tetany. Strong solutions of oxalic acid are corrosive. The mean adult lethal dose is about 15 to 30 g, although a fatality has been reported after the intravenous injection of only 1.2 g. Blood concentrations greater than 10 µg/ml are usually lethal. The maximum permissible atmospheric concentration is 1 mg/m³.

In a fatal poisoning case, a blood concentration of 110 µg/ml of oxalic acid was reported 6 hours after the ingestion of potassium hydrogen oxalate; postmortem tissue concentrations of 21 µg/g in the brain and 382 µg/g in the liver were also reported; a second subject who survived the ingestion of potassium hydrogen oxalate had a blood concentration of 3.7 µg/ml after 6 hours. Postmortem blood concentrations of 18 and 77 µg/ml were reported in 2 other fatalities (P. M. Zarembski and A. Hodgkinson, *J. clin. Path.*, 1967, *20*, 283–285).

In a fatality due to oxalic acid poisoning, a postmortem blood concentration of 370 µg/ml was reported (G. Gauthier *et al.*, *J. Can. Soc. forens. Sci.*, 1980, *13*(4), 1–9).

DISTRIBUTION IN BLOOD. Plasma: whole blood ratio, about 0.8.

PROTEIN BINDING. In plasma, not significantly bound at physiological pH values.

NOTE. For a review of oxalic acid metabolism in man, see A. Hodgkinson and P. M. Zarembski, *Calc. Tiss. Res.*, 1968, *2*, 115–132.

Oxazepam   *Tranquilliser*

Proprietary Names. Adumbran; Benzotran; Isodin; Murelax; Oxanid; Praxiten; Serax; Serenal; Serenid-D; Serepax; Seresta; Serpax; Sobril.
7-Chloro-1,3-dihydro-3-hydroxy-5-phenyl-2*H*-1,4-benzodiazepin-2-one
$C_{15}H_{11}ClN_2O_2 = 286.7$
CAS—604-75-1

A white to pale yellow crystalline powder. M.p. about 198°. Practically **insoluble** in water; soluble 1 in 220 of ethanol, 1 in 270 of chloroform, and 1 in 2200 of ether; soluble in dioxan.

Dissociation Constant. pK_a 1.7, 11.6 (20°).

Partition Coefficient. Log *P* (octanol/pH 7.4), 2.2.

Colour Test. Formaldehyde–Sulphuric Acid—orange.

Thin-layer Chromatography. *System TA*—Rf 56; *system TB*—Rf 00; *system TC*—Rf 40; *system TD*—Rf 22; *system TE*—Rf 44; *system TF*—Rf 37. (*Acidified iodoplatinate solution, positive; acidified potassium permanganate solution,* positive.)

Gas Chromatography. *System GA*—RI 2336; *system GG*—RI 2803.

High Pressure Liquid Chromatography. *System HI*—k' 4.62; *system HK*—k' 0.73.

Ultraviolet Spectrum. Aqueous acid—234 nm, 280 nm; aqueous alkali—233 nm, 344 nm; ethanol—230 nm ($A_1^1 = 1235$ a), 315 nm ($A_1^1 = 85$ a). (See below)

Infra-red Spectrum. Principal peaks at wavenumbers 1687, 1706, 693, 830, 1136, 1123 (KBr disk). (See below)

Mass Spectrum. Principal peaks at *m/z* 257, 77, 268, 239, 205, 267, 233, 259.

Quantification. GAS CHROMATOGRAPHY. In plasma: sensitivity 10 ng/ml, ECD—H. G. Giles *et al.*, *Can. J. pharm. Sci.*, 1978, *13*, 64–65.

HIGH PRESSURE LIQUID CHROMATOGRAPHY. In plasma or urine: sensitivity 30 ng/ml, UV detection—T. B. Vree *et al.*, *J. Chromat.*, 1979, *162*; *Biomed. Appl.*, *4*, 605–614.

Disposition in the Body. Readily absorbed after oral administration. About 70 to 80% of a single dose is excreted in the urine in 72 hours almost entirely as oxazepam glucuronide, with only traces of unchanged oxazepam and other minor metabolites. Up to 10% of a dose is eliminated in the faeces, mostly as unchanged drug.

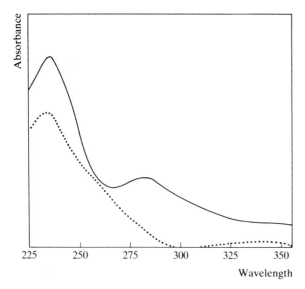

Absorbance

225   250   275   300   325   350

Wavelength

Wavelength

5   6   7   8   9   10 11 12 13 14 15

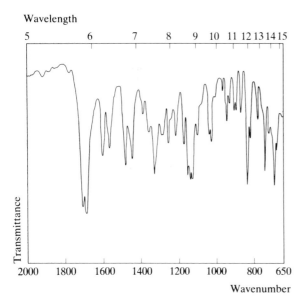

Transmittance

2000   1800   1600   1400   1200   1000   800   650

Wavenumber

Oxazepam is a metabolite of several benzodiazepines including chlordiazepoxide, clorazepate, demoxepam, desmethyldiazepam (nordazepam), diazepam, ketazolam, medazepam, prazepam, and temazepam.

THERAPEUTIC CONCENTRATION. In plasma, usually in the range 0.5 to 2 µg/ml.

A single oral dose of 45 mg administered to 8 subjects, produced serum concentrations of 0.88 to 1.44 µg/ml (mean 1.1) of oxazepam in about 2 hours, and concentrations of 0.7 to 1.4 µg/ml (mean 0.9) of oxazepam glucuronide in 2 to 4 hours. Daily oral doses of 10 mg every six hours administered to 6 subjects, produced serum concentrations of 0.14 to 0.56 µg/ml (mean 0.3) of oxazepam 2 hours after a dose, and concentrations of 0.22 to 0.40 µg/ml (mean 0.3) of oxazepam glucuronide 4 hours after a

dose (J. A. Knowles and H. W. Ruelius, *Arzneimittel-Forsch.*, 1972, *22*, 687–692).

TOXICITY. Blood concentrations greater than 2 µg/ml may produce toxic effects.

HALF-LIFE. Plasma half-life, 4 to 25 hours (mean 8).

VOLUME OF DISTRIBUTION. 0.5 to 2 litres/kg.

CLEARANCE. Plasma clearance, about 1 to 2 ml/min/kg.

DISTRIBUTION IN BLOOD. Plasma: whole blood ratio, about 0.9.

PROTEIN BINDING. In plasma, about 95%.

NOTE. For a review of the clinical pharmacokinetics of oxazepam see D. J. Greenblatt, *Clin. Pharmacokinet.*, 1981, *6*, 89–105.

Dose. 30 to 180 mg daily.

Oxedrine
Sympathomimetic

Synonyms. Oxyphenylmethylaminoethanol; Sympaethaminum; Synephrine.

Note. *m*-Synephrine has been used as a synonym for phenylephrine.

(±)-1-(4-Hydroxyphenyl)-2-methylaminoethanol
$C_9H_{13}NO_2 = 167.2$
CAS—94-07-5

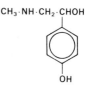

$CH_3 \cdot NH \cdot CH_2 \cdot CHOH$

OH

Crystals. M.p. 184° to 185°.

Oxedrine Tartrate

Synonym. Aethaphenum Tartaricum
Proprietary Names. Dulcidrine; Sympatol.
$(C_9H_{13}NO_2)_2, C_4H_6O_6 = 484.5$
CAS—16589-24-5; 67-04-9 (±)

Colourless crystals or white crystalline powder. M.p. about 185°, with decomposition.

Soluble 1 in 2 of water and 1 in 400 of ethanol; practically insoluble in chloroform and ether.

Dissociation Constant. pK_a 9.3 (—OH), 10.2 (—NH—), (25°).

Thin-layer Chromatography. *System TA*—Rf 25; *system TB*—Rf 04; *system TC*—Rf 01. (*Acidified potassium permanganate solution, positive.*)

High Pressure Liquid Chromatography. *System HB*—k' 0.27.

Ultraviolet Spectrum. Aqueous acid—273 nm ($A_1^1 = 81$ a); aqueous alkali—241 nm ($A_1^1 = 810$ b), 291 nm.

Infra-red Spectrum. Principal peaks at wavenumbers 835, 1510, 1054, 1271, 1098, 1611 (KBr disk).

Mass Spectrum. Principal peaks at *m/z* 44, 108, 42, 77, 107, 149, 95, 123.

Dose. Oxedrine tartrate has been given in doses of about 300 mg daily.

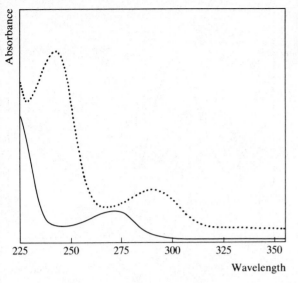

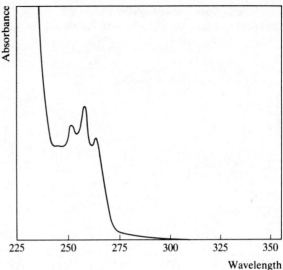

Oxeladin

Cough Suppressant

2-(2-Diethylaminoethoxy)ethyl 2-ethyl-2-phenylbutyrate
$C_{20}H_{33}NO_3 = 335.5$
CAS—468-61-1

$$C_6H_5 \cdot \underset{\underset{C_2H_5}{|}}{\overset{\overset{C_2H_5}{|}}{C}} \cdot CO \cdot O \cdot [CH_2]_2 \cdot O \cdot [CH_2]_2 \cdot N(C_2H_5)_2$$

A yellow oil.
Practically **insoluble** in water; soluble in ethanol, acetone, and ether.

Oxeladin Citrate

Proprietary Names. Dorex-retard; Paxeladine.
$C_{20}H_{33}NO_3, C_6H_8O_7 = 527.6$
CAS—52432-72-1
A white crystalline powder. M.p. 90° to 91°.
Soluble in water.

Colour Test. Marquis Test—orange.

Thin-layer Chromatography. *System TA*—Rf 50; *system TB*—Rf 51; *system TC*—Rf 22. (*Acidified iodoplatinate solution*, positive.)

Gas Chromatography. *System GA*—RI 2198.

High Pressure Liquid Chromatography. *System HA*—k' 3.0.

Ultraviolet Spectrum. Aqueous acid—252 nm, 258 nm, 264 nm.

Infra-red Spectrum. Principal peaks at wavenumbers 1731, 1128, 1221, 1100, 700, 1080 (KBr disk).

Mass Spectrum. Principal peaks at *m/z* 86, 91, 105, 87, 144, 58, 100, 56.

Dose. 80 to 120 mg of oxeladin citrate daily.

Oxethazaine

Local Anaesthetic

Synonym. Oxetacaine
Proprietary Names. It is an ingredient of Mucaine, Mucoxin, Mutesa, Muthesa, Oxaine, and Tepilta.
2,2'-(2-Hydroxyethylimino)bis[*N*-(αα-dimethylphenethyl)-*N*-methylacetamide]
$C_{28}H_{41}N_3O_3 = 467.7$
CAS—126-27-2

A white crystalline powder. M.p. about 104°.
Practically **insoluble** in water; soluble in ethanol and in dilute acids.

Oxethazaine Hydrochloride

Proprietary Name. Emoren
CAS—13930-31-9 (xHCl)
M.p. 146° to 147°.
Soluble in water.

Colour Tests. Mandelin's Test—violet-brown; Marquis Test—red-brown.

Thin-layer Chromatography. *System TA*—Rf 52; *system TB*—Rf 10; *system TC*—Rf 07; *system TL*—Rf 15. (*Acidified iodoplatinate solution*, positive.)

Gas Chromatography. *System GA*—RI 2525.

High Pressure Liquid Chromatography. *System HR—k′* 4.14.

Ultraviolet Spectrum. Aqueous acid—248 nm, 252 nm, 258 nm, 264 nm.

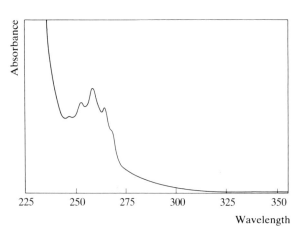

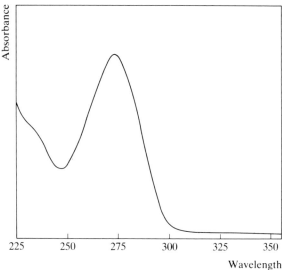

Infra-red Spectrum. Principal peaks at wavenumbers 1645, 756, 707, 1219, 1101, 1068.

Mass Spectrum. Principal peaks at *m/z* 72, 91, 114, 145, 75, 160, 117, 92.

Dose. 30 to 80 mg daily, by mouth.

Oxpentifylline   *Vasodilator*

Synonym. Pentoxifylline
Proprietary Names. Torental; Trental.
3,7-Dimethyl-1-(5-oxohexyl)xanthine
$C_{13}H_{18}N_4O_3 = 278.3$
CAS—6493-05-6

CH₃·CO·[CH₂]₃·CH₂— (structure)

A white crystalline powder. M.p. 102° to 105°.

Soluble in water; sparingly soluble in ethanol; freely soluble in chloroform and methanol; slightly soluble in ether.

Dissociation Constant. pK_a 0.3.

Colour Test. Amalic Acid Test—pink/violet.

Gas Chromatography. *System GA*—RI 2406.

Ultraviolet Spectrum. Aqueous acid—274 nm ($A_1^1 = 380$ a). No alkaline shift.

Infra-red Spectrum. Principal peaks at wavenumbers 1660, 1700, 1720, 1550, 762, 752 (KBr disk).

Quantification. GAS CHROMATOGRAPHY. In plasma: oxpentifylline and 5-hydroxyhexyl metabolite, sensitivity 3 to 10 ng/ml, AFID—T. A. Bryce and J. L. Burrows, *J. Chromat.*, 1980, *181*; *Biomed. Appl.*, 7, 355–361.

HIGH PRESSURE LIQUID CHROMATOGRAPHY. In plasma: oxpentifylline and 5-hydroxyhexyl metabolite, sensitivity 150 ng/ml, UV detection—W. Rieck and D. Platt, *J. Chromat.*, 1984, *305*; *Biomed. Appl.*, *30*, 419–427.

Disposition in the Body. Readily absorbed after oral administration. It is extensively metabolised and several metabolites have been identified in the urine. About 60% of a dose is excreted in the urine as metabolites in 24 hours, mostly in the first 4 hours; the major urinary metabolite, 1-(3-carboxypropyl)-3,7-dimethylxanthine (inactive), accounts for about 80% of the material excreted in the urine; less than 1% is excreted as unchanged drug. Other metabolites include 1-(5-hydroxyhexyl)-3,7-dimethylxanthine, which is active and is the major metabolite detected in blood, 1-(5,6-dihydroxyhexyl)-3,7-dimethylxanthine, 1-(4,5-dihydroxyhexyl)-3,7-dimethylxanthine, 1-(4-carboxybutyl)-3,7-dimethylxanthine, 3-methyl-1-(5-oxohexyl)xanthine, and 1-(5-hydroxyhexyl)-3-methylxanthine, all of which are inactive.

THERAPEUTIC CONCENTRATION.

Following a single oral dose of 400 mg to 16 fasting subjects, mean peak plasma concentrations of 1.3 μg/ml of oxpentifylline and 1.8 μg/ml of the 5-hydroxy metabolite were attained in 0.8 and 1.3 hours, respectively (R. J. Wills *et al.*, *Drug Dev. & ind. Pharm.*, 1981, 7, 385–396).

HALF-LIFE. Plasma half-life, oxpentifylline, about 1 hour, 5-hydroxy metabolite about 1 hour; 1-(3-carboxypropyl)-3,7-dimethylxanthine, derived from urinary excretion data, about 1.4 hours.

VOLUME OF DISTRIBUTION. About 5 litres/kg.

CLEARANCE. Plasma clearance, about 70 ml/min/kg.

DISTRIBUTION IN BLOOD. Plasma: whole blood ratio, about 1.2.

Dose. Usually 300 to 600 mg daily; sustained-release tablets are given in doses of 0.8 to 1.2 g daily.

Oxprenolol
Beta-adrenoceptor Blocking Agent

Synonym. Oxyprenolol
($\pm$)-1-(2-Allyloxyphenoxy)-3-isopropylaminopropan-2-ol
$C_{15}H_{23}NO_3 = 265.4$
CAS—6452-71-7; 22972-98-1 ($\pm$)

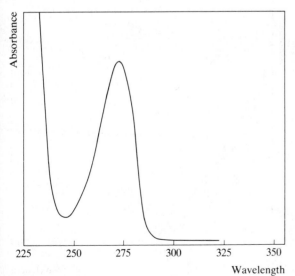

Crystals. M.p. 75° to 80°.

Oxprenolol Hydrochloride
Proprietary Names. Apsolox; Laracor; Slow-Pren; Slow-Trasicor; Trasicor. It is an ingredient of Trasidrex.
$C_{15}H_{23}NO_3,HCl = 301.8$
CAS—6452-73-9; 22972-97-0 ($\pm$)
A white to slightly cream-coloured crystalline powder. M.p. 106° to 109°.
Soluble 1 in less than 1 of water and 1 in 1.5 of ethanol; very slightly soluble in ether.

Dissociation Constant. pK_a 9.5.

Colour Tests. Liebermann's Test—black; Mandelin's Test—grey-violet; Marquis Test—violet; Sulphuric Acid—orange-red (fluoresces under ultraviolet light at 350 nm).

Thin-layer Chromatography. *System TA*—Rf 48; *system TB*—Rf 11; *system TC*—Rf 11. (*Acidified iodoplatinate solution*, positive.)

Gas Chromatography. *System GA*—RI 1870; *system GF*—RI 2270.

High Pressure Liquid Chromatography. *System HA*—k' 1.3.

Ultraviolet Spectrum. Aqueous acid—273 nm ($A_1^1 = 85$ a). No alkaline shift.

Infra-red Spectrum. Principal peaks at wavenumbers 1258, 750, 1500, 1120, 1092, 1037 (oxprenolol hydrochloride, KBr disk).

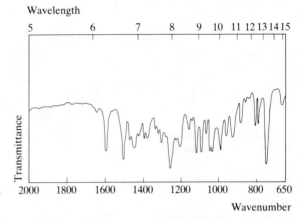

Mass Spectrum. Principal peaks at *m/z* 72, 41, 56, 43, 221, 73, 57, 45.

Quantification. GAS CHROMATOGRAPHY. In serum: detection limit 2 pg, ECD—D. DeBruyne *et al.*, *J. pharm. Sci.*, 1979, *68*, 511–512.

HIGH PRESSURE LIQUID CHROMATOGRAPHY. In plasma, blood or urine: sensitivity 10 ng/ml, UV detection—S. Tsuei *et al.*, *J. Chromat.*, 1980, *181*; *Biomed. Appl.*, *7*, 135–140.

THIN-LAYER CHROMATOGRAPHY–SPECTROFLUORIMETRY. In plasma: sensitivity 10 ng/ml—M. Schäefer and E. Mutschler, *J. Chromat.*, 1979, *164*; *Biomed. Appl.*, *6*, 247–252.

Disposition in the Body. Readily absorbed after oral administration but subject to extensive first-pass metabolism. The major metabolite is oxprenolol glucuronide. About 70 to 90% of a dose is excreted in the urine in 24 hours, with less than 5% as unchanged drug.

THERAPEUTIC CONCENTRATION.
Following a single oral dose of 40 mg to 7 subjects, peak blood concentrations of 0.09 to 0.24 µg/ml (mean 0.15) of oxprenolol and 0.11 to 0.35 µg/ml (mean 0.24) of oxprenolol glucuronide were attained in 0.5 to 1.5 hours and 1 to 2.5 hours respectively (P. Dayer *et al.*, *Eur. J. drug Met. Pharmacokinet.*, 1983, *8*, 181–188).
Following oral administration of 160 mg twice daily to 27 subjects, steady-state plasma concentrations of 0.1 to 1.8 µg/ml (mean 0.9) were reported, determined 1 hour after a dose (B. Silke *et al.*, *Eur. J. clin. Pharmac.*, 1983, *24*, 7–14).

TOXICITY.
In a fatality attributed to oxprenolol overdose, a postmortem liver concentration of 58 µg/g was reported (J. S. Oliver and A. A. Watson, *Medicine, Sci. Law*, 1977, *17*, 279–281).
In a fatality in which death occurred 2 hours after the ingestion of 4.5 g, the following postmortem concentrations were reported: blood 10 µg/ml, brain 71 µg/g, liver 230 µg/g (A. Khan and J. M. Muscat-Baron, *Br. med. J.*, 1977, *1*, 552).

HALF-LIFE. Plasma half-life, 1 to 3 hours.

VOLUME OF DISTRIBUTION. About 1 litre/kg.

PROTEIN BINDING. In plasma, about 80%.

Dose. 80 to 480 mg of oxprenolol hydrochloride daily.

Oxybuprocaine

Local Anaesthetic

Synonym. Benoxinate

2-Diethylaminoethyl 4-amino-3-butoxybenzoate

$C_{17}H_{28}N_2O_3 = 308.4$

CAS—99-43-4

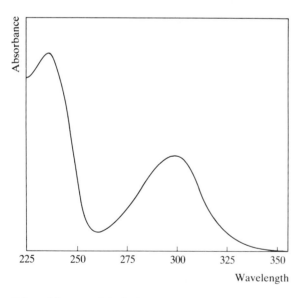

Oxybuprocaine Hydrochloride

Proprietary Names. Cébésine; Conjuncain; Novesine.

$C_{17}H_{28}N_2O_3,HCl = 344.9$

CAS—5987-82-6

White crystals or crystalline powder. M.p. about 158°.

Soluble 1 in 0.8 of water, 1 in 2.6 of ethanol, and 1 in 2.5 of chloroform; practically insoluble in ether.

Colour Tests. Coniferyl Alcohol—orange; Diazotisation—red.

Thin-layer Chromatography. *System TA*—Rf 62; *system TB*—Rf 23; *system TC*—Rf 41; *system TL*—Rf 36. (*Acidified iodoplatinate solution,* positive.)

Gas Chromatography. *System GA*—RI 2471.

High Pressure Liquid Chromatography. *System HQ*—k' 16.25; *system HR*—k' 0.86.

Ultraviolet Spectrum. Aqueous acid—235 nm $(A_1^1 = 437\,b)$, 298 nm; aqueous alkali—231 nm, 310 nm.

Infra-red Spectrum. Principal peaks at wavenumbers 1709, 1214, 1261, 1613, 1294, 1311 (oxybuprocaine hydrochloride, KBr disk).

Mass Spectrum. Principal peaks at *m/z* 86, 99, 29, 30, 100, 71, 87, 192.

Use. Oxybuprocaine hydrochloride is used as a 0.4% solution.

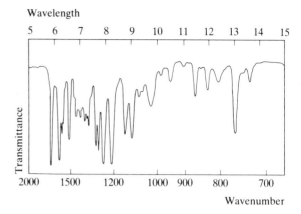

Oxyclozanide

Anthelmintic (Veterinary)

Proprietary Name. Zanil

3,3',5,5',6-Pentachloro-2'-hydroxysalicylanilide

$C_{13}H_6Cl_5NO_3 = 401.5$

CAS—2277-92-1

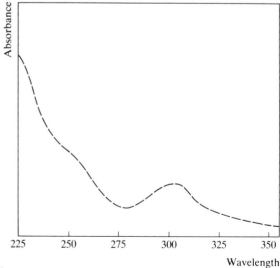

A cream-coloured powder. M.p. about 208°.

Very slightly **soluble** in water; soluble 1 in 20 of ethanol, 1 in 5 of acetone, and 1 in 600 of chloroform; soluble in solutions of alkali hydroxides and carbonates.

Colour Test. Mandelin's Test—violet → orange.

Thin-layer Chromatography. *System TA*—Rf 87. (*Acidified potassium permanganate solution,* positive.)

Gas Chromatography. *System GA*—not eluted.

Ultraviolet Spectrum. Aqueous alkali—324 nm $(A_1^1 = 338\,b)$; methanol—303 nm $(A_1^1 = 188\,b)$.

Infra-red Spectrum. Principal peaks at wavenumbers 1203, 1527, 1166, 1587, 1155, 1219 (KBr disk).

Oxycodone   *Narcotic Analgesic*

Synonyms.   7,8-Dihydro-14-hydroxycodeinone;   Dihydrone; Oxycone.

6-Deoxy-7,8-dihydro-14-hydroxy-3-*O*-methyl-6-oxomorphine

$C_{18}H_{21}NO_4 = 315.4$

CAS—76-42-6

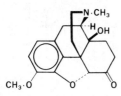

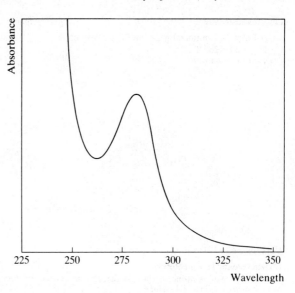

Wavelength

M.p. 218° to 220°.

Practically **insoluble** in water and ether; soluble in ethanol and chloroform.

Oxycodone Hydrochloride

Synonym. Thecodine

Proprietary Names. Endone; Eubine; Eukodal; Supeudol. It is an ingredient of Percocet and Percodan.

$C_{18}H_{21}NO_4,HCl,3H_2O = 405.9$

CAS—124-90-3 (anhydrous)

A white crystalline powder. M.p. about 275°.

Soluble 1 in 6 of water, 1 in 60 of ethanol, and 1 in 600 of chloroform; practically insoluble in ether.

Dissociation Constant. pK_a 8.9 (20°).

Colour Test. Marquis Test—yellow → brown → violet.

Thin-layer Chromatography. *System TA*—Rf 50; *system TB*—Rf 23; *system TC*—Rf 51. (*Dragendorff spray*, positive; *acidified iodoplatinate solution*, positive; *Marquis reagent*, violet.)

Gas Chromatography. *System GA*—oxycodone RI 2524, oxymorphone RI 2532.

High Pressure Liquid Chromatography. *System HA*—oxycodone k' 6.9 (tailing peak), oxymorphone k' 6.7 (tailing peak); *system HC*—k' 0.85.

Ultraviolet Spectrum. Aqueous acid—280 nm ($A_1^1 = 44$ a). No alkaline shift.

Infra-red Spectrum. Principal peaks at wavenumbers 1719, 1501, 1033, 1255, 934, 980 (KBr disk).

Mass Spectrum. Principal peaks at m/z 315, 230, 316, 70, 44, 42, 258, 140; oxymorphone 301, 216, 44, 42, 70, 302, 203, 57.

Quantification. GAS CHROMATOGRAPHY. In urine: oxycodone and oxymorphone, ECD—R. C. Baselt and C. B. Stewart, *J. analyt. Toxicol.*, 1978, *2*, 107–109. In plasma: sensitivity 2 ng/ml, AFID—N. L. Renzi and J. N. Tam, *J. pharm. Sci.*, 1979, *68*, 43–45. In plasma or urine: oxycodone and noroxycodone, sensitivity 1 ng/ml, ECD—S. H. Weinstein and J. C. Gaylord, *ibid.*, 527–528.

Disposition in the Body. Absorbed after oral administration. Metabolised to some extent by *O*-demethylation to oxymorphone which is active, and by *N*-demethylation to noroxycodone. About 30 to 60% of a dose is excreted in the urine in 24 hours as free and conjugated oxycodone, conjugated oxymorphone, and noroxycodone.

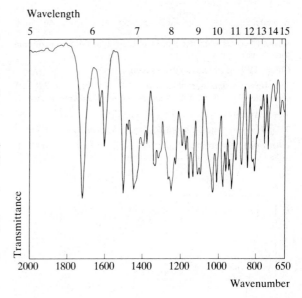

Wavelength

Wavenumber

THERAPEUTIC CONCENTRATION.

After a single oral dose containing 4.5 mg of oxycodone hydrochloride and 0.38 mg of oxycodone terephthalate, administered to 6 subjects, peak plasma concentrations of 0.017 to 0.037 µg/ml (mean 0.024) were attained in 1 to 2 hours (N. L. Renzi and J. N. Tam, *J. pharm. Sci.*, 1979, *68*, 43–45).

TOXICITY. The estimated minimum lethal dose is 500 mg. Prolonged use of oxycodone may lead to dependence of the morphine type.

The following postmortem concentrations were reported in a subject who died while underwater diving: blood 5 µg/ml, bile 28 µg/ml, brain 28 µg/g, liver 12 µg/g (P. Sedgwick, *Bull. int. Ass. forens. Toxicol.*, 1973, *9*(3&4), 16).

Dose. Oxycodone hydrochloride may be given by mouth in doses of 5 to 20 mg.

Oxymetazoline

Sympathomimetic

6-*tert*-Butyl-3-(2-imidazolin-2-ylmethyl)-2,4-xylenol
$C_{16}H_{24}N_2O = 260.4$
CAS—1491-59-4

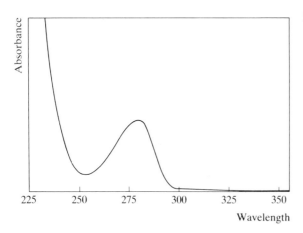

Crystals. M.p. 181° to 183°.

Oxymetazoline Hydrochloride

Proprietary Names. Afrazine; Afrin; Drixine; Durazol; Hazol; Iliadin-Mini; Nafrine; Nasivin; Rhinolitan.
$C_{16}H_{24}N_2O,HCl = 296.8$
CAS—2315-02-8
A white, hygroscopic, crystalline powder. M.p. about 300°, with decomposition.
Soluble 1 in 6.7 of water and 1 in 3.6 of ethanol; practically insoluble in chloroform and ether.

Colour Test. Mandelin's Test—green.

Thin-layer Chromatography. *System TA*—Rf 09; *system TB*—Rf 01; *system TC*—Rf 01. (*Acidified iodoplatinate solution*, positive.)

Gas Chromatography. *System GA*—RI 2168.

High Pressure Liquid Chromatography. *System HA*—k' 1.7.

Ultraviolet Spectrum. Aqueous acid—280 nm ($A_1^1 = 68$ a); aqueous alkali—303 nm ($A_1^1 = 164$ b).

Infra-red Spectrum. Principal peaks at wavenumbers 1595, 1199, 1285, 1250, 1070, 765 (oxymetazoline hydrochloride, KBr disk).

Mass Spectrum. Principal peaks at *m/z* 245, 260, 44, 217, 218, 246, 261, 259.

Use. Oxymetazoline hydrochloride is used as a 0.05% solution.

Oxymetholone

Anabolic Steroid

Proprietary Names. Adroyd; Anadrol-50; Anapolon; Anasteron; Nastenon; Pardroyd; Plenastril.

17β-Hydroxy-2-hydroxymethylene-17α-methyl-5α-androstan-3-one
$C_{21}H_{32}O_3 = 332.5$
CAS—434-07-1

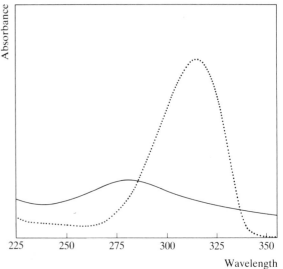

A white to creamy-white crystalline powder. M.p. 172° to 180°. Practically **insoluble** in water; soluble 1 in 50 of ethanol; freely soluble in chloroform; soluble in dioxan; slightly soluble in ether.

Colour Tests. Antimony Pentachloride—brown; Naphthol-Sulphuric Acid—brown/pink-orange; Sulphuric Acid—orange.

Thin-layer Chromatography. *System TP*—Rf 69; *system TQ*—Rf 23; *system TR*—Rf 85; *system TS*—Rf 82. (p-*Toluenesulphonic acid solution*, positive.)

Gas Chromatography. *System GA*—RI 2835.

Ultraviolet Spectrum. Methanolic acid—277 nm ($A_1^1 = 300$ b); methanolic alkali—315 nm ($A_1^1 = 547$ a).

Infra-red Spectrum. Principal peaks at wavenumbers 1612, 1204, 1219, 1306, 1157, 935 (KBr disk).

Dose. Usually 5 to 10 mg daily; doses of 100 to 350 mg daily may be given.

Oxymorphone
Narcotic Analgesic

Synonyms. 7,8-Dihydro-14-hydroxymorphinone; Oximorphone; Oxydimorphone.

6-Deoxy-7,8-dihydro-14-hydroxy-6-oxomorphine
$C_{17}H_{19}NO_4 = 301.3$
CAS—76-41-5

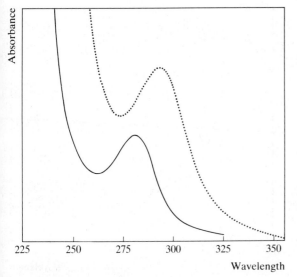

Crystals. M.p. 248° to 249°, with decomposition.
Soluble in boiling ethanol and in chloroform.

Oxymorphone Hydrochloride
Proprietary Name. Numorphan
$C_{17}H_{19}NO_4,HCl = 337.8$
CAS—357-07-1
A white powder which darkens on exposure to light.
Soluble 1 in 4 of water, 1 in 100 of ethanol, and 1 in 25 of methanol; very slightly soluble in chloroform and ether.

Dissociation Constant. pK_a 8.5, 9.3.

Partition Coefficient. Log P (octanol/pH 7.4), 0.

Colour Test. Marquis Test—grey-violet.

Thin-layer Chromatography. *System TA*—Rf 48; *system TB*—Rf 10; *system TC*—Rf 37. (*Dragendorff spray*, positive; *acidified iodoplatinate solution*, positive; *Marquis reagent*, grey.)

Gas Chromatography. *System GA*—RI 2532.

High Pressure Liquid Chromatography. *System HA*—k' 6.7 (tailing peak).

Ultraviolet Spectrum. Aqueous acid—281 nm ($A_1^1 = 34$ a); aqueous alkali—292 nm.

Infra-red Spectrum. Principal peaks at wavenumbers 1730, 1240, 1225, 1145, 941, 953 (KBr disk).

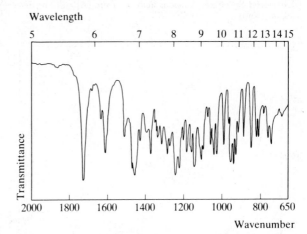

Mass Spectrum. Principal peaks at *m/z* 301, 216, 44, 42, 70, 302, 203, 57.

Disposition in the Body. Absorbed after oral administration. About 50% of an oral dose is excreted in the urine in 5 days (mostly in the first 24 hours), mainly as conjugated oxymorphone together with small quantities of unchanged drug and the conjugated 6α- and 6β-hydroxy metabolites.
Oxymorphone is a metabolite of oxycodone.

TOXICITY. The estimated minimum lethal dose is 50 mg. Prolonged use of oxymorphone may lead to dependence of the morphine type.

REFERENCE. E. J. Cone *et al.*, *Drug Met. Disp.*, 1983, *11*, 446–450.

Dose. 0.5 to 1.5 mg of oxymorphone hydrochloride given parenterally; doses of 5 to 10 mg have been given by mouth.

Oxypertine
Tranquilliser

Proprietary Names. Equipertine; Forit; Integrin; Opertil.
5,6 - Dimethoxy - 2 - methyl - 3 - [2 - (4 - phenylpiperazin - 1 - yl)ethyl]indole
$C_{23}H_{29}N_3O_2 = 379.5$
CAS—153-87-7

A white crystalline powder.
Slightly **soluble** in water and ethanol.

Colour Tests. Liebermann's Test—blue; Mandelin's Test—grey; Marquis Test—grey-green.

Thin-layer Chromatography. *System TA*—Rf 68; *system TB*—Rf 04; *system TC*—Rf 65. (*Acidified iodoplatinate solution*, positive.)

Gas Chromatography. *System GA*—RI 2355.

High Pressure Liquid Chromatography. *System HA*—k' 0.7; *system HF*—k' 1.33.

Ultraviolet Spectrum. Aqueous acid—301 nm (A$_1^1$ = 212 b). No alkaline shift.

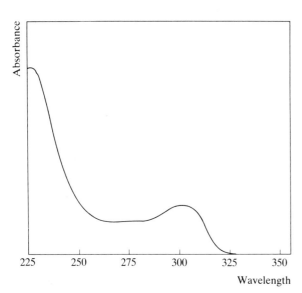

Infra-red Spectrum. Principal peaks at wavenumbers 1233, 1153, 1205, 1592, 762, 1003 (KBr disk).

Wavelength

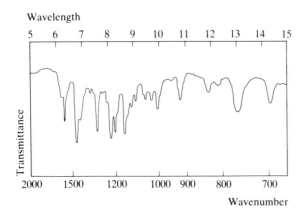

Wavenumber

Mass Spectrum. Principal peaks at *m/z* 175, 70, 176, 132, 379, 204, 56, 217.

Quantification. HIGH PRESSURE LIQUID CHROMATOGRAPHY. In serum: sensitivity 20 ng/ml, UV detection—Y. Minatogawa *et al., J. Chromat.*, 1983, *274*; *Biomed. Appl.*, *25*, 413–416.

Dose. Usually up to 300 mg daily.

Oxyphenbutazone   *Analgesic*

Synonym. Hydroxyphenylbutazone
Proprietary Names. Imbun; Isobutil; Oxalid; Oxybutazone; Phlogase; Rheumapax; Tandearil; Tanderil.

4 - Butyl - 1 - (4 - hydroxyphenyl) - 2 - phenylpyrazolidine - 3,5 - dione monohydrate
C$_{19}$H$_{20}$N$_2$O$_3$,H$_2$O = 342.4
CAS—*129-20-4* (anhydrous); *7081-38-1* (monohydrate)

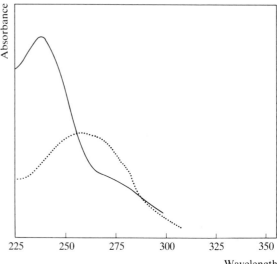

A white to yellowish-white crystalline powder. M.p. 85° to 100°. Practically **insoluble** in water; soluble 1 in 3 of ethanol, 1 in 6 of acetone, 1 in 20 of chloroform, and 1 in 20 of ether.

Dissociation Constant. pK$_a$ 4.7 (22°).

Partition Coefficient. Log *P* (octanol), 3.3.

Colour Test. Marquis Test—yellow.

Thin-layer Chromatography. *System TA*—Rf 77; *system TD*—Rf 52; *system TE*—Rf 07; *system TF*—Rf 62; *system TG*—Rf 25. (*Chromic acid solution*, yellow; *Ludy Tenger reagent*, orange; *mercurous nitrate spray*, positive; *acidified potassium permanganate solution*, positive.)

Gas Chromatography. *System GA*—RI 1630; *system GD*—retention time of methyl derivative 2.11 relative to *n*-C$_{16}$H$_{34}$.

High Pressure Liquid Chromatography. *System HD*—k' 1.95; *system HV*—retention time 0.69 relative to meclofenamic acid.

Ultraviolet Spectrum. Aqueous acid—237 nm; aqueous alkali—254 nm (A$_1^1$ = 750 a).

Infra-red Spectrum. Principal peaks at wavenumbers 1683, 1736, 1275, 1512, 765, 1600 (KBr disk).

Wavelength

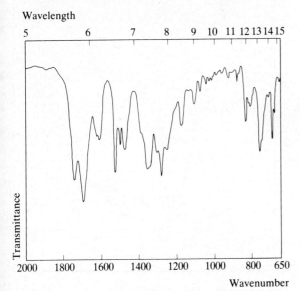

Mass Spectrum. Principal peaks at m/z 199, 324, 93, 77, 65, 55, 121, 135.

Quantification. GAS CHROMATOGRAPHY. In plasma: sensitivity 2.5 µg/ml, AFID—M. Bertrand *et al., J. Chromat.,* 1979, *171,* 377–383.

HIGH PRESSURE LIQUID CHROMATOGRAPHY. In plasma: sensitivity 250 ng/ml, UV detection—N. J. Pound and R. W. Sears, *J. pharm. Sci.,* 1975, *64,* 284–287.

Disposition in the Body. Almost completely absorbed after oral administration. It is slowly metabolised by glucuronide conjugation and by hydroxylation; it is slowly excreted in the urine, less than 2% of a dose being excreted as unchanged drug and about 1 to 5% as the *O*-glucuronide conjugate in 24 hours. Oxyphenbutazone is a major metabolite of phenylbutazone.

THERAPEUTIC CONCENTRATION.
Following a single oral dose of 200 mg to 10 subjects, peak plasma concentrations of 11.4 to 43.7 µg/ml were attained in 2 to 12 hours (M. Bertrand *et al., J. Chromat.,* 1979, *171,* 377–383).
Following daily oral doses of 300 to 400 mg to 6 subjects, steady-state plasma concentrations determined immediately before a dose ranged from 27 to 95 µg/ml (mean 62) (M. Weiner *et al., Proc. Soc. exp. Biol. Med.,* 1967, *124,* 1170–1173).

TOXICITY. The estimated minimum lethal dose is 5 g.

HALF-LIFE. Plasma half-life, about 2 to 3 days.

VOLUME OF DISTRIBUTION. About 0.1 litre/kg.

PROTEIN BINDING. In plasma, about 99%.

Dose. Oxyphenbutazone has been given in doses of 100 to 800 mg daily.

Oxyphencyclimine   *Anticholinergic*

1,4,5,6 - Tetrahydro - 1 - methylpyrimidin - 2 - ylmethyl α-cyclohexylmandelate
$C_{20}H_{28}N_2O_3 = 344.5$
CAS—125-53-1

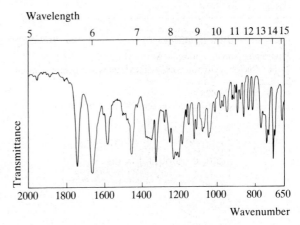

Oxyphencyclimine Hydrochloride
Proprietary Names. Daricon; Manir; Vagogastrin. It is an ingredient of Enarax and Vistrax.
$C_{20}H_{28}N_2O_3,HCl = 380.9$
CAS—125-52-0
A white crystalline powder. M.p. about 234°.
Soluble 1 in 100 of water, 1 in 75 of ethanol, 1 in 500 of chloroform, 1 in 3000 of ether, and 1 in 20 of methanol.

Partition Coefficient. Log *P* (heptane), 3.3.

Colour Test. Mandelin's Test—grey-green.

Thin-layer Chromatography. *System TA*—Rf 02; *system TB*—Rf 01; *system TC*—Rf 03. (*Acidified iodoplatinate solution,* positive.)

Gas Chromatography. *System GA*—RI 2550; *system GF*—RI 2900.

High Pressure Liquid Chromatography. *System HA*—k' 2.8.

Infra-red Spectrum. Principal peaks at wavenumbers 1656, 1737, 1227, 705, 1201, 1211 (oxyphencyclimine hydrochloride, KBr disk).

Wavelength

Mass Spectrum. Principal peaks at m/z 105, 129, 112, 77, 42, 313, 41, 55.

Dose. 10 to 20 mg of oxyphencyclimine hydrochloride daily; up to 50 mg daily has been given.

Oxyphenisatin   *Purgative*

Synonym. Dihydroxyphenylisatin
Proprietary Name. Veripaque
3,3-Bis(4-hydroxyphenyl)indolin-2-one
$C_{20}H_{15}NO_3 = 317.3$
CAS—125-13-3

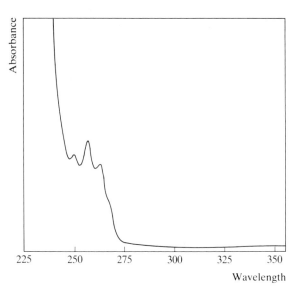

Oxyphenisatin Acetate

Synonyms. Acetphenolisatin; Bisatin; Diacetoxydiphenylisatin; Diacetyldiphenolisatin; Diasatin; Diphesatin; Isaphenin; Oxyphenisatin Diacetate.
$C_{24}H_{19}NO_5 = 401.4$
CAS—115-33-3
A white crystalline powder. M.p. about 245°.
Practically **insoluble** in water; soluble 1 in 70 of chloroform; very slightly soluble in ethanol and ether.

Colour Tests. Folin–Ciocalteu Reagent—blue; Koppanyi–Zwikker Test—violet; Liebermann's Test—black; Mandelin's Test—violet; Marquis Test—violet; Mercurous Nitrate—black.

Thin-layer Chromatography. *System TA—Rf 82. (Acidified potassium permanganate solution, positive.)*

Infra-red Spectrum. Principal peaks at wavenumbers 1188, 1727, 1495, 1232, 1162, 1011 (KBr disk).

Mass Spectrum. Principal peaks at m/z 317, 288, 359, 401, 43, 318, 289, 196 (oxyphenisatin acetate).

Dose. Oxyphenisatin acetate has been given in a dose of 5 to 20 mg.

Oxyphenonium Bromide   *Anticholinergic*

Proprietary Names. Antrenil; Antrenyl.
2 - (α - Cyclohexylmandeloyloxy)ethyldiethylmethylammonium bromide
$C_{21}H_{34}BrNO_3 = 428.4$
CAS—14214-84-7 (oxyphenonium); 50-10-2 (bromide)

A white crystalline powder. M.p. about 190°.
Freely **soluble** in water, ethanol, and chloroform.

Thin-layer Chromatography. *System TA—Rf 03. (Acidified iodoplatinate solution, positive.)*

High Pressure Liquid Chromatography. *System HA—k′ 2.6 (tailing peak).*

Ultraviolet Spectrum. Aqueous acid—252 nm, 258 nm ($A_1^1 = 5.3$ a), 264 nm.

Infra-red Spectrum. Principal peaks at wavenumbers 1225, 1719, 729, 704, 1030, 1111 (KBr disk).

Dose. 20 to 40 mg daily.

Oxytetracycline Dihydrate   *Antibiotic*

Synonyms. 5-Hydroxytetracycline; Oxytetracycline; Terrafungine.
Proprietary Names. Abbocin; Chemocycline (tablets); Galenomycin; Imperacin; Oxymed; Oxymycin; Terramycin (tablets).
5β-Hydroxytetracycline dihydrate
$C_{22}H_{24}N_2O_9,2H_2O = 496.5$
CAS—79-57-2 (anhydrous); 6153-64-6 (dihydrate)

A yellow to tan-coloured crystalline powder. Stable in air but darkens on exposure to strong sunlight.
Soluble 1 in 4150 of water, 1 in 66 of dehydrated alcohol, and 1 in 6250 of ether; sparingly soluble in ethanol; practically insoluble in chloroform; soluble in dilute acids and alkalis.

Oxytetracycline Calcium
Proprietary Names. Chemocycline (syrup); Terramycin (syrup).
$C_{44}H_{46}CaN_4O_{18} = 958.9$
CAS—15251-48-6 (xCa)
A yellow to light brown crystalline powder.
Practically **insoluble** in water; soluble in dilute solutions of sodium hydroxide.

Oxytetracycline Hydrochloride
Proprietary Names. Macocyn; Terramycin (capsules); Unimycin. It is an ingredient of Bisolvomycin and Terra-Cortril.
$C_{22}H_{24}N_2O_9,HCl = 496.9$
CAS—2058-46-0
A yellow, hygroscopic, crystalline powder, which darkens on exposure to sunlight or to moist air above 90°. It decomposes above 180°.

Soluble 1 in 2 of water, 1 in 45 of ethanol, and 1 in 45 of methanol; less soluble in dehydrated alcohol; practically insoluble in chloroform and ether. Solutions in water become turbid on standing owing to precipitation of oxytetracycline base.

Dissociation Constant. pK_a 3.3, 7.3, 9.1 (25°).

Partition Coefficient. Log P (octanol/pH 7.5), −1.6.

Colour Tests. Benedict's Reagent—red; Formaldehyde–Sulphuric Acid—brown-red; Liebermann's Test—red; Mandelin's Test—violet → red → orange; Marquis Test—orange; Sulphuric Acid—violet-red.

Thin-layer Chromatography. *System TA*—Rf 05, streaking. (Location under ultraviolet light, orange fluorescence; *acidified potassium permanganate solution*, positive.)

Ultraviolet Spectrum. Aqueous acid—268 nm ($A_1^1 = 400$ a), 352 nm; aqueous alkali—246 nm, 269 nm.

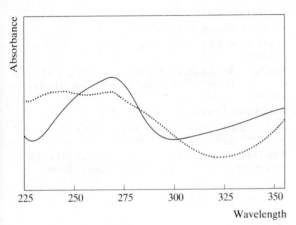

Infra-red Spectrum. Principal peaks at wavenumbers 1616, 1584, 1665, 1235, 1180, 1138 (oxytetracycline hydrochloride, KBr disk).

Quantification. SPECTROFLUORIMETRY. In blood or plasma: sensitivity < 100 ng/ml—B. Scales and D. A. Assinder, *J. pharm. Sci.*, 1973, *62*, 913–917.

Disposition in the Body. Incompletely and irregularly absorbed after oral administration and widely distributed throughout the body. About 70% of a dose is excreted in the urine; biliary excretion also occurs.

THERAPEUTIC CONCENTRATION.

Following oral doses of 500 mg to 4 subjects, peak plasma concentrations of 1.2 to 3.4 µg/ml (mean 2.1) were attained in 2 to 3 hours (B. Scales and D. A. Assinder, *ibid.*).

HALF-LIFE. Plasma half-life, about 9 hours, increased in renal impairment.

PROTEIN BINDING. In plasma, about 20 to 35%.

Dose. Up to 3 g of oxytetracycline hydrochloride daily.

Padimate   *Sunscreen Agent*

Synonyms. Amyl Dimethylaminobenzoate; Isoamyl Dimethylaminobenzoate; Padimate A.
Proprietary Names. Escalol 506; Pabafilm; SpectraBAN 4; Uvosan.

A mixture of pentyl, isopentyl, and 2-methylbutyl 4-dimethylaminobenzoates.
$C_{14}H_{21}NO_2 = 235.3$
CAS—14779-78-3
A yellow liquid.
Practically **insoluble** in water; soluble in ethanol, chloroform, and isopropyl alcohol.

Padimate O

Synonyms. 2-Ethylhexyl 4-(dimethylamino)benzoate; Octyl Dimethyl PABA.
Proprietary Names. Eclipse; Escalol 507; Phiasol; PreSun 4. It is an ingredient of Super Shade 15.
$C_{17}H_{27}NO_2 = 277.4$
CAS—21245-02-3
A light yellow, mobile liquid.
Practically **insoluble** in water; soluble in ethanol and isopropyl alcohol.

Colour Tests. Aromaticity (Method 2)—yellow/orange; Liebermann's Test (100°)—blue.

Thin-layer Chromatography. *System TA*—Rf 75. (*Acidified iodoplatinate solution*, positive.)

Gas Chromatography. *System GA*—RI 1964.

Use. Topically in a concentration of 2.5%.

Pancuronium Bromide   *Muscle Relaxant*

Synonym. Poncuronium Bromide
Proprietary Name. Pavulon
1,1' - (3α,17β - Diacetoxy - 5α - androstan - 2β,16β - ylene)bis(1 - methylpiperidinium) dibromide
$C_{35}H_{60}Br_2N_2O_4 = 732.7$
CAS—15500-66-0

White, hygroscopic crystals or crystalline powder. M.p. 215°, with decomposition. A solution in water is dextrorotatory.
Soluble 1 in 1 of water, 1 in 5 of ethanol, 1 in 5 of chloroform, and 1 in 1 of methanol; practically insoluble in ether.

Colour Test. Antimony Pentachloride—green.

Thin-layer Chromatography. *System TA*—Rf 01; *system TN*—Rf 80. (*Acidified iodoplatinate solution*, positive.)

Ultraviolet Spectrum. No significant absorption, 230 to 360 nm.

Infra-red Spectrum. Principal peaks at wavenumbers 1225, 1745, 1031, 1056, 1013, 907 (KBr disk). (See below)

Quantification. SPECTROFLUORIMETRY. In serum: sensitivity 50 ng/ml—L. B. Wingard *et al.*, *J. pharm. Sci.*, 1979, *68*, 914–916.

Disposition in the Body. Metabolised by hydroxylation to 3-hydroxypancuronium which is about half as active as pancuronium, and to a small extent to the 17-hydroxy and 3,17-dihydroxy derivatives which are virtually inactive. About 25% of a dose is

Wavelength

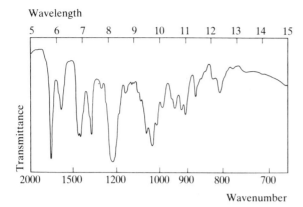

excreted in the urine unchanged and 15% as the 3-hydroxy metabolite, in about 30 hours; about 10% of a dose is excreted in the bile.

THERAPEUTIC CONCENTRATION.

After an intravenous injection of 4 mg to 6 subjects, plasma concentrations of about 0.6 µg/ml were reported at 5 minutes, decreasing to 0.07 µg/ml at 4 hours (K. McLeod et al., Br. J. Anaesth., 1976, 48, 341–345).

TOXICITY.

In a suicide case due to the intravenous administration of pancuronium bromide, postmortem concentrations were: blood 1.6 µg/ml, urine 1.5 µg/ml; thiopentone and thioridazine were also detected (A. Poklis and E. G. Melanson, J. analyt. Toxicol., 1980, 4, 275–280).

HALF-LIFE. Plasma half-life, about 2 hours.

VOLUME OF DISTRIBUTION. 0.1 to 0.4 litre/kg.

CLEARANCE. Plasma clearance, about 1 to 2 ml/min/kg.

PROTEIN BINDING. In plasma, about 87%.

NOTE. For a review of the pharmacokinetics of muscle relaxants see M. I. Ramzan et al., Clin. Pharmacokinet., 1981, 6, 25–60.

Dose. Initially 40 to 100 µg/kg intravenously.

Papaverine

Antispasmodic

Proprietary Name. It is an ingredient of Riddovydrin.
6,7-Dimethoxy-1-(3,4-dimethoxybenzyl)isoquinoline
$C_{20}H_{21}NO_4 = 339.4$
CAS—58-74-2

An alkaloid obtained from opium or prepared synthetically.
Crystals or white crystalline powder. M.p. 146° to 148°.
Practically **insoluble** in water; sparingly soluble in ethanol and ether.

Papaverine Hydrochloride

Proprietary Names. Cerebid; Cerespan; Dilaspan; Dipav; Dylate; Kavrin; Myobid; P-200; Panergon; Pava-2 Caps; Pavabid; Pavacap; Pavacen; Pavakey; Pavased; Pavatran; Pava-Wol; Pavine TD; Qua-Bid; Sustaverine; Therapav; Vasal; Vasocap; Vaso-Pav; Vasospan. It is an ingredient of Asma-Vydrin, Bepro, Brovon Inhalant Solution, Pavacol-D, Pholcomed (linctus), Riddobron Inhalant, Riddofan, and Rybarvin.
$C_{20}H_{21}NO_4,HCl = 375.9$
CAS—61-25-6
White crystals or crystalline powder. M.p. about 220°, with decomposition.
Soluble 1 in 30 to 1 in 40 of water, 1 in 120 of ethanol, and 1 in 10 of chloroform; practically insoluble in ether.

Papaverine Sulphate

$(C_{20}H_{21}NO_4)_2,H_2SO_4,5H_2O = 866.9$
CAS—32808-09-6 (anhydrous)
White crystals or crystalline powder.
Soluble 1 in 2 of water, 1 in 20 of ethanol, and 1 in 5000 of ether; slightly soluble in chloroform.

Dissociation Constant. pK_a 6.4 (25°).

Partition Coefficient. Log P (ether), 0.5.

Colour Tests. Liebermann's Test—black; Mandelin's Test—grey-green.

Thin-layer Chromatography. *System TA*—Rf 61; *system TB*—Rf 08; *system TC*—Rf 65. (*Dragendorff spray*, positive; *acidified iodoplatinate solution*, positive.)

Gas Chromatography. *System GA*—RI 2825.

High Pressure Liquid Chromatography. *System HA*—k′ 0.3; *system HC*—k′ 0.16; *system HS*—k′ 0.04.

Ultraviolet Spectrum. Aqueous acid—250 nm ($A_1^1 = 1830$ a); aqueous alkali—236 nm ($A_1^1 = 1994$ b), 277 nm, 326 nm.

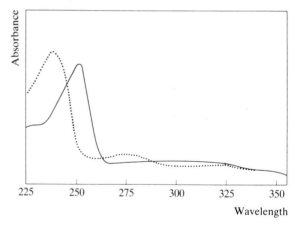

Infra-red Spectrum. Principal peaks at wavenumbers 1279, 1508, 1263, 1026, 1292, 1238 (papaverine hydrochloride, KBr disk).

Mass Spectrum. Principal peaks at m/z 339, 324, 338, 325, 340, 308, 154, 292.

Quantification. GAS CHROMATOGRAPHY. In blood: sensitivity 5 ng/ml, AFID—V. Bellia et al., J. Chromat., 1978, 161, 231–235.

GAS CHROMATOGRAPHY–MASS SPECTROMETRY. In blood: sensitivity 5 ng/ml—J. De Graeve et al., J. Chromat., 1977, 133, 153–160.

Wavelength

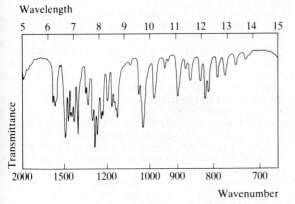

HIGH PRESSURE LIQUID CHROMATOGRAPHY. In plasma: sensitivity 2 ng/ml, UV detection—S. L. Pierson *et al.*, *J. pharm. Sci.*, 1979, *68*, 1550–1551. In blood: detection limit 5 ng/ml, UV detection—G. Hoogewijs *et al.*, *J. Chromat.*, 1981, *226*; *Biomed. Appl.*, *15*, 423–430.

Disposition in the Body. Readily and completely absorbed after oral administration but undergoes extensive first-pass metabolism; bioavailability about 30%. Metabolised by demethylation and glucuronic acid and sulphate conjugation of the resulting phenolic groups. About 50% to 80% of a dose is excreted in the urine in 48 hours as conjugated phenolic metabolites, mostly 6-hydroxypapaverine (37% of the dose) and 4'-hydroxypapaverine (about 8.5% of the dose). Less than 1% of a dose is excreted in the urine unchanged.

THERAPEUTIC CONCENTRATION.
After oral administration of single doses of 150 mg given as an elixir and tablets, respectively, to 6 subjects, mean peak plasma concentrations of 0.58 and 0.53 µg/ml were attained in about 1 hour (M. C. Meyer *et al.*, *J. clin. Pharmac.*, 1980, *19*, 435–444).

HALF-LIFE. Plasma half-life, about 7 hours.

PROTEIN BINDING. In plasma, about 90%.

Dose. Up to 600 mg of papaverine hydrochloride daily.

Paracetamol   *Analgesic*

Synonyms. Acetaminophen; *N*-Acetyl-*p*-aminophenol.
Proprietary Names. Acephen; Alba-Temp; Anuphen; Atasol; Bakese 2; Calpol; Campain; Capital; Datril; Dolanex; Exdol; Febrigesic; Febrilix; Fendon; Hedex; Korum; Liquiprin; Lyteca; Nebs; Oraphen-PD; Paldesic; Pamol (tablets); Panadol; Panaleve; Panasorb; Panets; Panofen; Phenaphen; Phendex; Placidex; Proval; Q-Panol; Robigesic; Rounox; Salzone; SK-APAP; Tapar; Tempra; Ticelgesic; Tivrin; Tylenol; Valadol.
Paracetamol is an ingredient of many proprietary preparations—see *Martindale, The Extra Pharmacopoeia*, 28th Edn.

4'-Hydroxyacetanilide
$C_8H_9NO_2 = 151.2$
CAS—103-90-2

White crystals or crystalline powder. M.p. 168° to 172°.
Soluble 1 in 70 of water, 1 in 7 to 1 in 10 of ethanol, and 1 in 13 of acetone; very slightly soluble in chloroform; practically insoluble in ether.

Dissociation Constant. pK_a 9.5 (25°).

Colour Tests. Ferric Chloride—blue; Folin–Ciocalteu Reagent—blue; Liebermann's Test—violet; Nessler's Reagent—brown (slow).
Boil 0.1 g with 1 ml of *hydrochloric acid* for 3 minutes, add 10 ml of water, cool, and add 0.05 ml of 0.02M potassium dichromate—violet, developing slowly (which in contrast to phenacetin does not become red).

Thin-layer Chromatography. *System TD*—Rf 15; *system TE*—Rf 45; *system TF*—Rf 34. (*Ferric chloride solution*, faint blue; *acidified potassium permanganate solution*, positive.)

Gas Chromatography. *System GA*—RI 1687.

High Pressure Liquid Chromatography. *System HD*—k' 0.1; *system HW*—k' 0.32.

Ultraviolet Spectrum. Aqueous acid—245 nm ($A_1^1 = 668$ a); aqueous alkali—257 nm ($A_1^1 = 715$ a).

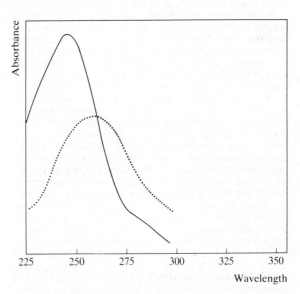

Infra-red Spectrum. Principal peaks at wavenumbers 1506, 1657, 1565, 1263, 1227, 1612 (KBr disk). (See below)

Mass Spectrum. Principal peaks at *m/z* 109, 151, 43, 80, 108, 81, 53, 52; cysteine conjugate 141, 43, 183, 44, 140, 80, 108, 52; mercapturic acid conjugate 43, 141, 183, 42, 87, 41, 140, 165.

Quantification. GAS CHROMATOGRAPHY. In serum: detection limit 7.5 µg/ml, FID—E. Kaa, *J. Chromat.*, 1980, *221*; *Biomed. Appl.*, *10*, 414–418.

Wavelength

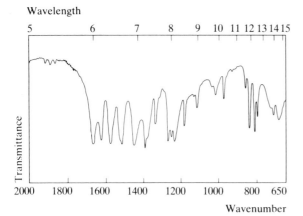

5   6   7   8   9   10 11 12 13 14 15

Transmittance

2000   1800   1600   1400   1200   1000   800   650

Wavenumber

HIGH PRESSURE LIQUID CHROMATOGRAPHY. In plasma: sensitivity 50 ng/ml, UV detection—J. N. Buskin et al., J. Chromat., 1982, 230; Biomed. Appl., 19, 443–447. In urine: paracetamol and 7 metabolites, electrochemical and UV detection—J. M. Wilson et al., J. Chromat., 1982, 227; Biomed. Appl., 16, 453–462. In blood or postmortem tissues: UV detection—J. C. West, J. analyt. Toxicol., 1981, 5, 118–121.

Disposition in the Body. Small doses are readily absorbed but the absorption of larger doses varies considerably and is influenced by gastric emptying rate, the presence of food, and the time of day; bioavailability 70 to 90%. Paracetamol is widely distributed throughout most body fluids and is present in the saliva at concentrations paralleling those in plasma. It undergoes first-pass metabolism and is metabolised mainly by conjugation to form glucuronides and ethereal sulphates; 3-hydroxylation also occurs followed by conjugation or O-methylation of the hydroxy group. Oxidation to a reactive metabolite thought to be acetylimino-p-benzoquinone occurs to a small extent after therapeutic doses but becomes more significant after larger doses, and this metabolite appears to be responsible for hepatic necrosis in paracetamol overdosage; it is normally detoxified by glutathione conjugation to form mercapturic acid and cysteine conjugates but once sources of glutathione are depleted, the free metabolite is available to bind covalently with liver cell protein; this binding occurs about 10 to 12 hours after dosing. About 90% of a therapeutic dose is excreted in the urine in 24 hours; of the excreted material, 1 to 4% is unchanged, 20 to 30% is conjugated with sulphate, 40 to 60% is conjugated with glucuronic acid, 5 to 10% consists of the 3-hydroxy-3-sulphate, the 3-methoxyglucuronide and the 3-methoxy-3-sulphate metabolites, and about 5 to 10% consists of the mercapturic acid and cysteine conjugates; 3-methylthio-4-hydroxyacetanilide has also been identified at concentrations of less than 1%. Larger amounts of the mercapturic acid and cysteine conjugates are excreted in overdose. Paracetamol is a metabolite of benorylate and phenacetin.

THERAPEUTIC CONCENTRATION. In plasma, usually in the range 10 to 20 µg/ml. Plasma concentrations vary considerably between subjects. The glucuronide and sulphate conjugates accumulate in subjects with impaired renal function.

After a single oral dose of 1.5 g to 14 subjects, peak plasma-paracetamol concentrations of 7.4 to 37 µg/ml (mean 24) were attained in 0.5 to 3 hours (mean 1.4) (R. C. Heading et al., Br. J. Pharmac., 1973, 47, 415–421).

Following daily oral doses of 1.8 to 3.6 g to 8 subjects, peak plasma concentrations obtained 1 to 2 hours after a dose ranged from 9.9 to 43.3 µg/ml (mean 23.7) (L. F. Prescott et al., Clin. Pharmac. Ther., 1968, 9, 605–614).

TOXICITY. The minimum lethal dose is about 10 g. Symptoms of hepatic damage do not occur for at least 12 hours after overdosage but may not appear until 4 to 6 days later. Plasma concentrations have been used to indicate possible hepatic necrosis; at 4 hours, hepatic necrosis is possible at concentrations of paracetamol of 120 to 300 µg/ml, probable at concentrations above 300 µg/ml, and unlikely at concentrations below 120 µg/ml. Similarly, at 12 hours, concentrations above 120 µg/ml indicate the probability of necrosis, concentrations of 50 to 120 µg/ml indicate that it is possible, and concentrations below 50 µg/ml indicate that it is unlikely.

The following postmortem tissue concentrations were reported in 3 fatalities: blood 160, 200 and 387 µg/ml, bile 180, –, 900 µg/ml, liver –, –, 385 µg/g, liver blood 200, –, 475 µg/ml, urine 180, 620, – µg/ml (A. E. Robinson et al., J. forens. Sci., 1977, 22, 708–717).

HALF-LIFE. Plasma half-life after therapeutic doses, adults about 1.5 to 3 hours, neonates, about 5 hours; plasma half-lives greater than about 4 hours in adults are indicative of possible liver damage.

VOLUME OF DISTRIBUTION. About 1 litre/kg.

CLEARANCE. Plasma clearance, about 5 ml/min/kg.

PROTEIN BINDING. In plasma, not bound at concentrations less than 60 µg/ml. In poisoned subjects, protein binding has been reported to vary between about 8% and 40%.

NOTE. For a review of the pharmacokinetics of paracetamol see J. A. H. Forrest et al., Clin. Pharmacokinet., 1982, 7, 93–107. For a review of paracetamol overdosage see L. F. Prescott, Drugs, 1983, 25, 290–314.

Dose. Up to 4 g daily.

Parachlorophenol   *Disinfectant*

Synonym. p-Chlorophenol
4-Chlorophenol
$C_6H_5ClO = 128.6$
CAS—106-48-9

White or pink crystals. M.p. about 42°.

Soluble 1 in 60 of water; very soluble in ethanol, chloroform, and ether.

Dissociation Constant. pK_a 9.2 (20°).

Colour Test. Ferric Chloride—blue.

Ultraviolet Spectrum. Aqueous alkali—298 nm ($A_1^1 = 194$ b); ethanol—284 nm ($A_1^1 = 149$ b), inflexion at 291 nm.

Mass Spectrum. Principal peaks at m/z 128, 130, 65, 39, 64, 63, 129, 99.

Paradichlorobenzene

Insecticide

Synonym. Dichlorbenzol
Proprietary Name. Santochlor
1,4-Dichlorobenzene
$C_6H_4Cl_2 = 147.0$
CAS—106-46-7

Colourless shining crystals; slowly volatile in air. M.p. 53° to 54°.

Practically **insoluble** in water; soluble in most organic solvents.

Ultraviolet Spectrum. Ethanol—272 nm ($A_1^1 = 27$ b), 265 nm ($A_1^1 = 20$ b), 282 nm ($A_1^1 = 17$ b).

Infra-red Spectrum. Principal peaks at wavenumbers 1012, 1091, 817, 1121, 951, 1000.

Mass Spectrum. Principal peaks at *m/z* 146, 148, 111, 75, 50, 150, 113, 147.

Disposition in the Body.

TOXICITY. The estimated minimum lethal dose is 25 g and the maximum permissible atmospheric concentration is 75 ppm or 450 mg/m³. Paradichlorobenzene is very irritant to the eyes, mucous membranes and skin, and it may cause narcosis.

Paraldehyde

Anticonvulsant/Hypnotic/Sedative

Synonym. Paracetaldehyde
Proprietary Name. Paral
The trimer of acetaldehyde; 2,4,6-trimethyl-1,3,5-trioxane.
$(C_2H_4O)_3 = 132.2$
CAS—123-63-7

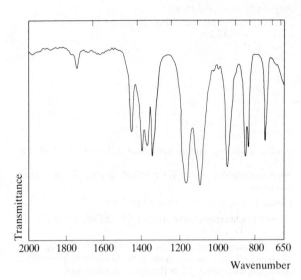

A clear colourless or pale yellow liquid which decomposes and increases in toxicity on storage. Relative density 0.993 to 0.996. F.p. 10° to 12°. B.p. 123° to 126°. At low temperatures it solidifies to form a crystalline mass.

Soluble 1 in 9 of water; miscible with ethanol, chloroform, and ether.

Gas Chromatography. *System GA*—paraldehyde RI 786, acetaldehyde RI 372; *system GI*—paraldehyde retention time 23.2 min, acetaldehyde retention time 0.70 min.

Infra-red Spectrum. Principal peaks at wavenumbers 1095, 1170, 946, 860, 846, 763 (thin film).

Mass Spectrum. Principal peaks at *m/z* 43, 44, 87, 31, 45, 42, 131, 71; acetaldehyde 29, 44, 43, 42, 26, 41, 28, 27.

Quantification. GAS CHROMATOGRAPHY. In blood, plasma or urine: headspace analysis; sensitivity 2 µg/ml—R. M. Anthony *et al.*, *J. analyt. Toxicol.*, 1978, *2*, 262–264. In blood or gastric fluid: headspace analysis after conversion to acetaldehyde—J. P. Hancock *et al.*, *J. analyt. Toxicol.*, 1977, *1*, 161–163.

Disposition in the Body. Readily absorbed after oral, rectal or intramuscular administration and distributed throughout the tissues. Probably metabolised by depolymerisation to acetaldehyde which is oxidised to acetic acid and ultimately to carbon dioxide. About 7% of an oral dose is exhaled unchanged in 4 hours.

THERAPEUTIC CONCENTRATION. In plasma, usually in the range 30 to 100 µg/ml. Concentrations in the cerebrospinal fluid are about 70% of those in plasma.

After oral doses of 100 mg/kg, peak blood concentrations of 100 to 150 µg/ml were attained in 0.5 hour; following rectal administration of 100 mg/kg, peak blood concentrations of 50 to 100 µg/ml were reported at 1.5 to 2 hours (R. M. Anthony *et al.*, *J. analyt. Toxicol.*, 1978, *2*, 262–264).

Following an intramuscular injection of 10 ml to 1 subject, a peak plasma concentration of 77 µg/ml was attained in 1.2 hours (R. Maes *et al.*, *J. forens. Sci.*, 1969, *14*, 235–254).

TOXICITY. The minimum lethal dose has been estimated as 25 ml orally and 12 ml rectally, although recovery has occurred after the ingestion of 125 ml. Toxic effects have been associated with blood concentrations of 200 to 400 µg/ml. Blood concentrations of about 500 µg/ml, or less if alcohol has also been ingested, may be lethal. On storage, paraldehyde may depolymerise to acetaldehyde and acetic acid; severe acidosis and fatalities may follow the use of partly depolymerised material.

In 15 fatalities attributed to paraldehyde overdose, blood concentrations of 490 to 1600 µg/ml were reported (J. N. Hayward and B. R. Boshell, *Am. J. Med.*, 1957, *23*, 965–976).

The following postmortem tissue concentrations were reported in 3 fatalities, 2 of which involved alcohol: blood 115, 480 and 140 µg/ml, brain 150, 300 and 370 µg/g, kidney 190, 50 and 260 µg/g, liver 210, 200 and 600 µg/g, urine –, –, 130 µg/ml (C. J. Rehling, Poison Residues in Human Tissues, in *Progress in Chemical Toxicology*, Vol. 3, A. Stolman (Ed.), New York, Academic Press Inc., 1967, pp. 363–386).

HALF-LIFE. Plasma half-life, 4 to 10 hours.

VOLUME OF DISTRIBUTION. About 1 litre/kg.

CLEARANCE. Plasma clearance, about 2 ml/min/kg.

Dose. 5 to 10 ml by mouth or by intramuscular injection.

Paramethadione

Anticonvulsant

Proprietary Name. Paradione
5-Ethyl-3,5-dimethyloxazolidine-2,4-dione
$C_7H_{11}NO_3 = 157.2$
CAS—115-67-3

A clear colourless liquid. Refractive index, at 25°, 1.4485 to 1.4505.
Sparingly **soluble** in water; freely soluble in ethanol, chloroform, and ether.

Colour Test. Koppanyi-Zwikker Test—violet.

Thin-layer Chromatography. *System TD*—Rf 00; *system TE*—Rf 07; *system TF*—Rf 60.

Gas Chromatography. *System GA*—RI 1120; *system GE*—paramethadione retention time 0.06, N-desmethylparametha-dione retention time 0.22, both relative to phenytoin.

Ultraviolet Spectrum. No significant absorption, 230 to 360 nm.

Infra-red Spectrum. Principal peaks at wavenumbers 1730, 1805, 1100, 1040, 1280, 1070 (thin film).

Mass Spectrum. Principal peaks at *m/z* 43, 129, 57, 56, 41, 72, 39, 58.

Quantification. GAS CHROMATOGRAPHY. In serum: parametha-dione and 5-ethyl-5-methyloxazolidine-2,4-dione, sensitivity 200 ng/ml, FID—D. J. Hoffman and A. H. C. Chun, *J. pharm. Sci.*, 1975, **64**, 1702–1703.

Disposition in the Body. Readily absorbed after oral administra-tion. Metabolised by N-demethylation to 5-ethyl-5-methyloxa-zolidine-2,4-dione which is active and accumulates during chronic administration; 30 to 80% of a dose is excreted slowly in the urine as the N-desmethyl metabolite with less than 1% as unchanged drug.

THERAPEUTIC CONCENTRATION.
After a single oral dose of 300 mg to 3 subjects, peak serum concentrations of parametha-dione of 5.4 to 7.6 µg/ml (mean 6.3) were attained in 0.5 to 1 hour; concentrations of the N-desmethyl metabolite gradually increased to a plateau of 8.1 to 8.6 µg/ml (mean 8.4) at 32 hours (D. J. Hoffman and A. H. C. Chun, *ibid.*).
Following oral administration of 900 mg daily to 2 subjects for 14 days, peak plasma concentrations of the N-desmethyl metabolite of about 240 µg/ml were reported (T. C. Butler, *J. Pharmac. exp. Ther.*, 1955, **113**, 178–185).

TOXICITY. The estimated minimum lethal dose is 5 g.

HALF-LIFE. Plasma half-life, parametha-dione about 16 hours after a single dose, N-desmethylparametha-dione about 7 to 14 days during chronic administration.

PROTEIN BINDING. In plasma, not significantly bound.

Dose. 0.9 to 1.8 g daily.

Paramethasone

Corticosteroid

6α-Fluoro-11β,17α,21-trihydroxy-16α-methylpregna-1,4-diene-3,20-dione
$C_{22}H_{29}FO_5 = 392.5$
CAS—53-33-8

Paramethasone Acetate

Synonym. 6α-Fluoro-16α-methylprednisolone 21-Acetate
Proprietary Names. Depodillar; Dilar; Haldrone; Metilar; Monocortin; Paramezone.
$C_{24}H_{31}FO_6 = 434.5$
CAS—1597-82-6
A white to creamy-white, fluffy, crystalline powder. M.p. about 240°, with decomposition.
Practically **insoluble** in water; soluble in ethanol, acetone, and ether; soluble 1 in 50 of chloroform.

Ultraviolet Spectrum. Parametha-sone acetate: methanol—241 nm ($A_1^1 = 500$ b).

Infra-red Spectrum. Principal peaks at wavenumbers 1658, 1227, 1600, 905, 1745, 1034 (Nujol mull).

Dose. Up to 12 mg of parametha-sone acetate daily.

Paraphenylenediamine

Dye

Synonyms. 'Para'; *p*-Phenylenediamine.
$C_6H_4(NH_2)_2 = 108.1$
CAS—106-50-3

White or reddish crystals. M.p. 145° to 147°.
Soluble 1 in 100 of water; soluble in ethanol, chloroform, and ether.

Colour Tests. Ferric Chloride—green; Mandelin's Test—yellow.

Thin-layer Chromatography. *System TA*—Rf 61. (*Acidified iodoplatinate solution*, positive.)

Paraquat

Herbicide

1,1'-Dimethyl-4,4'-bipyridyldiylium ion
$C_{12}H_{14}N_2 = 186.3$
CAS—4685-14-7

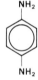

Paraquat Dichloride

Proprietary Names. Dextrone X; Gramoxone. It is an ingredient of Dexuron, Pathclear, and Weedol.

$C_{12}H_{14}Cl_2N_2 = 257.2$
CAS—1910-42-5

A white crystalline solid. Decomposes at about 300°.

Very **soluble** in water. Hydrolysed by alkalis.

Note. Unless otherwise stated, the analytical information given below refers to paraquat dichloride. For information on the monoene and diene reduction products for GC–MS analysis, see under Quaternary Ammonium Herbicides, p. 80.

Colour Test. Sodium Dithionite—blue.

Thin-layer Chromatography. *System TA*—Rf 00; *system TN*—Rf 22; *system TO*—Rf 10. (*Acidified iodoplatinate solution*, positive.)

Gas Chromatography. *System GK*—monoene reduction product retention time 0.36, diene reduction product retention time 0.58, both relative to caffeine.

Ultraviolet Spectrum. Aqueous acid—257 nm ($A_1^1 = 693$ b).

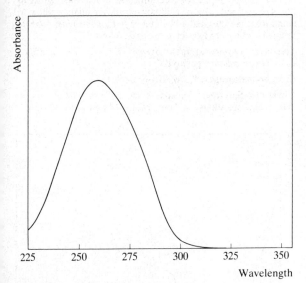

Infra-red Spectrum. Principal peaks at wavenumbers 1174, 1638, 1064, 1229, 1284, 850 (KBr disk).

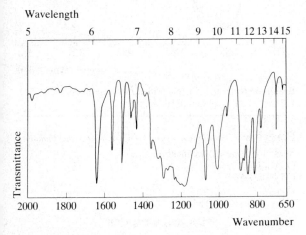

Mass Spectrum. Principal peaks at m/z 96, 42, 70, 72, 150, 122, 194, 43 (monoene reduction product); 96, 42, 148, 192, 94, 122, 134, 44 (diene reduction product).

Quantification. COLORIMETRY. In plasma or serum: sensitivity 50 ng/ml—D. R. Jarvie and M. J. Stewart—*Clinica chim. Acta*, 1979, *94*, 241–251.

GAS CHROMATOGRAPHY. In plasma: sensitivity 30 ng/ml, AFID—A. van Dijk *et al.*, *J. analyt. Toxicol.*, 1977, *1*, 151–154.

HIGH PRESSURE LIQUID CHROMATOGRAPHY. In postmortem blood or liver: detection limit 50 ng/ml and 100 ng/g respectively, UV detection— E. A. Querée *et al.*, *J. analyt. Toxicol.*, 1985, *9*, 10–14. In urine: paraquat and diquat, detection limit < 1 µg/ml, UV detection—R. Gill *et al.*, *J. Chromat.*, 1983, *255*, 483–490.

RADIOIMMUNOASSAY. In plasma: sensitivity 5 ng/ml—T. Levitt, *Proc. Analyt. Div. Chem. Soc.*, 1979, *16*, 72–76. In plasma—D. Fatori and W. M. Hunter, *Clinica chim. Acta*, 1980, *100*, 81–90.

Disposition in the Body. Less than 10% is absorbed after ingestion. It is slowly excreted unchanged in the urine and faeces, detectable concentrations have been found in the urine for up to 26 days after acute ingestion.

TOXICITY. Several hundred fatalities due to the accidental or suicidal ingestion of paraquat have occurred. The estimated minimum lethal dose is about 1 g. The maximum permissible atmospheric concentration is 0.1 mg/m³ and the maximum acceptable daily intake is 2 µg/kg as the dichloride. Large amounts of paraquat produce death in a few hours or days due to pulmonary oedema, haemorrhage, and toxic effects on the kidney, liver, and heart. Smaller doses may result in later mortality by progressive respiratory failure and death may still ensue even after concentrations in blood or urine are almost undetectable. Tissue concentrations in fatal cases therefore vary considerably according to the length of survival after ingestion. Blood concentrations greater than about 2 µg/ml at 4 hours and 0.1 µg/ml at 24 hours are likely to be lethal in most subjects but individual response is variable and some subjects with much higher concentrations have recovered.

In a review of 26 fatalities attributed to paraquat poisoning, the following postmortem tissue concentrations, µg/ml or µg/g (mean, *n*) were reported:

	Death within 24 hours	Death within 1 to 7 days	Death after 8 days or more
Blood	1.4–52 (14, *5*)	0.2–4.4 (1.3, *8*)	not detected
Kidney	22.5–279 (79, *6*)	1.4–74 (16, *10*)	0.6–2.8 (1.5, *5*)
Liver	8.8–141 (41, *6*)	0.3–57.6 (8, *10*)	0.2, 1.4 (*2*)
Lung	12.8–186 (78, *3*)	1.6–21.4 (7, *6*)	—
Urine	1210 (*1*)	4–15.8 (9, *3*)	trace, 2.2 (*2*)

(D. J. L. Carson and E. D. Carson, *Forens. Sci.*, 1976, *7*, 151–160).

NOTE. For a review of the toxicology of paraquat see T. J. Haley, *Clin. Toxicol.*, 1979, *14*, 1–46.

Parathion   *Pesticide*

Other Names. Alkron; Aphamite; Fosferno 20; Niran; Nitrostigmine; Paraphos; Thiophos.

OO-Diethyl *O*-4-nitrophenyl phosphorothioate
$C_{10}H_{14}NO_5PS = 291.3$
CAS—56-38-2

A pale yellow liquid which is decomposed by heat and darkens on exposure to light. M.p. 6°. B.p. 360° to 375°. Refractive index, at 25°, 1.5367.

Practically **insoluble** in water; miscible with most organic solvents. It is rapidly hydrolysed in alkaline solution.

Colour Tests. Palladium Chloride—brown; Phosphorus Test—yellow.

Thin-layer Chromatography. System TW—parathion Rf 81, parathion-methyl Rf 77.

Gas Chromatography. System GA—parathion RI 1942, aminoparathion RI 1885, paraoxon RI 1880; system GK—retention time 1.04 relative to caffeine.

Ultraviolet Spectrum. Ethanol—274 nm ($A_1^1 = 343$ b).

Infra-red Spectrum. Principal peaks at wavenumbers 1020, 925, 1515, 1219, 1587, 970.

Mass Spectrum. Principal peaks at m/z 97, 109, 291, 139, 125, 137, 155, 123.

Quantification. GAS CHROMATOGRAPHY. In urine: 4-nitrophenol, detection limit 20 ng/ml, ECD—D. E. Bradway and T. M. Shafik, *Bull. envir. Contam. Toxicol.*, 1973, *9*, 134–139.

RADIOIMMUNOASSAY. In plasma: sensitivity 100 ng/ml—C. D. Ercegovich et al., *J. agric. Fd Chem.*, 1981, *29*, 559–563.

Disposition in the Body. Parathion is activated in the liver by metabolism to paraoxon. Parathion and paraoxon are further metabolised to diethylthiophosphoric acid (DETP), diethylphosphoric acid (DEP), and 4-nitrophenol which are the major urinary excretion products although DETP and DEP are unstable in stored urine. Urinary 4-nitrophenol concentrations may be indicative of the extent of exposure to parathion. 4-Nitrophenol is rapidly excreted in the urine and is not detectable 48 hours after exposure by inhalation or ingestion, but excretion is more prolonged after exposure of intact skin due to the much slower absorption of parathion by this route. Aminoparathion has been detected in postmortem blood and tissues.

Urinary 4-nitrophenol concentrations ranged from 0.4 to 13.2 μg/ml in 23 occupationally exposed asymptomatic workers and correlated well with serum-parathion concentrations which were in the range 0.003 to 0.20 μg/ml (C. C. Roan et al., *Bull. envir. Contam. Toxicol.*, 1969, *4*, 362–369).

TOXICITY. The estimated minimum lethal dose by inhalation or ingestion is 20 mg and the maximum permissible atmospheric concentration is 0.1 mg/m³. Urinary concentrations of about 2 μg/ml or more of 4-nitrophenol may be associated with severe toxicity. Numerous fatalities have occurred due to contamination of food by parathion and also from suicidal ingestion.

The following postmortem tissue concentrations were reported in 19 fatalities due to parathion poisoning (determined by a bioassay based on cholinesterase inhibition): blood 0.5 to 34 μg/ml (mean 9.0, 11 cases); brain 0.9 to 12.5 μg/g (mean 4.9, 4 cases); kidney 0.2 to 11.9 μg/g (mean 3.3, 9 cases); liver 0.08 to 120 μg/g (mean 11, 13 cases); urine 0.4 to 78 μg/ml (mean 10, 10 cases) (A. Heyndrickx and F. De Clerc, *J. Pharm. Belg.*, 1977, *32*, 149–161).

In 2 fatalities due to parathion, the following postmortem tissue concentrations, μg/ml or μg/g, were reported:

	Parathion	Aminoparathion
Blood	0.01, 0.15	0.27, 6.7
Bile	—, 0.63	—, 0.31
Liver	ND, ND	0.47, 32
Urine	ND, —	0.02, —

(ND = not detected)
(L. T. F. Chan et al., *J. forens. Sci.*, 1983, *28*, 122–127).

HALF-LIFE. Derived from urinary excretion data, about 8 hours.

Parbendazole

Anthelmintic (Veterinary)

Proprietary Name. Helmatac
Methyl 5-butylbenzimidazol-2-ylcarbamate
$C_{13}H_{17}N_3O_2 = 247.3$
CAS—14255-87-9

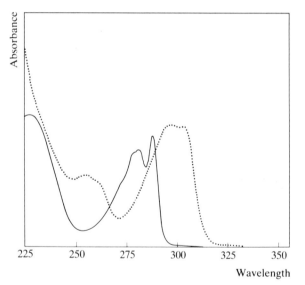

A white crystalline powder. M.p. 224° to 227°, with decomposition.

Practically **insoluble** in water; soluble 1 in 900 of ethanol and 1 in 300 of chloroform; very slightly soluble in ether; soluble in dilute mineral acids.

Colour Test. Dissolve 5 mg in 5 ml of 0.1M hydrochloric acid and add 3 mg of *p*-phenylenediamine dihydrochloride; shake to dissolve and add 0.1 g of zinc powder. After mixing, allow to stand for 2 minutes and add 10 ml of *ferric ammonium sulphate solution*—a blue or violet-blue colour develops.

Thin-layer Chromatography. System TA—Rf 70. (*Acidified iodoplatinate solution*, positive.)

Gas Chromatography. System GA—not eluted.

Ultraviolet Spectrum. Aqueous acid—281 nm, 288 nm ($A_1^1 = 760$ a); aqueous alkali—254 nm, 297 nm ($A_1^1 = 816$ b), 303 nm.

Infra-red Spectrum. Principal peaks at wavenumbers 1626, 1600, 1274, 1093, 1100, 1193 (KBr disk).

Pargyline

Antihypertensive (Monoamine Oxidase Inhibitor)

N-Methyl-*N*-prop-2-ynylbenzylamine
$C_{11}H_{13}N = 159.2$
CAS—555-57-7

Pargyline Hydrochloride

Proprietary Name. Eutonyl
$C_{11}H_{13}N,HCl = 195.7$
CAS—306-07-0
A white crystalline powder. M.p. 158° to 162°; sublimation occurs when kept at raised temperatures.
Soluble 1 in 0.6 of water, 1 in 5 of ethanol, and 1 in about 7 of chloroform. Aqueous solutions are unstable.

Dissociation Constant. pK_a 6.9.

Thin-layer Chromatography. *System TA*—Rf 70. (*Acidified iodoplatinate solution*, positive.)

Gas Chromatography. *System GA*—RI 1214; *system GB*—RI 1218; *system GC*—RI 1440.

High Pressure Liquid Chromatography. *System HA*—k' 0.2.

Ultraviolet Spectrum. Aqueous acid—251 nm, 256 nm, 261 nm ($A_1^1 = 16$ a), 268 nm; aqueous alkali—252 nm, 257 nm, 263 nm.

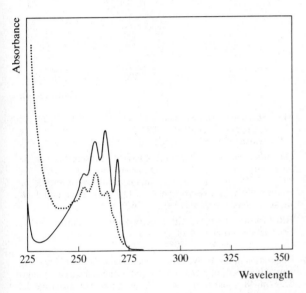

Infra-red Spectrum. Principal peaks at wavenumbers 697, 746, 714, 724, 1052, 1515 (KBr disk).

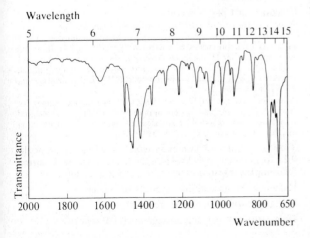

Mass Spectrum. Principal peaks at *m/z* 82, 68, 91, 159, 42, 158, 92, 65.

Dose. Usually 25 to 50 mg of pargyline hydrochloride daily; maximum of 200 mg daily.

Pecazine   *Tranquilliser*

Synonym. Mepazine
10-(1-Methyl-3-piperidylmethyl)phenothiazine
$C_{19}H_{22}N_2S = 310.5$
CAS—60-89-9

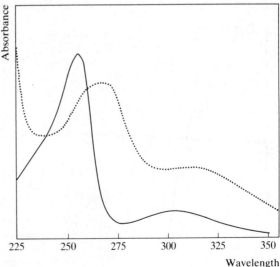

Pecazine Hydrochloride

$C_{19}H_{22}N_2S,HCl,H_2O = 364.9$
CAS—2975-36-2
A white crystalline powder. M.p. 171° to 174°, with decomposition.
Very slightly **soluble** in water; freely soluble in dehydrated alcohol; soluble in chloroform; practically insoluble in ether.

Dissociation Constant. pK_a 9.7 (24°).

Colour Tests. Mandelin's Test—green → violet; Marquis Test—violet.

Thin-layer Chromatography. *System TA*—Rf 53; *system TB*—Rf 46; *system TC*—Rf 44. (*Acidified iodoplatinate solution*, positive.)

Gas Chromatography. *System GA*—RI 2524.

High Pressure Liquid Chromatography. *System HA*—k' 3.9.

Ultraviolet Spectrum. Aqueous acid—253 nm ($A_1^1 = 892$ a), 300 nm; aqueous alkali—265 nm.

Infra-red Spectrum. Principal peaks at wavenumbers 750, 768, 1219, 1250, 1162, 1282 (pecazine hydrochloride, KBr disk).

Mass Spectrum. Principal peaks at m/z 310, 58, 199, 112, 311, 111, 212, 41.

Dose. Pecazine hydrochloride has been given in doses equivalent to 37.5 to 75 mg of the base daily.

Pemoline   *Central Stimulant*

Synonyms. Phenilone; 5-Phenylisohydantoin.

Proprietary Names. Cylert; Deltamine; Ronyl; Sigmadyn; Stimul; Tradon; Volital.

2-Imino-5-phenyloxazolidin-4-one
$C_9H_8N_2O_2 = 176.2$
CAS—2152-34-3

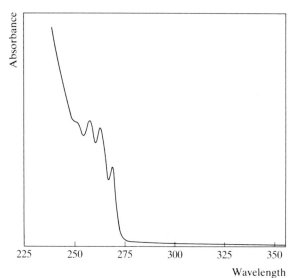

A white crystalline powder. M.p. 259°.
Practically **insoluble** in water, acetone, and ether; soluble 1 in 100 of propylene glycol.

Dissociation Constant. pK_a 10.5.

Colour Test. Koppanyi–Zwikker Test—violet.

Thin-layer Chromatography. *System TA*—Rf 60; *system TB*—Rf 00; *system TC*—Rf 23. (*Marquis reagent*, yellow-brown; *ninhydrin spray*, positive; *acidified potassium permanganate solution*, positive.)

Gas Chromatography. *System GA*—pemoline RI 2160, mandelic acid RI 1487.

High Pressure Liquid Chromatography. *System HA*—k' 0.2; *system HC*—k' 0.14.

Ultraviolet Spectrum. Aqueous acid—256 nm ($A_1^1 = 20$ a), 262 nm, 268 nm.

Infra-red Spectrum. Principal peaks at wavenumbers 1218, 1653, 695, 1560, 1137, 1275 (KBr disk).

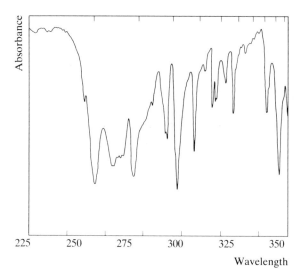

Wavelength

Mass Spectrum. Principal peaks at m/z 107, 176, 90, 77, 70, 105, 42, 79; mandelic acid 107, 79, 77, 51, 152, 105, 50, 78; 5-phenyloxazolidine-2,4-dione 90, 177, 105, 77, 106, 51, 89, 50.

Quantification. GAS CHROMATOGRAPHY. In serum or urine: sensitivity 50 ng/ml, AFID—D. J. Hoffman, *J. pharm. Sci.*, 1979, *68*, 445–447. In horse plasma or urine: sensitivity 50 ng/ml and 100 ng/ml, respectively, ECD—O. J. Igwe and J. W. Blake, *J. chromatogr. Sci.*, 1981, *19*, 617–624.

HIGH PRESSURE LIQUID CHROMATOGRAPHY. In plasma, saliva, or urine: detection limit 20 ng/ml, UV detection—K. Nishihara *et al.*, *Ther. Drug Monit.*, 1984, *6*, 232–237.

Disposition in the Body. Slowly absorbed after oral administration. About 50% of a dose is excreted in the urine as unchanged drug in 48 hours and about 4% as 5-phenyloxazolidine-2,4-dione; the remainder is excreted in the urine as conjugated pemoline and unidentified polar metabolites; mandelic acid is also a metabolite of pemoline. Less than 1% of a dose is eliminated in the faeces.

THERAPEUTIC CONCENTRATION.

After a single oral dose of 50 mg given to 3 subjects, peak plasma concentrations of 0.77 to 1.22 µg/ml (mean 1.0) were attained in about 2 to 3 hours; peak concentrations in saliva of 0.47 to 0.75 µg/ml (mean 0.59) were reported after 2 to 4 hours; following administration of 37.5 mg to 1 subject, peak plasma and saliva concentrations of 0.89 and 0.58 µg/ml, respectively, were attained in about 4 hours (N. P. E. Vermeulen *et al.*, *Br. J. clin. Pharmac.*, 1979, *8*, 459–463).

After daily oral doses of 37.5 and 75 mg to 28 hyperactive children for seven days, mean plasma concentrations of about 2 and 4 µg/ml respectively, were reported 3 hours after the last dose (C. P. Tomkins *et al.*, *Ther. Drug Monit.*, 1980, *2*, 255–260).

TOXICITY. Estimated minimum lethal dose, 2 g for an adult, 0.2 g for children up to 2 years, although recovery has occurred following the ingestion of up to 1.8 g by young children.

HALF-LIFE. Plasma half-life, about 10 to 18 hours.

PROTEIN BINDING. In plasma, about 30%.

Dose. Usually 40 mg daily; maximum of 120 mg daily.

Wavelength

Pempidine

Antihypertensive

1,2,2,6,6-Pentamethylpiperidine
$C_{10}H_{21}N = 155.3$
CAS—79-55-0

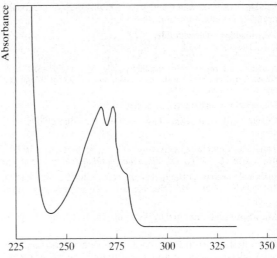

A liquid.

Pempidine Tartrate

$C_{10}H_{21}N, C_4H_6O_6 = 305.4$
CAS—546-48-5
A white crystalline powder. M.p. 160°.
Soluble 1 in 2 of water and 1 in 14 of ethanol; very slightly soluble in acetone; practically insoluble in chloroform and ether.

Thin-layer Chromatography. *System TA*—Rf 24; *system TB*—Rf 68; *system TC*—Rf 03. (*Acidified iodoplatinate solution*, positive.)

Infra-red Spectrum. Principal peaks at wavenumbers 1308, 1261, 1210, 1136, 1063, 675 (pempidine tartrate, KBr disk).

Mass Spectrum. Principal peaks at *m/z* 140, 84, 56, 41, 72, 69, 29, 39.

Dose. 7.5 to 80 mg of pempidine tartrate daily.

Penfluridol

Tranquilliser

Proprietary Name. Semap
1-[4,4-Bis(4-fluorophenyl)butyl]-4-(4-chloro-3-trifluoromethyl-phenyl)piperidin-4-ol
$C_{28}H_{27}ClF_5NO = 524.0$
CAS—26864-56-2

A white crystalline or microcrystalline powder. M.p. 104° to 109°.
Practically **insoluble** in water; very soluble in ethanol, acetone, and chloroform; freely soluble in ether.

Colour Test. Liebermann's Test—brown.

Thin-layer Chromatography. *System TA*—Rf 76; *system TB*—Rf 17; *system TC*—Rf 60. (*Dragendorff spray*.)

Gas Chromatography. *System GA*—RI 3380.

Ultraviolet Spectrum. Aqueous acid—267 nm $(A_1^1 = 47\text{ a})$, 273 nm. No alkaline shift.

Infra-red Spectrum. Principal peaks at wavenumbers 1500, 1138, 1225, 1315, 1157, 825 (KBr disk).

Mass Spectrum. Principal peaks at *m/z* 42, 292, 56, 294, 109, 203, 201, 44.

Quantification. GAS CHROMATOGRAPHY. In plasma: sensitivity 1 to 2 ng/ml, ECD—S. F. Cooper *et al.*, *Int. Pharmacopsychiat.*, 1975, *10*, 78–88.

Disposition in the Body. Incompletely absorbed after oral administration. It has a very long duration of action. About 5% of a dose is excreted in the urine in 7 days, mainly as 4,4′-bis(4-fluorophenyl)butyric acid; about 80% of a dose is eliminated in the faeces, mostly as unchanged drug.

THERAPEUTIC CONCENTRATION.
Following weekly oral administration of 30, 60 and 120 mg for 13 weeks to 7, 7 and 8 subjects, mean steady-state plasma concentrations of about 0.004 to 0.01, 0.006 to 0.012, and 0.008 to 0.025 µg/ml were reported. In all subjects maximum concentrations were attained within 12 hours of a dose; concentrations declined rapidly between 12 and 24 hours followed by a much slower decline during the next 120 hours and were still significant (about 0.001 µg/ml) 168 hours after the dose (S. F. Cooper *et al.*, *Clin. Pharmac. Ther.*, 1975, *18*, 325–329).

Dose. Usually 20 to 60 mg weekly, by mouth; doses of up to 120 mg weekly have been given.

Penicillamine

Chelating Agent

Synonyms. (−)-$\beta\beta$-Dimethylcysteine; D-3-Mercaptovaline; D-Penicillamine.
Proprietary Names. Cuprimine; Depen; Distamine; D-Pena-mine; Kelatin; Metalcaptase; Pemine; Pendramine; Trolovol.
3,3-Dimethyl-D-cysteine
$C_5H_{11}NO_2S = 149.2$
CAS—52-67-5

A white, finely crystalline powder. M.p. 201°, with decomposition.

Soluble 1 in 9 of water and 1 in 530 of ethanol; practically insoluble in chloroform and ether.

Penicillamine Hydrochloride

$C_5H_{11}NO_2S,HCl = 185.7$
CAS—2219-30-9
A white, hygroscopic, finely crystalline powder. M.p. 160° to 165°.
Soluble 1 in 1 of water, 1 in 1.5 of ethanol, and 1 in 230 of chloroform; practically insoluble in ether.

Dissociation Constant. pK_a 1.8, 7.9, 10.5.

Colour Tests. Mandelin's Test—yellow; Palladium Chloride—yellow.

Thin-layer Chromatography. *System TA*—Rf 36; *system TB*—Rf 01; *system TC*—Rf 03. (*Acidified iodoplatinate solution, positive.*)

Infra-red Spectrum. Principal peaks at wavenumbers 1595, 1525, 1615, 1550, 1090, 1055 (Nujol mull). Two polymorphic forms occur.

Mass Spectrum. Principal peaks at *m/z* 75, 41, 57, 70, 43, 59, 56, 47.

Quantification. HIGH PRESSURE LIQUID CHROMATOGRAPHY. In whole blood, plasma or urine: sensitivity 75 ng/ml for plasma and urine, 450 ng/ml for whole blood, electrochemical detection—R. F. Bergström *et al., J. Chromat.*, 1981, *222*; *Biomed. Appl.*, *11*, 445–452. In serum: sensitivity 130 ng/ml, fluorescence detection—E. P. Lankmayr *et al., J. Chromat.*, 1981, *222*; *Biomed. Appl.*, *11*, 249–255.

REVIEWS. For reviews of assay methods see D. R. Lecavalier and J. C. Crawhall, *J. Rheumatol.*, 1981, *Suppl.* 7, 20–27, and N. Kucharczyk and S. Shahinian, *ibid.*, 28–34.

Disposition in the Body. Readily but incompletely absorbed after oral administration. About 50% of an oral dose is excreted in the urine in 48 hours with about 10% as unchanged drug, up to 25% as cysteine-penicillamine disulphide, about 15% as penicillamine disulphide, and less than 10% as *S*-methyl-D-penicillamine; about 35% of an oral dose is eliminated in the faeces in 3 days. After intravenous administration, about 80% of the dose is excreted in the urine in 24 hours; traces of penicillamine remain in the plasma after 48 hours due to protein binding.

THERAPEUTIC CONCENTRATION.
Following daily oral doses of 500 to 750 mg to 10 subjects, peak plasma concentrations of 1.7 to 5.6 µg/ml (mean 3.7) were attained 1.5 to 3 hours after a dose (M. Butler *et al., Arthritis Rheum.*, 1982, *25*, 111–116).

HALF-LIFE. Plasma half-life, about 2 to 6 hours.

PROTEIN BINDING. In plasma, up to 90%.

NOTE. For further details of penicillamine metabolism and kinetics see R. F. Bergström *et al., Clin. Pharmac. Ther.*, 1981, *30*, 404–413, and J. C. Crawhall *et al., Biopharm. Drug Disp.*, 1979, *1*, 73–95.

Dose. 0.125 to 4 g daily.

Pentachlorophenol   *Preservative*

Synonym. PCP
$C_6HCl_5O = 266.3$
CAS—87-86-5

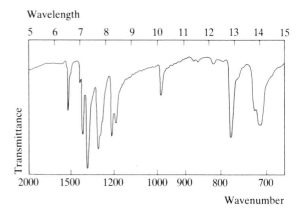

White crystals. M.p. about 191°.
Very slightly **soluble** in water; freely soluble in ethanol and ether.

Dissociation Constant. pK_a 4.8.

Colour Test. Fuming Nitric Acid—red/red/brown-violet.

Gas Chromatography. *System GA*—RI 1749.

Ultraviolet Spectrum. Aqueous alkali—319 nm $(A_1^1 = 194\ b)$; ethanol—295 nm $(A_1^1 = 89\ b)$, 303 nm $(A_1^1 = 115\ b)$.

Infra-red Spectrum. Principal peaks at wavenumbers 1307, 774, 1222, 711, 1196, 1553 (KBr disk).

Wavelength

[Infra-red spectrum chart with Wavelength axis (5, 6, 7, 8, 9, 10, 11, 12, 13, 14, 15) across the top, Transmittance on the vertical axis, and Wavenumber axis (2000, 1500, 1200, 1000, 900, 800, 700) across the bottom]

Wavenumber

Mass Spectrum. Principal peaks at *m/z* 266, 268, 264, 167, 165, 270, 202, 132.

Quantification. GAS CHROMATOGRAPHY. In serum, whole blood or urine: detection limit 1 ng/ml, ECD—L. L. Needham *et al., J. analyt. Toxicol.*, 1981, *5*, 283–286. In plasma or urine: sensitivity 10 ng/ml, ECD—D. L. Rick *et al., J. analyt. Toxicol.*, 1982, *6*, 297–300.

HIGH PRESSURE LIQUID CHROMATOGRAPHY. In urine: sensitivity 30 ng/ml, UV detection—K. Pekari and A. Aitio, *J. Chromat.*, 1982, *232*; *Biomed. Appl.*, *21*, 129–136.

Disposition in the Body. Readily absorbed after ingestion, inhalation or through intact skin. Pentachlorophenol and its oxidised metabolite, tetrachlorohydroquinone, are excreted in the urine in free and conjugated forms, with about 74% of a dose being excreted unchanged in 7 days. About 4% of a dose is eliminated in the faeces.

Urinary concentrations in 130 pest-control operators exposed to pentachlorophenol ranged from 0.003 to 35.7 µg/ml (mean 1.8) (A. Bevenue *et al., Bull. envir. Contam. Toxicol.*, 1967, *2*, 319–332).

BLOOD CONCENTRATION.
Plasma concentrations of 0.99 to 9.1 µg/ml were reported in 6 occupationally-exposed subjects and blood concentrations of 0.34 to 6.0 µg/ml were reported in 7 exposed workers (A. Bevenue *et al., J. Chromat.*, 1968, *38*, 467–472).

TOXICITY. The estimated minimum lethal dose is 1 g and the maximum permissible atmospheric concentration is 0.5 mg/m³. Blood concentrations greater than 30 µg/ml are usually toxic. Numerous fatalities after absorption, inhalation or ingestion have been reported.

In two fatalities, the following postmortem tissue concentrations (µg/ml or µg/g) were reported: blood 113, 156; brain 14, 35; kidney –, 123; liver 94, 134; urine –, 520 (M. F. Mason *et al., J. forens. Sci.*, 1965, *10*, 136–147).

In one fatality, the following postmortem tissue concentrations were reported: blood 173 μg/ml, kidney 116 μg/g, liver 225 μg/g, urine 75 μg/ml (M. J. Cretney, *Bull. int. Ass. forens. Toxicol.*, 1976, *12*(3), 10).

HALF-LIFE. Plasma half-life, about 30 hours.

DISTRIBUTION IN BLOOD. Plasma: whole blood ratio, 1.8.

PROTEIN BINDING. In plasma, about 99%.

Pentaerythritol Tetranitrate   *Anti-anginal Vasodilator*

Synonyms. Erynite; Nitropentaerythrol; Nitropenthrite; Pentanitrol.

Proprietary Names. Antime; Cardiacap; Dilcoran; Duotrate; El-Petn; Metranil; Mycardol; Mycartal; Nitrodex; Pentafin; Pentanitrine; Pentritol; Pentryate; Peritrate; Quintrate; Terpate; Tranite; Vasolate. It is an ingredient of Cartrax, Miltrate, and Pentoxylon.

2,2-Bis(hydroxymethyl)propane-1,3-diol tetranitrate
$C_5H_8N_4O_{12} = 316.1$
CAS—115-77-5 (pentaerythritol); *78-11-5* (tetranitrate)

$$CH_2 \cdot O \cdot NO_2$$
$$|$$
$$NO_2 \cdot O \cdot CH_2 \cdot C \cdot CH_2 \cdot O \cdot NO_2$$
$$|$$
$$CH_2 \cdot O \cdot NO_2$$

A white crystalline powder. M.p. 140°.
Practically **insoluble** in water; slightly soluble in ethanol; soluble in acetone.
Note. For medicinal purposes pentaerythritol tetranitrate is supplied diluted with an inert substance such as lactose, since the undiluted compound may explode upon percussion or on exposure to heat.

Ultraviolet Spectrum. Aqueous acid—255 nm; aqueous alkali—294 nm.

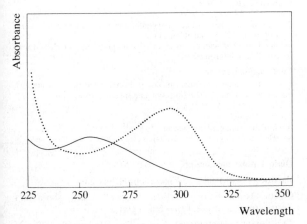

Mass Spectrum. Principal peaks at *m/z* 46, 76, 57, 55, 56, 60, 47, 97.

Quantification. GAS CHROMATOGRAPHY. In blood or urine: pentaerythritol tetranitrate and de-esterified metabolites, detec-

tion limits 100 pg/ml to 2 ng/ml in blood, ECD—G. B. Neurath and M. Dünger, *Arzneimittel-Forsch.*, 1977, *27*, 416–419.

HIGH PRESSURE LIQUID CHROMATOGRAPHY. In plasma: detection limit 100 pg—W. C. Yu and E. U. Goff, *Analyt. Chem.*, 1983, *55*, 29–32.

Disposition in the Body. Incompletely absorbed from the gastrointestinal tract; it may be absorbed through intact skin. The main metabolic reaction is stepwise de-esterification ultimately to pentaerythritol. The nitrate ester metabolites may be conjugated with glucuronic acid. About 50 to 60% of a dose is excreted in the urine in 48 hours, mainly as pentaerythritol and pentaerythritol mononitrate, with small amounts of the dinitrate ester. About 30 to 40% of a dose is eliminated in the faeces in 72 hours, partly as unchanged drug, with the main metabolite present being pentaerythritol, together with small quantities of the dinitrate and mononitrate esters.

HALF-LIFE. About 7 hours.

PROTEIN BINDING. In plasma, about 85%.

Dose. 30 to 240 mg daily.

Pentamidine   *Antiprotozoal*

4,4′-(Pentamethylenedioxy)dibenzamidine
$C_{19}H_{24}N_4O_2 = 340.4$
CAS—100-33-4

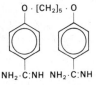

Pentamidine Isethionate
$C_{19}H_{24}N_4O_2, 2C_2H_6O_4S = 592.7$
CAS—140-64-7
White, hygroscopic crystals or powder. M.p. 188° to 192°.
Soluble 1 in 10 of water; slightly soluble in ethanol; practically insoluble in chloroform and ether.

Pentamidine Mesylate
Synonyms. Pentamidine Dimethylsulphonate; Pentamidine Methanesulphonate.
Proprietary Name. Lomidine
$C_{19}H_{24}N_4O_2, 2CH_3SO_3H = 532.6$
CAS—6823-79-6
A white or very faintly pink granular powder.
Slightly **soluble** in water and ethanol; practically insoluble in chloroform and ether.

Thin-layer Chromatography. *System TA*—Rf 01; *system TB*—Rf 01; *system TC*—Rf 00. (*Acidified iodoplatinate solution*, positive.)

Ultraviolet Spectrum. Aqueous acid—262 nm ($A_1^1 = 840$ a); aqueous alkali—249 nm. (See below)

Infra-red Spectrum. Principal peaks at wavenumbers 1188, 1604, 1260, 1028, 1676, 1003 (pentamidine isethionate, KBr disk). (See below)

Dose. Usually the equivalent of 2 to 4 mg/kg of pentamidine daily, by intramuscular injection.

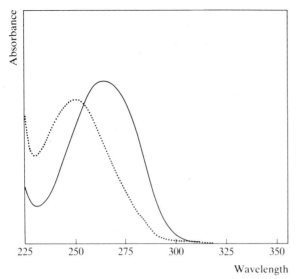

A white crystalline powder. M.p. 140° to 148°.

Freely **soluble** in water, chloroform, and methanol; soluble in ethanol.

Colour Tests. Liebermann's Test—red-orange; Marquis Test—orange.

Thin-layer Chromatography. *System TA*—Rf 01; *system TB*—Rf 00; *system TC*—Rf 01. (*Acidified iodoplatinate solution*, positive.)

Gas Chromatography. *System GA*—not eluted.

Ultraviolet Spectrum. Aqueous acid—253 nm, 258 nm, 265 nm.

Infra-red Spectrum. Principal peaks at wavenumbers 1210, 1730, 1252, 755, 1008, 1162 (Nujol mull).

Mass Spectrum. Principal peaks at m/z 96, 97, 98, 91, 136, 31, 29, 55.

Dose. 20 to 30 mg daily.

Pentazocine
Narcotic Analgesic

$(2R^*,6R^*,11R^*)$-1,2,3,4,5,6-Hexahydro-6,11-dimethyl-3-(3-methylbut-2-enyl)-2,6-methano-3-benzazocin-8-ol
$C_{19}H_{27}NO = 285.4$
CAS—359-83-1

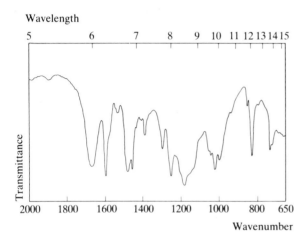

A white or pale tan-coloured powder. M.p. 147° to 158°.

Practically **insoluble** in water; soluble 1 in about 15 of ethanol, 1 in 2 of chloroform, and 1 in 33 of ether.

Pentazocine Hydrochloride

Proprietary Names. Algopent (tablets); Fortral (capsules and tablets); Talwin (tablets). It is an ingredient of Fortagesic.
$C_{19}H_{27}NO,HCl = 321.9$
CAS—2276-52-0; 64024-15-3

A white to pale cream-coloured crystalline powder. There are 2 forms, melting at about 218° and about 254°.

Soluble 1 in 30 of water, 1 in 16 of ethanol, and 1 in 4 of chloroform; practically insoluble in ether.

Pentazocine Lactate

Proprietary Names. Algopent (injection); Fortral (injection and suppositories); Pentalgina; Talwin (injection and suppositories).
$C_{19}H_{27}NO,C_3H_6O_3 = 375.5$
CAS—17146-95-1

A white to cream-coloured powder.

Soluble 1 in 25 of water, 1 in 12 of ethanol, 1 in 25 of chloroform, and 1 in 1500 of ether.

Dissociation Constant. pK_a 8.5, 10.0 (20°).

Partition Coefficient. Log P (octanol/pH 7.4), 2.0.

Colour Tests. Folin–Ciocalteu Reagent—blue; Mandelin's Test—green; Marquis Test—red → green.

Thin-layer Chromatography. *System TA*—Rf 61; *system TB*—Rf 15; *system TC*—Rf 12. (*Acidified iodoplatinate solution*, positive.)

Gas Chromatography. *System GA*—RI 2275; *system GB*—RI 1528; *system GC*—RI 2225; *system GF*—RI 3030.

High Pressure Liquid Chromatography. *System HA*—k' 1.8; *system HC*—k' 0.67.

Pentapiperide Methylsulphate
Anticholinergic

Synonyms. Pentapiperium Methylsulphate; Valpipamate Methylsulphate.

Proprietary Names. Crilin; Crylène.

Note. Pentapiperide methylsulphate and pentapiperium methylsulphate are identical but pentapiperide differs from pentapiperium in having one less methyl group.

1,1-Dimethyl-4-(3-methyl-2-phenylvaleryloxy)piperidinium methylsulphate
$C_{19}H_{30}NO_2,CH_3SO_4 = 415.5$
CAS—7009-54-3 (pentapiperide); *26372-86-1* (pentapiperium); *7681-80-3* (pentapiperide methylsulphate or pentapiperium methylsulphate)

Ultraviolet Spectrum. Aqueous acid—278 nm ($A_1^1 = 69$ a); aqueous alkali—240 nm ($A_1^1 = 330$ a), 300 nm ($A_1^1 = 106$ a).

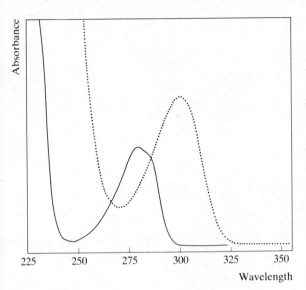

Wavelength

Infra-red Spectrum. Principal peaks at wavenumbers 1238, 1264, 1609, 1214, 854, 1054 (KBr disk). Polymorphism may occur.

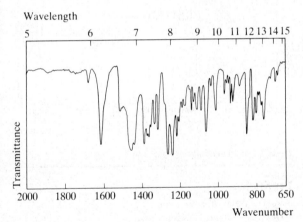

Wavenumber

Mass Spectrum. Principal peaks at m/z 45, 217, 70, 41, 69, 110, 285, 202.

Quantification. GAS CHROMATOGRAPHY. In blood: pentazocine and tripelennamine, AFID—M. A. Mackell and A. Poklis, *J. Chromat.*, 1982, *235*, 445–452. In blood, plasma or urine: sensitivity 5 ng, ECD—S. E. Swezey *et al.*, *J. Chromat.*, 1978, *154*, 256–260. In plasma or urine: pentazocine and metabolites, ECD and FID—K. A. Pittman and C. Davison, *J. pharm. Sci.*, 1973, *62*, 765–769.

RADIOIMMUNOASSAY. In plasma: detection limit 1 ng/ml—J. E. Peterson *et al.*, *J. pharm. Sci.*, 1979, *68*, 626–628.

Disposition in the Body. Well absorbed after oral, intramuscular, or rectal administration, but undergoes extensive first-pass metabolism after oral administration; bioavailability about 20%. Metabolism occurs mainly by extensive oxidation of the methyl groups of the dimethylallyl side-chain to produce the *cis*-hydroxy and the *trans*-carboxylic acid metabolites; the *trans*-hydroxy metabolite appears to be rapidly oxidised to the acid and is not detectable. Glucuronic acid conjugation of unchanged drug and metabolites also occurs; the 3-(3-hydroxy-3-methylbutyl) deriv- ative has also been detected in the urine after overdoses. There is considerable intersubject variation in the rate of metabolism, and smokers appear to metabolise 40% more pentazocine than non-smokers. After intramuscular administration, 65 to 76% of a dose is excreted in the urine in 48 hours. After an oral dose, up to 13% is excreted as unchanged drug and 12 to 30% as the conjugate in 24 hours, the major proportion being excreted in the first 12 hours. Less than 2% of a dose is eliminated in the faeces.

THERAPEUTIC CONCENTRATION. In plasma, usually in the range 0.05 to 0.20 µg/ml. Blood concentrations may be erratic and after intramuscular or oral administration, more than one peak may occur.

After an intramuscular dose of 45 mg given to 8 subjects, peak plasma concentrations of 0.11 to 0.24 µg/ml (mean 0.14) were attained in 1 hour. After a single oral dose of 75 mg given to 5 subjects, peak plasma concentrations of 0.11 to 0.30 µg/ml (mean 0.16) were attained in 1 to 3 hours (B. A. Berkowitz *et al.*, *Clin. Pharmac. Ther.*, 1969, *10*, 320–328).

TOXICITY. The estimated minimum lethal dose is 0.3 g, although recovery after ingestion of 1.2 g has been reported. Blood concentrations of 1 µg/ml or more may be lethal. Some cases of abuse have been reported resulting in a mild form of addiction. Pentazocine abuse has been reported to be widespread among 'street addicts' in the United States of America, in combination with tripelennamine ('T's and Blues').

In 2 fatalities due to pentazocine ingestion, the following postmortem tissue concentrations were reported: blood 9.2 and 3.3 µg/ml, liver 43 and 34 µg/g, urine, –, 4.5 µg/ml; ethanol was also detected in blood at concentrations of 200 and 1760 µg/ml. Blood- and liver-pentazocine concentrations in other cases taken from the literature were reported to range from 0.8 to 38 µg/ml and 3 to 197 µg/g respectively (A. Poklis and M. A. Mackell, *Forens. Sci. Int.*, 1982, *20*, 89–95).

In 17 fatalities involving intravenous abuse of pentazocine and tripelen- namine, pentazocine blood concentrations of 0 to 11 µg/ml (mean 3) were reported; tripelennamine concentrations ranged from 0 to 3.0 µg/ml (mean 0.5) (J. R. Monforte *et al.*, *J. forens. Sci.*, 1983, *28*, 90–101).

HALF-LIFE. Plasma half-life, about 2 to 4 hours.

VOLUME OF DISTRIBUTION. About 5 litres/kg.

CLEARANCE. Plasma clearance, about 18 ml/min/kg.

DISTRIBUTION IN BLOOD. Plasma: whole blood ratio, about 0.93.

PROTEIN BINDING. In plasma, about 60 to 70%.

NOTE. For a review of the pharmacokinetics of narcotic agonists- antagonists, see R. E. S. Bullingham *et al.*, *Clin. Pharmacokinet.*, 1983, *8*, 332–343.

Dose. The equivalent of up to 600 mg of pentazocine daily, by mouth; up to 360 mg daily, given parenterally.

Pentetrazol   *Respiratory Stimulant*

Synonyms. Corazol; Leptazol; Pentamethazol; 1,5-Pentamethy- lenetetrazole; Pentazol; Pentylenetetrazol.
Proprietary Names. Cardiazol; Metrazol.
6,7,8,9-Tetrahydro-5*H*-tetrazoloazepine
$C_6H_{10}N_4 = 138.2$
CAS—54-95-5

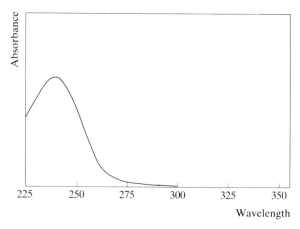

Colourless crystals or white crystalline powder. M.p. 57° to 60°.
Soluble 1 in less than 1 of water, of ethanol, and of chloroform, and 1 in less than 4 of ether.

Thin-layer Chromatography. *System TA*—Rf 72; *system TB*—Rf 07; *system TC*—Rf 64. (*Acidified iodoplatinate solution*, positive.)

Gas Chromatography. *System GA*—RI 1552; *system GB*—RI 1578; *system GC*—RI 2021.

Ultraviolet Spectrum. No significant absorption, 230 to 360 nm.

Infra-red Spectrum. Principal peaks at wavenumbers 1535, 1115, 1250, 1000, 900, 800 (KBr disk).

Mass Spectrum. Principal peaks at *m/z* 55, 82, 41, 39, 54, 42, 56, 109.

Quantification. GAS CHROMATOGRAPHY. In plasma: sensitivity 100 ng/ml, AFID—L. D. Bo *et al.*, *J. pharmacol. Methods*, 1979, *2*, 29–33. In plasma or urine: sensitivity 500 ng/ml, FID—H. W. Jun *et al.*, *J. pharm. Sci.*, 1975, *64*, 1843–1846.

Disposition in the Body. Readily absorbed after oral or parenteral administration and rapidly metabolised. About 60% of an oral dose is excreted in the urine in 24 hours with about 10% as unchanged drug and the remainder as metabolites.

THERAPEUTIC CONCENTRATION.
Following an oral dose of 100 mg to 3 subjects, who were taking the drug regularly, peak plasma concentrations of 1.5 to 3.1 μg/ml (mean 2.2) were attained in 1.3 to 5 hours (H. W. Jun *et al.*, *ibid.*).

Dose. Usually 100 mg parenterally.

Penthienate Methobromide   *Anticholinergic*

Synonym. Penthienate Bromide
Proprietary Name. Monodral
2-[2-Cyclopentyl-2-(2-thienyl)glycoloyloxy]ethyldiethylmethyl-ammonium bromide
$C_{18}H_{30}BrNO_3S = 420.4$
CAS—22064-27-3 ($C_{18}H_{30}NO_3S$); *60-44-6* (methobromide)

A white crystalline powder. M.p. 122° to 128°.
Soluble in water and ethanol; freely soluble in chloroform; practically insoluble in ether.

Colour Tests. The following tests are performed on the nitrate (see p. 128): Liebermann's Test—violet; Mandelin's Test—violet; Marquis Test—violet; Sulphuric Acid—orange.

Thin-layer Chromatography. *System TA*—Rf 02. (*Acidified iodoplatinate solution*, positive.)

High Pressure Liquid Chromatography. *System HA*—k′ 3.2.
Ultraviolet Spectrum. Aqueous acid—238 nm ($A_1^1 = 188$ a).

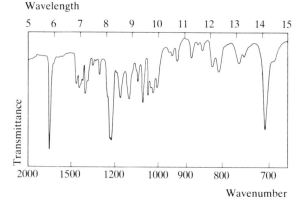

Infra-red Spectrum. Principal peaks at wavenumbers 1739, 1227, 1234, 704, 1064, 1130 (KBr disk).

Dose. 7.5 to 40 mg daily.

Pentifylline   *Vasodilator*

Synonym. 1-Hexyltheobromine
1-Hexyl-3,7-dimethylxanthine
$C_{13}H_{20}N_4O_2 = 264.3$
CAS—1028-33-7

A crystalline solid. M.p. about 82°.
Practically **insoluble** in water; soluble in ethanol, chloroform, and hydrochloric acid.

Colour Test. Amalic Acid Test—pink-orange/violet.

Thin-layer Chromatography. *System TA*—Rf 55; *system TB*—Rf 06; *system TC*—Rf 66. (*Acidified iodoplatinate solution*, positive.)

Gas Chromatography. *System GA*—RI 2195.

Ultraviolet Spectrum. Aqueous acid—275 nm ($A_1^1 = 335$ b).

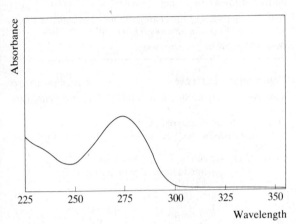

Infra-red Spectrum. Principal peaks at wavenumbers 1652, 1700, 1548, 1220, 760, 750 (KBr disk).

Mass Spectrum. Principal peaks at *m/z* 180, 264, 193, 109, 194, 181, 67, 42.

Dose. Pentifylline has been given in doses of up to 800 mg daily.

Pentobarbitone
Barbiturate

Synonyms. Mébubarbital; Mebumal; Pentobarbital.
Proprietary Names. Nembutal (elixir); Neodorm.
5-Ethyl-5-(1-methylbutyl)barbituric acid
$C_{11}H_{18}N_2O_3 = 226.3$
CAS—76-74-4

Colourless crystals or a white crystalline powder. M.p. 127° to 133°. A polymorphic form may occur, with a m.p. of about 115°; it gradually reverts to the more stable form on heating at about 110°.
Very slightly **soluble** in water; soluble 1 in 4.5 of ethanol, 1 in 4 of chloroform, and 1 in 10 of ether; very soluble in acetone and methanol.

Pentobarbitone Calcium
Synonym. Pentobarbital Calcium
Proprietary Name. Repocal
$(C_{11}H_{17}N_2O_3)_2Ca = 490.6$
CAS—7563-42-0 $(C_{11}H_{18}N_2O_3, xCa)$
A fine white crystalline powder.
Sparingly **soluble** in water; slightly soluble in ethanol; practically insoluble in ether.

Pentobarbitone Sodium
Synonyms. Ethaminal Sodium; Mebumalnatrium; Pentobarbital Sodium; Soluble Pentobarbitone.
Proprietary Names. Nembutal; Nova-Rectal; Penbon; Pentogen; Pentone; Petab. It is an ingredient of Carbrital.
$C_{11}H_{17}N_2NaO_3 = 248.3$
CAS—57-33-0
A white, hygroscopic, crystalline powder or granules.
Very **soluble** in water and ethanol; practically insoluble in ether. A solution in water slowly decomposes.

Dissociation Constant. pK_a 8.0 (20°).

Partition Coefficient. Log *P* (octanol/pH 7.4), 1.9.

Colour Tests. Koppanyi–Zwikker Test—violet; Mercurous Nitrate—black; Vanillin Reagent—brown-red/violet.

Thin-layer Chromatography. *System TD*—Rf 55; *system TE*—Rf 45; *system TF*—Rf 66; *system TH*—Rf 76. (*Mercuric chloride-diphenylcarbazone reagent*, positive; *mercurous nitrate spray*, black; *Zwikker's reagent*, pink.)

Gas Chromatography. *System GA*—RI 1740; *system GF*—RI 2465.

High Pressure Liquid Chromatography. *System HG*—k' 10.96; *system HH*—k' 8.07.

Ultraviolet Spectrum. *Borax buffer 0.05M* (pH 9.2)—239 nm ($A_1^1 = 438$ a); M sodium hydroxide (pH 13)—255 nm ($A_1^1 = 327$ b).

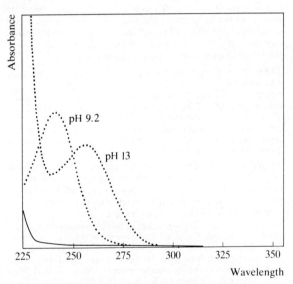

Infra-red Spectrum. Principal peaks at wavenumbers 1685, 1719, 1744, 1315, 1218, 845 (KBr disk). (See below)

Mass Spectrum. Principal peaks at *m/z* 141, 156, 43, 41, 157, 55, 39, 98; 3'-hydroxypentobarbitone 45, 156, 141, 69, 41, 43, 157, 55.

Quantification. See also under Amylobarbitone.

GAS CHROMATOGRAPHY. In serum: sensitivity 80 ng/ml, AFID—S.-R. Sun and D. J. Hoffman, *J. pharm. Sci.*, 1979, **68**, 386–388. In plasma: sensitivity 500 ng/ml, FID—A. Hulshoff *et al.*, *Analytica chim. Acta*, 1979, **105**, 139–146.

Disposition in the Body. More than 90% of the sodium salt is absorbed after oral administration. About 80% of a dose is excreted in the urine in 5 days, with about 7% as (+)-3'-

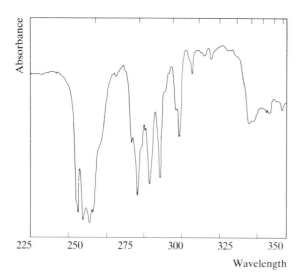

hydroxypentobarbitone, 30% as the (−)-3'-hydroxy isomer, up to 13% as the N-hydroxy metabolite, 7 to 14% as the 3'-oxo metabolite, and about 10 to 15% as the 3'-carboxy derivative. About 1% of a dose is excreted in the urine unchanged.
Pentobarbitone is a metabolite of thiopentone.

THERAPEUTIC CONCENTRATION. In plasma, usually in the range 1 to 10 µg/ml.

Following a single oral dose of 50 mg to 5 fasting subjects, peak plasma concentrations of 0.62 to 0.88 µg/ml (mean 0.73) were attained in 1 hour (R. B. Smith et al., J. Pharmacokinet. Biopharm., 1973, 1, 5–16).

After an intravenous injection of 100 mg to 7 subjects, mean plasma concentrations of 3 µg/ml were reported in 6 minutes (M. Ehrnebo, J. pharm. Sci., 1974, 63, 1114–1118).

TOXICITY. The estimated minimum lethal dose is 1 g. Toxic effects are usually associated with blood concentrations greater than about 8 µg/ml and concentrations of 12 µg/ml or more may produce coma. Fatalities have been associated with plasma concentrations of 8 to 24 to 73 µg/ml.

In 55 fatalities the following postmortem concentrations were reported: blood 5 to 169 µg/ml (mean 30), liver 23 to 550 µg/g (mean 130) (R. C. Baselt and R. H. Cravey, J. analyt. Toxicol., 1977, 1, 81–103).

The following postmortem tissue distribution (mean, n) was reported in 8 fatalities attributed to pentobarbitone: blood 19 to 90 µg/ml (46, 6), brain 21 to 117 µg/g (67, 7), kidney 16 to 156 µg/g (70, 6), liver 50 to 435 µg/g (198, 5), spleen 28 to 186 µg/g (120, 5), and urine 50 µg/ml (1 case) (C. J. Rehling, Poison Residues in Human Tissues, in Progress in Chemical Toxicology, Vol. 3, A. Stolman (Ed.), New York, Academic Press Inc., 1967, p. 370).

In 3 fatalities due to pentobarbitone, the following postmortem tissue distribution, µg/ml or µg/g, was reported:

	Pentobarbitone	3'-Hydroxy metabolite
Blood	51, 10, 25	ND, ND, 4
Bile	152, 148, 59	−, −, 13
Kidney (left)	46, 16, 38	4, 7, 7
Liver	165, 20, 46	5, 8, 9
Urine	7, 5, 62	−, 82, 65

(ND = not detected)
(A. E. Robinson and R. D. McDowall, J. Pharm. Pharmac., 1979, 31, 357–365).

HALF-LIFE. Plasma half-life, about 15 to 48 hours (mean 27).

VOLUME OF DISTRIBUTION. About 0.7 to 1 litre/kg.

CLEARANCE. Plasma clearance, about 0.3 to 0.5 ml/min/kg.

DISTRIBUTION IN BLOOD. Plasma : whole blood ratio, 0.93.

SALIVA. Plasma : saliva ratio, about 3.

PROTEIN BINDING. In plasma, about 65%.

NOTE. For a review of the pharmacokinetics of hypnotic drugs see D. D. Breimer, Clin. Pharmacokinet., 1977, 2, 93–109.

Dose. 100 to 200 mg, as a hypnotic.

Pentolinium Tartrate   Antihypertensive

Synonyms. Pentapyrrolidinium Bitartrate; Pentolonium Tartrate.
Proprietary Name. Ansolysen
NN'-Pentamethylenebis(1-methylpyrrolidinium) bis(hydrogen tartrate)
$C_{23}H_{42}N_2O_{12} = 538.6$
CAS—144-44-5 (pentolinium); 52-62-0 (tartrate)

A white powder. M.p. about 206°, with decomposition.
Soluble 1 in 0.4 of water and 1 in 800 of ethanol; practically insoluble in chloroform and ether.

Thin-layer Chromatography. System TA—Rf 00. (Acidified iodoplatinate solution, positive.)

Ultraviolet Spectrum. No significant absorption, 230 to 360 nm.

Infra-red Spectrum. Principal peaks at wavenumbers 1299, 1256, 1064, 1208, 1129, 676 (KBr disk).

Disposition in the Body. Incompletely and irregularly absorbed after oral administration. Excreted in the urine as unchanged drug.

Dose. 2.5 to 25 mg intravenously. Doses of 20 to 900 mg daily have been given by mouth.

Perazine   Tranquilliser

Synonym. Pemazine
10-[3-(4-Methylpiperazin-1-yl)propyl]phenothiazine
$C_{20}H_{25}N_3S = 339.5$
CAS—84-97-9

Crystals. M.p. 54° to 57°.

Perazine Dimalonate
Proprietary Name. Taxilan
$C_{20}H_{25}N_3S,2C_3H_4O_4 = 547.6$
CAS—14777-25-4
A white crystalline powder. M.p. 114° to 116°.
Soluble 1 in 1 of water, 1 in 33 of ethanol, and 1 in 250 of chloroform.

Partition Coefficient. Log P (octanol/pH 7.4), 2.9.

Colour Tests. Formaldehyde–Sulphuric Acid—red-violet; Forrest Reagent—brown-orange; FPN Reagent—brown-orange; Mandelin's Test—green → violet; Marquis Test—violet; Sulphuric Acid—violet.

Thin-layer Chromatography. *System TA*—Rf 48; *system TB*—Rf 24; *system TC*—Rf 37. (*Acidified iodoplatinate solution*, positive.)

Gas Chromatography. *System GA*—RI 2845.

Ultraviolet Spectrum. Aqueous acid—251 nm ($A_1^1 = 875$ a), 300 nm.

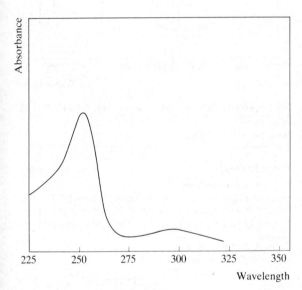

Absorbance / Wavelength

225   250   275   300   325   350

Infra-red Spectrum. Principal peaks at wavenumbers 748, 1279, 1244, 1163, 1143, 1570 (KBr disk).

Mass Spectrum. Principal peaks at m/z 113, 339, 44, 70, 141, 43, 60, 340.

Quantification. GAS CHROMATOGRAPHY. In serum: sensitivity 20 ng/ml, FID—J. Schley *et al.*, *J. clin. Chem. clin. Biochem.*, 1978, *16*, 307–311.

THIN-LAYER CHROMATOGRAPHY. In plasma: perazine and desmethylperazine, sensitivity 10 ng/ml—M. Kresse *et al.*, *J. Chromat.*, 1980, *183*; *Biomed. Appl.*, *9*, 475–482.

Disposition in the Body. Absorbed after oral administration but undergoes extensive metabolism by demethylation, sulphoxidation, *N*-oxidation and aromatic hydroxylation, followed by conjugation with glucuronic acid. About 15 to 30% of an oral dose is excreted in the urine mainly as conjugated phenolic metabolites.

THERAPEUTIC CONCENTRATION.
Following daily oral doses of 300 to 400 mg given to 14 subjects for at least 4 days, plasma concentrations of 0.02 to 0.34 µg/ml (mean 0.11) of

perazine and 0.04 to 0.54 µg/ml (mean 0.17) of the desmethyl metabolite were reported (U. Breyer and K. Villumsen, *Eur. J. clin. Pharmac.*, 1976, *9*, 457–465).

PROTEIN BINDING. In plasma, about 94 to 97%.

Dose. Usually the equivalent of 50 to 300 mg of perazine daily.

Perhexiline   *Anti-anginal*

2-(2,2-Dicyclohexylethyl)piperidine
$C_{19}H_{35}N = 277.5$
CAS—6621-47-2

Perhexiline Maleate
Proprietary Name. Pexid
$C_{19}H_{35}N,C_4H_4O_4 = 393.6$
CAS—6724-53-4
A white crystalline powder. M.p. about 189°.
Slightly **soluble** in water; soluble in chloroform and methanol.

Thin-layer Chromatography. *System TA*—Rf 41; *system TB*—Rf 57; *system TC*—Rf 08. (*Acidified iodoplatinate solution*, strong reaction.)

Gas Chromatography. *System GA*—RI 2153.

High Pressure Liquid Chromatography. *System HA*—k' 0.2.

Ultraviolet Spectrum. No significant absorption, 230 to 360 nm.

Infra-red Spectrum. Principal peaks at wavenumbers 1582, 873, 990, 730, 1029, 1081 (perhexiline maleate, KBr disk).

Mass Spectrum. Principal peaks at m/z 84, 194, 55, 85, 56, 41, 30, 99.

Quantification. GAS CHROMATOGRAPHY. In plasma: sensitivity 20 ng/ml, AFID—N. Grgurinovich, *J. Chromat.*, 1983, *274*; *Biomed. Appl.*, *25*, 361–365.

HIGH PRESSURE LIQUID CHROMATOGRAPHY. In plasma: sensitivity 5 ng/ml, fluorescence detection—J. D. Horowitz *et al.*, *J. pharm. Sci.*, 1981, *70*, 320–322.

Disposition in the Body. Incompletely absorbed after oral administration. It is metabolised by hydroxylation to mono- and dihydroxylated derivatives which are slowly excreted in the urine and faeces; very little unchanged drug is excreted in the urine.

THERAPEUTIC CONCENTRATION.
After a single oral dose of 150 mg given to 5 subjects, peak plasma concentrations of 0.02 to 0.12 µg/ml (mean 0.07) were attained in about 6 hours; following a single oral dose of 300 mg to the same subjects, peak plasma concentrations of 0.14 to 0.44 µg/ml (mean 0.27) were reported at 7 hours; absorption was considerably delayed in one subject with both doses (J. D. Horowitz *et al.*, *ibid.*).

Following chronic oral doses of 100 to 400 mg daily to 14 subjects, minimum steady-state plasma-perhexiline concentrations of 0.35 to 2.8 µg/ml (mean 1.07) were reported; steady-state plasma concentrations of the major monohydroxylated metabolite ranged from 1.25 to 7.4 µg/ml (mean 3.8). Steady-state plasma concentrations in 13 subjects who had been receiving similar daily doses but had developed toxic effects were:

perhexiline 2.2 to 6.5 µg/ml (mean 3.8), monohydroxy metabolite 0.6 to 3.8 µg/ml (mean 1.6) (E. Singlas *et al., Eur. J. clin. Pharmac.*, 1978, *14*, 195–201).

HALF-LIFE. Plasma half-life, about 2 to 6 days; the rate of elimination appears to be decreased in subjects with toxic effects, and may be dose-dependent.

Dose. 100 to 400 mg of perhexiline maleate daily.

Pericyazine   *Tranquilliser*

Synonyms. Periciazine; Propericiazine.
Proprietary Names. Aolept; Neulactil; Neuleptil.
10 - [3 - (4 - Hydroxypiperidino)propyl]phenothiazine - 2 - carbo-nitrile
$C_{21}H_{23}N_3OS = 365.5$
CAS—2622-26-6

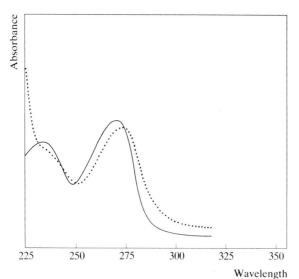

A yellow crystalline powder. M.p. 115°.
Practically **insoluble** in water; soluble in ethanol and acetone; freely soluble in chloroform; slightly soluble in ether.

Partition Coefficient. Log *P* (octanol), 3.5.

Colour Tests. Formaldehyde–Sulphuric Acid—red; Forrest Reagent—brown-orange; FPN Reagent—orange; Mandelin's Test—red; Marquis Test—red.

Thin-layer Chromatography. *System TA*—Rf 58; *system TB*—Rf 03; *system TC*—Rf 16. (*Acidified iodoplatinate solution*, positive.)

Gas Chromatography. *System GA*—RI 3285.

High Pressure Liquid Chromatography. *System HA*—k' 1.3.

Ultraviolet Spectrum. Aqueous acid—232 nm, 268 nm ($A_1^1 = 761$ a); aqueous alkali—272 nm.

Infra-red Spectrum. Principal peaks at wavenumbers 736, 1066, 811, 746, 1245, 1260 (KBr disk).

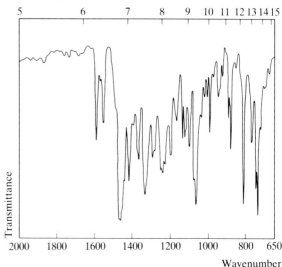

Mass Spectrum. Principal peaks at *m/z* 114, 44, 142, 365, 42, 223, 115, 205.

Dose. 10 to 75 mg daily.

Perphenazine   *Tranquilliser*

Synonym. Chlorpiprazine
Proprietary Names. Decentan; Fentazin; Phenazine; Trilafon; Trilifan. It is an ingredient of Etrafon, Triavil, and Triptafen.
2 - {4 - [3 - (2 - Chlorophenothiazin - 10 - yl)propyl]piperazin - 1 - yl}-ethanol
$C_{21}H_{26}ClN_3OS = 404.0$
CAS—58-39-9

A white or creamy-white powder. M.p. 94° to 100°.
Practically **insoluble** in water; soluble 1 in 20 of ethanol, 1 in 1 of chloroform, and 1 in 80 of ether.

Dissociation Constant. pK$_a$ 7.8 (24°).

Partition Coefficient. Log *P* (octanol/pH 7.0), 3.1.

Colour Tests. Formaldehyde–Sulphuric Acid—violet; Forrest Reagent—violet-red; FPN Reagent—violet-red; Liebermann's Test—red-brown; Mandelin's Test—violet; Marquis Test—violet.

Thin-layer Chromatography. *System TA*—Rf 55; *system TB*—Rf 07; *system TC*—Rf 29. (*Dragendorff spray*, positive; *FPN reagent*, pink; *acidified iodoplatinate solution*, positive; *Marquis reagent*, pink; *ninhydrin spray*, positive.)

Gas Chromatography. *System GA*—RI 2207.

High Pressure Liquid Chromatography. *System HA*—k' 1.9.

Ultraviolet Spectrum. Aqueous acid—254 nm ($A_1^1 = 805$ a), 307 nm; aqueous alkali—257 nm ($A_1^1 = 791$ a), 310 nm.

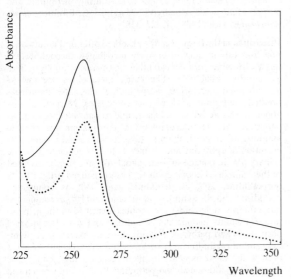

Infra-red Spectrum. Principal peaks at wavenumbers 757, 1294, 917, 1145, 1247, 1155 (KBr disk).

Wavelength

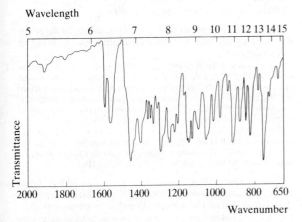

Mass Spectrum. Principal peaks at *m/z* 246, 143, 403, 70, 404, 42, 248, 113.

Quantification. GAS CHROMATOGRAPHY. In plasma: perphenazine and perphenazine sulphoxide, sensitivity 200 pg/ml, ECD—N.-E. Larsen and J. Naestoft, *J. Chromat.*, 1975, *109*, 259–264.

HIGH PRESSURE LIQUID CHROMATOGRAPHY. In serum: perphenazine and *N*-deshydroxyethylperphenazine, sensitivity 1 ng/ml, UV detection—M. Larsson and A. Forsman, *Ther. Drug Monit.*, 1983, *5*, 225–228.

RADIOIMMUNOASSAY. In plasma: detection limit 250 pg/ml—K. K. Midha *et al.*, *Br. J. clin. Pharmac.*, 1981, *11*, 85–88.

Disposition in the Body. Absorbed after oral administration but subject to first-pass metabolism. The main metabolic reactions are oxidation to the sulphoxide, which may have some pharmacological activity, *N*-dealkylation to form the *N*-deshydroxyethyl metabolite, *N*-oxidation, cleavage of the piperazine ring, and phenolic hydroxylation, followed by glucuronide conjugation. After oral administration, about 1 to 2% of the daily dose is excreted in the urine as unchanged drug, with about 13% as the sulphoxide and 30% as perphenazine glucuronide; after chronic administration of perphenazine enanthate intramuscularly, excretion of unchanged drug and the sulphoxide is increased to about 6% and 22% of the dose, respectively.

THERAPEUTIC CONCENTRATION.

After daily oral doses of 12 to 48 mg to 16 subjects, steady-state plasma concentrations of 0.0003 to 0.025 µg/ml (mean 0.004) of perphenazine and 0.0004 to 0.018 µg/ml (mean 0.004) of the sulphoxide were reported (L. B. Hansen and N.-E. Larsen, *Psychopharmacologia*, 1977, *53*, 127–130).

TOXICITY.

The following postmortem tissue concentrations were reported in a fatality due to the ingestion of about 1 g of perphenazine: blood 3 µg/ml, brain 11 µg/g, liver 149 µg/g; a blood-alcohol concentration of 1700 µg/ml was also reported (R. H. Cravey, per R. C. Baselt, *Disposition of Toxic Drugs and Chemicals in Man*, 2nd Edn, Davis, California, Biomedical Publications, 1982, pp. 610–612).

HALF-LIFE. Plasma half-life, about 8 to 12 hours.

VOLUME OF DISTRIBUTION. 10 to 35 litres/kg.

CLEARANCE. Plasma clearance, about 12 to 38 ml/min/kg.

Dose. Usually 12 to 24 mg daily; up to 64 mg daily has been given.

Pethidine
Narcotic Analgesic

Synonyms. Isonipecaine; Meperidine.
Ethyl 1-methyl-4-phenylpiperidine-4-carboxylate
$C_{15}H_{21}NO_2 = 247.3$
CAS—57-42-1

An oily liquid which slowly crystallises.

Pethidine Hydrochloride
Proprietary Names. Demer-Idine; Demerol; Dolantin(e); Dolosal; Pethoid. It is an ingredient of Mepergan and Pethilorfan.
$C_{15}H_{21}NO_2,HCl = 283.8$
CAS—50-13-5
A white crystalline powder. M.p. 186° to 190°.
Very **soluble** in water; soluble 1 in 20 of ethanol; soluble in chloroform; practically insoluble in ether.

Dissociation Constant. pK_a 8.7 (20°).

Partition Coefficient. Log *P* (octanol), 1.6.

Colour Tests. Liebermann's Test—red-orange; Marquis Test—orange.

Thin-layer Chromatography. *System TA*—Rf 52; *system TB*—Rf 37; *system TC*—Rf 34. (*Dragendorff spray*, positive; *acidified iodoplatinate solution*, positive; *Marquis reagent*, brown.)

Gas Chromatography. *System GA*—pethidine RI 1751, norpethidine RI 1745; *system GB*—RI 1753; *system GC*—RI 2025; *system GF*—RI 1995.

High Pressure Liquid Chromatography. *System HA*—pethidine k′ 2.8 (tailing peak), norpethidine k′ 1.7 (tailing peak), pethidinic acid k′ 2.8 (tailing peak); *system HC*—pethidine k′ 0.55, norpethidine k′ 2.04.

Ultraviolet Spectrum. Aqueous acid—251 nm, 257 nm ($A_1^1 =$ 8.5 a), 263 nm. No alkaline shift.

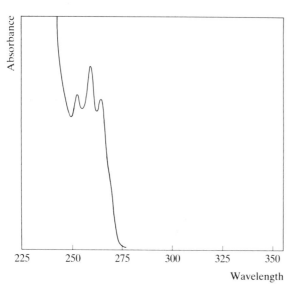

Wavelength

Infra-red Spectrum. Principal peaks at wavenumbers 1708, 1218, 1166, 1148, 688, 730 (pethidine hydrochloride, KBr disk).

Wavelength

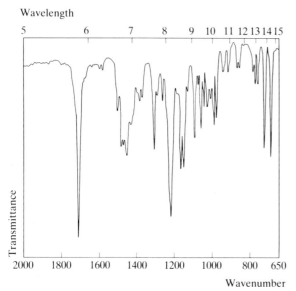

Wavenumber

Mass Spectrum. Principal peaks at *m/z* 71, 70, 44, 57, 42, 247, 43, 246; norpethidine 57, 233, 42, 56, 158, 43, 160, 103; pethidinic acid 71, 70, 57, 43, 219, 42, 218, 44.

Quantification. GAS CHROMATOGRAPHY. In blood, plasma or urine: pethidine and norpethidine, sensitivity 5 ng/ml for pethidine and 2.5 ng/ml for norpethidine, AFID—P. Jacob *et al.*, *J. pharm. Sci.*, 1982, *71*, 166–168. In plasma: pethidine and norpethidine, sensitivity 20 ng/ml, ECD—P. Hartvig and C. Fagerlund, *J. Chromat.*, 1983, *274*; *Biomed. Appl.*, *25*, 355–360.

GAS CHROMATOGRAPHY–MASS SPECTROMETRY. In plasma or serum: pethidine and norpethidine, detection limit 170 pg/ml for pethidine and 500 pg/ml for norpethidine—E. L. Todd *et al.*, *J. analyt. Toxicol.*, 1979, *3*, 256–259. In urine: pethidinic and norpethidinic acids, sensitivity 500 ng/ml—C. Lindberg *et al.*, *Acta pharm. suec.*, 1978, *15*, 327–336.

Disposition in the Body. Readily absorbed after oral administration and rapidly and extensively distributed throughout the tissues. It undergoes considerable first-pass metabolism; bioavailability about 55%. The major metabolites are the *N*-demethylated derivative, norpethidine, and the hydrolysis product, pethidinic acid, and its conjugates. Norpethidine is about half as active an analgesic and about twice as toxic as pethidine; it may accumulate in the plasma on chronic administration, particularly in subjects with renal failure. The excretion of pethidine and its metabolites is dependent on the urinary pH. In normal subjects, about 70% of a dose is excreted in the urine in 24 hours, up to 10% as unchanged drug, 10% as norpethidine, 20% as pethidinic acid, 16% as conjugated pethidinic acid, 8% as norpethidinic acid, and 10% as conjugated norpethidinic acid; other metabolites identified in the urine in minor amounts include the *N*-hydroxy and *N*-hydroxyphenyl derivatives and pethidine *N*-oxide. Urinary excretion of pethidine and norpethidine may both be enhanced to about 30% of a dose if the urine is acid; in alkaline urine, less than 5% is excreted as pethidine and norpethidine. In pregnant women and in women taking oral contraceptives, the excretion of unchanged pethidine appears to be increased; less unchanged drug is eliminated in older subjects and, in subjects with cirrhosis, excretion of pethidine is delayed.

Pethidine is a metabolite of phenoperidine.

THERAPEUTIC CONCENTRATION. In plasma, usually in the range 0.2 to 0.8 µg/ml. Higher plasma concentrations are found in elderly subjects.

Following a single oral dose of 50 mg to 6 subjects, a mean peak serum concentration of 0.14 µg/ml was attained in 2 hours; after an intramuscular injection of 50 mg to the same subjects, a mean peak serum concentration of 0.20 µg/ml in 1 hour was reported, and a mean serum concentration of 0.52 µg/ml was obtained one minute after an intravenous injection of 50 mg (J. E. Stambaugh *et al.*, *J. clin. Pharmac.*, 1976, *16*, 245–256).

Following multiple oral doses of 75 to 100 mg to 4 subjects, plasma concentrations of 0.16 to 0.54 µg/ml (mean 0.36) of pethidine and 0.13 to 0.48 µg/ml (mean 0.27) of norpethidine were reported 1 to 4 hours after a dose (H. H. Szeto *et al.*, *J. Chromat.*, 1976, *125*, 503–510).

TOXICITY. The estimated minimum lethal dose is 1 g. Toxic effects are usually associated with blood concentrations greater than 2 µg/ml but fatalities involving pethidine are uncommon.

The following postmortem tissue concentrations, µg/ml or µg/g, were reported in 6 fatalities due to the suicidal ingestion or accidental intravenous overdose of pethidine:

	Oral		Intravenous	
	Pethidine	Norpethidine	Pethidine	Norpethidine
Blood	8, 9, 20	18, 8, 30	1, 4, 8	7, 0.5, ND
Bile	13, –, –	16, –, –	–, –, –	–, –, –
Liver	7, 5, 10	66, 11, 15	2, 7, 16	12, 10, ND
Urine	–, 150, –	–, 50, –	20, 24, 2	69, 79, 0.1

(ND = not detected)
(T. J. Siek, *J. forens. Sci.*, 1978, *23*, 6–13).

HALF-LIFE. Plasma half-life, pethidine 3 to 10 hours (mean 5), increased in neonates and in renal impairment; norpethidine about 18 hours.

VOLUME OF DISTRIBUTION. About 4 litres/kg.

CLEARANCE. Plasma clearance, about 14 ml/min/kg, decreased in subjects with liver disease and in the elderly.

DISTRIBUTION IN BLOOD. Plasma:whole blood ratio, about 0.9.

PROTEIN BINDING. In plasma, about 40 to 50%.

NOTE. For reviews of the pharmacokinetics of pethidine see L. E. Mather and P. J. Meffin, *Clin. Pharmacokinet.*, 1978, *3*, 352–368, and D. J. Edwards *et al.*, *ibid.*, 1982, *7*, 421–433.

Dose. Usually 50 to 100 mg of pethidine hydrochloride, every 4 hours, by mouth or by intramuscular injection.

Phanquone   *Anti-amoebic/Antibacterial*

Synonym. Phanquinone
Proprietary Name. Entobex
4,7-Phenanthroline-5,6-dione
$C_{12}H_6N_2O_2 = 210.2$
CAS—84-12-8

An orange crystalline powder. M.p. 295°, with decomposition. Slightly **soluble** in water; practically insoluble in ethanol and chloroform.

Colour Tests. Marquis Test—yellow; Methanolic Potassium Hydroxide—yellow → brown-violet.

Thin-layer Chromatography. *System TA*—Rf 49; *system TB*—Rf 03; *system TC*—Rf 45. (*Acidified iodoplatinate solution*, positive.)

Ultraviolet Spectrum. Aqueous acid—265 nm ($A_1^1 = 500$ a), 272 nm ($A_1^1 = 500$ a), 292 nm ($A_1^1 = 480$ b).

Infra-red Spectrum. Principal peaks at wavenumbers 1700, 1283, 1584, 1275, 1683, 950 (KBr disk).

Dose. 150 to 300 mg daily.

Phenacaine   *Local Anaesthetic*

Synonym. Phenetidylphenacetin
NN'-Bis(4-ethoxyphenyl)acetamidine
$C_{18}H_{22}N_2O_2 = 298.4$
CAS—101-93-9

Phenacaine Hydrochloride
Proprietary Name. Holocaine
$C_{18}H_{22}N_2O_2, HCl, H_2O = 352.9$
CAS—620-99-5 (anhydrous); *6153-19-1* (monohydrate)
White crystals. M.p. about 190°.
Soluble 1 in 50 of water; freely soluble in ethanol and chloroform; practically insoluble in ether.

Gas Chromatography. *System GA*—RI 2617.

Infra-red Spectrum. Principal peaks at wavenumbers 1646, 1520, 1256, 1300, 1046, 815 (KBr disk).

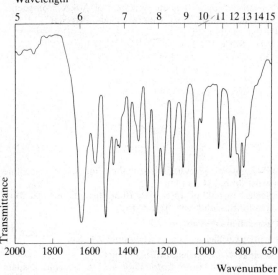

Uses. Phenacaine hydrochloride has been used as a 1% aqueous solution or as a 1 or 2% ointment.

Phenacemide   *Anticonvulsant*

Synonym. Carbamidum Phenylaceticum
Proprietary Name. Phenurone
(Phenylacetyl)urea
$C_9H_{10}N_2O_2 = 178.2$
CAS—63-98-9

$$C_6H_5 \cdot CH_2 \cdot CO \cdot NH \cdot CO \cdot NH_2$$

A white crystalline powder. M.p. about 213°.
Very slightly **soluble** in water, ethanol, chloroform, and ether; slightly soluble in acetone and methanol.

Colour Tests. Liebermann's Test—red-orange; Nessler's Reagent—brown-orange (slow).

Thin-layer Chromatography. *System TD*—Rf 22; *system TE*—Rf 65; *system TF*—Rf 40.

Gas Chromatography. *System GA*—RI 1473.

Ultraviolet Spectrum. Methanol—258 nm ($A_1^1 = 18$ a), 265 nm.

Infra-red Spectrum. Principal peaks at wavenumbers 1660, 1090, 716, 1618, 1170, 970 (KBr disk).

Mass Spectrum. Principal peaks at *m/z* 91, 92, 118, 44, 43, 135, 65, 178.

Disposition in the Body. Well absorbed after oral administration. It is extensively metabolised to inactive metabolites, principally by *p*-hydroxylation of the phenyl ring; the metabolites are excreted in the urine.

TOXICITY. The estimated minimum lethal dose is 5 g.

Dose. 1.5 to 3 g daily.

Phenacetin
Analgesic

Synonyms. Aceto-*p*-phenetidide; Acetophenetidin; Acetylphenetidin; Paracetophenetidin.

Proprietary Names. It is an ingredient of A.S.A. Compound, Coriforte, Fiorinal, P-A-C Compound, and Percodan.

4'-Ethoxyacetanilide
$C_{10}H_{13}NO_2 = 179.2$
CAS—62-44-2

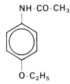

White glistening crystalline scales or fine white crystalline powder. M.p. 134° to 137°.

Soluble 1 in 1300 of water, 1 in 20 of ethanol, and 1 in 20 of chloroform; slightly soluble in ether.

Dissociation Constant. pK_a 2.2.

Partition Coefficient. Log *P* (octanol/pH 7.4), 1.6.

Colour Tests. Liebermann's Test—violet.

Boil 0.1 g with 1 ml of *hydrochloric acid* for 3 minutes, dilute with 10 ml of water, cool, filter, and add 1 drop of 0.02M potassium dichromate to the filtrate—violet → red.

Thin-layer Chromatography. *System TD*—Rf 38; *system TE*—Rf 68; *system TF*—Rf 38. (*Acidified potassium permanganate solution*, positive.)

Gas Chromatography. *System GA*—phenacetin RI 1675, paracetamol RI 1687; *system GF*—RI 2325.

High Pressure Liquid Chromatography. *System HD*—phenacetin k' 0.6, paracetamol k' 0.1; *system HW*—phenacetin k' 4.4, paracetamol k' 0.32.

Ultraviolet Spectrum. Aqueous acid—244 nm ($A_1^1 = 649$ a). No alkaline shift.

Infra-red Spectrum. Principal peaks at wavenumbers 1244, 1655, 1513, 1555, 1265, 836 (KBr disk).

Mass Spectrum. Principal peaks at *m/z* 108, 109, 179, 137, 43, 81, 80, 110; paracetamol 109, 151, 43, 80, 108, 81, 53, 52.

Quantification. See also under Paracetamol.

GAS CHROMATOGRAPHY. In plasma: phenacetin and paracetamol, detection limit < 100 ng/ml, FID—M. A. Evans and R. D. Harbison, *J. pharm. Sci.*, 1977, 66, 1628–1629.

GAS CHROMATOGRAPHY–MASS SPECTROMETRY. In plasma: phenacetin and paracetamol, sensitivity 1 ng/ml for phenacetin and 100 ng/ml for paracetamol—W. A. Garland *et al.*, *J. pharm. Sci.*, 1977, 66, 340–344.

HIGH PRESSURE LIQUID CHROMATOGRAPHY. In plasma: phenacetin and paracetamol, sensitivity 500 ng/ml, UV detection—G.R. Gotelli *et al.*, *Clin. Chem.*, 1977, 23, 957–959.

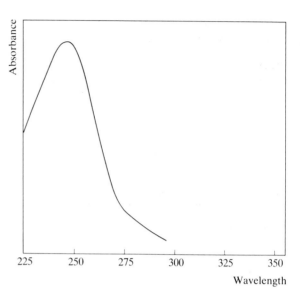

Absorbance

Wavelength

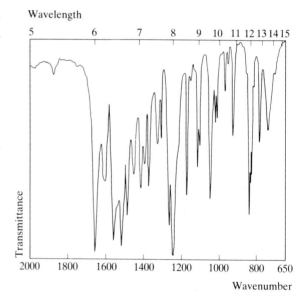

Wavelength

Transmittance

Wavenumber

Disposition in the Body. Readily absorbed after oral administration, but subject to extensive first-pass metabolism. It is metabolised mainly in the liver by *O*-dealkylation to paracetamol and acetaldehyde, followed by conjugation of the paracetamol with sulphate or glucuronic acid (see under Paracetamol); other reactions are deacetylation to phenetidine (*p*-ethoxyaniline), *N*-,2-, and α-hydroxylation forming mainly 2-hydroxyphenetidine and also 2-hydroxyphenacetin, sulphate conjugation of deacetylated metabolites, and glutathione conjugation to form *S*-(1-acetamido-4-hydroxyphenyl)cysteine and its corresponding mercapturic acid.

2-Hydroxyphenetidine appears to be the nephrotoxic metabolite and is possibly involved in the formation of methaemoglobinaemia. As the dose is increased so the percentage of the dose which is deacetylated is increased, producing proportionately more phenetidine and 2-hydroxyphenetidine; production of these metabolites is also increased by concomitant administration of aspirin, caffeine, and codeine. Phenacetin is not hepatotoxic despite being converted to paracetamol; this is because the enzyme systems which convert paracetamol to its toxic metabolite are also involved in the conversion of phenacetin to paracetamol and the two conversions therefore compete, resulting in reduced paracetamol oxidation. Phenacetin metabolism is stimulated by cigarette smoking. The extent of *O*-dealkylation appears to be genetically determined. About 80 to 90% of a dose is excreted in the urine in 24 hours with 50 to 80% of the dose as the sulphate and glucuronide conjugates of paracetamol, 6 to 8% as 2-hydroxyphenetidine sulphate, about 2% as *S*-(1-acetamido-4-hydroxyphenyl)cysteine, about 0.3% as phenetidine and 2-hydroxyphenacetin, 0.2% as unchanged drug, and 2 to 3% as unconjugated paracetamol.

THERAPEUTIC CONCENTRATION.
After a single oral dose of 0.9 g to 9 subjects, peak plasma-phenacetin concentrations of 0.2 to 7.4 μg/ml (mean 2.3) were attained in 1 to 2 hours, and peak plasma-paracetamol concentrations of 3.1 to 11.9 μg/ml (mean 7.9) were attained in 2 to 3.5 hours; plasma-phenacetin concentrations were reported to be lower in 9 smokers (E. J. Pantuck *et al.*, *Clin. Pharmac. Ther.*, 1974, *15*, 9–17).

TOXICITY. The estimated minimum lethal dose is 5 g. Prolonged use of phenacetin is associated with analgesic nephropathy; it may also produce haemolytic anaemia and methaemoglobinaemia.
In a fatality involving the intentional overdosage of a preparation containing codeine, aspirin, phenacetin and caffeine, a blood-phenacetin concentration of 136 μg/ml was reported; the codeine and salicylate blood concentrations were 5.3 and 265 μg/ml respectively (J. A. Wright *et al.*, *Clin. Toxicol.*, 1975, *8*, 457–463).

HALF-LIFE. Plasma half-life, phenacetin 0.7 to 1.5 hours, paracetamol 1.5 to 3 hours.

VOLUME OF DISTRIBUTION. About 1 to 2 litres/kg.

CLEARANCE. Plasma clearance, about 20 ml/min/kg.

DISTRIBUTION IN BLOOD. Plasma: whole blood ratio, 0.93.

PROTEIN BINDING. In plasma, about 30%.

Dose. Phenacetin has been given as a single dose of 300 to 600 mg; maximum daily dose of 3 g.

Phenaglycodol   *Tranquilliser*

Proprietary Name. Felixyn
2-(4-Chlorophenyl)-3-methylbutane-2,3-diol
$C_{11}H_{15}ClO_2 = 214.7$
CAS—79-93-6

A crystalline solid. M.p. 77° to 78°.
Practically **insoluble** in water; soluble in ethanol.

Colour Tests. Liebermann's Test—brown; Mandelin's Test—blue.

Ultraviolet Spectrum. Ethanol—259 nm, 266 nm ($A_1^1 = 13.5$ a), 275 nm.

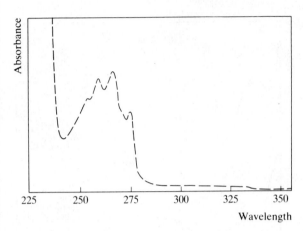

Infra-red Spectrum. Principal peaks at wavenumbers 1095, 1085, 1015, 1180, 807, 830 (KBr disk).

Mass Spectrum. Principal peaks at *m/z* 43, 59, 155, 121, 156, 31, 157, 158.

Quantification. ULTRAVIOLET SPECTROPHOTOMETRY. In blood or urine—J. E. Wallace, *J. pharm. Sci.*, 1968, *57*, 426–429.

Dose. 0.9 to 1.2 g daily.

Phenazocine   *Narcotic Analgesic*

Synonym. Phenethylazocine
1,2,3,4,5,6 - Hexahydro-6,11-dimethyl-3-phenethyl-2,6-methano-3-benzazocin-8-ol
$C_{22}H_{27}NO = 321.5$
CAS—127-35-5

Phenazocine Hydrobromide
Proprietary Name. Narphen
$C_{22}H_{27}NO,HBr,\frac{1}{2}H_2O = 411.4$
CAS—1239-04-9 (anhydrous)
A white microcrystalline powder, which can exist in 3 polymorphic forms. M.p. about 164°.
Soluble 1 in 350 of water, 1 in 45 of ethanol, and 1 in 140 of chloroform; practically insoluble in ether.

Dissociation Constant. pK_a 8.5.

Colour Test. Marquis Test—brown.

Thin-layer Chromatography. *System TA*—Rf 68; *system TB*—Rf 16; *system TC*—Rf 39. (*Dragendorff spray*, positive; *acidified iodoplatinate solution*, positive; *Marquis reagent*, brown.)

Gas Chromatography. *System GA*—RI 2684.

High Pressure Liquid Chromatography. *System HA*—k' 1.3; *system HC*—k' 0.30.

Ultraviolet Spectrum. Aqueous acid—278 nm ($A_1^1 = 64$ a); aqueous alkali—238 nm, 298 nm.

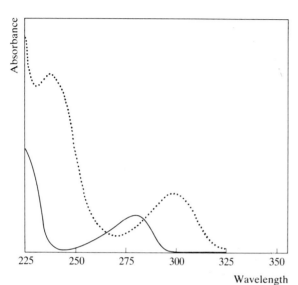

Infra-red Spectrum. Principal peaks at wavenumbers 1224, 1497, 1241, 705, 1613, 758 (phenazocine hydrobromide, Nujol mull).

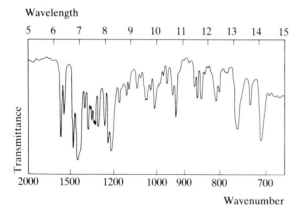

Mass Spectrum. Principal peaks at *m/z* 230, 231, 58, 44, 42, 105, 173, 159.

Disposition in the Body. Readily absorbed after oral, sublingual, or intramuscular administration; metabolised in the liver.

TOXICITY. The estimated minimum lethal dose is 0.2 g. Phenazocine is addictive although tolerance develops more slowly and to a lesser extent than with morphine.

Dose. Usually 5 mg of phenazocine hydrobromide every 4 to 6 hours; single doses of 20 mg may be given.

Phenazone
Analgesic

Synonyms. Analgésine; Antipyrin(e); Azophenum; Fenazona. *Proprietary Names.* It is an ingredient of Auralgan, Auralgicin, Auraltone, and Taumasthman.

1,5-Dimethyl-2-phenyl-4-pyrazolin-3-one
$C_{11}H_{12}N_2O = 188.2$
CAS—60-80-0

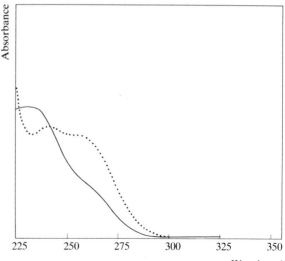

Small, colourless crystals or white crystalline powder. M.p. 110° to 113°.

Soluble 1 in 1 of water, 1 in 1 of ethanol, 1 in 1 of chloroform, and 1 in 50 of ether.

Dissociation Constant. pK_a 1.5 (25°).

Partition Coefficient. Log *P* (octanol/pH 7.4), 0.4.

Colour Tests. *p*-Dimethylaminobenzaldehyde (100°, 5 min)—red/violet; Ferric Chloride—red; Liebermann's Test (100°)—orange; Mandelin's Test—green; Nitrous Acid—green.

Thin-layer Chromatography. *System TA*—Rf 65; *system TD*—Rf 18; *system TE*—Rf 49; *system TF*—Rf 14. (*Ferric chloride solution*, red-brown; *acidified iodoplatinate solution*, positive; *mercuric chloride–diphenylcarbazone reagent*, positive; *acidified potassium permanganate solution*, positive; *Van Urk reagent*, pink.)

Gas Chromatography. *System GA*—phenazone RI 1848, 4-hydroxyphenazone RI 1874; *system GF*—RI 2445.

High Pressure Liquid Chromatography. *System HA*—k' 0.2; *system HD*—k' 0.1; *system HW*—k' 0.95.

Ultraviolet Spectrum. Aqueous acid—230 nm ($A_1^1 = 590$ a); aqueous alkali—242 nm ($A_1^1 = 494$ a), 256 nm.

Infra-red Spectrum. Principal peaks at wavenumbers 1660, 770, 1318, 1305, 1590, 1580, (KBr disk).

Wavelength

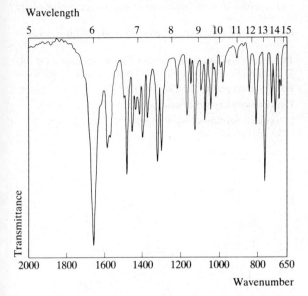

Mass Spectrum. Principal peaks at m/z 188, 96, 77, 56, 105, 189, 55, 51; norphenazone 174, 77, 91, 105, 132, –, –, –.

Quantification. GAS CHROMATOGRAPHY. In plasma: sensitivity 1 μg/ml, AFID—D. R. Abernethy et al., J. Chromat., 1981, 223; Biomed. Appl., 12, 432–437.

HIGH PRESSURE LIQUID CHROMATOGRAPHY. In plasma: sensitivity 500 ng/ml, UV detection—T. M. Campbell et al., J. Chromat., 1979, 163; Biomed. Appl., 5, 236–238. In urine: phenazone, 3-hydroxymethylphenazone, 4-hydroxyphenazone and norphenazone, sensitivity 1 to 2μg/ml, UV detection— M. Eichelbaum et al., Pharmacology, 1981, 23, 192–202.

RADIOIMMUNOASSAY. In plasma or saliva: sensitivity 10 ng/ml— R. L. Chang et al., Clin. Pharmac. Ther., 1976, 20, 219–226.

Disposition in the Body. Rapidly and completely absorbed after oral administration. Metabolised by 4-hydroxylation followed by glucuronic acid conjugation; demethylation also occurs. The rate of biotransformation is variable and appears to be genetically determined. Phenazone and its metabolites are excreted in the urine mainly as glucuronides, although sulphate conjugation has also been reported. About 30 to 40% of a dose is excreted in the urine in 48 hours as conjugated 4-hydroxyphenazone, 10 to 40% as the 3-hydroxymethyl derivative, up to about 20% as norphenazone, 3 to 6% as 4,4′-dihydroxyphenazone, 8 to 12% as 4,5-dioxypyrazoline, and less than 5% as unchanged drug; 3-carboxyphenazone has also been identified in the urine. A total of about 95% of a dose is excreted in the urine in 4 days.

THERAPEUTIC CONCENTRATION.
After a single oral dose of 10 mg/kg to 5 subjects, peak plasma concentrations of 10 to 15.5μg/ml (mean 13.4) were attained in 1 hour. Concentrations in saliva were similar to those in plasma (C. J. van Boxtel, et al. Eur. J. clin. Pharmac., 1976, 9, 327–332).

TOXICITY. The estimated minimum lethal dose is 5 g, but fatalities from acute poisoning are rare. Prolonged therapeutic administration may give rise to agranulocytosis.

In a suicide due to ingestion of phenazone, a postmortem blood concentration of 110 μg/ml was reported; alcohol was also detected in the blood at a concentration of 260 μg/ml (C. Péclet and M. Rousseau, Bull. int. Ass. forens. Toxicol., 1981, 16(1), 32).

HALF-LIFE. Plasma half-life, about 7 to 15 hours (mean 10); increased in subjects with renal impairment or hypothyroidism and in the elderly, decreased in subjects with hyperthyroidism; the half-life is also readily influenced by concomitant administration of other drugs.

VOLUME OF DISTRIBUTION. About 0.6 litre/kg.

CLEARANCE. Plasma clearance, about 0.7 ml/min/kg.

DISTRIBUTION IN BLOOD. Plasma: whole blood ratio, about 0.93.

PROTEIN BINDING. In plasma, less than 10%.

Dose. Phenazone has been given in doses of 300 to 600 mg; maximum daily dose of 4 g.

Phenazopyridine   Analgesic

3-Phenylazopyridine-2,6-diyldiamine
$C_{11}H_{11}N_5 = 213.2$
CAS—94-78-0

Phenazopyridine Hydrochloride
Proprietary Names. Phenazo; Pyridacil; Pyridium. It is an ingredient of Azo Gantanol, Azo Gantrisin, Azo-Mandelamine, Azotrex, and Uromide.
$C_{11}H_{11}N_5,HCl = 249.7$
CAS—136-40-3
A light or dark red to dark violet crystalline powder. M.p. about 235°, with decomposition.
Soluble 1 in 300 of cold water, 1 in 20 of boiling water, 1 in about 60 of ethanol, and 1 in about 330 of chloroform; very slightly soluble in ether; soluble in glacial acetic acid. Phenazopyridine hydrochloride readily forms supersaturated aqueous solutions which deposit slowly on storage.

Colour Tests. Mandelin's Test—green; Marquis Test—red.

Thin-layer Chromatography. System TA—Rf 59; system TB—Rf 01; system TC—Rf 50. (Acidified potassium permanganate solution, positive.)

Gas Chromatography. System GA—phenazopyridine RI 2245, 4-aminophenol RI 1265, aniline RI 1158.

Ultraviolet Spectrum. Ethanol—238 nm ($A_1^1 = 455$ a), 277 nm. (See below)

Infra-red Spectrum. Principal peaks at wavenumbers 1585, 1656, 762, 685, 1248, 1493 (Nujol mull). (See below)

Mass Spectrum. Principal peaks at m/z 108, 81, 213, 54, 77, 136, 51, 43; 4-aminophenol 109, 80, 53, 81, 108, 52, 54, 110.

Disposition in the Body. Absorbed after oral administration. Rapidly eliminated by the kidneys, giving an orange-red colour to the urine; about 90% of a dose is excreted in the urine in 24 hours, of which 7% is aniline, 20% is N-acetyl-4-aminophenol, 25% is 4-aminophenol, and 45% is unchanged drug.

TOXICITY. Methaemoglobinaemia and acute renal failure have been reported after overdoses.

Dose. Usually 600 mg of phenazopyridine hydrochloride daily.

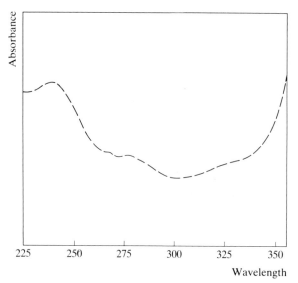

Absorbance / Wavelength

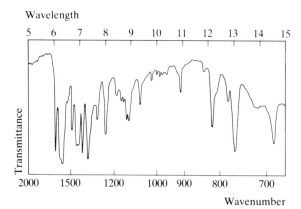

Transmittance / Wavenumber

Phenbutrazate Hydrochloride

$C_{23}H_{29}NO_3,HCl = 403.9$
CAS—6474-85-7
A fine white crystalline powder.
Slightly **soluble** in water; soluble in ethanol and acetone; practically insoluble in ether.

Colour Tests. Liebermann's Test—red-orange; Marquis Test—yellow (slow).

Thin-layer Chromatography. *System TA*—Rf 72; *system TB*—Rf 47; *system TC*—Rf 78. (*Acidified iodoplatinate solution*, positive.)

Gas Chromatography. *System GA*—RI 2670.

High Pressure Liquid Chromatography. *System HA*—k' 0.3.

Ultraviolet Spectrum. Aqueous acid—252 nm, 257 nm (A_1^1 = 10 b), 261 nm, 267 nm.

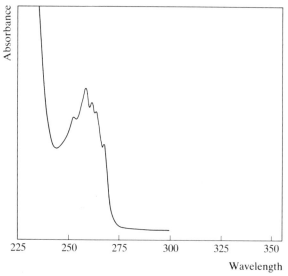

Absorbance / Wavelength

Infra-red Spectrum. Principal peaks at wavenumbers 1715, 1100, 1200, 690, 760, 1020 (KBr disk).

Mass Spectrum. Principal peaks at *m/z* 69, 56, 71, 91, 261, 84, 119, 70.

Dose. Phenbutrazate hydrochloride has been given in doses of 40 to 60 mg daily.

Phenbutrazate   *Anorectic*

Synonym. Fenbutrazate
2-(3-Methyl-2-phenylmorpholino)ethyl 2-phenylbutyrate
$C_{23}H_{29}NO_3 = 367.5$
CAS—4378-36-3

A viscous oil.
Soluble in methanol.

Phencyclidine   *Hallucinogen*

Synonym. PCP
1-(1-Phenylcyclohexyl)piperidine
$C_{17}H_{25}N = 243.4$
CAS—77-10-1

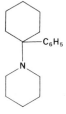

Crystals. M.p. 46°.

Phencyclidine Hydrochloride

$C_{17}H_{25}N,HCl = 279.9$

CAS—956-90-1

A white crystalline powder. M.p. about 228°.

Soluble 1 in 6 of water, 1 in 7 of ethanol, and 1 in 2 of chloroform; very slightly soluble in ether.

Dissociation Constant. pK_a 8.5.

Colour Test. *p*-Dimethylaminobenzaldehyde (100°, 3 min)—red.

Thin-layer Chromatography. *System TA*—Rf 59. (*Acidified iodoplatinate solution*, positive.)

Gas Chromatography. *System GA*—RI 1904; *system GF*—RI 2150.

High Pressure Liquid Chromatography. *System HA*—k' 2.4 (tailing peak).

Ultraviolet Spectrum. Aqueous acid—252 nm, 258 nm, 263 nm $(A_1^1 = 13.5 \text{ a})$, 270 nm.

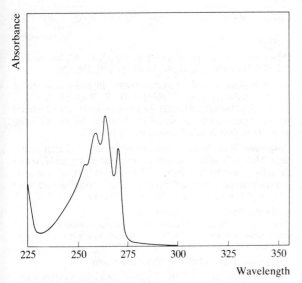

Infra-red Spectrum. Principal peaks at wavenumbers 700, 760, 1298, 1020, 892, 869 (phencyclidine hydrochloride, KBr disk).

Mass Spectrum. Principal peaks at *m/z* 200, 91, 243, 242, 84, 186, 166, 201; 1-(1-phenylcyclohexyl)-4-hydroxypiperidine 91, 216, 77, 259, –, –, –, –; 4-phenyl-4-piperidinocyclohexanol 200, 91, 84, 86, 186, 259, –, –.

Quantification. GAS CHROMATOGRAPHY. In cerebrospinal fluid, serum or urine: detection limit 5 ng/ml, AFID—J. N. Miceli *et al.*, *J. analyt. Toxicol.*, 1981, *5*, 29–32.

GAS CHROMATOGRAPHY (CAPILLARY COLUMN). In plasma, serum, saliva, tissues or urine: sensitivity 5 pg/ml, AFID—F. N. Pitts, jun. *et al.*, *J. Chromat.*, 1980, *193*, 157–159.

GAS CHROMATOGRAPHY–MASS SPECTROMETRY. In urine: phencyclidine and two monohydroxy metabolites, sensitivity for phencyclidine 10 ng/ml—E. J. Cone *et al.*, *J. Chromat.*, 1981, *223*; *Biomed. Appl.*, *12*, 331–339.

RADIOIMMUNOASSAY. In serum: sensitivity 500 pg/ml—S. M. Owens *et al.*, *Clin. Chem.*, 1982, *28*, 1509–1513.

Disposition in the Body. Phencyclidine is a drug of abuse which is self-administered orally, intravenously, by nasal insufflation,

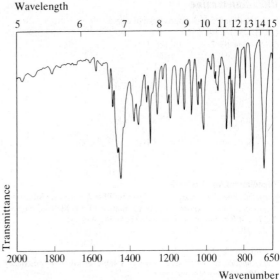

or by smoking impregnated plant material. The main metabolic reaction is hydroxylation and two metabolites have been identified in the urine as glucuronide conjugates: 4-phenyl-4-piperidinocyclohexanol and 1-(1-phenylcyclohexyl)-4-hydroxypiperidine. The product of *N*-dealkylation (1-phenylcyclohexylamine) has also been identified in urine, together with an oxidised derivative, 5-(1-phenylcyclohexylamino)valeric acid. About 73% of a dose is excreted in the urine and 5% is eliminated in the faeces in 10 days, of which about 16% of the dose is unchanged and 30% is conjugated hydroxylated metabolites; the rate of excretion of unchanged drug is increased in acidic urine.

BLOOD CONCENTRATION.

Following an oral dose of 1 mg, given to 5 subjects, a mean peak plasma concentration of 0.0027 µg/ml was reported at 2.5 hours (C. E. Cook *et al.*, *Clin. Pharmac. Ther.*, 1982, *31*, 625–634).

TOXICITY. Blood concentrations in the region of 0.1 µg/ml produce abnormal behaviour and concentrations of about 0.3 µg/ml or more cause severe toxic symptoms which may be followed by death although there is considerable intersubject variation. Many deaths have been due, not to the toxic effects of phencyclidine itself, but to the effects of irrational behaviour caused by the drug. In 53 cases of death reported in the literature as not directly due to phencyclidine, blood concentrations ranged from 0.01 to 2.1 µg/ml (mean 0.36); in 22 of these cases urine concentrations ranged from 0.1 to 10.6 µg/ml (mean 2.1); alcohol was also present in a number of these cases.

In 50 non-fatal cases of phencyclidine intoxication, blood concentrations were reported as 0.01 to 0.18 µg/ml (mean 0.07) (D. O. Clardy *et al.*, *J. analyt. Toxicol.*, 1979, *3*, 238–241).

In 9 fatalities directly attributable to phencyclidine overdose, the following postmortem concentrations were reported: blood 0.3 to 12 µg/ml (mean 2.4, 8 cases), brain 0.1 to 32 µg/g (mean 7.3, 6 cases), liver 0.9 to 80 µg/g (mean 20, 9 cases), urine 0.4 to 48.6 µg/ml (mean 21.7, 5 cases) (R. H. Cravey *et al.*, *J. analyt. Toxicol.*, 1979, *3*, 199–201).

HALF-LIFE. Plasma half-life, 7 to 46 hours (mean 17), increased up to 4 days in severe poisoning cases.

VOLUME OF DISTRIBUTION. About 6 litres/kg.

DISTRIBUTION IN BLOOD. Plasma: whole blood ratio, about 1.0.

PROTEIN BINDING. In plasma, about 65 to 80%.

Phendimetrazine

Anorectic

(+)-3,4-Dimethyl-2-phenylmorpholine
$C_{12}H_{17}NO = 191.3$
CAS—634-03-7

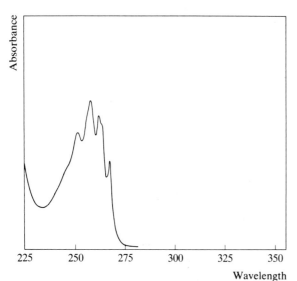

Phendimetrazine Tartrate

Synonyms. Phendimetrazine Acid Tartrate; Phendimetrazine Bitartrate.
Proprietary Names. Anorex; Bacarate; Bontril PDM; Melfiat; Plegine; Prelu-2; SPRX; Statobex; Trimstat; Trimtabs; Wehless.
$C_{12}H_{17}NO,C_4H_6O_6 = 341.4$
CAS—50-58-8
A white powder.
Freely **soluble** in water; very slightly soluble in ethanol; practically insoluble in chloroform and ether.

Dissociation Constant. pK_a 7.6.

Colour Test. Liebermann's Test—red-orange.

Thin-layer Chromatography. *System TA*—Rf 57; *system TB*—Rf 36; *system TC*—Rf 51. (*Dragendorff spray*, positive; *acidified iodoplatinate solution*, positive; *acidified potassium permanganate solution*, positive.)

Gas Chromatography. *System GA*—phendimetrazine RI 1444, phenmetrazine RI 1431; *system GB*—phendimetrazine RI 1513, phenmetrazine RI 1473; *system GC*—phendimetrazine RI 1735, phenmetrazine RI 1873.

High Pressure Liquid Chromatography. *System HA*—phendimetrazine k′ 0.9, phenmetrazine k′ 1.7; *system HC*—k′ 0.32.

Ultraviolet Spectrum. Aqueous acid—251 nm, 257 nm ($A_1^1 = 12.7$ a), 261 nm, 267 nm. No alkaline shift.

Infra-red Spectrum. Principal peaks at wavenumbers 1120, 1105, 697, 1083, 752, 1630 (K Br disk).

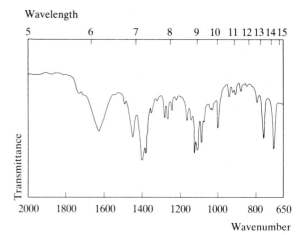

Mass Spectrum. Principal peaks at *m/z* 57, 85, 42, 56, 76, 191, 70, 77; phenmetrazine 71, 42, 56, 43, 177, 77, 178, 105.

Quantification. GAS CHROMATOGRAPHY. In plasma, serum or urine: sensitivity 2 ng/ml, AFID—G. R. Rudolph *et al., J. pharm. Sci.*, 1983, *72*, 519–521. In serum or urine: phendimetrazine and phenmetrazine, sensitivity 10 ng/ml, AFID—G. Long *et al., Drug Dev. & ind. Pharm.*, 1982, *8*, 203–213.

Disposition in the Body. Readily absorbed after oral administration. Metabolised by *N*-demethylation to phenmetrazine, which is active, and by *N*-oxidation. About 5 to 30% of a dose is excreted in the urine unchanged in 24 hours together with up to 30% as phenmetrazine and 20% as the *N*-oxide.

THERAPEUTIC CONCENTRATION.

Following a single oral dose of 35 mg to 20 subjects, a mean peak plasma concentration of about 0.07 μg/ml was attained in about 1 hour (G. R. Rudolph *et al., J. pharm. Sci.*, 1983, *72*, 519–521).

HALF-LIFE. Plasma half-life, about 2 to 3 hours.

Dose. Usually 70 to 105 mg of phendimetrazine tartrate daily; maximum of 210 mg daily.

Phenelzine

Antidepressant (Monoamine Oxidase Inhibitor)

Phenethylhydrazine
$C_8H_{12}N_2 = 136.2$
CAS—51-71-8

$$C_6H_5 \cdot [CH_2]_2 \cdot NH \cdot NH_2$$

Practically **insoluble** in water; soluble in chloroform and ether.

Phenelzine Sulphate

Proprietary Names. Nardelzine; Nardil.
$C_8H_{12}N_2,H_2SO_4 = 234.3$
CAS—156-51-4
A white or yellowish-white powder or pearly platelets. M.p. 164° to 168°.
Soluble 1 in 7 of water; practically insoluble in ethanol, chloroform, and ether.

Colour Tests. Benedict's Reagent—orange; Liebermann's Test—orange; Mandelin's Test—brown; Nessler's Reagent—black; Palladium Chloride—black.

Absorbance

225   250   275   300   325   350

Wavelength

Thin-layer Chromatography. *System TA*—Rf 77; *system TB*—Rf 37; *system TC*—Rf 12. (*Dragendorff spray*, positive; *acidified iodoplatinate solution*, positive; *Marquis reagent*, brown; *ninhydrin spray*, positive.)

Gas Chromatography. *System GA*—RI 1335; *system GC*—RI 1460.

High Pressure Liquid Chromatography. *System HA*—k' 1.0; *system HB*—k' 5.91; *system HC*—k' 0.37.

Ultraviolet Spectrum. Aqueous acid—247 nm, 252 nm, 257 nm ($A_1^1 = 12.9$ a), 263 nm.

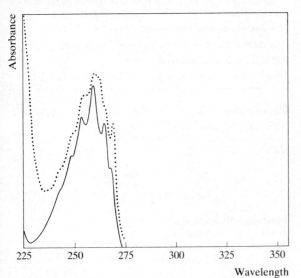

Infra-red Spectrum. Principal peaks at wavenumbers 1016, 1108, 1050, 1080, 940, 699 (phenelzine sulphate, KBr disk).

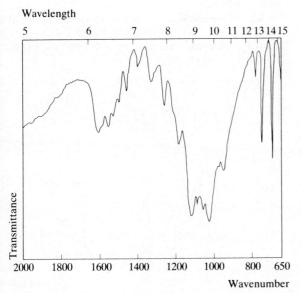

Mass Spectrum. Principal peaks at *m/z* 31, 45, 46, 29, 27, 59, 74, 43.

Quantification. GAS CHROMATOGRAPHY. In plasma: detection limit 2 ng/ml, AFID—I. J. McGilveray *et al.*, *J. Pharm. Pharmac.*, 1982, *34*, Suppl., 98P. In urine: detection limit 50 ng/ml, FID—B. Caddy and A. H. Stead, *Analyst, Lond.*, 1977, *102*, 42–49.

GAS CHROMATOGRAPHY–MASS SPECTROMETRY. In plasma: sensitivity 1 to 2 ng/ml—S. P. Jindal *et al.*, *J. Chromat.*, 1980, *221*; *Biomed. Appl.*, *10*, 301–308.

Disposition in the Body. Readily absorbed after oral administration and widely distributed throughout the body. It is believed to be metabolised by acetylation, followed by glutamine conjugation, producing phenylacetylglutamine. Aromatic hydroxylation and conjugation with glucuronic acid may also occur. Less than 5% of a dose is excreted in the urine unchanged.

THERAPEUTIC CONCENTRATION.

Following a single oral dose of 50 mg, given as a solution to 1 subject, a peak plasma concentration of 0.05 μg/ml was reported at 0.25 hour (I. J. McGilveray *et al.*, *J. Pharm. Pharmac.*, 1982, *34*, Suppl., 98P).

Following a single oral dose of 30 mg to 1 subject, a peak plasma concentration of 0.002 μg/ml was attained in 2 hours. In a subject who had been receiving daily oral doses of 30 mg for 6 weeks, a trough steady-state plasma concentration of 0.0002 μg/ml was reported (T. B. Cooper *et al.*, *Commun. Psychopharmacol.*, 1978, *2*, 505–512).

TOXICITY.

In a fatality attributed to phenelzine and alcohol, postmortem urine concentrations were: phenelzine 58 μg/ml, alcohol 1700 μg/ml; in a second non-fatal overdose subject, blood and plasma concentrations of 1.5 and 1.26 μg/ml were reported, 12 hours after ingestion (B. Caddy and A. H. Stead, *J. forens. Sci. Soc.*, 1978, *18*, 207–208).

HALF-LIFE. Plasma half-life, about 7 hours.

Dose. The equivalent of 45 to 60 mg of phenelzine daily.

Phenethicillin
Antibiotic

Synonyms. Penicillin B; α-Phenoxyethylpenicillin.
(6R)-6-(2-Phenoxypropionamido)penicillanic acid
$C_{17}H_{20}N_2O_5S = 364.4$
CAS—147-55-7

Phenethicillin Potassium

Proprietary Names. Altocillin; Broxil; Optipen; Penorale; Pensig; Syncillin.
$C_{17}H_{19}KN_2O_5S = 402.5$
CAS—132-93-4
A white, fine, crystalline powder.
Soluble 1 in 1.5 of water, 1 in 85 of ethanol, and 1 in 800 of dehydrated alcohol; slightly soluble in chloroform; practically insoluble in ether.

Dissociation Constant. pK_a 2.7 (25°).

Ultraviolet Spectrum. Phenethicillin potassium: aqueous acid—271 nm ($A_1^1 = 44$ b), 275 nm. No alkaline shift.

Infra-red Spectrum. Principal peaks at wavenumbers 1610, 1778, 1510, 1238, 1690, 752 (phenethicillin potassium, KBr disk).

Dose. The equivalent of 1 to 2 g of phenethicillin daily.

Phenethylamine

Putrefactive Base

Synonym. β-Aminoethylbenzene
2-Phenylethylamine
$C_8H_{11}N = 121.2$
CAS—64-04-0

$$C_6H_5 \cdot [CH_2]_2 \cdot NH_2$$

A strongly basic liquid which absorbs carbon dioxide from the air. B.p. 194° to 195°.
Soluble in water; freely soluble in ethanol and ether.

Colour Test. Marquis Test—orange.

Thin-layer Chromatography. *System TA*—Rf 49; *system TB*—Rf 28; *system TC*—Rf 28. (*Acidified iodoplatinate solution*, positive.)

Gas Chromatography. *System GA*—RI 1111.

High Pressure Liquid Chromatography. *System HA*—k' 1.2; *system HB*—k' 3.64; *system HC*—k' 1.31.

Ultraviolet Spectrum. Aqueous acid—242 nm ($A_1^1 = 15$ b), 247 nm ($A_1^1 = 17.2$ b), 252 nm ($A_1^1 = 19.8$ b), 257 nm ($A_1^1 = 21.3$ b), 263 nm ($A_1^1 = 16$ b).

Infra-red Spectrum. Principal peaks at wavenumbers 695, 745, 755, 942, 1146, 1608 (KBr disk).

Mass Spectrum. Principal peaks at m/z 30, 91, 65, 92, 51, 39, 121, 103.

Disposition in the Body. Phenethylamine is the putrefactive base obtained from phenylalanine by decarboxylation.

Pheneturide

Anticonvulsant

Synonym. Ethylphenacemide
Proprietary Name. Benuride
(2-Phenylbutyryl)urea
$C_{11}H_{14}N_2O_2 = 206.2$
CAS—90-49-3

$$\overset{\displaystyle C_6H_5}{\underset{\displaystyle}{|}}$$
$$CH_3 \cdot CH_2 \cdot CH \cdot CO \cdot NH \cdot CO \cdot NH_2$$

A white crystalline powder.
Practically **insoluble** in water and ether; slightly soluble in ethanol; very soluble in glacial acetic acid.

Colour Test. Nessler's Reagent—orange-brown (slow).

Thin-layer Chromatography. *System TA*—Rf 76; *system TD*—Rf 38; *system TE*—Rf 71; *system TF*—Rf 53.

Gas Chromatography. *System GA*—RI 1465.

High Pressure Liquid Chromatography. *System HE*—k' 6.84.

Ultraviolet Spectrum. Chloroform—259 nm ($A_1^1 = 18$ b), 265 nm ($A_1^1 = 11$ b).

Infra-red Spectrum. Principal peaks at wavenumbers 1672, 1700, 1093, 694, 1176, 1615 (KBr disk).

Mass Spectrum. Principal peaks at m/z 91, 146, 44, 119, 206, 41, 78, 77.

Quantification. HIGH PRESSURE LIQUID CHROMATOGRAPHY. In plasma or serum: pheneturide and other anticonvulsants, sensitivity 1.4 µg/ml, UV detection—J. A. Christofides and D. E. Fry, *Clin. Chem.*, 1980, *26*, 499–501.

THIN-LAYER CHROMATOGRAPHY–ULTRAVIOLET SPECTROPHOTO-METRY. In plasma, serum or urine: sensitivity 500 ng/ml in serum—R. L. Galeazzi *et al.*, *J. Pharmacokinet. Biopharm.*, 1979, *7*, 453–462.

Disposition in the Body. Slowly absorbed after oral administration. Pheneturide is thought to be completely metabolised as only traces of unchanged drug have been found in the urine. It may induce its own metabolism.

TOXICITY. Pheneturide has been reported to be less likely to cause toxic effects than phenacemide, to which it is chemically related.

HALF-LIFE. Plasma half-life, 30 to 90 hours (mean 54) after single doses and about 40 hours after chronic administration.

VOLUME OF DISTRIBUTION. About 3 litres/kg.

CLEARANCE. Plasma clearance, about 0.7 ml/min/kg.

REFERENCE. R. L. Galeazzi *et al.*, *ibid.*

Dose. Pheneturide has been given in doses of 0.6 to 1 g daily.

Phenformin

Antidiabetic

1-Phenethylbiguanide
$C_{10}H_{15}N_5 = 205.3$
CAS—114-86-3

$$C_6H_5 \cdot [CH_2]_2 \cdot NH \cdot \overset{\displaystyle NH}{\overset{\displaystyle \|}{C}} \cdot NH \cdot \overset{\displaystyle NH}{\overset{\displaystyle \|}{C}} \cdot NH_2$$

Phenformin Hydrochloride

Proprietary Names. Dibotin; Insoral.
Note. Insoral is also used as a proprietary name for carbutamide.
$C_{10}H_{15}N_5, HCl = 241.7$
CAS—834-28-6
A white crystalline powder. M.p. 176° to 179°.
Soluble 1 in 8 of water and 1 in 15 of ethanol; practically insoluble in chloroform and ether.

Dissociation Constant. pK$_a$ 2.7, 11.8 (32°).

Colour Tests. Mandelin's Test—green; Marquis Test—orange → brown.

Thin-layer Chromatography. *System TA*—Rf 03; *system TB*—Rf 00; *system TC*—Rf 00. (*Marquis reagent*, positive.)

Ultraviolet Spectrum. Aqueous acid—251 nm ($A_1^1 = 11$ a), 258 nm ($A_1^1 = 11$ a), 264 nm, 267 nm.

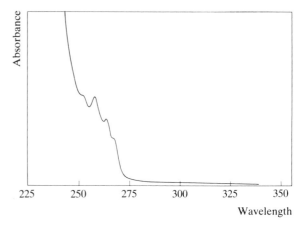

Infra-red Spectrum. Principal peaks at wavenumbers 1568, 1537, 1590, 1625, 1650, 1500 (phenformin hydrochloride, KBr disk).

Wavelength

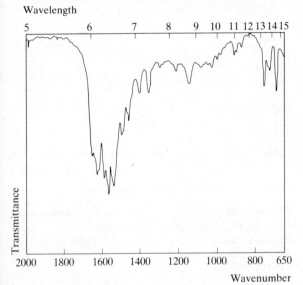

Mass Spectrum. Principal peaks at m/z 91, 30, 92, 42, 29, 146, 44, 104 (no peaks above 150).

Quantification. GAS CHROMATOGRAPHY. In plasma or urine: phenformin and other biguanides, detection limit <1 ng/ml in plasma, ECD—S. B. Matin *et al.*, *Analyt. Chem.*, 1975, *47*, 545–548.

HIGH PRESSURE LIQUID CHROMATOGRAPHY. In plasma or urine: sensitivity 10 ng/ml in plasma, UV detection—H. M. Hill and J. Chamberlain, *J. Chromat.*, 1978, *149*, 349–358. In urine: phenformin and 4-hydroxyphenformin, sensitivity 1 μg/ml for phenformin and 500 ng/ml for 4-hydroxyphenformin, UV detection—N. S. Oates *et al.*, *J. Pharm. Pharmac.*, 1980, *32*, 731–732.

Disposition in the Body. Well absorbed after oral administration. The major metabolic reaction is aromatic hydroxylation to form 4-hydroxyphenformin which is then conjugated with glucuronic acid. Up to about 50% of a dose is excreted in the urine in 24 hours, about two-thirds in the form of unchanged drug and one-third as the hydroxy metabolite.

THERAPEUTIC CONCENTRATION.
Following a single oral dose of 50 mg to 8 subjects, peak plasma concentrations of 0.08 to 0.18 μg/ml (mean 0.13) were attained in about 3 hours; plasma concentrations were higher in 4 subjects who were poor metabolisers of debrisoquine in comparison with the 4 extensive metabolisers (N. S. Oates *et al.*, *Clin. Pharmac. Ther.*, 1983, *34*, 827–834).
Following daily oral doses of 50 mg three times a day to 8 subjects, plasma concentrations of 0.10 to 0.24 μg/ml (mean 0.18) were reported 2 hours after a dose (J. Karam *et al.*, *Diabetes*, 1974, *23*, *Suppl.* 1, 375).

TOXICITY.
A 44-year-old woman ingested 1.5 g in slow-release capsules and died 30 hours later. A postmortem blood concentration of 3 μg/ml and liver concentration of 60 μg/g were reported (J. P. Bingle *et al.*, *Br. med. J.*, 1970, *3*, 752).

HALF-LIFE. Plasma half-life, 10 to 15 hours.

PROTEIN BINDING. In plasma, about 12% to 20%.

Dose. 50 to 100 mg of phenformin hydrochloride daily.

Phenglutarimide

Anticholinergic

2-(2-Diethylaminoethyl)-2-phenylglutarimide
$C_{17}H_{24}N_2O_2 = 288.4$
CAS—1156-05-4

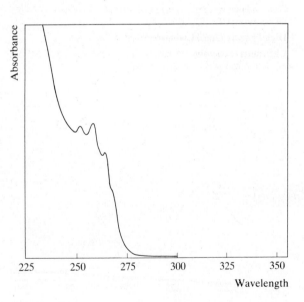

Crystals. M.p. 125° to 127°.

Phenglutarimide Hydrochloride
$C_{17}H_{24}N_2O_2,HCl = 324.8$
CAS—1674-96-0
A white crystalline powder. M.p. about 177°, with decomposition.
Soluble 1 in 1 of water and 1 in 1.5 of ethanol; very slightly soluble in ether.

Colour Tests. Koppanyi–Zwikker Test—violet; Liebermann's Test—red-orange.

Thin-layer Chromatography. *System TA*—Rf 40; *system TB*—Rf 17; *system TC*—Rf 08. (*Acidified iodoplatinate solution*, positive.)

Gas Chromatography. *System GA*—RI 2321.

High Pressure Liquid Chromatography. *System HA*—k' 2.9.

Ultraviolet Spectrum. Aqueous acid—251 nm, 257 nm ($A_1^1 = 13.3$ a), 263 nm.

Infra-red Spectrum. Principal peaks at wavenumbers 1698, 1194, 1181, 1250, 700, 1150 (phenglutarimide hydrochloride, KBr disk).

Mass Spectrum. Principal peaks at m/z 86, 30, 216, 87, 58, 100, 99, 56.

Dose. Phenglutarimide hydrochloride has been given in doses of 10 to 50 mg daily.

Phenindamine

Antihistamine

2,3,4,9 - Tetrahydro - 2 - methyl - 9 - phenyl - 1*H* - indeno[2,1-*c*]-pyridine
$C_{19}H_{19}N = 261.4$
CAS—82-88-2

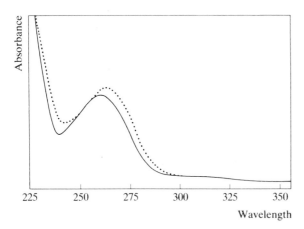

Crystals. M.p. 91°.

Phenindamine Tartrate

Proprietary Names. Nolahist; Thephorin.
$C_{19}H_{19}N,C_4H_6O_6 = 411.5$
CAS—569-59-5
A white voluminous powder. M.p. 160° to 162°; on further heating it solidifies and melts again at about 168°, with decomposition.
Soluble 1 in 70 of water and 1 in 300 of ethanol; practically insoluble in chloroform and ether.

Dissociation Constant. pK_a 8.3 (25°).

Colour Tests. Mandelin's Test—green; Marquis Test—grey-green.

Thin-layer Chromatography. *System TA*—Rf 63; *system TB*—Rf 45; *system TC*—Rf 57. (*Dragendorff spray*, positive; *acidified iodoplatinate solution*, positive; *Marquis reagent*, grey-brown.)

Gas Chromatography. *System GA*—RI 2167; *system GC*—RI 2926; *system GF*—RI 2515.

High Pressure Liquid Chromatography. *System HA*—k' 2.5.

Ultraviolet Spectrum. Aqueous acid—259 nm ($A_1^1 = 347$ a); aqueous alkali—263 nm ($A_1^1 = 385$ a).

Infra-red Spectrum. Principal peaks at wavenumbers 1751, 1302, 1585, 752, 1072, 693 (phenindamine tartrate, KBr disk).

Mass Spectrum. Principal peaks at *m/z* 260, 261, 42, 57, 184, 215, 217, 262.

Dose. Up to 150 mg of phenindamine tartrate daily.

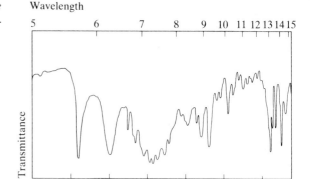

Wavelength

Wavenumber

Phenindione

Anticoagulant

Synonyms. Phenylindanedione; Phenylinium.
Proprietary Names. Danilone; Dindevan; Hedulin; Pindione.
2-Phenylindan-1,3-dione
$C_{15}H_{10}O_2 = 222.2$
CAS—83-12-5

Soft, white or creamy-white or pale yellow crystals or crystalline powder. M.p. 148° to 151°.
Very slightly **soluble** in water; soluble 1 in about 125 of ethanol, 1 in 6.5 of chloroform, and 1 in 110 of ether, forming yellow to red solutions.

Dissociation Constant. pK_a 4.1.

Colour Tests. Methanolic Potassium Hydroxide—red; Sulphuric Acid—violet.

Thin-layer Chromatography. *System TD*—Rf 65; *system TE*—Rf 21; *system TF*—Rf 56.

Gas Chromatography. *System GA*—RI 2055.

Ultraviolet Spectrum. Aqueous alkali—278 nm ($A_1^1 = 1310$ a), 330 nm ($A_1^1 = 400$ b).

Infra-red Spectrum. Principal peaks at wavenumbers 1700, 700, 766, 1219, 1740, 1280 (KBr disk).

Mass Spectrum. Principal peaks at *m/z* 222, 165, 76, 223, 166, 105, 104, 90.

Quantification. POLAROGRAPHY. In serum: sensitivity 4 µg/ml— E. Jacobsen and K. H. Klevan, *Analytica chim. Acta*, 1972, *62*, 405–413.

Disposition in the Body. Well absorbed after oral administration. The urine may be coloured red-orange due to the excretion of a metabolite.

TOXICITY. Fatalities have occurred after therapeutic doses.

HALF-LIFE. Plasma half-life, about 6 hours.

Dose. Maintenance, 25 to 150 mg daily.

Wavelength

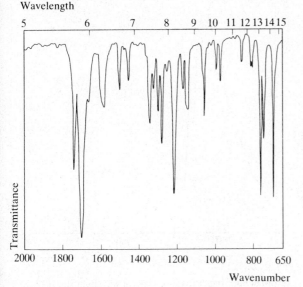

Thin-layer Chromatography. *System TA*—Rf 45; *system TB*—Rf 35; *system TC*—Rf 13. (*Dragendorff spray*, positive; *acidified iodoplatinate solution*, positive.)

Gas Chromatography. *System GA*—RI 1804; *system GB*—RI 1826; *system GF*—RI 2100.

High Pressure Liquid Chromatography. *System HA*—k' 4.1.

Ultraviolet Spectrum. Aqueous acid—261 nm ($A_1^1 = 305$ a), 266 nm ($A_1^1 = 310$ a); aqueous alkali—258 nm, 263 nm ($A_1^1 = 206$ a), 268 nm.

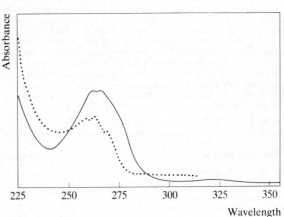

Pheniramine   *Antihistamine*

Synonym. Prophenpyridamine
Proprietary Name. Inhiston
NN-Dimethyl-3-phenyl-3-(2-pyridyl)propylamine
$C_{16}H_{20}N_2 = 240.3$
CAS—86-21-5

A slightly yellow oily liquid.
Practically **insoluble** in water; soluble in ethanol, chloroform, and ether.

Pheniramine Aminosalicylate
Proprietary Names. Avil (tablets); Aviletten; Avilettes; Fenamine (tablets).
$C_{16}H_{20}N_2,C_7H_7NO_3 = 393.5$
CAS—3269-83-8
Crystals. M.p. 142°, with decomposition.
Soluble 1 in 10 of water; freely soluble in ethanol; sparingly soluble in ether.

Pheniramine Maleate
Proprietary Names. Avil (syrup and sustained-release tablets); Daneral-SA; Fenamine (syrup and sustained-release tablets). It is an ingredient of Robitussin AC, Syrtussar, Triominic, and Triotussic.
$C_{16}H_{20}N_2,C_4H_4O_4 = 356.4$
CAS—132-20-7
A white crystalline powder. M.p. 106° to 109°.
Soluble 1 in 0.3 of water, 1 in 2.5 of ethanol, and 1 in 1.5 of chloroform; very slightly soluble in ether.

Dissociation Constant. pK_a 4.2, 9.3 (25°).

Colour Tests. Cyanogen Bromide—orange; Liebermann's Test—red-orange.

Infra-red Spectrum. Principal peaks at wavenumbers 1584, 690, 860, 870, 990, 1010 (pheniramine maleate, KBr disk).

Wavelength

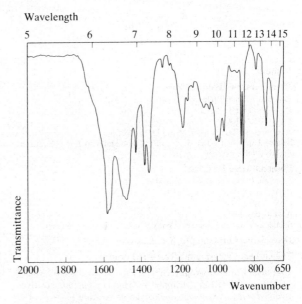

Mass Spectrum. Principal peaks at m/z 169, 58, 168, 170, 72, 167, 44, 42 (no peaks above 200).

Quantification. GAS CHROMATOGRAPHY. In blood, urine or tissues: sensitivity 50 ng/ml, AFID—E. A. Querée *et al.*, *J. analyt. Toxicol.*, 1979, *3*, 253–255.

Disposition in the Body. Absorbed after oral administration. About 17% of a dose is excreted in the urine as unchanged drug in 24 hours, increasing to 23% over a period of 6 days; after chronic oral administration about 24% is excreted daily as monodesmethylpheniramine, and 0.5% as didesmethylpheniramine.

THERAPEUTIC CONCENTRATION.

After a single oral dose of 75 mg to 6 subjects, blood concentrations of 0.01 to 0.19 μg/ml (mean 0.11) were reported at 2 hours (E. A. Querée *et al.*, *ibid.*).

TOXICITY. The estimated minimum lethal dose is 25 mg/kg.

In a fatality due to pheniramine overdose, the following postmortem tissue concentrations were reported: blood 1.9 μg/ml, brain 5.3 μg/g, kidney 4.0 μg/g, liver 6.6 μg/g, urine 149 μg/ml; in a second fatality in which methadone, pentobarbitone, phenobarbitone, and alcohol had also been ingested, postmortem blood and liver concentrations of 30 μg/ml and 115 μg/g, respectively, were reported (E. A. Querée *et al.*, *ibid.*).

In a fatality due to the ingestion of 3.75 g of pheniramine, the following postmortem tissue concentrations were reported: blood 10.7 μg/ml, bile 109 μg/ml, liver 33 μg/g, urine 362 μg/ml (L. F. T. Chan and W. J. Allender, *Bull. int. Ass. forens. Toxicol.*, 1983, *17*(2), 25–26).

Dose. Up to 150 mg of pheniramine maleate daily.

Phenmetrazine
Anorectic

Synonym. Oxazimédrine

(±)-*trans*-3-Methyl-2-phenylmorpholine

$C_{11}H_{15}NO = 177.2$

CAS—134-49-6

A liquid

Phenmetrazine Hydrochloride

Proprietary Name. Preludin

$C_{11}H_{15}NO,HCl = 213.7$

CAS—1707-14-8

A white crystalline powder. M.p. 172° to 182°.

Soluble 1 in 0.4 of water, 1 in 2 of ethanol, and 1 in 2 of chloroform; slightly soluble in ether.

Phenmetrazine Theoclate

Synonym. Phenmetrazine 8-Chlorotheophyllinate

$C_{11}H_{15}NO,C_7H_7ClN_4O_2 = 391.9$

CAS—13931-75-4

A white powder.

Soluble in water and ethanol; slightly soluble in acetone and ether.

Dissociation Constant. pK_a 8.4 (25°).

Colour Test. Liebermann's Test—red-orange.

Thin-layer Chromatography. *System TA*—Rf 50; *system TB*—Rf 14; *system TC*—Rf 21. (*Acidified iodoplatinate solution*, positive; *acidified potassium permanganate solution*, positive.)

Gas Chromatography. *System GA*—RI 1431; *system GB*—RI 1473; *system GC*—RI 1873.

High Pressure Liquid Chromatography. *System HA*—k′ 1.7.

Ultraviolet Spectrum. Aqueous acid—250 nm, 256 nm ($A_1^1 = 13.3$ a), 261 nm, 263 nm, 267 nm.

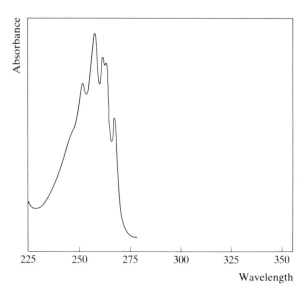

Infra-red Spectrum. Principal peaks at wavenumbers 1083, 757, 695, 965, 990, 1030 (phenmetrazine hydrochloride, KBr disk).

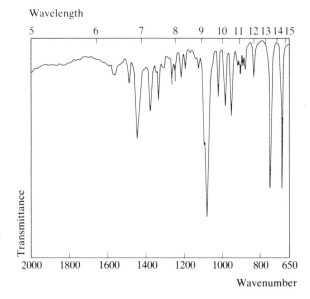

Mass Spectrum. Principal peaks at *m/z* 71, 42, 56, 43, 177, 77, 178, 105.

Quantification. GAS CHROMATOGRAPHY. In serum or urine: phendimetrazine and phenmetrazine, sensitivity 10 ng/ml, AFID—G. Long *et al.*, *Drug Dev. & ind. Pharm.*, 1982, *8*, 203–213.

Disposition in the Body. Readily absorbed after oral administration. About 70% of a dose is excreted in the urine in 24 hours with about 19% as unchanged drug, 19% as the lactam (5-methyl-3-oxo-6-phenylmorpholine), 12% as free 4-hydroxyphenmetrazine, 10% as conjugated 4-hydroxyphenmetrazine, and about 5% as the N-oxide.

Phenmetrazine is a metabolite of phendimetrazine.

THERAPEUTIC CONCENTRATION.
After a single oral dose of 75 mg given to 5 subjects, peak plasma concentrations of 0.10 to 0.24 μg/ml (mean 0.16) were attained in about 2 hours. Following a single oral dose of 75 mg of a slow-release preparation, average peak plasma concentrations of about 0.07 μg/ml were reported at 5 hours; concentrations remained almost constant over the period 5 to 24 hours (G. P. Quinn et al., Clin. Pharmac. Ther., 1967, 8, 369–373).

TOXICITY. Estimated minimum lethal dose for children up to 2 years of age, 200 mg. Large doses and prolonged treatment may lead to severe mental depression and dependence of the amphetamine type.

In a fatality following intravenous overdosage, the following postmortem distribution was reported: blood 4 μg/ml, bile 7 μg/ml, liver 5 μg/g, urine 24 μg/ml (G. Norheim, J. forens. Sci. Soc., 1973, 13, 287–289).

The following postmortem tissue concentrations were reported in 12 fatalities: blood 0.1 to 4.9 μg/ml (mean 1.1), bile 0.2 to 23 μg/ml (mean 5.5), brain 0.1 to 15 μg/g (mean 2.9), kidney 0.1 to 8 μg/g (mean 1.5), liver 0.1 to 20 μg/g (mean 3.1), urine 0.1 to 90 μg/ml (mean 21) (L. Gottschalk, per R. C. Baselt, Disposition of Toxic Drugs and Chemicals in Man, 2nd Edn, Davis, California, Biomedical Publications, 1982, pp. 625–627).

HALF-LIFE. Plasma half-life, about 8 hours.

Dose. 25 to 75 mg of phenmetrazine hydrochloride daily.

Phenobarbitone   *Barbiturate*

Synonyms. Fenobarbital; Phenemalum; Phenobarbital; Phenylethylbarbituric Acid; Phenylethylmalonylurea.

Proprietary Names. Gardenal; Luminal; Luminaletten; Nova-Pheno; Phenaemal; Sedadrops; Seda-Tablinen; Solfoton. It is an ingredient of Antrocol, Franol, Franyl, Phyldrox, Seominal, and Valpin 50-PB.

5-Ethyl-5-phenylbarbituric acid
$C_{12}H_{12}N_2O_3 = 232.2$
CAS—50-06-0

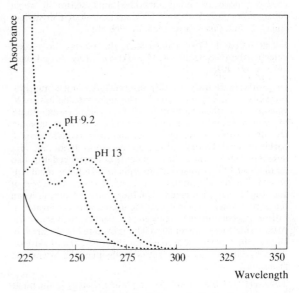

Colourless crystals or a white crystalline powder which may exhibit polymorphism. M.p. 174° to 178°.

Soluble 1 in 1000 of water, 1 in 10 of ethanol, 1 in 40 of chloroform, and 1 in 40 of ether.

Phenobarbitone Sodium

Synonyms. Phenemalnatrium; Phenobarbital Sodium; Sodium Phenylethylbarbiturate; Soluble Phenobarbitone.

Proprietary Names. Luminal Sodium. It is an ingredient of Garoin.

$C_{12}H_{11}N_2NaO_3 = 254.2$
CAS—57-30-7

A white hygroscopic powder, granules, or flakes. M.p. about 175°.

Soluble 1 in 3 of water and 1 in 25 of ethanol; practically insoluble in chloroform and ether.

Dissociation Constant. pK_a 7.4 (25°).

Partition Coefficient. Log P (octanol), 1.4.

Colour Tests. Koppanyi–Zwikker Test—violet; Liebermann's Test—red-orange; Mercurous Nitrate—black.

Thin-layer Chromatography. *System TD*—Rf 47; *system TE*—Rf 28; *system TF*—Rf 65; *system TH*—Rf 38. (*Mercuric chloride-diphenylcarbazone reagent,* positive; *mercurous nitrate spray,* black; *Zwikker's reagent,* pink.)

Gas Chromatography. *System GA*—phenobarbitone RI 1957, 4-hydroxyphenobarbitone RI 2415; *system GE*—retention time 0.74 relative to phenytoin; *system GF*—RI 2960.

High Pressure Liquid Chromatography. *System HE*—k' 2.76; *system HG*—k' 3.09; *system HH*—k' 1.23.

Ultraviolet Spectrum. *Borax buffer 0.05M* (pH 9.2)—239 nm (A_1^1 = 452 a); M sodium hydroxide (pH 13)—254 nm (A_1^1 = 342 b).

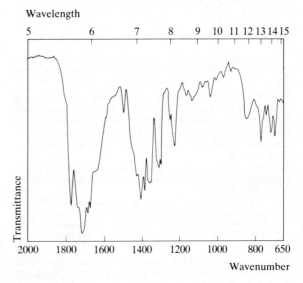

Infra-red Spectrum. Principal peaks at wavenumbers 1712, 1684, 1670, 1770, 1310, 1300 (KBr disk).

Mass Spectrum. Principal peaks at *m/z* 204, 117, 146, 161, 77, 103, 115, 118; 4-hydroxyphenobarbitone 219, 248, 148, 220, 120, 218, 133, 64.

Quantification. See also under Amylobarbitone.

GAS CHROMATOGRAPHY. In serum: sensitivity 500 ng/ml, FID—A. Di Corcia *et al.*, *J. Chromat.*, 1982, *229*; *Biomed. Appl.*, *18*, 365–372.

GAS CHROMATOGRAPHY-MASS SPECTROMETRY. In plasma or urine: phenobarbitone and 4-hydroxyphenobarbitone, detection limit 100 ng/ml—I. H. Patel *et al.*, *J. pharm. Sci.*, 1980, *69*, 1218–1219.

HIGH PRESSURE LIQUID CHROMATOGRAPHY. In plasma or serum: phenobarbitone and other anticonvulsants, sensitivity about 600 ng/ml for phenobarbitone, UV detection—J. A. Christofides and D. E. Fry, *Clin. Chem.*, 1980, *26*, 499–501.

POLARISATION FLUOROIMMUNOASSAY. In plasma or serum: detection limit 800 ng/ml—A. M. Sidki *et al.*, *Ther. Drug Monit.*, 1982, *4*, 397–403.

Disposition in the Body. Readily absorbed after oral administration; bioavailability almost 100%. The major metabolites are *N*-glucopyranosylphenobarbitone and 4-hydroxyphenobarbitone, together with its glucuronide conjugate. Other metabolites include two dihydrodiol compounds and hydroxymethylphenylbarbituric acid. During chronic dosing, up to about 25% of a dose is excreted in the urine in 24 hours as unchanged drug and up to about 17% as total 4-hydroxyphenobarbitone, about half of which is the glucuronide conjugate. Urinary excretion of unchanged drug is increased when the urine is alkaline or when the urinary volume is increased; the excretion of conjugated 4-hydroxyphenobarbitone is reduced in patients with liver disease. After a single dose, about 80 to 90% is excreted in the urine in 16 days; the *N*-glucoside accounts for about 30% of a single dose. Phenobarbitone is a metabolite of methylphenobarbitone and primidone.

THERAPEUTIC CONCENTRATION. In plasma, usually in the range 2 to 30 µg/ml. However, there is considerable intersubject variation and there does not appear to be any correlation between plasma concentration and clinical effect. Concentrations in cerebrospinal fluid reach about 50% of those in plasma.

Following a single oral dose of 100 mg to 6 subjects, peak serum concentrations of 2.1 to 3.8 µg/ml (mean 2.9) were attained in 0.5 to 4 hours (mean 1.5) (A. J. Wilensky *et al.*, *Eur. J. clin. Pharmac.*, 1982, *23*, 87–92).

Following daily oral doses of 100 mg to 10 subjects for 15 days, serum concentrations of 10.6 to 22.1 µg/ml (mean 17) were reported 12 hours after a dose (P. V. Luoma *et al.*, *Ther. Drug Monit.*, 1982, *4*, 65–68).

TOXICITY. The estimated minimum lethal dose is 1.5 g although recovery has occurred after ingestion of as much as 16 g. Toxic effects have been associated with blood concentrations of 4 to **17** to 90 µg/ml and fatalities with concentrations of 4 to **45** to 120 µg/ml. However, a degree of tolerance may develop in chronic dosing.

Blood concentrations ranged from 10 to 300 µg/ml (mean 86) in 113 fatalities attributed to phenobarbitone overdose (K. D. Parker *et al.*, *Clin. Toxicol.*, 1970, *3*, 131–145).

In 20 fatalities caused by phenobarbitone overdose, the following postmortem concentrations were reported: blood 15 to 540 µg/ml (mean 113), brain 0 to 833 µg/g (mean 135), kidney 17 to 867 µg/g (mean 152), liver 24 to 1450 µg/g (mean 236), spleen 0 to 850 µg/g (mean 137) (I. Sunshine and E. Hackett, *J. forens. Sci.*, 1957, *2*, 149–158).

HALF-LIFE. Plasma half-life, about 50 to 150 hours (mean 100) in adults, reduced to about 40 to 70 hours in children; increased in subjects with liver disease.

VOLUME OF DISTRIBUTION. About 0.5 litre/kg.

CLEARANCE. Plasma clearance, about 0.06 ml/min/kg.

DISTRIBUTION IN BLOOD. Plasma: whole blood ratio, 0.93.

SALIVA. Plasma: saliva ratio, about 3.

PROTEIN BINDING. In plasma, about 50%.

Dose. 45 to 180 mg daily.

Phenol   *Disinfectant*

Synonyms. Carbolic Acid; Fenol; Phenyl Hydrate.
Proprietary Name. It is an ingredient of Chloraseptic.
Hydroxybenzene
$C_6H_5 \cdot OH = 94.11$
CAS—108-95-2
Colourless or faintly pink, deliquescent crystals or crystalline masses, becoming pink on storage. F.p. 40° to 41°. B.p. about 181°.

Soluble 1 in about 13 of water, 6 in 1 of ethanol, 2 in 1 of chloroform, and 5 in 1 of ether.
Caution. Phenol is caustic to the skin.

Dissociation Constant. pK_a 10.0 (25°).

Partition Coefficient. Log *P* (octanol/pH 7.4), 0.6.

Colour Tests. *p*-Dimethylaminobenzaldehyde—orange/violet; Ferric Chloride—blue; Folin–Ciocalteu Reagent—blue; Liebermann's Test—green; Potassium Dichromate (Method 1)—yellow → brown (2 min).

Gas Chromatography. *System GA*—RI 981.

Ultraviolet Spectrum. Aqueous acid—270 nm $(A_1^1 = 172 \text{ b})$; aqueous alkali—287 nm $(A_1^1 = 281 \text{ a})$.

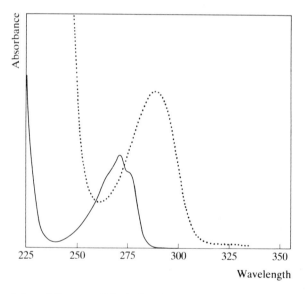

Infra-red Spectrum. Principal peaks at wavenumbers 690, 755, 1235, 1595, 1497, 811 (Nujol mull).

Mass Spectrum. Principal peaks at *m/z* 94, 66, 39, 65, 40, 55, 38, 95.

Quantification. GAS CHROMATOGRAPHY. In urine: FID—D. L. Rick *et al.*, *J. analyt. Toxicol.*, 1982, *6*, 297–300. In urine: FID—M. K. Baldwin *et al.*, *Analyst, Lond.*, 1981, *106*, 763–767.

HIGH PRESSURE LIQUID CHROMATOGRAPHY. In urine: detection limit < 500 ng/ml, UV detection—C. V. Eadsforth and P. C. Coveney, *Analyst, Lond.*, 1984, *109*, 175–176.

Wavelength

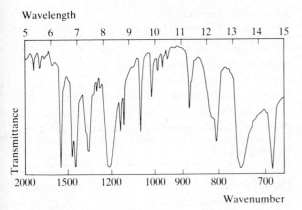

A white or yellowish-white crystalline or amorphous powder. M.p. 258° to 263°.

Practically **insoluble** in water; soluble 1 in 15 of ethanol, and 1 in 100 of ether; soluble in dilute solutions of alkali hydroxides.

Dissociation Constant. pK$_a$ 9.7 (25°).

Partition Coefficient. Log P (octanol/pH 7.4), 2.4.

Colour Test. Folin–Ciocalteu Reagent—blue.

Thin-layer Chromatography. *System TD*—Rf 38; *system TE*—Rf 51; *system TF*—Rf 59. (*Acidified potassium permanganate solution, positive.*)

Ultraviolet Spectrum. Methanol—277 nm (A$_1^1$ = 150 a).

Infra-red Spectrum. Principal peaks at wavenumbers 1740, 1178, 1230, 1265, 1278, 1510 (KBr disk).

Wavelength

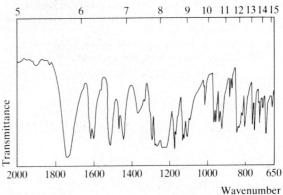

Disposition in the Body. Rapidly absorbed from the gastro-intestinal tract and readily penetrates the skin. It is metabolised by conjugation to yield phenyl glucuronide and phenyl sulphate; small amounts are oxidised to catechol and quinol which are also conjugated. Oxidation of these metabolites to quinones may tint the urine green. Acid-labile phenol conjugates are present endogenously in serum at concentrations of about 0.1 µg/ml. Phenol is a metabolite of benzene.

Endogenous phenol concentrations in urine average about 5 to 10 µg/ml.

TOXICITY. Phenol denatures and precipitates cellular proteins and thus may rapidly cause poisoning. The minimum lethal dose by mouth is about 1 g. Severe and even fatal poisoning may also arise from absorption of phenol from open wounds or through the intact skin. The maximum permissible atmospheric concentration is 5 ppm.

In a fatality due to the deliberate ingestion of a mixture containing phenol, the following postmortem tissue concentrations were reported: blood, phenol 56 µg/ml, alcohol 300 µg/ml; liver, phenol 74 µg/g. In a second fatality due to accidental percutaneous absorption, postmortem blood concentrations of 27 µg/ml of phenol and 300 µg/ml of alcohol were reported (E. R. Soares and J. P. Tift, *J. forens. Sci.*, 1982, *27*, 729–731).

In a fatality due to accidental dermal exposure to phenol, the following postmortem concentrations were reported: blood 4.7 µg/ml, unhydrolysed liver 3.3 µg/g, hydrolysed liver 7.1 µg/g (J. F. Lewin and W. T. Cleary, *Forens. Sci. Int.*, 1982, *19*, 177–179).

Mass Spectrum. Principal peaks at *m/z* 274, 225, 318, 273, 275, 226, 257, 121.

Quantification. COLORIMETRY. In serum or urine—S. M. Morris and D. W. Powell, *Analyt. Biochem.*, 1979, *95*, 465–471.

Disposition in the Body. Poorly absorbed after oral administration (up to about 15%), and partly excreted in the bile as the active glucuronide, and in the urine; if the urine is alkaline the excreted compound will impart a red colour. The greater part of the ingested material is eliminated in the faeces in both free and conjugated forms.

TOXICITY. Phenolphthalein is usually non-toxic even in relatively large doses, although fatalities have occurred in young children after ingestion of 0.6 to 1.8 g.

Dose. 50 to 300 mg.

Phenolphthalein   *Purgative*

Synonym. Dihydroxyphthalophenone

Proprietary Names. Darmol; Euchessina; Evac-U-Gen; Ex-Lax (pills); Prulet; Purganol. It is an ingredient of Agarol, Alophen, Anodyn, Kest, and Petrolagar (Red Label).

3,3-Bis(4-hydroxyphenyl)phthalide
C$_{20}$H$_{14}$O$_4$ = 318.3
CAS—77-09-8

Phenoperidine   *Narcotic Analgesic*

Ethyl 1-(3-hydroxy-3-phenylpropyl)-4-phenylpiperidine-4-carboxylate
C$_{23}$H$_{29}$NO$_3$ = 367.5
CAS—562-26-5

Phenoperidine Hydrochloride

Proprietary Name. Operidine

Note. Operidine is used as a synonym for pethidine hydrochloride in *Jap.P.*

$C_{23}H_{29}NO_3,HCl = 403.9$

CAS—2627-49-4

A white crystalline powder. M.p. 200° to 202°.

Soluble 1 in 50 of water, 1 in 10 of ethanol (90%), and 1 in 3 of chloroform; practically insoluble in ether.

Colour Test. Marquis Test—red.

Thin-layer Chromatography. *System TA*—Rf 71; *system TB*—Rf 26; *system TC*—Rf 64. (*Dragendorff spray*, positive; *acidified iodoplatinate solution*, positive; *Marquis reagent*, faint red.)

Gas Chromatography. *System GA*—phenoperidine RI 2872, norpethidine RI 1745, pethidine RI 1751.

High Pressure Liquid Chromatography. *System HA*—phenoperidine k' 0.8, norpethidine k' 1.7 (tailing peak), pethidine k' 2.8 (tailing peak); *system HC*—phenoperidine k' 0.10, norpethidine k' 2.04, pethidine k' 0.55.

Infra-red Spectrum. Principal peaks at wavenumbers 1710, 698, 1230, 1136, 1175, 1205 (phenoperidine hydrochloride, KBr disk).

Wavelength

5   6   7   8   9   10   11 12 13 14 15

Transmittance

2000 1800 1600 1400 1200 1000 800 650

Wavenumber

Mass Spectrum. Principal peaks at *m/z* 246, 42, 367, 247, 57, 56, 91, 77; norpethidine 57, 233, 42, 56, 158, 43, 160, 103; pethidine 71, 70, 44, 57, 42, 247, 43, 246.

Quantification. GAS CHROMATOGRAPHY. In plasma: sensitivity 2 ng/ml, AFID—K. Chan *et al., J. Chromat.*, 1981, *223*; *Biomed. Appl.*, *12*, 213–218.

Disposition in the Body. Absorbed from the gastro-intestinal tract but there is extensive first-pass metabolism; bioavailability about 30%. It is metabolised to pethidine and norpethidine. Up to about 5% of a dose is excreted unchanged in the urine, with about 18% as norpethidine and 2% as pethidine, in two to three days. The urinary excretion of unchanged phenoperidine is increased to about 7% when the urine is acidified.

THERAPEUTIC CONCENTRATION.

After a single intravenous dose of 2 mg administered to 5 patients during general anaesthesia, a mean plasma concentration of 0.02 μg/ml was reported at 2 minutes (L. Milne *et al., Br. J. Anaesth.*, 1980, *52*, 537–540).

HALF-LIFE. Plasma half-life, about 1 hour.

VOLUME OF DISTRIBUTION. About 2 litres/kg.

CLEARANCE. Plasma clearance, about 20 ml/min/kg.

PROTEIN BINDING. In plasma, about 80%.

Dose. 0.5 to 1 mg of phenoperidine hydrochloride intravenously. With assisted ventilation, an initial intravenous dose of 2 to 5 mg may be given.

Phenothiazine
Anthelmintic (Veterinary)

Synonym. Thiodiphenylamine

$C_{12}H_9NS = 199.3$

CAS—92-84-2

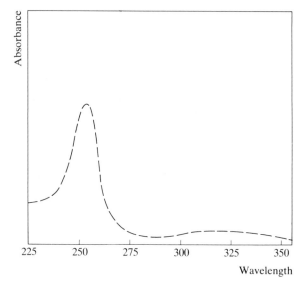

An olive-green or greyish-green, crystalline or amorphous powder. It is slowly oxidised in air and darkens on exposure to light. M.p. about 184°.

Practically **insoluble** in water; soluble 1 in 60 of ethanol, 1 in 5 of acetone, and 1 in 20 of chloroform.

Colour Tests. Ferric Chloride—green; Formaldehyde–Sulphuric Acid—red-violet; Forrest Reagent—orange; FPN Reagent—orange; Liebermann's Test—green; Sulphuric Acid—green.

Gas Chromatography. *System GA*—RI 2024; *system GF*—RI 2845.

High Pressure Liquid Chromatography. *System HA*—k' 0.1.

Ultraviolet Spectrum. Ethanol—254 nm ($A_1^1 = 2160$ b), 317 nm ($A_1^1 = 266$ b).

Absorbance

225   250   275   300   325   350

Wavelength

Infra-red Spectrum. Principal peaks at wavenumbers 735, 750, 1310, 710, 1300, 1590 (KBr disk).

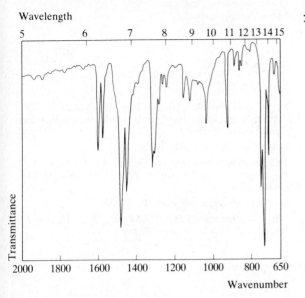

Wavelength

Mass Spectrum. Principal peaks at *m/z* 199, 167, 198, 166, 99, 154, 69, 77.

Phenoxybenzamine   *Antihypertensive*

N-(2-Chloroethyl)-*N*-(1-methyl-2-phenoxyethyl)benzylamine
$C_{18}H_{22}ClNO = 303.8$
CAS—59-96-1

$$C_6H_5 \cdot O \cdot CH_2 \cdot \overset{\displaystyle CH_3}{\underset{\displaystyle CH_2 \cdot C_6H_5}{CH \cdot N}} \cdot CH_2 \cdot CH_2 \cdot Cl$$

Crystals. M.p. 38° to 40°.
Soluble in benzene.

Phenoxybenzamine Hydrochloride

Proprietary Names. Dibenyline; Dibenzyline.
$C_{18}H_{22}ClNO,HCl = 340.3$
CAS—63-92-3
A white crystalline powder. M.p. 136° to 141°.
Soluble 1 in 25 of water, 1 in 9 of ethanol, and 1 in 9 of chloroform; practically insoluble in ether. Neutral and alkaline solutions are unstable.
Caution. Phenoxybenzamine hydrochloride in powder form should not be allowed to come into contact with eyes or skin, as it may cause irritation.

Colour Tests. Mandelin's Test—green → violet; Marquis Test—violet.

Thin-layer Chromatography. *System TA*—Rf 73; *system TB*—Rf 64; *system TC*—Rf 76. (*Acidified iodoplatinate solution*, positive.)

Gas Chromatography. *System GA*—RI 2233; *system GF*—RI 2600.

High Pressure Liquid Chromatography. *System HA*—k' 0.1.

Ultraviolet Spectrum. Aqueous acid—262 nm, 268 nm ($A_1^1 = 48$ a), 274 nm.

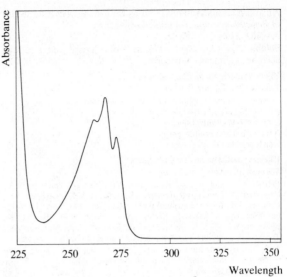

Infra-red Spectrum. Principal peaks at wavenumbers 1240, 750, 698, 1494, 1598, 1586 (phenoxybenzamine hydrochloride, KBr disk).

Wavelength

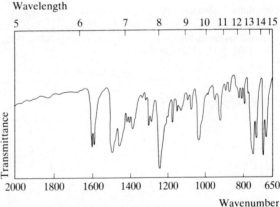

Mass Spectrum. Principal peaks at *m/z* 91, 196, 198, 92, 197, 65, 77, 56.

Dose. 10 to 60 mg of phenoxybenzamine hydrochloride daily; up to 200 mg daily has been given.

Phenoxymethylpenicillin   *Antibiotic*

Synonyms. Penicillin V; Phénomycilline.
Proprietary Names. Oracilline (powder and tablets); Penbec-V; V-Cillin.

(6*R*)-6-(2-Phenoxyacetamido)penicillanic acid
$C_{16}H_{18}N_2O_5S = 350.4$
CAS—87-08-1

An antimicrobial acid produced by the growth of certain strains of *Penicillium notatum* or related organisms.

A white crystalline powder.

Soluble 1 in 1700 of water, 1 in 7 of ethanol, and 1 in 6 of acetone; soluble in chloroform.

Phenoxymethylpenicillin Calcium

Synonym. Penicillin V Calcium

Proprietary Names. Calcipen; Crystapen V (suspension).

$(C_{16}H_{17}N_2O_5S)_2Ca,2H_2O = 774.9$

CAS—147-48-8 (anhydrous)

A white, finely crystalline powder.

Slowly **soluble** 1 in 20 of water.

Phenoxymethylpenicillin Potassium

Synonym. Penicillin V Potassium

Proprietary Names. Apsin VK; Betapen-VK; Co-Caps Penicillin V-K; Crystapen V (syrup and tablets); Distaquaine V-K; Dowpen VK; Econocil VK; Icipen; Ledercillin VK; Megacillin; Nadopen-V; Novopen-VK; Ospen (tablets); Paclin VK; Penapar VK; Pen-Vee-K; Pfizerpen VK; PVF K; Robicillin VK; Ro-Cillin VK; Stabillin V-K; Ticillin V-K; Uticillin VK; V-Cil-K; V-Cillin K; VC-K 500; Veetids.

Note. Megacillin is also used as a proprietary name for benzylpenicillin potassium, clemizol penicillin, and procaine penicillin.

$C_{16}H_{17}KN_2O_5S = 388.5$

CAS—132-98-9

A white crystalline powder.

Soluble 1 in 1.5 of water and 1 in 150 of ethanol; practically insoluble in ether.

Dissociation Constant. pK_a 2.7 (25°).

Ultraviolet Spectrum. Phenoxymethylpenicillin potassium: water—268 nm ($A_1^1 = 31$ b), 275 nm ($A_1^1 = 25$ b).

Infra-red Spectrum. Principal peaks at wavenumbers 1754, 1660, 1181, 1202, 1174, 1532 (KBr disk).

Wavelength

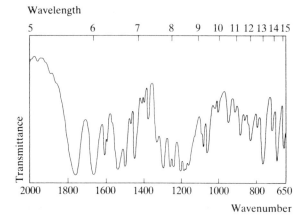

Wavenumber

Disposition in the Body. Rapidly but incompletely absorbed after oral administration; peak plasma concentrations are attained about 2 hours after a dose. About 20 to 35% of an oral dose is excreted in the urine unchanged in 24 hours and about 34% is excreted as penicilloic acid in the same period.

HALF-LIFE. Plasma half-life, about 0.5 hour.

PROTEIN BINDING. In plasma, about 80%.

Dose. 0.5 to 3 g daily.

Phenprobamate   *Tranquilliser*

Synonym. Proformiphen

Proprietary Name. Gamaquil

3-Phenylpropyl carbamate

$C_{10}H_{13}NO_2 = 179.2$

CAS—673-31-4

$$C_6H_5 \cdot [CH_2]_3 \cdot O \cdot CO \cdot NH_2$$

A fine, white, crystalline powder. M.p. 101° to 104°.

Practically **insoluble** in water; soluble in ethanol and chloroform; slightly soluble in ether.

Colour Test. Marquis Test—red-brown.

Thin-layer Chromatography. *System TA*—Rf 75; *system TD*—Rf 47; *system TE*—Rf 74; *system TF*—Rf 55. (*Furfuraldehyde reagent*, positive.)

Gas Chromatography. *System GA*—RI 1520.

Ultraviolet Spectrum. Ethanol—254 nm, 259 nm ($A_1^1 = 11.6$ b), 261 nm ($A_1^1 = 11.6$ b), 265 nm, 269 nm.

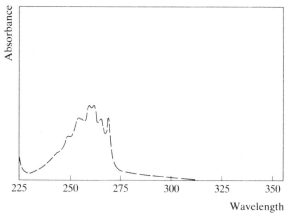

Infra-red Spectrum. Principal peaks at wavenumbers 1690, 1088, 1064, 700, 1605, 1623 (KBr disk).

Mass Spectrum. Principal peaks at m/z 118, 117, 91, 92, 119, 65, 77, 103.

Quantification. COLORIMETRY AND THIN-LAYER CHROMATOGRAPHY. In blood or urine: phenprobamate and metabolites—F. Schatz and U. Jahn, *Arzneimittel-Forsch.*, 1966, *16*, 866–870.

Disposition in the Body. Rapidly absorbed after oral administration and metabolised by oxidative degradation of the side chain and *p*-hydroxylation of the phenyl ring. About 7% of a dose is excreted unchanged in the urine in 48 hours and about 76% as metabolites, mostly as hippuric acid and free and conjugated 3-hydroxyphenprobamate. The 3-hydroxy metabolite, which is active, is present in blood at concentrations greater than those of unchanged drug.

HALF-LIFE. Plasma half-life, 5 to 8 hours.

REFERENCE. D. S. Farrier, *Arzneimittel-Forsch.*, 1975, *25*, 813–817.

Dose. 1.2 to 2.4 g daily.

Phenprocoumon

Anticoagulant

Synonym. Phenylpropylhydroxycoumarin
Proprietary Names. Liquamar; Marcoumar; Marcumar.
4-Hydroxy-3-(1-phenylpropyl)coumarin
$C_{18}H_{16}O_3 = 280.3$
CAS—435-97-2

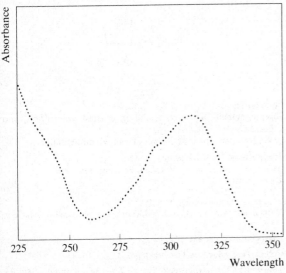

A fine white crystalline powder. M.p. 177° to 181°.
Practically **insoluble** in water; soluble in chloroform, methanol, and solutions of alkali hydroxides.

Thin-layer Chromatography. *System TD*—Rf 62; *system TE*—Rf 21; *system TF*—Rf 56.

Ultraviolet Spectrum. Aqueous alkali—310 nm $(A_1^1 = 540 \text{ b})$; methanol—285 nm $(A_1^1 = 394 \text{ a})$, 310 nm $(A_1^1 = 440 \text{ a})$.

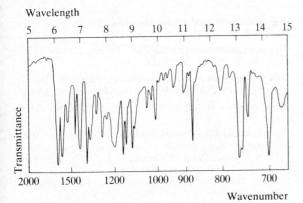

Infra-red Spectrum. Principal peaks at wavenumbers 1656, 759, 696, 1613, 1163, 1113 (Nujol mull).

Mass Spectrum. Principal peaks at *m/z* 251, 280, 118, 91, 121, 119, 252, 189.

Quantification. GAS CHROMATOGRAPHY. In plasma: sensitivity 125 ng/ml, FID—K. K. Midha *et al., J. pharm. Sci.*, 1976, *65*, 387–391.

HIGH PRESSURE LIQUID CHROMATOGRAPHY. In plasma or urine: sensitivity 100 ng/ml in plasma, UV detection—J. X. De Vries *et al., J. Chromat.*, 1982, *231*; *Biomed. Appl.*, *20*, 83–92.

THIN-LAYER CHROMATOGRAPHY–FLUORESCENCE DENSITOMETRY. In plasma: sensitivity 5 ng/ml—P. Haefelfinger, *J. Chromat.*, 1979, *162*; *Biomed. Appl.*, *4*, 215–222.

Disposition in the Body. Well absorbed after oral administration. The *S*-enantiomer is stated to be considerably more potent as an anticoagulant than the *R*-form but there appears to be little difference in pharmacokinetic properties. Phenprocoumon is thought to be excreted almost entirely as a glucuronide conjugate with less than 10% of the dose as unchanged drug.

THERAPEUTIC CONCENTRATION.

Following an intravenous injection of 3 mg to 1 subject, a plasma concentration of 0.8 µg/ml was reported at 5 minutes; in a subject receiving daily doses of 1.6 mg, a steady-state plasma concentration of 1.8 µg/ml was reported (P. Haefelfinger, *ibid.*).

HALF-LIFE. Plasma half-life, 3 to 9 days (mean 5).

VOLUME OF DISTRIBUTION. 0.1 to 0.2 litre/kg.

CLEARANCE. Plasma clearance, about 0.01 ml/min/kg.

PROTEIN BINDING. In plasma, more than 99%.

NOTE. For a review of the clinical pharmacokinetics of oral anticoagulants see J. G. Kelly and K. O'Malley, *Clin. Pharmacokinet.*, 1979, *4*, 1–15.

Dose. Maintenance, 0.75 to 4.5 mg daily.

Phensuximide

Anticonvulsant

Synonym. Fensuximid
Proprietary Name. Milontin
N-Methyl-2-phenylsuccinimide
$C_{11}H_{11}NO_2 = 189.2$
CAS—86-34-0

A white crystalline powder. M.p. 68° to 74°.
Soluble 1 in 250 of water, 1 in 20 of ethanol, 1 in 1.5 of chloroform, and 1 in 35 of ether.

Colour Test. Liebermann's Test—red-orange.

Thin-layer Chromatography. *System TA*—Rf 75; *system TD*—Rf 71; *system TE*—Rf 77; *system TF*—Rf 59. (*Acidified potassium permanganate solution*, positive.)

Gas Chromatography. *System GA*—RI 1634; *system GE*—retention time 0.39 relative to phenytoin.

Ultraviolet Spectrum. Ethanol—247 nm $(A_1^1 = 17.2 \text{ b})$, 252 nm $(A_1^1 = 16.2 \text{ b})$, 258 nm $(A_1^1 = 14.5 \text{ b})$, 264 nm $(A_1^1 = 9.6 \text{ b})$. (See below)

Infra-red Spectrum. Principal peaks at wavenumbers 1686, 1275, 1637, 1111, 695, 751 (KBr disk). (See below)

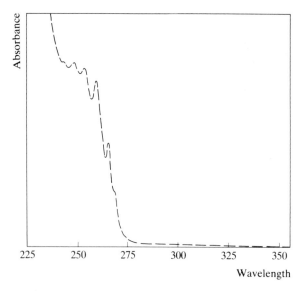

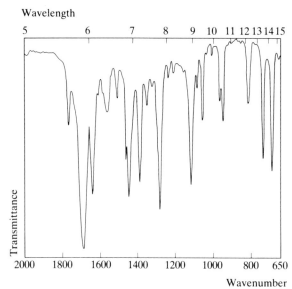

Mass Spectrum. Principal peaks at m/z 104, 189, 103, 78, 51, 77, 105, 52.

Quantification. GAS CHROMATOGRAPHY. In serum: phensuximide and other succinimide anticonvulsants, detection limit 1 to 5 µg/ml for phensuximide, FID—J. Bonitati, *Clin. Chem.*, 1976, *22*, 341–345. In plasma or urine: sensitivity 2.5 µg/ml, FID—E. van der Kleijn *et al.*, *J. Pharm. Pharmac.*, 1973, *25*, 324–327.

Disposition in the Body. Readily absorbed after oral administration and rapidly metabolised to the *N*-desmethyl derivative, which is active. About 27% of a dose is excreted in the urine in 48 hours, mostly as 4'-hydroxyphensuximide and its conjugate.

THERAPEUTIC CONCENTRATION.
After a single oral dose of 1 g to 12 subjects, peak plasma concentrations of 10.6 to 15.6 µg/ml were attained in 0.5 to 1.5 hours (A. J. Glazko and

W. A. Dill, Other Succinimides: Methsuximide and Phensuximide, in *Antiepileptic Drugs*, D. M. Woodbury *et al.* (Ed.), New York, Raven Press, 1972, pp. 455–464).
Following daily oral doses of 3 g to 5 subjects with intractable seizures, steady-state plasma concentrations of 3.9 to 7.9 µg/ml (mean 5.7) of phensuximide and 1.5 to 2.1 µg/ml (mean 1.7) of *N*-desmethylphensuximide, were reported (R. J. Porter *et al.*, *Neurology, Minneap.*, 1977, *27*, 375–376).

TOXICITY. The estimated minimum lethal dose is 5 g.

HALF-LIFE. Plasma half-life, 4 to 12 hours (mean 8).

PROTEIN BINDING. In plasma, not significantly bound.

Dose. 0.5 to 3 g daily.

Phentermine   *Anorectic*

Proprietary Names. Duromine; Ionamin; Linyl; Lipopill; Mirapront.
αα-Dimethylphenethylamine
$C_{10}H_{15}N = 149.2$
CAS—122-09-8

$$C_6H_5 \cdot CH_2 \cdot \overset{\displaystyle CH_3}{\underset{\displaystyle CH_3}{C}} \cdot NH_2$$

A colourless oily liquid.
Slightly **soluble** in water; soluble in ethanol, chloroform, and ether.
Note. Phentermine is an isomer of methylamphetamine.

Phentermine Hydrochloride
Proprietary Names. Adipex-P; Fastin; Pronidin; Teramine.
$C_{10}H_{15}N, HCl = 185.7$
CAS—1197-21-3
A white crystalline powder. M.p. 198°.
Very **soluble** in water, ethanol, and chloroform; practically insoluble in ether.

Dissociation Constant. pK_a 10.1.

Colour Test. Marquis Test—orange.

Thin-layer Chromatography. System *TA*—Rf 46; *system TB*—Rf 26; *system TC*—Rf 31. (*Acidified iodoplatinate solution, positive.*)

Gas Chromatography. System *GA*—RI 1147; *system GB*—RI 1182; *system GC*—RI 1450.

High Pressure Liquid Chromatography. System *HA*—k' 0.6; *system HB*—k' 19.46; *system HC*—k' 0.86.

Ultraviolet Spectrum. Aqueous acid—247 nm, 251 nm, 257 nm ($A_1^1 = 13.9$ b), 263 nm. No alkaline shift.

Infra-red Spectrum. Principal peaks at wavenumbers 730, 1285, 705, 1495, 1610, 1510 (phentermine hydrochloride, KCl disk).

Mass Spectrum. Principal peaks at m/z 58, 91, 42, 41, 134, 65, 59, 40.

Quantification. GAS CHROMATOGRAPHY. In blood or urine: amphetamine and phentermine, sensitivity 10 ng/ml in blood, FID—J. E. O'Brien *et al.*, *J. chromatogr. Sci.*, 1972, *10*, 336–341. In urine: phentermine, chlorphentermine and mephentermine, FID—A. H. Beckett and L. G. Brookes, *J. Pharm. Pharmac.*, 1971, *23*, 288–294.

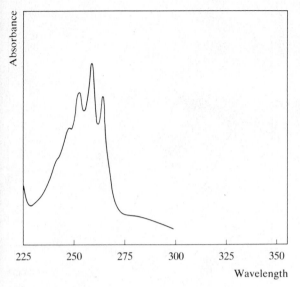

Wavelength

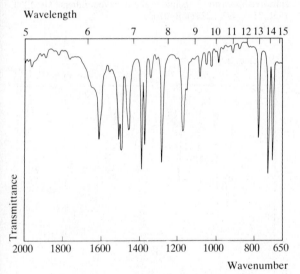

Disposition in the Body. Readily absorbed after oral administration. About 70 to 80% of a dose is excreted in the urine as unchanged drug in 24 hours together with small amounts of the *N*-hydroxy and nitroso metabolites and traces of free and conjugated 4-hydroxyphentermine.
Phentermine is a metabolite of mephentermine.

THERAPEUTIC CONCENTRATION.
The following postmortem tissue concentrations were reported in a subject who had been receiving daily oral doses of 40 mg of a slow-release preparation and who died of natural causes: blood 0.9 µg/ml, bile 6.5 µg/ml, liver 4 µg/g, urine 50 µg/ml (K. Price, *Bull. int. Ass. forens. Toxicol.*, 1974, *10*(1), 12–13).
Following single oral doses of 0.375 mg/kg, peak blood concentrations of about 0.1 µg/ml were attained in about 4 hours (O. N. Hinsvark *et al., J. Pharmacokinet. Biopharm.*, 1973, *1*, 319-328).

TOXICITY.
In a fatality involving the ingestion of phentermine, the following postmortem tissue concentrations were reported: blood 7.6 µg/ml, kidney 16 µg/g, liver 14 µg/g, urine 88 µg/ml; amylobarbitone and ethchlorvynol were also detected in blood at concentrations of 10 µg/ml and 12 µg/ml, respectively (B. Levine *et al., J. forens. Sci.*, 1984, *29*, 1242–1245).

HALF-LIFE. Plasma half-life, about 19 to 24 hours.

VOLUME OF DISTRIBUTION. About 3 to 4 litres/kg.

Dose. 15 to 30 mg daily.

Phentolamine   *Antihypertensive*

3-[*N*-(2-Imidazolin-2-ylmethyl)-*p*-toluidino]phenol
$C_{17}H_{19}N_3O = 281.4$
CAS—50-60-2

A white crystalline powder. M.p. 175°.

Phentolamine Hydrochloride
Proprietary Name. Regitin(e) (tablets)
$C_{17}H_{19}N_3O,HCl = 317.8$
CAS—73-05-2
A white or faintly cream-coloured crystalline powder. M.p. about 240°.
Soluble 1 in 50 of water and 1 in about 120 of ethanol; very slightly soluble in chloroform and ether. Solutions in water foam on shaking.

Phentolamine Mesylate
Synonym. Phentolamine Methanesulphonate
Proprietary Names. Regitin(e) (injection); Rogitine.
$C_{17}H_{19}N_3O,CH_3SO_3H = 377.5$
CAS—65-28-1
A white, slightly hygroscopic, crystalline powder. M.p. 177° to 181°.
Soluble 1 in 1 of water, 1 in 5 of ethanol, and 1 in 700 of chloroform.

Dissociation Constant. pK_a 7.7.

Colour Tests. Mandelin's Test—blue-green; Marquis Test—yellow.

Thin-layer Chromatography. *System TA*—Rf 32; *system TB*—Rf 01; *system TC*—Rf 03. (*Acidified iodoplatinate solution*, positive.)

Gas Chromatography. *System GA*—not eluted.

High Pressure Liquid Chromatography. *System HA*—k' 1.7.

Ultraviolet Spectrum. Aqueous acid—278 nm; aqueous alkali—291 nm.

Infra-red Spectrum. Principal peaks at wavenumbers 1195, 1508, 1610, 1580, 1592, 1247 (KBr disk). (See below)

Mass Spectrum. Principal peaks at *m/z* 281, 120, 91, 122, 280, 160, 68, 282.

Dose. 5 to 10 mg of phentolamine mesylate intravenously. Phentolamine hydrochloride has been given in doses of 200 to 300 mg daily, by mouth.

Wavelength

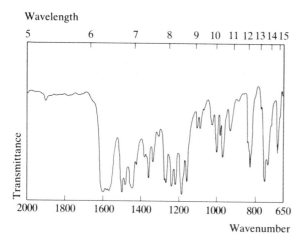

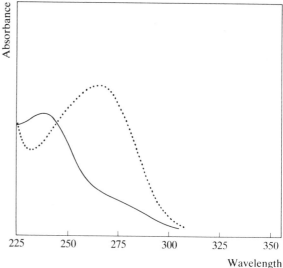

Wavelength

Phenylbutazone

Analgesic

Synonyms. Butadione; Fenilbutazona.

Proprietary Names. Algoverine; Artrizin; Azolid; Butacote; Butagesic; Butazolidin(e); Butazone; Intrabutazone; Malgesic; Nadozone; Neo-Zoline; Phenbutazone; Tibutazone.

4-Butyl-1,2-diphenylpyrazolidine-3,5-dione
$C_{19}H_{20}N_2O_2 = 308.4$
CAS—50-33-9

A fine, white, crystalline powder. M.p. 104° to 107°.
Practically **insoluble** in water; soluble 1 in 28 of ethanol, 1 in 1.25 of chloroform, and 1 in 15 of ether.

Dissociation Constant. pK_a 4.4 (20°).

Partition Coefficient. Log P (octanol/pH 7.4), 0.7.

Colour Tests. Liebermann's Test (100°)—brown; Mandelin's Test—violet.

Thin-layer Chromatography. *System TA*—Rf 79; *system TD*—Rf 78; *system TE*—Rf 66; *system TF*—Rf 68; *system TG*—Rf 23. (*Chromic acid solution*, brown; *Ludy Tenger reagent*, orange; *mercurous nitrate spray*, positive; *acidified potassium permanganate solution*, positive.)

Gas Chromatography. *System GA*—phenylbutazone RI 2365, oxyphenbutazone RI 1630; *system GD*—phenylbutazone retention times 2.05 and 1.81, oxyphenbutazone retention time 2.11, both as methyl derivatives relative to n-$C_{16}H_{34}$; *system GF*—RI 2860.

High Pressure Liquid Chromatography. *System HD*—phenylbutazone k' 6.5, oxyphenbutazone k' 1.95; *system HV*—phenylbutazone retention time 0.95, oxyphenbutazone retention time 0.69, both relative to meclofenamic acid.

Ultraviolet Spectrum. Aqueous acid—237 nm ($A_1^1 = 456$ a); aqueous alkali—264 nm ($A_1^1 = 660$ a).

Infra-red Spectrum. Principal peaks at wavenumbers 1714, 1300, 1755, 755, 1492, 1275 (KBr disk).

Wavelength

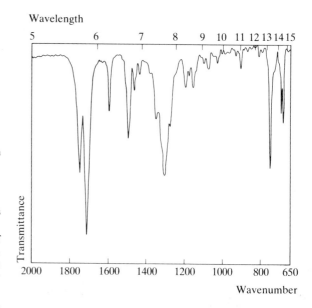

Wavenumber

Mass Spectrum. Principal peaks at m/z 77, 183, 308, 184, 105, 55, 51, 41; oxyphenbutazone 199, 324, 93, 77, 65, 55, 121, 135.

Quantification. GAS CHROMATOGRAPHY. In blood, plasma, bile, or urine: sensitivity 1 μg/ml—R. D. Budd, *J. Chromat.*, 1982, *243*, 368–371. In plasma: sensitivity 10 ng/ml, ECD—A. Sioufi *et al.*, *J. pharm. Sci.*, 1978, *67*, 243–245.

HIGH PRESSURE LIQUID CHROMATOGRAPHY. In plasma or urine: phenylbutazone, oxyphenbutazone and 3'-hydroxyphenylbutazone, detection limit 50 ng/ml, UV detection—T. Marunaka *et al., J. Chromat.*, 1980, *183*; *Biomed. Appl.*, *9*, 331–338. In plasma: phenylbutazone, oxyphenbutazone and 3'-hydroxyphenylbutazone, sensitivity 5.5 µg/ml for phenylbutazone, UV detection—L. Aarons and C. Higham, *Clinica chim. Acta*, 1980, *105*, 377–382.

Disposition in the Body. Readily absorbed after oral or rectal administration and slowly absorbed after intramuscular injection. The major metabolic reactions are *C*-glucuronidation at the 4-position of the pyrazolidine ring and 4-hydroxylation of one of the phenyl rings to form the active metabolite, oxyphenbutazone; 3-hydroxylation of the butyl side-chain to form 3'-hydroxyphenylbutazone, and formation of 4,3'-dihydroxyphenylbutazone also occur. About 61% of a dose is slowly excreted in the urine over a period of about 21 days, together with up to 27% in the faeces. Of the material excreted in the urine, the 4-*C*-glucuronide of phenylbutazone accounts for about 40%, free phenylbutazone and free oxyphenbutazone about 1%, 4,3'-dihydroxyphenylbutazone about 6%, 3'-hydroxyphenylbutazone about 3%, and the remainder consists of the *C*-glucuronide of 3'-hydroxyphenylbutazone (about 12%), oxyphenbutazone *O*-glucuronide and two other metabolites.

THERAPEUTIC CONCENTRATION. In plasma, usually in the range 50 to 100 µg/ml.

Following single oral doses of 100, 300 and 600 mg to 6 subjects, peak plasma concentrations of 12.5 to 17.1 µg/ml (mean 14), 30.8 to 46.3 µg/ml (mean 38), and 51.2 to 88.1 µg/ml (mean 75), respectively, were obtained in 1 to 7 hours (mean 3) (A. Sioufi *et al.*, *J. pharm. Sci.*, 1980, *69*, 1413–1416).

After daily oral doses of 100, 200, and 300 mg to 7 subjects, mean steady-state plasma concentrations of 52, 83, and 95 µg/ml respectively were reported; in 3 subjects given 400 mg daily, the mean steady-state concentration was 99 µg/ml (M. Orme *et al.*, *Br. J. clin. Pharmac.*, 1976, *3*, 185–191).

Following daily oral doses of 200 mg to 1 subject for 7 days, the following plasma concentrations were found: phenylbutazone about 50 µg/ml, oxyphenbutazone about 20 µg/ml, and 3'-hydroxyphenylbutazone about 12 µg/ml (K. K. Midha *et al.*, *J. pharm. Sci.*, 1974, *63*, 1751–1754).

TOXICITY. The estimated minimum lethal dose is 5 g. Toxic effects during treatment are frequent and may occur even when the dose does not exceed 400 mg daily; they are usually associated with plasma concentrations above 100 µg/ml. A considerable number of deaths have occurred, especially from blood disorders.

In a fatality due to an accidental overdose by a 5-year-old child, the following postmortem concentrations were reported: blood 400 µg/ml, bile 475 µg/ml, kidney 250 µg/g, liver 250 µg/g (K. L. Lam and K. Chien, *Bull. int. Ass. forens. Toxicol.*, 1976, *12*(2), 20).

A plasma concentration of 670 µg/ml was reported in one subject, 1 day after ingestion of 8 g. The concentration of phenylbutazone declined rapidly with a half-life of 23 hours but concentrations of 3'-hydroxyphenylbutazone were unusually high and exceeded those of unchanged drug after 48 hours; the subject recovered after about 3 days (L. F. Prescott *et al.*, *Br. med. J.*, 1980, *281*, 1106–1107).

HALF-LIFE. Plasma half-life, phenylbutazone 2 to 5 days (mean 3), but dose-dependent and increased in subjects with renal failure and in the elderly; oxyphenbutazone about 2 to 3 days, 3'-hydroxyphenylbutazone about 32 hours.

DISTRIBUTION IN BLOOD. Plasma: whole blood ratio, 1.8.

PROTEIN BINDING. In plasma, about 99% at therapeutic concentrations; decreased at higher concentrations when the binding sites become saturated.

NOTE. For a review of the pharmacokinetics of phenylbutazone see J. Aarbakke, *Clin. Pharmacokinet.*, 1978, *3*, 369–380.

Dose. Initially 300 to 600 mg daily; maintenance, 100 to 400 mg daily.

Phenylephrine   *Sympathomimetic*

Synonyms. Néosynéphrine; *m*-Synephrine.
Note. Synephrine has been used as a synonym for oxedrine.
Proprietary Name. It is an ingredient of Vibrocil.
(*R*)-1-(3-Hydroxyphenyl)-2-methylaminoethanol
$C_9H_{13}NO_2 = 167.2$
CAS—59-42-7

M.p. about 174°.

Phenylephrine Hydrochloride

Synonyms. Mesatonum; Metaoxedrini Chloridum.

Proprietary Names. Fenox; Isophrin; Mydfrin; Nazex; Neophryn; Optocrymal; Prefrin Liquifilm; Snef; Soothe; Visadron. It is an ingredient of Biomydrin, Bronchilator, Colrex Compound, Demazin, Dexylets, Dimotane (expectorant), Dimotapp, Dristan (tablets), Exyphen, Hayphryn, Isopto Frin, Naldecon, Neotep, Nethaprin Dospan, Tussils, Uniflu, and Zincfrin.

$C_9H_{13}NO_2,HCl = 203.7$
CAS—61-76-7

A white crystalline powder. M.p. 140° to 145°. A solution in water is laevorotatory.

Soluble 1 in 2 of water and 1 in 4 of ethanol.

Dissociation Constant. pK_a 8.9 (-OH), 10.1 (-NH-), (20°).

Colour Tests. Mandelin's Test—brown; Marquis Test—red.

Thin-layer Chromatography. *System TA*—Rf 33; *system TB*—Rf 01; *system TC*—Rf 01. (*Acidified potassium permanganate solution*, positive.)

Gas Chromatography. *System GC*—RI 1934.

High Pressure Liquid Chromatography. *System HA*—k' 1.3; *system HC*—k' 1.64.

Ultraviolet Spectrum. Aqueous acid—273 nm $(A_1^1 = 110\ a)$; aqueous alkali—238 nm $(A_1^1 = 534\ a)$, 291 nm $(A_1^1 = 182\ a)$. (See below)

Infra-red Spectrum. Principal peaks at wavenumbers 1594, 1273, 784, 696, 1304, 900 (phenylephrine hydrochloride, KBr disk). (See below)

Mass Spectrum. Principal peaks at *m/z* 44, 76, 77, 29, 45, 42, 95, 65.

Quantification. GAS CHROMATOGRAPHY. In plasma: sensitivity 12.5 ng/ml, ECD—L. J. Dombrowski *et al.*, *J. pharm. Sci.*, 1973, *62*, 1761–1763.

GAS CHROMATOGRAPHY–MASS SPECTROMETRY. In urine: phenylephrine and four metabolites—K. E. Ibrahim *et al.*, *J. Pharm. Pharmac.*, 1983, *35*, 144–147.

Disposition in the Body. Readily absorbed after oral administration, but undergoes extensive first-pass metabolism; bioavailability about 38%. It is metabolised by conjugation with sulphate and glucuronic acid and by oxidative deamination to *m*-hydroxymandelic acid (MHMA) and *m*-hydroxyphenylglycol (MHPG). About 80% of an oral dose is excreted in the urine in 24 hours, mainly as sulphate conjugates of phenylephrine and MHPG; about 30% of a dose is excreted as unconjugated MHMA.

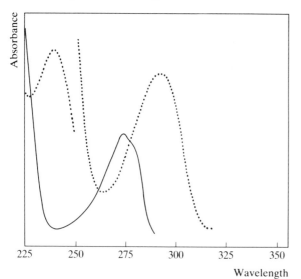

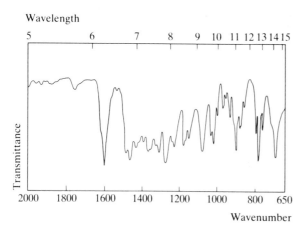

Phenylmethylbarbituric Acid   *Barbiturate*

Synonym. Heptobarbitalum (distinguish from Heptabarbital).
5-Methyl-5-phenylbarbituric acid
$C_{11}H_{10}N_2O_3 = 218.2$
CAS—76-94-8

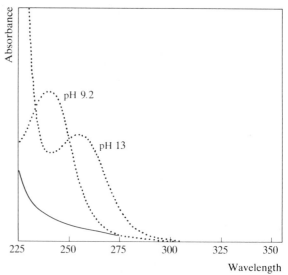

A white crystalline powder. M.p. about 226°.
Very slightly **soluble** in water; soluble 1 in 60 of ethanol; soluble in ether and aqueous solutions of alkalis.

Dissociation Constant. pK$_a$ 7.7 (25°).

Colour Test. Liebermann's Test—red-orange.

Thin-layer Chromatography. *System TD*—Rf 29; *system TE*—Rf 24; *system TF*—Rf 61; *system TH*—Rf 27. (*Mercurous nitrate spray*, black; *Zwikker's reagent*, pink.)

Gas Chromatography. *System GA*—RI 1880.

High Pressure Liquid Chromatography. *System HG*—k′ 1.48; *system HH*—k′ 0.94.

Ultraviolet Spectrum. *Borax buffer 0.05M* (pH 9.2)—238 nm (A$_1^1$ = 494 b); M sodium hydroxide (pH 13)—253 nm (A$_1^1$ = 350 b).

THERAPEUTIC CONCENTRATION.
After a single oral dose of 9 mg of ^{3}H-labelled phenylephrine hydrochloride to 6 subjects, peak plasma concentrations of 0.23 to 0.47 µg/ml (mean 0.31) of total phenylephrine and metabolites were attained in 1 to 2 hours (C. J. Cavallito *et al.*, *J. pharm. Sci.*, 1963, *52*, 259–263).

Following a single oral dose of 1 mg to 3 subjects, a mean peak plasma concentration of unconjugated phenylephrine of 0.0009 µg/ml was attained in about 1.3 hours (J. H. Hengstmann and J. Goronzy, *Eur. J. clin. Pharmac.*, 1982, *21*, 335–341).

TOXICITY. The estimated minimum lethal dose, for children up to 2 years is 100 mg intranasally and for adults is 1 g.

HALF-LIFE. Plasma half-life, about 2 to 3 hours.

VOLUME OF DISTRIBUTION. About 5 litres/kg.

CLEARANCE. Plasma clearance, about 30 ml/min/kg.

Dose. 30 to 40 mg of phenylephrine hydrochloride daily, by mouth.

Infra-red Spectrum. Principal peaks at wavenumbers 1702, 1720, 1751, 1240, 802, 716.

Mass Spectrum. Principal peaks at *m/z* 104, 132, 218, 51, 103, 77, 78, 52.

Dose. Phenylmethylbarbituric acid has been given in doses of 400 mg daily.

Wavelength

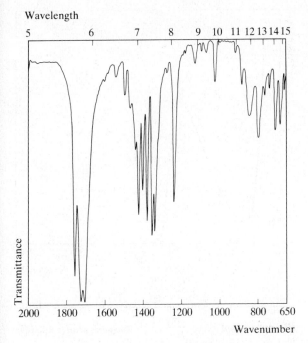

Wavenumber

Phenylpropanolamine

Sympathomimetic

*Synonym. dl-*Norephedrine
($\pm$)-2-Amino-1-phenylpropan-1-ol
$C_9H_{13}NO = 151.2$
CAS—14838-15-4

$$\underset{C_6H_5 \cdot CH \cdot CH \cdot CH_3}{\overset{OH \quad NH_2}{| \quad |}}$$

M.p. 101°.

Phenylpropanolamine Hydrochloride

Synonym. Mydriatin

Proprietary Names. Coldecon; Control; Monydrin; Propadrine; Rhindecon; Rinexin; Tepanil. It is an ingredient of Contac 400, Dimotane (expectorant), Dimotapp, Endecon, Eskornade, Exyphen, Hycomine, Naldecon, Nezcaam, Pholcolix, Rinurel, Sine-Off, Totolin, Triogesic, Triominic, Triotussic, and Vallex.

Note. The name Tepanil is also applied to diethylpropion hydrochloride.
$C_9H_{13}NO,HCl = 187.7$
CAS—154-41-6
A white to creamy-white crystalline powder. M.p. 191° to 196°.

Soluble 1 in 2.5 of water and 1 in 9 of ethanol; practically insoluble in chloroform and ether.

Dissociation Constant. pK_a 9.4 (20°).

Thin-layer Chromatography. *System TA*—Rf 44; *system TB*—Rf 04; *system TC*—Rf 04. (*Dragendorff spray,* positive; *FPN reagent,* violet; *acidified iodoplatinate solution,* positive; *Marquis reagent,* yellow; *ninhydrin spray,* positive; *acidified potassium permanganate solution,* positive.)

Gas Chromatography. *System GA*—RI 1313; *system GB*—RI 1353; *system GC*—RI 1383.

High Pressure Liquid Chromatography. *System HA*—k' 0.9; *system HB*—k' 3.87; *system HC*—k' 0.70.

Ultraviolet Spectrum. Aqueous acid—251 nm, 257 nm ($A_1^1 = 11.7$ a), 262 nm. No alkaline shift.

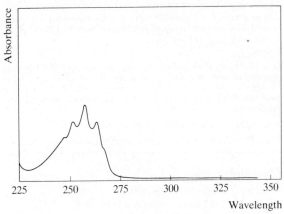

Wavelength

Infra-red Spectrum. Principal peaks at wavenumbers 700, 746, 1030, 1500, 1055, 1590 (phenylpropanolamine hydrochloride, KBr disk).

Wavelength

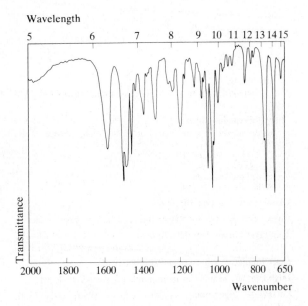

Wavenumber

Mass Spectrum. Principal peaks at *m/z* 44, 77, 79, 51, 45, 42, 107, 105.

Quantification. GAS CHROMATOGRAPHY (CAPILLARY COLUMN). In plasma: sensitivity 1 ng/ml, ECD—N. Crisologo *et al., J. pharm. Sci.,* 1984, *73,* 1313–1315.

HIGH PRESSURE LIQUID CHROMATOGRAPHY. In plasma: sensitivity 5 ng/ml, fluorescence detection—W. D. Mason and E. N. Amick, *J. pharm. Sci.*, 1981, *70*, 707–709.

Disposition in the Body. Absorbed after oral administration. More than 90% of a dose is excreted in the urine as unchanged drug in 24 hours, together with small amounts of hippuric acid. Phenylpropanolamine is a metabolite of amphetamine, diethylpropion, and ephedrine.

THERAPEUTIC CONCENTRATION.
Following a single oral dose of 25 mg to 12 subjects, a mean peak plasma concentration of about 0.08 µg/ml was attained in about 2 hours (W. D. Mason and E. N. Amick, *ibid.*).

TOXICITY.
In a fatality due to a phenylpropanolamine overdose, the following postmortem tissue concentrations were reported: blood 48 µg/ml, brain 86 µg/g, liver 460 µg/g (R. H. Cravey, per R. C. Baselt, *Disposition of Toxic Drugs and Chemicals in Man*, 2nd Edn, Davis, California, Biomedical Publications, 1982, pp. 641–643).

HALF-LIFE. Plasma half-life, about 4 hours.

Dose. 75 to 200 mg of phenylpropanolamine hydrochloride daily.

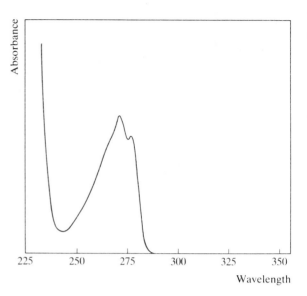

Phenyltoloxamine

Antihistamine

Synonyms. Phenyltolyloxamine; PRN.
Proprietary Name. It is an ingredient of Pholtex.
2-(2-Benzylphenoxy)-*NN*-dimethylethylamine
$C_{17}H_{21}NO = 255.4$
CAS—92-12-6

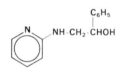

An oily liquid.
Note. Phenyltoloxamine is a structural isomer of diphenhydramine.

Phenyltoloxamine Citrate
Proprietary Names. It is an ingredient of Naldecon, Percogesic, and Rinurel.
$C_{17}H_{21}NO,C_6H_8O_7 = 447.5$
CAS—1176-08-5
Crystals. M.p. 138° to 140°.
Soluble in water.

Dissociation Constant. pK_a 9.1.

Colour Tests. Mandelin's Test—green; Marquis Test—violet.

Thin-layer Chromatography. *System TA*—Rf 53; *system TB*—Rf 39; *system TC*—Rf 48. (*Acidified iodoplatinate solution*, positive.)

Gas Chromatography. *System GA*—RI 1938.

High Pressure Liquid Chromatography. *System HA*—k' 3.1.

Ultraviolet Spectrum. Aqueous acid—270 nm ($A_1^1 = 73$ b), 276 nm.

Infra-red Spectrum. Principal peaks at wavenumbers 1245, 1491, 752, 1030, 697, 1111 (KBr disk).

Mass Spectrum. Principal peaks at *m/z* 58, 255, 42, 71, 59, 44, 181, 165.

Dose. 75 to 200 mg of phenyltoloxamine citrate daily.

Phenyramidol

Analgesic/Muscle Relaxant

1-Phenyl-2-(2-pyridylamino)ethanol
$C_{13}H_{14}N_2O = 214.3$
CAS—553-69-5

Crystals. M.p. 82° to 85°.

Phenyramidol Hydrochloride
Proprietary Names. Analexin; Cabral; Miodar.
$C_{13}H_{14}N_2O,HCl = 250.7$
CAS—326-43-2
A white crystalline powder. M.p. 140° to 142°.
Freely **soluble** in water; soluble in ethanol.

Dissociation Constant. pK_a 5.9.

Colour Tests. Cyanogen Bromide—orange-pink; Mandelin's Test—blue; Marquis Test—yellow.

Thin-layer Chromatography. *System TA*—Rf 69; *system TB*—Rf 09; *system TC*—Rf 52. (*Dragendorff spray*, positive; *acidified iodoplatinate solution*, positive; *acidified potassium permanganate solution*, positive.)

Gas Chromatography. *System GA*—RI 2006.

Ultraviolet Spectrum. Aqueous acid—237 nm ($A_1^1 = 666$ a), 309 nm.

Infra-red Spectrum. Principal peaks at wavenumbers 1613, 1524, 700, 768, 1058, 752 (KBr disk).

Mass Spectrum. Principal peaks at *m/z* 107, 108, 78, 79, 80, 77, 51, 52.

Dose. Up to 3.2 g of phenyramidol hydrochloride daily.

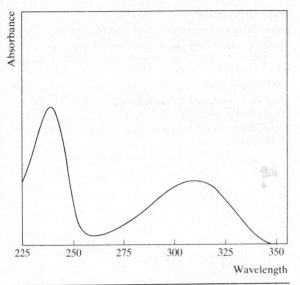

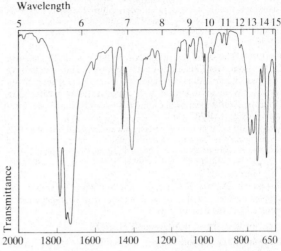

Infra-red Spectrum. Principal peaks at wavenumbers 1720, 1740, 1774, 748, 698, 785 (KBr disk).

Phenytoin   *Anticonvulsant*

Synonyms. Diphenylhydantoin; Fenitoína; Phenantoinum.
Proprietary Names of Phenytoin and Phenytoin Sodium. Dantoin; Di-Hydan; Dilantin; Diphenylan; Ditan; Epanutin; Phenhydan; Pyorédol; Solantyl; Zentropil. Phenytoin sodium is an ingredient of Garoin.

5,5-Diphenylimidazolidine-2,4-dione
$C_{15}H_{12}N_2O_2 = 252.3$
CAS—57-41-0

A white crystalline powder. M.p. about 295°, with decomposition.

Practically **insoluble** in water; slightly soluble in ethanol; soluble 1 in 500 of chloroform and 1 in 600 of ether; soluble in solutions of alkali hydroxides.

Phenytoin Sodium

Synonyms. Diphenin; Sodium Diphenylhydantoin; Soluble Phenytoin.
$C_{15}H_{11}N_2NaO_2 = 274.3$
CAS—630-93-3
A white, slightly hygroscopic, crystalline powder which on exposure to air absorbs carbon dioxide with the liberation of phenytoin.
Soluble in water and ethanol; practically insoluble in chloroform and ether. In aqueous solution it is partly hydrolysed to the base and turbidity develops.

Dissociation Constant. pK_a 8.3 (25°).

Colour Tests. Koppanyi–Zwikker Test—violet; Liebermann's Test—red-orange; Mercurous Nitrate—black.

Thin-layer Chromatography. *System TD*—Rf 33; *system TE*—Rf 36; *system TF*—Rf 53. (*Mercuric chloride–diphenylcarbazone reagent*, positive; *mercurous nitrate spray*, black.)

Gas Chromatography. *System GA*—RI 2330. Phenytoin is used as the reference substance in *System GE*.

High Pressure Liquid Chromatography. *System HE*—k' 9.71.

Ultraviolet Spectrum. Methanol—258 nm ($A_1^1 = 27$ a), 264 nm ($A_1^1 = 16$ a).

Mass Spectrum. Principal peaks at *m/z* 180, 104, 223, 77, 209, 252, 51, 165; 5-(4-hydroxyphenyl)-5-phenylhydantoin 239, 196, 268, 120, 197, 225, 77, 104.

Quantification. GAS CHROMATOGRAPHY. In plasma: sensitivity 0.5 to 1 μg/ml, FID—J. Gordos *et al.*, *J. Chromat.*, 1977, *143*; *Biomed. Appl.*, *1*, 171–181.

HIGH PRESSURE LIQUID CHROMATOGRAPHY. In plasma or serum: phenytoin and other anticonvulsants, sensitivity 1.3 μg/ml for phenytoin, UV detection—J. A. Christofides and D. E. Fry, *Clin. Chem.*, 1980, *26*, 499–501. In plasma or urine: phenytoin and 5-(4-hydroxyphenyl)-5-phenylhydantoin, sensitivity 100 ng/ml for phenytoin and 50 ng/ml for the metabolite, UV detection—R. J. Sawchuk and L. L. Cartier, *Clin. Chem.*, 1980, *26*, 835–839.

Disposition in the Body. Slowly but almost completely absorbed after oral administration; the rate of absorption is variable, being prolonged after large doses, and the bioavailability may vary considerably between different formulations. Aromatic hydroxylation is the major metabolic pathway and about 50 to 70% of a dose may be excreted as free or conjugated 5-(4-hydroxyphenyl)-5-phenylhydantoin (HPPH) in 24 hours; the excretion of this metabolite is dose-dependent and decreases as the dose is increased. Phenytoin hydroxylation is capacity-limited, and is therefore readily inhibited by agents which compete for its metabolic pathways. Less than 5% of a dose is excreted as unchanged drug. Minor metabolites include 5-(3-hydroxyphenyl)-5-phenylhydantoin, 3,4-dihydro-3,4-dihydroxyphenytoin, catechol, and 3-*O*-methylcatechol. Up to about 15% of a dose may be eliminated in the faeces.

THERAPEUTIC CONCENTRATION. In plasma, usually in the range 10 to 20 μg/ml.

A single oral dose of 100 mg given to 5 subjects produced peak plasma concentrations of 1.6 to 2.8 μg/ml (mean 2.2) in 2 to 4 hours; a second peak was observed at 10 to 12 hours (J. D. Robinson *et al.*, *Br. J. clin. Pharmac.*, 1975, *2*, 345–349).

Following daily oral doses of 300 mg, mean steady-state plasma concentrations of 1.3 to 6.6 μg/ml (mean 3.6) were reported in 5 subjects with short phenytoin half-lives, in comparison to mean steady-state plasma concentrations of 5.0 to 27.2 µg/ml (mean 13.4) in 4 subjects with long phenytoin half-lives; the corresponding concentrations of HPPH were 1.3 to 2.7 µg/ml (mean 2.0) and 0.7 to 1.3 µg/ml (mean 1.0), respectively (A. J. Glazko *et al.*, *Ther. Drug Monit.*, 1982, *4*, 281–292).

Following oral doses of 100 mg three times a day to 18 subjects, maximum steady-state plasma concentrations of 3.4 to 30.5 µg/ml (mean 11.8) were reported (R. J. Sawchuk *et al.*, *J. Pharmacokinet. Biopharm.*, 1982, *10*, 365–382).

TOXICITY. The estimated minimum lethal dose is 5 g but few deaths from overdosage have been reported. Side-effects have been associated with plasma concentrations greater than 20 µg/ml and severe toxic effects with concentrations greater than 40 µg/ml. Fatalities have been associated with blood concentrations greater than 70 µg/ml.

A 4½-year-old girl ingested 2 g of phenytoin and 24 hours later the blood concentration was found to be 94 µg/ml. She died on the third day and postmortem concentrations were: blood 45 µg/ml, brain 78 µg/g, kidney 112 µg/g, liver 272 µg/g (F. A. Laubscher, *J. Am. med. Ass.*, 1966, *198*, 1120–1121).

HALF-LIFE. Plasma half-life, varies considerably within the approximate range of 7 to 60 hours, and is dose-dependent, increasing as the dose increases.

VOLUME OF DISTRIBUTION. About 0.7 litre/kg.

DISTRIBUTION IN BLOOD. Plasma : whole blood ratio, about 1.6.

SALIVA. Plasma : saliva ratio, about 10.

PROTEIN BINDING. In plasma, about 90%.

NOTE. For a review of the pharmacokinetics of phenytoin see A. Richens, *Clin. Pharmacokinet.*, 1979, *4*, 153–169.

Dose. 300 to 600 mg of phenytoin sodium daily.

Pholcodine
Cough Suppressant

Synonyms. MEM; Morpholinylethylmorphine.

Proprietary Names. Adaphol; Dia-Tuss; Duro-Tuss; Pectolin; Sancos; Sedlingtus; Triopaed; Tussinol. It is an ingredient of Copholco, Copholcoids, Davenol, Expulin, Falcodyl, Pavacol-D, PEM, Pholcolix, Pholcomed (linctus), Pholtex, Rinurel (linctus), Rubelix, and Triocos.

3-*O*-(2-Morpholinoethyl)morphine monohydrate

$C_{23}H_{30}N_2O_4,H_2O = 416.5$

CAS—509-67-1 (anhydrous)

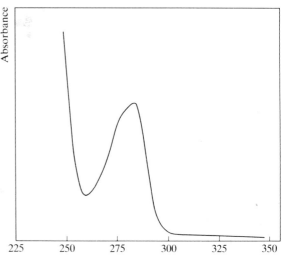

Colourless crystals or a white crystalline powder. M.p. about 99°.

Soluble 1 in 50 of water and 1 in 3 of dehydrated alcohol; very soluble in acetone and chloroform; slightly soluble in ether.

Pholcodine Tartrate

$C_{23}H_{30}N_2O_4,2C_4H_6O_6,3H_2O = 752.7$
A white crystalline powder.

Soluble 1 in 8 of water; very slightly soluble in ethanol; slightly soluble in chloroform and ether.

Dissociation Constant. pK_a 8.0, 9.3 (37°).

Colour Tests. Liebermann's Test—black; Marquis Test—violet.

Thin-layer Chromatography. *System TA*—Rf 36; *system TB*—Rf 03; *system TC*—Rf 18. (*Dragendorff spray*, positive; *acidified iodoplatinate solution*, positive; *Marquis reagent*, violet.)

Gas Chromatography. *System GA*—RI 3018.

High Pressure Liquid Chromatography. *System HA*—k′ 6.0 (tailing peak); *system HC*—k′ 1.63.

Ultraviolet Spectrum. Aqueous acid—283 nm ($A_1^1 = 40$ a). No alkaline shift.

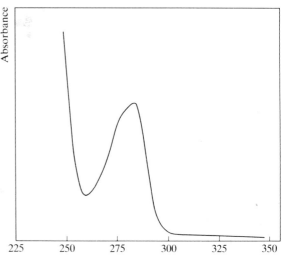

Infra-red Spectrum. Principal peaks at wavenumbers 1118, 969, 1250, 1043, 1500, 1098 (KBr disk).

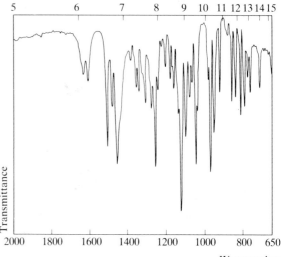

Mass Spectrum. Principal peaks at *m/z* 114, 100, 56, 42, 115, 101, 70, 398.

Dose. Up to 60 mg daily.

Pholedrine
Sympathomimetic

Synonyms. Isodrine; Sympropaminum.
4-(2-Methylaminopropyl)phenol
$C_{10}H_{15}NO = 165.2$
CAS—370-14-9

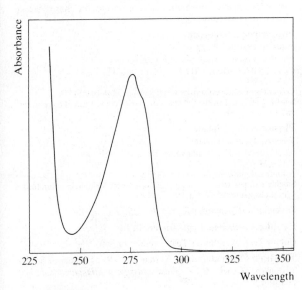

Crystals. M.p. 162°.
Slightly **soluble** in water; soluble in ethanol and ether.

Pholedrine Sulphate
Proprietary Name. Veritol
$(C_{10}H_{15}NO)_2,H_2SO_4 = 428.5$
CAS—6114-26-7
A white crystalline powder. M.p. about 321°, with decomposition.
Soluble 1 in 20 of water; practically insoluble in ethanol, chloroform, and ether.

Dissociation Constant. pK_a 9.4 (25°).

Colour Test. Marquis Test—grey → green.

Thin-layer Chromatography. *System TA*—Rf 29; *system TB*—Rf 04; *system TC*—Rf 03. (*Acidified potassium permanganate solution,* positive.)

Gas Chromatography. *System GA*—RI 1490.

Ultraviolet Spectrum. Aqueous acid—275 nm $(A_1^1 = 82$ a); aqueous alkali—238 nm $(A_1^1 = 640$ b), 295 nm $(A_1^1 = 150$ b).

Infra-red Spectrum. Principal peaks at wavenumbers 1258, 1513, 1274, 1590, 1610, 810 (KBr disk).

Mass Spectrum. Principal peaks at m/z 58, 30, 107, 59, 77, 56, 42, 43.

Disposition in the Body.

TOXICITY.
In a fatality involving the ingestion of pholedrine, the following postmortem concentrations were reported: blood 15 μg/g, kidney 122 μg/g, liver 73 μg/g (H.-J. Hammer *et al.*, *Dte GesundhWes.*, 1980, *35*, 1352–1354).

Dose. Pholedrine sulphate has been given parenterally in doses of up to 20 mg.

Phthalylsulphacetamide
Sulphonamide

Synonym. Sulfanilacetamidum Phthalylatum
Proprietary Names. Talecid; Thalacet.
4'-(Acetylsulphamoyl)phthalanilic acid
$C_{16}H_{14}N_2O_6S = 362.4$
CAS—131-69-1

White or creamy-white crystals or crystalline powder. M.p. 186° to 202°, with decomposition.
Very slightly **soluble** in water; slightly soluble in ethanol; soluble in acetone; freely soluble in solutions of alkali hydroxides.

Colour Test. Copper Sulphate (Method 1)—blue.

Thin-layer Chromatography. *System TD*—Rf 00; *system TE*—Rf 00; *system TF*—Rf 00.

Ultraviolet Spectrum. Aqueous acid—268 nm (broad); aqueous alkali—265 nm (broad).

Infra-red Spectrum. Principal peaks at wavenumbers 1170, 1681, 1527, 837, 1302, 1592.

Mass Spectrum. Principal peaks at m/z 109, 76, 104, 92, 239, 65, 108, 43.

Dose. 6 to 12 g daily.

Phthalylsulphathiazole
Sulphonamide

Synonyms. Ftalilsulfatiazol; Phthalazolum; Phthalylsulfathiazole.
Proprietary Names. Colicitina; Phthazol; Sulfathalidine; Talidine; Thalazole. It is an ingredient of Neo-Sulfazon.
4'-(Thiazol-2-ylsulphamoyl)phthalanilic acid
$C_{17}H_{13}N_3O_5S_2 = 403.4$
CAS—85-73-4

White or yellowish-white crystals, or powder, which darken on prolonged exposure to light. M.p. about 275°, with decomposition.

Practically **insoluble** in water, chloroform, and ether; soluble 1 in 600 of ethanol; freely soluble in dimethylformamide and solutions of alkali hydroxides and carbonates, and in hydrochloric acid.

Colour Test. Copper Sulphate (Method 1)—green.

Thin-layer Chromatography. *System TD*—Rf 00; *system TE*—Rf 00; *system TF*—Rf 00; *system TT*—Rf 02; *system TU*—Rf 04; *system TV*—Rf 04.

High Pressure Liquid Chromatography. *System HU*—k′ 14.0.

Ultraviolet Spectrum. Aqueous acid—282 nm; aqueous alkali—260 nm ($A_1^1 = 600$ a); methanol—260 nm ($A_1^1 = 497$ a), 288 nm ($A_1^1 = 648$ a).

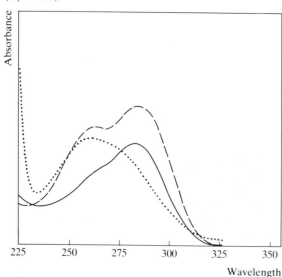

Infra-red Spectrum. Principal peaks at wavenumbers 1532, 1142, 1084, 1710, 1585, 1560 (KBr disk).

Mass Spectrum. Principal peaks at m/z 92, 156, 191, 65, 108, 76, 104, 50.

Disposition in the Body. Only about 5% of a dose is absorbed after oral administration and blood concentrations are therefore very low compared to other sulphonamides, usually less than 15 µg/ml. It is slowly hydrolysed to sulphathiazole in the gastrointestinal tract.

Dose. 2 to 12 g daily.

Physostigmine   *Anticholinesterase*

Synonyms. Eserine; Physostigmina.

$(3aS,8aR)$ - 1,2,3,3a,8,8a - Hexahydro - 1,3a,8 - trimethylpyrrolo [2,3-*b*]indol-5-yl methylcarbamate
$C_{15}H_{21}N_3O_2 = 275.3$
CAS—57-47-6

An alkaloid obtained from the calabar bean, the seed of *Physostigma venenosum* (Leguminosae).

Colourless crystals, or a white microcrystalline powder. M.p. not lower than 103°.

Soluble 1 in 75 of water, 1 in 10 of ethanol, 1 in 1 of chloroform, and 1 in 30 of ether.

Physostigmine, its salts and their aqueous solutions become red on exposure to heat, light, air, and on contact with traces of metals, owing to the formation of rubreserine; the change is less rapid in acid solution.

Physostigmine Salicylate
Synonym. Eserine Salicylate
Proprietary Names. Antilirium; Fisostin.
$C_{15}H_{21}N_3O_2,C_7H_6O_3 = 413.5$
CAS—57-64-7
Colourless or white crystals or white powder. M.p. 184° to 186°.
Soluble 1 in 75 to 1 in 90 of water, 1 in 25 of ethanol, 1 in 6 of chloroform, and 1 in 250 of ether.

Physostigmine Sulphate
Synonym. Eserine Sulphate
$(C_{15}H_{21}N_3O_2)_2,H_2SO_4 = 648.8$
CAS—64-47-1
A white deliquescent, microcrystalline powder. M.p. 143° to 147°.
Soluble 1 in less than 1 of water and of ethanol; soluble in chloroform; very slightly soluble in ether.

Dissociation Constant. pK_a 1.8, 7.9 (25°).

Partition Coefficient. Log P (octanol), 1.6.

Colour Test. Mandelin's Test—yellow-brown.

Thin-layer Chromatography. *System TA*—Rf 55; *system TB*—Rf 12; *system TC*—Rf 36. (*Acidified potassium permanganate solution, positive.*)

Gas Chromatography. *System GA*—RI 1804, 2035, and 2190.

High Pressure Liquid Chromatography. *System HA*—k′ 2.6.

Ultraviolet Spectrum. Aqueous acid—246 nm ($A_1^1 = 462$ a), 302 nm.

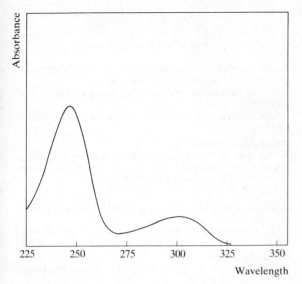

Infra-red Spectrum. Principal peaks at wavenumbers 1724, 1243, 1200, 1495, 1120, 1162 (KBr disk).

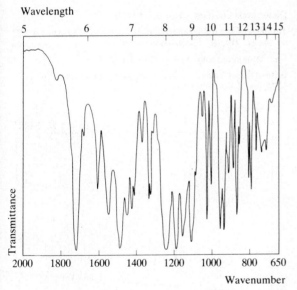

Mass Spectrum. Principal peaks at m/z 218, 174, 160, 161, 275, 219, 175, 162.

Quantification. HIGH PRESSURE LIQUID CHROMATOGRAPHY. In plasma: sensitivity 500 pg/ml, electrochemical detection—R. Whelpton, *J. Chromat.*, 1983, *272*; *Biomed. Appl.*, *23*, 216–220.

Disposition in the Body. Readily absorbed after oral or subcutaneous administration and from mucous membranes. Physostigmine readily penetrates the central nervous system. It is rapidly hydrolysed by cholinesterases and most of a dose is destroyed in 2 hours. Very little is excreted in the urine.

THERAPEUTIC CONCENTRATION.
After a single subcutaneous injection of 1 mg of physostigmine salicylate (equivalent to 0.67 mg base) to one subject, a peak plasma concentration of 0.0036 µg/ml was achieved after 15 minutes (R. Whelpton, *ibid.*).

After a single oral dose of 4 mg of physostigmine salicylate to one subject, a peak plasma concentration of about 0.001 µg/ml was attained in 0.75 hour (M. Gibson *et al.*, *Lancet*, 1985, *1*, 695–696).

TOXICITY. Fatalities have occurred following ingestion of 6 mg of physostigmine orally and administration of 1.2 mg intravenously. The ingestion of 6 calabar beans by a child has proved fatal.

Physostigmine Aminoxide   *Anticholinesterase*

Synonyms. Eseridine; Eserine Aminoxide; Physostigmine *N*-Oxide.
$C_{15}H_{21}N_3O_3 = 291.3$
CAS—25573-43-7
M.p. 129°.
Practically **insoluble** in water; soluble in ethanol, chloroform, and ether.

Physostigmine Aminoxide Salicylate
Synonym. Physostigmine *N*-Oxide Salicylate
Proprietary Name. Génésérine 3
$C_{15}H_{21}N_3O_3,C_7H_6O_3 = 429.5$
Crystals which become red on exposure to heat, light, and air. M.p. 90°.

Thin-layer Chromatography. *System TA*—Rf 31. (*Acidified potassium permanganate solution*, positive.)

Ultraviolet Spectrum. Aqueous acid—241 nm ($A_1^1 = 411$ b), 300 nm.

Infra-red Spectrum. Principal peaks at wavenumbers 1720, 1250, 1204, 1268, 1495, 1289 (KBr disk).

Dose. Physostigmine aminoxide salicylate has been given in doses of 9 mg daily.

Phytomenadione   *Vitamin*

Synonyms. Methylphytylnaphthochinonum; Phylloquinone; Phytonadione; Vitamin K_1.
Proprietary Names. Aquamephyton; Konakion; Mephyton.
2-Methyl-3-phytyl-1,4-naphthoquinone
$C_{31}H_{46}O_2 = 450.7$
CAS—84-80-0

A clear, deep yellow, very viscous oil which is stable in air but decomposes on exposure to light. Sp. gr. about 0.967. Refractive index 1.5255 to 1.5285.
Practically **insoluble** in water; soluble 1 in 70 of ethanol; more soluble in dehydrated alcohol; freely soluble in chloroform and ether.

Colour Test. Methanolic Potassium Hydroxide—green-yellow → violet → brown.

Gas Chromatography. *System GA*—RI 3287.

Ultraviolet Spectrum. Methanol—244 nm, 249 nm ($A_1^1 = 394$ a), 263 nm ($A_1^1 = 350$ b), 270 nm ($A_1^1 = 349$ a), 331 nm ($A_1^1 = 68$ a).

Infra-red Spectrum. Principal peaks at wavenumbers 1285, 1650, 714, 1587, 690, 1610.

Wavelength

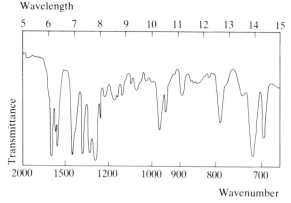

Quantification. HIGH PRESSURE LIQUID CHROMATOGRAPHY. In plasma: sensitivity 500 pg, UV detection—M. J. Shearer *et al.*, *Lancet*, 1982, *2*, 460–463.

Disposition in the Body. Absorbed from the gastro-intestinal tract in the presence of bile. Rapidly metabolised and excreted as conjugates in the urine, bile and faeces.
Endogenous plasma concentrations are usually in the range 0.0001 to 0.0007 µg/ml.

HALF-LIFE. Plasma half-life, about 2 hours.

Dose. Initially 2.5 to 25 mg by subcutaneous or intramuscular injection, or 5 to 20 mg by mouth.

Picrotoxin   *Respiratory Stimulant*

Synonym. Cocculin
$C_{30}H_{34}O_{13} = 602.6$
CAS—124-87-8
An active principle from the seeds of *Anamirta cocculus* (= *A. paniculata*) (Menispermaceae). The fruits of *A. cocculus* are sometimes known as 'fish berries' or 'Levant berries'.
Colourless, flexible, shining prismatic crystals or white micro-crystalline powder. M.p. about 199°.
Soluble 1 in 350 of water and 1 in 16 of ethanol; soluble in glacial acetic acid and solutions of acids and alkali hydroxides; slightly soluble in chloroform and ether.

Colour Tests. Dissolve in *sulphuric acid*—yellow → red-brown (slow). Add 1 drop of *fuming nitric acid* to the material—blue-green, discharged by excess acid.

Infra-red Spectrum. Principal peaks at wavenumbers 1780, 1755, 1795, 1123, 990, 1162 (KBr disk).

Mass Spectrum. Principal peaks at *m/z* 95, 55, 41, 43, 59, 27, 39, 67.

Dose. Picrotoxin was formerly given in doses of 3 to 6 mg intravenously.

Pilocarpine   *Parasympathomimetic*

Proprietary Name. Ocusert Pilo
(3S,4R) - 3 - Ethyldihydro - 4 - [(1 - methyl - 1*H* - imidazol - 5 - yl) - methyl]furan-2(3*H*)-one
$C_{11}H_{16}N_2O_2 = 208.3$
CAS—92-13-7

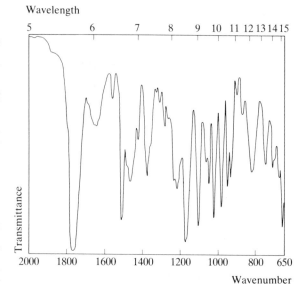

An alkaloid obtained from the leaflets of *Pilocarpus microphyllus* (Rutaceae) and other species of *Pilocarpus*.
A viscous, hygroscopic, colourless, oily liquid or crystals. M.p. about 34°.
Soluble in water, ethanol, and chloroform; sparingly soluble in ether.

Pilocarpine Hydrochloride
Proprietary Names. Adsorbocarpine; Isopto Carpine; Mi-Pilo; Neutra-carpine; Pilocar; Pilomann; Pilopt; Pilotonina; PV Carpine; Sno Pilo; Spersacarpin(e). It is an ingredient of E-Pilo and PE.
$C_{11}H_{16}N_2O_2,HCl = 244.7$
CAS—54-71-7
Hygroscopic, colourless crystals or white crystalline powder. M.p. 199° to 205°.
Soluble 1 in less than 1 of water, 1 in 3 of ethanol, and 1 in 360 of chloroform; practically insoluble in ether.

Pilocarpine Nitrate
Proprietary Names. Dulcicarpine; Marticarpine; Miopos; Pilo; Pilopos; PV Carpine; Vistacarpin.
$C_{11}H_{16}N_2O_2,HNO_3 = 271.3$
CAS—148-72-1
Colourless crystals or white crystalline powder. M.p. 171° to 179°, with decomposition.
Soluble 1 in 8 of water and 1 in 160 of ethanol; practically insoluble in chloroform and ether.

Dissociation Constant. pK_a 1.6, 7.1 (15°).

Thin-layer Chromatography. *System TA*—Rf 53; *system TB*—Rf 00; *system TC*—Rf 32. (*Acidified iodoplatinate solution*, positive.)

Gas Chromatography. *System GA*—RI 2014.

Infra-red Spectrum. Principal peaks at wavenumbers 1752, 1168, 1104, 660, 1505, 1020 (thin film).

Wavelength

Mass Spectrum. Principal peaks at *m/z* 95, 96, 42, 109, 41, 208, 54, 39.

Use. Pilocarpine hydrochloride is used as a 0.5 to 5% ophthalmic solution.

Piminodine

Narcotic Analgesic

Ethyl 1-(3-anilinopropyl)-4-phenylpiperidine-4-carboxylate
$C_{23}H_{30}N_2O_2 = 366.5$
CAS—13495-09-5

$$CH_2 \cdot [CH_2]_2 \cdot NH \cdot C_6H_5$$

$$C_6H_5 \quad CO \cdot O \cdot C_2H_5$$

Piminodine Esylate

Synonym. Piminodine Ethanesulphonate
$C_{23}H_{30}N_2O_2, C_2H_6O_3S = 476.6$
CAS—7081-52-9
A colourless crystalline powder. M.p. 128° to 135°.
Slightly **soluble** in water and ether; soluble 1 in 6 of ethanol and 1 in 2 of chloroform.

Colour Test. Marquis Test—orange.

Thin-layer Chromatography. *System TA*—Rf 67. (*Acidified iodoplatinate solution*, positive; *acidified potassium permanganate solution*, positive.)

High Pressure Liquid Chromatography. *System HA*—k' 1.0.

Ultraviolet Spectrum. Aqueous acid—247 nm, 253 nm, 257 nm, 263 nm.

Mass Spectrum. Principal peaks at m/z 246, 45, 42, 366, 58, 57, 43, 106.

Dose. Piminodine esylate has been given in doses of 25 to 50 mg by mouth and 10 to 20 mg parenterally.

Pimozide

Tranquilliser

Proprietary Names. Opiran; Orap.
1-{1-[4,4-Bis(4-fluorophenyl)butyl]-4-piperidyl}benzimidazolin-2-one
$C_{28}H_{29}F_2N_3O = 461.6$
CAS—2062-78-4

$$CH_2 \cdot CH_2 \cdot CH_2 \cdot CH$$

A colourless microcrystalline powder. M.p. 214° to 218°.
Practically **insoluble** in water; soluble 1 in 140 of ethanol, 1 in 5 of chloroform, and 1 in 500 of ether.

Dissociation Constant. pK$_a$ 7.3.

Colour Tests. Koppanyi–Zwikker Test—violet; Liebermann's Test—brown; Mandelin's Test—brown; Marquis Test—violet.

Thin-layer Chromatography. *System TA*—Rf 71; *system TB*—Rf 04; *system TC*—Rf 60. (*Acidified iodoplatinate solution*, positive.)

Gas Chromatography. *System GA*—not eluted.

High Pressure Liquid Chromatography. *System HA*—k' 0.7.

Ultraviolet Spectrum. Acid isopropyl alcohol—273 nm, 280 nm ($A_1^1 = 145$ a).

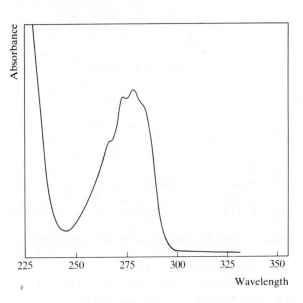

Infra-red Spectrum. Principal peaks at wavenumbers 1695, 1505, 753, 1220, 1230, 825 (KBr disk).

Mass Spectrum. Principal peaks at m/z 230, 187, 42, 217, 83, 82, 461, 96.

Quantification. GAS CHROMATOGRAPHY. In plasma: sensitivity 30 ng/ml, FID—M. P. Quaglio *et al.*, *Boll. chim.-farm.*, 1982, *121*, 276-284.

HIGH PRESSURE LIQUID CHROMATOGRAPHY. In plasma: sensitivity <5 ng/ml, fluorescence detection—Y. Miyao *et al.*, *J. Chromat.*, 1983, *275*; *Biomed. Appl.*, *26*, 443-449.

RADIOIMMUNOASSAY. In plasma: detection limit 50 pg—L. J. M. Michiels *et al.*, *Life Sci.*, 1975, *16*, 937-944.

Disposition in the Body. Readily but slowly absorbed after oral administration. About 40% of a dose is excreted in the urine in 4 days. Two metabolites which have been identified in the urine are 4-bis(4-fluorophenyl)butyric acid and 1-(4-piperidyl)-benzimidazolin-2-one. Very little unchanged drug is excreted in the urine. Both unchanged drug and the butyric acid metabolite are eliminated in the faeces.

THERAPEUTIC CONCENTRATION.
Following a single oral dose of 6 mg to 9 subjects, a mean peak plasma concentration of about 0.004 µg/ml was attained in 4 to 12 hours (mean 8) (R. G. McCreadie *et al.*, *Br. J. clin. Pharmac.*, 1979, *7*, 533-534).

HALF-LIFE. Plasma half-life, about 2 days.

NOTE. For a review of pimozide see R. M. Pinder *et al.*, *Drugs*, 1976, *12*, 1-39.

Dose. 2 to 20 mg daily.

Pindolol
Beta-adrenoceptor Blocking Agent

Synonyms. Prindolol; Prinodolol.
Proprietary Names. Visken. It is an ingredient of Viskaldix.

1-(Indol-4-yloxy)-3-isopropylaminopropan-2-ol
$C_{14}H_{20}N_2O_2 = 248.3$
CAS—13523-86-9

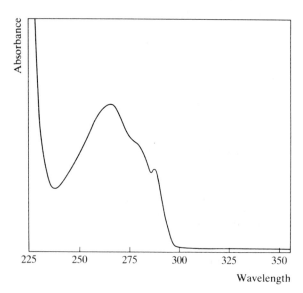

A white crystalline powder. M.p. 171° to 173°.
Practically **insoluble** in water; slightly soluble in dehydrated alcohol and chloroform; sparingly soluble in methanol.

Dissociation Constant. pK_a 9.7 (24°).

Partition Coefficient. Log *P* (octanol/pH 7.0), −0.9.

Colour Tests. *p*-Dimethylaminobenzaldehyde—red/violet; Liebermann's Test—blue-green; Mandelin's Test—green; Marquis Test—yellow → brown.

Thin-layer Chromatography. *System TA*—Rf 49; *system TB*—Rf 02; *system TC*—Rf 05.

Gas Chromatography. *System GA*—RI 2260.

High Pressure Liquid Chromatography. *System HA*—k′ 1.2.

Ultraviolet Spectrum. Aqueous acid—264 nm ($A_1^1 = 292$ b), 287 nm; methanol—264 nm ($A_1^1 = 330$ a), 287 nm ($A_1^1 = 182$ a). No alkaline shift.

Wavelength

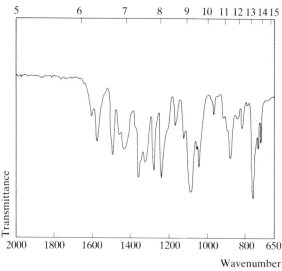

Mass Spectrum. Principal peaks at *m/z* 72, 133, 30, 116, 248, 134, 56, 41.

Quantification. GAS CHROMATOGRAPHY (CAPILLARY COLUMN). In plasma: sensitivity 500 pg/ml, ECD—M. Guerret, *J. Chromat.*, 1980, *221*; *Biomed. Appl.*, *10*, 387–392.

HIGH PRESSURE LIQUID CHROMATOGRAPHY. In plasma: sensitivity 2 ng/ml, fluorescence detection—M. Bangah *et al.*, *J. Chromat.*, 1980, *183*; *Biomed. Appl.*, *9*, 255–259.

Disposition in the Body. Well absorbed after oral administration. Metabolised by conjugation with glucuronic acid and sulphate. About 20 to 30% of an oral dose is excreted in the urine in 24 hours as unchanged drug.

THERAPEUTIC CONCENTRATION.

After a single oral dose of 5 mg given to 12 subjects, peak plasma concentrations of 0.02 to 0.08 μg/ml (mean 0.04) were attained in 0.5 to 3 hours (R. Gugler *et al.*, *Eur. J. clin. Pharmac.*, 1974, *7*, 17–24).

After daily oral dosing of 6 subjects with 5 mg three times a day, a mean steady-state plasma concentration of 0.015 μg/ml was reported (R. Gugler and G. Bodem, *Eur. J. clin. Pharmac.*, 1978, *13*, 13–16).

HALF-LIFE. Plasma half-life, 2 to 4 hours.

VOLUME OF DISTRIBUTION. About 1 to 2 litres/kg.

CLEARANCE. Plasma clearance, about 7 ml/min/kg.

DISTRIBUTION IN BLOOD. Plasma: whole blood ratio, 1.5.

PROTEIN BINDING. In plasma, 40 to 70%.

NOTE. For a review of the pharmacokinetics of the beta-blocking agents see G. Johnsson and C.-G. Regårdh, *Clin. Pharmacokinet.*, 1976, *1*, 233–263.

Dose. Up to 45 mg daily.

Infra-red Spectrum. Principal peaks at wavenumbers 768, 1096, 1250, 1288, 1053, 890.

Pipamperone
Tranquilliser

Synonym. Floropipamide

1-[3-(4-Fluorobenzoyl)propyl]-4-piperidinopiperidine-4-carboxamide
$C_{21}H_{30}FN_3O_2 = 375.5$
CAS—1893-33-0

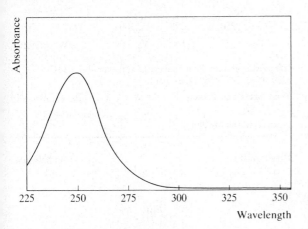

Pipamperone Hydrochloride

Proprietary Names. Dipiperon; Piperonil.
$C_{21}H_{30}FN_3O_2,2HCl = 448.4$
CAS—2448-68-2
Crystals. M.p. 125° to 126°.

Partition Coefficient. Log *P* (octanol), 2.4.

Thin-layer Chromatography. *System TA*—Rf 56; *system TB*—Rf 01; *system TC*—Rf 12. (*Acidified potassium permanganate solution*, positive.)

Gas Chromatography. *System GA*—RI 3070.

Ultraviolet Spectrum. Aqueous acid—248 nm ($A_1^1 = 315$ a).

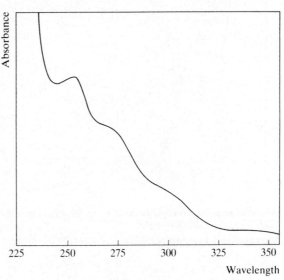

Infra-red Spectrum. Principal peaks at wavenumbers 1660, 1685, 1600, 1239, 1157, 1212 (KBr disk).

Mass Spectrum. Principal peaks at *m/z* 165, 138, 331, 123, 110, 194, 42, 41.

Dose. The equivalent of 120 to 360 mg of pipamperone daily.

Pipazethate   *Cough Suppressant*

Synonym. Piperestazine
2 - (2 - Piperidinoethoxy)ethyl pyrido[3,2 - *b*][1,4]benzothiazine-10-carboxylate
$C_{21}H_{25}N_3O_3S = 399.5$
CAS—2167-85-3

Pipazethate Hydrochloride

Proprietary Names. Selvigon; Selvjgon.
$C_{21}H_{25}N_3O_3S,HCl = 436.0$
CAS—6056-11-7
A white crystalline powder. M.p. about 162°.
Very **soluble** in water; soluble in ethanol and methanol.

Colour Tests. Aromaticity (Method 2)—colourless/yellow; Liebermann's Test—brown (→ red at 100°).

Thin-layer Chromatography. *System TA*—Rf 47; *system TB*—Rf 15; *system TC*—Rf 13. (*Acidified iodoplatinate solution*, positive.)

Gas Chromatography. *System GA*—RI 2037.

High Pressure Liquid Chromatography. *System HA*—k' 5.4.

Ultraviolet Spectrum. Aqueous acid—251 nm ($A_1^1 = 210$ a).

Infra-red Spectrum. Principal peaks at wavenumbers 1717, 1225, 1315, 1300, 1095, 1050 (KBr disk).

Mass Spectrum. Principal peaks at *m/z* 98, 111, 99, 199, 41, 288, 200, 55.

Dose. Pipazethate hydrochloride has been given in doses of 60 to 120 mg daily.

Pipenzolate Bromide   *Anticholinergic*

Synonym. Pipenzolate Methobromide
Proprietary Names. Piper; Piptal. It is an ingredient of Piptalin.
3-Benziloyloxy-1-ethyl-1-methylpiperidinium bromide
$C_{22}H_{28}BrNO_3 = 434.4$
CAS—13473-38-6 (pipenzolate); *125-51-9* (bromide)

A white crystalline powder. M.p. about 180°.
Freely **soluble** in water.

Colour Tests. The following tests are performed on pipenzolate nitrate (see p. 128): Mandelin's Test—orange → green; Marquis Test—orange → green → blue.

Thin-layer Chromatography. *System TA*—Rf 04. (*Acidified iodoplatinate solution*, positive.)

Ultraviolet Spectrum. Aqueous acid—252 nm, 258 nm ($A_1^1 = 11$ a), 262 nm.

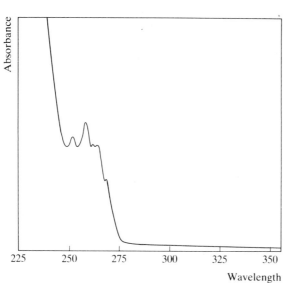

Wavelength

Infra-red Spectrum. Principal peaks at wavenumbers 1726, 698, 1220, 1160, 763, 1055 (KBr disk).

Mass Spectrum. Principal peaks at m/z 105, 111, 77, 96, 97, 183, 42, 51.

Dose. Usually 20 to 25 mg daily.

Piperacetazine   *Tranquilliser*

Proprietary Name. Quide

10 - {3 - [4 - (2 - Hydroxyethyl)piperidino]propyl}phenothiazin - 2-yl methyl ketone
$C_{24}H_{30}N_2O_2S = 410.6$
CAS—3819-00-9

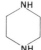

A yellow granular powder. M.p. 102° to 106°.

Practically **insoluble** in water; soluble 1 in 11 of ethanol, 1 in 1.3 of chloroform, and 1 in 1200 of ether.

Colour Tests. Formaldehyde–Sulphuric Acid—blue-violet; Forrest Reagent—red; FPN Reagent—brown-orange; Mandelin's Test—green → red → violet; Marquis Test—red; Sulphuric Acid—yellow → red.

Thin-layer Chromatography. *System TA*—Rf 56; *system TB*—Rf 06; *system TC*—Rf 19. (*Acidified iodoplatinate solution*, positive.)

Gas Chromatography. *System GA*—not eluted.

High Pressure Liquid Chromatography. *System HA*—k' 1.9.

Ultraviolet Spectrum. Aqueous acid—243 nm, 278 nm.

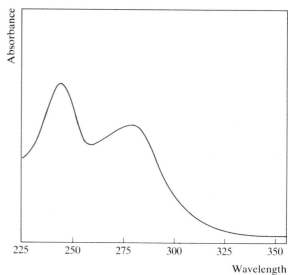

Wavelength

Infra-red Spectrum. Principal peaks at wavenumbers 1675, 1222, 1269, 1592, 748, 1560 (KBr disk).

Mass Spectrum. Principal peaks at m/z 142, 170, 44, 410, 42, 143, 43, 41.

Dose. 20 to 160 mg daily.

Piperazine   *Anthelmintic*

$C_4H_{10}N_2 = 86.14$
CAS—110-85-0

Crystals. M.p. 106°.
Soluble in water and ethanol; practically insoluble in ether.

Piperazine Adipate

Proprietary Names. Divermex; Entacyl; Ismiverm; Vermicompren.
$C_4H_{10}N_2, C_6H_{10}O_4 = 232.3$
CAS—142-88-1
A white crystalline powder. M.p. about 250°, with decomposition.
Soluble 1 in 18 of water; practically insoluble in ethanol, chloroform, and ether.

Piperazine Calcium Edetate

Synonym. Piperazine Calcium Edathamil
$C_4H_{10}N_2, C_{10}H_{14}CaN_2O_8 = 416.4$
CAS—12002-30-1
Freely **soluble** in water; very slightly soluble in ethanol and chloroform; practically insoluble in ether.

Piperazine Citrate

Synonym. Hydrous Tripiperazine Dicitrate
Proprietary Names. Antepar; Ascalix; Citrazine; Helmezine (elixir); Pipérol Fort.

$(C_4H_{10}N_2)_3,2C_6H_8O_7,xH_2O = 642.7$ (anhydrous)
CAS—144-29-6 (anhydrous); *41372-10-5* (hydrate)
A fine, white, crystalline or granular powder. M.p. about 190°.
Soluble 1 in 1.5 of water; practically insoluble in ethanol and ether.

Piperazine Hydrate
Synonyms. Diethylenediamine; Hexahydropyrazine; Piperazidine.
Proprietary Names. Antelmina; Antepar; Eraverm; Tasnon; Uvilon.
$C_4H_{10}N_2,6H_2O = 194.2$
CAS—142-63-2
Colourless, glassy, deliquescent crystals. M.p. about 43°.
Soluble 1 in 3 of water and 1 in 1 of ethanol; very slightly soluble in ether.

Piperazine Phosphate
Proprietary Names. Antepar; Helmezine (tablets); Tasnon. It is an ingredient of Pripsen.
$C_4H_{10}N_2,H_3PO_4,H_2O = 202.1$
CAS—14538-56-8 (anhydrous); *18534-18-4* (monohydrate)
A white crystalline powder.
Soluble 1 in about 60 of water; practically insoluble in ethanol, chloroform, and ether; soluble in dilute hydrochloric acid.

Dissociation Constant. pK_a 5.7, 9.8 (20°).

Partition Coefficient. Log *P* (octanol), −1.2.

Colour Test. Simon's Test—blue.

Thin-layer Chromatography. *System TA*—Rf 05; *system TB*—Rf 01; *system TC*—Rf 01. (*Acidified iodoplatinate solution*, positive.)

Gas Chromatography. *System GA*—RI 813.

Ultraviolet Spectrum. No significant absorption, 230 to 360 nm.

Infra-red Spectrum. Principal peaks at wavenumbers 1592, 955, 870, 1080, 1055, 1115 (piperazine citrate, KBr disk).

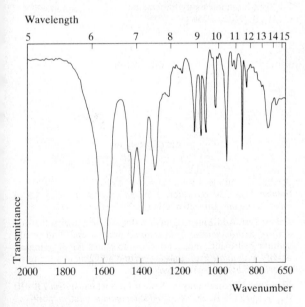

Mass Spectrum. Principal peaks at *m/z* 44, 100, 41, 60, 29, 27, 30, 86 (piperazine adipate).

Quantification. COLORIMETRY. In urine—S. Hanna and A. Tang, *J. pharm. Sci.*, 1973, **62**, 2024–2025.

Disposition in the Body. Readily absorbed after oral administration and excreted in the urine as unchanged drug and metabolites. There is wide variation in the rate of excretion between individuals, 15 to 75% of a dose being excreted in 24 hours.

TOXICITY. Toxic effects are rare and are usually due to accumulation after large doses. Three children had symptoms of toxicity after doses of 6, 9, and 12 g but they subsequently recovered.

Dose. The equivalent of 4 g of piperazine hydrate as a single dose, or 2 g daily for 7 days.

Piperidolate   *Anticholinergic*

1-Ethyl-3-piperidyl diphenylacetate
$C_{21}H_{25}NO_2 = 323.4$
CAS—82-98-4

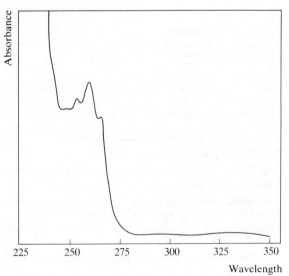

A liquid.

Piperidolate Hydrochloride
Proprietary Name. Dactil
$C_{21}H_{25}NO_2,HCl = 359.9$
CAS—129-77-1
A white or cream-coloured powder. M.p. 194° to 198°.
Soluble 1 in about 18 of water, 1 in about 52 of ethanol, 1 in about 4 of chloroform, and 1 in about 5 of methanol.

Colour Tests. Liebermann's Test—orange-brown; Mandelin's Test—brown; Marquis Test—orange.

Thin-layer Chromatography. *System TA*—Rf 69; *system TB*—Rf 55; *system TC*—Rf 81. (*Dragendorff spray*, positive; *acidified iodoplatinate solution*, positive; *Marquis reagent*, yellow.)

Gas Chromatography. *System GA*—RI 2318; *system GF*—RI 2660.

High Pressure Liquid Chromatography. *System HA*—k' 1.7.

Ultraviolet Spectrum. Aqueous acid—252 nm, 258 nm ($A_1^1 = 13.4$ a), 264 nm. No alkaline shift.

Infra-red Spectrum. Principal peaks at wavenumbers 1192, 1715, 1163, 1101, 700, 1149 (piperidolate hydrochloride, K Br disk).

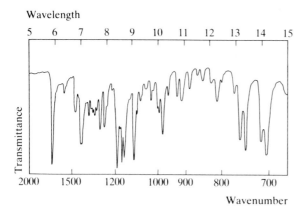

Wavelength

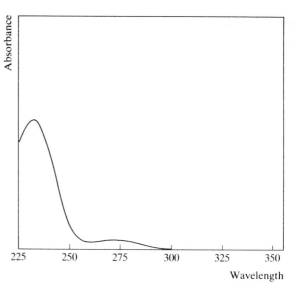

Wavelength

Mass Spectrum. Principal peaks at m/z 111, 96, 167, 112, 165, 71, 43, 42.

Dose. 200 mg of piperidolate hydrochloride daily.

Piperocaine   *Local Anaesthetic*

3-(2-Methylpiperidino)propyl benzoate
$C_{16}H_{23}NO_2 = 261.4$
CAS—136-82-3

CH$_2$·[CH$_2$]$_2$·O·CO·C$_6$H$_5$

CH$_3$

Piperocaine Hydrochloride
Proprietary Name. Metycaine Hydrochloride
$C_{16}H_{23}NO_2,HCl = 297.8$
CAS—24561-10-2
Small white crystals or white crystalline powder. M.p. 172° to 175°.
Soluble 1 in 1.5 of water and 1 in 4.5 of ethanol; soluble in chloroform; practically insoluble in ether.

Thin-layer Chromatography. *System TA*—Rf 55; *system TB*—Rf 53; *system TC*—Rf 37; *system TL*—Rf 27. (*Dragendorff spray*, positive; *acidified iodoplatinate solution*, positive.)

Gas Chromatography. *System GA*—RI 1980.

High Pressure Liquid Chromatography. *System HQ*—k' 4.59.

Ultraviolet Spectrum. Aqueous acid—231 nm, 274 nm.

Infra-red Spectrum. Principal peaks at wavenumbers 1278, 1703, 711, 1115, 1310, 1040 (piperocaine hydrochloride, K Br disk).

Mass Spectrum. Principal peaks at m/z 112, 246, 105, 77, 55, 41, 44, 247.

Use. Piperocaine hydrochloride is used in concentrations of 0.5 to 10%.

Pipobroman   *Antineoplastic*

Proprietary Names. Vercite 25; Vercyte.
1,4-Bis(3-bromopropionyl)piperazine
$C_{10}H_{16}Br_2N_2O_2 = 356.1$
CAS—54-91-1

CO·CH$_2$·CH$_2$·Br

N

N

CO·CH$_2$·CH$_2$·Br

A white crystalline powder. M.p. 101° to 105°.
Soluble 1 in 230 of water, 1 in 35 of ethanol, 1 in 4.8 of chloroform, and 1 in 530 of ether; soluble in acetone.

Colour Test. Add 2 mg to 2 ml of water and heat to dissolve; add 2 ml of *hydroxylamine hydrochloride solution* and 2 ml of 3M sodium hydroxide, mix, and allow to stand for 30 minutes; acidify with *dilute hydrochloric acid* and add 2 ml of a 9% ferric chloride solution—red-orange.

Thin-layer Chromatography. *System TA*—Rf 66; *system TB*—Rf 02; *system TC*—Rf 58. (*Acidified iodoplatinate solution*, positive.)

Gas Chromatography. *System GA*—RI 1811.

Ultraviolet Spectrum. No significant absorption, 230 to 360 nm.

Infra-red Spectrum. Principal peaks at wavenumbers 1626, 1219, 1003, 1266, 923, 892 (K Br disk).

Mass Spectrum. Principal peaks at m/z 85, 56, 69, 55, 27, 44, 42, 109.

Dose. Initially 1 to 1.5 mg/kg daily, by mouth; maintenance, 7 to 175 mg daily.

Pipothiazine

Tranquilliser

Synonym. Pipotiazine
Proprietary Name. Piportil

10-{3-[4-(2-Hydroxyethyl)piperidino]propyl} - *NN* - dimethyl-phenothiazine-2-sulphonamide
$C_{24}H_{33}N_3O_3S_2 = 475.7$
CAS—39860-99-6

Pipothiazine Palmitate

Proprietary Names. Piportil Depot; Piportil L4.
$C_{40}H_{63}N_3O_4S_2 = 714.1$
CAS—37517-26-3
A pale yellow crystalline powder.
Practically **insoluble** in water; sparingly soluble in ethanol; freely soluble in chloroform and ether.

Ultraviolet Spectrum. Pipothiazine palmitate: ethanol—265 nm $(A_1^1 = 500 \text{ b})$, 315 nm.

Infra-red Spectrum. Principal peaks at wavenumbers 1165, 1735, 710, 745, 1250, 955 (pipothiazine palmitate, solution in carbon tetrachloride-carbon disulphide).

Mass Spectrum. Principal peaks at *m/z* 142, 44, 140, 42, 198, 170, 41, 96.

Quantification. GAS CHROMATOGRAPHY. In plasma: detection limit 10 ng/ml, ECD—S. F. Cooper and Y. D. Lapierre, *J. Chromat.*, 1981, *222*; *Biomed. Appl.*, *11*, 291–296.

HIGH PRESSURE LIQUID CHROMATOGRAPHY. In plasma or urine: sensitivity 250 pg/ml for plasma and 2 ng/ml for urine, fluorescence detection—Y. Le Roux *et al.*, *J. Chromat.*, 1982, *230*; *Biomed. Appl.*, *19*, 401–408.

Disposition in the Body. Pipothiazine palmitate is very slowly absorbed from the site of intramuscular injections and gradually releases pipothiazine into the body. After oral administration of pipothiazine, about 1% of a dose is excreted in the urine unchanged in 24 hours.

THERAPEUTIC CONCENTRATION.
Following monthly intramuscular injections of 25 to 112.5 mg to 5 subjects, plasma concentrations of 0.018 to 0.058 µg/ml (mean 0.038) were reported immediately before a dose (S. F. Cooper and Y. D. Lapierre, *J. Chromat.*, 1981, *222*; *Biomed. Appl.*, *11*, 291–296).

Dose. Usually 10 to 20 mg of pipothiazine daily, by mouth. Pipothiazine palmitate is given intramuscularly in doses of 25 to 200 mg, at intervals of about 4 weeks.

Pipoxolan

Antispasmodic

5,5-Diphenyl-2-(2-piperidinoethyl)-1,3-dioxolan-4-one
$C_{22}H_{25}NO_3 = 351.4$
CAS—23744-24-3

Pipoxolan Hydrochloride

Proprietary Name. Rowapraxin
$C_{22}H_{25}NO_3,HCl = 387.9$
CAS—18174-58-8
A white crystalline powder. M.p. 207° to 209°.
Soluble in water.

Colour Tests. Liebermann's Test—brown; Mandelin's Test—green → brown; Marquis Test—violet → grey; Sulphuric Acid—red.

Thin-layer Chromatography. *System TA*—Rf 77; *system TB*—Rf 53; *system TC*—Rf 68. (*Acidified iodoplatinate solution*, positive.)

Infra-red Spectrum. Principal peaks at wavenumbers 1786, 1176, 1205, 1111, 1149, 698 (KBr disk).

Mass Spectrum. Principal peaks at *m/z* 98, 194, 166, 157, 55, 42, 165, 99.

Dose. Pipoxolan hydrochloride has been given in doses of 20 to 90 mg daily.

Pipradrol

Central Stimulant

α-(2-Piperidyl)benzhydrol
$C_{18}H_{21}NO = 267.4$
CAS—467-60-7

Pipradrol Hydrochloride

Proprietary Name. Detaril
$C_{18}H_{21}NO,HCl = 303.8$
CAS—71-78-3
Small white crystals or white crystalline powder. M.p. about 290°, with decomposition.
Soluble 1 in 30 of water, 1 in 35 of ethanol, 1 in 1000 of chloroform, and 1 in 8 of methanol; practically insoluble in ether.

Colour Test. Marquis Test—yellow-orange.

Thin-layer Chromatography. *System TA*—Rf 54; *system TB*—Rf 59; *system TC*—Rf 38. (*Dragendorff spray*, positive; *acidified iodoplatinate solution*, positive; *Marquis reagent*, red-brown; *ninhydrin spray*, positive.)

Gas Chromatography. *System GA*—RI 2145; *system GB*—RI 2215; *system GC*—RI 2478.

High Pressure Liquid Chromatography. *System HA*—k' 1.2; *system HC*—k' 0.69.

Ultraviolet Spectrum. Aqueous acid—252 nm, 258 nm $(A_1^1 = 17 \text{ a})$. No alkaline shift. (See below)

Infra-red Spectrum. Principal peaks at wavenumbers 701, 740, 690, 1585, 1300, 1065 (pipradrol hydrochloride, KBr disk).

Mass Spectrum. Principal peaks at *m/z* 84, 56, 85, 77, 105, 55, 30, 42.

Dose. Pipradrol hydrochloride has been given in doses of 2 to 6 mg daily.

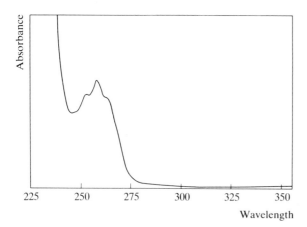

Pirenzepine

Treatment of Gastric Ulcers

5,11 - Dihydro - 11 - (4 - methylpiperazin - 1 - ylacetyl)pyrido[2, 3-*b*][1,4]benzodiazepin-6-one
$C_{19}H_{21}N_5O_2 = 351.4$
CAS—28797-61-7

Pirenzepine Hydrochloride

Proprietary Name. Gastrozepin
$C_{19}H_{21}N_5O_2,2HCl = 424.3$
CAS—29868-97-1

A white crystalline powder. M.p. 248° to 253°, with decomposition. Freely **soluble** in water; practically insoluble in ether; very slightly soluble in methanol.

Dissociation Constant. pK_a 2.1, 8.1.

High Pressure Liquid Chromatography. *System HA*—k' 2.7.

Ultraviolet Spectrum. Aqueous acid—280 nm ($A_1^1 = 237$ a); aqueous alkali—297 nm ($A_1^1 = 282$ b).

Infra-red Spectrum. Principal peaks at wavenumbers 1665, 1703, 1318, 1300, 1278, 1593 (pirenzepine hydrochloride, KBr disk).

Mass Spectrum. Principal peaks at *m/z* 113, 70, 42, 211, 351, 43, 71, 56.

Disposition in the Body. Incompletely absorbed after oral administration; bioavailability about 20 to 30%. Excreted in the urine and faeces largely as unchanged drug with less than 10% of a dose as the desmethyl metabolite.

THERAPEUTIC CONCENTRATION.
Following a single oral dose of 50 mg to 87 subjects, a mean peak plasma concentration of 0.05 µg/ml was attained in 2 hours (G. Bozler and R. Hammer, *Scand. J. Gastroenterol.*, 1980, *15*, *Suppl.* 66, 27–33).

HALF-LIFE. Plasma half-life, about 11 hours.

CLEARANCE. Plasma clearance, about 3.5 ml/min/kg.

PROTEIN BINDING. In plasma, about 10%.

Dose. 100 to 150 mg of pirenzepine hydrochloride daily.

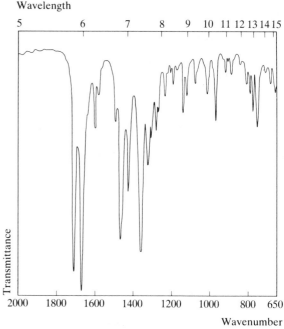

Piritramide

Narcotic Analgesic

Synonym. Pirinitramide
Proprietary Names. Dipidolor; Piridolan.
1 - (3 - Cyano - 3,3 - diphenylpropyl) - 4 - piperidinopiperidine - 4 - carboxamide
$C_{27}H_{34}N_4O = 430.6$
CAS—302-41-0

A crystalline powder. M.p. 149° to 150°.
Soluble in dilute acetic acid.

Thin-layer Chromatography. *System TA*—Rf 70; *system TB*—Rf 01; *system TC*—Rf 45. (*Dragendorff spray*, positive; *acidified iodoplatinate solution*, positive; *Marquis reagent*, orange; *ninhydrin spray*, positive.)

High Pressure Liquid Chromatography. *System HA*—k' 0.6; *system HC*—k' 0.14.

Infra-red Spectrum. Principal peaks at wavenumbers 1669, 701, 757, 1087, 1190, 1592 (KBr disk).
Mass Spectrum. Principal peaks at *m/z* 386, 138, 387, 84, 110, 42, 301, 263.

Dose. 20 mg by intramuscular injection.

Piroxicam

Analgesic

Proprietary Name. Feldene

4-Hydroxy-2-methyl-*N*-(2-pyridyl)-2*H*-1,2-benzothiazine-3-carboxamide 1,1-dioxide

$C_{15}H_{13}N_3O_4S = 331.3$

CAS—36322-90-4

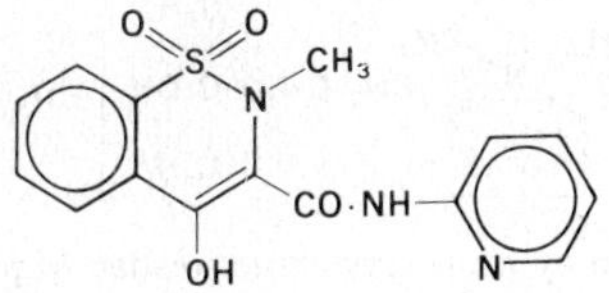

Crystals. M.p. 198° to 200°.

Colour Tests. Koppanyi–Zwikker Test (omit pyrrolidine)—orange; Liebermann's Test—yellow.

Thin-layer Chromatography. *System TD*—Rf 51; *system TE*—Rf 17; *system TF*—Rf 46.

High Pressure Liquid Chromatography. *System HD*—k' 0.6; *system HW*—k' 7.7.

Infra-red Spectrum. Principal peaks at wavenumbers 1524, 1180, 1298, 1147, 1573, 770.

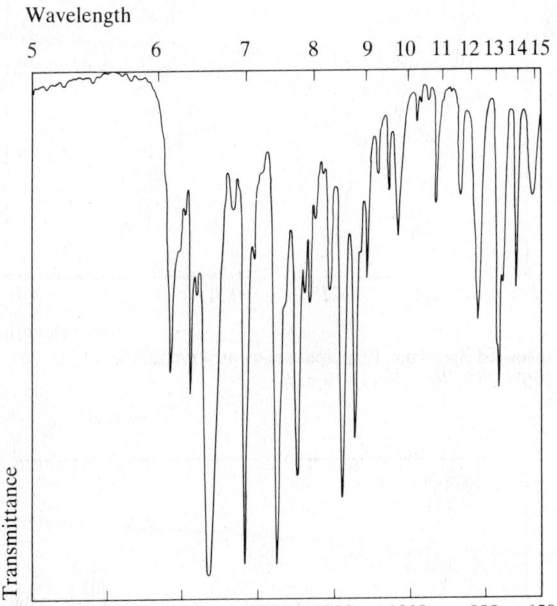

Mass Spectrum. Principal peaks at *m/z* 173, 117, 145, 78, 104, 94, 76, 147.

Quantification. HIGH PRESSURE LIQUID CHROMATOGRAPHY. In serum: sensitivity 500 ng/ml, UV detection—A. D. Fraser and J. F. L. Woodbury, *Ther. Drug Monit.*, 1983, *5*, 239–242.

Disposition in the Body. Readily absorbed after oral or rectal administration. It is extensively metabolised to inactive metabolites; the major metabolite is produced by hydroxylation of the pyridyl ring and exists free and conjugated with glucuronic acid. About 10% of an oral dose is excreted in the urine as unchanged drug in 8 days.

THERAPEUTIC CONCENTRATION. Piroxicam accumulates on repeated administration; steady-state plasma concentrations are attained after approximately 7 days.

Following oral administration of 40 mg to 20 subjects, peak plasma concentrations of 1.7 to 6.8 µg/ml (mean 4.3) were reported; multiple peak concentrations were observed in 16 subjects, suggesting possible enterohepatic circulation. After daily oral administration of 10, 20, and 30 mg to 5 subjects for 14 days, maximum steady-state plasma concentrations of 2.1 to 4.3 (mean 3.2), 3.6 to 6.5 (mean 4.5), and 9.0 to 16.5 (mean 11.7) µg/ml were reported (D. C. Hobbs and T. M. Twomey, *J. clin. Pharmac.*, 1979, *19*, 270–281).

HALF-LIFE. Plasma half-life, about 30 to 60 hours, increased in elderly subjects.

VOLUME OF DISTRIBUTION. About 0.1 litre/kg.

CLEARANCE. Plasma clearance, about 0.03 ml/min/kg.

PROTEIN BINDING. In plasma, about 99%.

NOTE. For a review of the pharmacokinetics of piroxicam see R. N. Brogden *et al.*, *Drugs*, 1984, *28*, 292–323.

Dose. Usually 20 mg daily; doses of 40 mg daily may be given for 7 days.

Pivampicillin

Antibiotic

Proprietary Names. Pondocil; Pondocillin.

Pivaloyloxymethyl(6*R*)-6-(α-D-phenylglycylamino)penicillanate

$C_{22}H_{29}N_3O_6S = 463.5$

CAS—33817-20-8

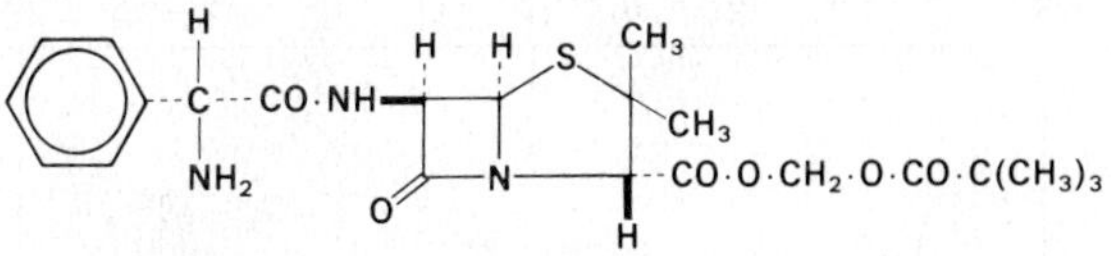

Pivampicillin Hydrochloride

Proprietary Name. Maxifen

$C_{22}H_{29}N_3O_6S,HCl = 500.0$

CAS—26309-95-5

A white, hygroscopic, crystalline powder.

Soluble 1 in 2 of water and 1 in 1.5 of chloroform; very slightly soluble in ether.

Dissociation Constant. pK_a 7.0.

Ultraviolet Spectrum. Aqueous acid—256 nm, 261 nm, 268 nm; aqueous alkali—257 nm, 311 nm.

Infra-red Spectrum. Principal peaks at wavenumbers 1760, 1742, 1104, 1683, 972, 1150 (KBr disk).

Dose. 1 to 2 g daily.

Pizotifen

Migraine Prophylactic

Synonym. Pizotyline

9,10 - Dihydro - 4 - (1 - methyl - 4 - piperidylidene) - 4*H* - benzo-[4,5]cyclohepta[1,2-*b*]thiophene

$C_{19}H_{21}NS = 295.4$

CAS—15574-96-6

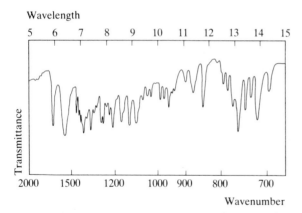

A white to yellow crystalline powder. M.p. 261° to 263°, with decomposition.

Soluble in dilute acetic acid and in chloroform:methanol (1:1).

Pizotifen Malate

Proprietary Names. Mosegor; Sandomigran; Sanmigran; Sanomigran.

$C_{19}H_{21}NS,C_4H_6O_5 = 429.5$

CAS—5189-11-7

Crystals. M.p. 185° to 186°, with decomposition.

Dissociation Constant. pK_a 7.0.

Colour Tests. Liebermann's Test—black; Mandelin's Test—violet → green; Marquis Test—orange → red; Sulphuric Acid—orange-yellow → violet.

Thin-layer Chromatography. *System TA*—Rf 48. (*Acidified iodoplatinate solution*, positive.)

Gas Chromatography. *System GA*—RI 2375.

High Pressure Liquid Chromatography. *System HA*—k' 3.4.

Infra-red Spectrum. Principal peaks at wavenumbers 1577, 756, 1212, 1703, 1124, 1274 (KBr disk).

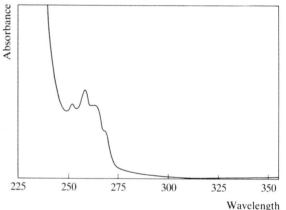

Disposition in the Body. Absorbed after oral administration. Peak blood concentrations of total radioactivity were attained in 5 to 7 hours after a single oral dose of 1 mg of ^{3}H-pizotifen. About 62% of a dose is excreted in the urine and 24% is eliminated in the faeces in 120 hours, with about 36% of the dose being excreted in the first 24 hours.

HALF-LIFE. Derived from urinary excretion data (total radioactivity), about 26 hours.

REFERENCE. T. M. Speight and S. Avery, *Drugs*, 1972, *3*, 159–203.

Dose. The equivalent of 0.5 to 6 mg of pizotifen daily.

Poldine Methylsulphate   *Anticholinergic*

Synonym. Poldine Methosulphate

Proprietary Names. Nactate; Nacton.

2 - Benziloyloxymethyl - 1,1 - dimethylpyrrolidinium methylsulphate

$C_{21}H_{26}NO_3,CH_3SO_4 = 451.5$

CAS—596-50-9 (poldine); *545-80-2* (methylsulphate)

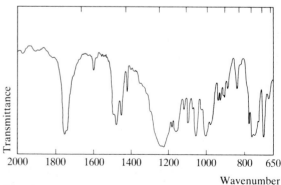

A white to creamy-white crystalline powder. M.p. 134° to 142°.

Soluble 1 in 1 of water, 1 in 20 of ethanol, and 1 in 1000 of chloroform; practically insoluble in ether.

Colour Tests. Mandelin's Test—orange → green → violet; Marquis Test—orange → green → blue.

Thin-layer Chromatography. *System TA*—Rf 02. (*Acidified iodoplatinate solution*, positive.)

High Pressure Liquid Chromatography. *System HA*—k' 3.3 (tailing peak).

Ultraviolet Spectrum. Aqueous acid—252 nm, 258 nm ($A_1^1 = 10.5$ a). No alkaline shift.

Infra-red Spectrum. Principal peaks at wavenumbers 1222, 701, 1061, 1008, 765, 1751 (KBr disk).

Dose. 8 to 16 mg daily.

Polythiazide

Diuretic

Proprietary Names. Drenusil; Nephril; Renese.

6-Chloro-3,4-dihydro-2-methyl-3-(2,2,2-trifluoroethylthio-methyl)-2*H*-1,2,4-benzothiadiazine-7-sulphonamide 1,1-dioxide

$C_{11}H_{13}ClF_3N_3O_4S_3 = 439.9$

CAS—346-18-9

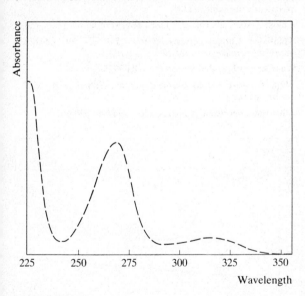

A white crystalline powder. M.p. 207° to 217°, with decomposition.

Practically **insoluble** in water and chloroform; soluble 1 in 40 of ethanol; soluble in acetone and methanol.

Colour Tests. Koppanyi–Zwikker Test—violet; Liebermann's Test—red-brown; Palladium Chloride—orange; Sulphuric Acid—orange.

Thin-layer Chromatography. *System TD*—Rf 22; *system TE*—Rf 63; *system TF*—Rf 60.

Gas Chromatography. *System GA*—RI 2380.

High Pressure Liquid Chromatography. *System HN*—k' 15.09.

Ultraviolet Spectrum. Methanol—268 nm ($A_1^1 = 500$ a), 317 nm.

Infra-red Spectrum. Principal peaks at wavenumbers 1162, 1120, 1597, 1071, 1240, 1500 (KBr disk).

Mass Spectrum. Principal peaks at *m/z* 310, 206, 42, 64, 312, 299, 45, 48.

Quantification. GAS CHROMATOGRAPHY. In plasma: sensitivity 200 pg/ml, ECD—D. C. Hobbs and T. M. Twomey, *Clin. Pharmac. Ther.*, 1978, **23**, 241–246.

Disposition in the Body. Well absorbed after oral administration. About 20% of a single oral dose is excreted in the urine as unchanged drug in 48 hours.

Wavelength

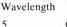

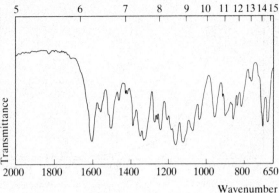

Wavenumber

THERAPEUTIC CONCENTRATION.

After a single oral dose of 1 mg to 18 subjects, peak plasma concentrations of 0.002 to 0.007 μg/ml (mean 0.004) were attained in 5 to 12 hours (D. C. Hobbs and T. M. Twomey, *ibid.*).

HALF-LIFE. Plasma half-life, about 26 hours.

PROTEIN BINDING. In plasma, about 80 to 85%.

Dose. 1 to 4 mg daily.

Practolol

Beta-adrenoceptor Blocking Agent

Proprietary Name. Eraldin

(±)-4'-(2-Hydroxy-3-isopropylaminopropoxy)acetanilide

$C_{14}H_{22}N_2O_3 = 266.3$

CAS—6673-35-4; 23313-50-0 (±)

A fine, white powder. M.p. 141° to 144°.

Soluble 1 in 400 of water, 1 in 40 of ethanol, and 1 in 200 of chloroform; very soluble in dilute solutions of acetic acid.

Dissociation Constant. pK$_a$ 9.5 (20°).

Partition Coefficient. Log *P* (octanol/pH 8.0), −1.3.

Colour Test. Liebermann's Test—black.

Thin-layer Chromatography. *System TA*—Rf 45; *system TB*—Rf 00; *system TC*—Rf 01. (*Acidified potassium permanganate solution*, positive.)

Gas Chromatography. *System GA*—not eluted.

High Pressure Liquid Chromatography. *System HA*—k' 0.5.

Ultraviolet Spectrum. Aqueous acid—243 nm ($A_1^1 = 467$ a); methanol—248 nm ($A_1^1 = 620$ a). (See below)

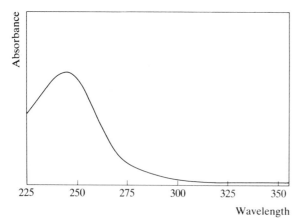

Infra-red Spectrum. Principal peaks at wavenumbers 1642, 1497, 1234, 1515, 822, 1019 (KBr disk).

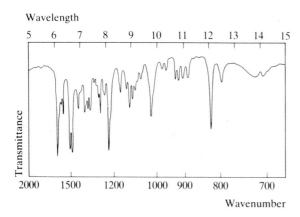

Mass Spectrum. Principal peaks at m/z 72, 30, 151, 43, 109, 56, 57, 108.

Quantification. SPECTROFLUORIMETRY. In blood or urine: sensitivity 200 ng/ml—G. Bodem and C. A. Chidsey, *Clin. Chem.*, 1972, *18*, 363–365.

GAS CHROMATOGRAPHY. In plasma or urine: sensitivity 10 ng/ml, ECD—J. P. Desager and C. Harvengt, *J. Pharm. Pharmac.*, 1975, *27*, 52-54.

HIGH PRESSURE LIQUID CHROMATOGRAPHY. In plasma: detection limit 30 ng/ml, UV detection—A. C. Mehta and R. T. Calvert, *J. Chromat.*, 1983, *276*; *Biomed. Appl.*, 27, 208–212.

Disposition in the Body. Completely absorbed after oral administration and almost entirely excreted in the urine as unchanged drug. Up to about 70% of a dose is excreted in the urine in 24 hours.

THERAPEUTIC CONCENTRATION.

After a single oral dose of 200 mg to 13 subjects, a mean peak plasma concentration of 1.3 µg/ml was attained in 2 hours (C. M. Castleden *et al.*, *Br. J. clin. Pharmac.*, 1975, *2*, 303–306).

Daily oral doses of 200 mg, 400 mg, and 800 mg to 8 subjects produced mean steady-state serum concentrations of 1.6, 2.9, and 4.5 µg/ml, respectively (E. L. Alderman *et al.*, *Clin. Pharmac. Ther.*, 1973, *14*, 175–181).

HALF-LIFE. Plasma half-life, 10 to 13 hours.

VOLUME OF DISTRIBUTION. About 1.6 litres/kg.

CLEARANCE. Plasma clearance, about 2 ml/min/kg.

PROTEIN BINDING. In plasma, less than 10%.

Dose. Practolol has been given in doses of 0.2 to 1.2 g daily.

Prajmalium Bitartrate   *Anti-arrhythmic*

Synonym. NPAB
Proprietary Names. Neo Aritmina; Neo-Gilurytmal.
N-Propylajmalinium hydrogen tartrate
$C_{23}H_{33}N_2O_2, C_4H_5O_6 = 518.6$
CAS—35080-11-6 (prajmalium); *2589-47-1* (bitartrate)

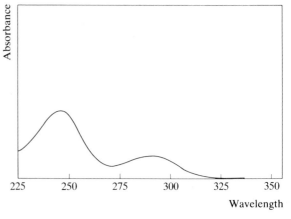

A white to pale yellow powder. M.p. about 133°, with decomposition.

Soluble in water; readily soluble in ethanol, glacial acetic acid, and dilute mineral acids; moderately soluble in chloroform; practically insoluble in ether.

Colour Tests. Liebermann's Test—red; Mandelin's Test—red.

Thin-layer Chromatography. *System TA*—Rf 59. (*Acidified potassium permanganate solution*, positive.)

Gas Chromatography. *System GA*—RI 2925.

High Pressure Liquid Chromatography. *System HA*—k' 2.2 (tailing peak).

Ultraviolet Spectrum. Aqueous acid—246 nm, 290 nm.

Quantification. GAS CHROMATOGRAPHY. In plasma: detection limit 5 ng/ml, AFID—M. Thoma *et al.*, *Arzneimittel-Forsch.*, 1981, *31*, 1020–1021.

HIGH PRESSURE LIQUID CHROMATOGRAPHY. In plasma: detection limit about 5 ng/ml, fluorescence detection—I. Grundevik and B. A. Persson, *J. liq. Chromat.*, 1982, *5*, 141–150.

Disposition in the Body.

THERAPEUTIC CONCENTRATION.
Following oral administration of 20 mg four times a day to 8 subjects, steady-state plasma concentrations of 0.08 to 0.55 µg/ml (mean 0.2) were reported (A. T. Trompler *et al.*, *Arzneimittel-Forsch.*, 1983, *33*, 436–439).

HALF-LIFE. Plasma half-life, about 7 hours.

Dose. 20 to 40 mg daily.

Pralidoxime Chloride   *Cholinesterase Reactivator*

Synonyms. 2-PAM Chloride; 2-PAMCl; Pyraloxime Chloride; 2-Pyridine Aldoxime Methochloride.
Proprietary Name. Protopam Chloride
2-Hydroxyiminomethyl-1-methylpyridinium chloride
$C_7H_9ClN_2O = 172.6$
CAS—6735-59-7 (pralidoxime); *51-15-0* (chloride)

A white or pale yellow crystalline powder. M.p. 215° to 225°, with decomposition.
Soluble 1 in less than 2 of water and 1 in 100 of ethanol.

Pralidoxime Iodide

Synonyms. PAM; P-2-AM; 2-PAM Iodide; 2-PAMI; Pamium; Pyraloxime Iodide; 2-Pyridine Aldoxime Methiodide.
$C_7H_9IN_2O = 264.1$
CAS—94-63-3
A yellow, hygroscopic, crystalline powder. M.p. about 220°, with decomposition.
Soluble 1 in 20 of water; practically insoluble in ethanol, chloroform, and ether. Aqueous solutions are unstable.

Pralidoxime Mesylate

Synonyms. 2-PAMM; Pralidoxime Methanesulphonate; P2S; 2-Pyridine Aldoxime Methyl Mesylate.
$C_8H_{12}N_2O_4S = 232.3$
CAS—154-97-2
A colourless or white, hygroscopic, crystalline or granular powder. M.p. 155°.
Soluble 1 in 2 of water and 1 in 12 of ethanol; practically insoluble in chloroform and ether.

Pralidoxime Methylsulphate

Proprietary Name. Contrathion
$C_8H_{12}N_2O_5S = 248.3$
CAS—1200-55-1
A white crystalline powder. M.p. about 111°.
Very soluble in water; slightly soluble in chloroform.

Dissociation Constant. pK_a 8.0 (20°).

Thin-layer Chromatography. *System TA*—Rf 05. (*Acidified iodoplatinate solution*, positive.)

Ultraviolet Spectrum. Aqueous acid—242 nm, 292 nm; aqueous alkali—332 nm, inflexion at 280 nm.

Disposition in the Body. Pralidoxime chloride is slowly absorbed from the gastro-intestinal tract; the mesylate is more readily absorbed. After intravenous administration as the chloride, about 86% of a dose is excreted in the urine in 24 hours, mostly in the first 3 hours. After oral administration as the mesylate, about 30% of a dose is excreted in the 24-hour urine. 1-Methyl-2-cyanopyridinium ion has been detected in urine as a metabolite.

HALF-LIFE. Plasma half-life, about 1 hour.

VOLUME OF DISTRIBUTION. About 0.6 litre/kg.

CLEARANCE. Plasma clearance, about 7 ml/min/kg.

PROTEIN BINDING. In plasma, not significantly bound.

REFERENCE. J. Josselson and F. R. Sidell, *Clin. Pharmac. Ther.*, 1978, *24*, 95–100.

Dose. 1 to 2 g of pralidoxime chloride parenterally, repeated if necessary; up to 15 g daily, by mouth.

Pramoxine   *Local Anaesthetic*

Synonym. Pramocaine
4-[3-(4-Butoxyphenoxy)propyl]morpholine
$C_{17}H_{27}NO_3 = 293.4$
CAS—140-65-8

Pramoxine Hydrochloride

Proprietary Names. Proctofoam/non steroid; Tronothane.
$C_{17}H_{27}NO_3,HCl = 329.9$
CAS—637-58-1
A white crystalline powder. M.p. 170° to 174°.
Freely soluble in water and ethanol; soluble 1 in 35 of chloroform; very slightly soluble in ether.

Colour Test. Marquis Test—yellow → green.

Thin-layer Chromatography. *System TA*—Rf 70; *system TB*—Rf 43; *system TC*—Rf 55; *system TL*—Rf 41. (*Dragendorff spray*, positive; *acidified iodoplatinate solution*, positive; *Marquis reagent*, green.)

Gas Chromatography. *System GA*—RI 2281; *system GF*—RI 2600.

High Pressure Liquid Chromatography. *System HA*—k' 0.6; *system HR*—k' 2.48.

Ultraviolet Spectrum. Aqueous acid—286 nm ($A_1^1 = 80$ c). No alkaline shift.

Infra-red Spectrum. Principal peaks at wavenumbers 1510, 1230, 1118, 1210, 824, 1635 (KBr disk).

Mass Spectrum. Principal peaks at *m/z* 100, 128, 70, 41, 42, 293, 56, 101.

Use. Pramoxine hydrochloride is used as a 1% cream or jelly.

Prazepam   *Tranquilliser*

Proprietary Names. Centrax: Demetrin; Lysanxia; Prazene.
7-Chloro-1-(cyclopropylmethyl)-1,3-dihydro-5-phenyl-2H-1,4-benzodiazepin-2-one
$C_{19}H_{17}ClN_2O = 324.8$
CAS—2955-38-6

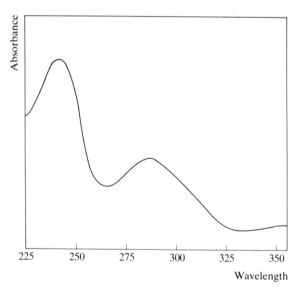

A white crystalline powder. M.p. 143° to 148°.
Soluble in ethanol, chloroform, and dilute mineral acids.

Dissociation Constant. pK_a 2.7.

Partition Coefficient. Log P (octanol/pH 7.4), 3.7.

Colour Test. Formaldehyde–Sulphuric Acid—orange.

Thin-layer Chromatography. *System TA*—Rf 65; *system TB*—Rf 36; *system TC*—Rf 74; *system TD*—Rf 64; *system TE*—Rf 81; *system TF*—Rf 55. (*Acidified iodoplatinate solution*, positive; *acidified potassium permanganate solution*, positive.)

Gas Chromatography. *System GA*—prazepam RI 2641, desmethyldiazepam RI 2496, 3-hydroxyprazepam RI 2860, oxazepam RI 2336; *system GG*—prazepam RI 3145, oxazepam RI 2803.

High Pressure Liquid Chromatography. *System HJ*—k' 4.60; *system HK*—prazepam k' 2.19, desmethyldiazepam k' 1.99, oxazepam k' 0.73.

Ultraviolet Spectrum. Aqueous acid—240 nm ($A_1^1 = 1760$ a), 285 nm, 360 nm.

Infra-red Spectrum. Principal peaks at wavenumbers 1667, 1316, 740, 694, 1602, 704 (K Br disk).

Mass Spectrum. Principal peaks at *m/z* 91, 269, 324, 55, 296, 295, 323, 297; desmethyldiazepam 242, 269, 270, 241, 243, 271, 244, 272; 3-hydroxyprazepam 257, 55, 311, 77, 259, 313, 44, 312; oxazepam 257, 77, 268, 239, 205, 267, 233, 259.

Quantification. GAS CHROMATOGRAPHY. In serum: prazepam, desmethyldiazepam, 3-hydroxyprazepam and oxazepam, sensitivity 1 ng/ml, ECD—H. Nau *et al.*, *J. Chromat.*, 1978, *146*; *Biomed. Appl.*, 3, 227–239.

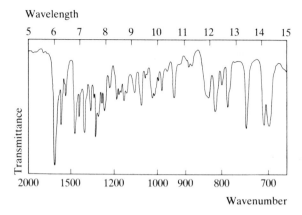

Disposition in the Body. Slowly and variably absorbed after oral administration. Desmethyldiazepam (nordazepam) is the major metabolite found in plasma and accounts for most of the activity. Prazepam is excreted in the urine mainly as glucuronide conjugates of oxazepam and 3-hydroxyprazepam with only trace amounts of desmethyldiazepam or unchanged drug. Up to about 20% of a dose is excreted in the urine in 24 hours and about 60% over a period of 7 days; about 7% of a dose is eliminated in the faeces in 48 hours.

THERAPEUTIC CONCENTRATION.

After a single oral dose of 30 mg to 10 subjects, peak plasma concentrations of 0.19 to 0.40 µg/ml (mean 0.3) of desmethyldiazepam were reported in 2 to 8 hours; a second peak plasma concentration was reported for each subject. Following oral administration of 20 mg three times a day for 3 days to 5 subjects, plasma concentrations averaged 0.8 µg/ml 12 hours after the final dose (R. R. Brodie *et al.*, *Biopharm. Drug Disp.*, 1981, *2*, 59–68).

HALF-LIFE. Plasma half-life, desmethyldiazepam about 40 to 100 hours but there is considerable intersubject variation—see under Nordazepam.

VOLUME OF DISTRIBUTION. Desmethyldiazepam, 0.5 to 2.5 litres/kg, increased in elderly subjects.

CLEARANCE. Plasma clearance, desmethyldiazepam about 0.1 to 0.3 ml/min/kg.

DISTRIBUTION IN BLOOD. Plasma:whole blood ratio, desmethyldiazepam about 1.7.

PROTEIN BINDING. In plasma, desmethyldiazepam about 97%.

Dose. 10 to 60 mg daily.

Prazosin   *Antihypertensive*

Synonym. Furazosin

1 - (4 - Amino - 6,7 - dimethoxyquinazolin - 2 - yl) - 4 - (2 - furoyl)piperazine
$C_{19}H_{21}N_5O_4 = 383.4$
CAS—19216-56-9

Crystals. M.p. 278° to 280°.

Prazosin Hydrochloride

Proprietary Names. Hypovase; Minipress; Peripress.
$C_{19}H_{21}N_5O_4,HCl = 419.9$
CAS—19237-84-4
A white to tan-coloured powder. M.p. about 264°, with decomposition.

Dissociation Constant. pK_a 6.5.

Colour Test. Liebermann's Test—brown-pink (→ red-orange at 100°).

Thin-layer Chromatography. *System TA*—Rf 60; *system TB*—Rf 01; *system TC*—Rf 47.

High Pressure Liquid Chromatography. *System HA*—k′ 0.8.

Ultraviolet Spectrum. Aqueous acid—247 nm ($A_1^1 = 1470$ b), 331 nm ($A_1^1 = 281$ b); aqueous alkali—252 nm ($A_1^1 = 1642$ b), 345 nm ($A_1^1 = 150$ b).

Infra-red Spectrum. Principal peaks at wavenumbers 1603, 1643, 1293, 1125, 1252, 1540 (prazosin hydrochloride).

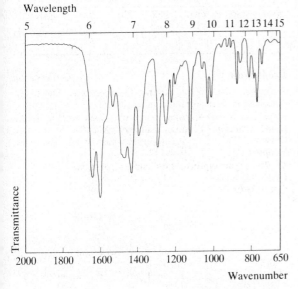

Wavelength

Mass Spectrum. Principal peaks at *m/z* 233, 383, 259, 245, 95, 56, 246, 234.

Quantification. HIGH PRESSURE LIQUID CHROMATOGRAPHY. In plasma, blood or urine: sensitivity 1 ng/ml, fluorescence detection—E. T. Lin *et al.*, *J. Chromat.*, 1980, *183*; *Biomed. Appl.*, *9*, 367–371. In plasma: sensitivity 500 pg/ml, fluoresence detection—P. A. Reece, *J. Chromat.*, 1980, *221*; *Biomed. Appl.*, *10*, 188–192.

Disposition in the Body. Readily absorbed after oral administration; bioavailability about 60%. Extensively metabolised by 6-*O*- and 7-*O*-demethylation and glucuronic acid conjugation; less than 5% of a dose is excreted in the urine as unchanged drug in 24 hours.

THERAPEUTIC CONCENTRATION.

After single oral doses of 0.5 mg and 1.5 mg given to 5 subjects, peak plasma concentrations of 0.001 to 0.005 μg/ml (mean 0.003) and 0.004 to 0.009 μg/ml (mean 0.006), respectively, were attained in 1 to 3 hours (M. K. Dynon *et al.*, *Clin. Pharmacokinet.*, 1980, *5*, 583–590).

Following oral administration of 0.5 mg three times a day to 8 subjects, mean steady-state plasma concentrations of 0.001 to 0.007 μg/ml (mean 0.003) were reported; after dosing with 2 mg three times a day in 7 subjects, mean steady-state plasma concentrations were 0.008 to 0.019 μg/ml (mean 0.013) (A. Grahnén *et al.*, *Clin. Pharmac. Ther.*, 1981, *30*, 439–446).

HALF-LIFE. Plasma half-life, about 3 hours.

VOLUME OF DISTRIBUTION. About 0.6 litre/kg.

CLEARANCE. Plasma clearance, about 3 ml/min/kg.

DISTRIBUTION IN BLOOD. Plasma:whole blood ratio, 1.4.

PROTEIN BINDING. In plasma, about 95%.

NOTE. For a review of the pharmacokinetics of prazosin see P. Jaillon, *Clin. Pharmacokinet.*, 1980, *5*, 365–376.

Dose. 0.5 to 20 mg of prazosin hydrochloride daily.

Prednisolone   *Corticosteroid*

Synonyms. 1,2-Dehydrohydrocortisone; Deltahydrocortisone; Metacortandralone.
Proprietary Names. Codelcortone; Delta Phoricol; Delta-Cortef; Deltacortril; Deltalone; Deltastab (tablets); Marsolone; Meti-Derm; Precortisyl; Prednis; Ropredlone; Sterane; Ulacort. It is an ingredient of Anacal and Hydromycin-D.
11β,17α,21-Trihydroxypregna-1,4-diene-3,20-dione
$C_{21}H_{28}O_5 = 360.4$
CAS—50-24-8 (anhydrous); *52438-85-4* (sesquihydrate)

A white, hygroscopic, crystalline powder. M.p. about 230° to 235°, with decomposition.
Soluble 1 in 1300 of water, 1 in 30 of ethanol, 1 in 27 of dehydrated alcohol, and 1 in 180 of chloroform; soluble in dioxan and methanol.

Prednisolone Acetate

Synonym. Prednisolone 21-Acetate
Proprietary Names. Deltastab (injection); Econopred; Meticortelone Aqueous; Pred Forte; Pred Mild; Savacort; Ultracortenol. It is an ingredient of Mydraped.
$C_{23}H_{30}O_6 = 402.5$
CAS—52-21-1
A white crystalline powder. M.p. about 235°, with decomposition.
Practically **insoluble** in water; soluble 1 in 120 of ethanol, 1 in 170 of dehydrated alcohol, and 1 in 150 of chloroform.

Prednisolone Pivalate

Synonyms. Prednisolone 21-Pivalate; Prednisolone Trimethylacetate.
Proprietary Name. Ultracortenol
$C_{26}H_{36}O_6 = 444.6$
CAS—1107-99-9
A white crystalline powder. M.p. about 229°.
Practically **insoluble** in water; soluble 1 in 150 of ethanol and 1 in 16 of chloroform.

Prednisolone Sodium Phosphate

Synonym. Prednisolone 21-(Disodium Phosphate)

Proprietary Names. Codelsol; Hydeltrasol; Inflamase; Metreton; Prednesol; Predsol; PSP-IV; Savacort-S; Sodasone.

$C_{21}H_{27}Na_2O_8P = 484.4$
CAS—125-02-0

A white or slightly yellow, hygroscopic powder or granules.

Soluble 1 in 3 or 1 in 4 of water, 1 in 1000 of dehydrated alcohol, and 1 in 13 of methanol; practically insoluble in chloroform.

Prednisolone Steaglate

Synonym. Prednisolone 21-Stearoylglycolate

Proprietary Name. Sintisone

$C_{41}H_{64}O_8 = 685.0$
CAS—5060-55-9

A white powder. M.p. about 105°.

Soluble in ethanol, acetone, and methanol.

Prednisolone Succinate

Synonym. Prednisolone 21-Hydrogen Succinate

Proprietary Name. Solu-Dacortin (sodium salt)

$C_{25}H_{32}O_8 = 460.5$
CAS—2920-86-7; 1715-33-9 (sodium salt)

A fine creamy-white powder with friable lumps. M.p. about 205°, with decomposition.

Very slightly **soluble** in water; soluble 1 in about 6 of ethanol and 1 in about 250 of ether; soluble in acetone; very slightly soluble in chloroform.

Prednisolone Tebutate

Synonyms. Prednisolone Butylacetate; Prednisolone 21-(3,3-Dimethylbutyrate); Prednisolone Tertiary-butylacetate.

Proprietary Names. Codelcortone TBA; Hydeltra-TBA.

$C_{27}H_{38}O_6, H_2O = 476.6$
CAS—7681-14-3 (anhydrous)

A white to slightly yellow, hygroscopic powder.

Very slightly **soluble** in water; sparingly soluble in ethanol; soluble in acetone; freely soluble in chloroform and dioxan.

Colour Tests. Naphthol–Sulphuric Acid—brown/brown; Sulphuric Acid—orange-pink.

Thin-layer Chromatography. Prednisolone: *system TP*—Rf 20; *system TQ*—Rf 00; *system TR*—Rf 02, streaking may occur; *system TS*—Rf 00. (*DPST solution.*) Prednisolone pivalate: *system TP*—Rf 69; *system TQ*—Rf 04; *system TR*—Rf 44; *system TS*—Rf 00. (*DPST solution.*) Prednisolone sodium phosphate: *system TP*—Rf 00; *system TQ*—Rf 00; *system TR*—Rf 00; *system TS*—Rf 00.

High Pressure Liquid Chromatography. *System HT*—k' 8.4.

Ultraviolet Spectrum. Ethanol—240 nm ($A_1^1 = 415$ a).

Infra-red Spectrum. Principal peaks at wavenumbers 1654, 1612, 1708, 887, 1112, 1085 (KBr disk).

Mass Spectrum. Principal peaks at *m/z* 121, 122, 91, 147, 225, 43, 135, 120.

Quantification. Gas Chromatography–Mass Spectrometry. In plasma: prednisolone and prednisone—S. B. Matin and B. Amos, *J. pharm. Sci.,* 1978, *67*, 923–926.

High Pressure Liquid Chromatography. In plasma: sensitivity 10 ng/ml, UV detection—R. Hartley and J. T. Brocklebank, *J. Chromat.,* 1982, *232*; *Biomed. Appl.,* *21*, 406–412. In plasma, saliva, or urine: prednisolone, prednisone and hydrocortisone, sensitivity 5 ng/ml, UV detection—J. Q. Rose and W. J. Jusko, *J. Chromat.,* 1979, *162*; *Biomed. Appl.,* *4*, 273–280.

Radioimmunoassay. In serum: sensitivity 10 ng/ml—A. Olivesi *et al., Clin. Chem.,* 1983, *29*, 1358–1362.

Dose. Usually 5 to 60 mg of prednisolone daily.

Wavelength

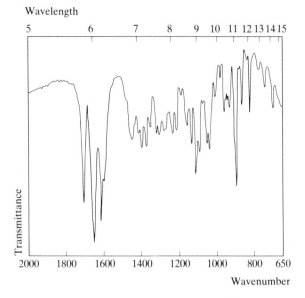

Prednisone   *Corticosteroid*

Synonyms. 1,2-Dehydrocortisone; Deltacortisone; Deltadehydrocortisone; Metacortandracin.

Proprietary Names. Colisone; Decortisyl; Deltacortone; Delta-Dome; Deltasone; Econosone; Lisacort; Marsone; Meticorten; Orasone; Paracort; Prednicen-M; Servisone; Sterapred; Winpred.

17α,21-Dihydroxypregna-1,4-diene-3,11,20-trione
$C_{21}H_{26}O_5 = 358.4$
CAS—53-03-2

A white crystalline powder. M.p. about 230°, with decomposition.

Practically **insoluble** in water; soluble 1 in about 190 of ethanol, 1 in 300 of dehydrated alcohol, and 1 in 200 of chloroform.

Prednisone Acetate

Synonym. Prednisone 21-Acetate

$C_{23}H_{28}O_6 = 400.5$
CAS—125-10-0

A white crystalline powder. M.p. about 240°, with decomposition.

Practically **insoluble** in water; soluble 1 in 120 of ethanol, 1 in 160 of dehydrated alcohol, and 1 in 6 of chloroform.

Colour Tests. Naphthol–Sulphuric Acid—brown/orange; Sulphuric Acid—yellow (green fluorescence under ultraviolet light).

Thin-layer Chromatography. *System TP*—Rf 41; *system TQ*—Rf 00; *system TR*—Rf 10; *system TS*—Rf 00. (*DPST solution.*)

High Pressure Liquid Chromatography. *System HT*—k' 3.4.

Ultraviolet Spectrum. Ethanol—240 nm ($A_1^1 = 420$ a).

Infra-red Spectrum. Principal peaks at wavenumbers 1668, 1707, 904, 1622, 1610, 1246 (KBr disk).

Wavelength

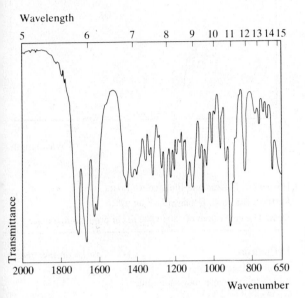

Dose. Usually 5 to 60 mg daily.

Prenalterol

Sympathomimetic

$(-)$-(S)-1-(4-Hydroxyphenoxy)-3-isopropylaminopropan-2-ol
$C_{12}H_{19}NO_3 = 225.3$
CAS—57526-81-5

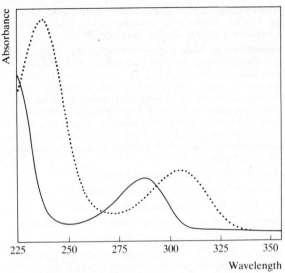

Infra-red Spectrum. Principal peaks at wavenumbers 1518, 1242, 1213, 1099, 840, 772 (prenalterol hydrochloride, KBr disk).

Wavelength

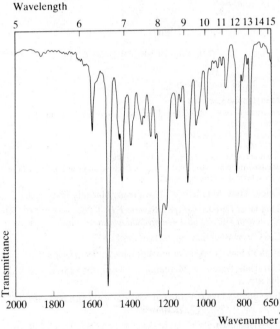

Prenalterol Hydrochloride
Proprietary Names. Hyprenan; Varbian.
$C_{12}H_{19}NO_3,HCl = 261.7$
CAS—61260-05-7
A white crystalline powder. M.p. about 128°.
Freely **soluble** in water and ethanol; slightly soluble in acetone; very slightly soluble in ether.

Dissociation Constant. pK_a 9.5 (ammonium ion), 10.0 (phenol).

Thin-layer Chromatography. *System TA*—Rf 47; *system TB*—Rf 01; *system TC*—Rf 09; *system TD*—Rf 02; *system TE*—Rf 25; *system TF*—Rf 02. (*Dragendorff spray*, positive; *ferric chloride solution*, violet; *acidified iodoplatinate solution*, positive; *Marquis reagent*, green → black; *acidified potassium permanganate solution*, positive.)

Gas Chromatography. *System GA*—RI 1933.

Ultraviolet Spectrum. Aqueous acid—287 nm ($A_1^1 = 105$ a); aqueous alkali—235 nm ($A_1^1 = 444$ b), 305 nm.

Mass Spectrum. Principal peaks at *m/z* 72, 30, 56, 43, 27, 41, 39, 110.

Quantification. GAS CHROMATOGRAPHY. In plasma or urine: sensitivity 2 ng/ml, ECD—P. H. Degen and M. Ervik, *J. Chromat.*, 1981, *222*; *Biomed. Appl.*, *11*, 437–444.

GAS CHROMATOGRAPHY–MASS SPECTROMETRY. In plasma or urine: sensitivity 1 ng/ml—M. Ervik *et al.*, *J. Chromat.*, 1982, *229*; *Biomed. Appl.*, *18*, 87–94.

HIGH PRESSURE LIQUID CHROMATOGRAPHY. In plasma: sensitivity 1 ng/ml, fluorescence detection—C. J. Oddie *et al.*, *J. Chromat.*, 1982, *231*; Biomed. Appl., *20*, 473–477.

Disposition in the Body. Rapidly and completely absorbed after oral administration, but subject to extensive first-pass metabolism; bioavailability about 25%. The main metabolic reaction is conjugation with sulphate at the phenol position; minor metabolites formed are β-(4-hydroxyphenoxy)lactic acid and prenalterol glucuronide. About 90% of a dose is excreted in the urine in 24 hours. After an intravenous dose, about 60% is excreted unchanged with about 35% as the sulphate; after oral administration, about 15% is excreted unchanged, with about 80% as the sulphate.

HALF-LIFE. Plasma half-life, about 2 hours.

VOLUME OF DISTRIBUTION. About 3.5 litres/kg.

CLEARANCE. Plasma clearance, about 20 ml/min/kg.

DISTRIBUTION IN BLOOD. Plasma: whole blood ratio, about 0.9.

PROTEIN BINDING. In plasma, less than 5%.

Dose. 0.5 mg of prenalterol hydrochloride per minute by intravenous infusion, to a total of not more than 20 mg.

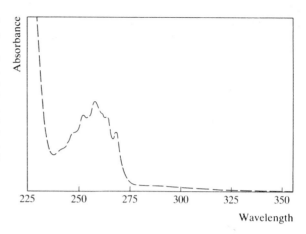

HALF-LIFE. Plasma half-life, about 7 hours.

PROTEIN BINDING. In plasma, about 97%.

Dose. The equivalent of 180 to 300 mg of prenylamine daily.

Prenylamine   *Anti-anginal*

N-(2-Benzhydrylethyl)-α-methylphenethylamine
$C_{24}H_{27}N = 329.5$
CAS—390-64-7

$$C_6H_5 \cdot CH_2 \cdot CH(CH_3) \cdot NH \cdot [CH_2]_2 \cdot CH(C_6H_5) \cdot C_6H_5$$

M.p. 36° to 38°.

Prenylamine Lactate
Proprietary Names. Angorsan; Eucardion; Reocorin; Segontin(e); Synadrin; Wasangor.
$C_{24}H_{27}N, C_3H_6O_3 = 419.6$
CAS—69-43-2
A white crystalline powder. M.p. 137° to 140°.
Soluble 1 in about 200 of water, 1 in 5 of ethanol, and 1 in 2 of chloroform; very soluble in glacial acetic acid.

Colour Tests. Mandelin's Test—green; Marquis Test—red.

Thin-layer Chromatography. *System TA*—Rf 68; *system TB*—Rf 55; *system TC*—Rf 68. (*Acidified iodoplatinate solution*, positive.)

Gas Chromatography. *System GA*—RI 2557.

High Pressure Liquid Chromatography. *System HA*—k' 1.0.

Ultraviolet Spectrum. Methanol—253 nm, 258 nm ($A_1^1 = 18.8$ a), 268 nm.

Infra-red Spectrum. Principal peaks at wavenumbers 700, 747, 1136, 1027, 1592, 1075 (KBr disk).

Mass Spectrum. Principal peaks at m/z 58, 238, 91, 45, 239, 167, 165, 56.

Quantification. GAS CHROMATOGRAPHY. In serum or urine: prenylamine and metabolites, detection limits 10 to 50 ng/ml, FID—M. Eichelbaum *et al.*, *Arzneimittel-Forsch.*, 1973, *23*, 74–77.

Disposition in the Body. Readily absorbed after oral administration but extensively metabolised. Numerous metabolites, including traces of amphetamine, have been detected in the urine; some unchanged drug is eliminated in the faeces.

Prilocaine   *Local Anaesthetic*

Synonym. Propitocaine
2-Propylaminopropiono-*o*-toluidide
$C_{13}H_{20}N_2O = 220.3$
CAS—721-50-6

$$NH \cdot CO \cdot CH(CH_3) \cdot NH \cdot [CH_2]_2 \cdot CH_3$$

A white crystalline powder. M.p. 36° to 38°.
Freely **soluble** in ethanol, chloroform, and ether.

Prilocaine Hydrochloride
Proprietary Names. Citanest; Xylonest.
$C_{13}H_{20}N_2O, HCl = 256.8$
CAS—1786-81-8
A white crystalline powder. M.p. 166° to 169°.
Soluble 1 in 5 of water, 1 in 6 of ethanol, and 1 in 175 of chloroform; practically insoluble in ether.

Dissociation Constant. pK_a 7.9 (25°).

Colour Test. Mandelin's Test—violet.

Thin-layer Chromatography. *System TA*—Rf 77; *system TB*—Rf 29; *system TC*—Rf 64; *system TL*—Rf 60.

Gas Chromatography. *System GA*—prilocaine RI 1825, *o*-toluidine RI 2356.

High Pressure Liquid Chromatography. *System HA*—k' 1.0; *system HQ*—k' 1.38.

Ultraviolet Spectrum. Methanol—230 nm ($A_1^1 = 295$ a).

Infra-red Spectrum. Principal peaks at wavenumbers 1695, 1543, 766, 754, 1299, 1258 (prilocaine hydrochloride, KBr disk).

Wavelength

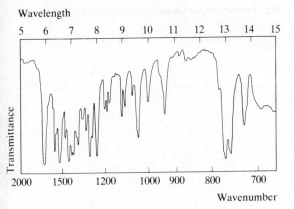

Transmittance

Wavenumber

Mass Spectrum. Principal peaks at *m/z* 86, 44, 87, 107, 43, 106, 56, 41.

Quantification. GAS CHROMATOGRAPHY. In blood: prilocaine and lignocaine, sensitivity < 500 ng/ml, FID—J. B. Keenaghan, *Anesthesiology*, 1968, *29*, 110–112.

Disposition in the Body. Metabolised by hydrolysis and hydroxylation resulting in deacetylated and hydroxylated metabolites which are excreted mainly as conjugates. About 35% of a dose is excreted in the urine as 4-hydroxy-2-methylaniline (*p*-hydroxytoluidine), 3% as 6-hydroxy-2-methylaniline, 1% as 2-methylaniline (*o*-toluidine), and less than 5% as unchanged drug.

THERAPEUTIC CONCENTRATION. In plasma, usually in the range 1 to 5 µg/ml. 4-Hydroxy-2-methylaniline has been detected in plasma at concentrations similar to those of prilocaine.

After the epidural administration of 200, 400, and 600 mg to 10 subjects, mean peak plasma concentrations determined within 10 to 20 minutes were 1.69, 2.67, and 4.47 µg/ml, respectively; after the intercostal administration of 20 ml of a 2% solution, the mean peak concentration was 4.5 µg/ml (D. B. Scott *et al.*, *Br. J. Anaesth.*, 1972, *44*, 1040–1049).

TOXICITY. Toxic effects are usually associated with plasma concentrations greater than 5 µg/ml. 4-Hydroxy-2-methylaniline is thought to be responsible for the methaemoglobinaemia which may occur after large doses.

HALF-LIFE. Plasma half-life, about 1 to 2 hours.

DISTRIBUTION IN BLOOD. Plasma:whole blood ratio, 0.80.

PROTEIN BINDING. In plasma, about 50%.

Dose. Maximum dose of prilocaine hydrochloride, 400 mg, or 600 mg in solutions with adrenaline.

Primaquine   *Antimalarial*

Synonym. Primachin

8-(4-Amino-1-methylbutylamino)-6-methoxyquinoline

$C_{15}H_{21}N_3O = 259.4$

CAS—90-34-6

A viscous liquid.
Moderately **soluble** in water.

Primaquine Phosphate

$C_{15}H_{21}N_3O,2H_3PO_4 = 455.3$

CAS—63-45-6

An orange-red crystalline powder. M.p. about 200°.

Soluble 1 in about 16 of water; practically insoluble in ethanol, chloroform, and ether.

Colour Tests. Mandelin's Test—violet → orange; Marquis Test—orange.

Dissolve 10 mg in 5 ml of water and add 1 ml of a 5% solution of ceric ammonium sulphate in *dilute nitric acid*—violet (distinction from chloroquine).

Thin-layer Chromatography. *System TA*—Rf 19; *system TB*—Rf 13; *system TC*—Rf 05. (*Acidified iodoplatinate solution*, positive.)

Gas Chromatography. *System GA*—RI 2314.

High Pressure Liquid Chromatography. *System HA*—k′ 1.4.

Ultraviolet Spectrum. Aqueous acid—265 nm ($A_1^1 = 579$ a), 282 nm ($A_1^1 = 574$ a), 334 nm.

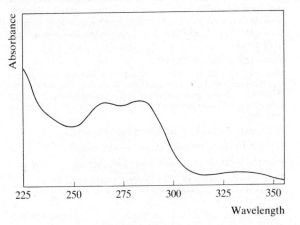

Absorbance

Wavelength

Infra-red Spectrum. Principal peaks at wavenumbers 1611, 1595, 815, 1230, 1572, 1170 (KBr disk).

Wavelength

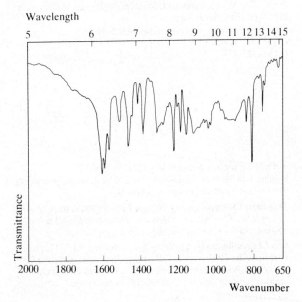

Transmittance

Wavenumber

Mass Spectrum. Principal peaks at m/z 201, 81, 98, 175, 259, 176, 202, 242.

Quantification. GAS CHROMATOGRAPHY. In blood: sensitivity 10 ng/ml, ECD—T. G. Rajagopalan *et al.*, *J. Chromat.*, 1981, *224*; *Biomed. Appl.*, *13*, 265–273.

GAS CHROMATOGRAPHY–MASS SPECTROMETRY. In plasma or urine—J. Greaves *et al.*, *Biomed. Mass Spectrom.*, 1979, *6*, 109–112.

HIGH PRESSURE LIQUID CHROMATOGRAPHY. In plasma: detection limit 1 ng/ml, UV detection—S. A. Ward *et al.*, *J. Chromat.*, 1983, *305*; *Biomed. Appl.*, *30*, 239–243. In plasma or urine: carboxyprimaquine and *N*-acetylprimaquine, sensitivity 75 ng/ml and 10 ng/ml, respectively, UV detection—G. W. Mihaly *et al.*, *Br. J. clin. Pharmac.*, 1984, *17*, 441–446.

Disposition in the Body. Readily absorbed after oral administration. It is extensively metabolised by oxidation to carboxyprimaquine which is the major plasma metabolite. Other reactions which may occur are demethylation and oxidation to the 5,6-diol, which is then converted to an active quinone, *N*-dealkylation to 8-amino-6-methoxyquinoline, and *N*-acetylation. Less than 5% of a dose is excreted in the urine unchanged in 24 hours.

THERAPEUTIC CONCENTRATION.

Following a single oral dose of 45 mg to 5 subjects, peak plasma concentrations of 0.13 to 0.18 µg/ml (mean 0.15) were attained in 2 to 3 hours; peak plasma concentrations of carboxyprimaquine of 1.1 to 1.8 µg/ml (mean 1.4) were attained in 2 to 12 hours (mean 7) (G. W. Mihaly *et al.*, *ibid.*).

HALF-LIFE. Plasma half-life, about 4 to 10 hours (mean 7).

VOLUME OF DISTRIBUTION. About 3 to 4 litres/kg.

PROTEIN BINDING. In plasma, extensively bound.

Dose. The equivalent of 15 to 45 mg of primaquine daily.

Primidone

Anticonvulsant

Synonyms. Hexamidinum; Primaclone.

Note. The name Hexamidine is applied to a compound with antibacterial and fungistatic properties.

Proprietary Names. Liskantin; Midone; Mylepsin; Mylepsinum; Mysoline; Resimatil; Sertan.

5-Ethylperhydro-5-phenylpyrimidine-4,6-dione
$C_{12}H_{14}N_2O_2 = 218.3$
CAS—125-33-7

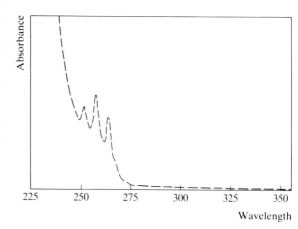

A white crystalline powder. M.p. 279° to 284°.
Soluble 1 in 2000 of water and 1 in 170 of ethanol; practically insoluble in most other organic solvents.

Thin-layer Chromatography. *System TD*—Rf 08; *system TE*—Rf 39; *system TF*—Rf 26. (*Mercuric chloride–diphenylcarbazone reagent*, positive; *mercurous nitrate spray*, positive.)

Gas Chromatography. *System GA*—primidone RI 2247, phenobarbitone RI 1957; *system GE*—primidone retention time 0.89, phenobarbitone retention time 0.74, and phenylethylmalondiamide retention time 0.65, all relative to phenytoin.

High Pressure Liquid Chromatography. *System HE*—primidone k' 1.35, phenobarbitone k' 2.76.

Ultraviolet Spectrum. Methanol—252 nm, 258 nm ($A_1^1 = 9.7$ c), 264 nm.

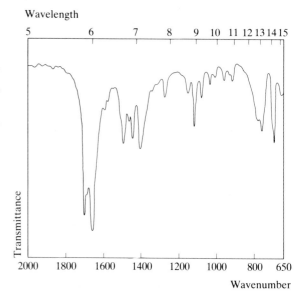

Infra-red Spectrum. Principal peaks at wavenumbers 1662, 1705, 1496, 700, 765, 1120 (KBr disk).

Mass Spectrum. Principal peaks at m/z 146, 190, 117, 118, 161, 189, 103, 91; phenobarbitone 204, 117, 146, 161, 77, 103, 115, 118; phenylethylmalondiamide 163, 148, 91, 103, 117, 120, 44, 77.

Quantification. GAS CHROMATOGRAPHY. In plasma: primidone, phenobarbitone and phenylethylmalondiamide, FID—K. W. Leal *et al.*, *J. analyt. Toxicol.*, 1978, *2*, 214–218.

GAS CHROMATOGRAPHY–MASS SPECTROMETRY. In serum, urine, saliva, breast-milk or tissues: primidone, phenobarbitone, 4-

hydroxyphenobarbitone and phenylethylmalondiamide, detection limits between 1.4 and 3.7 ng/ml—H. Nau *et al.*, *J. Chromat.*, 1980, *182*; *Biomed. Appl.*, *8*, 71–79.

HIGH PRESSURE LIQUID CHROMATOGRAPHY. In plasma or serum: primidone and phenobarbitone, sensitivity about 550 ng/ml for primidone, UV detection—J. A. Christofides and D. E. Fry, *Clin. Chem.*, 1980, *26*, 499–501.

Disposition in the Body. Readily absorbed after oral administration. Rapidly metabolised to phenylethylmalondiamide (PEMA) and more slowly metabolised to phenobarbitone; both metabolites are active anticonvulsants. Aromatic hydroxylation to form 4-hydroxyphenobarbitone also occurs followed by glucuronic acid conjugation. The formation of phenobarbitone is stimulated by phenytoin. During chronic treatment, about 92% of the daily dose is excreted in the urine in 24 hours, of which 15 to 65% (mean 42) is unchanged drug, 16 to 65% (mean 45) is PEMA, and 1 to 8% (mean 5) is phenobarbitone or its hydroxylated metabolites and conjugates.

THERAPEUTIC CONCENTRATION. In plasma, usually in the range 5 to 12 µg/ml but there is considerable intersubject variation. At the beginning of treatment there is a delay of several days before phenobarbitone appears in the plasma. Concentrations of phenobarbitone and PEMA accumulate during chronic treatment, and steady-state plasma-phenobarbitone concentrations are often used to monitor therapy.

After daily oral dosing of a number of subjects at various dose levels, steady-state plasma concentrations were as follows: 26 subjects at 250 mg per day, 0 to 13 µg/ml (mean 3.2); 26 subjects at 500 mg per day, 1 to 14 µg/ml (mean 6.7); 78 subjects at 750 mg per day, 2 to 23 µg/ml (mean 8.7); 52 subjects at 1000 mg per day, 3 to 20 µg/ml (mean 10.5); 9 subjects at 1250 mg per day, 10 to 19 µg/ml (mean 14.7). In 30 subjects given primidone but no barbiturate, the mean primidone concentration was 9.2 µg/ml and the mean phenobarbitone concentration was 31 µg/ml (H. E. Booker *et al.*, *Epilepsia*, 1970, *11*, 395–402).

Following oral doses of 75 to 250 mg three times a day to 7 subjects, the following steady-state serum concentrations were reported: primidone 5.0 to 13.4 µg/ml (mean 8.3), phenobarbitone 3.3 to 34.6 µg/ml (mean 12.6), PEMA 1.4 to 9.9 µg/ml (mean 4.6) (J. C. Cloyd *et al.*, *Clin. Pharmac. Ther.*, 1981, *29*, 402–407).

TOXICITY. The estimated minimum lethal dose is 5 g but instances of survival after the ingestion of 25 to 30 g have been reported. Toxic effects are usually associated with plasma concentrations greater than 10 µg/ml and concentrations greater than 50 µg/ml may be lethal.

In a fatality due to primidone ingestion, postmortem blood concentrations of 65 µg/ml of primidone and 3 µg/ml of phenobarbitone were reported (J. A. Wright per R. C. Baselt, *Disposition of Toxic Drugs and Chemicals in Man*, 2nd Edn, Davis, California, Biomedical Publications, 1982, pp. 657–661).

Serum concentrations of 95 µg/ml of primidone and 175 µg/ml of phenobarbitone were reported about 12 hours after a non-fatal suicide attempt by a 10-year-old epileptic subject; the corresponding urine concentrations were 1570 and 50 µg/ml, respectively (J. C. Cate and R. Tenser, *Clin. Toxicol.*, 1975, *8*, 385–389).

HALF-LIFE. Plasma half-life, primidone 3 to 20 hours (mean 10), phenobarbitone 50 to 150 hours, PEMA 24 to 48 hours.

VOLUME OF DISTRIBUTION. In children after oral dosing, about 0.6 litre/kg.

CLEARANCE. Plasma clearance, after oral administration, about 0.7 ml/min/kg.

SALIVA. Plasma:saliva ratio, about 1.0.

PROTEIN BINDING. In plasma, less than 20%.

Dose. Initially 125 to 250 mg daily, increasing to 0.75 to 2 g daily.

Probenecid   *Uricosuric*

Proprietary Names. Benemid(e); Benuryl; Procid; Urocid.

4-(Dipropylsulphamoyl)benzoic acid

$C_{13}H_{19}NO_4S = 285.4$

CAS—57-66-9

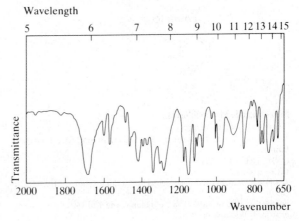

A white crystalline powder. M.p. 198° to 200°.

Practically **insoluble** in water; soluble 1 in 25 of ethanol and 1 in 12 of acetone; soluble in chloroform.

Dissociation Constant. pK_a 3.4 (20°).

Thin-layer Chromatography. *System TD*—Rf 13; *system TE*—Rf 05; *system TF*—Rf 23.

Gas Chromatography. *System GA*—RI 2336.

Ultraviolet Spectrum. Ethanolic acid—248 nm ($A_1^1 = 332$ a).

Infra-red Spectrum. Principal peaks at wavenumbers 1683, 1156, 1285, 1307, 1125, 1180 (KBr disk).

Wavelength

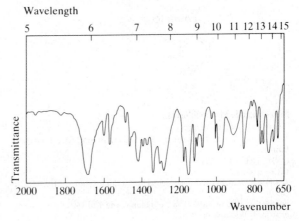

Mass Spectrum. Principal peaks at *m/z* 256, 121, 185, 43, 257, 65, 42, 214.

Quantification. SPECTROFLUORIMETRY. In plasma—R. F. Cunningham *et al.*, *J. pharm. Sci.*, 1978, *67*, 434–436.

GAS CHROMATOGRAPHY. In plasma or cerebrospinal fluid: sensitivity 20 ng/ml, ECD—B. E. Roos *et al.*, *Eur. J. clin. Pharmac.*, 1980, *17*, 223–226.

HIGH PRESSURE LIQUID CHROMATOGRAPHY. In plasma or urine: sensitivity 500 ng/ml, UV detection—P. Hekman *et al.*, *J. Chromat.*, 1980, *182*; *Biomed. Appl.*, *8*, 252–256.

Disposition in the Body. Readily absorbed after oral administration. Metabolised by side-chain oxidation, glucuronic acid conjugation, and *N*-dealkylation. Up to about 90% of a dose is excreted in the urine, the major urinary metabolite, probenecid acyl glucuronide, accounting for up to 50% of a dose; up to 25% of a dose is excreted as hydroxylated and carboxylic acid metabolites, and 5 to 15% as *N*-dealkylated metabolites. About 5 to 10% of a dose is excreted as unchanged drug but this appears to be variable, increasing with increasing urinary pH values and urinary flow.

THERAPEUTIC CONCENTRATION.
Following single oral doses of 0.5, 1.0, and 2.0 g to 5 subjects, mean peak plasma concentrations of 35.3, 69.6, and 149 µg/ml were reported at 3 to 4 hours (A. Selen *et al.*, *J. pharm. Sci.*, 1982, *71*, 1238–1242).

After daily oral administration of 0.5 g four times a day to 19 subjects for 4 weeks, a mean plasma concentration of 22.5 µg/ml was reported (R. F. Cunningham *et al.*, *Clin. Pharmacokinet.*, 1981, *6*, 135–151).

TOXICITY. Probenecid is relatively non-toxic and recovery has occurred after the ingestion of 47 g.

HALF-LIFE. Plasma half-life, 4 to 17 hours (dose-dependent).

VOLUME OF DISTRIBUTION. About 0.1 to 0.2 litre/kg.

PROTEIN BINDING. In plasma, about 90%.

NOTE. For a review of the clinical pharmacokinetics of probenecid see R. F. Cunningham *et al.*, *Clin. Pharmacokinet.*, 1981, *6*, 135–151.

Dose. 0.5 to 2 g daily.

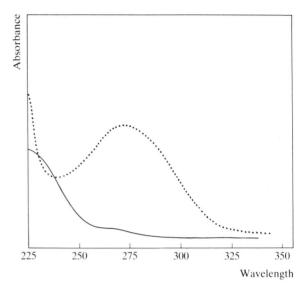

Procainamide   *Anti-arrhythmic*

4-Amino-*N*-(2-diethylaminoethyl)benzamide
$C_{13}H_{21}N_3O = 235.3$
CAS—51-06-9

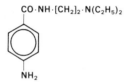

Procainamide Hydrochloride

Synonym. Novocainamidum
Proprietary Names. Novocamid; Procamide; Procan SR; Procapan; Pronestyl.
$C_{13}H_{21}N_3O,HCl = 271.8$
CAS—614-39-1
A white to tan-coloured, hygroscopic, crystalline powder. M.p. 165° to 169°.
Soluble 1 in 0.25 of water, 1 in 2 of ethanol, and 1 in 140 of chloroform; practically insoluble in ether.

Dissociation Constant. pK_a 9.2 (20°).

Partition Coefficient. Log *P* (ethyl acetate/pH 7.4), −1.5.

Colour Tests. Coniferyl Alcohol—orange; Diazotisation—red; Ninhydrin—yellow.

Thin-layer Chromatography. *System TA*—Rf 49; *system TB*—Rf 01; *system TC*—Rf 05. (*Acidified iodoplatinate solution*, positive.)

Gas Chromatography. *System GA*—procainamide RI 2248, *N*-acetylprocainamide RI 2698; *system GF*—RI 2965.

High Pressure Liquid Chromatography. *System HA*—procainamide k' 1.31, *N*-acetylprocainamide k' 3.0.

Ultraviolet Spectrum. Aqueous alkali—275 nm ($A_1^1 = 693$ a).

Infra-red Spectrum. Principal peaks at wavenumbers 1600, 1512, 1639, 1297, 1545, 1570 (procainamide hydrochloride, KBr disk).

Mass Spectrum. Principal peaks at *m/z* 86, 99, 120, 30, 92, 87, 58, 65; *N*-acetylprocainamide 86, 58, 99, 56, 162, 132, 149, 205.

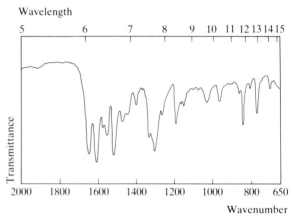

Quantification. GAS CHROMATOGRAPHY. In serum: sensitivity 100 ng, ECD—T. M. Ludden *et al.*, *J. pharm. Sci.*, 1978, *67*, 371–373.

HIGH PRESSURE LIQUID CHROMATOGRAPHY. In plasma: procainamide, *N*-acetylprocainamide, and other anti-arrhythmic agents, sensitivity 500 ng/ml, UV detection—R. R. Bridges and T. A. Jennison, *J. analyt. Toxicol.*, 1983, *7*, 65–68. In plasma: procainamide and *N*-acetylprocainamide, sensitivity 1 µg/ml, UV detection—K. Carr *et al.*, *J. Chromat.*, 1976, *129*, 363–368. In plasma or urine: procainamide and *N*-acetylprocainamide, sensitivity 50 ng/ml in plasma, UV detection—C.-M. Lai *et al.*, *J. pharm. Sci.*, 1980, *69*, 982–984.

Disposition in the Body. Readily absorbed after oral administration and widely distributed throughout the body; bioavailability 75 to 95%. The major metabolite, *N*-acetylprocainamide (acecainide), has similar pharmacological activity to procainamide; the acetylation of procainamide is subject to genetic polymorphism. Up to about 80% of a dose is excreted in the urine of normal subjects in 24 hours, about 50 to 60% as unchanged drug and up to about 30% as *N*-acetylprocainamide (less in slow acetylators). Other metabolites include monodesethylprocainamide and monodesethyl-*N*-acetylprocainamide.

THERAPEUTIC CONCENTRATION. There is considerable intersubject variation in plasma concentrations. The therapeutic effect has been correlated with plasma concentrations of about 4 to 10 μg/ml of procainamide and 5 to 30 μg/ml of combined procainamide and *N*-acetylprocainamide. *N*-Acetylprocainamide may accumulate during chronic administration in fast acetylators and in subjects with renal impairment.

After a single oral dose of 1 g to 5 normal subjects, peak plasma concentrations of 3.5 to 5.3 μg/ml of procainamide (mean 4.2) were attained in 1 to 2 hours; concentrations of *N*-acetylprocainamide reached a peak of 0.6 to 2.1 μg/ml (mean 1.6) in 3 to 8 hours (E.-G. V. Giardina *et al.*, *Clin. Pharmac. Ther.*, 1976, *19*, 339–351).

The following steady-state plasma concentrations were reported in 10 subjects receiving maintenance treatment: procainamide, 2.6 to 20.7 μg/ml (mean 10.6); *N*-acetylprocainamide, 4.6 to 43.6 μg/ml (mean 15.9); monodesethyl-*N*-acetylprocainamide 0.4 to 11.9 μg/ml (mean 2.7) (T. I. Ruo *et al.*, *J. Pharmac. exp. Ther.*, 1981, *216*, 357–362).

Following intravenous infusion of 84 to 374 mg/hour to 34 subjects, steady-state plasma concentrations of 1.7 to 17 μg/ml (mean 6.5) of procainamide and 1.1 to 20 μg/ml (mean 5.7) of *N*-acetylprocainamide were reported (J. J. Lima *et al.*, *Am. J. Cardiol.*, 1979, *43*, 98–105).

TOXICITY. Toxic effects are usually associated with plasma-procainamide concentrations of about 12 μg/ml or more and fatalities with concentrations greater than 20 μg/ml. As little as 200 mg intravenously can be fatal.

In 4 fatalities attributed to procainamide intoxication in subjects receiving therapeutic doses, plasma-procainamide concentrations shortly before death ranged from 17.6 to 25.2 μg/ml (J. Koch-Weser and S. W. Klein, *J. Am. med. Ass.*, 1971, *215*, 1454–1460).

The following postmortem concentrations were reported in a fatality attributed to procainamide: blood 114 μg/ml, liver 283 μg/g, urine 556 μg/ml (L. Kopjak and T. A. Jennison, *Bull. int. Ass. forens. Toxicol.*, 1976, *12*(1), 12–13).

HALF-LIFE. Plasma half-life, procainamide about 3 hours in normal subjects, increased in subjects with renal failure or with heart disease; *N*-acetylprocainamide about 6 to 9 hours.

VOLUME OF DISTRIBUTION. About 2 litres/kg.

CLEARANCE. Plasma clearance, about 5 to 15 ml/min/kg.

PROTEIN BINDING. In plasma, about 15%.

NOTE. For a review of the clinical pharmacokinetics of procainamide see E. Karlsson, *Clin. Pharmacokinet.*, 1978, *3*, 97–107.

Dose. Maintenance, 0.5 to 1 g of procainamide hydrochloride, by mouth, every 4 to 6 hours.

Procaine
Local Anaesthetic

Synonym. Ethocaine
2-Diethylaminoethyl 4-aminobenzoate
$C_{13}H_{20}N_2O_2 = 236.3$
CAS—59-46-1

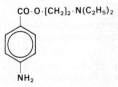

M.p. 61°.
Soluble in ethanol, chloroform, and ether.

Procaine Hydrochloride
Synonyms. Allocaine: Novocainum; Syncaine.
Proprietary Names. Gero H3 Aslan; Novocain; Recorcaina. It is an ingredient of Mydricaine.
$C_{13}H_{20}N_2O_2,HCl = 272.8$
CAS—51-05-8
Colourless crystals or a white crystalline powder. M.p. 153° to 158°.
Soluble 1 in 1 of water, 1 in 25 of ethanol, and 1 in 30 of dehydrated alcohol; slightly soluble in chloroform; practically insoluble in ether.

Dissociation Constant. pK_a 9.0 (20°).

Colour Test. Diazotisation—red-orange.

Thin-layer Chromatography. *System TA*—Rf 54; *system TB*—Rf 06; *system TC*—Rf 31; *system TL*—Rf 30. (*Dragendorff spray*, positive; *acidified iodoplatinate solution*, positive; *ninhydrin spray*, positive.)

Gas Chromatography. *System GA*—procaine RI 2018, 4-aminobenzoic acid RI 1547; *system GF*—RI 2580.

High Pressure Liquid Chromatography. *System HA*—k' 1.9; *system HQ*—k' 0.00.

Ultraviolet Spectrum. Aqueous acid—279 nm ($A_1^1 = 100$ a); methanol—296 nm ($A_1^1 = 954$ a).

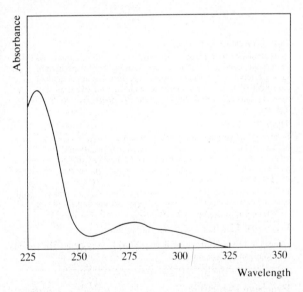

Infra-red Spectrum. Principal peaks at wavenumbers 1690, 1274, 1605, 1174, 1116, 772 (procaine hydrochloride, KBr disk). (See below)

Mass Spectrum. Principal peaks at *m/z* 86, 99, 120, 58, 87, 30, 92, 71; 4-aminobenzoic acid 137, 120, 92, 65, 39, 138, 121, 63.

Quantification. GAS CHROMATOGRAPHY. In plasma: procaine and chloroprocaine, sensitivity 100 ng/ml, FID—R. H. Smith *et al.*, *Clin. Chem.*, 1978, *24*, 1599–1601. In plasma: FID—R. L. Green *et al.*, *New Engl. J. Med.*, 1974, *291*, 223–226.

Disposition in the Body. Readily absorbed after parenteral administration and rapidly hydrolysed in the plasma to 4-aminobenzoic acid and diethylaminoethanol. About 80% of the 4-aminobenzoic acid is excreted unchanged or conjugated in the urine, together with about 30% of the diethylaminoethanol, the remainder being metabolised in the liver; about 2% of a dose is excreted in the urine as unchanged drug.

Wavelength

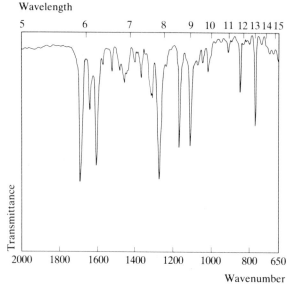

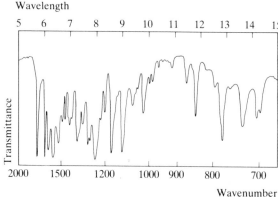

Ultraviolet Spectrum. Aqueous acid—278 nm ($A_1^1 = 53$ b); aqueous alkali—280 nm ($A_1^1 = 256$ b); methanol—295 nm ($A_1^1 = 367$ b).

Infra-red Spectrum. Principal peaks at wavenumbers 1266, 1600, 1779, 1692, 1176, 1120 (KBr disk).

Wavelength

THERAPEUTIC CONCENTRATION.

A mean steady-state plasma concentration of 12.7 µg/ml was reported during the continuous intravenous infusion of 1.0 mg/kg/min to 6 subjects; following continuous intravenous infusion of 1.5 mg/kg/min to a further 6 subjects, a mean steady-state plasma concentration of 42.7 µg/ml was reported (A. B. Seifen *et al.*, *Anesth. Analg. curr. Res.*, 1979, *58*, 382–386).

TOXICITY.

Following intravenous injection to 10 subjects until convulsions were induced (total dose 18 to 55 mg/kg), plasma concentrations of 21 to 86 µg/ml (mean 49) of procaine and 0.6 to 80 µg/ml (mean 23) of 4-aminobenzoic acid were reported (J. E. Usubiaga *et al.*, *Anesth. Analg. curr. Res.*, 1966, *45*, 611–620).

Following the accidental intravenous injection of 4 g to 1 subject, a peak blood concentration of 96 µg/ml was reported; the subject recovered (J. A. Wikinski *et al.*, *J. Am. med. Ass.*, 1970, *213*, 621–623).

HALF-LIFE. Plasma half-life, about 0.1 hour.

Dose. Up to 1 g of procaine hydrochloride may be administered by injection with adrenaline.

Procaine Penicillin   *Antibiotic*

Synonyms. Benzylpenicillin Novocaine; Penicillin G Procaine; Procaine Benzylpenicillin; Procaine Penicillin G.

Proprietary Names. Aquacaine G; Aquacillin; Ayercillin; Crysticillin AS; Depocillin; Duracillin AS; Megacillin; Pfizerpen AS; Wycillin. It is an ingredient of Bicillin and Triplopen.

Note. Bicillin is also used as a proprietary name for benzathine penicillin. Megacillin is also used for benzylpenicillin potassium, clemizole penicillin, and phenoxymethylpenicillin.

Procaine (6R)-6-(2-phenylacetamido)penicillanate monohydrate

$C_{13}H_{20}N_2O_2, C_{16}H_{18}N_2O_4S, H_2O = 588.7$

CAS—54-35-3 (anhydrous); *6130-64-9* (monohydrate)

A white crystalline powder. M.p. 106° to 110°, with decomposition.

Soluble 1 in 200 of water, 1 in 30 of ethanol, and 1 in 60 of chloroform; very slightly soluble in ether.

Dose. 300 to 600 mg daily, by deep intramuscular injection.

Procarbazine   *Antineoplastic*

Synonym. Ibenzmethyzin

N-Isopropyl-α-(2-methylhydrazino)-*p*-toluamide

$C_{12}H_{19}N_3O = 221.3$

CAS—671-16-9

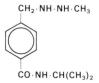

Procarbazine Hydrochloride

Proprietary Names. Matulane; Natulan.

$C_{12}H_{19}N_3O, HCl = 257.8$

CAS—366-70-1

A white to pale yellow, crystalline powder. M.p. about 223°, with decomposition.

Freely **soluble** in water; sparingly soluble in ethanol; slightly soluble in chloroform; practically insoluble in ether; soluble in methanol. Solutions in water are unstable.

Dissociation Constant. pK_a 6.8.

Colour Tests. Liebermann's Test (100°)—blue (15 s); Nessler's Reagent (room temperature)—black; Palladium Chloride—black.

Thin-layer Chromatography. System *TA*—Rf 49; system *TB*—Rf 02; system *TC*—Rf 10. (*Acidified potassium permanganate solution*, positive.)

Gas Chromatography. System *GA*—RI 1990.

Ultraviolet Spectrum. Aqueous acid—232 nm ($A_1^1 = 570$ a).

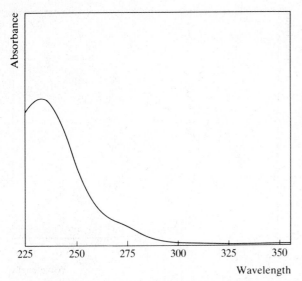

Infra-red Spectrum. Principal peaks at wavenumbers 1632, 1555, 1661, 1301, 861, 1176 (procarbazine hydrochloride, KBr disk).

Mass Spectrum. Principal peaks at m/z 177, 118, 45, 135, 90, 91, 221, 119.

Quantification. GAS CHROMATOGRAPHY–MASS SPECTROMETRY. In plasma: procarbazine and metabolites, sensitivity 10 ng/ml— R. M. Gorsen et al., J. Chromat., 1980, 221; Biomed. Appl., 10, 309–318.

HIGH PRESSURE LIQUID CHROMATOGRAPHY. In plasma or urine: sensitivity 10 ng, electrochemical detection—R. J. Rucki and S. A. Moros, J. Chromat., 1980, 190, 359–365. In plasma: procarbazine metabolites, UV detection—D. A. Shiba and R. J. Weinkam, J. Chromat., 1982, 229; Biomed. Appl., 18, 397–407.

Disposition in the Body. Readily absorbed after oral administration; peak plasma concentrations are attained in 0.5 to 1 hour. Rapidly metabolised to active azo derivatives and by oxidation to N-isopropylterephthalamic acid. Up to about 75% of a dose is excreted in the urine with about 5% of a dose consisting of unchanged drug.

Dose. Initially the equivalent of 50 mg of procarbazine daily, increasing to 250 or 300 mg daily.

Prochlorperazine   *Tranquilliser*

Synonym. Prochlorpemazine
Proprietary Names. Compazine; Stemetil (suppositories); Témentil. It is an ingredient of Eskatrol.
2-Chloro-10-[3-(4-methylpiperazin-1-yl)propyl]phenothiazine
$C_{20}H_{24}ClN_3S = 373.9$
CAS—58-38-8

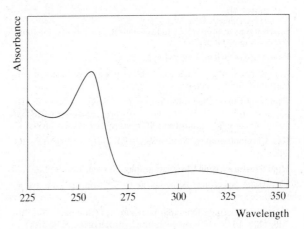

A clear, pale yellow, viscous liquid which is sensitive to light. Very slightly **soluble** in water; freely soluble in ethanol, chloroform, and ether.

Prochlorperazine Edisylate
Synonym. Prochlorperazine Ethanedisulphonate
Proprietary Name. Compazine
$C_{20}H_{24}ClN_3S,C_2H_6O_6S_2 = 564.1$
CAS—1257-78-9
A white to very light yellow, crystalline powder.
Soluble 1 in 2 of water and 1 in 1500 of ethanol; practically insoluble in chloroform and ether.

Prochlorperazine Maleate
Synonyms. Prochlorperazine Dihydrogen Maleate; Prochlorperazine Dimaleate.
Proprietary Names. Anti-Naus; Compazine; Stemetil (tablets); Vertigon. It is an ingredient of Combid.
$C_{20}H_{24}ClN_3S,2C_4H_4O_4 = 606.1$
CAS—84-02-6
A white or pale yellow, crystalline powder. M.p. 198° to 203°.
Practically **insoluble** in water, ethanol, and ether; slightly soluble in warm chloroform.

Prochlorperazine Mesylate
Synonyms. Prochlorperazine Dimethanesulphonate; Prochlorperazine Methanesulphonate.
Proprietary Name. Stemetil (injection and syrup)
$C_{20}H_{24}ClN_3S,2CH_3SO_3H = 566.1$
CAS—51888-09-6
A white powder. M.p. about 242°.
Soluble 1 in less than 0.5 of water and 1 in 40 of ethanol; slightly soluble in chloroform; practically insoluble in ether.

Dissociation Constant. pK_a 8.1 (24°).

Partition Coefficient. Log P (octanol/pH 7.0), 2.4.

Colour Tests. Formaldehyde–Sulphuric Acid—red-violet; Forrest Reagent—red; FPN Reagent—red; Mandelin's Test—brown → violet; Marquis Test—violet.

Thin-layer Chromatography. *System TA*—Rf 49; *system TB*—Rf 33; *system TC*—Rf 37. (*Acidified iodoplatinate solution*, positive.)

Gas Chromatography. *System GA*—RI 2954.

High Pressure Liquid Chromatography. *System HA*—k' 3.9.

Ultraviolet Spectrum. Aqueous acid—254 nm ($A_1^1 = 875$ a), 305 nm.

Infra-red Spectrum. Principal peaks at wavenumbers 752, 1280, 1569, 1165, 1242, 1145 (KBr disk).

Mass Spectrum. Principal peaks at *m/z* 113, 70, 373, 141, 43, 72, 42, 127.

Quantification. HIGH PRESSURE LIQUID CHROMATOGRAPHY. In plasma: detection limit about 200 pg/ml, electrochemical detection—M. G. Sankey *et al.*, *Br. J. clin. Pharmac.*, 1982, *13*, 578–580.

RADIOIMMUNOASSAY. In plasma: detection limit 156 pg/ml—K. K. Midha *et al.*, *Ther. Drug Monit.*, 1983, *5*, 117–121.

Disposition in the Body. Absorbed after oral administration but extensively metabolised.

THERAPEUTIC CONCENTRATION.
Following a single oral dose of 12.5 mg to 1 subject, a peak plasma concentration of about 0.0008 μg/ml was attained in 6 hours (M. G. Sankey *et al.*, *Br. J. clin Pharmac.*, 1982, *13*, 578–580).

TOXICITY.
Serum concentrations of 1.2 to 1.6 μg/ml were found in 4 cases of non-fatal overdose (S. L. Tompsett, *Acta pharmac. tox.*, 1968, *26*, 298–302).

Dose. Usually 15 to 30 mg of prochlorperazine maleate daily, as an anti-emetic; 50 to 100 mg daily for the treatment of psychoses.

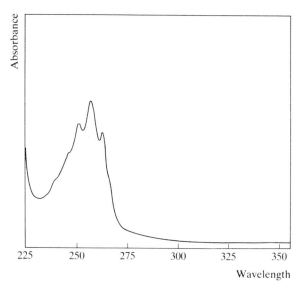
Wavelength

Procyclidine   *Anticholinergic*

1-Cyclohexyl-1-phenyl-3-(pyrrolidin-1-yl)propan-1-ol
$C_{19}H_{29}NO = 287.4$
CAS—77-37-2

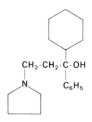

Crystals. M.p. 85° to 87°.

Procyclidine Hydrochloride
Proprietary Names. Arpicolin; Kemadrin(e); Osnervan; Procyclid.
$C_{19}H_{29}NO,HCl = 323.9$
CAS—1508-76-5
A white crystalline powder. M.p. 225° to 227°.
Soluble 1 in about 40 of water, 1 in 15 of ethanol, and 1 in 6 of chloroform; practically insoluble in ether.

Partition Coefficient. Log *P* (heptane), 1.7.

Colour Tests. Mandelin's Test—black; Marquis Test—violet; Sulphuric Acid—yellow.

Thin-layer Chromatography. *System TA*—Rf 48; *system TB*—Rf 63; *system TC*—Rf 31. (*Dragendorff spray*, positive; *acidified iodoplatinate solution*, positive; *Marquis reagent*, violet-brown.)

Gas Chromatography. *System GA*—RI 2156; *system GF*—RI 2485.

High Pressure Liquid Chromatography. *System HA*—k' 2.0.

Ultraviolet Spectrum. Aqueous acid—251 nm, 257 nm ($A_1^1 = 6.9$ a), 263 nm.

Infra-red Spectrum. Principal peaks at wavenumbers 700, 756, 746, 1128, 1075, 1175 (procyclidine hydrochloride, KBr disk).

Mass Spectrum. Principal peaks at *m/z* 84, 204, 205, 85, 42, 55, 105, 77.

Quantification. GAS CHROMATOGRAPHY. In plasma or urine: sensitivity 20 ng/ml, AFID—K. Dean *et al.*, *J. Chromat.*, 1980, *221*; *Biomed. Appl.*, *10*, 408–413. In blood: sensitivity 100 ng/ml, AFID—A. W. Missen *et al.*, *J. analyt. Toxicol.*, 1978, *2*, 238–240.

Disposition in the Body. Absorbed after oral administration; bioavailability about 75%. Metabolised by hydroxylation of the benzyl or cyclohexyl rings.

THERAPEUTIC CONCENTRATION.
Following a single oral dose of 10 mg to 6 subjects, a mean peak plasma concentration of 0.12 μg/ml was reported; in 5 of the subjects the peak concentrations were attained in about 1 hour, whereas in the sixth subject the time to peak concentration was 8 hours (P. D. Whiteman *et al.*, *Eur. J. clin. Pharmac.*, 1985, *28*, 73–78).

In 6 patients undergoing therapy with daily oral doses of 10 to 30 mg, mean steady-state blood concentrations of 0.15 to 0.63 μg/ml were reported (A. W. Missen *et al.*, *J. analyt. Toxicol.*, 1978, *2*, 238–240).

TOXICITY.
In 2 fatalities involving procyclidine, postmortem tissue concentrations were: blood 4 and 4.4 μg/ml, liver 15 and 11 μg/g, urine 7 and 1.8 μg/ml; in the second case benztropine and chlorpromazine were also detected (P. G. Ashton, *Bull. int. Ass. forens. Toxicol.*, 1980, *15*(2), 9–11).

HALF-LIFE. Plasma half-life, 8 to 16 hours (mean 12).

VOLUME OF DISTRIBUTION. About 1 litre/kg.

CLEARANCE. Plasma clearance, about 1 ml/min/kg.

Dose. 7.5 to 30 mg of procyclidine hydrochloride daily; up to 60 mg daily has been given.

Profadol
Narcotic Analgesic

3-(1-Methyl-3-propylpyrrolidin-3-yl)phenol
$C_{14}H_{21}NO = 219.3$
CAS—428-37-5

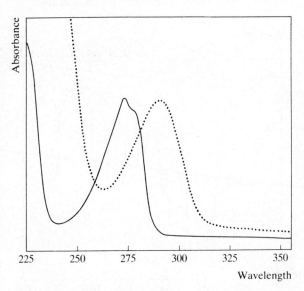

Profadol Hydrochloride
$C_{14}H_{21}NO,HCl = 255.8$
CAS—2324-94-9
A white solid. M.p. 145° to 146°.
Soluble in water and chloroform.

Colour Tests. Folin–Ciocalteu Reagent—blue; Liebermann's Test—black; Mandelin's Test—blue-green → green; Marquis Test—orange → red-brown.

Thin-layer Chromatography. *System TA*—Rf 42; *system TB*—Rf 08; *system TC*—Rf 06. (*Acidified iodoplatinate solution*, positive.)

Gas Chromatography. *System GA*—RI 1748.

Ultraviolet Spectrum. Aqueous acid—272 nm ($A_1^1 = 87$ b); aqueous alkali—237 nm, 290 nm.

Infra-red Spectrum. Principal peaks at wavenumbers 1575, 1590, 1234, 752, 702, 1267 (KBr disk).

Mass Spectrum. Principal peaks at *m/z* 57, 42, 44, 177, 58, 219, 133, 107.

Proflavine Hemisulphate
Disinfectant

Synonyms. Neutral Proflavine Sulphate; Proflavine.
3,6-Diaminoacridine sulphate dihydrate
$(C_{13}H_{11}N_3)_2,H_2SO_4,2H_2O = 552.6$
CAS—92-62-6 (proflavine); *553-30-0* (sulphate, anhydrous)

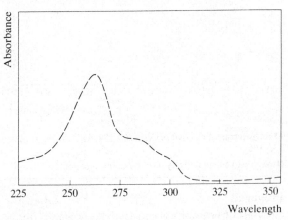

An orange to red, hygroscopic, crystalline powder.
Soluble 1 in 300 of water, 1 in 1 of boiling water, and 1 in 35 of glycerol; very slightly soluble in ethanol; practically insoluble in chloroform and ether. A saturated solution in water is deep orange in colour and gives a green fluorescence when freely diluted.

Colour Tests. Mandelin's Test—green; Marquis Test—yellow → orange.

Thin-layer Chromatography. *System TA*—Rf 16.

Ultraviolet Spectrum. Ethanol—261 nm ($A_1^1 = 1091$ b).

Infra-red Spectrum. Principal peaks at wavenumbers 1605, 1625, 1125, 1160, 1218, 1263 (KBr disk).

Progesterone
Progestational Steroid

Synonyms. Luteal Hormone; Luteine; Pregnenedione; Progestin.
Proprietary Names. Biograviplan; Cyclogest; Gesterol; Gestone; Lutogyl; Progestasert; Progestilin; Progestogel; Progestosol; Proluton.
Pregn-4-ene-3,20-dione
$C_{21}H_{30}O_2 = 314.5$
CAS—57-83-0

Colourless crystals or a white or slightly yellowish-white, crystalline powder. There are two forms, one melts at 126° to 131° and the other, known as β-progesterone, at about 121°. Practically **insoluble** in water; soluble 1 in 8 of ethanol, 1 in less than 1 of chloroform, and 1 in 16 of ether.

Colour Tests. Naphthol–Sulphuric Acid—brown/yellow; Sulphuric Acid—yellow (green fluorescence under ultraviolet light).

Thin-layer Chromatography. *System TP*—Rf 81; *system TQ*—Rf 20; *system TR*—Rf 99; *system TS*—Rf 95.

Gas Chromatography. *System GA*—RI 2793.

Ultraviolet Spectrum. Dehydrated alcohol—240 nm (A$_1^1$ = 540 a).

Infra-red Spectrum. Principal peaks at wavenumbers 1662, 1614, 1700, 872, 1209, 1232 (KBr disk).

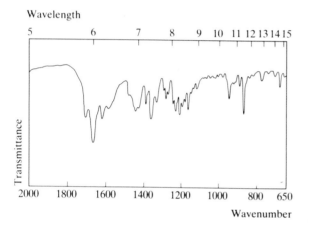

Mass Spectrum. Principal peaks at *m/z* 124, 43, 314, 79, 91, 229, 272, 105.

Dose. Up to 50 mg daily by intramuscular injection.

Proguanil
Antimalarial

Synonyms. Chloriguane; Chloroguanide; Proguanide.
1-(4-Chlorophenyl)-5-isopropylbiguanide
$C_{11}H_{16}ClN_5 = 253.7$
CAS—500-92-5

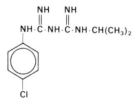

Colourless crystals. M.p. 130° to 131°.

Proguanil Hydrochloride
Synonym. Bigumalum
Proprietary Names. Paludrine; Paludrinol.
$C_{11}H_{16}ClN_5,HCl = 290.2$
CAS—637-32-1
A white crystalline powder. M.p. about 245°.
Soluble 1 in 110 of water and 1 in 40 of ethanol; practically insoluble in chloroform and ether.

Dissociation Constant. pK$_a$ 2.3, 10.4 (22.5°).

Colour Test. To 10 ml of a saturated solution of proguanil hydrochloride add 1 drop of 10% copper sulphate solution and 2.5 ml of *dilute ammonia solution* and shake well; add 5 ml of toluene and shake again—toluene layer is violet-red.

Thin-layer Chromatography. *System TA*—Rf 03; *system TB*—Rf 00; *system TC*—Rf 01. (*Acidified iodoplatinate solution*, positive.)

Ultraviolet Spectrum. Methanol—259 nm (A$_1^1$ = 886 b).

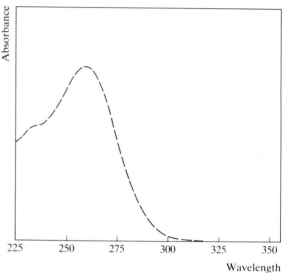

Infra-red Spectrum. Principal peaks at wavenumbers 1534, 1635, 1492, 1575, 1600, 1170 (proguanil hydrochloride, KBr disk).

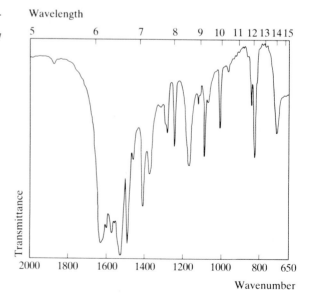

Mass Spectrum. Principal peaks at *m/z* 43, 127, 195, 85, 44, 36, 152, 58.

Quantification. HIGH PRESSURE LIQUID CHROMATOGRAPHY. In serum: proguanil, cycloguanil and 4-chlorophenylbiguanide, detection limit 60 ng/ml, UV detection—R. R. Moody *et al.*, *J. Chromat.*, 1980, *182*; *Biomed. Appl.*, *8*, 359–367.

Disposition in the Body. Readily absorbed after oral administration; peak plasma concentrations are attained in about 3 hours. About 60% of a dose is excreted in the urine unchanged, together with about 30% as the active metabolite cycloguanil; 4-chlorophenylbiguanide is also a metabolite.

PROTEIN BINDING. In plasma, about 75%.

Dose. 100 to 300 mg of proguanil hydrochloride daily.

Prolintane   *Central Stimulant*

1-(α-Propylphenethyl)pyrrolidine
$C_{15}H_{23}N = 217.4$
CAS—493-92-5

$$C_6H_5 \cdot CH_2 \cdot CH \cdot [CH_2]_2 \cdot CH_3$$

Prolintane Hydrochloride

Proprietary Names. Promotil. It is an ingredient of Villescon.
$C_{15}H_{23}N,HCl = 253.8$
CAS—1211-28-5
A white powder. M.p. about 133°.
Soluble in water, ethanol, and chloroform; practically insoluble in ether.

Colour Tests. Liebermann's Test—red-orange; Mandelin's Test—red; Marquis Test—orange → brown.

Thin-layer Chromatography. *System TA*—Rf 50; *system TB*—Rf 66; *system TC*—Rf 32. (*Dragendorff spray*, positive; *acidified iodoplatinate solution*, positive; *Marquis reagent*, orange-brown; *acidified potassium permanganate solution*, positive.)

Gas Chromatography. *System GA*—RI 1634; *system GB*—RI 1675; *system GC*—RI 1849.

High Pressure Liquid Chromatography. *System HA*—k' 2.0; *system HC*—k' 1.26.

Ultraviolet Spectrum. Aqueous acid—252 nm, 258 nm ($A_1^1 = 8.6$ a), 264 nm.

Infra-red Spectrum. Principal peaks at wavenumbers 776, 714, 752, 1501, 1141, 1020 (prolintane hydrochloride, KBr disk).

Mass Spectrum. Principal peaks at *m/z* 126, 127, 174, 91, 70, 69, 55, 42.

Dose. 20 mg of prolintane hydrochloride daily.

Promazine   *Tranquilliser*

NN-Dimethyl-3-(phenothiazin-10-yl)propylamine
$C_{17}H_{20}N_2S = 284.4$
CAS—58-40-2

$$CH_2 \cdot [CH_2]_2 \cdot N(CH_3)_2$$

An oily liquid.

Promazine Embonate

Synonym. Promazine Pamoate
Proprietary Names. Protactyl (suspension); Sparine (suspension).
$(C_{17}H_{20}N_2S)_2,C_{23}H_{16}O_6 = 957.2$

Promazine Hydrochloride

Synonym. Propazinum
Proprietary Names. Calmotal; Neuroplegil; Prazine; Promabec; Promanyl; Protactyl (injection and tablets); Sparine (injection and tablets); Talofen.
$C_{17}H_{20}N_2S,HCl = 320.9$
CAS—53-60-1
A white or slightly yellow, slightly hygroscopic, crystalline powder. It is affected by air and light and traces of heavy metals. Decomposed solutions may be coloured pink, red, or blue. M.p. 172° to 182°.
Soluble 1 in 1 of water, 1 in 2 of ethanol, and 1 in 2 of chloroform; practically insoluble in ether.

Dissociation Constant. pK_a 9.4 (25°).

Partition Coefficient. Log *P* (octanol/pH 7.4), 2.5.

Colour Tests. Formaldehyde–Sulphuric Acid—red; Forrest Reagent—red-brown; FPN Reagent—red-brown; Liebermann's Test—green-brown; Mandelin's Test—green → violet; Marquis Test—violet.

Thin-layer Chromatography. *System TA*—Rf 44; *system TB*—Rf 41; *system TC*—Rf 30. (*Dragendorff spray*, positive; *FPN reagent*, pink; *acidified iodoplatinate solution*, positive; *Marquis reagent*, red; *ninhydrin spray*, positive.)

Gas Chromatography. *System GA*—RI 2316; *system GF*—RI 2745.

High Pressure Liquid Chromatography. *System HA*—k' 5.9.

Ultraviolet Spectrum. Aqueous acid—251 nm ($A_1^1 = 1055$ a), 302 nm; aqueous alkali—254 nm, 306 nm.

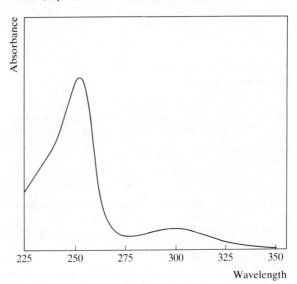

Infra-red Spectrum. Principal peaks at wavenumbers 751, 1250, 1234, 1287, 770, 1162 (promazine hydrochloride, KBr disk). (See below)

Mass Spectrum. Principal peaks at *m/z* 58, 284, 86, 238, 198, 199, 85, 42.

Dose. Usually up to 400 mg of promazine hydrochloride daily; maximum of 1 g daily.

Wavelength

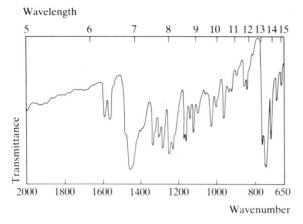

Thin-layer Chromatography. *System TA*—Rf 50; *system TB*—Rf 37; *system TC*—Rf 35. (*Dragendorff spray*, positive; *FPN reagent*, positive; *acidified iodoplatinate solution*, positive; *Marquis reagent*, violet; *ninhydrin spray*, positive.)

Gas Chromatography. *System GA*—RI 2259; *system GC*—RI 2546; *system GF*—RI 2675.

High Pressure Liquid Chromatography. *System HA*—k' 5.0.

Ultraviolet Spectrum. Aqueous acid—249 nm ($A_1^1 = 1032$ a), 298 nm; aqueous alkali—254 nm, 305 nm.

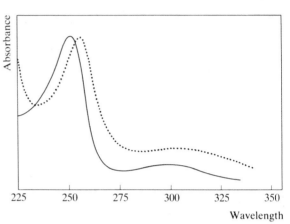

Promethazine   *Antihistamine*

Proprietary Name. Phenergan (cream)
1,*N*,*N*-Trimethyl-2-(phenothiazin-10-yl)ethylamine
$C_{17}H_{20}N_2S = 284.4$
CAS—60-87-7

A crystalline solid. M.p. about 60°.

Promethazine Hydrochloride

Synonyms. Diprazinum; Proazamine Chloride.
Proprietary Names. Atosil; Fellozine; Ganphen; Histantil; Phencen; Phenergan; Progan; Promine; Prothazine; Quadnite; Remsed; Sominex; V-Gan; ZiPan. It is an ingredient of Medised, Mepergan, Phensedyl, and Tixylix.
$C_{17}H_{20}N_2S,HCl = 320.9$
CAS—58-33-3
A white or faintly yellow, crystalline powder, which is slowly oxidised on prolonged exposure to air, becoming blue in colour. M.p. about 222°, with decomposition.
Soluble 1 in 0.6 of water, 1 in 9 of ethanol, and 1 in 2 of chloroform; practically insoluble in ether.

Promethazine Theoclate

Synonym. Promethazine Chlorotheophyllinate
Proprietary Names. Avomine; Meth-Zine.
$C_{17}H_{20}N_2S,C_7H_7ClN_4O_2 = 499.0$
CAS—17693-51-5
A white powder.
Very slightly **soluble** in water; soluble 1 in 70 of ethanol and 1 in 2.5 of chloroform; practically insoluble in ether.

Dissociation Constant. pK_a 9.1 (25°).

Partition Coefficient. Log *P* (octanol/pH 7.4), 2.9.

Colour Tests. Formaldehyde–Sulphuric Acid—blue-violet; Forrest Reagent—red; FPN Reagent—orange; Mandelin's Test—green → violet; Marquis Test—violet.

Infra-red Spectrum. Principal peaks at wavenumbers 758, 1229, 733, 1129, 1259, 1287 (promethazine hydrochloride, KBr disk).

Wavelength

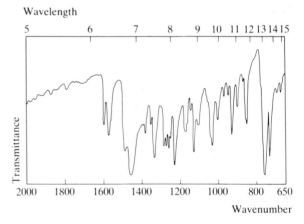

Mass Spectrum. Principal peaks at *m/z* 72, 73, 284, 198, 213, 199, 180, 56; *N*-monodesmethylpromethazine 58, 213, 198, 180, 214, 57, 212, 270.

Quantification. HIGH PRESSURE LIQUID CHROMATOGRAPHY. In blood: promethazine, *N*-monodesmethylpromethazine and promethazine sulphoxide, detection limit for promethazine 200 pg/ml, UV detection—G. Taylor and J. B. Houston, *J. Chromat.*, 1982, *230*; *Biomed. Appl.*, *19*, 194–198. In plasma or serum: detection limit 200 pg/ml, electrochemical detection—J. E. Wallace *et al.*, *Analyt. Chem.*, 1981, *53*, 960–962. In postmortem samples: promethazine and metabolites, UV detection—W. J. Allender and A. W. Archer, *J. forens. Sci.*, 1984, *29*, 515–526.

Disposition in the Body. Readily absorbed after oral administration but subject to extensive first-pass metabolism. About 2% of a dose is excreted in the urine unchanged. The major urinary metabolite is the sulphoxide; glucuronic acid conjugation also occurs. *N*-Monodesmethylpromethazine has been detected in plasma and urine.

THERAPEUTIC CONCENTRATION.
Following an oral dose of 25 mg to 10 subjects, a mean peak blood concentration of 0.005 µg/ml was attained in 2 hours; saliva concentrations averaged 0.008 µg/ml consistently from 1 to 6 hours after administration. After an intramuscular dose of 25 mg to the same subjects, mean peak concentrations of 0.022 µg/ml at 4 hours and 0.003 µg/ml at 2 hours were reported for blood and saliva, respectively (G. J. DiGregorio and E. Ruch, *J. pharm. Sci.*, 1980, *69*, 1457–1459).
Following single oral doses of 25 mg to 7 subjects, peak blood concentrations of 0.002 to 0.018 µg/ml were attained in 1.5 to 3 hours (G. Taylor *et al.*, *Br. J. clin. Pharmac.*, 1983, *15*, 287–293).

TOXICITY. The estimated minimum lethal dose is 200 mg/kg.
In 2 fatalities involving the ingestion of promethazine, the following postmortem tissue concentrations were reported (µg/ml or µg/g):

	Promethazine	Promethazine sulphoxide	*N*-Monodesmethyl-promethazine
Blood	5.2, 2.4	3.1, 0.8	0.8, 1.2
Bile	82.6, 11.6	23.5, 27.0	14.5, 3.0
Liver	30.6, 23.2	8.4, 5.4	6.3, 16.2
Urine	6.0, 14.0	26.0, 42.0	1.0, 3.0

Other drugs were detected in both cases (W. J. Allender and A. W. Archer, *J. forens. Sci.*, 1984, *29*, 515–526).

HALF-LIFE. Plasma half-life, 10 to 15 hours.

VOLUME OF DISTRIBUTION. About 13 litres/kg.

CLEARANCE. Plasma clearance, about 16 ml/min/kg.

DISTRIBUTION IN BLOOD. Plasma:whole blood ratio, 1.5.

PROTEIN BINDING. In plasma, about 75 to 93%.

Dose. 20 to 75 mg of promethazine hydrochloride daily.

Prometryne
Herbicide

Proprietary Name. Gesagard 50 WP
2,4-Bis(isopropylamino)-6-methylthio-1,3,5-triazine
$C_{10}H_{19}N_5S = 241.4$
CAS—7287-19-6

A white crystalline solid. M.p. 118° to 120°.
Practically **insoluble** in water; readily soluble in organic solvents.

Thin-layer Chromatography. *System TA*—Rf 76. (*Dragendorff spray*, positive.)

Gas Chromatography. *System GA*—RI 1853.

Infra-red Spectrum. Principal peaks at wavenumbers 1510, 1592, 1171, 1299, 809, 1217 (KBr disk).

Propamidine
Antibacterial/Antifungal

4,4′-Trimethylenedioxydibenzamidine
$C_{17}H_{20}N_4O_2 = 312.4$
CAS—104-32-5

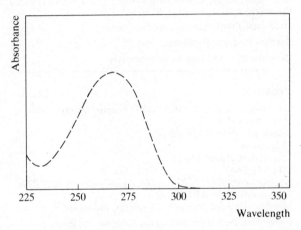

Propamidine Isethionate
Proprietary Names. Brolene (eye drops); M & B Antiseptic Cream.
$C_{17}H_{20}N_4O_2,2C_2H_6O_4S = 564.6$
CAS—140-63-6
A white, granular, hygroscopic powder. M.p. 235°.
Soluble 1 in 5 of water and 1 in 33 of ethanol; practically insoluble in organic solvents.

Thin-layer Chromatography. *System TA*—Rf 01; *system TB*—Rf 01; *system TC*—Rf 01. (*Acidified iodoplatinate solution*, positive.)

Ultraviolet Spectrum. Ethanol—267 nm ($A_1^1 = 1224$ b).

Infra-red Spectrum. Principal peaks at wavenumbers 1200, 1219, 1613, 1048, 1280, 1495 (propamidine isethionate, KBr disk).

Mass Spectrum. Principal peaks at *m/z* 41, 132, 102, 160, 96, 29, 27, 44.

Use. Propamidine isethionate is used in concentrations of 0.1 to 0.15%.

Propanidid
General Anaesthetic

Proprietary Name. Epontol
Propyl 4-diethylcarbamoylmethoxy-3-methoxyphenylacetate
$C_{18}H_{27}NO_5 = 337.4$
CAS—1421-14-3

A pale greenish-yellow, hygroscopic, viscous liquid. B.p. about 210°.
Very slightly **soluble** in water; miscible with ethanol, chloroform, and ether.

Colour Tests. Aromaticity (Method 2)—yellow/orange; Liebermann's Test—black.

Thin-layer Chromatography. *System TA*—Rf 66; *system TB*—Rf 20; *system TC*—Rf 70. (*Dragendorff spray*, positive.)

Gas Chromatography. *System GA*—RI 2433.

Ultraviolet Spectrum. Ethanol—280 nm ($A_1^1 = 82$ a).

Infra-red Spectrum. Principal peaks at wavenumbers 1258, 1508, 1637, 1142, 1724, 1220 (thin film).

Mass Spectrum. Principal peaks at m/z 114, 72, 43, 100, 29, 44, 337, 86.

Disposition in the Body. Rapidly metabolised by hydrolysis and demethylation to inactive metabolites which are excreted in the urine. About 90% of a dose is excreted in the urine in 2 hours and up to 6% is eliminated in the faeces.

THERAPEUTIC CONCENTRATION.
Following intravenous administration of 7 mg/kg to 10 subjects, a mean serum concentration of about 14 µg/ml was reported at 1 minute (A. Doenicke *et al.*, *Br. J. Anaesth.*, 1968, *40*, 415–428).

HALF-LIFE. Plasma half-life, about 0.2 hour.

PROTEIN BINDING. In plasma, about 75%.

Dose. Usually 5 to 10 mg/kg intravenously.

Propanol   *Solvent*

Synonyms. Normal Propyl Alcohol; Primary Propyl Alcohol; Propyl Alcohol.
Proprietary Name. Satinazid
Propan-1-ol
$CH_3 \cdot CH_2 \cdot CH_2OH = 60.10$
CAS—71-23-8
A clear, colourless, inflammable liquid. Wt per ml about 0.804 g. B.p. 96° to 100°.

Miscible with water, ethanol, chloroform, and ether.

Colour Test. Potassium Dichromate (Method 2)—green.

Gas Chromatography. *System GA*—RI 571; *system GI*—retention time 5.5 min.

Mass Spectrum. Principal peaks at m/z 31, 59, 42, 60, 27, 29, 45, 41.

Propantheline Bromide   *Anticholinergic*

Proprietary Names. Banlin; Pantheline; Pro-Banthine; Propanthel.
Di - isopropylmethyl[2 - (xanthen - 9 - ylcarbonyloxy)ethyl] - ammonium bromide
$C_{23}H_{30}BrNO_3 = 448.4$
CAS—298-50-0 (propantheline); *50-34-0* (bromide)

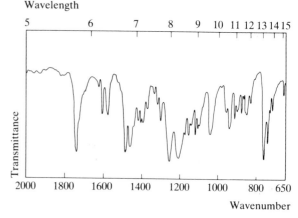

A white or yellowish-white powder. M.p. 156° to 162°, with decomposition.

Very **soluble** in water, ethanol, and chloroform; practically insoluble in ether.
Note. The dust is irritant to mucous membranes.

Colour Tests. The following tests are performed on the nitrate (see page 128): Mandelin's Test—orange; Marquis Test—orange.

Thin-layer Chromatography. *System TA*—Rf 04. (*Acidified iodoplatinate solution*, positive.)

High Pressure Liquid Chromatography. *System HA*—k' 4.4.

Ultraviolet Spectrum. Aqueous acid—243 nm ($A_1^1 = 103$ a), 281 nm; aqueous alkali—249 nm, 282 nm.

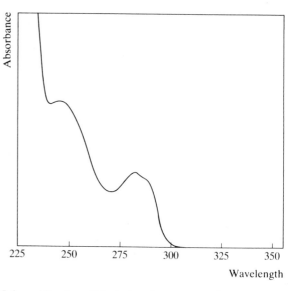

Infra-red Spectrum. Principal peaks at wavenumbers 1255, 761, 1208, 1733, 745, 1158 (KBr disk).

Mass Spectrum. Principal peaks at m/z 86, 181, 43, 44, 41, 114, 42, 152 (propantheline).

Quantification. GAS CHROMATOGRAPHY–MASS SPECTROMETRY. In plasma or urine: sensitivity 5 ng/ml and 10 ng/ml respectively—G. C. Ford *et al.*, *Biomed. Mass Spectrom.*, 1977, *4*, 94–97.

HIGH PRESSURE LIQUID CHROMATOGRAPHY. In serum: sensitivity 2 ng/ml, UV detection—D. K. Moses *et al.*, *Br. J. clin. Pharmac.*, 1983, *16*, 758–759.

Disposition in the Body. Poorly absorbed after oral administration due to decomposition in the small intestine. It undergoes extensive metabolism mainly by hydrolysis and glucuronide conjugation; aromatic hydroxylation also occurs. About 50 to 65% of an oral dose is excreted in the urine in 24 hours with less than 10% as unchanged drug. The major urinary metabolite is xanthanoic acid glucuronide conjugate; other metabolites include free xanthanoic acid, hydroxyxanthanoic acid, propantheline, and hydroxypropantheline.

THERAPEUTIC CONCENTRATION.
Following single oral doses of 30 mg and 60 mg to 6 subjects, peak plasma concentrations of 0.0 to 0.038 µg/ml (mean 0.024) and 0.033 to 0.162 µg/ml (mean 0.06), respectively, were attained in about 0.5 to 1 hour (C. W. Vose *et al.*, *Eur. J. drug Met. Pharmacokinet.*, 1980, *5*, 29–34).

HALF-LIFE. Plasma half-life, 1 to 3 hours.

CLEARANCE. Plasma clearance, about 20 ml/min/kg.

Dose. Usually 75 mg daily; maximum of 120 mg daily.

Propicillin   *Antibiotic*

Synonym. α-Phenoxypropylpenicillin
(6*R*)-6-(2-Phenoxybutyramido)penicillanic acid
$C_{18}H_{22}N_2O_5S = 378.4$
CAS—551-27-9

Propicillin Potassium
Proprietary Names. Baycillin; Oricillin.
$C_{18}H_{21}KN_2O_5S = 416.5$
CAS—1245-44-9
A white, hygroscopic, finely crystalline powder.
Soluble 1 in 1.2 of water, 1 in 25 of ethanol, and 1 in 65 of dehydrated alcohol; practically insoluble in chloroform and ether.

Dissociation Constant. pK_a 2.7 (25°).

Ultraviolet Spectrum. Propicillin potassium: water—269 nm ($A_1^1 = 27$ b), 276 nm ($A_1^1 = 21.5$ b).

Infra-red Spectrum. Principal peaks at wavenumbers 1600, 1757, 1669, 1224, 1314, 750 (propicillin potassium, KBr disk).

Dose. The equivalent of 0.5 to 1.5 g of propicillin daily.

Propiomazine   *Antihistamine/Sedative*

1-[10-(2-Dimethylaminopropyl)phenothiazin-2-yl]propan-1-one
$C_{20}H_{24}N_2OS = 340.5$
CAS—362-29-8

Propiomazine Hydrochloride
Proprietary Name. Largon
$C_{20}H_{24}N_2OS,HCl = 376.9$
CAS—1240-15-9
A yellow powder.
Soluble 1 in less than 1 of water, 1 in 6 of ethanol, and 1 in 2 of chloroform; practically insoluble in ether.

Propiomazine Maleate
Synonym. Propiomazine Hydrogen Maleate
Proprietary Name. Serentin
$C_{20}H_{24}N_2OS,C_4H_4O_4 = 456.6$
CAS—3568-23-8
A yellow microcrystalline powder. M.p. 160° to 161°.
Soluble 1 in 500 of water, 1 in 60 of ethanol, and 1 in 140 of dehydrated alcohol.

Dissociation Constant. pK_a 6.6.

Colour Tests. Formaldehyde–Sulphuric Acid—blue-violet; Forrest Reagent—red; FPN Reagent—pink-orange → red → fades; Liebermann's Test—violet; Mandelin's Test—violet; Marquis Test—red-violet.

Thin-layer Chromatography. *System TA*—Rf 55; *system TB*—Rf 34; *system TC*—Rf 42. (Location under ultraviolet light, pink fluorescence; *Dragendorff spray*, positive; *FPN reagent*, yellow; *acidified iodoplatinate solution*, positive; *Marquis reagent*, red.)

Gas Chromatography. *System GA*—RI 2738; *system GF*—RI 3225.

High Pressure Liquid Chromatography. *System HA*—k' 2.1.

Ultraviolet Spectrum. Aqueous acid—241 nm ($A_1^1 = 749$ a), 273 nm, 360 nm; aqueous alkali—243 nm, 283 nm.

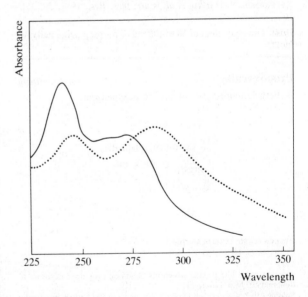

Infra-red Spectrum. Principal peaks at wavenumbers 754, 1653, 1221, 1186, 1575, 1316 (propiomazine hydrochloride, KBr disk). (See below)

Mass Spectrum. Principal peaks at *m/z* 72, 73, 340, 269, 197, 71, 70, 56.

Quantification. GAS CHROMATOGRAPHY. In plasma: propiomazine and *N*-monodesmethylpropiomazine, sensitivity 10 to 20 ng/ml, AFID—P. Hartvig *et al.*, *J. Chromat.*, 1980, *183*; *Biomed. Appl.*, 9, 229–233.

Wavelength

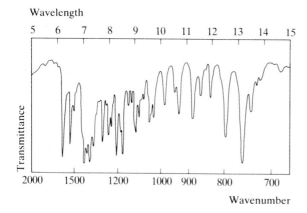

High Pressure Liquid Chromatography. *System HQ*—k' 1.09.

Ultraviolet Spectrum. Aqueous acid—235 nm (A_1^1 = 270 b), 298 nm.

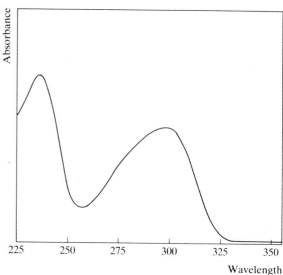

Wavelength

Disposition in the Body. Slowly absorbed after oral administration; bioavailability about 33%. Metabolised by *N*-demethylation.

THERAPEUTIC CONCENTRATION.

After a single oral dose of 50 mg to one subject, a peak serum concentration of about 0.05 µg/ml was attained in 2 to 3 hours. In several subjects, low concentrations (<0.01 µg/ml) of *N*-monodesmethylpropiomazine were also observed (P. Hartvig *et al., Curr. ther. Res.,* 1981, *29,* 351–362).

HALF-LIFE. Plasma half-life, 2 to 15 hours (mean 9).

VOLUME OF DISTRIBUTION. About 2 to 3 litres/kg.

CLEARANCE. Plasma clearance, 3 to 10 ml/min/kg (mean 5).

REFERENCE. P. Hartvig *et al., Curr. ther. Res.,* 1981, *29,* 351–362.

Dose. The equivalent of 50 to 100 mg of propiomazine daily, by mouth.

Infra-red Spectrum. Principal peaks at wavenumbers 1605, 1278, 1246, 1670, 1210, 1700 (KBr disk).

Mass Spectrum. Principal peaks at *m/z* 86, 99, 136, 30, 58, 178, 87, 71.

Use. Propoxycaine hydrochloride has been used as a 0.5% solution.

Propoxycaine   *Local Anaesthetic*

2-Diethylaminoethyl 4-amino-2-propoxybenzoate
$C_{16}H_{26}N_2O_3 = 294.4$
CAS—86-43-1

CO·O·[CH₂]₂·N(C₂H₅)₂
O·[CH₂]₂·CH₃
NH₂

Propoxycaine Hydrochloride

$C_{16}H_{26}N_2O_3,HCl = 330.9$
CAS—550-83-4
A white crystalline powder which discolours on prolonged exposure to light and air. M.p. 146° to 151°.
Soluble 1 in 2 of water, 1 in 10 of ethanol, and 1 in 80 of ether; practically insoluble in chloroform.

Dissociation Constant. pK_a 8.6.

Colour Tests. Coniferyl Alcohol—orange; Diazotisation—red; Mandelin's Test—brown.

Thin-layer Chromatography. *System TA*—Rf 58; *system TB*—Rf 03; *system TC*—Rf 33; *system TL*—Rf 28. (*Acidified iodoplatinate solution,* positive.)

Gas Chromatography. *System GA*—RI 2335.

Propranolol   *Beta-adrenoceptor Blocking Agent*

(±)-1-Isopropylamino-3-(1-naphthyloxy)propan-2-ol
$C_{16}H_{21}NO_2 = 259.3$
CAS—525-66-6; 13013-17-7 (±)

OH
O·CH₂·CH·CH₂·NH·CH(CH₃)₂

Crystals. M.p. 94° to 96°.

Propranolol Hydrochloride

Proprietary Names. Angilol; Apsolol; Avlocardyl; Bedranol; Berkolol; Beta-Neg; Cardinol; Dociton; Frekven; Inderal; Inderalici; Sloprolol; Tonum. It is an ingredient of Inderetic, Inderex, and Spiroprop.
$C_{16}H_{21}NO_2,HCl = 295.8$
CAS—318-98-9; 3506-09-0 (±)
A white powder. M.p. about 164°.
Soluble 1 in 20 of water and ethanol; slightly soluble in chloroform; practically insoluble in ether.

Dissociation Constant. pK_a 9.5 (24°).

Partition Coefficient. Log *P* (octanol/pH 7.4), 1.2.

Colour Tests. Mandelin's Test—green; Marquis Test—green.

Thin-layer Chromatography. *System TA*—Rf 50; *system TB*—Rf 07; *system TC*—Rf 10. (*Acidified iodoplatinate solution*, positive.)

Gas Chromatography. *System GA*—RI 2157.

High Pressure Liquid Chromatography. *System HA*—propranolol k' 1.3, 4-hydroxypropranolol k' 1.1.

Ultraviolet Spectrum. Aqueous acid—288 nm ($A_1^1 = 222$ a), 305 nm, 319 nm; methanol—290 nm ($A_1^1 = 240$ a), 306 nm ($A_1^1 = 143$ a), 319 nm ($A_1^1 = 86$ a). No alkaline shift.

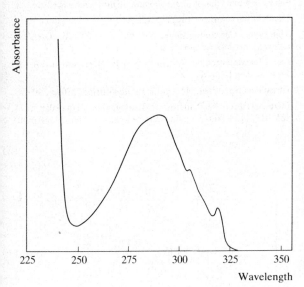

Infra-red Spectrum. Principal peaks at wavenumbers 1103, 1270, 772, 1580, 795, 1240 (propranolol hydrochloride, KBr disk).

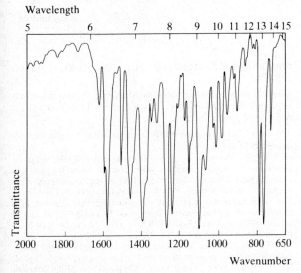

Mass Spectrum. Principal peaks at *m/z* 72, 56, 30, 43, 98, 115, 144, 41; 4-hydroxypropranolol 72, 30, 116, 56, 43, 160, 41, 158.

Quantification. Gas Chromatography. In plasma: sensitivity <1 ng/ml, ECD—R. E. Kates and C. L. Jones, *J. pharm. Sci.*, 1977, *66*, 1490–1492.

High Pressure Liquid Chromatography. In plasma: propranolol and 4-hydroxypropranolol, sensitivity 1 ng/ml for propranolol, fluorescence detection—R. L. Nation *et al.*, *J. Chromat.*, 1978, *145*; *Biomed. Appl.*, *2*, 429–436. In urine: propranolol and six metabolites, fluorescence and UV detection—J. F. Pritchard *et al.*, *J. Chromat.*, 1979, *162*; *Biomed. Appl.*, *4*, 47–58.

Radioimmunoassay. In plasma: sensitivity 600 pg/ml—G. P. Mould *et al.*, *Biopharm. Drug Disp.*, 1981, *2*, 49–57.

Disposition in the Body. Rapidly and almost completely absorbed after oral administration, but undergoes extensive first-pass metabolism with considerable intersubject variation; bioavailability 10 to 50% (mean 30). Metabolic reactions include ring hydroxylation, *N*-demethylation, oxidative deamination, and conjugation. In 48 hours, about 10% of a dose is excreted in the urine as propranolol glucuronide and less than 4% as unchanged drug. Metabolites found in the urine, in free and conjugated forms, include naphthoxylactic acid (14 to 22% of the dose in 48 hours) and the active metabolite, 4-hydroxypropranolol and its glucuronide (5 to 8% of the dose); propranolol glycol, *N*-desisopropylpropranolol, and naphthoxyacetic acid each account for less than 2% of the dose and 4-hydroxypropranolol sulphate accounts for about 18% of the dose. After intravenous doses, a greater proportion of naphthoxylactic acid (up to 40% of the dose) is excreted in the urine and 4-hydroxypropranolol is not found in the urine. Less than 5% of a dose is eliminated in the faeces.

Therapeutic Concentration. In plasma, usually in the range 0.05 to 1 µg/ml. However, there is considerable intersubject variation and a correlation between plasma concentration and therapeutic effect has not been established.

After a single oral dose of 80 mg administered to 6 subjects, the following mean peak concentrations of drug and metabolites were found in the plasma after 2 hours: propranolol 0.05 µg/ml, naphthoxylactic acid 0.53 µg/ml, 4-hydroxypropranolol 0.009 µg/ml, naphthoxyacetic acid 0.024 µg/ml, propranolol glycol 0.005 µg/ml (D. W. Schneck *et al.*, *Clin. Pharmac. Ther.*, 1980, *27*, 744–755).

Oral doses of 80 mg, administered twice daily to 24 subjects, produced steady-state plasma concentrations of 0.06 to 0.29 µg/ml (mean 0.16) (M. J. Serlin *et al.*, *Clin. Pharmac. Ther.*, 1980, *27*, 586–592).

Following oral administration of 160 mg twice a day to 12 subjects, mean steady-state plasma concentrations of 0.38 µg/ml of propranolol and 0.03 µg/ml of 4-hydroxypropranolol were reported (B. G. Charles *et al.*, *J. Pharm. Pharmac.*, 1982, *34*, 403–404).

Toxicity. Toxic effects have been associated with plasma concentrations greater than 2 µg/ml and fatalities with concentrations greater than 4 µg/ml.

In a case of suicide attributed to propranolol overdose, the following concentrations were found: blood 14 µg/ml, brain 67 µg/g, liver 171 µg/g, urine 0.9 µg/ml; alcohol was also present (J. Kristinsson and T. Johannesson, *Acta pharmac. tox.*, 1977, *41*, 190–192).

In two further cases of suicide, blood concentrations were 9 and 4 µg/ml and liver concentrations were 140 and 170 µg/g (N. Piper and D. Smith, *Bull. int. Ass. forens. Toxicol.*, 1976, *12*(1), 17–18).

In a fatality due to the ingestion of 9.6 g of propranolol, in which death occurred 8 hours after ingestion, the following postmortem tissue concentrations were reported: blood 20 µg/ml, brain 6 µg/g, kidney 26 µg/g, liver 10 µg/g, lung 69 µg/g (J. W. Jones *et al.*, *J. forens. Sci.*, 1982, *27*, 213–216).

Half-life. Plasma half-life, 2 to 6 hours (dose-dependent elimination has been reported).

Volume of Distribution. About 4 litres/kg.

CLEARANCE. Plasma clearance, about 10 to 20 ml/min/kg.

DISTRIBUTION IN BLOOD. Plasma: whole blood ratio, about 1.3.

PROTEIN BINDING. In plasma, about 90%.

NOTE. For a review of the clinical pharmacokinetics of propranolol see P. A. Routledge and D. G. Shand, *Clin. Pharmacokinet.*, 1979, *4*, 73–90. See also B. M. Silber *et al.*, *J. pharm. Sci.*, 1983, *72*, 725–732.

Dose. 30 to 400 mg of propranolol hydrochloride daily.

Propyl Hydroxybenzoate   *Preservative*

Synonyms. Propagin; Propyl Parahydroxybenzoate; Propyl-paraben.

Proprietary Names. Nipasol M. It is an ingredient of Nipasept and Nipastat.

Propyl 4-hydroxybenzoate
$C_{10}H_{12}O_3 = 180.2$
CAS—94-13-3

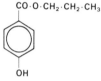

Colourless crystals or a white crystalline powder. M.p. 95° to 98°.

Soluble 1 in 2500 of cold water, 1 in 400 of boiling water, 1 in 3.5 of ethanol, 1 in 4 of chloroform, and 1 in 3 of ether.

Sodium Propyl Hydroxybenzoate

Synonyms. Sodium Propylparaben; Soluble Propyl Hydroxybenzoate.
Proprietary Name. Nipasol M Sodium
$C_{10}H_{11}NaO_3 = 202.2$
CAS—35285-69-9
A white, hygroscopic, crystalline powder.
Soluble 1 in 1 of water, 1 in 50 of ethanol, and 1 in 2 of ethanol (50%).

Dissociation Constant. pK_a 8.4 (22°).

Gas Chromatography. *System GA*—RI 1567.

Ultraviolet Spectrum. Aqueous acid—255 nm ($A_1^1 = 877$ b); aqueous alkali—296 nm ($A_1^1 = 1324$ b).

Infra-red Spectrum. Principal peaks at wavenumbers 1276, 1165, 1220, 1317, 1665, 1600 (KBr disk).

Propylhexedrine   *Sympathomimetic/Anorectic*

Proprietary Name. Benzedrex
$(\pm)$-2-Cyclohexyl-1,*N*-dimethylethylamine
$C_{10}H_{21}N = 155.3$
CAS—101-40-6; 3595-11-7 ($\pm$)

A clear colourless liquid which slowly volatilises at room temperature and absorbs carbon dioxide from the air. Wt per ml 0.853 to 0.861 g. B.p. about 204°.

Very slightly **soluble** in water; miscible with ethanol, chloroform, and ether.

Propylhexedrine Hydrochloride

Proprietary Name. Eventin(e)
$C_{10}H_{21}N,HCl = 191.7$
CAS—1007-33-6; 6192-95-6 ($\pm$)
A crystalline solid. M.p. about 127°, with decomposition.
Soluble in water, ethanol, and chloroform; slightly soluble in ether.

Dissociation Constant. pK_a 10.7 (25°).

Thin-layer Chromatography. *System TA*—Rf 26. (*Acidified iodoplatinate solution*, positive.)

Gas Chromatography. *System GA*—RI 1169; *system GB*—RI 1186; *system GC*—RI 1500.

Ultraviolet Spectrum. No significant absorption, 230 to 360 nm.

Infra-red Spectrum. Principal peaks at wavenumbers 1058, 1015, 885, 913, 1153, 966 (propylhexedrine hydrochloride, Nujol mull).

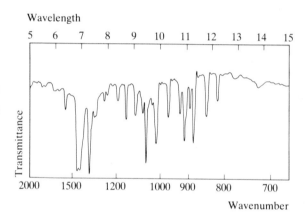

Mass Spectrum. Principal peaks at *m/z* 58, 140, 67, 72, 83, 81, 155, 156.

Disposition in the Body. Norpropylhexedrine, cyclohexylacetoxime, and *cis/trans*-4-hydroxypropylhexedrine have been identified as urinary metabolites.

TOXICITY. The estimated minimum lethal dose for children up to 2 years of age is 200 mg.

In a fatality attributed to propylhexedrine ingestion, the following postmortem tissue concentrations were reported: blood 35 µg/ml, bile 20 µg/ml, brain 24 µg/g, kidney 30 µg/g, liver 36 µg/g, lung 50 µg/g, urine 60 µg/ml (L. Riddick and R. Reisch, *J. forens. Sci.*, 1981, *26*, 834–839).

The following postmortem tissue concentrations were reported in 2 fatalities involving intravenous abuse: blood 1.8 and 2.7 µg/ml, kidney 1.5 and 9.5 µg/g, liver 2.8 and 11.8 µg/g, urine 12.6 µg/ml (first case) (W. Q. Sturner *et al.*, *J. forens. Sci.*, 1974, *19*, 572–574).

In a fatality attributed to acute intravenous propylhexedrine abuse, postmortem tissue concentrations were: blood 2 µg/ml, bile 9.4 µg/ml, kidney 4.0 µg/g, liver 7.4 µg/g, urine 69.5 µg/ml (V. J. M. DiMaio and J. C. Garriott, *J. forens. Sci.*, 1977, *22*, 152–158).

Dose. Usually 75 to 100 mg of propylhexedrine hydrochloride daily.

Propyliodone   *Contrast Medium*

Proprietary Name. Dionosil
Propyl 1,4-dihydro-3,5-di-iodo-4-oxo-1-pyridylacetate
$C_{10}H_{11}I_2NO_3 = 447.0$
CAS—587-61-1

CH₂·CO·O·CH₂·CH₂·CH₃

A white crystalline powder. M.p. 187° to 190°.
Practically **insoluble** in water; soluble 1 in 500 of ethanol and 1 in 150 of chloroform; soluble in acetone and ether.

Colour Test. Iodine Test—positive.

Thin-layer Chromatography. *System TA*—Rf 81. (*Acidified iodoplatinate solution*, positive.)

Gas Chromatography. *System GA*—not eluted.

Ultraviolet Spectrum. Dehydrated alcohol—239 nm ($A_1^1 =$ 320 a), 281 nm ($A_1^1 = 260$ a).

Infra-red Spectrum. Principal peaks at wavenumbers 1730, 1200, 1567, 1608, 751, 1227 (KBr disk).

Use. Administered as a 50% aqueous suspension or as a 60% oily suspension.

Propylthiouracil   *Antithyroid Agent*

Proprietary Names. Propycil; Propyl-Thyracil; Thyreostat II.
2,3-Dihydro-6-propyl-2-thioxopyrimidin-4(1*H*)-one
$C_7H_{10}N_2OS = 170.2$
CAS—51-52-5

CH₃·CH₂·CH₂

White or pale cream-coloured crystals or crystalline powder. M.p. 218° to 221°.
Soluble 1 in 700 of water, 1 in about 60 of ethanol, and 1 in 60 of acetone; slightly soluble in chloroform and ether; soluble in solutions of alkali hydroxides.

Dissociation Constant. pKₐ 8.3 (20°).

Ultraviolet Spectrum. Aqueous acid—275 nm ($A_1^1 = 987$ b); aqueous alkali—260 nm ($A_1^1 = 703$ a).

Infra-red Spectrum. Principal peaks at wavenumbers 1658, 1563, 1193, 1625, 1166, 1241 (KBr disk).

Quantification. HIGH PRESSURE LIQUID CHROMATOGRAPHY. In blood: sensitivity 300 ng/ml, UV detection—C. Kim, *J. Chromat.*, 1983, *272*; Biomed. Appl., *23*, 376–379.

RADIOIMMUNOASSAY. In serum: sensitivity 2.5 ng—D. S. Cooper *et al.*, *J. clin. Endocr. Metab.*, 1981, *52*, 204–213.

Disposition in the Body. Rapidly and almost completely absorbed after oral administration; concentrated in the thyroid. Metabolised by conjugation with glucuronic acid and sulphate. Less than 10% of a dose is excreted in the urine as unchanged drug.

THERAPEUTIC CONCENTRATION.
Following a single oral dose of 400 mg to 17 subjects, serum concentrations of 1.6 to 7.5 μg/ml (mean 4.2) were reported at 1 hour (J. P. Kampmann and J. E. M. Hansen, *Br. J. clin. Pharmac.*, 1981, *12*, 681–686).

HALF-LIFE. Plasma half-life, about 1 to 2 hours, increased in renal failure.

VOLUME OF DISTRIBUTION. About 0.4 litre/kg.

CLEARANCE. Plasma clearance, about 4 ml/min/kg.

PROTEIN BINDING. In plasma, about 80%.

NOTE. For a review of the pharmacokinetics of antithyroid drugs, see J. P. Kampmann and J. E. M. Hansen, *Clin. Pharmacokinet.*, 1981, *6*, 401–428.

Dose. Initially 200 to 600 mg daily; maintenance, 50 to 200 mg daily.

Propyphenazone   *Analgesic*

Synonyms. Isopropylantipyrine; Isopropylphenazone.
4-Isopropyl-1,5-dimethyl-2-phenyl-4-pyrazolin-3-one
$C_{14}H_{18}N_2O = 230.3$
CAS—479-92-5

White crystals or white crystalline powder. M.p. 101° to 103°.
Soluble 1 in 400 of water; freely soluble in ethanol and chloroform; soluble in ether.

Colour Tests. Ferric Chloride—orange; Liebermann's Test (100°)—blue (red with water).

Thin-layer Chromatography. *System TA*—Rf 71; *system TD*—Rf 61; *system TE*—Rf 73; *system TF*—Rf 50. (*Acidified potassium permanganate solution*, positive.)

Gas Chromatography. *System GA*—RI 1925; *system GF*—RI 2310.

High Pressure Liquid Chromatography. *System HD*—k' 1.25; *system HW*—k' 11.0.

Ultraviolet Spectrum. Aqueous acid—240 nm ($A_1^1 = 400$ a); aqueous alkali—245 nm ($A_1^1 = 385$ b), 265 nm. (See below)

Infra-red Spectrum. Principal peaks at wavenumbers 1650, 1618, 1131, 1590, 1500, 750 (KBr disk).

Mass Spectrum. Principal peaks at *m/z* 215, 230, 56, 77, 216, 96, 41, 39.

Dose. Propyphenazone has been given in doses of 0.3 to 1.5 g daily.

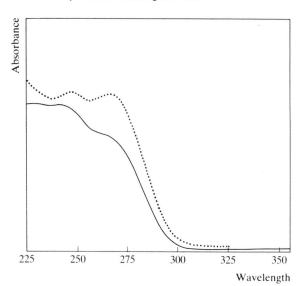

Proquamezine   *Antispasmodic (Veterinary)*

Synonyms. Aminopromazine; Tetrameprozine.
NNN'N' - Tetramethyl - 3 - (phenothiazin - 10 - yl)propane - 1,2 -
diamine
$C_{19}H_{25}N_3S = 327.5$
CAS—58-37-7

Proquamezine Fumarate
Proprietary Name. Myspamol
$(C_{19}H_{25}N_3S)_2,C_4H_4O_4 = 771.0$
CAS—3688-62-8
A white powder. M.p. about 168°, with decomposition.
Soluble 1 in 11 of water, 1 in 200 of ethanol, and 1 in 20 of methanol;
practically insoluble in ether.

Partition Coefficient. Log *P* (octanol), 4.8.

Colour Tests. Forrest Reagent—violet → red → orange; FPN
Reagent—violet-red → red → orange; Mandelin's Test—orange → violet; Marquis Test—violet.

Thin-layer Chromatography. *System TA*—Rf 50; *system TB*—Rf
43; *system TC*—Rf 19. (*Acidified iodoplatinate solution*, positive.)

Gas Chromatography. *System GA*—RI 2434.

Ultraviolet Spectrum. Aqueous acid—248 nm ($A_1^1 = 965$ a), 297
nm (broad) ($A_1^1 = 106$ a).

Infra-red Spectrum. Principal peaks at wavenumbers 1584, 745,
660, 1278, 1190, 765 (proquamezine fumarate, KBr disk).

Mass Spectrum. Principal peaks at *m/z* 198, 58, 115, 70, 269,
199, 72, 71.

Prothionamide   *Antituberculous Agent*

Proprietary Names. Ektebin; Trevintix.
2-Propylpyridine-4-carbothioamide
$C_9H_{12}N_2S = 180.3$
CAS—14222-60-7

Yellow crystals or crystalline powder. M.p. 140° to 143°.
Practically **insoluble** in water; soluble 1 in 30 of ethanol, 1 in 200
of chloroform, 1 in 300 of ether, and 1 in 16 of methanol; soluble
in acetone.

Colour Tests. Nessler's Reagent—brown-orange; Palladium
Chloride—brown.

Thin-layer Chromatography. *System TA*—Rf 66; *system TB*—Rf
01; *system TC*—Rf 38. (*Acidified iodoplatinate solution*, positive.)

Gas Chromatography. *System GA*—RI 1816.

Ultraviolet Spectrum. Ethanol—291 nm ($A_1^1 = 390$ b).

Infra-red Spectrum. Principal peaks at wavenumbers 828, 1590,
1284, 902, 1148, 710 (KBr disk).

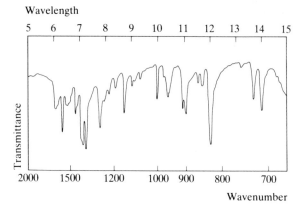

Mass Spectrum. Principal peaks at *m/z* 152, 119, 165, 163, 180,
60, 179, 153.

Quantification. HIGH PRESSURE LIQUID CHROMATOGRAPHY. In
plasma, serum or urine: detection limit 10 ng/ml, UV detection—
P. J. Jenner and G. A. Ellard, *J. Chromat.*, 1981, *225*; *Biomed.
Appl.*, *14*, 245–251.

Disposition in the Body. Readily absorbed after oral administration. Metabolised to the sulphoxide and excreted in the urine
mainly as metabolites.

THERAPEUTIC CONCENTRATION.

Following a single oral dose of 500 mg to 10 subjects, mean peak plasma
concentrations of 3 µg/ml of unchanged drug and 2.7 µg/ml of the
sulphoxide were attained in 1 hour (J. Pütter, *Arzneimittel-Forsch.*, 1972,
22, 1027–1031).

Dose. Usually 0.5 to 1 g daily.

Prothipendyl

Tranquilliser

Synonym. Phrenotropin
NN - Dimethyl - 3 - (pyrido[3,2 - *b*][1,4]benzothiazin - 10 - yl) -
propylamine
$C_{16}H_{19}N_3S = 285.4$
CAS—303-69-5

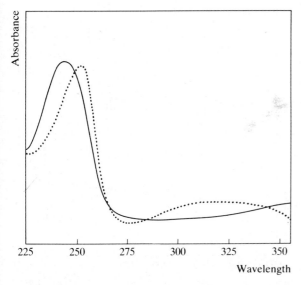

Prothipendyl Hydrochloride

Proprietary Name. Dominal
$C_{16}H_{19}N_3S,HCl,H_2O = 339.9$
CAS—1225-65-6 (anhydrous)
A crystalline powder. M.p. 108° to 112°.
Freely **soluble** in water and methanol; practically insoluble in ether.

Dissociation Constant. pK_a 2.3 (25°).

Partition Coefficient. Log P (octanol), 5.5.

Colour Test. Marquis Test—orange.

Thin-layer Chromatography. *System TA*—Rf 47; *system TB*—Rf
45; *system TC*—Rf 23. (*Dragendorff spray*, positive; *FPN reagent*,
yellow; *acidified iodoplatinate solution*, positive; *Marquis reagent*,
orange.)

Gas Chromatography. *System GA*—RI 2339; *system GF*—RI
2800.

High Pressure Liquid Chromatography. *System HA*—k' 4.4.

Ultraviolet Spectrum. Aqueous acid—242 nm ($A_1^1 = 928$ a);
aqueous alkali—250 nm ($A_1^1 = 909$ a), 320 nm ($A_1^1 = 163$ b).

Infra-red Spectrum. Principal peaks at wavenumbers 757, 1295,
780, 1592, 1162, 1110 (prothipendyl hydrochloride, KBr disk).

Mass Spectrum. Principal peaks at *m/z* 58, 285, 214, 200, 86,
227, 85, 213.

Dose. The equivalent of up to 960 mg of prothipendyl daily.

Protokylol

Sympathomimetic

Synonym. Protochylol
1 - (3,4 - Dihydroxyphenyl) - 2 - (α - methyl - 3,4 - methylenedioxy-
phenethylamino)ethanol
$C_{18}H_{21}NO_5 = 331.4$
CAS—136-70-9

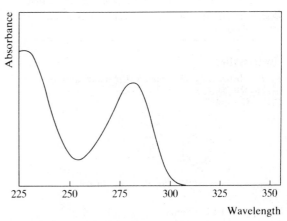

Protokylol Hydrochloride

Proprietary Names. Asmetil; Beres.
$C_{18}H_{21}NO_5,HCl = 367.8$
CAS—136-69-6
A white crystalline powder. M.p. about 126°.
Soluble in water.

Colour Tests. Ammoniacal Silver Nitrate—red-grey/brown;
Ferric Chloride—green; Folin–Ciocalteu Reagent—blue; Liebermann's Test—black; Mandelin's Test—yellow → brown;
Marquis Test—grey-green; Methanolic Potassium Hydroxide—
orange → yellow; Nessler's Reagent—black; Potassium Dichromate—brown → red-brown (on warming).

Thin-layer Chromatography. *System TA*—Rf 65; *system TB*—Rf
01; *system TC*—Rf 03. (*Acidified potassium permanganate solution*,
positive.)

Gas Chromatography. *System GA*—RI 1487.

High Pressure Liquid Chromatography. *System HA*—k' 3.1
(tailing peak).

Ultraviolet Spectrum. Aqueous acid—281 nm ($A_1^1 = 168$ b).

Infra-red Spectrum. Principal peaks at wavenumbers 1492, 1250,
1271, 1227, 1036, 1128 (KBr disk).

Mass Spectrum. Principal peaks at *m/z* 178, 44, 163, 135, 77,
196, 176, 179.

Dose. Protokylol hydrochloride has been given in doses of 8 to
16 mg daily.

Protoveratrine A   *Antihypertensive*

Proprietary Name. Pro-Amid
Protoverine 6,7-diacetate 3(*S*)-(2-hydroxy-2-methylbutyrate) 15(*R*)-(2-methylbutyrate)
$C_{41}H_{63}NO_{14} = 793.5$
CAS—143-57-7
An alkaloid obtained from white veratrum, *Veratrum album* (Liliaceae).
White crystals. M.p. 259° to 262°; or 302° to 304°, with decomposition.
Practically **insoluble** in water; soluble in hot ethanol and in chloroform.

Protoveratrine B

Synonym. Neoprotoveratrine
Protoverine 6,7-diacetate 3(*S*)-(2,3-dihydroxy-2-methylbutyrate) 15(*R*)-(2-methylbutyrate)
$C_{41}H_{63}NO_{15} = 809.9$
CAS—124-97-0
An alkaloid obtained from white veratrum.
White crystals. M.p. 254° to 255°; or 285° to 290°, with decomposition.
Practically **insoluble** in water; soluble in hot ethanol and in chloroform.

Protoveratrines A and B
CAS—8053-18-7
A white crystalline powder with a strong sternutatory action. M.p. 256° to 262°, with decomposition.
Practically **insoluble** in water; soluble in chloroform; very slightly soluble in ether. It is rapidly decomposed in alkaline and alcoholic solutions.

Thin-layer Chromatography. Protoveratrine A: *system TA*—Rf 72. Protoveratrine B: *system TA*—Rf 70. (*Acidified iodoplatinate solution*, positive; *acidified potassium permanganate solution*, positive.)

Gas Chromatography. *System GA*—protoveratrines A and B, RI 2465.

Infra-red Spectrum. Principal peaks at wavenumbers 1742, 1200, 1182, 1240, 1150, 1055 (protoveratrines A and B, KCl disk).

Dose. Protoveratrines A and B have been given in a dose of 1.6 to 6 mg daily.

Protriptyline   *Antidepressant*

3-(5*H*-Dibenzo[*a,d*]cyclohepten-5-yl)-*N*-methylpropylamine
$C_{19}H_{21}N = 263.4$
CAS—438-60-8

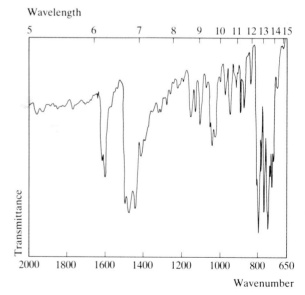

Protriptyline Hydrochloride
Proprietary Names. Concordin(e); Maximed; Triptil; Vivactil.
Note. The name Vivactil is also applied to a vitamin/amino acid preparation.
$C_{19}H_{21}N,HCl = 299.8$
CAS—1225-55-4
A white to yellowish powder. M.p. about 168°.
Soluble 1 in 2 of water, 1 in 3.5 of ethanol, and 1 in 2.5 of chloroform; practically insoluble in ether.

Partition Coefficient. Log *P* (octanol/pH 7.4), 1.2.

Colour Tests. Mandelin's Test—violet-brown; Marquis Test—green; Sulphuric Acid—green.

Thin-layer Chromatography. *System TA*—Rf 19; *system TB*—Rf 17; *system TC*—Rf 07. (*Acidified iodoplatinate solution*, positive.)

Gas Chromatography. *System GA*—RI 2261; *system GF*—RI 2590.

High Pressure Liquid Chromatography. *System HA*—k' 2.1; *system HF*—k' 3.60.

Ultraviolet Spectrum. Methanolic acid—292 nm ($A_1^1 = 530$ a). No alkaline shift.

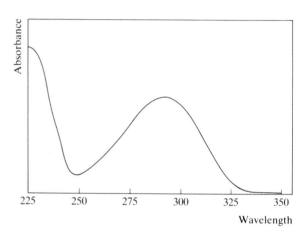

Infra-red Spectrum. Principal peaks at wavenumbers 792, 750, 768, 1490, 730, 1595 (protriptyline hydrochloride, KBr disk).

Mass Spectrum. Principal peaks at *m/z* 70, 44, 191, 192, 188, 59, 165, 71; 10,11-dihydro-10,11-dihydroxyprotriptyline 44, 70, 179, 178, 207, 280, 250, 236; 10-hydroxyprotriptyline 70, 44, 207, 178, 279, 249, –, –.

Quantification. GAS CHROMATOGRAPHY. In serum: protriptyline and other tricyclic antidepressants, detection limit 10 to 20 ng/ml, AFID—J. Kristinsson, *Acta pharmac. tox.*, 1981, *49*, 390–398.

GAS CHROMATOGRAPHY–MASS SPECTROMETRY. In plasma: protriptyline and other tricyclic antidepressants, sensitivity 10 ng/ml—J. T. Biggs *et al.*, *J. pharm. Sci.*, 1976, *65*, 261–268.

HIGH PRESSURE LIQUID CHROMATOGRAPHY. In plasma: sensitivity 60 ng/ml, UV detection—L. P. Hackett and L. J. Dusci, *Clin. Toxicol.*, 1979, *15*, 55–61.

Disposition in the Body. Slowly but well absorbed after oral administration; bioavailability about 75 to 90% (10 to 25% first-pass metabolism). Metabolised by oxidation to form the 10-hydroxy and 10,11-dihydro-10,11-dihydroxy derivatives and 5,10-dihydro-10-formylanthracen-5-ylpropylamine; glucuronic acid conjugation also occurs. About 50% of a dose is excreted in the urine in 16 days with only small amounts of unchanged drug; about 2% of a dose is eliminated in the faeces.

THERAPEUTIC CONCENTRATION. In plasma, usually in the range 0.07 to 0.25 µg/ml.

After a single oral dose of 30 mg to 8 subjects, peak plasma concentrations of 0.010 to 0.022 µg/ml (mean 0.014) were attained in 6 to 12 hours (V. E. Ziegler *et al.*, *Clin. Pharmac. Ther.*, 1978, *23*, 580–584).

Following daily oral doses of 40 mg to 30 subjects, steady-state plasma concentrations of 0.11 to 0.38 µg/ml (mean 0.22) were reported (J. P. Moody *et al.*, *Eur. J. clin. Pharmac.*, 1977, *11*, 51–56).

TOXICITY. Toxic effects are associated with plasma concentrations greater than 0.5 µg/ml; concentrations above 1 µg/ml may be lethal.

HALF-LIFE. Plasma half-life, during chronic dosing, about 3 to 8 days (mean 4).

VOLUME OF DISTRIBUTION. About 22 litres/kg.

CLEARANCE. Plasma clearance, 2 to 5 ml/min/kg.

PROTEIN BINDING. In plasma, about 92%.

NOTE. For a review of tricyclic antidepressants see G. Molnar and R. N. Gupta, *Biopharm. Drug Disp.*, 1980, *1*, 283–305.

Dose. 15 to 60 mg of protriptyline hydrochloride daily.

Proxymetacaine
Local Anaesthetic

Synonym. Proparacaine
2-Diethylaminoethyl 3-amino-4-propoxybenzoate
$C_{16}H_{26}N_2O_3 = 294.4$
CAS—499-67-2

Proxymetacaine Hydrochloride
Proprietary Names. Alcaine; Kéracaine; Ophthaine; Ophthetic; Piloptic.
$C_{16}H_{26}N_2O_3, HCl = 330.9$
CAS—5875-06-9
A white or faintly buff-coloured crystalline powder. It discolours on heating or exposure to air and solutions exposed to air become yellow and then dark brown. M.p. 178° to 185°.
Soluble 1 in 30 of water and 1 in 50 of ethanol; practically insoluble in ether; soluble in methanol.

Colour Tests. Coniferyl Alcohol—orange; Diazotisation—red; Ninhydrin—yellow.

Thin-layer Chromatography. *System TA*—Rf 62; *system TB*—Rf 26; *system TC*—Rf 41; *system TL*—Rf 35. (*Acidified iodoplatinate solution,* positive; *Van Urk reagent,* yellow.)

Gas Chromatography. *System GA*—RI 2323.

High Pressure Liquid Chromatography. *System HA*—k′ 2.1; *system HQ*—k′ 1.38.

Ultraviolet Spectrum. Water—231 nm, 268 nm ($A_1^1 = 326$ b), 310 nm ($A_1^1 = 182$ a).

Infra-red Spectrum. Principal peaks at wavenumbers 1213, 1708, 1305, 1104, 1590, 1520 (proxymetacaine hydrochloride, KCl disk).

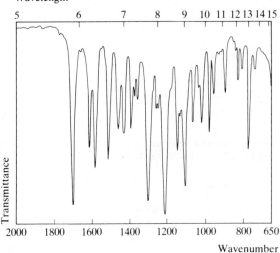

Mass Spectrum. Principal peaks at *m/z* 86, 99, 30, 87, 58, 71, 136, 100.

Use. Proxymetacaine hydrochloride is used as a 0.5% ophthalmic solution.

Proxyphylline
Xanthine Bronchodilator

Proprietary Names. Pantafillina; Spantin; Spasmolysin; Thean.
7-(2-Hydroxypropyl)theophylline
$C_{10}H_{14}N_4O_3 = 238.2$
CAS—603-00-9

A white crystalline powder. M.p. 134° to 136°.

Soluble 1 in 1.5 of water, 1 in 12 of ethanol, 1 in 6 of chloroform, and 1 in 500 of ether.

Colour Test. Amalic Acid Test—yellow/violet.

Thin-layer Chromatography. *System TA*—Rf 58; *system TB*—Rf 02; *system TC*—Rf 33. (*Acidified potassium permanganate solution, positive.*)

Gas Chromatography. *System GA*—RI 2103.

High Pressure Liquid Chromatography. *System HA*—k′ 0.1.

Ultraviolet Spectrum. Aqueous acid—273 nm ($A_1^1 = 372$ a). No alkaline shift.

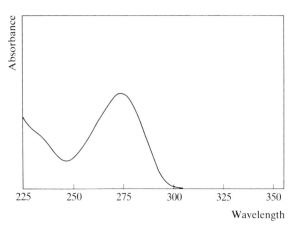

Infra-red Spectrum. Principal peaks at wavenumbers 1656, 1690, 750, 1538, 763, 1282 (KBr disk).

Wavelength

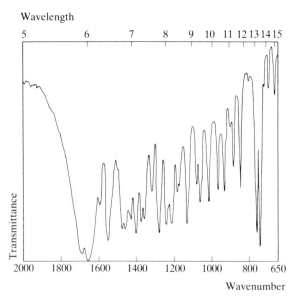

Wavenumber

Mass Spectrum. Principal peaks at m/z 194, 180, 109, 193, 238, 95, 137, 81.

Quantification. GAS CHROMATOGRAPHY. In plasma: sensitivity 100 ng/ml, ECD—A. Arbin *et al.*, *Acta pharm. suec.*, 1976, *13*, 235–240.

HIGH PRESSURE LIQUID CHROMATOGRAPHY. In serum: detection limit 12 ng/ml, UV detection—K. Selvig and K. S. Bjerve, *Scand. J. clin. Lab. Invest.*, 1977, *37*, 373–378.

Disposition in the Body. Rapidly and completely absorbed after oral administration. More than 95% of a dose is excreted in the urine in 96 hours with about 30% as unchanged drug, 58% as 1-methyl-7-(2-hydroxypropyl)xanthine, 10% as proxyphylline glucuronide, and 2% as 1-methyl-7-(2-hydroxypropyl)uric acid.

THERAPEUTIC CONCENTRATION.

After a single oral dose of 400 mg given to 5 subjects, plasma concentrations of 7 to 13 μg/ml (mean 10) were attained in 1 hour. Oral dosing of 5 subjects with 400 mg three times a day for 5 days, produced peak plasma concentrations of 12 to 25 μg/ml (mean 18) on the 5th day (C. Graffner *et al.*, *Acta pharm. suec.*, 1973, *10*, 425–434).

HALF-LIFE. Plasma half-life, 8 to 12 hours (mean 9).

VOLUME OF DISTRIBUTION. About 0.6 litre/kg.

CLEARANCE. Plasma clearance, about 0.8 ml/min/kg.

Dose. Usually 900 mg daily.

Pseudoephedrine   *Sympathomimetic*

Synonyms. d-ψ-Ephedrine; d-Isoephedrine.
Proprietary Name. It is an ingredient of Extil.
(1S,2S)-2-Methylamino-1-phenylpropan-1-ol
$C_{10}H_{15}NO = 165.2$
CAS—90-82-4

$$C_6H_5-\underset{\underset{OH}{|}}{\overset{\overset{H}{|}}{C}}-\underset{\underset{H}{|}}{\overset{\overset{NH\cdot CH_3}{|}}{C}}-CH_3$$

An alkaloid obtained from *Ephedra* spp. It is a stereoisomer of ephedrine. M.p. 118° to 119°.
Sparingly **soluble** in water; soluble in ethanol and ether.

Pseudoephedrine Hydrochloride

Proprietary Names. D-Feda; Eltor; Novafed; Robidrine; Sinufed; Sudafed; Sudelix. It is an ingredient of Actifed, Benafed, Benylin Decongestant, CoTylenol, Deconamine, Fedahist, Fedrazil, Intensin, Linctifed, Naldegesic, Paragesic, Rondec, Sancos Co, and Triocos.
$C_{10}H_{15}NO, HCl = 201.7$
CAS—345-78-8
White crystals or powder. M.p. 182° to 186°. A solution in water is dextrorotatory.
Soluble 1 in 1.6 of water, 1 in 4 of ethanol, and 1 in 60 of chloroform; very slightly soluble in ether.

Pseudoephedrine Sulphate

Proprietary Names. Afrinol; Drixora Repetabs. It is an ingredient of Congesteze, Disophrol, Drixoral, and Halin.
$(C_{10}H_{15}NO)_2, H_2SO_4 = 428.5$
CAS—7460-12-0
A white crystalline powder. M.p. 174° to 179°. A solution in water is dextrorotatory.
Soluble in water.

Dissociation Constant. pK_a 9.8.

Thin-layer Chromatography. *System TA*—Rf 33; *system TB*—Rf 54; *system TC*—Rf 04. (*Acidified potassium permanganate solution, positive.*)

Gas Chromatography. *System GA*—RI 1354; *system GB*—RI 1399; *system GC*—RI 1543.

High Pressure Liquid Chromatography. *System HA*—pseudoephedrine k′ 1.2, norpseudoephedrine k′ 1.0; *system HB*—k′ 5.90; *system HC*—k′ 1.77.

Ultraviolet Spectrum. Aqueous acid—251 nm, 257 nm ($A_1^1 =$ 11.9 a), 263 nm. No alkaline shift.

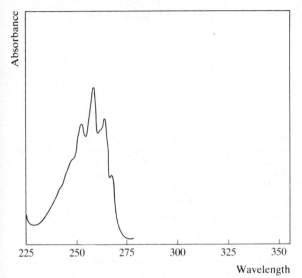

Infra-red Spectrum. Principal peaks at wavenumbers 704, 1036, 764, 1005, 1210, 1595 (pseudoephedrine hydrochloride, KBr disk).

Mass Spectrum. Principal peaks at m/z 58, 77, 59, 56, 51, 42, 105, 91.

Quantification. GAS CHROMATOGRAPHY. In plasma or urine: pseudoephedrine and norpseudoephedrine, sensitivity 20 ng/ml for pseudoephedrine in plasma, ECD—L. Y. Lo *et al.*, *J. Chromat.*, 1981, *222*; *Biomed. Appl.*, *11*, 297–302. In serum: detection limit 20 ng/ml, ECD—S.-R. Sun and M. J. Leveque, *J. pharm. Sci.*, 1979, *68*, 1567–1568.

HIGH PRESSURE LIQUID CHROMATOGRAPHY. In urine: pseudoephedrine and norpseudoephedrine, sensitivity 1.5 μg/ml for pseudoephedrine, UV detection—C. M. Lai *et al.*, *J. pharm. Sci.*, 1979, *68*, 1243–1246.

RADIOIMMUNOASSAY. In plasma: sensitivity 0.2 to 2.5 ng/ml depending on the method—J. W. A. Findlay *et al.*, *J. pharm. Sci.*, 1981, *70*, 624–631.

Disposition in the Body. Rapidly and completely absorbed after oral administration. Up to about 90% of a dose is excreted unchanged in the urine in 24 hours with less than 1% as norpseudoephedrine (cathine) (pH-dependent).

THERAPEUTIC CONCENTRATION.
After a single oral dose of 180 mg to 3 subjects, peak plasma concentrations of 0.72 to 0.81 μg/ml were attained in 2 to 3 hours (R. G. Kuntzman *et al.*, *Clin. Pharmac. Ther.*, 1971, *12*, 62–67).

Following oral administration of 60 mg 4 times a day to 17 subjects, maximum steady-state plasma concentrations of 0.41 to 0.79 μg/ml (mean 0.55) were reported about 1.5 hours after a dose (J. G. Perkins *et al.*, *Curr. ther. Res.*, 1980, *28*, 650–668).

TOXICITY. Toxic effects have occurred after single doses of 60 mg.
The following postmortem tissue concentrations were reported in a fatality involving pseudoephedrine: blood 19 μg/ml, brain 22 μg/g, liver 33 μg/g, urine 105 μg/ml (*Registry of Human Toxicology*, American Academy of Forensic Sciences, 1978).

HALF-LIFE. Plasma half-life, 5 to 8 hours but may be increased when the urine is alkaline and decreased when it is acid.

VOLUME OF DISTRIBUTION. About 3 litres/kg.

Dose. Usually 180 to 240 mg of pseudoephedrine hydrochloride daily.

Pseudomorphine

Synonym. Oxydimorphine
2,2′-Bimorphine
$C_{34}H_{36}N_2O_6,3H_2O = 622.7$
CAS—125-24-6 (anhydrous); *6472-73-7* (trihydrate)
White crystals. M.p. 327°, with decomposition.
Practically **insoluble** in water, ethanol, and ether; soluble in dilute hydrochloric acid, dilute acetic acid, and pyridine.

Colour Test. Marquis Test—green.

Thin-layer Chromatography. *System TA*—Rf 46; *system TB*—Rf 00; *system TC*—Rf 00. (*Acidified iodoplatinate solution*, positive.)

Gas Chromatography. *System GA*—RI 2770.

Ultraviolet Spectrum. Aqueous acid—231 nm ($A_1^1 = 308$ b).

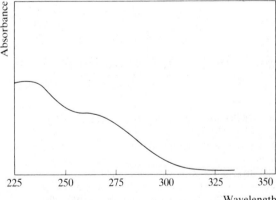

Infra-red Spectrum. Principal peaks at wavenumbers 1118, 1098, 1069, 1044, 1195, 1210 (KBr disk).

Mass Spectrum. Principal peaks at m/z 30, 44, 42, 568, 31, 58, 27, 81.

NOTE. Pseudomorphine may be found as an oxidation product of morphine in decomposed viscera.

Psilocin   *Hallucinogen*

Synonym. 4-Hydroxy-*NN*-dimethyltryptamine
3-(2-Dimethylaminoethyl)indol-4-ol
$C_{12}H_{16}N_2O = 204.3$
CAS—520-53-6

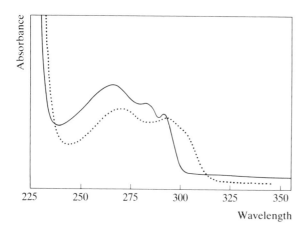

An indole alkaloid obtained from the mushroom *Psilocybe mexicana* (Agaricaceae).
White crystals. M.p. 173° to 176°.
Soluble in ethanol and dilute acetic acid.

Colour Test. Marquis Test—green-brown.

Thin-layer Chromatography. *System TA*—Rf 39; *system TB*—Rf 05; *system TC*—Rf 09. (*Van Urk reagent*, faint blue.)

Gas Chromatography. *System GA*—RI 1980.

High Pressure Liquid Chromatography. *System HA*—k' 3.1 (tailing peak).

Ultraviolet Spectrum. Aqueous acid—266 nm, 283 nm, 292 nm; aqueous alkali—270 nm, 293 nm.

Infra-red Spectrum. Principal peaks at wavenumbers 836, 1261, 1236, 1042, 1061, 733.

Mass Spectrum. Principal peaks at *m/z* 58, 204, 59, 42, 30, 146, 77, 44.

Disposition in the Body. Absorbed from the gastro-intestinal tract. It is a metabolite of psilocybin. An oral dose of several milligrams may produce hallucinations and related effects.

Psilocybin   *Hallucinogen*

Synonym. 4-Phosphoryloxy-*NN*-dimethyltryptamine
3-(2-Dimethylaminoethyl)indol-4-yl dihydrogen phosphate
$C_{12}H_{17}N_2O_4P = 284.3$
CAS—520-52-5

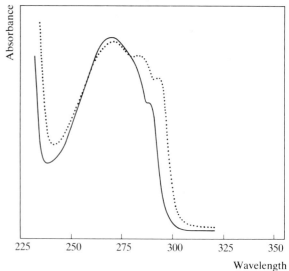

The main indole alkaloid present in the mushroom *Psilocybe mexicana* (Agaricaceae). Psilocybin is also present in the mushrooms *Stropharia cubensis* and *Conocybe* spp.
White crystals. M.p. 185° to 195°, with decomposition.
Soluble in dilute acetic acid.

Colour Test. Marquis Test—orange.

Thin-layer Chromatography. *System TA*—Rf 05. (*Van Urk reagent*, grey-violet.)

Gas Chromatography. *System GA*—RI 2059.

Ultraviolet Spectrum. Aqueous acid—268 nm; aqueous alkali—269 nm, 282 nm, 292 nm.

Infra-red Spectrum. Principal peaks at wavenumbers 1105, 1045, 1062, 1183, 1160, 932 (KBr disk).

Mass Spectrum. Principal peaks at *m/z* 58, 42, 30, 51, 204, 146, 77, 44.

Disposition in the Body. Absorbed from the gastro-intestinal tract; hallucinogenic effects usually occur within 30 minutes of ingestion with a duration of effect of about 6 hours. It is rapidly dephosphorylated to psilocin which appears to be the psycho-active compound.

Wavelength

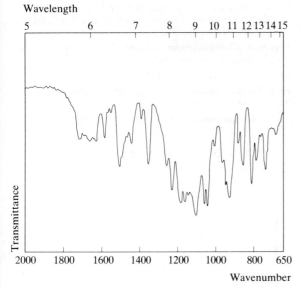

Transmittance

Wavenumber

Putrescine

Putrefactive Base

Synonym. Tetramethylenediamine
Butane-1,4-diamine
$NH_2 \cdot [CH_2]_4 \cdot NH_2 = 88.15$
CAS—110-60-1
Crystals with a strong odour. M.p. 27° to 28°. B.p. 158° to 159°.
Very **soluble** in water.

Colour Test. Ninhydrin—violet.

Thin-layer Chromatography. *System TA*—Rf 02. (*Acidified iodoplatinate solution*, positive.)

Gas Chromatography. *System GA*—RI 930.

Infra-red Spectrum. Principal peaks at wavenumbers 1118, 874, 1288, 923, 1026, 1036 (KBr disk).

Pyrantel

Anthelmintic

Synonym. Pirantel
1,4,5,6 - Tetrahydro - 1 - methyl - 2 - [(E) - 2 - (2 - thienyl) - vinyl]pyrimidine
$C_{11}H_{14}N_2S = 206.3$
CAS—15686-83-6

Crystals. M.p. 178° to 179°.

Pyrantel Embonate

Synonym. Pyrantel Pamoate
Proprietary Names. Antiminth; Combantrin; Helmex; Strongid-P (vet.).
$C_{11}H_{14}N_2S, C_{23}H_{16}O_6 = 594.7$
CAS—22204-24-6
A yellow to tan-coloured crystalline powder.
Practically **insoluble** in water, ethanol, and methanol; soluble in dimethyl sulphoxide.

Pyrantel Tartrate

$C_{11}H_{14}N_2S, C_4H_6O_6 = 356.4$
CAS—33401-94-4
A white to pale greenish-yellow, crystalline powder. M.p. 147° to 151°.
Soluble 1 in 5 of water and 1 in 9 of methanol; slightly soluble in chloroform; practically insoluble in ether.

Dissociation Constant. pK_a 11.0 (20°).

Colour Tests. Liebermann's Test—black; Mandelin's Test—violet; Marquis Test—blue-violet; Sulphuric Acid—orange → violet.

Thin-layer Chromatography. *System TA*—Rf 06. (*Acidified iodoplatinate solution*, positive.)

Gas Chromatography. *System GA*—not eluted.

Ultraviolet Spectrum. Methanolic acid—315 nm ($A_1^1 = 920$ a).

Infra-red Spectrum. Principal peaks at wavenumbers 1640, 1605, 1305, 1208, 1132, 1065 (pyrantel tartrate, KBr disk).

Mass Spectrum. Principal peaks at m/z 205, 42, 135, 173, 206, 123, 145, 45.

Dose. The equivalent of 10 to 20 mg/kg of pyrantel, as a single dose.

Pyrazinamide

Antituberculous Agent

Synonym. Pyrazinoic Acid Amide
Proprietary Names. Piraldina; Pyrafat; Tebrazid; Zinamide.
Pyrazine-2-carboxamide
$C_5H_5N_3O = 123.1$
CAS—98-96-4

A white crystalline powder. M.p. 188° to 191°.
Soluble 1 in 60 of water and 1 in 110 of ethanol; soluble in chloroform and ether.

Dissociation Constant. pK_a 0.5.

Colour Test. Nessler's Reagent—brown-orange.

Thin-layer Chromatography. *System TA*—Rf 63.

Gas Chromatography. *System GA*—RI 1250.

Ultraviolet Spectrum. Aqueous acid—269 nm ($A_1^1 = 659$ a), 312 nm. No alkaline shift. (See below)

Infra-red Spectrum. Principal peaks at wavenumbers 1685, 1020, 1600, 1584, 1050, 1165 (KBr disk). (See below)

Quantification. GAS CHROMATOGRAPHY–MASS SPECTROMETRY. In serum or urine: pyrazinamide, pyrazine-2-carboxylic acid and 5-hydroxypyrazine-2-carboxylic acid, sensitivity 10 ng/ml for pyrazinamide—J. Roboz *et al.*, *J. Chromat.*, 1978, *147*, 337–347.

Disposition in the Body. Well absorbed after oral administration. Metabolised by hydrolysis to pyrazine-2-carboxylic acid and subsequent hydroxylation to 5-hydroxypyrazine-2-carboxylic acid. In 24 hours, about 30 to 40% of a dose is excreted in the urine as pyrazine-2-carboxylic acid and less than 4% as unchanged drug; the 5-hydroxy metabolite is also excreted in the urine.

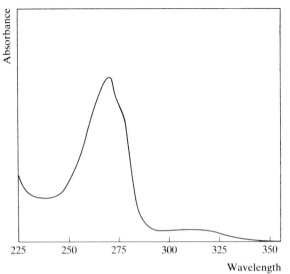

A white, deliquescent, crystalline powder. M.p. 153° to 157°.

Soluble 1 in less than 1 of water, 1 in less than 1 of ethanol, and 1 in 1 of chloroform; practically insoluble in ether.

Thin-layer Chromatography. *System TA*—Rf 04. (*Acidified iodoplatinate solution*, positive.)

Gas Chromatography. *System GA*—RI 1515.

High Pressure Liquid Chromatography. *System HA*—k' 6.3 (tailing peak).

Ultraviolet Spectrum. Aqueous acid—270 nm (A_1^1 = 186 a).

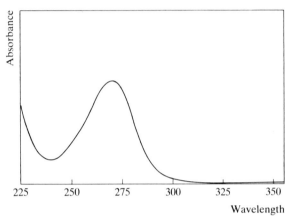

Infra-red Spectrum. Principal peaks at wavenumbers 1728, 1156, 1249, 1500, 1630, 1010 (KBr disk).

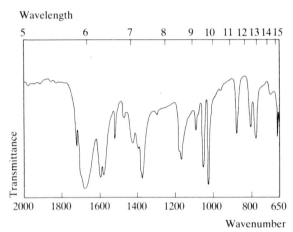

THERAPEUTIC CONCENTRATION.
After an oral dose of 3 g to one subject, a peak serum concentration of 134 µg/ml was attained in 1 hour; the serum concentration of pyrazine-2-carboxylic acid was 20 to 30 µg/ml after the first hour and the concentration of 5-hydroxypyrazine-2-carboxylic acid ranged between 3 and 8 µg/ml over a period of 12 hours (J. Roboz *et al.*, *ibid.*).

HALF-LIFE. Plasma half-life, 4 to 10 hours.

PROTEIN BINDING. In plasma, about 50%.

Dose. 20 to 35 mg/kg to a maximum of 3 g daily.

Pyridostigmine Bromide   *Anticholinesterase*

Proprietary Names. Mestinon; Regonol.
3-Dimethylcarbamoyloxy-1-methylpyridinium bromide
$C_9H_{13}BrN_2O_2$ = 261.1
CAS—*155-97-5* (pyridostigmine); *101-26-8* (bromide)

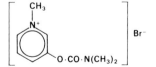

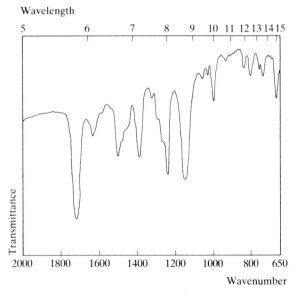

Mass Spectrum. Principal peaks at *m/z* 72, 39, 42, 38, 94, 56, 51, 81.

Quantification. GAS CHROMATOGRAPHY. In plasma: detection limit 5 ng/ml, AFID—K. Chan *et al.*, *J. Chromat.*, 1976, *120*, 349–358.

GAS CHROMATOGRAPHY–MASS SPECTROMETRY. In plasma: sensitivity 50 ng/ml—S. M. Aquilonius *et al.*, *Eur. J. clin. Pharmac.*, 1980, *18*, 423–428.

HIGH PRESSURE LIQUID CHROMATOGRAPHY. In blood or urine: sensitivity 40 ng/ml—R. I. Ellin *et al.*, *J. Chromat.*, 1982, *228*; *Biomed. Appl.*, *17*, 235–244.

Disposition in the Body. Poorly and irregularly absorbed after oral administration and may undergo significant first-pass metabolism. Up to about 16% of an oral dose is excreted in the urine unchanged, together with small amounts of 3-hydroxy-*N*-methylpyridinium. After intravenous administration, up to about 90% is excreted in the urine unchanged.

THERAPEUTIC CONCENTRATION. In plasma, usually in the range 0.05 to 0.1 µg/ml.

After a single oral dose of 120 mg to 5 subjects, peak plasma concentrations of about 0.04 to 0.07 µg/ml were attained in 1 to 2 hours (S. M. Aquilonius *et al.*, *Eur. J. clin. Pharmac.*, 1980, *18*, 423–428).

Following daily oral doses of 60 to 660 mg to 6 subjects, maximum steady-state plasma concentrations of 0.04 to 0.08 µg/ml were reported (T. N. Calvey and K. Chan, *Clin. Pharmac. Ther.*, 1977, *21*, 187–193).

HALF-LIFE. Plasma half-life, 0.3 to 2 hours, increased in subjects with renal disease.

VOLUME OF DISTRIBUTION. About 1 litre/kg.

CLEARANCE. Plasma clearance, about 8 to 16 ml/min/kg.

Dose. Usually 0.3 to 1.2 g daily.

Pyridoxine   *Vitamin*

Synonyms. Adermine; Pyridoxol; Vitamin B_6.
3-Hydroxy-4,5-bis(hydroxymethyl)-2-methylpyridine
$C_8H_{11}NO_3 = 169.2$
CAS—65-23-6

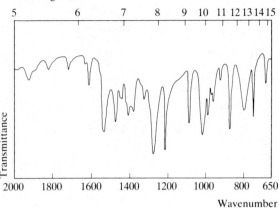

Pyridoxine Hydrochloride
Proprietary Names. Bécilan; Benadon; Comploment; Dermo 6; Hexa-Betalin; Hexavibex; Hexobion; Paxadon; Pydox; Pyroxin; Seibion. It is an ingredient of Ancoloxin, Apisate, Bendectin, Debendox, and Optimax.
$C_8H_{11}NO_3,HCl = 205.6$
CAS—58-56-0
A white crystalline powder, or crystals. M.p. 202° to 206°, with decomposition.
Soluble 1 in 5 of water and 1 in about 115 of ethanol; practically insoluble in chloroform and ether.

Dissociation Constant. pK_a 5.0 (—N=), 9.0 (—OH), (25°).

Colour Test. Mandelin's Test—blue → grey-green.

Thin-layer Chromatography. *System TA*—Rf 59. (*Acidified potassium permanganate solution*, positive.)

Ultraviolet Spectrum. Aqueous acid—290 nm ($A_1^1 = 523$ a); *phosphate buffer (pH 6.88)*—254 nm ($A_1^1 = 219$ a), 324 nm ($A_1^1 = 426$ a).

Infra-red Spectrum. Principal peaks at wavenumbers 1277, 1212, 1015, 1540, 870, 1086 (pyridoxine hydrochloride, KBr disk).

Mass Spectrum. Principal peaks at *m/z* 151, 94, 122, 106, 51, 53, 149, 150.

Wavelength

Quantification. HIGH PRESSURE LIQUID CHROMATOGRAPHY. In plasma or urine: pyridoxine, pyridoxal and 4-pyridoxic acid, sensitivity 300 ng/ml for plasma, 500 ng/ml for urine, UV detection—W. J. O'Reilly *et al.*, *J. Chromat.*, 1980, *183*; *Biomed. Appl.*, *9*, 492–498.

Disposition in the Body. Absorbed from the gastro-intestinal tract and converted to the active form, pyridoxal phosphate. Excreted in the urine mainly as 4-pyridoxic acid.

PROTEIN BINDING. In plasma, pyridoxine not significantly bound, pyridoxal phosphate almost completely bound.

Dose. 20 to 200 mg of pyridoxine hydrochloride daily.

Pyrimethamine   *Antimalarial*

Proprietary Names. Daraprim; Erbaprelina. It is an ingredient of Fansidar, Maloprim, Supacox (vet.), and Whitsyn S (vet.).
5-(4-Chlorophenyl)-6-ethylpyrimidine-2,4-diamine
$C_{12}H_{13}ClN_4 = 248.7$
CAS—58-14-0

A white crystalline powder. M.p. 238° to 242°.
Practically **insoluble** in water; soluble 1 in 200 of ethanol and 1 in 125 of chloroform; soluble in warm dilute mineral acids.

Dissociation Constant. pK_a 7.0 (20°).

Thin-layer Chromatography. *System TA*—Rf 61; *system TB*—Rf 02; *system TC*—Rf 31. (*Acidified iodoplatinate solution*, positive.)

Gas Chromatography. *System GA*—RI 2138.

High Pressure Liquid Chromatography. *System HA*—k' 1.0.

Ultraviolet Spectrum. Aqueous acid—272 nm ($A_1^1 = 320$ a); aqueous alkali—286 nm ($A_1^1 = 381$ b). (See below)

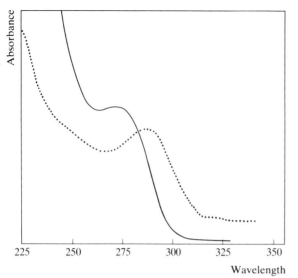

225   250   275   300   325   350

Wavelength

Infra-red Spectrum. Principal peaks at wavenumbers 1628, 1575, 1640, 1075, 835, 805 (K Br disk).

Wavelength

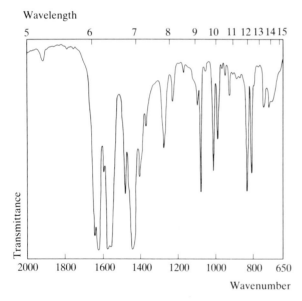

5   6   7   8   9   10 11 12 13 14 15

2000   1800   1600   1400   1200   1000   800   650

Wavenumber

Mass Spectrum. Principal peaks at m/z 247, 248, 249, 250, 219, 212, 106, 221.

Quantification. GAS CHROMATOGRAPHY. In plasma or urine: sensitivity 5 ng/ml, ECD—C. Midskov, *J. Chromat.*, 1984, *306*; *Biomed. Appl.*, *31*, 388–393.

HIGH PRESSURE LIQUID CHROMATOGRAPHY. In plasma: sensitivity 10 ng/ml, fluorescence detection—U. Timm and E. Weidekamm, *J. Chromat.*, 1982, *230*; *Biomed. Appl.*, *19*, 107–114.

Disposition in the Body. Well absorbed after oral administration, and very slowly excreted in the urine, about 20% of a dose being excreted in 7 days.

THERAPEUTIC CONCENTRATION.
A single oral dose of 50 mg given to 5 subjects produced a peak plasma concentration of 0.21 to 0.43 µg/ml (mean 0.34) in 2 to 4 hours, followed by a slow decline over several days (L. Donno *et al.*, *Curr. ther. Res.*, 1980, *27*, 346–355).

TOXICITY. Children have died following ingestion of 0.4 to 1 g.

HALF-LIFE. Plasma half-life, about 4 days.

Dose. Up to 75 mg daily.

Pyrithidium Bromide   *Trypanocide (Veterinary)*

Synonym. Pyritidium Bromide
3-Amino-8-(2-amino-1,6-dimethylpyrimidinium-4-ylamino)-6-(4-aminophenyl)-5-methylphenanthridinium dibromide
$C_{26}H_{27}Br_2N_7 = 597.4$
CAS—3616-05-5 (pyrithidium); *14222-46-9* (bromide)

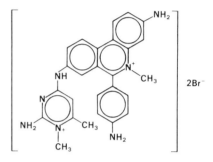

A brick-red to reddish-purple, hygroscopic powder.
Soluble 1 in 40 of water and 1 in 1900 of ethanol.

Thin-layer Chromatography. *System TA*—Rf 01. (Location under ultraviolet light, yellow fluorescence; *acidified iodoplatinate solution*, positive.)

Ultraviolet Spectrum. Aqueous acid—256 nm ($A_1^1 = 425$ a), 313 nm ($A_1^1 = 813$ a).

Infra-red Spectrum. Principal peaks at wavenumbers 1615, 1642, 1515, 1250, 1562, 1298 (K Br disk).

Pyrrobutamine   *Antihistamine*

1-[4-(4-Chlorophenyl)-3-phenylbut-2-enyl]pyrrolidine
$C_{20}H_{22}ClN = 311.9$
CAS—91-82-7

An oily liquid. On standing gives crystals. M.p. 48° to 49°.

Pyrrobutamine Phosphate
Proprietary Name. It is an ingredient of Co-Pyronil.
$C_{20}H_{22}ClN,2H_3PO_4 = 507.8$
CAS—135-31-9
A white crystalline powder. M.p. 127° to 131°.
Soluble in water; soluble 1 in 20 of ethanol; practically insoluble in chloroform and ether.

Dissociation Constant. pK$_a$ 8.8 (25°).

Colour Tests. Liebermann's Test—brown; Mandelin's Test—violet; Marquis Test—grey-violet.

Thin-layer Chromatography. *System TA*—Rf 54; *system TB*—Rf 55; *system TC*—Rf 37. (*Dragendorff spray*, positive; *acidified iodoplatinate solution*, positive; *Marquis reagent*, grey.)

Gas Chromatography. *System GA*—RI 2419; *system GF*—RI 2815.

High Pressure Liquid Chromatography. *System HA*—k' 2.8.

Infra-red Spectrum. Principal peaks at wavenumbers 995, 1018, 1087, 772, 1492, 820 (pyrrobutamine phosphate, KBr disk).

Mass Spectrum. Principal peaks at *m/z* 205, 240, 91, 84, 125, 242, 206, 186.

Dose. 30 to 90 mg of pyrrobutamine phosphate daily.

Quinalbarbitone   *Barbiturate*

Synonyms. Meballymal; Secobarbital.
Proprietary Name. Seconal
5-Allyl-5-(1-methylbutyl)barbituric acid
C$_{12}$H$_{18}$N$_2$O$_3$ = 238.3
CAS—76-73-3

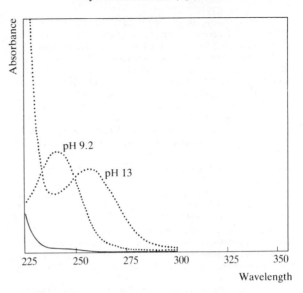

A white amorphous or crystalline powder. M.p. 100°.
Very slightly **soluble** in water; freely soluble in ethanol and ether; soluble in chloroform.

Quinalbarbitone Sodium

Synonyms. Meballymalnatrium; Secobarbital Sodium; Secobarbitone Sodium.
Proprietary Names. Imménoctal; Immenox; Proquinal; Quinbar; Secogen; Seconal Sodium; Seral. It is an ingredient of Tuinal.
C$_{12}$H$_{17}$N$_2$NaO$_3$ = 260.3
CAS—309-43-3
A white hygroscopic powder.
Soluble 1 in 3 of water and 1 in 5 of ethanol; practically insoluble in chloroform and ether.

Dissociation Constant. pK$_a$ 7.9 (20°).

Colour Tests. Koppanyi–Zwikker Test—violet; Mercurous Nitrate—black; Vanillin Reagent—brown-red/violet.

Thin-layer Chromatography. *System TD*—Rf 55; *system TE*—Rf 44; *system TF*—Rf 68; *system TH*—Rf 78. (*Mercuric chloride–diphenylcarbazone reagent*, positive; *mercurous nitrate spray*, black; *acidified potassium permanganate solution*, yellow-brown; *Zwikker's reagent*, pink.)

Gas Chromatography. *System GA*—quinalbarbitone RI 1791; 3'-hydroxyquinalbarbitone RI 1965; *system GF*—RI 2510.

High Pressure Liquid Chromatography. *System HG*—k' 16.28; *system HH*—k' 11.47.

Ultraviolet Spectrum. *Borax buffer 0.05M* (pH 9.2)—239 nm (A$_1^1$ = 393 a); M sodium hydroxide (pH 13)—254 nm (A$_1^1$ = 330 b).

Infra-red Spectrum. Principal peaks at wavenumbers 1559, 1648, 1690, 1298, 1270, 925 (quinalbarbitone sodium, KBr disk).

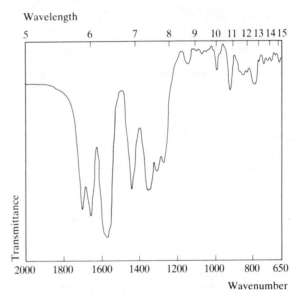

Mass Spectrum. Principal peaks at *m/z* 167, 168, 41, 43, 97, 124, 39, 55; 5-(2,3-dihydroxypropyl)quinalbarbitone 171, 43, 143, 41, 128, 55, 141, 159; 3'-hydroxyquinalbarbitone 41, 45, 43, 168, 39, 70, 69, 167; 3'-ketoquinalbarbitone 43, 69, 168, 41, 85, 167, 86, 169.

Quantification. See also under Amylobarbitone.

GAS CHROMATOGRAPHY. In plasma or urine: sensitivity 200 ng/ml in plasma, FID—J. L. Valentine *et al.*, *Analyt. Lett. (Part B)*, 1982, *15*, 343–361.

HIGH PRESSURE LIQUID CHROMATOGRAPHY. In serum: detection limit 20 ng/ml, UV detection—H. L. Levine *et al.*, *J. pharm. Sci.*, 1982, *71*, 1281–1283.

Disposition in the Body. About 90% of a dose is absorbed after oral administration. The major metabolic reactions are hydroxylation of both side-chains at the C$_5$-position with further oxidation of the ω-position on the butyl side-chain. Less than 5% of an oral dose is excreted unchanged in the urine. Two diastereoisomeric forms of the following metabolites have been found in the urine, each metabolite accounting for about 4% of the dose in 24 hours: 5-allyl-5-(3-hydroxy-1-methylbutyl)-barbituric acid (3'-hydroxyquinalbarbitone), 5-allyl-5-(3-carboxy-1-methylpropyl)barbituric acid, and 5-(2,3-dihydroxy-propyl)quinalbarbitone; an additional metabolite, 5-allyl-5-(1-methyl-3-oxobutyl)barbituric acid (3'-ketoquinalbarbitone), accounts for about 3% of the dose in 96 hours. A total of about 45% of the dose is excreted in the urine over a period of 108 hours.

THERAPEUTIC CONCENTRATION. In plasma, usually in the range 2 to 10 µg/ml.

After an oral dose of 3.3 mg/kg to 6 subjects, peak blood concentrations of 2.0 to 2.2 µg/ml (mean 2.1) were attained in about 3 hours (J. M. Clifford et al., Clin. Pharmac. Ther., 1974, 16, 376–389).

TOXICITY. The estimated minimum lethal dose is 2 g. Toxic effects are usually associated with blood concentrations greater than about 8 µg/ml. In 276 reported fatalities attributed to quinalbarbitone, blood concentrations ranged from 4 to 132 µg/ml (mean 30).

The following postmortem tissue distribution was reported in 5 fatalities: blood 35 to 123 µg/ml (mean 66), brain 109 µg/g (1 case), kidney 67 to 270 µg/g (mean 152, 3 cases), liver 25 to 605 µg/g (mean 271, 4 cases), spleen 42 µg/g (1 case), urine 12 to 182 µg/ml (mean 72, 3 cases) (C. J. Rehling, Poison Residues in Human Tissues, in Progress in Chemical Toxicology, Vol. 3, A. Stolman (Ed.), New York, Academic Press Inc., 1967, p. 371).

The following postmortem tissue concentrations (µg/ml or µg/g) were reported in 3 fatalities due to quinalbarbitone:

	Quinalbarbitone	3'-Hydroxyquinalbarbitone
Blood	12, 9, 13	0, —, 2
Bile	—, 42, 79	—, —, 0
Left Kidney	37, 25, 25	3, —, 17
Right Kidney	69, 24, 28	4, —, 16
Liver	77, 51, 44	4, —, 25
Urine	6, 3, 32	0, —, 33

(A. E. Robinson and R. D. McDowall, J. Pharm. Pharmac., 1979, 31, 357–365).

HALF-LIFE. Plasma half-life, 19 to 34 hours (mean 25).

VOLUME OF DISTRIBUTION. About 1.5 litres/kg.

CLEARANCE. Plasma clearance, about 0.8 ml/min/kg.

SALIVA. Plasma: saliva ratio, about 3.3.

PROTEIN BINDING. In plasma, about 70%.

Dose. 50 to 200 mg daily.

Quinethazone   *Diuretic*

Synonym. Chinethazonum
Proprietary Names. Aquamox; Hydromox.
7 - Chloro - 2 - ethyl - 1,2,3,4 - tetrahydro - 4 - oxoquinazoline - 6 - sulphonamide
$C_{10}H_{12}ClN_3O_3S = 289.7$
CAS—73-49-4

A white to yellowish-white, crystalline powder. M.p. 245° to 252°.

Very slightly **soluble** in water; slightly soluble in ethanol; freely soluble in solutions of alkali hydroxides and carbonates.

Dissociation Constant. pK_a 9.3, 10.7.

Colour Test. Koppanyi–Zwikker Test—violet.

Thin-layer Chromatography. System TA—Rf 75; system TD—Rf 04; system TE—Rf 41; system TF—Rf 21. (Location under ultraviolet light, blue fluorescence; acidified iodoplatinate solution, positive.)

High Pressure Liquid Chromatography. System HN—k' 0.67.

Ultraviolet Spectrum. Ethanol—234 nm ($A_1^1 = 1532$ a), 278 nm, 345 nm.

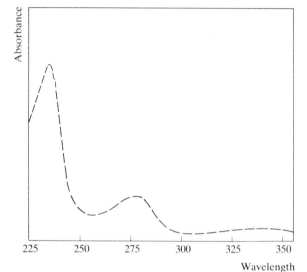

Infra-red Spectrum. Principal peaks at wavenumbers 1600, 1650, 1160, 960, 1510, 1040 (KBr disk).

Mass Spectrum. Principal peaks at m/z 260, 262, 180, 287, 261, 145, 286, 124.

Dose. 50 to 200 mg daily.

Quinidine   *Anti-arrhythmic*

Synonyms. Chinidinum; Quinidina.
(8R,9S)-6'-Methoxycinchonan-9-ol dihydrate
$C_{20}H_{24}N_2O_2,2H_2O = 360.5$
CAS—56-54-2 (anhydrous); 63717-04-4 (dihydrate)

A dextrorotatory stereoisomer of quinine, obtained from the bark of species of Cinchona (Rubiaceae). Commercial samples may contain 20 to 30% of hydroquinidine.
A white amorphous powder or acicular crystals.

Soluble 1 in 2000 of water and 1 in 70 of ether. The anhydrous alkaloid is soluble 1 in 1.6 of chloroform.

Quinidine Bisulphate
Proprietary Names. Biquin; Kiditard; Kinidin Durules; Quinidurile.
$C_{20}H_{24}N_2O_2,H_2SO_4 = 422.5$
CAS—747-45-5
Colourless crystals.
Soluble 1 in 8 of water and 1 in 3 of ethanol; practically insoluble in ether.

Quinidine Gluconate
Proprietary Names. Duraquin; Quinaglute; Quinate.
$C_{20}H_{24}N_2O_2,C_6H_{12}O_7 = 520.6$
CAS—7054-25-3
A white powder. M.p. 175° to 177°.
Freely **soluble** in water; slightly soluble in ethanol.

Quinidine Polygalacturonate
Proprietary Names. Cardioquin; Galactoquin.
$C_{20}H_{24}N_2O_2,(C_6H_{10}O_7)_x,xH_2O$
CAS—27555-34-6 (anhydrous); 65484-56-2 (hydrate)
An amorphous powder. M.p. 180°, with decomposition.
The anhydrous product is sparingly **soluble** in water; practically insoluble in ethanol, chloroform, ether, and methanol.

Quinidine Sulphate
Proprietary Names. Cin-Quin; Kinidine; Quinicardine; Quinidex; Quinidoxin; Quinora; Systodin.
$(C_{20}H_{24}N_2O_2)_2,H_2SO_4,2H_2O = 782.9$
CAS—50-54-4 (anhydrous); 6591-63-5 (dihydrate)
White acicular crystals or fine white powder, darkening on exposure to light. M.p. about 207°, with decomposition.
Soluble 1 in 80 of water, 1 in 10 of ethanol, and 1 in 15 of chloroform; practically insoluble in ether.

Dissociation Constant. pK_a 4.2, 8.8 (20°).

Colour Tests. Sulphuric Acid—yellow (fluoresces under ultraviolet light); Thalleioquin Test—green.

Thin-layer Chromatography. *System TA*—Rf 51; *system TB*—Rf 03; *system TC*—Rf 11. (Location under ultraviolet light, blue fluorescence; *Dragendorff spray*, positive; *acidified iodoplatinate solution*, positive.)

Gas Chromatography. *System GA*—RI 2798.

High Pressure Liquid Chromatography. *System HA*—k' 2.1.

Ultraviolet Spectrum. Aqueous acid—250 nm ($A_1^1 = 959$ a), 317 nm, 345 nm; aqueous alkali—280 nm, 330 nm.

Infra-red Spectrum. Principal peaks at wavenumbers 1258, 1514, 1619, 1040, 860, 820 (KBr disk).

Mass Spectrum. Principal peaks at *m/z* 136, 81, 322, 188, 55, 42, 41, 172.

Quantification. GAS CHROMATOGRAPHY. In serum: quinidine and other anti-arrhythmic agents, AFID—K. M. Kessler *et al.*, *Clin. Chem.*, 1982, *28*, 1187–1190.

HIGH PRESSURE LIQUID CHROMATOGRAPHY. In plasma: quinidine and other anti-arrhythmic agents, sensitivity 500 ng/ml, UV detection—R. R. Bridges and T. A. Jennison, *J. analyt. Toxicol.*, 1983, *7*, 65–68. In plasma: quinidine, hydroquinidine, and 2 quinidine metabolites, sensitivity 50 ng/ml for quinidine, fluorescence detection—L. K. Pershing *et al.*, *J. analyt. Toxicol.*, 1982, *6*, 153–156. In plasma or urine: quinidine, hydroquinidine and quinidine metabolites, detection limit 10 ng/ml for quinidine, fluorescence and UV detection—T. W. Guentert *et al.*, *J. Chromat.*, 1980, *183*; *Biomed. Appl.*, *9*, 514–518.

Disposition in the Body. Readily absorbed after oral administration; bioavailability about 70 to 80% but there is considerable intersubject variation. Extensively metabolised, mainly by hydroxylation. The major metabolites, 3-hydroxyquinidine and

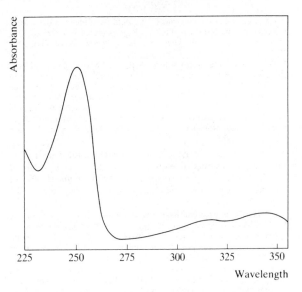

Wavelength

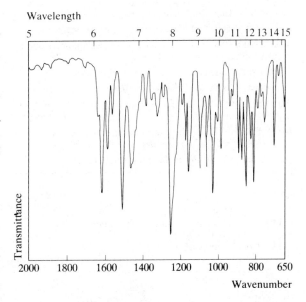

Wavenumber

quinidin-2'-one appear to be pharmacologically active. Hydroquinidine which may occur in quinidine as an impurity, at concentrations of up to about 30%, has similar pharmacological activity to quinidine. About 10 to 30% of a dose is excreted in the urine as unchanged drug in 48 hours and the remainder is mostly excreted in the urine as metabolites; O-desmethylquinidine accounts for about 2% of a dose; quinidine-10,11-dihydrodiol and an N-oxide metabolite have been detected in plasma and urine. The proportion of unchanged drug is dependent on the urinary pH, being decreased if the urine is alkaline.

THERAPEUTIC CONCENTRATION. In plasma, usually in the range 2 to 6 µg/ml; there is, however, considerable intersubject variation. Concentrations appear to be higher in subjects with congestive heart failure.

After single oral doses of 4.5 mg/kg of quinidine sulphate to 10 subjects, peak plasma concentrations of 0.9 to 1.8 μg/ml (mean 1.2) were attained in about 50 minutes (T. W. Guentert *et al.*, *J. Pharmacokinet. Biopharm.*, 1979, *7*, 315–330).

Following daily oral doses of 8 to 19 mg/kg (mean 12) to 5 subjects, steady-state serum concentrations of 0.5 to 2.5 μg/ml (mean 1.8) of quinidine, 0.38 to 0.94 μg/ml (mean 0.55) of 3-hydroxyquinidine, and 0.02 to 0.12 μg/ml (mean 0.07) of quinidin-2'-one, were reported; following daily oral doses of 8.6 to 13.3 mg/kg (mean 10.7) to 8 subjects with mild renal dysfunction, steady-state serum-quinidine concentrations ranged from 1.4 to 3.6 μg/ml (mean 2.3) (D. E. Drayer *et al.*, *Clin. Pharmac. Ther.*, 1978, *24*, 31–39).

TOXICITY. Plasma concentrations greater than 6 μg/ml are progressively associated with toxicity, and concentrations of about 15 μg/ml may cause toxic reactions in about 50% of patients; concentrations in excess of about 30 μg/ml may be lethal.

The following postmortem tissue concentrations were reported in one fatality: blood 75 μg/ml, brain 11 μg/g, kidney 89 μg/g, liver 145 μg/g, spleen 136 μg/g, urine 52 μg/ml; 3-hydroxyquinidine, and lactone conjugates of quinidine and 3-hydroxyquinidine were also detected (J. G. Leferink *et al.*, *J. analyt. Toxicol.*, 1977, *1*, 62–65).

In a fatality involving the ingestion of about 5 g of a sustained-release preparation by a 2-year-old child, the following postmortem tissue concentrations were reported: blood 45 μg/ml, kidney 180 μg/g, liver 220 μg/g; death occurred 28 hours after ingestion (A. J. McBay and R. F. Turk, *Bull. int. Ass. forens. Toxicol.*, 1972, *8*(4), 2–3).

HALF-LIFE. Plasma half-life, about 4 to 12 hours (mean 7).

VOLUME OF DISTRIBUTION. About 2 to 3 litres/kg, decreased in subjects with congestive heart failure.

CLEARANCE. Plasma clearance, about 4 ml/min/kg.

DISTRIBUTION IN BLOOD. Plasma: whole blood ratio, about 1.0.

PROTEIN BINDING. In plasma, quinidine about 75 to 90%, 3-hydroxyquinidine about 70%, and quinidin-2'-one about 55%.

NOTE. For a review of the pharmacokinetics of quinidine see H. R. Ochs *et al.*, *Clin. Pharmacokinet.*, 1980, *5*, 150–168.

Dose. Usually 0.6 to 1.6 g of quinidine sulphate daily.

Quinine   *Antimalarial*

Synonym. Chininum
(8*S*,9*R*)-6'-Methoxycinchonan-9-ol trihydrate
$C_{20}H_{24}N_2O_2,3H_2O = 378.5$
CAS—130-95-0 (anhydrous)

The chief alkaloid of various species of *Cinchona* (Rubiaceae). It is a laevorotatory stereoisomer of quinidine.

A white, slightly efflorescent, flaky, granular or microcrystalline powder. M.p. about 173°.

Very slightly **soluble** in water; soluble 1 in 1 of ethanol (90%), 1 in 3 of chloroform, and 1 in 4 of ether saturated with water.

Quinine Bisulphate

Synonyms. Neutral Quinine Sulphate; Quinine Acid Sulphate.
Proprietary Names. Biquin; Biquinate; Dentojel; Myoquin; Quinbisan.
$C_{20}H_{24}N_2O_2,H_2SO_4,7H_2O = 548.6$
CAS—549-56-4 (anhydrous)
Colourless crystals or white crystalline powder. It effloresces in dry air and becomes yellow when exposed to light.
Soluble 1 in 8 of water, 1 in 50 of ethanol, and 1 in 625 of chloroform.

Quinine Dihydrobromide

Synonyms. Neutral Quinine Hydrobromide; Quinine Acid Hydrobromide.
$C_{20}H_{24}N_2O_2,2HBr,3H_2O = 540.3$
CAS—549-47-3 (anhydrous)
Yellowish or white crystals or powder.
Soluble 1 in 7 of water; soluble in ethanol; practically insoluble in ether.

Quinine Dihydrochloride

Synonyms. Neutral Quinine Hydrochloride; Quinine Acid Hydrochloride.
$C_{20}H_{24}N_2O_2,2HCl = 397.3$
CAS—60-93-5
A white powder.
Soluble 1 in 0.5 of water, 1 in 14 of ethanol, and 1 in 7 of chloroform; practically insoluble in ether.

Quinine Ethyl Carbonate

Synonym. Euquinina
$C_{23}H_{28}N_2O_4 = 396.5$
CAS—83-75-0
White masses of silky crystals which darken on exposure to light. M.p. 91° to 95°.
Very slightly **soluble** in water; soluble 1 in 2 of ethanol, 1 in 1 of chloroform, and 1 in 10 of ether.

Quinine Hydrobromide

Synonym. Basic Quinine Hydrobromide
Proprietary Name. Coquelusédal Quinine
$C_{20}H_{24}N_2O_2,HBr,2H_2O = 441.4$
CAS—549-49-5 (anhydrous)
White, silky, efflorescent crystals which darken on exposure to light.
Soluble 1 in about 55 of water, 1 in 0.7 of ethanol, and 1 in 1 of chloroform, the solution in chloroform being turbid due to separation of water.

Quinine Hydrochloride

Synonym. Basic Quinine Hydrochloride
Proprietary Name. Kinin
$C_{20}H_{24}N_2O_2,HCl,2H_2O = 396.9$
CAS—130-89-2 (anhydrous); *6119-47-7* (dihydrate)
Colourless, fine, silky, acicular crystals which effloresce in dry air and gradually become yellowish on exposure to light.
Soluble 1 in 23 of water, 1 in 0.9 of ethanol, and 1 in 2 of chloroform to give a turbid solution; very slightly soluble in ether.

Quinine Salicylate

$C_{20}H_{24}N_2O_2,C_7H_6O_3,H_2O = 480.6$
CAS—750-90-3 (anhydrous)
White silky crystals or a crystalline powder; it becomes pink on storage.
Very slightly **soluble** in water; soluble 1 in 24 of ethanol and 1 in 25 of chloroform.

Quinine Sulphate

Synonym. Basic Quinine Sulphate
Proprietary Names. Adquin; Kinine; Quinamm; Quinate; Quine; Quinite; Quinoctal; Quinsan.
$(C_{20}H_{24}N_2O_2)_2,H_2SO_4,2H_2O = 782.9$
CAS—804-63-7 (anhydrous); *6119-70-6* (dihydrate)
Colourless acicular crystals or a white crystalline powder, becoming brown on exposure to light.
Soluble 1 in about 810 of water and 1 in about 95 of ethanol; slightly soluble in chloroform and ether; readily soluble in a 2:1 mixture of chloroform and dehydrated alcohol.

Dissociation Constant. pK_a 4.1, 8.5 (20°).

Colour Tests. Sulphuric Acid—yellow (fluoresces under ultraviolet light); Thalleioquin Test—green.

Thin-layer Chromatography. *System TA*—Rf 51; *system TB*—Rf 03; *system TC*—Rf 11. (Location under ultraviolet light, blue fluorescence; *Dragendorff spray*, positive; *acidified iodoplatinate solution*, positive.)

Gas Chromatography. *System GA*—RI 2798.

High Pressure Liquid Chromatography. *System HA*—k' 2.4; *system HS*—k' 2.02.

Ultraviolet Spectrum. Aqueous acid—250 nm ($A_1^1 = 959$ a), 317 nm, 346 nm; aqueous alkali—280 nm, 330 nm.

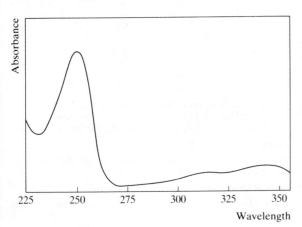

Infra-red Spectrum. Principal peaks at wavenumbers 1235, 1215, 1510, 1619, 1030, 1105 (KBr disk).

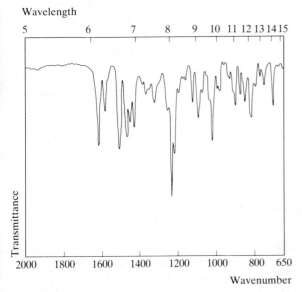

Mass Spectrum. Principal peaks at m/z 136, 137, 81, 42, 41, 189, 55, 117.

Quantification. SPECTROFLUORIMETRY. In plasma or urine— A. P. Hall *et al.*, *Clin. Pharmac. Ther.*, 1973, *14*, 580–585.

GAS CHROMATOGRAPHY–MASS SPECTROMETRY. In urine: sensitivity 50 pg—R. L. Furner *et al.*, *J. analyt. Toxicol.*, 1981, *5*, 275–278.

Disposition in the Body. Readily absorbed after oral administration but more slowly absorbed after intramuscular or subcutaneous doses. Hydroquinine may occur in quinine as an impurity at concentrations up to about 10%. Metabolised by oxidation to hydroxylated metabolites, mainly the 2-hydroxyquinoline and 6-hydroxyquinoline derivatives, 3-hydroxyquinine, and the corresponding dihydro compounds; quinine-10,11-epoxide and quinine-10,11-dihydrodiol have also been detected in urine. Up to about 20% of a single dose is excreted in the urine in 24 hours with less than 5% as unchanged drug. Less than 5% of a dose is eliminated in the faeces. The urinary excretion of quinine is increased when the urine is acid; quinine is excreted to some extent in the bile.

THERAPEUTIC CONCENTRATION. In plasma, usually in the range 3 to 7 µg/ml. Malarial infection inhibits hepatic metabolism and thus plasma concentrations resulting from a given dose will vary according to the severity of the infection.

Oral doses of 540 mg, given 8-hourly for 3 days to 11 subjects, resulted in a mean peak plasma concentration of 4 µg/ml after 72 hours (A. P. Hall *et al.*, *Clin. Pharmac. Ther.*, 1973, *14*, 580–585).

Oral doses of 650 mg, given 8-hourly to 15 subjects, resulted in a mean steady-state plasma concentration of 11 µg/ml during the first 5 days; thereafter the concentration declined slowly to about 8 µg/ml after 14 days (M. H. Brooks *et al.*, *Clin. Pharmac. Ther.*, 1969, *10*, 85–91).

TOXICITY. The estimated minimum lethal dose is 8 g. Blood concentrations greater than about 10 µg/ml may cause toxic effects and can be lethal.

Fatal quinine poisoning occurred in three young females, and the following postmortem concentrations (µg/ml or µg/g) were reported: blood –, 11, –; kidney 300, 96, 410; liver 1500, 39, 150; spleen 600, 87, –; urine –, –, 860 (G. W. Walker, personal communication, 1964).

In a fatality involving the ingestion of 32.5 g of quinine sulphate, postmortem brain and liver concentrations of 292 and 3000 µg/g, respectively, were reported (S. Andrtauskas *et al.*, *Bull. int. Ass. forens. Toxicol.*, 1974, *10*(3), 7–8).

HALF-LIFE. Plasma half-life, 4 to 15 hours (mean 9); it appears to increase during malarial infection.

VOLUME OF DISTRIBUTION. About 2 litres/kg.

DISTRIBUTION IN BLOOD. Plasma: whole blood ratio, about 0.93 in normal subjects. In malarial subjects, the plasma concentration rises but this does not seem to be accompanied by a rise in the amount taken up by erythrocytes; under these conditions there may be twice as much in the plasma as in the erythrocytes.

PROTEIN BINDING. In plasma, 70 to 90%.

Dose. 2 g of quinine sulphate or other salt, daily, for 14 days.

Quinuronium Sulphate   *Antiprotozoal (Veterinary)*

Synonym. Quinolyl Urea
Proprietary Names. Ludobal; Pirevan V.
6,6'-Ureylenebis(1-methylquinolinium) bis(methyl sulphate)
$C_{23}H_{26}N_4O_9S_2 = 566.6$
CAS—135-14-8

A creamy-white to yellow, crystalline powder. M.p. 235°, with decomposition.

Very **soluble** in water; very slightly soluble in organic solvents. On heating, aqueous solutions darken and some decomposition may occur.

Colour Test. Aromaticity (Method 2)—yellow/orange.

Thin-layer Chromatography. *System TA*—Rf 00. (*Acidified iodoplatinate solution*, positive.)

Ultraviolet Spectrum. Aqueous acid—274 nm ($A_1^1 = 1527$ a), 323 nm, 359 nm.

Infra-red Spectrum. Principal peaks at wavenumbers 1210, 1248, 1276, 1572, 1025, 1525 (KBr disk).

Racemorphan   *Narcotic Analgesic*

($\pm$)-9a-Methylmorphinan-3-ol
$C_{17}H_{23}NO = 257.4$
CAS—297-90-5

A white powder. M.p. 251° to 253°.
Soluble in dilute acetic acid.

Thin-layer Chromatography. *System TA*—Rf 35; *system TB*—Rf 13; *system TC*—Rf 07. (*Dragendorff spray*, positive; *acidified iodoplatinate solution*, positive.)

Gas Chromatography. *System GA*—RI 2230.

Ultraviolet Spectrum. Aqueous acid—279 nm ($A_1^1 = 79$ a); aqueous alkali—240 nm ($A_1^1 = 339$ a), 299 nm ($A_1^1 = 119$ a).

Infra-red Spectrum. Principal peaks at wavenumbers 1242, 1280, 1580, 1495, 1505, 760 (KBr disk).

Mass Spectrum. Principal peaks at *m/z* 257, 59, 150, 256, 31, 157, 42, 200.

Racephedrine   *Sympathomimetic*

Synonyms. dl-Ephedrine; Racemic Ephedrine.
Proprietary Name. It is an ingredient of Riddofan.
($\pm$)-2-Methylamino-1-phenylpropan-1-ol
$C_{10}H_{15}NO = 165.2$
CAS—90-81-3

Crystals. M.p. 79°.
Soluble in water, ethanol, chloroform, and ether.

Racephedrine Hydrochloride
Proprietary Names. Efetonina; Ephetonin.
$C_{10}H_{15}NO,HCl = 201.7$
CAS—134-71-4
Fine, white, crystals or powder. M.p. 187° to 188°.
Soluble 1 in about 4 of water and 1 in about 25 of ethanol; practically insoluble in ether.
For analytical data see under Ephedrine.

Dose. 50 to 200 mg of racephedrine hydrochloride daily.

Rafoxanide   *Anthelmintic (Veterinary)*

Proprietary Names. Flukanide. It is an ingredient of Ranizole.
3'-Chloro-4'-(4-chlorophenoxy)-3,5-di-iodosalicylanilide
$C_{19}H_{11}Cl_2I_2NO_3 = 626.0$
CAS—22662-39-1

A greyish-white to brown powder. M.p. about 175°.
Practically **insoluble** in water; soluble 1 in 25 of acetone, 1 in 40 of chloroform, 1 in 35 of ethyl acetate, and 1 in 200 of methanol.

Colour Test. Iodine Test—positive.

Thin-layer Chromatography. *System TA*—Rf 89. (*Acidified potassium permanganate solution*, positive.)

Gas Chromatography. *System GA*—not eluted.

Ultraviolet Spectrum. Methanolic acid—280 nm ($A_1^1 = 243$ b), 335 nm ($A_1^1 = 149$ a).

Infra-red Spectrum. Principal peaks at wavenumbers 1215, 1562, 1592, 1257, 1087, 1275 (KBr disk).

Ranitidine   *Histamine H_2-Receptor Antagonist*

NN - Dimethyl - 5 - [2 - (1 - methylamino - 2 - nitrovinylamino) - ethylthiomethyl]furfurylamine
$C_{13}H_{22}N_4O_3S = 314.4$
CAS—66357-35-5

Ranitidine Hydrochloride
Proprietary Name. Zantac
$C_{13}H_{22}N_4O_3S,HCl = 350.9$
CAS—71130-06-8
A yellowish-grey powder. M.p. about 130°.
Freely **soluble** in water.

Dissociation Constant. pK_a 2.3, 8.2.

High Pressure Liquid Chromatography. *System HA*—k' 2.3.

Ultraviolet Spectrum. Water—313 nm ($A_1^1 = 499$ a).

Infra-red Spectrum. Principal peaks at wavenumbers 1220, 1620, 1192, 1570, 1590, 1260 (ranitidine hydrochloride, KBr disk).

Quantification. HIGH PRESSURE LIQUID CHROMATOGRAPHY. In plasma or urine: sensitivity 5 ng/ml for ranitidine, 15 ng/ml for desmethylranitidine, UV detection—G. W. Mihaly *et al., J.*

Wavelength

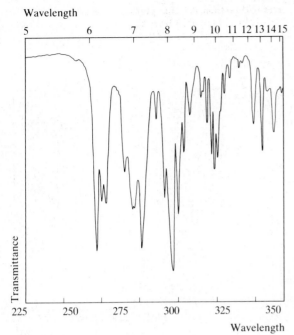

Transmittance

pharm. Sci., 1980, *69*, 1155–1157. In urine: ranitidine and metabolites, UV detection—P. F. Carey *et al.*, *J. Chromat.*, 1981, *225*; *Biomed. Appl.*, *14*, 161–168.

RADIOIMMUNOASSAY. In biological fluids: sensitivity 2 ng/ml—W. N. Jenner *et al.*, *Life Sci.*, 1981, *28*, 1323–1329.

Disposition in the Body. Readily absorbed after oral administration; bioavailability about 50%, but there is considerable intersubject variation. It is metabolised by *N*-oxidation, *S*-oxidation, and demethylation, but is excreted mainly as unchanged drug. After oral administration, about 30 to 70% is excreted unchanged in the urine in 24 hours (dose-dependent), together with small amounts of the metabolites; after an intravenous dose, about 70 to 80% is excreted unchanged in the urine in 24 hours.

THERAPEUTIC CONCENTRATION.
Following a single oral dose of 150 mg to 5 subjects, peak plasma concentrations of 0.24 to 0.63 µg/ml (mean 0.5) were reported; plasma concentrations initially peaked at 0.5 to 1.5 hours but a second peak at 3 hours was reported in 4 subjects (A. M. van Hecken *et al.*, *Br. J. clin. Pharmac.*, 1982, *14*, 195–200).
Following oral administration of 150 mg twice daily to 10 subjects, maximum steady-state plasma concentrations of 0.31 to 0.82 µg/ml (mean 0.6) were reported at 0.5 to 2 hours compared with peak concentrations of 0.21 to 0.54 µg/ml (mean 0.37), 1 to 3 hours after a single 150-mg dose given to the same subjects (M. L. McFadyen *et al.*, *Eur. J. clin. Pharmac.*, 1983, *24*, 441–447).

HALF-LIFE. Plasma half-life, about 2 to 3 hours, increased in elderly subjects, and in renal impairment.

VOLUME OF DISTRIBUTION. 1 to 2 litres/kg.

CLEARANCE. Plasma clearance, about 10 ml/min/kg.

PROTEIN BINDING. In plasma, about 15%.

NOTE. For a review of ranitidine pharmacokinetics see C. J. C. Roberts, *Clin. Pharmacokinet.*, 1984, *9*, 211–221.

Dose. The equivalent of 150 to 900 mg of ranitidine daily.

Rescinnamine   *Antihypertensive*

Proprietary Names. Cinnasil; Moderil.
Methyl 18-*O*-(3,4,5-trimethoxycinnamoyl)reserpate
$C_{35}H_{42}N_2O_9 = 634.7$
CAS—24815-24-5

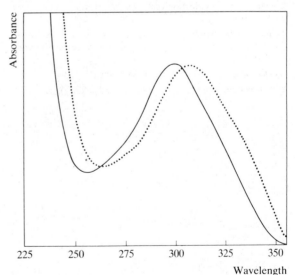

An alkaloid obtained from the roots of certain species of *Rauwolfia* (Apocynaceae), mainly *R. serpentina* and *R. vomitoria*, or by synthesis.
A white or pale buff to cream-coloured, crystalline powder. It slowly darkens on exposure to light but more rapidly when in solution. M.p. about 226°.
Practically **insoluble** in water; soluble in ethanol, acetic acid, and chloroform.

Colour Tests. Mandelin's Test—brown; Marquis Test—grey-green.

Thin-layer Chromatography. *System TA*—Rf 73; *system TB*—Rf 01; *system TC*—Rf 75. (*Acidified potassium permanganate solution, positive.*)

Gas Chromatography. *System GA*—RI 2180.

High Pressure Liquid Chromatography. *System HA*—k' 0.6.

Ultraviolet Spectrum. Aqueous acid—299 nm; aqueous alkali—306 nm.

Infra-red Spectrum. Principal peaks at wavenumbers 1266, 1147, 1124, 1165, 1233, 1715 (KBr disk).

Mass Spectrum. Principal peaks at *m/z* 221, 199, 200, 186, 395, 251, 77, 214.

Dose. 0.25 to 1 mg daily.

Reserpine
Antihypertensive

Proprietary Names. Lemiserp; Neo-Serp; Rau-Sed; Resercen; Reserfia; Reserpanca; Reserpoid; Sandril; Sedaraupin; Serpasil; Serpate; Vio-Serpine. It is an ingredient of Abicol, Diupres, Hydropres, Metatensin, Naquival, Regroton, Renese-R, Salutensin, and Seominal.

Methyl 18-*O*-(3,4,5-trimethoxybenzoyl)reserpate
$C_{33}H_{40}N_2O_9 = 608.7$
CAS—50-55-5

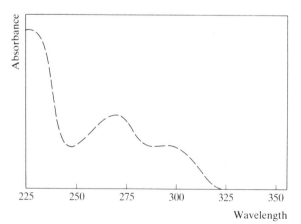

An alkaloid obtained from the roots of certain species of *Rauwolfia* (Apocynaceae), mainly *R. serpentina* and *R. vomitoria*, or by synthesis.

Fine, white or pale buff to slightly yellow-coloured crystals or crystalline powder. It darkens slowly on exposure to light, but more rapidly when in solution. M.p. about 270°, with decomposition.

Practically **insoluble** in water and ether; soluble 1 in 2000 of ethanol and 1 in 6 of chloroform; freely soluble in acetic acid.

Dissociation Constant. pK_a 6.6 (25°).

Colour Tests. Mandelin's Test—green; Marquis Test—grey-green → brown.

Thin-layer Chromatography. *System TA*—Rf 69; *system TB*—Rf 02; *system TC*—Rf 74. (*Acidified potassium permanganate solution*, positive.)

Gas Chromatography. *System GA*—not eluted.

Ultraviolet Spectrum. Ethanol—267 nm ($A_1^1 = 272$ a), 295 nm.

Infra-red Spectrum. Principal peaks at wavenumbers 1220, 1120, 1700, 1240, 1720, 1265 (KBr disk).

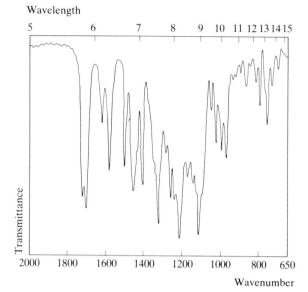

Mass Spectrum. Principal peaks at *m/z* 608, 606, 195, 609, 395, 397, 212, 396.

Quantification. HIGH PRESSURE LIQUID CHROMATOGRAPHY. In plasma: sensitivity 300 pg/ml, fluorescence detection—R. F. Suckow *et al.*, *J. liq. Chromat.*, 1983, 6, 1111–1122.

THIN-LAYER CHROMATOGRAPHY. In plasma: sensitivity 50 pg/ml—S. L. Tripp *et al.*, *Life Sci.*, 1975, *16*, 1167–1177.

Disposition in the Body. Readily but somewhat erratically absorbed after oral administration. Rapidly and extensively metabolised by hydrolysis and *O*-demethylation; the major metabolites are trimethoxybenzoic acid and methyl reserpate, together with reserpic acid, syringomethyl reserpate, and syringic acid; metabolites may be conjugated with glucuronic acid or sulphate. About 6% of an oral dose is excreted in the urine in 24 hours and about 8% in the first 4 days, mainly as trimethoxybenzoic acid; less than 3% of a dose is excreted in the urine unchanged. About 60% of the dose is eliminated in the faeces in 4 days, mainly as unchanged drug.

THERAPEUTIC CONCENTRATION.

After a single oral dose of 1 mg to 2 subjects, peak plasma concentrations of 0.0004 to 0.0006 µg/ml were attained in 2 to 3 hours (S. L. Tripp *et al.*, *ibid.*).

TOXICITY. High dosage may occasionally cause a parkinsonian-like syndrome and severe depression; several cases of accidental poisoning have been reported in children but fatalities are unlikely.

HALF-LIFE. Plasma half-life, extremely variable and may be up to 11 days.

DISTRIBUTION IN BLOOD. Plasma: whole blood ratio, 1.1.

PROTEIN BINDING. In plasma, about 40%.

Dose. Usually 250 to 500 µg daily, for hypertension. Doses of 0.1 to 1 mg or more daily have been given as a sedative.

Resorcinol

Dermatological Agent

Synonyms. m-Dihydroxybenzene; Dioxybenzolum; Resorcin.
Proprietary Names. Castel-Minus; Egosol R. It is an ingredient of Acnil, Acnomel, and Eskamel.
Benzene-1,3-diol
$C_6H_6O_2 = 110.1$
CAS—108-46-3

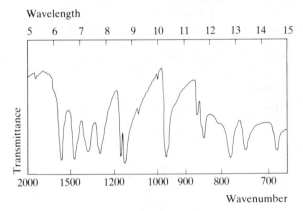

Colourless or slightly pinkish-grey, acicular crystals or crystalline powder. It becomes red on exposure to air and light. M.p. 109° to 112°; it sublimes on further heating.

Soluble 1 in less than 1 of water and 1 in 1 of ethanol; slightly soluble in chloroform; freely soluble in ether.

Resorcinol Monoacetate

Synonyms. 3-Acetoxyphenol; Resorcin Acetate.
Proprietary Name. Euresol
$C_8H_8O_3 = 152.1$
CAS—102-29-4
A pale yellow or amber, viscous liquid. Sp. gr. 1.203 to 1.207. B.p. about 283°, with decomposition.
Sparingly **soluble** in water; soluble in ethanol and most organic solvents.

Dissociation Constant. pK_a 9.5, 10.1 (20°).

Colour Test. Liebermann's Test—violet.

Gas Chromatography. *System GA*—RI 1258.

Ultraviolet Spectrum. Aqueous acid—273 nm ($A_1^1 = 172$ a); aqueous alkali—290 nm ($A_1^1 = 315$ a).

Infra-red Spectrum. Principal peaks at wavenumbers 1149, 1603, 774, 962, 1164, 1289 (KBr disk).

Wavelength

5 6 7 8 9 10 11 12 13 14 15

Transmittance

2000 1500 1200 1000 900 800 700

Wavenumber

Mass Spectrum. Principal peaks at m/z 110, 82, 39, 81, 53, 69, 55, 111.

Quantification. HIGH PRESSURE LIQUID CHROMATOGRAPHY. In plasma or urine: sensitivity 500 ng/ml, UV detection—D. Yeung *et al.*, *J. Chromat.*, 1981, *224*; *Biomed. Appl.*, *13*, 513–518.

Disposition in the Body. Resorcinol may be absorbed through the skin or from ulcerated surfaces.

TOXICITY. The estimated minimum lethal dose is 2 g and the maximum permissible atmospheric concentration is 10 ppm. The systemic effects of resorcinol are similar to those of phenol but convulsions may be more frequent.

Use. Topically in concentrations of 2 to 5%.

Riboflavine

Vitamin

Synonyms. Lactoflavin; Riboflavin; Vitamin B_2; Vitamin G.
Proprietary Names. Beflavin(e). It is an ingredient of Apisate.
3,10 - Dihydro - 7,8 - dimethyl - 10 - (D - *ribo* - 2,3,4,5 - tetra - hydroxypentyl)benzopteridine-2,4-dione
$C_{17}H_{20}N_4O_6 = 376.4$
CAS—83-88-5

A yellow or orange-yellow, crystalline powder. M.p. about 280°, with decomposition. Solutions deteriorate on exposure to light.
Soluble 1 in 3000 to 1 in 20 000 of water, the variation in solubility being due to the variation in the internal crystalline structure; practically insoluble in ethanol, acetone, chloroform, and ether; very soluble in dilute solutions of alkali hydroxides.

Dissociation Constant. pK_a 1.9, 10.2 (20°).

Colour Test. Dissolve 1 mg in 100 ml of water—the solution is green-yellow when viewed by transmitted light and shows an intense yellow-green fluorescence which disappears on adding mineral acids, alkalis, and reducing agents such as sodium dithionite.

Ultraviolet Spectrum. Aqueous acid—267 nm ($A_1^1 = 820$ a); aqueous alkali—270 nm, 356 nm.

Infra-red Spectrum. Principal peaks at wavenumbers 1544, 1575, 1641, 1715, 1235, 1070 (KBr disk).

Quantification. HIGH PRESSURE LIQUID CHROMATOGRAPHY. In urine: sensitivity 50 ng/ml, fluorescence detection—M. D. Smith, *J. Chromat.*, 1980, *182*; *Biomed. Appl.*, *8*, 285–291.

Disposition in the Body. Readily absorbed after oral administration. Widely distributed throughout the body but little is stored, and amounts in excess of the body's requirements are excreted in the urine. Metabolised by phosphorylation to flavine mononucleotide (FMN) and then to flavine adenine dinucleotide (FAD). The recommended daily intake is up to 500 µg/kg. Endogenous plasma concentrations are usually less than 0.1 µg/ml.

HALF-LIFE. Plasma half-life, about 1 hour.

PROTEIN BINDING. In plasma, about 60%.

Dose. 2 to 10 mg daily.

Rifampicin
Antituberculous Agent

Synonyms. Rifaldazine; Rifampin; Rifamycin AMP.
Proprietary Names. Rifa; Rifadin(e); Rimactan(e); Rofact. It is an ingredient of Rifinah and Rimactazid.
3-(4-Methylpiperazin-1-yliminomethyl)rifamycin SV
$C_{43}H_{58}N_4O_{12} = 823.0$
CAS—13292-46-1
A brick-red to reddish-brown, crystalline powder. M.p. about 185°, with decomposition.
Slightly **soluble** in water, ethanol, and ether; freely soluble in chloroform; soluble in ethyl acetate and methanol.

Dissociation Constant. pK_a 1.7, 7.9.

Colour Test. Mandelin's Test—orange-brown.

Thin-layer Chromatography. *System TA*—Rf 79. (Visible red-brown spot; *acidified potassium permanganate solution*, positive.)

Ultraviolet Spectrum. Aqueous acid—231 nm ($A_1^1 = 320$ a), 263 nm, 336 nm ($A_1^1 = 250$ a).

Infra-red Spectrum. Principal peaks at wavenumbers 1250, 1567, 976, 1098, 1064, 1650 (KBr disk).

Mass Spectrum. Principal peaks at m/z 43, 45, 60, 58, 95, 99, 398, 206.

Quantification. HIGH PRESSURE LIQUID CHROMATOGRAPHY. In plasma, urine or saliva: rifampicin and metabolites, sensitivity 100 ng/ml, UV detection—J. B. Lecaillon *et al.*, *J. Chromat.*, 1978, *145*; *Biomed. Appl.*, 2, 319–324. In serum: rifampicin and desacetylrifampicin, detection limits 17 ng/ml and 10 ng/ml, respectively—M. Guillaumont *et al.*, *J. Chromat.*, 1982, *232*; *Biomed. Appl.*, 21, 369–376.

Disposition in the Body. Readily absorbed after oral administration; peak plasma concentrations are attained in about 2 hours after a single dose. Widely distributed in the tissues and fluids and undergoes enterohepatic circulation. Metabolised to desacetylrifampicin, which is active; excreted in the urine and bile.

HALF-LIFE. Plasma half-life, about 2 to 6 hours (dose-dependent), decreased during chronic dosing; prolonged in subjects with liver disease.

VOLUME OF DISTRIBUTION. About 1 litre/kg.

PROTEIN BINDING. In plasma, about 80%.

NOTE. For a review of the pharmacokinetics of rifampicin see G. Acocella, *Clin. Pharmacokinet.*, 1978, *3*, 108–127.

Dose. Usually 600 mg daily.

Rifamycin SV
Antibiotic

Synonym. Rifomycin SV
$C_{37}H_{47}NO_{12} = 697.8$
CAS—6998-60-3
Rifamycin SV is a semi-synthetic antibiotic derived from rifamycin B, a substance produced during growth of certain strains of *Streptomyces mediterranei*.
Dark yellow crystals.
Practically **insoluble** in water; very soluble in ethanol; soluble in acetone, chloroform, ether, ethyl acetate, and methanol.

Rifamycin Sodium
Synonym. Rifamycin SV Sodium
Proprietary Name. Rifocin(e)
$C_{37}H_{46}NNaO_{12} = 719.8$
CAS—15105-92-7
A brick-red, fine or slightly granular powder.

Soluble in water and chloroform; freely soluble in dehydrated alcohol and methanol; practically insoluble in ether.

Colour Test. Mandelin's Test—yellow-brown.

Thin-layer Chromatography. *System TA*—Rf 84. (Visible orange spot.)

Ultraviolet Spectrum. Ethanol—315 nm ($A_1^1 = 420$ b).

Dose. 0.5 to 1 g of rifamycin sodium daily, by intramuscular injection.

Rimantadine
Antiviral

Synonym. α-Methyl-1-adamantanemethylamine
1-(Tricyclo[3.3.1.1^{3,7}]dec-1-yl)ethylamine
$C_{12}H_{21}N = 179.3$
CAS—13392-28-4

Rimantadine Hydrochloride
$C_{12}H_{21}N,HCl = 215.8$
CAS—1501-84-4
A white crystalline powder. M.p. above 300°.
Soluble 1 in 17 of water, 1 in 20 of ethanol, and 1 in 6 of chloroform.

Colour Test. Ninhydrin—pink-violet.

Thin-layer Chromatography. *System TA*—Rf 37; *system TB*—Rf 50; *system TC*—Rf 11. (*Acidified iodoplatinate solution*, strong reaction.)

Gas Chromatography. *System GA*—RI 1388.

Infra-red Spectrum. Principal peaks at wavenumbers 1538, 1600, 1266, 1277, 1160, 1117 (KBr disk).

Mass Spectrum. Principal peaks at m/z 44, 43, 79, 93, 41, 135, 91, 81.

Dose. 300 to 400 mg of rimantadine hydrochloride daily.

Rimiterol
Sympathomimetic

erythro-3,4-Dihydroxy-α-(2-piperidyl)benzyl alcohol
$C_{12}H_{17}NO_3 = 223.3$
CAS—32953-89-2

Crystals. M.p. 203° to 204°.

Rimiterol Hydrobromide

Proprietary Name. Pulmadil
$C_{12}H_{17}NO_3,HBr = 304.2$
CAS—31842-61-2
A white or pale grey, crystalline powder. M.p. about 220°, with decomposition.
Soluble 1 in 10 of water and 1 in 20 of methanol.

Dissociation Constant. pK_a 8.7, 10.3 (25°).

Colour Tests. Ammoniacal Silver Nitrate—red/brown; Ferric Chloride—green; Liebermann's Test—black; Marquis Test—brown→black; Methanolic Potassium Hydroxide—orange-pink; Nessler's Reagent—black; Palladium Chloride—orange; Potassium Dichromate—green→brown; Sulphuric Acid—yellow.

Ultraviolet Spectrum. Aqueous acid—280 nm ($A_1^1 = 131$ a).

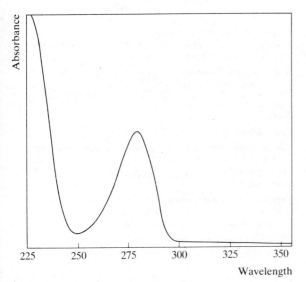

Infra-red Spectrum. Principal peaks at wavenumbers 1020, 1230, 1290, 1210, 1530, 1605 (rimiterol hydrobromide, KCl disk).

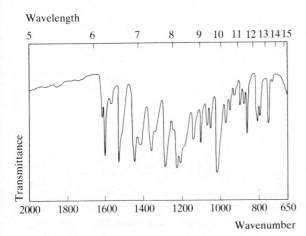

Disposition in the Body. Rapidly absorbed from the lungs, but most of an inhaled dose is swallowed; readily absorbed from the gastro-intestinal tract. It is subject not only to extensive first-pass metabolism by sulphate and glucuronide conjugation, but also to metabolism by catechol-*O*-methyltransferase (COMT) forming 3-*O*-methylrimiterol. It also appears to be metabolised by COMT in the lungs. After intrabronchial administration, about 70% of a dose is excreted in the urine in 24 hours, mainly as free and conjugated 3-*O*-methylrimiterol, together with some free and conjugated rimiterol. A proportion of a dose is excreted in the bile. After oral or aerosol administration, less than 50% of a dose is excreted in the urine, mainly as conjugates of rimiterol.

HALF-LIFE. Plasma half-life, about 3 minutes after intravenous administration.

Dose. 200 to 600 µg of rimiterol hydrobromide, by aerosol inhalation; maximum of 8 doses daily.

Ritodrine   *Sympathomimetic*

erythro - 2 - (4 - Hydroxyphenethylamino) - 1 - (4 - hydroxyphenyl)propan-1-ol
$C_{17}H_{21}NO_3 = 287.4$
CAS—26652-09-5

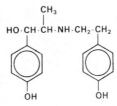

M.p. 88° to 90°.

Ritodrine Hydrochloride

Proprietary Names. Pre-Par; Utopar; Yutopar.
$C_{17}H_{21}NO_3,HCl = 323.8$
CAS—23239-51-2
A white crystalline powder. M.p. 193° to 195°, with decomposition.
Soluble in chloroform and dilute acetic acid.

Colour Tests. Folin–Ciocalteu Reagent—blue; Liebermann's Test—black; Mandelin's Test—green; Marquis Test—yellow-brown.

Thin-layer Chromatography. *System TA*—Rf 73. (*Acidified iodoplatinate solution*, positive.)

Gas Chromatography. *System GA*—not eluted.

Ultraviolet Spectrum. Aqueous acid—274 nm ($A_1^1 = 98$ a). (See below)

Infra-red Spectrum. Principal peaks at wavenumbers 1510, 1209, 1256, 1610, 833, 1170 (KBr disk). (See below)

Mass Spectrum. Principal peaks at *m/z* 121, 164, 77, 57, 56, 165, 162, 122.

Quantification. HIGH PRESSURE LIQUID CHROMATOGRAPHY. In serum: sensitivity 2 ng/ml, electrochemical detection—L. S. Lin *et al.*, *J. pharm. Sci.*, 1984, *73*, 131–133.

RADIOIMMUNOASSAY. In plasma or serum: sensitivity 300 pg/ml—R. Gandar *et al.*, *Eur. J. clin. Pharmac.*, 1980, *17*, 117–122.

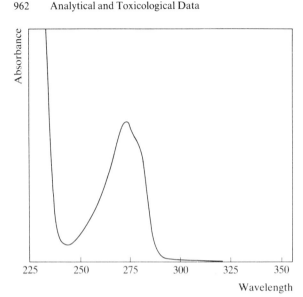

Wavelength

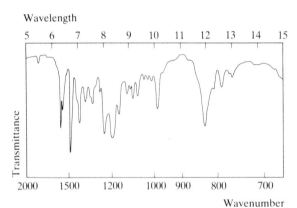

Wavenumber

Disposition in the Body. Readily absorbed after oral administration but subject to considerable first-pass metabolism; bioavailability about 30%. About 70 to 90% of an oral dose is excreted in the urine in 24 hours, mainly as sulphate and glucuronide conjugates with about 5% of the dose as unchanged drug.

THERAPEUTIC CONCENTRATION.

Following oral and intramuscular administration of 10 mg to 4 subjects, mean peak serum concentrations of 0.01 μg/ml and 0.02 μg/ml were attained in 20 to 40 minutes and 10 minutes, respectively (R. Gandar *et al.*, *ibid.*).

HALF-LIFE. Plasma half-life, about 1 to 2 hours; a longer elimination half-life of about 15 to 20 hours has also been reported.

PROTEIN BINDING. In plasma, about 32%.

NOTE. For a review of ritodrine see B. W. Finklestein, *Drug Intell. & clin. Pharm.*, 1981, *15*, 425–433.

Dose. 50 to 350 μg/min of ritodrine hydrochloride by intravenous infusion; up to 120 mg daily, by mouth.

Rolitetracycline   *Antibiotic*

Synonyms. PMT; Pyrrolidinomethyltetracycline.
Proprietary Names. Reverin; Tetralidina; Transcycline.
N^2-(Pyrrolidin-1-ylmethyl)tetracycline
$C_{27}H_{33}N_3O_8 = 527.6$
CAS—751-97-3

A light yellow crystalline powder. M.p. about 163°.
Soluble 1 in 1.1 of water and 1 in 200 of ethanol; soluble in acetone; very slightly soluble in ether.

Rolitetracycline Nitrate
$C_{27}H_{33}N_3O_8,HNO_3,1\tfrac{1}{2}H_2O = 617.6$
CAS—20685-78-3 (anhydrous); *26657-13-6* (sesquihydrate)
A yellow crystalline powder.
Soluble 1 in 40 of water.

Dissociation Constant. pK_a 7.4.

Colour Tests. Benedict's Reagent—red; Formaldehyde–Sulphuric Acid—green-yellow (→ yellow-brown); Mandelin's Test—violet → red → orange; Marquis Test—orange; Sulphuric Acid—violet.

Thin-layer Chromatography. *System TA*—Rf 05, streaking. (Location under ultraviolet light, orange fluorescence; *acidified potassium permanganate solution*, positive.)

Ultraviolet Spectrum. Aqueous acid—272 nm ($A_1^1 = 325$ a), 357 nm; aqueous alkali—248 nm ($A_1^1 = 261$ b), 268 nm ($A_1^1 = 266$ b).

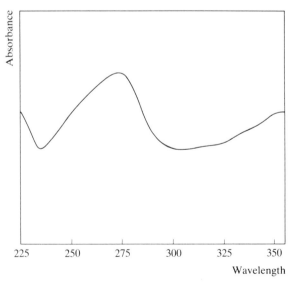

Wavelength

Dose. Up to 700 mg daily, given parenterally.

Rotenone
Pesticide

$(-)$-1,2,12,12a-Tetrahydro-2-isopropenyl-8,9-dimethoxy-6aH-furo[2,3-h][1]benzopyrano[3,4-b][1]benzopyran-6-one
$C_{23}H_{22}O_6 = 394.4$
CAS—83-79-4

Rotenone is the principal active insecticidal constituent of derris, the dried rhizome and roots of *Derris elliptica*, *D. malaccensis* (Leguminosae) and other species of *Derris*, and of lonchocarpus, the dried root of *Lonchocarpus utilis*, *L. urucu* and other species of *Lonchocarpus* (Leguminosae).

Colourless to brownish crystals, or a white to brownish-white, crystalline powder; it decomposes on exposure to light and air. M.p. about 163°. A dimorphic form melts at 181°.

Practically **insoluble** in water; soluble 1 in 300 of ethanol, 1 in 12 of acetone, 1 in 3 of chloroform, and 1 in 200 of ether.

Colour Tests. Antimony Pentachloride—brown; Liebermann's Test—black; Sulphuric Acid—orange.

Gas Chromatography. *System GA*—RI 3242.

Ultraviolet Spectrum. Aqueous acid—235 nm ($A_1^1 = 480$ b), 292 nm ($A_1^1 = 550$ b).

Saccharin
Sweetening Agent

Synonyms. Benzosulphimide; Garantose; Gluside; Sacarina; Saccarina; Zaharina.
1,2-Benzisothiazolin-3-one 1,1-dioxide
$C_7H_5NO_3S = 183.2$
CAS—81-07-2

White crystals or crystalline powder. M.p. 226° to 230°.
Soluble 1 in 290 of water, 1 in 30 of ethanol, and 1 in 12 of acetone; slightly soluble in chloroform and ether; readily soluble in dilute ammonia solution and in solutions of alkali hydroxides and, with the evolution of carbon dioxide, in solutions of alkali bicarbonates and carbonates.

Saccharin Calcium
Synonym. Calcium Benzosulphimide
$C_{14}H_8CaN_2O_6S_2,3\frac{1}{2}H_2O = 467.5$
CAS—6485-34-3 (anhydrous); *6381-91-5* (hydrate)
White crystals or crystalline powder.
Soluble 1 in about 2.5 of water and 1 in about 5 of ethanol.

Saccharin Sodium

Synonyms. Saccharoidum Natricum; Sodium Benzosulphimide; Soluble Gluside; Soluble Saccharin.
$C_7H_4NNaO_3S,2H_2O = 241.2$
CAS—128-44-9 (anhydrous); *6155-57-3* (dihydrate)
White efflorescent crystals or a white crystalline powder.
Soluble 1 in 1.5 of water and 1 in 50 of ethanol; practically insoluble in chloroform and ether.

Dissociation Constant. pK_a 1.6 (20°).

Colour Tests. Koppanyi–Zwikker Test—violet; Mercurous Nitrate—black.

Thin-layer Chromatography. *System TD*—Rf 01; *system TE*—Rf 07; *system TF*—Rf 01.

Gas Chromatography. *System GA*—RI 1819.

Ultraviolet Spectrum. Aqueous alkali—235 nm ($A_1^1 = 351$ b), 268 nm ($A_1^1 = 82$ a).

Infra-red Spectrum. Principal peaks at wavenumbers 1260, 1154, 1646, 750, 678, 1120 (saccharin sodium, KBr disk).

Mass Spectrum. Principal peaks at m/z 183, 76, 90, 50, 91, 120, 106, 92.

Quantification. GAS CHROMATOGRAPHY. In urine: detection limit 10 ng/ml, ECD—P. Hartvig *et al.*, *J. Chromat.*, 1978, *151*, 232–236.

GAS CHROMATOGRAPHY–MASS SPECTROMETRY. In plasma or urine: sensitivity 50 ng/ml—C. Pantarotto *et al.*, *J. pharm. Sci.*, 1981, *70*, 871–874.

Disposition in the Body. Rapidly absorbed after oral administration; peak plasma concentrations are attained in 0.5 to 1 hour. About 60% of a dose is excreted in the urine unchanged in 6 hours and 80% in 24 hours.

HALF-LIFE. Plasma half-life, about 5 to 9 hours in regular saccharin users.

Salbutamol
Sympathomimetic

Synonym. Albuterol
Proprietary Names. Asmaven (inhaler); Broncovaleas; Cobutolin (inhaler); Proventil (inhaler); Salbulin (inhaler); Sultanol (aerosol); Ventolin(e) (inhaler). It is an ingredient of Ventide.
2 - *tert* - Butylamino - 1 - (4 - hydroxy - 3 - hydroxymethylphenyl)-ethanol
$C_{13}H_{21}NO_3 = 239.3$
CAS—18559-94-9

A white crystalline powder. M.p. about 156°.
Soluble 1 in 70 of water and 1 in 25 of ethanol; slightly soluble in ether.

Salbutamol Sulphate
Proprietary Names. Asmaven (tablets); Cobutolin (tablets); Proventil (tablets); Salbulin (tablets and syrup); Sultanol; Ventolin(e).
$C_{13}H_{21}NO_3,\frac{1}{2}H_2SO_4 = 288.4$
CAS—51022-70-9
A white powder.
Soluble 1 in 4 of water; slightly soluble in ethanol, chloroform, and ether.

Dissociation Constant. pK$_a$ 9.3, 10.3.

Colour Tests. Liebermann's Test—black; Mandelin's Test—blue rim → brown rim; Marquis Test—yellow; Sulphuric Acid—yellow.

Thin-layer Chromatography. *System TA*—Rf 46; *system TB*—Rf 01; *system TC*—Rf 01. (*Acidified potassium permanganate solution*, positive.)

High Pressure Liquid Chromatography. *System HA*—k′ 1.0.

Ultraviolet Spectrum. Aqueous acid—276 nm (A$_1^1$ = 71 a); aqueous alkali—245 nm (A$_1^1$ = 510 a), 295 nm (A$_1^1$ = 133 a).

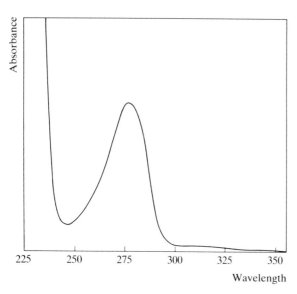

Infra-red Spectrum. Principal peaks at wavenumbers 1075, 1038, 1263, 1228, 1213, 822 (KBr disk).

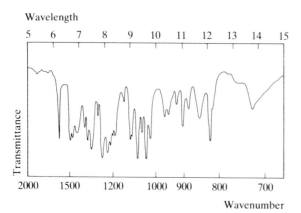

Mass Spectrum. Principal peaks at *m/z* 30, 86, 57, 41, 77, 135, 29, 206.

Quantification. Gas Chromatography (Capillary Column)–Mass Spectrometry. In serum: detection limit 1 ng/ml—J. G. Leferink *et al.*, *J. Chromat.*, 1982, *229*; *Biomed. Appl.*, 18, 217–221.

High Pressure Liquid Chromatography. In plasma: detection limit 500 pg/ml, electrochemical detection—B. Oosterhuis and C. J. van Boxtel, *J. Chromat.*, 1982, *232*; *Biomed. Appl.*, 21, 327–334.

Disposition in the Body. Rapidly absorbed after oral administration and after inhalation. About 60 to 90% of a dose is excreted in the urine in 24 hours, of which approximately 50% is unchanged salbutamol and 50% is the 4′-O-sulphate of salbutamol. Up to about 12% is eliminated in the faeces.

Therapeutic Concentration.

After a single oral dose of 8 mg given to 3 subjects, peak plasma concentrations of 0.096 to 0.117 µg/ml were attained in 1 to 3 hours. An inhaled dose of 0.04 to 0.1 mg given to 6 subjects produced peak plasma concentrations of 0.0006 to 0.0014 µg/ml in 3 to 5 hours. The ratio of salbutamol to an unidentified metabolite in the plasma was found to be 1:4 (S. R. Walker *et al.*, *Clin. Pharmac. Ther.*, 1972, *13*, 861–867).

Toxicity. Hypokalaemia has been reported after overdosage; recovery has occurred after the ingestion of up to 240 mg.

Half-life. Plasma half-life, 2 to 7 hours.

Protein Binding. In plasma, not significantly bound.

Dose. Usually the equivalent of 6 to 16 mg of salbutamol daily.

Salicylamide

Analgesic

Proprietary Names. Amid-Sal; Salamide; Salizell. It is an ingredient of Anodyne, Coriforte, and Delimon.

2-Hydroxybenzamide
C$_7$H$_7$NO$_2$ = 137.1
CAS—65-45-2

A white crystalline powder. M.p. 139° to 142°.

Soluble 1 in 500 of water, 1 in 15 of ethanol, 1 in 100 of chloroform, and 1 in 35 of ether; soluble in solutions of alkalis.

Dissociation Constant. pK$_a$ 8.2 (37°).

Colour Tests. Ferric Chloride—blue-violet (after hydrolysis); McNally's Test—orange; Nessler's Reagent—brown-orange (weak).

Thin-layer Chromatography. *System TD*—Rf 38; *system TE*—Rf 46; *system TF*—Rf 55. (Location under ultraviolet light, violet fluorescence; *ferric chloride solution*, violet; *acidified potassium permanganate solution*, positive.)

Gas Chromatography. *System GA*—RI 1455.

High Pressure Liquid Chromatography. *System HD*—k′ 0.4; *system HW*—k′ 2.5.

Ultraviolet Spectrum. Aqueous acid—235 nm (A$_1^1$ = 572 a), 298 nm; aqueous alkali—241 nm (A$_1^1$ = 547 a), 328 nm.

Infra-red Spectrum. Principal peaks at wavenumbers 1250, 752, 758, 1670, 1626, 1587 (Nujol mull).

Mass Spectrum. Principal peaks at *m/z* 120, 92, 137, 65, 121, 39, 64, 53.

Quantification. Spectrofluorimetry. In blood, serum or urine: sensitivity 100 ng/ml—S. A. Varesh *et al.*, *J. pharm. Sci.*, 1971, *60*, 1092–1095.

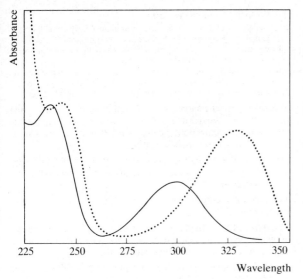

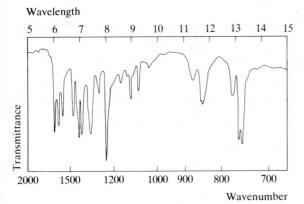

Following a single oral dose of 1.5 g of sodium salicylamide given as an aqueous solution to 5 subjects, peak plasma concentrations of 21.8 to 44.6 µg/ml (mean 31) of salicylamide were attained in 5 to 10 minutes (A. G. de Boer *et al.*, *Biopharm. Drug Disp.*, 1983, *4*, 321–330).

HALF-LIFE. Derived from urinary excretion data, about 1 hour.

Dose. Salicylamide has been given in doses of 1.5 to 10 g daily.

Salicylic Acid   *Dermatological Agent/Analgesic*

Proprietary Names. Egocappol; Fomac; Keralyt; Saligel; Xseb. It is an ingredient of Aserbine, Cuplex, Dithrolan, Duofilm, Malatex, Monphytol, Pragmatar, Psorin, Salactol, and Stie-Lasan.

2-Hydroxybenzoic acid
$C_7H_6O_3 = 138.1$
CAS—69-72-7

Colourless, feathery crystals or a white crystalline powder. M.p. 158° to 161°.
Soluble 1 in about 550 of water, 1 in about 4 of ethanol, 1 in 45 of chloroform, and 1 in 3 of ether.

Choline Salicylate

Synonym. (2-Hydroxyethyl)trimethylammonium Salicylate
Proprietary Names. Arthropan; Syrap. It is an ingredient of Audax, Bonjela, and Teejel.
$C_{12}H_{19}NO_4 = 241.3$
CAS—2016-36-6
A white, crystalline, very hygroscopic powder. M.p. about 50°.
Very **soluble** in water, ethanol, and acetone; practically insoluble in ether.

Sodium Salicylate

Synonym. Sodium 2-Hydroxybenzoate
Proprietary Names. Ancosal; Ensalate; Entérosalicyl; Entrosalyl (Standard); Rhumax. It is an ingredient of Bronchotone.
$C_7H_5NaO_3 = 160.1$
CAS—54-21-7
Colourless crystals, crystalline flakes, or white or faintly pink powder.
Soluble 1 in 1 of water and 1 in 11 of ethanol; practically insoluble in chloroform and ether. Concentrated aqueous solutions are liable to deposit crystals of the hexahydrate on standing.

Dissociation Constant. pK_a 3.0, 13.4 (25°).

Colour Tests. Ferric Chloride—blue-violet; Folin–Ciocalteu Reagent—blue; McNally's Test—red.

Thin-layer Chromatography. *System TD*—salicylic acid Rf 07, salicyluric acid Rf 00; *system TE*—salicylic acid Rf 11, salicyluric acid Rf 00; *system TF*—salicylic acid Rf 25, salicyluric acid Rf 00. (Location under ultraviolet light, violet fluorescence; *ferric chloride solution*, violet; *acidified potassium permanganate solution*, positive.)

Gas Chromatography. *System GA*—RI 1308.

High Pressure Liquid Chromatography. *System HD*—salicylic acid k' 0.7, choline salicylate k' 0.7; *system HW*—salicylic acid k' 4.6, choline salicylate k' 4.8.

Ultraviolet Spectrum. Aqueous acid—236 nm ($A_1^1 = 647a$), 303 nm; aqueous alkali—298 nm ($A_1^1 = 259$ a). Choline salicylate: methanol—298 nm ($A_1^1 = 170$ b). (See below)

GAS CHROMATOGRAPHY. In plasma, saliva or urine: sensitivity 1 µg/ml in plasma and saliva, 5 µg/ml in urine, AFID—A. G. de Boer *et al.*, *J. Chromat.*, 1979, *162*; *Biomed. Appl.*, *4*, 457–460.

HIGH PRESSURE LIQUID CHROMATOGRAPHY. In plasma: limit of detection 500 pg, fluorescence detection—S. R. Gautam *et al.*, *Analyt. Lett. (Part B)*, 1981, *14*, 577–582. In serum, saliva or urine: salicylamide and metabolites, sensitivity 1 to 2 µg/ml, UV detection—M. E. Morris and G. Levy, *J. pharm. Sci.*, 1983, *72*, 612–617.

Disposition in the Body. Readily absorbed after oral administration but undergoes significant first-pass metabolism; widely distributed throughout the body. It is rapidly excreted in the urine mainly as the sulphate and glucuronide conjugates together with small amounts of gentisamide glucuronide and traces of gentisamide and gentisamide sulphate; only traces are excreted unchanged.

THERAPEUTIC CONCENTRATION.

After a single oral dose of 1.3 g given to 5 subjects, mean peak plasma concentrations of about 2 µg/ml of free salicylamide and about 18 µg/ml of total (free + conjugated) salicylamide were attained in 0.3 and 2 hours respectively; following similar doses of a solution of sodium salicylamide, peak plasma concentrations were higher and were attained more rapidly (L. Fleckenstein *et al.*, *Clin. Pharmac. Ther.*, 1976, *19*, 451–458).

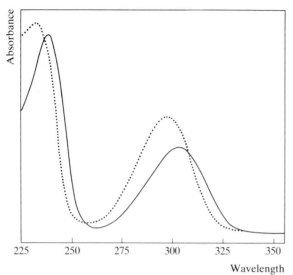

Infra-red Spectrum. Principal peaks at wavenumbers 758, 1657, 1288, 1210, 1250, 1150 (salicylic acid, KBr disk); 1587, 1724, 1176, 1515, 699, 1041 (choline salicylate).

Wavelength

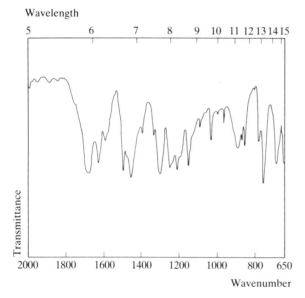

Wavenumber

Mass Spectrum. Principal peaks at m/z 120, 92, 138, 64, 39, 63, 121, 65; salicyluric acid 121, 120, 69, 92, 195, 39, 93, 45.

Quantification. See under Aspirin.

Disposition in the Body. Rapidly absorbed and distributed throughout the body. Metabolised by conjugation with glucuronic acid and glycine to give salicyluric acid, salicyl O-glucuronide, and salicyl ester glucuronide; hydroxylation to gentisic acid, gentisuric acid, and dihydroxy and trihydroxy derivatives also occurs. Excreted in the urine as unchanged drug and metabolites.
Salicylic acid is the major metabolite of aspirin, methyl salicylate, and salsalate.

THERAPEUTIC CONCENTRATION.
Following daily oral doses of 9 mg/kg of sodium salicylate to 20 female and 20 male subjects, mean peak plasma concentrations of 57 and 58 µg/ml were attained in 0.9 and 0.5 hours respectively (S. L. Miaskiewicz et al., Clin. Pharmac. Ther., 1982, 31, 30–37).
After daily oral doses of choline salicylate, equivalent to 3.8 g of aspirin, a mean steady-state serum concentration of 166 µg/ml was reported (P. D. Hansten and W. L. Hayton, J. clin. Pharmac., 1980, 20, 326–331).

TOXICITY. The estimated minimum lethal dose is 15 g. Plasma concentrations greater than 300 µg/ml are likely to produce toxic effects and concentrations greater than 500 µg/ml are associated with moderate to severe intoxication.

HALF-LIFE. Plasma half-life, dose-dependent (2 to 4 hours after salicylate doses of less than 3 g, increasing to about 19 hours after large doses).

VOLUME OF DISTRIBUTION. About 0.1 to 0.2 litre/kg (dose-dependent).

PROTEIN BINDING. In plasma, about 50 to 90% (dose-dependent, about 90% bound at concentrations below 100 µg/ml, decreasing to 50% at concentrations above 400 µg/ml).

NOTE. For a review of the pharmacokinetics of salicylates see M. Mandelli and G. Tognoni, Clin. Pharmacokinet., 1980, 5, 424–440.

Uses. Salicylic acid is applied topically in concentrations ranging from 1 to 50%. Sodium salicylate has been given by mouth in doses of up to 10 g daily.

Salinazid   *Antituberculous Agent*

Synonyms. o-Hydroxybenzal Isonicotinyl Hydrazone; INSH; SAH; Salizid.
2'-Salicylideneisonicotinohydrazide
$C_{13}H_{11}N_3O_2 = 241.2$
CAS—495-84-1

A pale cream-coloured powder.
Very slightly **soluble** in water; soluble in dilute acids and alkalis.

Colour Tests. Aromaticity (Method 2)—yellow/orange; Ferric Chloride—yellow-brown; Folin–Ciocalteu Reagent—blue; Liebermann's Test—orange; Mandelin's Test—brown; Marquis Test—yellow; Nessler's Reagent (100°)—black; Sulphuric Acid—yellow.

Thin-layer Chromatography. *System TA*—Rf 84; *system TB*—Rf 01; *system TC*—Rf 20. (*Acidified iodoplatinate solution*, positive.)

Ultraviolet Spectrum. Aqueous acid—257 nm ($A_1^1 = 697$ a), 327 nm (broad); aqueous alkali—264 nm.

Infra-red Spectrum. Principal peaks at wavenumbers 1290, 1680, 1565, 1270, 687, 772 (KBr disk).

Mass Spectrum. Principal peaks at m/z 106, 123, 78, 51, 119, 79, 77, 107.

Dose. Salinazid was formerly given in doses of 0.2 to 3 g daily.

Salol   *Sunscreen Agent*

Proprietary Name. Sola-Stick
Phenyl salicylate
$C_{13}H_{10}O_3 = 214.2$
CAS—118-55-8

Colourless acicular crystals, or white crystalline powder. M.p. 42° to 44°.

Soluble 1 in 7000 of water, 1 in 9 of ethanol, and 1 in 0.3 of chloroform and of ether.

Gas Chromatography. *System GA*—RI 1685.

High Pressure Liquid Chromatography. *System HD*—k' 15.6.

Ultraviolet Spectrum. Ethanol—242 nm ($A_1^1 = 664$ a), 310 nm ($A_1^1 = 248$ a).

Use. Topically in concentrations of 5 to 10%.

Salsalate   *Analgesic*

Synonyms. Salicyl Salicylate; Salicylosalicylic Acid; Salysal; Sasapyrine.
Proprietary Names. Arcylate; Disalcid.
O-(2-Hydroxybenzoyl)salicylic acid
$C_{14}H_{10}O_5 = 258.2$
CAS—552-94-3

Colourless crystals or white crystalline powder. M.p. about 145°. Practically **insoluble** in water but gradually hydrolysed to 2 molecules of salicylic acid; soluble in ethanol and ether.

Dissociation Constant. pK_a 3.5, 9.8 (25°).

Thin-layer Chromatography. *System TG*—Rf 23. (*Chromic acid solution*, brown.)

Gas Chromatography. *System GD*—retention time of methyl derivative 0.4 and 0.6 relative to n-$C_{16}H_{34}$.

High Pressure Liquid Chromatography. *System HD*—k' 3.6; *system HV*—retention time 0.69 relative to meclofenamic acid.

Ultraviolet Spectrum. Aqueous acid—310 nm; aqueous alkali—341 nm.

Infra-red Spectrum. Principal peaks at wavenumbers 1690, 1205, 1170, 1310, 1620, 1270 (KBr disk).

Quantification. HIGH PRESSURE LIQUID CHROMATOGRAPHY. In plasma or urine: sensitivity 1 μg/ml for salsalate and salicylic acid, UV detection—L. I. Harrison *et al.*, *J. pharm. Sci.*, 1980, 69, 1268–1271.

Disposition in the Body. Rapidly absorbed after oral administration and extensively hydrolysed to salicylic acid. Less than 1% of a dose is excreted in the urine as unchanged salsalate in 24 hours, and the remainder is excreted in the urine by the normal metabolic route for salicylic acid.

THERAPEUTIC CONCENTRATION.
Following a single oral dose of 1 g of salsalate to 12 subjects, a mean peak plasma concentration of 21 μg/ml of salsalate was attained in 1.5 hours and peak plasma-salicylic acid concentrations of 38 to 77 μg/ml (mean 54) were reported at 2 to 4 hours (L. I. Harrison *et al.*, *J. clin. Pharmac.*, 1981, *21*, 401–404).

HALF-LIFE. Plasma half-life, about 1 hour.

Dose. Up to 4 g daily.

Santonin   *Anthelmintic*

Synonym. Santolactone
(3*S*,3a*S*,5a*S*,9b*S*) - 3a,5,5a,9b - Tetrahydro - 3,5a,9 - trimethyl-naphtho[1,2-*b*]furan-2,8(3*H*,4*H*)-dione
$C_{15}H_{18}O_3 = 246.3$
CAS—481-06-1

A crystalline lactone obtained from the dried unexpanded flowerheads of *Artemisia cina* and other species of *Artemisia* (Compositae).

Colourless crystals, or white crystalline powder, becoming yellow on exposure to light. M.p. about 173°.

Practically **insoluble** in water; soluble 1 in 50 of ethanol and 1 in 3 of chloroform; slightly soluble in ether.

Thin-layer Chromatography. *System TD*—Rf 64; *system TE*—Rf 75; *system TF*—Rf 50. (*Acidified iodoplatinate solution*, positive; *acidified potassium permanganate solution*, positive.)

Gas Chromatography. *System GA*—RI 2174.

Ultraviolet Spectrum. Methanol—239 nm ($A_1^1 = 493$ a).

Mass Spectrum. Principal peaks at *m/z* 41, 173, 91, 135, 77, 55, 44, 69.

Dose. Santonin was formerly given in doses of 60 to 200 mg daily for 3 days.

Secbutobarbitone   *Barbiturate*

Synonyms. Butabarbital; Secbutobarbital.
Proprietary Names. Neo-Barb. It is an ingredient of Quibron Plus.
5-*sec*-Butyl-5-ethylbarbituric acid
$C_{10}H_{16}N_2O_3 = 212.2$
CAS—125-40-6

A fine, white, microcrystalline powder. M.p. 165° to 168°.
Soluble 1 in 1400 of water, 1 in 12 of ethanol, 1 in 30 of chloroform, and 1 in 30 of ether.

Secbutobarbitone Sodium

Synonyms. Butabarbital Sodium; Butabarbitone Sodium (distinguish from Butobarbitone); Secumalnatrium; Sodium Butabarbital.

Proprietary Names. Buticaps; Butisol Sodium.

$C_{10}H_{15}N_2NaO_3 = 234.2$
CAS—143-81-7
A white powder.

Soluble 1 in 2 of water and 1 in 7 of ethanol; very slightly soluble in chloroform; practically insoluble in ether.

Dissociation Constant. pK_a 8.0 (20°).

Partition Coefficient. Log P (octanol/pH 7.4), 1.3.

Colour Tests. Koppanyi–Zwikker Test—violet; Mercurous Nitrate—black; Vanillin Reagent—orange/violet.

Thin-layer Chromatography. *System TD*—Rf 50; *system TE*—Rf 41; *system TF*—Rf 63; *system TH*—Rf 69. (*Mercurous nitrate spray,* black.)

Gas Chromatography. *System GA*—secbutobarbitone RI 1662, 2'-hydroxysecbutobarbitone RI 1928.

High Pressure Liquid Chromatography. *System HG*—k' 4.89; *system HH*—k' 3.32.

Ultraviolet Spectrum. *Borax buffer 0.05M* (pH 9.2)—239 nm ($A_1^1 = 428$ a); M sodium hydroxide (pH 13)—254 nm ($A_1^1 = 354$ b).

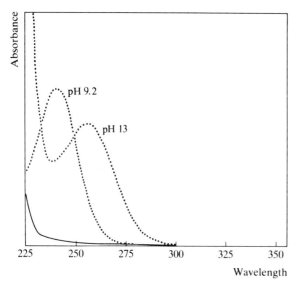

Wavelength

Infra-red Spectrum. Principal peaks at wavenumbers 1675, 1760, 1317, 1303, 1230, 853 (KBr disk).

Mass Spectrum. Principal peaks at m/z 141, 156, 41, 57, 39, 98, 157, 47.

Quantification. See under Amylobarbitone.

Disposition in the Body. Well absorbed after oral administration. Rapidly metabolised by ω- and ($\omega - 1$)-oxidation of the methyl-propyl side-chain. About 40 to 60% of a dose is slowly excreted in the urine, 5 to 9% as unchanged drug, 30% as 5-(2-carboxy-1-methylethyl)-5-ethylbarbituric acid, 3% as 2'-hydroxysecbutobarbitone, and 1% as 2'-oxosecbutobarbitone; greater amounts of unchanged drug may be excreted after excessive doses.

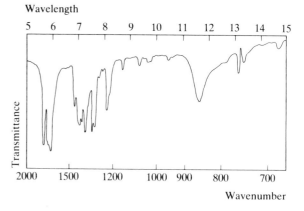

Wavelength

TOXICITY. The estimated minimum lethal dose is 2 g. Blood concentrations greater than about 10 μg/ml are likely to cause toxic reactions, and concentrations greater than 30 μg/ml may be fatal.

Following oral administration of 600 mg, given in 3 doses over a period of 3 hours to 5 subjects, peak blood concentrations of 7.6 to 16.9 μg/ml (mean 12.3) were reported, 0.5 hour after the third dose. Tests 2 hours after the first dose indicated depression of the central nervous system in all subjects (K. D. Parker *et al., Clin. Toxicol.,* 1970, *3,* 131–145).

In 4 fatalities attributed to secbutobarbitone overdose, blood concentrations of 30 to 88 μg/ml (mean 58) and liver concentrations of 51 to 250 μg/g (mean 112) were reported (R. C. Baselt and R. H. Cravey, *J. analyt. Toxicol.,* 1977, *1,* 81–102).

HALF-LIFE. Plasma half-life, 34 to 42 hours.

PROTEIN BINDING. In plasma, about 26%.

Dose. Usually 45 to 120 mg daily.

Selegiline   *Antiparkinsonian*

Synonyms. Synonyms used in the literature are confusing and include (−)-Deprenil, L-Deprenil, Deprenyl, (−)-Deprenyl, L-Deprenyl, L-Deprenaline, and E-250. It is the (−)-isomer which is active.

(−)-(R)-N,α-Dimethyl-N-(prop-2-ynyl)phenethylamine
$C_{13}H_{17}N = 187.3$
CAS—14611-51-9

$$C_6H_5 \cdot CH_2 \cdots \overset{\overset{\displaystyle H}{|}}{\underset{\underset{\displaystyle CH_3}{|}}{C}} \cdot \overset{\overset{\displaystyle CH_3}{|}}{N} \cdot CH_2 \cdot C{\equiv}CH$$

An oil.

Selegiline Hydrochloride

Proprietary Name. Eldepryl
$C_{13}H_{17}N,HCl = 223.7$
CAS—14611-52-0
A white crystalline solid.

Thin-layer Chromatography. *System TA*—Rf 74; *system TB*—Rf 57; *system TC*—Rf 69. (*Dragendorff spray,* positive; *acidified iodoplatinate solution,* positive; *Marquis reagent,* orange.)

Gas Chromatography. *System GA*—selegiline RI 1436, amphetamine RI 1123, methylamphetamine RI 1176.

Ultraviolet Spectrum. Aqueous acid—252 nm, 258 nm ($A_1^1 = 9.1$ b), 264 nm; aqueous alkali—259 nm, 269 nm.

Infra-red Spectrum. Principal peaks at wavenumbers 704, 765, 740, 1492, 1092, 981 (selegiline hydrochloride, KBr disk).

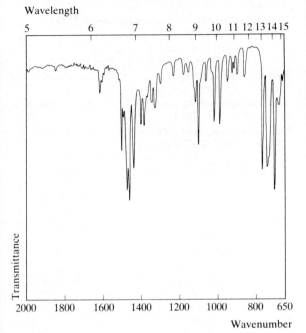

Wavelength

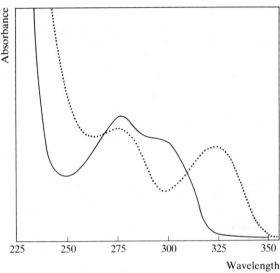

Wavelength

Mass Spectrum. Principal peaks at m/z 96, 56, 42, 91, 97, 39, 65, 58; amphetamine 44, 91, 40, 42, 65, 45, 39, 43; methylamphetamine 58, 91, 59, 134, 65, 56, 42, 57.

Quantification. See under Amphetamine and Methylamphetamine.

Disposition in the Body. Rapidly absorbed after oral administration and distributed to the tissues. Selegiline is almost completely metabolised to form methylamphetamine and amphetamine. About 50% of a dose is excreted in the urine in 24 hours and 75% in 72 hours; excreted mainly as methylamphetamine with lesser amounts of amphetamine. The excretion of metabolites is increased in acid urine. About 15% of a dose is eliminated in the faeces in 72 hours.

HALF-LIFE. Derived from urinary excretion data (total radio-activity), about 39 hours.

Dose. 5 to 10 mg of selegiline hydrochloride daily.

Serotonin

Synonyms. Enteramine; 5-HT; 5-Hydroxytryptamine.
3-(2-Aminoethyl)-1H-indol-5-ol
$C_{10}H_{12}N_2O = 176.2$
CAS—50-67-9

White crystals.

Soluble in water.

Dissociation Constant. pK_a 9.1, 9.8.

Colour Test. Marquis Test—brown (slow).

Thin-layer Chromatography. *System TA*—Rf 25. (*Acidified potassium permanganate solution*, positive.)

Ultraviolet Spectrum. Aqueous acid—276 nm; aqueous alkali—274 nm, 323 nm.

Infra-red Spectrum. Principal peaks at wavenumbers 1195, 1225, 1582, 1627, 720, 1105 (serotonin oxalate, KBr disk).

Disposition in the Body. Widely distributed in the body, arising from the hydroxylation and subsequent decarboxylation of tryptophan. It is metabolised chiefly by oxidative deamination to 5-hydroxyindol-3-ylacetic acid; N-methylation of the side-chain may also occur.

Simazine   *Herbicide*

Proprietary Names. Gesatop; Herbazin 50; Simadex SC; Simflow; Weedex S2 G. It is an ingredient of Pathclear.
2-Chloro-4,6-bis(ethylamino)-1,3,5-triazine
$C_7H_{12}ClN_5 = 201.7$
CAS—122-34-9

A white crystalline powder. M.p. 224° to 227°.
Practically **insoluble** in water; very slightly soluble in chloroform and ether.

Thin-layer Chromatography. *System TA*—Rf 73.

Gas Chromatography. *System GA*—RI 1690; *system GK*—retention time 0.79 relative to caffeine.

Ultraviolet Spectrum. Ethanol—262 nm ($A_1^1 = 162$ b). (See below)

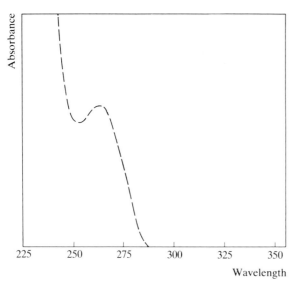

Wavelength

Infra-red Spectrum. Principal peaks at wavenumbers 1553, 1621, 1289, 797, 1103, 1129 (KBr disk).

Wavelength

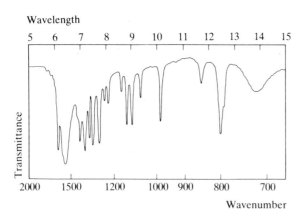

Wavenumber

Mass Spectrum. Principal peaks at m/z 201, 44, 186, 68, 173, 96, 158, 203.

Sodium Cromoglycate

Anti-allergic

Synonyms. Cromolyn Sodium; Disodium Cromoglycate.

Proprietary Names. Colimune; Frenal; Intal; Lomudal; Lomusol; Nalcrom; Opticrom; Rynacrom.

Disodium 4,4'-dioxo-5,5'-(2-hydroxytrimethylenedioxy)di(4*H*-chromene-2-carboxylate)
$C_{23}H_{14}Na_2O_{11} = 512.3$
CAS—16110-51-3 (cromoglycic acid); *15826-37-6* (disodium salt)

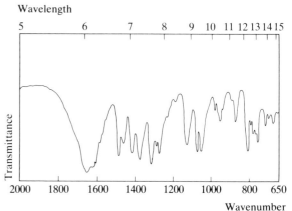

A white, hygroscopic, crystalline powder. M.p. 241° to 242°, with decomposition.

Soluble 1 in 20 of water; practically insoluble in ethanol and chloroform.

Dissociation Constant. Cromoglycic acid: pK$_a$ 2.5 (20°).

Colour Tests. Copper Sulphate (Method 2)—blue (1 to 2 min); Mandelin's Test—red; Marquis Test—yellow; Methanolic Potassium Hydroxide—yellow; Sulphuric Acid—yellow.

Thin-layer Chromatography. Cromoglycic acid: *system TD*—Rf 00; *system TE*—Rf 00; *system TF*—Rf 00.

Ultraviolet Spectrum. *Phosphate buffer (pH 7.4)*—238 nm (A$_1^1$ = 600 b), 326 nm (A$_1^1$ = 164 a).

Infra-red Spectrum. Principal peaks at wavenumbers 1635, 1305, 1264, 805, 1069, 1047 (KBr disk).

Wavelength

Wavenumber

Mass Spectrum. Principal peaks at m/z 44, 206, 162, 108, 51, 207, 201, 178 (cromoglycic acid).

Quantification. SPECTROFLUORIMETRY. In plasma: sensitivity 100 ng/ml—G. F. Moss *et al.*, *Toxic. appl. Pharmac.*, 1971, *20*, 147–156.

HIGH PRESSURE LIQUID CHROMATOGRAPHY. In urine: sensitivity 50 ng/ml, UV detection—J. J. Gardner, *J. Chromat.*, 1984, *305*; *Biomed. Appl.*, *30*, 228–232.

POLAROGRAPHY. In urine: limit of detection 500 ng/ml—A. G. Fogg and N. Fayad, *Analytica chim. Acta*, 1978, *102*, 205–210.

Disposition in the Body. Poorly absorbed after oral or subcutaneous administration. After inhalation most of a dose is swallowed with less than 10% reaching the lungs, from where it is rapidly absorbed; the amount absorbed after inhalation is dependent on particle size, smaller particles being absorbed better than large ones. It does not appear to be metabolised. Up to about 3% of an inhaled dose is excreted unchanged in the urine in 24 hours and up to about 87% is eliminated unchanged in the faeces in 3 days. After oral administration less than 1% is excreted in the urine, and after an intravenous dose about 50% is excreted in the urine and 50% is eliminated in the faeces.

THERAPEUTIC CONCENTRATION.

Following inhalation of a ^{14}C-labelled 20-mg dose by 12 asthmatic subjects, peak plasma concentrations of 0.006 to 0.012 µg/ml (mean 0.009) were attained in 15 minutes (S. R. Walker *et al.*, *J. Pharm. Pharmac.*, 1972, *24*, 525–531).

After inhalation of a single 60-mg dose by 3 subjects, peak plasma concentrations of about 0.2 to 0.3 µg/ml were reported in 10 to 15 minutes (G. F. Moss *et al.*, *Toxic. appl. Pharmac.*, 1971, *20*, 147–156).

HALF-LIFE. Plasma half-life, about 1 to 1.5 hours.

CLEARANCE. Plasma clearance, about 8 ml/min/kg.

PROTEIN BINDING. In plasma, about 60 to 70%.

Dose. 20 mg inhaled as a dry powder 4 times daily; 800 mg daily, by mouth.

Solanidine   *Alkaloid*

Synonym. Solatubine
$C_{27}H_{43}NO = 397.6$
CAS—80-78-4

An alkaloid present in various species of *Solanum* (Solanaceae). It is the aglycone of solanine.
A white crystalline powder. M.p. 218° to 219°, with decomposition.
Practically **insoluble** in water and ether; slightly soluble in ethanol; freely soluble in chloroform; soluble in dilute acids.

Colour Tests. Mandelin's Test—orange → violet → blue; Marquis Test—violet.

Thin-layer Chromatography. *System TA*—Rf 68.

Quantification. RADIOIMMUNOASSAY. In plasma: sensitivity 200 pg/ml—J. A. Matthew *et al., Food Chem. Toxicol.,* 1983, *21,* 637–640.

Solanine   *Alkaloid*

Synonym. Solatunine
$C_{45}H_{73}NO_{15} = 868.1$
CAS—20562-02-1
A glycoalkaloid present in various species of *Solanum,* particularly *S. tuberosum* (Solanaceae).
A white crystalline powder which decomposes at about 285°.
Practically **insoluble** in water, chloroform, and ether; soluble in hot ethanol, dilute acids, and amyl alcohol.

Colour Tests. Mandelin's Test—orange → violet → blue; Marquis Test—yellow → violet.

Thin-layer Chromatography. *System TA*—Rf 52. (*Marquis reagent,* positive.)

Sorbic Acid   *Preservative*

Proprietary Name. Sorbistat
(E,E)-Hexa-2,4-dienoic acid
$C_6H_8O_2 = 112.1$
CAS—110-44-1; 22500-92-1

A white or creamy-white crystalline powder. M.p. 132° to 137°.
Soluble 1 in 700 of water, 1 in 10 of ethanol, 1 in 16 of chloroform, 1 in 20 of ether, and 1 in 8 of methanol.
Caution. Sorbic acid is irritant to the eyes and possibly also to the skin.

Potassium Sorbate
Proprietary Name. Sorbistat-K
$C_6H_7KO_2 = 150.2$
CAS—590-00-1; 24634-61-5
White or creamy-white crystals or powder. M.p. about 270°, with decomposition.
Soluble 1 in less than 1 of water and 1 in 70 of ethanol; very slightly soluble in acetone, chloroform, and ether; soluble in propylene glycol.

Dissociation Constant. pK_a 4.8.

Ultraviolet Spectrum. Aqueous acid—264 nm ($A_1^1 = 2343$ a); aqueous alkali—254 nm ($A_1^1 = 2211$ b).

Infra-red Spectrum. Principal peaks at wavenumbers 1550, 1005, 1616, 1602, 1647, 882 (potassium sorbate, K Br disk).

Use. In concentrations of 0.1 to 0.2%.

Sotalol   *Beta-adrenoceptor Blocking Agent*

4′-(1-Hydroxy-2-isopropylaminoethyl)methanesulphonanilide
$C_{12}H_{20}N_2O_3S = 272.4$
CAS—3930-20-9

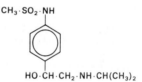

Sotalol Hydrochloride
Proprietary Names. Beta-Cardone; Sotacor; Sotalex. It is an ingredient of Sotazide and Tolerzide.
$C_{12}H_{20}N_2O_3S,HCl = 308.8$
CAS—959-24-0
An off-white to pale cream crystalline powder. M.p. 206° to 207°, with decomposition.
Freely **soluble** in water; sparingly soluble in chloroform.

Dissociation Constant. pK_a 8.3, 9.8.

Colour Tests. Liebermann's Test (100°)—brown; Mercurous Nitrate—black.

Thin-layer Chromatography. *System TA*—Rf 53; *system TB*—Rf 01; *system TC*—Rf 03.

Gas Chromatography. *System GA*—RI 2413.

High Pressure Liquid Chromatography. *System HA*—k′ 1.2.

Ultraviolet Spectrum. Aqueous acid—269 nm ($A_1^1 = 16$ a); aqueous alkali—249 nm ($A_1^1 = 552$ b). (See below)

Infra-red Spectrum. Principal peaks at wavenumbers 1160, 992, 785, 1512, 1230, 1585 (sotalol hydrochloride, K Br disk). (See below)

Mass Spectrum. Principal peaks at *m/z* 72, 30, 43, 122, 73, 41, 106, 121.

Quantification. HIGH PRESSURE LIQUID CHROMATOGRAPHY. In plasma: detection limit 20 ng/ml, fluorescence detection—M. A. Lefebvre *et al., J. pharm. Sci.,* 1980, *69,* 1216–1217.

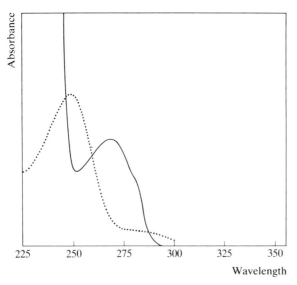

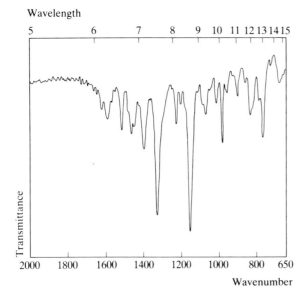

0.59 µg/g, heart 42.7 µg/g, kidney 116 µg/g, liver 88 µg/g, lung 59.7 µg/g, urine 416 µg/ml (M. Montagna and A. Groppi, *Arch. Tox.*, 1980, *43*, 221–226).

HALF-LIFE. Plasma half-life, 10 to 17 hours, increased in renal insufficiency and in elderly subjects.

VOLUME OF DISTRIBUTION. About 1 to 2 litres/kg.

CLEARANCE. Plasma clearance, about 1 to 2 ml/min/kg.

PROTEIN BINDING. In plasma, not significantly bound.

Dose. Usually 120 to 600 mg of sotalol hydrochloride daily.

Sparteine
Oxytocic

Synonyms. Lupinidine; (−)-Sparteine; *l*-Sparteine.
Dodecahydro - 7,14 - methano - 2*H*,6*H* - dipyrido[1,2 - *a*:1′,2′ - *e*][1,5]diazocine
$C_{15}H_{26}N_2 = 234.4$
CAS—90-39-1

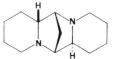

A dibasic alkaloid obtained from scoparium, the dried tops of broom, *Sarothamnus scoparius* (= *Cytisus scoparius*) (Leguminosae).
A viscous oily liquid.
Soluble 1 in 325 of water; very soluble in ethanol, chloroform, and ether.

Sparteine Sulphate
Proprietary Name. Depasan
$C_{15}H_{26}N_2, H_2SO_4, 5H_2O = 422.5$
CAS—299-39-8 (anhydrous); *6160-12-9* (pentahydrate)
Colourless crystals or white crystalline granules or powder which decompose at 136°.
Soluble 1 in 2 of water and 1 in 5 of ethanol; practically insoluble in chloroform and ether.

Thin-layer Chromatography. *System TA*—Rf 05; *system TB*—Rf 67; *system TC*—Rf 03. (*Acidified iodoplatinate solution*, positive.)

Gas Chromatography. *System GA*—RI 1801.

Ultraviolet Spectrum. No significant absorption, 230 to 360 nm.

Infra-red Spectrum. Principal peaks at wavenumbers 1118, 1070, 1045, 980, 962, 1015 (sparteine sulphate, KBr disk).

Mass Spectrum. Principal peaks at m/z 98, 137, 97, 136, 41, 193, 84, 110.

Quantification. GAS CHROMATOGRAPHY. In urine: sparteine and metabolites, sensitivity 50 ng/ml, FID—M. Eichelbaum *et al.*, *Eur. J. clin. Pharmac.*, 1979, *16*, 183–187. In plasma: sparteine and metabolites, sensitivity 30 ng/ml, FID—*idem.*, 189–194.

Disposition in the Body. Metabolised by *N*-oxidation followed by rearrangement to 2- and 5-dehydrosparteine. About 5% of the population are non-metabolisers (greater than 90% of a dose excreted in the urine unchanged in 24 hours). In metabolisers, about 55% of a dose is excreted in the urine in 24 hours, about 30% of the dose as unchanged drug, 7% as 5-dehydrosparteine, and 18% as 2-dehydrosparteine.

HALF-LIFE. Plasma half-life, about 3 hours in metabolisers, and 7 hours in non-metabolisers.

Dose. Sparteine sulphate has been given intramuscularly in a dose of 150 mg.

Wavelength

Wavelength

Disposition in the Body. Almost completely absorbed after oral administration; bioavailability about 90%. It is excreted almost entirely in the urine as unchanged drug, 50 to 80% of a dose being excreted in 24 hours. Less than 10% is eliminated in the faeces.

THERAPEUTIC CONCENTRATION.

A single oral dose of 160 mg given to 8 subjects produced peak plasma concentrations of 1.1 to 1.4 µg/ml in about 3 hours (M. Anttila *et al.*, *Acta pharmac. tox.*, 1976, *39*, 118–128).

Following daily oral doses of 400 mg for 5 days to 5 subjects, a mean plasma concentration of 6 µg/ml was reported 3 hours after the last dose (D. G. McDevitt and R. G. Shanks, *Br. J. clin. Pharmac.*, 1977, *4*, 153–156).

TOXICITY.

A man ingested about 3 g of sotalol and subsequently died; the following postmortem concentrations were reported: blood 40 µg/ml, brain

Spiramycin
Antibiotic

Proprietary Names. Rovamycin(e); Selectomycin.

A mixture of basic antimicrobial substances produced by the growth of *Streptomyces ambofaciens* and consisting of Spiramycin I, $C_{45}H_{78}N_2O_{15} = 887.1$ (about 63%), Spiramycin II, $C_{47}H_{80}N_2O_{16} = 929.2$ (about 24%), and Spiramycin III, $C_{48}H_{82}N_2O_{16} = 943.2$ (about 13%).

Note. The stated molecular formulae for the spiramycins may vary.

CAS—8025-81-8

A white or slightly yellowish amorphous powder.

Soluble 1 in 50 of water; very soluble in ethanol and chloroform.

Dissociation Constant. pK_a 8.0.

Colour Tests. Mandelin's Test—orange-brown; Marquis Test—orange.

Thin-layer Chromatography. *System TA*—Rf 42. (*Acidified potassium permanganate solution*, positive.)

Ultraviolet Spectrum. Aqueous acid—233 nm ($A_1^1 = 160$ b). No alkaline shift.

Infra-red Spectrum. Principal peaks at wavenumbers 1052, 1163, 1122, 994, 1016, 1730 (KBr disk).

Dose. 2 to 4 g daily.

Spironolactone
Diuretic

Synonyms. Espironolactona; Spirolactone.

Proprietary Names. Aldactone; Aldopur; Altex; Diatensec; Laractone; Sincomen; Spiretic; Spiro; Spiroctan; Spirolang; Spirolone; Spirotone. It is an ingredient of Aldactide, Lasilactone, and Spiroprop.

Note. The name Aldactone is also used in some countries as a proprietary name for canrenoate potassium.

7α-Acetylthio-3-oxo-17α-pregn-4-ene-21,17β-carbolactone
$C_{24}H_{32}O_4S = 416.6$
CAS—52-01-7

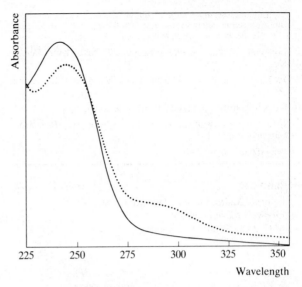

A white to light tan powder. M.p. 198° to 207°.

Practically **insoluble** in water; soluble 1 in 80 of ethanol, 1 in 3 of chloroform, and 1 in 100 of ether.

Colour Tests. Palladium Chloride—brown; Sulphuric Acid—orange → yellow-green (yellow-green fluorescence under ultraviolet light).

Thin-layer Chromatography. *System TD*—Rf 66; *system TE*—Rf 79; *system TF*—Rf 51.

Gas Chromatography. *System GA*—RI 3280.

Ultraviolet Spectrum. Aqueous acid—242 nm ($A_1^1 = 464$ a); aqueous alkali—247 nm ($A_1^1 = 405$ a).

Infra-red Spectrum. Principal peaks at wavenumbers 1773, 1676, 1170, 1127, 1115, 1185 (KBr disk).

Mass Spectrum. Principal peaks at m/z 341, 43, 340, 374, 267, 107, 55, 342.

Quantification. GAS CHROMATOGRAPHY. In urine: canrenone, detection limit 20 ng, FID—T. Fehér *et al.*, *J. Chromat.*, 1976, *123*, 460–462.

HIGH PRESSURE LIQUID CHROMATOGRAPHY. In serum: canrenone, sensitivity 5 ng/ml, UV detection—E. Besenfelder and R. Endele, *J. High Resolut. Chromat., Chromat. Commun.*, 1981, *4*, 419–421. In serum or urine: canrenone, detection limit 5 ng/ml in serum, UV detection—G. B. Neurath and D. Ambrosius, *J. Chromat.*, 1979, *163*; *Biomed. Appl.*, 5, 230–235.

NOTE. Plasma-canrenone concentrations are apparently overestimated when determined by spectrofluorimetry in comparison to HPLC methods (U. Abshagen *et al.*, *Eur. J. clin. Pharmac.*, 1979, *16*, 255–262).

Disposition in the Body. Rapidly but incompletely absorbed after oral administration; subject to extensive first-pass metabolism and enterohepatic circulation. The metabolism of spironolactone is very complex and there are a large number of metabolites; the initial step appears to be the formation of a thiol intermediate which is subsequently hydrolysed to canrenone, and which may also be methylated to thiomethylspironolactone. The transformation is rapid and spironolactone cannot be measured in the plasma. Canrenone, which is an active metabolite, is in enzymatic equilibrium with canrenoic acid, which may be conjugated with glucuronic acid; canrenone may also be hydroxylated to 15α-hydroxycanrenone. Other active sulphur-containing metabolites are thought to be formed from hydroxylation and sulphoxidation of thiomethylspironolactone. About 25 to 55% of a dose is excreted in the urine in 6 days and up to 40% may be eliminated in the faeces. About 11% of a dose is excreted in the urine as canrenone, canrenoic acid and its glucuronide conjugate, and about 6% as the 6β-hydroxysulphoxide metabolite; the 6β-hydroxysulphone derivative has also been detected in the urine.

THERAPEUTIC CONCENTRATION.

Following a single oral dose of 100 mg to 20 subjects, a mean peak serum-canrenone concentration of 0.13 µg/ml was attained in 2.5 to 3 hours;

after daily oral doses of 100 mg to 20 subjects, the mean maximum steady-state serum concentration was reported to be 0.20 µg/ml (U. Abshagen *et al.*, *Eur. J. clin. Pharmac.*, 1979, *16*, 255–262).

HALF-LIFE. Plasma half-life, canrenone 13 to 24 hours (mean 18).

DISTRIBUTION IN BLOOD. Plasma: whole blood ratio, canrenone 1.85.

PROTEIN BINDING. In plasma, canrenone, about 98%.

NOTE. For a review of spironolactone see A. Karim, *Drug Met. Rev.*, 1978, *8*, 151–188.

Dose. 100 to 400 mg daily.

Stanolone
Anabolic Steroid

Synonyms. Androstanolone; Dihydrotestosterone.
Proprietary Name. Anabolex
17β-Hydroxy-5α-androstan-3-one
$C_{19}H_{30}O_2 = 290.4$
CAS—521-18-6

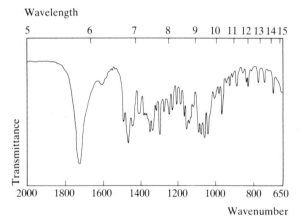

A white crystalline powder. M.p. 178° to 183°.
Practically **insoluble** in water; soluble 1 in 20 of ethanol and 1 in 70 of ether.

Thin-layer Chromatography. *System TP*—Rf 78; *system TQ*—Rf 11; *system TR*—Rf 90; *system TS*—Rf 72.

Infra-red Spectrum. Principal peaks at wavenumbers 1698, 1046, 1277, 1027, 1064, 1079 (KBr disk).

Wavelength

Dose. Stanolone has been given sublingually or sublabially in doses of 50 to 75 mg daily.

Stanozolol
Anabolic Steroid

Synonyms. Androstanazole; Methylstanazole; Stanazolol.
Proprietary Names. Stromba; Winstrol.
17α-Methyl-2'*H*-5α-androst-2-eno[3,2-*c*] pyrazol-17β-ol
$C_{21}H_{32}N_2O = 328.5$
CAS—10418-03-8

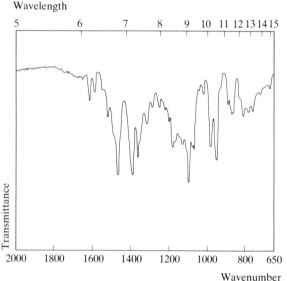

A white crystalline powder. It exists as needles, m.p. 155° or prisms, m.p. about 235°.
Practically **insoluble** in water; soluble 1 in about 40 of ethanol, 1 in about 75 of chloroform, and 1 in 370 of ether; soluble in dimethylformamide.

Colour Tests. Mandelin's Test—brown; Marquis Test—orange-yellow.

Thin-layer Chromatography. *System TA*—Rf 78. (*Acidified iodoplatinate solution*, positive.)

Ultraviolet Spectrum. Methanolic acid—230 nm ($A_1^1 = 200$ b).

Infra-red Spectrum. Principal peaks at wavenumbers 1096, 950, 1068, 982, 1175, 1125 (KCl disk).

Wavelength

Quantification. GAS CHROMATOGRAPHY–MASS SPECTROMETRY. In urine: detection limit 2 ng/ml—O. Lantto *et al.*, *J. Steroid Biochem.*, 1981, *14*, 721–727.

Dose. 5 to 10 mg daily.

Stilbazium Iodide   *Anthelmintic*

1-Ethyl-2,6-bis[4-(pyrrolidin-1-yl)styryl]pyridinium iodide
$C_{31}H_{36}IN_3 = 577.6$
CAS—3784-99-4

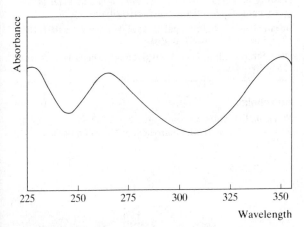

M.p. about 282°.
Soluble in ethanol and dilute acetic acid.

Thin-layer Chromatography. *System TA*—Rf 10. (*Acidified iodoplatinate solution*, positive.)

Ultraviolet Spectrum. Aqueous acid—264 nm ($A_1^1 = 274$ b), 355 nm ($A_1^1 = 310$ b).

Infra-red Spectrum. Principal peaks at wavenumbers 1175, 1538, 1582, 1510, 1307, 1274 (KBr disk).

Dose. Stilbazium iodide has been given in doses of 10 mg/kg once or twice daily for up to 3 days.

Stilboestrol   *Oestrogen*

Synonyms. Diethylstilboestrol; Stilbol.
Proprietary Names. Cyren-A; Desma; Dicorvin; Distilbene; Stibilium.
(*E*)-αβ-Diethylstilbene-4, 4'-diol
$C_{18}H_{20}O_2 = 268.4$
CAS—56-53-1

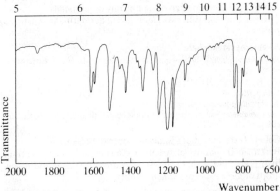

A white crystalline powder. M.p. 169° to 175°.
Practically **insoluble** in water; soluble 1 in 5 of ethanol, 1 in 200 of chloroform, and 1 in 3 of ether; soluble in acetone and methanol.

Caution. Stilboestrol is a powerful oestrogen. Contact with the skin or inhalation should be avoided.

Stilboestrol Diphosphate

Synonyms. Diethylstilboestrol Diphosphate; Fosfestrol; Phosphoestrolum.
Proprietary Name. Stilphostrol (tablets)
Note. Fosfestrol Sodium (the tetra-sodium salt of stilboestrol diphosphate) is available under the proprietary names Honvan, Honvol, ST-52, and Stilphostrol (injection).
$C_{18}H_{22}O_8P_2 = 428.3$
CAS—522-40-7
An off-white crystalline powder which decomposes at about 205°.
Sparingly **soluble** in water; soluble in ethanol and dilute alkalis.

Stilboestrol Dipropionate

Proprietary Name. Stilbocream
$C_{24}H_{28}O_4 = 380.5$
CAS—130-80-3
Colourless crystals or white crystalline powder. M.p. 104° to 108°.
Slightly **soluble** in water and dilute mineral acids; soluble 1 in 100 of ethanol (90%) and 1 in 6 of ether; freely soluble in acetone and chloroform.

Colour Tests. Antimony Pentachloride—red; Naphthol–Sulphuric Acid—yellow/orange; Sulphuric Acid—orange.
Dissolve about 0.5 mg in 0.2 ml of *acetic acid*, add 1 ml of *phosphoric acid*, and heat on a water-bath for 3 minutes—yellow, disappearing on dilution with 3 ml of *acetic acid*. (This test distinguishes stilboestrol from dienoestrol, which produces a violet colour.)

Thin-layer Chromatography. *System TP*—Rf 65, streaking may occur; *system TQ*—Rf 10, streaking may occur; *system TR*—Rf 18, streaking may occur; *system TS*—Rf 03.

Gas Chromatography. *System GA*—RI 2298.

Ultraviolet Spectrum. Ethanol—241 nm ($A_1^1 = 600$ a).

Infra-red Spectrum. Principal peaks at wavenumbers 1205, 1176, 833, 1250, 1512, 1610 (KBr disk).

Mass Spectrum. Principal peaks at *m/z* 107, 145, 268, 238, 121, 133, 159, 224.

Quantification. GAS CHROMATOGRAPHY. In blood, plasma, serum, bile or tissues: FID—K. A. Kohrman and J. MacGee, *J. Ass. off. analyt. Chem.*, 1977, *60*, 5–8.

HIGH PRESSURE LIQUID CHROMATOGRAPHY. In plasma, urine or tissues: UV detection—G. D. Newport *et al.*, *J. liq. Chromat.*, 1980, *3*, 1053–1070.

Dose. 0.1 to 2 mg daily; doses of 15 mg daily may be given.

Streptomycin   *Antibiotic*

Synonym. Estreptomicina
4-*O*-[2-*O*-(2-deoxy-2-methylamino-α-L-glucopyranosyl)-5-deoxy-3-*C*-formyl-α-L-lyxofuranosyl]-*NN'*-diamidino-D-streptamine
$C_{21}H_{39}N_7O_{12} = 581.6$
CAS—57-92-1

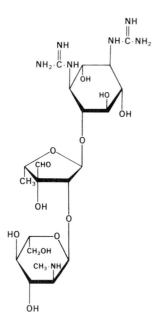

An antimicrobial organic base produced by the growth of certain strains of *Streptomyces griseus*, or by any other means.
Caution. Streptomycin may cause severe dermatitis in sensitised persons.

Streptomycin Sulphate
Proprietary Names. Solvo-strept S; Strycin. It is an ingredient of Streptotriad.
$(C_{21}H_{39}N_7O_{12})_2,3H_2SO_4 = 1457$
CAS—3810-74-0
A white hygroscopic powder.
Very **soluble** in water; practically insoluble in ethanol, chloroform, and ether.

Colour Tests. Benedict's Reagent—orange-brown.
Boil a small quantity of streptomycin sulphate with M sodium hydroxide, add a slight excess of *hydrochloric acid* and a few drops of *ferric chloride solution*—violet.

Thin-layer Chromatography. *System TA*—Rf 00. (*Acidified potassium permanganate solution*, positive.)

Disposition in the Body. Poorly and irregularly absorbed from the gastro-intestinal tract. Rapidly absorbed after intramuscular administration and widely distributed throughout the body. About 30 to 90% of a parenteral dose is excreted unchanged in the urine in 24 hours.

HALF-LIFE. Plasma half-life, about 2 to 4 hours, increased in neonates, in elderly subjects, and in renal impairment.

DISTRIBUTION IN BLOOD. Plasma: whole blood ratio, about 1.9.

PROTEIN BINDING. In plasma, about 20 to 30%.

Dose. The equivalent of 0.5 to 1 g of streptomycin daily, by intramuscular injection.

Strophanthin-K   *Cardiac Glycoside*

Synonyms. Estrofantina; Kombé Strophanthin; K-Strophanthin; Strophanthoside-K.
Proprietary Names. Kombetin; Myokombin; Strofopan; Trauphantin.
A mixture of glycosides from strophanthus, the dried ripe seeds of *Strophanthus kombe* (Apocynaceae), adjusted by admixture with a suitable diluent such as lactose so as to possess 40% of the activity of anhydrous ouabain.
CAS—11005-63-3
A white or yellowish-white powder containing microscopic crystals.
Soluble in water and ethanol; very slightly soluble in chloroform; practically insoluble in ether.

Colour Tests. Antimony Pentachloride—orange → red.
Dissolve in a cold mixture of *sulphuric acid* and water (4:1)—green, immediately (distinction from ouabain).

Infra-red Spectrum. Principal peaks at wavenumbers 1071, 1035, 1733, 1140, 1165, 1640 (KBr disk).

Dose. Strophanthin-K has been given intravenously in doses of 125 to 500 µg daily.

Strychnine   *Alkaloid*

Synonym. Estricnina
Proprietary Name. It is an ingredient of Neuro Phosphates.
Strychnidin-10-one
$C_{21}H_{22}N_2O_2 = 334.4$
CAS—57-24-9

An alkaloid obtained from nux vomica and the seeds of other species of *Strychnos*.
Translucent colourless crystals or white crystalline powder. M.p. about 268°.
Very slightly **soluble** in water; soluble 1 in 250 of ethanol and 1 in 6 of chloroform; practically insoluble in ether.

Strychnine Hydrochloride
Proprietary Name. It is an ingredient of Aneurone.
$C_{21}H_{22}N_2O_2,HCl,2H_2O = 406.9$
CAS—1421-86-9 (anhydrous); *6101-04-8* (dihydrate)
Colourless crystals or white crystalline powder.
Soluble 1 in 40 of water and 1 in 85 of ethanol; practically insoluble in ether.

Strychnine Nitrate

$C_{21}H_{22}N_2O_2,HNO_3 = 397.4$
CAS—66-32-0
Colourless glistening crystals.
Soluble 1 in 50 of water, 1 in 150 of ethanol, and 1 in 110 of chloroform; practically insoluble in ether.

Strychnine Sulphate

$(C_{21}H_{22}N_2O_2)_2,H_2SO_4,5H_2O = 857.0$
CAS—60-41-3 (anhydrous); *60491-10-3* (pentahydrate)
Colourless crystals or white crystalline powder. It is efflorescent in dry air. Melts when anhydrous at about 200°, with decomposition.
Soluble 1 in 50 of water and 1 in 135 of ethanol; slightly soluble in chloroform; practically insoluble in ether.

Dissociation Constant. pK_a 2.3, 8.0 (25°).

Colour Test. Mandelin's Test—violet.

Thin-layer Chromatography. *System TA*—Rf 26; *system TB*—Rf 08; *system TC*—Rf 19. (*Dragendorff spray*, positive; *acidified iodoplatinate solution*, positive.)

Gas Chromatography. *System GA*—RI 3119.

High Pressure Liquid Chromatography. *System HA*—k' 13.0 (tailing peak); *system HS*—k' 2.43.

Ultraviolet Spectrum. Aqueous acid—254 nm $(A_1^1 = 373$ a); aqueous alkali—255 nm, 278 nm.

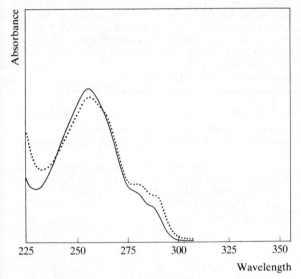

Infra-red Spectrum. Principal peaks at wavenumbers 1664, 764, 1050, 1110, 1282, 775 (KBr disk).

Mass Spectrum. Principal peaks at *m/z* 334, 335, 162, 120, 107, 144, 143, 130.

Quantification. GAS CHROMATOGRAPHY. In postmortem tissues: FID—J. S. Oliver *et al.*, *Medicine, Sci. Law*, 1979, *19*, 134–137.

HIGH PRESSURE LIQUID CHROMATOGRAPHY. In plasma or urine: sensitivity 625 ng/ml, UV detection—L. Alliot *et al.*, *J. Chromat.*, 1982, *232*; *Biomed. Appl.*, *21*, 440–442.

Disposition in the Body. Readily absorbed after oral or parenteral administration and rapidly oxidised. It is taken up to some extent by the red blood cells. About 20% of a dose is excreted unchanged in the urine.

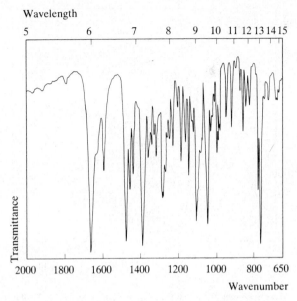

TOXICITY. The minimum lethal dose is about 15 to 30 mg for children and 50 to 100 mg for adults, although with adequate treatment recovery may occur after the ingestion of 250 mg or more.
From a review of nine fatalities due to strychnine poisoning, the following postmortem tissue concentrations were reported: blood 0 to 61 µg/g (mean 25, 5 cases), brain 0.47, 4.2, 5 µg/g (3 cases), kidney 0.07 to 90 µg/g (mean 36, 6 cases), liver 0 to 209 µg/g (mean 95.5, 8 cases), spinal cord 0.1, 1.8, 1.9 µg/g (3 cases), urine 1, 2.5, 7.7 µg/g (3 cases) (J. S. Oliver *et al.*, *Medicine, Sci. Law*, 1979, *19*, 134–137).

Dose. Strychnine has been given, as a bitter and analeptic, in doses of 2 to 8 mg, usually as its salts.

Styramate   *Muscle Relaxant*

Proprietary Name. Sinaxar
β-Hydroxyphenethyl carbamate
$C_9H_{11}NO_3 = 181.2$
CAS—94-35-9

$$\underset{NH_2 \cdot CO \cdot O \cdot CH_2 \cdot \overset{\displaystyle \overset{C_6H_5}{|}}{C}HOH}{}$$

A crystalline powder. M.p. 108° to 110°.
Sparingly **soluble** in water; soluble in ethanol, chloroform, and ether.

Thin-layer Chromatography. *System TA*—Rf 62; *system TB*—Rf 01; *system TC*—Rf 20; *system TD*—Rf 13; *system TE*—Rf 53; *system TF*—Rf 39. (*Furfuraldehyde reagent*, positive; *Van Urk reagent*, positive.)

Gas Chromatography. *System GA*—RI 1667.

Ultraviolet Spectrum. Aqueous acid—251 nm, 257 nm $(A_1^1 = 11$ b), 263 nm. (See below)

Infra-red Spectrum. Principal peaks at wavenumbers 1660, 1059, 1630, 750, 699, 1115 (KBr disk).

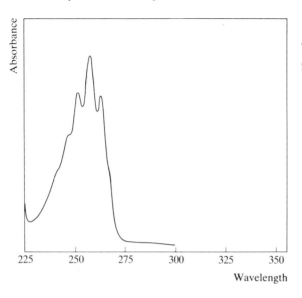

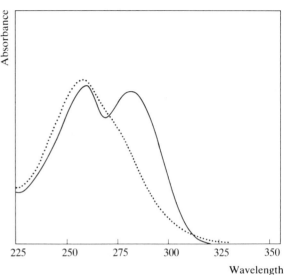

Mass Spectrum. Principal peaks at m/z 107, 120, 79, 75, 77, 44, 91, 45.

Dose. Usually 0.8 to 1.6 g daily.

Succinylsulphathiazole   *Sulphonamide*

Synonyms. Succinylsulfathiazole; Sulfasuccithiazole.
Proprietary Names. SS Thiazole; Sulfasuxidine; Thiacyl.
4′-(Thiazol-2-ylsulphamoyl)succinanilic acid monohydrate
$C_{13}H_{13}N_3O_5S_2,H_2O = 373.4$
CAS—116-43-8 (anhydrous)

White or yellowish-white crystals or powder which darken on exposure to light. M.p. about 190°, with decomposition.
Soluble 1 in 5000 of water, 1 in 200 of ethanol, and 1 in 150 of acetone; practically insoluble in chloroform and ether; soluble in aqueous solutions of alkali hydroxides and carbonates.

Dissociation Constant. pK_a 4.5.

Colour Tests. Copper Sulphate (Method 1)—green (→ violet); Koppanyi–Zwikker Test—red-violet; Mercurous Nitrate—black.

Thin-layer Chromatography. *System TD*—Rf 00; *system TE*—Rf 00; *system TF*—Rf 00; *system TT*—Rf 02; *system TU*—Rf 01; *system TV*—Rf 01.

High Pressure Liquid Chromatography. *System HU*—k′ 16.8.

Ultraviolet Spectrum. Aqueous acid—258 nm ($A_1^1 = 570$ a), 281 nm; aqueous alkali—257 nm ($A_1^1 = 651$ a).

Infra-red Spectrum. Principal peaks at wavenumbers 1143, 1585, 1091, 840, 1529, 1667 (Nujol mull).

Mass Spectrum. Principal peaks at m/z 92, 156, 65, 191, 108, 55, 45, 174.

Disposition in the Body. Only about 5% of a dose is absorbed after oral administration and blood concentrations are therefore very low compared to other sulphonamides, usually less than 40 μg/ml. It is slowly hydrolysed to sulphathiazole in the gastro-intestinal tract. Considerable amounts of sulphathiazole are eliminated in the faeces.

Dose. Usually 10 to 20 g daily.

Sulfadoxine   *Sulphonamide*

Synonyms. Sulfadimoxinum; Sulformethoxine; Sulforthomidine; Sulphadoxine; Sulphormethoxine; Sulphorthodimethoxine.
Proprietary Names. Fanaril; Fanasil; Fanasulf; Fanzil; Fontasul. It is an ingredient of Borgal (vet.), Fansidar, and Trivetrin (vet.).
N^1-(5,6-Dimethoxypyrimidin-4-yl)sulphanilamide
$C_{12}H_{14}N_4O_4S = 310.3$
CAS—2447-57-6

A white or creamy-white crystalline powder. M.p. 197° to 200°. Very slightly **soluble** in water; slightly soluble in ethanol and in methanol; practically insoluble in ether.

Colour Tests. Coniferyl Alcohol—orange; Copper Sulphate (Method 1)—green; Mercurous Nitrate—black; Nitrous Acid—yellow.

Thin-layer Chromatography. *System TA*—Rf 67; *system TD*—Rf 37; *system TE*—Rf 08; *system TF*—Rf 51.

High Pressure Liquid Chromatography. *System HU*—k' 4.4.

Ultraviolet Spectrum. Aqueous acid—264 nm; aqueous alkali—272 nm ($A_1^1 = 762$ a).

Infra-red Spectrum. Principal peaks at wavenumbers 1583, 1161, 1596, 1315, 1091, 1305 (KBr disk).

Quantification. HIGH PRESSURE LIQUID CHROMATOGRAPHY. The method referred to under Sulphamethoxazole may be used.

Disposition in the Body. Sulfadoxine·is a long-acting sulphonamide which is readily absorbed after oral administration. The main metabolic reaction is N^4-acetylation together with glucuronidation. High concentrations of sulfadoxine are attained in the blood in about 4 hours with about 5% as the acetyl derivative and 2% as the glucuronide. It is excreted very slowly in the urine, about 8% of a dose being excreted in 24 hours and 30% in 7 days. The excreted material consists of 30 to 60% acetyl derivative and 30 to 60% unchanged sulfadoxine of which up to 40% may be conjugated with glucuronic acid and up to 10% with sulphate.

THERAPEUTIC CONCENTRATION.
Blood concentrations of 130 to 200 µg/ml were attained by 31 patients receiving 1.5 to 2 g weekly (V. Haegi, *Schweiz. med. Wschr.*, 1966, *96*, 1308, per *Int. pharm. Abstr.*, 1967, *4*, 93).

HALF-LIFE. Plasma half-life, about 4 to 8 days.

PROTEIN BINDING. In plasma, about 90%.

Dose. Initially 2 g, followed by 1 to 1.5 g weekly.

Sulfamerazine   *Sulphonamide*

Synonyms. Sulfamethyldiazine; Sulfamethylpyrimidine; Sulphamerazine.

Proprietary Names. It is an ingredient of Sulphatriad and Trinamide (vet.).

N^1-(4-Methylpyrimidin-2-yl)sulphanilamide
$C_{11}H_{12}N_4O_2S = 264.3$
CAS—127-79-7

A white or faintly yellowish-white crystalline powder which slowly darkens on exposure to light. M.p. 234° to 239°, with decomposition.

Soluble 1 in 6250 of water, 1 in 550 of ethanol, and 1 in 60 of acetone; slightly soluble in chloroform; very slightly soluble in ether; soluble in dilute mineral acids and in solutions of alkali hydroxides and carbonates.

Sulfamerazine Sodium

Synonyms. Soluble Sulphamerazine; Sulphamerazine Sodium.
$C_{11}H_{11}N_4NaO_2S = 286.3$
CAS—127-58-2
A white or yellowish-white powder. It slowly darkens on exposure to light; on exposure to moist air it absorbs carbon dioxide and becomes less soluble in water.
Soluble 1 in 3.5 of water; slightly soluble in ethanol; practically insoluble in chloroform and ether.

Dissociation Constant. pK_a 7.1 (20°).

Partition Coefficient. Log *P* (octanol/pH 7.5), −0.1.

Colour Tests. Coniferyl Alcohol—orange; Copper Sulphate (Method 1)—green → brown; Koppanyi–Zwikker Test—pink; Mercurous Nitrate—black.

Thin-layer Chromatography. *System TA*—Rf 65; *system TD*—Rf 23; *system TE*—Rf 08; *system TF*—Rf 41; *system TT*—Rf 33; *system TU*—Rf 18; *system TV*—Rf 07.

Gas Chromatography. *System GJ*—retention time of methyl derivative 0.69 relative to griseofulvin.

High Pressure Liquid Chromatography. *System HU*—k' 8.1.

Ultraviolet Spectrum. Aqueous acid—242 nm ($A_1^1 = 596$ a), 304 nm; aqueous alkali—242 nm ($A_1^1 = 820$ b), 255 nm ($A_1^1 = 828$ b).

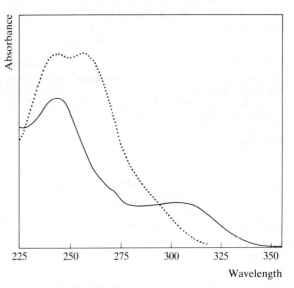

Infra-red Spectrum. Principal peaks at wavenumbers 1149, 1590, 1560, 1316, 1088, 1618 (KBr disk).

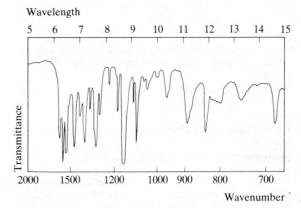

Mass Spectrum. Principal peaks at *m/z* 199, 200, 92, 65, 108, 39, 66, 201.

Quantification. HIGH PRESSURE LIQUID CHROMATOGRAPHY. In plasma or urine: sulfamerazine and acetylsulfamerazine, detection limit 300 ng/ml, UV detection—T. B. Vree *et al.*, *Biopharm. Drug Disp.*, 1983, *4*, 271–291.

Disposition in the Body. Rapidly absorbed after oral administration. It penetrates into the cerebrospinal fluid to produce concentrations about one-half of those in blood. Metabolised by N^4-acetylation, the extent of which is genetically determined; in slow acetylators about 15% of the sulfamerazine in the blood is in the form of the acetyl derivative compared with 35% in rapid acetylators. About 60% of a dose is excreted in the urine in 48 hours; approximately half of the excreted material is in the form of the acetyl derivative.

TOXICITY. Serious toxic effects, sometimes fatal, have occurred in young children, after therapeutic doses.

HALF-LIFE. Plasma half-life, 9 to 14 hours in rapid acetylators and about 24 hours in slow acetylators.

VOLUME OF DISTRIBUTION. About 0.4 litre/kg.

PROTEIN BINDING. In plasma, about 80 to 90%.

Dose. 4 g daily.

Sulfametopyrazine   *Sulphonamide*

Synonyms. Sulfalene; Sulfamethoxypyrazine; Sulfapyrazin Methoxyne; Sulphalene.
Proprietary Names. Kelfizine W; Longum.
N^1-(3-Methoxypyrazin-2-yl)sulphanilamide
$C_{11}H_{12}N_4O_3S = 280.3$
CAS—152-47-6

A white or yellowish-white crystalline powder. M.p. 175° to 178°.
Practically **insoluble** in water; slightly soluble in ethanol and chloroform; freely soluble in acetone and in dilute mineral acids and solutions of alkali hydroxides.

Dissociation Constant. pK_a 7.0.

Colour Tests. Coniferyl Alcohol—orange; Copper Sulphate (Method 1)—green; Mercurous Nitrate—black; Nitrous Acid—yellow.

Thin-layer Chromatography. *System TA*—Rf 67; *system TD*—Rf 40; *system TE*—Rf 08; *system TF*—Rf 50. (*Van Urk reagent*, positive.)

Infra-red Spectrum. Principal peaks at wavenumbers 1145, 1315, 1162, 1601, 1642, 1085 (KBr disk).

Disposition in the Body. Sulfametopyrazine is a long-acting sulphonamide and is readily absorbed after oral administration. It is acetylated in the body, 5 to 10% of the sulfametopyrazine in the blood being in the form of the N^4-acetyl derivative which is inactive. It is slowly excreted in the urine, about 70% of the excreted material being the acetyl derivative and about 14 to 20% being unchanged drug.

THERAPEUTIC CONCENTRATION.
After a single oral dose of 500 mg to 3 subjects, peak plasma concentrations of 25 to 33 µg/ml (mean 29) were attained in 2 to 4 hours (R. L. Herting *et al.*, *Antimicrob. Ag. Chemother.*, 1964, 554–561).

Maximum steady-state plasma concentrations of 51 to 69 µg/ml (mean 58) were reported on the seventh day after 6 subjects had received an initial dose of 600 mg followed by 200 mg daily (D. S. Reeves *et al.*, *J. antimicrob. Chemother.*, 1980, *6*, 647–656).

HALF-LIFE. Plasma half-life, 2 to 4 days.

VOLUME OF DISTRIBUTION. About 0.2 to 0.3 litre/kg.

PROTEIN BINDING. In plasma, 65 to 80%.

Dose. 2 g once a week.

Sulfaquinoxaline   *Coccidiostat (Veterinary)*

Synonyms. Sulfabenzpyrazine; Sulphaquinoxaline.
Proprietary Names. It is an ingredient of Pancoxin, Saquadil, Supacox, and Whitsyn S.
N^1-(Quinoxalin-2-yl)sulphanilamide
$C_{14}H_{12}N_4O_2S = 300.3$
CAS—59-40-5

A yellow powder. M.p. about 250°, with decomposition.
Practically **insoluble** in water and ether; very slightly soluble in ethanol and chloroform; soluble in dilute solutions of mineral acids and in solutions of alkalis.

Dissociation Constant. pK_a 5.5 (20°).

Colour Test. Copper Sulphate (Method 1)—green.

Thin-layer Chromatography. *System TA*—Rf 71.

High Pressure Liquid Chromatography. *System HU*—k' 4.8.

Ultraviolet Spectrum. Aqueous acid—248 nm ($A_1^1 = 648$ b), 263 nm ($A_1^1 = 540$ b), 348 nm ($A_1^1 = 263$ b); aqueous alkali—252 nm ($A_1^1 = 1085$ a), 357 nm ($A_1^1 = 265$ b).

Sulforidazine   *Tranquilliser*

Synonym. Sulphoridazine
Proprietary Name. Inofal
10-[2-(1-Methyl-2-piperidyl)ethyl]-2-methylsulphonylphenothiazine
$C_{21}H_{26}N_2O_2S_2 = 402.6$
CAS—14759-06-9

Crystals. M.p. 121° to 123°.

Ultraviolet Spectrum. Aqueous acid—265 nm ($A_1^1 = 700$ b), 311 nm ($A_1^1 = 75$ b); aqueous alkali—266 nm ($A_1^1 = 659$ b).

Quantification. See under Thioridazine.

Disposition in the Body. Sulforidazine is an active metabolite of mesoridazine and thioridazine.

Dose. Sulforidazine has been given in doses of 150 to 300 mg daily.

Sulindac
Analgesic

Proprietary Names. Arthrocine; Clinoril; Imbaral.
(Z)-[5-Fluoro-2-methyl-1-(4-methylsulphinylbenzylidene)-inden-3-yl]acetic acid
$C_{20}H_{17}FO_3S = 356.4$
CAS—38194-50-2

A yellow crystalline powder. M.p. about 182° to 185°.
Practically **insoluble** in water; slightly soluble in ethanol, chloroform, and methanol.

Colour Tests. Liebermann's Test—brown; Mandelin's Test—orange; Marquis Test—green (slow); Sulphuric Acid—brown.

Thin-layer Chromatography. *System TD*—Rf 14; *system TE*—Rf 01; *system TF*—Rf 10; *system TG*—Rf 13. (*Chromic acid solution*, white; *Ludy Tenger reagent*, orange-brown.)

Gas Chromatography. *System GA*—RI 2690, 2750, and 2820; *system GD*—retention time of methyl derivative 0.49 relative to $n\text{-}C_{16}H_{34}$.

High Pressure Liquid Chromatography. *System HD*—k' 1.25; *system HV*—retention time 0.78 relative to meclofenamic acid.

Ultraviolet Spectrum. Methanolic acid—284 nm ($A_1^1 = 420$ a), 327 nm ($A_1^1 = 373$ a); aqueous alkali—280 nm ($A_1^1 = 442$ b), 327 nm ($A_1^1 = 364$ b).

Infra-red Spectrum. Principal peaks at wavenumbers 1704, 1006, 1018, 1160, 1270, 1603 (KBr disk).

Mass Spectrum. Principal peaks at *m/z* 341, 233, 356, 246, 247, 248, 234, 281.

Quantification. HIGH PRESSURE LIQUID CHROMATOGRAPHY. In plasma or urine: sulindac and its sulphide and sulphone metabolites, sensitivity 100 ng/ml in plasma, UV detection—B. N. Swanson and V. K. Boppana, *J. Chromat.*, 1981, *225*; *Biomed. Appl.*, *14*, 123–130. In plasma, urine, bile, or gastric fluid: sulindac and its sulphide and sulphone metabolites, sensitivity 250 ng/ml for plasma, UV detection—D. G. Musson *et al.*, *J. pharm Sci.*, 1984, *73*, 1270–1273.

Disposition in the Body. Readily absorbed after oral administration. It is metabolised by oxidation to the sulphone and by reduction to the sulphide which is thought to be responsible for most of the pharmacological activity. A total of about 36% of a dose is excreted in the urine in 24 hours and about 75% in 4 days. In four days, about 30% of a dose is excreted as the sulphone and its conjugate, and 20% as unchanged drug and its conjugate; no significant amount of the sulphide or its conjugate is found in the urine. Sulindac and its metabolites are excreted in the bile

and undergo extensive enterohepatic circulation. Up to about 25% of a dose is eliminated in the faeces in 4 days, with less than 2% as unchanged drug.

THERAPEUTIC CONCENTRATION.

A single dose of 200 mg to 14 subjects produced a mean peak plasma concentration of about 4 µg/ml after 1 hour; mean peak plasma concentrations for the sulphide and sulphone were about 3 and about 2 µg/ml, respectively, after 2 hours (D. F. Duggan *et al.*, *Clin. Pharmac. Ther.*, 1977, *21*, 326–335).

Following daily oral doses of 200 mg, twice a day to 12 subjects, mean maximum steady-state plasma concentrations were: sulindac 5.0 µg/ml, sulphide 6.9 µg/ml, sulphone 2.6 µg/ml; a diurnal variation in plasma concentrations was reported with lower concentrations being attained after the evening dose. After oral administration of 400 mg once daily to 12 subjects, maximum steady-state plasma concentrations were: sulindac 8.7 µg/ml, sulphide 8.8 µg/ml, sulphone 3.9 µg/ml (B. N. Swanson *et al.*, *Clin. Pharmac. Ther.*, 1982, *32*, 397–403).

HALF-LIFE. Plasma half-life, sulindac about 7 hours, sulphide metabolite about 16 to 18 hours.

PROTEIN BINDING. In plasma, sulindac, sulphone, and sulphide, about 95%.

NOTE. For a review of the pharmacokinetics of sulindac see R. N. Brogden *et al.*, *Drugs*, 1978, *16*, 97–114.

Dose. 200 to 400 mg daily.

Sulphacetamide
Sulphonamide

Synonyms. Acetosulfaminum; Sulfacetamide.
Proprietary Name. It is an ingredient of Sultrin.
N-Sulphanilylacetamide
$C_8H_{10}N_2O_3S = 214.2$
CAS—144-80-9

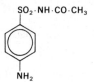

A white or yellowish-white crystalline powder. M.p. 181° to 184°.
Soluble 1 in 150 of water, 1 in 15 of ethanol, and 1 in 7 of acetone; very slightly soluble in chloroform; slightly soluble in ether.

Sulphacetamide Sodium

Synonyms. Soluble Sulphacetamide; Sulfacetamide Sodium; Sulfacylum Natrium.
Proprietary Names. Acetopt; Albucid; Antebor; Bleph-10; Cetamide; Optamide; Optosulfex; Sebizon; Sodium Sulamyd; Sulf-10; Sulphacalyre. It is an ingredient of Ocusol.
$C_8H_9N_2NaO_3S,H_2O = 254.2$
CAS—127-56-0 (anhydrous); *6209-17-2* (monohydrate)
White or yellowish-white crystals or crystalline powder. It slowly darkens on exposure to light; on exposure to moist air it absorbs carbon dioxide and becomes less soluble.
Soluble 1 in 1.5 of water; slightly soluble in ethanol; sparingly soluble in acetone; practically insoluble in chloroform and ether.

Dissociation Constant. pK_a 1.8, 5.4.

Colour Tests. Coniferyl Alcohol—orange; Copper Sulphate (Method 1)—blue; Koppanyi-Zwikker Test—blue-violet.

Thin-layer Chromatography. *System TA*—Rf 70; *system TD*—Rf 17; *system TE*—Rf 05; *system TF*—Rf 42; *system TT*—Rf 53; *system TU*—Rf 37; *system TV*—Rf 04. (*Mercuric chloride-diphenylcarbazone reagent*, blue; *acidified potassium permanganate solution*, positive; *Van Urk reagent*, yellow.)

Gas Chromatography. *System GJ*—retention time of methyl derivative 0.16 relative to griseofulvin.

High Pressure Liquid Chromatography. *System HU*—k' 7.7.

Ultraviolet Spectrum. Aqueous acid—271 nm $(A_1^1 = 260 \text{ a})$; aqueous alkali—256 nm $(A_1^1 = 750 \text{ a})$.

Infra-red Spectrum. Principal peaks at wavenumbers 1145, 1264, 1552, 1090, 825, 1600 (sulphacetamide sodium, KBr disk).

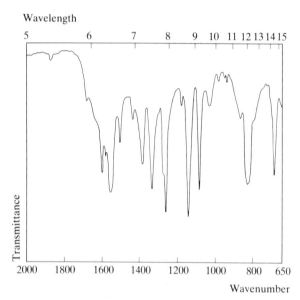

Wavelength

Transmittance

Wavenumber

Mass Spectrum. Principal peaks at *m/z* 172, 92, 156, 65, 108, 39, 44, 41.

Quantification. HIGH PRESSURE LIQUID CHROMATOGRAPHY. The method referred to under Sulphamethoxazole may be used.

Disposition in the Body. After oral administration sulphacetamide is readily absorbed and rapidly excreted in the urine, mainly as unchanged drug. However, it is usually only used topically in the treatment of eye infections; absorption into the blood may occur after application to the eye if the conjunctiva is inflamed.

HALF-LIFE. Plasma half-life, 7 to 14 hours.

PROTEIN BINDING. In plasma, 15 to 18%.

Use. Sulphacetamide sodium is used as a 10 to 30% ophthalmic solution.

Sulphachlorpyridazine   *Sulphonamide*

Synonym. Sulfachlorpyridazine
Proprietary Names. Nefrosul; Sonilyn.
N^1-(6-Chloropyridazin-3-yl)sulphanilamide
$C_{10}H_9ClN_4O_2S = 284.7$
CAS—80-32-0

A yellowish crystalline powder.
Soluble in bicarbonate solutions.

Colour Tests. Coniferyl Alcohol—orange; Copper Sulphate (Method 1)—green; Koppanyi–Zwikker Test—pink; Mercurous Nitrate—black; Nitrous Acid—yellow.

Thin-layer Chromatography. *System TA*—Rf 70. (*Van Urk reagent*, positive.)

High Pressure Liquid Chromatography. *System HU*—k' 3.3.

Ultraviolet Spectrum. Aqueous acid—256 nm; aqueous alkali—257 nm.

Infra-red Spectrum. Principal peaks at wavenumbers 1124, 1220, 1087, 1208, 963, 1618 (KBr disk).

Disposition in the Body. Readily absorbed after oral administration and rapidly excreted in the urine.

THERAPEUTIC CONCENTRATION.

After a single oral dose of 500 mg to 10 subjects, peak plasma concentrations of 39.7 to 85.5 µg/ml (mean 59.6) were attained in about 1 hour (E. L. Marino *et al., Int. J. clin. Pharmac. Ther. Toxicol.*, 1980, *18*, 10–14).

HALF-LIFE. Plasma half-life, about 3 to 4 hours.

VOLUME OF DISTRIBUTION. About 0.1 litre/kg.

CLEARANCE. Plasma clearance, about 0.5 ml/min/kg.

PROTEIN BINDING. In plasma, about 94 to 99%.

REFERENCE. E. L. Marino *et al., ibid.*

Dose. Sulphachlorpyridazine has been given in an initial dose of 4 g, followed by 2 to 4 g daily.

Sulphadiazine   *Sulphonamide*

Synonyms. Solfadiazina; Solfapirimidina; Sulfadiazine. It is an ingredient of Co-tetroxazine and Co-trimazine.
Proprietary Names. Adiazine; Diazyl Dulcet; S-Diazine. It is an ingredient of Streptotriad, Sulphatriad, Tibirox, Triglobe, and Trinamide (vet.).
N^1-(Pyrimidin-2-yl)sulphanilamide
$C_{10}H_{10}N_4O_2S = 250.3$
CAS—68-35-9

White, yellowish-white, or pinkish-white crystals or powder, slowly darkening on exposure to light. M.p. about 255°, with decomposition.

Practically **insoluble** in water, chloroform, and ether; very slightly soluble in ethanol; soluble 1 in 300 of acetone; soluble in dilute mineral acids and in solutions of alkali hydroxides and carbonates.

Sulphadiazine Sodium

Synonyms. Soluble Sulphadiazine; Sulfadiazine Sodium.
$C_{10}H_9N_4NaO_2S = 272.3$
CAS—547-32-0

A white or yellowish-white powder. It slowly darkens on exposure to light; on exposure to moist air it absorbs carbon dioxide with the liberation of sulphadiazine and becomes incompletely soluble in water. **Soluble** 1 in 2 of water; slightly soluble in ethanol; practically insoluble in chloroform and ether.

Dissociation Constant. pK_a 6.5 (25°).

Partition Coefficient. Log P (octanol/pH 7.5), −1.3.

Colour Tests. Coniferyl Alcohol—orange; Copper Sulphate (Method 1)—violet-brown; Koppanyi-Zwikker Test—violet-pink; Mercurous Nitrate—black.

Thin-layer Chromatography. *System TA*—Rf 64; *system TD*—Rf 22; *system TE*—Rf 04; *system TF*—Rf 39; *system TT*—Rf 24; *system TU*—Rf 22; *system TV*—Rf 03.

Gas Chromatography. *System GJ*—retention time of the methyl derivative of sulphadiazine 0.66 and of N^4-acetylsulphadiazine 1.69, both relative to griseofulvin.

High Pressure Liquid Chromatography. *System HU*—k' 8.7.

Ultraviolet Spectrum. Aqueous acid—242 nm $(A_1^1 = 587 a)$; aqueous alkali—240 nm $(A_1^1 = 867 a)$, 254 nm $(A_1^1 = 868 a)$.

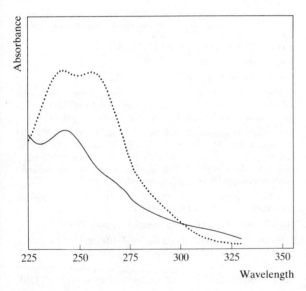

Infra-red Spectrum. Principal peaks at wavenumbers 1580, 1159, 1494, 682, 940, 797 (KBr disk).

Mass Spectrum. Principal peaks at m/z 186, 185, 92, 65, 108, 39, 93, 187.

Quantification. GAS CHROMATOGRAPHY. In plasma or urine: sulphadiazine and acetyl derivative, sensitivity 1 ng, ECD—A. Bye and G. Land, *J. Chromat.*, 1977, *139*, 181–185.

HIGH PRESSURE LIQUID CHROMATOGRAPHY. In plasma or urine: detection limit 400 ng/ml for sulphadiazine in plasma, 5 and 7 μg/ml for sulphadiazine and the acetyl derivative, respectively, in urine, UV detection—D. Westerlund and A. Wijkström, *J. pharm. Sci.*, 1982, *71*, 1142–1145.

Disposition in the Body. Readily absorbed after oral administration. It is acetylated in the body and up to 15% of the sulphadiazine in the blood is in the form of the inactive N^4-acetyl derivative. About 50% of a dose is excreted in the urine in 24 hours; up to about 40% of the excreted material is the acetyl derivative and up to about 50% is unchanged drug. Excretion is influenced by the pH of the urine, the rate being increased when the urine is alkaline.

THERAPEUTIC CONCENTRATION.

After a single oral dose of 820 mg to 5 subjects, peak serum concentrations of sulphadiazine plus metabolites of 19 to 40 μg/ml (mean 33) were attained in 4 hours (T. Bergan *et al.*, *Clin. Pharmac. Ther.*, 1977, *22*, 211–224).

HALF-LIFE. Plasma half-life, 6 to 17 hours.

VOLUME OF DISTRIBUTION. About 0.3 litre/kg.

CLEARANCE. Plasma clearance, about 0.3 ml/min/kg.

DISTRIBUTION IN BLOOD. Plasma: whole blood ratio, 0.93.

PROTEIN BINDING. In plasma, about 50%.

Dose. An initial dose of 2 to 4 g, followed by 1 g every 4 to 6 hours.

Sulphadimethoxine   *Sulphonamide*

Synonym. Sulfadimethoxine
Proprietary Names. Crozinal; Ipersulfa; Madribon; Risulpir; Sulfabon; Sulfaduran.
N^1-(2,6-Dimethoxypyrimidin-4-yl)sulphanilamide
$C_{12}H_{14}N_4O_4S = 310.3$
CAS—122-11-2

A white or creamy-white crystalline powder. M.p. 198° to 204°. Very slightly **soluble** in water; soluble 1 in 200 of ethanol, 1 in 800 of chloroform, and 1 in 2000 of ether; soluble in dilute mineral acids and in solutions of alkali hydroxides and carbonates.

Dissociation Constant. pK_a 5.9 (25°).

Colour Tests. Coniferyl Alcohol—orange; Copper Sulphate (Method 1)—green; Koppanyi-Zwikker Test—violet-pink; Mercurous Nitrate—black.

Thin-layer Chromatography. *System TA*—Rf 65; *system TD*—Rf 31; *system TE*—Rf 10; *system TF*—Rf 51; *system TT*—Rf 85; *system TU*—Rf 52; *system TV*—Rf 34.

Ultraviolet Spectrum. Aqueous acid—275 nm $(A_1^1 = 449\ a)$; aqueous alkali—269 nm $(A_1^1 = 845\ a)$.

Infra-red Spectrum. Principal peaks at wavenumbers 1590, 1147, 1090, 1314, 685, 1066 (KBr disk).

Wavelength

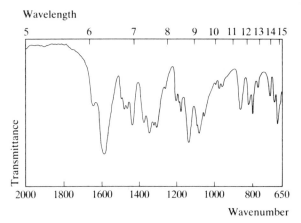

Mass Spectrum. Principal peaks at *m/z* 246, 92, 65, 245, 108, 247, 39, 260.

Disposition in the Body. Sulphadimethoxine is a long-acting sulphonamide which is readily absorbed after oral administration. After a single dose, peak blood concentrations are attained in about 4 to 6 hours. It is acetylated in the body and about 10% of the sulphadimethoxine in the blood is present as the inactive N^4-acetyl derivative, and about 5% as the N^1-glucuronide. About 50% of a dose is excreted in the urine in 48 hours, about 20% of the excreted material being the acetyl derivative, about 5% unchanged drug, and 60 to 80% the N^1-glucuronide. Both unchanged drug and the N^1-glucuronide are excreted in the bile.

THERAPEUTIC CONCENTRATION. In plasma, usually in the range 50 to 100 µg/ml.

Following an oral dose of 2 g, peak blood concentrations of 120 to 180 µg/ml were attained (H. Seneca, *J. Am. med. Ass.*, 1966, *198*, 975–980).

HALF-LIFE. Plasma half-life, 20 to 40 hours.

VOLUME OF DISTRIBUTION. About 0.1 to 0.2 litre/kg.

PROTEIN BINDING. In plasma, 90 to 99%.

Dose. An initial dose of 1 or 2 g, followed by 0.5 to 1 g daily.

Sulphadimidine   *Sulphonamide*

Synonyms. Sulfadimérazine; Sulfadimezinum; Sulfadimidine; Sulfamethazine; Sulphadimethylpyrimidine; Sulphamethazine.

Note. Sulfadimethylpyrimidine has been used as a synonym for sulphasomidine. Care should be taken to avoid confusion between the two compounds, which are isomeric.

Proprietary Names. Diazil; S-Dimidine. It is an ingredient of Streptotriad.

N^1-(4,6-Dimethylpyrimidin-2-yl)sulphanilamide
$C_{12}H_{14}N_4O_2S = 278.3$
CAS—57-68-1

White or yellowish-white crystals or powder which darken and decompose on exposure to light. M.p. 197° to 200°.

Very slightly **soluble** in water; soluble 1 in 120 of ethanol, 1 in 30 of acetone, 1 in 600 of chloroform, and 1 in 2500 of ether; soluble in dilute mineral acids and in aqueous solutions of alkali hydroxides and carbonates.

Sulphadimidine Sodium

Synonyms. Soluble Sulphadimethylpyrimidine; Soluble Sulphadimidine; Soluble Sulphamethazine.

Proprietary Name. Sulphamezathine

$C_{12}H_{13}N_4NaO_2S = 300.3$
CAS—1981-58-4

White or creamy-white hygroscopic crystals or powder. It slowly discolours and decomposes on exposure to light; on exposure to air it absorbs carbon dioxide and becomes less soluble in water.

Soluble 1 in 2.5 of water and 1 in 60 of ethanol.

Dissociation Constant. pK_a 7.4 (25°).

Partition Coefficient. Log *P* (octanol), 0.3.

Colour Tests. Coniferyl Alcohol—orange; Copper Sulphate (Method 1)—green → brown; Koppanyi-Zwikker Test—violet-pink; Mercurous Nitrate—black; Nitrous Acid—yellow.

Thin-layer Chromatography. *System TA*—Rf 62; *system TD*—Rf 23; *system TE*—Rf 13; *system TF*—Rf 45; *system TT*—Rf 50; *system TU*—Rf 27; *system TV*—Rf 62. (*Mercuric chloride-diphenylcarbazone reagent*, blue; *acidified potassium permanganate solution*, positive; *Van Urk reagent*, yellow.)

Gas Chromatography. *System GJ*—retention time of methyl derivative 0.71 relative to griseofulvin.

High Pressure Liquid Chromatography. *System HU*—k' 7.1.

Ultraviolet Spectrum. Aqueous acid—243 nm $(A_1^1 = 541\ a)$, 301 nm; aqueous alkali—242 nm $(A_1^1 = 760\ a)$, 258 nm $(A_1^1 = 783\ a)$.

Infra-red Spectrum. Principal peaks at wavenumbers 1145, 1595, 1304, 1635, 682, 1090 (KCl disk).

Mass Spectrum. Principal peaks at *m/z* 214, 213, 92, 65, 215, 108, 39, 42.

Quantification. HIGH PRESSURE LIQUID CHROMATOGRAPHY. In plasma or blood: sulphadimidine and acetyl metabolite, sensitivity 6 µg/ml, UV detection—R. Whelpton *et al.*, *Clin. Chem.*, 1981, *27*, 1911–1914.

Disposition in the Body. Readily absorbed after oral administration. It is acetylated in the body, the degree of acetylation being dependent on the acetylator status of the subject. In rapid

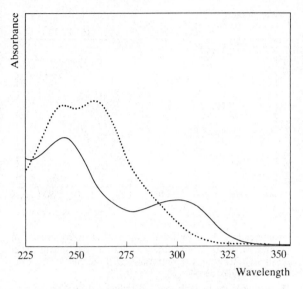

Absorbance

225   250   275   300   325   350

Wavelength

Wavelength

5   6   7   8   9   10   11 12 13 14 15

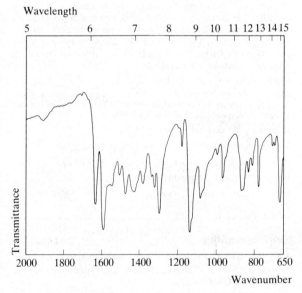

Transmittance

2000   1800   1600   1400   1200   1000   800   650

Wavenumber

HALF-LIFE. Derived from urinary excretion data, 1 to 5 hours for rapid acetylators and 3 to 11 hours (mean 6) for slow acetylators.

VOLUME OF DISTRIBUTION. About 0.6 litre/kg.

PROTEIN BINDING. In plasma, 60 to 90%.

Dose. An initial dose of up to 3 g, followed by 0.5 to 1.5 g every 6 hours.

Sulphaethidole   *Sulphonamide*

Synonyms. Aethazolum; Ethazol; SETD; Sulfaethidole; Sulphaethylthiadiazole.
Proprietary Name. Sulfa-Perlongit
N^1-(5-Ethyl-1,3,4-thiadiazol-2-yl)sulphanilamide
$C_{10}H_{12}N_4O_2S_2 = 284.4$
CAS—94-19-9

A white or yellowish-white crystalline powder. M.p. 186° to 190°.
Very slightly **soluble** in water; soluble 1 in 75 of ethanol, 1 in 13 of acetone, 1 in 1300 of chloroform, and 1 in 1700 of ether; freely soluble in solutions of alkali hydroxides.

Dissociation Constant. pK_a 5.6.

Colour Tests. Coniferyl Alcohol—orange; Copper Sulphate (Method 1)—green; Koppanyi–Zwikker Test—violet; Mercurous Nitrate—black; Nitrous Acid—yellow.

Thin-layer Chromatography. *System TA*—Rf 67; *system TD*—Rf 14; *system TE*—Rf 08; *system TF*—Rf 35.

Infra-red Spectrum. Principal peaks at wavenumbers 1086, 1298, 1538, 1149, 689, 917.

Mass Spectrum. Principal peaks at *m/z* 92, 284, 156, 108, 65, 106, 93, 220.

Quantification. HIGH PRESSURE LIQUID CHROMATOGRAPHY. The method referred to under Sulphamethoxazole may be used.

Disposition in the Body. Readily absorbed after oral administration and only slightly acetylated in the body. More than 75% of a dose is excreted in the urine in 48 hours as unchanged drug.

THERAPEUTIC CONCENTRATION.
Following oral administration of 3.9 g to 6 subjects, peak blood concentrations of 138 to 275 µg/ml (mean 227) were attained in about 2 hours (A. E. Nicholson *et al.*, *J. Am. pharm. Ass.*, 1960, *49*, 40–44).

HALF-LIFE. Plasma half-life, about 10 to 12 hours.

VOLUME OF DISTRIBUTION. About 0.1 litre/kg.

PROTEIN BINDING. In plasma, 96 to 99%.

Dose. Sulphaethidole has been given in sustained-release form in a dose of up to 3.9 g.

acetylators, 60 to 90% of the sulphadimidine in the blood is present as the N^4-acetyl derivative whereas, in slow acetylators, the proportion is only about 16 to 37%. About 50% of a dose is excreted in the urine in 48 hours. Of the excreted material, up to about 15% is unchanged drug and up to about 95% may be the acetyl derivative.

THERAPEUTIC CONCENTRATION. In plasma, free sulphadimidine, usually in the range 50 to 100 µg/ml.
Following a single oral dose of 1.5 g to 8 slow acetylators, plasma-sulphadimidine concentrations of 64.0 to 88.4 µg/ml (mean 80.7) were attained in 3 to 4 hours; after a similar dose to 8 rapid acetylators, peak plasma concentrations ranged from 38.8 to 64.1 µg/ml (mean 45.7) at 3 hours (U. M. Woolhouse and L. C. Atu-Taylor, *Clin. Pharmac. Ther.*, 1982, *31*, 377–383).

Sulphafurazole
Sulphonamide

Synonyms. Sulfafurazolum; Sulfisoxazole.

Proprietary Names. Chemovag; Gantrisin (tablets); Koro-Sulf; Novosoxazole; SK-Soxazole; Sosol; Soxa; Sulfagan; Sulfazole; Sulfizin; Urizole; Urogan; Velmatrol. It is an ingredient of Azo Gantrisin.

N^1-(3,4-Dimethylisoxazol-5-yl)sulphanilamide
$C_{11}H_{13}N_3O_3S = 267.3$
CAS—127-69-5

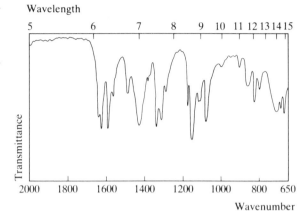

A white or yellowish-white crystalline powder. M.p. 194° to 199°.

Soluble 1 in 7700 of water, 1 in 50 of ethanol, 1 in 1000 of chloroform, and 1 in 800 of ether; freely soluble in acetone; soluble in methanol.

Acetyl Sulphafurazole

Synonym. Sulfisoxazole Acetyl

Proprietary Names. Gantrisin (suspension and syrup); Lipo-Gantrisin.

Note. Acetyl sulphafurazole [N-(3,4-dimethylisoxazol-5-yl)-N-sulphanilyl-acetamide] should be distinguished from the N^4-acetyl derivative formed from sulphafurazole by acetylation in the body.
$C_{13}H_{15}N_3O_4S = 309.3$
CAS—80-74-0
A white to slightly yellow crystalline powder. M.p. 192° to 195°.
Practically **insoluble** in water; soluble 1 in about 180 of ethanol, 1 in 35 of chloroform, 1 in about 1100 of ether, and 1 in about 200 of methanol.

Sulphafurazole Diethanolamine

Synonyms. Sulfisoxazole Diolamine; Sulphafurazole Diolamine.

Proprietary Name. Gantrisin (injection)
$C_{11}H_{13}N_3O_3S,C_4H_{11}NO_2 = 372.4$
CAS—4299-60-9
A white, fine, crystalline powder. M.p. 119° to 124°.
Soluble 1 in 2 of water, 1 in 16 of ethanol, 1 in 1000 of chloroform, and 1 in 4 of methanol; practically insoluble in ether.

Dissociation Constant. pK_a 5.0 (20°).

Partition Coefficient. Log P (octanol/pH 7.5), -0.9.

Colour Tests. Coniferyl Alcohol—orange; Copper Sulphate (Method 1)—brown; Koppanyi–Zwikker Test—blue-violet; Mercurous Nitrate—black; Nitrous Acid—orange.

Thin-layer Chromatography. *System TA*—Rf 65; *system TD*—Rf 25; *system TE*—Rf 08; *system TF*—Rf 52; *system TT*—Rf 74; *system TU*—Rf 48; *system TV*—Rf 04. (*Mercuric chloride-diphenylcarbazone reagent*, blue; *acidified potassium permanganate solution*, positive; *Van Urk reagent*, yellow.)

Gas Chromatography. *System GA*—RI 1212; *system GJ*—retention time of methyl derivative 0.42 relative to griseofulvin.

High Pressure Liquid Chromatography. *System HU*—k' 6.0.

Ultraviolet Spectrum. Aqueous acid—265 nm; aqueous alkali—253 nm ($A_1^1 = 783$ a).

Infra-red Spectrum. Principal peaks at wavenumbers 1166, 1633, 1598, 1092, 1647, 690 (KBr disk).

Mass Spectrum. Principal peaks at m/z 156, 92, 108, 65, 140, 43, 157, 42.

Wavelength

Transmittance / *Wavenumber*

Quantification. HIGH PRESSURE LIQUID CHROMATOGRAPHY. In plasma or urine: sulphafurazole and acetylsulphafurazole, sensitivity 50 ng/ml, UV detection—D. Jung and S. Øie, *Clin. Chem.*, 1980, *26*, 51–54.

Disposition in the Body. Rapidly absorbed after oral administration. It is acetylated in the body, about 30% of the sulphafurazole in the blood being in the form of the inactive N^4-acetyl derivative. It is rapidly excreted in the urine, almost the entire dose being excreted within 48 hours, with up to about 60% as unchanged drug and up to about 30% as the acetyl derivative. Excretion is influenced by the pH of the urine, the rate being increased when the urine is alkaline.

THERAPEUTIC CONCENTRATION.

After a single oral dose of 2 g to 7 subjects, peak plasma concentrations of sulphafurazole of 127 to 210 μg/ml (mean 169) were attained in 1 to 4 hours (S. A. Kaplan *et al.*, *J. pharm. Sci.*, 1972, *61*, 773–778).

HALF-LIFE. Plasma half-life, 4 to 7 hours.

VOLUME OF DISTRIBUTION. About 0.1 to 0.2 litre/kg.

CLEARANCE. Plasma clearance, about 0.3 ml/min/kg.

PROTEIN BINDING. In plasma, 85 to 95%.

Dose. An initial dose of 2 to 4 g, followed by 1 to 2 g every 4 to 6 hours.

Sulphaguanidine
Sulphonamide

Synonyms. Sulfaguanidine; Sulfamidinum; Sulginum.

Proprietary Names. Ganidan; Resulfon; S-Guanidine. It is an ingredient of Guanimycin.

N^1-Amidinosulphanilamide monohydrate
$C_7H_{10}N_4O_2S,H_2O = 232.3$
CAS—57-67-0 (anhydrous); *6190-55-2* (monohydrate)

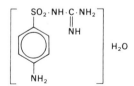

White crystals or powder, slowly darkening on exposure to light. M.p. 188° to 193°.

Soluble 1 in 1000 of water and 1 in 250 of ethanol; practically insoluble in ether; readily soluble in dilute mineral acids.

Partition Coefficient. Log *P* (octanol), −1.2.

Colour Tests. Coniferyl Alcohol—orange; Copper Sulphate (Method 1)—blue; Koppanyi–Zwikker Test—violet (transient).

Thin-layer Chromatography. *System TA*—Rf 65; *system TD*—Rf 01; *system TE*—Rf 25; *system TF*—Rf 06; *system TT*—Rf 21; *system TU*—Rf 90; *system TV*—Rf 48.

Gas Chromatography. *System GA*—not eluted.

Ultraviolet Spectrum. Aqueous acid—264 nm ($A_1^1 = 115$ a), 271 nm ($A_1^1 = 107$ c); aqueous alkali—259 nm ($A_1^1 = 758$ a).

Infra-red Spectrum. Principal peaks at wavenumbers 1620, 1129, 1230, 1537, 1075, 1176 (KBr disk).

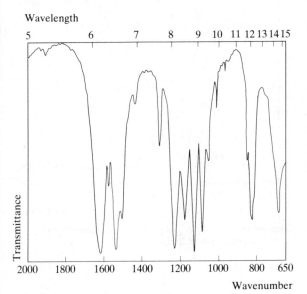

Wavelength

Transmittance / Wavenumber

Mass Spectrum. Principal peaks at *m/z* 92, 65, 108, 214, 156, 39, 109, 43.

Quantification. HIGH PRESSURE LIQUID CHROMATOGRAPHY. In plasma: sensitivity 10 ng/ml, UV detection—R. L. Suber and G. T. Edds, *J. liq. Chromat.*, 1980, *3*, 257–268.

Disposition in the Body. Absorption is variable after oral administration. It is rapidly excreted in the urine, about 30% of the excreted material being in the form of the inactive N^4-acetyl derivative. Large amounts are also eliminated in the faeces.

THERAPEUTIC CONCENTRATION. In plasma, usually in the range 15 to 40 µg/ml.

PROTEIN BINDING. In plasma, about 8%.

Dose. Sulphaguanidine has been given in doses of 9 g daily for 3 days.

Sulphamethizole   *Sulphonamide*

Synonyms. Sulfamethizole; Sulfamethylthiadiazole.
Proprietary Names. Microsul; Proklar-M; Rufol; S-Methizole; Thiosulfil; Urolex; Urolucosil; Uroz. It is an ingredient of Azotrex.

N^1-(5-Methyl-1,3,4-thiadiazol-2-yl)sulphanilamide
$C_9H_{10}N_4O_2S_2 = 270.3$
CAS—144-82-1

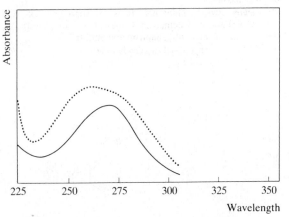

Colourless crystals or white or creamy-white crystalline powder. M.p. 208° to 212°.

Soluble 1 in 2000 of water, 1 in 25 of ethanol, 1 in 13 to 1 in 15 of acetone, and 1 in 1900 of chloroform and ether; soluble in solutions of alkali hydroxides and in dilute mineral acids.

Dissociation Constant. pK_a 5.5 (25°).

Partition Coefficient. Log *P* (octanol/pH 7.5), −1.1.

Colour Tests. Coniferyl Alcohol—orange; Copper Sulphate (Method 1)—green; Koppanyi–Zwikker Test—red-violet; Mercurous Nitrate—black; Nitrous Acid—yellow.

Thin-layer Chromatography. *System TA*—Rf 65; *system TD*—Rf 12; *system TE*—Rf 04; *system TF*—Rf 23; *system TT*—Rf 46; *system TU*—Rf 36; *system TV*—Rf 02. (*Mercuric chloride-diphenylcarbazone reagent*, blue; *acidified potassium permanganate solution*, positive; *Van Urk reagent*, yellow.)

Gas Chromatography. *System GJ*—retention time of methyl derivative 0.98 relative to griseofulvin.

Ultraviolet Spectrum. Aqueous acid—268 nm ($A_1^1 = 542$ a); aqueous alkali—260 nm.

Absorbance / Wavelength

Infra-red Spectrum. Principal peaks at wavenumbers 1549, 1134, 699, 1084, 1152, 1600 (KBr disk). (See below)

Mass Spectrum. Principal peaks at *m/z* 92, 270, 65, 156, 108, 106, 93, 59.

Quantification. HIGH PRESSURE LIQUID CHROMATOGRAPHY. The method referred to under Sulphamethoxazole may be used.

Disposition in the Body. Readily absorbed after oral administration and only slightly acetylated in the body. It is rapidly excreted in the urine, up to 90% of a dose being excreted within 24 hours, mainly as unchanged drug.

THERAPEUTIC CONCENTRATION.
Following oral administration of 0.5 g of sulphamethizole to 5 subjects, a mean peak blood concentration of 20 µg/ml was attained in about 2 hours (G. L. Mattock and I. J. McGilveray, *J. pharm. Sci.*, 1972, *61*, 746–749).

Wavelength

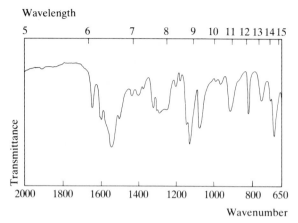

HALF-LIFE. Plasma half-life, 1 to 2 hours.

VOLUME OF DISTRIBUTION. About 0.3 litre/kg.

CLEARANCE. Blood clearance, about 3 ml/min/kg.

PROTEIN BINDING. In plasma, about 90%.

Dose. 1 to 4 g daily.

Sulphamethoxazole   *Sulphonamide*

Synonyms. Sulfamethoxazole; Sulfisomezole. It is an ingredient of Co-trimoxazole.

Proprietary Names. Gantanol. It is an ingredient of Azo Gantanol, Bactrim, Chemotrim, Comox, Cotrimox, Eusaprim, Fectrim, Laratrim, Septra, Septrin, and Sulfotrimin.

N^1-(5-Methylisoxazol-3-yl)sulphanilamide
$C_{10}H_{11}N_3O_3S = 253.3$
CAS—723-46-6

CH₃ structure: N^1-(5-Methylisoxazol-3-yl)sulphanilamide with CH₃, O, N in isoxazole ring, NH·SO₂ linked to benzene ring with NH₂

A white or yellowish-white crystalline powder. M.p. 168° to 172°.

Very slightly **soluble** in water; soluble 1 in 50 of ethanol and 1 in 3 of acetone; practically insoluble in chloroform and ether; soluble in solutions of alkali hydroxides.

Dissociation Constant. pK_a 5.6 (25°).

Colour Tests. Coniferyl Alcohol—orange; Copper Sulphate (Method 1)—green; Koppanyi–Zwikker Test—blue-violet; Mercurous Nitrate—black; Nitrous Acid—yellow.

Thin-layer Chromatography. *System TA*—Rf 65; *system TD*—Rf 26; *system TE*—Rf 05; *system TF*—Rf 54; *system TT*—Rf 88; *system TU*—Rf 33; *system TV*—Rf 02. (*Mercuric chloride-diphenylcarbazone reagent*, blue; *acidified potassium permanganate solution*, positive; *Van Urk reagent*, yellow.)

Gas Chromatography. *System GJ*—retention time of the methyl derivative of sulphamethoxazole 0.40 and of N^4-acetylsulphamethoxazole 0.91, both relative to griseofulvin.

High Pressure Liquid Chromatography. *System HU*—sulphamethoxazole k′ 4.8, N^4-acetylsulphamethoxazole k′ 4.9.

Ultraviolet Spectrum. Aqueous acid—265 nm $(A_1^1 = 175\ a)$; aqueous alkali—256 nm $(A_1^1 = 673\ a)$.

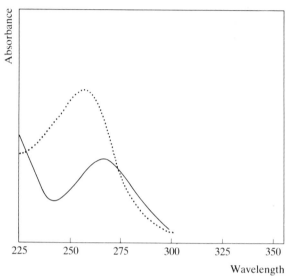

Infra-red Spectrum. Principal peaks at wavenumbers 1145, 1160, 1599, 1621, 685, 1306 (KBr disk).

Wavelength

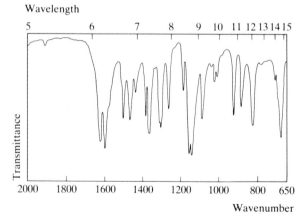

Mass Spectrum. Principal peaks at m/z 156, 92, 108, 65, 140, 253, 157, 43.

Quantification. COLORIMETRY. In plasma—P. Heizmann and P. Haefelfinger, *Experientia*, 1981, *37*, 806–807.

HIGH PRESSURE LIQUID CHROMATOGRAPHY. In serum or urine: detection limit 500 ng/ml, UV detection—T. B. Vree *et al.*, *J. Chromat.*, 1978, *146*; *Biomed. Appl.*, *3*, 103–112.

Disposition in the Body. Readily absorbed after oral administration. It is metabolised mainly by acetylation with the formation of the N^1-acetyl and N^4-acetyl derivatives; about 15% of the sulphamethoxazole in the blood is present as acetylated metabolites. Excreted in the urine mostly as the N^4-acetyl derivative and unchanged sulphamethoxazole together with some glucuronide conjugates. Urinary excretion is variable and is dependent on the pH of the urine, the proportion of unchanged drug excreted being increased when the urine is alkaline. Up to about 25% of the dose is excreted unchanged when the urine is acid, rising to 40% or more in alkaline urine. The amount of the N^4-acetyl derivative excreted may be 30 to 70% of the dose. Sulphamethoxazole is frequently administered together with trimethoprim but this does not affect its metabolism.

THERAPEUTIC CONCENTRATION.

After a single oral dose containing 800 mg of sulphamethoxazole and 160 mg of trimethoprim given to 8 subjects, peak serum concentrations of 28 to 45 µg/ml (mean 39) of sulphamethoxazole were attained in 2 to 4 hours. Peak concentrations of trimethoprim of 0.9 to 1.5 µg/ml (mean 1.3) were attained in 1 to 2 hours (W. A. Craig and C. M. Kunin, *Ann. intern. Med.*, 1973, *78*, 491–497).

Oral dosing of 5 subjects with 800 mg of sulphamethoxazole and 160 mg of trimethoprim twice daily, produced minimum steady-state plasma concentrations of about 55 µg/ml of sulphamethoxazole and 1.7 µg/ml of trimethoprim, on the ninth day (P. Kremers *et al.*, *J. clin. Pharmac.*, 1974, *14*, 112–117).

TOXICITY. Plasma concentrations greater than 400 µg/ml may be associated with toxic effects.

HALF-LIFE. Plasma half-life, 9 to 12 hours.

VOLUME OF DISTRIBUTION. About 0.2 litre/kg.

CLEARANCE. Plasma clearance, about 0.2 ml/min/kg.

DISTRIBUTION IN BLOOD. Plasma: whole blood ratio, about 1.35.

SALIVA. Plasma: saliva ratio, about 14.

PROTEIN BINDING. In plasma, 60 to 70%.

NOTE. For a review of the clinical pharmacokinetics of sulphamethoxazole and trimethoprim see R. B. Patel and P. G. Welling, *Clin. Pharmacokinet.*, 1980, *5*, 405–423.

Dose. Usually 2 g initially, followed by 1 g twice daily; maximum of 3 g daily.

Sulphamethoxydiazine   *Sulphonamide*

Synonyms. Sulfameter; Sulfamethoxydiazine; Sulfametin; Sulfametorinum; Sulphamethoxydin.

Proprietary Names. Bayrena; Durenat; Kirocid; Sullá.

N^1-(5-Methoxypyrimidin-2-yl)sulphanilamide

$C_{11}H_{12}N_4O_3S = 280.3$

CAS—651-06-9

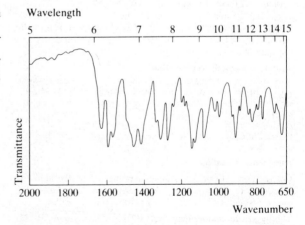

A white or yellowish-white crystalline powder. M.p. 209° to 213°.

Practically **insoluble** in water; slightly soluble in ethanol; sparingly soluble in acetone; freely soluble in aqueous solutions of alkali hydroxides and carbonates.

Dissociation Constant. pK$_a$ 7.0.

Colour Tests. Coniferyl Alcohol—orange; Copper Sulphate (Method 1)—violet-brown; Koppanyi–Zwikker Test—pink; Mercurous Nitrate—black; Nitrous Acid—yellow.

Thin-layer Chromatography. *System TA*—Rf 60; *system TD*—Rf 24; *system TE*—Rf 12; *system TF*—Rf 43; *system TT*—Rf 55; *system TU*—Rf 17; *system TV*—Rf 15.

Gas Chromatography. *System GJ*—retention time of methyl derivative 1.38 relative to griseofulvin.

High Pressure Liquid Chromatography. *System HU*—k′ 8.2.

Ultraviolet Spectrum. Aqueous alkali—245 nm (A$^1_1$ = 920 a).

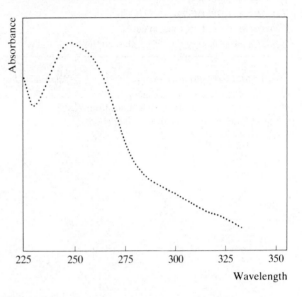

Infra-red Spectrum. Principal peaks at wavenumbers 1153, 1597, 1140, 1284, 1090, 925 (KBr disk).

Mass Spectrum. Principal peaks at *m/z* 216, 215, 92, 65, 108, 54, 125, 39.

Disposition in the Body. Sulphamethoxydiazine is a long-acting sulphonamide which is readily absorbed after oral administration. It is acetylated in the body, about 10% being present in the blood as the inactive N^4-acetyl derivative. It is excreted slowly in the urine, 20 to 40% of a dose being excreted in 24 hours and about 70% in 3 days. About 50% of the excreted material is unchanged drug, about 25% is the acetyl derivative, and about 20% is a glucuronide conjugate.

THERAPEUTIC CONCENTRATION.
After a single oral dose of 1 g to 4 subjects, peak serum concentrations of 62 to 90 µg/ml (mean 80) were attained in about 6 to 8 hours; following a single oral dose of 2 g to a further 4 subjects, peak serum concentrations of 113 to 148 µg/ml (mean 134) were reported at 6 to 8 hours; mean peak serum concentrations of 86 µg/ml and 166 µg/ml respectively were reported following daily oral doses of 0.5 and 1 g for 3 days (W. H. Chew et al., Clin. Pharmac. Ther., 1965, 6, 307–315).

HALF-LIFE. Plasma half-life, 29 to 59 hours (mean 37).

VOLUME OF DISTRIBUTION. About 0.3 litre/kg.

PROTEIN BINDING. In plasma, about 80%.

Dose. An initial dose of 1 or 1.5 g, followed by 500 mg daily.

Sulphamethoxypyridazine   *Sulphonamide*

Synonym. Sulfamethoxypyridazine
Proprietary Names. Lederkyn; Microcid; Midicel.
N^1-(6-Methoxypyridazin-3-yl)sulphanilamide
$C_{11}H_{12}N_4O_3S = 280.3$
CAS—80-35-3

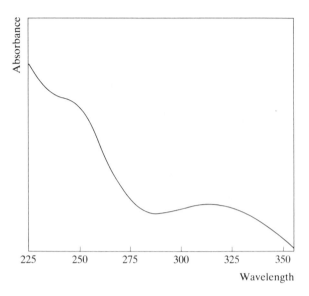

A white or yellowish-white crystalline powder which slowly darkens on exposure to light. M.p. 180° to 183°.
Very slightly **soluble** in water; sparingly soluble in ethanol; soluble 1 in 25 of acetone and 1 in 400 of chloroform; practically insoluble in ether; freely **soluble** in dilute mineral acids and solutions of alkali hydroxides.

Acetyl Sulphamethoxypyridazine

Note. Acetyl sulphamethoxypyridazine [N-(6-methoxypyridazin-3-yl)-N-sulphanilylacetamide] should be distinguished from the N^4-acetyl derivative formed from sulphamethoxypyridazine by acetylation in the body.
$C_{13}H_{14}N_4O_4S = 322.3$
CAS—3568-43-2
Crystals. M.p. 186° to 187°, with decomposition.
Very **soluble** in water.

Dissociation Constant. pK_a 7.2 (20°).

Colour Tests. Coniferyl Alcohol—orange; Copper Sulphate (Method 1)—green-brown; Koppanyi-Zwikker Test—red-violet; Mercurous Nitrate—black; Nitrous Acid—yellow.

Thin-layer Chromatography. *System TA*—Rf 65; *system TD*—Rf 19; *system TE*—Rf 11; *system TF*—Rf 39; *system TT*—Rf 53; *system TU*—Rf 26; *system TV*—Rf 50.

Gas Chromatography. *System GJ*—retention time of methyl derivative 0.93 relative to griseofulvin.

High Pressure Liquid Chromatography. *System HU*—k' 7.5.

Ultraviolet Spectrum. Aqueous acid—316 nm ($A_1^1 = 163$ b); aqueous alkali—250 nm ($A_1^1 = 712$ a).

Infra-red Spectrum. Principal peaks at wavenumbers 1159, 1599, 1130, 1305, 1630, 1088 (KBr disk).

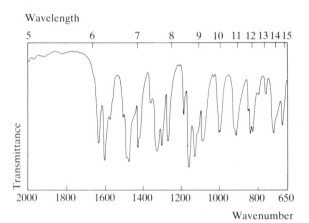

Mass Spectrum. Principal peaks at m/z 215, 92, 216, 65, 108, 53, 69, 39.

Quantification. HIGH PRESSURE LIQUID CHROMATOGRAPHY. The method referred to under Sulphamethoxazole may be used.

Disposition in the Body. Sulphamethoxypyridazine is a long-acting sulphonamide which is readily absorbed after oral administration and may be detected in blood for up to 7 days after discontinuation of treatment. It is acetylated in the body and 10 to 15% of the sulphamethoxypyridazine in the blood is present as the inactive N^4-acetyl derivative. About 45% of a dose is excreted in the urine in 48 hours, with 40 to 70% of the excreted material as the acetyl derivative, about 20% as unchanged drug, and about 13% as glucuronide conjugates. Excretion is influenced by the pH of the urine, the rate being increased when the urine is alkaline.

THERAPEUTIC CONCENTRATION.
Blood concentrations of 110 to 180 µg/ml were attained in 5 hours following an oral dose of 4 g (H. Seneca, J. Am. med. Ass., 1966, 198, 975–980).

HALF-LIFE. Plasma half-life, 1 to 3 days.

VOLUME OF DISTRIBUTION. About 0.2 litre/kg.

DISTRIBUTION IN BLOOD. Small amounts are taken up by the erythrocytes.

PROTEIN BINDING. In plasma, 80 to 90%.

Dose. An initial dose of 1 to 2 g, followed by 500 mg daily.

Sulphamoxole
Sulphonamide

Synonyms. SDMO; Sulfamoxole; Sulphadimethyloxazole. It is an ingredient of Co-trifamole.
Proprietary Names. Justamil; Sulfuno. It is an ingredient of Co-Fram and Supristol.
N^1-(4,5-Dimethyloxazol-2-yl)sulphanilamide
$C_{11}H_{13}N_3O_3S = 267.3$
CAS—729-99-7

A white crystalline powder. M.p. about 193°.
Slightly **soluble** in water.

Dissociation Constant. pK_a 7.4.

Partition Coefficient. Log P (chloroform/pH 7.4), −0.3.

Colour Tests. Coniferyl Alcohol—orange; Copper Sulphate (Method 1)—green-brown; Mercurous Nitrate—black; Nitrous Acid—yellow.

Thin-layer Chromatography. *System TA*—Rf 67. (*Van Urk reagent*, positive.)

Gas Chromatography. *System GA*—not eluted; *system GJ*—retention time of methyl derivative 0.40 relative to griseofulvin.

High Pressure Liquid Chromatography. *System HU*—k' 12.6.

Ultraviolet Spectrum. Aqueous acid—249 nm ($A_1^1 = 375$ b); aqueous alkali—250 nm ($A_1^1 = 685$ b).

Infra-red Spectrum. Principal peaks at wavenumbers 1605, 1626, 1127, 1145, 1276, 1094 (KBr disk).

Disposition in the Body. Rapidly absorbed after oral administration. About 65 to 71% of a dose is excreted in the urine, mainly as unchanged drug, the N^4-acetyl conjugate, and sulphanilamide.

THERAPEUTIC CONCENTRATION.
Following single oral doses of 1, 2, and 4 g to 4 subjects, peak serum concentrations of 73.5 to 94.8 (mean 88), 138 to 182 (mean 157), and 215 to 290 µg/ml (mean 241), respectively, were attained in about 2 hours (C. G. vom Bruck *et al., Arzneimittel-Forsch.*, 1960, *10*, 621–626).

Following oral administration of 400 mg twice a day to 10 subjects (in combination with trimethoprim 80 mg), a mean maximum steady-state plasma concentration of 75 µg/ml and a mean trough concentration of 42 µg/ml were reported (I. D. Watson *et al., Br. J. clin. Pharmac.*, 1982, *14*, 437–443).

HALF-LIFE. Plasma half-life, 4 to 11 hours.

VOLUME OF DISTRIBUTION. About 0.1 litre/kg.

DISTRIBUTION IN BLOOD. Plasma : whole blood ratio, about 1.8.

PROTEIN BINDING. In plasma, about 25%.

Dose. 2 g daily for 1 or 2 days, followed by 1 g daily.

Sulphanilamide
Sulphonamide

Synonyms. Solfammide; Streptocidum; Sulfaminum; Sulfanilamide.
Proprietary Names. Exoseptoplix; Streptosil; Sulfonamid-Spuman; Tablamide. It is an ingredient of Rhinamid.
4-Aminobenzenesulphonamide
$C_6H_8N_2O_2S = 172.2$
CAS—63-74-1

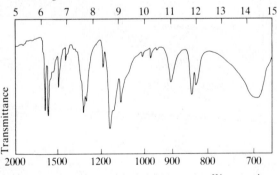

A white crystalline powder. On heating the dry powder it becomes violet-blue and eventually aniline and ammonia are produced. M.p. about 165°.

Soluble 1 in 170 of water, 1 in 30 of ethanol, and 1 in 4 of acetone; practically insoluble in chloroform and ether; soluble in hydrochloric acid and solutions of alkali hydroxides.

Dissociation Constant. pK_a 10.4 (20°).

Partition Coefficient. Log P (octanol/pH 7.5), −0.9.

Colour Tests. Coniferyl Alcohol—orange; Copper Sulphate (Method 1)—blue; Koppanyi–Zwikker Test—blue-violet; Mercurous Nitrate—black.

Thin-layer Chromatography. *System TA*—Rf 67; *system TD*—Rf 13; *system TE*—Rf 52; *system TF*—Rf 46; *system TT*—Rf 61; *system TU*—Rf 96; *system TV*—Rf 66. (*Mercuric chloride-diphenylcarbazone reagent*, blue; *acidified potassium permanganate solution*, positive; *Van Urk reagent*, yellow.)

Gas Chromatography. *System GA*—RI 2166.

High Pressure Liquid Chromatography. *System HU*—sulphanilamide k' 8.9, N^4-acetylsulphanilamide k' 9.6.

Ultraviolet Spectrum. Aqueous acid—262 nm ($A_1^1 = 106$ a), 269 nm ($A_1^1 = 85$ a); aqueous alkali—250 nm ($A_1^1 = 932$ b).

Infra-red Spectrum. Principal peaks at wavenumbers 1149, 1603, 1316, 1637, 1099, 1294 (KBr disk).

Wavelength

Transmittance

Wavenumber

Mass Spectrum. Principal peaks at *m/z* 172, 92, 156, 65, 108, 173, 39, 174.

Dose. Sulphanilamide has been given in an initial dose of 3 g, followed by 1 to 1.5 g every 4 hours.

Sulphaphenazole   *Sulphonamide*

Synonyms. Sulfaphenazole; Sulphaphenylpyrazol.
Proprietary Names. Fenazolo; Orisul; Sulforal.
N^1-(1-Phenylpyrazol-5-yl)sulphanilamide
$C_{15}H_{14}N_4O_2S = 314.4$
CAS—526-08-9

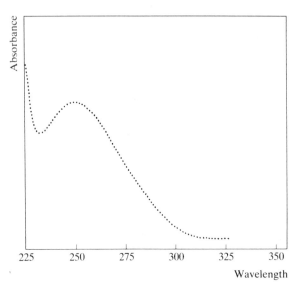

A white crystalline powder. When heated, the powder becomes brown; when further heated, it produces yellow fumes and an odour of sulphur dioxide. M.p. 179° to 183°.
Very slightly **soluble** in water, ethanol, chloroform, and ether; soluble in acetone, mineral acids, and solutions of alkali hydroxides.

Dissociation Constant. pK_a 6.5.

Partition Coefficient. Log P (octanol/pH 7.5), 0.1.

Colour Tests. Coniferyl Alcohol—orange; Copper Sulphate (Method 1)—blue; Koppanyi–Zwikker Test—blue-violet; Mercurous Nitrate—black; Nitrous Acid—yellow.

Thin-layer Chromatography. *System TA*—Rf 69; *system TD*—Rf 29; *system TE*—Rf 09; *system TF*—Rf 51; *system TT*—Rf 89; *system TU*—Rf 70; *system TV*—Rf 13.

Gas Chromatography. *System GJ*—retention time of methyl derivative 1.71 relative to griseofulvin.

Ultraviolet Spectrum. Aqueous alkali—249 nm ($A_1^1 = 700$ b).

Infra-red Spectrum. Principal peaks at wavenumbers 1148, 1507, 1313, 1592, 675, 1630 (KBr disk).

Wavelength

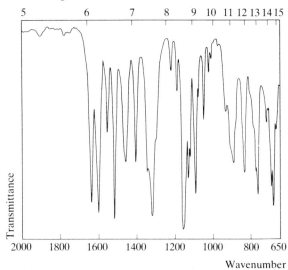

Mass Spectrum. Principal peaks at *m/z* 156, 158, 92, 77, 157, 314, 108, 65.

Quantification. HIGH PRESSURE LIQUID CHROMATOGRAPHY. The method referred to under Sulphamethoxazole may be used.

Disposition in the Body. Readily absorbed after oral administration. It is acetylated in the body and slowly excreted in the urine, about 70 to 80% of a dose being excreted in 72 hours, 30% as the acetyl derivative.

HALF-LIFE. Plasma half-life, 8 to 12 hours.

PROTEIN BINDING. In plasma, about 90 to 99%.

Dose. 2 to 3 g daily for 2 days, followed by 1 g daily.

Sulphapyridine   *Sulphonamide*

Synonym. Sulfapyridine
Proprietary Names. Dagenan; M & B 693. It is an ingredient of Trinamide (vet.).
N^1-(2-Pyridyl)sulphanilamide
$C_{11}H_{11}N_3O_2S = 249.3$
CAS—144-83-2

A white or yellowish-white crystalline powder or granules. It slowly darkens on exposure to light. M.p. 190° to 193°.
Soluble 1 in 3500 of water, 1 in about 440 of ethanol, and 1 in 65 of acetone; practically insoluble in chloroform and ether; soluble in dilute mineral acids and aqueous solutions of alkali hydroxides.

Sulphapyridine Sodium

Synonym. Soluble Sulphapyridine

$C_{11}H_{10}N_3NaO_2S = 271.3$ (or with $1H_2O = 289.3$)

CAS—127-57-1 (anhydrous); *6101-41-3* (monohydrate)

A white or yellowish-white crystalline powder. On exposure to air, it slowly absorbs carbon dioxide with the liberation of sulphapyridine and becomes incompletely soluble in water.

Soluble 1 in 3 of water and 1 in 10 of ethanol.

Dissociation Constant. pK_a 8.4 (25°).

Partition Coefficient. Log P (octanol/pH 7.5), 0.9.

Colour Tests. Coniferyl Alcohol—orange; Copper Sulphate (Method 1)—green → brown-green; Koppanyi–Zwikker Test—pink; Mercurous Nitrate—black; Nitrous Acid—yellow.

Thin-layer Chromatography. *System TA*—Rf 67; *system TD*—Rf 16; *system TE*—Rf 24; *system TF*—Rf 42; *system TT*—Rf 47; *system TU*—Rf 43; *system TV*—Rf 73.

Gas Chromatography. *System GJ*—retention time of methyl derivative 0.47 relative to griseofulvin.

High Pressure Liquid Chromatography. *System HU*—k' 3.8.

Ultraviolet Spectrum. Aqueous acid—240 nm ($A_1^1 = 392$ a); aqueous alkali—247 nm.

Infra-red Spectrum. Principal peaks at wavenumbers 1585, 1264, 1127, 1078, 1639, 950 (KBr disk).

Mass Spectrum. Principal peaks at m/z 184, 92, 185, 65, 39, 108, 66, 186.

Quantification. COLORIMETRY. In serum, saliva or plasma: sensitivity 1.5 μg/ml for sulphapyridine or the acetyl metabolite—T. R. Bates and H. J. Pieniaszek, *Analyt. Lett. (Part B)*, 1978, *11*, 709–720.

HIGH PRESSURE LIQUID CHROMATOGRAPHY. In plasma: sulphapyridine and metabolites, detection limit 1 μg/ml, UV detection—C. Fischer and U. Klotz, *J. Chromat.*, 1978, *146*; *Biomed. Appl.*, *3*, 157–162. In plasma, saliva or urine: comparison with GC, detection limits 50 ng for HPLC (fluorescence detection), 10 ng for GC (ECD)—M. E. Sharp *et al.*, *Can. J. pharm. Sci.*, 1980, *15*, 35–38.

Disposition in the Body. Irregularly absorbed after oral administration. It is acetylated in the body, about 30 to 70% of the sulphapyridine in the blood being present as the inactive N^4-acetyl derivative; the extent of acetylation is genetically determined. The rate of excretion appears to be irregular but about 25% of a dose may be excreted in the urine as the acetyl derivative and about 20% as unchanged drug in 60 hours. Other metabolites include the 5-hydroxy derivative and its glucuronide conjugate.

Sulphapyridine is a metabolite of sulphasalazine.

THERAPEUTIC CONCENTRATION.

After an oral dose of 2.5 g given to 5 subjects, peak serum concentrations of sulphapyridine plus metabolites of about 35 to 60 μg/ml were attained in 3 to 5 hours (H. Schröder and D. E. S. Campbell, *Clin. Pharmac. Ther.*, 1972, *13*, 539–551).

TOXICITY. Toxic effects are associated with plasma concentrations greater than 50 μg/ml.

HALF-LIFE. Plasma half-life, about 6 hours in rapid acetylators, increased in slow acetylators to about 13 hours.

VOLUME OF DISTRIBUTION. About 0.4 litre/kg.

SALIVA. Plasma: saliva ratio, about 1.8.

PROTEIN BINDING. In plasma, about 40 to 60%.

Dose. Initially 3 or 4 g daily, followed by 0.5 to 1 g daily.

Sulphasalazine   *Sulphonamide*

Synonyms. Salazosulfapyridine; Salicylazosulphapyridine; Sulfasalazine.

Proprietary Names. Azulfidine; Colo-Pleon; Salazopyrin(e); Salisulf; SAS-500.

4 - Hydroxy - 4' - (2-pyridylsulphamoyl)azobenzene - 3 - carboxylic acid

$C_{18}H_{14}N_4O_5S = 398.4$

CAS—599-79-1

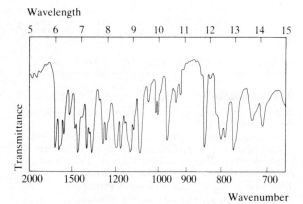

A fine bright yellow to brownish-yellow powder. M.p. about 255°, with decomposition.

Practically **insoluble** in water, chloroform, and ether; soluble 1 in 2900 of ethanol; soluble in aqueous solutions of alkali hydroxides.

Dissociation Constant. pK_a 0.6, 2.4, 9.7, 11.8.

Colour Tests. Copper Sulphate (Method 1)—orange-brown; Palladium Chloride—black.

Thin-layer Chromatography. *System TA*—Rf 66; *system TD*—Rf 00; *system TE*—Rf 00; *system TF*—Rf 00. (Visible orange spot.)

Infra-red Spectrum. Principal peaks at wavenumbers 1078, 1123, 772, 1634, 1175, 1672 (Nujol mull).

Wavelength

Infra-red spectrum with axes: Wavelength (top, 5 to 15), Wavenumber (bottom, 2000 to 700), Transmittance (vertical).

Wavenumber

Mass Spectrum. Principal peaks at m/z 169, 92, 289, 65, 290, 39, 333, 184.

Quantification. HIGH PRESSURE LIQUID CHROMATOGRAPHY. In plasma: sulphapyridine, acetylsulphapyridine, 5-aminosalicylic acid, and 5-acetamidosalicylic acid, sensitivity 500 ng/ml, UV and fluorescence detection—P. N. Shaw *et al.*, *J. Chromat.*, 1983, *274*; *Biomed. Appl.*, *25*, 393–397. In plasma or urine: 5-aminosalicylic acid and 5-acetamidosalicylic acid, sensitivity 20 ng/ml, fluorescence detection—C. Fischer *et al.*, *J. Chromat.*,

1981, *225*; *Biomed. Appl.*, *14*, 498–503. In bile: 5-aminosalicylic acid and 5-acetamidosalicylic acid, fluorescence detection—C. Fischer *et al.*, *Br. J. clin. Pharmac.*, 1983, *15*, 273–274.

Disposition in the Body. Partially and irregularly absorbed after oral administration. The absorbed material is not metabolised but is excreted unchanged in the urine and accounts for up to about 10% of the dose. The greater part of the dose passes unchanged into the colon where it is metabolised by bacteria to sulphapyridine and 5-aminosalicylic acid, which is thought to be the active moiety. The sulphapyridine so formed is absorbed, and metabolised by N^4-acetylation, ring hydroxylation, and glucuronidation. The degree of acetylation is dependent on the acetylator status of the subject. About 60% of the dose is excreted in the urine as free and acetylated sulphapyridine and their glucuronides, and about 25% of the dose is eliminated as sulphapyridine in the faeces. The 5-aminosalicylic acid is partially absorbed and metabolised by *N*-acetylation; about 30% is excreted in the urine as unchanged drug and 5-acetamidosalicylic acid, and most of the remainder is eliminated unchanged in the faeces.

THERAPEUTIC CONCENTRATION.

Following a single oral dose of 2 g to 8 subjects, peak plasma concentrations of 7 to 32 μg/ml (mean 17) of sulphasalazine were attained in about 3 hours; peak plasma concentrations of sulphapyridine averaged about 20 μg/ml (E. M. Ryde and J. J. Lima, *Curr. ther. Res.*, 1981, *29*, 728–737). Following daily oral doses of 3 g to 6 subjects, minimum steady-state plasma concentrations of 0.04 to 0.34 μg/ml of 5-aminosalicylic acid and 0.2 to 1.4 μg/ml of 5-acetamidosalicylic acid were reported (C. Fischer *et al.*, *J. Chromat.*, 1981, 225; *Biomed. Appl.*, 14, 498–503). After daily oral doses of 4 g to 9 subjects, steady-state serum concentrations of 37 to 92 μg/ml (median 50) for total sulphapyridine and its metabolites, 4.7 to 45 μg/ml (median 12) for sulphasalazine, and less than 2 μg/ml for 5-aminosalicylic acid metabolites were reported on the 5th day (H. Schröder and D. E. S. Campbell, *Clin. Pharmac. Ther.*, 1972, *13*, 539–551).

TOXICITY. Toxic effects are associated with plasma concentrations of sulphapyridine greater than 50 μg/ml.

HALF-LIFE. Plasma half-life, sulphasalazine, 6 to 17 hours (mean 10).

NOTE. For a review of the pharmacokinetics of sulphasalazine see K. M. Das and R. Dubin, *Clin. Pharmacokinet.*, 1976, *1*, 406–425.

Dose. Initially 4 to 8 g daily; maintenance, 1.5 to 2 g daily.

Sulphasomidine

Sulphonamide

Synonyms. Sulfa-isodimérazine; Sulfaisodimidine; Sulfasomidine; Sulfisomidine.

Note. Sulfadimethylpyrimidine has been used as a synonym for sulphasomidine and is sometimes used as a synonym for sulphadimidine. Care should be taken to avoid confusion between the two compounds, which are isomeric.

Proprietary Names. Elcosine; Elkosin(e); Pepsilphen.

N^1-(2,6-Dimethylpyrimidin-4-yl)sulphanilamide

$C_{12}H_{14}N_4O_2S = 278.3$

CAS—515-64-0

A white or creamy-white finely crystalline powder which slowly darkens on exposure to light. M.p. 244° to 246°.

Slightly **soluble** in water and ethanol; very slightly soluble in chloroform and ether; readily soluble in dilute mineral acids and solutions of alkali hydroxides.

Dissociation Constant. pK_a 7.5 (27°).

Colour Tests. Coniferyl Alcohol—orange; Copper Sulphate (Method 1)—green; Koppanyi-Zwikker Test—blue-violet (transient); Mercurous Nitrate—black; Nitrous Acid—yellow.

Thin-layer Chromatography. *System TA*—Rf 64; *system TD*—Rf 05; *system TE*—Rf 05; *system TF*—Rf 16; *system TT*—Rf 11; *system TU*—Rf 49; *system TV*—Rf 20.

Ultraviolet Spectrum. Aqueous acid—262 nm; aqueous alkali—262 nm ($A_1^1 = 764$ b); methanol—272 nm ($A_1^1 = 745$ a).

Infra-red Spectrum. Principal peaks at wavenumbers 1125, 1260, 1138, 1595, 1650, 1070 (KBr disk).

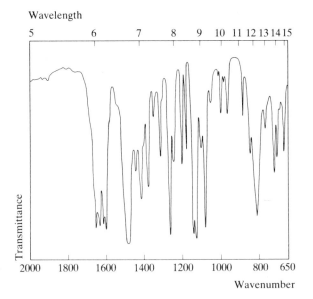

Wavelength

Mass Spectrum. Principal peaks at *m/z* 214, 92, 65, 213, 108, 42, 215, 39.

Quantification. HIGH PRESSURE LIQUID CHROMATOGRAPHY. The method referred to under Sulphamethoxazole may be used.

Disposition in the Body. Absorbed after oral administration. It is acetylated in the body to only a small extent, about 10 to 25% of the material in the blood being in the form of the inactive N^4-acetyl derivative. It is rapidly excreted in the urine, about 87% of the dose being excreted within 48 hours as unchanged drug together with about 6% as the acetyl derivative.

HALF-LIFE. Plasma half-life, 6 to 8 hours.

PROTEIN BINDING. In plasma, 40 to 90% (dose-dependent).

Dose. Sulphasomidine has been given in an initial dose of 2 to 4 g, followed by 6 g daily.

Sulphathiazole   *Sulphonamide*

Synonyms. Norsulfazolum; Sulfanilamidothiazolum; Sulfathiazole; Sulfonazolum.

Proprietary Names. Cibazol: Sulfamul; Thiazamide. It is an ingredient of Streptotriad, Sulphatriad, and Sultrin.

N^1-(Thiazol-2-yl)sulphanilamide

$C_9H_9N_3O_2S_2 = 255.3$

CAS—72-14-0

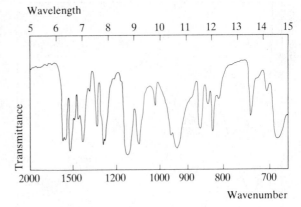

Wavelength

A white crystalline powder which slowly darkens on exposure to light. M.p. 200° to 203°.

Soluble 1 in 2500 of water and 1 in 120 of ethanol; practically insoluble in chloroform and ether; soluble in dilute mineral acids and solutions of alkali hydroxides and carbonates.

Sulphathiazole Sodium

Synonym. Soluble Sulphathiazole

Proprietary Name. It is an ingredient of Tylasul Soluble (vet.).

$C_9H_8N_3NaO_2S_2,5H_2O = 367.4$

CAS—144-74-1 (anhydrous); *6791-71-5* (pentahydrate)

A white or yellowish-white microcrystalline powder. It slowly darkens on exposure to light; on exposure to moist air it absorbs carbon dioxide and becomes incompletely soluble in water.

Soluble 1 in 3 of water and 1 in 20 of ethanol.

Dissociation Constant. pK_a 7.1 (25°).

Partition Coefficient. Log P (octanol/pH 7.5), −0.4.

Colour Tests. Coniferyl Alcohol—orange; Copper Sulphate (Method 1)—violet-brown; Koppanyi–Zwikker Test—red-violet; Mercurous Nitrate—black; Nitrous Acid—yellow.

Thin-layer Chromatography. *System TA*—Rf 66; *system TD*—Rf 09; *system TE*—Rf 09; *system TF*—Rf 20; *system TT*—Rf 53; *system TU*—Rf 40; *system TV*—Rf 05. (*Mercuric chloride–diphenylcarbazone reagent*, blue; *acidified potassium permanganate solution*, positive; *Van Urk reagent*, yellow.)

Gas Chromatography. *System GA*—not eluted; *system GJ*—retention time of methyl derivative 0.49 relative to griseofulvin.

High Pressure Liquid Chromatography. *System HU*—k′ 13.4.

Ultraviolet Spectrum. Aqueous acid—280 nm ($A_1^1 = 498$ a); aqueous alkali—256 nm ($A_1^1 = 716$ b).

Infra-red Spectrum. Principal peaks at wavenumbers 1130, 1527, 929, 1274, 1082, 1592 (Nujol mull).

Mass Spectrum. Principal peaks at *m/z* 92, 156, 65, 108, 191, 45, 39, 55.

Quantification. HIGH PRESSURE LIQUID CHROMATOGRAPHY. In plasma or urine: sensitivity, 250 ng/ml in plasma, 2.5 µg/ml in urine, UV detection—A. Sioufi *et al.*, *J. Chromat.*, 1980, *221*; *Biomed. Appl.*, *10*, 419–424.

Disposition in the Body. Readily absorbed after oral administration and acetylated in the body, about 20% of the sulphathiazole in the blood being in the form of the inactive N^4-acetyl derivative. It is rapidly excreted in the urine, about 60 to 90% of a dose being excreted in 24 hours; about 20% of the excreted material is the acetyl derivative.

Sulphathiazole is a metabolite of phthalylsulphathiazole and succinylsulphathiazole.

HALF-LIFE. Plasma half-life, about 4 hours.

PROTEIN BINDING. In plasma, 55 to 80%.

Dose. An initial dose of 2 to 3 g, followed by 1 g every 4 to 6 hours.

Sulphaurea   *Sulphonamide*

Synonyms. Sulfacarbamide; Sulfanilcarbamide; Sulphacarbamide; Sulphanilylurea; Urosulphanum.

Proprietary Names. Euvernil. It is an ingredient of Uromide.

Sulphanilylurea monohydrate

$C_7H_9N_3O_3S,H_2O = 233.2$

CAS—547-44-4 (anhydrous); *6101-35-5* (monohydrate)

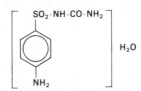

A white crystalline powder. M.p. 125° to 127°.

Soluble 1 in 430 of water; slightly soluble in ethanol; practically insoluble in chloroform and ether; soluble in acetone, dilute mineral acids, and solutions of alkali hydroxides.

Colour Tests. Copper Sulphate (Method 1)—blue; Koppanyi–Zwikker Test—violet; Palladium Chloride—black.

Thin-layer Chromatography. *System TA*—Rf 76; *system TB*—Rf 00; *system TC*—Rf 01.

Ultraviolet Spectrum. Aqueous acid—266 nm ($A_1^1 = 188$ b), 272 nm; aqueous alkali—255 nm. (See below)

Infra-red Spectrum. Principal peaks at wavenumbers 1694, 1149, 1587, 1086, 1612, 684.

Disposition in the Body. Readily absorbed after oral administration. It is rapidly excreted in the urine, most of a single dose being eliminated in 12 hours. About 10 to 15% of the material in the urine is the inactive N^4-acetyl metabolite and the remainder is unchanged drug.

HALF-LIFE. Plasma half-life, about 2.5 hours.

Dose. 3 g daily.

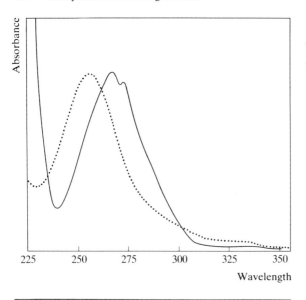

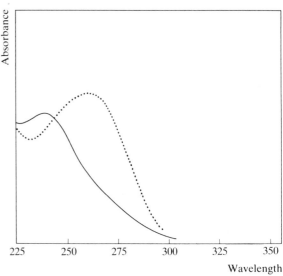

Sulphinpyrazone

Uricosuric

Synonyms. Sulfinpyrazone; Sulphoxyphenylpyrazolidine.

Proprietary Names. Anturan(e); Enturen; Zynol.

1,2-Diphenyl-4-(2-phenylsulphinylethyl)pyrazolidine-3,5-dione
$C_{23}H_{20}N_2O_3S = 404.5$
CAS—57-96-5

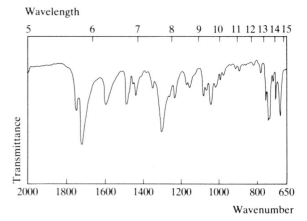

A white powder. M.p. 131° to 135°.

Practically **insoluble** in water; soluble 1 in 40 of ethanol, 1 in about 10 of acetone, 1 in 2 of chloroform, and 1 in 750 of ether.

Dissociation Constant. pK_a 2.8 (22°).

Partition Coefficient. Log P (octanol), 2.3.

Colour Tests. Copper Sulphate (Method 1)—blue; Koppanyi–Zwikker Test—violet (transient); Liebermann's Test—orange; Nitrous Acid—yellow.

Thin-layer Chromatography. *System TD*—Rf 04; *system TE*—Rf 16; *system TF*—Rf 04.

Gas Chromatography. *System GA*—RI 2253.

Ultraviolet Spectrum. Aqueous acid—237 nm ($A_1^1 = 436$ a); aqueous alkali—260 nm ($A_1^1 = 559$ a).

Infra-red Spectrum. Principal peaks at wavenumbers 1716, 1305, 750, 688, 1750, 1595 (KBr disk).

Mass Spectrum. Principal peaks at m/z 77, 278, 105, 78, 51, 279, 252, 130.

Quantification. GAS CHROMATOGRAPHY. In plasma or urine: sulphinpyrazone and its *p*-hydroxy and sulphone metabolites, detection limit for sulphinpyrazone 100 ng/ml using AFID or 10 ng/ml using ECD—P. Jakobsen and A. Kirstein Pedersen, *J. Chromat.*, 1979, *163*; *Biomed. Appl.*, 5, 259–269.

GAS CHROMATOGRAPHY–MASS SPECTROMETRY. In plasma or urine: sulphide and *p*-hydroxysulphide metabolites, detection limit 5 ng/ml for sulphide and 30 ng/ml for *p*-hydroxysulphide—P. Jakobsen and A. Kirstein Pedersen, *J. Pharm. Pharmac.*, 1981, *33*, 89–92.

HIGH PRESSURE LIQUID CHROMATOGRAPHY. In plasma or urine: sulphinpyrazone and its *p*-hydroxy and sulphone metabolites, sensitivity 50 ng/ml for sulphinpyrazone, UV detection—T. D. Bjornsson *et al.*, *J. Chromat.*, 1980, *181*; *Biomed. Appl.*, 7, 417–425. In plasma: sulphinpyrazone and metabolites, sensitivity 30 ng/ml, UV detection—B.-S. Kuo *et al.*, *Arzneimittel-Forsch.*, 1984, *34*, 548–550.

Disposition in the Body. Readily absorbed after oral administration. It is metabolised by reduction to the sulphide which is active and is the predominant circulating metabolite, reaching a concentration about 25% of that of sulphinpyrazone. It is also oxidised to the sulphone (active) and there are several hydroxy metabolites. All metabolites are excreted in the urine as the *C*-glucuronides, only a small proportion being excreted in *O*-glucuronidated or unconjugated form. Up to 50% of a dose is excreted in the urine as unchanged drug or its glucuronide.

About 80% of a single dose is recovered within the first 24 hours and more than 95% within 4 days (85% from urine and 10% from faeces).

THERAPEUTIC CONCENTRATION.

Following single oral doses of 200 mg to 6 subjects, peak plasma concentrations of 6.0 to 17.0 µg/ml (mean 13) of sulphinpyrazone were attained in 1 to 4 hours; peak plasma concentrations of the metabolites attained in about 4, 4, and 11 hours, respectively, were: sulphone 0.2 to 1.1 µg/ml, p-hydroxysulphinpyrazone 0.1 to 0.48 µg/ml, sulphide 0.6 to 8.9 µg/ml (C. Mahony et al., Clin. Pharmac. Ther., 1983, 33, 491–497).

Following oral administration of 200 mg four times a day to 6 subjects, mean maximum steady-state plasma concentrations were: sulphinpyrazone 20.7 µg/ml about 2 hours after a dose, sulphide 13.9 µg/ml about 7 hours after a dose, sulphone 3.4 µg/ml 2 hours after a dose (B. Rosenkranz et al., Eur. J. clin. Pharmac., 1983, 24, 231–235).

Daily oral doses of 600 to 800 mg to 8 diabetics, treated for 2.5 years or more, produced sulphinpyrazone plasma concentrations of 2.5 to 13.2 µg/ml (mean 7) before the first morning dose of 200 mg and 9.1 to 23.2 µg/ml (mean 16) 2 hours later. The corresponding sulphide plasma concentrations were 1.0 to 6.0 µg/ml (mean 2.8) and 1.5 to 8.6 µg/ml (mean 4.3) (A. Kirstein-Pedersen et al., Br. J. clin. Pharmac., 1981, 11, 597–603).

HALF-LIFE. Plasma half-life, about 3 to 5 hours, sulphide metabolite about 14 to 21 hours.

VOLUME OF DISTRIBUTION. About 0.06 litre/kg.

CLEARANCE. Plasma clearance, about 0.3 ml/min/kg.

DISTRIBUTION IN BLOOD. Plasma: whole blood ratio, 1.8.

PROTEIN BINDING. In plasma, about 98%.

NOTE. For a review of the pharmacokinetics of sulphinpyrazone see A. Kirstein Pedersen et al., Clin. Pharmacokinet., 1982, 7, 42–56.

Dose. 100 to 800 mg daily.

Sulpiride   Tranquilliser

Proprietary Names. Championyl; Dogmatil; Dolmatil; Equilid; Sursumid.

N-(1-Ethylpyrrolidin-2-ylmethyl)-2-methoxy-5-sulphamoyl-benzamide
$C_{15}H_{23}N_3O_4S = 341.4$
CAS—15676-16-1

A white crystalline powder. M.p. 175° to 182°, with decomposition.

Soluble 1 in about 2200 of water, 1 in 100 of ethanol, 1 in about 220 of chloroform, 1 in about 2600 of ether, and 1 in 50 of methanol.

Dissociation Constant. pK$_a$ 8.9.

Thin-layer Chromatography. System TA—Rf 38.

Ultraviolet Spectrum. Aqueous acid—292 nm (A$_1^1$ = 70 a). No alkaline shift.

Mass Spectrum. Principal peaks at m/z 98, 70, 214, 111, 134, 341, 199, 326.

Quantification. HIGH PRESSURE LIQUID CHROMATOGRAPHY. In serum, cerebrospinal fluid or urine: detection limits 10 ng/ml in serum or CSF, 200 ng/ml in urine, fluorescence detection—G. Alfredsson et al., J. Chromat., 1979, 164; Biomed. Appl., 6, 187–193.

RADIOIMMUNOASSAY. In serum: sensitivity 100 pg—A. Mizuchi et al., Archs int. Pharmacodyn. Thér., 1981, 254, 317–326.

Disposition in the Body. Slowly and incompletely absorbed after oral administration. About 70% of an intravenous dose is excreted as unchanged drug in the urine in 36 hours; up to about 20% of an oral dose is excreted in the urine as unchanged drug.

THERAPEUTIC CONCENTRATION.

After a single oral dose of 200 mg given to 10 subjects, peak plasma concentrations of 0.18 to 0.32 µg/ml (mean 0.24) were attained in 3 to 4 hours (F. R. Sugnaux et al., Eur. J. drug Met. Pharmacokinet., 1983, 8, 189–200).

Following oral administration of 50 mg, three times a day to 14 subjects, steady-state plasma concentrations of 0.03 to 0.6 µg/ml (mean 0.18) were reported, 4 to 7 hours after the final dose (J. K. Salminen et al., Curr. ther. Res., 1980, 27, 109–115).

HALF-LIFE. Plasma half-life, after intravenous administration 4 to 13 hours; after oral administration variously reported as 6 to 15 hours (mean 10) and 13 to 41 hours (mean 25).

VOLUME OF DISTRIBUTION. About 2 to 3 litres/kg.

CLEARANCE. Plasma clearance, about 6 ml/min/kg.

Dose. For psychoses, 0.4 to 2.4 g daily.

Sulthiame   Anticonvulsant

Synonym. Sultiame
Proprietary Name. Ospolot
4-(Tetrahydro-2H-1,2-thiazin-2-yl)benzenesulphonamide SS-dioxide
$C_{10}H_{14}N_2O_4S_2 = 290.4$
CAS—61-56-3

A white crystalline powder. M.p. 185° to 188°.

Soluble 1 in 2000 of water, 1 in 350 of ethanol, 1 in 700 of chloroform, and 1 in 500 of ether; readily soluble in alkaline solutions.

Dissociation Constant. pK$_a$ 10.0.

Colour Tests. Copper Sulphate (Method 1)—blue; Koppanyi-Zwikker Test—violet-blue.

Thin-layer Chromatography. System TD—Rf 23; system TE—Rf 53; system TF—Rf 43.

High Pressure Liquid Chromatography. System HE—k' 1.57.

Ultraviolet Spectrum. Methanol—246 nm (A$_1^1$ = 390 a).

Infra-red Spectrum. Principal peaks at wavenumbers 1138, 1158, 1172, 1293, 889, 1192 (KBr disk). (See below)

Mass Spectrum. Principal peaks at m/z 290, 184, 185, 104, 77, 168, 291, 198.

Wavelength

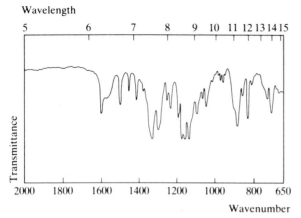

Infra-red Spectrum. Principal peaks at wavenumbers 1590, 1220, 1722, 1050, 1308, 743 (KBr disk).

Quantification. HIGH PRESSURE LIQUID CHROMATOGRAPHY. In plasma: sensitivity 100ng/ml, UV detection—K. B. Alton and J. E. Patrick, *J. pharm. Sci.*, 1978, *67*, 985–987.

Disposition in the Body. Rapidly and well absorbed after oral administration. About 72% of a dose is excreted in the urine in 6 hours, mainly as dihydrosuprofen glucuronide.

THERAPEUTIC CONCENTRATION.

After a single oral dose of 200 mg to 6 subjects, peak plasma concentrations of 4.5 to 28.9 µg/ml (mean 17.5) were attained in 0.25 to 2 hours (H. W. Zulliger and A. Fassolt, *Arzneimittel-Forsch.*, 1983, *33*, 1322–1326).

HALF-LIFE. Plasma half-life, about 2 hours.

PROTEIN BINDING. In plasma, about 99.5%.

Dose. 600 to 800 mg daily.

Quantification. HIGH PRESSURE LIQUID CHROMATOGRAPHY. In plasma: UV detection—D. J. Berry *et al.*, *J. Chromat.*, 1979, *171*, 363–370. In plasma: sensitivity 150 ng/ml, UV detection— T. Sadanaga *et al.*, *Chem. pharm. Bull.*, 1981, *29*, 872–874.

Disposition in the Body. Readily but variably absorbed after oral administration. During long-term therapy 17 to 70% (mean 32) of the daily dose is excreted in 24 hours, of which about 60% is unchanged drug and the remainder is an inactive metabolite. Up to 15% of a dose may be eliminated in the faeces.

THERAPEUTIC CONCENTRATION.

Following daily oral doses of 3 to 14.5 mg/kg to 36 subjects, serum concentrations ranged from 0.5 to 12.5 µg/ml; peak concentrations were attained 1 to 5 hours after a dose (O. V. Olesen, *Acta pharmac. tox.*, 1968, *26*, 22–28).

TOXICITY. Recovery has occurred after the ingestion of 4 to 5 g. Blood concentrations of 12 to 26 µg/ml have been reported in fatalities.

Dose. 200 to 600 mg daily.

Suprofen   *Analgesic*

Synonym. Sutoprofen
Proprietary Name. Suprol
2-[4-(2-Thenoyl)phenyl]propionic acid
$C_{14}H_{12}O_3S = 260.3$
CAS—40828-46-4

CH₃·CH·COOH

A white to slightly yellowish powder. M.p. 120° to 125°.
Soluble 1 in 5 of ethanol, 1 to 3 of acetone, 1 in about 4 of chloroform, and 1 in about 20 of ether.

Dissociation Constant. pK_a 3.9.

Ultraviolet Spectrum. Isopropyl alcohol—265 nm ($A_1^1 = 550$ b), 291 nm ($A_1^1 = 550$ b).

Suxamethonium Chloride   *Muscle Relaxant*

Synonyms. Choline Chloride Succinate; Succicurarium Chloride; Succinylcholine Chloride.
Proprietary Names. Anectine; Celocurin; Lysthenon; Midarine; Myotenlis; Pantolax; Quelicin; Scoline; Succinyl-Asta; Sucostrin; Sux-Cert.
2,2′-Succinyldioxybis(ethyltrimethylammonium) dichloride dihydrate
$C_{14}H_{30}Cl_2N_2O_4, 2H_2O = 397.3$
CAS—306-40-1 (suxamethonium); *71-27-2* (chloride, anhydrous); *6101-15-1* (chloride, dihydrate)

$[(CH_3)_3N^+ \cdot [CH_2]_2 \cdot O \cdot CO \cdot [CH_2]_2 \cdot CO \cdot O \cdot [CH_2]_2 \cdot N^+(CH_3)_3]$ $2Cl^-, 2H_2O$

A white, hygroscopic, crystalline powder. M.p. about 160°.
Soluble 1 in 1 of water and 1 in 350 of ethanol; practically insoluble in chloroform and ether; soluble in methanol.

Suxamethonium Bromide
Synonyms. Choline Bromide Succinate; Succinylcholine Bromide.
Proprietary Name. Brevidil M
$C_{14}H_{30}Br_2N_2O_4, 2H_2O = 486.2$
CAS—55-94-7
A white or creamy-white powder. M.p. about 225°.
Soluble 1 in 0.3 of water and 1 in 5 of ethanol; practically insoluble in chloroform and ether.

Suxamethonium Iodide
Synonym. Dithylinum
Proprietary Name. Célocurine
$C_{14}H_{30}I_2N_2O_4 = 544.2$
CAS—541-19-5
A white, slightly hygroscopic, crystalline powder. M.p. about 250°.
Freely **soluble** in water; very slightly soluble in ethanol; practically insoluble in ether.

Thin-layer Chromatography. *System TA*—Rf 01; *system TN*—Rf 35; *system TO*—Rf 10. (*Acidified iodoplatinate solution*, positive.)

Gas Chromatography. *System GA*—not eluted.

Ultraviolet Spectrum. No significant absorption, 230 to 360 nm.

Infra-red Spectrum. Principal peaks at wavenumbers 1724, 1148, 1308, 961, 952, 1612 (KBr disk).

Wavelength

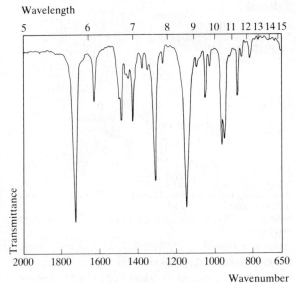

Transmittance

Wavenumber

Disposition in the Body. Slowly and incompletely absorbed after oral administration; absorbed after intramuscular administration but generally given by the intravenous route. Rapidly distributed into the extracellular fluids throughout the body. Suxamethonium is rapidly hydrolysed in plasma and body tissues to succinylmonocholine (weak activity) and choline. Succinylmonocholine is then slowly hydrolysed to succinic acid and choline. Less than 3% of a dose is excreted unchanged in the urine.

HALF-LIFE. Plasma half-life, about 3 minutes.

Dose. Usually 20 to 100 mg of suxamethonium chloride, intravenously.

Suxethonium Bromide   *Muscle Relaxant*

Proprietary Name. Brevidil E
2,2'-Succinyldioxybis(diethyldimethylammonium) dibromide
$C_{16}H_{34}Br_2N_2O_4 = 478.3$
CAS—111-00-2

$$[(CH_3)_2\overset{+}{N}\cdot[CH_2]_2\cdot O\cdot CO\cdot[CH_2]_2\cdot CO\cdot O\cdot[CH_2]_2\cdot \overset{+}{N}(CH_3)_2]\ 2Br^-$$
$$\underset{C_2H_5}{|}\qquad\qquad\qquad\qquad\qquad\underset{C_2H_5}{|}$$

A slightly hygroscopic, white or slightly cream, crystalline powder. M.p. 158°.
Readily **soluble** in water, yielding weakly acidic solutions.

Thin-layer Chromatography. *System TA*—Rf 01; *system TN*—Rf 40; *system TO*—Rf 23. (*Acidified iodoplatinate solution*, positive.)

Ultraviolet Spectrum. No significant absorption, 230 to 360 nm.

Infra-red Spectrum. Principal peaks at wavenumbers 1740, 1163, 1638, 1270, 962, 1012 (KBr disk).

Disposition in the Body. After intravenous administration it is rapidly hydrolysed in plasma and body tissues to succinic acid and choline.

Dose. 1.5 to 1.9 mg/kg intravenously.

Syrosingopine   *Antihypertensive*

Synonym. Methyl Carbethoxysyringoyl Reserpate
Proprietary Names. Neoreserpan; Raunova.
Methyl   18-*O*-(4-ethoxycarbonyloxy-3,5-dimethoxybenzoyl)-reserpate
$C_{35}H_{42}N_2O_{11} = 666.7$
CAS—84-36-6

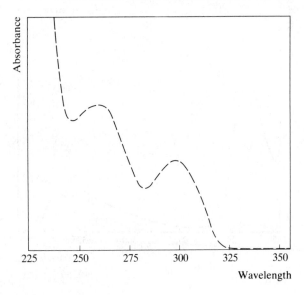

A white or slightly yellowish crystalline powder. M.p. 220° to 225°.
Practically **insoluble** in water; freely soluble in chloroform and acetic acid; slightly soluble in ether.

Colour Tests. Mandelin's Test—green-brown; Marquis Test—brown.

Thin-layer Chromatography. *System TA*—Rf 78. (*Acidified potassium permanganate solution*, positive.)

Ultraviolet Spectrum. Ethanol—258 nm ($A_1^1 = 242$ a), 298 nm.

Absorbance

Wavelength

Infra-red Spectrum. Principal peaks at wavenumbers 1209, 1130, 1247, 1180, 1770, 1727 (KBr disk).

Mass Spectrum. Principal peaks at *m/z* 181, 395, 198, 251, 397, 396, 199, 666.

Dose. 0.5 to 3 mg daily.

Tacrine
Anticholinesterase/Central Stimulant

Synonym. Tetrahydroaminacrine
1,2,3,4-Tetrahydroacridin-9-ylamine
$C_{13}H_{14}N_2 = 198.3$
CAS—321-64-2

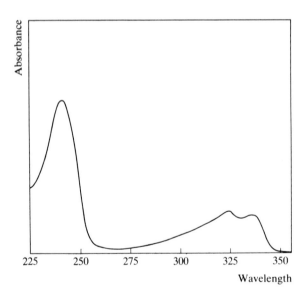

M.p. 183° to 184°.

Tacrine Hydrochloride
Proprietary Name. THA
$C_{13}H_{14}N_2,HCl = 234.7$
CAS—1684-40-8
A pale yellow crystalline powder. M.p. 283° to 284°.
Readily **soluble** in water.

Thin-layer Chromatography. *System TA*—Rf 43; *system TB*—Rf 05; *system TC*—Rf 04. (*Acidified iodoplatinate solution*, positive.)

Gas Chromatography. *System GA*—RI 2165.

High Pressure Liquid Chromatography. *System HA*—k' 1.6.

Ultraviolet Spectrum. Aqueous acid—240 nm ($A_1^1 = 2032$ a), 323 nm, 336 nm; aqueous alkali—237 nm, 317 nm.

Infra-red Spectrum. Principal peaks at wavenumbers 1650, 1590, 765, 1496, 774, 1176 (KBr disk).

Mass Spectrum. Principal peaks at *m/z* 198, 197, 170, 199, 182, 169, 77, 183.

Dose. Tacrine hydrochloride has been given in doses of 10 to 60 mg, intravenously.

Talbutal
Barbiturate

Proprietary Name. Lotusate
5-Allyl-5-*sec*-butylbarbituric acid
$C_{11}H_{16}N_2O_3 = 224.3$
CAS—115-44-6

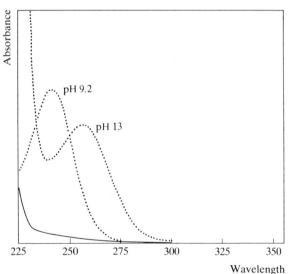

A white crystalline powder. It occurs in 2 polymorphic forms with m.p. about 108° and 111°.
Soluble 1 in 500 of water, 1 in 1 of ethanol, 1 in 2 of chloroform, and 1 in 40 of ether.

Dissociation Constant. pK_a 7.9 (20°).

Partition Coefficient. Log *P* (octanol/pH 7.4), 1.3.

Colour Tests. Koppanyi–Zwikker Test—violet; Mercurous Nitrate—black; Vanillin Reagent—brown-orange/violet.

Thin-layer Chromatography. *System TD*—Rf 53; *system TE*—Rf 41; *system TF*—Rf 67; *system TH*—Rf 71.

Gas Chromatography. *System GA*—RI 1701.

High Pressure Liquid Chromatography. *System HG*—k' 7.25; *system HH*—k' 4.67.

Ultraviolet Spectrum. *Borax buffer 0.05M* (pH 9.2)—239 nm ($A_1^1 = 415$ a); M sodium hydroxide (pH 13)—255 nm ($A_1^1 = 313$ b).

Infra-red Spectrum. Principal peaks at wavenumbers 1703, 1728, 1752, 1315, 1211, 829 (KBr disk).

Mass Spectrum. Principal peaks at *m/z* 167, 168, 41, 97, 124, 39, 57, 53.

Disposition in the Body.

TOXICITY. The estimated minimum lethal dose is 2 g.

In one fatality involving talbutal, a blood concentration of 13 µg/ml and a liver concentration of 305 µg/g was reported (R. C. Baselt and R. H. Cravey, *J. analyt. Toxicol.*, 1977, *1*, 81–102).

Dose. 60 to 150 mg daily.

Temazepam   *Hypnotic*

Synonym. 3-Hydroxydiazepam

Proprietary Names. Euhypnos; Levanxol; Maeva; Normison; Restoril.

7-Chloro-1,3-dihydro-3-hydroxy-1-methyl-5-phenyl-2*H*-1,4-benzodiazepin-2-one

$C_{16}H_{13}ClN_2O_2 = 300.7$

CAS—846-50-4

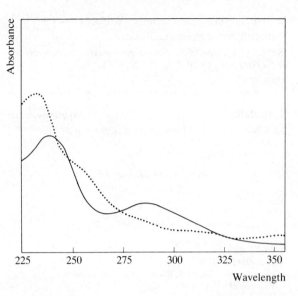

A white crystalline powder. M.p. 156° to 159°.

Practically **insoluble** in water; soluble 1 in 10 of ethanol and 1 in 10 of chloroform.

Dissociation Constant. pK_a 1.6.

Colour Test. Formaldehyde–Sulphuric Acid—orange.

Thin-layer Chromatography. *System TA*—Rf 53; *system TB*—Rf 08; *system TC*—Rf 59; *system TD*—Rf 51; *system TE*—Rf 63; *system TF*—Rf 47. (*Dragendorff spray*, positive; *acidified iodoplatinate solution*, positive; *acidified potassium permanganate solution*, positive.)

Gas Chromatography. *System GA*—temazepam RI 2633, oxazepam RI 2336; *system GG*—temazepam RI 3125, oxazepam RI 2803.

High Pressure Liquid Chromatography. *System HI*—temazepam k′ 5.68, oxazepam k′ 4.62; *system HK*—temazepam k′ 0.60, oxazepam k′ 0.73.

Ultraviolet Spectrum. Aqueous acid—237 nm ($A_1^1 = 980$ b), 284 nm ($A_1^1 = 283$ b), 358 nm ($A_1^1 = 68$ b); aqueous alkali—231 nm, 313 nm; methanol—230 nm ($A_1^1 = 1090$ a), 314 nm ($A_1^1 = 76$ b).

Infra-red Spectrum. Principal peaks at wavenumbers 1687, 1670, 1112, 1603, 705, 1150 (KBr disk).

Mass Spectrum. Principal peaks at *m/z* 271, 273, 300, 272, 256, 77, 255, 257; oxazepam 257, 77, 268, 239, 205, 267, 233, 259.

Quantification. GAS CHROMATOGRAPHY. In plasma: sensitivity 5 ng/ml, ECD—M. Divoll and D. J. Greenblatt, *J. Chromat.*, 1981, *222*; *Biomed. Appl.*, *11*, 125–128.

Disposition in the Body. Rapidly absorbed after oral administration. Metabolised principally by glucuronic acid conjugation; demethylation to oxazepam occurs to a small extent. About 80% of a dose is excreted in the urine, mostly as conjugates; less than 2% of a dose is excreted as unchanged drug. About 12% of a dose is eliminated in the faeces.

Temazepam is a metabolite of several benzodiazepines, including diazepam, ketazolam, and medazepam.

THERAPEUTIC CONCENTRATION.

After a single oral dose of 30 mg given to 14 subjects, peak plasma concentrations of 0.29 to 0.75 µg/ml (mean 0.5) were attained in about 2 hours (M. Divoll *et al.*, *J. pharm. Sci.*, 1981, *70*, 1104–1107).

Following daily oral doses of 20 mg to 10 subjects for 6 days, trough steady-state serum concentrations of 0.017 to 0.132 µg/ml (mean 0.05) were reported (H. R. Ochs *et al.*, *J. clin. Pharmac.*, 1984, *24*, 58–64).

HALF-LIFE. Plasma half-life, about 3 to 38 hours (mean 10); there is considerable intersubject variation, and sex differences have been reported.

VOLUME OF DISTRIBUTION. About 1 litre/kg.

CLEARANCE. Plasma clearance, about 1 to 2 ml/min/kg.

DISTRIBUTION IN BLOOD. Plasma: whole blood ratio, 1.9.

PROTEIN BINDING. In plasma, about 97%.

NOTE. For a review of the pharmacokinetics of temazepam see R. C. Heel *et al.*, *Drugs*, 1981, *21*, 321–340.

Dose. 10 to 60 mg.

Terbutaline
Sympathomimetic

2-*tert*-Butylamino-1-(3,5-dihydroxyphenyl)ethanol
$C_{12}H_{19}NO_3 = 225.3$
CAS—23031-25-6

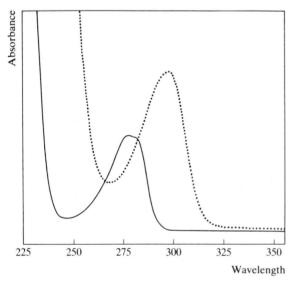

$(CH_3)_3C \cdot NH \cdot CH_2 \cdot CH \cdot OH$

Crystals. M.p. 119° to 122°.

Terbutaline Sulphate

Proprietary Names. Brethine; Bricanyl; Feevone; Terbasmin.
$C_{12}H_{19}NO_3, \frac{1}{2}H_2SO_4 = 274.3$
CAS—23031-32-5
A white to greyish-white crystalline powder. M.p. about 255°.
Soluble 1 in 4 of water; slightly soluble in ethanol; practically insoluble in chloroform and ether.

Dissociation Constant. pK_a 8.7, 10.0, 11.0 (20°).

Colour Tests. *p*-Dimethylaminobenzaldehyde—orange/violet; Folin–Ciocalteu Reagent—blue; Liebermann's Test—black; Mandelin's Test—grey-green; Marquis Test—yellow; Potassium Dichromate (Method 1)—brown (slow).

Thin-layer Chromatography. *System TA*—Rf 47; *system TB*—Rf 01; *system TC*—Rf 01. (*Acidified potassium permanganate solution*, strong reaction.)

High Pressure Liquid Chromatography. *System HA*—k′ 0.9.

Ultraviolet Spectrum. Aqueous acid—276nm ($A_1^1 = 85$ a); aqueous alkali—297 nm ($A_1^1 = 150$ b).

Infra-red Spectrum. Principal peaks at wavenumbers 1210, 1231, 1155, 1069, 1610, 1042 (terbutaline sulphate, KBr disk).

Mass Spectrum. Principal peaks at *m/z* 30, 86, 57, 41, 29, 39, 192, 42.

Quantification. GAS CHROMATOGRAPHY–MASS SPECTROMETRY. In plasma: unconjugated terbutaline, detection limit 100 pg/ml—S.-E. Jacobsson *et al.*, *Biomed. Mass Spectrom.*, 1980, 7, 265–268. In plasma or urine: unconjugated and total terbutaline, detection limit 300 pg/ml—R. A. Clare *et al.*, *Biomed. Mass Spectrom.*,1979, 6, 31–37. In postmortem tissues: unconjugated terbutaline, detection limit 1.5 ng/g—J. G. Leferink *et al.*, *J. analyt. Toxicol.*, 1978, 2, 86–88.

HIGH PRESSURE LIQUID CHROMATOGRAPHY. In plasma: sensitivity about 1 ng/ml, electrochemical detection—S. Bergquist and L.-E. Edholm, *J. liq. Chromat.*, 1983, 6, 559–574.

Disposition in the Body. Incompletely absorbed after oral administration. Extensive first-pass metabolism occurs in the liver and gut wall to produce the sulphate conjugate (the main metabolite) but some glucuronic acid conjugation also occurs. Less than 15% of an oral dose is present as free drug in the plasma. It is excreted in the urine as unchanged drug and the inactive conjugates, the concentration of each being dependent upon the route of administration. After oral administration, up to about 50% of a dose is excreted in the urine, predominantly as the sulphate conjugate, with up to 10% as unchanged drug. Up to about 60% of a dose is eliminated in the faeces, mainly in unchanged form. After intravenous or subcutaneous administration, more than 80% of a dose is excreted in the urine, with up to about 60% as unchanged drug and only about 2 to 3% is eliminated in the faeces.

THERAPEUTIC CONCENTRATION.

After single oral doses of 5 mg to 8 subjects, peak serum concentrations of 0.002 to 0.005 μg/ml (mean 0.003) were attained in 2 to 4 hours. In 3 subjects there were 2 peaks, the first occurred in 1 to 2 hours and the second in 3 to 4 hours. After single subcutaneous doses of 0.5 mg to the same subjects, peak serum concentrations of 0.005 to 0.011 μg/ml (mean 0.007) were attained in 0.2 to 0.6 hour (J. G. Leferink *et al.*, *Arzneimittel-Forsch.*, 1982, *32*, 159–164).

TOXICITY.

A female subject took several tablets of terbutaline during a severe night attack of asthma and died the next morning. The following postmortem tissue concentrations were reported: serum 0.014 μg/ml, heart 0.036 μg/g, kidney 0.054 μg/g, liver 0.055 μg/g, lung 0.026 μg/g, muscle 0.063 μg/g (J. G. Leferink *et al.*, *J. analyt. Toxicol.*, 1978, 2, 86–88).

HALF-LIFE. Plasma half-life, about 3 to 4 hours.

VOLUME OF DISTRIBUTION. About 1 litre/kg.

CLEARANCE. Plasma clearance, about 4 ml/min/kg.

PROTEIN BINDING. In plasma, about 15 to 25%.

Dose. 10 to 15 mg of terbutaline sulphate daily.

Terbutryne
Herbicide

Proprietary Names. Clarosan; Prebane. It is an ingredient of Opogard.

2-*tert*-Butylamino-4-ethylamino-6-methylthio-1,3,5-triazine
$C_{10}H_{19}N_5S = 241.4$
CAS—886-50-0

A white crystalline powder. M.p. 104° to 105°.

Practically **insoluble** in water; readily soluble in chloroform, ether, and methanol.

Thin-layer Chromatography. *System TA*—Rf 77. (*Dragendorff spray*, positive.)

Gas Chromatography. *System GA*—RI 1940; *system GK*—retention time 0.99 relative to caffeine.

Infra-red Spectrum. Principal peaks at wavenumbers 1520, 1587, 1215, 806, 1266, 1133 (KBr disk).

Testosterone   *Androgen*

Proprietary Names. Andronaq; Hydrotest; Malogen; Oreton; Percutacrine Androgénique Forte; Testoral Sublings.

Note. Testoral is also used as a proprietary name for Fluoxymesterone.

17β-Hydroxyandrost-4-en-3-one
$C_{19}H_{28}O_2 = 288.4$
CAS—58-22-0

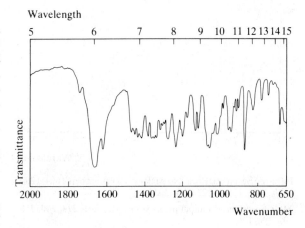

White or creamy-white crystals or crystalline powder. M.p. 152° to 157°.

Practically **insoluble** in water; soluble 1 in 6 of dehydrated alcohol, 1 in 2 of chloroform, and 1 in 100 of ether.

Testosterone Cypionate

Synonym. Testosterone Cyclopentylpropionate

Proprietary Names. Andronate; Ciclosterone; Jectatest-LA.

$C_{27}H_{40}O_3 = 412.6$
CAS—58-20-8

A white or creamy-white crystalline powder. M.p. 98° to 104°.

Practically **insoluble** in water; freely soluble in ethanol, chloroform, and ether.

Testosterone Enanthate

Synonyms. Testosterone Heptanoate; Testosterone Oenanthate.

Proprietary Names. Androtardyl; Delatestryl; Malogen LA; Malogex; Primoteston-Depot; Testate; Testone LA; Testostroval-PA; Testoviron-Depot.

$C_{26}H_{40}O_3 = 400.6$
CAS—315-37-7

A white or creamy-white crystalline powder. M.p. 34° to 39°.

Practically **insoluble** in water; soluble 1 in 0.3 of ethanol, chloroform, and ether.

Testosterone Isocaproate

Synonym. Testosterone Isohexanoate

Proprietary Names. It is an ingredient of Mixogen (injection) and Sustanon.

$C_{25}H_{38}O_3 = 386.6$
CAS—15262-86-9

White to creamy-white crystals or crystalline powder. M.p. about 80°.

Practically **insoluble** in water; very soluble in ethanol and chloroform.

Testosterone Phenylpropionate

Proprietary Names. It is an ingredient of Mixogen (injection) and Sustanon.

$C_{28}H_{36}O_3 = 420.6$
CAS—1255-49-8

A white crystalline powder. M.p. 114° to 117°.

Practically **insoluble** in water; soluble 1 in 40 of ethanol.

Testosterone Propionate

Proprietary Names. Stérandryl; Testoviron (injection); Virormone. It is an ingredient of Mixogen (injection), Plex-Hormone (injection), and Sustanon.

$C_{22}H_{32}O_3 = 344.5$
CAS—57-85-2

Colourless or yellowish-white crystals or a white or creamy-white crystalline powder. M.p. 118° to 123°.

Practically **insoluble** in water; soluble 1 in 6 of ethanol and 1 in 4 of acetone; very soluble in chloroform; freely soluble in ether.

Colour Tests. Naphthol–Sulphuric Acid—yellow/green, brown dichroism; Sulphuric Acid—no initial colour (green fluorescence under ultraviolet light).

Thin-layer Chromatography. Testosterone: *system TP*—Rf 60; *system TQ*—Rf 07; *system TR*—Rf 90; *system TS*—Rf 63. Testosterone phenylpropionate: *system TP*—Rf 86; *system TQ*—Rf 28; *system TR*—Rf 99; *system TS*—Rf 98. Testosterone propionate: *system TP*—Rf 78; *system TQ*—Rf 12; *system TR*—Rf 99; *system TS*—Rf 98.

Gas Chromatography. *System GA*—RI 2620.

Ultraviolet Spectrum. Dehydrated alcohol—240 nm ($A_1^1 = 560$ a).

Infra-red Spectrum. Principal peaks at wavenumbers 1660, 871, 1615, 1057, 1236, 1066 (KBr disk).

Quantification. RADIOIMMUNOASSAY. In plasma or other biological fluids: sensitivity 8 pg—C. S. Corker and D. W. Davidson, *J. Steroid Biochem.*, 1978, 9, 373–374.

ENZYME IMMUNOASSAY. In plasma or saliva: detection limit 4 pg—A. Turkes *et al.*, *Steroids*, 1979, 33, 347–359.

Disposition in the Body. Testosterone is the androgenic hormone formed in the testes. In man, it is metabolised to 5α-androstane-3α,17β-diol, androsterone, etiocholanolone, and 5α-androstene-3,17-dione. In the horse, the major metabolites are 5α-androstane-3β,17α-diol, which is excreted in the urine as the glucuronide conjugate, and the 17β-epimer which is excreted in the urine as the sulphate conjugate.

Dose. 10 to 30 mg daily, sublingually; 200 to 600 mg by implantation.

Tetrabenazine
Tranquilliser

Synonym. TBZ
Proprietary Name. Nitoman
1,3,4,6,7,11b - Hexahydro - 3 - isobutyl - 9,10 - dimethoxy - 2*H* - benzo[*a*]quinolizin-2-one
$C_{19}H_{27}NO_3 = 317.4$
CAS—58-46-8

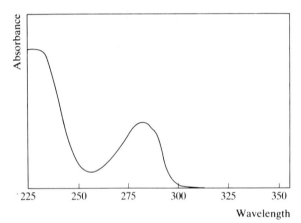

A white crystalline powder. M.p. 126° to 131°.
Soluble in hot water, ethanol, and chloroform.

Colour Tests. Liebermann's Test—black; Mandelin's Test—brown; Marquis Test—yellow.

Thin-layer Chromatography. *System TA*—Rf 69; *system TB*—Rf 41; *system TC*—Rf 78. (*Acidified iodoplatinate solution*, positive.)

Ultraviolet Spectrum. Aqueous acid—282 nm ($A_1^1 = 108$ a). No alkaline shift.

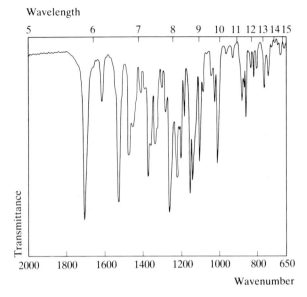

Infra-red Spectrum. Principal peaks at wavenumbers 1694, 1260, 1520, 1155, 1140, 1222 (KBr disk).

Mass Spectrum. Principal peaks at *m/z* 191, 261, 274, 260, 316, 192, 190, 176.

Quantification. HIGH PRESSURE LIQUID CHROMATOGRAPHY. In plasma: tetrabenazine and 2-hydroxy metabolite, detection limits 100 pg/ml and 1 ng/ml, respectively, fluorescence detection—M. S. Roberts *et al.*, *J. Chromat.*, 1981, *226*; *Biomed. Appl.*, *15*, 175–182.

Disposition in the Body. Absorbed after oral administration. It is extensively metabolised and excreted in the urine as free and conjugated metabolites; nine metabolites have been identified in the urine. 2-Hydroxytetrabenazine is an active metabolite.

THERAPEUTIC CONCENTRATION.
Following a single oral dose of 50 mg to 1 subject, peak plasma concentrations of about 0.015 μg/ml of tetrabenazine and 0.085 μg/ml of the 2-hydroxy metabolite were attained in 1 hour and 2 hours, respectively (M. S. Roberts *et al.*, *ibid.*).

Dose. 75 to 200 mg daily.

Tetrachloroethane
Solvent

Synonym. Acetylene Tetrachloride
1,1,2,2-Tetrachloroethane
$CHCl_2 \cdot CHCl_2 = 167.8$
CAS—79-34-5
A clear, colourless, heavy, non-inflammable, mobile liquid. Wt per ml 1.590 to 1.595 g. B.p. 142° to 147°. Refractive index, at 25°, 1.4918.
Soluble 1 in 400 of water; miscible with ethanol, chloroform, and ether.

Gas Chromatography. *System GA*—RI 910; *system GI*—retention time 24.9 min.

Disposition in the Body. Absorbed from the gastro-intestinal tract, lungs, and through the skin.

TOXICITY. Tetrachloroethane is probably the most toxic of the chlorinated hydrocarbons. The estimated lethal dose is 3 ml.

Tetrachloroethylene
Anthelmintic/Solvent

Synonym. Perchloroethylene
Proprietary Name. Perklone
$CCl_2 : CCl_2 = 165.8$
CAS—127-18-4
A colourless, heavy, non-inflammable, mobile liquid. Wt per ml 1.620 to 1.626 g. F.p. −22°. B.p. 118° to 122°.
Tetrachloroethylene (*B.P.*) contains thymol 0.01% w/w as a preservative.
Practically **insoluble** in water; soluble in ethanol; miscible with chloroform and ether.

Colour Test. Tetrachloroethylene may be distinguished from carbon tetrachloride and chloroform by the following test: to 5 ml in a stoppered cylinder add 5 ml of *bromine solution* and shake vigorously at intervals of 15 minutes for 1 hour—bromine colour fades and there is a white turbidity in the lower layer.

Gas Chromatography. *System GA*—RI 789; *system GI*—retention time 24.3 min.

Mass Spectrum. Principal peaks at m/z 166, 164, 129, 131, 168, 94, 133, 96.

Quantification. GAS CHROMATOGRAPHY. In blood or tissues: ECD—B. Levine *et al.*, *J. forens. Sci.*, 1981, *26*, 206–209.

GAS CHROMATOGRAPHY–MASS SPECTROMETRY. In blood or tissues—T. Lukaszewski, *Clin. Toxicol.*, 1979, *15*, 411–415.

Disposition in the Body. Slightly absorbed from the gastro-intestinal tract and through the skin; well absorbed from the lungs. It has an affinity for lipid-rich tissues from which it is slowly released. About 25% of an inhaled dose is excreted unchanged in expired air in 40 hours and this is thought to be the major route of excretion; small amounts are eliminated through the skin. Less than about 3% of a dose is metabolised and excreted in the urine, partly as trichloroacetic acid, in 3 days.

TOXICITY. The maximum permissible atmospheric concentration is 100 ppm. Exposure to air concentrations of more than 1000 ppm may cause unconsciousness within a short time.

Exposure to a concentration of 194 ppm of tetrachloroethylene for 3 hours produced peak blood concentrations of about 2 to 3 µg/ml (mean 2.6) in 6 subjects, at the end of the exposure period (R. D. Stewart *et al.*, *Archs envir. Hlth*, 1961, *2*, 516–522).

A 53-year-old man was found dead after exposure to tetrachloroethylene vapour. The following postmortem concentrations were reported: blood 4.5 µg/ml, brain 69 µg/g, kidney 71 µg/g, liver 240 µg/g, and lung 30 µg/g (B. Levine *et al.*, *J. forens. Sci.*, 1981, *26*, 206–209).

In a case of fatal exposure to tetrachloroethylene vapour, a 33-year-old man had the following postmortem concentrations: blood 44 µg/ml, brain 360 µg/g, and lung 3 µg/g (T. Lukaszewski, *Clin. Toxicol.*, 1979, *15*, 411–415).

HALF-LIFE. About 72 hours.

Dose. Usually 0.1 ml/kg, to a maximum of 5 ml, as a single dose.

Tetracycline   *Antibiotic*

Proprietary Names. Tetracycline and Tetracycline Hydrochloride are ingredients of many proprietary preparations—see *Martindale, The Extra Pharmacopoeia*, 28th Edn.

A hydrated form of (4*S*,4a*S*,5a*S*,6*S*,12a*S*)-4-dimethylamino-1,4,4a,5,5a,6,11,12a-octahydro-3,6,10,12,12a-pentahydroxy-6-methyl-1,11-dioxonaphthacene-2-carboxamide

$C_{22}H_{24}N_2O_8 = 444.4$

CAS—60-54-8 (anhydrous); *6416-04-2* (trihydrate)

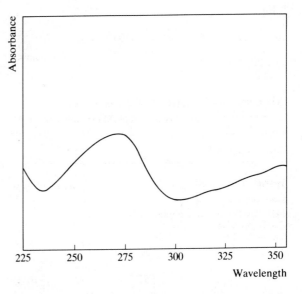

A yellow, crystalline, amphoteric powder which darkens in moist air on exposure to strong sunlight.
Soluble 1 in 2500 of water and 1 in 50 of ethanol; practically insoluble in chloroform and ether; freely soluble in dilute acids and, with decomposition, in solutions of alkali hydroxides.

Tetracycline Hydrochloride

$C_{22}H_{24}N_2O_8,HCl = 480.9$

CAS—64-75-5

A yellow, hygroscopic, crystalline, amphoteric powder which darkens in moist air on exposure to strong sunlight. M.p. about 214°, with decomposition.

Soluble 1 in 10 of water and 1 in 100 of ethanol; practically insoluble in chloroform and ether; soluble in methanol and in aqueous solutions of alkali hydroxides and carbonates. Solutions in water become turbid on standing owing to hydrolysis and precipitation of tetracycline.

Dissociation Constant. pK_a 3.3, 7.7, 9.7 (25°).

Partition Coefficient. Log *P* (octanol/pH 7.4), −1.4.

Colour Tests. Benedict's Reagent—red; Formaldehyde-Sulphuric Acid—green-yellow → yellow-brown; Liebermann's Test—black; Mandelin's Test—violet → red → orange; Marquis Test—orange; Sulphuric Acid—violet.

Thin-layer Chromatography. *System TA*—Rf 05, streaking. (Location under ultraviolet light, orange fluorescence; *acidified potassium permanganate solution*, positive.)

Gas Chromatography. *System GA*—RI 1950.

Ultraviolet Spectrum. Aqueous acid—270 nm ($A_1^1 = 417$ a), 356 nm.

Infra-red Spectrum. Principal peaks at wavenumbers 1612, 1580, 1660, 1226, 1248, 1530 (tetracycline hydrochloride, KCl disk). (See below)

Quantification. HIGH PRESSURE LIQUID CHROMATOGRAPHY. In plasma or urine: sensitivity 100 ng/ml, UV detection—J. Hermansson, *J. Chromat.*, 1982, *232*; *Biomed. Appl.*, *21*, 385–393.

RADIOIMMUNOASSAY. In plasma or urine: detection limit about 20 ng/ml—B. A. Faraj and F. M. Ali, *J. Pharmac. exp. Ther.*, 1981, *217*, 10–14.

Disposition in the Body. Irregularly and incompletely absorbed after oral administration; widely distributed throughout the body. Up to about 60% of an intravenous dose and 20 to 50% of an oral dose is excreted in the urine unchanged in 48 hours. Excreted in the bile and undergoes some enterohepatic circulation.

THERAPEUTIC CONCENTRATION. In plasma, usually in the range 1 to 5 µg/ml.

HALF-LIFE. Plasma half-life, about 9 hours.

VOLUME OF DISTRIBUTION. About 1.3 litres/kg.

Wavelength

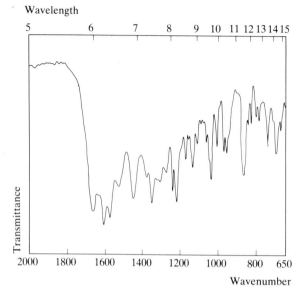

CLEARANCE. Plasma clearance, about 2 ml/min/kg.

DISTRIBUTION IN BLOOD. Plasma: whole blood ratio, about 0.97.

PROTEIN BINDING. In plasma, 25 to 65%.

Dose. 1 to 2 g daily.

Tetrahydrozoline   *Sympathomimetic*

Synonym. Tetryzoline
2-(1,2,3,4-Tetrahydro-1-naphthyl)-2-imidazoline
$C_{13}H_{16}N_2 = 200.3$
CAS—84-22-0

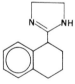

A white crystalline powder.
Soluble in water and chloroform.

Tetrahydrozoline Hydrochloride
Proprietary Names. Murine Plus; Tyzine; Visine; Yxin.
$C_{13}H_{16}N_2,HCl = 236.7$
CAS—522-48-5
A white crystalline powder. M.p. about 256°, with decomposition.
Soluble 1 in 3.5 of water and 1 in 7.5 of ethanol; very slightly soluble in chloroform; practically insoluble in ether.

Colour Tests. Aromaticity (Method 2)—colourless/yellow; Liebermann's Test—brown-orange.

Thin-layer Chromatography. *System TA*—Rf 13; *system TB*—Rf 07; *system TC*—Rf 02. (*Acidified iodoplatinate solution*, positive.)

Gas Chromatography. *System GA*—RI 1833.

Ultraviolet Spectrum. Aqueous acid—265 nm $(A_1^1 = 21\ a)$, 272 nm. No alkaline shift.

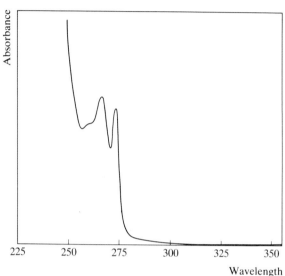

Infra-red Spectrum. Principal peaks at wavenumbers 1600, 742, 1293, 1250, 763, 1500 (tetrahydrozoline hydrochloride, KBr disk).

Mass Spectrum. Principal peaks at *m/z* 200, 185, 199, 171, 44, 84, 71, 131.

Use. Tetrahydrozoline hydrochloride is used as a 0.1% nasal solution.

Tetramisole   *Anthelmintic*

(±)-2,3,5,6-Tetrahydro-6-phenylimidazo[2,1-*b*]thiazole
$C_{11}H_{12}N_2S = 204.3$
CAS—5036-02-2

Crystals. M.p. 87° to 89°.
Practically **insoluble** in water; soluble in chloroform.

Tetramisole Hydrochloride
Proprietary Name. Nilverm (pig wormer)
$C_{11}H_{12}N_2S,HCl = 240.8$
CAS—5086-74-8
A white to pale cream-coloured crystalline powder. M.p. 264° to 265°.
Soluble 1 in 5 of water, 1 in 50 of ethanol, 1 in 3000 of chloroform, and 1 in 10 of methanol; very slightly soluble in ether.

For analytical data see under Levamisole.

Dose. 2.5 to 5 mg/kg of tetramisole hydrochloride as a single dose.

Tetrazepam
Muscle Relaxant/Tranquilliser

Proprietary Name. Myolastan
7-Chloro-5-(cyclohex-1-enyl)-1,3-dihydro-1-methyl-2*H*-1,4-benzodiazepin-2-one
$C_{16}H_{17}ClN_2O = 288.8$
CAS—10379-14-3

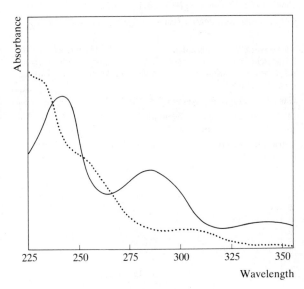

Yellow-brown crystals. M.p. 144°.

Colour Test. Formaldehyde–Sulphuric Acid—orange.

Ultraviolet Spectrum. Aqueous acid—239 nm ($A_1^1 = 940$ b), 284 nm, 345 nm; aqueous alkali—305 nm ($A_1^1 = 84$ b).

Infra-red Spectrum. Principal peaks at wavenumbers 1678, 1602, 825, 1132, 1310, 800 (KBr disk).

Mass Spectrum. Principal peaks at *m/z* 253, 288, 287, 289, 225, 259, 254, 41.

Quantification. HIGH PRESSURE LIQUID CHROMATOGRAPHY. In serum: detection limit 100 pg/ml for tetrazepam and 500 pg/ml for desmethyltetrazepam, UV detection—M. G. Baumgärtner *et al., Arzneimittel-Forsch.,* 1984, *34*, 724–729.

Disposition in the Body. Rapidly absorbed after oral administration. Extensively metabolised by *N*-demethylation and hydroxylation. Urinary metabolites include 3-hydroxytetrazepam, 3-hydroxydesmethyltetrazepam, 3'-hydroxytetrazepam, and 3'-hydroxydesmethyltetrazepam.

THERAPEUTIC CONCENTRATION.
Following a single oral dose of 50 mg to 12 subjects, peak serum concentrations of 0.49 to 0.63 µg/ml (mean 0.57) of tetrazepam and 0.005 to 0.008 µg/ml of desmethyltetrazepam were attained in about 2 hours and 4 hours respectively (M. G. Baumgärtner *et al., ibid.*).

HALF-LIFE. Plasma half-life, 10 to 25 hours (mean 15).

REFERENCE. M. G. Baumgärtner *et al., ibid.*

Dose. 25 to 150 mg daily.

Thalidomide
Hypnotic/Immunosuppressant

2-Phthalimidoglutarimide
$C_{13}H_{10}N_2O_4 = 258.2$
CAS—50-35-1

A white crystalline powder. M.p. 269° to 271°.
Slightly **soluble** in water and ethanol; practically insoluble in chloroform and ether.

Ultraviolet Spectrum. Aqueous acid—240 nm ($A_1^1 = 385$ b), 300 nm ($A_1^1 = 94$ b).

Infra-red Spectrum. Principal peaks at wavenumbers 1681, 727, 1205, 1250, 1316, 1110 (Nujol mull).

Mass Spectrum. Principal peaks at *m/z* 76, 173, 104, 111, 148, 50, 169, 130.

Quantification. ULTRAVIOLET SPECTROPHOTOMETRY. In blood, plasma or urine—J. N. Green and B. C. Benson, *J. Pharm. Pharmac.,* 1961, *13*, 117T–121T.

Disposition in the Body. Absorbed from the gastro-intestinal tract. Thalidomide is hydrolysed in the body, forming mainly 2-(*o*-carboxybenzamido)glutarimide, although many other hydrolysis products are also detectable.

TOXICITY. Thalidomide has a low acute toxicity; in 2 cases of reported overdose there was no evidence of respiratory or cardiac depression. Thalidomide has teratogenic effects when administered to women early in pregnancy.

Dose. 50 to 400 mg daily, in the treatment of lepra reactions.

Thebacon
Narcotic Analgesic

Synonyms. Acethydrocodone; Acetyldihydrocodeinone; Dihydrocodeinone Enol Acetate.
(−)-(5*R*)-4,5-Epoxy-3-methoxy-9a-methylmorphin-6-en-6-yl acetate
$C_{20}H_{23}NO_4 = 341.4$
CAS—466-90-0

A white powder. M.p. 154°.
Practically **insoluble** in water; soluble in ethanol, chloroform, and ether.

Thebacon Hydrochloride

Proprietary Name. Acedicon
$C_{20}H_{23}NO_4, HCl = 377.9$
CAS—20236-82-2
White crystals. M.p. 132° to 135°, with decomposition.
Soluble in water.

Colour Test. Marquis Test—yellow → violet.

Thin-layer Chromatography. *System TA*—Rf 45; *system TB*—Rf 19; *system TC*—Rf 34. (*Acidified iodoplatinate solution*, positive.)

Gas Chromatography. *System GA*—RI 2533.

High Pressure Liquid Chromatography. *System HA*—k′ 3.7 (tailing peak); *system HC*—k′ 0.85.

Ultraviolet Spectrum. Aqueous acid—281 nm ($A_1^1 = 41$ b).

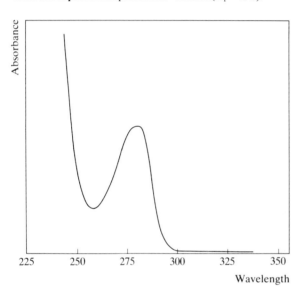

Infra-red Spectrum. Principal peaks at wavenumbers 1208, 1138, 1744, 1500, 905, 1194 (KBr disk).

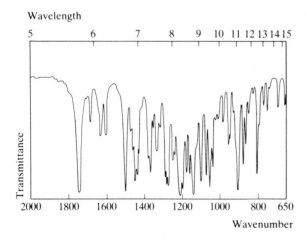

Mass Spectrum. Principal peaks at m/z 341, 298, 43, 44, 55, 284, 242.

Dose. Usually 10 mg of thebacon hydrochloride daily.

Thebaine   *Alkaloid*

Synonym. Paramorphine
3,6-Dimethoxy-4,5-epoxy-9a-methylmorphin-6,8-diene
$C_{19}H_{21}NO_3 = 311.4$
CAS—115-37-7

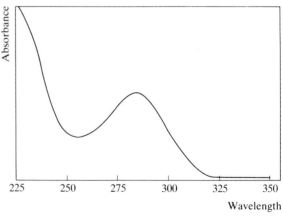

An alkaloid present in opium.
A white powder. M.p. 193°.
Soluble 1 in 1500 of water, 1 in 10 of ethanol, 1 in 13 of chloroform, and 1 in 200 of ether.

Dissociation Constant. pK_a 8.2 (20°).

Partition Coefficient. Log P (octanol/pH 7.5), 0.3.

Colour Tests. Mandelin's Test—orange-brown; Marquis Test—red → orange.

Thin-layer Chromatography. *System TA*—Rf 45; *system TB*—Rf 23; *system TC*—Rf 37. (*Dragendorff spray*, positive; *FPN reagent*, faint brown; *acidified iodoplatinate solution*, positive; *Marquis reagent*, yellow.)

Gas Chromatography. *System GA*—RI 2517.

High Pressure Liquid Chromatography. *System HA*—k′ 4.6 (tailing peak); *system HC*—k′ 0.94; *system HS*—k′ 0.79.

Ultraviolet Spectrum. Aqueous acid—284 nm ($A_1^1 = 253$ a). No alkaline shift.

Infra-red Spectrum. Principal peaks at wavenumbers 1234, 1605, 1144, 1270, 1030, 910 (KBr disk).

Mass Spectrum. Principal peaks at m/z 311, 255, 42, 44, 296, 310, 312, 174.

Thenalidine
Antihistamine

Synonyms. Thenophenopiperidine; Thenopiperidine.
N-(1-Methyl-4-piperidyl)-*N*-(2-thenyl)aniline
$C_{17}H_{22}N_2S = 286.4$
CAS—86-12-4

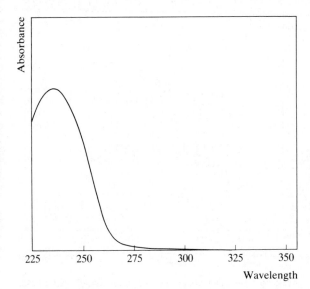

M.p. 95° to 97°.
Practically **insoluble** in water; soluble in chloroform.

Thenalidine Tartrate
$C_{17}H_{22}N_2S,C_4H_6O_6 = 436.5$
CAS—16509-35-6
A white crystalline powder. M.p. 170° to 172°.
Soluble in water.

Colour Tests. Mandelin's Test—orange → brown; Marquis Test—grey-violet.

Thin-layer Chromatography. *System TA*—Rf 50; *system TB*—Rf 38; *system TC*—Rf 44. (*Acidified iodoplatinate solution*, positive.)

Gas Chromatography. *System GA*—RI 2318.

High Pressure Liquid Chromatography. *System HA*—k' 3.5.

Ultraviolet Spectrum. Aqueous acid—234 nm ($A_1^1 = 280$ b).

(graph: Absorbance vs Wavelength, x-axis 225, 250, 275, 300, 325, 350)

Infra-red Spectrum. Principal peaks at wavenumbers 1505, 748, 1600, 693, 1279, 755 (KBr disk).

Mass Spectrum. Principal peaks at *m/z* 97, 70, 99, 43, 98, 44, 42, 188.

Dose. Thenalidine tartrate has been given in doses of 100 to 150 mg daily.

Thenium Closylate
Anthelmintic (Veterinary)

Dimethyl(2-phenoxyethyl)(2-thenyl)ammonium 4-chloroben-zenesulphonate
$C_{21}H_{24}ClNO_4S_2 = 454.0$
CAS—16776-64-0 (thenium); *4304-40-9* (closylate)

A white crystalline powder. M.p. 156° to 162°.
Soluble 1 in 200 of water, 1 in 25 of ethanol, and 1 in 35 of chloroform.

Colour Tests. Mandelin's Test—green; Marquis Test—violet.

Thin-layer Chromatography. *System TA*—Rf 02. (*Acidified iodoplatinate solution*, positive.)

Ultraviolet Spectrum. Aqueous acid—268 nm ($A_1^1 = 45$ b), 275 nm ($A_1^1 = 36$ b).

Infra-red Spectrum. Principal peaks at wavenumbers 1210, 1174, 1042, 1135, 760, 1010 (KBr disk).

Thenyldiamine
Antihistamine

NN-Dimethyl-*N'*-(2-pyridyl)-*N'*-(3-thenyl)ethylenediamine
$C_{14}H_{19}N_3S = 261.4$
CAS—91-79-2

A liquid.
Practically **insoluble** in water; soluble in chloroform.

Thenyldiamine Hydrochloride
Proprietary Names. It is an ingredient of Bronchilator, Franol Plus, and Hayphryn.
$C_{14}H_{19}N_3S,HCl = 297.8$
CAS—958-93-0
A white crystalline powder. M.p. 167° to 171°.
Soluble 1 in 5 of water, 1 in 5 of ethanol, and 1 in 5 of chloroform; practically insoluble in ether.

Dissociation Constant. pK_a 3.9, 8.9 (25°).

Colour Tests. Mandelin's Test—green; Marquis Test—black-violet.

Thin-layer Chromatography. *System TA*—Rf 53; *system TB*—Rf 42; *system TC*—Rf 25. (*Dragendorff spray*, positive; *acidified iodoplatinate solution*, positive; *Marquis reagent*, violet.)

Gas Chromatography. *System GA*—RI 1999; *system GB*—RI 2034; *system GC*—RI 2300; *system GF*—RI 2340.

High Pressure Liquid Chromatography. *System HA*—k' 4.0.

Ultraviolet Spectrum. Aqueous acid—239 nm ($A_1^1 = 703$ a), 315 nm; aqueous alkali—246 nm, 310 nm.

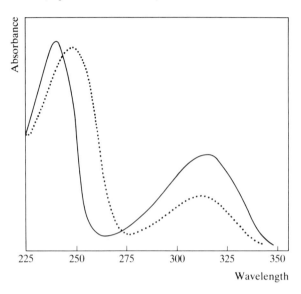

Infra-red Spectrum. Principal peaks at wavenumbers 1597, 766, 1242, 976, 1159, 1311.

Mass Spectrum. Principal peaks at m/z 58, 97, 72, 71, 203, 191, 190, 42.

Dose. Thenyldiamine hydrochloride has been given in doses of up to 90 mg daily.

Theobromine   *Xanthine Derivative*

Synonyms. 3,7-Dimethylxanthine; Santheose.
Proprietary Names. It is an ingredient of Seominal.
3,7-Dihydro-3,7-dimethylpurine-2,6(1*H*)-dione
$C_7H_8N_4O_2 = 180.2$
CAS—83-67-0

An alkaloid contained in the seeds of *Theobroma cacao* (Sterculiaceae).
A white microcrystalline powder which sublimes at about 290°.
Soluble 1 in 2000 of water, 1 in 2500 of ethanol, and 1 in 6000 of chloroform; practically insoluble in ether; freely soluble in dilute mineral acids and aqueous solutions of alkali hydroxides.

Dissociation Constant. $pK_a < 1$, 10.0 (25°).

Partition Coefficient. Log *P* (octanol), -0.8.

Colour Test. Amalic Acid Test—yellow/violet.

Thin-layer Chromatography. *System TA*—Rf 53; *system TB*—Rf 01; *system TC*—Rf 31; *system TG*—Rf 47. (*Ludy Tenger reagent*, orange.)

High Pressure Liquid Chromatography. *System HA*—k' 0.1.

Ultraviolet Spectrum. Aqueous acid—272 nm ($A_1^1 = 563$ a); aqueous alkali—274 nm.

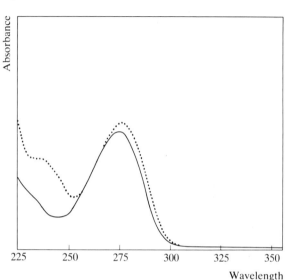

Infra-red Spectrum. Principal peaks at wavenumbers 1690, 1665, 1221, 1550, 1595, 680 (KBr disk).

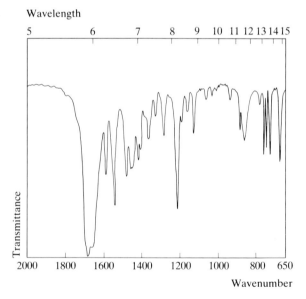

Mass Spectrum. Principal peaks at m/z 180, 55, 67, 109, 82, 42, 137, 70; 3-methylxanthine 166, 68, 95, 41, 53, 123, -, -; 7-methylxanthine 166, 68, 123, 53, 42, 41, 95, -.

Disposition in the Body. Well absorbed after oral administration. It is metabolised by demethylation, mainly to 7-methylxanthine, together with some 3-methylxanthine. The 7-methylxanthine is further oxidised to 7-methyluric acid. About 90% of a dose is excreted in the urine in 48 hours, of which about 40% is 7-methylxanthine, 20% is 3-methylxanthine, 11% is 7-methyluric acid, and 15% is unchanged drug. An additional metabolite, 6-amino-5-(*N*-methylformylamino)-1-methyluracil, accounts for about 7% of a dose.

Theobromine is a metabolite of caffeine.

HALF-LIFE. Plasma half-life, 5 to 11 hours (mean 8) after a single dose, increased on chronic administration.

VOLUME OF DISTRIBUTION. About 0.5 to 1 litre/kg.

CLEARANCE. Plasma clearance, about 0.8 ml/min/kg.

SALIVA. Plasma : saliva ratio, about 1.0.

Dose. 300 to 600 mg.

Theophylline   *Xanthine Bronchodilator*

Synonyms. Anhydrous Theophylline, 1,3-Dimethylxanthine; Teofilina.

Proprietary Names. Accurbron; Aerolate; Asthmophylline; Bronkodyl; Elixicon; Elixophyllin; LāBID; Lasma; Nuelin (tablets); Physpan; Pro-vent; Slo-Phyllin; Somophyllin-T; Sustaire; Theobid; Theoclear; Theocontin; Theo-Dur; Theograd; Theolair; Theolixir; Theon-300; Theophyl; Theospan; Theovent; Uniphyllin Unicontin. It is an ingredient of Franol, Franyl, Labophylline, Phyldrox, Quibron, Tancolin, Taumasthman, and Tedral.

3,7-Dihydro-1,3-dimethylpurine-2,6(1*H*)-dione
$C_7H_8N_4O_2 = 180.2$
CAS—58-55-9

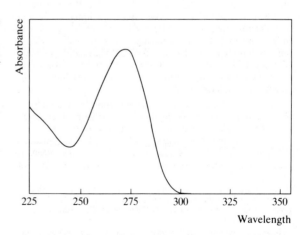

A white crystalline powder. M.p. 270° to 274°.
Soluble 1 in 120 of water, 1 in 80 of ethanol, and 1 in about 200 of chloroform; very slightly soluble in ether; freely soluble in dilute acids, ammonia and alkali hydroxide solutions.

Aminophylline

Synonyms. Euphyllinum; Metaphyllin; Theophyllaminum; Theophylline and Ethylenediamine; Theophylline Ethylenediamine Compound.

Proprietary Names. Aminodur; Aminophyl; Androphyllin; Cardophyllin; Carine; Corophyllin; Euphyllin; Inophyline (injection); Lixaminol; Minilix; Phyllocontin; Phyllotemp; Somophyllin. It is an ingredient of Amesec, and Theodrox.

A stable mixture containing 78 to 84% of anhydrous theophylline and 13 to 14% of ethylenediamine with a variable quantity of water.
Its composition approximately corresponds to the formula $(C_7H_8N_4O_2)_2,C_2H_4(NH_2)_2,2H_2O = 456.5$
CAS—317-34-0 (anhydrous)
White or slightly yellowish granules or powder.
Soluble 1 in 5 of water at 25°, but the addition of ethylenediamine or ammonia solution may be necessary to give complete solution. Practically insoluble in ethanol and ether.

Choline Theophyllinate

Synonyms. Oxtriphylline; Theophylline Cholinate.
Proprietary Names. Choledyl; Euspirax; Sabidal.
$C_{12}H_{21}N_5O_3 = 283.3$
CAS—4499-40-5
A white crystalline powder. M.p. 185° to 192°.
Soluble 1 in less than 1 of water and 1 in 10 of ethanol; very slightly soluble in chloroform and ether.

Theophylline Hydrate

Synonym. Theophylline Monohydrate
Proprietary Names. It is an ingredient of Asmapax and Franol Expect.
$C_7H_8N_4O_2,H_2O = 198.2$
CAS—5967-84-0
A white crystalline powder. M.p. about 272°, after drying.
Soluble 1 in 120 of water and 1 in 80 of ethanol; very slightly soluble in ether; soluble in solutions of alkali hydroxides.

Theophylline Monoethanolamine

Synonym. Theophylline Olamine
Proprietary Names. Inophyline (tablets); Monotheamin.
An equimolecular compound of anhydrous theophylline and monoethanolamine.
$C_7H_8N_4O_2,C_2H_7NO = 241.2$
CAS—573-41-1
A white crystalline powder.
Soluble 1 in 20 of water.

Theophylline Sodium Glycinate

Synonym. Theophylline Sodium Aminoacetate
Proprietary Names. Acet-Am (liquid); Nuelin (liquid); Synophylate; Theocyne.
An equilibrium mixture of theophylline sodium ($C_7H_7N_4NaO_2 = 202.1$) and glycine ($C_2H_5NO_2 = 75.07$) in approximately equimolecular proportions, buffered with an additional mole of glycine.
CAS—8000-10-0
A white crystalline powder.
Soluble 1 in 6 of water; very slightly soluble in ethanol; practically insoluble in chloroform.

Dissociation Constant. $pK_a < 1$, 8.6 (25°).

Partition Coefficient. Log *P* (octanol), 0.0.

Colour Tests. Amalic Acid Test—yellow/violet; Folin–Ciocalteu Reagent—blue.

Thin-layer Chromatography. *System TA*—Rf 75; *system TB*—Rf 01; *system TC*—Rf 30; *system TG*—Rf 33. (*Ludy Tenger reagent, orange.*)

Gas Chromatography. *System GA*—RI 1999; *system GF*—RI 2745.

High Pressure Liquid Chromatography. *System HA*—k' 0.1.

Ultraviolet Spectrum. Aqueous acid—270 nm ($A_1^1 = 536$ a); aqueous alkali—275 nm ($A_1^1 = 650$ a).

Infra-red Spectrum. Principal peaks at wavenumbers 1670, 1717, 1567, 745, 980, 1190 (KBr disk). (See below)

Wavelength

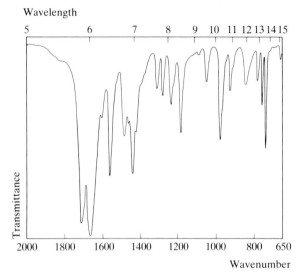

Wavenumber

Mass Spectrum. Principal peaks at m/z 180, 95, 68, 41, 53, 181, 96, 40; 3-methylxanthine 166, 68, 95, 41, 53, 123, –, –.

Quantification. GAS CHROMATOGRAPHY. In serum: sensitivity 2.5 µg/ml, FID—H. A. Schwertner, *Clin. Chem.*, 1979, *25*, 212–214.

HIGH PRESSURE LIQUID CHROMATOGRAPHY. In plasma or saliva: sensitivity 500 ng/ml, UV detection—K. T. Muir *et al.*, *J. Chromat.*, 1982, *231*; *Biomed. Appl.*, *20*, 73–82. In serum: UV detection—S. J. Soldin and J. G. Hill, *Clin. Biochem.*, 1977, *10*, 74–77. In urine: theophylline and major metabolites, UV detection—K. T. Muir *et al.*, *J. Chromat.*, 1980, *221*; *Biomed. Appl.*, *10*, 85–95.

FLUOROIMMUNOASSAY. In serum—T. M. Li *et al.*, *Clin. Chem.*, 1981, *27*, 22–26.

Disposition in the Body. Readily absorbed after oral administration of aminophylline; less rapidly absorbed when given as theophylline; irregularly absorbed after rectal administration. Rapidly and widely distributed throughout the tissues. Metabolised by N-demethylation to form 3-methylxanthine (which is active but less potent than theophylline), 1,3-dimethyluric acid, and 1-methyluric acid. In adults, about 13% of a dose is excreted in the urine in 24 hours as unchanged drug, with about 15% as 3-methylxanthine, 35 to 50% as 1,3-dimethyluric acid, and about 20% as 1-methyluric acid. In premature neonates, most of a dose is excreted as unchanged drug with up to 10% as caffeine. Theophylline is a metabolite of caffeine.

THERAPEUTIC CONCENTRATION. There is considerable intersubject variation in serum-theophylline concentrations; therapeutic effect has been correlated with concentrations of 10 to 15 µg/ml. 3-Methylxanthine accumulates in the serum to concentrations of about 25% of those of theophylline. Diurnal variations in plasma concentrations have been reported with higher concentrations in the morning.

After oral doses of 200 to 300 mg of aminophylline every 6 hours to 83 subjects, trough serum-theophylline concentrations of 2.9 to 32.6 µg/ml (mean about 13) were reported (J. W. Jenne *et al.*, *Clin. Pharmac. Ther.*, 1972, *13*, 349–360).

Following a single oral dose of 5 mg/kg of an elixir containing theophylline, administered to 12 subjects, peak serum concentrations of 11.0 to 16.8 µg/ml (mean 13.9) were attained in 0.5 to 2 hours (R. L. Manfredi and E. S. Vessell, *Clin. Pharmac. Ther.*, 1981, *29*, 224–229).

Following single oral doses of 250 mg and 500 mg of theophylline to 8 subjects, peak plasma concentrations of 5.0 to 12.1 µg/ml (mean 8.0) and 10.7 to 20.5 µg/ml (mean 15), respectively, were attained in 0.5 to 3 hours (V. Rovei *et al.*, *Br. J. clin. Pharmac.*, 1982, *14*, 769–778).

Following daily oral doses of 6.9 to 18.2 mg/kg of aminophylline to 14 subjects, trough steady-state serum concentrations of 6.6 to 15 µg/ml (mean 11) were reported in the morning, in comparison with trough serum concentrations of 5.0 to 13 µg/ml (mean 9.6) in the afternoon (L. J. Lesko *et al.*, *J. pharm. Sci.*, 1980, *69*, 358–359).

TOXICITY. The estimated minimum lethal dose after intravenous administration is 0.1 g; fatalities have occurred after oral doses of 8.4 mg/kg in a child and after 25 to 100 mg/kg of aminophylline given as a suppository. Recovery has been reported after ingestion of choline theophyllinate equivalent to 12.8 g of theophylline. Toxic effects are usually associated with plasma concentrations greater than 30 µg/ml and fatalities with concentrations above 50 µg/ml; premature neonates appear to be relatively resistant to theophylline poisoning.

In a review of nine cases of theophylline poisoning, plasma concentrations on admission to hospital ranged from 24.5 to 120 µg/ml. Convulsions followed by death occurred in three of these cases, the amounts of drug taken being 11.5 g (intravenously over 36 hours), 10.5 g (oral) and 11.2 g (oral); the respective plasma concentrations were 66, 85, and 120 µg/ml (M. Helliwell and D. Berry, *Br. med. J.*, 1979, *2*, 1114).

In a fatality due to the ingestion of theophylline, the following postmortem tissue concentrations were reported: blood 250 µg/ml, bile 275 µg/ml, brain 231 µg/g, kidney 212 µg/g, liver 200 µg/g (C. L. Winek *et al.*, *Forens. Sci. Int.*, 1980, *15*, 233–236).

The following postmortem concentrations were reported in a fatality due to theophylline overdose: blood 63 µg/ml, brain 120 µg/g, liver 275 µg/g; death occurred 23 hours after the subject was discovered comatose (M. R. Loveland, *Bull. int. Ass. forens. Toxicol.*, 1974, *10*(1), 16).

HALF-LIFE. Plasma half-life, 3 to 13 hours in normal subjects (mean 7) but decreased in smokers and in children, and increased in premature neonates and in certain disease states such as hepatic disease, heart failure, and chronic obstructive pulmonary disease. The half-life may also be affected by the amount of dietary methylxanthines ingested.

VOLUME OF DISTRIBUTION. About 0.5 litre/kg.

CLEARANCE. Plasma clearance, about 0.5 to 2 ml/min/kg in normal subjects.

DISTRIBUTION IN BLOOD. Plasma: whole blood ratio, 1.2.

SALIVA. Plasma: saliva ratio, about 2, but there is considerable intersubject variation.

PROTEIN BINDING. In plasma, about 40% (temperature and pH-dependent); decreased in neonates and in subjects with hepatic cirrhosis.

NOTE. For reviews of the clinical pharmacokinetics of theophylline see R. I. Ogilvie, *Clin. Pharmacokinet.*, 1978, *3*, 267–293 and T. J. Haley, *Drug Met. Rev.*, 1983, *14*, 295–335).

Dose. 0.18 to 1 g daily.

Thiabendazole
Anthelmintic

Proprietary Names. Equizole (vet.); Mintezol; Thiprazole (vet.). It is an ingredient of Ranizole (vet.).

2-(Thiazol-4-yl)-1H-benzimidazole
$C_{10}H_7N_3S = 201.3$
CAS—148-79-8

A white or cream-coloured powder. M.p. 296° to 303°.
Practically **insoluble** in water; soluble 1 in 150 of ethanol, 1 in 300 of chloroform, and 1 in 2000 of ether; soluble in dilute mineral acids.

Thin-layer Chromatography. *System TA*—Rf 67; *system TB*—Rf 07; *system TC*—Rf 54. (*Acidified iodoplatinate solution*, positive.)

Gas Chromatography. *System GA*—RI 2040; *system GK*—retention time 1.18 relative to caffeine.

Ultraviolet Spectrum. Aqueous acid—243 nm, 302 nm ($A_1^1 = 1230\ a$).

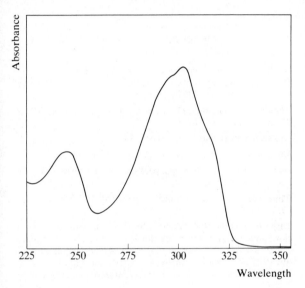

Absorbance

Wavelength

Infra-red Spectrum. Principal peaks at wavenumbers 740, 1306, 902, 1095, 1279, 1231 (KBr disk).

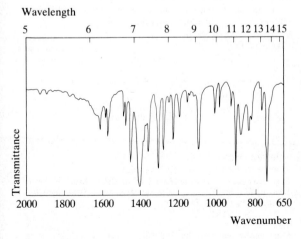

Wavelength

Transmittance

Wavenumber

Mass Spectrum. Principal peaks at *m/z* 201, 174, 63, 202, 64, 65, 175, 90.

Quantification. HIGH PRESSURE LIQUID CHROMATOGRAPHY. In serum: thiabendazole and 5-hydroxythiabendazole, detection limit 100 ng/ml and 400 ng/ml, respectively, fluorescence detection—M. T. Watts *et al.*, *J. Chromat.*, 1982, *230*; *Biomed. Appl.*, *19*, 79–86.

Disposition in the Body. Readily absorbed after oral administration; peak plasma concentrations are attained in 1 to 2 hours. Metabolised to the 5-hydroxy derivative and excreted in the urine as conjugates. About 90% of a dose is excreted in the urine in 48 hours and 5% is eliminated in the faeces. Less than 1% of a dose is excreted in the urine unchanged.

HALF-LIFE. Plasma half-life, about 1 hour.

Dose. Usually 25 mg/kg twice daily, to a maximum daily dose of 3 g.

Thiacetazone   *Antituberculous Agent/Antileprotic*

Synonyms. Amithiozone; Tebezonum; Thioacetazone.
4-Acetamidobenzaldehyde thiosemicarbazone
$C_{10}H_{12}N_4OS = 236.3$
CAS—104-06-3

CH:N·NH·CS·NH₂

NH·CO·CH₃

Pale yellow crystals or crystalline powder. M.p. 225° to 230°, with decompostion.
Very slightly **soluble** in water; soluble 1 in 500 of ethanol and 1 in 100 of propylene glycol; practically insoluble in chloroform and ether.

Colour Tests. Nessler's Reagent (100°)—black; Palladium Chloride—orange.

Thin-layer Chromatography. *System TA*—Rf 78. (*Acidified iodoplatinate solution*, positive.)

Gas Chromatography. *System GA*—RI 2038.

Ultraviolet Spectrum. Ethanol—328 nm ($A_1^1 = 1870\ a$).

Infra-red Spectrum. Principal peaks at wavenumbers 1515, 1603, 1580, 1661, 1250, 1305 (KBr disk).

Quantification. HIGH PRESSURE LIQUID CHROMATOGRAPHY. In plasma or urine: detection limit 3 ng/ml, UV detection—P. J. Jenner, *J. Chromat.*, 1983, *276*; *Biomed. Appl.*, *27*, 463–470.

Disposition in the Body. Slowly absorbed after oral administration. Most of a dose is metabolised and excreted in the urine; about 20% of a dose is excreted in the urine unchanged.

THERAPEUTIC CONCENTRATION.
Following a single oral dose of 4 mg/kg to 10 subjects, peak serum concentrations of 1.3 to 4.0 µg/ml (mean 3.1) were attained in about 5 hours (P. K. Sen *et al.*, *J. Indian med. Ass.*, 1973, *61*, 306–308).

HALF-LIFE. About 8 to 12 hours.

Dose. Up to 150 mg daily.

Thialbarbitone   *Barbiturate*

Synonym. Thialbarbital
5-Allyl-5-(cyclohex-2-enyl)-2-thiobarbituric acid
$C_{13}H_{16}N_2O_2S = 264.3$
CAS—467-36-7

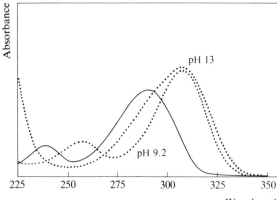

Crystals. M.p. 148° to 150°.
Sparingly **soluble** in water; readily soluble in most organic solvents.

Thialbarbitone Sodium

Synonyms. Natrium Cyclohexenylallylthiobarbituricum; Thiohexallymalnatrium.
$C_{13}H_{15}N_2NaO_2S = 286.3$
CAS—3546-29-0
A pale yellow hygroscopic powder. M.p. 130° to 132°.
Very **soluble** in water and ethanol; slightly soluble in chloroform; practically insoluble in ether.

Colour Tests. Palladium Chloride—orange-yellow; Vanillin Reagent—brown-orange/violet (transient).

Thin-layer Chromatography. *System TD*—Rf 77; *system TE*—Rf 44; *system TF*—Rf 74; *system TH*—Rf 75. (*Mercurous nitrate spray*, black; *acidified potassium permanganate solution*, yellowbrown; *Zwikker's reagent*, green.)

Gas Chromatography. *System GA*—RI 2116.

Ultraviolet Spectrum. *Borax buffer 0.05M* (pH 9.2)—256 nm, 307 nm ($A_1^1 = 1236$ b); M sodium hydroxide (pH 13)—306 nm ($A_1^1 = 1271$ b).

[Graph: Absorbance vs Wavelength, showing curves labelled pH 13 and pH 9.2, x-axis from 225 to 350]

Infra-red Spectrum. Principal peaks at wavenumbers 1685, 1610, 1300, 1130, 1270, 1000 (thialbarbitone sodium, KBr disk).

Mass Spectrum. Principal peaks at m/z 81, 223, 79, 41, 80, 157, 185, 77.

Dose. Thialbarbitone sodium has been given in doses of 0.2 to 1 g intravenously.

Thiambutosine   *Antileprotic*

Synonym. DPT
Proprietary Name. Ciba-1906
1-(4-Butoxyphenyl)-3-(4-dimethylaminophenyl)thiourea
$C_{19}H_{25}N_3OS = 343.5$
CAS—500-89-0

A white or creamy-white crystalline powder. M.p. 123° to 127°.
Practically **insoluble** in water; soluble 1 in 1.5 of chloroform and 1 in 300 of ether; soluble in acetone.

Thin-layer Chromatography. *System TA*—Rf 76; *system TB*—Rf 06; *system TC*—Rf 77.

Gas Chromatography. *System GA*—RI 1715.

Ultraviolet Spectrum. Ethanol—270 nm ($A_1^1 = 720$ a).

Infra-red Spectrum. Principal peaks at wavenumbers 1234, 720, 1307, 1499, 813, 1093.

Mass Spectrum. Principal peaks at m/z 151, 109, 136, 178, 177, 29, 207, 135.

Disposition in the Body. Poorly absorbed after oral administration; aqueous suspensions are slowly and possibly incompletely absorbed after intramuscular injection. About 10% of a dose is metabolised to water-soluble compounds and rapidly excreted in the urine; about 75% of a dose is eliminated unchanged in the faeces.

Dose. 1 to 3 g daily.

Thiamine   *Vitamin*

Synonyms. Aneurine; Vitamin B_1.
3-(4-Amino-2-methylpyrimidin-5-ylmethyl)-5-(2-hydroxyethyl)-4-methylthiazolium chloride
$C_{12}H_{17}ClN_4OS = 300.8$
CAS—59-43-8

Thiamine Hydrochloride

Synonym. Aneurine Chloride Hydrochloride
Proprietary Names. Benerva; Betabion; Betalin S; Betamin; Beta-Sol; Betaxin; Bévitine; Bewon; Invite B_1; Megamin. It is an ingredient of Aneurone, Apisate and Effico.
$C_{12}H_{17}ClN_4OS,HCl = 337.3$
CAS—67-03-8
Colourless crystals or white crystalline powder. M.p. about 248°, with decomposition.
Soluble 1 in 1 of water and 1 in 100 of ethanol; practically insoluble in dehydrated alcohol and ether; soluble in methanol.

Thiamine Mononitrate

Synonyms. Aneurine Mononitrate; Thiamine Nitrate; Vitamin B_1 Mononitrate.
Proprietary Name. B_1-Vicotrat
$C_{12}H_{17}N_5O_4S = 327.4$
CAS—532-43-4
White crystals or crystalline powder. M.p. about 193°, with decomposition.
Soluble 1 in 44 of water; slightly soluble in ethanol and chloroform.

Dissociation Constant. pK_a 4.8 (20°).

Colour Test. Dissolve about 5 mg of thiamine hydrochloride in a mixture of 1 ml of *lead acetate solution* and 1 ml of 10% sodium hydroxide solution—yellow; after heating on a steam-bath—brown; on standing—a black precipitate of lead sulphide.

Thin-layer Chromatography. *System TA*—Rf 01. (*Acidified iodoplatinate solution*, positive.)

High Pressure Liquid Chromatography. *System HA*—k' 2.0.

Ultraviolet Spectrum. Aqueous acid—246 nm ($A_1^1 = 450$ a); aqueous alkali—232 nm ($A_1^1 = 566$ b), 336 nm.

Infra-red Spectrum. Principal peaks at wavenumbers 1660, 1618, 1048, 1237, 1595, 1228 (thiamine hydrochloride, KBr disk).

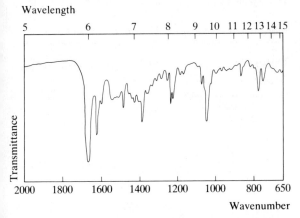

Wavelength

Thiamylal   *Barbiturate*

5-Allyl-5-(1-methylbutyl)-2-thiobarbituric acid
$C_{12}H_{18}N_2O_2S = 254.3$
CAS—77-27-0

Crystals. M.p. 132° to 133°.

Sodium Thiamylal

Proprietary Name. Surital
$C_{12}H_{17}N_2NaO_2S = 276.3$
CAS—337-47-3
Thiamylal sodium for injection is a mixture of sodium thiamylal with anhydrous sodium carbonate. It is a pale yellow hygroscopic powder.
Soluble in water.

Dissociation Constant. pK_a 7.5.

Gas Chromatography. *System GA*—RI 1899.

Ultraviolet Spectrum. Aqueous acid—238 nm, 287 nm; aqueous alkali—305 nm.

Infra-red Spectrum. Principal peaks at wavenumbers 1668, 1541, 1731, 1170, 1318, 1291 (KBr disk).

Mass Spectrum. Principal peaks at m/z 43, 41, 184, 168, 167, 97, 55, 53.

Dose. Initially 3 to 6 ml of a 2.5% solution of sodium thiamylal intravenously.

Thiazinamium Methylsulphate   *Antihistamine*

Synonym. Methylpromethazinium Methylsulfuricum
Proprietary Name. Multergan
Trimethyl[1-methyl-2-(phenothiazin-10-yl)ethyl]ammonium methylsulphate
$C_{19}H_{26}N_2O_4S_2 = 410.5$
CAS—2338-21-8 (thiazinamium); *58-34-4* (methylsulphate)

Quantification. HIGH PRESSURE LIQUID CHROMATOGRAPHY. In plasma: detection limit 150 pg/ml, fluorescence detection—W. Weber and H. Kewitz, *Eur. J. clin. Pharmac.*, 1985, 28, 213–219.

Disposition in the Body. Well absorbed from the gastro-intestinal tract and widely distributed throughout the body. It is converted in the body to thiamine pyrophosphate. Thiamine is not stored to any appreciable extent in the body and amounts in excess of the body's requirements are excreted in the urine unchanged or as metabolites. About 1 mg of thiamine is metabolised in the body daily.
Endogenous blood concentrations are about 0.010 to 0.015 µg/ml and concentrations of thiamine pyrophosphate in erythrocytes are usually 0.03 to 0.11 µg/ml.
Endogenous plasma concentrations in 91 subjects ranged from 0.002 to 0.013 µg/ml (median 0.004) (W. Weber and H. Kewitz, *ibid.*).

Dose. 10 to 100 mg daily.

A white crystalline powder which discolours on exposure to light. M.p. 206° to 210°, with decomposition.
Soluble 1 in 10 of water; very soluble in ethanol; practically insoluble in ether.

Colour Tests. Formaldehyde–Sulphuric Acid—brown-violet; Forrest Reagent—red; FPN Reagent—red; Liebermann's Test—red.

Thin-layer Chromatography. *System TA*—Rf 02. (*Acidified iodoplatinate solution*, positive.)

Ultraviolet Spectrum. Aqueous acid—251 nm ($A_1^1 = 450$ b), 299 nm. (See below)

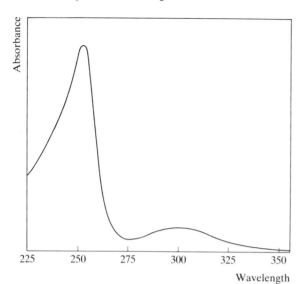

Absorbance

225   250   275   300   325   350

Wavelength

Infra-red Spectrum. Principal peaks at wavenumbers 1224, 1010, 1059, 764, 743, 1036.

Quantification. GAS CHROMATOGRAPHY. In plasma or urine: sensitivity 20 ng/ml, AFID—J. H. G. Jonkman et al., *J. Pharm. Pharmac.*, 1975, *27*, 849–854.

Disposition in the Body. Incompletely absorbed after oral administration and undergoes considerable first-pass metabolism to thiazinamium sulphoxide; well absorbed after intramuscular administration. About 40% of a parenteral dose is excreted in the urine unchanged in 8 hours, together with 9% of the dose as the sulphoxide.

THERAPEUTIC CONCENTRATION.

Following single oral doses equivalent to 300 mg and 900 mg of thiazinamium to 10 subjects, peak plasma concentrations of 0.03 to 0.13 μg/ml (mean 0.07) and 0.06 to 0.36 μg/ml (mean 0.17) were attained in about 2.4 hours and 5 hours, respectively (J. H. G. Jonkman et al., *Clin. Pharmac. Ther.*, 1977, *21*, 457–463).

Dose. 0.6 to 1.2 g daily.

Thiethylperazine   *Anti-emetic*

2 - Ethylthio - 10 - [3 - (4 - methylpiperazin - 1 - yl)propyl]-phenothiazine
$C_{22}H_{29}N_3S_2 = 399.6$
CAS—1420-55-9

Crystals. M.p. 62° to 64°.
Practically **insoluble** in water.

Thiethylperazine Malate

Proprietary Name. Torecan (injection)
$C_{22}H_{29}N_3S_2, 2C_4H_6O_5 = 667.8$
CAS—52239-63-1
A white to faintly yellow crystalline powder. M.p. 139°.
Soluble 1 in 40 of water, 1 in 90 of ethanol, 1 in 525 of chloroform, and 1 in 3400 of ether.

Thiethylperazine Maleate

Proprietary Name. Torecan (suppositories and tablets)
$C_{22}H_{29}N_3S_2, 2C_4H_4O_4 = 631.8$
CAS—1179-69-7
A yellowish granular powder. M.p. about 183°, with decomposition.
Soluble 1 in 1700 of water and 1 in 530 of ethanol; practically insoluble in chloroform and ether.

Colour Tests. Formaldehyde–Sulphuric Acid—green; Forrest Reagent—blue; FPN Reagent—blue; Mandelin's Test—violet; Marquis Test—red → green.

Thin-layer Chromatography. *System TA*—Rf 51; *system TB*—Rf 30; *system TC*—Rf 41. (*Acidified iodoplatinate solution*, positive.)

Gas Chromatography. *System GA*—RI 3247.

High Pressure Liquid Chromatography. *System HA*—k' 3.8.

Ultraviolet Spectrum. Aqueous acid—255 nm ($A_1^1 = 857$ b), 309 nm ($A_1^1 = 98$ b).

Infra-red Spectrum. Principal peaks at wavenumbers 1563, 864, 1613, 1212, 1105, 1067 (KBr disk).

Mass Spectrum. Principal peaks at *m/z* 70, 113, 141, 399, 43, 26, 72, 42.

Dose. Usually 20 to 30 mg of thiethylperazine maleate daily.

Thiocarlide   *Antituberculous Agent*

Synonym. Tiocarlide
Proprietary Name. Isoxyl
1,3-Bis(4-isopentyloxyphenyl)thiourea
$C_{23}H_{32}N_2O_2S = 400.6$
CAS—910-86-1

$(CH_3)_2CH \cdot CH_2 \cdot CH_2 \cdot O$ $O \cdot CH_2 \cdot CH_2 \cdot CH(CH_3)_2$

A white crystalline powder. M.p. 134° to 145°.
Practically **insoluble** in water; soluble in ethanol and chloroform.

Colour Tests. Liebermann's Test—green; Mandelin's Test—green → yellow.

Thin-layer Chromatography. *System TA*—Rf 80; *system TB*—Rf 07; *system TC*—Rf 78. (*Acidified iodoplatinate solution*, positive.)

Gas Chromatography. *System GA*—RI 2005.

Infra-red Spectrum. Principal peaks at wavenumbers 1228, 1499, 1534, 823, 1163, 1285 (KBr disk).

Mass Spectrum. Principal peaks at *m/z* 109, 151, 43, 41, 221, 179, 29, 108.

Dose. 6 g daily.

Thioguanine

Antineoplastic

Synonyms. 6-TG; 6-Thioguanine.
Proprietary Name. Lanvis
2-Aminopurine-6(1*H*)-thione
$C_5H_5N_5S = 167.2$
CAS—154-42-7 (anhydrous); *5580-03-0* (hemihydrate)

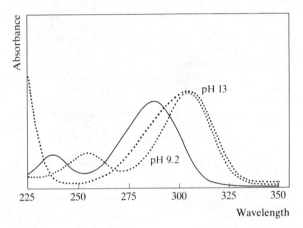

A pale yellow crystalline powder.
Practically **insoluble** in water, ethanol, and chloroform; freely soluble in dilute solutions of alkali hydroxides.

Ultraviolet Spectrum. Aqueous acid—258 nm ($A_1^1 = 490$ b), 348 nm ($A_1^1 = 1240$ a); aqueous alkali—320 nm ($A_1^1 = 1015$ b).

Infra-red Spectrum. Principal peaks at wavenumbers 1625, 1668, 1257, 1539, 1231, 971 (KBr disk).

Quantification. SPECTROFLUORIMETRY. In plasma: sensitivity 5 ng/ml—T. Dooley and J. L. Maddocks, *Br. J. clin. Pharmac.*, 1980, *9*, 77–82.

HIGH PRESSURE LIQUID CHROMATOGRAPHY. In plasma or urine: sensitivity 200 ng/ml, UV detection—H. Breithaupt and G. Goebel, *J. chromatogr. Sci.*, 1981, *19*, 496–499. In plasma: thioguanine and metabolites, sensitivity about 130 ng/ml, UV detection—P. A. Andrews *et al.*, *J. Chromat.*, 1982, *227*; *Biomed. Appl.*, *16*, 83–91.

Disposition in the Body. Incompletely and variably absorbed after oral administration. Rapidly activated by intracellular conversion to thioguanylic acid. Inactivated by methylation to aminomethylthiopurine and by deamination to thioxanthine. About 40% of an oral dose is excreted in the urine as metabolites in 24 hours; only traces of thioguanine have been detected.

Dose. Initially 2 to 2.5 mg/kg daily.

Thiopentone

Barbiturate

Synonyms. Penthiobarbital; Thiomebumal; Thiopental.
5-Ethyl-5-(1-methylbutyl)-2-thiobarbituric acid
$C_{11}H_{18}N_2O_2S = 242.3$
CAS—76-75-5

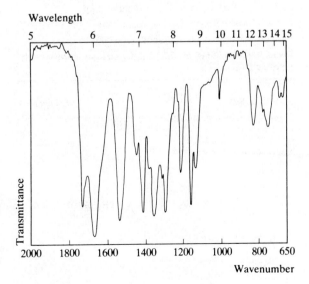

Thiopentone Sodium
Synonyms. Soluble Thiopentone; Thiopental Sodium.
Proprietary Names. Farmotal; Intraval Sodium; Nesdonal; Pentothal; Trapanal.
$C_{11}H_{17}N_2NaO_2S = 264.3$
CAS—71-73-8
A white to yellowish-white to pale green, hygroscopic powder. It usually contains anhydrous sodium carbonate in the proportion of 6 parts to each 100 parts of thiopentone sodium.

Soluble 1 in 1.5 of water; partly soluble in ethanol; practically insoluble in ether.

Dissociation Constant. pK_a 7.6 (20°).

Colour Tests. Koppanyi–Zwikker Test—violet; Palladium Chloride—orange; Vanillin Reagent—brown-red/violet.

Thin-layer Chromatography. *System TD*—Rf 77; *system TE*—Rf 49; *system TF*—Rf 74; *system TH*—Rf 80. (*Mercuric chloride-diphenylcarbazone reagent*, positive; *mercurous nitrate spray*, black; *acidified potassium permanganate solution*, yellow-brown; *Zwikker's reagent*, green.)

Gas Chromatography. *System GA*—RI 1859; *system GF*—RI 2600.

Ultraviolet Spectrum. *Borax buffer 0.05M* (pH 9.2)—255 nm, 304 nm ($A_1^1 = 1138$ b); M sodium hydroxide (pH 13)—303 nm ($A_1^1 = 1170$ b).

Infra-red Spectrum. Principal peaks at wavenumbers 1670, 1540, 1300, 1170, 1735, 1220 (KBr disk).

Mass Spectrum. Principal peaks at m/z 172, 157, 173, 43, 41, 55, 69, 71.

Quantification. See also under Amylobarbitone.

GAS CHROMATOGRAPHY. In plasma: sensitivity 25 ng/ml, AFID—D. Jung *et al.*, *Clin. Chem.*, 1981, *27*, 113–115.

HIGH PRESSURE LIQUID CHROMATOGRAPHY. In plasma: detection limit 200 ng/ml, UV detection—C. Salvadori *et al.*, *Ther. Drug Monit.*, 1981, *3*, 171–176. In blood or tissues: sensitivity 1 µg/ml, UV detection—B. Levine *et al.*, *J. analyt. Toxicol.*, 1983, *7*, 207–208.

Disposition in the Body. About 10% of a dose is concentrated in the brain within 1 minute of an intravenous injection and it is then rapidly distributed throughout the body, eventually accumulating in body fat; about 50% of a dose accumulates in this way after 30 to 90 minutes. The very short action of thiopentone is due to the brief α-phase half-life and the redistribution of the drug from the brain to other fatty tissues. Metabolic reactions include ω-hydroxylation, further oxidation and, to a lesser extent, desulphuration to pentobarbitone. Less than 1% of a dose is excreted in the urine as unchanged drug. 5-(3-Carboxy-1-methylpropyl)-5-ethyl-2-thiobarbituric acid has been reported to be a urinary metabolite.

THERAPEUTIC CONCENTRATION.

Plasma concentrations of 4.2 to 134 µg/ml (mean 28) were reported in 22 patients after intravenous injections (K. E. Becker, *Anesthesiology*, 1976, *45*, 656–660).

TOXICITY. The estimated minimum lethal dose is 1 g. Numerous fatalities have occurred due to accidental or intentional overdosage, and blood concentrations from 6 to 392 µg/ml have been reported in fatalities.

The following postmortem tissue distribution was reported in one suicide case: blood 6 µg/ml, brain 24 µg/g, heart 22 µg/g, kidney 31 µg/g, and liver 63 µg/g (A. M. Bruce *et al.*, *Forens. Sci.*, 1977, *9*, 205–207).

In a fatality due to intravenous self-administration of thiopentone, the following postmortem tissue concentrations were reported: blood 285 µg/ml, brain 414 µg/g, kidney 195 µg/g, liver 440 µg/g (E. Reed and J. R. Monforte, *Bull. int. Ass. forens. Toxicol.*, 1973, *9* (3&4), 12).

HALF-LIFE. Plasma half-life, 4 to 20 hours (mean 9), increased after high doses (25 mg/min), up to 60 hours.

VOLUME OF DISTRIBUTION. 0.5 to 4 litres/kg.

CLEARANCE. Plasma clearance, 1 to 4 ml/min/kg.

DISTRIBUTION IN BLOOD. Plasma: whole blood ratio, 1.0.

PROTEIN BINDING. In plasma, about 75 to 90%.

Dose. 100 to 150 mg of thiopentone sodium intravenously, repeated if necessary.

Thiopropazate
Tranquilliser

2-{4-[3-(2-Chlorophenothiazin-10-yl)propyl]piperazin-1-yl}-ethyl acetate
$C_{23}H_{28}ClN_3O_2S = 446.0$
CAS—84-06-0

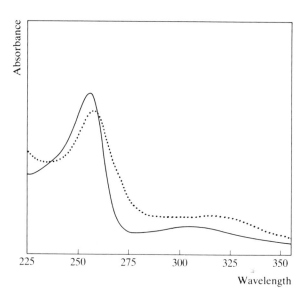

Practically **insoluble** in water; soluble in chloroform and ether.

Thiopropazate Hydrochloride
Proprietary Names. Dartal; Dartalan.
$C_{23}H_{28}ClN_3O_2S,2HCl = 518.9$
CAS—146-28-1
A white or pale yellow crystalline powder. M.p. 228° to 232°.
Soluble 1 in 4 of water, 1 in 130 of ethanol, and 1 in 65 of chloroform; practically insoluble in ether.
Caution. Thiopropazate hydrochloride may cause severe dermatitis in sensitised persons.

Dissociation Constant. pK_a 7.3 (24°).

Colour Tests. Formaldehyde–Sulphuric Acid—red-violet; Forrest Reagent—red; FPN Reagent—red; Liebermann's Test—green-brown; Mandelin's Test—violet; Marquis Test—violet.

Thin-layer Chromatography. *System TA*—Rf 61; *system TB*—Rf 35; *system TC*—Rf 53. (*Dragendorff spray*, positive; *FPN reagent*, pink; *acidified iodoplatinate solution*, positive; *Marquis reagent*, red; *ninhydrin spray*, positive.)

Gas Chromatography. *System GA*—RI 3465.

High Pressure Liquid Chromatography. *System HA*—k' 1.0.

Ultraviolet Spectrum. Aqueous acid—255 nm ($A_1^1 = 733$ a), 305 nm; aqueous alkali—257 nm.

Infra-red Spectrum. Principal peaks at wavenumbers 1222, 1728, 746, 1265, 1250, 1200 (thiopropazate hydrochloride, KBr disk).

Mass Spectrum. Principal peaks at m/z 42, 43, 70, 246, 185, 55, 56, 445.

Dose. Initially 15 to 30 mg of thiopropazate hydrochloride daily; maximum of 100 mg daily.

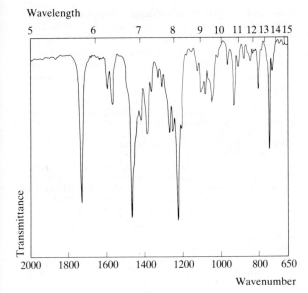

Wavelength

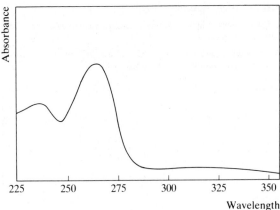

Infra-red Spectrum. Principal peaks at wavenumbers 1156, 1042, 1212, 720, 960, 762 (thioproperazine mesylate, Nujol mull).

Mass Spectrum. Principal peaks at m/z 79, 96, 31, 113, 81, 70, 127, 78.

Dose. Usually 15 to 30 mg of thioproperazine mesylate daily; up to 90 mg daily has been given.

Thioproperazine   *Tranquilliser*

NN - Dimethyl - 10 - [3 - (4 - methylpiperazin - 1 - yl)propyl]-phenothiazine-2-sulphonamide
$C_{22}H_{30}N_4O_2S_2 = 446.6$
CAS—316-81-4

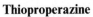

Crystals. M.p. 140°.
Practically **insoluble** in water.

Thioproperazine Mesylate

Synonyms. Thioproperazine Dimethanesulphonate; Thioproperazine Methanesulphonate.
Proprietary Name. Majeptil
$C_{22}H_{30}N_4O_2S_2,2CH_4O_3S = 638.8$
CAS—2347-80-0
A fine, white or pale cream powder, which becomes coloured on exposure to light. M.p. about 227°.
Soluble in water; slightly soluble in ethanol.

Colour Tests. Formaldehyde–Sulphuric Acid—pink; Forrest Reagent—red; FPN Reagent—orange; Mandelin's Test—brown → green → violet; Marquis Test—red.

Thin-layer Chromatography. *System TA*—Rf 46; *system TB*—Rf 07; *system TC*—Rf 34. (*Acidified iodoplatinate solution*, positive.)

Gas Chromatography. *System GA*—not eluted.

High Pressure Liquid Chromatography. *System HA*—k′ 4.1.

Ultraviolet Spectrum. Aqueous acid—234 nm, 263 nm ($A_1^1 = 668$ a), 312 nm. No alkaline shift.

Thioridazine   *Tranquilliser*

Proprietary Names. Mellaril-S; Melleretten; Melleril.
10-[2-(1-Methyl-2-piperidyl)ethyl]-2-methylthiophenothiazine
$C_{21}H_{26}N_2S_2 = 370.6$
CAS—50-52-2

A white or slightly yellow crystalline powder which darkens on exposure to light. M.p. 69° to 74°.
Practically **insoluble** in water; soluble 1 in 6 of ethanol, 1 in 0.8 of chloroform, and 1 in 3 of ether.

Thioridazine Hydrochloride

Proprietary Names. Mellaril; Melleretten (tablets); Melleril (tablets); Novoridazine; Thioril.
$C_{21}H_{26}N_2S_2,HCl = 407.0$
CAS—130-61-0
A white or slightly yellow crystalline powder. M.p. 157° to 163°.
Soluble 1 in 9 of water, 1 in 10 of ethanol, and 1 in 1.5 of chloroform; practically insoluble in ether.

Dissociation Constant. pK_a 9.5 (24°).

Colour Tests. Formaldehyde–Sulphuric Acid—blue; Forrest Reagent—blue; FPN Reagent—blue; Mandelin's Test—blue → violet; Marquis Test—violet-red → blue-green.

Thin-layer Chromatography. *System TA*—Rf 48; *system TB*—Rf 43; *system TC*—Rf 30. (*Dragendorff spray*, positive; *FPN reagent*, blue; *acidified iodoplatinate solution*, positive; *Marquis reagent*, grey-violet.)

Gas Chromatography. *System GA*—RI 3114.

High Pressure Liquid Chromatography. *System HA*—thioridazine k' 5.2, mesoridazine k' 5.0.

Ultraviolet Spectrum. Aqueous acid—262 nm $(A_1^1 = 987$ a), 310 nm; aqueous alkali—275 nm.

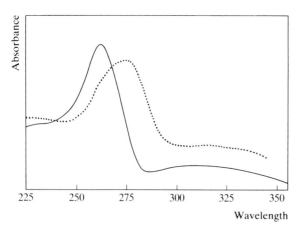

Infra-red Spectrum. Principal peaks at wavenumbers 754, 1248, 796, 1234, 1281, 1211 (thioridazine hydrochloride, KBr disk).

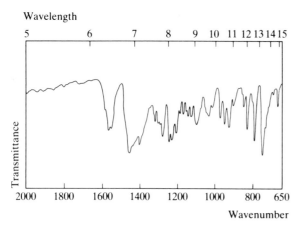

Mass Spectrum. Principal peaks at *m/z* 98, 370, 126, 99, 40, 70, 371, 258; mesoridazine 98, 70, 99, 42, 386, 126, 55, 41.

Quantification. GAS CHROMATOGRAPHY. In plasma: detection limit for thioridazine 100 ng/ml and for mesoridazine and sulforidazine 150 ng/ml, FID—F. A. J. Vanderheeren *et al.*, *J. Chromat.*, 1976, *120*, 123–128.

HIGH PRESSURE LIQUID CHROMATOGRAPHY. In plasma: thioridazine and metabolites, sensitivity 2 ng/ml, fluorescence detection—C. E. Wells *et al.*, *J. pharm. Sci.*, 1983, *72*, 622–625.

Disposition in the Body. Readily absorbed after oral administration. It is metabolised mainly by sulphoxidation to give the side-chain sulphoxide (mesoridazine), the side-chain sulphone (sulforidazine), both of which are active, and the ring sulphoxide and sulphone; *N*-demethylation also occurs. Other metabolites are produced by combinations of these metabolic reactions. It is metabolised in the liver, secreted in the bile, and excreted mainly in the faeces. Less than about 10% of a dose is excreted in the

urine, with less than 1% as unchanged drug; mesoridazine and sulforidazine are also excreted in the urine in amounts slightly greater than unchanged drug.

THERAPEUTIC CONCENTRATION. Plasma concentrations of drug and metabolites show considerable intersubject variation. Concentrations appear to be independent of dose and tend to decrease during chronic treatment.

After a single oral dose of 100 mg administered to 5 subjects, the following peak serum concentrations were found: thioridazine 0.05 to 0.50 µg/ml (mean 0.24) in 1 to 4 hours, mesoridazine 0.10 to 0.51 µg/ml (mean 0.32) in 2 to 6 hours, sulforidazine 0.02 to 0.11 µg/ml (mean 0.07) in 5 to 8 hours, ring sulphoxide 0.07 to 0.38 µg/ml (mean 0.18) in 4 to 8 hours (R. Axelsson and E. Martensson, *Curr. ther. Res.*, 1977, *21*, 561–586).

Following daily oral doses of 100 to 800 mg (mean 382) to 17 subjects, serum concentrations, determined 12 hours after a dose, were: thioridazine 0.4 to 2.0 µg/ml (mean 0.9), mesoridazine 0.2 to 1.6 µg/ml (mean 0.8), sulforidazine 0 to 0.6 µg/ml (mean 0.2), ring sulphoxide 0.06 to 4.0 µg/ml (mean 1.5) (R. Axelsson *et al.*, *Eur. J. clin. Pharmac.*, 1982, *23*, 359–363).

TOXICITY. The estimated minimum lethal dose is 1 g. Blood concentrations greater than about 2 µg/ml may produce toxic effects and can be lethal.

Six cases of non-fatal overdose were found to have blood concentrations in the range 2.4 to 11.8 µg/ml (mean 4.6) (S. L. Tompsett, *Acta pharmac. tox.*, 1968, *26*, 298–302).

In 12 cases of death attributed to thioridazine overdose, postmortem concentrations (total thioridazine and metabolites) were: blood 1 to 18 µg/ml (mean 4.7), kidney 18 to 70 µg/g (mean 47, 4 cases), liver 25 to 513 µg/g (mean 100), urine 5 to 236 µg/ml (mean 62, 5 cases). In 4 subjects who were undergoing chronic treatment and who died from causes other than drug overdose, postmortem concentrations were: blood 0.6 to 3.6 µg/ml (mean 1.6), liver 1 to 12 µg/g (mean 5.2) (R. C. Baselt *et al.*, *J. analyt. Toxicol.*, 1978, *2*, 41–43).

In 2 fatalities attributed to thioridazine overdose, the following postmortem concentrations were reported, µg/ml or µg/g:

	Blood	Liver*
Thioridazine	8.85, 2.43	138, 50
Mesoridazine	26.8, 0.29	—
Sulforidazine	0.87, 0	—

*Total thioridazine plus metabolites determined by a non-specific fluorimetric assay.

The determination of two stereoisomeric ring sulphoxides is also discussed (A. Poklis *et al.*, *J. analyt. Toxicol.*, 1982, *6*, 250–252).

HALF-LIFE. Plasma half-life, 10 to 36 hours.

DISTRIBUTION IN BLOOD. Plasma: whole blood ratio, 0.79.

PROTEIN BINDING. In plasma, thioridazine greater than 99.5%; mesoridazine and sulforidazine, about 99%.

Dose. 30 to 300 mg of thioridazine hydrochloride daily; maximum of 800 mg daily.

Thiotepa
Antineoplastic

Synonyms. TESPA; Thiophosphamide; Triethylene Thiophosphoramide; TSPA.
Proprietary Names. Ledertepa; Tifosyl.
Phosphorothioic tri(ethyleneamide)
$C_6H_{12}N_3PS = 189.2$
CAS—52-24-4

Fine white crystalline flakes. M.p. 52° to 57°.

Soluble 1 in 8 of water, 1 in 2 of ethanol, 1 in 2 of chloroform, and 1 in about 4 of ether.

Caution. Thiotepa is irritant; avoid contact with skin and mucous membranes.

Gas Chromatography. *System GA*—RI 1504.

Ultraviolet Spectrum. No significant absorption, 230 to 360 nm.

Infra-red Spectrum. Principal peaks at wavenumbers 932, 1255, 729, 718, 669, 815 (solution in carbon disulphide).

Dose. Up to 60 mg in single or divided doses by injection or by instillation.

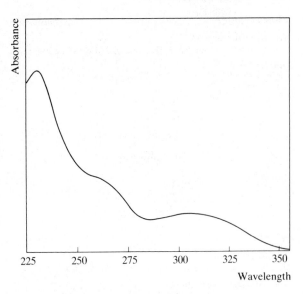

Thiothixene

Tranquilliser

Synonym. Tiotixene
Proprietary Names. Navane (capsules and tablets); Orbinamon.

(*Z*) - *NN* - Dimethyl - 9 - [3 - (4 - methylpiperazin - 1 - yl)pro-pylidene]thioxanthene-2-sulphonamide
$C_{23}H_{29}N_3O_2S_2 = 443.6$
CAS—5591-45-7; 3313-26-6 (Z)

A white to tan-coloured crystalline powder. M.p. 147° to 152°. Practically **insoluble** in water; soluble 1 in 110 of dehydrated alcohol, 1 in 2 of chloroform, and 1 in 120 of ether.

Thiothixene Hydrochloride

Proprietary Name. Navane (oral concentrate)
$C_{23}H_{29}N_3O_2S_2,2HCl,2H_2O = 552.6$
CAS—58513-59-0 (anhydrous); *49746-04-5* (anhydrous, *Z*); *22189-31-7* (dihydrate); *49746-09-0* (dihydrate, *Z*)
A white crystalline powder.
Soluble 1 in 8 of water, 1 in 270 of dehydrated alcohol, and 1 in 280 of chloroform; practically insoluble in ether.

Colour Tests. Formaldehyde–Sulphuric Acid—red; Lieber-mann's Test—red; Mandelin's Test—red; Marquis Test—red; Sulphuric Acid—orange.

Thin-layer Chromatography. *System TA*—Rf 49; *system TB*—Rf 09; *system TC*—Rf 40. (*Acidified iodoplatinate solution,* positive.)

Gas Chromatography. *System GA*—RI 3060.

High Pressure Liquid Chromatography. *System HA*—k' 3.8.

Ultraviolet Spectrum. Aqueous acid—308 nm ($A_1^1 = 191$ a).

Infra-red Spectrum. Principal peaks at wavenumbers 1156, 719, 765, 1176, 957, 747 (KBr disk).

Mass Spectrum. Principal peaks at *m/z* 113, 70, 114, 42, 221, 222, 56, 43.

Quantification. GAS CHROMATOGRAPHY–MASS SPECTROMETRY. In plasma: sensitivity <1 ng/ml—D. C. Hobbs *et al., Clin. Pharmac. Ther.,* 1974, *16*, 473–478.

HIGH PRESSURE LIQUID CHROMATOGRAPHY. In plasma: *cis-* and *trans*-thiothixene, UV detection—S. C. Bogema *et al., J. Chromat.,* 1982, *233*; *Biomed. Appl., 22,* 257–267.

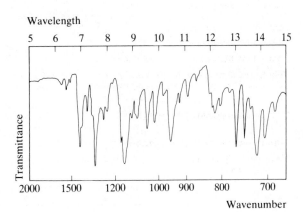

Disposition in the Body. Rapidly absorbed after oral administration. The *N*-desmethyl derivative accounts for about 10% of the plasma concentration; other unidentified metabolites may accumulate on chronic administration.

THERAPEUTIC CONCENTRATION.

Following chronic oral administration of 15 to 60 mg daily in divided doses to 15 subjects, plasma concentrations, determined 2 to 2½ hours after the last daily dose, were in the range 0.010 to 0.023 μg/ml (mean 0.016) (D. C. Hobbs *et al., Clin. Pharmac. Ther.,* 1974, *16*, 473–478).

TOXICITY.

In a fatality involving the ingestion of 250 mg of thiothixene and an unknown quantity of doxepin, a postmortem blood concentration of 0.13 μg/ml of thiothixene was reported (R. C. Baselt, *Disposition of Toxic Drugs and Chemicals in Man,* 2nd Edn, Davis, California, Biomedical Publications, 1982, pp. 734–736).

HALF-LIFE. Plasma half-life, about 34 hours.

Dose. Usually 10 to 30 mg daily; up to 60 mg daily may be given.

Thonzylamine

Antihistamine

Synonym. Histylamine
N-*p*-Anisyl-*N′N′*-dimethyl-*N*-(pyrimidin-2-yl)ethylenediamine
$C_{16}H_{22}N_4O = 286.4$
CAS—91-85-0

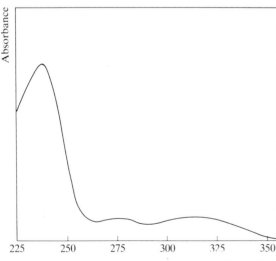

An oily liquid.
Practically **insoluble** in water; soluble in chloroform.

Thonzylamine Hydrochloride

Proprietary Names. Tonamil. It is an ingredient of Biomydrin.
$C_{16}H_{22}N_4O,HCl = 322.8$
CAS—63-56-9
A white crystalline powder. M.p. 173° to 176°.
Soluble 1 in 1 of water, 1 in 6 of ethanol, and 1 in 4 of chloroform; practically insoluble in ether.

Dissociation Constant. pK_a 2.1, 8.8 (25°).

Colour Test. Mandelin's Test—red-violet.

Thin-layer Chromatography. *System TA*—Rf 55; *system TB*—Rf 38; *system TC*—Rf 28. (*Dragendorff spray*, positive; *acidified iodoplatinate solution*, positive.)

Gas Chromatography. *System GA*—RI 2203; *system GC*—RI 2576.

High Pressure Liquid Chromatography. *System HA*—k′ 3.2.

Ultraviolet Spectrum. Aqueous acid—236 nm ($A_1^1 = 857$ a), 274 nm, 316 nm.

Infra-red Spectrum. Principal peaks at wavenumbers 1515, 1593, 1550, 1250, 1613, 1175 (KBr disk).

Mass Spectrum. Principal peaks at *m/z* 58, 121, 72, 71, 216, 215, 122, 78.

Dose. Usually 50 to 100 mg of thonzylamine hydrochloride daily.

Thymol

Disinfectant

Synonyms. Acido Timico; Isopropylmetacresol; Timol.
2-Isopropyl-5-methylphenol
$C_{10}H_{14}O = 150.2$
CAS—89-83-8

Colourless crystals or white crystalline powder. M.p. 48° to 51°; when melted it remains liquid at a considerably lower temperature.
Soluble 1 in 1000 of water, 1 in 0.3 of ethanol, 1 in 0.6 of chloroform, and 1 in 0.7 of ether.

Colour Test. Liebermann's Test—black.

Thin-layer Chromatography. *System TD*—Rf 73; *system TE*—Rf 81; *system TF*—Rf 68.

Gas Chromatography. *System GA*—RI 1260.

Ultraviolet Spectrum. Aqueous acid—272 nm ($A_1^1 = 137$ b); aqueous alkali—292 nm ($A_1^1 = 257$ b).

Infra-red Spectrum. Principal peaks at wavenumbers 817, 1248, 1290, 1095, 1160, 952.

Mass Spectrum. Principal peaks at *m/z* 135, 150, 91, 107, 117, –, –, –.

Thymoxamine

Vasodilator

Synonym. Moxisylyte
4 - (2 - Dimethylaminoethoxy) - 5 - isopropyl - 2 - methylphenyl acetate
$C_{16}H_{25}NO_3 = 279.4$
CAS—54-32-0

Practically **insoluble** in water; soluble in chloroform.

Thymoxamine Hydrochloride

Proprietary Names. Arlitene; Carlytène Fort; Opilon.
$C_{16}H_{25}NO_3,HCl = 315.8$
CAS—964-52-3
A white crystalline powder. M.p. about 212°.
Soluble 1 in 2.5 of water, 1 in 11 of ethanol, and 1 in 3 of chloroform; practically insoluble in ether.

Colour Test. Marquis Test—yellow-brown.

Absorbance

225   250   275   300   325   350

Wavelength

Thin-layer Chromatography. *System TA*—Rf 52; *system TB*—Rf 31; *system TC*—Rf 44. (*Acidified iodoplatinate solution*, positive.)

Gas Chromatography. *System GA*—RI 1832.

High Pressure Liquid Chromatography. *System HA*—thymoxamine k' 2.9, desacetylthymoxamine k' 2.3.

Ultraviolet Spectrum. Aqueous acid—275 nm ($A_1^1 = 80$ a); aqueous alkali—235 nm, 301 nm ($A_1^1 = 146$ b).

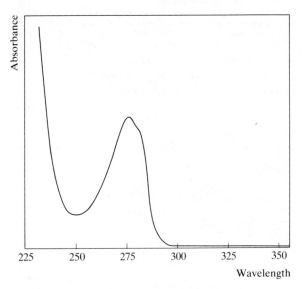

Infra-red Spectrum. Principal peaks at wavenumbers 1184, 1212, 1761, 1261, 1504, 931 (thymoxamine hydrochloride, KBr disk).

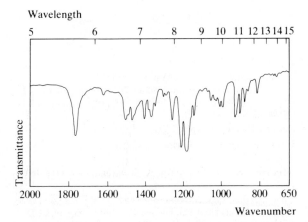

Mass Spectrum. Principal peaks at m/z 58, 72, 279, 234, 151, 192, 166, 165.

Quantification. SPECTROFLUORIMETRY. In plasma—A. G. Arbab and P. Turner. *J. Pharm. Pharmac.*, 1971, *23*, 719–721.

HIGH PRESSURE LIQUID CHROMATOGRAPHY. In monkey plasma: metabolites of thymoxamine, detection limits 2 ng for desacetylthymoxamine and 4 ng for desmethyldesacetylthymoxamine, fluorescence detection—A. E. Geahchan and P. L. Chambon, *Analyt. Chem.*, 1980, *52*, 999–1001.

Disposition in the Body. Poorly absorbed after oral administration. Deacetylation to give desacetylthymoxamine and subsequent demethylation to give desmethyldesacetylthymoxamine may occur.

THERAPEUTIC CONCENTRATION.

After single oral doses of 150 mg to 4 female subjects, plasma concentrations of about 0.06 µg/ml were achieved after 30 to 60 minutes in 2 subjects; the drug was not detected in the other two subjects. After an intravenous injection of 0.2 mg/kg over 2 minutes to 2 male subjects, plasma concentrations at 2, 7 and 15 minutes were 0.14, 0.08 and 0.05 µg/ml in the first subject and 0.1, 0.04 and 0.03 µg/ml in the other (A. G. Arbab and P. Turner., *J. Pharm. Pharmac.*, 1971, *23*, 719–721).

Dose. The equivalent of 160 mg of thymoxamine daily.

Thyroxine   *Thyroid Agent*

Synonyms. Levothyroxine; L-Thyroxine. The abbreviation T_4 is often used for thyroxine in medical and biochemical reports.
4-*O*-(4-Hydroxy-3,5-di-iodophenyl)-3,5-di-iodo-L-tyrosine
$C_{15}H_{11}I_4NO_4 = 776.9$
CAS—51-48-9

Crystals. M.p. 235° to 236°, with decomposition.

Thyroxine Sodium

Proprietary Names. Cytolen; Eltroxin; Euthyrox; Levoid; Levothroid; Oroxine; Percutacrine Thyroxinique; Synthroid; Thyroxinal. It is an ingredient of Euthroid and Thyrolar.
$C_{15}H_{10}I_4NNaO_4, xH_2O = 798.9$ (anhydrous)
CAS—55-03-8 (anhydrous); *25416-65-3* (hydrate)
A white to pale brownish-yellow, hygroscopic, amorphous or crystalline powder. It may assume a slight pink colour on exposure to light.
Soluble 1 in 700 of water and 1 in 300 of ethanol; practically insoluble in chloroform and ether; soluble in solutions of alkali hydroxides. Alkaline solutions are unstable.

Dissociation Constant. pK_a 2.2, 6.7, 10.1.

Ultraviolet Spectrum. Aqueous alkali—325 nm ($A_1^1 = 78$ a).

Infra-red Spectrum. Principal peaks at wavenumbers 1628, 1585, 1308, 1185, 1240, 1148 (KBr disk).

Quantification. GAS CHROMATOGRAPHY. In serum: thyroxine and liothyronine, sensitivity 10 ng/ml and 2.7 ng/ml, respectively, ECD—N. N. Nihei *et al.*, *Analyt. Biochem.*, 1971, *43*, 433–445.

RADIOIMMUNOASSAY. In serum: thyroxine and liothyronine, detection limit 10 ng/ml and 260 pg/ml, respectively—C. E. Denning *et al.*, *Clinica chim. Acta*, 1979, *98*, 5–18.

Disposition in the Body. Incompletely and variably absorbed after oral administration. It is metabolised by de-iodination to liothyronine (tri-iodothyronine) which is the principal active form of thyroxine; further de-iodination to thyroacetic acid (4-*p*-hydroxyphenoxyphenylacetic acid), and conjugation with glucuronic acid and sulphate also occur. About 30 to 55% of a dose is excreted in the urine and 20 to 40% is eliminated in the faeces; of the urinary material about 40% is thyroacetic acid and 20% is liothyronine.
Endogenous serum-thyroxine concentrations range from 0.05 to 0.12 µg/ml in normal subjects.

HALF-LIFE. Plasma half-life, 6 to 7 days which may be increased in pregnancy or myxoedema and decreased in hyperthyroidism.

PROTEIN BINDING. In plasma, more than 99.9%.

Dose. 50 to 300 µg of anhydrous thyroxine sodium daily.

Tiaprofenic Acid   *Analgesic*

Proprietary Name. Surgam
2-(5-Benzoyl-2-thienyl)propionic acid
$C_{14}H_{12}O_3S = 260.3$
CAS—33005-95-7

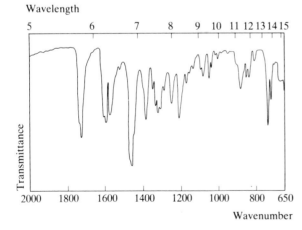

A white microcrystalline powder. M.p. about 95°.
Slightly **soluble** in water; soluble in ethanol, chloroform, and ether.

Dissociation Constant. pK_a 3.0.

Ultraviolet Spectrum. Ethanolic acid—260 nm ($A_1^1 = 370$ a), 305 nm ($A_1^1 = 575$ a).

Infra-red Spectrum. Principal peaks at wavenumbers 1727, 718, 1593, 1198, 1605, 1572 (Nujol mull).

Wavelength

5   6   7   8   9   10 11 12 13 14 15

Transmittance

2000   1800   1600   1400   1200   1000   800 650

Wavenumber

Quantification. HIGH PRESSURE LIQUID CHROMATOGRAPHY. In plasma: detection limit 500 ng/ml, UV detection—G. T. Ward *et al., J. liq. Chromat.*, 1982, *5*, 165–174.

Disposition in the Body. Rapidly and almost completely absorbed after oral administration. Metabolised by reduction to 2-(5-α-hydroxybenzyl-2-thienyl)propionic acid, oxidation to 2-(5-*p*-hydroxybenzoyl-2-thienyl)propionic acid, and conjugation with glucuronic acid. About 60% of an oral dose is excreted in the urine in 24 hours, about 55% as tiaprofenic acid (excreted mainly as an acylglucuronide conjugate), and about 5% as the two metabolites, excreted partly as acylglucuronides.

THERAPEUTIC CONCENTRATION.
Following daily oral administration of 300 mg twice a day to 6 subjects, maximum steady-state serum concentrations of 18.6 to 73.3 µg/ml (mean 48) were reported 0.5 to 1.5 hour after a dose (T. J. Daymond and R. Herbert, *Br. J. clin. Pharmac.*, 1983, *15*, 157P–158P).

HALF-LIFE. Plasma half-life, 1 to 2 hours.

CLEARANCE. Plasma clearance, about 1.4 ml/min/kg.

PROTEIN BINDING. In plasma, about 98%.

NOTE. For a review of tiaprofenic acid see E. M. Sorkin and R. N. Brogden, *Drugs*, 1985, *29*, 208–235.

Dose. 600 mg daily.

Tienilic Acid   *Diuretic*

Synonym. Ticrynafen
Proprietary Name. Diflurex
[2,3-Dichloro-4-(2-thenoyl)phenoxy]acetic acid
$C_{13}H_8Cl_2O_4S = 331.2$
CAS—40180-04-9

A white crystalline powder. M.p. 152° to 156°.
Very slightly **soluble** in water; soluble 1 in 14 of ethanol, 1 in about 5 of acetone, 1 in 77 of chloroform, and 1 in about 6 of methanol.

Dissociation Constant. pK_a 2.7 (25°).

Ultraviolet Spectrum. Ethanol—267 nm ($A_1^1 = 343$ a), 296 nm ($A_1^1 = 384$ a).

Infra-red Spectrum. Principal peaks at wavenumbers 1185, 1620, 1075, 1762, 1580, 1290 (KBr disk).

Quantification. GAS CHROMATOGRAPHY. In plasma, serum or urine: tienilic acid and metabolites, sensitivity 10 ng/ml, ECD—B. Hwang *et al., J. pharm. Sci.*, 1978, *67*, 1095–1098.

HIGH PRESSURE LIQUID CHROMATOGRAPHY. In plasma or urine: tienilic acid and monohydroxy metabolite, detection limit 200 ng/ml, UV detection—A. L. M. Kerremans *et al., Eur. J. clin. Pharmac.*, 1982, *22*, 515–521.

Disposition in the Body. Absorbed after oral administration. It is metabolised by hydroxylation and oxidation. About 40% of a dose is excreted in the urine in 24 hours; about 20% of the dose is excreted in the urine as unchanged drug, up to 10% as [2,3-dichloro-4-(α-hydroxy-2-thenyl)phenoxy]acetic acid, about 15%

Wavelength

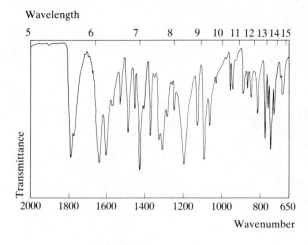

as a dihydroxylated metabolite, and 1 to 2% as (2,3-dichloro-4-carboxyphenoxy)acetic acid.

THERAPEUTIC CONCENTRATION.

After a single oral dose of 250 mg to 8 subjects, mean peak plasma concentrations of 11 µg/ml of tienilic acid, 0.7 µg/ml of the monohydroxylated metabolite, and 0.07 µg/ml of the *p*-carboxy metabolite were attained in 3 to 4 hours (B. Hwang *et al., J. pharm. Sci.,* 1978, *67,* 1095–1098).

Following a single oral dose of 250 mg to 8 subjects, peak plasma concentrations of 7.7 to 27.4 µg/ml (mean 16) of tienilic acid were attained in 1 to 2 hours (A. L. M. Kerremans *et al., Eur. J. clin. Pharmac.,* 1982, *22,* 515–521).

HALF-LIFE. Plasma half-life, 1.5 to 4 hours.

DISTRIBUTION IN BLOOD. Plasma: whole blood ratio, about 1.6.

PROTEIN BINDING. In plasma, about 99%.

Dose. Tienilic acid has been given in doses of 0.25 to 1 g daily.

Tigloidine   *Anticholinergic*

Synonym. Tiglylpseudotropeine
(1*R*,3*s*,5*S*)-3-(3-Methylmethacryloyloxy)tropane
$C_{13}H_{21}NO_2 = 223.3$
CAS—495-83-0

Tigloidine Hydrobromide

Proprietary Name. Tiglyssin
$C_{13}H_{21}NO_2,HBr = 304.2$
CAS—22846-83-9
A white crystalline solid. M.p. 234° to 235°.
Soluble in water and chloroform.

Tigloidine was first isolated from *Duboisia myoporoides* (Solanaceae) but is now synthesised.
A thin syrupy liquid.

Thin-layer Chromatography. *System TA*—Rf 42; *system TB*—Rf 39; *system TC*—Rf 21. (*Acidified iodoplatinate solution,* positive.)

Gas Chromatography. *System GA*—RI 1687.

High Pressure Liquid Chromatography. *System HA*—k' 3.6 (tailing peak).

Infra-red Spectrum. Principal peaks at wavenumbers 1700, 1266, 1136, 1036, 1156, 1073 (thin film).

Mass Spectrum. Principal peaks at *m/z* 124, 82, 83, 94, 55, 42, 67, 96.

Dose. 1 to 2 g of tigloidine hydrobromide daily.

Tilidate   *Narcotic Analgesic*

Synonym. Tilidine
(±)-Ethyl *trans*-2-dimethylamino-1-phenylcyclohex-3-ene-1-carboxylate
$C_{17}H_{23}NO_2 = 273.4$
CAS—20380-58-9

Tilidate Hydrochloride

Proprietary Name. Valoron
$C_{17}H_{23}NO_2,HCl,\frac{1}{2}H_2O = 318.8$
CAS—27107-79-5 (anhydrous)
A white crystalline powder. M.p. 162°.
Soluble in water.

Gas Chromatography. *System GA*—tilidate RI 1840, bisnortilidate RI 1825, nortilidate RI 1835.

Ultraviolet Spectrum. Aqueous acid—251 nm ($A_1^1 = 6.2$ b), 257 nm ($A_1^1 = 7.6$ b), 262 nm ($A_1^1 = 6.1$ b).

Infra-red Spectrum. Principal peaks at wavenumbers 1714, 1238, 1182, 1263, 1167, 703 (tilidate hydrochloride). (See below)

Mass Spectrum. Principal peaks at *m/z* 103, 77, 82, 29, 97, 42, 51, 104; bisnortilidate 69, 68, 70, 77, 103, 56, 54, 51; nortilidate 83, 68, 82, 72, 84, 77, 103, 115.

Quantification. GAS CHROMATOGRAPHY. In plasma or urine: tilidate, nortilidate and bisnortilidate, sensitivity 1 ng/ml, AFID—H. Hengy *et al., J. pharm. Sci.,* 1978, *67,* 1765–1768.

Disposition in the Body. Rapidly and almost completely absorbed after oral administration. It is rapidly metabolised by *N*-demethylation to form nortilidate and bisnortilidate; these metabolites may then be conjugated with glucuronic acid. About 80% of an oral dose is excreted in the urine in 24 hours, with less than 0.1% of a dose as unchanged drug, about 1.5% as nortilidate, 2.5% as bisnortilidate, and the rest as unknown metabolites. Up to 10% may be eliminated in the faeces.

THERAPEUTIC CONCENTRATION.

Following a single oral dose of 50 mg to 1 subject, peak plasma concentrations of 0.127 µg/ml of (+)-nortilidate and 0.121 µg/ml of (−)-nortilidate were attained in about 2 hours (H. Hengy *et al., Clin. Chem.,* 1978, *24,* 692–697).

Dose. The equivalent of up to 400 mg of the anhydrous hydrochloride daily.

Wavelength

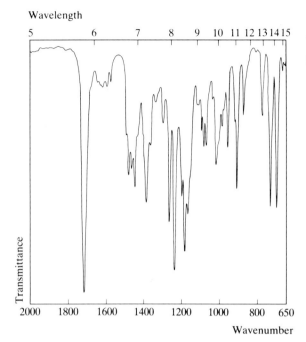

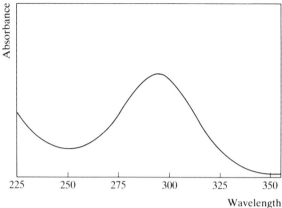

Wavelength

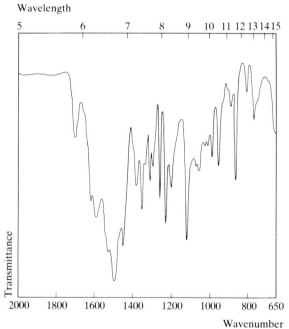

Timolol

Beta-adrenoceptor Blocking Agent

$(-)$-(S)-1-*tert*-Butylamino-3-(4-morpholino-1,2,5-thiadiazol-3-yloxy)propan-2-ol
$C_{13}H_{24}N_4O_3S = 316.4$
CAS—26839-75-8

Timolol Maleate

Proprietary Names. Betim; Blocadren; Temserin; Timacor; Timoptic; Timoptol. It is an ingredient of Moducren and Prestim.
$C_{13}H_{24}N_4O_3S,C_4H_4O_4 = 432.5$
CAS—26921-17-5
A white crystalline powder. M.p. about 200°.

Soluble in water, ethanol, and methanol; sparingly soluble in chloroform; practically insoluble in ether.

Colour Test. Liebermann's Test (100°)—violet.

Thin-layer Chromatography. *System TA*—Rf 52; *system TB*—Rf 06; *system TC*—Rf 11.

Gas Chromatography. *System GA*—RI 2270.

High Pressure Liquid Chromatography. *System HA*—k' 1.2.

Ultraviolet Spectrum. Aqueous acid—295 nm ($A_1^1 = 279$ a). No alkaline shift.

Infra-red Spectrum. Principal peaks at wavenumbers 1497, 1527, 1120, 1230, 1590, 1620 (timolol maleate, KBr disk).

Mass Spectrum. Principal peaks at *m/z* 30, 86, 57, 129, 74, 56, 41, 114.

Quantification. GAS CHROMATOGRAPHY. In plasma or urine: sensitivity 2 ng/ml and 20 ng/ml, respectively, ECD—D. J. Tocco *et al.*, *J. pharm. Sci.*, 1975, *64*, 1879–1881.

GAS CHROMATOGRAPHY–MASS SPECTROMETRY. In plasma or urine: sensitivity 5 ng/ml—J. B. Fourtillan *et al.*, *J. pharm. Sci.*, 1981, *70*, 573–575.

HIGH PRESSURE LIQUID CHROMATOGRAPHY. In plasma or urine: detection limit 40 ng/ml, UV detection—M. A. Lefebvre *et al.*, *J. liq. Chromat.*, 1981, *4*, 483–500.

Disposition in the Body. Almost completely absorbed after oral administration; bioavailability 50 to 75%. Metabolised mainly by oxidation and hydrolytic cleavage of the morpholine ring. About 70% of a dose is excreted in the urine in 24 hours, with about 20% of the dose as unchanged drug.

THERAPEUTIC CONCENTRATION.
After a single oral dose of 20 mg to 5 subjects, peak plasma concentrations of 0.05 to 0.11 µg/ml (mean 0.08) were attained in 0.5 to 3 hours (J. B. Fourtillan *et al.*, *Eur. J. clin. Pharmac.*, 1981, *19*, 193–196).

Following daily oral administration of 15 mg three times a day to 8 subjects, maximum steady-state plasma concentrations of 0.04 to 0.23 µg/ml (mean 0.11) were reported (B. N. Singh *et al.*, *Clin. Pharmac. Ther.*, 1980, *28*, 159–166).

HALF-LIFE. Plasma half-life, about 2 to 6 hours.

VOLUME OF DISTRIBUTION. 1 to 3 litres/kg.

CLEARANCE. Plasma clearance, about 5 to 10 ml/min/kg.

Dose. 10 to 60 mg of timolol maleate daily.

Tinidazole

Antiprotozoal

Proprietary Names. Fasigyn; Simplotan.
1-[2-(Ethylsulphonyl)ethyl]-2-methyl-5-nitroimidazole
$C_8H_{13}N_3O_4S = 247.3$
CAS—19387-91-8

Colourless crystals. M.p. about 127°.

Gas Chromatography. *System GA*—RI 2024.

Ultraviolet Spectrum. Aqueous acid—277 nm ($A_1^1 = 245$ b); methanol—230 nm ($A_1^1 = 148$ b), 311 nm ($A_1^1 = 354$ b).

Quantification. GAS CHROMATOGRAPHY. In plasma or tissues: sensitivity 100 ng/ml and 50 ng/g, respectively, AFID—H. Laufen *et al*, *J. Chromat.*, 1979, *163*; *Biomed. Appl.*, *5*, 217–220.

HIGH PRESSURE LIQUID CHROMATOGRAPHY. In serum or urine: sensitivity 300 ng/ml and 600 ng/ml, respectively, UV detection—I. Nilsson-Ehle *et al.*, *Antimicrob. Ag. Chemother.*, 1981, *19*, 754–760.

Disposition in the Body. Well absorbed after oral administration; bioavailability greater than 90%. It is excreted in the bile. About 25% of a dose is excreted in the urine unchanged in 72 hours together with small amounts of 2-hydroxymethyltinidazole and its glucuronide.

THERAPEUTIC CONCENTRATION.
Following a single oral dose of 2 g to 3 subjects, peak serum concentrations of 35.7, 35.7 and 46.3 µg/ml were attained in 2 to 3 hours; serum concentrations of 0.19, 0.24 and 0.46 µg/ml of the hydroxymethyl metabolite were reported, 6 hours after the dose (R. A. Robson *et al.*, *Clin. Pharmacokinet.*, 1984, *9*, 88–94).

HALF-LIFE. Plasma half-life, about 12 to 17 hours.

VOLUME OF DISTRIBUTION. About 0.7 litre/kg.

CLEARANCE. Plasma clearance, about 0.6 ml/min/kg.

PROTEIN BINDING. In plasma, about 12%.

NOTE. For a review of tinidazole see A. A. Carmine *et al.*, *Drugs*, 1982, *24*, 85–117.

Dose. Usually 2 g initially, by mouth, followed by 1 g daily.

Tobramycin

Antibiotic

Synonym. Nebramycin Factor 6
Proprietary Names. Gernebcin (sulphate); Nebcin(e) (sulphate); Obracin (sulphate); Tobralex; Tobrex.
6-*O*-(3-Amino-3-deoxy-α-D-glucopyranosyl)-2-deoxy-4-*O*-(2,6-diamino-2,3,6-trideoxy-α-D-*ribo*-hexopyranosyl)-D-streptamine
$C_{18}H_{37}N_5O_9 = 467.5$
CAS—32986-56-4; 49842-07-1 (sulphate)

A white hygroscopic powder. A solution in water is dextro-rotatory.
Soluble 1 in 1.5 of water and 1 in 2000 of ethanol; practically insoluble in chloroform and ether.

Dissociation Constant. pK_a 6.7, 8.3, 9.9.

Ultraviolet Spectrum. No significant absorption, 230 to 360 nm.

Infra-red Spectrum. Principal peaks at wavenumbers 1040, 1590, 845, 770, 660, 1260 (KBr disk).

Quantification. See also under Amikacin.

HIGH PRESSURE LIQUID CHROMATOGRAPHY. In serum or urine: sensitivity 200 ng/ml, fluorescence detection—D. B. Haughey *et al.*, *Antimicrob. Ag. Chemother.*, 1980, *17*, 649–653.

Disposition in the Body. Poorly absorbed after oral administration, but rapidly absorbed after intramuscular injection. Up to 90% of a dose is excreted unchanged in the urine in 24 hours, most being excreted within the first 6 hours. It accumulates in the tissues and may be detected in serum and urine for several days after cessation of treatment.

THERAPEUTIC CONCENTRATION. During treatment, the serum concentration should be in the range 4 to 10 µg/ml and should be monitored regularly, especially in patients who have renal insufficiency. During multiple dosing the trough concentration immediately preceding a dose should not exceed 2 µg/ml.

After an intravenous infusion of 100 mg administered over 1 hour to 4 subjects, peak serum concentrations of 4.1 to 5.1 µg/ml (mean 4.6) were achieved at the end of the infusion. After a single intramuscular injection of 100 mg administered to 3 subjects, a mean peak serum concentration of 5.16 µg/ml was achieved after 0.3 to 0.75 hour (C. Regamey *et al.*, *Clin. Pharmac. Ther.*, 1973, *14*, 396–403).

TOXICITY. Toxic effects may be produced at serum concentrations of 12 µg/ml or more or, during chronic treatment, if the trough serum concentration exceeds 2 µg/ml.

HALF-LIFE. Plasma half-life, about 2 to 3 hours, increased in renal failure; a long terminal elimination phase of about 6 days has also been reported.

VOLUME OF DISTRIBUTION. About 0.3 litre/kg.

CLEARANCE. Plasma clearance, about 1.5 ml/min/kg.

PROTEIN BINDING. In plasma, up to 10%.

Dose. Usually the equivalent of 3 to 5 mg/kg of tobramycin daily, given parenterally.

Tocainide   *Anti-arrhythmic*

2-Aminopropiono-2',6'-xylidide
$C_{11}H_{16}N_2O = 193.2$
CAS—41708-72-9

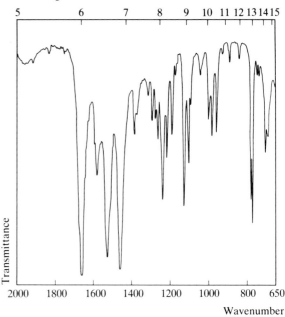

Wavelength

A white waxy solid. M.p. 53° to 55°.
Sparingly **soluble** in water; freely soluble in organic solvents.

Tocainide Hydrochloride
Proprietary Name. Tonocard
$C_{11}H_{16}N_2O,HCl = 228.7$
CAS—35891-93-1
A white crystalline powder. M.p. about 245°, with decomposition.
Freely **soluble** in water and ethanol; practically insoluble in chloroform and ether.

Dissociation Constant. pK_a 7.8.

High Pressure Liquid Chromatography. *System HA*—k' 1.2.

Ultraviolet Spectrum. Aqueous acid—262 nm $(A_1^1 = 22$ a), 270 nm $(A_1^1 = 18$ b).

Infra-red Spectrum. Principal peaks at wavenumbers 1675, 1540, 765, 1128, 772, 1240 (tocainide hydrochloride, KBr disk).

Mass Spectrum. Principal peaks at m/z 44, 121, 77, 120, 42, 106, 91, 39.

Quantification. GAS CHROMATOGRAPHY. In plasma or urine: detection limit 2 pg, ECD—G. K. Pillai *et al., J. Chromat.,* 1982, *229; Biomed. Appl., 18,* 103–109. In plasma or serum: sensitivity 200 ng/ml, FID—S. D. Gettings *et al., J. Chromat.,* 1981, *225; Biomed. Appl., 14,* 469–475.

HIGH PRESSURE LIQUID CHROMATOGRAPHY. In plasma: sensitivity 100 ng/ml, fluorescence detection—A. J. Sedman and J. Gal, *J. Chromat.,* 1982, *232; Biomed. Appl., 21,* 315–326.

Disposition in the Body. Almost completely absorbed after oral administration. About 20 to 50% of a dose is excreted in the urine as unchanged drug in 24 hours, and about 20 to 30% as a glucuronide conjugate, which is thought to be tocainide carbamoyl *O-β*-D-glucuronide (TOCG); an additional metabolite, lactoxylidide has also been detected in urine.

THERAPEUTIC CONCENTRATION. In plasma, usually in the range 4 to 12 µg/ml.

Following a single oral dose of 400 mg to 3 subjects, peak plasma concentrations of 1.6 to 1.8 µg/ml were attained in 0.5 to 2 hours. After oral administration of 400 mg three times a day to 4 subjects, steady-state plasma concentrations of 4.9 to 7.1 µg/ml (mean 5.9) were reported (C. Graffner *et al., Clin. Pharmac. Ther.,* 1980, *27,* 64–71).

HALF-LIFE. Plasma half-life, 8 to 25 hours (mean 14).

VOLUME OF DISTRIBUTION. About 1 to 3 litres/kg.

CLEARANCE. Plasma clearance, about 2 to 3 ml/min/kg.

PROTEIN BINDING. In plasma, variously reported as 10 to 50%.

NOTE. For a review of tocainide see B. Holmes *et al., Drugs,* 1983, *26,* 93–123.

Dose. 1.2 to 2.4 g of tocainide hydrochloride daily, by mouth.

Tofenacin   *Antidepressant*

Synonyms. N-Demethylorphenadrine; Desmethylorphenadrine.
N-Methyl-2-(2-methylbenzhydryloxy)ethylamine
$C_{17}H_{21}NO = 255.4$
CAS—15301-93-6

A liquid.

Tofenacin Hydrochloride
Proprietary Name. Elamol
$C_{17}H_{21}NO,HCl = 291.8$
CAS—10488-36-5
A white crystalline powder. M.p. 143° to 147°.
Soluble 1 in about 3 of water, 1 in 8 of ethanol, and 1 in 3 of chloroform; practically insoluble in ether.

Colour Tests. Liebermann's Test—red-orange; Mandelin's Test—yellow; Marquis Test—yellow; Sulphuric Acid—orange.

Thin-layer Chromatography. *System TA*—Rf 45; *system TB*—Rf 25; *system TC*—Rf 21. (*Acidified potassium permanganate solution*, positive.)

Gas Chromatography. *System GA*—RI 1920.

High Pressure Liquid Chromatography. *System HA*—k' 1.7.

Ultraviolet Spectrum. Ethanol—259 nm, 265 nm, 272 nm.

Infra-red Spectrum. Principal peaks at wavenumbers 1102, 704, 757, 1117, 1042, 917 (tofenacin hydrochloride, KBr disk).

Mass Spectrum. Principal peaks at *m/z* 44, 59, 165, 166, 181, 179, 178, 43.

Quantification. See under Orphenadrine.

Disposition in the Body. Tofenacin is a metabolite of orphenadrine.

Dose. Up to 240 mg of tofenacin hydrochloride daily.

Tolazamide
Antidiabetic

Proprietary Names. Diabewas; Norglycin; Tolanase; Tolinase.

1-(Perhydroazepin-1-yl)-3-*p*-tolylsulphonylurea

$C_{14}H_{21}N_3O_3S = 311.4$

CAS—1156-19-0

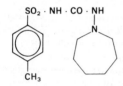

A white crystalline powder. M.p. 161° to 169°, with decomposition.

Very slightly **soluble** in water; slightly soluble in ethanol; soluble in acetone; freely soluble in chloroform.

Dissociation Constant. pK_a 3.5, 5.7.

Thin-layer Chromatography. *System TD*—Rf 52; *system TE*—Rf 06; *system TF*—Rf 50. (*Acidified potassium permanganate solution*, positive.)

Gas Chromatography. *System GA*—RI 1651.

Ultraviolet Spectrum. Methanol—257 nm, 263 nm ($A_1^1 = 21$ a), 268 nm, 275 nm.

Infra-red Spectrum. Principal peaks at wavenumbers 1694, 1176, 884, 819, 675, 1086 (KBr disk). Polymorphism may occur.

Mass Spectrum. Principal peaks at *m/z* 91, 155, 114, 65, 197, 42, 41, 85.

Quantification. HIGH PRESSURE LIQUID CHROMATOGRAPHY. In serum: sensitivity 1 µg/ml, UV detection—P. G. Welling *et al.*, *J. pharm. Sci.*, 1982, *71*, 1259–1263.

Disposition in the Body. Slowly absorbed after oral administration. About 85% of a dose is excreted in the urine in 5 days, mostly in the first 24 hours. Of the urinary material, about 17% is the *p*-carboxy derivative, 25% is 4-hydroxytolazamide, 10% is *p*-hydroxymethyltolazamide, 26% is *p*-toluenesulphonamide, and 7% is unchanged drug.

THERAPEUTIC CONCENTRATION.

Following a single oral dose of 500 mg to 20 subjects, a mean peak serum concentration of 27.8 µg/ml was attained in 3 hours (P. G. Welling *et al.*, *J. pharm. Sci.*, 1982, *71*, 1259–1263).

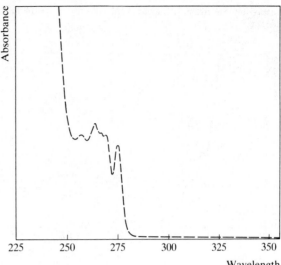

HALF-LIFE. Plasma half-life, about 5 hours.

PROTEIN BINDING. In plasma, about 94%.

NOTE. For a review of the pharmacokinetics of sulphonylurea hypoglycaemic drugs see J. E. Jackson and R. Bressler, *Drugs*, 1981, *22*, 211–245.

Dose. 0.1 to 1 g daily.

Tolazoline
Vasodilator

Synonym. Benzazoline

2-Benzyl-2-imidazoline

$C_{10}H_{12}N_2 = 160.2$

CAS—59-98-3

Soluble in water and chloroform.

Tolazoline Hydrochloride

Proprietary Names. Priscol; Priscoline; Zoline.

$C_{10}H_{12}N_2,HCl = 196.7$

CAS—59-97-2

A white or creamy-white crystalline powder. M.p. 172° to 176°.

Soluble 1 in 0.5 of water, 1 in 2 of ethanol, and 1 in 3 of chloroform; practically insoluble in ether.

Dissociation Constant. pK_a 10.6 (20°).

Colour Tests. Aromaticity (Method 2)—colourless/orange; Liebermann's Test—orange.

Thin-layer Chromatography. *System TA*—Rf 13; *system TB*—Rf 02; *system TC*—Rf 02. (*Acidified iodoplatinate solution*, positive.)

Gas Chromatography. *System GA*—RI 1598.

High Pressure Liquid Chromatography. *System HA*—k' 2.1.

Ultraviolet Spectrum. Aqueous acid—257 nm $(A_1^1 = 14.7$ a), 263 nm.

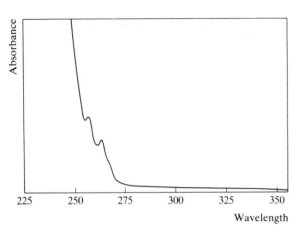

Infra-red Spectrum. Principal peaks at wavenumbers 1608, 1296, 721, 1580, 690, 775 (KBr disk).

Wavelength

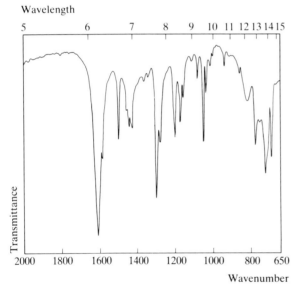

Wavenumber

Mass Spectrum. Principal peaks at m/z 91, 159, 160, 131, 65, 92, 81, 39.

Quantification. HIGH PRESSURE LIQUID CHROMATOGRAPHY. In plasma: detection limit 200 ng/ml, UV detection—V. Rovei *et al.*, *J. Chromat.*, 1982, *231*; *Biomed Appl.*, *20*, 210–215.

Disposition in the Body. Well absorbed after oral or parenteral administration. It is excreted in the urine, about 90% of an oral dose being eliminated unchanged in 12 hours.

THERAPEUTIC CONCENTRATION.

After a bolus intravenous injection of 2 mg/kg followed by continuous intravenous infusion to provide a maintenance dose of 2 mg/kg to 1 neonate, plasma concentrations attained a steady-state of 7 to 8 µg/ml and declined with a half-life of 5 hours at the end of the infusion (V. Rovei *et al.*, *J. Chromat.*, 1982, *231*; *Biomed. Appl.*, *20*, 210–215).

TOXICITY.

A 54-year-old woman found comatose after ingesting 2.5 g of tolazoline hydrochloride died about 3 hours later. Postmortem concentrations were: femoral blood 130 µg/ml, liver 102 µg/g (L. K. Turner, personal communication, 1964).

Dose. 12.5 to 200 mg of tolazoline hydrochloride daily.

Tolbutamide   *Antidiabetic*

Synonyms. Butamidum; Tolglybutamide.

Proprietary Names. Artosin; Chembutamide; Dolipol; Glyconon; Guabeta N; Mellitol; Mobenol; Neo-Dibetic; Novobutamide; Oramide; Orinase; Pramidex; Rastinon (tablets); Tolbutone.

1-Butyl-3-*p*-tolylsulphonylurea
$C_{12}H_{18}N_2O_3S = 270.3$
CAS—64-77-7

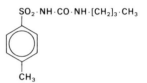

A white crystalline powder. M.p. 126° to 132°.
Practically **insoluble** in water; soluble 1 in 10 of ethanol and 1 in 3 of acetone; soluble in chloroform; slightly soluble in ether.

Tolbutamide Sodium

Proprietary Names. Orinase Diagnostic; Rastinon (injection).
$C_{12}H_{17}N_2NaO_3S = 292.3$
CAS—473-41-6
A white crystalline powder.
Freely **soluble** in water; soluble in ethanol and chloroform; very slightly soluble in ether.

Dissociation Constant. pK$_a$ 5.3 (20°).

Colour Tests. Koppanyi–Zwikker Test—violet; Mercurous Nitrate—black.

Thin-layer Chromatography. *System TA*—Rf 76; *system TD*—Rf 51; *system TE*—Rf 12; *system TF*—Rf 55; *system TT*—Rf 98; *system TU*—Rf 35; *system TV*—Rf 04.

Gas Chromatography. *System GA*—RI 1683.

Ultraviolet Spectrum. Methanol—257 nm, 263 nm $(A_1^1 = 22$ a), 268 nm, 275 nm.

Infra-red Spectrum. Principal peaks at wavenumbers 1658, 1157, 1552, 668, 1090, 905 (KBr disk). Polymorphism may occur.

Mass Spectrum. Principal peaks at m/z 91, 30, 155, 108, 65, 197, 39, 107.

Quantification. See also under Chlorpropamide.

GAS CHROMATOGRAPHY. In plasma or urine: tolbutamide and two metabolites, sensitivity 1 µg/ml, ECD—S. B. Matin and M. Rowland, *Analyt. Lett. (Part B)*, 1973, *6*, 865–876.

HIGH PRESSURE LIQUID CHROMATOGRAPHY. In plasma: tolbutamide and carboxytolbutamide, sensitivity 2 µg/ml for tolbutamide and 100 ng/ml for the carboxy metabolite, UV detection—G. Raghow and M. C. Meyer, *J. pharm. Sci.*, 1981, *70*, 1166–1168. In plasma: sensitivity 200 ng/ml, UV detection—H. M. Hill and J. Chamberlain, *J. Chromat.*, 1978, *149*, 349–358.

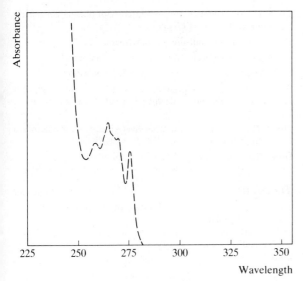

Absorbance

225 250 275 300 325 350

Wavelength

Wavelength

5 6 7 8 9 10 11 12 13 14 15

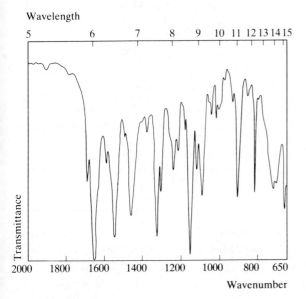

Transmittance

2000 1800 1600 1400 1200 1000 800 650

Wavenumber

Disposition in the Body. Readily absorbed after oral administration. About 85% of an oral dose is excreted in the urine in 48 hours, of which about two-thirds is the 4-carboxy metabolite and about one-third is the 4-hydroxymethyl metabolite; less than 5% is excreted as unchanged drug. About 9% of a dose is eliminated in the faeces in 48 hours.

THERAPEUTIC CONCENTRATION.
Following a single oral dose of 500 mg to 1 subject, a peak plasma-tolbutamide concentration of 49 μg/ml was attained in about 4 hours and a peak plasma concentration of the 4-carboxy metabolite of about 2.2 μg/ml was attained in 6 hours (G. Raghow and M. C. Meyer, *J. pharm. Sci.*, 1981, *70*, 1166–1168).

TOXICITY. Several fatalities from hypoglycaemia have been reported.
The following postmortem tissue distribution was reported in one suicide after the ingestion of 50 g: blood 640 μg/ml, kidney 1073 μg/g, liver 930 μg/g, urine 3510 μg/ml (O. Pribilla, *Arch. Tox.*, 1968, *23*, 153–159).

HALF-LIFE. Plasma half-life, usually in the range 4 to 12 hours (mean 7) but may vary up to 70 hours during concomitant administration of other drugs such as sulphonamides, phenylbutazone, or dicoumarol.

VOLUME OF DISTRIBUTION. 0.1 to 0.2 litre/kg.

CLEARANCE. Plasma clearance, about 0.3 ml/min/kg.

PROTEIN BINDING. In plasma, about 95% at concentrations up to 100 μg/ml, decreasing to about 90% at plasma concentrations of 200 μg/ml.

NOTE. For a review of sulphonylurea hypoglycaemic drugs see J. E. Jackson and R. Bressler, *Drugs*, 1981, *22*, 211–245.

Dose. 0.25 to 3 g daily.

Tolfenamic Acid   *Analgesic*

Proprietary Name. Clotam
N-(3-Chloro-*o*-tolyl)anthranilic acid
$C_{14}H_{12}ClNO_2 = 261.7$
CAS—13710-19-5

A white crystalline powder. M.p. 210° to 214°.
Practically **insoluble** in water; soluble 1 in 70 of ethanol, 1 in 140 of chloroform, 1 in 15 of dimethylformamide, and 1 in 45 of ether.

Ultraviolet Spectrum. Dehydrated alcohol—294 nm, 330 nm.

Infra-red Spectrum. Principal peaks at wavenumbers 1670, 1270, 1590, 755, 1500, 1575 (KBr disk).

Quantification. HIGH PRESSURE LIQUID CHROMATOGRAPHY. In plasma or urine: sensitivity 20 ng/ml, UV detection—P. J. Pentikäinen *et al.*, *Eur. J. clin. Pharmac.*, 1981, *19*, 359–365.

Disposition in the Body. Readily absorbed after oral administration; bioavailability about 60%. It is metabolised by hydroxylation to *N*-(2-hydroxymethyl-3-chlorophenyl)anthranilic acid and *N*-(2-methyl-3-chloro-4-hydroxyphenyl)anthranilic acid, which are the major metabolites. About 50% of an oral dose is excreted in the urine in 48 hours mainly as glucuronide conjugates of the two hydroxylated metabolites. Less than 10% of a dose is excreted in the urine as unchanged drug or its glucuronide conjugate. Tolfenamic acid and its metabolites are excreted in the bile.

THERAPEUTIC CONCENTRATION.
Following single oral doses of 100 mg and 200 mg to 6 subjects, mean peak plasma concentrations of 2.0 and 3.0 μg/ml were attained in 1.3 and 1.5 hours respectively (P. J. Pentikäinen *et al.*, *ibid.*).

HALF-LIFE. Plasma half-life, about 2.5 hours.

VOLUME OF DISTRIBUTION. About 0.5 litre/kg.

CLEARANCE. Plasma clearance about 2.5 ml/min/kg.

PROTEIN BINDING. In plasma, more than 99.5%.

Dose. Tolfenamic acid has been given in doses of 300 to 600 mg daily.

Tolmetin

Analgesic

(1-Methyl-5-*p*-toluoylpyrrol-2-yl)acetic acid
$C_{15}H_{15}NO_3 = 257.3$
CAS—26171-23-3

Crystals. M.p. 155° to 157°, with decomposition.

Tolmetin Sodium

Proprietary Names. Tolectin; Tolmex.
$C_{15}H_{14}NNaO_3,2H_2O = 315.3$
CAS—35711-34-3 (anhydrous); *64490-92-2* (dihydrate)

Dissociation Constant. pK_a 3.5.

Colour Tests. Formaldehyde–Sulphuric Acid—brown-red; Liebermann's Test (100°)—red.

Thin-layer Chromatography. *System TD*—Rf 13; *system TE*—Rf 07; *system TF*—Rf 20; *system TG*—Rf 10. (*Ludy Tenger reagent,* black.)

Gas Chromatography. *System GD*—retention times of methyl derivative 1.77 and 1.36, relative to $n\text{-}C_{16}H_{34}$.

High Pressure Liquid Chromatography. *System HD*—k' 2.05; *system HV*—retention times 0.60 and 0.99 relative to meclofenamic acid.

Ultraviolet Spectrum. Aqueous acid—262 nm $(A_1^1 = 345 \text{ b})$, 315 nm $(A_1^1 = 735 \text{ b})$; aqueous alkali—260 nm $(A_1^1 = 333 \text{ b})$, 323 nm $(A_1^1 = 762 \text{ b})$.

Mass Spectrum. Principal peaks at *m/z* 212, 213, 122, 198, 44, 53, 91, 65.

Quantification. GAS CHROMATOGRAPHY. In plasma: sensitivity 100 ng/ml, ECD—K.-T. Ng, *J. Chromat.*, 1978, *166*, 527–535.

HIGH PRESSURE LIQUID CHROMATOGRAPHY. In plasma or urine: sensitivity for tolmetin and the dicarboxylated metabolite, 40 ng/ml in plasma, UV detection—R. K. Desiraju *et al.*, *J. Chromat.*, 1982, *232*; *Biomed. Appl.*, *21*, 119–128.

Disposition in the Body. Rapidly and almost completely absorbed after oral administration. Metabolised mainly by oxidation to inactive metabolites. More than 90% of a dose is excreted in the urine in 24 hours, mostly in the first 8 hours. The urinary material consists mostly of free and conjugated (glucuronide) 5-(4-carboxybenzoyl)-1-methylpyrrol-2-ylacetic acid and conjugated (glucuronide) tolmetin; up to 15% is excreted in the urine as unchanged drug.

THERAPEUTIC CONCENTRATION.

After a single oral dose of 300 mg to 5 subjects, a mean peak plasma concentration of 29.3 μg/ml of tolmetin was attained in 0.25 to 1 hour; plasma concentrations of the dicarboxylated metabolite reached a peak of about 5 μg/ml in 1.5 to 3 hours (M. L. Selley *et al.*, *Clin. Pharmac. Ther.*, 1975, *17*, 599–605).

Following oral administration of 400 mg four times a day to 5 subjects for 7 days, maximum steady-state plasma concentrations of 8.3 to 78.9 μg/ml (mean 45) of tolmetin and 4.1 to 13.6 μg/ml (mean 10) of the dicarboxylated metabolite were reported about 0.75 and 1.75 hour after a dose, respectively (S. H. Dromgoole *et al.*, *Clin. Pharmac. Ther.*, 1982, *32*, 371–377).

TOXICITY. Toxic effects are associated with plasma concentrations greater than about 60 μg/ml.

HALF-LIFE. Plasma half-life, about 6 hours.

CLEARANCE. Plasma clearance, about 1 to 2 ml/min/kg.

DISTRIBUTION IN BLOOD. Plasma:whole blood ratio, 1.8.

PROTEIN BINDING. In plasma, tolmetin more than 99% but displaced by salicylic acid; dicarboxylated metabolite about 70%.

NOTE. For a review of the pharmacokinetics of tolmetin see R. N. Brogden *et al.*, *Drugs*, 1978, *15*, 429–450.

Dose. The equivalent of 0.6 to 1.8 g of tolmetin daily.

Tolnaftate

Antifungal

Proprietary Names. Aftate; Sporiderm; Sporiline; Tinactin; Tinaderm; Tonoftal.
O-2-Naphthyl *m,N*-dimethylthiocarbanilate
$C_{19}H_{17}NOS = 307.4$
CAS—2398-96-1

A white to creamy-white powder. M.p. 109° to 113°. Practically **insoluble** in water; soluble 1 in 4000 of ethanol, 1 in 9 of acetone, 1 in 3 of chloroform, and 1 in 55 of ether.

Colour Tests. Mandelin's Test—brown; Marquis Test—blue-green.

Ultraviolet Spectrum. Methanol—257 nm $(A_1^1 = 708 \text{ a})$.

Infra-red Spectrum. Principal peaks at wavenumbers 1211, 1170, 1156, 754, 1234, 810 (KBr disk).

Use. Topically as a 1% solution, powder, or cream.

Tolpropamine

Antihistamine

NN-Dimethyl-3-phenyl-3-*p*-tolylpropylamine
$C_{18}H_{23}N = 253.4$
CAS—5632-44-0

Practically **insoluble** in water; soluble in chloroform.

Tolpropamine Hydrochloride

Proprietary Name. Pragman
$C_{18}H_{23}N,HCl = 289.8$
CAS—3339-11-5
A white crystalline powder. M.p. 182° to 184°.
Soluble in water and ethanol; practically insoluble in chloroform and ether.

Colour Tests. Mandelin's Test—brown; Marquis Test—red.

Thin-layer Chromatography. *System TA*—Rf 51; *system TB*—Rf 52; *system TC*—Rf 32. (*Acidified iodoplatinate solution*, positive.)

High Pressure Liquid Chromatography. *System HA*—k′ 2.9.

Ultraviolet Spectrum. Aqueous acid—260 nm $(A_1^1 = 25 \, a)$, 265 nm $(A_1^1 = 25 \, a)$, 273 nm.

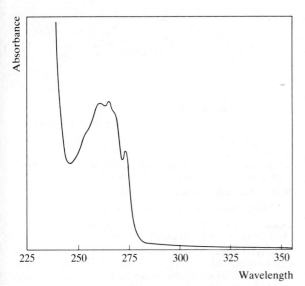

Infra-red Spectrum. Principal peaks at wavenumbers 727, 776, 700, 802, 1515, 970 (tolpropamine hydrochloride, KBr disk).

Use. Topically in a concentration of 1% of the hydrochloride.

Toluene
Solvent

Synonyms. Methylbenzene; Toluol(e).

$C_6H_5 \cdot CH_3 = 92.14$
CAS—108-88-3

A colourless, mobile, highly inflammable liquid which burns with a smoky flame. Wt per ml about 0.87 g. B.p. 109° to 111°. Practically **insoluble** in water; miscible with organic solvents and glacial acetic acid.

Gas Chromatography. *System GA*—RI 756; *system GI*—retention time 24.8 min.

Mass Spectrum. Principal peaks at *m/z* 91, 92, 65, 39, 63, 93, 51, 89.

Quantification. GAS CHROMATOGRAPHY. In blood or breath: sensitivity 1 µg/ml, FID—J. C. Garriott *et al.*, *Clin. Toxicol.*, 1981, *18*, 471–479.

GAS CHROMATOGRAPHY AND GAS CHROMATOGRAPHY–MASS SPECTROMETRY. In blood or tissues: toluene and other volatile compounds, using head-space analysis—J. A. Bellanca *et al.*, *J. analyt. Toxicol.*, 1982, *6*, 238–240.

HIGH PRESSURE LIQUID CHROMATOGRAPHY. In urine: hippuric acid and *o*-cresol, detection limits hippuric acid 50 µg/ml and *o*-cresol 5 ng/ml, fluorescence and UV detection—S. H. Hansen and M. Døssing, *J. Chromat.*, 1982, *229*; *Biomed. Appl.*, *18*, 141–148.

Disposition in the Body. Toluene is absorbed from the gastro-intestinal tract, through the skin and mucous membranes, and from the lungs. It has an affinity for lipid-rich tissues from which it is slowly released. About 80% of an inhaled dose is oxidised to benzoic acid which is conjugated with glycine to give hippuric acid and excreted in the urine. Conjugation with glucuronic acid also occurs when large amounts of toluene are absorbed. About 20% of the dose is excreted unchanged in expired air with less than 0.1% in the urine.

TOXICITY. Toluene has about the same acute toxicity as benzene but is a less serious industrial hazard. The maximum permissible atmospheric concentration of toluene is 100 ppm. Exposure to air concentrations of 10 000 to 30 000 ppm may cause unconsciousness within a few minutes. A blood concentration of more than 10 µg/ml may be lethal although higher concentrations have been found in habitual abusers.

Exposure to a concentration of 100 ppm of toluene produced a mean venous-blood concentration of about 0.39 µg/ml in 6 healthy subjects at rest and about 1.16 µg/ml in 6 subjects during light exercise, after 20 to 30 minutes. Exposure to 200 ppm for the same time, produced a mean blood concentration of about 0.55 µg/ml in 4 subjects at rest (I. Astrand *et al.*, *Work envir. Hlth*, 1972, *9*, 119–130).

Seven children aged from 9 to 13 years, with an acute encephalopathy due to toluene intoxication from glue-sniffing were found to have blood-toluene concentrations of 0.8 to 7.7 µg/g (mean 2.3) (M. D. King *et al.*, *Br. med. J.*, 1981, *283*, 663–665).

A boy of 13 years found dead after sniffing glue had the following postmortem concentrations of toluene in body tissues: blood 11 µg/ml, brain 44 µg/g, kidney 39 µg/g, liver 47 µg/g (W. D. Collom and C. L. Winek, *Clin. Toxicol.*, 1970, *3*, 125–130).

The following postmortem tissue concentrations of toluene were reported in a 16-year-old boy found dead with a plastic bag over his head: blood 20.6 µg/ml, brain 297 µg/g, liver 89 µg/g; acetone was also detected in blood at a concentration of 3 µg/ml (S. C. Paterson and R. Sarvesvaran, *Medicine, Sci. Law*, 1983, *23*, 64–66).

HALF-LIFE. Blood half-life about 7.5 hours.

Tramadol
Narcotic Analgesic

$(\pm)$ - *trans* - 2 - Dimethylaminomethyl - 1 - (3 - methoxyphenyl)-cyclohexanol
$C_{16}H_{25}NO_2 = 263.4$
CAS—27203-92-5

Tramadol Hydrochloride
Proprietary Name. Tramal
$C_{16}H_{25}NO_2, HCl = 299.8$
CAS—36282-47-0
A white crystalline powder. M.p. 179° to 180°.
Readily **soluble** in water.

Dissociation Constant. pK$_a$ 8.3.

Ultraviolet Spectrum. Aqueous acid—272 nm $(A_1^1 = 70 \, a)$, shoulder at 279 nm. No alkaline shift.

Infra-red Spectrum. Principal peaks at wavenumbers 1284, 1601, 1042, 1238, 1575, 702 (tramadol hydrochloride, KBr disk).

Disposition in the Body. Rapidly absorbed after oral or parenteral administration; bioavailability about 65%. Peak serum concentrations are achieved in about 2 hours. The main metabolic reactions are *N*- and *O*-demethylation and conjugation with glucuronic acid and sulphate. The major metabolites formed are *O*-monodesmethyltramadol, *N,O*-didesmethyltramadol and their conjugates, and *N*-monodesmethyltramadol. *O*-Monodesmethyltramadol is an active metabolite and has a greater analgesic activity than the parent drug. About 90% of an oral dose is excreted in the urine in 3 days, about 30% of the dose as unchanged drug, and the rest as metabolites. The remainder of the dose is eliminated in the faeces.

HALF-LIFE. Plasma half-life, tramadol about 6 hours, *O*-monodesmethyltramadol, about 9 hours.

VOLUME OF DISTRIBUTION. About 3 litres/kg.

CLEARANCE. Plasma clearance, about 6 ml/min/kg.

PROTEIN BINDING. In plasma, less than 5%.

Dose. Tramadol hydrochloride is given parenterally in doses of 50 to 100 mg.

Tramazoline   *Sympathomimetic*

2-(5,6,7,8-Tetrahydro-1-naphthylamino)-2-imidazoline
$C_{13}H_{17}N_3 = 215.3$
CAS—1082-57-1

Crystals. M.p. 142° to 143°.

Tramazoline Hydrochloride
Proprietary Names. Biciron; Rhinogutt; Rhinospray; Spray-Tish. It is an ingredient of Dexa-Rhinaspray.
$C_{13}H_{17}N_3,HCl = 251.8$
CAS—3715-90-0
A white crystalline solid. M.p. 171°.
Soluble 1 in 6 of water.

Partition Coefficient. Log *P* (chloroform/pH 7.4), −0.8.

Colour Tests. Mandelin's Test—brown; Marquis Test—red-violet.

Thin-layer Chromatography. *System TA*—Rf 06; *system TB*—Rf 04; *system TC*—Rf 02. (*Acidified potassium permanganate solution*, positive.)

Gas Chromatography. *System GA*—RI 2440.

High Pressure Liquid Chromatography. *System HA*—k' 1.8.

Ultraviolet Spectrum. Aqueous acid—267 nm, 275 nm.

Infra-red Spectrum. Principal peaks at wavenumbers 1667, 1626, 1590, 1302, 797, 1289 (tramazoline hydrochloride, KBr disk).

Mass Spectrum. Principal peaks at *m/z* 215, 214, 44, 185, 200, 216, 157, 186.

Tranylcypromine

Antidepressant (Monoamine Oxidase Inhibitor)

Synonyms. Tranilcipromina; Transamine.
(±)-*trans*-2-Phenylcyclopropylamine
$C_9H_{11}N = 133.2$
CAS—155-09-9

A liquid.

Tranylcypromine Sulphate
Proprietary Names. Parnate; Tylciprine. It is an ingredient of Parstelin.
$(C_9H_{11}N)_2,H_2SO_4 = 364.5$
CAS—13492-01-8
A white crystalline powder.
Soluble 1 in 20 to 1 in 25 of water and 1 in 2000 of ether; very slightly soluble in ethanol; practically insoluble in chloroform.

Dissociation Constant. pK_a 8.2.

Partition Coefficient. Log *P* (octanol/chloroform), 0.6.

Colour Tests. Liebermann's Test—red-orange; Mandelin's Test—green → violet; Marquis Test—red → brown.

Thin-layer Chromatography. *System TA*—Rf 54; *system TB*—Rf 33; *system TC*—Rf 33. (*Dragendorff spray*, positive; *FPN reagent*, yellow; *acidified iodoplatinate solution*, positive; *Marquis reagent*, orange-brown; *ninhydrin spray*, positive.)

Gas Chromatography. *System GA*—RI 1223; *system GB*—RI 1245; *system GC*—RI 1759; *system GF*—RI 1455.

High Pressure Liquid Chromatography. *System HA*—k' 1.0; *system HC*—k' 0.26.

Ultraviolet Spectrum. Aqueous acid—258 nm, 264 nm ($A_1^1 = $ 22 a), 271 nm; aqueous alkali—260 nm, 266 nm, 273 nm.

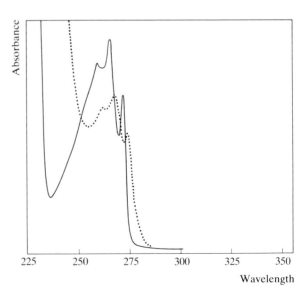

Wavelength

Infra-red Spectrum. Principal peaks at wavenumbers 1023, 1112, 695, 963, 1153, 743 (tranylcypromine sulphate, Nujol mull).

Wavelength

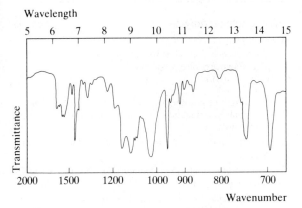

Mass Spectrum. Principal peaks at *m/z* 133, 132, 56, 115, 30, 117, 91, 77.

Quantification. GAS CHROMATOGRAPHY. In serum or urine: sensitivity 1 ng/ml, ECD—R. C. Baselt *et al.*, *J. analyt. Toxicol.*, 1977, *1*, 215–217. In plasma or urine: sensitivity 2.5 ng/ml, AFID—E. Bailey and E. J. Barron, *J. Chromat.*, 1980, *183*; *Biomed. Appl.*, 9, 25–31.

Disposition in the Body. Readily absorbed after oral administration and extensively metabolised. Less than 2% of a dose is excreted as unchanged drug in the urine in 24 hours; this increases to about 8% if the urine is maintained at an acid pH.

THERAPEUTIC CONCENTRATION.
A single oral dose of 30 mg administered to 2 subjects produced a peak serum concentration of about 0.04 μg/ml in 1 hour. During chronic treatment of 42 patients with 10 to 30 mg daily, serum concentrations of 0.005 to 0.01 μg/ml were found when measured 12 hours after the last dose (R. C. Baselt *et al.*, *J. analyt. Toxicol.*, 1977, *1*, 215–217).

TOXICITY. Several cases of addiction to tranylcypromine have been reported.
A woman died 24 hours after taking 850 mg of tranylcypromine; the postmortem liver concentration was 0.5 μg/g and the urine concentration 3 μg/ml (G. J. Griffiths, *Medicine, Sci. Law*, 1973, *13*, 93–94).
In a fatality attributed to ingestion of 850 mg of tranylcypromine, a postmortem blood concentration of 0.25 μg/ml and a liver concentration of 13 μg/g were reported (M. A. Mackell *et al.*, *Medicine, Sci. Law*, 1979, *19*, 66–68).
The following postmortem tissue concentrations were reported in a fatality involving the ingestion of 300 mg of tranylcypromine: blood 3.7 μg/ml, brain 1.0 μg/g, liver 7.3 μg/g, urine 25 μg/ml; several other drugs were detected (R. C. Baselt *et al.*, *J. analyt. Toxicol.*, 1977, *1*, 168–170).

HALF-LIFE. Plasma half-life, about 2 hours.

Dose. The equivalent of 10 to 30 mg of tranylcypromine daily.

Trazodone   *Antidepressant*

2-{3-[4-(3-Chlorophenyl)piperazin-1-yl]propyl}-1,2,4-triazolo-[4,3-*a*]pyridin-3(2*H*)-one
$C_{19}H_{22}ClN_5O = 371.9$
CAS—19794-93-5

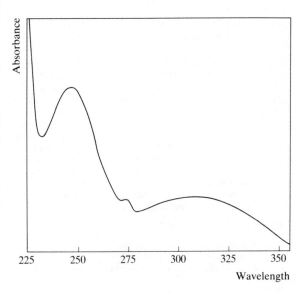

Crystals. M.p. 96°.
Soluble 1 in 50 of ethanol and methanol; freely soluble in acetone and benzene; slightly soluble in ether.

Trazodone Hydrochloride
Proprietary Names. Desyrel; Molipaxin; Thombran; Trittico.
$C_{19}H_{22}ClN_5O,HCl = 408.3$
CAS—25332-39-2
White crystals. M.p. about 225°.
Sparingly **soluble** in water, ethanol, and methanol; soluble in chloroform.

Colour Tests. Liebermann's Test—violet (transient); Mandelin's Test—grey → violet.

Thin-layer Chromatography. System *TA*—Rf 63; *system TB*—Rf 09; *system TC*—Rf 58. (Location under ultraviolet light, violet fluorescence; *Dragendorff spray*, positive; *acidified iodoplatinate solution*, positive.)

Gas Chromatography. System *GA*—RI 3250.

High Pressure Liquid Chromatography. System *HA*—k′ 0.6.

Ultraviolet Spectrum. Aqueous acid—246 nm ($A_1^1 = 314$ a), 274 nm, 310 nm. No alkaline shift.

Infra-red Spectrum. Principal peaks at wavenumbers 1705, 1595, 943, 1640, 742, 1272 (trazodone hydrochloride, KBr disk). (See below)

Mass Spectrum. Principal peaks at *m/z* 205, 70, 231, 78, 135, 136, 42, 166.

Quantification. GAS CHROMATOGRAPHY. In plasma or brain: trazodone and 1-(3-chlorophenyl)piperazine, detection limits 50 ng/ml and 10 ng/ml, respectively, AFID—S. Caccia *et al.*, *J. Chromat.*, 1981, *210*, 311–318.

Wavelength

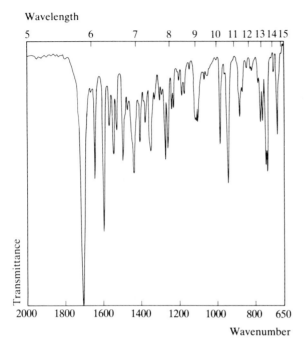

HIGH PRESSURE LIQUID CHROMATOGRAPHY. In plasma: sensitivity 20 ng/ml, UV detection—S. I. Ankier et al., Br. J. clin. Pharmac., 1981, 11, 505–509.

Disposition in the Body. Rapidly and almost completely absorbed after oral administration. It is extensively metabolised by hydroxylation and oxidation. About 75% of a dose is excreted in the urine as metabolites and 15% is eliminated in the faeces, in 72 hours. Less than 1% of a dose is excreted in the urine as unchanged drug. The major urinary metabolites are a propionic acid derivative (3-oxo-1,2,4-triazolo[4,3-a]pyridine-2-propionic acid), p-hydroxytrazodone, and a dihydrodiol derivative and its glucuronide and sulphate conjugates, which account for about 35%, 20%, and 15% of the urinary material respectively; an N-oxide has also been identified. In plasma, the major metabolite is 1-(3-chlorophenyl)piperazine (active), but this accounts for less than 1% of a dose in the urine.

THERAPEUTIC CONCENTRATION.
After an oral dose of 50 mg to 13 subjects, peak plasma concentrations of 0.49 to 2.3 µg/ml (mean 1.1) were attained in 0.5 to 2.5 hours (S. I. Ankier et al., Br. J. clin. Pharmac., 1981, 11, 505–509).
Following a single oral dose of 150 mg to 4 subjects, mean peak plasma concentrations of 2.05 µg/ml of trazodone and 0.01 µg/ml of 1-(3-chlorophenyl)piperazine were reported at about 2 hours and 2 to 4 hours, respectively (S. Caccia et al., J. Pharm. Pharmac., 1982, 34, 605–606).
Following oral administration of 25 mg three times a day to 10 subjects, steady-state serum concentrations averaged 0.7 µg/ml on the twelfth day (B. Catanese et al., Boll. chim.-farm., 1978, 117, 424–427).

TOXICITY.
In a fatality in which a woman was found drowned in a bath following the ingestion of about 2 to 4 g of trazodone, the following postmortem concentrations were reported: blood 15 µg/ml, bile 45 µg/ml, liver 57 µg/g, urine 2.5 µg/ml (D. Demorest, J. analyt. Toxicol., 1983, 7, 63).

HALF-LIFE. Plasma half-life, about 4 to 7 hours.

PROTEIN BINDING. In plasma, about 90%.

NOTE. For a review of the pharmacokinetics of trazodone see R. N. Brogden et al., Drugs, 1981, 21, 401–429.

Dose. 100 to 300 mg of trazodone hydrochloride daily; maximum of 600 mg daily.

Triacetyloleandomycin   *Antibiotic*

Synonym. Troleandomycin
Proprietary Names. Cetilmin; Isotriacin; TAO.
The triacetyl ester of oleandomycin.
$C_{41}H_{67}NO_{15} = 814.0$
CAS—2751-09-9
A white crystalline powder. M.p. 176°, with decomposition.
Slightly **soluble** in water and ether; soluble 1 in 10 of ethanol and 1 in 1 of chloroform.

Colour Tests. Mandelin's Test—violet (slow); Marquis Test—yellow-brown.

Thin-layer Chromatography. *System TA*—Rf 65. (*Acidified iodoplatinate solution,* positive.)

Infra-red Spectrum. Principal peaks at wavenumbers 1744, 1239, 1735, 1053, 1004, 1123 (KBr disk).

Dose. The equivalent of 1 to 2 g of oleandomycin daily.

Triamcinolone   *Corticosteroid*

Synonyms. 9α-Fluoro-16α-hydroxyprednisolone; Fluoxiprednisolonum.
Proprietary Names. Aristocort (tablets); Kenacort (tablets); Ledercort (tablets); Triamcort.
9α-Fluoro-11β,16α,17α,21-tetrahydroxypregna-1,4-diene-3,20-dione
$C_{21}H_{27}FO_6 = 394.4$
CAS—124-94-7

A white, slightly hygroscopic, crystalline powder. M.p. about 262°.
Soluble 1 in 500 of water and 1 in 240 of ethanol; slightly soluble in methanol; very slightly soluble in chloroform and ether.

Triamcinolone Acetonide

Proprietary Names. Adcortyl; Aristocort A; Aristogel; Cenocort A; Kenacort-A; Kenalog; Ledercort (cream and ointment); Tédarol (cream); Tramacin; Triaderm; Triam-A; Trimacort. It is an ingredient of Audicort, Aureocort, Nystadermal, and Silderm.
$C_{24}H_{31}FO_6 = 434.5$
CAS—76-25-5
A white or cream-coloured crystalline powder. M.p. about 277°.
Very slightly **soluble** in water; soluble 1 in 150 of ethanol, 1 in 11 of acetone, and 1 in 40 of chloroform; very soluble in dehydrated alcohol and methanol.

Triamcinolone Diacetate

Proprietary Names. Aristocort (injection and syrup); Cenocort Forte; Cino-40; Kenacort (syrup); Ledercort diacetat; Tédarol (injection and syrup); Tracilon.

$C_{25}H_{31}FO_8 = 478.5$

CAS—67-78-7

A fine, white, crystalline powder.

Practically **insoluble** in water; soluble 1 in 13 of ethanol, 1 in 80 of chloroform, and 1 in 40 of methanol; slightly soluble in ether.

Triamcinolone Hexacetonide

Synonym. Triamcinolone Acetonide 21-(3,3-Dimethylbutyrate)

Proprietary Names. Aristospan; Hexatrione; Lederspan.

$C_{30}H_{41}FO_7 = 532.6$

CAS—5611-51-8

A white to cream-coloured powder. M.p. 295° to 296°, with decomposition. Practically **insoluble** in water; soluble in chloroform; slightly soluble in methanol.

Colour Tests. Naphthol–Sulphuric Acid—green, yellow dichroism/yellow; Sulphuric Acid—orange.

Thin-layer Chromatography. Triamcinolone: *system TP*—Rf 09; *system TQ*—Rf 00; *system TR*—Rf 00; *system TS*—Rf 00. (*DPST solution.*) Triamcinolone acetonide: *system TP*—Rf 32; *system TQ*—Rf 00; *system TR*—Rf 20; *system TS*—Rf 06. (*DPST solution.*)

Gas Chromatography. *System GA*—RI 2970 and 3107.

High Pressure Liquid Chromatography. Triamcinolone acetonide: *system HT*—k' 2.5.

Ultraviolet Spectrum. Methanol—238 nm ($A_1^1 = 390$ a).

Infra-red Spectrum. Principal peaks at wavenumbers 1663, 1057, 1618, 1609, 902, 1080 (triamcinolone acetonide, KBr disk).

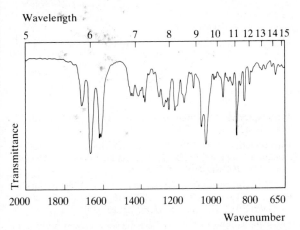

Quantification. RADIOIMMUNOASSAY. In plasma: sensitivity < 12.5 ng/ml—J. C. K. Loo and N. Jordan, *Res. Commun. chem. Path. Pharmac.*, 1979, **23**, 493–504.

Dose. 4 to 48 mg daily.

Triamterene   *Diuretic*

Proprietary Names. Dyrenium; Dytac; Jatropur; Tériam. It is an ingredient of Dyazide, Dytenzide, Dytide, Frusene, and Kalspare.

6-Phenylpteridine-2,4,7-triamine

$C_{12}H_{11}N_7 = 253.3$

CAS—396-01-0

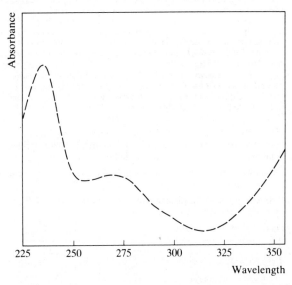

A yellow crystalline powder. Acidified solutions give a blue fluorescence.

Soluble 1 in 1000 of water, 1 in 3000 of ethanol, 1 in 4000 of chloroform, and 1 in 30 of formic acid; very slightly soluble in acetic acid and dilute mineral acids; practically insoluble in ether.

Dissociation Constant. pK_a 6.2.

Colour Tests. Liebermann's Test—red-orange; Marquis Test—yellow.

Thin-layer Chromatography. *System TA*—Rf 51; *system TB*—Rf 01; *system TC*—Rf 08. (Location under ultraviolet light, blue fluorescence.)

Ultraviolet Spectrum. Aqueous acid—250 nm ($A_1^1 = 634$ b), 360 nm ($A_1^1 = 840$ a); aqueous alkali—232 nm, 270 nm ($A_1^1 = 555$ a); methanol—233 nm ($A_1^1 = 1570$ a), 267 nm ($A_1^1 = 580$ a).

Infra-red Spectrum. Principal peaks at wavenumbers 1574, 1610, 1584, 1536, 761, 822 (KBr disk). (See below)

Mass Spectrum. Principal peaks at *m/z* 253, 252, 43, 104, 254, 235, 77, 89.

Quantification. HIGH PRESSURE LIQUID CHROMATOGRAPHY. In plasma: triamterene and *p*-hydroxytriamterene, detection limit 20 ng/ml, UV detection—G. J. Yakatan and J. E. Cruz, *J. pharm. Sci.*, 1981, **70**, 949–951. In plasma, whole blood, or urine: triamterene and *p*-hydroxytriamterene sulphate, sensitivity, for blood, 1 ng/ml and 2 ng/ml, respectively, for urine, 40 ng/ml and 100 ng/ml, respectively, fluorescence detection—F. Sörgel *et al.*, *J. pharm. Sci.*, 1984, **73**, 831–833.

Disposition in the Body. Rapidly but incompletely absorbed after oral administration and extensively metabolised; bioavailability

Wavelength

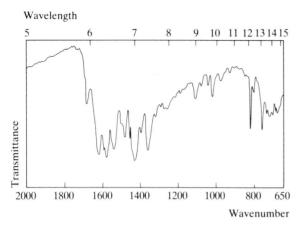

30 to 70%. After oral administration, about 30 to 70% of a dose is excreted in the urine, mainly as the sulphate conjugate of p-hydroxytriamterene, with about 5 to 10% of a dose as unchanged drug; variable amounts are excreted in the bile. p-Hydroxytriamterene sulphate is an active metabolite.

THERAPEUTIC CONCENTRATION.

After single oral doses of 150 to 300 mg to 7 subjects, peak plasma-triamterene concentrations of 0.03 to 0.15 µg/ml (mean about 0.1) were attained in 1 to 2 hours; peak plasma concentrations of p-hydroxytriamterene sulphate averaged about 1 µg/ml at 2 to 4 hours; both unchanged drug and the metabolite exhibited a second peak concentration several hours later, possibly due to enterohepatic circulation (U. Gundert-Remy et al., Eur. J. clin. Pharmac., 1979, 16, 39–44).

Following a single oral dose of 100 mg to 6 subjects, peak plasma concentrations of 0.06 to 0.18 µg/ml (mean 0.13) of triamterene and 1.3 to 3.2 µg/ml (mean 1.8) of p-hydroxytriamterene sulphate were attained in about 1 to 2 hours (J. Hasegawa et al., J. Pharmacokinet. Biopharm., 1982, 10, 507–523).

HALF-LIFE. Plasma half-life, triamterene about 2 to 4 hours, p-hydroxytriamterene sulphate, about 3 hours; half-life derived from urinary excretion data, 6 to 12 hours.

DISTRIBUTION IN BLOOD. Plasma : whole blood ratio, triamterene 0.97, p-hydroxytriamterene sulphate, 1.7.

PROTEIN BINDING. In plasma, triamterene about 45 to 70%, p-hydroxytriamterene sulphate about 90%.

Dose. 150 to 300 mg daily.

Triazolam   Hypnotic

Synonym. Clorazolam

Proprietary Name. Halcion

8-Chloro-6-(2-chlorophenyl)-1-methyl-4H-1,2,4-triazolo[4,3-a]-1,4-benzodiazepine

$C_{17}H_{12}Cl_2N_4 = 343.2$

CAS—28911-01-5

A white or pale yellow crystalline powder. M.p. 233° to 235°. Slightly **soluble** in water; soluble in ethanol.

Thin-layer Chromatography. System TA—Rf 60; system TB—Rf 01; system TC—Rf 40; system TD—Rf 05; system TE—Rf 45; system TF—Rf 02.

Gas Chromatography. System GA—RI 2965.

High Pressure Liquid Chromatography. System HI—k' 4.38; system HK—k' 1.83.

Infra-red Spectrum. Principal peaks at wavenumbers 761, 842, 1618, 1003, 1310, 827 (K Br disk).

Wavelength

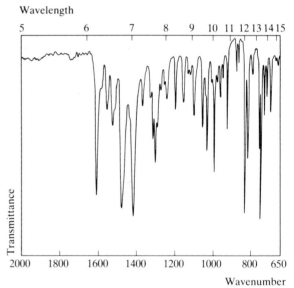

Mass Spectrum. Principal peaks at m/z 313, 238, 342, 315, 75, 344, 239, 137.

Quantification. GAS CHROMATOGRAPHY. In plasma: limit of detection 250 pg/ml, ECD—D. J. Greenblatt et al., J. Chromat., 1981, 225; Biomed. Appl., 14, 202–207.

GAS CHROMATOGRAPHY (CAPILLARY COLUMN). In plasma or urine: sensitivity 500 pg/ml, ECD—P. Coassolo et al., J. Chromat., 1983, 274; Biomed. Appl., 25, 161–170.

HIGH PRESSURE LIQUID CHROMATOGRAPHY. In serum: limit of detection 1 ng, UV detection—W. J. Adams et al., Analyt. Lett. (Part B), 1980, 13, 149–161.

RADIOIMMUNOASSAY. In serum or plasma: sensitivity 1 ng/ml—H. Ko et al., Analyt. Lett. (Part B), 1977, 10, 1019–1040.

Disposition in the Body. Rapidly and almost completely absorbed after oral administration. It is metabolised mainly by hydroxylation. The major metabolite, 1-hydroxymethyltriazolam, has a hypnotic potency approximately equivalent to that of triazolam. Other metabolites include 4-hydroxytriazolam, 1-hydroxymethyl-4-hydroxytriazolam, and three dichlorotriazolylbenzophenone derivatives. About 80% of a dose is excreted in the urine in 48 hours and about 7% is eliminated in the faeces in 72 hours.

THERAPEUTIC CONCENTRATION.

Following oral administration of 0.88 mg of ^{14}C-labelled triazolam to 6 subjects, peak plasma concentrations of 0.006 to 0.017 µg/ml (mean 0.009) of triazolam were attained in 0.75 to 3 hours; peak plasma concentrations of the glucuronide conjugates of the 1-hydroxymethyl and 4-hydroxy metabolites of 0.003 to 0.010 µg/ml (mean 0.006) and 0.002 to 0.009 µg/ml (mean 0.006) were attained in 0.75 to 2.5 hours and 1.5 to 5 hours respectively (F. S. Eberts *et al.*, *Clin. Pharmac. Ther.*, 1981, *29*, 81–93).

HALF-LIFE. Plasma half-life, triazolam 1.5 to 3 hours, 1-hydroxymethyltriazolam about 4 hours.

VOLUME OF DISTRIBUTION. About 1 to 2 litres/kg.

CLEARANCE. Plasma clearance, about 10 ml/min/kg.

PROTEIN BINDING. In plasma, about 78%.

NOTE. For a review of the pharmacokinetics of triazolam see G. E. Pakes *et al.*, *Drugs*, 1981, *22*, 81–110.

Dose. 125 to 250 µg, as a hypnotic.

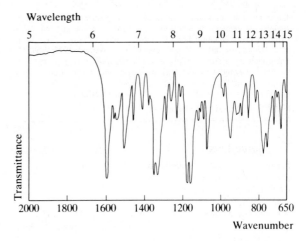

Wavelength

Transmittance / Wavenumber

Trichlormethiazide   *Diuretic*

Proprietary Names. Esmarin; Fluitran; Metahydrin; Naqua. It is an ingredient of Metatensin and Naquival.

6-Chloro-3-dichloromethyl-3,4-dihydro-2*H*-1,2,4-benzothiadiazine-7-sulphonamide 1,1-dioxide

$C_8H_8Cl_3N_3O_4S_2 = 380.6$

CAS—133-67-5

NH$_2$·SO$_2$ — (ring structure) — NH, Cl, NH, CHCl$_2$, O=S=O

A white crystalline powder. M.p. about 274°, with decomposition.

Very slightly **soluble** in water, chloroform, and ether; soluble 1 in 48 of ethanol, 1 in about 9 of dioxan, and 1 in about 5 of dimethylformamide; freely soluble in acetone.

Dissociation Constant. pK$_a$ 8.6.

Colour Test. Sulphuric Acid—yellow.

Thin-layer Chromatography. *System TA*—Rf 80; *system TD*—Rf 15; *system TE*—Rf 14; *system TF*—Rf 60. (*Acidified potassium permanganate solution*, positive.)

High Pressure Liquid Chromatography. *System HN*—k' 3.10.

Infra-red Spectrum. Principal peaks at wavenumbers 1158, 1177, 1597, 772, 1073, 1509 (KBr disk).

Mass Spectrum. Principal peaks at *m/z* 296, 298, 279, 205, 36, 64, 117, 62.

Quantification. HIGH PRESSURE LIQUID CHROMATOGRAPHY. In plasma or urine: sensitivity 10 ng/ml for plasma, UV detection—M. C. Meyer and P. T. R. Hwang, *J. Chromat.*, 1981, *223*; *Biomed. Appl.*, *12*, 466–472.

Disposition in the Body. Readily absorbed after oral administration. About 70% of a dose is excreted in the urine unchanged in 48 hours, mostly in the first 8 hours.

THERAPEUTIC CONCENTRATION.

Following a single oral dose of 4 mg to 7 subjects, peak plasma concentrations of 0.027 to 0.067 µg/ml (mean 0.04) were attained in 1 to 3.5 hours (mean 2) (I. S. Sketris *et al.*, *Eur. J. clin. Pharmac.*, 1981, *20*, 453–457).

HALF-LIFE. Plasma half-life, about 1 to 4 hours (mean 2), increased in renal impairment.

Dose. Usually 2 to 4 mg daily; initial doses of 4 to 8 mg daily may be given.

Trichloroethane   *Solvent*

Synonyms. Methylchloroform; α-Trichloroethane.

Proprietary Name. Genklene

1,1,1-Trichloroethane

$CCl_3 \cdot CH_3 = 133.4$

CAS—71-55-6

A colourless non-inflammable liquid. F.p. −32.5° to −32.7°. B.p. 71° to 81°.

Practically **insoluble** in water; soluble in organic solvents.

Colour Test. Fujiwara Test—red.

Gas Chromatography. *System GA*—RI 634; *system GI*—retention time 8.2 min.

Mass Spectrum. Principal peaks at *m/z* 97, 99, 61, 117, 119, 63, 101, 62.

Quantification. GAS CHROMATOGRAPHY. In blood, bile or tissues: using head space analysis and FID—Y. H. Caplan *et al.*, *Clin. Toxicol.*, 1976, *9*, 69–74.

Disposition in the Body. Rapidly absorbed from the gastro-intestinal tract and the lungs; poorly absorbed through the skin. It is metabolised by oxidation and conjugation; only a small proportion of an absorbed dose is excreted in the urine as trichloroethanol glucuronide (urochloralic acid) and trichloro-acetic acid. About 60 to 80% of a dose is excreted unchanged in expired air in one week.

TOXICITY. The estimated minimum lethal dose by ingestion or inhalation is 5 ml and the maximum permissible atmospheric concentration is 350 ppm. Exposure to air concentrations of more than 5000 ppm may cause unconsciousness within a short time. Fatalities have been associated with blood concentrations greater than 15 µg/ml.

During exposure to a concentration of 250 ppm trichloroethane for 30 minutes, mean blood concentrations of 1.4 µg/g were reported in 12 subjects at rest, and 3.1 µg/g in 9 subjects who performed light exercise. During exposure to 350 ppm for the same time, a mean blood concentration of 3 µg/g was produced in 5 subjects at rest (I. Astrand *et al.*, *Scand. J. Work Envir. & Hlth*, 1973, *10*, 69–81).

A woman of 40 years was found dead after exposure to trichloroethane vapour; the following postmortem concentrations were reported: blood 20 µg/ml, bile < 10 µg/ml, brain 360 µg/ml, kidney 120 µg/ml, liver 50 µg/ml, and lung 10 µg/ml (Y. H. Caplan *et al.*, *Clin. Toxicol.*, 1976, *9*, 69–74). The following postmortem tissue concentrations were reported in a fatality involving the accidental inhalation of trichloroethane: blood 18 µg/ml, brain 80 µg/g, liver 80 µg/g, lungs 31 µg/g, urine 0.9 µg/ml (A. Franc, *Bull. int. Ass. forens. Toxicol.*, 1983, *17*(2), 22–25).

HALF-LIFE. Blood half-life, about 10 to 12 hours.

Trichloroethanol   *Hypnotic*

Synonym. 2,2,2-Trichloroethyl Alcohol
2,2,2-Trichloroethanol
$CCl_3 \cdot CH_2OH = 149.4$
CAS—115-20-8

A hygroscopic liquid or crystals. M.p. 18°. B.p. 151° to 153°.

Soluble 1 in about 12 of water; miscible with ethanol and ether.

Colour Test. Fujiwara Test—yellow.

Gas Chromatography. *System GA*—RI 857; *system GI*—retention time 25.5 min.

Mass Spectrum. Principal peaks at *m/z* 31, 49, 77, 113, 115, 82, 51, 117.

Quantification. See under Chloral Hydrate.

Disposition in the Body. Trichloroethanol is a metabolite of chloral hydrate, trichloroethane, trichloroethylene, and triclofos; it has hypnotic activity. It is further metabolised by conjugation with glucuronic acid to form urochloralic acid and by oxidation to trichloroacetic acid.

TOXICITY. See under Chloral Hydrate.

HALF-LIFE. Plasma half-life, about 8 hours.

VOLUME OF DISTRIBUTION. About 0.6 litre/kg.

DISTRIBUTION IN BLOOD. Plasma:whole blood ratio, about 0.9.

PROTEIN BINDING. In plasma, about 35%.

Trichloroethylene   *General Anaesthetic/Solvent*

Synonym. Trichlorethylene
Proprietary Names. Triklone (solvent); Trilene.
$CHCl:CCl_2 = 131.4$
CAS—79-01-6

A clear, colourless or pale blue, mobile, non-inflammable liquid. It decomposes in light in the presence of air with the formation of hydrochloric acid. Relative density 1.464 to 1.470. B.p. 85° to 88°.

Trichloroethylene (*B.P.*) contains thymol 0.01% w/w as a preservative and may contain not more than 0.001% w/w of a suitable blue colouring matter to distinguish it from chloroform. Practically **insoluble** in water; miscible with dehydrated alcohol, chloroform, and ether.

Colour Test. Fujiwara Test—red.

Gas Chromatography. *System GA*—RI 710; *system GI*—retention time 14.8 min.

Mass Spectrum. Principal peaks at *m/z* 95, 130, 132, 60, 97, 35, 134, 47; trichloroacetic acid 44, 83, 85, 36, 28, –, –, –.

Quantification. GAS CHROMATOGRAPHY. In blood: using headspace analysis, FID—F. N. Prior, *Anaesthesia*, 1972, *27*, 379–389. In blood or urine: trichloroethanol and trichloroacetic acid, using headspace analysis, detection limit 500 ng/ml for trichlo-

roethanol, ECD—D. D. Breimer *et al.*, *J. Chromat.*, 1974, *88*, 55–63.

Disposition in the Body. Rapidly absorbed from the lungs; about 50 to 65% of an inhaled dose is retained. Absorbed from the gastro-intestinal tract and through the skin. It is highly soluble in lipid-rich tissues, from which it is slowly released. Chloral hydrate is a transient metabolite which is further metabolised by reduction to trichloroethanol and oxidation to trichloroacetic acid. Trichloroethanol is mainly excreted as its glucuronide conjugate (urochloralic acid). Monochloroacetic acid is a minor metabolite. About 45% of an absorbed dose is excreted as urochloralic acid and about 30% as trichloroacetic acid in the urine in 3 weeks; small amounts are eliminated in the faeces. About 16% is excreted unchanged in expired air.

THERAPEUTIC CONCENTRATION. In blood, for anaesthesia, usually in the range 26 to 82 µg/ml.

During anaesthesia, exposure to an induction level of 1% of trichloroethylene for 30 minutes to 20 patients, produced blood concentrations of 34 to 90 µg/ml (mean 65) (F. N. Prior, *Anaesthesia*, 1972, *27*, 379–389).

TOXICITY. The estimated minimum lethal dose by ingestion or inhalation is 5 ml and the maximum permissible atmospheric concentration is 100 ppm.

Exposure of 5 subjects to a concentration of 100 ppm of trichloroethylene for 6 hours produced mean peak blood concentrations of about 1 µg/ml of trichloroethylene 2 hours after the start of exposure, and about 6 µg/ml of trichloroethanol at the end of the exposure period (G. Müller *et al.*, *Arch. Tox.*, 1974, *32*, 283–295).

A man of 56 years was found dead after exposure to trichloroethylene fumes. The following postmortem concentrations of trichloroethylene were reported: blood about 90 µg/ml, brain about 270 µg/g, lung about 40 µg/g (A. Alha *et al.*, *Bull. int. Ass. forens. Toxicol.*, 1974, *10*(1), 14–15).

In 19 cases of fatal trichloroethylene poisoning, the following postmortem concentrations were reported: blood 1 to 41 µg/ml (mean 14, 15 cases), brain 4 to 74 µg/g (mean 31, 5 cases), kidney 4 to 140 µg/g (mean 30, 8 cases), liver 1 to 250 µg/g (mean 64, 9 cases), lung 1 to 15 µg/g (mean 7, 6 cases), urine a trace to 91 µg/ml (mean 35, 5 cases) (R. Bonnichsen and A. C. Maehly, *J. forens. Sci.*, 1966, *11*, 414–427).

HALF-LIFE. About 30 to 38 hours.

Dose. To produce light anaesthesia, 0.5 to 2% of the vapour by inhalation.

Trichlorofluoromethane   *Aerosol Propellant/Refrigerant*

Synonyms. Fluorotrichloromethane; Propellent 11; Refrigerant 11; Trichloromonofluoromethane.
Proprietary Names. It is an ingredient of PR Spray and Skefron.
$CCl_3F = 137.4$
CAS—75-69-4

A clear, colourless, non-inflammable volatile liquid. B.p. about 24°.

In the liquid state it is practically **immiscible** with water but miscible with dehydrated alcohol.

Gas Chromatography. *System GA*—RI 484; *system GI*—retention time 3.0 min.

Mass Spectrum. Principal peaks at *m/z* 101, 103, 105, 66, 47, 35, 31, 82.

Trichlorophenoxyacetic Acid   *Herbicide*

Synonym. 2,4,5-T

Proprietary Names. Boots Nettle Killer; Marks Brushwood Killer; Phortox; Silvapron T; Trioxone 50. It is an ingredient of Econal, Nettle Ban, Spontox, and Stancide BWK 75.

2,4,5-Trichlorophenoxyacetic acid
$C_8H_5Cl_3O_3 = 255.5$
CAS—93-76-5; 35915-18-5

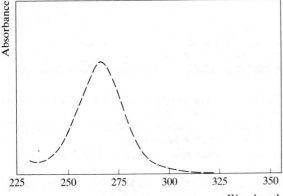

A white crystalline solid. M.p. 154° to 155°.
Very slightly **soluble** in water; soluble in ethanol, acetone, and ether.

Colour Test. Liebermann's Test—pink($\rightarrow$ brown).

Gas Chromatography. Trichlorophenoxyacetic acid methyl ester: *system GA*—RI 1740; *system GK*—retention time 0.80 relative to caffeine. Trichlorophenoxyacetic acid iso-octyl ester: *system GK*—retention times 1.24 and 1.31, relative to caffeine.

Mass Spectrum. Principal peaks at *m/z* 233, 45, 42, 59, 179, 146, 109, 235 (methyl ester); 43, 57, 41, 55, 71, 69, 56, 70 (iso-octyl ester).

Triclocarban   *Disinfectant*

Synonym. 3,4,4'-Trichlorocarbanilide
Proprietary Names. Cutisan; Nobacter; Septivon-Lavril; Solu-bacter; TCC.
1-(4-Chlorophenyl)-3-(3,4-dichlorophenyl)urea
$C_{13}H_9Cl_3N_2O = 315.6$
CAS—101-20-2

A fine white powder. M.p. 250° to 256°.
Practically **insoluble** in water; soluble 1 in 25 of acetone and 1 in 100 of propylene glycol.

Thin-layer Chromatography. *System TD*—Rf 60; *system TE*—Rf 75; *system TF*—Rf 59.

Ultraviolet Spectrum. Ethanol—265 nm ($A_1^1 = 1391$ b).

Infra-red Spectrum. Principal peaks at wavenumbers 1634, 1587, 1550, 820, 1089, 1232 (KBr disk).

Mass Spectrum. Principal peaks at *m/z* 127, 161, 163, 153, 129, 187, 90, 189.

Quantification. GAS CHROMATOGRAPHY. In blood: sensitivity 12.5 ng/ml, ECD—D. R. Hoar and M. H. Bowen, *J. pharm. Sci.*, 1977, *66*, 725–726.

Use. In concentrations of 1 to 2%.

Triclofos Sodium   *Hypnotic*

Proprietary Name. Triclos
Sodium hydrogen 2,2,2-trichloroethyl phosphate
$C_2H_3Cl_3NaO_4P = 251.4$
CAS—306-52-5 (triclofos); *7246-20-0* (sodium salt)

A white hygroscopic powder.
Soluble 1 in 2 of water and 1 in 250 of ethanol; practically insoluble in ether.

Colour Test. Phosphorus Test—yellow precipitate.

Infra-red Spectrum. Principal peaks at wavenumbers 1107, 1227, 926, 1124, 709, 876 (triclofos sodium, Nujol mull).

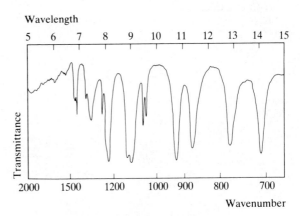

Mass Spectrum. Principal peaks at *m/z* 31, 49, 77, 29, 113, 51, 48, 115, no peaks above 120 (triclofos); trichloroacetic acid 44, 83, 85, 36, 28, –, –, –; trichloroethanol 31, 49, 77, 113, 115, 82, 51, 117.

Quantification. Determination of trichloroethanol—see under Chloral Hydrate.

Disposition in the Body. Rapidly hydrolysed in the stomach to trichloroethanol which is readily absorbed. Trichloroethanol, the active metabolite, is conjugated with glucuronic acid to give urochloralic acid, and oxidised to trichloroacetic acid. About 12% of a dose is excreted in the urine in 24 hours as metabolites.

THERAPEUTIC CONCENTRATION. In plasma, trichloroethanol, usually in the range 1.5 to 15 µg/ml.

After an oral dose of 22 mg/kg given to 7 subjects, peak plasma concentrations of trichloroethanol and urochloralic acid of about 8 µg/ml and 2 µg/ml, respectively, were reported; no unchanged triclofos was detectable in plasma (E. M. Sellers *et al.*, *Clin. Pharmac. Ther.*, 1973, *14*, 147).

TOXICITY. Plasma concentrations greater than 40 µg/ml of trichloroethanol are likely to produce toxic effects, and concentrations greater than 100 µg/ml may be fatal.

The following postmortem tissue concentrations of trichloroethanol were reported in a fatality due to triclofos ingestion: blood 335 µg/ml, bile 696 µg/ml, brain 326 µg/g, kidney 928 µg/g, liver 690 µg/g, urine 195 µg/ ml; other drugs were also detected (D. J. Doedens and J. A. Benz, *Bull. int. Ass. forens. Toxicol.*, 1976, *12*(2), 10–11).

HALF-LIFE. Plasma half-life, trichloroethanol about 8 hours, urochloralic acid about 7 hours, trichloroacetic acid about 4 days.

VOLUME OF DISTRIBUTION. Trichloroethanol, about 0.6 litre/kg.

DISTRIBUTION IN BLOOD. Plasma:whole blood ratio, trichloroethanol about 0.9.

PROTEIN BINDING. In plasma, trichloroethanol about 35% and trichloroacetic acid about 94%.

Dose. 1 to 2 g, as a hypnotic.

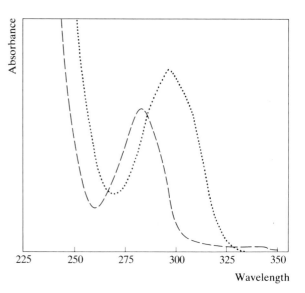

Triclosan   *Disinfectant*

Synonym. Cloxifenol

Proprietary Names. Adasept; Gamophen (antiseptic soap); Irgasan DP300; Ster-Zac (bath concentrate); Tersaseptic; Zalclense. It is an ingredient of Manusept.

5-Chloro-2-(2,4-dichlorophenoxy)phenol
$C_{12}H_7Cl_3O_2 = 289.5$
CAS—3380-34-5

A white crystalline powder or soft agglomerates. M.p. 55° to 57°.

Practically **insoluble** in water; very soluble in most organic solvents.

Ultraviolet Spectrum. Ethanol—283 nm ($A_1^1 = 179$ b); alkaline ethanol—295 nm.

Mass Spectrum. Principal peaks at *m/z* 288, 290, 218, 146, 114, 63, 51, 148.

Quantification. GAS CHROMATOGRAPHY. In plasma or urine: sensitivity 2 ng/ml, ECD—A. Sioufi *et al.*, *J. pharm. Sci.*, 1977, *66*, 1166–1168.

Use. In concentrations of 0.05 to 2%.

Tricyclamol Chloride   *Anticholinergic*

1-(3-Cyclohexyl-3-hydroxy-3-phenylpropyl)-1-methylpyrrolidinium chloride
$C_{20}H_{32}ClNO = 337.9$
CAS—3818-88-0

A white crystalline powder. M.p. 165° to 168°.

Soluble 1 in 3 of water, 1 in 3 of ethanol, and 1 in 25 of chloroform; practically insoluble in ether.

Colour Tests. Mandelin's Test—grey-violet; Marquis Test—violet.

Thin-layer Chromatography. *System TA*—Rf 06. (*Acidified iodoplatinate solution*, positive.)

Ultraviolet Spectrum. Aqueous acid—251 nm, 257 nm ($A_1^1 = 5.7$ a), 263 nm. No alkaline shift.

Infra-red Spectrum. Principal peaks at wavenumbers 705, 920, 1115, 772, 1045, 1061 (KBr disk).

Dose. Tricyclamol chloride has been given in doses of 50 to 100 mg.

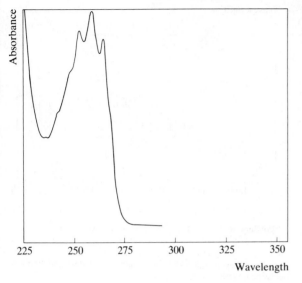

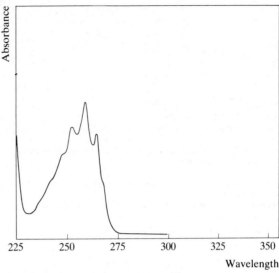

Tridihexethyl Chloride   *Anticholinergic*

Proprietary Names. Pathilon. It is an ingredient of Milpath.
(3 - Cyclohexyl - 3 - hydroxy - 3 - phenylpropyl)triethyl-
ammonium chloride
$C_{21}H_{36}ClNO = 354.0$
CAS—60-49-1 (tridihexethyl); *4310-35-4* (chloride)

A white crystalline powder. M.p. 196° to 202°.
Soluble 1 in 3 of water, 1 in 3 of ethanol, and 1 in 2 of chloroform;
practically insoluble in ether.

Colour Tests. Mandelin's Test—violet; Marquis Test—brown-
violet.

Thin-layer Chromatography. *System TA*—Rf 07. (*Acidified
iodoplatinate solution*, positive.)

Ultraviolet Spectrum. Aqueous acid—251 nm, 257 nm, 263 nm.
No alkaline shift.

Infra-red Spectrum. Principal peaks at wavenumbers 717, 1492,
710, 769, 1162, 729 (KBr disk).

Mass Spectrum. Principal peaks at m/z 86, 58, 88, 105, 206, 87,
55, 77.

Dose. 75 to 300 mg daily.

Trifluomeprazine   *Tranquilliser (Veterinary)*

Synonym. Triflutrimeprazine
2,N,N - Trimethyl - 3 - (2 - trifluoromethylphenothiazin - 10 - yl)-
propylamine
$C_{19}H_{21}F_3N_2S = 366.4$
CAS—2622-37-9

Trifluomeprazine Maleate

$C_{19}H_{21}F_3N_2S,C_4H_4O_4 = 482.5$
A white crystalline powder. M.p. about 178°.
Very slightly **soluble** in water; soluble 1 in 25 of ethanol and 1 in 25 of
chloroform; practically insoluble in ether.

Colour Tests. Mandelin's Test—green → red-violet; Marquis
Test—red-violet; Sulphuric Acid—red-violet.

Thin-layer Chromatography. *System TA*—Rf 65; *system TB*—Rf
60; *system TC*—Rf 58. (*Acidified iodoplatinate solution*, positive.)

Gas Chromatography. *System GA*—RI 2250.

Ultraviolet Spectrum. Aqueous acid—255 nm ($A_1^1 = 803$ a),
305 nm, less well-defined.

Mass Spectrum. Principal peaks at m/z 58, 366, 59, 100, 266,
248, 84, 44.

Trifluoperazine   *Tranquilliser*

10-[3-(4-Methylpiperazin-1-yl)propyl]-2-trifluoromethylpheno-
thiazine
$C_{21}H_{24}F_3N_3S = 407.5$
CAS—117-89-5

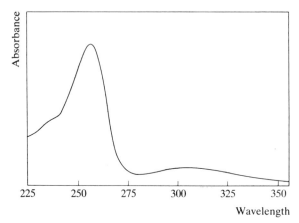

Trifluoperazine Hydrochloride

Synonym. Triphthazinum

Proprietary Names. Calmazine; Clinazine; Jatroneural; Modalina; Novoflurazine; Pentazine; Solazine; Stelazine; Terfluzin(e); Triflurin; Tripazine. It is an ingredient of Expansyl, Parstelin, and Stelabid.

$C_{21}H_{24}F_3N_3S,2HCl = 480.4$

CAS—440-17-5

A white to pale yellow, hygroscopic, crystalline powder. M.p. 242°, with decomposition.

Soluble 1 in 2 of water, 1 in 11 of ethanol, and 1 in 100 of chloroform; practically insoluble in ether.

Dissociation Constant. pK_a 8.1 (24°).

Partition Coefficient. Log P (octanol/pH 7.0), 3.9.

Colour Tests. Formaldehyde–Sulphuric Acid—pink; Forrest Reagent—orange; FPN Reagent—orange; Liebermann's Test—red; Mandelin's Test—red-brown; Marquis Test—red-violet.

Thin-layer Chromatography. *System TA*—Rf 53; *system TB*—Rf 33; *system TC*—Rf 30. (*Dragendorff spray*, positive; *FPN reagent*, pink; *acidified iodoplatinate solution*, positive; *Marquis reagent*, pink.)

Gas Chromatography. *System GA*—RI 2683; *system GF*—RI 3050.

High Pressure Liquid Chromatography. *System HA*—k' 3.0.

Ultraviolet Spectrum. Aqueous acid—256 nm ($A_1^1 = 743$ a), 305 nm; aqueous alkali—258 nm, 308 nm.

Infra-red Spectrum. Principal peaks at wavenumbers 1114, 1316, 1145, 1081, 755, 1255 (trifluoperazine hydrochloride, KBr disk).

Mass Spectrum. Principal peaks at *m/z* 113, 70, 407, 43, 141, 42, 127, 71.

Quantification. GAS CHROMATOGRAPHY. In plasma: sensitivity 200 pg/ml, AFID—J. I. Javaid *et al.*, *J. pharm. Sci.*, 1982, *71*, 63–66.

RADIOIMMUNOASSAY. In plasma: sensitivity 250 pg/ml—K. K. Midha *et al.*, *Br. J. clin. Pharmac.*, 1981, *12*, 189–193.

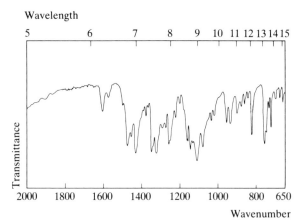

Disposition in the Body. Absorbed after oral administration. About 1% of a daily dose is excreted in the 24-hour urine as unchanged drug and up to 6% of a dose as the sulphoxide. Metabolism to 7-hydroxytrifluoperazine and desmethyltrifluoperazine has been reported.

THERAPEUTIC CONCENTRATION.

Following a single oral dose of 20 mg to 4 subjects, peak plasma concentrations of 0.001 to 0.004 µg/ml (mean 0.002) were attained in 3 to 6 hours (T. J. Gillespie and I. Sipes, *J. Chromat.*, 1981, *223*; *Biomed. Appl., 12*, 95–102).

Following daily oral doses of 80 mg to 1 subject, a peak plasma concentration of 0.028 µg/ml was reported 8 hours after a dose (S. H. Curry *et al.*, *Lancet*, 1981, *1*, 395–396).

TOXICITY.

Postmortem blood and liver concentrations of 0.06 µg/ml and 0.31 µg/g respectively were reported in a woman who died of suspected trifluoperazine overdose whilst receiving daily oral doses of 40 mg (E. Street, per R. C. Baselt, *Disposition of Toxic Drugs and Chemicals in Man*, 2nd Edn, Davis, California, Biomedical Publications, 1982, pp. 759–760).

The following postmortem concentrations were reported in a fatality attributed to trifluoperazine ingestion: blood 0.4 µg/ml, kidney 83 µg/g, liver 198 µg/g; 7-hydroxytrifluoperazine, kidney 61 µg/g, liver 161 µg/g; desmethyltrifluoperazine, kidney 89 µg/g, liver 205 µg/g (I. Quai *et al.*, *J. analyt. Toxicol.*, 1985, *9*, 43–44).

HALF-LIFE. Plasma half-life, 7 to 18 hours (mean 12).

Dose. For psychoses, the equivalent of 10 to 20 mg of trifluoperazine daily; more than 40 mg daily has been given.

Trifluperidol   *Tranquilliser*

Synonym. Flumoperone

4′ - Fluoro - 4 - [4 - hydroxy - 4 - (3 - trifluoromethylphenyl)-piperidino]butyrophenone

$C_{22}H_{23}F_4NO_2 = 409.4$

CAS—749-13-3

A white crystalline powder. M.p. 93° to 95°.

Trifluperidol Hydrochloride

Proprietary Names. Psicoperidol; Triperidol.

$C_{22}H_{23}F_4NO_2,HCl = 445.9$
CAS—2062-77-3

A white, amorphous or crystalline, flocculent powder which is stable in air but darkens slowly on exposure to light. M.p. about 205°.

Slightly **soluble** in water and chloroform; soluble in ethanol; practically insoluble in ether; freely soluble in methanol.

Thin-layer Chromatography. *System TA*—Rf 73; *system TD*—Rf 02; *system TE*—Rf 80; *system TF*—Rf 05. (*Acidified iodoplatinate solution,* positive.)

High Pressure Liquid Chromatography. *System HA*—k' 1.2.

Ultraviolet Spectrum. Aqueous acid—248 nm ($A_1^1 = 308$ a).

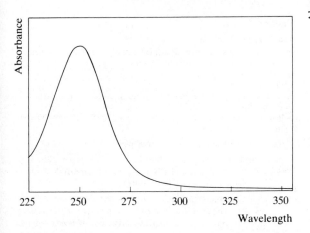

Infra-red Spectrum. Principal peaks at wavenumbers 1317, 1150, 1665, 1170, 1110, 1595 (trifluperidol hydrochloride, KBr disk).

Mass Spectrum. Principal peaks at *m/z* 42, 271, 258, 123, 56, 83, 240, 95.

Quantification. GAS CHROMATOGRAPHY. In plasma or tissues: ECD—F. Marcucci *et al., J. Chromat.,* 1971, *59,* 174–177.

Dose. Initially the equivalent of 500 μg of trifluperidol daily, increased to a maximum dose of 8 mg daily.

Trilostane   *Adrenocortical Suppressant*

Proprietary Name. Modrenal

4α,5α-Epoxy-17β-hydroxy-3-oxoandrostane-2α-carbonitrile
$C_{20}H_{27}NO_3 = 329.4$
CAS—13647-35-3

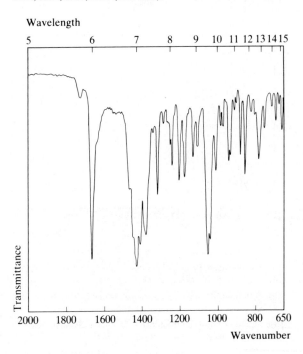

A white powder. M.p. not less than 260°, with some decomposition.

Practically **insoluble** in water, chloroform, and ether; slightly soluble in a mixture of equal parts of chloroform and methanol.

Thin-layer Chromatography. *System TA*—Rf 88; *system TB*—Rf 00; *system TC*—Rf 18; *system TD*—Rf 30; *system TE*—Rf 07; *system TF*—Rf 45. (*Marquis reagent,* red; *mercuric chloride-diphenylcarbazone reagent,* violet, fades to pink; *acidified potassium permanganate solution,* positive.)

Gas Chromatography. *System GA*—RI 3075, decomposition occurs.

Ultraviolet Spectrum. Aqueous alkali—281 nm; ethanol—253 nm ($A_1^1 = 234$ b).

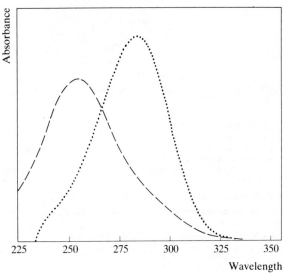

Infra-red Spectrum. Principal peaks at wavenumbers 1665, 1060, 1050, 1320, 1205, 1180 (KBr disk).

Mass Spectrum. Principal peaks at m/z 41, 147, 79, 93, 55, 105, 67, 91.

Dose. 120 to 480 mg daily.

Trimeperidine   *Narcotic Analgesic*

Synonym. Promedolum
1,2,5-Trimethyl-4-phenyl-4-piperidyl propionate
$C_{17}H_{25}NO_2 = 275.4$
CAS—64-39-1

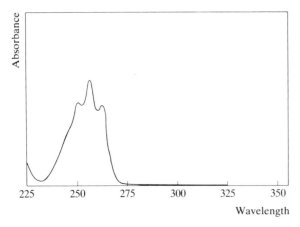

Trimeperidine Hydrochloride

$C_{17}H_{25}NO_2,HCl = 311.9$
CAS—125-80-4
A white crystalline powder.
Freely **soluble** in water and chloroform; soluble in ethanol; practically insoluble in ether.

Colour Test. Marquis Test—red-violet.

Thin-layer Chromatography. *System TA*—Rf 58; *system TB*—Rf 41; *system TC*—Rf 41. (*Dragendorff spray*, positive; *acidified iodoplatinate solution*, positive; *Marquis reagent*, red-violet.)

Gas Chromatography. *System GA*—RI 1652, 1737, 1808, and 1851.

High Pressure Liquid Chromatography. *System HA*—k' 2.1.

Ultraviolet Spectrum. Aqueous acid—251 nm, 257 nm ($A_1^1 = 7.6$ b), 263 nm. No alkaline shift.

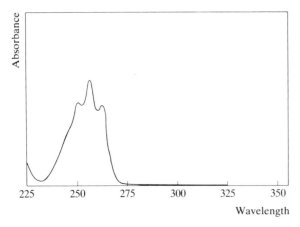

Infra-red Spectrum. Principal peaks at wavenumbers 1738, 1181, 1141, 1162, 1195, 1077 (KBr disk).

Mass Spectrum. Principal peaks at m/z 186, 42, 201, 56, 57, 187, 202, 71.

Dose. Trimeperidine hydrochloride has been given in doses of up to 200 mg daily.

Trimeprazine   *Antihistamine/Sedative*

Synonym. Alimemazine
NN-Dimethyl-2-methyl-3-(phenothiazin-10-yl)propylamine
$C_{18}H_{22}N_2S = 298.4$
CAS—84-96-8

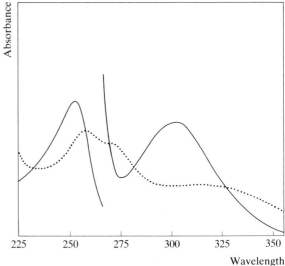

Crystals. M.p. 68°.

Trimeprazine Tartrate

Proprietary Names. Panectyl; Repeltin; Temaril; Theralene; Vallergan. It is an ingredient of Valledrine and Vallex.
$(C_{18}H_{22}N_2S)_2,C_4H_6O_6 = 747.0$
CAS—4330-99-8
A white or slightly cream-coloured crystalline powder which darkens in colour on exposure to light. M.p. 159° to 163°.
Soluble 1 in 4 of water, 1 in 30 of ethanol, and 1 in 5 of chloroform; very slightly soluble in ether.

Partition Coefficient. Log *P* (octanol/pH 7.4), 2.9.

Colour Tests. Formaldehyde–Sulphuric Acid—red-violet; Forrest Reagent—brown-red; FPN Reagent—brown-red; Mandelin's Test—violet; Marquis Test—violet.

Thin-layer Chromatography. *System TA*—Rf 58; *system TB*—Rf 55; *system TC*—Rf 39. (*Dragendorff spray*, positive; *FPN reagent*, pink; *acidified iodoplatinate solution*, positive; *Marquis reagent*, pink; *ninhydrin spray*, positive.)

Gas Chromatography. *System GA*—RI 2309; *system GC*—RI 2646; *system GF*—RI 2715.

High Pressure Liquid Chromatography. *System HA*—k' 3.1.

Ultraviolet Spectrum. Aqueous acid—251 nm ($A_1^1 = 926$ a), 300 nm; aqueous alkali—256 nm, 310 nm.

Infra-red Spectrum. Principal peaks at wavenumbers 748, 1248, 1260, 1305, 1590, 1275 (trimeprazine tartrate, KBr disk).

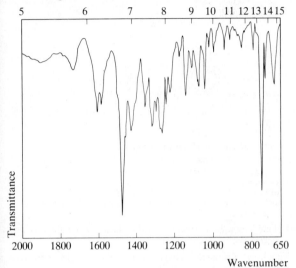

Wavelength

Mass Spectrum. Principal peaks at *m/z* 58, 298, 212, 198, 100, 299, 252, 199.

Quantification. HIGH PRESSURE LIQUID CHROMATOGRAPHY. In plasma: detection limit 100 pg/ml, electrochemical detection—J. E. Holt *et al.*, *Br. J. clin. Pharmac.*, 1983, *15*, 604P–605P.

Disposition in the Body. Readily absorbed after oral administration and widely distributed throughout the body. About 70% of an oral dose is excreted in the urine in 48 hours mostly as sulphoxides and glucuronides.

THERAPEUTIC CONCENTRATION.
Following single oral doses of 5 mg to 2 subjects, peak plasma concentrations of 0.0008 and 0.0018 μg/ml were reported at 4 hours (G. McKay *et al.*, *J. Chromat.*, 1982, *233*; *Biomed. Appl.*, *22*, 417–422).

Dose. Usually 10 to 40 mg of trimeprazine tartrate daily; up to 100 mg daily has been given.

Trimetaphan Camsylate

Antihypertensive

Synonyms. Méthioplégium; Trimetaphan Camphorsulphonate; Trimethaphan Camsylate.
Proprietary Name. Arfonad

1,3 - Dibenzylperhydro - 2 - oxoimidazo[4,5 - *c*]thieno[1,2 - *a*]thiolium (+)-camphor-10-sulphonate
$C_{22}H_{25}N_2OS, C_{10}H_{15}O_4S = 596.8$
CAS—7187-66-8 (trimetaphan); *68-91-7* (camsylate)

Colourless crystals or white crystalline powder. M.p. about 232°, with decomposition.
Soluble 1 in less than 5 of water and 1 in 2 of ethanol; freely soluble in chloroform; practically insoluble in ether.

Colour Tests. Aromaticity (Method 2)—colourless/yellow; Liebermann's Test—orange.

Thin-layer Chromatography. *System TA*—Rf 02. (*Acidified iodoplatinate solution*, positive.)

Ultraviolet Spectrum. Aqueous acid—252 nm $(A_1^1 = 8.2 \text{ a})$, 258 nm $(A_1^1 = 8.3 \text{ a})$, 264 nm. No alkaline shift.

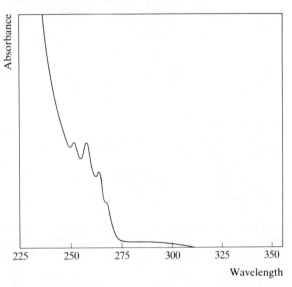

Wavelength

Infra-red Spectrum. Principal peaks at wavenumbers 1701, 1220, 1184, 1735, 1052, 1672 (KBr disk).

Wavelength

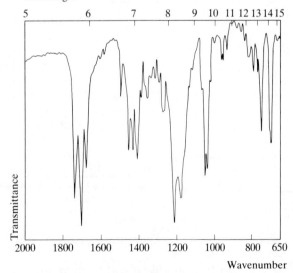

Mass Spectrum. Principal peaks at *m/z* 91, 65, 187, 92, 277, 259, 90, 273.

Dose. Initially 3 to 4 mg/minute by intravenous infusion.

Trimetazidine

Anti-anginal Vasodilator

Synonym. Trimetazine
1-(2,3,4-Trimethoxybenzyl)piperazine
$C_{14}H_{22}N_2O_3 = 266.3$
CAS—5011-34-7

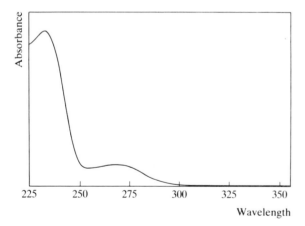

Trimetazidine Hydrochloride

Proprietary Name. Vastarel
$C_{14}H_{22}N_2O_3,2HCl = 339.3$
CAS—13171-25-0
A white crystalline powder. M.p. 222° to 228°.
Soluble in water; very slightly soluble in ethanol.

Colour Tests. Mandelin's Test—violet; Marquis Test—yellow (fades).

Thin-layer Chromatography. *System TA*—Rf 22; *system TB*—Rf 05; *system TC*—Rf 04. (*Acidified iodoplatinate solution*, positive.)

High Pressure Liquid Chromatography. *System HA*—k' 3.0 (tailing peak).

Ultraviolet Spectrum. Aqueous acid—231 nm ($A_1^1 = 424$ a), 269 nm.

Infra-red Spectrum. Principal peaks at wavenumbers 1093, 1494, 1280, 1011, 1042, 1600 (KBr disk).

Mass Spectrum. Principal peaks at *m/z* 181, 85, 56, 166, 266, 182, 179, 91.

Dose. Trimetazidine hydrochloride has been given in doses of 40 to 60 mg daily.

Trimethobenzamide

Antihistamine

N-[4-(2-Dimethylaminoethoxy)benzyl]-3,4,5-trimethoxybenz-amide
$C_{21}H_{28}N_2O_5 = 388.5$
CAS—138-56-7

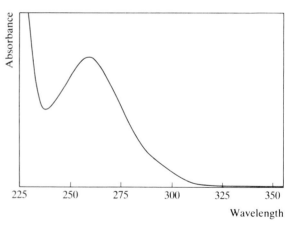

Trimethobenzamide Hydrochloride

Proprietary Names. Ibikin; Tigan.
$C_{21}H_{28}N_2O_5,HCl = 424.9$
CAS—554-92-7
A white crystalline powder. M.p. 186° to 190°.
Soluble 1 in 2 of water, 1 in about 60 of ethanol, 1 in 67 of chloroform, and 1 in 720 of ether.

Colour Tests. Liebermann's Test—black; Mandelin's Test—violet-brown.

Thin-layer Chromatography. *System TA*—Rf 42. (*Acidified iodoplatinate solution*, positive.)

Gas Chromatography. *System GA*—RI 3287.

High Pressure Liquid Chromatography. *System HA*—k' 4.7.

Ultraviolet Spectrum. Aqueous acid—258 nm ($A_1^1 = 312$ b). No alkaline shift.

Infra-red Spectrum. Principal peaks at wavenumbers 1123, 1230, 1575, 1505, 1616, 990 (KBr disk).

Mass Spectrum. Principal peaks at *m/z* 58, 195, 59, 72, 388, 89, 315, 42.

Quantification. GAS CHROMATOGRAPHY–MASS SPECTROMETRY. In saliva: sensitivity <100 ng/ml—T. A. Robert *et al.*, *J. Chromat.*, 1981, *224*; *Biomed. Appl.*, *13*, 116–121.

HIGH PRESSURE LIQUID CHROMATOGRAPHY. In serum: UV detection—T. A. Robert *et al.*, *J. clin. Pharmac.*, 1982, *22*, 53–58.

Disposition in the Body.

THERAPEUTIC CONCENTRATION.
Following a single oral dose of 250 mg to 4 subjects, peak blood concentrations of 1.3 to 2.4 µg/ml (mean 1.7) were attained in 1.5 hours (R. C. Baselt and R. H. Cravey, *J. analyt. Toxicol.*, 1977, *1*, 81–103).

TOXICITY.
In a fatality involving the ingestion of trimethobenzamide, postmortem blood and bile concentrations of 184 µg/ml and 1150 µg/ml, respectively, were reported; a postmortem blood-alcohol concentration of 1100 µg/ml was also reported (J. C. Harrill, *Bull. int. Ass. forens. Toxicol.*, 1976, *12*(2), 29–30).

Dose. 0.75 to 1 g daily.

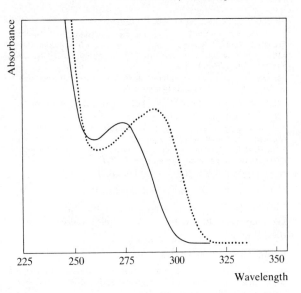

Trimethoprim   *Antimicrobial*

Synonyms. Trimethoxyprim. It is an ingredient of Co-trifamole, Co-trimazine, and Co-trimoxazole.
Proprietary Names. Ipral; Monotrim; Proloprim; Syraprim; Tiempe; Trimogal; Trimopan; Trimpex; Unitrim. It is an ingredient of Bactrim, Borgal (vet.), Chemotrim, Co-Fram, Comox, Cotrimox, Eusaprim, Fectrim, Laratrim, Polytrim, Septra, Septrin, Supristol, Triglobe and Trivetrin (vet.).
5-(3,4,5-Trimethoxybenzyl)pyrimidine-2,4-diyldiamine
$C_{14}H_{18}N_4O_3 = 290.3$
CAS—738-70-5

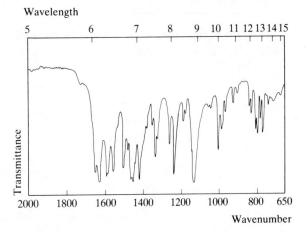

White or yellowish-white crystals or crystalline powder. M.p. 199° to 203°.
Soluble 1 in 2500 of water, 1 in 300 of ethanol, 1 in 55 of chloroform, and 1 in 80 of methanol; practically insoluble in ether.

Dissociation Constant. pK_a 7.2.

Colour Tests. Aromaticity (Method 2)—yellow/red; Mandelin's Test—yellow-brown; Marquis Test—orange.
Cold *nitric acid* gives a red colour which fades to yellow on heating.

Thin-layer Chromatography. *System TA*—Rf 55; *system TB*—Rf 00; *system TC*—Rf 22. (*Acidified iodoplatinate solution*, positive.)

Gas Chromatography. *System GA*—RI 2638.

High Pressure Liquid Chromatography. *System HA*—k' 1.2.

Ultraviolet Spectrum. Aqueous acid—271 nm ($A_1^1 = 218$ a); aqueous alkali—287 nm ($A_1^1 = 250$ a).

Infra-red Spectrum. Principal peaks at wavenumbers 1126, 1630, 1596, 1235, 1650, 1565 (KBr disk).

Mass Spectrum. Principal peaks at *m/z* 290, 259, 275, 291, 243, 123, 200, 43.

Quantification. GAS CHROMATOGRAPHY. In plasma or urine: detection limit 100 ng/ml, AFID—G. Land *et al.*, *J. Chromat.*, 1978, *146*; *Biomed. Appl.*, *3*, 143–147.

HIGH PRESSURE LIQUID CHROMATOGRAPHY. In serum or urine: detection limit 10 ng/ml, electrochemical detection—L. Nordholm and L. Dalgaard, *J. Chromat.*, 1982, *233*; *Biomed. Appl.*, *22*, 427–431. In serum or urine: detection limit 100 ng/ml, UV detection—R. Gochin *et al.*, *J. Chromat.*, 1981, *223*; *Biomed. Appl.*, *12*, 139–145.

Disposition in the Body. Readily absorbed after oral administration. Metabolic reactions include oxidation of the methylene group to a hydroxymethyl group, *N*-oxidation, *O*-demethylation, hydroxylation, and conjugation with glucuronic acid or sulphate. Metabolites are excreted in the urine as conjugates but the greater part of the dose is excreted as unchanged drug. Urinary excretion is pH-dependent and is increased in acid urine. About 40 to 75% of a dose is excreted in 24 hours, up to 60% being in the form of unchanged drug, with about 4% each as the 3'-hydroxymethyl and 4'-hydroxymethyl metabolites, and 2% as the N^1-oxide. Less than 4% is eliminated in the faeces.

THERAPEUTIC CONCENTRATION.
Following oral administration of 300 mg once daily to 6 subjects, maximum steady-state plasma concentrations of 3.1 to 9.5 µg/ml (mean 6.0) were attained in 1 to 4 hours (mean 2) (B. Odlind *et al.*, *Eur. J. clin. Pharmac.*, 1984, *26*, 393–397).
For further references to trimethoprim when administered with sulpha-methoxazole, see under Sulphamethoxazole.

TOXICITY. Toxic effects have been associated with plasma concentrations greater than 20 µg/ml.
A 28-year-old man ingested 8 g of trimethoprim and 14 hours later the plasma concentration was 19.6 µg/ml. It was estimated that the actual amount of trimethoprim absorbed was about 3 g. The patient subsequently recovered (K. Hoppu *et al.*, *Lancet*, 1980, *1*, 778).

HALF-LIFE. Plasma half-life, 8 to 17 hours (mean 11).

VOLUME OF DISTRIBUTION. About 1.4 litres/kg.

CLEARANCE. Plasma clearance, about 2 ml/min/kg.

DISTRIBUTION IN BLOOD. Plasma:whole blood ratio, about 0.78.

SALIVA. Plasma:saliva ratio, about 1.3.

PROTEIN BINDING. In plasma, 40 to 70%.

NOTE. For a review of the clinical pharmacokinetics of sulphamethoxazole and trimethoprim see R. B. Patel and P. G. Welling, *Clin. Pharmacokinet.*, 1980, *5*, 405–423.

Dose. Usually 400 mg daily; doses of 1.5 g daily for 3 days have been given for malaria.

Trimethoxyamphetamine   *Hallucinogen*

α-Methyl-3,4,5-trimethoxyphenethylamine
$C_{12}H_{19}NO_3 = 225.3$
CAS—1082-88-8

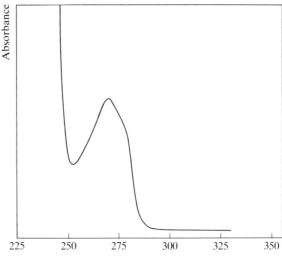

Trimethoxyamphetamine is the α-methyl homologue of mescaline.
An oil.
Practically **insoluble** in water; soluble in chloroform.
The hydrochloride is soluble in water; m.p. 219° to 220°.

Colour Test. Marquis Test—orange.

Thin-layer Chromatography. *System TA*—Rf 33; *system TB*—Rf 08; *system TC*—Rf 11. (*Acidified iodoplatinate solution*, positive.)

Gas Chromatography. *System GA*—RI 1748.

High Pressure Liquid Chromatography. *System HC*—k' 1.48.

Ultraviolet Spectrum. Aqueous acid—269 nm ($A_1^1 = 26$ b). No alkaline shift.

Infra-red Spectrum. Principal peaks at wavenumbers 1130, 1595, 1510, 1240, 1000, 1151 (KBr disk).

Mass Spectrum. Principal peaks at *m/z* 43, 182, 167, 225, 181, 183, 151, 142.

Trimetozine   *Tranquilliser*

Synonyms. Trimethoxazine; Trimolide.
Proprietary Name. Opalene
4-(3,4,5-Trimethoxybenzoyl)morpholine
$C_{14}H_{19}NO_5 = 281.3$
CAS—635-41-6

A white crystalline powder. M.p. about 121°.

Slightly **soluble** in water and ethanol; freely soluble in chloroform and methanol.

Colour Tests. Liebermann's Test—black; Marquis Test—red-brown.

Thin-layer Chromatography. *System TA*—Rf 61; *system TB*—Rf 11; *system TC*—Rf 72. (*Acidified iodoplatinate solution*, positive.)

Gas Chromatography. *System GA*—RI 2198.

Ultraviolet Spectrum. Methanol—245 nm (A_1^1 = 259 b).

Infra-red Spectrum. Principal peaks at wavenumbers 1131, 1642, 1229, 1110, 1592, 1001 (KBr disk).

Mass Spectrum. Principal peaks at *m/z* 195, 281, 196, 152, 280, 81, 77, 66.

Dose. Usually 0.6 to 1.8 g daily; maximum of 3 g daily.

Trimipramine   *Antidepressant*

Synonym. Trimeprimine

3 - (10,11 - Dihydro - 5*H* - dibenz[*b*, *f*]azepin - 5 - yl) - 2,*N*,*N* - tri-methylpropylamine

$C_{20}H_{26}N_2 = 294.4$

CAS—739-71-9

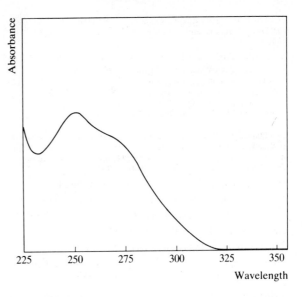

A pale yellowish-white waxy solid. M.p. about 45°.

Practically **insoluble** in water; readily soluble in ethanol.

Trimipramine Maleate

Proprietary Name. Surmontil

$C_{20}H_{26}N_2,C_4H_4O_4 = 410.5$

CAS—521-78-8

A white crystalline powder. M.p. 140° to 144°.

Slightly **soluble** in water and ethanol; freely soluble in chloroform; practically insoluble in ether.

Colour Tests. Forrest Reagent—blue; FPN Reagent—blue; Mandelin's Test (add water)—blue.

Thin-layer Chromatography. *System TA*—Rf 59; *system TB*—Rf 62; *system TC*—Rf 54. (*Acidified iodoplatinate solution*, positive.)

Gas Chromatography. *System GA*—trimipramine RI 2201, *N*-monodesmethyltrimipramine RI 2250; *system GF*—RI 2505.

High Pressure Liquid Chromatography. *System HA*—trimipramine k' 2.7, *N*-monodesmethyltrimipramine k' 1.8; *system HF*—k' 6.17.

Ultraviolet Spectrum. Aqueous acid—250 nm (A_1^1 = 300 a).

Infra-red Spectrum. Principal peaks at wavenumbers 1490, 762, 1240, 1230, 741, 749 (KBr disk).

Mass Spectrum. Principal peaks at *m/z* 58, 249, 208, 99, 193, 234, 84, 248.

Quantification. GAS CHROMATOGRAPHY. In plasma: trimipramine and *N*-monodesmethyltrimipramine, sensitivity 500 pg/ml, AFID—D. R. Abernethy *et al.*, *Clin. Pharmac. Ther.*, 1984, *35*, 348–353. In plasma: sensitivity 5 ng/ml, AFID—G. Caillé

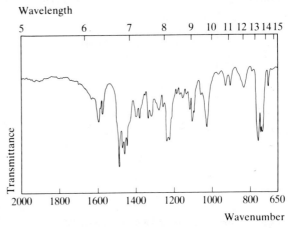

et al., *Biopharm. Drug Disp.*, 1980, *1*, 187–194. In postmortem tissues: sensitivity 500 ng/ml, FID—N. B. Wu Chen *et al.*, *J. forens. Sci.*, 1983, *28*, 116–121.

HIGH PRESSURE LIQUID CHROMATOGRAPHY. In plasma: trimipramine and metabolites, sensitivity 3 ng/ml, electrochemical detection—R. F. Suckow and T. B. Cooper, *J. pharm. Sci.*, 1984, *73*, 1745–1748.

Disposition in the Body. Readily absorbed after oral administration but undergoes considerable first-pass metabolism to *N*-monodesmethyltrimipramine; bioavailability about 40% with wide intersubject variation. Excreted in the urine mainly as metabolites.

THERAPEUTIC CONCENTRATION.

A single oral dose of 50 mg administered to 9 subjects, resulted in peak plasma concentrations of 0.015 to 0.051 µg/ml (mean 0.028) in 1 to 6 hours (D. R. Abernethy *et al.*, *Clin. Pharmac. Ther.*, 1984, *35*, 348–353). Following daily oral doses of 75 or 150 mg to 29 subjects, the following steady-state plasma concentrations were reported: trimipramine 0.01 to 0.24 µg/ml (mean 0.09), *N*-monodesmethyltrimipramine 0.003 to 0.38 µg/ml (mean 0.07), 2-hydroxytrimipramine 0.003 to 0.04 µg/ml (mean 0.016), and 2-hydroxy-*N*-monodesmethyltrimipramine 0.003 to 0.05 μg/ml (mean 0.017) (R. F. Suckow and T. B. Cooper, *J. pharm. Sci.*, 1984, *73*, 1745–1748).

TOXICITY. Toxic effects have been associated with plasma concentrations greater than 1 μg/ml.

In a fatality involving the ingestion of up to 6 g of trimipramine, the following postmortem tissue concentrations were reported: blood 9.5 μg/ml, brain 27 μg/g, kidney 42 μg/g, liver 224 μg/g, spleen 31 μg/g (J. J. Rousseau and M. Rousseau, *Bull. int. Ass. forens. Toxicol.*, 1970, *7*(3), 5–6).

In a fatality involving the ingestion of trimipramine and clomipramine, postmortem concentrations were: blood, trimipramine 11.6 μg/ml, clomipramine 2.1 μg/ml; liver, trimipramine 544 μg/g, clomipramine 56 μg/g (R. S. Hucker, *Bull. int. Ass. forens. Toxicol.*, 1983, *17*(2), 20–22).

HALF-LIFE. Plasma half-life, 16 to 40 hours (mean 24).

VOLUME OF DISTRIBUTION. About 20 to 50 litres/kg (mean 30).

CLEARANCE. Plasma clearance, 10 to 25 ml/min/kg (mean 16).

DISTRIBUTION IN BLOOD. Plasma: whole blood ratio, 1.2.

PROTEIN BINDING. In plasma, about 94%.

Dose. The equivalent of 50 to 300 mg of trimipramine daily.

Trioxsalen   *Pigmenting Agent*

Synonyms. 4,5′,8-Trimethylpsoralen; Trioxysalen.
Proprietary Name. Trisoralen
2,5,9-Trimethyl-7*H*-furo[3,2-*g*]chromen-7-one
$C_{14}H_{12}O_3 = 228.2$
CAS—3902-71-4

A white or greyish crystalline solid. M.p. about 230°.
Practically **insoluble** in water; soluble 1 in 1150 of ethanol, 1 in 84 of chloroform, and 1 in 43 of methylene chloride.

Gas Chromatography. *System GA*—RI 2155.

Ultraviolet Spectrum. Methanol—248 nm ($A_1^1 = 981$ b), 296 nm ($A_1^1 = 428$ b), 338 nm ($A_1^1 = 276$ b).

Infra-red Spectrum. Principal peaks at wavenumbers 1710, 1600, 1110, 880, 930, 1620 (Nujol mull).

Mass Spectrum. Principal peaks at *m/z* 228, 200, 199, 128, 229, 185, 115, 201.

Quantification. HIGH PRESSURE LIQUID CHROMATOGRAPHY. In blood, ophthalmic fluid or skin: detection limit 2 ng/ml, UV detection—S. G. Chakrabarti *et al.*, *J. invest. Derm.*, 1982, *79*, 374–377.

Dose. 5 to 10 mg daily.

Tripelennamine   *Antihistamine*

N-Benzyl-*N′N′*-dimethyl-*N*-(2-pyridyl)ethylenediamine
$C_{16}H_{21}N_3 = 255.4$
CAS—91-81-6

An oily liquid.
Miscible with water.

Tripelennamine Citrate
Proprietary Name. PBZ (elixir)
$C_{16}H_{21}N_3,C_6H_8O_7 = 447.5$
CAS—6138-56-3
A white crystalline powder. M.p. about 107°.
Soluble 1 in 1 of water; freely soluble in ethanol; practically insoluble in chloroform; very slightly soluble in ether.

Tripelennamine Hydrochloride
Proprietary Names. PBZ (tablets); Pyribenzamine.
$C_{16}H_{21}N_3,HCl = 291.8$
CAS—154-69-8
A white crystalline powder which slowly darkens on exposure to light. M.p. 188° to 192°.
Soluble 1 in 1 of water, 1 in 6 of ethanol, and 1 in 6 of chloroform; practically insoluble in ether.

Dissociation Constant. pK_a 3.9, 9.0 (25°).

Colour Tests. Cyanogen Bromide—yellow; Liebermann's Test—orange → brown; Mandelin's Test—yellow-brown; Marquis Test—red-brown.

Thin-layer Chromatography. *System TA*—Rf 55; *system TB*—Rf 44; *system TC*—Rf 27. (*Dragendorff spray*, positive; *acidified iodoplatinate solution*, positive; *Marquis reagent*, brown.)

Gas Chromatography. *System GA*—RI 1980.

High Pressure Liquid Chromatography. *System HA*—k′ 3.6.

Ultraviolet Spectrum. Aqueous acid—239 nm ($A_1^1 = 562$ a), 314 nm; aqueous alkali—249 nm, 312 nm.

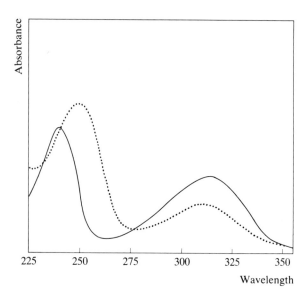

Infra-red Spectrum. Principal peaks at wavenumbers 1496, 1592, 770, 1250, 955, 735 (tripelennamine hydrochloride, KBr disk).

Wavelength

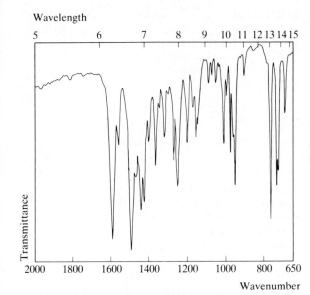

Transmittance

Wavenumber

Mass Spectrum. Principal peaks at m/z 58, 91, 72, 71, 197, 185, 184, 92.

Quantification. GAS CHROMATOGRAPHY. In postmortem tissues: FID—J. R. Monforte *et al.*, *J. forens. Sci.*, 1983, *28*, 90–101.

Disposition in the Body. Rapidly absorbed after oral administration. Metabolised by ring hydroxylation and demethylation followed by conjugation with glucuronic acid. It is excreted in the urine, mainly as metabolites, and in the bile, and appears to undergo enterohepatic circulation. The major urinary metabolites are tripelennamine-*N*-glucuronide, conjugated hydroxytripelennamine, and the conjugated hydroxydesmethyl metabolite; the *N*-oxide is a minor metabolite.

THERAPEUTIC CONCENTRATION.
After a single oral dose of 100 mg, a peak plasma concentration of 0.06 μg/ml was reportedly attained in 2 to 3 hours (per M. Bayley *et al.*, *J. forens. Sci.*, 1975, *20*, 539–543).

TOXICITY.
In one fatality arising from the ingestion of about 1 g, in which death occurred about 7 hours after ingestion, the following postmortem tissue distribution was reported: blood 10 μg/ml, brain 43 μg/g, kidney 35 μg/g, liver 83 μg/g, urine 287 μg/ml (M. Bayley *et al.*, *ibid.*).
In 17 fatalities involving the intravenous abuse of tripelennamine and pentazocine, tripelennamine blood concentrations of 0 to 3.0 μg/ml (mean 0.5) were reported; kidney concentrations of 0.4 to 2.0 μg/g (mean 1.1) were reported in 4 subjects and liver concentrations of 1.0 to 6.5 μg/g (mean 3.1) in 5 subjects; pentazocine blood concentrations ranged from 0 to 11 μg/ml (mean 3) (J. R. Monforte *et al.*, *J. forens. Sci.*, 1983, *28*, 90–101).

Dose. 25 to 50 mg of tripelennamine hydrochloride every 4 to 6 hours; up to 600 mg daily has been given.

Triphenyltetrazolium Chloride   *Diagnostic Agent*

Synonyms. Red Tetrazolium; RT; TPTZ; TTC.
Proprietary Name. Uroscreen
2,3,5-Triphenyl-2*H*-tetrazolium chloride
$C_{19}H_{15}ClN_4 = 334.8$
CAS—298-96-4

A white crystalline powder. M.p. 243°, with decomposition.
Soluble in water, ethanol, and acetone; practically insoluble in ether.

Colour Tests. Liebermann's Test—red-orange; Mandelin's Test—blue (slow).

Thin-layer Chromatography. *System TA*—Rf 61. (*Acidified iodoplatinate solution*, positive.)

Ultraviolet Spectrum. Aqueous acid—246 nm ($A_1^1 = 680$ b).

Infra-red Spectrum. Principal peaks at wavenumbers 691, 769, 1529, 720, 1164, 998 (KBr disk).

Triprolidine   *Antihistamine*

(*E*)-2-[3-(Pyrrolidin-1-yl)-1-*p*-tolylprop-1-enyl]pyridine
$C_{19}H_{22}N_2 = 278.4$
CAS—486-12-4

Crystals. M.p. 59° to 61°.

Triprolidine Hydrochloride

Proprietary Names. Actidil; Actidilon; Pro-Actidil; Pro-Actidilon. It is an ingredient of Actifed and Linctifed.
$C_{19}H_{22}N_2,HCl,H_2O = 332.9$
CAS—550-70-9 (anhydrous); *6138-79-0* (monohydrate)
A white crystalline powder. M.p. 118° to 121°.
Soluble 1 in about 2 of water, 1 in about 1.5 of ethanol, 1 in less than 1 of chloroform, and 1 in 2000 of ether.

Dissociation Constant. pK_a 6.5.

Partition Coefficient. Log *P* (octanol), 3.9.

Colour Tests. Cyanogen Bromide—orange-pink (after 1 to 2 min); Liebermann's Test—orange.

Thin-layer Chromatography. *System TA*—Rf 51; *system TB*—Rf 39; *system TC*—Rf 20. (*Dragendorff spray*, positive; *acidified iodoplatinate solution*, positive.)

Gas Chromatography. *System GA*—RI 2253; *system GC*—RI 2954; *system GF*—RI 2600.

High Pressure Liquid Chromatography. *System HA*—k' 3.2.

Ultraviolet Spectrum. Aqueous acid—290 nm ($A_1^1 = 347$ a). (See below)

Infra-red Spectrum. Principal peaks at wavenumbers 775, 1580, 825, 990, 1509, 1146 (triprolidine hydrochloride, KBr disk). (See below)

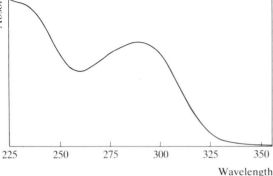

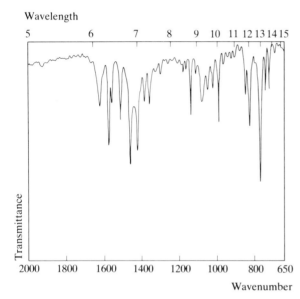

Mass Spectrum. Principal peaks at *m/z* 208, 209, 278, 207, 193, 200, 194, 84.

Quantification. THIN-LAYER CHROMATOGRAPHY–DENSITOMETRY. In plasma: sensitivity 800 pg/ml—R. L. DeAngelis *et al.*, *J. pharm. Sci.*, 1977, *66*, 841–843.

Disposition in the Body. Irregularly absorbed after oral administration.

THERAPEUTIC CONCENTRATION.

Following oral administration of 15 ml of a syrup containing 3.75 mg of triprolidine hydrochloride to 16 subjects, peak plasma concentrations of 0.004 to 0.017 µg/ml (mean 0.009) were attained in about 2 hours (R. L. DeAngelis *et al.*, *J. pharm. Sci.*, 1977, *66*, 841–843).
Following oral administration of 2.5 mg of triprolidine hydrochloride and 60 mg of pseudoephedrine hydrochloride four times a day to 17 subjects for 5 days, peak plasma-triprolidine concentrations of 0.004 to 0.044 µg/ml (mean 0.013) were reported about 1.6 hours after a dose (J. G. Perkins *et al.*, *Curr. ther. Res.*, 1980, *28*, 650–668).

HALF-LIFE. Plasma half-life, 1.5 to 20 hours (mean 5).

Dose. Usually 7.5 to 15 mg of triprolidine hydrochloride daily.

Trometamol   *Treatment of Acidosis*

Synonyms. THAM; Trihydroxymethylaminomethane; TRIS; Tris(hydroxymethyl)aminomethane; Tromethamine.
Proprietary Names. Alcaphor; Thamesol; Trisaminol.
2-Amino-2-hydroxymethylpropane-1,3-diol
$C_4H_{11}NO_3 = 121.1$
CAS—77-86-1

$$HOCH_2 \cdot \overset{\displaystyle NH_2}{\underset{\displaystyle CH_2OH}{C}} \cdot CH_2OH$$

A white crystalline powder. M.p. 168° to 172°.
Soluble 1 in 1.3 of water and 1 in about 45 of ethanol; practically insoluble in chloroform; slightly soluble in ether.

Dissociation Constant. pK_a 8.2 (20°).

Thin-layer Chromatography. *System TA*—Rf 57. (*Ninhydrin spray*, positive.)

Gas Chromatography. *System GA*—RI 1645.

Infra-red Spectrum. Principal peaks at wavenumbers 1031, 1018, 1076, 975, 1582, 1279 (KBr disk).

Quantification. GAS CHROMATOGRAPHY. In plasma: sensitivity 5 ng/ml, FID—A. Hulshoff and H. B. Kostenbauder, *J. Chromat.*, 1978, *145*; *Biomed. Appl.*, *2*, 155–159.

THIN-LAYER CHROMATOGRAPHY. In serum: detection limit 20 µg—G. Andermann and C. Andermann, *J. High Resolut. Chromat. Chromat. Commun.*, 1980, *3*, 36–37.

Disposition in the Body. About 75% of a dose is excreted in the urine as unchanged drug in 8 hours and the remainder is excreted over a period of 3 days. Trometamol may accumulate in the body if large doses are given frequently.

THERAPEUTIC CONCENTRATION.

Following an intravenous injection of 109 mg to an infant, a plasma concentration of 430 µg/ml was reported at 0.5 hour, declining to 86 µg/ml at 4.5 hours (A. Hulshoff and H. B. Kostenbauder, *J. Chromat.*, 1978, *145*; *Biomed. Appl.*, *2*, 155–159).

Dose. Up to 500 mg/kg by intravenous infusion.

Tropicamide   *Anticholinergic*

Synonym. Bistropamide
Proprietary Names. Mydriacyl; Mydriaticum; Visumidriatic.
N-Ethyl-*N*-(4-pyridylmethyl)tropamide
$C_{17}H_{20}N_2O_2 = 284.4$
CAS—1508-75-4

A white crystalline powder. M.p. 95° to 100°.
Soluble 1 in 160 of water, 1 in 3.5 of ethanol, and 1 in 2 of chloroform.

Dissociation Constant. pK_a 5.2.

Colour Tests. Cyanogen Bromide—violet-pink; Liebermann's Test—yellow.

Thin-layer Chromatography. *System TA*—Rf 65. (*Acidified iodoplatinate solution*, positive.)

Gas Chromatography. *System GA*—RI 2330.

Ultraviolet Spectrum. Aqueous acid—254 nm ($A_1^1 = 180$ a); aqueous alkali—256 nm.

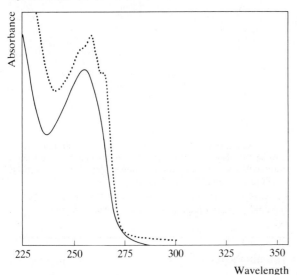

Wavelength

Infra-red Spectrum. Principal peaks at wavenumbers 1627, 1601, 709, 1266, 761, 1070 (KBr disk).

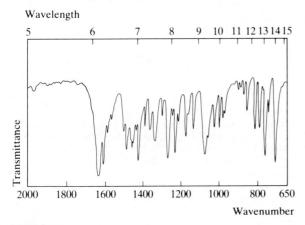

Wavelength

Mass Spectrum. Principal peaks at *m/z* 92, 91, 65, 103, 93, 39, 163, 77.

Use. As a 0.5 to 1% ophthalmic solution.

Troxidone   *Anticonvulsant*

Synonyms. Trimethadione; Trimethinum.
Proprietary Names. Tridione; Trimedone.
3,5,5-Trimethyloxazolidine-2,4-dione
$C_6H_9NO_3 = 143.1$
CAS—127-48-0

Colourless or white granular crystals. M.p. 45° to 47°.
Soluble 1 in 13 of water and 1 in 2 of ethanol; freely soluble in chloroform and ether.

Gas Chromatography. *System GA*—RI 1100; *system GE*—retention time 0.04 relative to phenytoin.

Infra-red Spectrum. Principal peaks at wavenumbers 1730, 1802, 1098, 1200, 770, 1295 (KBr disk).

Wavelength

Mass Spectrum. Principal peaks at *m/z* 43, 58, 143, 42, 41, 40, 39, 128.

Quantification. GAS CHROMATOGRAPHY. In plasma: troxidone and dimethadione, FID—D. L. Bius *et al.*, *Ther. Drug Monit.*, 1979, *1*, 495–505.

Disposition in the Body. Readily absorbed after oral administration and extensively metabolised in the liver to the active metabolite, dimethadione, which is thought to be primarily responsible for the pharmacological activity. It is very slowly excreted in the urine over a period of several days, almost entirely in the form of dimethadione; the excretion of dimethadione is increased in alkaline urine.

THERAPEUTIC CONCENTRATION. Dimethadione attains plasma concentrations about 20 times greater than those of troxidone and accumulates on chronic administration; there is considerable intersubject variation in plasma concentrations.

Steady-state plasma concentrations of 19 to 41 µg/ml (mean 25) of troxidone and 350 to 1033 µg/ml (mean 550) of dimethadione were reported in 5 subjects during chronic treatment with troxidone (D. L. Bius *et al.*, *Ther. Drug Monit.*, 1979, *1*, 495–505).

TOXICITY. The estimated minimum lethal dose is 5 g. Toxic effects may be associated with plasma-dimethadione concentrations greater than 1000 µg/ml.

HALF-LIFE. Plasma half-life, troxidone about 16 hours; dimethadione, half-life derived from urinary excretion data, 6 to 13 days.

PROTEIN BINDING. In plasma, not significantly bound.

Dose. Initially 900 mg daily, increasing to 1.8 g daily.

Tryptamine   *Putrefactive Base*

2-(Indol-3-yl)ethylamine
$C_{10}H_{12}N_2 = 160.2$
CAS—61-54-1

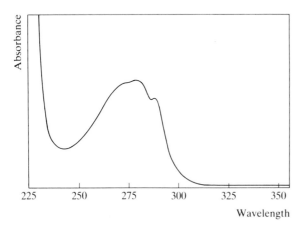

A white crystalline powder. M.p. 116°.
Practically **insoluble** in water, chloroform, and ether; soluble in ethanol.

Tryptamine Hydrochloride

$C_{10}H_{12}N_2,HCl = 196.7$
CAS—343-94-2
A white crystalline powder. M.p. 252°.
Soluble in water.

Colour Tests. *p*-Dimethylaminobenzaldehyde—red/violet; Formaldehyde–Sulphuric Acid—brown; Marquis Test—orange.

Thin-layer Chromatography. *System TA*—Rf 23; *system TB*—Rf 01; *system TC*—Rf 02. (*Acidified iodoplatinate solution*, positive.)

Gas Chromatography. *System GA*—RI 1742.

High Pressure Liquid Chromatography. *System HA*—k' 1.2.

Ultraviolet Spectrum. Aqueous acid—278 nm ($A_1^1 = 353$ a), 287 nm.

Infra-red Spectrum. Principal peaks at wavenumbers 742, 1585, 1233, 1035, 909, 1494 (KBr disk).

Mass Spectrum. Principal peaks at *m/z* 130, 131, 30, 160, 77, 103, 132, 102.

Tryptophan   *Amino Acid*

Synonyms. L-Trp; L-Tryptophan.
Proprietary Names. Pacitron; Trofan; Tryptacin. It is an ingredient of Optimax.
L-2-Amino-3-(indol-3-yl)propionic acid
$C_{11}H_{12}N_2O_2 = 204.2$
CAS—73-22-3

White to slightly yellowish-white crystals or crystalline powder.
Soluble 1 in about 100 of water; very slightly soluble in ethanol; practically insoluble in chloroform and ether; soluble in solutions of dilute acids and alkali hydroxides.

Ultraviolet Spectrum. Aqueous acid—278 nm ($A_1^1 = 290$ b), 286 nm ($A_1^1 = 234$ b); aqueous alkali—280 nm, 288 nm.

Dose. 3 to 6 g daily.

Tuaminoheptane   *Sympathomimetic*

1-Methylhexylamine
$C_7H_{17}N = 115.2$
CAS—123-82-0

$$CH_3 \cdot [CH_2]_4 \cdot \overset{\overset{\displaystyle CH_3}{|}}{CH} \cdot NH_2$$

A colourless or pale yellow volatile liquid.
It absorbs carbon dioxide on exposure to air, forming a white precipitate of tuaminoheptane carbonate. Sp. gr. 0.760 to 0.763.
Soluble 1 in 100 of water, 1 in 25 of ethanol, and 1 in 20 of chloroform; freely soluble in ether.

Tuaminoheptane Sulphate

Proprietary Name. Tuamine Sulfate
$(C_7H_{17}N)_2,H_2SO_4 = 328.5$
CAS—6411-75-2
A white powder.
Freely **soluble** in water; soluble in ethanol; sparingly soluble in ether.

Dissociation Constant. pK_a 10.5.

Thin-layer Chromatography. *System TA*—Rf 33; *system TB*—Rf 01; *system TC*—Rf 07. (*Acidified iodoplatinate solution*, positive.)

Gas Chromatography. *System GA*—RI 888; *system GB*—RI 849; *system GC*—RI 1287.

Ultraviolet Spectrum. No significant absorption, 230 to 360 nm.

Mass Spectrum. Principal peaks at *m/z* 44, 30, 42, 41, 29, 27, 100, 55.

Use. As a 1% solution of the sulphate for nasal drops or spray.

Tubocurarine Chloride

Muscle Relaxant

Synonym. d-Tubocurarine Chloride
Proprietary Names. Curarin; Intocostrin-T; Jexin; Tubarine.
(+) - 7′,12′ - Dihydroxy-6,6′ - dimethoxy - 2,2′,2′ - trimethyltubo-curaranium dichloride pentahydrate
$C_{37}H_{42}Cl_2N_2O_6,5H_2O = 771.7$
Note. The empirical formula of tubocurarine chloride was formerly considered to be $C_{38}H_{44}Cl_2N_2O_6,5H_2O$.
CAS—57-95-4 (tubocurarine); *57-94-3* (chloride, anhydrous); *6989-98-6* (chloride, pentahydrate)

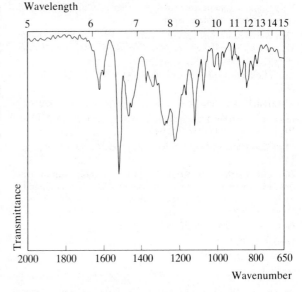

The chloride of an alkaloid, (+)-tubocurarine. It may be obtained from extracts of the stems of *Chondodendron tomentosum* (Menispermaceae).
A white or slightly yellowish-white or greyish-white crystalline powder. M.p. about 270°, with decomposition.
Soluble 1 in 20 of water and 1 in about 30 of ethanol; practically insoluble in chloroform and ether.

Dissociation Constant. pK_a 8.0, 9.2 (22°).

Colour Tests. Aromaticity (Method 2)—yellow/brown; Folin–Ciocalteu Reagent—blue; Liebermann's Test—black; Mandelin's Test—brown; Millon's Reagent (hot)—red.
Cold *nitric acid* gives a black colour.

Thin-layer Chromatography. System *TA*—Rf 00; *system TN*—Rf 85; *system TO*—Rf 40. (*Acidified iodoplatinate solution*, positive.)

Gas Chromatography. System *GA*—RI 2495.

Ultraviolet Spectrum. Water—280 nm (A_1^1 = 119 a).

Infra-red Spectrum. Principal peaks at wavenumbers 1516, 1228, 1120, 1280, 1265, 1165 (KBr disk).

Mass Spectrum. Principal peaks at *m/z* 298, 594, 58, 593, 299, 609, 595, 564.

Quantification. ULTRAVIOLET SPECTROPHOTOMETRY. In postmortem tissues—H. M. Stevens and R. H. Fox, *J. forens. Sci. Soc.*, 1971, *11*, 177–182.

HIGH PRESSURE LIQUID CHROMATOGRAPHY. In plasma: sensitivity 25 ng/ml, UV detection—A. Meulemans *et al.*, *J. Chromat.*, 1981, *226*; *Biomed. Appl.*, *15*, 255–258.

RADIOIMMUNOASSAY. In serum or urine: sensitivity 5 ng/ml—P. E. Horowitz and S. Spector, *J. Pharmac. exp. Ther.*, 1973, *185*, 94–100.

Disposition in the Body. After intravenous administration it is widely distributed throughout the tissues and is concentrated at the neuromuscular junctions; slowly and irregularly absorbed

following intramuscular injection. About 45% of a dose is excreted in the urine unchanged in 24 hours.

THERAPEUTIC CONCENTRATION. In plasma, usually in the range 0.7 to 1 µg/ml.
After an intravenous bolus of 540 µg/kg followed by constant intravenous infusion of 2.9 µg/kg/min to 9 subjects, a mean steady-state plasma concentration of 1.1 µg/ml was attained in about 1 hour (M. I. Ramzan *et al.*, *Br. J. Anaesth.*, 1980, *52*, 893–899).

TOXICITY.
In a fatality due to tubocurarine, a postmortem liver concentration of about 0.8 µg/g was reported (H. M. Stevens and R. H. Fox, *J. forens. Sci. Soc.*, 1971, *11*, 177–182).

HALF-LIFE. Plasma half-life, about 2 to 4 hours.

VOLUME OF DISTRIBUTION. About 0.3 to 0.6 litre/kg.

CLEARANCE. Plasma clearance, about 2 ml/min/kg.

DISTRIBUTION IN BLOOD. Plasma: whole blood ratio, 1.9.

PROTEIN BINDING. In plasma, 33 to 50%.

NOTE. For a review of the pharmacokinetics of neuromuscular blocking agents see M. I. Ramzan *et al.*, *Clin. Pharmacokinet.*, 1981, *6*, 25–60.

Dose. Initially 10 to 15 mg intravenously, with additional doses of 5 mg.

Tybamate

Tranquilliser

Proprietary Name. Tybatran
2-Methyl-2-propyltrimethylene butylcarbamate carbamate
$C_{13}H_{26}N_2O_4 = 274.4$
CAS—4268-36-4

$$NH_2 \cdot CO \cdot O \cdot CH_2 \cdot \overset{\overset{\textstyle CH_3}{|}}{\underset{\underset{\textstyle CH_2 \cdot CH_2 \cdot CH_3}{|}}{C}} \cdot CH_2 \cdot O \cdot CO \cdot NH \cdot [CH_2]_3 \cdot CH_3$$

A white crystalline powder or clear viscous liquid which may congeal to a solid form on standing. M.p. of the powder 49° to 54°.

Very slightly **soluble** in water; very soluble in ethanol and acetone; freely soluble in ether.

Thin-layer Chromatography. *System TA*—Rf 77; *system TD*—Rf 35; *system TE*—Rf 68; *system TF*—Rf 65. (*Furfuraldehyde reagent*, positive.)

Gas Chromatography. *System GA*—RI 1725; *system GF*—RI 2130.

Ultraviolet Spectrum. No significant absorption, 230 to 360 nm.

Infra-red Spectrum. Principal peaks at wavenumbers 1695, 1250, 1065, 1538, 1600, 1140 (KBr disk).

Mass Spectrum. Principal peaks at m/z 55, 72, 97, 41, 56, 158, 118, 57.

Disposition in the Body. Readily absorbed after oral administration. Metabolised in the liver and excreted in the urine, mainly as hydroxylated compounds. Meprobamate can appear as a minor metabolite.

HALF-LIFE. Plasma half-life, about 3 hours.

Dose. Usually 0.75 to 2 g daily; maximum of 3 g daily.

Tylosin   *Antibiotic (Veterinary)*

Proprietary Names of Tylosin and its Salts. Tylamix; Tylan. Tylosin tartrate is an ingredient of Tylasul Soluble.

CAS—1401-69-0

An antimicrobial substance with a macrolide structure, produced by a strain of *Streptomyces fradiae*.

An almost white to buff-coloured powder. M.p. 128° to 132°.

Soluble 1 in 400 of water, 1 in 15 of ethanol, 1 in 30 of chloroform, and 1 in 6 of methanol.

Tylosin Tartrate

CAS—1405-54-5

A white to buff-coloured powder. M.p. 140° to 146°.

Soluble 1 in 10 of water; slightly soluble in ethanol; very slightly soluble in chloroform; practically insoluble in ether.

Colour Tests. Mandelin's Test—yellow → yellow-brown; Marquis Test—yellow-brown; Sulphuric Acid—yellow-brown (slow).

Thin-layer Chromatography. *System TA*—Rf 72. (*Acidified iodoplatinate solution*, positive.)

Ultraviolet Spectrum. Aqueous acid—290 nm ($A_1^1 = 225$ b).

Infra-red Spectrum. Principal peaks at wavenumbers 1075, 1052, 1162, 1111, 1010, 1587.

Tyramine   *Diagnostic Agent/Sympathomimetic*

Synonyms. *p*-Tyramine; Tyrosamine.

4-(2-Aminoethyl)phenol

$C_8H_{11}NO = 137.2$

CAS—51-67-2

CH₂·CH₂·NH₂ — OH

Colourless crystals. M.p. 164° to 165°.

Soluble 1 in 95 of water and 1 in 10 of boiling ethanol.

Tyramine Hydrochloride

Proprietary Name. Mydrial

$C_8H_{11}NO,HCl = 173.6$

CAS—60-19-5

Crystals. M.p. about 270°, with decomposition.

Soluble in water.

Dissociation Constant. pK_a 9.5 (phenol), 10.8 (—NH₂).

Colour Tests. *p*-Dimethylaminobenzaldehyde—orange/violet; Marquis Test—brown → green.

Thin-layer Chromatography. *System TA*—Rf 31. (*Acidified potassium permanganate solution*, positive.)

Gas Chromatography. *System GA*—RI 1436.

High Pressure Liquid Chromatography. *System HA*—k' 1.2; *system HB*—k' 0.81; *system HC*—k' 1.47.

Ultraviolet Spectrum. Aqueous acid—274 nm ($A_1^1 = 110$ a); aqueous alkali—294 nm ($A_1^1 = 182$ b).

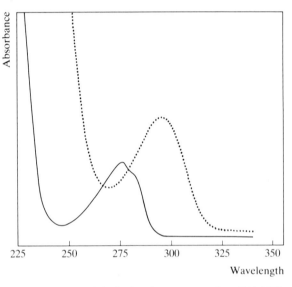

Infra-red Spectrum. Principal peaks at wavenumbers 1266, 1518, 1595, 822, 1495, 1612 (KBr disk).

Mass Spectrum. Principal peaks at m/z 30, 108, 107, 77, 39, 51, 137, 27.

Quantification. GAS CHROMATOGRAPHY. In urine: sensitivity 25 ng, ECD—R. T. Coutts *et al.*, *Res. Commun. chem. Path. Pharmac.*, 1980, *28*, 177–184.

Dose. Tyramine hydrochloride has been given by mouth in doses of up to 250 mg daily, in the investigation of migraine.

Urea   *Diuretic*

Synonyms. Carbamide; Ureum.

Proprietary Names. Aquacare; Aquadrate; Calmurid; Carmol; Gormel; Nutraplus; Ultra-Mide; Ureaphil. It is an ingredient of Psoradrate.

$NH_2 \cdot CO \cdot NH_2 = 60.06$

CAS—57-13-6

Colourless, slightly hygroscopic, prismatic crystals or pellets, or white crystalline powder. M.p. 132° to 135°.

Soluble 1 in about 1.5 of water and 1 in about 11 of ethanol; practically insoluble in chloroform and ether.

Dissociation Constant. pK_a 0.2 (25°).

Colour Test. Nessler's Reagent—brown-orange.

Gas Chromatography. *System GA*—not eluted.

Mass Spectrum. Principal peaks at m/z 60, 44, 28, -, -, -, -, -.

Disposition in the Body. Rapidly absorbed after oral administration. Excreted in the urine as unchanged drug and also metabolised to ammonium salts in the colon. Endogenous urinary excretion is in the range 10 to 35 g in 24 hours; urea is not usually found in the faeces.

THERAPEUTIC CONCENTRATION. Endogenous concentrations in blood are about 300 µg/ml in adults and lower in infants.

After intravenous infusion of 0.6 to 1.2 g/kg of a solution containing 30% urea and 10% invert sugar to 7 subjects over a period of 0.5 to 2 hours, plasma concentrations at the end of the infusion were reported to range from 1160 to 3400 µg/ml (mean 2430) (P. R. Yarnell *et al.*, *Clin. Pharmac. Ther.*, 1972, *13*, 558–562).

HALF-LIFE. Biological half-life, about 1 hour.

Dose. 40 to 80 g by intravenous infusion, not exceeding 1.5 g/kg daily.

Urethane   *Antineoplastic*

Synonyms. Ethylurethane; Urethan.

Ethyl carbamate
$NH_2 \cdot CO \cdot O \cdot C_2H_5 = 89.09$
CAS—51-79-6
Colourless crystals or white granular powder. M.p. 48° to 50°.
Soluble 1 in 1.5 of water, 1 in 1 of ethanol, 1 in 1 of chloroform, and 1 in 2 of ether.

Gas Chromatography. *System GA*—RI 838.

Infra-red Spectrum. Principal peaks at wavenumbers 1713, 1075, 1610, 805, 1010 (KBr disk).

Dose. Formerly given in doses of 3 g daily; maximum of 6 g daily.

Valethamate Bromide   *Anticholinergic*

Proprietary Name. Epidosin

Diethylmethyl[2-(3-methyl-2-phenylvaleryloxy)ethyl]ammonium bromide
$C_{19}H_{32}BrNO_2 = 386.4$
CAS—16376-74-2 (valethamate); *90-22-2* (bromide)

A white crystalline powder. M.p. 100° to 101°.
Freely **soluble** in water; very soluble in ethanol; practically insoluble in ether.

Thin-layer Chromatography. *System TA*—Rf 02. (*Acidified iodoplatinate solution*, positive.)

Ultraviolet Spectrum. Aqueous acid—253 nm, 259 nm ($A_1^1 = 5.4$ b), 265 nm.

Infra-red Spectrum. Principal peaks at wavenumbers 1730, 1230, 695, 726, 1163, 1265 (KBr disk).

Dose. 30 to 80 mg daily.

Valproic Acid   *Anticonvulsant*

Proprietary Names. Convulex (capsules); Depakene (capsules).
2-Propylvaleric acid
$C_8H_{16}O_2 = 144.2$
CAS—99-66-1

A colourless liquid.
Very slightly **soluble** in water.

Sodium Valproate

Proprietary Names. Convulex (solution and tablets); Depakene (syrup); Depakin(e); Epilim; Ergenyl; Orfiril.
$C_8H_{15}NaO_2 = 166.2$
CAS—1069-66-5
A white, crystalline, deliquescent powder.
Soluble 1 in 5 of water and of ethanol.

Dissociation Constant. pK_a 5.0.

Colour Test. Ferric Chloride—orange.

Thin-layer Chromatography. *System TD*—Rf 00; *system TE*—Rf 00; *system TF*—Rf 00.

Gas Chromatography. *System GE*—retention time 0.09 relative to phenytoin.

Infra-red Spectrum. Principal peaks at wavenumbers 1708, 1213, 1250, 1278, 946, 1107 (thin film).

Mass Spectrum. Principal peaks at m/z 73, 102, 41, 57, 43, 27, 55, 29.

Quantification. GAS CHROMATOGRAPHY. In plasma: detection limit 1 to 2 µg/ml, FID—R. Riva *et al.*, *J. pharm. Sci.*, 1982, *71*, 110–111.

GAS CHROMATOGRAPHY–MASS SPECTROMETRY. In serum, urine, or breast-milk: valproic acid and several metabolites, detection limits between 2.8 and 18 ng/ml in serum—H. Nau *et al.*, *J. Chromat.*, 1981, *226*; *Biomed. Appl.*, *15*, 69–78.

HIGH PRESSURE LIQUID CHROMATOGRAPHY. In serum: detection limit 9 µg/ml, UV detection—J. P. Moody and S. M. Allan, *Clinica chim. Acta*, 1983, *127*, 263–269.

Disposition in the Body. Well absorbed after oral administration; bioavailability almost 100%. Metabolised mainly by oxidation to a number of metabolites, including 3-oxovalproic acid, 2-propylglutaric acid, 3-hydroxyvalproic acid, 4-hydroxyvalproic acid, 5-hydroxyvalproic acid, and valpro-1,4-lactone. About 20% of a dose is excreted in the urine as the glucuronide of valproic acid in 72 hours; most of the remainder is excreted as glucuronides of metabolites, less than 5% of a dose being excreted as unchanged drug.

THERAPEUTIC CONCENTRATION. In plasma, usually in the range 40 to 100 µg/ml, but there is no clear correlation with therapeutic effect.

Following a single oral dose of 500 mg to 6 subjects, peak plasma concentrations of 36 to 73 µg/ml (mean 58) were attained in 1 to 5 hours (mean 3) (C. A. May and W. R. Garnett, *Clin. Pharm.*, 1983, *2*, 143–147). Daily oral doses in the range 1 to 3.75 g were administered to 20 patients; at the end of 10 weeks, minimum serum concentrations were 30 to 135 µg/ml (mean 82) and maximum concentrations were 70 to 190 µg/ml (mean 109). About 75% of the patients had serum concentrations within 55 to 100 µg/ml (J. Bruni *et al.*, *Clin. Pharmac. Ther.*, 1978, *24*, 324–332).

TOXICITY. Plasma concentrations greater than 200 µg/ml are associated with toxic effects but valproic acid is relatively non-toxic after overdose, and recovery after the ingestion of up to 75 g has been reported. Hepatotoxicity has been reported during therapeutic administration.

A patient whose death was attributed to an overdose of valproic acid had ingested 2.25 g each day for 5 days; the postmortem blood concentration was 52 µg/ml and therapeutic concentrations of phenobarbitone and phenytoin were also present; death was thought to be due to the high initial dose of valproic acid (J. P. Tift, *New Engl. J. Med.*, 1980, *303*, 394).

HALF-LIFE. Plasma half-life, about 6 to 20 hours, reduced when administered in combination with other anticonvulsants.

VOLUME OF DISTRIBUTION. About 0.1 to 0.2 litre/kg.

CLEARANCE. Plasma clearance, about 0.1 to 0.3 ml/min/kg.

DISTRIBUTION IN BLOOD. Plasma: whole blood ratio, about 1.8.

PROTEIN BINDING. In plasma, about 90% (concentration-dependent; decreased at plasma concentrations > 100 µg/ml).

NOTE. For a review of the clinical pharmacokinetics of valproic acid see R. Gugler and G. E. von Unruh, *Clin. Pharmacokinet.*, 1980, *5*, 67–83.

Dose. Initially 600 mg of sodium valproate daily, increasing to 2.6 g daily.

Vancomycin   *Antibiotic*

CAS—1404-90-6

An amphoteric glycopeptide antimicrobial substance produced by the growth of certain strains of *Streptomyces orientalis*.

Vancomycin Hydrochloride

Proprietary Name. Vancocin
CAS—1404-93-9
A light brown powder.
Soluble 1 in 10 of water and 1 in 700 of ethanol; practically insoluble in chloroform; slightly soluble in ether.

Colour Test. Marquis Test—yellow.

Thin-layer Chromatography. *System TA*—Rf 22. (*Acidified potassium permanganate solution*, positive.)

Ultraviolet Spectrum. Vancomycin hydrochloride: aqueous acid—281 nm (A_1^1 = 34 b).

Quantification. HIGH PRESSURE LIQUID CHROMATOGRAPHY. In serum: sensitivity 2 µg/ml, UV detection—R. J. Hoagland *et al.*, *J. analyt. Toxicol.*, 1984, *8*, 75–77.

RADIOIMMUNOASSAY. In serum or urine: sensitivity 40 pg/ml—K.-L. L. Fong *et al.*, *Antimicrob. Ag. Chemother.*, 1981, *19*, 139–143.

Disposition in the Body. Not absorbed from the gastro-intestinal tract. About 90% of an intravenous dose is excreted in the urine with about 50% of the dose being excreted in 4 hours.

THERAPEUTIC CONCENTRATION. In plasma, usually in the range 10 to 40 µg/ml.

HALF-LIFE. Plasma half-life, about 4 to 10 hours.

VOLUME OF DISTRIBUTION. About 0.4 to 1 litre/kg.

CLEARANCE. Plasma clearance, about 1 ml/min/kg.

PROTEIN BINDING. In plasma, about 55%.

NOTE. For a review of vancomycin see B. A. Cunha and A. M. Ristuccia, *Clin. Pharm.*, 1983, *2*, 417–424.

Dose. The equivalent of up to 2 g of vancomycin daily, by mouth or by intravenous infusion.

Vanillin   *Flavouring Agent*

Synonyms. Vainillina; Vanillic Aldehyde.
4-Hydroxy-3-methoxybenzaldehyde
$C_8H_8O_3 = 152.1$
CAS—121-33-5

White or slightly yellow crystalline needles or powder. M.p. 81° to 83°.

Soluble 1 in 100 of water; soluble in ethanol, chloroform, and ether.

Dissociation Constant. pK_a 7.4 (20°).

Ultraviolet Spectrum. Aqueous acid—230 nm, 278 nm (A_1^1 = 685 b), 309 nm; aqueous alkali—248 nm, 348 nm (A_1^1 = 1640 b).

Infra-red Spectrum. Principal peaks at wavenumbers 1660, 1153, 1267, 735, 1590, 1300 (KCl disk).

Mass Spectrum. Principal peaks at *m/z* 152, 151, 81, 109, 51, –, –, –.

Verapamil   *Anti-arrhythmic*

Synonym. Iproveratril
5-[*N*-(3,4-Dimethoxyphenethyl)-*N*-methylamino]-2-(3,4-dimethoxyphenyl)-2-isopropylvaleronitrile
$C_{27}H_{38}N_2O_4 = 454.6$
CAS—52-53-9

A pale yellow viscous oil.
Practically **insoluble** in water; soluble in ethanol, chloroform, and ether.

Verapamil Hydrochloride

Proprietary Names. Berkatens; Calan; Cordilox; Isoptin(e); Securon.
$C_{27}H_{38}N_2O_4,HCl = 491.1$
CAS—152-11-4
A white crystalline powder. M.p. 141° to 144°.
Soluble 1 in 20 of water, 1 in 25 of ethanol, and 1 in 1.5 of chloroform; practically insoluble in ether.

Colour Tests. Liebermann's Test—black; Marquis Test—yellow-green → grey.

Thin-layer Chromatography. *System TA*—Rf 59; *system TB*—Rf 23; *system TC*—Rf 70. (*Acidified iodoplatinate solution*, positive.)

High Pressure Liquid Chromatography. *System HA*—verapamil k' 2.6, norverapamil k' 1.7.

Ultraviolet Spectrum. Aqueous acid—278 nm (A_1^1 = 127 a).

Infra-red Spectrum. Principal peaks at wavenumbers 1510, 1253, 1026, 1232, 1149, 1587 (thin film).

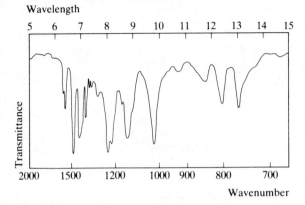

Wavelength

Mass Spectrum. Principal peaks at m/z 303, 58, 43, 304, 151, 44, 42, 57.

Quantification. GAS CHROMATOGRAPHY. In plasma: sensitivity 25 ng/ml, FID—R. G. McAllister *et al.*, *J. pharm. Sci.*, 1979, *68*, 574–577. In postmortem tissues—B. M. Thomson and L. K. Pannell, *J. analyt. Toxicol.*, 1981, *5*, 105–109.

HIGH PRESSURE LIQUID CHROMATOGRAPHY. In serum, saliva or urine: sensitivity 10 ng/ml, fluorescence detection—V. K. Piotrovskii *et al.*, *J. Chromat.*, 1983, *275*; *Biomed. Appl.*, *26*, 195–200. In plasma: verapamil and metabolites, sensitivity 2.5 ng/ml, fluorescence detection—M. Kuwada *et al.*, *J. Chromat.*, 1981, *222*; *Biomed. Appl.*, *11*, 507–511. In postmortem tissues: see B. M. Thomson and L. K. Pannell, *J. analyt. Toxicol.*, 1981, *5*, 105–109.

Disposition in the Body. Almost completely absorbed after oral administration but undergoes extensive first-pass metabolism; bioavailability about 20%. The main metabolic reactions are *N*-dealkylation (*N*-demethylation gives norverapamil which is thought to be active), and *O*-demethylation of the resulting compounds. About 70% of a dose is excreted in the urine in 5 days with about 50% in the first 24 hours; less than 5% is excreted as unchanged drug. The urinary metabolites consist mainly of *N*-dealkylated compounds together with about 10% of the dose as norverapamil or its *O*-demethylated derivative; conjugated *O*-demethylated products account for about 17% of the urinary material. About 16% of a dose is eliminated in the faeces.

THERAPEUTIC CONCENTRATION.
Following single oral doses of 80 mg to 20 subjects, mean peak plasma concentrations of 0.038 µg/ml of verapamil and 0.026 µg/ml of norverapamil were attained in about 3 hours; after oral doses of 120 mg to the same subjects, mean peak plasma concentrations of 0.068 µg/ml of verapamil and 0.059 µg/ml of norverapamil were reported at 2 hours (R. G. McAllister and E. B. Kirsten, *Clin. Pharmac. Ther.*, 1982, *31*, 418–426).

Following chronic oral doses of 80 mg 6-hourly to 16 subjects, steady-state trough plasma concentrations of 0.031 to 0.168 µg/ml (mean 0.105) of verapamil, and 0.078 to 0.279 µg/ml (mean 0.171) of norverapamil were reported; maximum steady-state plasma concentrations were 0.135 to 0.447 µg/ml (mean 0.255) and 0.134 to 0.361 µg/ml (mean 0.226) for verapamil and norverapamil respectively, attained 1 hour after a dose (S. B. Freedman *et al.*, *Clin. Pharmac. Ther.*, 1981, *30*, 644–652).

TOXICITY.
In a fatality due to verapamil ingestion, the following postmortem tissue concentrations were reported: blood 8.8 µg/ml, kidney 28 µg/g, liver

165 µg/g (B. M. Thomson and L. K. Pannell, *J. analyt. Toxicol.*, 1981, *5*, 105–109).

Serum concentrations of 3 µg/ml of verapamil and 2.5 µg/ml of norverapamil were reported in a 17-year-old girl 12 hours after ingestion of an unknown overdose of verapamil; death occurred after 19 hours (G. M. Orr *et al.*, *Lancet*, 1982, *2*, 1218–1219).

HALF-LIFE. Plasma half-life, verapamil about 2 to 7 hours, increased during long term oral dosing and in subjects with liver disease; norverapamil about 5 to 13 hours.

VOLUME OF DISTRIBUTION. About 2 to 6 litres/kg.

CLEARANCE. Plasma clearance, about 10 to 20 ml/min/kg.

DISTRIBUTION IN BLOOD. Plasma: whole blood ratio, about 1.2.

PROTEIN BINDING. In plasma, about 90%.

NOTE. For a review of the pharmacokinetics of verapamil see S. R. Hamann *et al.*, *Clin. Pharmacokinet.*, 1984, *9*, 26–41.

Dose. 120 to 480 mg of verapamil hydrochloride daily.

Veratrine

A mixture of alkaloids from sabadilla, the dried ripe seeds of *Schoenocaulon officinale* (Liliaceae).
Note. Veratrine should be distinguished from protoveratrines obtained from veratrum.
CAS—8051-02-3 (mixture)
A white or greyish-white powder. M.p. 145° to 155°.
Practically **insoluble** in water; soluble 1 in 3 of ethanol, 1 in 3 of chloroform, and 1 in 6 of ether.
Caution. Veratrine has a violent irritant action on mucous membranes, even in minute doses, and must be handled with great care.

Colour Tests. Liebermann's Test—brown; Mandelin's Test—yellow → orange → violet-brown; Marquis Test—orange; Sulphuric Acid—yellow → violet.

Thin-layer Chromatography. *System TA*—Rf 59; *system TB*—Rf 04; *system TC*—Rf 35.

Ultraviolet Spectrum. Aqueous acid—262 nm ($A_1^1 = 67$ b), 292 nm.

Infra-red Spectrum. Principal peaks at wavenumbers 1270, 1085, 1111, 1136, 1234, 1035 (KBr disk).

Viloxazine   *Antidepressant*

2-(2-Ethoxyphenoxymethyl)morpholine
$C_{13}H_{19}NO_3 = 237.3$
CAS—46817-91-8

Viloxazine Hydrochloride
Proprietary Names. Vicilan; Vivalan.
$C_{13}H_{19}NO_3,HCl = 273.8$
CAS—35604-67-2
M.p. 185° to 186°.

Dissociation Constant. pK$_a$ 8.1.

Colour Tests. Liebermann's Test—black; Mandelin's Test—blue-green; Marquis Test—violet.

Thin-layer Chromatography. *System TA*—Rf 42; *system TB*—Rf 07; *system TC*—Rf 23.

Gas Chromatography. *System GA*—RI 2005.

High Pressure Liquid Chromatography. *System HF*—k' 2.7.

Ultraviolet Spectrum. Aqueous acid—273 nm ($A_1^1 = 92$ b). No alkaline shift.

Infra-red Spectrum. Principal peaks at wavenumbers 1217, 1121, 1252, 739, 1511, 1031 (viloxazine hydrochloride, KBr disk).

Wavelength

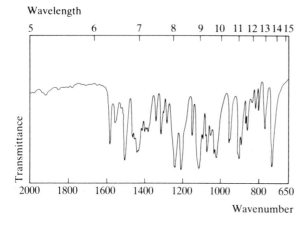

Wavenumber

Mass Spectrum. Principal peaks at *m/z* 56, 100, 138, 110, 57, 237, 70, 41.

Quantification. GAS CHROMATOGRAPHY. In plasma: detection limit 200 ng/ml, FID—T. R. Norman *et al., Br. J. clin. Pharmac.,* 1979, *8*, 169–171.

HIGH PRESSURE LIQUID CHROMATOGRAPHY. In plasma or urine: sensitivity 25 ng/ml and 1 µg/ml, respectively, fluorescence detection—R. Gillilan and W. D. Mason, *J. pharm. Sci.,* 1981, *70*, 220–221.

Disposition in the Body. Rapidly and completely absorbed after oral administration and crosses the blood-brain barrier. It is extensively metabolised by hydroxylation. About 90% of an oral dose is excreted in the urine in 24 hours, of which 12 to 15% is unchanged drug, 3% is the free 4- and 5-hydroxy metabolites, and more than 40% is the glucuronide conjugate of 5-hydroxyviloxazine; about 16% is excreted as the glucuronide of a hydroxylated 5-oxo metabolite.

THERAPEUTIC CONCENTRATION.
Following single oral doses of 100 mg to 10 subjects, peak plasma concentrations of 1.11 to 2.93 µg/ml (mean 1.7) were attained in about 1.5 hours (B. Vandel *et al., Eur. J. drug Met. Pharmacokinet.,* 1982, *7*, 65–68).
Following oral doses of 400 mg daily in divided doses to 13 subjects, a mean steady-state blood concentration of about 1.3 µg/ml was reported (P. F. C. Bayliss and D. E. Case, *Br. J. clin. Pharmac.,* 1975, *2*, 209–214).

TOXICITY. A number of attempted suicides have been reported but recovery has occurred after the ingestion of up to 6.5 g of viloxazine together with other drugs.
The following postmortem tissue concentrations were reported in a fatality attributed to viloxazine: blood 45 µg/ml, liver 185 µg/g, urine 640 µg/ml; death occurred about 8 to 12 hours after ingestion (M. Bailey, *Bull. int. Ass. forens. Toxicol.,* 1976, *12*(3), 22).

HALF-LIFE. Plasma half-life, 2 to 5 hours.

VOLUME OF DISTRIBUTION. About 0.5 to 1.5 litres/kg.

PROTEIN BINDING. In plasma, about 85 to 90%.

NOTE. For a review of viloxazine see R. M. Pinder *et al., Drugs,* 1977, *13,* 401–421.

Dose. The equivalent of 100 to 400 mg of viloxazine daily.

Vinbarbitone   *Barbiturate*

Synonyms. Butenemal; Vinbarbital.
5-Ethyl-5-(1-methylbut-1-enyl)barbituric acid
$C_{11}H_{16}N_2O_3 = 224.3$
CAS—125-42-8

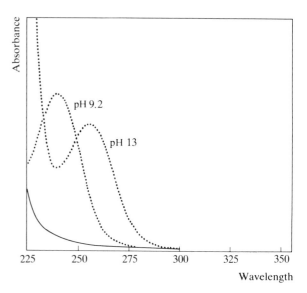

A white powder. M.p. 160° to 163°.
Very slightly **soluble** in water; soluble in ethanol; sparingly soluble in ether.

Dissociation Constant. pK$_a$ 7.5 (20°).

Colour Tests. Koppanyi-Zwikker Test—violet; Mercurous Nitrate—black; Vanillin Reagent—violet-brown/colourless.

Thin-layer Chromatography. *System TD*—Rf 50; *system TE*—Rf 32; *system TF*—Rf 64; *system TH*—Rf 56. (*Mercurous nitrate spray,* black; *acidified potassium permanganate solution,* yellow-brown; *Zwikker's reagent,* pink.)

Gas Chromatography. *System GA*—RI 1740; *system GF*—RI 2495.

High Pressure Liquid Chromatography. *System HG*—k' 4.83; *system HH*—k' 2.32.

Ultraviolet Spectrum. *Borax buffer 0.05 M* (pH 9.2)—238 nm ($A_1^1 = 452$ a); M sodium hydroxide (pH 13)—254 nm ($A_1^1 = 374$ b).

Wavelength

Infra-red Spectrum. Principal peaks at wavenumbers 1675, 1760, 1725, 1234, 1282, 1298 (KBr disk).

Mass Spectrum. Principal peaks at m/z 195, 41, 141, 69, 39, 152, 135, 196.

Quantification. See under Amylobarbitone.

Dose. 100 to 200 mg daily.

Vinblastine
Antineoplastic

Synonyms. Vincaleucoblastine; Vincaleukoblastine.
$C_{46}H_{58}N_4O_9 = 811.0$
CAS—865-21-4
An alkaloid extracted from *Vinca rosea* (*Catharanthus roseus*) (Apocynaceae).
Crystals. M.p. 211° to 216°.
Practically **insoluble** in water; soluble in ethanol and chloroform.

Vinblastine Sulphate
Proprietary Names. Velban; Velbe.
$C_{46}H_{58}N_4O_9,H_2SO_4 = 909.1$
CAS—143-67-9
A white to slightly yellow, very hygroscopic, amorphous or crystalline powder. M.p. about 284°, with decomposition.
Soluble 1 in 10 of water, 1 in 1200 of ethanol, and 1 in 50 of chloroform; practically insoluble in ether; soluble in methanol.

Dissociation Constant. pK_a 5.4, 7.4.

Colour Test. Marquis Test—red.

Thin-layer Chromatography. *System TA*—Rf 60; *system TB*—Rf 01; *system TC*—Rf 60.

Ultraviolet Spectrum. Aqueous acid—268 nm ($A_1^1 = 176$ b).

Infra-red Spectrum. Principal peaks at wavenumbers 1227, 1136, 1111, 1724, 1176, 1613 (vinblastine sulphate, KBr disk).

Quantification. RADIOIMMUNOASSAY. In plasma: vinblastine and vincristine, sensitivity 2.1 ng/ml and 3.8 ng/ml, respectively— J. D. Teale *et al.*, *Br. J. clin. Pharmac.*, 1977, *4*, 169–172.

Disposition in the Body. Poorly absorbed after oral administration. After intravenous administration, it is metabolised to desacetylvinblastine which is active. About 14% of a radioactively-labelled dose is excreted in the urine in 72 hours and 10% is eliminated in the faeces in the same period.

HALF-LIFE. Plasma half-life (total radioactivity), about 20 hours.

PROTEIN BINDING. In plasma, about 99%.

Dose. Initially 100 µg/kg of vinblastine sulphate weekly, by intravenous injection.

Vincristine
Antineoplastic

Synonym. Leurocristine
22-Oxovincaleukoblastine
$C_{46}H_{56}N_4O_{10} = 825.0$
CAS—57-22-7
An alkaloid obtained from *Vinca rosea* (*Catharanthus roseus*) (Apocynaceae).
Crystals. M.p. 218° to 220°.

Vincristine Sulphate
Proprietary Name. Oncovin
$C_{46}H_{56}N_4O_{10},H_2SO_4 = 923.0$
CAS—2068-78-2
A white to slightly yellow, very hygroscopic, amorphous or crystalline powder. M.p. about 277°.
Soluble 1 in 2 of water, 1 in 600 of ethanol, and 1 in 30 of chloroform; practically insoluble in ether; soluble in methanol.

Dissociation Constant. pK_a 5.0, 7.4.

Ultraviolet Spectrum. Aqueous acid—256 nm ($A_1^1 = 181$ b), 297 nm ($A_1^1 = 179$ b).

Infra-red Spectrum. Principal peaks at wavenumbers 1230, 1745, 1170, 1685, 1030, 1130 (vincristine sulphate, KBr disk).

Quantification. See under Vinblastine.

Disposition in the Body. Poorly absorbed after oral administration. After intravenous injection it disappears rapidly from the blood and is excreted mainly in the bile. About 12% of a dose is excreted in the urine in 72 hours, and 70% is eliminated in the faeces in the same period.

HALF-LIFE. Plasma half-life, about 3 hours; a terminal elimination half-life of about 23 hours has also been reported.

Dose. Initially 25 to 75 µg/kg of vincristine sulphate weekly, by intravenous injection.

Vindesine
Antineoplastic

Synonym. Desacetyl Vinblastine Amide
3 - Carbamoyl - O^4-deacetyl - 3 - de(methoxycarbonyl)vincaleu-koblastine
$C_{43}H_{55}N_5O_7 = 753.9$
CAS—53643-48-4
Crystals. M.p. 230° to 232°.

Vindesine Sulphate
Proprietary Name. Eldisine
$C_{43}H_{55}N_5O_7,H_2SO_4 = 852.0$
CAS—59917-39-4
An amorphous solid.
Freely **soluble** in water.

Dissociation Constant. pK_a 5.4, 7.4.

Ultraviolet Spectrum. Methanol—270 nm ($A_1^1 = 235$ b).

Infra-red Spectrum. Principal peaks at wavenumbers 1120, 1230, 1680, 1175, 1610, 1038 (vindesine sulphate, KBr disk).

Quantification. RADIOIMMUNOASSAY. In plasma: sensitivity 50 pg/ml—R. Rahmani *et al.*, *Clinica chim. Acta*, 1983, *129*, 57–69.

Disposition in the Body. Poorly absorbed after oral administration. After intravenous injection, about 13% of a dose is excreted in the urine in 24 hours.

HALF-LIFE. Plasma half-life, about 24 hours.

Dose. Initially 3 mg/m^2 of vindesine sulphate weekly, by intravenous injection.

Vinylbitone
Barbiturate

Synonyms. Butylvinal; Butyvinal; Vinylbital; Vinylmalum.
Proprietary Names. Bykonox; Optanox; Speda; Suppoptanox.
5-(1-Methylbutyl)-5-vinylbarbituric acid
$C_{11}H_{16}N_2O_3 = 224.3$
CAS—2430-49-1

Crystals. M.p. 90° to 92°.

Gas Chromatography. *System GA*—RI 1720.

Ultraviolet Spectrum. Aqueous alkali—247 nm ($A_1^1 = 298$ b).

Infra-red Spectrum. Principal peaks at wavenumbers 1692, 1730, 1750, 1318, 1220, 1630.

Quantification. See also under Amylobarbitone.

GAS CHROMATOGRAPHY. In plasma: sensitivity < 125 ng/ml, AFID—D. D. Breimer and A. G. de Boer, *Arzneimittel-Forsch.*, 1976, *26*, 448–454.

Disposition in the Body. Readily absorbed after oral administration. Metabolites which have been identified in urine are 3′-hydroxyvinylbitone and the corresponding desvinyl derivative, 5-(3-hydroxy-1-methylbutyl)barbituric acid. Less than 5% of a dose is excreted in the urine unchanged in 72 hours.

THERAPEUTIC CONCENTRATION.

Following a single oral dose of 150 mg to 6 subjects, peak plasma concentrations of 2.2 to 3.9 µg/ml were attained in 1 to 2 hours (D. D. Breimer and A. G. de Boer, *ibid.*).

HALF-LIFE. Plasma half-life, 18 to 34 hours (mean 24).

VOLUME OF DISTRIBUTION. About 0.7 litre/kg.

REFERENCE. D. D. Breimer and A. G. de Boer, *ibid.*

Dose. 100 to 200 mg, as a hypnotic.

Viprynium Embonate
Anthelmintic

Synonyms. Pyrvinium Pamoate; Viprynium Pamoate.

Proprietary Names. Molevac; Pamovin; Povan; Povanyl; Pyr-Pam; Vanquin.

Bis{6-dimethylamino-2-[2-(2,5-dimethyl-1-phenylpyrrol-3-yl)vinyl]-1-methylquinolinium} 4,4′-methylenebis(3-hydroxy-2-naphthoate)

$C_{52}H_{56}N_6, C_{23}H_{14}O_6 = 1152$

CAS—3546-41-6

A bright orange or orange-red to almost black, crystalline powder. M.p. about 206°, with decomposition.

Practically **insoluble** in water and ether; very slightly soluble in ethanol; soluble 1 in 1000 of chloroform; freely soluble in glacial acetic acid.

Colour Tests. Mandelin's Test—yellow; Marquis Test—yellow.

Thin-layer Chromatography. *System TA*—Rf 67. (*Acidified potassium permanganate solution*, weak reaction.)

Ultraviolet Spectrum. 2-Methoxyethanol—239 nm, 358 nm ($A_1^1 = 380$ b).

Infra-red Spectrum. Principal peaks at wavenumbers 1592, 1618, 1294, 1188, 1500, 1513 (KBr disk).

Dose. The equivalent of 5 mg/kg of viprynium as a single dose.

Warfarin
Anticoagulant/Rodenticide

Proprietary Names. Biotrol; Dethmor; Sorexa (all rodenticides).

4-Hydroxy-3-(3-oxo-1-phenylbutyl)coumarin

$C_{19}H_{16}O_4 = 308.3$

CAS—81-81-2

Colourless crystals. M.p. of the purified compound 159° to 160°; of the technical grade 157°.

Practically **insoluble** in water; moderately soluble in alcohols; readily soluble in acetone.

Warfarin Potassium

Proprietary Name. Athrombin-K

$C_{19}H_{15}KO_4 = 346.4$

CAS—2610-86-8

A white crystalline powder which discolours on exposure to light.

Soluble 1 in 1.5 of water and 1 in 1.9 of ethanol; very slightly soluble in chloroform and ether.

Warfarin Sodium

Proprietary Names. Coumadin(e); Marevan; Panwarfin; Warfilone; Warnerin.

$C_{19}H_{15}NaO_4 = 330.3$

CAS—129-06-6

A white amorphous or crystalline powder which discolours on exposure to light.

Soluble 1 in less than 1 of water and ethanol; slightly soluble in chloroform and ether.

Dissociation Constant. pK_a 5.0 (20°).

Partition Coefficient. Log P (octanol/pH 8.0), 0.0.

Colour Test. Liebermann's Test—red-orange.

Thin-layer Chromatography. *System TD*—Rf 64; *system TE*—Rf 18; *system TF*—Rf 62. (*Acidified potassium permanganate solution*, positive.)

Gas Chromatography. *System GA*—RI 1432.

Ultraviolet Spectrum. Aqueous acid—270 nm, 280 nm, 303 nm; aqueous alkali—293 nm, 308 nm ($A_1^1 = 462$ a).

Infra-red Spectrum. Principal peaks at wavenumbers 1517, 1599, 1640, 750, 1700, 692 (warfarin sodium, KBr disk).

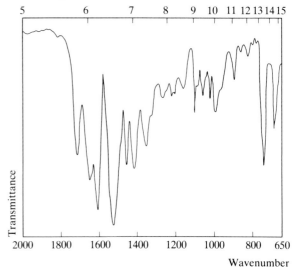

Wavelength

Mass Spectrum. Principal peaks at m/z 265, 308, 121, 43, 266, 187, 213, 251.

Quantification. GAS CHROMATOGRAPHY. In plasma: sensitivity 300 ng/ml, FID—S. Hanna et al., J. pharm. Sci., 1978, 67, 84–86.

HIGH PRESSURE LIQUID CHROMATOGRAPHY. In plasma or urine: (R)- and (S)-warfarin and metabolites, fluorescence detection—C. Banfield and M. Rowland, J. pharm. Sci., 1984, 73, 1392–1396. In plasma or serum: sensitivity 50 ng/ml, UV detection—R. A. R. Tasker and K. Nakatsu, J. Chromat., 1982, 228; Biomed. Appl., 17, 346–349. In plasma or urine: warfarin and metabolites, fluorescence detection—S. H. Lee et al., Analyt. Chem., 1981, 53, 467–471.

Disposition in the Body. Readily absorbed after oral administration. The (R)-enantiomer of warfarin is metabolised mainly by reduction to (RS)-3'-hydroxywarfarin although 6-hydroxylation also occurs. The (S)-enantiomer is metabolised mainly by 6- and 7-hydroxylation with smaller amounts of the (SS)-3'-hydroxy metabolite; the reduced metabolites are less active than warfarin; the 6- and 7-hydroxy metabolites are inactive. Less than 1% of a dose is excreted in the urine as unchanged drug. About 16 to 43% of a single dose is excreted in the urine as free or conjugated metabolites in 6 days.

THERAPEUTIC CONCENTRATION. In plasma, usually in the range 1 to 3 µg/ml but there are considerable intersubject variations in sensitivity to warfarin and measurement of the plasma concentration is generally of little value since the pharmacological effect can be easily measured.

Following a single oral dose of 50 mg to 8 subjects, peak plasma concentrations of 5.2 to 10.9 µg/ml (mean 7.2) were attained in 0.3 to 3 hours (mean 1.5) (A. Welle-Watne et al., Meddr norsk farm. Selsk., 1980, 42, 103–113).

In 6 subjects receiving daily oral doses of 5 to 11 mg, steady-state plasma concentrations of 1.2 to 2.6 µg/ml were attained (M. L'E. Orme et al., Br. med. J., 1977, 1, 1564–1565).

TOXICITY. Toxic effects are associated with plasma concentrations greater than 10 µg/ml. The maximum permissible atmospheric concentration is 0.1 mg/m^3.

HALF-LIFE. Plasma half-life, 15 to 85 hours (mean 42), decreased in subjects with renal disease. The half-life of the R-enantiomer (mean about 45 hours) appears to be longer than that of the S-enantiomer (mean, about 30 hours).

VOLUME OF DISTRIBUTION. 0.05 to 0.25 litre/kg (mean 0.15).

CLEARANCE. Plasma clearance, 0.02 to 0.08 ml/min/kg (mean 0.04).

DISTRIBUTION IN BLOOD. Plasma: whole blood ratio, about 1.8.

PROTEIN BINDING. In plasma, 97 to 99%, reduced in renal impairment.

Dose. Maintenance, 3 to 12 mg of warfarin sodium daily.

Xanthinol Nicotinate   *Vasodilator*

Synonym. Xanthinol Niacinate
Proprietary Names. Complamin(e); Emodinamin; Vasoprin.
7-{2-Hydroxy-3-[(2-hydroxyethyl)methylamino]propyl}theophylline nicotinate
$C_{13}H_{21}N_5O_4$,$C_6H_5NO_2 = 434.5$
CAS—2530-97-4 (xanthinol); *437-74-1* (nicotinate)

Colourless crystals. M.p. 180°.
Soluble in water.

Colour Tests. Amalic Acid Test—orange/violet; Cyanogen Bromide—orange.

Thin-layer Chromatography. *System TA*—Rf 41. (*Acidified potassium permanganate solution*, positive.)

Ultraviolet Spectrum. Aqueous acid—267 nm ($A_1^1 = 300$ a). Xanthinol: aqueous acid—273 nm ($A_1^1 = 270$ b).

Infra-red Spectrum. Principal peaks at wavenumbers 1658, 1695, 1548, 763, 750, 1029 (xanthinol, KBr disk).

Dose. 450 to 900 mg daily.

Xipamide   *Diuretic*

Proprietary Name. Diurexan
4-Chloro-5-sulphamoylsalicylo-2',6'-xylidide
$C_{15}H_{15}ClN_2O_4S = 354.8$
CAS—14293-44-8

A white crystalline substance. M.p. about 260°, with decomposition.
Practically **insoluble** in water; soluble in ethanol; very soluble in acetone; slightly soluble in chloroform and ether.

Dissociation Constant. pK_a 4.8 (phenol), 10.0 (sulphonamide).

Colour Tests. Koppanyi–Zwikker Test—violet; Liebermann's Test—orange; Mandelin's Test—blue; Mercurous Nitrate—black.

Thin-layer Chromatography. *System TD*—Rf 38; *system TE*—Rf 11; *system TF*—Rf 64.

Ultraviolet Spectrum. Aqueous acid—296 nm ($A_1^1 = 92$ b); aqueous alkali—330 nm ($A_1^1 = 160$ b).

Infra-red Spectrum. Principal peaks at wavenumbers 1163, 1635, 1578, 1560, 975, 1525 (KBr disk). (See below)

Mass Spectrum. Principal peaks at m/z 121, 120, 354, 122, 43, 234, 106, 64.

Quantification. HIGH PRESSURE LIQUID CHROMATOGRAPHY. In urine: UV detection—W. Diembeck et al., Arzneimittel-Forsch., 1982, 32, 1482–1485.

Wavelength

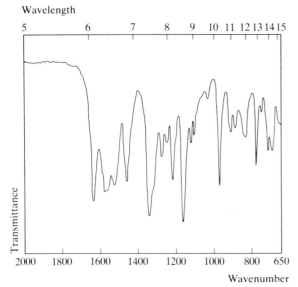

THIN-LAYER CHROMATOGRAPHY-SPECTROFLUORIMETRY. In plasma or urine: detection limit <10 ng/ml in plasma—M. Sobel and E. Mutschler, *J. Chromat.*, 1980, *183*; *Biomed. Appl.*, 9, 124–130.

Disposition in the Body. Completely and fairly rapidly absorbed after oral administration. About 88% of a dose is excreted in the urine in 48 hours with about 50% as unchanged drug and 30% as xipamide-*O*-glucuronide; free amine metabolites have also been detected. In normal subjects, only traces are excreted in the bile, but biliary excretion may be extensive in renal failure.

HALF-LIFE. Plasma half-life, about 5 to 8 hours.

PROTEIN BINDING. In plasma, about 99%.

Dose. Usually 20 to 40 mg daily; doses of 80 mg daily have been given.

Xylazine   *Sedative/Analgesic (Veterinary)*

Proprietary Name. Rompun
N-(5,6-Dihydro-4*H*-1,3-thiazin-2-yl)-2,6-xylidine
$C_{12}H_{16}N_2S = 220.3$
CAS—7361-61-7

Colourless crystals. M.p. about 138°.
Practically **insoluble** in water; soluble in acetone and chloroform.

Xylazine Hydrochloride
$C_{12}H_{16}N_2S,HCl = 256.8$
CAS—23076-35-9
A white powder. M.p. 164° to 167°.
Readily **soluble** in water, ethanol, and methanol; very slightly soluble in chloroform and ether.

Colour Tests. Liebermann's Test—red; Mandelin's Test—blue.
Thin-layer Chromatography. *System TA*—Rf 60. (*Acidified iodoplatinate solution*, positive.)
Infra-red Spectrum. Principal peaks at wavenumbers 1613, 1585, 1164, 1314, 1085, 1099 (KBr disk).
Mass Spectrum. Principal peaks at *m/z* 205, 77, 41, 39, 220, 130, 145, 131.
Disposition in the Body.
TOXICITY.

Coma and severe respiratory depression occurred in a 34-year-old man after the intramuscular injection of about 10 mg of xylazine hydrochloride; the subject recovered (S. G. Carruthers *et al.*, *Clin. Toxicol.*, 1979, *15*, 281–285).

Xylazine was detected in the urine but not in plasma (<100 ng/ml) in a non-fatal poisoning case following the ingestion of 400 mg (A. G. Gallanosa *et al.*, *Clin. Toxicol.*, 1981, *18*, 663–678).

Xylene   *Solvent*

Synonym. Xylol(e)
Proprietary Name. Cerulyse
A mixture of *o*-, *m*- and *p*-dimethylbenzene in which the *m*-isomer predominates.
$C_8H_{10} = 106.2$
CAS—1330-20-7; *108-38-3* (*m*-xylene); *95-47-6* (*o*-xylene); *106-42-3* (*p*-xylene)
A colourless, inflammable liquid. Wt per ml 0.85 to 0.86 g. B.p. 136° to 142°.
Practically **insoluble** in water; miscible with ethanol, ether, and other organic solvents.

Gas Chromatography. *System GA*—*o*-xylene RI 884, *m*-xylene RI 863, *p*-xylene RI 860; *system GI*—*o*-xylene retention time 34.5 min, *m*-xylene retention time 33.2 min, *p*-xylene retention time 34.2 min.

Mass Spectrum. Principal peaks at *m/z* 91, 106, 105, 77, 51, 39, 29, 92 (*m*-xylene).

Quantification. GAS CHROMATOGRAPHY. In urine: *m* and *p*-methylhippuric acids, sensitivity 1.0 μg/ml, AFID—M. Morin *et al.*, *J. Chromat.*, 1981, *210*, 346–349.

GAS CHROMATOGRAPHY AND GAS CHROMATOGRAPHY–MASS SPECTROMETRY. In blood or tissues: xylenes and other volatile compounds, using headspace analysis—J. A. Bellanca *et al.*, *J. analyt. Toxicol.*, 1982, 6, 238–240.

Disposition in the Body. The three isomers of xylene are absorbed from the gastro-intestinal tract, through the skin, and from the lungs. The main metabolic reactions are oxidation of a methyl group to give the corresponding *o*-, *m*-, or *p*-toluic acid and conjugation with glycine to *o*-, *m*-, or *p*-methylhippuric acid; about 70% of the absorbed material is excreted as these conjugates in the urine in 18 hours. Hydroxylation of the xylenes to the corresponding xylenols also occurs and these may be excreted in the urine as conjugates. About 5% of a dose is excreted unchanged in expired air and less than 0.01% in the urine.

TOXICITY. Xylene has about the same acute toxicity as benzene or toluene. The maximum permissible atmospheric concentration is 100 ppm. Exposure to air concentrations of 10 000 ppm has been reported to cause unconsciousness or death.

Exposure to a concentration of 100 ppm of *m*-xylene, for 6 hours, produced a mean peak blood-xylene concentration of about 1.0 μg/ml in 4 subjects at rest; when the concentration was increased to 200 ppm for 3 hours, the mean peak blood concentration was about 2.1 μg/ml (K. Savolainen *et al.*, *Int. Archs occup. Envir. Hlth*, 1979, *44*, 201–211).

Two men, aged 51 and 55 years, died in two separate incidents after ingestion of petrol which contained xylenes. The following postmortem concentrations of xylene in body tissues were reported: blood 20 and 3.0 µg/ml, and liver 1.0 µg/g for both subjects. A woman of 55, found dead, had the following postmortem concentrations of xylene in body tissues: blood 40 µg/ml, liver 1.0 µg/g (R. Bonnichsen *et al.*, *J. forens. Sci.*, 1966, *11*, 186–204).

HALF-LIFE. Blood half-life, about 20 to 30 hours.

Xylometazoline

Sympathomimetic

2-(4-*tert*-Butyl-2,6-dimethylbenzyl)-2-imidazoline
$C_{16}H_{24}N_2 = 244.4$
CAS—526-36-3

M.p. 131° to 133°.

Xylometazoline Hydrochloride
Proprietary Names. Long Acting Neo-Synephrine; Otrivin(e); Otrix; Sinex Long-Acting; 4-Way.
Note. The name Otrivin has also been applied to a preparation containing naphazoline hydrochloride.
$C_{16}H_{24}N_2,HCl = 280.8$
CAS—1218-35-5
A white crystalline powder. M.p. above 300°, with decomposition.
Soluble 1 in 12 of water, 1 in 4 of ethanol, and 1 in 25 of chloroform; practically insoluble in ether.

Partition Coefficient. Log P (chloroform/pH 7.4), 0.6.

Colour Tests. Mandelin's Test—red; Marquis Test—orange.

Thin-layer Chromatography. *System TA*—Rf 13; *system TB*—Rf 08; *system TC*—Rf 05. (*Acidified iodoplatinate solution*, positive.)

Gas Chromatography. *System GA*—RI 1940.

High Pressure Liquid Chromatography. *System HA*—k' 1.6.

Ultraviolet Spectrum. Aqueous acid—265 nm ($A_1^1 = 11.5$ a).

Infra-red Spectrum. Principal peaks at wavenumbers 1602, 1253, 1298, 871, 1237, 800 (xylometazoline hydrochloride, KBr disk).

Mass Spectrum. Principal peaks at m/z 244, 229, 44, 173, 40, 230, 243, 245.

Disposition in the Body.

TOXICITY.
The following postmortem concentrations were reported in a 23-year-old man who died after the intravenous self-administration of xylometazoline: blood 0.14 µg/ml, liver blood 0.37 µg/ml (P. Vanezis and P. A. Toseland, *Medicine, Sci. Law*, 1980, *20*, 35–36).

Use. In concentrations of 0.05 to 0.1% of the hydrochloride, as nasal drops or spray.

Yohimbine

Alkaloid

Synonyms. Aphrodine; Corynine; Québrachine.
Methyl 17α-hydroxy-yohimban-16α-carboxylate
$C_{21}H_{26}N_2O_3 = 354.4$
CAS—146-48-5

The principal alkaloid of the bark of the yohimbe tree, *Pausinystalia yohimbe* (= *Corynanthe yohimbi*) (Rubiaceae). Crystals. M.p. about 234°.
Very slightly **soluble** in water; soluble in ethanol and chloroform; sparingly soluble in ether.

Yohimbine Hydrochloride
Proprietary Name. It is an ingredient of Vikonon.
$C_{21}H_{26}N_2O_3,HCl = 390.9$
CAS—65-19-0
A white crystalline powder. M.p. about 302°, with decomposition.
Soluble 1 in 100 of water; more soluble in hot water and ethanol.

Colour Tests. Liebermann's Test—blue; Mandelin's Test—blue → green.

Thin-layer Chromatography. *System TA*—Rf 63; *system TB*—Rf 05; *system TC*—Rf 38. (*Dragendorff spray*, positive; *acidified iodoplatinate solution*, positive; *Marquis reagent*, grey.)

Gas Chromatography. *System GA*—RI 3269.

Ultraviolet Spectrum. Aqueous acid—271 nm ($A_1^1 = 211$ a), 277 nm ($A_1^1 = 207$ a), 287 nm; aqueous alkali—280 nm.

Infra-red Spectrum. Principal peaks at wavenumbers 1705, 741, 1197, 1160, 1290, 1135 (yohimbine hydrochloride, KBr disk).

Mass Spectrum. Principal peaks at m/z 353, 354, 169, 170, 355, 156, 184, 144.

Quantification. HIGH PRESSURE LIQUID CHROMATOGRAPHY. In plasma: sensitivity 10 ng/ml, electrochemical detection—M. R. Goldberg *et al.*, *J. liq. Chromat.*, 1984, *7*, 1003–1012.

Dose. Yohimbine hydrochloride has been given in doses of up to 30 mg daily.

Zimeldine

Antidepressant

Note. Zimeldine was previously known as zimelidine.
(Z)-4-Bromo-*NN*-dimethyl-γ-(3-pyridyl)cinnamylamine
$C_{16}H_{17}BrN_2 = 317.2$
CAS—56775-88-3

A white crystalline solid.

Zimeldine Hydrochloride
Proprietary Name. Zelmid
$C_{16}H_{17}BrN_2,2HCl,H_2O = 408.2$
CAS—60525-15-7 (anhydrous); *61129-30-4* (monohydrate)
A white to yellowish-white crystalline substance. M.p. 195° to 200°, with decomposition.
Soluble 1 in less than 1 of water and 1 in 1000 of ethanol; practically insoluble in chloroform and ether.

Dissociation Constant. pK_a 3.8, 8.6.

Colour Tests. Cyanogen Bromide (30 s)—red; Liebermann's Test—brown.

Thin-layer Chromatography. *System TA*—Rf 47; *system TB*—Rf 27; *system TC*—Rf 25. (Location under ultraviolet light, violet fluorescence; *Dragendorff spray*, positive.)

Gas Chromatography. *System GA*—RI 2213.

High Pressure Liquid Chromatography. *System HA*—zimeldine k' 3.2 (tailing peak), norzimeldine k' 2.9 (tailing peak); *system HF*—k' 0.67.

Ultraviolet Spectrum. Aqueous acid—250 nm ($A_1^1 = 630$ a); aqueous alkali—258 nm.

Infra-red Spectrum. Principal peaks at wavenumbers 815, 1492, 699, 953, 1075, 840 (KBr disk).

Mass Spectrum. Principal peaks at m/z 58, 70, 318, 316, 317, 193, 319, 161.

Quantification. Gas Chromatography. In plasma: zimeldine and norzimeldine, sensitivity 5 ng/ml, ECD—G. Caillé *et al.*, *Clin. Pharmacokinet.*, 1983, *8*, 530–540.

High Pressure Liquid Chromatography. In plasma: zimeldine and norzimeldine, detection limits 1.5 ng/ml and 700 pg/ml, respectively, UV detection—D. Westerlund and E. Erixson, *J. Chromat.*, 1979, *185*, 593–603.

Disposition in the Body. Readily absorbed after oral administration and rapidly demethylated by first-pass metabolism to norzimeldine which is active; bioavailability 20 to 50%. Other metabolites include zimeldine N'-oxide and 3-(4-bromophenyl)-3-(3-pyridyl)acrylic acid; very little unchanged drug is excreted in the urine.

Therapeutic Concentration.

Following a single oral dose of 100 mg to 10 subjects, peak plasma-zimeldine concentrations of 0.048 to 0.164 µg/ml (mean 0.10) were attained in 2 to 3 hours and peak plasma-norzimeldine concentrations of 0.012 to 0.092 µg/ml (mean 0.04) were attained in 1.5 to 8 hours (G. Caillé *et al., Clin. Pharmacokinet.*, 1983, *8*, 530–540).

Following oral doses averaging 225 mg daily, given twice a day to 8 subjects, steady-state plasma concentrations of 0.029 to 0.102 µg/ml (mean 0.07) of zimeldine and 0.145 to 0.554 µg/ml (mean 0.25) of norzimeldine were reported. The corresponding steady-state concentrations in cerebrospinal fluid were 0.003 to 0.007 (mean 0.006) and 0.027 to 0.072 (mean 0.043) for zimeldine and norzimeldine respectively (H. M. Calil *et al., Clin. Pharmac. Ther.*, 1982, *31*, 522–527).

Toxicity. Zimeldine has been withdrawn from use because of potentially severe neurological side-effects. Recovery within 48 hours of ingestion of 3 g of zimeldine together with half a bottle of vodka has been reported.

The following postmortem tissue distribution was reported in a female subject who had been receiving 300 mg of zimeldine daily and had been found drowned: blood, zimeldine 0.3 µg/ml, norzimeldine 0.9 µg/ml; bile, zimeldine 5.0 µg/ml, norzimeldine 15 µg/ml; liver, zimeldine 4.0 µg/g, norzimeldine 16 µg/g (R. Geyer, *Bull. int. Ass. forens. Toxicol.*, 1981, *16*(2), 30–31).

Half-life. Plasma half-life, zimeldine about 4 to 9 hours, norzimeldine about 15 to 25 hours.

Volume of Distribution. Zimeldine, about 4 litres/kg, norzimeldine, about 9 litres/kg.

Clearance. Plasma clearance, zimeldine about 7 to 11 ml/min/kg, norzimeldine about 8 ml/min/kg.

Protein Binding. In plasma, zimeldine about 90%, norzimeldine about 80%.

Note. For a review of the pharmacokinetics of zimeldine see R. C. Heel *et al., Drugs*, 1982, *24*, 169–206.

Dose. Zimeldine hydrochloride has been given in doses of 100 to 300 mg daily.

Zomepirac   *Analgesic*

5-(4-Chlorobenzoyl)-1,4-dimethylpyrrol-2-ylacetic acid
$C_{15}H_{14}ClNO_3 = 291.7$
CAS—33369-31-2

White crystals. M.p. 178° to 179°, with decomposition.

Zomepirac Sodium

Proprietary Name. Zomax
$C_{15}H_{13}ClNNaO_3, 2H_2O = 349.7$
CAS—64092-48-4 (anhydrous); *64092-49-5* (dihydrate)
A pale yellow crystalline powder. M.p. 303° to 305°.

Colour Tests. Formaldehyde–Sulphuric Acid—red; Liebermann's Test (100°)—orange; Marquis Test—yellow (→ orange at 100°); Sulphuric Acid—yellow.

Thin-layer Chromatography. *System TD*—Rf 12; *system TE*—Rf 04; *system TF*—Rf 12. (*Marquis reagent*, yellow → green, slow; *mercuric chloride–diphenylcarbazone reagent*, blue, pink after heating; *acidified potassium permanganate solution*, positive; *Van Urk reagent*, positive, red after heating.)

Gas Chromatography. *System GA*—zomepirac RI 2048, zomepirac decomposition product RI 1870.

High Pressure Liquid Chromatography. *System HD*—k' 3.7.

Ultraviolet Spectrum. Aqueous acid—262 nm ($A_1^1 = 418$ b), 324 nm ($A_1^1 = 492$ b); aqueous alkali—261 nm, 330 nm ($A_1^1 = 525$ a).

Infra-red Spectrum. Principal peaks at wavenumbers 1587, 1560, 760, 1275, 958, 1493 (zomepirac sodium, KBr disk).

Mass Spectrum. Principal peaks at m/z 246, 291, 248, 290, 247, 139, 111, 292.

Quantification. Gas Chromatography. In plasma: sensitivity 5 ng/ml, ECD—K.-T. Ng and J. J. Kalbron, *J. Chromat.*, 1983, *276*; *Biomed. Appl.*, 27, 311–318.

High Pressure Liquid Chromatography. In serum or plasma: sensitivity 50 ng/ml, UV detection—C. L. Welch *et al.*, *Clin. Chem.*, 1982, *28*, 481–484. In urine: zomepirac and zomepirac glucuronide, detection limit about 100 ng/ml, UV detection—P. Pietta and A. Calatroni, *J. Chromat.*, 1983, *275*; *Biomed. Appl.*, *26*, 217–222.

Disposition in the Body. Rapidly and completely absorbed after oral administration. About 90% of a dose is excreted in the urine in 48 hours with about 5 to 20% as unchanged drug and about 60 to 80% as a glucuronide conjugate; about 5% of the dose is excreted as a hydroxylated metabolite; 4-chlorobenzoic acid has been reported to be a minor metabolite. Less than 2% of a dose is eliminated in the faeces.

THERAPEUTIC CONCENTRATION.

After a single oral dose of 100 mg to 21 subjects, peak plasma concentrations averaged 4.7 µg/ml at about 1 hour; following oral administration of 100 mg four times a day to 10 subjects, steady-state plasma concentrations of about 3 to 4 µg/ml were reported (R. K. Nayak et al., Clin. Pharmac. Ther., 1980, 27, 395–401).

Following a single oral dose of 200 mg to 5 subjects, peak plasma concentrations of 4.5 to 11.3 µg/ml (mean 9) were attained in about 1 hour; mean peak plasma concentrations of zomepirac glucuronide and hydroxyzomepirac of 3.9 µg/ml and 0.2 µg/ml, respectively, were attained in 0.5 to 3 hours (P. J. O'Neill et al., J. clin. Pharmac., 1982, 22, 470–476).

TOXICITY. Zomepirac has been withdrawn from use because of reports of allergic anaphylactoid reactions.

In a fatality due to the ingestion of 9 g of zomepirac sodium, a postmortem blood concentration of 152 µg/ml and an antemortem blood concentration, obtained 9 hours prior to death, of 286 µg/ml were reported (R. C. Backer et al., J. analyt. Toxicol., 1983, 7, 223–224).

HALF-LIFE. Plasma half-life, about 4 to 10 hours.

DISTRIBUTION IN BLOOD. Plasma: whole blood ratio, 1.9.

PROTEIN BINDING. In plasma, 98 to 99%.

NOTE. For a review of zomepirac see P. A. Morley et al., Drugs, 1982, 23, 250–275.

Dose. Zomepirac sodium has been given in doses equivalent to 400 to 600 mg of zomepirac daily.

PART 3: Indexes to Analytical Data

Molecular Weights

Mol. Wt.	Compound	Mol. Wt.	Compound	Mol. Wt.	Compound
30.03	Formaldehyde	123.1	Nicotinic Acid	151.2	Cathine
32.04	Methanol		Nitrobenzene		Ethyl Nicotinate
44.05	Acetaldehyde		Pyrazinamide		Hydroxyamphetamine
46.03	Formic Acid	124.2	Dimercaprol		Paracetamol
46.07	Ethanol	126.1	Oxalic Acid		Phenylpropanolamine
58.08	Acetone	127.2	Coniine	151.3	Amantadine
60.05	Acetic Acid	128.1	Barbituric Acid	152.1	Mandelic Acid
60.06	Urea	128.2	Naphthalene		Methyl Hydroxybenzoate
60.10	Isopropyl Alcohol	128.6	Parachlorophenol		Methyl Salicylate
	Propanol	129.1	Dimethadione		Resorcinol Monoacetate
61.08	Ethanolamine		Flucytosine		Vanillin
62.07	Ethylene Glycol	129.2	Metformin	152.2	Camphor
72.11	Methyl Ethyl Ketone	130.1	Fluorouracil	153.1	Aminosalicylic Acid
73.89	Lithium Carbonate	130.2	Amyl Acetate	153.2	Dopamine
74.12	Ether	131.2	Aminocaproic Acid	153.6	Betaine Hydrochloride
76.05	Hydroxyurea	131.4	Trichloroethylene	153.8	Carbon Tetrachloride
76.10	Propylene Glycol	132.2	Paraldehyde	154.2	Diphenyl
77.06	Fluoroacetamide	133.2	Tranylcypromine	154.3	Cineole
78.04	Fluoroacetic Acid	133.4	Trichloroethane	155.2	Arecoline
78.11	Benzene	135.2	Acetanilide		Bemegride
	Ethylenediamine Hydrate		Amphetamine	155.3	Pempidine
78.13	Dimethyl Sulphoxide		Dexamphetamine		Propylhexedrine
84.1	Aminotriazole		Levamphetamine	156.3	Menthol
84.93	Methylene Chloride	136.1	Allopurinol	156.6	Chloroxylenol
86.14	Piperazine	136.2	Betahistine	157.2	Buformin
88.11	Ethyl Acetate		Mebanazine	157.2	Paramethadione
88.15	Amyl Alcohol		Phenelzine	159.2	Pargyline
	Putrescine	137.1	Aminobenzoic Acid	160.1	Sodium Salicylate
89.09	Urethane		Isoniazid	160.2	Hydralazine
92.14	Toluene		Methyl Nicotinate		Tolazoline
93.13	Aniline		Salicylamide		Tryptamine
94.11	Phenol	137.2	Tyramine	161.2	Aletamine
98.14	Methylpentynol	137.4	Trichlorofluoromethane	161.6	Chlormethiazole
100.0	Sodium Fluoroacetate	138.1	Salicylic Acid	162.2	Nicotine
102.1	Cycloserine	138.2	Pentetrazol	163.2	Acetylcysteine
102.2	Cadaverine	139.6	Choline Chloride	163.3	Dimethylamphetamine
106.1	Benzaldehyde	140.2	Hexamine		Mephentermine
106.2	Xylene	141.1	Dimetridazole	164.2	Eugenol
108.1	Benzyl Alcohol	141.2	Ethosuximide	165.0	Methoxyflurane
	Cresol		Methylpentynol Carbamate	165.2	Benzocaine
	Paraphenylenediamine	141.3	Cyclopentamine		Ephedrine (anhydrous)
109.1	4-Aminophenol		Isometheptene		Etenzamide
	Nicotinyl Alcohol	142.2	Methylthiouracil		Hordenine
110.1	Hydroquinone	142.6	Chlorocresol		Methoxyamphetamine
	Resorcinol	143.1	Troxidone		Pholedrine
111.1	Ametazole	144.1	Sodium Benzoate		Pseudoephedrine
	Histamine	144.2	Betanaphthol		Racephedrine
112.1	Sorbic Acid		Valproic Acid	165.4	Chloral Hydrate
114.2	Methimazole	144.6	Ethchlorvynol	165.6	Metformin Hydrochloride
115.2	Tuaminoheptane	145.1	Aminonitrothiazole	165.8	Tetrachloroethylene
117.1	Amyl Nitrite	145.2	Emylcamate	166.2	Ethionamide
	Betaine		Heptaminol		Ethyl Hydroxybenzoate
119.4	Chloroform		Hydroxyquinoline		Sodium Valproate
120.2	Noxythiolin	147.0	Paradichlorobenzene	167.2	Ethinamate
120.9	Dichlorodifluoromethane	149.2	Methylamphetamine		Metaraminol
121.1	Trometamol		Penicillamine		Oxedrine
121.2	Choline		Phentermine		Phenylephrine
	Phenethylamine	149.4	Trichloroethanol		Thioguanine
122.1	Benzoic Acid	150.2	Potassium Sorbate	167.3	Mecamylamine
	Nicotinamide		Thymol	167.8	Tetrachloroethane

Mol. Wt.	Compound
168.2	Norharman
169.2	Ammonium Mandelate
	Noradrenaline
	Pyridoxine
169.6	Chlorzoxazone
170.2	Mercaptopurine
	Propylthiouracil
170.9	Dichlorotetrafluoroethane
171.2	Metronidazole
172.2	Menadione
	Sulphanilamide
172.6	Pralidoxime Chloride
173.6	Tyramine Hydrochloride
174.1	Sodium Methyl Hydroxy-benzoate
174.2	Ephedrine
	5-Methyltryptamine
	α-Methyltryptamine
	N-Methyltryptamine
175.2	Debrisoquine
	Potassium Aminobenzoate
176.1	Ascorbic Acid
176.2	Pemoline
	Serotonin
177.2	Bemegride Sodium
	Bethanidine
	Phenmetrazine
177.6	Dimetridazole Hydrochloride
177.7	Cyclopentamine Hydrochloride
	Isometheptene Hydrochloride
178.2	Nikethamide
	Phenacemide
178.3	Amylmetacresol
	Etisazole
179.2	Iproniazid
	Methylenedioxyamphetamine
	Phenacetin
	Phenprobamate
179.3	Methoxyphenamine
	Methylephedrine
	Mexiletine
	Rimantadine
180.2	Aspirin
	Butylated Hydroxyanisole
	Propyl Hydroxybenzoate
	Theobromine
	Theophylline
180.3	Prothionamide
181.2	Etilefrine
	Hydroxyephedrine
	Styramate
181.7	Acetylcholine Chloride
	Heptaminol Hydrochloride
182.2	Harman
	Mephenesin
182.6	Carbachol
183.2	Adrenaline
	Methyprylone
	Normetanephrine
	Saccharin
183.7	Chlorphentermine
184.1	Ametazole Hydrochloride
	Histamine Hydrochloride
184.2	Apronal

Mol. Wt.	Compound
	Barbitone
	Diquat
184.5	Enflurane
185.2	Ecgonine
185.7	Methylamphetamine Hydro-chloride
	Penicillamine Hydrochloride
	Phentermine Hydrochloride
186.2	Carbimazole
	Mafenide
186.3	Paraquat
186.5	Chlorbutol
187.2	Acinitrazole
187.3	Selegiline
187.7	Amantadine Hydrochloride
	Cathine Hydrochloride
	Phenylpropanolamine Hydro-chloride
188.2	Phenazone
	Sodium Ethyl Hydroxy-benzoate
188.3	Dimethyltryptamine
	Fenproporex
189.2	Phensuximide
	Thiotepa
189.6	Dopamine Hydrochloride
190.2	Cytisine
	Dihydralazine
	Nitroxoline
191.1	Isosorbide Mononitrate
191.2	Potassium Aminosalicylate
191.3	Amiphenazole
	Diethyltoluamide
	Phendimetrazine
191.7	Propylhexedrine Hydro-chloride
192.0	Clopidol
192.2	Myristicin
192.3	Bitoscanate
	Tocainide
193.2	Butyl Aminobenzoate
193.3	Etafedrine
193.5	Butylchloral Hydrate
193.7	Buformin Hydrochloride
194.2	Aminacrine
	Aminohippuric Acid
	Caffeine
	Dimethyl Phthalate
	Piperazine Hydrate
194.3	Hexylresorcinol
195.7	Methacholine Chloride
	Pargyline Hydrochloride
196.2	Cantharidin
196.6	Hydralazine Hydrochloride
196.7	Bethanechol Chloride
	Tolazoline Hydrochloride
	Tryptamine Hydrochloride
197.2	Ethylnoradrenaline
	Levodopa
	Metanephrine
197.4	Halothane
197.7	Aletamine Hydrochloride
	Beclamide
198.1	Dinitro-orthocresol

Mol. Wt.	Compound
	Nitrofurazone
	Sodium Ascorbate
198.2	Ethyl Gallate
	Guaiphenesin
	Metharbitone
	Theophylline Hydrate
198.3	Guanethidine
	Tacrine
199.3	Diethylcarbamazine
	Phenothiazine
199.4	Octamylamine
200.3	Amantadine Sulphate
	Tetrahydrozoline
200.6	Methylchlorophenoxyacetic Acid
201.2	Carbaryl
201.3	Thiabendazole
201.7	Edrophonium Chloride
	Ephedrine Hydrochloride
	Methoxyamphetamine Hydro-chloride
	Pseudoephedrine Hydro-chloride
	Racephedrine Hydrochloride
	Simazine
202.1	Piperazine Phosphate
202.2	Sodium Propyl Hydroxy-benzoate
202.6	Chlorphenesin
203.2	Methsuximide
203.3	Crotamiton
203.7	Phenylephrine Hydrochloride
203.8	Mecamylamine Hydrochloride
204.2	Ethotoin
	Tryptophan
204.3	Bufotenine
	Ethambutol
	Levamisole
	Psilocin
	Tetramisole
205.3	Dexpanthenol
	Diethylpropion
	Phenformin
205.6	Noradrenaline Hydrochloride
	Pyridoxine Hydrochloride
206.2	Barbitone Sodium
	Pheneturide
206.3	Ibuprofen
	Pyrantel
207.2	Guanoxan
	Hydrastinine
207.3	Hexyl Nicotinate
208.1	Coniine Hydrobromide
208.2	Allobarbitone
208.3	Pilocarpine
209.1	Betahistine Hydrochloride
209.2	Hydroxyphenamate
209.3	Bamethan
	DOM
	Minoxidil
210.2	Aprobarbitone
	Phanquone
210.3	Naphazoline

Mol. Wt.	Compound	Mol. Wt.	Compound	Mol. Wt.	Compound
210.7	5-Methyltryptamine Hydro-chloride	222.7	Mafenide Hydrochloride		Dexamphetamine Phosphate
		223.1	Bromvaletone		Sulphaurea
211.1	Sodium Aminosalicylate	223.3	Bufexamac	233.3	Methylphenidate
211.3	Benethamine		Butoxyethyl Nicotinate	233.4	Meptazinol
	Isoprenaline		Ethamivan	233.7	Ethylnoradrenaline Hydro-chloride
	Mescaline		Rimiterol		
	Methoxamine		Tigloidine	234.1	Diloxanide
	Orciprenaline	223.7	Selegiline Hydrochloride	234.2	Secbutobarbitone Sodium
212.2	Benzyl Benzoate	224.1	Mevinphos	234.3	Cyclopentobarbitone
	Butobarbitone	224.2	Etofylline		Lignocaine
	Caffeine Hydrate	224.3	Butalbital		Methisazone
	Secbutobarbitone		Enallylpropymal		Phenelzine Sulphate
212.3	Harmine		Idobutal	234.4	Sparteine
213.2	Benzyl Nicotinate		Talbutal	234.7	Tacrine Hydrochloride
	Phenazopyridine		Vinbarbitone	235.3	Azapetine
213.3	Desmetryne		Vinylbitone		Meprylcaine
213.7	Baclofen	225.2	Dinitolmide		Padimate
	Clorprenaline		Furazolidone		Procainamide
	Phenmetrazine Hydrochloride		Mephenesin Carbamate	235.8	Octamylamine Hydrochloride
214.2	Niridazole	225.3	Dimethoxyamphetamine	236.1	Arecoline Hydrobromide
	Salol		Prenalterol		Isosorbide Dinitrate
	Sulphacetamide		Terbutaline	236.2	Carbazochrome
214.3	Harmaline	225.7	Hydrastinine Hydrochloride	236.3	Carbamazepine
	Phenyramidol	226.1	Acetylcholine Bromide		Cyclobarbitone
214.7	Etisazole Hydrochloride	226.2	Dithranol		Dropropizine
	Phenaglycodol		Nimorazole		Hexobarbitone
215.3	Fencamfamin	226.3	Amylobarbitone		Methazolamide
	Tramazoline		Crotethamide		Procaine
215.7	Atrazine		Metyrapone		Thiacetazone
	Methoxyphenamine Hydro-chloride		Pentobarbitone	236.7	Tetrahydrozoline Hydro-chloride
		226.7	Alclofenac		
	Methylephedrine Hydro-chloride	227.1	Glyceryl Trinitrate	237.1	Carbromal
		227.3	Ametryne	237.3	Cotarnine
	Mexiletine Hydrochloride	227.7	Amiphenazole Hydrochloride		Viloxazine
215.8	Rimantadine Hydrochloride		Buclosamide	237.7	Ketamine
216.2	Methoxsalen	228.1	Chlorquinaldol	238.2	Methyldopa
	Sodium Aminohippurate	228.2	Trioxsalen		Nitrofurantoin
216.3	Diethyltryptamine	228.7	Tocainide Hydrochloride		Proxyphylline
217.3	Captopril	229.2	Dimethoate	238.3	Nealbarbitone
	Glutethimide		Phenyl Aminosalicylate		Nomifensine
217.4	Prolintane	229.6	Amiloride		Quinalbarbitone
217.7	Etilefrine Hydrochloride	229.7	Etafedrine Hydrochloride	239.3	Isoetharine
	Hydroxyephedrine Hydro-chloride	230.1	Clonidine		Methyldopate
		230.3	Demeton-S-methyl		Salbutamol
218.2	Phenylmethylbarbituric Acid		Metomidate	239.4	Benzphetamine
218.3	Meprobamate		Naproxen	240.1	Methacholine Bromide
	Methallibure		Propyphenazone	240.2	Danthron
	Methoin	230.7	Diazoxide	240.3	Cropropamide
	Primidone	231.3	Amidopyrine		Hexethal
219.3	Profadol		Fenfluramine		Pheniramine
219.7	Adrenaline Hydrochloride		Isocarboxazid	240.8	Levamisole Hydrochloride
220.1	Chlorphentermine Hydro-chloride	232.1	Hydroxyamphetamine Hydro-bromide		Tetramisole Hydrochloride
				241.2	Methocarbamol
220.3	Morantel	232.2	Aprobarbitone Sodium		Saccharin Sodium
	Prilocaine		Nalidixic Acid		Salinazid
	Xylazine		Phenobarbitone		Theophylline Monoethanol-amine
220.4	Butylated Hydroxytoluene	232.3	Aminoglutethimide		
221.0	Dichlorophenoxyacetic Acid		Mebutamate	241.3	Choline Salicylate
221.3	Procarbazine		Piperazine Adipate		Mefenamic Acid
222.2	Acetazolamide		Pralidoxime Mesylate	241.4	Prometryne
	Diethyl Phthalate		Sulphaguanidine		Terbutryne
	Morinamide	233.1	Diuron	241.7	Phenformin Hydrochloride
	Phenindione	233.2	Amphetamine Phosphate	241.8	Diethylpropion Hydrochloride
222.3	Nicametate			242.3	Fenoprofen

Mol. Wt.	Compound	Mol. Wt.	Compound	Mol. Wt.	Compound
	Mexenone		Sulphacetamide Sodium	264.3	Pentifylline
	Thiopentone	254.3	Fenbufen		Sulfamerazine
242.7	Clofibrate		Ketoprofen		Thialbarbitone
243.2	Cytarabine		Thiamylal		Thiopentone Sodium
243.4	Phencyclidine	254.8	Butanilicaine	264.4	Amethocaine
244.2	Acetazolamide Sodium	255.3	Ambazone		Mianserin
	Carbidopa		Sulphathiazole	264.5	Monosulfiram
244.3	Amidephrine	255.4	Diphenhydramine	265.3	Albendazole
	Etomidate		Phenyltoloxamine	265.4	Antazoline
	Flurbiprofen		Tofenacin		Ethomoxane
244.4	Isoaminile		Tripelennamine		Oxprenolol
	Xylometazoline	255.5	Trichlorophenoxyacetic Acid	266.3	Atenolol
244.7	Pilocarpine Hydrochloride	255.8	Profadol Hydrochloride		Dienoestrol
245.3	Isopropylaminophenazone	256.3	Ethoxazene		Pentachlorophenol
245.7	Chlorphenesin Carbamate	256.8	Prilocaine Hydrochloride		Practolol
246.3	Busulphan		Xylazine Hydrochloride		Trimetazidine
	Mafenide Acetate	257.2	Benserazide	266.4	Cyclizine
	Methylphenobarbitone		Paraquat Dichloride		Desipramine
	Santonin	257.3	Ethebenecid	266.6	Clonidine Hydrochloride
246.4	Mepivacaine		Tolmetin	266.7	Metomidate Hydrochloride
246.7	Naphazoline Hydrochloride	257.4	Dextrorphan	267.3	Apomorphine
247.3	Ketobemidone		Levorphanol		Lysergamide
	Parbendazole		Racemorphan		Sulphafurazole
	Pethidine	257.7	Meclofenoxate		Sulphamoxole
	Tinidazole	257.8	Procarbazine Hydrochloride	267.4	Azacyclonol
247.7	Isoprenaline Hydrochloride	258.2	Salsalate		Metoprolol
	Methoxamine Hydrochloride		Thalidomide		Pipradrol
248.3	Amylobarbitone Sodium	258.3	Acetomenaphthone	267.7	Fenfluramine Hydrochloride
	Bunitrolol		Demeton-S	268.2	Clorprenaline Hydrochloride
	Dapsone		Ethoxzolamide	268.3	Lysergic Acid
	Pentobarbitone Sodium		Hexobarbitone Sodium	268.4	Stilboestrol
	Pindolol	258.7	Morinamide Hydrochloride	269.1	Dichlorophen
	Pralidoxime Methylsulphate	259.2	Nicotinyl Tartrate	269.3	Bufylline
248.7	Aminacrine Hydrochloride	259.3	Propranolol	269.4	Orphenadrine
	Pyrimethamine	259.4	Primaquine	269.8	Meptazinol Hydrochloride
249.3	Cinchophen	260.1	Carbarsone		Methylphenidate Hydro-
	Sulphapyridine		Nitrofurantoin Sodium		chloride
249.4	Alprenolol	260.3	Carisoprodol	270.1	Halazone
	Benzoctamine		Diaveridine	270.3	Sulphamethizole
249.7	Phenazopyridine Hydro-		Imolamine		Tolbutamide
	chloride		Mafenide Propionate	270.4	Doxylamine
250.2	Diflunisal		Quinalbarbitone Sodium		Hexoestrol
250.3	Heptabarbitone		Suprofen		Oestrone
	Methaqualone		Tiaprofenic Acid	270.7	Mecloqualone
	Sulphadiazine	260.4	Oxymetazoline		Nordazepam
250.7	Phenyramidol Hydrochloride	261.1	Pyridostigmine Bromide	270.8	Chloroprocaine
251.4	Triclofos Sodium	261.4	Alphaprodine		Medazepam
251.7	Cycloguanil		Ethoheptazine	271.3	Carbutamide
251.8	Fencamfamin Hydrochloride		Hexylcaine		Normorphine
	Tramazoline Hydrochloride		Methapyrilene		Pilocarpine Nitrate
252.2	Naproxen Sodium		Phenindamine		Sulphapyridine Sodium
252.3	Anisindione		Piperocaine	271.4	Cyclazocine
	Cimetidine		Thenyldiamine		Dextromethorphan
	Phenytoin	261.7	Prenalterol Hydrochloride		Methoprotryne
253.3	Choline Bitartrate		Tolfenamic Acid	271.8	Meprylcaine Hydrochloride
	Ethacridine	262.3	Hexethal Sodium		Procainamide Hydrochloride
	Nefopam		Methohexitone	272.1	Muzolimine
	Sulphamethoxazole	262.7	Clonixin	272.2	Clorgyline
	Triamterene	263.1	Guanoclor	272.3	Sulphadiazine Sodium
253.4	Tolpropamine	263.4	Butethamate	272.4	Dimethisoquin
253.7	Proguanil		Nortriptyline		Oestradiol
253.8	Prolintane Hydrochloride		Protriptyline		Sotalol
254.2	Diprophylline		Tramadol	272.8	Procaine Hydrochloride
	Phenobarbitone Sodium	264.1	Pralidoxime Iodide	273.3	Hexamethonium Chloride

Mol. Wt.	Compound	Mol. Wt.	Compound	Mol. Wt.	Compound
	Naphazoline Nitrate	281.7	Chloramine	289.7	Quinethazone
273.4	Tilidate	282.0	Lithium Citrate	289.8	Chlophedianol
273.7	Chlormezanone	282.2	Acriflavine		Halopyramine
273.8	Viloxazine Hydrochloride		Niflumic Acid		Nefopam Hydrochloride
274.2	Ketamine Hydrochloride	282.6	Chloral Betaine		Tolpropamine Hydrochloride
274.3	Phenytoin Sodium	282.8	Mepivacaine Hydrochloride	290.0	Nitroxynil
	Terbutaline Sulphate	283.3	Choline Theophyllinate	290.2	Proguanil Hydrochloride
274.4	Nandrolone	283.4	Levallorphan	290.3	Isoniazid Aminosalicylate
	Tybamate	283.8	Pethidine Hydrochloride		Trimethoprim
274.8	Chlorpheniramine	284.3	Methohexitone Sodium	290.4	Androsterone
	Dexchlorpheniramine		Psilocybin		Azatadine
275.1	Acetarsol	284.4	Iprindole		Stanolone
275.3	Homatropine		Lynoestrenol		Sulthiame
	Physostigmine		Promazine	290.8	Benzene Hexachloride
275.4	Cyclobenzaprine		Promethazine		Carbinoxamine
	Trimeperidine		Sulphaethidole		Lindane
275.7	Methyldopate Hydrochloride		Tropicamide	291.3	Parathion
275.8	Benzphetamine Hydrochloride	284.7	Diazepam		Physostigmine Aminoxide
	Isoetharine Hydrochloride		Disulphamide	291.4	Cyclopentolate
276.3	Sodium Thiamylal		Mazindol		Eucatropine
276.4	Cyclandelate		Sulphachlorpyridazine	291.5	Diethylthiambutene
	Etidocaine	285.3	Hydromorphone	291.7	Cotarnine Chloride
	Gloxazone		Nifuratel		Zomepirac
	Mebhydrolin		Norcodeine	291.8	Diphenhydramine Hydro-
	Molindone	285.4	Isothipendyl		chloride
276.7	Chlorpropamide		Mepyramine		Tofenacin Hydrochloride
277.2	Ethambutol Hydrochloride		Pentazocine		Tripelennamine Hydrochloride
	Iproniazid Phosphate		Probenecid	292.3	Coumatetralyl
277.3	Azathioprine		Prothipendyl		Hexamine Mandelate
277.4	Acecainide	285.8	Alprenolol Hydrochloride		Tolbutamide Sodium
	Amitriptyline		Benzoctamine Hydrochloride	292.4	Ambucetamide
	Maprotiline	286.3	Sulfamerazine Sodium		Dimethindene
	Padimate O		Thialbarbitone Sodium	292.8	Ethoxazene Hydrochloride
277.5	Perhexiline	286.4	Methallenoestril	293.4	Diamthazole
278.3	Dibutyl Phthalate		Thenalidine		Embutramide
	Oxpentifylline		Thonzylamine		Pramoxine
	Sulphadimidine	286.7	Demoxepam	293.5	Butriptyline
	Sulphasomidine		Oxazepam	293.7	Benserazide Hydrochloride
278.4	Triprolidine	286.8	Methaqualone Hydrochloride	294.2	Meclofenoxate Hydrochloride
279.1	Acetylcarbromal	287.1	Brallobarbitone	294.4	Cinchonidine
	Cyclophosphamide	287.2	Fenticlor		Cinchonine
279.3	Etamiphylline	287.4	Cycrimine		Noxiptyline
279.4	Doxepin		Cyproheptadine		Propoxycaine
	Fenpiprane		Dihydromorphine		Proxymetacaine
	Thymoxamine		Procyclidine		Trimipramine
279.7	Cytarabine Hydrochloride		Ritodrine	295.3	Choline Dihydrogen Citrate
279.9	Phencyclidine Hydrochloride	288.2	Chlorproguanil		Mebendazole
280.3	Hydroxystilbamidine	288.3	Dihydralazine Sulphate	295.4	Dibenzepin
	Phenprocoumon	288.4	Bupivacaine		Dothiepin
	Sulfametopyrazine		Oestriol		Normethadone
	Sulphamethoxydiazine		Phenglutarimide		Pizotifen
	Sulphamethoxypyridazine		Salbutamol Sulphate	295.7	Chlorothiazide
280.4	Bamipine		Testosterone	295.8	Chloropyrilene
	Histapyrrodine	288.5	Ethyloestrenol		Propranolol Hydrochloride
	Imipramine	288.8	Lignocaine Hydrochloride	296.2	Acriflavine
280.8	Xylometazoline Hydrochloride		Tetrazepam		Diclofenac
281.2	Flufenamic Acid	289.1	Ibomal		Flunixin
281.3	Diminazene	289.3	Benzoylecgonine		Meclofenamic Acid
	Indoprofen		Sulphapyridine Sodium	296.3	Amicarbalide
	Nitrazepam	289.4	Atropine	296.4	Ethinyloestradiol
	Trimetozine		Caramiphen		Guanethidine Monosulphate
281.4	Alverine		Dyclonine		Methdilazine
	Diphenylpyraline		Hyoscyamine	296.5	Disulfiram
	Phentolamine	289.5	Triclosan	296.8	Imolamine Hydrochloride

Mol. Wt.	Compound	Mol. Wt.	Compound	Mol. Wt.	Compound
	Oxymetazoline Hydrochloride	305.2	Dichlorphenamide		Δ^9-Tetrahydrocannabinol
297.1	Fenclofenac		Mannomustine	314.7	Clorazepic Acid
297.7	Hydrochlorothiazide		Melphalan	314.9	Clomipramine
297.8	Alphaprodine Hydrochloride	305.4	Atropine Oxide		Homochlorcyclizine
	Hexylcaine Hydrochloride		Pempidine Tartrate	315.2	Amprolium Hydrochloride
	Methapyrilene Hydrochloride	305.5	Clioquinol	315.3	Tolmetin Sodium
	Piperocaine Hydrochloride	305.8	Orphenadrine Hydrochloride	315.4	Oxycodone
	Thenyldiamine Hydrochloride	306.4	Butacaine	315.6	Triclocarban
298.3	Nialamide	307.1	Histamine Acid Phosphate	315.7	Clonazepam
298.4	Diethazine	307.2	Chloroprocaine Hydrochloride	315.8	Doxepin Hydrochloride
	Norethisterone	307.4	Benztropine		Thymoxamine Hydrochloride
	Norethynodrel		Tolnaftate	315.9	Chlorprothixene
	Phenacaine	308.3	Nifenazone		Fenpiprane Hydrochloride
	Trimeprazine		Warfarin	316.1	Pentaerythritol Tetranitrate
299.3	Fenbendazole	308.4	Oxybuprocaine	316.2	Bromazepam
299.4	Buphenine		Phenylbutazone	316.4	Butalamine
	Hydrocodone	308.6	Clorgyline Hydrochloride		Timolol
	Neopine	308.8	Alprazolam	316.9	Histapyrrodine Hydrochloride
299.8	Chlordiazepoxide		Sotalol Hydrochloride		Imipramine Hydrochloride
	Metoclopramide	308.9	Dimethisoquin Hydrochloride	317.2	Zimeldine
	Nortriptyline Hydrochloride	309.3	Acetyl Sulphafurazole	317.3	Azinphos-methyl
	Protriptyline Hydrochloride	309.4	Benzydamine		Metaraminol Tartrate
	Tramadol Hydrochloride		Ketotifen		Oxyphenisatin
300.3	Sulfaquinoxaline		Metipranolol	317.4	Codeine
	Sulphadimidine Sodium		Nadolol		Tetrabenazine
300.4	Methandienone	309.5	Dicyclomine	317.7	Chlorothiazide Sodium
300.5	Allyloestrenol		Diphenidol	317.8	Phentolamine Hydrochloride
300.7	Clobazam		Methadone	317.9	Diphenylpyraline Hydro-
	Temazepam		Methixene		chloride
300.8	Amethocaine Hydrochloride	310.3	Sulfadoxine	318.1	Diclofenac Sodium
	Chlorcyclizine		Sulphadimethoxine		Meclofenamate Sodium
	Mianserin Hydrochloride	310.4	Cannabinol	318.3	Phenolphthalein
	Thiamine		Ibogaine	318.8	Tilidate Hydrochloride
301.3	Oxymorphone		Mestranol	318.9	Chlorpromazine
301.4	Dihydrocodeine	310.5	Pecazine	319.2	Brompheniramine
	Dobutamine	311.4	Adiphenine		Dexbrompheniramine
	Isoxsuprine		Nalorphine	319.4	Hexamine Hippurate
301.5	Benzhexol		Thebaine	319.9	Chloroquine
301.7	Benoxaprofen		Tolazamide	320.4	Feprazone
301.8	Antazoline Hydrochloride	311.5	Biperiden	320.9	Iprindole Hydrochloride
	Ethomoxane Hydrochloride	311.9	Cyclobenzaprine Hydro-		Promazine Hydrochloride
	Oxprenolol Hydrochloride		chloride		Promethazine Hydrochloride
302.1	Amiloride Hydrochloride		Pyrrobutamine	321.2	Lorazepam
302.4	Cambendazole		Trimeperidine Hydrochloride	321.5	Fenchlorphos
302.5	Methyltestosterone	312.4	Propamidine		Phenazocine
	Norethandrolone	312.5	Dydrogesterone	321.8	Hydromorphone Hydro-
302.8	Cyclizine Hydrochloride		Ethisterone		chloride
	Desipramine Hydrochloride		Ethopropazine	321.9	Isothipendyl Hydrochloride
303.0	Broxyquinoline	312.8	Apomorphine Hydrochloride		Pentazocine Hydrochloride
303.1	Ethacrynic Acid		Molindone Hydrochloride	322.3	Acetyl Sulphamethoxy-
303.2	Neostigmine Bromide	312.9	Etidocaine Hydrochloride		pyridazine
303.4	Cocaine	313.3	Benorylate		Carbazochrome Sodium
	Fenoterol		Flunitrazepam		Sulphonate
	Hyoscine	313.4	Ethylmorphine	322.4	Fenpipramide
	Morphine	313.8	Acecainide Hydrochloride		Gelsemine
303.8	Azacyclonol Hydrochloride		Amoxapine	322.5	Aprindine
	Chlorphenoxamine	313.9	Amitriptyline Hydrochloride		Mequitazine
	Phenoxybenzamine		Maprotiline Hydrochloride	322.8	Thonzylamine Hydrochloride
	Pipradrol Hydrochloride	314.3	Dantrolene	323.1	Chloramphenicol
304.2	Chlorambucil	314.4	Ranitidine	323.4	Dimefline
	Rimiterol Hydrobromide		Sulphaphenazole		Gliclazide
	Tigloidine Hydrobromide	314.5	Cannabidiol		Lysergide
304.3	Diazinon		Progesterone		Piperidolate
304.5	Mesterolone		Δ^8-Tetrahydrocannabinol		

Mol. Wt.	Compound	Mol. Wt.	Compound	Mol. Wt.	Compound
323.8	Dihydromorphine Hydrochloride	331.8	Dibenzepin Hydrochloride		Fenethylline
		331.9	Dothiepin Hydrochloride		Naltrexone
	Ritodrine Hydrochloride		Normethadone Hydrochloride		Phendimetrazine Tartrate
323.9	Cycrimine Hydrochloride	332.5	Alphaxalone		Sulpiride
	Procyclidine Hydrochloride		Oxymetholone		Thebacon
324.3	Furaltadone	332.9	Methdilazine Hydrochloride	341.8	Atropine Oxide Hydrochloride
324.4	Acetohexamide		Triprolidine Hydrochloride	342.4	Calcium Mandelate
324.6	Chlorproguanil Hydrochloride	333.3	Adrenaline Acid Tartrate		Oxyphenbutazone
324.8	Phenglutarimide Hydrochloride		Azapetine Phosphate	342.9	Bupivacaine Hydrochloride
		333.5	Carbetapentane	343.2	Triazolam
	Prazepam		Deptropine	343.4	Ethacridine Lactate
325.1	Ethacrynate Sodium	334.3	Bromodiphenhydramine	343.5	Cinchocaine
325.4	Ergometrine	334.4	Benzylpenicillin		Thiambutosine
	Methylpiperidyl Benzilate		Neostigmine Methylsulphate	343.9	Clemastine
	Monocrotaline		Strychnine		Clothiapine
325.8	Clemizole	334.8	Triphenyltetrazolium Chloride	344.0	Diquat Dibromide
	Ethiazide	334.9	Diethazine Hydrochloride	344.5	Oxyphencyclimine
	Midazolam	335.2	Lormetazepam		Testosterone Propionate
325.9	Caramiphen Hydrochloride	335.4	Isoetharine Mesylate	344.8	Clotrimazole
	Dyclonine Hydrochloride	335.5	Norpipanone	344.9	Oxybuprocaine Hydrochloride
326.3	Chlophedianol Hydrochloride		Oxeladin	345.7	Methoxychlor
	Halopyramine Hydrochloride	335.9	Buphenine Hydrochloride	345.8	Clopamide
326.4	Ajmaline		Hydroxychloroquine	345.9	Benzydamine Hydrochloride
	Hydroquinidine	336.2	Chlordiazepoxide Hydrochloride		Diphenidol Hydrochloride
	Hydroquinine				Methadone Hydrochloride
326.5	Acepromazine	336.3	Dicoumarol		Methixene Hydrochloride
326.8	Clozapine	336.4	Acebutolol	346.0	Dicyclomine Hydrochloride
327.1	Niclosamide		Azapropazone	346.3	Nifedipine
327.4	Azaperone		Fluoxymesterone	346.4	Warfarin Potassium
	Benactyzine	336.5	Fentanyl	346.9	Ibogaine Hydrochloride
	6-Monoacetylmorphine	337.3	Chlorcyclizine Hydrochloride	347.5	Indoramin
	Naloxone		Noradrenaline Acid Tartrate	347.7	Chlordantoin
	Thiamine Mononitrate		Thiamine Hydrochloride	347.8	Nalorphine Hydrochloride
327.5	Butorphanol	337.4	Propanidid	347.9	Adiphenine Hydrochloride
	Proquamezine	337.5	Lobeline		Biperiden Hydrochloride
327.8	Loxapine	337.8	Dobutamine Hydrochloride	348.5	Alphadolone
327.9	Cyclopentolate Hydrochloride		Isoxsuprine Hydrochloride	348.9	Ethopropazine Hydrochloride
	Diethylthiambutene Hydrochloride		Oxymorphone Hydrochloride	349.4	Ampicillin
		337.9	Benapryzine Hydrochloride		Cephradine
	Eucatropine Hydrochloride		Benzhexol Hydrochloride	349.5	Dipipanone
328.2	Diloxanide Furoate		Tricyclamol Chloride	349.7	Zomepirac Sodium
328.4	Labetalol	338.4	Dodecyl Gallate	350.4	Phenoxymethylpenicillin
328.5	Methotrimeprazine	338.8	Chlorthalidone	350.9	Cyproheptadine Hydrochloride
	Stanozolol	339.3	Trimetazidine Hydrochloride		Ranitidine Hydrochloride
	Tuaminoheptane Sulphate	339.4	Methylergometrine	351.3	Clomipramine Hydrochloride
328.8	Clorexolone		Papaverine	351.4	Dipyrone
329.4	Trilostane	339.5	Dextropropoxyphene		Pipoxolan
329.5	Prenylamine		Disopyramide		Pirenzepine
329.9	Butriptyline Hydrochloride		Levopropoxyphene	352.3	Dithranol Triacetate
	Pramoxine Hydrochloride		Perazine	352.4	Fluopromazine
330.3	Menadione Sodium Bisulphite	339.6	Hexetidine	352.5	Anileridine
	Warfarin Sodium	339.8	Cocaine Hydrochloride	352.8	Butanilicaine Phosphate
330.4	Malathion	339.9	Prothipendyl Hydrochloride		Clorazepate Monopotassium
330.5	Deoxycortone	340.3	Chlorphenoxamine Hydrochloride		Griseofulvin
	Hydroxyprogesterone			352.9	Butalamine Hydrochloride
330.7	Frusemide		Phenoxybenzamine Hydrochloride		Phenacaine Hydrochloride
330.9	Noxiptyline Hydrochloride			353.3	Bamipine Hydrochloride
	Propoxycaine Hydrochloride	340.4	Amidephrine Mesylate		Nicoumalone
	Proxymetacaine Hydrochloride		Diphenadione	353.4	Berberine
331.2	Tienilic Acid		Pentamidine		Chelidonine
331.3	Glymidine	340.5	Norethisterone Acetate	353.5	Levomethadyl Acetate
	Hydroflumethiazide		Propiomazine		Methysergide
	Piroxicam	341.4	Acetylcodeine	354.0	Tridihexethyl Chloride
331.4	Protokylol		Benapryzine	354.1	Idoxuridine

Mol. Wt.	Compound	Mol. Wt.	Compound	Mol. Wt.	Compound
354.3	Metoclopramide Hydro-chloride		Methotrimeprazine Hydro-chloride		Papaverine Hydrochloride
354.4	Nomifensine Maleate		Pecazine Hydrochloride	376.1	Bromhexine
	Yohimbine	365.2	Nifursol	376.4	Riboflavine
354.5	Dicophane	365.4	Amoxycillin	376.5	Fluocortolone
354.8	Xipamide		Cephalexin		Fluorometholone
355.3	Chlorpromazine Hydrochloride		Methyl Benzoquate		Oestradiol Benzoate
355.9	Amodiaquine	365.5	Pericyazine	376.9	Fenpipramide Hydrochloride
356.1	Pipobroman	365.8	Metolazone		Propiomazine Hydrochloride
356.3	Homatropine Hydrobromide	366.3	Diamthazole Hydrochloride	377.5	Famprofazone
356.4	Benzylpenicillin Sodium	366.4	Atropine Methonitrate		Morazone
	Fluanisone		Trifluomeprazine		Phentolamine Mesylate
	Pheniramine Maleate	366.5	Glibornuride	377.9	Fenethylline Hydrochloride
	Pyrantel Tartrate		Piminodine		Naltrexone Hydrochloride
	Sulindac	366.9	Cinchonine Hydrochloride		Thebacon Hydrochloride
356.5	Cyclizine Lactate		Dimoxyline	378.1	Mannomustine Hydrochloride
	Oestradiol Valerate		Sulphathiazole Sodium	378.4	Carbenicillin
356.6	Conessine	367.5	Phenbutrazate		Propicillin
357.4	Nalbuphine		Phenoperidine	378.5	Doxapram
357.8	Indomethacin	367.8	Protokylol Hydrochloride		Quinine
358.0	Cetylpyridinium Chloride	368.5	Amphetamine Sulphate	379.4	Droperidol
358.4	Prednisone		Cinnarizine	379.5	Oxypertine
358.5	Dimethisterone		Dexamphetamine Sulphate	379.9	Cinchocaine Hydrochloride
	Dimethoxanate	368.8	Ketazolam		Cyclopenthiazide
	Δ^9-Tetrahydrocannabinolic	369.3	Etofenamate	380.3	Neopine Hydrobromide
	Acid	369.4	Diamorphine	380.4	Hyoscine Methonitrate
359.0	Aprindine Hydrochloride	370.3	Dextromethorphan Hydro-bromide		Methicillin
359.2	Obidoxime Chloride			380.5	Fludrocortisone
359.5	Cyclomethycaine		Homatropine Methobromide		Stilboestrol Dipropionate
359.6	Captodiame		Hyoscyamine Hydrobromide	380.6	Trichlormethiazide
359.9	Dimefline Hydrochloride	370.4	Morantel Tartrate	380.9	Chlorotrianisene
	Piperidolate Hydrochloride	370.6	Thioridazine		Dieldrin
360.2	Methyclothiazide	370.7	Bromodiphenhydramine Hydrochloride		Endrin
360.4	Aldosterone				Hydrocodone Hydrochloride
	Cortisone	370.9	Lorcainide		Oxyphencyclimine Hydro-chloride
	Prednisolone	371.4	Ampicillin Sodium		
360.5	Drostanolone Propionate	371.8	Camazepam	381.4	Benperidol
	Quinidine	371.9	Codeine Hydrochloride		Fendosal
361.4	Bisacodyl		Norpipanone Hydrochloride	381.7	Econazole
	Chromonar		Trazodone	382.5	Hexoestrol Dipropionate
361.5	Antazoline Mesylate	372.4	Diamphenethide	382.6	Bunamidine
361.8	Bezafibrate		Sulphafurazole Diethanol-amine	382.9	Mefruside
362.2	Hexamethonium Bromide			383.2	Ecothiopate Iodide
362.3	Clemizole Hydrochloride	372.5	Ajmaline Monoethanolate	383.4	Hydrastine
	Octatropine Methylbromide		Benzylpenicillin Potassium		Prazosin
362.4	Emepronium Bromide		Deoxycortone Acetate	383.9	Indoramin Hydrochloride
	Phthalylsulphacetamide		Nabilone	384.3	Atropine Methobromide
362.5	Hydrocortisone	372.8	Glafenine		Fenoterol Hydrobromide
362.9	Hydroquinidine Hydrochloride	372.9	Acebutolol Hydrochloride	384.5	Caramiphen Edisylate
363.4	Antazoline Phosphate	373.3	Heptachlor		Ethynodiol Diacetate
363.5	Opipramol	373.4	Succinylsulphathiazole		Megestrol Acetate
363.8	6-Monoacetylmorphine Hydro-chloride	373.9	Lobeline Hydrochloride	384.6	Cholecalciferol
			Prochlorperazine	385.5	Bamifylline
	Naloxone Hydrochloride	374.5	Methylprednisolone	385.9	Ethylmorphine Hydrochloride
363.9	Benactyzine Hydrochloride	374.8	Indapamide	386.3	Caffeine Citrate
	Lachesine Chloride	374.9	Hydroxyzine	386.4	Valethamate Bromide
364.3	Bibenzonium Bromide	375.5	Benzylmorphine	386.5	Medroxyprogesterone Acetate
364.4	Bumetanide		Pentazocine Lactate	386.6	Mesoridazine
	Cyclofenil		Pipamperone		Testosterone Isocaproate
	Phenethicillin	375.8	Morphine Hydrochloride	386.7	Cholesterol
364.5	Flugestone		Norcodeine Hydrochloride	387.2	Acetarsol Sodium
	Tranylcypromine Sulphate	375.9	Dextropropoxyphene Hydro-chloride	387.4	Amoxycillin Sodium
364.9	Aldrin			387.9	Flurazepam
	Labetalol Hydrochloride		Haloperidol		Pipoxolan Hydrochloride
				388.4	Hydroxyquinoline Sulphate

Mol. Wt.	Compound	Mol. Wt.	Compound	Mol. Wt.	Compound
388.5	Aminacrine Hexylresorcinate	401.5	Biperiden Lactate		Diperodon
	Doxylamine Succinate		Mepyramine Maleate		Pentapiperide Methylsulphate
	Phenoxymethylpenicillin		Oxyclozanide	415.6	Haloxon
	Potassium	402.5	Cortisone Acetate	416.1	Miconazole
	Trimethobenzamide		Phenethicillin Potassium	416.4	Piperazine Calcium Edetate
388.9	Fluopromazine Hydrochloride		Prednisolone Acetate	416.5	Alfentanil
389.5	Diphemanil Methylsulphate	402.6	Sulforidazine		Desonide
389.9	Cyclothiazide	403.4	Ampicillin Trihydrate		Methylprednisolone Acetate
390.0	Levomethadyl Acetate Hydro-		Phthalylsulphathiazole		Pholcodine
	chloride	403.5	Benztropine Mesylate		Propicillin Potassium
390.5	Alphadolone Acetate	403.9	Phenbutrazate Hydrochloride	416.6	Spironolactone
390.9	Chlorpheniramine Maleate		Phenoperidine Hydrochloride	417.5	Decoquinate
	Dexchlorpheniramine Maleate	404.0	Dipipanone Hydrochloride	418.3	Decamethonium Bromide
	Yohimbine Hydrochloride		Perphenazine	418.4	Barbaloin
391.0	Meclozine	404.5	Benzquinamide		Cephalothin Sodium
391.4	Ambutonium Bromide		Hydrocortisone Acetate	419.0	Bunamidine Hydrochloride
	Diethylcarbamazine Citrate		Sulphinpyrazone		Lofepramine
391.5	Dimethothiazine	404.9	Chlormadinone Acetate	419.4	Amoxycillin Trihydrate
	Flavoxate	405.9	Oxycodone Hydrochloride	419.6	Prenylamine Lactate
391.9	Phenmetrazine Theoclate	406.0	Clomiphene	419.9	Hydrastine Hydrochloride
392.3	Nalorphine Hydrobromide	406.4	Codeine Phosphate		Prazosin Hydrochloride
392.5	Betamethasone		Floctafenine	420.3	Mepenzolate Bromide
	Dexamethasone	406.5	Flugestone Acetate		Methanthelinium Bromide
	Dextromoramide		Lincomycin	420.4	Methicillin Sodium
	Paramethasone	406.6	Nandrolone Phenylpropionate		Penthienate Methobromide
393.5	Methindizate	406.9	Carbinoxamine Maleate	420.5	Hexoprenaline
	Pheniramine Aminosalicylate		Endosulfan	420.6	Testosterone Phenylpropionate
393.6	Perhexiline Maleate		Hexachlorophane	421.1	Broxaldine
393.9	Nalbuphine Hydrochloride		Strychnine Hydrochloride	421.4	Bendrofluazide
394.3	Homidium Bromide	407.0	Thioridazine Hydrochloride	421.9	Bamifylline Hydrochloride
394.4	Rotenone	407.4	Lorcainide Hydrochloride	422.4	Carbenicillin Sodium
	Triamcinolone	407.5	Trifluoperazine	422.5	Fludrocortisone Acetate
394.9	Dimethoxanate Hydrochloride	407.8	Berberine Hydrochloride		Quinidine Bisulphate
396.0	Captodiame Hydrochloride	408.2	Zimeldine Hydrochloride		Sparteine Sulphate
396.1	Cetalkonium Chloride	408.3	Trazodone Hydrochloride	423.9	Diamorphine Hydrochloride
396.4	Cephalothin	408.4	Ethyl Biscoumacetate	424.1	Benzbromarone
396.5	Quinine Ethyl Carbonate	408.5	Dimethindene Maleate	424.3	Dibenzepin Hydrochloride
396.6	Oestradiol Cypionate	408.9	Beclomethasone		Flurazepam Monohydro-
396.7	Ergocalciferol		Clorazepate Dipotassium		chloride
396.9	Quinine Hydrochloride	409.4	Trifluperidol	424.9	Trimethobenzamide Hydro-
397.0	Di-iodohydroxyquinoline	409.6	Butaperazine		chloride
397.3	Quinine Dihydrochloride	409.8	Chlordane	425.0	Clindamycin
	Suxamethonium Chloride	410.5	Flumethasone	425.4	Anileridine Hydrochloride
397.4	Strychnine Nitrate		Thiazinamium Methylsulphate	425.5	Ketotifen Fumarate
397.6	Solanidine		Trimipramine Maleate	425.6	Carphenazine
397.9	Chromonar Hydrochloride	410.6	Piperacetazine		Diprenorphine
398.3	Glycopyrronium Bromide	411.4	Phenazocine Hydrobromide	425.8	Epithiazide
	Hyoscine Methobromide	411.5	Etorphine	427.6	Dixyrazine
398.4	Calcium Aminosalicylate		Phenindamine Tartrate	427.9	Flavoxate Hydrochloride
	Sulphasalazine	411.6	Acetophenazine	428.3	Stilboestrol Diphosphate
398.7	Dihydrotachysterol	411.9	Benzylmorphine Hydro-	428.4	Oxyphenonium Bromide
399.2	Clefamide		chloride	428.5	Ephedrine Sulphate
399.3	Dantrolene Sodium	412.3	Heteronium Bromide		Pholedrine Sulphate
399.4	Colchicine	412.6	Bromhexine Hydrochloride		Pseudoephedrine Sulphate
	Dihydrocodeine Phosphate		Testosterone Cypionate	428.6	Hexocyclium Methylsulphate
	Morphine Acetate	413.4	Noscapine		Hydroxyprogesterone
399.5	Pipazethate	413.5	Physostigmine Salicylate		Hexanoate
399.6	Thiethylperazine	413.9	Morazone Hydrochloride	428.7	Nandrolone Decanoate
400.0	Mepacrine	414.4	Bretylium Tosylate	429.5	Physostigmine Aminoxide
400.5	Prednisone Acetate		Nicametate Citrate		Salicylate
400.6	Testosterone Enanthate	414.5	Domiphen Bromide		Pizotifen Malate
	Thiocarlide	414.6	Deoxycortone Pivalate	429.6	Mebeverine
401.0	Clopenthixol		Gestronol Hexanoate	430.0	Methindizate Hydrochloride
401.4	Oxyphenisatin Acetate	415.5	Cephaloridine	430.6	Piritramide

Mol. Wt.	Compound	Mol. Wt.	Compound	Mol. Wt.	Compound
431.9	Benzthiazide		Tripelennamine Citrate	469.5	Methysergide Maleate
432.4	Clidinium Bromide	447.8	Hydroxyzine Hydrochloride	470.0	Dimenhydrinate
432.5	Timolol Maleate	448.0	Etorphine Hydrochloride	470.2	Dibromopropamidine
432.6	Hydrocortisone Butyrate	448.1	Benzethonium Chloride	470.7	Enoxolone
433.0	Buclizine	448.4	Pipamperone Hydrochloride	471.0	Alfentanil Hydrochloride
	Doxapram Hydrochloride		Propantheline Bromide	472.8	Alpha Tocopheryl Acetate
433.4	Berberine Sulphate	448.5	Debrisoquine Sulphate	473.4	Clofazimine
433.5	Levallorphan Tartrate	450.1	Octaphonium Chloride	473.6	Alverine Citrate
433.9	Diperodon Hydrochloride	450.5	Anileridine Phosphate		Naftidrofuryl Oxalate
	Hydroxychloroquine Sulphate	450.7	Phytomenadione	473.9	Clopenthixol Hydrochloride
434.4	Benzilonium Bromide	451.5	Dihydrocodeine Tartrate	474.5	Methylprednisolone Hemi-
	Pipenzolate Bromide		Poldine Methylsulphate		succinate
434.5	Betamethasone Acetate	452.5	Fluocinolone Acetonide	474.6	Fluocortolone Hexanoate
	Dexamethasone Acetate	452.6	Bethanidine Sulphate	475.6	Fluspirilene
	Flupenthixol		Diphenoxylate	475.7	Pipothiazine
	Paramethasone Acetate	453.3	Chloramphenicol Cinnamate	475.9	Cloxacillin Sodium
	Triamcinolone Acetonide	453.5	Ethoheptazine Citrate	476.6	Betamethasone Valerate
	Xanthinol Nicotinate	453.6	Acetorphine		Piminodine Esylate
435.3	Brompheniramine Maleate	453.9	Flucloxacillin		Prednisolone Tebutate
	Dexbrompheniramine Maleate	454.0	Thenium Closylate	477.0	Loperamide
435.4	Ajmaline Hydrochloride	454.1	Dofamium Chloride	477.6	Butorphanol Tartrate
435.9	Cloxacillin	454.4	Methotrexate	478.3	Suxethonium Bromide
436.0	Chloroquine Sulphate	454.6	Verapamil	478.5	Triamcinolone Diacetate
	Pipazethate Hydrochloride	455.0	Halcinonide	478.6	Dehydroemetine
436.4	Opipramol Hydrochloride	455.3	Primaquine Phosphate	478.9	Chlortetracycline
436.5	Flurandrenolone	455.4	Lofepramine Hydrochloride		Methacycline Hydrochloride
	Isoaminile Citrate	455.5	Butethamate Citrate	479.0	Clobetasone Butyrate
	Thenalidine Tartrate		Methylergometrine Maleate	479.1	Miconazole Nitrate
436.6	Bialamicol	456.2	Hexamethonium Iodide	479.5	Clindamycin Hydrochloride
437.5	Disopyramide Phosphate	456.5	Aminophylline	480.4	Isopropamide Iodide
	Fluphenazine	456.6	Propiomazine Maleate		Trifluoperazine Hydrochloride
438.3	Hyoscine Hydrobromide	457.4	Amygdalin	480.6	Emetine
439.9	Polythiazide	457.5	Minocycline		Quinine Salicylate
440.4	Hyoscine Butylbromide	457.6	Cyclomethycaine Sulphate	480.9	Tetracycline Hydrochloride
440.7	Oestradiol Undecanoate	460.0	Clemastine Fumarate	481.9	Narceine Hydrochloride
441.0	Benzquinamide Hydrochloride	460.5	Prednisolone Succinate	482.5	Trifluomeprazine Maleate
441.4	Folic Acid	460.6	Fluocortolone Pivalate	483.9	Mersalyl Acid
	Quinine Hydrobromide		Mephentermine Sulphate	484.4	Nicergoline
441.5	Ergometrine Maleate	460.7	Docusate Potassium		Prednisolone Sodium
442.4	Methacycline	460.8	Flurazepam Hydrochloride		Phosphate
442.5	Acepromazine Maleate	461.0	Lincomycin Hydrochloride	484.5	Hydrocortisone Sodium
443.5	Bephenium Hydroxy-	461.5	Orphenadrine Citrate		Succinate
	naphthoate	461.6	Pimozide		Kanamycin
	Levorphanol Tartrate	462.0	Diprenorphine Hydrochloride		Oxedrine Tartrate
443.6	Thiothixene	462.5	Doxycycline	486.2	Suxamethonium Bromide
444.4	Tetracycline		Hydrocortisone Hydrogen	486.4	Hydrocortisone Sodium
444.5	Methotrimeprazine Maleate		Succinate		Phosphate
444.6	Docusate Sodium	463.5	Pivampicillin	486.6	Hydrocortisone Cypionate
	Prednisolone Pivalate	463.9	Meclozine Hydrochloride	487.4	Fluclorolone Acetonide
444.7	Econazole Nitrate	464.6	Hordenine Sulphate	487.6	Dimethothiazine Mesylate
445.2	Chloramphenicol Sodium	464.8	Amodiaquine Hydrochloride	488.0	Chloropyrilene Citrate
	Succinate	464.9	Demeclocycline	489.1	Diphenoxylate Hydrochloride
445.5	Glipizide		Loprazolam	490.0	Acetorphine Hydrochloride
445.6	Metopimazine	465.4	Dimoxyline Phosphate	490.6	Dexamethasone Tebutate
445.9	Cycloguanil Embonate	465.5	Bacampicillin		Pentobarbitone Calcium
	Loxapine Succinate	466.0	Mebeverine Hydrochloride	491.1	Verapamil Hydrochloride
	Trifluperidol Hydrochloride	466.5	Brucine	491.5	Flunixin Meglumine
446.0	Thiopropazate	466.6	Cephaëline	491.6	Lidoflazine
446.4	Hydrocodone Phosphate	467.0	Clobetasol Propionate	492.6	Bezitramide
446.6	Denatonium Benzoate	467.5	Saccharin Calcium	492.7	Isometheptene Mucate
	Hydrocortisone Valerate		Tobramycin	493.4	Hexoprenaline Hydrochloride
	Thioproperazine	467.6	Buprenorphine	493.9	Flucloxacillin Sodium
447.0	Propyliodone	467.7	Oxethazaine		Minocycline Hydrochloride
447.5	Phenyltoloxamine Citrate	467.9	Noscapine Hydrochloride	494.0	Glibenclamide

Mol. Wt.	Compound	Mol. Wt.	Compound	Mol. Wt.	Compound
494.5	Fluocinonide	530.9	Clomocycline Sodium	597.4	Pyrithidium Bromide
	Hydrocodone Tartrate	531.4	Ketoconazole	598.1	Clomiphene Citrate
494.6	Flumethasone Pivalate	532.6	Hydroxystilbamidine	600.5	Nicofuranose
496.5	Methylprednisolone Sodium		Isethionate	602.6	Picrotoxin
	Succinate		Pentamidine Mesylate	603	Lymecycline
	Oxytetracycline Dihydrate		Triamcinolone Hexacetonide	604.3	Fazadinium Bromide
496.6	Betamethasone Benzoate	538.6	Pentolinium Tartrate	605.6	Butaperazine Phosphate
496.9	Oxytetracycline Hydrochloride	538.7	Sodium Fusidate	606.1	Prochlorperazine Maleate
497.6	Dexamethasone Isonicotinate	539.5	Cephaëline Hydrochloride	608.5	Ambenonium Chloride
499.0	Promethazine Theoclate	540.3	Quinine Dihydrobromide	608.7	Methoserpidine
499.3	Nitroxynil (Eglumine Salt)	541.5	Clioxanide		Reserpine
499.5	Narceine	542.6	Dextromoramide Tartrate	610.2	Mepacrine Mesylate
500.0	Pivampicillin Hydrochloride	543.5	Doxorubicin	614.6	Neomycin B
500.5	Hexamethonium Tartrate	544.2	Suxamethonium Iodide	614.7	Carbenoxolone Sodium
501.3	Demeclocycline Hydrochloride	544.7	Mesoridazine Benzene-	615.6	Butyl Aminobenzoate Picrate
502.0	Bacampicillin Hydrochloride		sulphonate	617.6	Rolitetracycline Nitrate
504.1	Buprenorphine Hydrochloride	547.6	Perazine Dimalonate	622.7	Pseudomorphine
504.6	Betamethasone Dipropionate	548.6	Amicarbalide Isethionate	624.3	Guanoclor Sulphate
	Dipyridamole		Quinine Bisulphate	625.6	Chlorhexidine Acetate
505.0	Clindamycin Phosphate	549.7	Fluphenazine Enanthate	626.0	Rafoxanide
505.5	Chlorhexidine	550.3	Mebezonium Iodide	631.8	Thiethylperazine Maleate
505.9	Mersalyl Sodium	551.6	Dehydroemetine Hydro-	634.7	Rescinnamine
506.0	Buclizine Hydrochloride		chloride	638.8	Thioproperazine Mesylate
507.4	Flupenthixol Hydrochloride	552.6	Proflavine Hemisulphate	641.7	Butaperazine Maleate
507.8	Pyrrobutamine Phosphate		Thiothixene Hydrochloride	642.7	Piperazine Citrate
508.9	Clomocycline	554.7	Ethopropazine Hybenzate	643.7	Acetophenazine Maleate
	Mepacrine Hydrochloride	555.2	Clopenthixol Decanoate	645.3	Amiodarone
509.6	Bialamicol Hydrochloride	556.6	Isoprenaline Sulphate	645.7	Aconitine
510.4	Fluphenazine Hydrochloride	558.6	Fenoprofen Calcium	648.8	Physostigmine Sulphate
510.6	Cyclobarbitone Calcium	560.7	Desferrioxamine	651.0	Liothyronine
511.6	Etamiphylline Camsylate	561.5	Chloramphenicol Palmitate	651.2	Kanamycin Acid Sulphate
	Norbormide	561.7	Ergotoxine	654.6	Bromocriptine
512.3	Sodium Cromoglycate	562.5	Acepifylline	656.8	Desferrioxamine Mesylate
512.5	Guanoxan Sulphate	564.1	Prochlorperazine Edisylate	657.7	Carphenazine Maleate
512.9	Doxycycline Hydrochloride	564.6	Propamidine Isethionate	659.8	Dihydroergocornine Mesylate
513.5	Chlormethiazole Edisylate	565.7	Dextropropoxyphene	665.6	Hexobendine Hydrochloride
	Loperamide Hydrochloride		Napsylate	665.7	Natamycin
515.3	Chlortetracycline Hydro-		Levopropoxyphene Napsylate	666.7	Syrosingopine
	chloride	566.1	Prochlorperazine Mesylate	667.8	Diethylperazine Malate
515.9	Chloroquine Phosphate	566.6	Quinuronium Sulphate	671.8	Ergotoxine Esylate
516.4	Betamethasone Sodium	570.8	Bunamidine Hydroxy-	673.0	Liothyronine Sodium
	Phosphate		naphthoate	673.8	Dihydroergocryptine Mesylate
	Dexamethasone Sodium		Carbenoxolone	679.7	Emetine Hydrochloride
	Phosphate	574.8	Dequalinium Acetate	679.8	Dihydroergotamine Mesylate
516.6	Bamethan Sulphate	576.3	Distigmine Bromide	681.8	Amiodarone Hydrochloride
518.1	Benziodarone	577.6	Stilbazium Iodide	684.8	Metoprolol Tartrate
518.4	Conessine Hydrobromide	578.4	Chlorhexidine Hydrochloride	685.0	Prednisolone Steaglate
518.6	Hexoprenaline Sulphate	578.7	Deserpidine	687.9	Oleandomycin
	Prajmalium Bitartrate	579.0	Loprazolam Mesylate	694.8	Atropine Sulphate
518.9	Thiopropazate Hydrochloride	580.0	Doxorubicin Hydrochloride	697.8	Rifamycin SV
519.0	Dichloralphenazone	581.6	Streptomycin	699.9	Clindamycin Palmitate Hydro-
520.6	Orciprenaline Sulphate	581.7	Ergotamine		chloride
	Quinidine Gluconate	582.6	Kanamycin Sulphate	707.8	Dihydroergocristine Mesylate
521.0	Beclomethasone Dipropionate	583.6	Dihydrostreptomycin	708.8	Aconitine Nitrate
522.6	Azatadine Maleate	583.7	Dihydroergotamine	711.0	Butacaine Sulphate
524.0	Penfluridol	585.6	Amikacin	712.9	Hyoscyamine Sulphate
525.6	Carbetapentane Citrate	587.6	Diminazene Aceturate	714.1	Pipothiazine Palmitate
	Deptropine Citrate	588.7	Procaine Penicillin	716.6	Demecarium Bromide
525.7	Fusidic Acid	588.8	Flupenthixol Decanoate	719.8	Rifamycin Sodium
527.6	Dequalinium Chloride	591.8	Fluphenazine Decanoate	722.4	Dibromopropamidine
	Gliquidone	592.7	Hexobendine		Isethionate
	Oxeladin Citrate		Pentamidine Isethionate	728.8	Ouabain
	Rolitetracycline	594.7	Pyrantel Embonate	731.8	Diphenhydramine
528.6	Fentanyl Citrate	596.8	Trimetaphan Camsylate		Di(acefyllinate)

Mol. Wt.	Compound	Mol. Wt.	Compound	Mol. Wt.	Compound
732.7	Pancuronium Bromide	798.9	Thyroxine Sodium	923.0	Vincristine Sulphate
733.9	Erythromycin	800.9	Ergometrine Tartrate	924.1	Amphotericin
747.0	Trimeprazine Tartrate	807.0	Acetyldigitoxin	926.1	Nystatin
750.7	Bromocriptine Mesylate	809.9	Protoveratrine B	929.2	Spiramycin II
750.9	Codeine Sulphate	810.7	Inositol Nicotinate	943.1	Deslanoside
752.7	Pholcodine Tartrate	811.0	Vinblastine	943.2	Amitriptyline Embonate
753.9	Vindesine	813.0	Cinchonidine Sulphate		Spiramycin III
758.8	Morphine Sulphate	814.0	Triacetyloleandomycin	949.2	Imipramine Embonate
763.3	Hydroxyzine Embonate	823.0	Rifampicin	957.2	Promazine Embonate
764.9	Digitoxin	825.0	Vincristine	958.9	Oxytetracycline Calcium
771.0	Proquamezine Fumarate	827.9	Alcuronium Chloride	960.1	Erythromycin Gluceptate
771.7	Tubocurarine Chloride	841.1	Mebhydrolin Napadisylate	985.1	Lanatoside C
773.0	Lobeline Sulphate	852.0	Vindesine Sulphate	1013	Brucine Sulphate
774.8	Morphine Tartrate	857.0	Strychnine Sulphate	1018	Erythromycin Stearate
774.9	Phenoxymethylpenicillin	862.1	Erythromycin Ethylsuccinate	1026	Chlorpromazine Embonate
	Calcium	866.9	Papaverine Sulphate	1056	Erythromycin Estolate
776.9	Thyroxine	868.1	Solanine	1092	Erythromycin Lactobionate
780.9	Digoxin	871.0	Methapyrilene Fumarate	1152	Viprynium Embonate
781.8	Amikacin Sulphate	883.2	Docusate Calcium	1313	Ergotamine Tartrate
782.9	Quinidine Sulphate	887.1	Spiramycin I	1317	Dihydroergotamine Tartrate
	Quinine Sulphate	891.5	Gallamine Triethiodide	1346	Hydroxocobalamin
785.9	Oleandomycin Phosphate	897.8	Chlorhexidine Gluconate	1355	Cyanocobalamin
790.0	Erythromycin Propionate		Sodium	1457	Streptomycin Sulphate
793.5	Protoveratrine A	906.6	Metocurine Iodide	1461	Dihydrostreptomycin Sulphate
795.0	Medigoxin	909.1	Vinblastine Sulphate		

Melting Points

d = 'with decomposition'

°C	Compound	°C	Compound	°C	Compound
18	Trichloroethanol	59	DOM	80	Allyloestrenol
24	Amylmetacresol		Hyoscine		Anileridine
27–28	Menthol (racemic)	59–61	Triprolidine		Bamifylline
	Putrescine	<60	Cyclandelate		Isopropylaminophenazone
28.5–32	Monosulfiram	60	Promethazine		Naphthalene
33–35	Fluoroacetic Acid	60–62	Levamisole		Testosterone Isocaproate
33–37	Nandrolone Decanoate	61	Procaine	80–85	Lysergide
34	Pilocarpine	62–64	Thiethylperazine	81–83	Vanillin
34–39	Testosterone Enanthate	62–65	Butylated Hydroxyanisole	82	Pentifylline
35–36	Mescaline	62–65.5	Cinchocaine	82–85	Phenyramidol
36–38	Prenylamine	62–68	Hexylresorcinol	83–84	Fentanyl
	Prilocaine	63–64	Isoaminile Citrate		Histamine
38	Ephedrine, Anhydrous	64–66	Chlorocresol	83–88	Methdilazine
38–39	Benzydamine	64–67	Dichloralphenazone	84	Cholecalciferol
38–40	Phenoxybenzamine	64–69	Chlorambucil	84–86	Ametryne
40–41	Phenol	66–67	Cannabidiol		Desmetryne
40–42	Methyl Nicotinate	66–69	Lignocaine	85–87	Procyclidine
40–43	Ephedrine	67	Etomidate	85–89	Glutethimide
41–43	Fenpiprane	68	Isometheptene Hydrochloride	85–100	Oxyphenbutazone
41–44	Menthol (−)		Trimeprazine	86	Benzoylecgonine (hydrated)
41–46	Amethocaine	68–70	Methoprotryne		Dinitro-orthocresol
42	Parachlorophenol	68–74	Phensuximide	87	Econazole
42–44	Salol	69	Diphenyl	87–89	Diethyltryptamine Hydro-
43	Piperazine Hydrate	69–73	Disulfiram		chloride
44–47	Dimethyltryptamine	69–74	Thioridazine		Tetramisole
45	Trimipramine	70	DOM	87–91	Etidocaine
45–46	Butanilicaine		Embutramide	87–92	Chloroquine
45–47	Troxidone		Isosorbide Dinitrate	87–95	Chloramphenicol Palmitate
46	Phencyclidine		Levomethadyl Acetate	88	Ethambutol
46–52	Ethosuximide	70–73	Mephenesin	88–90	Ritodrine
46–74	Heptachlor (technical)	70–80	Barbaloin (monohydrate)	88–92	Benzocaine
48–49	Pyrrobutamine	70–100	Endosulfan	88–93	Haloxon
48–50	Urethane	72–76	Fluanisone	89	Anileridine
48–51	Thymol	73–74	Azinphos-methyl		Methoxychlor (pure)
49	Diethylcarbamazine	74	Emetine		Ethyloestrenol
49–53	Cyclophosphamide	74–75	Methylphenidate	89–91	Hydroxychloroquine
49–54	Tybamate	74–78	Methyprylone		Isosorbide Mononitrate
49–60	Aldrin (technical)	74–79	Lignocaine Hydrochloride	90	Chlorphenesin Carbamate
50	Choline Salicylate	75	Etamiphylline		Ethotoin
50–53	Metyrapone	75–76	Dextropropoxyphene		Physostigmine Aminoxide
50–56	Methsuximide		Levopropoxyphene		Salicylate
50–58	Chloral Hydrate	75–77	Hexobendine	90–91	Oxeladin Citrate
51	Benactyzine	75–78	Ibuprofen	90–92	Vinylbitone
51–52	Dimethoate	75–80	Oxprenolol	90–94	Methocarbamol
52–57	Thiotepa	76	Hydroxyquinoline	90–95	Azaperone
53–54	Paradichlorobenzene	76–77	Cannabinol		Carbetapentane Citrate
53–55	Ethopropazine		Dimethadione	90–96	Cycrimine
	Tocainide	76–79	Chlorbutol	90–100	Clobetasone Butyrate
53–56	Methylpentynol Carbamate	77	Methoxychlor (technical)	91	Alclofenac
54–57	Perazine	77–78	Cathine		Buclosamide
55–57	Hydroxyphenamate		Phenaglycodol		Phenindamine
	Triclosan	77–79	Mebutamate	91–94	Beclamide
56–57	Enallylpropymal	77–82	Flurazepam	91–95	Quinine Ethyl Carbonate
56–58	Emylcamate	78	Butylchloral Hydrate	92–93	Ketamine
56–60	Chlorpromazine		Etisazole	92–94	Carisoprodol
57–59	Alprenolol	78–81	Chlorphenesin		Maprotiline
	Butyl Aminobenzoate	78–82	Guaiphenesin	92–96	Methohexitone
57–60	Pentetrazol	79	Racephedrine	93	Mephenesin Carbamate
58–60	Cetalkonium Chloride	79–84	Cetylpyridinium Chloride	93–95	Trifluperidol

°C	Compound
93–96	Ketoprofen
94–96	Propranolol
94–98	Ethinamate
94–99	Ethamivan
94–100	Perphenazine
95	Disopyramide
	Mebhydrolin
	Tiaprofenic Acid
95–96	Heptachlor (pure)
95–97	Thenalidine
95–98	Propyl Hydroxybenzoate
95–99	Nandrolone Phenylpropionate
95–100	Cinchocaine Hydrochloride
	Tropicamide
96	Trazodone
96–97.5	Dodecyl Gallate
96–98	Cocaine
96.5–101.5	Chlorprothixene
98	Bretylium Tosylate
98–104	Testosterone Cypionate
98–104d	Noradrenaline Acid Tartrate
98–108	α-Methyltryptamine
99	Pholcodine
99–100	Homatropine
99–102	Mexenone
99–103	Mepyramine Maleate
100	Butacaine Sulphate
	Orciprenaline
	Quinalbarbitone
100d	Dimethisterone
100–101	Opipramol
	Valethamate Bromide
100–103	Alverine Citrate
	Medazepam
100–115	Methylchlorophenoxyacetic Acid (technical)
101	Phenylpropanolamine
101–103	Propyphenazone
101–104	Phenprobamate
101–105	Pipobroman
102–103	Clorgyline Hydrochloride
102–105	Oxpentifylline
102–106	Piperacetazine
102–107	Dimenhydrinate
102–108	Gentamicin
<103	Physostigmine
103	Isoxsuprine
103–104	Diphenidol
103–107	Meprobamate
103–108	Choline Dihydrogen Citrate
	Doxylamine Succinate
103–113	Dexbrompheniramine Maleate
104	Aldrin (pure)
	Oxethazaine
104–105	Terbutryne
104–107	Phenylbutazone
104–108	Stilboestrol Dipropionate
104–109	Penfluridol
104–110	Acetylcysteine
105	Brucine (hydrated)
	Prednisolone Steaglate
105–107	Menadione

°C	Compound
105–108	Isocarboxazid
105–109	Metipranolol
105–110	Fenoprofen Calcium
	Hexamine Hippurate
106	Captopril
	Lofepramine
	Piperazine
106–109	Cyclizine
	Hyoscyamine
	Oxprenolol Hydrochloride
	Pheniramine Maleate
106–110d	Procaine Penicillin
106–116	Domiphen Bromide
107	Tripelennamine Citrate
107–108	Bupivacaine
107–110	Butethamate Citrate
108	Amidopyrine
	Naftidrofuryl Oxalate
	Talbutal
108–109	Dropropizine
108–110	Styramate
108–111	Alprenolol Hydrochloride
108–112	Prothipendyl Hydrochloride
109	Acetylcarbromal
	Dicophane
	α-Endosulfan
109–110	Butyl Aminobenzoate Picrate
	Loxapine
109–112	Resorcinol
109–113	Dextromethorphan
	Tolnaftate
110	Flurbiprofen
	Nimorazole
110–113	Phenazone
110–115	Dexchlorpheniramine Maleate
111	Pralidoxime Methylsulphate
	Talbutal
111–112	Buphenine
	Nandrolone
111–115	Clomiphene
111–117	Cyclopentamine Hydrochloride
112	Lindane
112–113	Dihydrocodeine
112–115	Acetomenaphthone
	Adiphenine Hydrochloride
112–116	Biperiden
	Chloropyrilene Citrate
113	Chlorquinaldol
	Cyproheptadine
	Dihydrotachysterol
	Iproniazid
113–115	Acetanilide
113–119	Ergocalciferol
114	Benzhexol
114–116	Chloroxylenol
	Diloxanide Furoate
	Perazine Dimalonate
114–117	Levorphanol Tartrate
	Methaqualone
	Testosterone Phenylpropionate
114–118	Atropine
115	Bamipine
	Chlormezanone

°C	Compound
	Pentobarbitone (polymorphic form)
	Pericyazine
115–116	Caramiphen Edisylate
	Cephaëline
115–118	Busulphan
	Ethyl Hydroxybenzoate
116	Hydrastine Hydrochloride
	Tryptamine
116–117	Dibenzepin
116–121	Carbinoxamine Maleate
116–122	Clothiapine
117	Hydrastinine
117–118	Hordenine
117–120	Carbromal
	Ethoxazene
118	Chlorotrianisene
118–119	Methylchlorophenoxyacetic Acid (pure)
	Pseudoephedrine
118–120	Morinamide
	Prometryne
118–121	Triprolidine Hydrochloride
118–123	Testosterone Propionate
119	Chloramphenicol Cinnamate
119d	Ecothiopate Iodide
119–121	Mandelic Acid
119–122	Terbutaline
119–123	Acebutolol
	Gestronol Hexanoate
119–124	Sulphafurazole Diethanolamine
120	Metoprolol Tartrate
	Naphazoline
120–124	Hydroxyprogesterone Hexanoate
120–125	Suprofen
121	Antazoline
	Etilefrine Hydrochloride
	Octamylamine Hydrochloride
	β-Progesterone
	Trimetozine
121–123	Betanaphthol
	Sulforidazine
121–124	Benzoic Acid
122–125	Carbimazole
122–127	Butobarbitone
122–128	Penthienate Methobromide
123	Ethacrynic Acid
123d	Ethylmorphine Hydrochloride
123–127	Thiambutosine
123–129	Dihydrotachysterol
123.5–125	Bamethan
124	Nandrolone
124d	Chloral Betaine
124–125	Dimoxyline
	Flufenamic Acid
124–127	Dipipanone Hydrochloride
124–130	Gestronol Hexanoate
124–136	Nadolol
125d	Dextromethorphan Hydrobromide
125–126	Hydroxyamphetamine
	Pipamperone Hydrochloride

°C	Compound
125–127	Phenglutarimide
	Sulphaurea
125–128	Mecloqualone
	Methyl Hydroxybenzoate
125–140d	Chloropyrilene Citrate
126	Methotrimeprazine
	Protokylol Hydrochloride
126–127	Butanilicaine Phosphate
126–128	Bemegride
126–129	Chlormethiazole Edisylate
126–130	Chlorpropamide
126–131	Ethynodiol Diacetate
	Progesterone
	Tetrabenazine
126–132	Tolbutamide
127	Neopine
	Tinidazole
127d	Hexamine Mandelate
	Propylhexedrine Hydro-
	chloride
127–128	Atropine Oxide
	Hexoestrol Dipropionate
127–129	Conessine
127–130	Aprindine Hydrochloride
127–131	Pyrrobutamine Phosphate
127–133	Drostanolone Propionate
	Meptazinol
	Pentobarbitone
128	Idobutal
	Prenalterol Hydrochloride
128d	Isoprenaline Sulphate
128–131	Nicotinamide
128–132	Tylosin
128–135	Piminodine Esylate
129	Physostigmine Aminoxide
130	Methoxyphenamine Hydro-
	chloride
	Ranitidine Hydrochloride
130–131	Lobeline
	Proguanil
130–131.5	Benzquinamide
130–132	Bitoscanate
	Thialbarbitone Sodium
130–133	Histamine Acid Phosphate
130–135	Brompheniramine Maleate
	Chlorpheniramine Maleate
	Chlorphenoxamine Hydro-
	chloride
131	Benzphetamine Hydrochloride
131–132	Captodiame Hydrochloride
131–133	Xylometazoline
131–134	Etenzamide
	Morazone
131–135	Bisacodyl
	Diazepam
	Sulphinpyrazone
131–136	Mebeverine Hydrochloride
132	Benzylmorphine
	Hydrastine
132–133	Famprofazone
	Thiamylal
132–135	Urea
132–135d	Thebacon Hydrochloride
132–137	Sorbic Acid

°C	Compound
132–137d	Cotarnine
132–143	Nicofuranose
133	Prolintane Hydrochloride
133d	Hydroxyurea
	Prajmalium Bitartrate
133–137	Methapyrilene Fumarate
134	Ambucetamide
	Amethocaine Hydrochloride
	Chlorhexidine
134–135	Acetylcodeine
134–136	Flufenamic Acid
	Proxyphylline
134–137	Clefamide
	Muzolimine
	Phenacetin
134–138	Orphenadrine Citrate
134–142	Poldine Methylsulphate
134–145	Thiocarlide
134–147	Amethocaine Hydrochloride
135	Erythromycin
	Norethandrolone
135–136	Chelidonine
135–137	Flunixin Meglumine
135–138	Cyclopentolate Hydrochloride
	Erythromycin Estolate
135–140	Alfentanil Hydrochloride
135–141	Butalamine Hydrochloride
136	Fenclofenac
	Meclofenoxate Hydrochloride
136–138	Nicergoline
136–139	Acepromazine Maleate
	Nitroxynil
136–140	Methoin
136–141	Diethylcarbamazine Citrate
	Phenoxybenzamine Hydro-
	chloride
137–140	Cyclofenil
	Prenylamine Lactate
138	δ-Benzene Hexachloride
	Methallenoestril
	Narceine (anhydrous)
	Xylazine
138–140	Bufotenine
	Phenyltoloxamine Citrate
138–141	Butalbital
	Dimetridazole
139	Amethocaine Hydrochloride
	Thiethylperazine Malate
139–140	Cyclopentobarbitone
139–142	Salicylamide
140	Ajmaline Hydrochloride
	Amitriptyline Embonate
	Dichlorophenoxyacetic Acid
	Ethoheptazine Citrate
	Pentaerythritol Tetranitrate
	Thioproperazine
140–142	Isoniazid Aminosalicylate
	Phenyramidol Hydrochloride
140–143	Clonidine
	Prothionamide
140–144	Hyoscine Butylbromide
	Trimipramine Maleate
140–145	Phenylephrine Hydrochloride
140–146	Tylosin Tartrate

°C	Compound
140–148	Pentapiperide Methylsulphate
141–142	Deoxycortone
141–143	Clindamycin Hydrochloride
141–144	Acebutolol Hydrochloride
	Practolol
	Verapamil Hydrochloride
141–145	Benztropine Mesylate
141–146	Ethinyloestradiol
142	Aprobarbitone
	Carbaryl
	Cimetidine
142d	Clotrimazole
	Pheniramine Aminosalicylate
142–143	Tramazoline
142–144	Bibenzonium Bromide
142–146	Caramiphen Hydrochloride
143	Acetylcholine Bromide
	Aspirin
	Mequitazine
143–147	Physostigmine Sulphate
	Tofenacin Hydrochloride
143–148	Methoxsalen
	Prazepam
143–150	Oestradiol Valerate
144	Berberine
	Iprindole Hydrochloride
	Tetrazepam
144–145	Carbutamide
144–147	Methimazole
144–148	Dimethisoquin Hydrochloride
	Droperidol
	Hexobarbitone
144–149	Neostigmine Methylsulphate
144–150	Diphenadione
145	Salsalate
145d	Clomiphene Citrate
145–146	Noradrenaline Hydrochloride
	Profadol Hydrochloride
145–147	Paraphenylenediamine
145–149	Bezitramide
145–154	Azatadine Maleate
145–155	Veratrine
146	Cycloguanil
	Ketoconazole
146–147	Oxethazaine Hydrochloride
146–148	Atenolol
	Papaverine
146–149	Nicotinyl Tartrate
146–151	Propoxycaine Hydrochloride
146–154	Mestranol
147–148	Etilefrine
147–150	Cholesterol
147–151	Pyrantel Tartrate
147–152	Fentanyl Citrate
	Haloperidol
	Thiothixene
147–152d	Adrenaline Acid Tartrate
147–158	Pentazocine
148	Amethocaine Hydrochloride
	Barbaloin
	Methacholine Bromide
	Metoclopramide
148d	Isometheptene Mucate
148–149	Mefruside

°C	Compound	°C	Compound	°C	Compound
148–150	Thialbarbitone	158–160	Midazolam	164–167	Dipyridamole
148–151	Phenindione	158–160d	Bufexamac		Xylazine Hydrochloride
148–152	Bromodiphenhydramine	158–161	Lidoflazine	164–168	Phenelzine Sulphate
	Hydrochloride		Salicylic Acid	165	Betamethasone Acetate
149	Hyoscyamine Hydrobromide	158–162	Indomethacin		Glafenine
149–150	Piritramide		Pargyline Hydrochloride		Sulphanilamide
149–153	Chloramphenicol	158–163	Benzethonium Chloride	165d	Acetophenazine Maleate
	Mepivacaine	158–165	Dextropropoxyphene	165–167.5	Dimethyltryptamine Hydro-
	Oestradiol Cypionate		Napsylate		chloride
150	Acetylcholine Chloride		Ethionamide	165–168	Antazoline Mesylate
	Bromvaletone		Levopropoxyphene Napsylate		Secbutobarbitone
150–151	Aminosalicylic Acid	159	Aminotriazole		Tricyclamol Chloride
150–153	Meprylcaine Hydrochloride		α-Benzene Hexachloride	165–169	Procainamide Hydrochloride
151	Aminoglutethimide		Benzydamine Hydrochloride	165–170d	Edrophonium Chloride
	Benzbromarone		Chromonar Hydrochloride		Isoprenaline Hydrochloride
151–153	Ketotifen	159–160	Methindizate Hydrochloride	165–171	Alphaxalone
	Nialamide		Warfarin (pure)	166	Benapryzine Hydrochloride
151–154	Diethylthiambutene Hydro-	159–161	Amidephrine	166–168	Lorazepam
	chloride	159–162	Orphenadrine Hydrochloride	166–169	Prilocaine Hydrochloride
	Ethyl Gallate	159–163	Metronidazole	166–170	Denatonium Benzoate
	Mafenide		Trimeprazine Tartrate	167	Atropine Methonitrate
151–155	Metharbitone	160	Cephalothin		Benziodarone
152	Betahistine Hydrochloride		Pempidine Tartrate		Clemizole
152–153	Ibogaine		Suxamethonium Chloride	167–170	Alphadolone
152–154	Hydroxyephedrine	160–161	Azacyclonol		Morantel Tartrate
	Lofepramine Hydrochloride		Propiomazine Maleate	167–171	Dydrogesterone
152–156	Tienilic Acid	160–162	Phenindamine Tartrate		Heptabarbitone
152–157	Testosterone	160–163	Vinbarbitone		Thenyldiamine Hydrochloride
152–158	Anisindione	160–164	Lynoestrenol	167–172	Diphenhydramine Hydro-
153	Phenyl Aminosalicylate	160–165	Diprophylline		chloride
153–155	Cycloserine		Penicillamine Hydrochloride	167–174	Naltrexone
153–157	Pyridostigmine Bromide	161	Amiodarone Hydrochloride	168	Naphazoline Nitrate
153–158	Procaine Hydrochloride	161d	Dimethindene Maleate		Protriptyline Hydrochloride
154	Thebacon	161–162	Butaperazine Phosphate	168d	Phenindamine Tartrate
154–155	Imolamine		Clorprenaline Hydrochloride		Proquamezine Fumarate
	Trichlorophenoxyacetic Acid	161–163d	Dimethoxanate Hydrochloride	168–169	Brallobarbitone
154–157	Cytisine	161–165	Methapyrilene Hydrochloride		Chlortetracycline
154–158	Codeine	161–166	Etofylline	168–172	Fenfluramine Hydrochloride
155	Ethyl Biscoumacetate	161–167	Hexachlorophane		Paracetamol
	Isoprenaline	161–169d	Tolazamide		Sulphamethoxazole
	Pralidoxime Mesylate	162	Ergometrine		Trometamol
	Stanozolol		Pholedrine	168–173d	Bephenium Hydroxy-
155–157	Nealbarbitone		Pipazethate Hydrochloride		naphthoate
155–157d	Tolmetin		Tilidate Hydrochloride	169	Hydroquinidine
155–161	Amylobarbitone	162–166	Cyclomethycaine Sulphate	169–171	Hydrocortisone Sodium
	Deoxycortone Acetate	162–168	Isoetharine Mesylate		Succinate
156	Amylobarbitone Sodium		Medigoxin	169–174	Dicyclomine Hydrochloride
	Naproxen		Methyltestosterone	169–175	Stilboestrol
	Salbutamol	162–171	Mafenide Acetate	170	Diamorphine
156–157	Ketobemidone	163	Norethisterone Acetate		Flunitrazepam
156–158	Diclofenac		Rolitetracycline	170–171	Metopimazine
156–159	Temazepam		Rotenone		Narceine
156–162	Thenium Closylate	163–164d	Amiphenazole	170–172	Thenalidine Tartrate
156–162d	Propantheline Bromide	163–167	Methandienone	170–173	Hydrocortisone Hydrogen
157	Colchicine	163–168d	Demecarium Bromide		Succinate
	Feprazone	163–169	Dextropropoxyphene Hydro-		Methacholine Chloride
	Warfarin (technical)		chloride	170–174	Hexobendine Hydrochloride
157d	Dihydromorphine (hydrated)	164	Aldosterone		Imipramine Hydrochloride
157–163	Thioridazine Hydrochloride		Bunitrolol		Isoniazid
158	Amodiaquine Hydrochloride		Phenazocine		Pramoxine Hydrochloride
	Mafenide Propionate		Propranolol Hydrochloride	170–175	Benperidol
	Oxybuprocaine Hydrochloride	164d	Econazole Nitrate		Bunamidine Hydroxy-
	Suxethonium Bromide	164–165	Guanoxan		naphthoate
158–159	Diuron		Tyramine	170–178	Fluopromazine Hydrochloride

°C	Compound	°C	Compound	°C	Compound
170–179d	Betamethasone Dipropionate	176	Fenticlor	183–184	Etafedrine Hydrochloride
171	Tramazoline Hydrochloride	176d	Triacetyloleandomycin		Tacrine
171d	Methoserpidine	176–179	Phenformin Hydrochloride	183–186	Bezafibrate
171–172d	Morazone Hydrochloride	176–181	Methylphenobarbitone		Eucatropine Hydrochloride
171–173	Pindolol	176–185d	Carphenazine Maleate	183–187	Meptazinol Hydrochloride
171–174d	Pecazine Hydrochloride	177d	Phenglutarimide Hydro-	184	Dextromoramide
171–175	Cyclobarbitone		chloride		Phenothiazine
	Nifedipine	177–180	Naloxone	184–185	Oxedrine
171–176d	Neostigmine Bromide	177–180d	Melphalan	184–186	Physostigmine Salicylate
171–177	Methanthelinium Bromide	177–181	Benactyzine Hydrochloride	184–190	Methdilazine Hydrochloride
171–178	Metaraminol Tartrate		Dinitolmide	185	Androsterone
171–179d	Pilocarpine Nitrate		Phenprocoumon		Bamifylline Hydrochloride
172	Dipyrone		Phentolamine Mesylate		Metoclopramide Hydro-
	Halopyramine Hydrochloride	178	Brucine (anhydrous)		chloride
	Metomidate Hydrochloride		Gelsemine		Norcodeine
172d	Methylergometrine		Gliquidone	185d	Ergometrine Maleate
172–173	Hydralazine		Hydroxyquinoline Sulphate		Oxedrine Tartrate
172–174	Glibenclamide		Trifluomeprazine Maleate		Rifampicin
	Hydroquinone	178d	Mesoridazine Benzene-	185–186	Viloxazine Hydrochloride
	Methylamphetamine Hydro-		sulphonate	185–186d	Pizotifen Malate
	chloride	178–179	Pyrantel	185–188	Diethazine Hydrochloride
172–175	Arecoline Hydrobromide	178–179d	Zomepirac		Hexoestrol
	Piperocaine Hydrochloride	178–181	Benorylate		Sulthiame
172–176	Coumatetralyl	178–183	Stanolone	185–191	Doxepin Hydrochloride
	Tolazoline Hydrochloride	178–185	Proxymetacaine Hydrochloride	185–192	Choline Theophyllinate
172–180	Oxymetholone	179–180	Tramadol Hydrochloride	185–195d	Methylergometrine Maleate
172–182	Phenmetrazine Hydrochloride	179–181	Nomifensine		Psilocybin
	Promazine Hydrochloride	179–182	Ibomal	186	4-Aminophenol (commercial)
173	Allobarbitone		Nitroxoline		Butriptyline Hydrochloride
	Hydroquinine	179–183	Sulphaphenazole	186d	Hexamethonium Tartrate
	Quinine	180	Ethyl Biscoumacetate	186–187d	Acetyl Sulphamethoxy-
	Santonin		Fenbufen		pyridazine
173–174	Camazepam		Labetalol Hydrochloride	186–188	Nifuratel
173–175	Atrazine		Lobeline Hydrochloride	186–189	Aminobenzoic Acid
173–176	Chloroprocaine Hydrochloride		Pipenzolate Bromide		Glibornuride
	Psilocin		Xanthinol Nicotinate	186–190	Pethidine Hydrochloride
	Thonzylamine Hydrochloride	180d	Clioquinol		Sulphaethidole
173–178	Dyclonine Hydrochloride		Ergotamine Tartrate		Trimethobenzamide Hydro-
173–179	Oestradiol		Quinidine Polygalacturonate		chloride
174	Carbarsone	180–181	Cathine Hydrochloride	186–202d	Phthalylsulphacetamide
	Phenylephrine		Molindone	187	Fluocortolone Pivalate
174–176d	Noscapine	180–182	Clobazam		Methallibure
174–177	Buformin		Levallorphan	187d	Methotrimeprazine Maleate
	Levallorphan Tartrate	180–183	Sulphamethoxypyridazine	187–188	Racephedrine Hydrochloride
	Normethadone Hydrochloride	180–186	Ethinyloestradiol	187–190	Propyliodone
174–178	Phenobarbitone	181	Gliclazide	188	Fenpipramide
174–179	Pseudoephedrine Sulphate		Isopropamide Iodide	188d	Ethopropazine Hybenzate
174–181	Camphor		Rotenone	188–191	Fluocortolone
174–184	Norethynodrel	181–182	Norpipanone		Pyrazinamide
175	Dichlorophen	181–183	Oxymetazoline	188–192	Barbitone
	Diloxanide	181–184	Sulphacetamide		Pentamidine Isethionate
	Dimethothiazine Mesylate	182	Miconazole Nitrate		Tripelennamine Hydrochloride
	Phenobarbitone Sodium	182–184	Heteronium Bromide	188–193	Sulphaguanidine
	Phentolamine		Hexylcaine	189	Perhexiline
	Rafoxanide		Tolpropamine Hydrochloride	189–190	Benoxaprofen
175d	Diethylpropion Hydrochloride	182–185	Sulindac	189–191	Dobutamine Hydrochloride
175–176	Amoxapine	182–186	Etisazole Hydrochloride		Noxiptyline Hydrochloride
175–177	Quinidine Gluconate		Pseudoephedrine Hydro-	189–192	Hydroxyamphetamine Hydro-
175–178	Sulfametopyrazine		chloride		bromide
175–179	Floctafenine	182–187	Acetohexamide	189–193	Carbamazepine
175–181	Alphadolone Acetate	182–189	Methotrexate	189–194	Ethylnoradrenaline Hydro-
	Dapsone	183	Clozapine		chloride
	Dithranol		Ketazolam	189–195	Ethoxzolamide
175–182d	Sulpiride	183d	Thiethylperazine Maleate	189–196	Diphemanil Methylsulphate

°C	Compound
	Cinchonidine
	Ethopropazine Hydrochloride
	Opipramol Hydrochloride
210–214	Hydrocortisone Hydrogen Succinate (recrystallised)
	Tolfenamic Acid
210–215	Chloroquine Phosphate
211	Bethanechol Chloride
	Coniine Hydrobromide
211–213	Fenpiprane Hydrochloride
211–215d	Azapetine
211–216	Vinblastine
212	Diflunisal
	Indoprofen
	Thymoxamine Hydrochloride
212d	Adrenaline
	Beclomethasone Dipropionate
	Flurazepam Hydrochloride
	Hydrastinine Hydrochloride
	Isothipendyl Hydrochloride
212–213	Cytarabine
212–214	Lachesine Chloride
212–214d	Ergotamine
212–218	Chlordiazepoxide Hydrochloride
212–218d	Methylpiperidyl Benzilate Hydrochloride
213	β-Endosulfan
	Methazolamide
	Phenacemide
213–216	Cinchophen
214	Desipramine Hydrochloride
214d	Hexoprenaline Sulphate
	Hydrocortisone
	Tetracycline Hydrochloride
214–215	Etorphine
	Loprazolam
214–216d	Cyproheptadine Hydrochloride
214–217d	Benzylpenicillin Potassium
	Homatropine Hydrobromide
214–218	Pimozide
214–219	Methoxamine Hydrochloride
214–221d	Diphenidol Hydrochloride
214–225d	Nifursol
215	Atropine Methobromide
	Clofazimine
	Fazadinium Bromide
	Levomethadyl Acetate Hydrochloride
215d	Cinchonine Hydrochloride (anhydrous)
	Pancuronium Bromide
215–216	Clioxanide
215–218d	Bromocriptine
215–219	Cyclobenzaprine Hydrochloride
215–220	Nortriptyline Hydrochloride
215–225d	Pralidoxime Chloride
216	Methixene Hydrochloride
	Methyclothiazide
	Nordazepam
216–218	Cantharidin
217	Megestrol Acetate
217d	Diminazene Aceturate

°C	Compound
	Noradrenaline
217–219d	Butorphanol Tartrate
217–220	Ephedrine Hydrochloride
217–221	Acetyldigitoxin
217–224	Griseofulvin
	Meclozine Hydrochloride
217–224d	Cortisone
217–225	Cyclothiazide
218	Pentazocine Hydrochloride
218–219d	Solanidine
218–220	Alphaprodine Hydrochloride
	Oxycodone
	Vincristine
218–221	Propylthiouracil
219	ε-Benzene Hexachloride
	Bethanechol Chloride
219–220	Trimethoxyamphetamine Hydrochloride
220	Amygdalin
	Deslanoside
	Doxapram Hydrochloride
220d	Bendrofluazide
	Betamethasone Benzoate
	Chlorthalidone
	Hydrocortisone Acetate
	Papaverine Hydrochloride
	Pralidoxime Iodide
	Rimiterol Hydrobromide
220–225	Syrosingopine
220–226	Diphenoxylate Hydrochloride
222d	Carbazochrome
	Promethazine Hydrochloride
222–223	Hydroxyprogesterone
222–228	Trimetazidine Hydrochloride
223	Glymidine
223d	Procarbazine Hydrochloride
223–226	Buphenine Hydrochloride
224d	Dothiepin Hydrochloride
224–227	Simazine
224–227d	Parbendazole
225	Chlorcyclizine Hydrochloride
	Fludrocortisone Acetate
	Metformin Hydrochloride
	Suxamethonium Bromide
	Trazodone Hydrochloride
225d	Dexamethasone Acetate
	Hyoscine Methobromide
	Loperamide Hydrochloride
	Methylprednisolone Acetate
	Minoxidil
	Obidoxime Chloride
225–227	Procyclidine Hydrochloride
225–230d	Thiacetazone
225–231	Alprazolam
	Nalidixic Acid
226	Dibromopropamidine Isethionate
	Ethacridine
	Phenylmethylbarbituric Acid
	Rescinnamine
226–228	Flunixin
226–230	Nitrazepam
	Saccharin
227	Metolazone

°C	Compound
	Thioproperazine Mesylate
227–228d	Carbazochrome Sodium Sulphonate
227–229	Levamisole Hydrochloride
227–234	Dienoestrol
228	Azapropazone (anhydrous)
	Niclosamide
	Phencyclidine Hydrochloride
228–229d	Ambutonium Bromide
228–232	Thiopropazate Hydrochloride
229	Prednisolone Pivalate
229–233	Diamorphine Hydrochloride
230	Bumetanide
	Fluphenazine Hydrochloride
	Mefenamic Acid
	Trioxsalen
230d	Betaine Hydrochloride
	Endrin
	Fenoterol Hydrobromide
	Mepenzolate Bromide
	Prednisone
230–232	Maprotiline Hydrochloride
	Vindesine
230–234d	Deserpidine
230–235d	Prednisolone
230–236	Flavoxate Hydrochloride
230–240	Buclizine Hydrochloride
	Flupenthixol Hydrochloride
231	Nalbuphine
231–234	Cycloguanil Embonate
232d	Trimetaphan Camsylate
232–247	Cetrimide
233	Diaveridine
233d	Fenbendazole
233–235	Triazolam
233–236	Methadone Hydrochloride
234	Chlorphentermine Hydrochloride
	Clonixin
	Oxyphencyclimine Hydrochloride
	Yohimbine
234–235	Tigloidine Hydrobromide
234–237	Nicotinic Acid
234–239	Caffeine
234–239d	Sulfamerazine
235	Aminacrine Hydrochloride
	Bromhexine Hydrochloride
	Hydroxystilbamidine
	Propamidine Isethionate
	Stanozolol
235d	Cyclopenthiazide
	Gallamine Triethiodide
	Phenazopyridine Hydrochloride
	Prednisolone Acetate
	Quinuronium Sulphate
235–236d	Thyroxine
235–255	Emetine Hydrochloride (dried)
236	Amiphenazole Hydrochloride
236d	Liothyronine
	Nitrofurazone
237	Dibenzepin Hydrochloride
238	Harman

°C	Compound	°C	Compound	°C	Compound
238d	Azathioprine		Guanethidine Monosulphate		Fluocinolone Acetonide
238–240d	Cambendazole		Mepacrine Hydrochloride		Potassium Sorbate
238–242	Pyrimethamine		Methaqualone Hydrochloride		Reserpine
239	Clonazepam		Morphine Sulphate		Tubocurarine Chloride
	Dihydroergotamine		Piperazine Adipate		Tyramine Hydrochloride
239–241	Fendosal		Sulfaquinoxaline	270–274	Theophylline
	Morantel	250–253	Indoramin Hydrochloride	270–275	Hydroflumethiazide
240	Ametazole Hydrochloride	250–253d	Dexamethasone	270–281	Azacyclonol Hydrochloride
	Benzthiazide	250–256	Triclocarban	271	Nitrofurantoin
	Chlordiazepoxide	251–253	Racemorphan	272	Theophylline Hydrate
	Dichlorphenamide	252	Tryptamine Hydrochloride	272–276	Ethisterone
	Hydroxychloroquine Sulphate	252d	Nefopam Hydrochloride	273–274	Hydroquinidine Hydrochloride
	Methacycline Hydrochloride	254	Pentazocine Hydrochloride	273–277	Normorphine
	Phentolamine Hydrochloride	254–255	Protoveratrine B	274d	Debrisoquine Sulphate
240d	Acetarsol	254–256d	Morphine		Trichlormethiazide
	Antazoline Hydrochloride	255	Bufylline	274–276	Naltrexone Hydrochloride
	Betamethasone		Inositol Nicotinate	275	Oxycodone Hydrochloride
	Cortisone Acetate		Terbutaline Sulphate	275d	Biperiden Hydrochloride
	Digoxin	255d	Chlorhexidine Hydrochloride		Hydralazine Hydrochloride
	Lanatoside C		Naphazoline Hydrochloride		Levodopa
	Lysergic Acid		Sulphadiazine		Phthalylsulphathiazole
	Paramethasone Acetate		Sulphasalazine	276	Hydroxyprogesterone
	Prednisone Acetate	255–262d	Mepivacaine Hydrochloride	277	Triamcinolone Acetonide
240–242	Amiloride	256	Digitoxin		Vincristine Sulphate
240–243d	Methylprednisolone	256d	Tetrahydrozoline Hydro-	278	Fluoxymesterone
241	Aminacrine		chloride	278d	Mannomustine
241d	Dopamine Hydrochloride	256–262d	Protoveratrines A and B	278–280	Prazosin
	Mannomustine Hydrochloride	257d	Clopenthixol Hydrochloride	279–280	Dantrolene
241–242d	Sodium Cromoglycate	258d	Ephedrine Sulphate	279–284	Primidone
242	Clidinium Bromide	258–261	Ketamine Hydrochloride	280	Bethanidine Sulphate
	Decoquinate	258–263	Phenolphthalein		Hydroxystilbamidine
	Prochlorperazine Mesylate	259	Pemoline		Isethionate
242d	Cycrimine Hydrochloride	259d	Furazolidone		Oestriol
	Trifluoperazine	259–262	Protoveratrine A	280d	Codeine Hydrochloride
242–245d	Loprazolam Mesylate	260	Acepifylline		Dequalinium Acetate
243d	Triphenyltetrazolium Chloride		Disulphamide		Fluorometholone
244	Fluocortolone Hexanoate		Mafenide Hydrochloride		Hexamethonium Bromide
244–246	Sulphasomidine	260d	Acetazolamide		Riboflavine
245	Dihydralazine Sulphate		Hydromorphone	282	Stilbazium Iodide
	Oxyphenisatin Acetate		Mebezonium Iodide	282–284	Mianserin Hydrochloride
	Proguanil Hydrochloride		Oestrone	283–284	Tacrine Hydrochloride
245d	Ethacridine Lactate		Xipamide	283–285	Diclofenac Sodium
	Fluclorolone Acetonide	>260d	Trilostane	284d	Vinblastine Sulphate
	Histamine Hydrochloride	260–263	Nalorphine Hydrochloride	285d	Cyclizine Hydrochloride
	Homidium Bromide	260–264	Niridazole	285–288d	Amiloride Hydrochloride
	Mecamylamine	261d	Harmine	285–290d	Protoveratrine B
	Tocainide Hydrochloride	261–263d	Pizotifen	289–291	Meclofenamate Sodium
245–252	Quinethazone	262	Triamcinolone	289–292	5-Methyltryptamine Hydro-
246	Clemizole Hydrochloride	263	Lorcainide Hydrochloride		chloride
	Clopamide	264	Cinchonine	290	Dicoumarol
246–247	Chlorproguanil Hydrochloride	264d	Prazosin Hydrochloride		Mebendazole
247	Bromazepam	264–265	Tetramisole Hydrochloride	290d	Pipradrol Hydrochloride
247d	Amprolium Hydrochloride	264–265d	Acinitrazole	291–294	Carbenoxolone
247–248	Azapropazone (dihydrate)		Halcinonide	295d	Flucytosine
247–255	Flurandrenolone	265d	Decamethonium Bromide		Phanquone
248d	Barbituric Acid	266	Clorexolone		Phenytoin
	Methisazone	266–267	Etorphine Hydrochloride	295–296d	Triamcinolone Hexacetonide
	Thiamine Hydrochloride	266–269	Flugestone Acetate	295–300	Dexamphetamine Sulphate
248–249d	Oxymorphone	268	Strychnine	296	Enoxolone
248–250d	Bupivacaine Hydrochloride	268d	Hydrochlorothiazide	296–303	Thiabendazole
248–253d	Pirenzepine Hydrochloride	269–270	Ethiazide	299–300d	Ibogaine Hydrochloride
249–250d	Harmaline	269–271	Thalidomide	300d	Amphetamine Sulphate
250	Suxamethonium Iodide	270	Metolazone		Fluocinonide
250d	Benzhexol Hydrochloride	270d	Anileridine Hydrochloride		Oxymetazoline Hydrochloride

°C	Compound	°C	Compound	°C	Compound
	Xylometazoline Hydrochloride	310d	Betaine	330d	Methylthiouracil
>300	Rimantadine Hydrochloride	312	β-Benzene Hexachloride	330–331	Diazoxide
302d	Yohimbine Hydrochloride	313	Clonidine Hydrochloride	335	Diquat Dibromide
302–304d	Protoveratrine A	315d	Benzoctamine Hydrochloride	340d	Chlorothiazide
303–305	Zomepirac Sodium		Dequalinium Chloride		Conessine Hydrobromide
305–315d	Hydromorphone Hydro-	>320	Clopidol	360d	Amantadine Hydrochloride
	chloride	321d	Pholedrine Sulphate	618	Lithium Carbonate
308d	Mercaptopurine	327d	Pseudomorphine		
310	Methyldopa	329	Octatropine Methylbromide		

Thin-layer Chromatographic Data

s = 'with streaking'

System TA (p. 167)—Rf Values

Rf	Compound
00	Adrenaline
	Decamethonium Bromide
	Demecarium Bromide
	Diminazene
	Diquat Dibromide
	Distigmine Bromide
	Ethyl Nicotinate
	Gallamine Triethiodide
	Hexamethonium Bromide
	Hydrastinine
	Mebezonium Iodide
	Neomycin
	Noradrenaline
	Paraquat Dichloride
	Pentolinium Tartrate
	Quinuronium Sulphate
	Streptomycin
	Tubocurarine Chloride
01	Alcuronium Chloride
	Benserazide
	Bethanidine
	Bretylium Tosylate
	Carbachol
	Debrisoquine
	Dibromopropamidine
	Dihydrostreptomycin
	Guanethidine
	Guanoxan
	Hexylcaine
	Homatropine
	Hydroxystilbamidine
	Hyoscine
	Kanamycin
	Mepenzolate Bromide
	Metformin
	Obidoxime Chloride
	Pancuronium Bromide
	Pentamidine
	Pentapiperide
	Propamidine
	Pyrithidium Bromide
	Suxamethonium Chloride
	Suxethonium Bromide
	Thiamine
02	Acetylcholine Chloride
	Ambenonium Chloride
	Amprolium Hydrochloride
	Atropine Methonitrate
	Bethanechol Chloride
	Bibenzonium Bromide
	Buformin
	Cadaverine
	Cetrimide
	Choline
	Clidinium Bromide

Rf	Compound
	Cotarnine
	Diphemanil Methylsulphate
	Ecothiopate Iodide
	Hexocyclium Methylsulphate
	Homatropine Methobromide
	Hyoscine Methonitrate
	Lachesine Chloride
	Methacholine Chloride
	Methanthelinium Bromide
	Neostigmine Bromide
	Octatropine Methylbromide
	Oxyphencyclimine
	Penthienate Methobromide
	Poldine Methylsulphate
	Putrescine
	Thenium Closylate
	Thiazinamium Methylsulphate
	Trimetaphan Camsylate
	Valethamate Bromide
03	Ambutonium Bromide
	Benzethonium Chloride
	Benzilonium Bromide
	Chlorproguanil
	Dequalinium Chloride
	Dofamium Chloride
	Glycopyrronium Bromide
	Guanoclor
	Heteronium Bromide
	Hexoprenaline
	Oxyphenonium Bromide
	Phenformin
	Proguanil
04	Acepifylline
	Pipenzolate Bromide
	Propantheline Bromide
	Pyridostigmine Bromide
05	Cytarabine
	Domiphen Bromide
	Emepronium Bromide
	Isopropamide Iodide
	Piperazine
	Pralidoxime Chloride
	Psilocybin
	Sparteine
05s	Amicarbalide
	Chlortetracycline
	Clomocycline
	Demeclocycline
	Lymecycline
	Methacycline
	Oxytetracycline
	Rolitetracycline
	Tetracycline
06	Pyrantel
	Tramazoline

Rf	Compound
	Tricyclamol Chloride
07	Acriflavine
	Berberine
	Edrophonium Chloride
	Tridihexethyl Chloride
08	Hyoscine Butylbromide
08s	Desferrioxamine
09	Oxymetazoline
10	Azacyclonol
	Betahistine
	Denatonium Benzoate
	Mequitazine
	Stilbazium Iodide
12	Doxorubicin
	Doxycycline
12s	Cetalkonium Chloride
13	Benztropine
	Deptropine
	Histamine
	Nitroxoline
	Norcodeine
	Tetrahydrozoline
	Tolazoline
	Xylometazoline
14	Naphazoline
15	Amidephrine
	Maprotiline
15s	Octaphonium Chloride
16	Brucine
	Mecamylamine
	Proflavine Hemisulphate
17	Ecgonine
	Normorphine
18	Atropine
	Hyoscyamine
	N-Methyltryptamine
18s	Dopamine
19	Primaquine
	Protriptyline
19s	Halquinol
20	Cetylpyridinium Chloride
	Cyclopentamine
	Mescaline
21	Atropine Oxide
	Benzoylecgonine
	Metanephrine
22	Acriflavine
	Octamylamine
	Trimetazidine
	Vancomycin
23	Amantadine
	Betaine
	Heptaminol
	Hydromorphone
	Methoxyphenamine

Rf	Compound
	Tryptamine
24	Amiloride
	Isometheptene
	Mersalyl Acid
	Pempidine
25	Dihydromorphine
	Hydrocodone
	Mephentermine
	Oxedrine
	Serotonin
26	Ametazole
	Coniine
	Desipramine
	Dihydrocodeine
	Propylhexedrine
	Strychnine
28	Acriflavine
	Conessine
	Homochlorcyclizine
29	Methdilazine
	Pholedrine
30	Ephedrine
	Ethambutol
	Hexamine
31	Antazoline
	Methylamphetamine
	Physostigmine Aminoxide
	Tyramine
32	Methylephedrine
	Phentolamine
32s	Hydroxyquinoline
33	Chlorhexidine
	Codeine
	Normetanephrine
	Phenylephrine
	Pseudoephedrine
	Trimethoxyamphetamine
	Tuaminoheptane
34	Dextromethorphan
	Nortriptyline
35	Bufotenine
	Dextrorphan
	Hydroxyamphetamine
	Levorphanol
	Neopine
	Racemorphan
35s	Hydroxyephedrine
36	Methindizate
	Monocrotaline
	Penicillamine
	Pholcodine
37	Morphine
	Rimantadine
38	Chloroquine
	Harmaline
	Mesoridazine
	Sulpiride
39	Azatadine
	Dimethoxanate
	Methylenedioxyamphetamine
	Psilocin
40	Cytisine
	Dimethyltryptamine
	Ethoheptazine

Rf	Compound
	Ethylmorphine
	Hordenine
	Isoprenaline
	Mexiletine
	Phenglutarimide
41	Benzylmorphine
	Etilefrine
	Perhexiline
	Xanthinol Nicotinate
42	Cathine
	Dimethindene
	Ethylnoradrenaline
	Metaraminol
	Nadolol
	Profadol
	Spiramycin
	Tigloidine
	Trimethobenzamide
	Viloxazine
43	Amphetamine
	Dehydroemetine
	Furaltadone
	Mepacrine
	Tacrine
44	Benzydamine
	Chlorphentermine
	Cycloserine
	Etafedrine
	Furazolidone
	Hydroquinine
	Phenylpropanolamine
	Promazine
45	Atenolol
	Brompheniramine
	Chlorpheniramine
	Disopyramide
	Hydroquinidine
	Hydroxychloroquine
	Oleandomycin
	Pheniramine
	Practolol
	Thebacon
	Thebaine
	Tofenacin
46	Clemastine
	Diethyltryptamine
	Diphenylpyraline
	Eucatropine
	6-Monoacetylmorphine
	Phentermine
	Pseudomorphine
	Salbutamol
	Thioproperazine
47	Acebutolol
	Diamorphine
	Hexobendine
	Iprindole
	Isoniazid
	Ketobemidone
	Metoclopramide
	Pipazethate
	Prenalterol
	Prothipendyl
	Terbutaline

Rf	Compound
	Zimeldine
48	Acepromazine
	Carbetapentane
	Carbinoxamine
	Chromonar
	Diprophylline
	Doxylamine
	Fenfluramine
	Imipramine
	Methadone
	Orciprenaline
	Oxprenolol
	Oxymorphone
	Perazine
	Pizotifen
	Procyclidine
	Thioridazine
49	Bamipine
	Chlorpromazine
	Cinchonidine
	Cinchonine
	Gelsemine
	Mafenide
	Methyldopa
	Metoprolol
	Phanquone
	Phenethylamine
	Pindolol
	Procainamide
	Procarbazine
	Prochlorperazine
	Thiothixene
50	Alphaprodine
	Methixene
	Nefopam
	Oxeladin
	Oxycodone
	Phenmetrazine
	Prolintane
	Promethazine
	Propranolol
	Proquamezine
	Thenalidine
51	Amitriptyline
	Broxyquinoline
	Clomipramine
	Cyproheptadine
	DOM
	Dothiepin
	Doxepin
	Hydralazine
	Mepyramine
	Minoxidil
	Quinidine
	Quinine
	Thiethylperazine
	Tolpropamine
	Triamterene
	Triprolidine
52	Alprenolol
	Caffeine
	Chlophedianol
	Diamthazole
	Diethylcarbamazine

Rf	Compound
	Mebeverine
	Phenindamine
	Pyrazinamide
	Trazodone
	Yohimbine
64	Adiphenine
	Benethamine
	Biperiden
	Bunamidine
	Chlormethiazole
	Cropropamide
	Doxapram
	Etenzamide
	Mephenesin
	Naftidrofuryl Oxalate
	Nicergoline
	Norharman
	Noscapine
	Sulphadiazine
	Sulphasomidine
65	Bamifylline
	Beclamide
	Benzquinamide
	Bitoscanate
	Cocaine
	Dropropizine
	Ethionamide
	Ethoxazene
	Ibogaine
	Mebendazole
	Mepivacaine
	Methisazone
	Methyldopate
	Methysergide
	Naloxone
	Phenazone
	Prazepam
	Protokylol
	Sulfamerazine
	Sulphadimethoxine
	Sulphafurazole
	Sulphaguanidine
	Sulphamethizole
	Sulphamethoxazole
	Sulphamethoxypyridazine
	Triacetyloleandomycin
	Trifluomeprazine
	Tropicamide
66	Alverine
	Amidopyrine
	Azaperone
	Benactyzine
	Captodiame
	Caramiphen
	Chlormezanone
	Co-dergocrine
	Cycrimine
	Diloxanide
	Dipipanone
	Ergotoxine
	Ketazolam
	Pipobroman
	Propanidid
	Prothionamide

Rf	Compound
	Sulphasalazine
	Sulphathiazole
67	Benorylate
	Benzocaine
	Clorgyline
	Droperidol
	Ethopropazine
	Etomidate
	Haloperidol
	Levallorphan
	Lincomycin
	Medazepam
	Piminodine
	Sulfadoxine
	Sulfametopyrazine
	Sulphaethidole
	Sulphamoxole
	Sulphanilamide
	Sulphapyridine
	Thiabendazole
	Viprynium Embonate
68	Aconitine
	Aminotriazole
	Azapropazone
	Benzhexol
	Butalamine
	Dextropropoxyphene
	Dicyclomine
	Dimoxyline
	Dipyridamole
	Hydroxyzine
	Isoaminile
	Nifedipine
	Nitrazepam
	Norpipanone
	Oxypertine
	Phenazocine
	Prenylamine
	Solanidine
69	Bupivacaine
	Butethamate
	Clefamide
	Fluspirilene
	Iproniazid
	Phenyramidol
	Piperidolate
	Reserpine
	Sulphaphenazole
	Tetrabenazine
70	Aminosalicylic Acid
	Azapetine
	Clofazimine
	Dexpanthenol
	Diethylthiambutene
	Diperodon
	Diprenorphine
	Ethosuximide
	Fentanyl
	Harman
	Hexetidine
	Hexyl Nicotinate
	Lidoflazine
	Lignocaine
	Loperamide

Rf	Compound
	Mebanazine
	Methaqualone
	Methocarbamol
	Nialamide
	Norbormide
	Parbendazole
	Pargyline
	Piritramide
	Pramoxine
	Protoveratrine B
	Sulphacetamide
	Sulphachlorpyridazine
71	Bezitramide
	Butacaine
	Chlorquinaldol
	Disulfiram
	Isocarboxazid
	Phenoperidine
	Pimozide
	Propyphenazone
	Sulfaquinoxaline
72	Acetorphine
	Amiodarone
	Aniline
	Bromocriptine
	Carbimazole
	Chelidonine
	Chlorpropamide
	Clindamycin
	Clonazepam
	Deserpidine
	Embutramide
	Famprofazone
	Methazolamide
	Methoserpidine
	Pentetrazol
	Phenbutrazate
	Protoveratrine A
	Tylosin
73	Ambucetamide
	Anileridine
	Benzphetamine
	Cephaloridine
	Desmetryne
	Diethyltoluamide
	Etorphine
	Fluanisone
	Methoxyamphetamine
	Metomidate
	Miconazole
	Nifuratel
	Phenoxybenzamine
	Rescinnamine
	Ritodrine
	Simazine
	Trifluperidol
74	Bialamicol
	Bisacodyl
	Broxaldine
	Buphenine
	Diphenoxylate
	Etisazole
	Hydroxyphenamate
	Methoprotryne

Rf	Compound	Rf	Compound	Rf	Compound
	Noxythiolin		Penfluridol		Rifampicin
	Selegiline		Pheneturide	80	Acinitrazole
75	Aminonitrothiazole		Prometryne		Glibenclamide
	Bromhexine		Sulphaurea		Thiocarlide
	Buclizine		Thiambutosine		Trichlormethiazide
	Cinchophen		Tolbutamide	81	Diamphenethide
	Diazepam	77	Atrazine		Piperidolate
	Dinitolmide		Bephenium Hydroxynaphthoate		Propyliodone
	Glutethimide		Cyclothiazide	82	Chlorphenesin
	Monosulfiram		Gloxazone		Diazoxide
	Padimate		Meclofenoxate		Dichlorphenamide
	Phenprobamate		Oxyphenbutazone		Oxyphenisatin
	Phensuximide		Phenelzine	83	Apomorphine
	Quinethazone		Pipoxolan		Crotamiton
	Theophylline		Prilocaine		Nitroxynil
76	Ametryne		Terbutryne	84	Clorazepic Acid
	Buprenorphine		Tybamate		Dipyrone
	Butanilicaine	78	Carbutamide		Rifamycin SV
	Cinnarizine		Clemizole		Salinazid
	Clorexolone		Isoxsuprine	86	Nifursol
	Dextromoramide		Stanozolol	87	Glipizide
	Diethylpropion		Syrosingopine		Oxyclozanide
	Ethinamate		Thiacetazone	88	Trilostane
	Ethoxzolamide	79	Clioxanide	89	Rafoxanide
	Glymidine		Clopamide	90	Buclosamide
	Meclozine		Methallibure	91	Niclosamide
	Methsuximide		Phenylbutazone		

System TB (p. 167)—Rf Values

Rf	Compound	Rf	Compound	Rf	Compound
00	Acebutolol		Debrisoquine		Metopimazine
	Adrenaline		Demoxepam		Minoxidil
	Ambazone		Diminazene		Morphine
	Amidephrine		Diprophylline		Narceine
	Amiloride		Dipyridamole		Nitrazepam
	Apomorphine		Dipyrone		Noradrenaline
	Atenolol		Dobutamine		Norbormide
	Azacyclonol		Ergometrine		Norcodeine
	Bamifylline		Ethionamide		Norharman
	Benorylate		Ethoxazene		Oxazepam
	Benserazide		Furaltadone		Pemoline
	Benzoylecgonine		Furazolidone		Pentapiperide
	Bethanidine		Glipizide		Phenformin
	Bromocriptine		Glymidine		Pilocarpine
	Broxyquinoline		Guanethidine		Practolol
	Brucine		Guanoclor		Proguanil
	Buformin		Guanoxan		Pseudomorphine
	Bufotenine		Harmine		Sulphaurea
	Chlorproguanil		Hydroxychloroquine		Trilostane
	Cimetidine		Hydroxystilbamidine		Trimethoprim
	Clefamide		Isoetharine	01	Acepifylline
	Clioquinol		Isoprenaline		Cephaëline
	Clonazepam		Mebendazole		Chlormezanone
	Colchicine		Metformin		Co-dergocrine
	Cytarabine		Methylergometrine		Cycloserine

Rf	Compound
	Cytisine
	Diazoxide
	Dihydroergotamine
	Dihydromorphine
	Ergotamine
	Ergotoxine
	Ethylnoradrenaline
	Heptaminol
	Hexoprenaline
	Homatropine
	Inositol Nicotinate
	Iproniazid
	Isoniazid
	Lorazepam
	Metaraminol
	Methimazole
	Methyldopa
	Methysergide
	Metoclopramide
	Nadolol
	Nalorphine
	Nifedipine
	Niridazole
	Orciprenaline
	Oxymetazoline
	Oxyphencyclimine
	Penicillamine
	Pentamidine
	Phenazopyridine
	Phentolamine
	Phenylephrine
	Pipamperone
	Piperazine
	Piritramide
	Prazosin
	Prenalterol
	Procainamide
	Propamidine
	Prothionamide
	Protokylol
	Rescinnamine
	Salbutamol
	Salinazid
	Sotalol
	Styramate
	Terbutaline
	Theobromine
	Theophylline
	Triamterene
	Triazolam
	Tryptamine
	Tuaminoheptane
	Vinblastine
02	Amiphenazole
	Buclosamide
	Chlordiazepoxide
	Droperidol
	Hydroquinine
	Hydroxyamphetamine
	Isoxsuprine
	Ketobemidone
	Mephenesin
	Metronidazole
	Nialamide

Rf	Compound
	Pindolol
	Pipobroman
	Procarbazine
	Proxyphylline
	Pyrimethamine
	Reserpine
	Tolazoline
03	Acetophenazine
	Azathioprine
	Buphenine
	Caffeine
	Clorazepic Acid
	Deserpidine
	Etenzamide
	Ethambutol
	Etilefrine
	Fenethylline
	Hydromorphone
	Hydroquinidine
	Lysergide
	Mesoridazine
	Methisazone
	Naphazoline
	Nimorazole
	Pericyazine
	Phanquone
	Pholcodine
	Propoxycaine
	Quinidine
	Quinine
04	Bamethan
	Carbamazepine
	Clozapine
	Fluspirilene
	Hexamine
	Hydrocodone
	Mescaline
	Methoserpidine
	Mexiletine
	Nicotinyl Alcohol
	Nordazepam
	Oxedrine
	Oxypertine
	Phenylpropanolamine
	Pholedrine
	Pimozide
	Tramazoline
	Veratrine
05	Ambucetamide
	Carphenazine
	Chloroprocaine
	Ephedrine
	Fenpipramide
	Flupenthixol
	Hordenine
	Neopine
	Psilocin
	Tacrine
	Trimetazidine
	Yohimbine
06	Atropine
	Benzocaine
	Benzylmorphine
	Cinchonidine

Rf	Compound
	Cinchonine
	Codeine
	Dehydroemetine
	Fluphenazine
	Hyoscine
	Mazindol
	Mequitazine
	6-Monoacetylmorphine
	Opipramol
	Pentifylline
	Piperacetazine
	Procaine
	Thiambutosine
	Timolol
07	Antazoline
	Benzquinamide
	Clopenthixol
	Disopyramide
	Ethylmorphine
	Etorphine
	Lormetazepam
	Pentetrazol
	Perphenazine
	Propranolol
	Tetrahydrozoline
	Thiabendazole
	Thiocarlide
	Thioproperazine
	Viloxazine
08	Aconitine
	Amodiaquine
	Beclamide
	Clonidine
	Dihydrocodeine
	Ketazolam
	Metoprolol
	Morazone
	Morinamide
	Nomifensine
	Papaverine
	Profadol
	Strychnine
	Temazepam
	Trimethoxyamphetamine
	Xylometazoline
09	Buprenorphine
	Butacaine
	Clobazam
	Dimethyltryptamine
	Emetine
	Hydroxyzine
	Loperamide
	Naloxone
	Phenyramidol
	Thiothixene
	Trazodone
10	Flunitrazepam
	Haloperidol
	Hexobendine
	Oxethazaine
	Oxymorphone
11	Alprenolol
	Ametazole
	Lidoflazine

Rf	Compound
	Miconazole
	Oxprenolol
	Trimetozine
12	Bromazepam
	Etamiphylline
	Physostigmine
13	Dextrorphan
	Dimethothiazine
	Levorphanol
	Primaquine
	Racemorphan
14	Butanilicaine
	Chloroquine
	Phenmetrazine
15	Amethocaine
	Amphetamine
	Bisacodyl
	Cyclazocine
	Diamorphine
	Diethyltryptamine
	Dimefline
	Diperodon
	Mepacrine
	Nikethamide
	Pentazocine
	Pipazethate
16	Diloxanide
	Dimoxyline
	DOM
	Metyrapone
	Phenazocine
17	Chromonar
	Diethylcarbamazine
	Isocarboxazid
	Lobeline
	Maprotiline
	Methylenedioxyamphetamine
	Penfluridol
	Phenglutarimide
	Protriptyline
18	Chlorphentermine
	Clorprenaline
	Dimethoxanate
	Eucatropine
	Levamisole
19	Amantadine
	Levallorphan
	Thebacon
20	Desipramine
	Dibenzepin
	Doxapram
	Propanidid
22	Noscapine
23	Diazepam
	Oxybuprocaine
	Oxycodone
	Thebaine
	Verapamil
24	Butaperazine
	Deptropine
	Methoxyphenamine
	Perazine
25	Carbinoxamine
	Cathine

Rf	Compound
	Cinchocaine
	Tofenacin
26	Acepromazine
	Benztropine
	Etomidate
	Meclofenoxate
	Phenoperidine
	Phentermine
	Proxymetacaine
27	Cyclopentolate
	Mepivacaine
	Nortriptyline
	Zimeldine
28	Crotethamide
	Ibogaine
	Mebhydrolin
	Methylamphetamine
	Octamylamine
	Phenethylamine
29	Cropropamide
	Prilocaine
30	Alphaprodine
	Diamthazole
	Flurazepam
	Thiethylperazine
31	Clemizole
	Thymoxamine
32	Cyclopentamine
	Methdilazine
33	Brompheniramine
	Chlorpheniramine
	Nefopam
	Prochlorperazine
	Tranylcypromine
	Trifluoperazine
34	Ethomoxane
	Mephentermine
	Methylphenidate
	Propiomazine
35	Etafedrine
	Lignocaine
	Pheniramine
	Thiopropazate
36	Benzydamine
	Dihydralazine
	Dimethindene
	Flavoxate
	Methoxyamphetamine
	Phendimetrazine
	Prazepam
37	Aletamine
	Diphenylpyraline
	Famprofazone
	Ketamine
	Methaqualone
	Methyl Nicotinate
	Pethidine
	Phenelzine
	Promethazine
38	Disulfiram
	Hydralazine
	Thenalidine
	Thonzylamine
39	Mepyramine

Rf	Compound
	Mianserin
	Nicotine
	Phenyltoloxamine
	Tigloidine
	Triprolidine
40	Bamipine
	Benactyzine
	Dextromoramide
	Mebeverine
	Medazepam
	Normethadone
41	Bezitramide
	Chlophedianol
	Clothiapine
	Doxylamine
	Fenfluramine
	Halopyramine
	Isothipendyl
	Nicametate
	Promazine
	Tetrabenazine
	Trimeperidine
42	Benzyl Nicotinate
	Bupivacaine
	Chlorcyclizine
	Clorgyline
	Diphenoxylate
	Nicofuranose
	Thenyldiamine
43	Methapyrilene
	Noxiptyline
	Pramoxine
	Proquamezine
	Thioridazine
44	Bromodiphenhydramine
	Chlormethiazole
	Dextromethorphan
	Tripelennamine
45	Butoxyethyl Nicotinate
	Cyproheptadine
	Diphenhydramine
	Ethoheptazine
	Fentanyl
	Phenindamine
	Prothipendyl
46	Pecazine
47	Chlorphenoxamine
	Cocaine
	Phenbutrazate
48	Benethamine
	Carbetapentane
	Clemastine
	Mebanazine
	Methixene
	Orphenadrine
49	Chlorpromazine
	Conessine
	Cyclizine
	Dyclonine
	Fluopromazine
	Imipramine
	Iprindole
	Methotrimeprazine
50	Dothiepin

Rf	Compound	Rf	Compound	Rf	Compound
	Rimantadine	56	Adiphenine		Bialamicol
51	Chlorprothixene		Clomiphene		Diethylpropion
	Cinnarizine		Diphenidol		Fencamfamin
	Mecamylamine	57	Azapetine		Levomethadyl Acetate
	Oxeladin		Benzoctamine		Trimipramine
52	Broxaldine		Clofazimine	63	Procyclidine
	Doxepin		Diethazine	64	Ethopropazine
	Naftidrofuryl Oxalate		Perhexiline		Phenoxybenzamine
	Tolpropamine		Selegiline	65	Alverine
53	Azapropazone	58	Isoaminile		Benzhexol
	Piperocaine		Meclozine	66	Dipipanone
	Pipoxolan	59	Butethamate		Prolintane
54	Clomipramine		Dextropropoxyphene	67	Benzphetamine
	Pseudoephedrine		Norpipanone		Bromhexine
55	Amitriptyline		Pipradrol		Cycrimine
	Cyclomethycaine	60	Trifluomeprazine		Dicyclomine
	Dimethisoquin	61	Buclizine		Sparteine
	Piperidolate		Butriptyline	68	Biperiden
	Prenylamine		Diethylthiambutene		Pempidine
	Pyrrobutamine		Methadone		
	Trimeprazine	62	Amiodarone		

System TC (p. 167)—Rf Values

Rf	Compound	Rf	Compound	Rf	Compound
00	Ametazole		Practolol		Chloroquine
	Bethanidine		Proguanil		Deptropine
	Buformin		Propamidine		Methoxyphenamine
	Debrisoquine		Salbutamol		Mexiletine
	Diminazene		Sulphaurea		Phenylpropanolamine
	Guanoclor		Terbutaline		Pseudoephedrine
	Guanoxan	02	Atenolol		Tacrine
	Hexoprenaline		Dihydralazine		Trimetazidine
	Hydroxystilbamidine		Ethambutol	05	Azapropazone
	Isoetharine		Ethylnoradrenaline		Cathine
	Metformin		Etilefrine		Clioquinol
	Noradrenaline		Guanethidine		Ephedrine
	Pentamidine		Heptaminol		Maprotiline
	Phenformin		Hydroxyamphetamine		Mepacrine
	Pseudomorphine		Hydroxychloroquine		Norcodeine
01	Acepifylline		Mecamylamine		Pindolol
	Adrenaline		Tetrahydrozoline		Primaquine
	Amidephrine		Tolazoline		Procainamide
	Amiloride		Tramazoline		Xylometazoline
	Benserazide		Tryptamine	06	Bamethan
	Benzoylecgonine	03	Acebutolol		Benztropine
	Bufotenine		Atropine		Broxyquinoline
	Chlorproguanil		Azacyclonol		Hordenine
	Cycloserine		Conessine		Mequitazine
	Cytarabine		Dihydromorphine		Mesoridazine
	Dipyrone		Minoxidil		Naphazoline
	Dobutamine		Narceine		Profadol
	Homatropine		Orciprenaline	07	Amantadine
	Isoprenaline		Oxyphencyclimine		Antazoline
	Metaraminol		Pempidine		Dextrorphan
	Methyldopa		Penicillamine		Hydroquinine
	Nadolol		Phentolamine		Levorphanol
	Oxedrine		Pholedrine		Metoclopramide
	Oxymetazoline		Protokylol		Oxethazaine
	Pentapiperide		Sotalol		Protriptyline
	Phenylephrine		Sparteine		Racemorphan
	Piperazine	04	Ambazone		Tuaminoheptane

Rf	Compound
08	Azathioprine
	Disopyramide
	Hydroquinidine
	Mephentermine
	Metoprolol
	Perhexiline
	Phenglutarimide
	Triamterene
09	Amphetamine
	Cimetidine
	Dimethyltryptamine
	Etafedrine
	Hydromorphone
	Ketobemidone
	Morphine
	Prenalterol
	Psilocin
10	Cinchonidine
	Cinchonine
	Cyclopentamine
	Cytisine
	Diethyltryptamine
	Doxylamine
	Mescaline
	Procarbazine
	Propranolol
11	Desipramine
	Hydralazine
	Isoniazid
	Metopimazine
	Octamylamine
	Oxprenolol
	Quinidine
	Quinine
	Rimantadine
	Timolol
	Trimethoxyamphetamine
12	Alprenolol
	Diprophylline
	Ergometrine
	Methylenedioxyamphetamine
	Neopine
	Pentazocine
	Phenelzine
	Pipamperone
13	Cyclazocine
	Dihydrocodeine
	Dimethindene
	Eucatropine
	Hexamine
	Mazindol
	Methylamphetamine
	Pheniramine
	Pipazethate
14	Buphenine
	Methylergometrine
15	Clorprenaline
	Methdilazine
16	Brompheniramine
	Fenfluramine
	Fenpipramide
	Nortriptyline
	Pericyazine
17	Brucine

Rf	Compound
	Chlorphentermine
	Dextromethorphan
	DOM
	Nicotinyl Alcohol
18	Chlorpheniramine
	Codeine
	Pholcodine
	Trilostane
19	Carbinoxamine
	Cephaëline
	Ethoheptazine
	6-Monoacetylmorphine
	Piperacetazine
	Proquamezine
	Strychnine
20	Hydrocodone
	Methadone
	Salinazid
	Styramate
	Triprolidine
21	Apomorphine
	Dehydroemetine
	Methysergide
	Phenmetrazine
	Tigloidine
	Tofenacin
22	Benzydamine
	Carbetapentane
	Ethylmorphine
	Harmine
	Opipramol
	Oxeladin
	Trimethoprim
23	Benzylmorphine
	Chloroprocaine
	Fluphenazine
	Imipramine
	Iproniazid
	Nalorphine
	Pemoline
	Prothipendyl
	Viloxazine
24	Acepromazine
	Chromonar
	Dimethoxanate
	Levallorphan
25	Acetophenazine
	Clemastine
	Mepyramine
	Methixene
	Nialamide
	Thenyldiamine
	Zimeldine
26	Diethylcarbamazine
	Methapyrilene
27	Carphenazine
	Haloperidol
	Tripelennamine
28	Diazoxide
	Dihydroergotamine
	Diphenylpyraline
	Halopyramine
	Phenethylamine
	Thonzylamine

Rf	Compound
29	Nomifensine
	Perphenazine
30	Butacaine
	Diamthazole
	Isothipendyl
	Norharman
	Promazine
	Theophylline
	Thioridazine
	Trifluoperazine
31	Clonidine
	Phentermine
	Procaine
	Procyclidine
	Pyrimethamine
	Theobromine
32	Amethocaine
	Amitriptyline
	Clopenthixol
	Isoxsuprine
	Loperamide
	Nefopam
	Pilocarpine
	Prolintane
	Tolpropamine
33	Amiphenazole
	Diphenhydramine
	Dipipanone
	Flupenthixol
	Orphenadrine
	Propoxycaine
	Proxyphylline
	Tranylcypromine
34	Cinchocaine
	Clomipramine
	Emetine
	Ergotamine
	Fencamfamin
	Iprindole
	Methylphenidate
	Normethadone
	Pethidine
	Thebacon
	Thioproperazine
35	Alphaprodine
	Chlorpromazine
	Demoxepam
	Dibenzepin
	Fluopromazine
	Lobeline
	Nicametate
	Nicotine
	Noxiptyline
	Promethazine
	Veratrine
36	Chlorphenoxamine
	Cyclomethycaine
	Ethionamide
	Lorazepam
	Metronidazole
	Nitrazepam
	Physostigmine
37	Butaperazine
	Chlophedianol

Rf	Compound
	Colchicine
	Dipyridamole
	Doxepin
	Oxymorphone
	Perazine
	Piperocaine
	Prochlorperazine
	Pyrrobutamine
	Thebaine
38	Clozapine
	Diamorphine
	Methotrimeprazine
	Pipradrol
	Prothionamide
	Yohimbine
39	Aconitine
	Alverine
	Cyclopentolate
	Etamiphylline
	Hyoscine
	Levomethadyl Acetate
	Lysergide
	Phenazocine
	Trimeprazine
40	Aletamine
	Amodiaquine
	Dyclonine
	Furaltadone
	Oxazepam
	Thiothixene
	Triazolam
41	Bromazepam
	Cyclizine
	Glipizide
	Naftidrofuryl Oxalate
	Oxybuprocaine
	Proxymetacaine
	Thiethylperazine
	Trimeperidine
42	Dothiepin
	Meclofenoxate
	Propiomazine
43	Bamipine
	Bromodiphenhydramine
	Diethylthiambutene
	Inositol Nicotinate
	Mephenesin
44	Cyproheptadine
	Hexobendine
	Nimorazole
	Niridazole
	Pecazine
	Thenalidine
	Thymoxamine
45	Diphenidol
	Fenethylline
	Mebhydrolin
	Phanquone
	Piritramide
46	Chlorcyclizine
	Dimethisoquin
	Morazone
47	Cocaine
	Ethomoxane

Rf	Compound
	Ethopropazine
	Furazolidone
	Prazosin
48	Butriptyline
	Co-dergocrine
	Dimefline
	Dimethothiazine
	Droperidol
	Flurazepam
	Levamisole
	Phenyltoloxamine
49	Morinamide
50	Chlordiazepoxide
	Ibogaine
	Norpipanone
	Phenazopyridine
51	Benorylate
	Chlorprothixene
	Diethazine
	Oxycodone
	Phendimetrazine
52	Benzoctamine
	Clomiphene
	Methimazole
	Phenyramidol
53	Benactyzine
	Clonazepam
	Mebeverine
	Thiopropazate
54	Bamifylline
	Butanilicaine
	Hydroxyzine
	Isoaminile
	Thiabendazole
	Trimipramine
55	Dextropropoxyphene
	Nordazepam
	Pramoxine
56	Carbamazepine
	Clefamide
	Clorazepic Acid
	Ethoxazene
	Nikethamide
57	Benzocaine
	Butethamate
	Phenindamine
58	Caffeine
	Diperodon
	Metyrapone
	Mianserin
	Pipobroman
	Trazodone
	Trifluomeprazine
59	Benethamine
	Clofazimine
	Clothiapine
	Etenzamide
	Fluspirilene
	Mebendazole
	Temazepam
60	Adiphenine
	Penfluridol
	Pimozide
	Vinblastine

Rf	Compound
61	Benzhexol
	Cycrimine
	Etorphine
62	Ergotoxine
	Lormetazepam
	Mepivacaine
	Norbormide
63	Chlormezanone
	Diethylpropion
	Ketamine
	Lidoflazine
64	Biperiden
	Dicyclomine
	Ketazolam
	Pentetrazol
	Phenoperidine
	Prilocaine
65	Beclamide
	Glymidine
	Nifedipine
	Oxypertine
	Papaverine
66	Methyl Nicotinate
	Naloxone
	Pentifylline
67	Azapetine
	Buclosamide
	Crotethamide
	Flavoxate
	Miconazole
68	Ambucetamide
	Amiodarone
	Buprenorphine
	Methisazone
	Pipoxolan
	Prenylamine
69	Benzquinamide
	Bromocriptine
	Butoxyethyl Nicotinate
	Chlormethiazole
	Clemizole
	Cropropamide
	Mebanazine
	Selegiline
70	Benzphetamine
	Clobazam
	Clorgyline
	Doxapram
	Nicofuranose
	Propanidid
	Verapamil
71	Benzyl Nicotinate
	Dextromoramide
	Etomidate
72	Flunitrazepam
	Trimetozine
73	Bupivacaine
	Diazepam
	Lignocaine
74	Diloxanide
	Famprofazone
	Fentanyl
	Isocarboxazid
	Medazepam

Rf	Compound	Rf	Compound	Rf	Compound
	Noscapine		Methoserpidine	79	Bezitramide
	Prazepam		Methoxyamphetamine		Bromhexine
	Reserpine		Thiambutosine		Broxaldine
75	Dimoxyline	78	Cinnarizine		Meclozine
	Rescinnamine		Disulfiram	80	Bialamicol
76	Bisacodyl		Phenbutrazate		Methaqualone
	Phenoxybenzamine		Tetrabenazine	81	Diphenoxylate
77	Deserpidine		Thiocarlide	83	Buclizine

System TD (p. 168)—Rf Values

Rf	Compound	Rf	Compound	Rf	Compound
00	Barbituric Acid		Butalamine		Diclofenac
	Carbazochrome		Chlorphenesin Carbamate		Sulphafurazole
	Carbidopa		Diphenadione	26	Benzoic Acid
	Cromoglycic Acid		Ethiazide		Sulphamethoxazole
	Lysergic Acid		Guaiphenesin	27	Ketoprofen
	Paramethadione	12	Sulphamethizole	29	Phenylmethylbarbituric Acid
	Phthalylsulphacetamide		Zomepirac		Sulphaphenazole
	Phthalylsulphathiazole	13	Bromazepam	30	Flurbiprofen
	Salicyluric Acid		Probenecid		Trilostane
	Succinylsulphathiazole		Styramate	31	Clorexolone
	Sulphasalazine		Sulphanilamide		Methyprylone
	Valproic Acid		Tolmetin		Sulphadimethoxine
01	Baclofen	14	Benzthiazide	32	Aminoglutethimide
	Bumetanide		Dichlorphenamide	33	Apronal
	Digoxin		Mephenesin Carbamate		Chlorambucil
	Frusemide		Sulindac		Naproxen
	Mafenide		Sulphaethidole		Phenytoin
	Nicotinic Acid	15	Demoxepam	34	Clorazepic Acid
	Saccharin		Paracetamol		Nordazepam
	Sulphaguanidine		Trichlormethiazide	35	Alphadolone Acetate
02	Chlorothiazide	16	Indomethacin		Clonazepam
	Prenalterol		Sulphapyridine		Nitrazepam
	Trifluperidol	17	Di-iodohydroxyquinoline		Tybamate
03	Ethacrynic Acid		Sulphacetamide	36	Carisoprodol
	Flurazepam	18	Alclofenac	37	Sulfadoxine
04	Acetazolamide		Aspirin	38	Chlorpropamide
	Aloxiprin		Cyclothiazide		Ethamivan
	Chlorthalidone		Dicoumarol		Indapamide
	Clozapine		Fenbufen		Phenacetin
	Dichlorophenoxyacetic Acid		Phenazone		Pheneturide
	Ethyl Biscoumacetate	19	Aminobenzoic Acid		Phenolphthalein
	Hydrochlorothiazide		Clopamide		Salicylamide
	Quinethazone		Dantrolene		Xipamide
	Sulphinpyrazone		Methyclothiazide	39	Acetohexamide
05	Aminosalicylic Acid		Sulphamethoxypyridazine		Nalidixic Acid
	Captopril	21	4-Aminophenol	40	Glibornuride
	Sulphasomidine		Cyclopenthiazide		Sulfametopyrazine
	Triazolam		Enoxolone	41	Barbitone
07	Carbenoxolone	22	Oxazepam		Mefenamic Acid
	Hydroflumethiazide		Phenacemide	42	Fenoprofen
	Methocarbamol		Polythiazide	43	Ethoxzolamide
	Salicylic Acid		Sulphadiazine		Lormetazepam
08	Diflunisal	23	Lorazepam	45	Acetanilide
	Primidone		Metolazone		Ketazolam
09	Meprobamate		Sulfamerazine		Mefruside
	Methylchlorophenoxyacetic Acid		Sulphadimidine	46	Ibuprofen
	Sulphathiazole		Sulthiame	47	Phenobarbitone
10	Chlordiazepoxide	24	Sulphamethoxydiazine		Phenprobamate
	Mebutamate	25	Amidopyrine	48	Aprobarbitone
11	Bufexamac		Bendrofluazide	49	Acetylcarbromal

Rf	Compound	Rf	Compound	Rf	Compound
	Ethinamate		Ethotoin		Santonin
	Methylpentynol Carbamate		Hexethal		Warfarin
50	Allobarbitone		Talbutal	65	Hexobarbitone
	Butobarbitone	54	Butalbital		Phenindione
	Cyclobarbitone		Flunitrazepam	66	Metharbitone
	Cyclopentobarbitone	55	Idobutal		Spironolactone
	Ethosuximide		Pentobarbitone	70	Methylphenobarbitone
	Heptabarbitone		Quinalbarbitone	71	Enallylpropymal
	Ibomal	56	Benzocaine		Glyceryl Trinitrate
	Secbutobarbitone		Medazepam		Phensuximide
	Vinbarbitone	58	Diazepam	73	Coumatetralyl
51	Piroxicam		Dichlorophen		Methohexitone
	Temazepam		Nealbarbitone		Thymol
	Tolbutamide	60	Triclocarban	74	Cyclandelate
52	Amylobarbitone	61	Propyphenazone	75	Clofibrate
	Bemegride	62	Benziodarone	77	Thialbarbitone
	Brallobarbitone		Methoin		Thiopentone
	Nicoumalone		Phenprocoumon	78	Phenylbutazone
	Oxyphenbutazone	63	Carbimazole	80	Danthron
	Tolazamide		Glutethimide	82	Dicophane
53	Carbromal		Methaqualone		
	Clobazam	64	Prazepam		

System TE (p. 168)—Rf Values

Rf	Compound	Rf	Compound	Rf	Compound
00	Baclofen	07	Aminosalicylic Acid		Trichlormethiazide
	Barbituric Acid		Benzoic Acid	15	Nicoumalone
	Carbenoxolone		Enoxolone	16	Aspirin
	Carbidopa		Flurbiprofen		Carbazochrome
	Cromoglycic Acid		Frusemide		Diflunisal
	Lysergic Acid		Ibuprofen		Sulphinpyrazone
	Nicotinic Acid		Ketoprofen	17	Piroxicam
	Phthalylsulphacetamide		Naproxen	18	Bufexamac
	Phthalylsulphathiazole		Paramethadione		Warfarin
	Salicyluric Acid		Oxyphenbutazone	21	Phenindione
	Succinylsulphathiazole		Saccharin		Phenprocoumon
	Sulphasalazine		Tolmetin	23	Benziodarone
	Valproic Acid		Trilostane	24	Ethyl Biscoumacetate
01	Aminobenzoic Acid	08	Sulfadoxine		Phenylmethylbarbituric Acid
	Sulindac		Sulfamerazine		Sulphapyridine
02	Captopril		Sulfametopyrazine	25	Prenalterol
	Chlorothiazide		Sulphaethidole		Sulphaguanidine
	Nalidixic Acid		Sulphafurazole	27	Mafenide
03	Acetazolamide	09	Aloxiprin	28	Di-iodohydroxyquinoline
	Bumetanide		Benzthiazide		Phenobarbitone
04	Alclofenac		Dantrolene	30	Brallobarbitone
	Dichlorophenoxyacetic Acid		Fenoprofen		Heptabarbitone
	Ethacrynic Acid		Sulphaphenazole	31	Allobarbitone
	Fenbufen		Sulphathiazole		Barbitone
	Sulphadiazine	10	Sulphadimethoxine		Ibomal
	Sulphamethizole	11	Chlorpropamide	32	Dicoumarol
	Zomepirac		Salicylic Acid		Vinbarbitone
05	Glibornuride		Sulphamethoxypyridazine	33	Dichlorphenamide
	Methylchlorophenoxyacetic Acid		Xipamide		Digoxin
	Probenecid	12	Acetohexamide	34	Dichlorophen
	Sulphacetamide		Sulphamethoxydiazine		Hydrochlorothiazide
	Sulphamethoxazole		Tolbutamide	35	Cyclobarbitone
	Sulphasomidine	13	Coumatetralyl	36	Amylobarbitone
06	Chlorambucil		Diclofenac		Aprobarbitone
	Indomethacin		Sulphadimidine		Phenytoin
	Tolazamide	14	Mefenamic Acid	37	Cyclopentobarbitone

Rf	Compound	Rf	Compound	Rf	Compound
	Guaiphenesin		Clopamide		Nordazepam
38	Butalbital		Sulphanilamide	68	Bemegride
	Butobarbitone	53	Chlorphenesin Carbamate		Phenacetin
39	Nealbarbitone		Metharbitone		Tybamate
	Primidone		Methyclothiazide	70	Acetanilide
40	Ethamivan		Styramate	71	Alphadolone Acetate
	Hydroflumethiazide		Sulthiame		Pheneturide
41	Idobutal	55	Mephenesin Carbamate	73	Carisoprodol
	Quinethazone	57	Acetylcarbromal		Clobazam
	Secbutobarbitone		Ethosuximide		Ketazolam
	Talbutal		Metolazone		Propyphenazone
42	Chlorthalidone	58	Clorexolone	74	Carbromal
43	Danthron		Enallylpropymal		Ethinamate
	Ethoxzolamide		Methohexitone		Flurazepam
	Methylphenobarbitone	59	4-Aminophenol		Methylpentynol Carbamate
44	Demoxepam		Cyclothiazide		Phenprobamate
	Hexethal		Mebutamate	75	Santonin
	Oxazepam		Nitrazepam		Triclocarban
	Quinalbarbitone	60	Clonazepam	76	Methoin
	Thialbarbitone		Meprobamate	77	Benzocaine
45	Lorazepam	61	Lormetazepam		Diazepam
	Paracetamol		Methyprylone		Flunitrazepam
	Pentobarbitone	62	Bromazepam		Phensuximide
	Triazolam	63	Amidopyrine	78	Glutethimide
46	Diphenadione		Clorazepic Acid	79	Medazepam
	Salicylamide		Clozapine		Spironolactone
47	Carbimazole		Polythiazide	80	Trifluperidol
48	Hexobarbitone		Temazepam	81	Cyclandelate
49	Methocarbamol	65	Aminoglutethimide		Prazepam
	Phenazone		Mefruside		Thymol
	Thiopentone		Phenacemide	82	Clofibrate
50	Ethiazide	66	Cyclopenthiazide	86	Butalamine
51	Chlordiazepoxide		Phenylbutazone		Glyceryl Trinitrate
	Phenolphthalein	67	Apronal	87	Dicophane
52	Bendrofluazide		Indapamide		

System TF (p. 168)—Rf Values

Rf	Compound	Rf	Compound	Rf	Compound
00	Baclofen	06	Dichlorophenoxyacetic Acid	21	Quinethazone
	Barbituric Acid		Ethacrynic Acid	22	Demoxepam
	Carbazochrome		Sulphaguanidine	23	Methocarbamol
	Cromoglycic Acid	10	Aloxiprin		Probenecid
	Lysergic Acid		Bumetanide		Sulphamethizole
	Nicotinic Acid		Diflunisal	24	Aminosalicylic Acid
	Phthalylsulphacetamide		Sulindac	25	Methyprylone
	Phthalylsulphathiazole	11	Chlordiazepoxide		Salicylic Acid
	Salicyluric Acid		Methylchlorophenoxyacetic Acid	26	Primidone
	Succinylsulphathiazole	12	Frusemide	28	Alclofenac
	Sulphasalazine		Zomepirac	29	Butalamine
	Valproic Acid	14	Phenazone	30	Aspirin
01	Mafenide	15	Amidopyrine		Fenbufen
	Saccharin	16	Chlorothiazide	31	Acetazolamide
02	Captopril		Sulphasomidine		Nalidixic Acid
	Carbidopa	17	Carbenoxolone	32	Dicoumarol
	Prenalterol		Guaiphenesin		Ethyl Biscoumacetate
	Triazolam	19	Bufexamac	33	Diphenadione
03	Flurazepam		Di-iodohydroxyquinoline	34	Chlorphenesin Carbamate
04	Sulphinpyrazone	20	Bromazepam		Meprobamate
05	Clozapine		Indomethacin		Paracetamol
	Digoxin		Sulphathiazole	35	Ethamivan
	Trifluperidol		Tolmetin		Mebutamate

Rf	Compound	Rf	Compound	Rf	Compound
	Sulphaethidole		Flunitrazepam	62	Benzocaine
36	Dantrolene	49	Clobazam		Cyclopenthiazide
	Mephenesin Carbamate	50	Ethiazide		Glutethimide
37	Oxazepam		Methyclothiazide		Methylpentynol Carbamate
38	Clopamide		Propyphenazone		Oxyphenbutazone
	Phenacetin		Santonin		Warfarin
39	Benzoic Acid		Sulfametopyrazine	63	Secbutobarbitone
	Hydrochlorothiazide		Tolazamide	64	Apronal
	Lorazepam	51	Benzthiazide		Cyclobarbitone
	Styramate		Clorexolone		Cyclopentobarbitone
	Sulphadiazine		Metolazone		Dichlorphenamide
	Sulphamethoxypyridazine		Nicoumalone		Vinbarbitone
40	Alphadolone Acetate		Spironolactone		Xipamide
	4-Aminophenol		Sulfadoxine	65	Amylobarbitone
	Chlorambucil		Sulphadimethoxine		Aprobarbitone
	Diclofenac		Sulphaphenazole		Butobarbitone
	Ketoprofen	52	Sulphafurazole		Ethoxzolamide
	Medazepam	53	Bemegride		Heptabarbitone
	Phenacemide		Carisoprodol		Hexobarbitone
41	Flurbiprofen		Fenoprofen		Phenobarbitone
	Sulfamerazine		Pheneturide		Tybamate
42	Sulphacetamide		Phenytoin	66	Allobarbitone
	Sulphapyridine	54	Ibuprofen		Clofibrate
43	Acetohexamide		Mefenamic Acid		Pentobarbitone
	Aminobenzoic Acid		Sulphamethoxazole	67	Butalbital
	Chlorpropamide	55	Phenprobamate		Dichlorophen
	Chlorthalidone		Prazepam		Hexethal
	Sulphamethoxydiazine		Salicylamide		Ibomal
	Sulthiame		Tolbutamide		Metharbitone
45	Acetanilide	56	Carbromal		Talbutal
	Clonazepam		Ethosuximide	68	Phenylbutazone
	Clorazepic Acid		Phenindione		Quinalbarbitone
	Ketazolam		Phenprocoumon		Thymol
	Naproxen	58	Benziodarone	69	Brallobarbitone
	Nitrazepam		Mefruside		Danthron
	Nordazepam		Methoin		Idobutal
	Sulphadimidine	59	Ethinamate		Methylphenobarbitone
	Trilostane		Phenolphthalein		Nealbarbitone
46	Enoxolone		Phensuximide	71	Bendrofluazide
	Piroxicam		Triclocarban		Cyclandelate
	Sulphanilamide	60	Cyclothiazide		Enallylpropymal
47	Aminoglutethimide		Glibornuride	72	Glyceryl Trinitrate
	Hydroflumethiazide		Paramethadione		Methohexitone
	Lormetazepam		Polythiazide	74	Coumatetralyl
	Temazepam		Trichlormethiazide		Dicophane
48	Acetylcarbromal	61	Barbitone		Thialbarbitone
	Carbimazole		Indapamide		Thiopentone
	Diazepam		Phenylmethylbarbituric Acid		

System TG (p. 169)—Rf Values

Rf	Compound	Rf	Compound	Rf	Compound
08	Indoprofen	18	Ibuprofen	32	Mefenamic Acid
09	Fenbufen	19	Frusemide	33	Flunixin
10	Tolmetin	20	Fenclofenac		Theophylline
12	Alclofenac		Indomethacin	36	Bufexamac
13	Sulindac	23	Phenylbutazone	37	Diflunisal
14	Benoxaprofen		Salsalate		Flufenamic Acid
	Ketoprofen	25	Oxyphenbutazone	38	Meclofenamic Acid
	Naproxen	28	Niflumic Acid	45	Feprazone
16	Fenoprofen	29	Diclofenac	47	Theobromine
	Flurbiprofen	30	Clonixin		

System TH (p. 171)—Rf Values

Rf	Compound	Rf	Compound	Rf	Compound
03	Barbituric Acid		Heptabarbitone	75	Thialbarbitone
27	Phenylmethylbarbituric Acid	66	Aprobarbitone	76	Pentobarbitone
38	Phenobarbitone	67	Butalbital	78	Nealbarbitone
47	Brallobarbitone	68	Butobarbitone		Quinalbarbitone
51	Barbitone	69	Secbutobarbitone	80	Thiopentone
53	Allobarbitone	71	Idobutal	85	Hexobarbitone
56	Vinbarbitone		Talbutal	86	Metharbitone
59	Cyclobarbitone	72	Methylphenobarbitone	87	Enallylpropymal
61	Ibomal	74	Amylobarbitone	93	Methohexitone
62	Cyclopentobarbitone		Hexethal		

System TI (p. 172)—Rf Values

Rf	Compound
05	Cannabidiol
30	Δ^9-Tetrahydrocannabinol
52	Cannabinol

System TJ (p. 172)—Rf Values

Rf	Compound
20	Cannabinol
29	Δ^9-Tetrahydrocannabinol
36	Cannabidiol

System TK (p. 172)—Rf Values

Rf	Compound
09	Ouabain
27	Deslanoside
36	Lanatoside C
62	Digoxin
72	Digitoxin
82	Acetyldigitoxin

System TL (p. 173)—Rf Values

Rf	Compound	Rf	Compound	Rf	Compound
00	Lysergic Acid		Dyclonine	48	Ergotoxine
06	Lysergamide	27	Piperocaine		Mepivacaine
08	Ergometrine	28	Dimethisoquin	54	Cocaine
12	Methylergometrine		Propoxycaine	60	Prilocaine
	Methysergide	29	Co-dergocrine	61	Butanilicaine
14	Dihydroergotamine	30	Procaine	63	Lignocaine
15	Oxethazaine	35	Cinchocaine	64	Butacaine
16	Amethocaine		Proxymetacaine	65	Bupivacaine
23	Ergotamine	36	Oxybuprocaine	66	Benzocaine
24	Lysergide	37	Chloroprocaine		Diperodon
25	Cyclomethycaine	41	Pramoxine		

System TM (p. 173)—Rf Values

Rf	Compound	Rf	Compound	Rf	Compound
00	Lysergic Acid	33	Methysergide	64	Co-dergocrine
26	Ergometrine	40	Dihydroergotamine	67	Ergotoxine
27	Lysergamide	48	Ergotamine	70	Lysergide
31	Methylergometrine				

System TN (p. 175)—Rf Values

Rf	Compound	Rf	Compound	Rf	Compound
22	Paraquat Dichloride	56	Decamethonium Bromide	85	Tubocurarine Chloride
34	Gallamine Triethiodide		Guanethidine	94	Bretylium Tosylate
35	Suxamethonium Chloride	60	Choline	95	Atropine Methonitrate
36	Hexamethonium Bromide	70	Acetylcholine Chloride	100	Cetrimide
40	Suxethonium Bromide	80	Pancuronium Bromide		

System TO (p. 175)—Rf Values

Rf	Compound	Rf	Compound
05	Gallamine Triethiodide	40	Bretylium Tosylate
10	Hexamethonium Bromide		Tubocurarine Chloride
	Paraquat Dichloride	50	Cetrimide
	Suxamethonium Chloride		Guanethidine
16	Decamethonium Bromide	60	Acetylcholine Chloride
23	Suxethonium Bromide		Choline
35	Atropine Methonitrate		

System TP (p. 175)—Rf Values

Rf	Compound	Rf	Compound	Rf	Compound
00	Betamethasone Sodium Phosphate		Testosterone		Methallenoestril
	Hydrocortisone Sodium Phosphate	65	Methandienone		Norethynodrel
	Prednisolone Sodium Phosphate	65s	Stilboestrol		Oestradiol Benzoate
08	Hydrocortisone Hydrogen Succinate	69	Oxymetholone	80	Dimethisterone
09	Triamcinolone		Prednisolone Pivalate		Medroxyprogesterone Acetate
20	Prednisolone	70	Methyltestosterone		Megesterol Acetate
23	Methylprednisolone	71	Norethandrolone	81	Hydroxyprogesterone Hexanoate
27	Hydrocortisone		Norethisterone		Progesterone
30	Betamethasone	72	Cortisone Acetate	83	Ethynodiol Diacetate
32	Dexamethasone		Dienoestrol	86	Deoxycortone Acetate
	Triamcinolone Acetonide		Ethinyloestradiol		Dydrogesterone
41	Prednisone	75	Beclomethasone Dipropionate		Mestranol
42	Fluocinolone Acetonide	77	Lynoestrenol		Testosterone Phenylpropionate
51	Fluoxymesterone	78	Ethisterone	87	Nandrolone Phenylpropionate
	Hydrocortisone Acetate		Fluocortolone Pivalate		Norethisterone Acetate
58	Betamethasone Valerate		Stanolone	88	Chlorotrianisene
	Fludrocortisone Acetate		Testosterone Propionate		Nandrolone Decanoate
59	Alphadolone Acetate	79	Ethyloestrenol		
60	Alphaxalone		Fluocortolone Hexanoate		

System TQ (p. 175)—Rf Values

Rf	Compound	Rf	Compound	Rf	Compound
00	Betamethasone	09	Fluoxymesterone	23	Oxymetholone
	Betamethasone Sodium Phosphate	10	Methandienone	25	Dienoestrol
	Hydrocortisone Hydrogen Succinate	10s	Stilboestrol	27	Betamethasone Valerate
	Hydrocortisone Sodium Phosphate	11	Hydrocortisone Acetate	28	Cortisone Acetate
	Prednisolone		Stanolone		Testosterone Phenylpropionate
	Prednisolone Sodium Phosphate	12	Fludrocortisone Acetate	30	Ethinyloestradiol
	Prednisone		Testosterone Propionate	32	Norethynodrel
	Triamcinolone	16	Methyltestosterone		Oestradiol Benzoate
	Triamcinolone Acetonide	18	Methallenoestril	35	Fluocortolone Pivalate
02	Hydrocortisone	20	Norethandrolone	38	Beclomethasone Dipropionate
04	Prednisolone Pivalate		Progesterone	39	Ethisterone
07	Testosterone	22	Alphadolone Acetate		Fluocortolone Hexanoate
08	Dexamethasone		Alphaxalone		Norethisterone Acetate
	Fluocinolone Acetonide		Norethisterone	42	Dimethisterone

Rf	Compound
48	Nandrolone Phenylpropionate
49	Nandrolone Decanoate
50	Ethyloestrenol
	Medroxyprogesterone Acetate
	Megestrol Acetate

Rf	Compound
52	Deoxycortone Acetate
	Mestranol
53	Dydrogesterone
55	Hydroxyprogesterone Hexanoate
	Lynoestrenol

Rf	Compound
61	Ethynodiol Diacetate
77	Chlorotrianisene
80	Methylprednisolone

System TR (p. 175)—Rf Values

Rf	Compound
00	Betamethasone
	Betamethasone Sodium Phosphate
	Dexamethasone
	Hydrocortisone Hydrogen Succinate
	Hydrocortisone Sodium Phosphate
	Prednisolone Sodium Phosphate
	Triamcinolone
02s	Prednisolone
03	Methylprednisolone
08	Hydrocortisone
10	Fluocinolone Acetonide
	Prednisone
18s	Stilboestrol
20	Betamethasone Valerate
	Triamcinolone Acetonide
30	Fludrocortisone Acetate
34	Dienoestrol
38	Fluoxymesterone
	Hydrocortisone Acetate

Rf	Compound
40	Ethinyloestradiol
44	Prednisolone Pivalate
55	Cortisone Acetate
70	Methallenoestril
80	Alphadolone Acetate
	Ethisterone
85	Oxymetholone
87	Methandienone
	Norethisterone
88	Fluocortolone Hexanoate
89	Beclomethasone Dipropionate
	Fluocortolone Pivalate
90	Alphaxalone
	Mestranol
	Stanolone
	Testosterone
91	Dimethisterone
	Methyltestosterone
	Norethynodrel

Rf	Compound
94	Ethyloestrenol
95	Ethynodiol Diacetate
	Norethandrolone
96	Dydrogesterone
	Oestradiol Benzoate
97	Nandrolone Decanoate
	Nandrolone Phenylpropionate
98	Chlorotrianisene
	Deoxycortone Acetate
	Medroxyprogesterone Acetate
	Megestrol Acetate
	Norethisterone Acetate
99	Hydroxyprogesterone Hexanoate
	Lynoestrenol
	Progesterone
	Testosterone Phenylpropionate
	Testosterone Propionate

System TS (p. 175)—Rf Values

Rf	Compound
00	Betamethasone
	Betamethasone Sodium Phosphate
	Cortisone Acetate
	Dexamethasone
	Ethisterone
	Fludrocortisone Acetate
	Fluocortolone Hexanoate
	Hydrocortisone
	Hydrocortisone Acetate
	Hydrocortisone Hydrogen Succinate
	Hydrocortisone Sodium Phosphate
	Methylprednisolone
	Prednisolone
	Prednisolone Pivalate
	Prednisolone Sodium Phosphate
	Prednisone
	Triamcinolone
01	Fluocinolone Acetonide
02s	Betamethasone Valerate

Rf	Compound
03	Stilboestrol
05s	Dienoestrol
06	Triamcinolone Acetonide
16s	Fluoxymesterone
40s	Ethinyloestradiol
42s	Beclomethasone Dipropionate
45s	Alphadolone Acetate
54s	Methallenoestril
58	Fluocortolone Pivalate
61	Methandienone
63	Testosterone
63s	Norethisterone
71	Methyltestosterone
	Norethynodrel
72	Stanolone
72s	Alphaxalone
78	Norethandrolone
79	Oestradiol Benzoate
82	Oxymetholone

Rf	Compound
85s	Medroxyprogesterone Acetate
	Megestrol Acetate
90	Hydroxyprogesterone Hexanoate
	Mestranol
	Norethisterone Acetate
92	Chlorotrianisene
95	Deoxycortone Acetate
	Dimethisterone
	Nandrolone Decanoate
	Nandrolone Phenylpropionate
	Progesterone
97	Lynoestrenol
98	Dydrogesterone
	Testosterone Phenylpropionate
	Testosterone Propionate
99	Ethyloestrenol
	Ethynodiol Diacetate

System TT (p. 176)—Rf Values

Rf	Compound
02	Phthalylsulphathiazole
	Succinylsulphathiazole
11	Sulphasomidine
21	Sulphaguanidine
24	Sulphadiazine
33	Sulfamerazine
46	Sulphamethizole

Rf	Compound
47	Sulphapyridine
50	Sulphadimidine
53	Sulphacetamide
	Sulphamethoxypyridazine
	Sulphathiazole
55	Sulphamethoxydiazine
61	Sulphanilamide

Rf	Compound
74	Sulphafurazole
84	Chlorpropamide
85	Sulphadimethoxine
88	Sulphamethoxazole
89	Sulphaphenazole
90	Carbutamide
98	Tolbutamide

System TU (p. 176)—Rf Values

Rf	Compound
01	Succinylsulphathiazole
04	Phthalylsulphathiazole
17	Sulphamethoxydiazine
18	Sulfamerazine
22	Sulphadiazine
26	Sulphamethoxypyridazine
27	Carbutamide

Rf	Compound
	Sulphadimidine
33	Sulphamethoxazole
35	Tolbutamide
36	Sulphamethizole
37	Sulphacetamide
40	Sulphathiazole
43	Chlorpropamide

Rf	Compound
	Sulphapyridine
48	Sulphafurazole
49	Sulphasomidine
52	Sulphadimethoxine
70	Sulphaphenazole
90	Sulphaguanidine
96	Sulphanilamide

SystemTV (p. 176)—Rf Values

Rf	Compound
01	Succinylsulphathiazole
02	Sulphamethizole
	Sulphamethoxazole
03	Chlorpropamide
	Sulphadiazine
04	Phthalylsulphathiazole
	Sulphacetamide

Rf	Compound
	Sulphafurazole
	Tolbutamide
05	Sulphathiazole
07	Carbutamide
	Sulfamerazine
13	Sulphaphenazole
15	Sulphamethoxydiazine

Rf	Compound
20	Sulphasomidine
34	Sulphadimethoxine
48	Sulphaguanidine
50	Sulphamethoxypyridazine
62	Sulphadimidine
66	Sulphanilamide
73	Sulphapyridine

System TW (p. 177)—Rf Values

Rf	Compound
00	Oxydemeton-methyl
09	Trichlorphon
19	Dimethoate
23	Mevinphos
68	Azinphos-methyl
74	Malathion

Rf	Compound
77	Parathion-methyl
81	Parathion
82	Diazinon
100	Disulfoton
	Phorate

Gas Chromatographic Data

System GA (p. 192)—Retention Index

RI	Compound
300	Propane
305	Dichlorodifluoromethane
361	Dichlorotetrafluoroethane
372	Acetaldehyde
400	Butane
405	Bromochlorodifluoromethane
421	Ethanol
462	Enflurane
469	Acetone
484	Trichlorofluoromethane
491	Methanol
515	Ether
	Methylene Chloride
530	Isopropyl Alcohol
533	Halothane
571	Propanol
579	Methyl Ethyl Ketone
596	Ethyl Acetate
600	Hexane
605	Chloroform
634	1,1,1-Trichloroethane
659	Carbon Tetrachloride
660	Benzene
680	Amyl Nitrite
693	Isopropyl Nitrate
695	Chloral Hydrate
701	Methoxyflurane
710	Trichloroethylene
715	Methylpentynol
724	Isobutyl Methyl Ketone
748	1,1,2-Trichloroethane
756	Toluene
780	Ethanolamine
786	Paraldehyde
789	Tetrachloroethylene
798	Ethylene Glycol
813	Piperazine
838	Urethane
849	Ethylbenzene
857	Trichloroethanol
860	*p*-Xylene
863	*m*-Xylene
882	Allopurinol
884	*o*-Xylene
888	Tuaminoheptane
910	Tetrachloroethane
930	Putrescine
947	Benzaldehyde
949	Chlorbutol
981	Phenol
1000	Acepifylline
1017	Fluspirilene
1030	Ethchlorvynol
1035	Cadaverine
1046	Benzyl Alcohol
1052	Isometheptene
1087	Cyclopentamine
1100	4-Chloroaniline

RI	Compound
	Methyl Nicotinate
	Troxidone
1105	Emylcamate
1111	Phenethylamine
1118	Heptaminol
1120	Paramethadione
1123	Amphetamine
1133	Norfenfluramine
1136	Camphor
1147	Phentermine
1158	Aniline
1169	Propylhexedrine
1176	Methylamphetamine
1180	Benzoic Acid
1186	Naphthalene
1193	Methyl Salicylate
1205	2-Bromo-2-ethylbutyramide
1206	Ethosuximide
1210	Hexamine
1212	Sulphafurazole
1214	Pargyline
1215	Acetylcarbromal
	Nicotinyl Alcohol
1220	Hydroquinone
1222	Fenfluramine
1223	Tranylcypromine
1230	Chlormethiazole
1235	Betahistine
1236	Dimethylamphetamine
1239	Mephentermine
1240	Mebanazine
1250	Pyrazinamide
1257	Amantadine
1258	Resorcinol
1260	Thymol
1265	4-Aminophenol
1280	Labetalol
1293	Aletamine
1302	Cathine
1303	Octamylamine
1308	Salicylic Acid
1309	Aminosalicylic Acid
	Aspirin
1313	Phenylpropanolamine (norephedrine)
1320	Hydroxyamphetamine
	3-Hydroxyethosuximide
1323	3,4-Dichloroaniline
1335	Nicotinic Acid
	Phenelzine
1340	2-Bromo-2-ethyl-3-hydroxybutyramide
	Mexiletine
1342	Chlorphentermine
1348	Nicotine
1353	Dimetridazole
1354	Pseudoephedrine
1358	Acetanilide

RI	Compound
1361	Methoxyphenamine
1363	Ephedrine
	Ethinamate
1368	Eugenol
1370	1-Hydroxyethylethosuximide
1373	Bemegride
1380	2-Ethylbutyrylurea
1385	Methoxyamphetamine
1388	Rimantadine
1389	Diphenyl
1390	Ametazole
1400	Methylephedrine
1406	Dimethyl Phthalate
1419	Methyl Hydroxybenzoate
1431	Phenmetrazine
1432	Warfarin
1436	Nicotinamide
	Selegiline
	Tyramine
1444	Phendimetrazine
1450	Hydroquinine
	Mevinphos
1455	Salicylamide
1462	Butylated Hydroxyanisole
1465	Pheneturide
1472	Metharbitone
	Methylenedioxyamphetamine
1473	Phenacemide
1480	Beclamide
1486	Diethylpropion
1487	Mandelic Acid
	Protokylol
1490	Alphanaphthol
	Butylated Hydroxytoluene
	Cantharidin
	Pholedrine
1497	Barbitone
	Diethylcarbamazine
	Histamine
1504	Thiotepa
1513	Carbromal
1515	Pyridostigmine Bromide
1517	Mercaptopurine
1519	Etafedrine
1520	Glibornuride
	Phenprobamate
1525	Nikethamide
1528	Hydralazine
1529	Methyprylone
1542	Etenzamide
1547	Acetylcysteine
	Aminobenzoic Acid
1549	Clofibrate
1550	Crotamiton
	Methimazole
1552	Pentetrazol
1555	Benzocaine
1561	Enallylpropymal

RI	Compound
1564	Diethyl Phthalate
1567	Propyl Hydroxybenzoate
1568	Mephenesin
1583	Diethyltoluamide
1590	Hydrastinine
1592	Metronidazole
1593	Iproniazid
1598	Tolazoline
1604	Clorprenaline
1605	Dichlorophenoxyacetic Acid (methyl ester)
1606	Allobarbitone
1608	Nicametate
	Nifenazone
1616	DOM
1617	Dinitro-orthocresol
1619	Fenproporex
1621	Chlorproguanil
1622	Aprobarbitone
	Methsuximide
1628	Demeton-S-methyl
1630	Oxyphenbutazone
1631	Ibuprofen
1632	3'-Hydroxyamylobarbitone
1634	Phensuximide
	Prolintane
1640	Butoxyethyl Nicotinate
	Dipyridamole
1645	Trometamol
1650	Guaiphenesin
1651	Tolazamide
1652	Trimeperidine
1655	Atrazine
1662	Secbutobarbitone
1665	Butobarbitone
1667	Styramate
1668	Butalbital
	Etisazole
1670	Isoniazid
1675	Phenacetin
	Phorate
1676	Dofamium Chloride
1677	Chlorphenesin
	Fencamfamin
1678	Beclamide
	Carbimazole
	Cotinine
	Dyclonine
1682	Hydroxyephedrine
1683	Tolbutamide
1685	Etilefrine
	Salol
1687	Paracetamol
	Tigloidine
1688	Crotethamide
	Mescaline
1690	α-Benzene Hexachloride
	Glibornuride
	Simazine
1698	Idobutal
1701	Talbutal
1710	β-Benzene Hexachloride
1715	Thiambutosine
1718	Amylobarbitone

RI	Compound
	Morazone
1720	Nealbarbitone
	Vinylbitone
1724	Hydroxyphenamate
1725	Dimethirimol (methyl ether)
	Dimethoate
	Tybamate
1726	Methoxamine
1728	Chlorzoxazone
1730	Isoprenaline
1737	Methylphenidate
	Trimeperidine
1738	Benzyl Benzoate
	Cropropamide
1740	α-Methyltryptamine
	Pentobarbitone
	Trichlorophenoxyacetic Acid (methyl ester)
	Vinbarbitone
1742	Butyl Aminobenzoate
	Tryptamine
1743	Halquinol
1745	Lindane
	Norpethidine
1748	Profadol
	Trimethoxyamphetamine
1749	Pentachlorophenol
1751	Pethidine
1754	Butethamate
	Nitroxynil
1755	δ-Benzene Hexachloride
1756	Ethionamide
1758	Diazinon
1760	Alprenolol
1766	Methohexitone
1770	5-(2-Acetonyl)-5-isopropyl-barbituric Acid
	Meclofenoxate
	N-Methyltryptamine
	Neostigmine Bromide
1775	Ametryne
1777	Hexylresorcinol
1778	2-Phenylglutarimide
1779	Nicoumalone
1780	Glibornuride
	Lobeline
1791	Chlorpropamide
	Methoin
	Quinalbarbitone
1792	Alphaprodine
1795	5-Acetonyl-5-allylbarbituric Acid
	Desmetryne
	5-Methyltryptamine
1796	Meprobamate
1798	Benethamine
1800	Ethotoin
1801	Sparteine
1802	Chlorquinaldol
1803	Nimorazole
1804	Pheniramine
	Physostigmine
1807	Dexpanthenol
1808	Cotarnine
	Trimeperidine

RI	Compound
1810	Caffeine
	Dimethyltryptamine
1811	Pipobroman
1815	Parathion-methyl
1816	Prothionamide
1819	Saccharin
1825	Bisnortilidate
	Prilocaine
1830	Carisoprodol
	Isoaminile
1832	Thymoxamine
1833	Tetrahydrozoline
1835	Nortilidate
1836	Glutethimide
1840	Benorylate
	Tilidate
1843	Ketamine
1844	Dimenhydrinate
1848	Phenazone
1851	Trimeperidine
1852	Lachesine Chloride
1853	Prometryne
1855	Benzphetamine
1857	Ethoheptazine
	Hexobarbitone
1858	Brallobarbitone
	Hexethal
1859	Thiopentone
1860	Metyrapone
1862	Cyclopentobarbitone
1870	Lignocaine
	Oxprenolol
	Zomepirac (decomposition product)
1873	Diphenhydramine
1874	4-Hydroxyphenazone
1875	4-Hydroxyglutethimide
1880	Heptachlor
	Paraoxon
	Phenylmethylbarbituric Acid
1883	Clorgyline
	Ibomal
1885	Aminoparathion
1889	Mebutamate
1891	Methylphenobarbitone
1898	Dofamium Chloride
1899	Thiamylal
1902	Digitoxin
1903	Amidopyrine
	Cyclandelate
1904	Phencyclidine
1906	Doxylamine
	Morinamide
1910	Diethyltryptamine
1913	Dibutyl Phthalate
1917	Malathion
1920	Bamethan
	Tofenacin (N-monodesmethyl-orphenadrine)
1923	Bibenzonium Bromide
1925	Bethanidine
	Propyphenazone
1928	2'-Hydroxysecbutobarbitone
	Levamisole

RI	Compound	RI	Compound	RI	Compound
1930	Iminostilbene	2038	Thiacetazone	2187	Cocaine ·
1933	Prenalterol	2040	Thiabendazole		Levomethadyl Acetate
1936	Orphenadrine	2048	Zomepirac		Methazolamide
1938	Phenyltoloxamine	2050	Norbormide	2188	Dextropropoxyphene
1939	Azapetine		Norcyclizine	2190	Ketocyclobarbitone
1940	Terbutryne	2055	Phenindione		Physostigmine
	Xylometazoline	2057	Naphazoline	2191	Cyclophosphamide
1942	Parathion	2058	Heptabarbitone	2192	Hyoscyamine
1943	Aldrin	2059	Psilocybin	2195	Pentifylline
1945	Nystatin	2070	Berberine	2196	Amitriptyline
1949	Isocarboxazid		op'-DDE	2198	Oxeladin
1950	Flufenamic Acid	2071	Mepivacaine		Trimetozine
	2-Ethyl-5-methyl-3,3-diphenyl-1-	2072	Chlorphenoxamine	2199	Atropine
	pyrroline		Homatropine	2201	Mefenamic Acid
	Tetracycline	2080	Carbinoxamine		Trimipramine
1952	Harman		Chlophedianol	2203	Thonzylamine
1957	Phenobarbitone	2082	Benzoctamine	2207	Perphenazine
1963	Cyclobarbitone	2085	Endosulfan	2210	Nortriptyline
1964	Padimate	2090	Etofylline	2211	Bamipine
1965	Hexylcaine	2091	Normethadone		Fluopromazine
	3'-Hydroxyquinalbarbitone	2093	Hexetidine		Mianserin
1971	Caramiphen	2096	Brompheniramine	2213	Zimeldine
1973	Emepronium Bromide	2097	Dicyclomine	2217	Doxepin
1974	Dofamium Chloride	2098	Methoprotryne	2218	op'-DDT
1975	Ethomoxane	2099	Diphenylpyraline	2219	Amethocaine
1980	Methoxsalen	2100	Clotrimazole		Benzhexol
	Piperocaine	2103	Proxyphylline	2220	Mepyramine
	Psilocin	2110	Dieldrin	2223	Imipramine
	Tripelennamine	2112	Dropropizine	2225	Chlorcyclizine
1981	Methapyrilene	2114	Cycrimine	2226	Medazepam
1983	Dipyrone	2116	Thialbarbitone	2227	Aminoglutethimide
1990	Procarbazine	2120	Glycopyrronium Bromide	2229	Chloroprocaine
1999	Thenyldiamine	2122	Nomifensine	2230	Dextrorphan
	Theophylline	2125	Methaqualone		Levorphanol
2000	Captan	2130	pp'-DDE		Racemorphan
	Nefopam		Naproxen	2232	Carbetapentane
2002	Chlorpheniramine	2133	Chloropyrilene	2233	Phenoxybenzamine
2005	Thiocarlide	2138	Pyrimethamine	2234	Halopyramine
	Viloxazine	2140	Dextromethorphan	2235	Ambucetamide
2006	Phenyramidol		Dichlorophen		Monodesmethyldoxepin
2008	Diethylthiambutene	2141	Disulfiram	2238	Chlormezanone
	Etomidate	2142	Alverine	2240	Aminacrine
2010	Baclofen	2145	Chlorthalidone		N^1-Desalkyl-3-hydroxyflurazepam
	Metoprolol		Pipradrol	2242	Desipramine
2013	Octaphonium Chloride	2148	Methadone	2243	Azacyclonol
2014	Pilocarpine	2153	Perhexiline	2245	Phenazopyridine
2018	Procaine	2155	Bromodiphenhydramine	2247	Primidone
2020	Cyclizine		Trioxsalen	2248	Benactyzine
	Cyclopentolate	2156	Procyclidine		Clonidine
2021	Fenoprofen	2157	Propranolol		Procainamide
2024	Phenothiazine	2160	Pemoline	2250	N-Monodesmethyltrimipramine
	Tinidazole	2165	Tacrine		Trifluomeprazine
2025	Butanilicaine	2166	Sulphanilamide	2253	Sulphinpyrazone
2026	Eucatropine	2167	Phenindamine		Triprolidine
2029	Dimethoxanate	2168	Oxymetazoline	2255	Mecloqualone
2030	Bufotenine	2170	Nifedipine	2258	Dimethindene
	Carbamazepine-10,11-epoxide	2174	Santonin	2259	Promethazine
	Dimethisoquin	2175	Dopamine	2260	Pindolol
	2-Ethylidene-1,5-dimethyl-3,3-di-	2177	Imolamine	2261	Protriptyline
	phenylpyrrolidine	2180	Rescinnamine	2266	Biperiden
2032	Flurbiprofen	2181	Butriptyline	2267	Isothipendyl
2035	Ketobemidone	2183	Endrin		Noxiptyline
	Physostigmine	2184	Ergocryptine	2270	Timolol
2037	Pipazethate	2186	Adiphenine	2271	Diclofenac

RI	Compound
2273	Anisindione
	Bupivacaine
2274	Clopenthixol
2275	3′-Hydroxyheptabarbitone
	Pentazocine
2281	Pramoxine
2290	Carbamazepine
2291	Harmine
2298	Stilboestrol
2299	pp′-DDT
2300	Isoxsuprine
2301	Bufylline
2303	Hyoscine
2309	Trimeprazine
2310	Chloramphenicol
	Domiphen Bromide
2314	Benztropine
	Buphenine
	Primaquine
2315	Dihydroergotamine
2316	Promazine
2318	Piperidolate
	Thenalidine
2320	3′-Oxoheptabarbitone
2321	Phenglutarimide
2323	Proxymetacaine
2327	Mepenzolate Bromide
2328	Antazoline
2330	Phenytoin
	Tropicamide
2335	Iprindole
	Propoxycaine
2336	Oxazepam
	Probenecid
2337	Bromhexine
2339	Prothipendyl
2355	Atenolol
	Mazindol
	Oxypertine
2356	Maprotiline
	o-Toluidine
2357	Ethopropazine
2359	Levallorphan
2360	10-Hydroxyamitriptyline
	2-Hydroxymethylmethaqualone
2363	Dihydrocodeine
2365	Phenylbutazone
2366	Cyproheptadine
	Ergotamine
2368	Benzydamine
2370	Diperodon
	Noxythiolin
2375	Pizotifen
2376	Codeine
2377	Diethazine
2380	Dothiepin
	Feprazone
	Polythiazide
2382	Cannabidiol
2384	Diphenidol
2385	10-Hydroxynortriptyline
2388	2-Amino-5-nitrobenzophenone
	Norcodeine
2390	Monodesmethyldothiepin

RI	Compound
2395	Neopine
	Norpropoxyphene
2402	Hexoestrol
	Lorazepam
2406	Clomipramine
	Oxpentifylline
2410	2′-Hydroxymethylmethaqualone
2411	Ethylmorphine
2413	Sotalol
2415	Azatadine
	Clemastine
	4-Hydroxyphenobarbitone
2417	op′-Methoxychlor
2419	Pyrrobutamine
2420	Diloxanide
	Meclofenamic Acid
2425	Diazepam
2430	Azinphos-methyl
2433	Propanidid
2434	Proquamezine
2438	Normorphine
2440	Acebutolol
	Hydrocodone
	Tramazoline
2443	Dibenzepin
	Diphenoxylate
2445	Ethynodiol Diacetate
2450	Dothiepin Sulphoxide
2451	Dihydromorphine
2453	Chlordiazepoxide
2454	Morphine
2457	Butacaine
	Clorazepic Acid
2461	Azapropazone
	Methixene
2465	Mebhydrolin
	Molindone
	Protoveratrines A and B
2467	Hydromorphone
	Methdilazine
2471	N^1-Desalkylflurazepam
	Oxybuprocaine
2473	Δ^9-Tetrahydrocannabinol
2474	Dipipanone
2475	Aprindine
2480	Didesmethylchlorpromazine
	Monodesmethylchlorpromazine
2486	Chlorpromazine
2487	Chlorprothixene
2488	Androsterone
	Norpipanone
2490	Butalamine
	3′-Hydroxymethaqualone
2495	Disopyramide
	Ergocristine
	Tubocurarine Chloride
2496	Nordazepam (desmethyldiazepam)
2505	Emetine
2510	Acetylcodeine
2514	Methotrimeprazine
2517	Thebaine
2520	Cannabinol
	4′-Hydroxymethaqualone
2524	Oxycodone

RI	Compound
	Pecazine
2525	6-Hydroxymethaqualone
	Oxethazaine
2529	Demoxepam
2530	Apomorphine
	Chlordiazepoxide
	Loxapine
2532	Oxymorphone
2533	Thebacon
2537	3-Hydroxybromazepam
	6-Monoacetylmorphine
2540	2-Hydroxyimipramine
2550	Nadolol
	Oxyphencyclimine
2551	Norethynodrel
2555	Dimefline
2557	Prenylamine
2570	Benzoylecgonine
2577	Nalorphine
2578	Ethoxzolamide
2590	Amiodarone (decomposition product)
	Chloroquine
	Cinchonidine
	Cinchonine
	Nifuratel
2607	Ketotifen
2612	Mestranol
	Oestrone
2614	Diamorphine
2615	Deptropine
2617	Phenacaine
2620	Testosterone
2625	Gallamine Triethiodide
	Norethisterone
2630	Metoclopramide
2633	Temazepam
2638	Trimethoprim
2640	Naloxone
2641	Prazepam
2643	Methyltestosterone
2645	Flunitrazepam
2650	Fentanyl
2659	Amoxapine
	Oestradiol
2663	Bromazepam
2670	Phenbutrazate
2672	Methandienone
2674	Lormetazepam
2675	Clemizole
2680	Benzthiazide
2683	Trifluoperazine
2684	Phenazocine
2685	Indomethacin
2686	Broxaldine
2688	N^1-(2-Hydroxyethyl)flurazepam
2690	Sulindac
2694	Acepromazine
	Clobazam
2698	Acecainide
2700	Griseofulvin
2701	Cinchocaine
2705	Ajmaline
	Azaperone

RI	Compound	RI	Compound	RI	Compound
2719	Ethinyloestradiol	2835	Oxymetholone	3059	Famprofazone
2723	7-Aminoflunitrazepam	2845	Perazine	3060	Thiothixene
2727	Lormetazepam (decomposition product)	2849	Hydroxyzine	3065	Cinnarizine
		2850	Anileridine		Fluphenazine
2732	Fluanisone		Gelsemine	3070	Pipamperone
2738	Propiomazine	2860	3-Hydroxyprazepam	3075	Trilostane
2740	Desmethylflunitrazepam	2872	Hydroxychloroquine	3078	Dimethothiazine
2748	Naftidrofuryl Oxalate		Ibogaine	3086	Cholesterol
2750	Nitrazepam		Phenoperidine	3089	Methysergide
	Sulindac	2880	Dapsone	3107	Triamcinolone
2755	Desmethylclobazam	2885	Clonazepam	3114	Thioridazine
2760	Mequitazine	2890	7-Amino-3-hydroxyclonazepam	3119	Strychnine
2770	Pseudomorphine	2895	Dimoxyline	3120	Noscapine
2774	Captodiame	2900	7-Aminoclonazepam	3205	7-Acetamidonitrazepam
2775	Acebutolol	2906	Doxapram	3242	Rotenone
2779	Ethynodiol Diacetate	2925	Prajmalium Bitartrate	3247	Thiethylperazine
2780	Amiodarone (decomposition product)	2930	Clomiphene	3250	Trazodone
		2934	Diphenadione	3263	7-Acetamidoclonazepam
2785	Flurazepam	2940	Dextromoramide	3269	Yohimbine
2793	Progesterone	2942	Haloperidol	3280	Brucine
2798	Quinidine	2950	Mefruside		Spironolactone
	Quinine	2954	Camazepam	3285	Pericyazine
2799	Chlordiazepoxide		Prochlorperazine	3286	Buclizine
2807	Hexachlorophane	2965	Triazolam	3287	Phytomenadione
2810	Hydroquinidine	2967	Clozapine		Trimethobenzamide
2820	Bisacodyl	2970	Dexamethasone	3335	Amiodarone
	Chromonar		Oestriol	3380	Penfluridol
	Sulindac		Triamcinolone	3430	Droperidol
2825	7-Amino-1-desmethyl-flunitrazepam	2980	Miconazole	3445	Lysergide
		2988	Hydrastine	3465	Thiopropazate
	Papaverine	3015	Benzylmorphine	3590	Carphenazine
2828	7-Aminonitrazepam	3018	Pholcodine		
2830	Fenethylline	3033	Meclozine		

System GB (p. 193)—Retention Index

RI	Compound	RI	Compound	RI	Compound
849	Tuaminoheptane	1375	Nicotine	1804	Meclofenoxate
994	Isometheptene	1386	Ephedrine	1826	Pheniramine
1066	Norfenfluramine	1399	Pseudoephedrine	1862	Caffeine
1084	Heptaminol	1410	Chlorphentermine	1872	Diphenhydramine
1095	Cyclopentamine	1440	Methylephedrine	1875	Dimenhydrinate
1134	Amphetamine	1473	Phenmetrazine	1882	Ethoheptazine
1150	Amiphenazole	1507	Diethylpropion	1895	Benzphetamine
1158	Fenfluramine	1510	Etafedrine	1938	Dextropropoxyphene
1182	Phentermine	1513	Nikethamide	2034	Thenyldiamine
1186	Propylhexedrine		Phendimetrazine	2038	Chlorpheniramine
1200	Methylamphetamine	1528	Pentazocine	2081	Cyclizine
1218	Pargyline	1578	Pentetrazol	2090	Carbinoxamine
1245	Tranylcypromine	1600	Codeine	2122	Naphazoline
1261	Dimethylamphetamine	1614	Clorprenaline	2124	Methadone
1278	Mephentermine	1675	Prolintane	2136	Diphenylpyraline
1353	Phenylpropanolamine (norephedrine)	1735	Methoxamine	2159	Brompheniramine
		1736	Cotinine	2215	Pipradrol
1362	Cathine	1745	Fencamfamin		
1370	Methoxyphenamine	1753	Pethidine		

System GC (p. 193)—**Retention Index**

The values given are those of the tertiary bases or of trifluoroacetyl derivatives.

RI	Compound	RI	Compound	RI	Compound
1253	Bemegride	1737	Etafedrine	2430	Carbinoxamine
1287	Tuaminoheptane	1759	Tranylcypromine	2447	Diphenylpyraline
1383	Cathine	1849	Prolintane	2457	Brompheniramine
	Phenylpropanolamine	1852	Nikethamide		Naphazoline
	(norephedrine)	1873	Phenmetrazine	2470	Methadone
1429	Dimethylamphetamine	1880	Clorprenaline	2478	Pipradrol
1440	Pargyline	1934	Phenylephrine	2504	Dihydromorphine
1450	Phentermine	2021	Pentetrazol	2542	Morphine
1460	Phenelzine	2025	Pethidine	2546	Promethazine
1467	Ephedrine	2111	Cotinine	2563	Amiphenazole
1470	Norfenfluramine	2172	Benzphetamine	2576	Thonzylamine
1480	Methylephedrine	2173	Dextropropoxyphene	2586	Chlorpheniramine
1500	Propylhexedrine	2180	Fencamfamin	2646	Trimeprazine
1536	Amphetamine	2200	Meclofenoxate	2669	Dimethindene
1543	Pseudoephedrine		Methylphenidate	2681	Codeine
1573	Nicotine	2225	Pentazocine	2702	Dihydrocodeine
1621	Fenfluramine	2230	Doxapram	2739	Mebhydrolin
1630	Ethoheptazine		Levorphanol	2749	Antazoline
1668	Mephentermine	2300	Thenyldiamine	2894	Dipipanone
1670	Methoxyphenamine	2307	Cyproheptadine	2926	Phenindamine
1715	Diethylpropion	2348	Cyclizine	2954	Triprolidine
1722	Methylamphetamine	2376	Caffeine	3028	Hydrocodone
1725	Chlorphentermine	2378	Diphenhydramine	3469	Anileridine
1735	Phendimetrazine	2409	Ethamivan	3625	Dextromoramide

System GD (p. 194)—**Retention Time Relative to n-$C_{16}H_{34}$**

The values given are of the methyl derivatives.

RRT	Compound	RRT	Compound	RRT	Compound
0.4	Salsalate	1.31	Fenoprofen	1.77	Tolmetin
0.49	Indomethacin	1.36	Tolmetin	1.79	Fenbufen
	Sulindac	1.37	Naproxen	1.81	Feprazone
0.6	Salsalate	1.38	Niflumic Acid		Phenylbutazone
0.89	Ibuprofen	1.39	Flunixin	1.98	Benoxaprofen
1.12	Bufexamac	1.42	Diclofenac	2.05	Phenylbutazone
1.13	Alclofenac	1.45	Ketoprofen	2.07	Indoprofen
1.18	Naproxen		Mefenamic Acid	2.11	Oxyphenbutazone
1.20	Diflunisal	1.55	Fenclofenac	2.27	Indoprofen
1.26	Fenclofenac		Indomethacin	2.64	Frusemide
	Flufenamic Acid	1.61	Clonixin		
1.30	Flurbiprofen	1.62	Meclofenamic Acid		

System GE (p. 194)—**Retention Time Relative to Phenytoin**

RRT	Compound	RRT	Compound	RRT	Compound
0.04	Troxidone	0.39	Phensuximide	0.74	Phenobarbitone
0.06	Paramethadione	0.50	N-Desmethylmethsuximide	0.83	Carbamazepine
0.09	Valproic Acid	0.55	Methoin	0.89	Primidone
0.18	Ethosuximide	0.57	Ethotoin	1.35	Cholesterol
0.22	N-Desmethylparamethadione	0.65	Phenylethylmalondiamide		
0.35	Methsuximide	0.73	5-Ethyl-5-phenylhydantoin		

System GF (p. 195)—**Retention Index**

RI	Compound	RI	Compound	RI	Compound
1315	Amphetamine	1525	Nicotine	1935	Methylphenidate
1335	Methylamphetamine	1655	Diethylpropion	1995	Pethidine
1455	Tranylcypromine	1895	Nikethamide	2050	Benzphetamine

RI	Compound	RI	Compound	RI	Compound
2090	Methyprylone	2455	Carbetapentane		Theophylline
2100	Benzocaine	2460	Meprobamate	2765	Brallobarbitone
	Pheniramine		Nealbarbitone	2770	Dothiepin
2105	Diphenhydramine	2465	Butriptyline	2775	Ethopropazine
2110	Ethoheptazine		Pentobarbitone	2795	Clomipramine
2130	Tybamate	2470	Brompheniramine	2800	Feprazone
2150	Phencyclidine	2480	Bromodiphenhydramine		Prothipendyl
2170	Doxylamine	2485	Procyclidine	2815	Pyrrobutamine
2185	Orphenadrine	2495	Vinbarbitone	2820	Dothiepin Sulphoxide
2190	2-Ethyl-5-methyl-3,3-diphenyl-1-	2505	Trimipramine	2825	Cyclobarbitone
	pyrroline	2510	Amitriptyline	2830	10-Hydroxyamitriptyline
2195	Cotinine		Quinalbarbitone	2840	Dihydrocodeine
2230	Barbitone	2515	Phenindamine	2845	Phenothiazine
2240	Lignocaine	2540	Imipramine	2860	Codeine
2265	Amidopyrine	2550	Cocaine		Phenylbutazone
	Dicyclomine		Fluopromazine	2880	10-Hydroxyamitriptyline
2270	Oxprenolol	2560	Chlorcyclizine	2885	Dibenzepin
2280	2-Ethylidene-1,5-dimethyl-3,3-di-		Mepyramine		Hyoscine
	phenylpyrrolidine	2570	Doxepin	2895	Methixene
2305	Methapyrilene	2580	Methaqualone	2900	Oxyphencyclimine
2310	Propyphenazone		Procaine	2910	Chlorprothixene
2315	Glutethimide	2590	Protriptyline		Disopyramide
2320	Cyclizine	2595	Mianserin	2920	Mebhydrolin
2325	Phenacetin	2600	Phenoxybenzamine		Methdilazine
2335	Chlorpheniramine		Pramoxine	2930	Hydrocodone
2340	Allobarbitone		Thiopentone	2940	Chlorpromazine
	Caffeine		Triprolidine		Heptabarbitone
	Thenyldiamine	2610	Carbamazepine	2960	Phenobarbitone
2345	Mepivacaine	2620	Iminostilbene	2965	Methotrimeprazine
2365	Chlorphenoxamine	2640	Medazepam		Procainamide
2370	Dextropropoxyphene	2660	Atropine	3010	Azapropazone
	Methadone		Piperidolate	3025	Norpropoxyphene
2380	Hexobarbitone	2670	Nomifensine	3030	Pentazocine
	Nefopam	2675	Promethazine	3045	Diazepam
2390	Butobarbitone	2710	Clemastine	3050	Trifluoperazine
2395	Butalbital		Cyproheptadine	3210	Flurazepam
2405	Diphenylpyraline		Dipipanone	3225	Propiomazine
2430	Amylobarbitone	2715	Amethocaine	3230	Acepromazine
2445	Benzoctamine		Trimeprazine	3245	Chloroquine
	Phenazone	2745	Promazine		

System GG (p. 196)—Retention Index

RI	Compound	RI	Compound	RI	Compound
2620	Medazepam	3043	Demoxepam	3190	Flunitrazepam
2803	Oxazepam	3065	Chlordiazepoxide	3220	Flurazepam
2910	Lorazepam	3125	Clorazepic Acid	3280	Bromazepam
2940	Diazepam		Temazepam	3450	Nitrazepam
	Ketazolam	3145	Prazepam	3455	Clozapine
3041	Nordazepam (desmethyldiazepam)	3147	Clobazam	3600	Clonazepam

System GH (p. 197)—Retention Index

The values given are of the trimethylsilyl esters or ethers.

RI	Compound	RI	Compound	RI	Compound
2110	Propylcannabidiol	2350	Δ^9-THC	2620	11-Hydroxy-THC
2170	Propyl-Δ^9-THC	2430	Cannabinol	2710	8α,11-Dihydroxy-THC
2270	Cannabidiol	2440	Cannabigerol	2756	11-Nor-Δ^9-THC-9-carboxylic Acid
2280	Cannabicyclol	2580	8α-Hydroxy-THC		

System GI (p. 199)—Retention Time (min)

RT	Compound	RT	Compound	RT	Compound
0.6	Propane	7.3	Methyl Ethyl Ketone	20.3	Amyl Nitrite
0.7	Acetaldehyde	8.2	1,1,1-Trichloroethane	21.1	Isobutyl Methyl Ketone
	Methanol	8.3	Enflurane	23.2	Paraldehyde
0.9	Dichlorodifluoromethane	8.5	Halothane	24.3	Tetrachloroethylene
1.6	Bromochlorodifluoromethane	8.6	Carbon Tetrachloride	24.8	Toluene
1.9	Ethanol	9.4	Ethyl Acetate	24.9	Tetrachloroethane
	Methylene Chloride	12.0	Isopropyl Nitrate	25.5	Trichloroethanol
2.0	Dichlorotetrafluoroethane	12.5	Chloral Hydrate (tailing)	29.5	Ethylbenzene
2.3	Butane	14.8	Benzene	29.8	Chlorbutol
2.5	Acetone		Trichloroethylene	33.2	m-Xylene
3.0	Trichlorofluoromethane	16.4	1,1,2-Trichloroethane	34.2	Benzaldehyde
4.0	Isopropyl Alcohol	17.0	Ethylene Glycol (tailing)		p-Xylene
5.5	Propanol	17.4	Hexane	34.5	o-Xylene
5.9	Ether	17.6	Methoxyflurane	35.2	Ethchlorvynol
6.2	Chloroform	20.1	Methylpentynol	38.2	Camphor

System GJ (p. 200)—Retention Time Relative to Griseofulvin

The values given are of the methyl derivatives.

RRT	Compound	RRT	Compound	RRT	Compound
0.16	Sulphacetamide	0.53	Glymidine	0.98	Sulphamethizole
0.40	Sulphamethoxazole	0.66	Sulphadiazine	1.38	Sulphamethoxydiazine
	Sulphamoxole	0.69	Sulfamerazine	1.69	N^4-Acetylsulphadiazine
0.42	Sulphafurazole	0.71	Sulphadimidine	1.71	Sulphaphenazole
0.47	Sulphapyridine	0.91	N^4-Acetylsulphamethoxazole		
0.49	Sulphathiazole	0.93	Sulphamethoxypyridazine		

System GK (p. 73)—Retention Time Relative to Caffeine

GCDP = Gas chromatography
decomposition product

RRT	Compound	RRT	Compound	RRT	Compound
0.02	Phenyl isocyanate (GCDP of fenuron)		4-Isopropylphenyl isocyanate (GCDP of propoxur)	0.29	2-Ethylthiomethylphenol (GCDP of ethiofencarb)
0.05	N-Hydroxythioacetimidate (GCDP of methomyl)	0.18	3,3-Dimethyl-1-(methylthio)butan-2-one oxime (GCDP of thiofanox)	0.31	Dichlobenil
0.06	Aniline (GCDP of fenuron)				2,5-Dichloro-4-bromophenol (bromophos impurity)
	m-Tolyl isocyanate (GCDP of phenmedipham)	0.19	4-Chloroaniline (GCDP of monolinuron)		2,2-Dimethyl-1,3-benzodioxol-4-ol (GCDP of bendiocarb)
0.07	2-Methyl-2-(methylthio)-propionaldehyde oxime (GCDP of aldicarb)	0.20	4-Bromoaniline (GCDP of metobromuron)		Nicotine
		0.23	3-Chloro-4-methylaniline (GCDP of chlortoluron)	0.35	3-Chloro-4-methoxyphenyl isocyanate (GCDP of metoxuron)
0.08	4-Bromophenyl isocyanate (GCDP of metobromuron)		Dichlorvos		Propham
	4-Chlorophenyl isocyanate (GCDP of monolinuron)		2,3-Dihydro-2,2-dimethylbenzo-furan-7-ol (GCDP of carbofuran)	0.36	3,4-Dichloroaniline (GCDP of diuron, linuron)
0.09	o-Isopropoxyphenol (GCDP of propoxur)	0.26	3-Chloro-4-bromophenyl isocyanate (GCDP of chlorbromuron)		Paraquat (reduction product I—monoene)
0.13	3-Chloro-4-methylphenyl isocyanate (GCDP of chlortoluron)	0.27	Trichlorphon	0.40	Diquat (reduction product I—monoene)
	3,4-Dichlorophenyl isocyanate (GCDP of diuron, linuron)	0.28	2-(1,3-Dioxolan-2-yl)phenol (GCDP of dioxacarb)	0.45	Mecoprop (methyl ester)
				0.47	Alphanaphthol (GCDP of carbaryl)

High Pressure Liquid Chromatographic Data

System HA (p. 214)—*k′* Values

t = 'tailing peak'

k′	Compound
0.1	Acetanilide
	Acetazolamide
	Benzocaine
	Chlormethiazole
	N^1-Desalkylflurazepam
	Diazepam
	Diazoxide
	Indapamide
	Indole
	Lorazepam
	Methocarbamol
	Nitrazepam
	Phenothiazine
	Phenoxybenzamine
	Proxyphylline
	Theobromine
	Theophylline
0.2	Bezitramide
	Caffeine
	Colchicine
	Cotinine
	Diphenoxylate
	Dipyridamole
	2-Ethyl-5-methyl-3,3-diphenyl-1-pyrroline
	Mebanazine
	Medazepam
	Mephenesin
	Methaqualone
	Nifedipine
	Nordazepam
	Pargyline
	Pemoline
	Perhexiline
	Phenazone
0.3	Amidopyrine
	Benzquinamide
	Ergocristine
	Ergosine
	Ergosinine
	Noscapine
	Papaverine
	Phenbutrazate
0.4	Acetorphine
	Bromhexine
	Buprenorphine
	Cimetidine
	Deserpidine
	Doxapram
	Ergocornine
	Ergocryptine
	Ergometrine
	Ergotamine
	Methylergometrine
	Methysergide
0.5	Lysergamide
	Methoserpidine

k′	Compound
	Practolol
0.6	Dihydroergotamine
	Diprenorphine
	Droperidol
	Etorphine
	Lidoflazine
	Lignocaine
	Lofepramine
	Phentermine
	Piritramide
	Pramoxine
	Rescinnamine
	Trazodone
0.6t	Diphenoxylic Acid
0.7	Buclizine
	Dextromoramide
	Fenoterol
	Lysergide
	Meclozine
	Morazone
	Narceine
	Oxypertine
	Pimozide
0.8	Cinnarizine
	Fentanyl
	Harmine
	Isoxsuprine
	Phenoperidine
	Prazosin
0.8t	Lysergic Acid
0.9	Amphetamine
	Bamethan
	Buphenine
	Bupivacaine
	Chlorphentermine
	Mepivacaine
	Metaraminol
	Methoxamine
	Nomifensine
	Phendimetrazine
	Phenylpropanolamine
	Terbutaline
0.9t	Benzoylecgonine
1.0	Cathine
	Ephedrine
	Nalorphine
	Norfenfluramine
	Phenelzine
	Piminodine
	Prenylamine
	Prilocaine
	Pyrimethamine
	Salbutamol
	Thiopropazate
	Tranylcypromine
1.1	Anileridine
	Benperidol

k′	Compound
	Clorprenaline
	Desmethylmaprotiline
	Dicyclomine
	Ecgonine
	4-Hydroxypropranolol
	Hyoscine
	Loxapine
	Lysergol
	3-Methoxy-4, 5-methylenedioxy-amphetamine
	Nicotine
1.1t	Orphenadrine *N*-oxide
1.2	Alprenolol
	Azacyclonal
	Benzphetamine
	Butacaine
	Clonidine
	Debrisoquine
	Etamiphylline
	Flupenthixol
	Fluphenazine
	Haloperidol
	2-Hydroxydesipramine
	Mexiletine
	Monoethylglycinexylidide
	Nadolol
	Phenethylamine
	Pindolol
	Pipradrol
	Pseudoephedrine
	Sotalol
	Timolol
	Tocainide
	Trifluperidol
	Trimethoprim
	Tryptamine
	Tyramine
1.2t	Nialamide
1.3	Atenolol
	Didesmethylimipramine
	Fencamfamin
	Fenfluramine
	Flupenthixol Sulphoxide
	Flurazepam
	Mescaline
	Metoprolol
	Norpropoxyphene
	Oxprenolol
	Pericyazine
	Phenazocine
	Phenylephrine
	Propranolol
1.4	Acebutolol
	Diethylcarbamazine
	Hydroxyzine
	Metopimazine
	Naloxone

k'	Compound		k'	Compound		k'	Compound
4.2t	Homatropine			Codeine		6.0t	Pholcodine
4.3t	Bretylium Tosylate		5.0	Mesoridazine		6.3t	Pyridostigmine Bromide
4.4	Doxylamine			Metoclopramide		6.7t	Oxymorphone
	Propantheline Bromide			Promethazine		6.9t	Oxycodone
	Prothipendyl		5.0t	Deptropine		7.1t	Emetine
4.4t	Benzylmorphine		5.1	Dimethindene			Hydrocodone
	Levorphanol		5.2	Emepronium Bromide		7.2t	Dihydrocodeine
4.6t	Dothiepin Sulphoxide			Thioridazine		7.7t	Cephaëline
	Thebaine		5.4	Pipazethate		7.9t	Hydromorphone
4.7	Trimethobenzamide		5.6t	Dextromethorphan		8.2t	Cotarnine
4.7t	Carbinoxamine		5.7t	Dihydromorphine		8.3t	Mequitazine
	Dextrorphan		5.8t	Dimethoxanate		11.1t	Brucine
	Neostigmine Bromide		5.9	Promazine		13.0t	Strychnine
4.8t	Clemizole		6.0	Methdilazine		15.2t	Chloroquine

System HB (p. 214)—k' Values

k'	Compound		k'	Compound		k'	Compound
0.10	Noradrenaline		3.64	Phenethylamine		8.48	Amphetamine
0.27	Oxedrine		3.87	Phenylpropanolamine		10.52	Methylamphetamine
0.73	Hydroxyephedrine		4.39	Cathine		11.08	Dimethylamphetamine
0.81	Tyramine		5.68	Ephedrine		16.82	Mescaline
2.00	Hordenine		5.90	Pseudoephedrine		19.46	Phentermine
2.24	Hydroxyamphetamine		5.91	Phenelzine		32.17	Methoxyphenamine

System HC (p. 214)—k' Values

k'	Compound		k'	Compound		k'	Compound
0.05	Buprenorphine		0.67	Pentazocine		1.30	Morphine
0.09	Dextromoramide		0.69	Pipradrol		1.31	Phenethylamine
0.10	Phenoperidine		0.70	Phenylpropanolamine		1.46	Levallorphan
0.14	Pemoline		0.72	Fencamfamin		1.47	Tyramine
	Piritramide		0.78	Acetylcodeine		1.48	Trimethoxyamphetamine
0.15	Benzphetamine		0.80	6-Monoacetylmorphine		1.55	Ethoheptazine
	Noscapine		0.82	Chlorphentermine		1.56	Morphine-3-glucuronide
0.16	Diethylpropion		0.83	Cathine		1.61	Dipipanone
	Papaverine		0.85	Oxycodone		1.63	Pholcodine
0.17	Naloxone			Thebacon		1.64	Phenylephrine
0.19	Dextropropoxyphene		0.86	Phentermine		1.77	Pseudoephedrine
0.20	Mazindol		0.88	Fenfluramine		1.79	Ephedrine
0.26	Caffeine		0.94	Thebaine		1.83	Methylephedrine
	Tranylcypromine		0.98	Amphetamine		1.89	Dimethylamphetamine
0.27	Fenethylline			Methylenedioxyamphetamine		2.04	Norpethidine
0.29	Nalorphine		1.03	Benzylmorphine		2.07	Methylamphetamine
0.30	Phenazocine			Methadone		2.17	Hydrocodone
0.32	Phendimetrazine		1.06	Ethylmorphine			Mescaline
0.35	Norpipanone		1.08	Normetanephrine		2.48	Mephentermine
0.36	Methylphenidate		1.11	Etorphine		2.50	Dihydrocodeine
0.37	Phenelzine			Fentanyl		2.75	Dihydromorphine
0.53	Normethadone			Hydroxyamphetamine		3.20	Levorphanol
0.55	Pethidine		1.13	DOM		3.51	Norcodeine
0.63	Adrenaline		1.21	Codeine		3.92	Normorphine
0.66	Diamorphine		1.26	Prolintane			

System HD (p. 214)—k' Values

k'	Compound		k'	Compound		k'	Compound
0.1	Dipyrone			Phenazone			Salicylamide
	Nifenazone		0.2	Amidopyrine		0.5	Acetanilide
	Paracetamol		0.4	Morazone			Aspirin

k'	Compound
0.55	Etenzamide
0.6	Phenacetin
	Piroxicam
0.7	Benorylate
	Choline Salicylate
	Salicylic Acid
1.2	Indoprofen
1.25	Propyphenazone
	Sulindac
1.95	Bufexamac

k'	Compound
	Oxyphenbutazone
2.05	Tolmetin
2.4	Ketoprofen
2.5	Famprofazone
2.6	Alclofenac
3.3	Naproxen
3.6	Salsalate
3.7	Zomepirac
3.9	Methyl Salicylate
4.0	Fenbufen

k'	Compound
4.1	Diflunisal
6.5	Phenylbutazone
6.95	Indomethacin
7.9	Fenoprofen
11.3	Benoxaprofen
11.5	Diclofenac
15.1	Ibuprofen
15.6	Salol
19.7	Flufenamic Acid
21.2	Mefenamic Acid

System HE (p. 215)—k' Values

k'	Compound
0.91	Ethosuximide
1.35	Primidone
1.57	Sulthiame
2.76	Phenobarbitone
2.81	Ethotoin

k'	Compound
6.02	Methsuximide
6.84	Pheneturide
7.97	Glutethimide
8.30	Carbamazepine
9.71	Phenytoin

System HF (p. 215)—k' Values

k'	Compound
0.17	Viloxazine
0.42	Nomifensine
0.50	Dibenzepin
0.67	Zimeldine
1.33	Oxypertine
1.63	Noxiptyline
	Opipramol

k'	Compound
2.27	Doxepin
3.60	Desipramine
	Dothiepin
	Protriptyline
4.17	Imipramine
4.58	Nortriptyline
4.92	Maprotiline

k'	Compound
5.42	Amitriptyline
6.17	Trimipramine
7.33	Butriptyline
9.92	Clomipramine
10.83	Iprindole

System HG (p. 216)—k' Values

k'	Compound
1.11	Barbitone
1.48	Phenylmethylbarbituric Acid
2.46	Allobarbitone
2.69	Metharbitone
3.09	Brallobarbitone
	Phenobarbitone
3.42	Aprobarbitone
4.01	Ibomal
4.83	Vinbarbitone

k'	Compound
4.89	Secbutobarbitone
5.25	Cyclobarbitone
5.43	Butobarbitone
6.00	Cyclopentobarbitone
6.17	Butalbital
7.25	Talbutal
7.27	Methylphenobarbitone
7.37	Hexobarbitone
8.12	Idobutal

k'	Compound
8.65	Enallylpropymal
9.90	Heptabarbitone
10.22	Nealbarbitone
10.91	Amylobarbitone
10.96	Pentobarbitone
16.28	Quinalbarbitone
27.61	Methohexitone
34.28	Hexethal

System HH (p. 216)—k' Values

k'	Compound
0.63	Barbitone
0.94	Phenylmethylbarbituric Acid
1.23	Phenobarbitone
1.33	Allobarbitone
1.72	Brallobarbitone
1.99	Metharbitone
2.22	Aprobarbitone
2.32	Vinbarbitone
2.58	Ibomal

k'	Compound
2.61	Cyclobarbitone
3.32	Secbutobarbitone
3.42	Butobarbitone
3.48	Butalbital
3.84	Cyclopentobarbitone
	Methylphenobarbitone
4.67	Talbutal
4.77	Idobutal
4.93	Heptabarbitone

k'	Compound
5.67	Hexobarbitone
6.19	Nealbarbitone
6.96	Enallylpropymal
7.05	Amylobarbitone
8.07	Pentobarbitone
11.47	Quinalbarbitone
20.39	Hexethal
20.48	Methohexitone

System HI (p. 216)—k' Values

k'	Compound	k'	Compound	k'	Compound
0.46	7-Aminonitrazepam	3.15	Flunitrazepam	5.19	N^1-Desalkylflurazepam
0.68	7-Acetamidonitrazepam	3.91	Clobazam	5.68	Temazepam
1.17	Clorazepic Acid	4.27	N^1-(2-Hydroxyethyl)flurazepam	6.32	Lormetazepam
2.32	Bromazepam	4.38	Triazolam	6.41	Chlordiazepoxide
2.42	Demoxepam	4.47	Desmethylchlordiazepoxide	8.00	Nordazepam (desmethyldiazepam)
2.85	Clonazepam	4.60	Lorazepam	9.47	Diazepam
2.96	Nitrazepam	4.62	Oxazepam	9.75	Midazolam
3.06	Desmethylclobazam	4.70	Alprazolam	12.81	Ketazolam

System HJ (p. 217)—k' Values

k'	Compound
2.10	Midazolam
2.29	Diazepam
2.45	Ketazolam
3.19	Flurazepam
4.60	Prazepam
7.05	Medazepam

System HK (p. 217)—k' Values

k'	Compound	k'	Compound	k'	Compound
0.00	7-Aminonitrazepam	0.60	Temazepam	2.19	Prazepam
0.01	Desmethylclobazam	0.73	Oxazepam	2.39	Desmethylchlordiazepoxide
0.03	Clobazam	1.43	N^1-(2-Hydroxyethyl)flurazepam	2.49	Diazepam
	Demoxepam	1.49	Nitrazepam	2.79	Alprazolam
0.04	Ketazolam	1.52	N^1-Desalkylflurazepam	2.87	Chlordiazepoxide
0.08	Lormetazepam	1.83	Triazolam	2.99	Bromazepam
0.14	Lorazepam	1.93	7-Acetamidonitrazepam	4.44	Medazepam
0.35	Clonazepam	1.99	Nordazepam (desmethyldiazepam)	5.90	Midazolam
0.47	Flunitrazepam	2.00	Clorazepic Acid	6.50	Flurazepam

System HL (p. 217)—k' Values

k'	Compound	k'	Compound
7.47	Cannabidiol	13.35	Δ^9-Tetrahydrocannabinol
	Cannabivarin	14.07	Δ^8-Tetrahydrocannabinol
8.18	Cannabigerol	14.64	Tetrahydrocannabivaric Acid
	Tetrahydrocannabivarin	14.78	Cannabicyclol
8.76	Cannabidiolic Acid	19.09	Cannabichromene
11.77	Cannabinol	25.83	Tetrahydrocannabinolic Acid

System HM (p. 217)—k' Values

k'	Compound	k'	Compound	k'	Compound
2.0	Digitoxigenin	5.4	Digitoxin	11.3	Digoxin
2.8	Digitoxigenin Monodigitoxoside	5.5	Digoxigenin Monodigitoxoside	17.9	Lanatoside A
3.7	Gitoxigenin	6.5	Gitoxigenin Bisdigitoxoside	31.8	Lanatoside B
3.9	Digitoxigenin Bisdigitoxoside	6.8	Gitaloxin	39.5	Lanatoside C
4.5	Digoxigenin	8.2	Digoxigenin Bisdigitoxoside		
	Gitoxigenin Monodigitoxoside	8.6	Gitoxin		

System HN (p. 217)—*k'* Values

k'	Compound	*k'*	Compound	*k'*	Compound
0.54	Chlorothiazide	3.82	Methyclothiazide	10.78	Cyclothiazide
0.67	Quinethazone	4.01	Clopamide	11.91	Cyclothiazide
0.70	Hydrochlorothiazide	4.89	Metolazone	12.81	Cyclothiazide
1.28	Chlorthalidone	7.26	Clorexolone	15.09	Polythiazide
1.30	Hydroflumethiazide	8.67	Mefruside	15.35	Bendrofluazide
3.10	Trichlormethiazide	9.32	Benzthiazide	16.45	Cyclopenthiazide

System HP (p. 218)—*k'* Values

k'	Compound	*k'*	Compound	*k'*	Compound
0.00	Iso-lysergide	0.92	2-Oxylysergide	11.4	Dihydroergotamine
	Lysergic Acid	1.83	Lysergide	15.2	Ergocryptine
0.33	Lysergamide	1.98	Lysergic Acid Methylpropylamide	15.9	Dihydroergocryptine
0.50	Ergometrine	2.33	Methysergide	17.3	Ergocristine
0.83	Iso-lysergic Acid	7.08	Ergosine	17.7	Ergosinine
	Lysergol	9.58	Ergotamine	18.3	Dihydroergocristine
	Methylergometrine	10.2	Ergocornine	44.3	Bromocriptine

System HQ (p. 218)—*k'* Values

k'	Compound	*k'*	Compound	*k'*	Compound
0.00	Procaine		Proxymetacaine	8.97	Butacaine
0.24	Chloroprocaine	2.68	Cocaine	16.25	Amethocaine
0.79	Lignocaine	4.42	Butanilicaine		Oxybuprocaine
1.09	Mepivacaine	4.59	Piperocaine	20.06	Benzocaine
	Propoxycaine	5.68	Benzoylecgonine		
1.38	Prilocaine	7.19	Bupivacaine		

System HR (p. 218)—*k'* Values

k'	Compound	*k'*	Compound
0.86	Bupivacaine	2.78	Dyclonine
	Oxybuprocaine	4.14	Oxethazaine
1.33	Amethocaine	5.51	Cinchocaine
1.61	Benzocaine	10.31	Cyclomethycaine
2.48	Diperodon	11.24	Dimethisoquin
	Pramoxine		

System HS (p. 219)—*k'* Values

k'	Compound	*k'*	Compound
0.01	Noscapine	1.00	6-Monoacetylmorphine
0.04	Papaverine	1.45	Ethylmorphine
0.21	Caffeine	1.90	Codeine
0.35	Diamorphine	2.02	Quinine
0.50	Acetylcodeine	2.43	Strychnine
0.79	Thebaine	5.16	Morphine

System HT (p. 219)—*k'* Values

k'	Compound	*k'*	Compound
2.4	Cortisone	4.8	Dexamethasone
2.5	Triamcinolone Acetonide	5.8	Hydrocortisone
3.4	Prednisone	7.5	Methylprednisolone
4.2	Beclomethasone	8.4	Prednisolone

System HU (p. 220)—k' Values

k'	Compound	k'	Compound	k'	Compound
3.3	Sulphachlorpyridazine	7.1	Sulphadimidine	9.6	N^4-Acetylsulphanilamide
3.8	Sulphapyridine	7.5	Sulphamethoxypyridazine	12.6	Sulphamoxole
4.4	Sulfadoxine	7.7	Sulphacetamide	13.4	Sulphathiazole
4.8	Sulfaquinoxaline	8.1	Sulfamerazine	14.0	Phthalylsulphathiazole
	Sulphamethoxazole	8.2	Sulphamethoxydiazine	16.8	Succinylsulphathiazole
4.9	N^4-Acetylsulphamethoxazole	8.7	Sulphadiazine		
6.0	Sulphafurazole	8.9	Sulphanilamide		

System HV (p. 97)—Retention Times Relative to Meclofenamic Acid

RRT	Compound	RRT	Compound	RRT	Compound
0.45	Frusemide	0.77	Diflunisal	0.92	Feprazone
0.52	Indoprofen	0.78	Sulindac	0.93	Niflumic Acid
0.60	Tolmetin	0.81	Fenbufen	0.95	Mefenamic Acid
0.61	Alclofenac	0.85	Diclofenac		Phenylbutazone
0.66	Ketoprofen	0.87	Clonixin	0.98	Benoxaprofen
0.67	Naproxen		Indomethacin	0.99	Flunixin
0.69	Oxyphenbutazone	0.89	Flurbiprofen		Tolmetin
	Salsalate	0.91	Fenclofenac	1.00	Flufenamic Acid

System HW (p. 215)—k' Values

k'	Compound	k'	Compound	k'	Compound
0.32	Amidopyrine	2.3	Acetanilide	4.8	Choline Salicylate
	Paracetamol	2.5	Salicylamide	7.7	Piroxicam
0.45	Dipyrone	2.7	Aspirin	11.0	Propyphenazone
	Nifenazone	4.4	Phenacetin	22.4	Benorylate
0.95	Phenazone	4.6	Etenzamide		
2.05	Morazone		Salicylic Acid		

Ultraviolet Absorption Maxima

In the following tables no values below 230 nm have been included although some have been recorded in the monographs in Part 2. Details of A(1%, 1 cm) values are given in the monographs in Part 2.

Table A gives the wavelengths of maximum absorption, together with the wavelengths of any subsidiary peaks in the range 230 to 360 nm, for the compounds in **acid** solution. Table B gives the wavelengths of maximum absorption in **alkaline** solution when values in acid solution are not recorded in the monographs in Part 2 or when the values in alkaline solution differ significantly from the values in acid solution. Table C gives the values in **neutral** solution for compounds for which values in acid or alkaline solution are not recorded in the monographs in Part 2 or when the values in neutral solution differ significantly from those in acid or alkaline solution.

For an unknown compound, the wavelength of maximum absorption should be compared with the tables using a tolerance of $\pm$ 2 nm to give a list of possible compounds; reference may then be made to the monographs in Part 2.

A. In Acid Solution—Wavelengths of Maximum Absorption

λ max nm	Compound	Subsidiary Peaks nm	λ max nm	Compound	Subsidiary Peaks nm
230	Amiphenazole	261		Spiramycin	
	Amoxycillin	272	234	Acebutolol	320
	Aspirin	278		Aconitine	275
	Benzoic Acid	273		Aminosalicylic Acid	300
	Bromodiphenhydramine			Benzoylecgonine	274
	Chloroprocaine	288		Etenzamide	293
	Chlorprothixene	268, 324		Heteronium Bromide	
	Clobazam	289		Mebendazole	288
	Dehydroemetine	283		Methaqualone	269
	Dichloralphenazone			Oxazepam	280
	Diprenorphine	286		Thenalidine	
	Dothiepin	303	235	Ambucetamide	
	Emetine	282		Cinchonine	315
	Ethionamide	275		Clomiphene	292
	Flupenthixol			Disulphamide	276, 285
	Gliclazide			Frusemide	274, 342
	Phenazone			Hydroxychloroquine	256, 329, 343
	Stanozolol			Oxybuprocaine	298
231	Aloxiprin			Propoxycaine	298
	Amicarbalide			Salicylamide	298
	Clopenthixol	269, 325	236	Cinchonidine	316
	Lormetazepam	311		Flurazepam	284
	Piperocaine	274		Salicylic Acid	303
	Pseudomorphine			Thonzylamine	274, 316
	Rifampicin	263, 336	237	Amodiaquine	343
	Trimetazidine	269		Benzbromarone	281
232	Bunitrolol	292		Chloropyrilene	312
	Chlorcyclizine			Clorazepic Acid	287
	Chlorpropamide			Demoxepam	305
	Diperodon			Halazone	
	Etisazole	323		Methapyrilene	314
	Hexylcaine	275		Metolazone	271, 344
	Hydroxyzine	258, 263, 270		Oxyphenbutazone	
	Meprylcaine			Phenylbutazone	
	Procarbazine			Phenyramidol	309
233	Cocaine	275		Sulphinpyrazone	
	Doxorubicin	253, 290		Temazepam	284, 358
	Floctafenine	348	238	Dropropizine	
	Homochlorcyclizine	258, 263, 270		Nifedipine	338
	Methylenedioxyamphetamine	285		Nordazepam	283, 361

λ max nm	Compound	Subsidiary Peaks nm
	Penthienate Methobromide	
239	Acetanilide	
	Amitriptyline	
	Bromazepam	345
	Chlorpromazine Sulphoxide	274, 300, 341
	Halopyramine	315
	Mepyramine	316
	Niridazole	
	Nortriptyline	
	Tetrazepam	284, 345
	Thenyldiamine	315
	Tripelennamine	314
240	Muzolimine	
	Prazepam	285, 360
	Propyphenazone	
	Sulphapyridine	
	Tacrine	323, 336
	Thalidomide	300
241	Amiodarone	
	Antazoline	291
	Cephaloridine	254
	Dequalinium Chloride	330
	Flavoxate	293, 320
	Physostigmine Aminoxide	300
	Propiomazine	273, 360
242	Azaperone	312
	Butaperazine	277
	Clopamide	
	Diazepam	284, 366
	Oleandomycin	
	Prothipendyl	
	Spironolactone	
	Sulfamerazine	304
	Sulphadiazine	
243	Acepromazine	279
	Acetophenazine	278
	Ascorbic Acid	
	Carphenazine	277
	Cinchophen	268, 344
	Fluanisone	
	Methacycline	340
	Methallibure	
	Nitroxynil	350
	Piperacetazine	278
	Practolol	
	Propantheline Bromide	281
	Sulphadimidine	301
244	Diamphenethide	
	Dofamium Chloride	
	Ethosuximide	
	Phenacetin	
245	Ajmaline	289
	Bromhexine	310
	Buclosamide	297
	Chlorhexidine	
	Clozapine	297
	Haloperidol	
	Harman	300
	Isothipendyl	
	Paracetamol	
246	Amprolium	262
	Chlordiazepoxide	308
	Physostigmine	302

λ max nm	Compound	Subsidiary Peaks nm
	Prajmalium Bitartrate	290
	Thiamine	
	Trazodone	274, 310
	Triphenyltetrazolium Chloride	
247	Acetohexamide	
	Cinchocaine	319
	Cyclofenil	
	Flurbiprofen	
	Gentamicin	
	Harmine	319
	Methoxsalen	304
	Norharman	300
	Prazosin	331
248	Azapetine	
	Carbenoxolone	
	Droperidol	276
	Lobeline	
	Pipamperone	
	Probenecid	
	Proquamezine	297
	Sulfaquinoxaline	263, 348
	Trifluperidol	
249	Benperidol	231, 279
	Hydrastinine	306, 363
	Kanamycin	306
	Menadione	244, 261, 340
	Nitroxoline	293
	Promethazine	298
	Sulphamoxole	
250	Allopurinol	
	Azapropazone	
	Chlorproguanil	
	Desipramine	
	Diethazine	298
	Ethopropazine	299
	Histapyrrodine	295
	Hydroquinidine	316, 345
	Hydroquinine	316, 345
	Methotrimeprazine	302
	Noxiptyline	
	Papaverine	
	Quinidine	317, 345
	Quinine	317, 346
	Trimipramine	
	Zimeldine	
251	Aminoglutethimide	257
	Bezitramide	
	Clomipramine	
	Diflunisal	315
	Hydroxyquinoline	308, 318, 356
	Imipramine	
	Loxapine	292
	Perazine	300
	Phenformin	258, 264, 267
	Pipazethate	
	Promazine	302
	Thiazinamium Methylsulphate	299
	Trimeprazine	300
252	Amoxapine	293
	Bacitracin Zinc	
	Caramiphen	259, 265
	Flunixin	327
	Gelsemine	

λ max nm	Compound	Subsidiary Peaks nm	λ max nm	Compound	Subsidiary Peaks nm
	Methimazole			Methylephedrine	251, 263
253	Diethylpropion			Methylphenidate	251, 264
	Medazepam			Methylpiperidyl Benzilate	251
	Methdilazine	302		Nalidixic Acid	315
	Opipramol			Paraquat Dichloride	
	Pecazine	300		Pethidine	251, 263
	Piminodine	247, 257, 263		Phenbutrazate	252, 261, 267
254	Cinnarizine			Phendimetrazine	251, 261, 267
	Dimethoxanate			Phenelzine	247, 252, 263
	Enoxolone			Phenethylamine	242, 247, 252, 263
	Ethyl Hydroxybenzoate			Phenglutarimide	251, 263
	Perphenazine	307		Phentermine	247, 251, 263
	Prochlorperazine	305		Phenylpropanolamine	251, 262
	Strychnine			Procyclidine	251, 263
	Tropicamide			Pseudoephedrine	251, 263
255	Aniline	249, 261		Salinazid	327
	Chlorpromazine			Styramate	251, 263
	Molindone	299		Tilidate	251, 262
	Niflumic Acid	329		Tolazoline	263
	Pentaerythritol Tetranitrate			Tricyclamol Chloride	251, 263
	Propyl Hydroxybenzoate			Tridihexethyl Chloride	251, 263
	Thiethylperazine	309		Trimeperidine	251, 263
	Thiopropazate	305	258	Adiphenine	253, 264
	Triflumeprazine	305		Anileridine	252, 264
256	Cycrimine	251, 263		Atropine	252, 264
	Fluopromazine	305		Atropine Methonitrate	252, 264
	Fluphenazine	306		Beclamide	252, 264
	Harmaline			Benactyzine	252, 262, 264
	Mequitazine	307		Benzhexol	252, 264
	Pemoline	262, 268		Benzilonium Bromide	252, 264
	Phenmetrazine	250, 261, 263, 267		Benzphetamine	252, 262, 268
	Pivampicillin	261, 268		Bethanidine	252, 264
	Sulphachlorpyridazine			Bibenzonium Bromide	253, 264, 268
	Trifluoperazine	305		Butethamate	253, 264
	Vincristine	297		Carbetapentane	252, 264
257	Aletamine	251, 263		Cathine	252, 263
	Alphaprodine	251, 263		Cephalexin	
	Amidopyrine			Chlormethiazole	
	Amphetamine	251, 263		Desmetryne	
	Ampicillin	262, 268		Diphenidol	252
	Bamipine			Diphenylpyraline	253
	Benapryzine	251, 261, 264		Dipyrone	
	Carbarsone			Emepronium Bromide	253, 268
	Cephradine			Eucatropine	252, 264
	Clemastine			Glycopyrronium Bromide	252, 264
	Dextropropoxyphene	252, 263		Halquinol	
	Diminazene Aceturate			Homatropine	252, 264
	Diphenhydramine	252		Homatropine Methobromide	252, 264
	Ephedrine	251, 263		Hyoscine Butylbromide	252, 264
	Etafedrine	251, 263		Hyoscine Methobromide	253, 264
	Ethoheptazine	251, 263		Hyoscyamine	252, 264
	Fenproporex	252, 263		Isoaminile	252, 264
	Fentanyl	251, 263		Lachesine Chloride	252, 264
	Hexamine	251, 263		Levomethadyl Acetate	253
	Hexocyclium	252, 264		Mepenzolate Bromide	252, 261, 263
	Hydroxyphenamate	251, 263		Morazone	
	Hyoscine	251, 263		Oxeladin	252, 264
	Hyoscine Methonitrate	251, 263		Oxethazaine	248, 252, 264
	Mandelic Acid	251, 262		Oxyphenonium Bromide	252, 264
	Mebanazine	251, 261, 267		Pentapiperide	253, 265
	Mephentermine	251, 263		Pipenzolate Bromide	252, 262
	Methindizate	251		Piperidolate	252, 264
	Methylamphetamine	252, 263		Pipradrol	252

λ max nm	Compound	Subsidiary Peaks nm
	Poldine Methylsulphate	252
	Prolintane	252, 264
	Selegiline	252, 264
	Succinylsulphathiazole	281
	Trimetaphan Camsylate	252, 264
	Trimethobenzamide	
259	Alverine	253, 264, 268
	Ambutonium Bromide	253, 265
	Azacyclonol	253
	Benztropine	253
	Biperiden	252, 264
	Carbenicillin	265, 327
	Chlophedianol	265
	Chlorphenoxamine	
	Clidinium Bromide	253
	Demecarium Bromide	265
	Dextromoramide	254, 264
	Doxapram	253, 265
	Fencamfamin	253, 265, 269
	Fenpipramide	253, 265
	Fenpiprane	268
	Nicotine	
	Nifuratel	367
	Phenindamine	
	Valethamate Bromide	253, 265
260	Alprazolam	
	Aminacrine	313, 326
	Cetylpyridinium Chloride	
	Dimethindene	
	Hexyl Nicotinate	
	Isopropylaminophenazone	
	Ketoprofen	
	Loperamide	254, 266
	Metyrapone	
	Mexiletine	
	Neostigmine Bromide	266
	Nicotinyl Alcohol	
	Norpipanone	294
	Tolpropamine	265, 273
261	Betahistine	
	Cyclomethycaine	
	Dibromopropamidine	
	Doxylamine	
	Ethoxazene	310
	Ethyl Nicotinate	
	Inositol Nicotinate	
	Methyl Benzoquate	
	Nicametate	
	Nicotinamide	
	Nitrofurazone	
	Pargyline	251, 256, 268
262	Acriflavine	
	Cyclizine	257, 268
	Diloxanide Furoate	
	Dimethothiazine	235
	Etidocaine	271
	Mebeverine	
	Mesoridazine	238, 310
	Nicofuranose	
	Nifenazone	
	Pentamidine	
	Sulphanilamide	269
	Sulphasomidine	

λ max nm	Compound	Subsidiary Peaks nm
	Thioridazine	310
	Tocainide	270
	Veratrine	292
263	Broxyquinoline	
	Bupivacaine	271
	Carbinoxamine	
	Chlorquinaldol	330
	Denatonium Benzoate	269
	Lignocaine	272
	Mepivacaine	271
	Phencyclidine	252, 258, 270
	Thioproperazine	234, 312
264	Berberine	345
	Bisacodyl	
	Cetalkonium Chloride	258, 270
	Fenfluramine	271
	Metopimazine	310
	Nikethamide	
	Orphenadrine	258
	Pindolol	287
	Sorbic Acid	
	Sulfadoxine	
	Sulphaguanidine	271
	Tranylcypromine	258, 271
265	Acetazolamide	
	Acetone	
	Brompheniramine	
	Brucine	300
	Butriptyline	
	Chlormezanone	258, 272
	Chlorpheniramine	
	Decoquinate	
	Hexobendine	
	Minocycline	354
	Phanquone	272, 292
	Primaquine	282, 334
	Sulforidazine	311
	Sulphafurazole	
	Sulphamethoxazole	
	Tetrahydrozoline	272
	Xylometazoline	
266	Acecainide	
	Aprindine	260, 272
	Baclofen	259, 274
	Bialamicol	
	Captodiame	
	Carbutamide	
	Chlortetracycline	359
	Clorprenaline	262
	Coniine	
	Fluorouracil	
	Gallamine Triethiodide	
	Iproniazid	
	Isoniazid	
	Lidoflazine	272
	Nialamide	
	Pheniramine	261
	Psilocin	283, 292
	Sulphaurea	272
267	Butanilicaine	275
	Chlorphentermine	259, 274
	Ethomoxane	
	Mafenide	274

λ max nm	Compound	Subsidiary Peaks nm	λ max nm	Compound	Subsidiary Peaks nm
	Nefopam	275		Cyclothiazide	314
	Penfluridol	273		Epithiazide	315
	Riboflavine			Ethiazide	
	Tramazoline	275		Etilefrine	
	Xanthinol Nicotinate			Fenoprofen	
268	Clomocycline	229		Guanoclor	278
	Demeclocycline			Hydrochlorothiazide	318
	Ethacridine			Maprotiline	265
	Flucloxacillin	274, 344		Metaraminol	
	Mescaline			Naproxen	262, 315, 328
	Methixene			Profadol	
	Oxytetracycline	352		Pyrimethamine	
	Pericyazine	232		Rolitetracycline	357
	Phthalylsulphacetamide			Theobromine	
	Psilocybin			Thymol	
	Sulphamethiazole			Tramadol	
	Thenium Closylate	275	273	Anisindione	
	Vinblastine			Bendrofluazide	325
269	Benzethonium Chloride	263, 274		Buphenine	
	Deserpidine			Caffeine	
	Dimethisoquin	261, 331		Clonazepam	
	Disopyramide	263		Diclofenac	
	Doxycycline	346		Diprophylline	
	Ketamine	276		Edrophonium Chloride	
	Ketoconazole			Guaiphenesin	
	Lymecycline	356		Hydroflumethiazide	325
	Morinamide	314		Hydroxyephedrine	
	Octaphonium Chloride	274, 281		Metoclopramide	309
	Pyrazinamide	312		Oxedrine	
	Sotalol			Oxprenolol	
	Trimethoxyamphetamine			Phenylephrine	
270	Alprenolol	276		Proxyphylline	
	Aminobenzoic Acid			Resorcinol	
	Diamthazole	293		Viloxazine	
	Distigmine Bromide			Xanthinol	
	Ethacrynic Acid		274	Acepifylline	
	Etofylline			Atenolol	280
	Mephenesin	276		Cyclopenthiazide	319
	Methyclothiazide	314		Hordenine	
	Phenol			Isoxsuprine	269
	Phenyltoloxamine	276		Methoxyamphetamine	
	Pyridostigmine Bromide			Metoprolol	
	Tetracycline	356		Oxpentifylline	
	Theophylline			Quinuronium Sulphate	323, 359
271	Ambenonium Chloride	277		Ritodrine	
	4-Aminophenol			Tyramine	
	Benzoctamine	264	275	Bamethan	
	Bufylline			Clemizole	
	Clonidine	278		Fenethylline	
	Dinitro-orthocresol			Fenoterol	
	Econazole	265, 280		Guanoxan	
	Embutramide	276		Hydroxyamphetamine	
	Mazindol			Pentifylline	
	Methoxyphenamine			Pholedrine	
	Phenethicillin Potassium	275		Propylthiouracil	
	Sulphacetamide			Sulphadimethoxine	
	Trimethoprim			Thymoxamine	
	Yohimbine	277, 287	276	Diaveridine	
272	Amidephrine			Dimenhydrinate	
	Apomorphine			Glipizide	
	Benserazide			Insulin	
	Benzocaine	278		Methylthiouracil	
	Bretylium Tosylate	263, 278		Nadolol	269

λ max nm	Compound	Subsidiary Peaks nm	λ max nm	Compound	Subsidiary Peaks nm
	Orciprenaline			Ketobemidone	
	Salbutamol			Levodopa	
	Serotonin			Methyldopate	
	Terbutaline			Metocurine Iodide	
277	Alclofenac			Nitrazepam	
	Cyclazocine			Oxycodone	
	Dimetridazole			Oxymetazoline	
	Meclofenoxate			Pimozide	273
	Metanephrine			Pirenzepine	
	Metronidazole			Rafoxanide	335
	Narceine			Rimiterol	
	Oxymetholone			Sulphathiazole	
	Tinidazole			Warfarin	270, 303
278	Amylmetacresol	286	281	Acetarsol	
	Bamifylline			Minoxidil	230
	Bufotenine	297		Naloxone	
	Butacaine	272		Naltrexone	
	Butorphanol			Naphazoline	271, 288, 291
	Chlorothiazide			Oxymorphone	
	Dextromethorphan			Protokylol	
	Diethyltryptamine	287		Thebacon	
	Ethylnoradrenaline			Vancomycin Hydrochloride	
	Ibogaine		282	Benzquinamide	
	Isoetharine			Carbidopa	
	Metipranolol			Clorgyline	
	Normetanephrine			Dichlorophen	
	Pentazocine			Dyclonine	
	Phenazocine			Methanthelinium Bromide	
	Phentolamine			Phthalylsulphathiazole	
	Procaine Penicillin			Pralidoxime Chloride	242
	Tryptamine	287		Tetrabenazine	
	Tryptophan	286	283	Azatadine	
	Vanillin	230, 309		Benzthiazide	
	Verapamil			Cephaëline	
279	Butyl Aminobenzoate			Clofazimine	
	Chlorocresol			Dihydrocodeine	
	Chloroxylenol			Dihydromorphine	
	Dextrorphan			Fazadinium Bromide	
	Diamorphine			Homidium Bromide	242
	Dimethyltryptamine	288		Naftidrofuryl Oxalate	273
	Dobutamine			Pholcodine	
	Famprofazone	243	284	Acetorphine	
	Isoprenaline			Acetylcodeine	
	Levallorphan			Benzylmorphine	
	Levorphanol			Ethylmorphine	
	Mefenamic Acid	350		Etofenamate	349
	Mepacrine	343		Norcodeine	
	Methyldopa			Sulindac	327
	α-Methyltryptamine	288		Thebaine	
	Mianserin		285	Amiloride	361
	Noradrenaline			Codeine	
	Procaine			Coumatetralyl	275, 309
	Racemorphan			Dipyridamole	230
280	Adrenaline			Morphine	
	Azathioprine			Nalorphine	
	Chlorzoxazone			Neopine	
	Cytarabine			Normorphine	
	Dihydroergotamine			Obidoxime Chloride	
	Dopamine		286	Buprenorphine	
	Ethamivan			Cyproheptadine	
	Hexoprenaline			Dichlorphenamide	296
	Hydrocodone			Flucytosine	
	Hydromorphone			Mebhydrolin	320

λ max nm	Compound	Subsidiary Peaks nm	λ max nm	Compound	Subsidiary Peaks nm
	Mersalyl Acid			Thiabendazole	243
	Nicergoline		303	Natamycin	290, 318
	Pramoxine		304	Ethoxzolamide	253
287	Iprindole	293	305	Lysergic Acid	
	6-Monoacetylmorphine			Tiaprofenic Acid	260
	Prenalterol		306	Bromocriptine	
	Thiamylal	238		Dihydralazine	240, 274
288	Dapsone		307	Benzydamine	
	Diethylthiambutene	268		Methotrexate	243
	Idoxuridine		308	Thiothixene	
	Parbendazole	281	309	Dimefline	
	Propranolol	305, 319		Dimoxyline	285, 335
289	DOM		310	Diquat Dibromide	
	Etorphine			Salsalate	
290	Cyclobenzaprine		312	Amethocaine	281
	Methazolamide	255		Haloxon	290
	Methoxamine			Noscapine	290
	Pyridoxine		313	Ergometrine	
	Triprolidine			Lysergamide	
	Tylosin			Methylergometrine	
291	Alcuronium Chloride	255		Pyrithidium Bromide	256
	Carbimazole		315	Lysergide	
292	Albendazole			Pyrantel	
	Butylated Hydroxyanisole			Tolmetin	262
	Doxepin		316	Ergotamine	
	Methadone	253, 259, 264		Sulphamethoxypyridazine	
	Normethadone	253, 259, 265	318	Indomethacin	
	Protriptyline		319	Cambendazole	235
	Rotenone	235	321	Chromonar	
	Sulpiride		322	Methysergide	230
293	Dipipanone	259, 265	324	Zomepirac	262
294	Hydrastine		325	Mercaptopurine	
295	Timolol		329	Gloxazone	
296	Xipamide		332	Cotarnine	253
297	Ketotifen		336	Diphenadione	
	Nimorazole		340	Bumetanide	
298	Bunamidine		343	Chloroquine	257, 329
299	Glymidine	273	344	Hydroxystilbamidine	
	Rescinnamine		345	Acinitrazole	237
300	Aloin	245, 253		Glafenine	
	Norbormide	238	348	Thioguanine	258
301	Oxypertine		352	Cloxacillin	
302	Cytisine	232	355	Stilbazium Iodide	264
	Fenbendazole	289	360	Triamterene	250
	Labetalol		362	Furaltadone	255

B. In Alkaline Solution—Wavelengths of Maximum Absorption

In this table wavelengths of maximum absorption in alkaline solution are given only for those compounds for which maxima in acid solution are not recorded in the monographs in Part 2, or for which the maxima in alkaline solution differ significantly from the maxima in acid solution.

λ max nm	Compound	Subsidiary peaks nm	λ max nm	Compound	Subsidiary peaks nm
230	Buformin		233	Bromvaletone	
231	Aspirin	298		Niridazole	282
	Flurazepam	312		Oxazepam	344
	Temazepam	313	235	Prenalterol	305
232	Chlorhexidine (pH 10)	253		Saccharin	268
	Harman	284	236	Dobutamine	292
	Thiamine	336		Papaverine	277, 326

λ max nm	Compound	Subsidiary Peaks nm
237	Bromazepam	348
	Cambendazole	314
	Cyclazocine	298
	Etilefrine	290
	Profadol	290
	Tacrine	317
238	Captopril	
	Cinchocaine	325
	Clozapine	261, 297
	Fenbendazole	312
	Hexethal (pH 9.2)	
	Hydroxyamphetamine	294
	Metaraminol	292
	Phenazocine	298
	Phenylephrine	291
	Phenylmethylbarbituric Acid (pH 9.2)	
	Pholedrine	295
	Vinbarbitone (pH 9.2)	
239	Barbitone (pH 9.2)	
	Bromocriptine	300
	Butobarbitone (pH 9.2)	
	Cresol	290
	Cyclobarbitone (pH 9.2)	
	Heptabarbitone (pH 9.2)	
	Idobutal (pH 9.2)	
	Lymecycline	267
	Pentobarbitone (pH 9.2)	
	Phenobarbitone (pH 9.2)	
	Quinalbarbitone (pH 9.2)	
	Secbutobarbitone (pH 9.2)	
	Talbutal (pH 9.2)	
240	Amylobarbitone (pH 9.2)	
	Brallobarbitone (pH 9.2)	
	Butalbital (pH 9.2)	
	Clioxanide	282, 362
	Dextrorphan	299
	Edrophonium Chloride	294
	Ibomal (pH 9.2)	
	Levallorphan	299
	Levorphanol	299
	Nealbarbitone (pH 9.2)	
	Nordazepam	340
	Pentazocine	300
	Racemorphan	299
241	Allobarbitone (pH 9.2)	
	Aprobarbitone (pH 9.2)	
	Cyclopentobarbitone (pH 9.2)	
	Demeclocycline	276
	Methapyrilene	312
	Oxedrine	291
	Salicylamide	328
242	Bamethan	290
	Buphenine	291
	Chloroxylenol	296
	Dichloralphenazone	256
	Hexoestrol	297
	Hydroxyephedrine	290
	Phenazone	256
243	Chloropyrilene	308
	Chlorzoxazone	287
	Demoxepam	255, 310
	Glymidine	317

λ max nm	Compound	Subsidiary Peaks nm
	Harmine	275, 300
	Hexobarbitone (pH 9.2 & 13)	
	Isoxsuprine·	270, 277, 292
	Methylphenobarbitone (pH 13)	
	Methysergide	320
	Minocycline	
	Propiomazine	283
244	Carbimazole	
	Chlorocresol	299
	Enallylpropymal (pH 13)	
	Metharbitone (pH 9.2 & 13)	
	Methylphenobarbitone (pH 9.2)	
245	Acepromazine	283
	Dichlorophen	304
	Enallylpropymal (pH 9)	
	Metanephrine	291
	Propyphenazone	265
	Salbutamol	295
	Sulphamethoxydiazine	
246	Diethylpropion	
	Diprenorphine	299
	Droperidol	288
	Eugenol	296
	Labetalol	333
	Methohexitone (pH 9.2 & 13)	
	Oxytetracycline	269
	Thenyldiamine	310
247	Amoxycillin	291
	Antazoline	295
	Buclosamide	325
	Diminazene Aceturate	
	Spironolactone	
	Sulphapyridine	
	Vinylbitone	
248	Benperidol	288
	Bisacodyl	
	Carbarsone	
	Halopyramine	313
	Loxapine	298
	Mepyramine	312
249	Acetohexamide	
	Floctafenine	359
	Hexachlorophane	320
	Pentamidine	
	Propantheline Bromide	282
	Sotalol	
	Sulphaphenazole	
	Tripelennamine	312
250	Acetarsol	299
	Amoxapine	299
	Chlormethiazole	
	Isothipendyl	
	Prothipendyl	320
	Sulphamethoxypyridazine	
	Sulphamoxole	
	Sulphanilamide	
251	Amiodarone	
	Clomocycline	283
	Gentamicin	
	Nalorphine	298
252	Imipramine	
	Prazosin	345
	Sulfaquinoxaline	357

λ max nm	Compound	Subsidiary Peaks nm	λ max nm	Compound	Subsidiary Peaks nm
253	Apomorphine			Chlormezanone	
	Chlortetracycline	284, 346		Cinchophen	330
	Ethopropazine	302		Halquinol	343
	Hexethal (pH 13)			Methotrimeprazine	323
	Hydroxychloroquine	330		Selegiline	269
	Phenylmethylbarbituric Acid			Sulphaguanidine	
	(pH 13)		260	Cyclizine	
	Sulphafurazole			Enoxolone	
254	Barbitone (pH 13)			Phthalylsulphathiazole	
	Butobarbitone (pH 13)			Propylthiouracil	
	Chloroquine	330		Sulphamethizole	
	Clemizole	269, 275, 283		Sulphinpyrazone	
	Cyclopentobarbitone (pH 13)		261	Carbinoxamine	
	Idobutal (pH 13)			Cephaloridine	
	Oxyphenbutazone			Disopyramide	
	Phenobarbitone (pH 13)			Naproxen	271, 316, 330
	Promazine	306		Nicotine	
	Promethazine	305		Nikethamide	256
	Quinalbarbitone (pH 13)		262	Bromhexine	317
	Secbutobarbitone (pH 13)			Brompheniramine	269
	Sorbic Acid			Chlordiazepoxide	
	Sulphadiazine	240		Chlorpheniramine	
	Vinbarbitone (pH 13)			Coniine	268
255	Amylobarbitone (pH 13)			Cyclofenil	
	Azapropazone	325		Debrisoquine	270
	Butalbital (pH 13)			Ketoprofen	
	Carbutamide			Sulphasomidine	
	Heptabarbitone (pH 13)		263	Chlorquinaldol	345
	Methdilazine	308		Gliclazide	
	Nealbarbitone (pH 13)			Morazone	244
	Pentobarbitone (pH 13)			Nicofuranose	
	Strychnine	278		Phenindamine	
	Sulfamerazine	242		Pheniramine	258, 268
	Sulphaurea		264	Amidopyrine	
	Talbutal (pH 13)			Methyclothiazide	300
256	Allobarbitone (pH 13)			Phenylbutazone	
	Brallobarbitone (pH 13)			Salinazid	
	Cyclobarbitone (pH 13)		265	Aminobenzoic Acid	
	Folic Acid	283		Aminosalicylic Acid	300
	Methylthiouracil			Diethazine	
	Sulphacetamide			Dinitro-orthocresol	
	Sulphamethoxazole			Ibuprofen	273
	Sulphathiazole			Methaqualone	306
	Trimeprazine	310		Pecazine	
	Tropicamide			Phthalylsulphacetamide	
257	Allopurinol		266	Acecainide	
	Aprobarbitone (pH 13)			4-Aminophenol	
	Barbituric Acid (pH 9.2)			Brucine	304
	Carbenoxolone			Feprazone	
	Ibomal (pH 13)			Sulforidazine	
	Paracetamol			Tranylcypromine	260, 273
	Pargyline	252, 263	268	Aloin	
	Perphenazine	310		Dimethothiazine	
	Succinylsulphathiazole			Flucloxacillin	274, 318
	Sulphachlorpyridazine			Gelsemine	
	Thiopropazate			Phenoxybenzamine	262, 274
258	Cyclopentolate	252, 264		Rolitetracycline	248
	Methotrexate	303	269	Mebeverine	290
	Nalidixic Acid	334		Psilocybin	282, 292
	Sulphadimidine	242		Sulphadimethoxine	
	Trifluoperazine	308	270	Mebendazole	355
	Zimeldine			Mepacrine	345
259	Barbituric Acid (pH 13)			Psilocin	293

λ max nm	Compound	Subsidiary Peaks nm	λ max nm	Compound	Subsidiary Peaks nm
	Riboflavine	356	290	Hydromorphone	
	Triamterene	232		Mersalyl Acid	
271	Frusemide	333		Resorcinol	
	Isopropylaminophenazone		291	Acetazolamide	240
	Nitroxynil			Carbidopa	
272	Pericyazine			Phentolamine	
	Sulfadoxine		292	Chlorothiazide	
273	Amodiaquine	287		Dapsone	256
	Bendrofluazide	330		Fendosal	
	Captodiame			Hydrastine	
274	Cytarabine			Oxymorphone	
	Hydrochlorothiazide	324		Thymol	
	Hydroflumethiazide	333	293	Flucytosine	
	Isocarboxazid			Methallibure	
	Serotonin	323		Naltrexone	
	Theobromine		294	Pentaerythritol Tetranitrate	
275	Bufexamac			Tyramine	
	Deserpidine		295	Diethylthiambutene	
	Diclofenac			Dipyridamole	
	Mazindol	269		Ethyl Hydroxybenzoate	
	Meclofenamic Acid	319		Fenoterol	
	Procainamide			Triclosan	
	Theophylline		296	Noradrenaline	
	Thioridazine			Propyl Hydroxybenzoate	
276	Dithranol		297	Adrenaline	242
	Gliquidone			Benzthiazide	
277	Diflunisal			Dihydromorphine	
	Ethionamide			Isoprenaline	
278	Dimenhydrinate			Orciprenaline	
	Phenindione	330		Parbendazole	254, 303
279	Idoxuridine			Pirenzepine	
	Indomethacin	230		Terbutaline	
280	Danthron		298	Aloxiprin	
	Diazoxide			Isoniazid	
	Nicergoline			Morphine	
	Procaine Penicillin			Parachlorophenol	
	Sulindac	327		Salicylic Acid	
	Tryptophan	288	299	Butorphanol	
	Yohimbine			Diamorphine	
281	Ethylmorphine		300	Buprenorphine	
	Flunixin			Ketobemidone	
	Noscapine	315	301	Thymoxamine	235
	Trilostane		302	Etorphine	
282	Butacaine			Iprindole	
284	Cyproheptadine			Ketotifen	237
	Nitrofurazone			Methyldopa	
	Nomifensine		303	Amethocaine	
285	Azathioprine			Gloxazone	
	Benzocaine			Oxymetazoline	
	Butyl Aminobenzoate			Thiopentone (pH 13)	
	Fenbufen		304	Thiopentone (pH 9.2)	255
	Mefenamic Acid	332	305	Nimorazole	
286	Ambucetamide	279		Nystatin	291, 319
	Clobazam			Tetrazepam	
	Cotarnine	330		Thiamylal	
	Pyrimethamine		306	Rescinnamine	
287	Ketoconazole			Thialbarbitone (pH 13)	
	Phenol		307	Iproniazid	242
	Trimethoprim			Nialamide	
288	Cinchonine	302, 315		Thialbarbitone (pH 9.2)	256
	Methazolamide		308	Lysergic Acid	
	Minoxidil	262		Warfarin	293
	Niflumic Acid		309	Albendazole	

λ max nm	Compound	Subsidiary Peaks nm	λ max nm	Compound	Subsidiary Peaks nm
	Benoxaprofen	244		Metronidazole	
	Lysergamide			Pentachlorophenol	
310	Bacampicillin		320	Thioguanine	
	Ergometrine		322	Dimetridazole	
	Ergotamine		323	Tolmetin	260
	Hydroxystilbamidine		324	Oxyclozanide	
	Lysergide		325	Thyroxine	
	Mercaptopurine	231	330	Harmaline	
	Methylergometrine			Quinidine	280
	Oxybuprocaine	231		Quinine	280
	Phenprocoumon			Xipamide	
311	Coumatetralyl			Zomepirac	261
	Ethyl Biscoumacetate		332	Pralidoxime Chloride	
	Pivampicillin	257	341	Salsalate	
314	Dantrolene		348	Vanillin	248
	Dicoumarol		353	Obidoxime Chloride	
315	Oxymetholone		355	Benzbromarone	240
317	Bumetanide		377	Niclosamide	334
319	Liothyronine Sodium				

C. In Neutral Solution—Wavelengths of Maximum Absorption

The compounds listed below are those whose wavelengths of maximum absorption in acid or alkaline solution are not given in the monographs in Part 2 or for which the maxima in neutral solution differ significantly from those in acid or alkaline solution.

λ max nm	Compound	Subsidiary peaks nm	λ max nm	Compound	Subsidiary peaks nm
230	Benzyl Benzoate			Triamcinolone	
	Bezafibrate		239	Beclomethasone Dipropionate	
	Hexoestrol	280		Clobetasol Propionate	
	Lorazepam	316		Propyliodone	281
	Meclozine	266, 273		Santonin	
	Oxazepam	315	240	Benorylate	
	Prilocaine			Benziodarone	275, 357
	Temazepam	314		Betamethasone	
231	Camazepam	315		Cortisone Acetate	
	Oestradiol Benzoate			Deoxycortone Acetate	
232	Eugenol	282		Dequalinium Chloride	326, 335
233	4-Aminophenol	303		Dexamethasone	
	Bromazepam	320		Dimethisterone	
	Clioxanide			Ethisterone	
	Doxorubicin	253, 290		Fludrocortisone Acetate	
	Triamterene	267		Fluocinolone Acetonide	
234	Bephenium Hydroxynaphthoate	263, 270, 283, 295, 352		Fluocinonide	
	Cephaloridine			Fluoxymesterone	
	Quinethazone	278, 345		Gestronol Hexanoate	
235	Acebutolol	328		Hydralazine	260, 304, 315
	Aniline	286		Hydrocortisone	
	Flurandrenolone			Hydroxyprogesterone Hexanoate	
236	Clobetasone Butyrate			Methylprednisolone	
	Demoxepam	310		Metomidate	
	Dicophane	267		Nandrolone Decanoate	
	Fluclorolone Acetonide			Nandrolone Phenylpropionate	
	Metformin			Norethandrolone	
237	Cephalothin Sodium	265		Norethisterone	
	Cycloguanil	278, 289, 301		Prednisolone	
238	Flugestone Acetate			Prednisone	
	Flumethasone			Progesterone	
	Methyl Salicylate	306		Testosterone	
	Phenazopyridine	277	241	Aldosterone	
	Sodium Cromoglycate	326		Betamethasone Sodium Phosphate	

λ max nm	Compound	Subsidiary peaks nm
	Fluorometholone	
	Medroxyprogesterone Acetate	
	Methyltestosterone	
	Nomifensine	292
	Paramethasone	
	Stilboestrol	
242	Etomidate	
	Fluocortolone	
	Indapamide	288
	Ketazolam	
	Meclofenamic Acid	282, 331
	Salol	310
243	Buclosamide	301
	Colchicine	350
	Desonide	
244	Ketoconazole	296
	Noxythiolin	
245	Benzaldehyde	279, 289
	Clonazepam	309
	Methandienone	
	Trimetozine	
246	Ethebenecid	
	Sulthiame	
247	Azaperone	300
	Chlorotrianisene	307
	Methsuximide	252, 258, 264
	Phensuximide	252, 258, 264
248	Diazinon	
	Halquinol	263, 334
	Practolol	
	Trioxsalen	296, 338
249	Broxyquinoline	325
	Phytomenadione	244, 263, 270, 331
250	Diuron	287
251	Bamipine	298
	Chlorquinaldol	315
	Dihydrotachysterol	242
252	Clorexolone	
	Danthron	283
	Flunitrazepam	308
	Fluspirilene	273, 293
253	Trilostane	
254	Phenothiazine	317
255	Benzene	
	Clioquinol	325
	Dixyrazine	305
	Lofepramine	
256	Busulphan	
	Dithranol	288, 360
257	Benzylpenicillin Sodium	264, 325
	Lorcainide	263
	Methoin	264
	Methyl Hydroxybenzoate	
	Tolnaftate	
258	Alfentanil	264, 268
	Aprindine	296
	Beclamide	252, 264, 268
	Benethamine	
	Benzyl Alcohol	252, 264
	Chlorambucil	303
	Clidinium Bromide	252, 264
	Cyclandelate	252, 264
	Di-iodohydroxyquinoline	

λ max nm	Compound	Subsidiary peaks nm
	Diloxanide Furoate	
	Diphenoxylate	252, 264
	Glutethimide	252, 264
	Nitrobenzene	
	Phenacemide	265
	Phenytoin	264
	Prenylamine	253, 268
	Primidone	252, 264
	Syrosingopine	298
259	Ethotoin	265
	Isopropamide Iodide	265
	Pheneturide	265
	Phenprobamate	254, 261, 265, 269
	Proguanil	
260	Aminacrine	311, 325
	Buclizine	255
	Cephalexin	
	Chlorproguanil	
	Clotrimazole	254
	Melphalan	301
261	Proflavine Hemisulphate	
262	Benzalkonium Chloride	256, 268
	Benzyl Nicotinate	
	Simazine	
263	Atrazine	
	Bacampicillin	258, 269
	Cetalkonium Chloride	253, 258, 270
	Nicotinic Acid	
	Tolazamide	257, 268, 275
	Tolbutamide	257, 268, 275
264	Glibornuride	257, 275
	Methallenoestril	253, 273, 317, 332
	Methyl Nicotinate	
	Pindolol	287
265	Cholecalciferol	
	Ergocalciferol	
	Pipothiazine	315
	Suprofen	291
	Tofenacin	259, 272
	Triclocarban	
266	Deptropine	272
	Phenaglycodol	259, 275
267	Propamidine	
	Reserpine	295
268	Domiphen Bromide	277
	Phenoxymethylpenicillin	275
	Polythiazide	317
	Proxymetacaine	231, 310
269	Clopidol	
	Isopropylaminophenazone	243
	Octaphonium Chloride	263, 274, 282
	Propicillin	276
270	Fenclofenac	276
	Thiambutosine	
	Vindesine	
271	Benzoic Acid	280
	Chloramphenicol Palmitate	
	Paradichlorobenzene	265, 282
	Sulphasomidine	
272	Miconazole	264, 280
273	Fenoprofen	280
	Methoserpidine	
274	Betanaphthol	285, 322, 330

λ max nm	*Compound*	*Subsidiary peaks* nm	λ max nm	*Compound*	*Subsidiary peaks* nm
	Dibutyl Phthalate			Cannabinol	
	Etamiphylline			Carbamazepine	237
	Methisazone	241		Chlormadinone Acetate	
	Parathion		286	Anisindione	340
275	Chlorthalidone	284		Dydrogesterone	
	Cresol	279	287	Megestrol Acetate	
	Dimethyl Phthalate			Mexenone	243, 325
	Dodecyl Gallate			Nicergoline	
	Ecgonine		288	Flufenamic Acid	339
	Ethyl Biscoumacetate	303		Phthalylsulphathiazole	260
	Ethyl Gallate		289	Camphor	
	Methocarbamol			Clonixin	335
	Nabilone	282		Indoramin	273, 289
	Naphthalene	266, 286	290	Alphadolone Acetate	
276	Cephaëline	235		Alphaxalone	
	Mefruside	284		Methoxamine	
	Methoxychlor			Propranolol	306, 319
277	Bamifylline		291	Griseofulvin	236
	Clopamide	232, 286		Prothionamide	
	Meptazinol		293	Benzocaine	
	Phenolphthalein		294	Butyl Aminobenzoate	
278	Butylated Hydroxytoluene			Tolfenamic Acid	330
	Cannabidiol		295	Hydroquinone	
	Chloramphenicol			Procaine Penicillin	
	Diloxanide		296	Fenbendazole	
	Mestranol	287		Procaine	
	Nadolol	270		Tienilic Acid	267
	Δ⁹-Tetrahydrocannabinol		298	Choline Salicylate	
279	Butoxyethyl Nicotinate		299	Hexachlorophane	
	Carbaryl		300	Glibenclamide	275
280	Aminohippuric Acid		303	Clefamide	
	Chlorphenesin Carbamate	288		Oxyclozanide	
	Clofibrate	288		Pentachlorophenol	295
	Methicillin		308	Benzonatate	
	Methylchlorophenoxyacetic Acid		310	Phenprocoumon	285
	Oestriol		311	Bitoscanate	296
	Oestrone			Gliquidone	
	Propanidid			Tinidazole	230
	Tubocurarine Chloride		313	Ranitidine	
281	Chlorphenesin	289	315	Rifamycin SV	
	Ethinyloestradiol		322	Morantel	
	Monosulfiram		324	Pyridoxine	254
282	Alclofenac	290	328	Thiacetazone	
	Hexylresorcinol		330	Loprazolam	
	Indoprofen		333	Niclosamide	
283	Nicoumalone	306	351	Hydroxocobalamin	274
	Δ⁹-Tetrahydrocannabinolic Acid	278	344	Harmaline	260
	Triclosan		356	Carbazochrome	
284	Alpha Tocopheryl Acetate		358	Viprynium Embonate	239
	Dichlorophenoxyacetic Acid	292	361	Cyanocobalamin	278
	Parachlorophenol		367	Furazolidone	259
285	Acetomenaphthone	322		Nitrofurantoin	266
	Azinphos-methyl	302, 315	386	Aminonitrothiazole	

Infra-red Peaks

The table below lists the six major absorption bands which have been selected from recorded spectra over the range 2000 to 650 cm^{-1} (5 to 15 μm). The selected peaks are the six most intense peaks, except that peaks in the region where Nujol absorbs (1490 to 1320 cm^{-1}, 6.7 to 7.6 μm) have been omitted. The peaks are arranged in descending order of amplitude. Shoulders have been chosen only if they are clearly resolved and the point of maximum absorption can be easily determined. Where there is more than one peak of the same intensity at the sixth intensity level, the choice has been arbitrary. It should be noted that, because of variations in instruments and conditions, other determinations of the spectrum may not give peaks with the same relative intensities. In particular, the order of the two most intense peaks may be reversed and this should be taken into consideration when using the index.

To identify an unknown compound, the wavenumbers of the two most intense peaks should be compared with the table, initially allowing a tolerance of ± 4 cm^{-1}, to produce a list of possible compounds. Comparison of the six most intense peaks with this list may allow a tentative identification; reference should then be made to the spectra given in the monographs in Part 2.

If a tentative identification cannot be made it may be necessary to use a wider coverage, or to search on the 3rd most intense peak.

Principal Peaks in Descending Order of Amplitude

Wavenumbers cm^{-1}					Compound
675	1262	1305	1556	1215 788	Nicotinyl Alcohol
680	665	695	778	840 950	Lindane
683	1040	1014	1053	813 1266	Lynoestrenol
685	1629	776	1174	715 1205	Cetylpyridinium Chloride
688	855	704	781	917 957	Benzene Hexachloride
690	755	1235	1595	1497 811	Phenol
691	769	1529	720	1164 998	Triphenyltetrazolium Chloride
694	1190	740	1075	1020 1694	Alverine
694	751	1086	1041	1010 714	Captodiame
695	1723	1231	1054	1162 751	Benactyzine
695	745	755	942	1146 1608	Phenethylamine
696	1036	835	723	1255 893	Aldrin
696	745	1111	1022	1592 1067	Benethamine
696	1117	755	751	1030 1298	Cycrimine
697	701	749	773	1123 1219	Diphenidol
697	1051	1020	1000	740 1115	Etafedrine
697	746	714	724	1052 1515	Pargyline
699	1175	760	1199	1292 1070	Mebanazine
700	1664	764	1590	1315 979	Ambutonium Bromide
700	740	1495	1090	1605 825	Amphetamine
700	1590	1123	1086	1041 751	Doxylamine
700	720	760	940	805 1491	Meclozine Hydrochloride
700	1040	762	1025	1605 1200	N-Methyltryptamine
700	760	1298	1020	892 869	Phencyclidine Hydrochloride
700	746	1030	1500	1055 1590	Phenylpropanolamine Hydrochloride
700	747	1136	1027	1592 1075	Prenylamine
700	756	746	1128	1075 1175	Procyclidine Hydrochloride
701	1230	1682	1287	973 1594	Diethylpropion Hydrochloride
701	740	690	1585	1300 1065	Pipradrol Hydrochloride
702	745	1316	1063	971 1155	Azacyclonol
702	726	780	875	1618 1211	Benzalkonium Chloride
702	756	973	1206	1196 935	Benzhexol Hydrochloride
702	735	1121	997	760 1153	Biperiden
702	691	1138	964	740 1000	Cinnarizine
704	1265	1020	1075	1612 826	Chlordane
704	1036	764	1005	1210 1595	Pseudoephedrine Hydrochloride
704	765	740	1492	1092 981	Selegiline Hydrochloride
705	1095	749	759	1020 952	Bibenzonium Bromide
705	920	1115	772	1045 1061	Tricyclamol Chloride
708	1250	1230	1010	765 699	Diphemanil Methylsulphate
708	699	752	1102	742 1134	Emepronium Bromide
708	756	1042	797	738 1492	Fencamfamin Hydrochloride
709	1689	1296	667	935 685	Benzoic Acid
710	1709	769	1107	943 1133	Methadone Hydrochloride
712	1022	810	1575	1310 1040	Nicotine
713	754	1103	1017	1180 991	Diphenhydramine Hydrochloride
714	787	1205	1220	928 1515	Chloroform
716	756	701	984	1125 1496	Cyclizine Hydrochloride
716	743	851	833	1244 1618	Diethylthiambutene Hydrochloride
717	1492	710	769	1162 729	Tridihexethyl Chloride
720	760	775	1112	1130 1038	Nefopam Hydrochloride
722	698	1612	1204	875 790	Cetalkonium Chloride
727	776	700	802	1515 970	Tolpropamine Hydrochloride
728	1695	833	1086	1050 1010	Benoxaprofen
730	1285	705	1495	1610 1510	Phentermine Hydrochloride
735	750	1310	710	1300 1590	Phenothiazine
736	1066	811	746	1245 1260	Pericyazine
737	1134	1316	695	1122 1212	Mebhydrolin
738	1650	1612	1145	1173 1040	Iprindole
740	1111	1063	1086	1234 724	Diethyltryptamine
740	710	1573	1175	1018 918	Diphenyl
740	747	765	1230	1110 756	Imipramine Hydrochloride
740	1306	902	1095	1279 1231	Thiabendazole
742	1039	702	1052	990 1162	Methylephedrine
742	1585	1233	1035	909 1494	Tryptamine
743	1113	1235	1050	812 1010	Dimethyltryptamine
745	1510	1602	1187	1258 1035	Aprindine Hydrochloride

	Wavenumbers cm^{-1}				*Compound*
745	1593	725	1495	690	1275	Bamipine
745	1583	697	1019	707	1139	Fenproporex Hydrochloride
746	741	763	1230	1590	1104	Desipramine Hydrochloride
747	1240	1561	1125	1095	1220	Chlorpromazine
747	698	1060	1491	1590	1085	Methylamphetamine Hydrochloride
748	918	1063	990	1111	1639	Azapetine
748	765	740	833	1111	1010	Clemizole
748	1245	1587	1282	1562	1219	Diethazine
748	1248	1590	1282	1568	1125	Ethopropazine
748	1279	1244	1163	1143	1570	Perazine
748	1248	1260	1305	1590	1275	Trimeprazine Tartrate
750	1006	768	1198	1290	1219	Doxepin Hydrochloride
750	729	1052	1162	1086	1280	Methixene
750	768	1219	1250	1162	1282	Pecazine Hydrochloride
751	1317	1235	1504	1245	1567	Harman
751	1250	742	1220	729	1042	Mequitazine
751	1250	1234	1287	770	1162	Promazine Hydrochloride
752	1271	1124	803	984	795	Azatadine
752	1225	805	842	1212	1237	Clomipramine Hydrochloride
752	1280	1569	1165	1242	1145	Prochlorperazine
753	1242	1319	1222	1277	1031	Methdilazine Hydrochloride
754	899	1090	800	877	1587	Cinchonidine
754	1656	700	1492	1590	1117	Morazone
754	1653	1221	1186	1575	1316	Propiomazine Hydrochloride
754	1248	796	1234	1281	1211	Thioridazine Hydrochloride
755	1155	790	1237	1115	1126	Opipramol
756	741	1103	1092	1046	1280	Ajmaline
756	770	746	969	1014	1258	Amitriptyline Hydrochloride
756	700	1035	770	1190	735	Chlophedianol
756	742	768	720	775	1590	Nortriptyline Hydrochloride
757	743	732	1134	1060	1020	Benzoctamine
757	1033	1265	740	1098	1149	Butriptyline
757	1294	917	1145	1247	1155	Perphenazine
757	1295	780	1592	1162	1110	Prothipendyl Hydrochloride
758	1229	733	1129	1259	1287	Promethazine Hydrochloride
758	1657	1288	1210	1250	1150	Salicylic Acid
759	1250	1698	699	731	1199	Cinchophen
759	1271	747	1575	1242	932	Levallorphan
759	1140	1592	1032	1308	935	Maprotiline Hydrochloride
760	1556	1645	1655	750	1612	Aminacrine
760	1110	1505	1590	990	909	Cinchonine
761	842	1618	1003	1310	827	Triazolam
763	1590	724	747	1570	1050	Dimethindene
763	727	747	1252	963	717	Dothiepin Hydrochloride
763	1656	1063	1175	674	1093	Mazindol
764	778	800	968	988	880	Cyclobenzaprine
764	1674	1708	1242	1268	829	Fenbufen
765	752	708	1075	741	1205	Clotrimazole
768	1096	1250	1288	1053	890	Pindolol
775	790	1500	1100	1022	850	Dicophane
775	1580	825	990	1509	1146	Triprolidine Hydrochloride
776	1104	832	746	1030	1170	Chlorprothixene
776	714	752	1501	1141	1020	Prolintane Hydrochloride
777	756	815	786	1640	960	Cyproheptadine Hydrochloride
787	772	1138	1254	1314	742	Mianserin Hydrochloride

	Wavenumbers cm^{-1}				*Compound*
790	833	1145	1186	917	980	Chlorbutol
792	750	768	1490	730	1595	Protriptyline Hydrochloride
800	1515	1612	1587	1234	1315	5-Methyltryptamine Hydrochloride
800	1515	1065	1130	1290	1205	Norcodeine
805	1243	1118	945	1086	833	Morphine
815	1492	699	953	1075	840	Zimeldine
817	1248	1290	1095	1160	952	Thymol
818	1493	1092	1020	848	754	Chlorphentermine Hydrochloride
828	1590	1284	902	1148	710	Prothionamide
830	1090	1051	1020	690	1300	Butylchloral Hydrate
832	1228	1066	1264	1494	1108	Bamethan
832	1151	1673	1217	1136	1598	Haloperidol
835	1083	1300	970	1620		Chloral Hydrate
835	1510	1054	1271	1098	1611	Oxedrine
836	1261	1236	1042	1061	733	Psilocin
840	1630	1085	1130	730	1500	Chloral Betaine
840	1622	1522	1084	802	1577	Histamine Hydrochloride
848	811	1038	700	1005	912	Dieldrin
851	750	724	1049	889	1010	Endrin
887	1538	784	823	1297	1584	Acetarsol
905	1008	999	1020	1101	985	Allyloestrenol
913	970	1630	945	1063	1000	Hexamethonium Bromide
917	1126	1156	995	1030	1050	Methylpentynol
932	1255	729	718	669	815	Thiotepa
935	950	830	1010	1063	980	Ethchlorvynol
949	1089	869	1231	1000	1740	Acetylcholine Chloride
952	1123	1162	819	1111	1298	Isopropyl Alcohol
953	1198	808	784	1266	728	Clioquinol
961	909	952	719	970	724	Cetrimide
961	888	831	1621	985	1020	Mebezonium Iodide
970	980	1185	1616	1150	1205	Hexylresorcinol
973	1059	1079	1712	893	1000	Ergocalciferol
975	994	964	1299	1142	1165	Ethyloestranol
975	1090	1672	1110	1065	1025	Iproniazid
980	1075	1219	847	1162	1052	Cineole
980	1238	835	1157	1129	792	Hydroxyephedrine
988	725	760	706	1087	870	Chlorcyclizine Hydrochloride
994	699	754	1049	1242	670	Ephedrine Hydrochloride
995	1018	1087	772	1492	820	Pyrrobutamine Phosphate
996	1090	1637	1600	1282	847	Obidoxime Chloride
1000	1666	833	781	1041	775	Azinphos-methyl
1002	1131	754	800	1075	694	Buclizine
1010	1065	1038	1103	1183	1126	Amphotericin
1010	1666	819	666	1538	1176	Dimethoate
1012	1091	817	1121	951	1000	Paradichlorobenzene
1015	1041	667	1548	1602	1190	Diamthazole
1016	1108	1050	1080	940	699	Phenelzine Sulphate
1017	1030	1070	987	1090	1080	Isothipendyl
1018	1748	1174	1209	824	1250	Malathion
1020	1250	775	793	826	1190	Demeton-S-methyl
1020	1587	971	1562	823	1159	Diazinon
1020	925	1515	1219	1587	970	Parathion
1020	1230	1290	1210	1530	1605	Rimiterol Hydrobromide
1022	1050	990	1270	1235	1170	Dimercaprol
1023	1250	1200	970	1718	1585	Nitrofurazone
1023	1112	695	963	1153	743	Tranylcypromine Sulphate
1026	1111	1312	1136	1653	990	Ascorbic Acid
1030	1143	1127	1070	1050	1630	Guanethidine Sulphate
1031	1018	1076	975	1582	1279	Trometamol
1033	1007	1575	1300	1078	1139	Coniine Hydrobromide

Wavenumbers cm⁻¹						*Compound*

Wavenumbers cm^{-1} — *Compound*

1033	1068	1143	1123	980	1516	Kanamycin Sulphate
1035	1257	1222	1497	748	1070	Chelidonine
1033	1068	1143	1123	980	1516	Kanamycin Sulphate
1035	1257	1222	1497	748	1070	Chelidonine
1040	1590	845	770	660	1260	Tobramycin
1045	695	754	704	1091	976	Cathine
1046	1026	995	1102	1078	979	Menthol
1047	1248	1124	1493	756	748	Mephenesin
1050	1630	1120	1145	1545	940	Amikacin
1050	1168	1074	1010	1108	1734	Erythromycin
1050	752	1239	1282	1562	1091	Mesoridazine
1052	894	901	967	862	1075	Cholecalciferol
1052	1268	1500	1111	793	934	Codeine
1052	1163	1122	994	1016	1730	Spiramycin
1054	700	742	1191	1204	1075	Benztropine
1056	967	1018	1009	870	980	Dihydrotachysterol
1058	1015	885	913	1153	966	Propylhexedrine Hydrochloride
1059	1022	800	959	952	839	Cholesterol
1059	1040	751	760	738	1114	Deptropine
1062	1618	862	1266	1653	1089	Isosorbide
1062	1002	1563	1709	1101	1258	Natamycin
1064	1045	1129	1499	1185	1264	Ethylmorphine Hydrochloride
1065	1025	695	758	1272	890	Amygdalin
1065	1013	1298	1284	1102	1581	Mannomustine Hydrochloride
1066	1690	1729	1140	1008	1242	Norethynodrel
1067	1094	1007	696	1041	746	Bromodiphenhydramine
1067	1000	1570	1175	1316	847	Nystatin
1070	709	1050	696	765	1101	Diphenylpyraline Hydrochloride
1071	1035	1733	1140	1165	1640	Strophanthin-K
1072	1058	1010	1740	1168	990	Digitoxin
1075	775	1587	1041	1030	1123	Clorprenaline
1075	1027	1145	1109	1178	1002	Cytarabine
1075	1709	1055	1020	1160	1110	Digoxin
1075	1038	1263	1228	1213	822	Salbutamol
1075	1052	1162	1111	1010	1587	Tylosin
1078	1123	772	1634	1175	1672	Sulphasalazine
1082	1130	1005	1149	1063	800	Hydroxyzine
1083	757	695	965	990	1030	Phenmetrazine Hydrochloride
1084	1110	1584	1041	763	1010	Carbinoxamine
1085	1014	1730	1163	1130	864	Medigoxin
1085	1319	827	1302	1038	812	Miconazole Nitrate
1086	1173	1605	1010	1305	995	Orciprenaline Sulphate
1086	1298	1538	1149	689	917	Sulphaethidole
1088	1490	1010	760	700	990	Chlorphenoxamine Hydrochloride
1090	1011	700	763	1121	1210	Clemastine
1090	1230	795	1264	1247	1724	Dichlorophenoxyacetic Acid
1090	1310	805	825	1010	1040	Econazole Nitrate
1090	1061	1142	987	1050	1009	Ethambutol
1092	1273	1713	1235	710	1020	Aconitine
1092	1070	1248	1262	1582	1217	Nadolol
1093	854	1300	910	1176	1234	Hexetidine
1093	1494	1280	1011	1042	1600	Trimetazidine
1094	1113	1163	1074	975	1205	Metaldehyde
1095	1605	1266	1172	1698	1527	Benzonatate
1095	1170	946	860	846	763	Paraldehyde
1095	1085	1015	1180	807	830	Phenaglycodol

1096	950	1068	982	1175	1125	Stanozolol
1100	1120	1260	1000	780	1600	Gallamine Triethiodide
1101	1153	1270	799	1207	1316	Amidephrine
1102	1242	1190	1605	1517	1280	Hexoprenaline Sulphate
1102	704	757	1117	1042	917	Tofenacin Hydrochloride
1103	1270	772	1580	795	1240	Propranolol Hydrochloride
1105	1045	1062	1183	1160	932	Psilocybin
1107	1227	926	1124	709	876	Triclofos Sodium
1111	1666	1052	1724	1250	1515	Dihydrostreptomycin
1111	1068	1078	1592	1098	890	Mecamylamine Hydrochloride
1111	711	1162	696	763	1587	Mephentermine
1111	1052	1075	1010	1162	1190	Oleandomycin Phosphate
1113	1630	1495	1226	1591	1034	Ethacridine
1113	1195	1205	1155	1088	1005	Etorphine
1114	1316	1145	1081	755	1255	Trifluoperazine Hydrochloride
1115	1176	1653	1284	1265	1600	Flufenamic Acid
1115	1495	1264	1665	1592	748	Guanoxan
1116	767	1245	1144	1084	836	Fluphenazine Hydrochloride
1117	1316	1159	1237	1075	1030	Fluopromazine
1118	969	1250	1043	1500	1098	Pholcodine
1118	1098	1069	1044	1195	1210	Pseudomorphine
1118	874	1288	923	1026	1036	Putrescine
1118	1070	1045	980	962	1015	Sparteine Sulphate
1119	1320	1160	1081	1253	1287	Flupenthixol
1120	1225	1272	805	1584	938	Amylmetacresol
1120	1279	1594	1493	1097	1252	Ethomoxane
1120	1060	1625	1525	1290	880	Gentamicin
1120	1220	1710	1088	1180	1740	Methoserpidine
1120	1105	697	1083	752	1630	Phendimetrazine
1120	1230	1680	1175	1610	1038	Vindesine Sulphate
1121	1222	1508	1252	1205	1022	Dehydroemetine Hydrochloride
1122	1315	1572	1237	1142	1165	Flunixin
1123	1219	1703	1585	1497	1171	Hexobendine
1123	1230	1575	1505	1616	990	Trimethobenzamide
1124	1220	1087	1208	963	1618	Sulphachlorpyridazine
1125	1260	1138	1595	1650	1070	Sulphasomidine
1126	1630	1596	1235	1650	1565	Trimethoprim
1127	1242	1592	996	1513	834	Mescaline Hydrochloride
1130	1515	1587	1612	1639	1315	Ambazone
1130	1092	1267	1247	691	1220	Glymidine
1130	1527	929	1274	1082	1592	Sulphathiazole
1130	1595	1510	1240	1000	1151	Trimethoxyamphetamine
1131	1642	1229	1110	1592	1001	Trimetozine
1135	1010	1600	1618	1630	720	Homochlorcyclizine
1138	1158	1172	1293	889	1192	Sulthiame
1139	1294	1166	1495	1112	812	Diazoxide
1140	1238	1735	1175	1282	1090	Clofibrate
1143	1668	1565	1240	1590	1260	Frusemide
1143	1585	1091	840	1529	1667	Succinylsulphathiazole
1145	1315	1162	1601	1642	1085	Sulfametopyrazine
1145	1264	1552	1090	825	1600	Sulphacetamide Sodium
1145	1595	1304	1635	682	1090	Sulphadimidine
1145	1160	1599	1621	685	1306	Sulphamethoxazole
1148	1733	704	1199	735	990	Cyclopentolate Hydrochloride
1148	1507	1313	1592	675	1630	Sulphaphenazole
1149	1603	774	962	1164	1289	Resorcinol
1149	1590	1560	1316	1088	1618	Sulfamerazine

Wavenumbers
cm^{-1} *Compound*

1149	1603	1316	1637	1099	1294	Sulphanilamide
1150	1090	757	740	1052	1123	Clopenthixol
1150	1276	1592	1107	685	1633	Dapsone
1150	1310	750	1665	1102	1248	Metopimazine
1151	1180	1125	1052	1300	1525	Hydroflumethiazide
1151	1316	1299	897	1089	1592	Mafenide
1153	1597	1140	1284	1090	925	Sulphamethoxydiazine
1155	1248	1724	761	1200	755	Methanthelinium Bromide
1156	1042	1212	720	960	762	Thioproperazine Mesylate
1156	719	765	1176	957	747	Thiothixene
1157	1305	1595	1090	1123	1620	Chlorothiazide
1158	1317	1590	1020	858	848	Chloroxylenol
1158	1595	715	1063	1515	1300	Methyclothiazide
1158	1177	1597	772	1073	1509	Trichlormethiazide
1159	1045	1718	1176	700	1212	Atropine Methonitrate
1159	1599	1130	1305	1630	1088	Sulphamethoxypyridazine
1160	947	1311	1092	1078	934	Diprenorphine
1160	992	785	1512	1230	1585	Sotalol Hydrochloride
1162	1176	882	702	907	1123	Dichlorphenamide
1162	1176	819	1041	746	909	Mefruside
1162	1120	1597	1071	1240	1500	Polythiazide
1163	1172	1603	1312	781	1510	Ethiazide
1163	1635	1578	1560	975	1525	Xipamide
1164	1599	1042	1508	750	700	Antazoline Mesylate
1164	1730	1118	1026	1056	1195	Atropine *N*-Oxide
1165	1031	1681	1531	905	1264	Acetohexamide
1165	1316	1105	825	710	920	Chloramine
1165	1116	1070	698	793	1202	Fenfluramine Hydro-chloride
1165	817	1629	1200	1282	1239	Harmine
1165	1735	710	745	1250	955	Pipothiazine Palmitate
1166	1633	1598	1092	1647	690	Sulphafurazole
1167	1548	1316	1665	671	1115	Acetazolamide
1167	1183	1742	1080	833	1768	Meclofenoxate
1168	1138	1605	1309	1511	1060	Cyclopenthiazide
1170	1155	1306	1518	1621	750	Bendrofluazide
1170	1633	1217	1660	1715	1045	Bromocriptine Mesylate
1170	1490	1263	824	1224	1036	Ethoxzolamide
1170	1682	1520	1710	1050	1100	Glibornuride
1170	1681	1527	837	1302	1592	Phthalylsulphacetamide
1174	1638	1064	1229	1284	850	Paraquat Dichloride
1175	1523	1220	840	857	1615	Hexoestrol
1175	1721	1052	874	1072	709	Hyoscine Butylbromide
1175	1538	1582	1510	1307	1274	Stilbazium Iodide
1176	1730	1183	1267	1149	1236	Acetylcarbromal
1176	1314	1167	1126	1603	1269	Epithiazide
1178	934	861	980	962	773	Busulphan
1178	1605	1229	1672	1575	965	Dyclonine Hydrochloride
1180	1160	1310	1502	1620	1590	Benzthiazide
1181	1258	1515	825	746	1119	Dimetridazole
1182	1050	1661	1730	1248	1194	Benorylate
1183	1688	1305	1755	925	1219	Aspirin
1184	1212	1761	1261	1504	931	Thymoxamine Hydro-chloride
1185	1620	1075	1762	1580	1290	Tienilic Acid
1187	1535	1070	1265	745	1160	Metronidazole
1188	1012	1032	1120	680	815	Bretylium Tosylate
1188	1727	1495	1232	1162	1011	Oxyphenisatin
1188	1604	1260	1028	1676	1003	Pentamidine Isethionate
1190	1658	1730	1608	890	1053	Beclomethasone Di-propionate
1190	1227	1041	1031	779	823	Chlormethiazole Edisylate
1190	1647	1520	1309	1764	816	Clioxanide

Wavenumbers
cm^{-1} *Compound*

1190	1654	1266	1047	1600	1306	Dibromopropamidine Isethionate
1192	1715	1163	1101	700	1149	Piperidolate Hydrochloride
1195	1590	1672	1250	1562	1052	Amicarbalide
1195	1508	1610	1580	1592	1247	Phentolamine
1195	1225	1582	1627	720	1105	Serotonin Oxalate
1196	1028	1667	1597	742	1053	Hydroxystilbamidine Isethionate
1200	1218	1168	1760	1150	1122	Acetorphine Hydrochloride
1200	1623	1176	1504	1515	1252	Aminonitrothiazole
1200	1287	1075	1114	1518	1160	Isoetharine
1200	1040	770	760	1595	1090	Mexiletine Hydrochloride
1200	1219	1613	1048	1280	1495	Propamidine Isethionate
1202	1220	1050	805	1185	1294	Butylated Hydroxyanisole
1203	1527	1166	1587	1155	1219	Oxyclozanide
1204	1219	1754	917	1162	1492	Cyclofenil
1204	781	806	920	1265	869	Di-iodohydroxyquinoline
1205	1190	1057	1160	1220	717	Dimethothiazine Mesylate
1205	1176	833	1250	1512	1610	Stilboestrol
1206	827	1173	1510	1248	775	Dienoestrol
1208	1041	1541	1515	1634	1094	DOM
1208	1138	1744	1500	905	1194	Thebacon
1209	816	1515	741	1176	1105	*p*-Cresol
1209	1130	1247	1180	1770	1727	Syrosingopine
1210	1760	1163	1070	775	1030	Acetomenaphthone
1210	1755	1075	1105	1160	1250	Alpha Tocopheryl Acetate
1210	1705	1530	1600	1305	1050	Diperodon
1210	1192	1520	760	1240	813	Hydroquinone
1210	1730	1252	755	1008	1162	Pentapiperide
1210	1248	1276	1572	1025	1525	Quinuronium Sulphate
1210	1231	1155	1069	1610	1042	Terbutaline Sulphate
1210	1174	1042	1135	760	1010	Thenium Closylate
1211	1170	1156	754	1234	810	Tolnaftate
1212	1198	1754	1162	1500	909	Bisacodyl
1212	1708	712	1112	1132	664	Etomidate
1213	1708	1305	1104	1590	1520	Proxymetacaine Hydro-chloride
1215	1170	1050	750	1520	790	α-Methyltryptamine Esylate
1215	1562	1592	1257	1087	1275	Rafoxanide
1216	1266	1132	1510	1715	1174	Mebeverine Hydrochloride
1217	1121	1252	739	1511	1031	Viloxazine Hydrochloride
1218	1653	695	1560	1137	1275	Pemoline
1220	1611	1210	1583	1135	800	Griseofulvin
1220	1727	1163	763	1062	1093	Mepenzolate Bromide
1220	1620	1192	1570	1590	1260	Ranitidine Hydrochloride
1220	1120	1700	1240	1720	1265	Reserpine
1222	701	1061	1008	765	1751	Poldine Methylsulphate
1222	1728	746	1265	1250	1200	Thiopropazate Hydro-chloride
1224	1005	748	1052	700	770	Hexocyclium Methyl-sulphate
1224	1497	1241	705	1613	758	Phenazocine Hydro-bromide
1224	1010	1059	764	743	1036	Thiazinamium Methyl-sulphate
1225	1044	975	1088	945	1128	Cyclophosphamide
1225	1127	1715	1100	1184	1590	Deserpidine
1225	1719	729	704	1030	1111	Oxyphenonium Bromide
1225	1745	1031	1056	1013	907	Pancuronium Bromide
1226	817	1111	1162	1245	1170	Dichlorophen
1227	1739	1015	1250	1101	738	Furazolidone
1227	1136	1111	1724	1176	1613	Vinblastine Sulphate
1228	1758	1710	1278	1010	1043	Alphadolone Acetate

Wavenumbers cm⁻¹					Compound

1228	752	1500	1600	689	1080	Domiphen Bromide
1228	1067	917	1147	1250	1605	Oestriol
1228	1499	1534	823	1163	1285	Thiocarlide
1230	1745	1170	1685	1030	1130	Vincristine Sulphate
1232	824	1493	1615	792	1052	Bufotenine
1232	1043	818	1109	1490	710	Chlorphenesin
1232	812	671	1010	1044	724	Hexamine
1233	1731	1272	1042	1055	1501	Acetylcodeine
1233	768	1653	1590	858	726	Bephenium Hydroxy-naphthoate
1233	1153	1205	1592	762	1003	Oxypertine
1234	1605	1144	1270	1030	910	Thebaine
1234	720	1307	1499	813	1093	Thiambutosine
1235	1032	1499	925	1075	934	Hydrastinine
1235	1215	1510	1619	1030	1105	Quinine
1236	749	1047	1125	1026	1175	Methoxyphenamine
1237	1306	1580	832	1500	1531	Azathioprine
1238	1724	1646	1219	881	1597	Chlormadinone Acetate
1238	1495	753	1278	1578	1608	Levorphanol
1238	1730	1213	1050	1030	1131	6-Monoacetylmorphine
1238	1264	1609	1214	854	1054	Pentazocine
1240	1505	1120	826	1063	769	Benzethonium Chloride
1240	1495	1280	1580	756	1610	Dextrorphan
1240	1225	1507	1623	1026	1132	Hydroquinine
1240	1735	702	1496	1015	1031	Levomethadyl Acetate
1240	840	760	1515	708	1185	Octaphonium Chloride
1240	750	698	1494	1598	1586	Phenoxybenzamine Hydrochloride
1242	746	1031	1492	1079	916	Alprenolol
1242	962	900	1786	1852	1002	Cantharidin
1242	1667	1744	1718	1203	1610	Deoxycortone Acetate
1242	1258	1707	1215	1100	772	Fenclofenac
1242	1280	1580	1495	1505	760	Racemorphan
1244	1733	1633	1204	1515	1123	Benzquinamide
1244	1666	1510	1595	1078	880	Clefamide
1244	1728	940	1230	922	1050	Naloxone
1244	1655	1513	1555	1265	836	Phenacetin
1245	1624	1635	1600	1185	1501	Ethoxazene
1245	1764	1178	1215	911	1736	Diamorphine Hydrochloride
1245	760	940	747	1085	1145	Dihydromorphine
1245	1627	1587	1500	1560	1522	Mepacrine Hydrochloride
1245	1054	1227	1493	1276	821	Oestradiol
1245	1491	752	1030	697	1111	Phenyltoloxamine
1246	1293	1535	1230	1040	1607	Isoprenaline Hydrochloride
1247	1198	1748	1499	1143	806	Methylchlorophenoxyacetic Acid
1247	731	747	1630	813	1280	Norharman
1250	1510	1606	1174	813	1184	Chlorotrianisene
1250	1550	1588	1610	1090	1655	Colchicine
1250	1567	976	1098	1064	1650	Rifampicin
1250	752	758	1670	1626	1587	Salicylamide
1251	1281	1606	1176	1674	1566	Nifursol
1252	1505	1298	1285	1020	1060	Ethinyloestradiol
1252	1226	1746	1737	1012	1028	Ethynodiol Diacetate
1252	1512	820	1612	1270	869	Hordenine
1253	1274	1500	945	1224	871	Adrenaline
1253	1582	1060	1090	1000	1047	Narceine
1255	1510	740	1230	1125	1020	Guaiphenesin
1255	1647	1572	1504	757	1163	Mefenamic Acid
1255	1060	1035	1612	1291	1241	Mestranol
1255	761	1208	1733	745	1158	Propantheline Bromide
1258	1689	1235	933	1016	1500	Alclofenac

Wavenumbers cm⁻¹					Compound

1258	750	1500	1120	1092	1037	Oxprenolol Hydrochloride
1258	1513	1274	1590	1610	810	Pholedrine
1258	1508	1637	1142	1724	1220	Propanidid
1258	1514	1619	1040	860	820	Quinidine
1259	1517	1599	1102	813	1111	Hydroxyamphetamine
1260	1598	1637	1211	1613	920	Mexenone
1260	1154	1646	750	678	1120	Saccharin Sodium
1263	1706	1106	713	698	1067	Benzyl Benzoate
1263	1249	1733	1662	1712	1630	Megestrol Acetate
1263	1304	1216	1591	1136	1063	Metaraminol
1264	1515	1116	1229	1213	1616	Cephaëline Hydrochloride
1264	740	1620	1597	1152	1197	Danthron
1265	1298	1204	752	985	790	Apomorphine
1265	1293	1216	1200	1066	1137	Noradrenaline Acid Tartrate
1266	1600	1779	1692	1176	1120	Procaine Penicillin
1266	1147	1124	1165	1233	1715	Rescinnamine
1266	1518	1595	822	1495	1612	Tyramine
1267	1193	1492	1147	966	913	Disulfiram
1267	1547	1706	1238	1020	966	Sodium Fusidate
1269	1130	1233	1575	1249	1303	Butorphanol Tartrate
1269	825	1209	818	889	1104	Fenticlor
1270	1718	1105	710	1068	1022	Hexylcaine
1270	1490	1198	1142	968	915	Monosulfiram
1270	1085	1111	1136	1234	1035	Veratrine
1272	1734	1102	1593	1025	718	Inositol Nicotinate
1273	1595	1681	1630	1111	1163	Butyl Aminobenzoate
1274	1040	1502	1017	763	1056	Benzylmorphine
1275	1720	1618	717	1116	1316	Benzoylecgonine
1275	1165	1598	1694	1639	1111	Butacaine
1275	1500	1118	1050	1250	782	Neopine
1276	1182	737	1139	960	1213	Hexachlorophane
1276	1165	1220	1317	1665	1600	Propyl Hydroxybenzoate
1277	1212	1015	1540	870	1086	Pyridoxine Hydrochloride
1278	1724	1108	740	699	1587	Benzyl Nicotinate
1278	1703	711	1115	1310	1040	Piperocaine Hydrochloride
1279	1508	1263	1026	1292	1238	Papaverine Hydrochloride
1280	1680	1598	1170	1315	1634	Benzocaine
1280	1250	1055	1099	801	1124	Clorgyline
1280	1220	1160	1250	760	780	Fazadinium Bromide
1280	1650	1635	852	1090	968	Isosorbide Mononitrate
1281	751	1718	1306	1075	1103	Nicergoline
1282	1724	1111	740	1020	1587	Butoxyethyl Nicotinate
1282	990	1010	1587	1612	1204	Doxorubicin Hydrochloride
1282	1718	1111	741	1022	703	Methyl Nicotinate
1282	820	1709	1244	921	1493	Oestrone
1284	1601	1042	1238	1575	702	Tramadol Hydrochloride
1285	1650	714	1587	690	1610	Phytomenadione
1286	1724	1110	740	1591	1025	Ethyl Nicotinate
1290	1673	1170	1240	1610	1590	Ethyl Hydroxybenzoate
1290	1680	1565	1270	687	772	Salinazid
1299	1256	1064	1208	1129	676	Pentolinium Tartrate
1300	744	1710	1042	694	1180	Nicotinic Acid
1301	1638	1595	1510	805	1180	Aminosalicylic Acid
1307	774	1222	711	1196	1553	Pentachlorophenol
1308	1261	1210	1136	1063	675	Pempidine Tartrate
1312	790	1258	1066	1275	1030	Normorphine
1314	1176	1709	1215	818	740	Acinitrazole
1315	1063	1136	833	1204	1234	Methoxyflurane
1316	1190	930	806	1258	782	Broxyquinoline
1317	1150	1665	1170	1110	1595	Trifluperidol Hydrochloride
1318	1180	1150	1168	1602	1060	Hydrochlorothiazide

Wavenumbers cm⁻¹					*Compound*
1320	1077	1503	1155	1120	947	Buprenorphine Hydrochloride
1320	1172	1552	965	675	1550	Disulphamide
1490	1610	697	1316	1540	827	Alprazolam
1490	1210	1140	810	1020	835	Ibogaine Hydrochloride
1490	1257	1038	1504	799	1188	Methylenedioxyamphetamine
1490	762	1240	1230	741	749	Trimipramine
1492	1631	1092	698	1010	1600	Fenpiprane
1492	1512	1598	1247	1175	1035	Mepyramine
1492	1250	1271	1227	1036	1128	Protokylol
1494	1598	769	1562	1010	1098	Halopyramine
1495	1592	1283	1650	1030	757	Alcuronium Chloride
1495	1637	688	750	1665	1050	Amiphenazole
1495	1694	770	1136	1562	1587	Butanilicaine
1495	1271	1040	1250	1055	1149	Dihydrocodeine
1496	1242	1040	1300	1280	1070	Dextromethorphan Hydrobromide
1496	1219	1022	1276	1179	1050	Methoxamine Hydrochloride
1496	1592	770	1250	955	735	Tripelennamine Hydrochloride
1497	740	698	1028	1125	1220	Benzphetamine
1497	1527	1120	1230	1590	1620	Timolol Maleate
1500	1665	1593	1195	1570	1265	Benserazide
1500	1660	1280	1195	1120	1212	Brucine
1500	1529	1280	1265	1052	1600	Ethylnoradrenaline
1500	1138	1225	1315	1157	825	Penfluridol
1503	1497	1316	1603	1089	1517	Amantadine Hydrochloride
1503	1287	1190	1174	813	1115	Dopamine
1504	1247	1208	1145	1225	865	Dimoxyline
1504	1277	1307	1189	1149	1565	Nitroxoline
1505	1271	1234	1030	1587	1098	Berberine
1505	1645	1220	1155	835	775	Lidoflazine
1505	1121	1155	1304	805	945	Nalorphine Hydrobromide
1505	748	1600	693	1279	755	Thenalidine
1506	1657	1565	1263	1227	1612	Paracetamol
1507	1640	1240	1258	1200	1221	Ketoconazole
1508	1580	1101	903	1681	1248	Carbarsone
1508	1560	1205	1587	747	1083	Clofazimine
1509	1261	1620	1234	854	1030	Hydroquinidine
1509	779	709	1282	1219	1190	Hydroxyquinoline
1510	1220	1265	1280	1125	1240	Metocurine Iodide
1510	1245	1108	1028	1175	810	Metoprolol
1510	1230	1118	1210	824	1635	Pramoxine
1510	1592	1171	1299	809	1217	Prometryne
1510	1209	1256	1610	833	1170	Ritodrine
1510	1253	1026	1232	1149	1587	Verapamil
1512	1220	750	695	1182	837	Buphenine
1512	1282	812	1200	950	785	Halquinol
1512	1259	1033	808	1190	1623	Methoxyamphetamine Hydrochloride
1513	1664	1080	1050	1302	1250	Clindamycin
1513	1604	750	698	1500	732	Histapyrrodine
1514	1256	1228	1110	1200	1150	Emetine
1514	1240	745	1220	1043	1500	Isoxsuprine
1515	1595	1294	1166	806	1140	Ametryne
1515	1603	1580	1661	1563	1305	Thiacetazone
1515	1593	1550	1250	1613	1175	Thonzylamine
1516	1228	1120	1280	1265	1165	Tubocurarine Chloride
1517	1599	1640	750	1700	692	Warfarin Sodium
1518	1242	1213	1099	840	772	Prenalterol Hydrochloride

Wavenumbers cm⁻¹					*Compound*
1520	1562	1620	1600	1128	1290	Chlorproguanil Hydrochloride
1520	1280	1266	1190	1200	1220	Dobutamine Hydrochloride
1520	1587	1215	806	1266	1133	Terbutryne
1522	1498	1140	1166	1097	1632	Diquat Dibromide
1524	1160	1623	1718	1276	823	Glibenclamide
1524	1577	1209	1025	1147	1258	Methallibure
1524	1180	1298	1147	1573	770	Piroxicam
1526	1214	1010	1076	1041	1251	Dipyridamole
1527	835	1574	1495	1624	1095	Baclofen
1527	1628	1575	1235	820	1080	Chlorhexidine
1527	1672	1612	738	1595	1289	Dinitolmide
1527	1726	1516	1290	1240	1215	Methyldopate
1528	1690	1650	1159	1032	900	Glipizide
1529	740	1491	1613	1182	1141	Benzydamine
1529	1537	896	1622	1153	1614	Heptaminol
1529	1245	1123	730	1309	1600	Nitroxynil
1529	1162	1250	1037	1290	1123	Normetanephrine Hydrochloride
1530	1300	1230	1275	1580	1715	Acetylcysteine
1530	1634	1666	1562	1587	1149	Buformin
1531	1587	1258	806	1292	1163	Desmetryne
1532	1142	1084	1710	1585	1560	Phthalylsulphathiazole
1534	1635	1492	1575	1600	1170	Proguanil Hydrochloride
1535	1115	1250	1000	900	800	Pentetrazol
1538	1613	1098	1319	1258	1203	Aminocaproic Acid
1538	1504	753	1618	762	1095	Clopidol
1538	811	1304	1121	1272	1175	Methoprotryne
1538	1600	1266	1277	1160	1117	Rimantadine
1539	1612	1295	804	1161	1121	Atrazine
1543	898	1190	1590	1201	1506	Buclosamide
1544	1575	1641	1715	1235	1070	Riboflavine
1549	1134	699	1084	1152	1600	Sulphamethizole
1550	1596	1680	719	704	757	Denatonium Benzoate
1550	1005	1616	1602	1647	882	Potassium Sorbate
1553	1621	1289	797	1103	1129	Simazine
1558	1042	1230	987	1026	1517	Noxythiolin
1559	1648	1690	1298	1270	925	Quinalbarbitone Sodium
1562	1642	1715	1289	1261	1210	Carbenoxolone Sodium
1562	1225	696	1211	1268	1248	Fenoprofen Calcium
1563	1316	1647	775	928	1044	Ametazole
1563	864	1613	1212	1105	1067	Thiethylperazine
1565	815	1535	1255	869	847	Amodiaquine
1565	1508	1600	1120	1173	923	Cadaverine
1566	1650	863	1615	1190	740	Methysergide Maleate
1568	1537	1590	1625	1650	1500	Phenformin Hydrochloride
1570	1255	1304	754	1227	1241	Cyclazocine
1570	1271	740	1250	765	675	Methimazole
1572	1079	1263	1234	763	1511	Bunamidine
1572	756	1504	775	1286	1308	Diclofenac Sodium
1572	1515	1613	1285	1650	1218	Niclosamide
1573	1538	1612	1155	800	870	Chloroquine
1574	1275	740	1246	1150	767	Carbimazole
1574	1610	1584	1536	761	822	Triamterene
1575	1590	1234	752	702	1267	Profadol
1576	1631	1499	1155	1115	751	Dimethisoquin
1577	1550	1526	1620	934	877	Cycloserine
1577	756	1212	1703	1124	1274	Pizotifen
1579	1608	1530	1050	1150	810	Hydroxychloroquine
1580	1613	1660	1244	1220	1040	Doxycycline Hydrochloride
1580	708	795	1225	1205	1300	Meptazinol Hydrochloride
1580	1620	1063	1075	935	740	Metformin
1580	1270	1175	1030	1205	752	Methotrimeprazine

Wavenumbers cm⁻¹						Compound
1580	1490	1650	1620	1065	1103	Methylergometrine
1580	877	741	1000	708	775	Nomifensine Maleate
1580	1159	1494	682	940	797	Sulphadiazine
1580	1030	1620	1180	1080	1260	Δ^8-Tetrahydrocannabinol
1580	1040	1620	1180	1130	1050	Δ^9-Tetrahydrocannabinol
1582	873	990	730	1029	1081	Perhexiline Maleate
1583	1161	1596	1315	1091	1305	Sulfadoxine
1584	690	860	870	990	1010	Pheniramine Maleate
1584	745	660	1278	1190	765	Proquamezine Fumarate
1585	1560	1290	762	1238	1145	Betahistine
1585	750	1003	1067	1565	1040	Brompheniramine
1585	1630	1020	1210	1240	1050	Cannabidiol
1585	1557	1666	1204	751	1298	Carphenazine
1585	1086	746	1010	830	1562	Chlorpheniramine
1585	1020	1050	1100	1082	1158	Cyclopentamine
1585	1305	1252	1131	1605	1070	Floctafenine
1585	1656	762	685	1248	1493	Phenazopyridine
1585	1264	1127	1078	1639	950	Sulphapyridine
1587	1669	775	1236	1222	1152	Azaperone
1587	1724	1176	1515	699	1041	Choline Salicylate
1587	1079	1228	1259	1575	1022	Gloxazone
1587	1575	1197	699	1150	1248	Levamisole
1587	1560	760	1275	958	1493	Zomepirac Sodium
1588	1620	1208	1082	1160	1503	Cimetidine
1588	808	865	1275	1140	880	Ethionamide
1589	1742	1202	1192	1229	1245	Captopril
1590	1640	1500	1133	1270	1695	Azapropazone
1590	1111	700	1245	1505	1170	Clomiphene
1590	1603	1564	1109	1188	1248	Loxapine
1590	1614	1530	1496	1254	1311	Metoclopramide Hydrochloride
1590	1147	1090	1314	685	1066	Sulphadimethoxine
1590	1220	1722	1050	1308	743	Suprofen
1592	787	758	1308	691	1015	Lysergic Acid
1592	765	1558	1250	1158	1316	Methapyrilene
1592	955	870	1080	1055	1115	Piperazine Citrate
1592	1618	1294	1188	1500	1513	Viprynium Embonate
1594	1273	784	696	1304	900	Phenylephrine Hydrochloride
1595	1698	1240	1625	1111	1315	Chloroprocaine
1595	767	990	1562	1149	1234	Chloropyrilene
1595	1238	1500	760	1060	925	Dropropizine
1595	1650	1114	914	1313	1248	Methylprednisolone
1595	1199	1285	1250	1070	765	Oxymetazoline Hydrochloride
1595	1525	1615	1550	1090	1055	Penicillamine
1596	1570	1548	1295	757	1234	Clothiapine
1596	1153	1168	1307	1500	1075	Cyclothiazide
1597	1198	1562	1220	1745	760	Aloxiprin
1597	1168	1290	1665	1305	1625	Aminobenzoic Acid
1597	1548	1300	702	1230	830	Clorazepate Dipotassium
1597	1068	797	1305	1279	1222	Etilefrine Hydrochloride
1597	766	1242	976	1159	1311	Thenyldiamine
1598	1643	1540	766	1236	1574	Cinchocaine
1598	1620	1765	1495	1659	771	Cloxacillin Sodium
1598	1278	1615	1222	1168	1635	Dithranol
1600	1286	1174	1688	1126	1532	Amethocaine Hydrochloride
1600	1764	1656	1538	715	1143	Cephaloridine
1600	1634	1501	1307	1205	1053	Clomocycline Sodium
1600	1560	758	1136	1101	1117	Clozapine
1600	1225	1510	850	1713	1108	Dantrolene Sodium
1600	700	830	765	964	986	Loperamide Hydrochloride

Wavenumbers cm⁻¹						Compound
1600	1511	1634	1305	1200	1538	Methotrexate
1600	1288	1261	1530	1123	1219	Methyldopa
1600	1645	1525	1225	1310	1050	Minocycline Hydrochloride
1600	1512	1639	1297	1545	1570	Procainamide Hydrochloride
1600	1757	1669	1224	1314	750	Propicillin Potassium
1600	1650	1160	960	1510	1040	Quinethazone
1600	742	1293	1250	763	1500	Tetrahydrozoline Hydrochloride
1602	1031	1074	1548	1122	857	Bromhexine
1602	1253	1298	871	1237	800	Xylometazoline Hydrochloride
1603	1767	1622	1495	1660	794	Flucloxacillin Sodium
1603	1643	1293	1125	1252	1540	Prazosin Hydrochloride
1604	1592	752	1181	1246	1107	Amoxapine
1605	1086	1490	1655	1505	1300	Cotarnine Hydrochloride
1605	1660	765	1560	1540	1307	Dequalinium Chloride
1605	1232	1090	1218	1546	1156	Dinitro-orthocresol
1605	1510	700	1160	1575	1200	Fenoterol Hydrobromide
1605	1493	1097	1673	1040	826	Methisazone
1605	1625	1125	1160	1218	1263	Proflavine Hemisulphate
1605	1278	1246	1670	1210	1700	Propoxycaine
1605	1626	1127	1145	1276	1094	Sulphamoxole
1607	1766	1673	1500	1093	1260	Methicillin Sodium
1608	1633	1575	1537	1136	769	Dihydralazine
1608	1270	1585	1240	1300	1543	Ethamivan
1608	1314	1292	772	706	1111	Etisazole
1608	1180	1493	1250	1535	1320	Liothyronine
1608	820	767	1310	1210	995	Midazolam
1608	1296	721	1580	690	775	Tolazoline
1609	690	1217	1495	934	1280	Edrophonium Chloride
1610	1635	1588	1171	1267	1198	Diminazene
1610	1178	1298	700	1255	815	Medazepam
1610	1220	1570	1010	865	780	Mercaptopurine
1610	1660	1165	1145	962	1012	Metolazone
1610	1778	1510	1238	1690	752	Phenethicillin Potassium
1611	1595	815	1230	1572	1170	Primaquine
1612	1234	1515	980	1052	1176	Bufexamac
1612	1754	1315	1123	1030	1000	Carbenicillin
1612	1204	1219	1306	1157	935	Oxymetholone
1612	1580	1660	1226	1248	1530	Tetracycline Hydrochloride
1613	1704	809	1250	1225	1515	Nalidixic Acid
1613	1524	700	768	1058	752	Phenyramidol
1613	1585	1164	1314	1085	1099	Xylazine
1614	1090	1650	1583	750	715	Debrisoquine Sulphate
1615	762	740	1685	1250	1570	Coumatetralyl
1615	1575	1658	1224	1258	1206	Methacycline
1615	780	1499	791	1211	800	Naphazoline
1615	1642	1515	1250	1562	1298	Pyrithidium Bromide
1616	1573	1660	1190	1298	1315	Demeclocycline
1616	1584	1665	1235	1180	1138	Oxytetracycline Hydrochloride
1618	756	1577	1135	1293	1176	Benziodarone
1618	1258	1217	1712	1105	1149	Diethylcarbamazine
1618	1684	695	712	702	764	Fenpipramide
1620	1777	1500	1310	1700	703	Benzylpenicillin Sodium
1620	1050	1580	1030	1120	1228	Cannabinol
1620	1630	1540	1560	740	1317	Indoramin Hydrochloride (form II)
1620	1129	1230	1537	1075	1176	Sulphaguanidine
1621	1513	1186	1160	1250	1205	Melphalan
1621	1689	1250	1089	1211	1550	Methyl Benzoquate

Wavenumbers
cm⁻¹ · *Compound*

1622	1580	1666	1311	1041	1227	Chlortetracycline Hydrochloride
1623	703	1107	717	858	1002	Dextromoramide
1625	1121	1260	1525	1290	875	Carbidopa
1625	760	1260	690	1590	850	Chlordiazepoxide
1625	1520	1547	698	670	1600	Nialamide
1625	1668	1257	1539	1231	971	Thioguanine
1626	1307	1136	1066	1212	749	Lysergide
1626	1577	1319	1305	1148	955	Morantel
1626	1600	1274	1093	1100	1193	Parbendazole
1626	1219	1003	1266	923	892	Pipobroman
1627	910	965	1030	1136	1063	Decamethonium Bromide
1627	1601	709	1266	761	1070	Tropicamide
1628	1195	1562	1265	1149	1041	Desferrioxamine
1628	1492	1260	1312	836	1077	Homidium Bromide
1628	1610	1045	1182	1192	1518	Loprazolam Mesylate
1628	1575	1640	1075	835	805	Pyrimethamine
1628	1585	1308	1185	1240	1148	Thyroxine
1629	1035	1064	1520	1282	1250	Dexpanthenol
1629	1284	794	1305	1581	1095	Diethyltoluamide
1630	748	1245	1558	1170	998	Amiodarone Hydrochloride
1630	1111	1174	701	1192	1066	Bethanidine Sulphate
1630	1645	1598	1250	1510	1570	Diaveridine
1631	1590	1171	1181	1316	1242	Acriflavine
1631	1712	750	1208	1136	1160	Ergotamine
1632	1555	1661	1301	861	1176	Procarbazine Hydrochloride
1633	1245	1510	1184	805	820	Atenolol
1633	1662	1720	1705	1558	768	Dihydroergocornine
1633	1210	1172	1048	1675	1732	Dihydroergocryptine Mesylate
1633	1121	1718	1255	759	1272	Flavoxate
1634	1602	1504	1686	1238	1538	Amiloride Hydrochloride
1634	754	748	1044	1212	1541	Ergometrine
1634	1233	753	1276	1114	1587	Etenzamide
1634	1587	1550	820	1089	1232	Triclocarban
1635	1728	1510	1215	760	1540	Dihydroergocristine
1635	1260	1590	1730	1230	705	Mebendazole
1635	1590	1291	1103	1316	712	Nikethamide
1635	1305	1264	805	1069	1047	Sodium Cromoglycate
1636	1620	953	1075	1040	860	Choline Chloride
1637	1278	1602	1081	699	1136	Dimefline
1638	1522	1593	787	1562	1149	Amprolium
1638	698	752	1610	1500	1070	Imolamine
1639	1509	1527	1696	1600	1259	Acecainide Hydrochloride
1639	1047	1534	1595	1211	971	Aminotriazole
1639	751	1603	694	1492	1170	Butalamine
1639	1052	1612	1086	1265	1694	Desonide
1639	775	761	1603	1250	1316	Dibenzepin Hydrochloride
1639	1721	758	1534	1212	1294	Ergotoxine
1639	1592	1111	1492	812	758	Hydroxyurea
1640	696	736	1558	1275	1290	Beclamide
1640	1685	1118	755	712	1255	Dimenhydrinate
1640	1702	1610	1232	1042	1115	Hydrocortisone
1640	1535	1316	745	1575	715	Indoramin Hydrochloride (form I)
1640	1610	1550	1231	1210	758	Minoxidil
1640	1605	1305	1208	1132	1065	Pyrantel Tartrate
1642	1497	1234	1515	822	1019	Practolol
1645	1170	1564	1198	850	1240	Methylthiouracil
1645	756	707	1219	1101	1068	Oxethazaine
1646	1520	1256	1300	1046	815	Phenacaine
1647	1279	843	1013	903	754	Glyceryl Trinitrate

Wavenumbers
cm⁻¹ · *Compound*

1647	1562	1117	1241	1274	1520	Levodopa
1648	1670	1588	1511	1302	1495	Nifenazone
1649	716	1094	1298	1153	1016	Lorcainide Hydrochloride
1649	1068	1617	689	1272	660	Norethisterone
1650	986	1020	999	1062	1075	Aldosterone
1650	1698	1538	729	1041	1205	Bamifylline
1650	1150	1130	1315	880	1090	Chlormezanone
1650	1540	1565	1140	790	1311	Cytisine
1650	1520	765	1235	1272	1180	Etidocaine
1650	1576	705	769	757	1500	Isopropamide Iodide
1650	1280	1255	1302	1720	1180	Ketotifen Fumarate
1650	1523	760	1220	1123	1265	Mepivacaine
1650	1263	1612	1210	894	1185	Norethandrolone
1650	1618	1131	1590	1500	750	Propyphenazone
1650	1590	765	1496	774	1176	Tacrine
1651	1271	1714	1736	1246	1041	Fludrocortisone Acetate
1652	1248	1037	1595	1562	1063	Embutramide
1652	1700	1548	1220	760	750	Pentifylline
1653	1610	778	795	1295	1568	Clonidine Hydrochloride
1653	1508	1529	1238	1136	1597	Diamphenethide
1653	1600	768	1560	754	1730	Ethyl Biscoumacetate
1653	1242	1718	816	1220	1495	Fluorouracil
1653	1541	1621	676	992	845	Isoniazid
1654	1617	1219	1282	1098	1123	Cropropamide
1654	867	1036	1247	926	1282	Fluoxymesterone
1654	1612	1708	887	1112	1085	Prednisolone
1655	1617	1234	1098	1282	1123	Crotethamide
1655	1104	1075	1564	1040	1262	Lincomycin Hydrochloride
1655	1699	1755	1275	1205	815	Metharbitone
1656	1513	1176	1250	1026	820	Ambucetamide
1656	1739	1605	758	1111	1153	Chlorquinaldol
1656	1623	1235	1280	1316	1590	Crotamiton
1656	767	1587	1562	1315	1298	Dichloralphenazone
1656	1706	748	1543	1220	1600	Etamiphylline
1656	1693	1284	714	690	1226	Ketoprofen
1656	1737	1227	705	1201	1211	Oxyphencyclimine Hydrochloride
1656	759	696	1613	1163	1113	Phenprocoumon
1656	1690	750	1538	763	1282	Proxyphylline
1658	1698	747	1548	1242	760	Caffeine
1658	1605	1275	876	1281	1241	Dimethisterone
1658	1163	1622	1722	1176	1747	Fluocortolone Hexanoate
1658	1227	1600	905	1745	1034	Paramethasone
1658	1563	1193	1625	1166	1241	Propylthiouracil
1658	1157	1552	668	1090	905	Tolbutamide
1658	1695	1548	763	750	1029	Xanthinol
1660	1598	752	1538	1315	1500	Acetanilide
1660	1315	1126	750	700	1620	Amidopyrine
1660	1617	1606	1710	1056	907	Betamethasone
1660	1497	1575	1070	1150	1220	Cyanocobalamin
1660	1210	1712	1053	1140	768	Dihydroergotamine
1660	1700	1039	747	1562	1234	Diprophylline
1660	1622	1697	1581	1232	1197	Dydrogesterone
1660	1060	1235	1612	1127	723	Ethisterone
1660	701	1493	1263	1273	1236	Fentanyl
1660	1060	1730	1080	1250	1175	Halcinonide
1660	1620	886	1601	1160	1240	Methandienone
1660	1160	1239	950	1612	1090	Methyltestosterone
1660	1693	1085	1310	750	869	Methyprylone
1660	1700	1720	1550	762	752	Oxpentifylline
1660	1090	716	1618	1170	970	Phenacemide
1660	770	1318	1305	1590	1580	Phenazone
1660	1685	1600	1239	1157	1212	Pipamperone

Wavenumbers cm⁻¹					Compound

Wavenumbers cm⁻¹ / *Compound*

1660	1059	1630	750	699	1115	Styramate
1660	871	1615	1057	1236	1066	Testosterone
1660	1717	1567	745	980	1190	Theophylline
1660	1618	1048	1237	1595	1228	Thiamine Hydrochloride
1660	1153	1267	735	1590	1300	Vanillin
1661	1147	1599	1089	1635	1310	Carbutamide
1661	1159	1553	757	1086	909	Chlorpropamide
1661	1172	1234	1149	978	1613	Clorexolone
1662	1159	1725	1619	1605	1285	Fluocortolone Pivalate
1662	1495	762	1204	1290	1086	Lignocaine
1662	1705	1496	700	765	1120	Primidone
1662	1614	1700	872	1209	1232	Progesterone
1663	1172	1038	1532	1285	928	Clopamide
1663	896	1622	1695	1052	1603	Dexamethasone
1663	1057	1618	1609	902	1080	Triamcinolone Acetonide
1664	1585	697	1163	1562	760	Disopyramide
1664	1705	1600	1546	746	1219	Fenethylline
1664	1623	901	1733	1139	1160	Flumethasone Pivalate
1664	764	1050	1110	1282	775	Strychnine
1665	1245	1525	1495	1217	1285	Acebutolol Hydrochloride
1665	1712	1636	1562	740	1180	Bufylline
1665	790	1582	1000	810	1175	Hydralazine Hydrochloride
1665	1703	1318	1300	1278	1593	Pirenzepine Hydrochloride
1665	1060	1050	1320	1205	1180	Trilostane
1666	1612	1724	884	1063	1010	Clobetasol Propionate
1666	1086	1052	1063	1724	1639	Fluclorolone Acetonide
1666	1250	1123	724			Oxalic Acid
1667	1522	1279	1222	787	944	Bupivacaine Hydrochloride
1667	1036	1117	1020	810	1239	Fluoroacetamide
1667	1259	1096	1605	1289	1070	Idoxuridine
1667	1248	1119	1215	1010	1080	Methocarbamol
1667	1101	1499	1125	1002	1019	Morinamide
1667	1316	740	694	1602	704	Prazepam
1667	1626	1590	1302	797	1289	Tramazoline Hydrochloride
1668	1707	904	1622	1610	1246	Prednisone
1668	1541	1731	1170	1318	1291	Thiamylal
1669	1074	1629	910	1056	1615	Fluocinolone Acetonide
1669	701	757	1087	1190	1592	Piritramide
1670	1220	1265	1587	746	1149	Acetophenazine
1670	1626	760	1538	1592	1298	Dofamium Chloride
1670	1240	1730	1750	1070	1635	Fluocinonide
1670	750	705	870	815	1595	Isocarboxazid
1670	760	783	1618	1158	1270	Lysergamide
1670	1540	1300	1170	1735	1220	Thiopentone
1670	1270	1590	755	1500	1575	Tolfenamic Acid
1672	1064	1179	1163	1208	1639	Dipyrone
1672	1613	1316	1211	1171	1100	Flurazepam
1672	1134	1652	1050	765	1243	Guanoclor
1672	1578	1255	714	699	970	Metyrapone
1672	1700	1093	694	1176	1615	Pheneturide
1673	1515	1628	1570	760	1224	Cycloguanil
1673	1761	1718	1237	1292	1303	Heptabarbitone
1675	1220	1265	1587	746	1562	Acepromazine
1675	1505	767	806	1136	1190	Ambenonium Chloride
1675	749	1279	1193	1163	1143	Butaperazine
1675	1242	1500	1615	1298	765	Fendosal
1675	1701	1059	1045	1095	1079	Flurandrenolone
1675	820	1105	1195	1308	1242	Ketazolam
1675	1222	1269	1592	748	1560	Piperacetazine
1675	1760	1317	1303	1230	835	Secbutobarbitone
1675	1540	765	1128	772	1240	Tocainide Hydrochloride
1675	1760	1725	1234	1282	1298	Vinbarbitone
1676	1704	1092	1620	1185	750	Apronal

1676	1638	1548	1230	1516	1211	Flucytosine
1678	1594	800	769	787	1298	Carbamazepine
1678	690	1240	1265	755	717	Demoxepam
1678	1197	1093	1290	1727	1167	Diloxanide
1678	1602	825	1132	1310	800	Tetrazepam
1679	1733	1205	1178	1255	692	Nandrolone Phenyl-propionate
1680	1720	1767	1320	1245	875	Barbitone
1680	1277	1730	860	1160	1145	Bemegride
1680	1718	1193	1318	1110	703	Camazepam
1680	1510	730	1300	1220	1605	Indoprofen
1680	1643	1502	1270	820	1250	Labetalol Hydrochloride
1680	1709	1316	1193	1253	1040	Methohexitone Sodium
1680	705	1310	1220	760	1255	Methyl Salicylate
1680	1698	703	1618	1594	1026	Nicotinamide
1680	700	1602	820	738	790	Nordazepam
1681	847	1072	1515	816	1562	Chloramphenicol
1681	1313	705	840	1125	740	Diazepam
1681	1228	1218	1706	1299	1065	Indomethacin
1681	727	1205	1250	1316	1110	Thalidomide
1682	1153	1121	1315	1610	843	Lormetazepam
1682	1070	1710	1601	1140	788	Mebutamate
1682	1605	768	782	1282	1583	Mecloqualone
1682	1599	1565	770	1265	697	Methaqualone
1683	1492	1248	1220	1150	978	Diflunisal
1683	753	710	1253	696	764	Doxapram Hydrochloride
1683	1736	1275	1512	765	1600	Oxyphenbutazone
1683	1156	1285	1307	1125	1180	Probenecid
1684	1664	704	1490	764	845	Clobazam
1685	825	750	802	1315	1230	Bromazepam
1685	1033	1160	845	1190	1310	Chlorthalidone
1685	1610	748	1255	1578	1532	Clonazepam
1685	1705	1595	1230	752	1156	Droperidol
1685	1149	1317	1120	1605	826	Lorazepam
1685	1719	1744	1315	1218	845	Pentobarbitone
1685	1020	1600	1584	1050	1165	Pyrazinamide
1685	1610	1300	1130	1270	1000	Thialbarbitone Sodium
1686	1602	1636	1191	1567	1225	Folic Acid
1686	1710	1200	1270	1281	704	Glutethimide
1686	1616	1508	1070	762	1570	Nicoumalone
1686	1275	1637	1111	695	751	Phensuximide
1687	1315	925	1219	847	1640	Allobarbitone
1687	700	1211	1115	1052	769	Lobeline
1687	1706	693	830	1136	1123	Oxazepam
1687	1670	1112	1603	705	1150	Temazepam
1688	1210	1200	1223	1134	1179	Ecgonine Hydrochloride
1688	1069	1090	1590	1310	1140	Meprobamate
1689	1718	1550	1640	1285	672	Enallylpropymal
1689	1232	1270	857	1606	1149	Methallenoestril
1690	1720	1740	1310	1290	1200	Butalbital
1690	1610	1041	1170	1150	1010	Emylcamate
1690	1235	1497	1598	1155	750	Fluanisone
1690	1640	1602	835	665	880	Muzolimine
1690	1225	1527	1120	1496	1310	Nifedipine
1690	1610	698	1536	745	784	Nitrazepam
1690	1088	1064	700	1605	1623	Phenprobamate
1690	1274	1605	1174	1116	772	Procaine Hydrochloride
1690	1205	1170	1310	1620	1270	Salsalate
1690	1665	1221	1550	1595	680	Theobromine
1692	1587	916	1224	1235	956	Allopurinol
1692	1730	1750	1318	1220	1630	Vinylbitone
1693	1720	1745	1316	1255	860	Aprobarbitone
1693	1725	1745	1300	1210	830	Cyclobarbitone

Wavenumbers
cm⁻¹   *Compound*

1728	697	1183	1120	1215	1495	Diphenoxylate
1728	1670	1177	1188	1716	1224	Hydroxyprogesterone Hexanoate
1728	1156	1249	1500	1630	1010	Pyridostigmine Bromide
1729	1283	1594	1130	1116	743	Nicametate
1730	1158	1194	694	1265	1219	Butethamate
1730	1047	1025	1277	1095	755	Camphor
1730	1083	1056	930	1102	1200	Carbachol
1730	1786	730	1059	766	1309	Chlordantoin
1730	1240	769	1190	712	1011	Clidinium Bromide
1730	1175	725	704	776	1026	Dextropropoxyphene
1730	1172	1030	735	1063	1125	Homatropine
1730	853	1166	736	705	1047	Hyoscine Hydrobromide
1730	1230	725	770	1288	1200	Metomidate Hydrochloride
1730	1165	722	1280	1620	1070	Naftidrofuryl Oxalate
1730	1240	1225	1145	941	953	Oxymorphone
1730	1805	1100	1040	1280	1070	Paramethadione
1730	1200	1567	1608	751	1227	Propyliodone
1730	1802	1098	1200	770	1295	Troxidone
1730	1230	695	726	1163	1265	Valethamate Bromide
1731	1206	885	994	902	1250	Betaine
1731	1128	1221	1100	700	1080	Oxeladin
1733	755	1708	700	1286	1054	Bezitramide
1733	1287	1086	1132	744	1044	Diethyl Phthalate
1733	1667	1715	1266	1250	1618	Gestronol Hexanoate
1734	1192	1212	1274	1104	1074	Cyclandelate
1734	1195	965	685	1160	720	Methylpiperidyl Benzilate Hydrochloride
1735	1255	1170	1507	1135	1295	Distigmine Bromide
1735	1219	1085	1234	1063	700	Heteronium Bromide
1735	1175	1185	1317	860	923	Hyoscine Methonitrate
1735	1175	1210	1150	705	740	Methylphenidate Hydrochloride
1735	1155	1178	1040	1237	1203	Octatropine Methylbromide
1736	1145	700	1190	1500	746	Adiphenine

1736	1064	1110	1183	1242	1174	Monocrotaline
1738	1225	1164	1178	1115	1192	Glycopyrronium Bromide
1738	1010	1070	1036	1277	1605	Haloxon
1738	1160	1025	1145	1225	1050	Hyoscyamine Hydrobromide
1738	1181	1141	1162	1195	1077	Trimeperidine
1739	1241	699	743	1176	1191	Lachesine Chloride
1739	1248	1066	1632	972	1128	Methacholine Chloride
1739	1238	1227	702	1058	1093	Methindizate
1739	1227	1234	704	1064	1130	Penthienate Methobromide
1740	1178	1134	694	1030	1055	Alphaprodine
1740	1760	1815	1188	1280	1007	Dimethadione
1740	1178	1230	1265	1278	1510	Phenolphthalein
1740	1163	1638	1270	962	1012	Suxethonium Bromide
1742	1200	1182	1240	1150	1055	Protoveratrines A and B
1744	1239	1735	1053	1004	1123	Triacetyloleandomycin
1745	1276	1038	1010	1498	1080	Noscapine
1748	1253	1232	1520	1027	1126	Nifuratel
1751	1302	1585	752	1072	693	Phenindamine Tartrate
1752	1168	1104	660	1505	1020	Pilocarpine
1753	1215	700	690	1180	1020	Benapryzine Hydrochloride
1754	1582	1681	1271	695	1186	Cephalexin
1754	1582	1678	1271	1235	1190	Cephradine
1754	1660	1181	1202	1174	1532	Phenoxymethylpenicillin
1755	1226	1250	1110	1020	1315	Furaltadone
1760	1501	1037	1260	1020	1111	Hydrastine
1760	1742	1104	1683	972	1150	Pivampicillin
1762	801	962	1149	840	1300	Chlorzoxazone
1770	1075	1788	1263	1687	1744	Bacampicillin Hydrochloride
1773	1676	1170	1127	1115	1185	Spironolactone
1775	1583	1684	1248	1613	1313	Amoxycillin Trihydrate
1775	1693	1526	1308	1497	1583	Ampicillin
1780	1755	1795	1123	990	1162	Picrotoxin
1786	1176	1205	1111	1149	698	Pipoxolan

Mass Spectral Data of Drugs

In the following table the *m/z* values of the eight most intense ions are listed in descending order of intensity for drugs and other compounds of forensic interest. To identify an unknown compound, the *m/z* values of the two most intense ions should be compared with the table in order to produce a list of possible compounds. The eight most intense ions of the unknown can then be compared with this list. Comparison with standard spectra should then be made. Complete mass spectra for about 1000 drugs, metabolites, and other compounds of forensic and pharmaceutical interest are reproduced in *Pharmaceutical Mass Spectra* (London, Pharmaceutical Press, 1985).

Principal peaks at m/z								Compound
29	30	28	31	32	–	–	–	Formaldehyde
29	41	39	42	69	116	167	168	Ascorbic Acid
29	44	43	42	26	41	28	27	Acetaldehyde
29	46	45	28	44	30	47	–	Formic Acid
30	27	124	56	123	87	78	41	Hexoprenaline
30	42	43	27	44	29	31	41	Ethylenediamine Hydrate
30	43	72	102	73	42	118	99	Diminazene
30	44	41	45	86	55	43	69	Octamylamine
30	44	42	568	31	58	27	81	Pseudomorphine
30	57	82	116	99	53	55	42	Cimetidine
30	72	43	135	121	148	52	56	Guanoxan
30	86	57	41	29	39	192	42	Terbutaline
30	86	57	41	77	135	29	206	Salbutamol
30	86	57	129	74	56	41	114	Timolol
30	86	57	294	71	310	70	87	Nadolol
30	91	65	92	51	39	121	103	Phenethylamine
30	108	107	77	39	51	137	27	Tyramine
30	138	195	140	103	197	77	196	Baclofen
30	167	45	168	165	183	166	152	Didesmethyldiphenhydramine
30	313	246	211	273	274	302	183	Didesethylflurazepam
31	32	29	30	28	33	34	27	Methanol
31	33	29	32	43	28	27	42	Ethylene Glycol
31	45	29	27	46	43	30	42	Ethanol
31	45	46	29	27	59	74	43	Phenelzine
31	49	77	29	113	51	48	115	Triclofos
31	49	77	113	115	82	51	117	Trichloroethanol
31	59	29	45	74	27	41	43	Ether
31	59	42	60	27	29	45	41	Propanol
41	43	29	55	39	57	73	81	Lanatoside C
41	43	183	167	140	184	124	109	N-Hydroxyaprobarbitone
41	45	43	168	39	70	69	167	3'-Hydroxyquinalbarbitone
41	81	53	221	79	39	178	233	Methohexitone
41	132	102	160	96	29	27	44	Propamidine
41	147	79	93	55	105	67	91	Trilostane
41	167	124	39	80	53	68	141	Allobarbitone
41	167	168	39	124	97	141	181	Butalbital
41	226	77	143	181	141	39	145	Alclofenac
41	229	43	329	69	344	29	283	Δ⁹-THC-11-oic Acid
42	31	61	43	29	27	44	41	Ethanolamine
42	43	70	246	185	55	56	445	Thiopropazate
42	128	85	43	44	41	70	69	Barbituric Acid
42	140	112	41	85	43	71	141	Hexamine
42	271	258	123	56	83	240	95	Trifluperidol
42	292	56	294	109	203	201	44	Penfluridol
43	29	27	72	57	42	44	41	Methyl Ethyl Ketone
43	29	28	59	30	42	74	102	Cycloserine
43	29	39	41	45	57	68	58	Digitoxin
43	31	29	61	60	85	73	44	Isosorbide Dinitrate

Principal peaks at m/z								Compound
43	31	57	73	60	29	55	44	Amygdalin
43	41	184	168	167	97	55	53	Thiamylal
43	44	85	86	42	129	68	30	Metformin
43	44	87	31	45	42	131	71	Paraldehyde
43	45	60	58	95	99	398	206	Rifampicin
43	45	60	120	42	92	138	44	Aloxiprin
43	55	299	91	147	79	253	271	Deoxycortone Acetate
43	58	42	44	30	129	36	143	Carbachol
43	58	42	143	85	171	157	102	Bethanechol Chloride
43	58	59	27	42	26	39	29	Acetone
43	58	143	42	41	40	39	128	Troxidone
43	59	155	121	156	31	157	158	Phenaglycodol
43	61	45	70	29	27	73	42	Ethyl Acetate
43	69	168	41	85	167	86	169	3'-Ketoquinalbarbitone
43	70	29	71	27	154	41	267	Ergotoxine
43	70	55	42	41	73	61	87	Amyl Acetate
43	70	71	54	44	154	267	55	Ergocornine
43	70	71	154	41	209	69	267	Ergocryptine
43	71	55	79	91	109	123	336	Fluoxymesterone
43	91	134	92	65	39	63	135	Phenylacetone
43	91	227	268	312	79	55	77	Dydrogesterone
43	114	85	30	101	86	44	72	Buformin
43	127	195	85	44	36	152	58	Proguanil
43	129	57	56	41	72	39	58	Paramethadione
43	129	69	41	86	97	55	44	Acetylcarbromal
43	141	183	42	87	41	140	165	Paracetamol Mercapturic Acid Conjugate
43	180	42	45	44	64	100	222	Acetazolamide
43	182	167	225	181	183	151	142	Trimethoxyamphetamine
43	187	42	171	229	86	144	170	Amiloride
43	221	83	236	56	223	222	55	Methazolamide
43	327	299	298	292	329	328	256	7-Acetamidoclonazepam
43	340	298	325	91	41	231	280	Norethisterone Acetate
44	30	42	41	29	27	100	55	Tuaminoheptane
44	42	124	165	163	123	93	65	Adrenaline
44	42	147	120	65	43	45	39	Amidephrine
44	42	159	43	45	184	41	109	Norfenfluramine
44	43	59	56	69	55	41	113	Heptaminol
44	43	79	93	41	135	91	81	Rimantadine
44	45	26	218	215	203	202	42	10-Hydroxynortriptyline
44	45	58	76	60	43	42	46	Noradrenaline
44	57	43	40	55	41	79	77	Cathine
44	59	165	166	181	179	178	43	Tofenacin
44	69	41	208	210	55	71	43	Carbromal
44	70	59	277	71	191	278	203	Maprotiline
44	70	179	178	207	280	250	236	10,11-Dihydro-10,11-dihydroxyprotriptyline
44	71	268	227	193	42	269	229	Monodesmethylclomipramine
44	76	77	29	45	42	95	65	Phenylephrine

Principal peaks at m/z — *Compound*

								Compound
44	77	76	29	95	39	58	42	Metaraminol
44	77	79	51	45	42	107	105	Phenylpropanolamine (norephedrine)
44	82	80	107	77	108	81	79	Hydroxyamphetamine
44	83	85	36	28	–	–	–	Trichloroacetic Acid
44	83	180	182	137	143	139	41	Bromvaletone
44	91	40	42	65	45	39	43	Amphetamine
44	100	41	60	29	27	30	86	Piperazine Adipate
44	108	42	77	107	149	95	123	Oxedrine
44	121	77	120	42	106	91	39	Tocainide
44	122	121	78	77	42	51	52	Methoxyamphetamine
44	136	51	135	77	42	78	45	Methylenedioxy-amphetamine
44	146	147	39	41	190	42	148	Cytisine
44	166	151	57	43	91	135	209	DOM
44	167	168	165	183	105	152	77	Monodesmethyl-diphenhydramine
44	180	209	227	223	77	208	179	3'-Carboxymefenamic Acid
44	194	109	67	86	238	56	85	Acepifylline
44	202	45	220	218	215	91	–	Nortriptyline
44	204	203	202	41	221	57	55	Desmethyldothiepin
44	206	162	108	51	207	201	178	Cromoglycic Acid
44	208	117	58	193	130	57	29	Norpropoxyphene
44	209	211	250	210	224	42	251	2-Hydroxydesipramine
44	215	411	324	45	164	42	216	Etorphine
45	29	43	60	42	28	44	41	Acetic Acid
45	43	27	41	39	29	59	44	Isopropyl Alcohol
45	130	44	71	42	61	115	55	2-Ethylbutyrylurea
45	156	141	69	41	43	157	55	3'-Hydroxypentobarbitone
45	217	70	41	69	110	285	202	Pentazocine
46	76	57	55	56	60	47	97	Pentaerythritol Tetranitrate
49	84	86	51	47	35	88	41	Methylene Chloride
55	41	42	43	70	57	29	31	Amyl Alcohol
55	44	142	141	41	61	81	82	Apronal
55	57	43	97	41	56	158	44	Carisoprodol
55	72	97	41	56	158	118	57	Tybamate
55	82	41	39	54	42	56	109	Pentetrazol
55	83	82	41	113	70	29	69	Bemegride
55	378	43	29	57	410	379	84	Buprenorphine
56	42	83	57	77	51	97	54	Dipyrone
56	55	41	43	45	85	42	84	Cadaverine
56	100	138	110	57	237	70	41	Viloxazine
56	231	97	111	112	42	77	71	Amidopyrine
57	41	141	167	39	83	55	182	Nealbarbitone
57	42	44	177	58	219	133	107	Profadol
57	58	70	42	44	188	84	43	Ethoheptazine
57	85	42	56	76	191	70	77	Phendimetrazine
57	233	42	56	158	43	160	103	Norpethidine
58	30	59	56	77	–	–	–	Hydroxyephedrine
58	30	59	77	29	95	65	57	Etilefrine
58	30	107	59	77	56	42	43	Pholedrine
58	30	363	44	72	29	27	364	Bialamicol
58	41	30	126	59	69	56	44	Cyclopentamine
58	41	56	30	124	65	59	93	Ethylnoradrenaline
58	42	30	51	204	146	77	44	Psilocybin
58	42	41	125	59	30	89	168	Chlorphentermine
58	42	59	30	77	107	57	51	Hordenine
58	42	69	41	30	215	202	59	10-Hydroxyamitriptyline
58	43	57	149	71	42	41	55	Acetylcholine
58	44	31	59	57	42	45	40	Dothiepin Sulphoxide
58	44	41	83	77	69	85	43	Mexiletine
58	55	41	44	43	128	59	56	Isometheptene
58	59	42	215	202	57	189	43	Cyclobenzaprine
58	59	72	45	292	218	42	–	Dimethindene
58	59	179	42	178	72	77	30	Chlorphenoxamine
58	59	202	42	203	214	217	–	Amitriptyline
58	59	221	30	42	222	255	43	Chlorprothixene
58	70	318	316	317	193	319	161	Zimeldine
58	71	26	54	167	72	42	44	Carbinoxamine
58	71	72	167	182	42	180	59	Doxylamine
58	71	72	207	42	91	59	118	Cyclopentolate
58	71	150	176	72	193	105	59	Amethocaine
58	71	208	72	59	42	89	57	Noxiptyline
58	72	29	42	71	57	59	224	Normethadone
58	72	30	77	56	44	42	73	Methylephedrine
58	72	43	78	271	57	44	77	Camazepam
58	72	279	234	151	192	166	165	Thymoxamine
58	73	44	45	165	42	40	181	Orphenadrine
58	73	45	43	57	167	44	165	Dimenhydrinate
58	73	45	165	59	42	166	149	Bromodiphenhydramine
58	73	45	167	165	166	44	152	Diphenhydramine
58	77	59	56	51	42	105	91	Pseudoephedrine
58	85	86	57	84	70	43	268	8-Hydroxyclomipramine
58	85	269	268	270	271	314	242	Clomipramine
58	86	318	85	320	272	319	273	Chlorpromazine
58	91	42	41	134	65	59	40	Phentermine
58	91	59	56	30	42	121	78	Methoxyphenamine
58	91	59	134	65	56	42	57	Methylamphetamine
58	91	72	71	197	185	184	92	Tripelennamine
58	97	72	71	42	191	79	78	Methapyrilene
58	97	72	71	203	191	190	42	Thenyldiamine
58	107	30	178	77	56	57	137	Dobutamine
58	111	71	42	75	59	141	113	Meclofenoxate
58	116	198	199	72	59	42	44	Dimethoxanate
58	117	208	115	193	91	179	130	Dextropropoxyphene
58	121	72	71	216	215	122	78	Thonzylamine
58	125	71	72	36	127	79	219	Halopyramine
58	131	72	71	79	42	30	78	Chloropyrilene
58	140	67	72	83	81	155	156	Propylhexedrine
58	146	56	105	77	42	106	40	Ephedrine
58	165	255	359	166	73	199	45	Captodiame
58	170	284	213	145	212	159	144	Iprindole
58	179	180	225	178	165	42	210	Nefopam
58	181	43	45	60	44	165	73	Orphenadrine N-Oxide
58	188	130	59	42	143	129	115	Dimethyltryptamine
58	195	59	72	388	89	315	42	Trimethobenzamide
58	204	59	42	30	146	77	44	Psilocin
58	204	146	59	42	160	43	159	Bufotenine
58	213	198	180	214	57	212	270	N-Monodesmethyl-promethazine
58	220	219	59	191	189	42	205	Doxepin
58	224	209	71	225	72	210	180	Dibenzepin
58	234	193	192	42	235	194	59	Lofepramine
58	235	85	234	236	195	193	208	Imipramine
58	236	40	202	235	203	42	44	Dothiepin
58	238	91	45	239	167	165	56	Prenylamine
58	249	208	99	193	234	84	248	Trimipramine
58	251	250	211	85	42	209	296	2-Hydroxyimipramine
58	254	45	44	77	42	59	72	Chlophedianol
58	255	42	71	59	44	181	165	Phenyltoloxamine
58	282	30	284	355	73	283	44	Amodiaquine
58	284	86	238	198	199	85	42	Promazine
58	285	214	200	86	227	85	213	Prothipendyl
58	293	45	59	193	100	178	294	Butriptyline
58	298	212	198	100	299	252	199	Trimeprazine

Principal peaks at m/z								*Compound*
58	328	100	228	185	329	242	229	Methotrimeprazine
58	352	86	353	85	306	42	266	Fluopromazine
58	366	59	100	266	248	84	44	Trifluomeprazine
58	427	234	59	50	42	428	91	Narceine
59	157	156	141	43	41	71	69	3'-Hydroxyamylobarb- itone
59	257	150	256	31	76	42	157	Dextrorphan
59	257	150	256	44	31	200	157	Levorphanol
59	271	150	270	31	214	42	171	Dextromethorphan
60	42	88	30	31	43	29	70	Benserazide
60	44	28	–	–	–	–	–	Urea
63	78	45	61	46	62	48	47	Dimethyl Sulphoxide
66	120	39	65	269	205	118	77	Cyclothiazide
67	193	66	41	169	39	65	77	Cyclopentobarbitone
67	137	91	138	55	79	41	95	Dimethisterone
69	43	41	44	71	167	165	55	2-Bromo-2-ethylbutyr- amide
69	56	71	91	261	84	119	70	Phenbutrazate
69	68	70	77	103	56	54	51	Bisnortilidate
69	83	43	79	41	81	53	80	Methylpentynol Carb- amate
70	41	69	75	114	42	217	68	Captopril
70	43	55	41	57	42	71	–	Amyl Nitrite
70	43	154	71	41	209	86	195	Bromocriptine
70	44	191	192	188	59	165	71	Protriptyline
70	44	207	178	279	249	–	–	10-Hydroxyprotriptyline
70	71	42	44	57	190	29	247	Ketobemidone
70	71	269	154	195	55	59	57	Dihydroergocornine
70	83	42	257	193	56	228	164	Loxapine
70	112	293	264	44	42	305	41	Bromhexine
70	113	141	399	43	26	72	42	Thiethylperazine
70	120	43	91	39	103	71	65	Aletamine
70	125	71	91	153	267	154	221	Ergocristine
70	125	91	153	43	41	44	244	Dihydroergotamine
70	150	151	153	77	51	118	60	Chloramphenicol
70	154	125	41	43	155	42	225	Co-dergocrine
71	42	56	43	177	77	178	105	Phenmetrazine
71	58	72	43	159	56	42	201	Dimethisoquin
71	70	44	57	42	247	43	246	Pethidine
71	70	57	43	219	42	218	44	Pethidinic Acid
71	72	58	100	83	56	70	44	Diethylcarbamazine
71	91	106	177	57	72	65	30	Bethanidine
72	30	43	77	73	51	41	27	Clorprenaline
72	30	43	122	73	41	106	121	Sotalol
72	30	56	43	27	41	39	110	Prenalterol
72	30	56	73	249	98	234	102	Alprenolol
72	30	56	98	43	107	41	73	Atenolol
72	30	107	56	45	41	44	43	Metoprolol
72	30	116	56	43	160	41	158	4-Hydroxypropranolol
72	30	151	43	109	56	57	108	Practolol
72	39	42	38	94	56	51	81	Pyridostigmine Bromide
72	41	56	43	221	73	57	45	Oxprenolol
72	42	208	108	65	73	66	39	Neostigmine Bromide
72	43	30	56	151	221	41	98	Acebutolol
72	43	73	41	70	65	40	39	Orciprenaline
72	44	43	124	123	30	42	41	Isoprenaline
72	44	159	73	58	42	109	56	Fenfluramine
72	56	30	43	98	115	144	41	Propranolol
72	58	71	42	73	70	56	44	Isoaminile
72	73	43	91	224	56	71	129	Levomethadyl Acetate
72	73	91	293	223	165	85	71	Methadone
72	73	214	200	44	285	86	56	Isothipendyl
72	73	284	198	213	199	180	56	Promethazine
72	73	320	71	70	56	210	198	Dimethothiazine

Principal peaks at m/z								*Compound*
72	73	340	269	197	71	70	56	Propiomazine
72	91	73	44	42	56	70	65	Dimethylamphetamine
72	91	73	56	148	65	57	42	Mephentermine
72	91	114	145	75	160	117	92	Oxethazaine
72	133	30	116	248	134	56	41	Pindolol
72	176	91	58	177	41	42	30	Alverine
72	181	85	152	42	44	58	43	Methanthelinium Bromide
73	43	84	55	69	41	44	85	Emylcamate
73	58	57	43	41	39	29	45	Digoxin
73	102	41	57	43	27	55	29	Valproic Acid
75	41	57	70	43	59	56	47	Penicillamine
76	173	104	111	148	50	169	130	Thalidomide
76	239	104	240	285	241	50	75	Chlorthalidone
77	51	123	50	65	93	30	78	Nitrobenzene
77	105	91	51	65	212	50	78	Benzyl Benzoate
77	106	105	51	50	78	52	39	Benzaldehyde
77	183	308	184	105	55	51	41	Phenylbutazone
77	278	105	78	51	279	252	130	Sulphinpyrazone
78	77	52	51	50	39	79	74	Benzene
78	106	51	137	50	136	107	79	Methyl Nicotinate
78	106	135	136	51	50	79	52	N-Methylnicotinamide
79	77	108	101	51	50	39	40	Benzyl Alcohol
79	78	52	105	304	314	316	51	3-Hydroxybromazepam
79	96	31	113	81	70	127	78	Thioproperazine
79	105	104	51	78	52	50	77	Betahistine
81	53	330	96	82	332	64	63	Frusemide
81	83	46	110	82	112	84	117	Chloral Betaine
81	95	71	41	67	55	138	123	Menthol
81	124	54	53	125	171	45	42	Metronidazole
81	223	79	41	80	157	185	77	Thialbarbitone
82	30	81	54	28	55	83	41	Histamine
82	30	81	83	55	54	42	27	Ametazole
82	47	84	29	111	83	113	85	Chloral Hydrate
82	68	91	159	42	158	92	65	Pargyline
82	97	42	83	96	57	94	55	Ecgonine
82	182	83	105	303	77	94	96	Cocaine
83	68	82	72	84	77	103	115	Nortilidate
83	70	273	244	209	42	71	43	Clothiapine
83	84	55	56	43	71	41	62	Meprobamate
83	85	47	87	48	49	35	82	Chloroform
83	140	82	124	43	96	97	42	Deptropine
83	140	82	124	96	97	42	125	Benztropine
84	56	85	77	105	55	30	42	Pipradrol
84	71	85	82	80	341	70	356	Conessine
84	82	80	56	43	28	30	41	Coniine
84	91	77	55	182	85	65	104	Antazoline
84	91	85	56	55	150	41	118	Methylphenidate
84	128	179	42	85	178	214	98	Clemastine
84	133	42	162	161	105	77	119	Nicotine
84	178	161	133	118	–	–	–	Nicotine-1'-N-oxide
84	194	55	85	56	41	30	99	Perhexiline
84	204	205	85	42	55	105	77	Procyclidine
84	209	67	43	110	41	192	164	Minoxidil
85	43	42	86	44	41	75	110	Mefruside
85	56	69	55	27	44	42	109	Pipobroman
85	58	86	91	84	70	42	225	Benzydamine
85	84	183	105	56	77	55	30	Azacyclonol
85	87	101	50	103	31	66	35	Dichlorodifluoromethane
85	135	87	137	31	101	100	50	Dichlorotetrafluoro- ethane
86	30	57	108	44	29	84	41	Bamethan
86	30	58	29	130	87	77	42	Diethyltryptamine
86	30	58	123	78	51	29	42	Nicametate

Principal peaks at m/z								Compound		Principal peaks at m/z								Compound
86	30	72	44	141	42	29	57	Butanilicaine		91	269	324	55	296	295	323	297	Prazepam
86	30	167	99	87	58	165	29	Adiphenine		92	65	108	214	156	39	109	43	Sulphaguanidine
86	30	216	87	58	100	99	56	Phenglutarimide		92	91	65	103	93	39	163	77	Tropicamide
86	36	87	84	58	56	44	38	Amiodarone		92	156	65	108	191	45	39	55	Sulphathiazole
86	36	126	30	58	38	112	99	Mepacrine		92	156	65	191	108	55	45	174	Succinylsulphathiazole
86	44	30	265	41	180	29	87	Ethomoxane		92	156	191	65	108	76	104	50	Phthalylsulphathiazole
86	44	87	107	43	106	56	41	Prilocaine		92	270	65	156	108	106	93	59	Sulphamethizole
86	58	87	42	56	77	44	43	Etafedrine		92	284	156	108	65	106	93	220	Sulphaethidole
86	58	88	105	206	87	55	77	Tridihexethyl Chloride		93	135	43	66	65	39	94	92	Acetanilide
86	58	99	56	162	132	149	205	Acecainide (N-acetyl-procainamide)		94	66	39	65	40	55	38	95	Phenol
86	58	319	87	73	247	245	112	Chloroquine		94	138	42	108	136	41	96	97	Hyoscine
86	71	99	58	55	56	100	87	Dicyclomine		94	151	57	95	40	41	58	108	Amantadine
86	87	58	30	29	84	56	42	Chromonar		95	55	41	43	59	27	39	67	Picrotoxin
86	87	58	44	72	42	120	85	Lignocaine		95	81	41	69	55	83	67	137	Camphor
86	87	58	149	111	99	57	41	Cinchocaine		95	96	42	109	41	208	54	39	Pilocarpine
86	87	99	58	84	387	315	56	Flurazepam		95	130	132	60	97	35	134	47	Trichloroethylene
86	87	100	30	58	44	42	29	Clomiphene		95	327	39	329	96	122	244	67	Diloxanide Furoate
86	91	87	145	58	144	30	44	Carbetapentane		96	44	43	31	45	27	78	264	Hydroxystilbamidine
86	91	105	87	144	58	100	56	Oxeladin		96	56	42	91	97	39	65	58	Selegiline
86	99	29	30	100	71	87	192	Oxybuprocaine		96	97	98	91	136	31	29	55	Pentapiperide
86	99	30	87	58	71	136	100	Proxymetacaine		96	105	77	97	216	42	218	51	Lobeline
86	99	91	144	58	56	41	87	Caramiphen		97	43	71	70	96	91	98	42	Bamipine
86	99	91	191	87	119	58	248	Butethamate		97	55	69	72	71	98	43	62	Mebutamate
86	99	100	141	87	71	44	58	Naftidrofuryl		97	70	99	43	98	44	42	188	Thenalidine
86	99	120	30	92	87	58	65	Procainamide		97	98	296	199	55	212	96	198	Methdilazine
86	99	120	58	87	30	92	71	Procaine		97	99	61	117	119	63	101	62	Trichloroethane
86	99	136	30	58	178	87	71	Propoxycaine		97	105	77	96	42	183	98	82	Mepenzolate Bromide
86	99	154	30	87	58	29	156	Chloroprocaine		97	105	77	183	84	36	42	51	Methylpiperidyl Benzilate
86	99	184	58	30	87	201	186	Metoclopramide		98	41	42	55	99	77	69	44	Cycrimine
86	100	44	30	29	42	58	56	Diamthazole		98	70	99	42	386	126	55	41	Mesoridazine
86	105	77	87	182	99	183	58	Benactyzine		98	70	214	111	134	341	199	326	Sulpiride
86	109	30	151	87	81	99	58	Etamiphylline		98	84	71	56	41	42	99	124	Mecamylamine
86	114	100	44	238	115	56	72	Isopropamide Iodide		98	99	70	42	96	55	41	40	Mepivacaine
86	181	43	44	41	114	42	152	Propantheline		98	99	105	77	55	41	127	111	Diphenidol
86	298	87	30	58	299	212	180	Diethazine		98	105	55	41	99	77	218	84	Benzhexol
87	79	51	225	42	50	86	80	Furazolidone		98	111	99	42	55	41	29	112	Norpipanone
88	42	123	124	89	77	51	44	Methyldopa		98	111	99	147	55	41	42	96	Flavoxate
90	177	105	77	106	51	89	50	5-Phenyloxazolidine-2,4-dione		98	111	99	199	41	288	200	55	Pipazethate
91	30	92	42	29	146	44	104	Phenformin		98	112	99	55	42	41	211	84	Fenpipramide
91	30	155	108	65	197	39	107	Tolbutamide		98	119	91	99	124	64	41	55	Diperodon
91	65	187	92	277	259	90	273	Trimetaphan Camsylate		98	137	97	136	41	193	84	110	Sparteine
91	79	67	201	77	105	93	120	Lynoestrenol		98	152	154	42	69	174	208	153	Chlormezanone
91	81	106	78	39	95	68	43	Ethinamate		98	176	42	118	41	119	51	175	Cotinine
91	92	65	39	63	93	51	89	Toluene		98	194	166	157	55	42	165	99	Pipoxolan
91	92	118	44	43	135	65	178	Phenacemide		98	215	58	84	91	56	71	186	Fencamfamin
91	106	105	77	51	39	29	92	m-Xylene		98	218	99	55	41	42	77	84	Biperiden
91	106	197	162	107	148	27	63	Beclamide		98	370	126	99	40	70	371	258	Thioridazine
91	120	65	121	92	105	77	118	Benethamine		99	56	72	165	300	228	229	242	Chlorcyclizine
91	121	65	122	309	64	230	123	Benzthiazide		99	56	167	207	194	266	195	165	Cyclizine
91	127	106	110	43	92	65	120	Isocarboxazid		99	114	98	167	70	165	57	43	Diphenylpyraline
91	133	176	174	44	107	92	177	Buphenine		99	197	44	58	112	309	41	42	Methixene
91	146	44	119	206	41	78	77	Pheneturide		100	44	72	101	77	56	42	105	Diethylpropion
91	148	149	65	92	42	56	39	Benzphetamine		100	56	42	101	55	54	41	30	Nimorazole
91	155	114	65	197	42	41	85	Tolazamide		100	56	42	176	98	120	70	189	Molindone
91	155	197	65	84	39	95	41	Glibornuride		100	56	101	42	185	184	41	128	Furaltadone
91	159	160	131	65	92	81	39	Tolazoline		100	58	41	101	43	56	65	30	Isoetharine
91	177	44	106	45	78	123	51	Nialamide		100	58	105	77	56	101	41	70	Meprylcaine
91	196	198	92	197	65	77	56	Phenoxybenzamine		100	72	240	340	44	197	254	43	Acepromazine Maleate
91	215	79	105	77	55	41	298	Norethynodrel		100	101	44	72	198	180	42	29	Ethopropazine
91	216	77	259	-	-	-	-	1-(1-Phenylcyclohexyl)-4-hydroxypiperidine		100	113	56	101	87	378	194	91	Doxapram
										100	128	70	41	42	293	56	101	Pramoxine
										100	265	128	266	44	98	56	101	Dextromoramide
91	233	30	232	31	276	275	65	Mebhydrolin		101	103	105	66	47	35	31	82	Trichlorofluoromethane

Principal peaks at m/z							Compound	Principal peaks at m/z							Compound
102	30	72	44	116	55	173	71	Ethambutol	116	88	29	44	60	148	56	27	Disulfiram
102	84	58	56	42	30	103	91	Bamifylline	117	119	47	35	121	82	84	49	Carbon Tetrachloride
102	245	247	304	305	306	58	126	Hydroxychloroquine	117	198	196	119	129	67	127	98	Halothane
103	77	82	29	97	42	51	104	Tilidate	118	108	182	91	225	107	57	75	Mephenesin Carbamate
104	105	204	77	78	133	51	132	Ethotoin	118	117	91	92	119	65	77	103	Phenprobamate
104	132	218	51	103	77	78	52	Phenylmethylbarbituric Acid	118	117	203	103	77	78	119	91	Methsuximide
104	189	103	78	51	77	105	52	Phensuximide	120	43	138	92	121	39	64	63	Aspirin
104	189	103	117	78	91	51	146	2-Phenylglutarimide	120	92	105	148	150	121	133	65	Etenzamide
105	77	51	122	50	39	74	76	Benzoic Acid	120	92	137	65	121	39	64	53	Salicylamide
105	77	96	183	51	42	182	94	Clidinium Bromide	120	92	138	64	39	63	121	65	Salicylic Acid
105	77	106	44	51	128	78	40	Broxaldine	120	92	152	121	65	64	93	63	Methyl Salicylate
105	104	77	79	244	106	103	27	Etomidate	120	106	78	92	51	226	41	39	Metyrapone
105	111	77	96	97	183	42	51	Pipenzolate Bromide	120	137	193	92	65	121	138	41	Butyl Aminobenzoate
105	129	112	77	42	313	41	55	Oxyphencyclimine	120	165	92	65	137	39	121	93	Benzocaine
105	135	51	134	77	106	50	78	Hippuric Acid	120	263	142	178	100	264	41	29	Butacaine
105	177	77	209	254	210	103	181	Ketoprofen	121	43	122	223	147	91	41	135	Betamethasone
105	554	540	43	45	77	31	29	Aconitine	121	58	72	71	214	122	215	78	Mepyramine
106	30	77	185	105	104	89	141	Mafenide	121	65	36	185	50	38	76	39	Halazone
106	78	51	137	50	79	107	31	Isoniazid	121	120	69	92	195	39	93	45	Salicyluric Acid
106	78	177	51	178	107	149	40	Nikethamide	121	120	354	122	43	234	106	64	Xipamide
106	123	78	51	119	79	77	107	Salinazid	121	122	91	147	225	43	135	120	Prednisolone
107	69	125	83	79	55	41	77	Cyclandelate	121	122	315	43	147	223	135	41	Dexamethasone
107	79	77	51	152	105	50	78	Mandelic Acid	121	152	40	93	65	–	–	–	Methyl Hydroxybenzoate
107	108	77	79	51	39	53	50	p-Cresol	121	163	151	109	43	122	108	65	Benorylate
107	108	78	79	80	77	51	52	Phenyramidol	121	164	77	57	56	165	162	122	Ritodrine
107	120	79	75	77	44	91	45	Styramate	121	318	317	173	120	362	44	31	Ethyl Biscoumacetate
107	145	268	238	121	133	159	224	Stilboestrol	122	78	106	51	50	52	44	123	Nicotinamide
107	163	223	108	29	164	41	57	Bufexamac	122	121	91	147	161	43	107	120	Ethisterone
107	165	123	95	121	–	–	–	Azaperone	123	31	58	106	79	43	78	51	Iproniazid
107	176	90	77	70	105	42	79	Pemoline	123	51	78	106	50	52	105	39	Isonicotinic Acid
108	81	213	54	77	136	51	43	Phenazopyridine	123	57	42	103	44	85	124	51	Carbidopa
108	107	91	182	109	77	79	31	Mephenesin	123	105	78	51	106	77	124	50	Nicotinic Acid
108	109	179	137	43	81	80	110	Phenacetin	123	106	78	51	105	50	77	52	Nicofuranose
108	248	140	65	92	141	109	80	Dapsone	123	124	77	44	51	74	53	39	Levodopa
109	76	104	92	239	65	108	43	Phthalylsulphacetamide	124	43	314	79	91	229	272	105	Progesterone
109	80	44	81	53	39	52	54	Aminosalicylic Acid	124	82	83	94	55	42	67	96	Tigloidine
109	80	53	81	108	52	54	110	4-Aminophenol	124	82	94	83	42	96	103	67	Atropine
109	108	80	53	51	39	91	27	Nicotinyl Alcohol	124	82	168	77	105	42	94	83	Benzoylecgonine
109	151	43	41	221	179	29	108	Thiocarlide	124	107	82	83	42	77	79	94	Homatropine
109	151	43	80	108	81	53	52	Paracetamol	124	109	198	81	77	125	52	31	Guaiphenesin
110	82	39	81	53	69	55	111	Resorcinol	124	118	198	109	43	57	125	77	Methocarbamol
111	96	167	112	165	71	43	42	Piperidolate	124	276	58	140	56	72	125	41	Eucatropine
111	127	55	83	59	41	112	42	Clopamide	125	44	70	91	41	40	244	153	Ergotamine
111	175	75	85	30	276	127	113	Chlorpropamide	125	70	91	153	41	244	43	71	Dihydroergocristine
112	77	105	139	55	41	96	56	Hexylcaine	125	93	127	173	158	99	55	79	Malathion
112	161	85	45	163	113	114	59	Chlormethiazole	125	189	230	127	191	63	232	90	Diazoxide
112	246	105	77	55	41	44	247	Piperocaine	126	44	30	42	41	55	43	58	Guanethidine
112	264	113	91	179	110	178	115	Dipipanone	126	127	174	91	70	69	55	42	Prolintane
112	344	121	41	67	55	54	345	Cyclomethycaine	127	43	229	44	161	231	85	186	Chlorproguanil
113	70	42	211	351	43	71	56	Pirenzepine	127	161	163	153	129	187	90	189	Triclocarban
113	70	55	42	41	39	85	69	Ethosuximide	128	96	70	39	41	27	42	29	Cantharidin
113	70	114	42	221	222	56	43	Thiothixene	128	130	65	39	64	63	129	99	Parachlorophenol
113	70	373	141	43	72	42	127	Prochlorperazine	128	130	169	87	41	129	242	171	Clofibrate
113	70	407	43	141	42	127	71	Trifluoperazine	128	130	202	31	29	65	43	111	Chlorphenesin
113	70	409	43	141	283	42	127	Butaperazine	128	130	202	43	129	111	75	204	Chlorphenesin Carb-amate
113	86	116	98	117	115	58	84	Aprindine	128	141	268	130	270	77	143	233	Dichlorophen
113	339	44	70	141	43	60	340	Perazine	130	131	30	160	77	103	132	102	Tryptamine
114	42	72	113	69	81	54	115	Methimazole	131	256	125	42	255	89	258	257	Clemizole
114	44	142	365	42	223	115	205	Pericyazine	132	104	44	175	103	117	43	130	Debrisoquine
114	72	43	100	29	44	337	86	Propanidid	133	132	56	115	30	117	91	77	Tranylcypromine
114	100	56	42	115	101	70	398	Pholcodine	135	57	91	77	43	119	105	180	Hydroxyphenamate
115	86	79	57	56	107	100	52	Morinamide	135	150	91	107	117	–	–	–	Thymol
115	117	89	53	109	51	91	39	Ethchlorvynol	136	81	137	42	41	55	130	128	Cinchonidine

Principal peaks at m/z								Compound
136	81	322	188	55	42	41	172	Quinidine
136	135	52	28	137	109	29	18	Allopurinol
136	137	81	42	41	189	55	117	Quinine
136	294	81	159	55	42	41	143	Cinchonine
136	310	135	225	149	122	155	311	Ibogaine
137	120	92	65	39	138	121	63	Aminobenzoic Acid
138	55	189	82	41	110	326	42	Hydroquinine
138	326	55	110	189	82	160	139	Hydroquinidine
138	352	215	310	214	69	321	354	Griseofulvin
139	141	357	111	359	140	113	75	Indomethacin
140	84	56	41	72	69	29	39	Pempidine
140	141	84	41	29	96	56	55	Bupivacaine
141	43	183	44	140	80	108	52	Paracetamol Cysteine Conjugate
141	156	41	55	98	39	142	155	Butobarbitone
141	156	41	57	39	98	157	47	Secbutobarbitone
141	156	43	41	157	55	39	98	Pentobarbitone
141	445	169	123	155	96	42	317	Metopimazine
142	44	140	42	198	170	41	96	Pipothiazine
142	57	42	197	185	339	240	226	Hexetidine
142	143	100	155	44	112	57	29	Butalamine
142	170	44	410	42	143	43	41	Piperacetazine
143	70	100	144	42	56	98	221	Clopenthixol
143	70	100	144	42	98	58	56	Flupenthixol
145	117	122	89	105	90	63	146	Hydroxyquinoline
146	148	111	75	50	150	113	147	Paradichlorobenzene
146	190	117	118	161	189	103	91	Primidone
146	233	103	133	91	117	115	77	4-Hydroxyglutethimide
147	43	146	42	193	118	164	44	Carbazochrome
147	131	130	132	119	148	365	218	Indapamide
149	41	29	57	56	104	32	65	Dibutyl Phthalate
149	177	150	65	76	105	176	104	Diethyl Phthalate
150	121	56	93	39	151	66	94	Glipizide
150	152	165	41	167	43	44	130	2-Bromo-2-ethyl-3-hydroxybutyramide
151	72	223	123	222	152	52	29	Ethamivan
151	94	122	106	51	53	149	150	Pyridoxine
151	109	136	178	177	29	207	135	Thiambutosine
152	119	165	163	180	60	179	153	Prothionamide
152	151	81	109	51	–	–	–	Vanillin
153	93	30	65	152	154	125	110	Normetanephrine
154	70	155	167	223	225	349	153	Dihydroergocryptine
155	96	140	43	42	81	94	53	Arecoline
155	140	83	98	55	41	84	69	Methyprylone
155	157	227	154	185	44	30	156	Buclosamide
155	170	112	169	55	82	41	39	Metharbitone
156	92	108	65	140	43	157	42	Sulphafurazole
156	92	108	65	140	253	157	43	Sulphamethoxazole
156	141	45	157	41	29	55	27	3'-Hydroxybutobarbitone
156	141	55	41	157	43	98	39	Hexethal
156	141	55	155	98	39	82	43	Barbitone
156	141	157	41	55	142	98	39	Amylobarbitone
156	158	92	77	157	314	108	65	Sulphaphenazole
158	214	57	145	124	45	70	96	Niridazole
159	161	81	335	333	163	337	205	Miconazole
160	103	89	131	115	76	161	104	Hydralazine
160	300	189	145	188	301	161	42	Azapropazone
162	43	63	164	30	44	98	42	Guanoclor
163	77	164	135	194	76	92	50	Dimethyl Phthalate
163	148	91	103	117	120	44	77	Phenylethylmalondiamide
163	161	119	91	206	117	107	164	Ibuprofen
164	149	131	137	103	77	133	165	Eugenol
165	138	331	123	110	194	42	41	Pipamperone
165	234	194	235	193	196	166	179	Azapetine
166	68	95	41	53	123	–	–	3-Methylxanthine
166	68	123	53	42	41	95	–	7-Methylxanthine
166	164	129	131	168	94	133	96	Tetrachloroethylene
166	165	167	138	133	105	60	106	Ethionamide
167	41	124	168	97	39	169	45	Aprobarbitone
167	41	168	124	39	97	141	67	Idobutal
167	168	41	43	97	124	39	55	Quinalbarbitone
167	168	41	97	124	39	57	53	Talbutal
167	209	43	124	39	41	53	140	Ibomal
168	137	44	139	43	152	124	167	Methoxamine
168	140	169	114	141	167	113	63	Norharman
169	58	168	170	72	167	44	42	Pheniramine
169	78	171	113	115	63	51	170	Chlorzoxazone
169	92	289	65	290	39	333	184	Sulphasalazine
171	43	143	41	128	55	141	159	5-(2,3-Dihydroxypropyl)-quinalbarbitone
172	92	156	65	108	39	44	41	Sulphacetamide
172	92	156	65	108	173	39	174	Sulphanilamide
172	157	173	43	41	55	69	71	Thiopentone
172	187	84	57	42	188	44	43	Alphaprodine
173	117	145	78	104	94	76	147	Piroxicam
173	340	168	167	165	341	174	322	Diphenadione
174	77	91	105	132	–	–	–	Norphenazone
175	70	176	132	379	204	56	217	Oxypertine
176	59	132	150	45	193	105	29	Benzonatate
177	118	45	135	90	91	221	119	Procarbazine
178	44	135	179	77	84	107	41	Isoxsuprine
178	44	163	135	77	196	176	179	Protokylol
178	192	272	466	244	288	191	273	Cephaëline
180	55	67	109	82	42	137	70	Theobromine
180	77	181	44	179	51	209	167	trans-10,11-Dihydro-10,11-dihydroxy-carbamazepine
180	95	68	41	53	181	96	40	Theophylline
180	95	68	41	58	53	123	96	Bufylline
180	104	223	77	209	252	51	165	Phenytoin
180	179	178	152	44	181	223	51	Carbamazepine-10,11-epoxide
180	209	182	152	181	30	211	138	Ketamine
180	223	194	254	109	95	193	166	Diprophylline
180	264	193	109	194	181	67	42	Pentifylline
181	41	182	39	124	53	138	97	Enallylpropymal
181	85	56	166	266	182	179	91	Trimetazidine
181	152	153	254	182	151	76	127	Fenbufen
181	183	109	219	111	217	51	221	Lindane
181	395	198	251	397	396	199	666	Syrosingopine
182	30	181	167	211	183	151	148	Mescaline
182	57	43	55	40	69	41	181	Harman
183	43	29	60	41	129	91	73	Ouabain
183	76	90	50	91	120	106	92	Saccharin
183	77	252	320	184	41	69	51	Feprazone
184	92	185	65	39	108	66	186	Sulphapyridine
185	230	141	186	184	115	170	153	Naproxen
186	42	201	56	57	187	202	71	Trimeperidine
186	114	29	72	42	113	27	109	Carbimazole
186	185	92	65	108	39	93	187	Sulphadiazine
186	218	77	295	263	105	51	158	Mebendazole
188	47	82	96	29	77	84	56	Dichloralphenazone
188	96	77	56	105	189	55	51	Phenazone
188	189	159	132	53	173	131	145	Nalidixic Acid
189	104	190	77	44	105	132	103	Methoin
189	105	201	285	165	166	190	134	Meclozine
189	132	117	160	91	115	103	77	Glutethimide

Principal peaks at m/z								Compound
251	280	118	91	121	119	252	189	Phenprocoumon
252	237	253	181	238	77	76	209	Anisindione
253	252	43	104	254	235	77	89	Triamterene
253	288	287	289	225	259	254	41	Tetrazepam
254	143	42	70	411	113	56	157	Acetophenazine
254	256	118	255	303	305	63	45	Chlorambucil
256	121	185	43	257	65	42	214	Probenecid
256	283	284	285	257	255	258	286	Diazepam
256	284	283	285	84	257	258	255	Ketazolam
256	301	91	258	119	65	257	303	Benoxaprofen
257	55	311	77	259	313	44	312	3-Hydroxyprazepam
257	59	150	256	31	157	42	200	Racemorphan
257	77	268	239	205	267	233	259	Oxazepam
260	259	288	287	261	289	262	290	N^1-Desalkylflurazepam
260	261	42	57	184	215	217	262	Phenindamine
260	262	180	287	261	145	286	124	Quinethazone
260	302	216	215	243	189	242	188	Cambendazole
263	281	166	92	145	167	235	139	Flufenamic Acid
265	308	121	43	266	187	213	251	Warfarin
266	267	224	220	268	44	250	248	Apomorphine
266	268	264	167	165	270	202	132	Pentachlorophenol
266	268	267	255	231	102	88	176	Mazindol
267	221	207	180	223	154	196	268	Lysergamide
267	299	266	31	51	268	29	77	Fenbendazole
268	143	425	70	269	42	394	157	Carphenazine
268	224	154	180	207	223	192	179	Lysergic Acid
269	205	221	297	271	62	285	124	Hydrochlorothiazide
269	240	241	268	270	107	121	213	7-Amino-1-desmethyl-flunitrazepam
271	43	41	311	295	312	297	91	8α-Hydroxy-Δ⁹-THC
271	43	295	41	297	29	330	272	8β-Hydroxy-Δ⁹-THC
271	81	150	201	148	110	272	82	Normorphine
271	273	300	272	256	77	255	257	Temazepam
272	273	41	327	145	76	42	29	Butorphanol
274	225	318	273	275	226	257	121	Phenolphthalein
276	111	219	42	277	97	29	100	Diethylthiambutene
277	279	165	278	241	239	242	240	Clotrimazole
279	163	323	58	277	308	280	322	Dimefline
280	143	42	70	437	406	113	56	Fluphenazine
280	253	281	206	234	252	254	264	Nitrazepam
280	314	315	286	234	288	316	240	Clonazepam
281	43	282	187	107	91	55	105	Megestrol Acetate
281	120	91	122	280	160	68	282	Phentolamine
282	236	237	281	263	145	44	93	Niflumic Acid
282	299	284	283	241	56	301	253	Chlordiazepoxide
283	44	255	282	254	284	264	256	7-Aminoflunitrazepam
283	282	256	176	157	43	41	57	Levallorphan
284	91	375	81	42	36	285	175	Benzylmorphine
285	81	215	148	286	164	110	115	Norcodeine
285	96	229	228	70	214	115	200	Hydromorphone
285	162	42	215	286	124	44	284	Morphine
285	256	257	258	44	287	110	220	7-Aminoclonazepam
285	268	284	77	286	42	287	233	Desmethyl-chlordiazepoxide
285	286	269	287	241	242	77	270	Demoxepam
285	312	313	286	266	238	294	284	Flunitrazepam
286	229	91	81	287	41	77	228	Famprofazone
286	244	77	218	51	217	288	215	Desmethylclobazam
286	300	96	42	244	230	301	82	Bezitramide
287	70	44	164	42	288	59	230	Dihydromorphine
287	96	286	215	70	44	58	42	Cyproheptadine
288	69	178	41	287	43	289	55	Nabilone
288	273	331	287	304	290	289	275	N^1-(2-Hydroxy-ethyl)flurazepam

Principal peaks at m/z								Compound
288	290	218	146	114	63	51	148	Triclosan
290	67	108	107	79	55	41	93	Androsterone
290	184	185	104	77	168	291	198	Sulthiame
290	259	275	291	243	123	200	43	Trimethoprim
291	239	274	293	75	302	276	138	Lorazepam
293	265	264	292	43	222	223	294	7-Acetamidonitrazepam
295	296	238	310	119	43	251	239	Cannabinol
296	41	44	110	298	285	55	268	Cyclopenthiazide
296	195	58	297	253	196	212	84	Hexobendine
296	215	217	298	216	152	181	251	Fenclofenac
296	298	205	221	64	63	41	125	Ethiazide
296	298	279	205	36	64	117	62	Trichlormethiazide
298	271	299	224	272	270	252	280	Desmethylflunitrazepam
298	594	58	593	299	609	595	564	Tubocurarine Chloride
299	42	162	124	229	59	300	69	Codeine
299	43	41	67	300	69	231	29	11-Hydroxy-Δ⁹-THC
299	162	229	123	59	42	44	300	Neopine
299	231	314	43	41	295	55	271	Δ⁹-THC
299	242	59	243	42	96	70	214	Hydrocodone
300	258	77	259	283	302	231	256	Clobazam
301	44	42	59	164	70	302	242	Dihydrocodeine
301	216	44	42	70	302	203	57	Oxymorphone
302	57	85	231	91	110	79	215	Norethandrolone
302	124	43	91	79	121	105	122	Methyltestosterone
303	58	43	304	151	44	42	57	Verapamil
303	262	135	175	41	55	43	95	Enoxolone
303	301	305	115	194	196	114	87	Broxyquinoline
303	331	239	255	30	158	64	159	Hydroflumethiazide
304	306	64	74	109	177	176	48	Dichlorphenamide
305	150	307	115	152	114	306	123	Clioquinol
305	307	306	309	308	334	102	75	Lormetazepam
308	165	309	121	55	154	98	56	Mebeverine
308	279	204	273	77	307	310	309	Alprazolam
309	96	42	58	98	70	57	44	Ketotifen
310	58	199	112	311	111	212	41	Pecazine
310	64	36	312	42	43	62	63	Methyclothiazide
310	121	353	311	43	120	92	296	Nicoumalone
310	206	42	64	312	299	45	48	Polythiazide
310	312	311	163	325	75	39	297	Midazolam
311	255	42	44	296	310	312	174	Thebaine
311	312	41	188	80	82	81	241	Nalorphine
312	43	299	297	356	281	371	311	Colchicine
313	162	314	124	284	59	42	243	Ethylmorphine
313	238	342	315	75	344	239	137	Triazolam
315	230	316	70	44	42	258	140	Oxycodone
317	43	271	147	289	390	95	81	Alphadolone Acetate
317	288	359	401	43	318	289	196	Oxyphenisatin Acetate
321	278	320	292	306	191	322	304	Berberine
321	364	304	240	168	91	322	365	Bumetanide
323	221	181	222	207	72	223	324	Lysergide
327	43	369	268	310	42	215	204	Diamorphine
327	268	42	43	215	44	328	269	6-Monoacetylmorphine
327	328	41	242	286	96	229	70	Naloxone
329	284	224	268	330	285	225	270	Nifedipine
330	118	91	319	219	64	92	421	Bendrofluazide
331	43	71	332	121	147	131	41	Clobetasone
332	333	304	335	176	303	334	162	Chelidonine
334	335	162	120	107	144	143	130	Strychnine
336	121	120	215	162	92	337	187	Dicoumarol
339	221	196	181	207	223	222	72	Methylergometrine
339	324	338	325	340	308	154	292	Papaverine
341	43	340	374	267	107	55	342	Spironolactone
341	55	36	300	342	110	243	256	Naltrexone
341	233	356	246	247	248	234	281	Sulindac

Principal peaks at m/z								Compound
341	282	229	42	43	59	342	204	Acetylcodeine
341	298	43	42	44	55	284	242	Thebacon
343	70	344	109	42	113	491	56	Lidoflazine
350	91	259	352	348	65	351	107	Metolazone
352	367	338	366	29	368	353	339	Dimoxyline
353	210	235	336	72	54	236	195	Methysergide
353	354	169	170	355	156	184	144	Yohimbine
361	277	319	276	199	318	362	43	Bisacodyl
363	206	143	42	70	207	218	113	Opipramol
377	43	55	246	278	59	378	41	Halcinonide
380	223	382	238	152	345	215	113	Chlorotrianisene

Principal peaks at m/z								Compound
386	138	387	84	110	42	301	263	Piritramide
386	368	43	55	275	81	57	95	Cholesterol
394	395	379	392	120	197	203	393	Brucine
397	115	242	398	88	143	271	62	Di-iodohydroxyquinoline
455	457	472	474	459	456	458	473	Clofazimine
504	473	429	505	221	474	84	430	Dipyridamole
518	173	264	519	373	376	520	249	Benziodarone
578	195	577	367	351	579	366	365	Deserpidine
608	195	607	397	609	395	381	396	Methoserpidine
608	606	195	609	395	397	212	396	Reserpine

Mass Spectral Data of Pesticides and Gas Chromatographic Decomposition Products (GCDP)

In the following table the m/z values of the eight most intense ions are listed in descending order of intensity; the table should be used as described under Mass Spectral Data of Drugs.

The values for m/z in this table were obtained using a quadrupole spectrometer, after gas chromatography unless otherwise stated, except for those substances marked † the data for which were obtained on a magnetic sector instrument.

Principal peaks at m/z (percentage relative abundance)								Compound
41(100)	44(82)	45(42)	48(31)	47(29)	86(28)	87(26)	42(22)	2-Methyl-2-(methylthio)-propionaldehyde oxime (GCDP of Aldicarb)
41(100)	86(89)	58(85)	85(61)	87(50)	44(50)	55(45)	76(43)	Aldicarb (probe)
41(100)	140(85)	196(72)	74(64)	106(64)	168(53)	45(40)	227(37)	Mephosfolan
41(100)	173(83)	91(65)	135(49)	77(45)	55(43)	44(42)	69(59)	Santonin
42(100)	115(61)	61(55)	57(46)	55(43)	68(38)	161(38)	45(37)	3,3-Dimethyl-1-(methylthio)butan-2-one oxime (GCDP of Thiofanox)
43(100)	44(88)	136(80)	94(58)	47(56)	95(32)	46(30)	47(27)	Acephate (probe)
43(100)	45(99)	46(91)	94(54)	47(50)	199(49)	139(48)	68(46)	Aziprotryne
43(100)	57(98)	41(76)	55(54)	71(41)	69(27)	56(27)	42(26)	Dichlorophenoxyacetic Acid (2,4-D) (iso-octyl ester)
43(100)	57(96)	41(79)	55(47)	71(44)	69(35)	56(31)	70(28)	Trichlorophenoxyacetic Acid (2,4,5-T) (iso-octyl ester)
43(100)	57(83)	41(61)	71(48)	55(47)	162(41)	164(30)	69(29)	Dichlorprop (iso-octyl ester)
43(100)	57(94)	169(77)	41(70)	142(69)	55(52)	71(33)	56(29)	Mecoprop (iso-octyl ester)
43(100)	58(84)	44(75)	200(69)	68(43)	215(40)	41(38)	42(37)	Atrazine
43(100)	61(81)	62(67)	97(59)	45(59)	44(47)	89(47)	106(38)	Dalapon (probe)
43(100)	73(80)	59(52)	55(47)	72(46)	100(46)	44(45)	86(40)	Dodine (probe)
43(100)	86(73)	41(43)	42(31)	70(23)	44(21)	143(20)	128(19)	Tri-allate
43(100)	86(62)	41(38)	44(25)	42(24)	70(19)	128(13)	234(13)	Di-allate
43(100)	93(88)	41(42)	120(24)	65(24)	137(23)	179(21)	119(15)	Propham
43(100)	127(49)	41(35)	45(20)	44(18)	129(16)	63(12)	153(12)	Chlorpropham
43(100)	175(92)	57(84)	177(60)	42(35)	258(22)	302(18)	112(15)	Oxadiazon
43(100)	211(80)	41(71)	44(57)	205(31)	163(29)	42(28)	45(25)	Dinobuton
43(100)	264(33)	306(32)	57(7)	42(6)	290(5)	145(4)	307(4)	Trifluralin
44(100)	43(60)	68(60)	212(48)	41(47)	42(34)	173(28)	172(25)	Cyanazine
44(100)	58(81)	105(69)	45(59)	42(55)	47(52)	57(36)	56(31)	Methomyl (probe)
44(100)	73(97)	159(89)	191(80)	86(72)	150(71)	72(68)	59(56)	Thiophanate-methyl (probe)
44(100)	161(44)	124(36)	187(31)	159(24)	163(23)	189(20)	216(20)	Methazole (probe)
45(100)	47(91)	58(78)	48(74)	105(71)	46(54)	42(50)	88(38)	N-Hydroxythioacetimidate (GCDP of Methomyl)
45(100)	188(23)	160(18)	77(7)	146(6)	224(6)	237(6)	91(5)	Alachlor
51(100)	153(76)	87(66)	222(44)	52(43)	63(43)	41(42)	69(39)	Barban
53(100)	127(20)	51(13)	164(13)	223(13)	70(10)	153(10)	50(10)	Chlorbufam
54(100)	53(93)	43(82)	124(65)	212(63)	187(61)	198(59)	285(49)	Vinclozolin
54(100)	108(89)	81(33)	190(31)	111(26)	135(25)	83(25)	80(25)	Diquat (reduction product II—diene)
56(100)	174(79)	175(31)	57(24)	176(23)	41(20)	131(16)	132(12)	Terbacil (N-methyl derivative)
57(100)	42(75)	68(39)	61(38)	55(34)	47(33)	115(31)	45(30)	Thiofanox
57(100)	43(94)	41(85)	196(63)	71(60)	198(59)	55(56)	223(35)	Fenoprop (iso-octyl ester)
57(100)	127(83)	43(78)	55(52)	42(25)	88(15)	128(14)	58(12)	Bromoxynil Octanoate
61(100)	46(43)	60(15)	91(13)	258(13)	170(12)	260(11)	172(9)	Metobromuron
61(100)	46(24)	62(11)	63(10)	60(9)	124(8)	45(8)	233(6)	Chlorbromuron
61(100)	126(63)	153(42)	214(34)	46(29)	125(25)	99(22)	127(21)	Monolinuron
61(100)	187(43)	189(29)	124(28)	46(28)	44(23)	161(18)	160(13)	Linuron
66(100)	91(50)	79(47)	263(42)	65(35)	101(34)	261(25)	265(24)	Aldrin†
67(100)	81(67)	263(59)	36(58)	79(47)	82(41)	261(36)	265(33)	Endrin†
72(100)	44(34)	73(25)	42(20)	232(19)	187(13)	124(13)	45(12)	Diuron (probe)
72(100)	44(29)	167(28)	132(25)	45(20)	77(11)	42(10)	212(10)	Chlortoluron
72(100)	44(27)	183(23)	228(22)	45(21)	73(15)	168(14)	42(12)	Metoxuron (probe)

Principal peaks at m/z (percentage relative abundance)								*Compound*
72(100)	100(81)	128(62)	44(55)	115(41)	127(36)	57(30)	55(20)	Napropamide
72(100)	164(27)	119(24)	91(22)	42(14)	44(11)	64(11)	45(10)	Fenuron
72(100)	166(85)	42(63)	44(44)	43(24)	238(23)	69(21)	167(19)	Pirimicarb
72(100)	167(86)	165(42)	239(21)	152(17)	168(14)	166(13)	73(5)	Diphenamid
72(100)	245(37)	44(31)	75(21)	45(19)	63(16)	90(14)	247(13)	Chloroxuron (probe)
75(100)	47(54)	121(43)	97(43)	65(37)	45(30)	93(27)	79(17)	Phorate
77(100)	160(77)	132(67)	44(30)	105(29)	104(27)	93(24)	76(22)	Azinphos-methyl
77(100)	221(60)	88(37)	220(35)	51(26)	105(24)	223(20)	222(18)	Chloridazon
79(100)	80(61)	77(56)	44(44)	78(37)	149(34)	51(31)	117(28)	Captan
79(100)	80(42)	77(28)	78(19)	151(17)	51(13)	57(13)	92(12)	Captafol
79(100)	82(32)	81(30)	263(17)	77(17)	108(14)	265(12)	80(12)	Dieldrin†
81(100)	267(73)	109(55)	269(47)	323(26)	91(23)	170(21)	173(18)	Chlorfenvinphos
83(100)	108(73)	96(50)	54(47)	111(44)	192(44)	84(34)	55(33)	Diquat (reduction product I—monoene)
84(100)	58(49)	43(32)	44(24)	42(10)	53(8)	55(8)	86(4)	Aminotriazole (probe)
84(100)	133(21)	42(18)	162(17)	161(15)	105(9)	77(8)	119(6)	Nicotine†
85(100)	145(90)	93(32)	125(22)	47(21)	58(20)	63(14)	75(11)	Methidathion
87(100)	57(81)	43(62)	71(45)	41(42)	69(29)	77(19)	42(17)	MCPB (iso-octyl ester)
87(100)	58(47)	44(40)	61(29)	59(26)	60(25)	45(22)	145(20)	Vamidothion
87(100)	93(76)	125(56)	58(40)	47(39)	63(33)	79(22)	42(21)	Dimethoate
88(100)	42(25)	44(20)	208(18)	73(15)	45(10)	89(10)	76(9)	Thiram
88(100)	60(50)	109(24)	142(17)	79(14)	47(11)	111(11)	61(10)	Demeton-S-methyl
88(100)	60(63)	125(56)	61(52)	47(49)	93(47)	89(47)	63(34)	Thiometon
88(100)	89(43)	61(40)	60(39)	97(36)	65(23)	59(19)	47(19)	Disulfoton†
90(100)	153(89)	125(82)	44(67)	63(40)	127(36)	155(32)	62(24)	4-Chlorophenyl isocyanate (GCDP of Monolinuron)
91(100)	133(70)	161(55)	117(48)	107(47)	160(43)	105(42)	115(35)	Pyrethrin II
93(100)	66(52)	94(6)	67(4)	78(3)	46(3)	54(3)	–	Aniline (GCDP of Fenuron)
93(100)	125(89)	126(68)	42(49)	47(48)	87(40)	63(31)	45(29)	Formothion
96(100)	42(53)	70(50)	72(26)	150(23)	122(21)	194(14)	43(11)	Paraquat (reduction product I—monoene)
96(100)	42(64)	148(35)	192(35)	94(22)	122(22)	134(21)	44(15)	Paraquat (reduction product II—diene)
97(100)	65(35)	303(32)	125(28)	359(27)	109(27)	301(25)	357(22)	Bromophos-ethyl
97(100)	109(90)	291(57)	139(47)	125(41)	137(39)	155(32)	123(24)	Parathion†
97(100)	195(59)	199(53)	65(27)	47(23)	314(21)	201(19)	125(19)	Chlorpyrifos
97(100)	279(92)	223(90)	109(67)	162(53)	251(46)	65(45)	281(42)	Dichlofenthion
100(100)	272(81)	274(65)	270(42)	237(33)	102(33)	65(30)	276(28)	Heptachlor†
101(100)	59(95)	41(39)	162(36)	69(28)	63(25)	42(23)	164(23)	2,4-DB (methyl ester)
101(100)	59(70)	77(40)	107(25)	41(22)	142(20)	42(15)	89(15)	MCPB (methyl ester)
104(100)	202(66)	42(42)	174(35)	77(24)	103(19)	173(18)	76(16)	Metamitron
105(100)	77(47)	106(10)	292(10)	145(7)	51(7)	294(6)	172(6)	Benzoylprop-ethyl
105(100)	77(46)	276(20)	106(14)	230(12)	44(11)	156(7)	129(7)	Flamprop-methyl
105(100)	77(44)	276(21)	106(18)	278(7)	51(5)	129(4)	156(4)	Flamprop-isopropyl
107(100)	69(48)	77(29)	41(26)	81(21)	45(17)	78(16)	57(16)	Ethiofencarb
107(100)	91(69)	135(69)	93(67)	55(66)	121(58)	43(52)	163(48)	Jasmolin II
107(100)	93(57)	121(53)	91(50)	149(35)	105(33)	79(27)	77(26)	Cinerin II
107(100)	168(37)	77(24)	108(15)	78(15)	79(10)	45(9)	51(8)	2-Ethylthiomethylphenol (GCDP of Ethiofencarb)
107(100)	235(91)	203(85)	139(60)	123(46)	95(35)	237(32)	314(29)	Nuarimol
108(100)	219(61)	80(31)	221(22)	65(16)	53(12)	109(6)	156(5)	4-(4-Chlorophenoxy)aniline (GCDP of Chloroxuron)
109(100)	79(34)	47(26)	44(20)	185(17)	80(8)	48(7)	83(7)	Trichlorphon
109(100)	110(72)	79(69)	59(67)	58(38)	47(38)	63(37)	45(37)	Oxydemeton-methyl
109(100)	125(80)	263(56)	79(26)	63(18)	93(18)	47(13)	247(8)	Parathion-methyl
109(100)	185(18)	79(17)	187(6)	145(6)	47(5)	220(4)	110(3)	Dichlorvos†
109(100)	329(48)	331(42)	79(20)	333(14)	93(9)	240(8)	238(6)	Tetrachlorvinphos (probe)
110(100)	41(20)	43(19)	152(13)	81(11)	53(10)	64(10)	111(10)	o-Isopropoxyphenol (GCDP of Propoxur)
110(100)	152(47)	43(28)	58(27)	41(21)	111(20)	81(15)	64(13)	Propoxur (probe)
110(100)	156(83)	79(39)	109(32)	58(30)	47(21)	80(19)	44(17)	Omethoate
115(100)	144(78)	116(42)	89(16)	63(15)	145(8)	62(7)	50(7)	Alphanaphthol (GCDP of Carbaryl)
119(100)	72(54)	91(44)	45(38)	64(37)	74(29)	44(28)	73(24)	Carbetamide (probe)
119(100)	91(62)	64(34)	41(16)	63(16)	44(15)	43(11)	50(10)	Phenyl isocyanate (GCDP of Fenuron)
120(100)	77(66)	93(36)	43(35)	51(30)	41(27)	176(23)	104(18)	Propachlor

Principal peaks at m/z (percentage relative abundance)								Compound
121(100)	122(47)	45(43)	73(39)	166(38)	165(37)	65(22)	107(21)	2-(1,3-Dioxolan-2-yl)phenol (GCDP of Dioxacarb)
121(100)	122(62)	166(46)	165(42)	73(35)	45(31)	162(21)	51(18)	Dioxacarb (probe)
121(100)	227(94)	228(15)	114(9)	152(9)	122(8)	63(5)	165(5)	Methoxychlor (*op'*)
123(100)	43(52)	55(34)	93(25)	91(24)	81(23)	164(23)	107(20)	Jasmolin I
123(100)	43(62)	91(58)	81(47)	105(45)	55(43)	133(40)	77(33)	Pyrethrin I
123(100)	43(35)	93(33)	121(27)	81(27)	150(27)	107(24)	91(24)	Cinerin I
123(100)	79(40)	43(32)*	81(31)	91(29)	136(27)	107(23)	55(19)	Allethrin
123(100)	92(33)	224(29)	167(27)	63(23)	77(22)	226(22)	64(21)	Dichlofluanid
123(100)	171(67)	128(52)	143(49)	81(38)	91(28)	172(25)	45(23)	Resmethrin
125(100)	93(96)	127(75)	173(55)	158(37)	99(35)	55(23)	79(20)	Malathion†
125(100)	109(92)	79(62)	47(57)	63(44)	93(40)	51(26)	277(25)	Fenitrothion
125(100)	127(61)	44(50)	90(50)	99(33)	237(24)	63(23)	43(22)	Drazoxolon (probe)
125(100)	165(64)	75(46)	196(43)	51(43)	101(37)	127(36)	102(35)	Chlorfenprop-methyl
125(100)	292(91)	181(90)	47(84)	153(84)	56(73)	79(61)	93(48)	Etrimfos
125(100)	377(78)	47(64)	79(59)	93(54)	109(49)	63(38)	97(37)	Iodofenphos
126(100)	151(91)	166(50)	43(39)	41(32)	51(30)	52(24)	108(16)	2,2-Dimethyl-1,3-benzodioxol-4-ol (GCDP of Bendiocarb)
127(100)	57(96)	41(34)	43(33)	55(26)	371(16)	88(13)	128(12)	Ioxynil (iso-octyl ester)
127(100)	65(48)	63(27)	129(27)	92(23)	52(20)	64(13)	128(13)	4-Chloroaniline (GCDP of Mono-linuron)
127(100)	67(25)	97(23)	109(14)	58(14)	192(13)	43(8)	193(8)	Monocrotophos
127(100)	192(30)	109(27)	67(20)	43(8)	193(7)	39(6)	79(5)	Mevinphos†
128(100)	43(26)	42(18)	44(13)	129(11)	55(5)	115(4)	57(4)	Tridemorph
128(100)	43(17)	42(16)	129(10)	70(4)	117(4)	57(4)	91(4)	Fenpropiomorph
133(100)	104(46)	132(45)	78(27)	105(21)	44(20)	91(17)	77(17)	*m*-Tolyl isocyanate (GCDP of Phen-medipham)
133(100)	104(52)	132(34)	91(34)	165(31)	44(27)	78(26)	77(23)	Phenmedipham
137(100)	179(74)	152(65)	93(47)	153(42)	199(39)	97(38)	43(37)	Diazinon
139(100)	107(95)	111(40)	219(39)	141(33)	251(31)	75(30)	53(26)	Fenarimol
139(100)	111(39)	141(33)	75(18)	83(17)	251(16)	113(12)	253(12)	Dicofol (probe)
139(100)	111(66)	141(43)	75(40)	250(26)	44(23)	113(20)	252(17)	*pp*-Dichlorobenzophenone (GCDP of Dicofol)
141(100)	43(93)	71(74)	143(44)	41(42)	77(33)	140(25)	142(24)	Pentanochlor
141(100)	140(37)	106(68)	142(36)	143(28)	77(25)	78(10)	54(8)	3-Chloro-4-methylaniline (GCDP of Chlortoluron)
141(100)	200(51)	115(24)	142(11)	139(10)	201(7)	140(3)	116(2)	2-(1-Naphthyl)acetic Acid (methyl ester)
141(100)	214(84)	125(68)	155(65)	46(60)	77(50)	89(47)	143(38)	Methylchlorophenoxyacetic Acid (MCPA) (methyl ester)
142(100)	114(41)	157(35)	144(32)	52(20)	116(14)	159(13)	78(13)	3-Chloro-4-methoxyaniline (GCDP of Metoxuron)
142(100)	237(96)	44(75)	214(67)	107(62)	212(61)	144(61)	249(56)	Quintozene
144(100)	115(82)	116(48)	57(31)	58(20)	63(20)	145(19)	89(14)	Carbaryl (probe)
146(100)	72(54)	44(35)	128(29)	45(28)	161(25)	42(11)	147(11)	Isoproturon
146(100)	128(34)	44(30)	161(30)	147(10)	91(4)	118(3)	117(3)	4-Isopropylphenyl isocyanate (GCDP of Propoxur)
151(100)	126(58)	166(48)	51(19)	58(18)	43(17)	41(14)	223(9)	Bendiocarb (probe)
153(100)	154(20)	110(15)	109(15)	152(13)	136(10)	82(9)	80(8)	Lenacil
154(100)	55(45)	42(44)	43(35)	141(20)	128(20)	155(19)	56(16)	Dodemorph
159(100)	191(57)	103(38)	104(37)	52(32)	51(29)	77(22)	90(21)	Carbendazim (probe)
160(100)	161(99)	117(69)	42(45)	41(41)	162(37)	163(33)	57(31)	Terbacil
161(100)	163(70)	57(64)	217(16)	165(11)	219(9)	162(9)	63(8)	Propanil
161(100)	163(66)	99(26)	90(24)	63(23)	73(13)	62(13)	126(13)	3,4-Dichloroaniline (GCDP of Diuron and Linuron)
161(100)	207(82)	83(52)	137(45)	105(41)	179(41)	133(39)	79(30)	Ethofumesate
162(100)	42(87)	89(79)	44(73)	76(59)	43(53)	73(39)	45(22)	Dazomet
162(100)	164(80)	59(62)	189(56)	63(39)	191(35)	55(31)	248(27)	Dichlorprop (methyl ester)
163(100)	181(79)	165(68)	91(41)	77(33)	51(29)	127(28)	115(17)	Cypermethrin
164(100)	136(84)	135(81)	108(42)	163(35)	69(30)	82(24)	96(22)	2-Methylaminobenzthiazole (GCDP of Methabenzthiazuron)
164(100)	136(73)	135(69)	163(42)	69(30)	58(25)	45(25)	57(25)	Methabenzthiazuron (probe)
164(100)	149(70)	41(27)	58(25)	131(25)	122(25)	51(23)	123(22)	Carbofuran

Principal peaks at m/z (percentage relative abundance) — *Compound*

								Compound
164(100)	149(86)	131(41)	103(36)	51(35)	122(35)	77(34)	123(33)	2,3-Dihydro-2,2-dimethylbenzofuran-7-ol (GCDP of Carbofuran)
165(100)	311(51)	77(37)	233(31)	69(26)	241(20)	239(20)	166(18)	Fluotrimazole
166(100)	209(17)	167(14)	96(12)	194(4)	55(2)	71(2)	210(2)	Ethirimol
167(100)	132(97)	169(29)	166(26)	168(16)	77(16)	76(12)	51(12)	3-Chloro-4-methylphenyl isocyanate (GCDP of Chlortoluron)
167(100)	135(93)	122(49)	43(41)	68(31)	81(31)	65(27)	149(24)	3-Methoxycarbonylaminophenol (GCDP of Phenmedipham)
167(100)	166(45)	168(12)	165(12)	124(9)	123(6)	122(5)	67(4)	Lenacil (*N*-methyl derivative)
168(100)	153(84)	45(40)	109(37)	91(31)	58(21)	57(15)	169(14)	Methiocarb (probe)
168(100)	153(70)	109(62)	45(44)	91(36)	77(18)	107(14)	65(13)	4-Methylthio-3,5-xylenol (GCDP of Methiocarb)
168(100)	183(72)	140(67)	76(40)	170(33)	112(36)	185(26)	142(25)	3-Chloro-4-methoxyphenyl isocyanate (GCDP of Metoxuron)
168(100)	318(94)	152(88)	304(79)	180(73)	42(71)	109(71)	333(69)	Pirimiphos-ethyl
169(100)	143(79)	59(58)	141(57)	228(54)	107(50)	77(47)	125(35)	Mecoprop (methyl ester)
170(100)	60(61)	171(50)	172(49)	205(35)	173(29)	100(24)	207(24)	Chlorthiamid (probe)
170(100)	134(75)	198(74)	257(73)	172(40)	200(31)	108(30)	259(28)	Benazolin (methyl ester)
171(100)	44(26)	128(21)	83(20)	71(18)	98(13)	56(13)	172(11)	Hexazinone
171(100)	65(99)	173(93)	92(43)	52(12)	63(12)	141(11)	106(8)	4-Bromoaniline (GCDP of Metobromuron)
171(100)	173(62)	100(31)	136(24)	75(24)	50(19)	99(12)	74(11)	Dichlobenil
180(100)	223(23)	85(14)	181(12)	55(10)	96(9)	42(8)	43(6)	Ethirimol (methyl ether)
180(100)	223(23)	181(10)	224(3)	42(2)	109(2)	150(2)	71(1)	Dimethirimol (methyl ether)
181(100)	183(97)	109(89)	219(86)	111(75)	217(68)	51(43)	221(41)	Lindane†
182(100)	121(48)	97(36)	184(32)	154(24)	111(24)	65(22)	138(20)	Phosalone†
182(100)	165(74)	89(69)	90(57)	212(48)	51(47)	65(45)	91(38)	Dinitro-orthocresol (methyl ether)
183(100)	163(29)	165(25)	44(15)	184(15)	91(13)	77(13)	127(9)	Permethrin
187(100)	124(65)	189(64)	159(28)	126(21)	161(19)	97(10)	191(10)	3,4-Dichlorophenyl isocyanate (GCDP of Diuron and Linuron)
191(100)	193(61)	206(60)	53(57)	208(39)	141(35)	113(29)	85(16)	Chloroneb
195(100)	36(95)	237(91)	41(89)	241(79)	75(78)	239(76)	170(76)	Endosulfan†
196(100)	198(89)	59(82)	55(36)	87(34)	223(31)	200(29)	225(29)	Fenoprop (methyl ester)
198(100)	41(78)	57(54)	43(39)	47(38)	74(36)	61(34)	103(32)	Metribuzin
198(100)	196(97)	197(37)	200(34)	195(32)	170(21)	225(17)	125(16)	Picloram (methyl ester)
199(100)	45(97)	175(94)	145(70)	111(69)	109(68)	234(64)	133(62)	Dichlorophenoxyacetic Acid (2,4-D) (methyl ester)
199(100)	197(97)	90(72)	171(35)	169(31)	65(17)	62(9)	50(8)	4-Bromophenyl isocyanate (GCDP of Metobromuron)
200(100)	43(81)	186(52)	229(52)	214(50)	42(48)	68(48)	44(46)	Trietazine
201(100)	44(96)	186(72)	68(63)	173(57)	96(40)	158(38)	203(35)	Simazine†
201(100)	174(72)	63(12)	202(11)	64(11)	65(9)	175(8)	90(8)	Thiabendazole†
203(100)	201(69)	108(69)	215(60)	44(57)	213(51)	178(45)	205(41)	Tecnazene
203(100)	205(60)	234(27)	188(26)	97(21)	201(20)	190(18)	236(17)	Dicamba (methyl ester)
205(100)	207(75)	42(25)	70(16)	206(16)	162(12)	41(11)	188(11)	Bromacil
206(100)	234(67)	116(51)	174(22)	148(22)	173(19)	89(15)	88(14)	Quinomethionate
207(100)	205(89)	90(27)	63(26)	209(24)	99(24)	126(21)	62(13)	3-Chloro-4-bromoaniline (GCDP of Chlorbromuron)
208(100)	210(31)	76(20)	173(17)	209(12)	357(10)	104(9)	172(9)	Dialifos
209(100)	207(94)	211(32)	238(24)	240(23)	74(20)	109(18)	179(17)	Trichlorobenzoic Acid (2,3,6-TBA) (methyl ester)
213(100)	57(67)	58(66)	198(58)	82(44)	171(39)	43(38)	99(25)	Desmetryne
216(100)	127(27)	115(27)	157(20)	217(15)	129(11)	143(10)	126(6)	2-Naphthyloxyacetic Acid (methyl ester)
219(100)	221(68)	41(45)	188(41)	190(40)	56(37)	220(32)	42(31)	Bromacil (*N*-methyl derivative)
227(100)	228(15)	114(10)	152(5)	212(4)	63(3)	169(3)	115(3)	Methoxychlor (*pp'*)
233(100)	45(99)	42(86)	59(79)	179(69)	146(65)	109(65)	235(64)	Trichlorophenoxyacetic Acid (2,4,5-T) (methyl ester)
233(100)	231(82)	44(75)	124(74)	207(72)	73(30)	235(30)	205(26)	3-Chloro-4-bromophenyl isocyanate (GCDP of Chlorbromuron)
235(100)	237(58)	165(37)	236(16)	75(12)	239(11)	82(10)	199(10)	Dicophane (*pp'*-DDT)
235(100)	237(59)	165(33)	236(16)	199(12)	75(12)	239(11)	176(10)	Dicophane (*op'*-DDT)
239(100)	209(41)	43(36)	91(35)	77(33)	254(33)	51(27)	131(26)	Dinoterb (methyl ether)

Principal peaks at m/z (percentage relative abundance)								Compound
242(100)	240(62)	244(48)	97(35)	62(33)	61(18)	178(16)	135(13)	2,5-Dichloro-4-bromophenol (Bromophos impurity)
245(100)	182(49)	90(46)	75(45)	63(41)	247(34)	50(32)	51(32)	4-(4-Chlorophenoxy)phenyl isocyanate (GCDP of Chloroxuron)
252(100)	43(53)	57(43)	41(41)	281(37)	253(34)	162(22)	77(22)	Pendimethalin
252(100)	254(67)	324(51)	108(49)	75(40)	322(40)	326(26)	50(22)	Tetrasul
273(100)	76(53)	228(35)	50(29)	229(25)	274(19)	140(13)	104(12)	Naptalam (methyl ester)
283(100)	285(67)	202(55)	50(55)	139(37)	63(37)	76(31)	75(28)	Nitrofen
290(100)	276(93)	125(69)	305(53)	233(44)	42(41)	109(38)	93(37)	Pirimiphos-methyl
291(100)	88(77)	276(67)	289(55)	293(53)	248(50)	274(37)	278(32)	Bromoxynil (methyl ether)
301(100)	299(81)	303(47)	332(29)	142(26)	221(24)	330(23)	223(22)	Chlorthal Dimethyl
305(100)	43(49)	261(38)	307(37)	216(16)	306(15)	42(13)	232(13)	Dinitramine
331(100)	125(91)	329(80)	79(57)	109(53)	93(45)	47(34)	333(29)	Bromophos
373(100)	375(84)	377(46)	371(39)	44(36)	109(36)	75(35)	272(35)	*cis*-Chlordane
373(100)	375(93)	377(53)	371(47)	272(36)	237(30)	75(29)	65(28)	*trans*-Chlordane
385(100)	243(56)	370(41)	127(13)	386(10)	88(9)	228(8)	101(7)	Ioxynil (methyl ether)

PART 4: Appendix of Reagents and Proprietary Test Materials

Reagents

The names of all the reagents listed and defined below are printed in *italic type* wherever they occur in descriptions of tests in Part 1 or Part 2.

Acetate Buffer (pH 5): dissolve 13.6 g of sodium acetate and 6 ml of *acetic acid* in sufficient water to produce 1000 ml.

Acetic Acid: Glacial Acetic Acid: contains not less than 99% w/w of $CH_3 \cdot CO_2H$.

Acetic Acid, Dilute: contains approximately 6% w/w of $CH_3 \cdot CO_2H$.

Ammonia Buffer (pH 9.5): dissolve 10.7 g of ammonium chloride in 40 ml of 5M ammonia and dilute with water to 1000 ml.

Ammonia Solution, Dilute: dilute 37.5 ml of *strong ammonia solution* to 100 ml with water. It contains about 10% w/w of NH_3.

Ammonia Solution, Strong: contains 27 to 30% w/w of NH_3.

Ammonium Polysulphide Solution: dissolve a sufficient quantity of precipitated sulphur in *ammonium sulphide solution* to produce a deep orange solution.

Ammonium Sulphide Solution: saturate 120 ml of 5M ammonia with washed hydrogen sulphide and add 80 ml of 5M ammonia. It should be recently prepared.

p-Anisaldehyde Reagent: dissolve 0.5 ml of *p*-anisaldehyde in 50 ml of *acetic acid* and 1 ml of *hydrochloric acid*.

Ascorbic Acid Reagent: a 2% solution of ascorbic acid.

Barium Chloride Solution: a 10% solution of barium chloride.

Benzalkonium Chloride Solution: a solution containing 50% of a mixture of alkylbenzyldimethylammonium chlorides.

Borax Buffer 0.05M: dissolve 19.07 g of borax in sufficient water to produce 1000 ml.

Bromine Solution: Bromine Water: a freshly-prepared, saturated solution of bromine.

Chlorine Solution: a freshly-prepared, saturated solution of chlorine.

Chromic Acid Solution: dissolve 3 g of potassium dichromate in 10 ml of water, then carefully dilute to 100 ml with *sulphuric acid* with continuous stirring. The solution is stable for one month.

Cobalt Thiocyanate Solution: dissolve 6 g of cobalt nitrate and 18 g of potassium thiocyanate in 100 ml of water.

Copper Sulphate Solution: a 5% solution of copper sulphate.

Dimethyl Yellow Solution: a 0.2% solution of dimethyl yellow in ethanol (90%).

Dithiobisnitrobenzoic Acid Solution: dissolve 10 mg of 5,5'-dithiobis-2-nitrobenzoic acid in 100 ml of *phosphate buffer (pH 7.4)*.

DPST Solution: dissolve 0.5 g of 2,5-diphenyl-3-(4-styrylphenyl)-tetrazolium chloride in 100 ml of ethanol; dilute 5 ml of this solution to 50 ml with 2M sodium hydroxide immediately before use.

Dragendorff Spray: (a) mix together 2 g of bismuth subnitrate, 25 ml of *acetic acid*, and 100 ml of water; (b) dissolve 40 g of potassium iodide in 100 ml of water. Mix together 10 ml of (a), 10 ml of (b), 20 ml of *acetic acid*, and 100 ml of water. Prepare every 2 days.

Duquenois Reagent: dissolve 2 g of vanillin and 0.3 ml of acetaldehyde in 100 ml of ethanol. The reagent should be stored in the dark.

Fast Blue B Solution: a 1% solution of fast blue B salt (diazotised *o*-dianisidine). It should be freshly prepared.

Ferric Ammonium Sulphate Solution: a 10% solution of ferric ammonium sulphate.

Ferric Chloride Solution: a 5% solution of ferric chloride.

Fluorescein Solution: mix 10 ml of a saturated solution of fluorescein in *acetic acid* with 15 ml of *acetic acid* and 25 ml of *strong hydrogen peroxide solution*. This solution must be freshly prepared.

Formaldehyde Solution: Formalin: contains 34 to 38% w/w of formaldehyde.

Forrest Reagent: mix together equal volumes of a 0.2% solution of potassium dichromate, a 30% v/v solution of *sulphuric acid*, a 20% w/w solution of *perchloric acid*, and a 50% v/v solution of *nitric acid*.

FPN Reagent: mix together 5 ml of *ferric chloride solution*, 45 ml of a 20% w/w solution of *perchloric acid*, and 50 ml of a 50% v/v solution of *nitric acid*.

Furfuraldehyde Reagent: (a) dilute 2 ml of redistilled furfuraldehyde to 100 ml with acetone; (b) dilute 4 ml of *sulphuric acid* to 100 ml with acetone; prepare immediately before use. Spray with (a) first, followed by (b).

Furfuraldehyde Solution: a 10% solution of furfuraldehyde in ethanol.

Hydriodic Acid: contains about 55% w/w of HI.

Hydrochloric Acid: Concentrated: contains 35 to 39% w/w of HCl.

Hydrochloric Acid, Dilute: mix 274 g of *hydrochloric acid* with 726 g of water. It contains about 10% w/w of HCl.

Hydrogen Peroxide Solution, Strong: 100 volume: contains 29 to 31% w/v of H_2O_2.

Hydroxylamine Hydrochloride Solution: dissolve 3.5 g of hydroxylamine hydrochloride in 95 ml of ethanol (60%), add 0.5 ml of a 0.1% solution of bromophenol blue followed by 0.5M potassium hydroxide in ethanol until a green tint develops in the solution, then add sufficient ethanol (60%) to produce 100 ml.

Iodine Solution: dissolve 2 g of iodine and 3 g of potassium iodide in sufficient water to produce 100 ml.

Iodobismuthous Acid Solution: mix 40 mg of bismuth subcarbonate with 0.5 ml of 0.5M sulphuric acid and add 5 ml of a 10% solution of potassium iodide, 1 ml of 0.5M sulphuric acid, and 25 ml of water.

Iodoplatinate Solution: dissolve 0.25 g of platinic chloride and 5 g of potassium iodide in sufficient water to produce 100 ml.

Iodoplatinate Solution, Acidified: add 5 ml of *hydrochloric acid* to 100 ml of *iodoplatinate solution*.

Lead Acetate Paper: immerse white filter paper in a mixture of 10 volumes of *lead acetate solution* and 1 volume of 2M acetic acid. After drying, cut the paper into strips. Store in a well-closed container.

Lead Acetate Solution: a 10% solution of lead acetate in carbon dioxide-free water.

Ludy Tenger Reagent: dissolve 5 g of bismuth subcarbonate in 15 ml of *hydrochloric acid*, add 30 g of potassium iodide and then add 85 ml of water very slowly and with constant stirring. For use as a TLC spray, dilute 1 volume with 4 volumes of water.

Mandelin's Reagent: dissolve 0.5 g of ammonium vanadate in 1.5 ml of water and dilute to 100 ml with *sulphuric acid*. Filter the solution through glass wool.

Marquis Reagent: mix 1 ml of *formaldehyde solution* with 9 ml of *sulphuric acid*. Prepare daily.

Mercuric Chloride–Diphenylcarbazone Reagent: (a) dissolve 0.1 g of diphenylcarbazone in 50 ml of ethanol; (b) dissolve 1 g of mercuric chloride in 50 ml of ethanol; prepare the solutions daily. Mix (a) and (b) just before spraying.

Mercuric Nitrate Solution: dissolve 40 g of mercuric oxide (red or yellow) in a mixture of 32 ml of *nitric acid* and 15 ml of water. Store in glass containers protected from light.

Mercurous Nitrate Spray: a saturated solution of mercurous nitrate.

Molybdate–Antimony Reagent: dissolve 10 g of ammonium molybdate in 40 ml of 2M sulphuric acid; dissolve 0.1 g of sodium antimony tartrate in 50 ml of 2M sulphuric acid. Mix the two solutions and dilute to 500 ml with 2M sulphuric acid.

Naphthoquinone Sulphonate Solution: dissolve 0.3 g of sodium 1,2-naphthoquinone-4-sulphonate in 100 ml of ethanol:water (1:1).

N-(1-Naphthyl)ethylenediamine Solution: a 0.5% solution of N-(1-naphthyl)ethylenediamine hydrochloride.

Ninhydrin Spray: add 0.5 g of ninhydrin to 10 ml of *hydrochloric acid* and dilute to 100 ml with acetone. Prepare daily.

Nitric Acid: Concentrated: contains 69 to 71% w/w of HNO_3.

Nitric Acid, Dilute: mix 106 ml of *nitric acid* with sufficient water to produce 1000 ml. It contains about 10% w/w of HNO_3.

Nitric Acid, Fuming: contains not less than 95% w/w of HNO_3.

Nitrogen Dioxide Vapour: produced by the action of *nitric acid* on copper turnings. For location in thin-layer chromatography the TLC plate is exposed to the nitrous fumes which are evolved.

Nitroso-naphthol Solution: a 0.2% solution of 2-nitroso-1-naphthol in ethanol.

Perchloric Acid: contains about 72% w/w of $HClO_4$.

Perchloric Acid Solution: add 15 ml of *perchloric acid* to sufficient water to produce 100 ml.

Phosphate Buffer (pH 5.6): dissolve 62.4 g of sodium dihydrogen phosphate in sufficient water to produce 100 ml.

Phosphate Buffer (pH 6.88): dissolve 3.40 g (0.025M) of potassium dihydrogen phosphate and 3.53 g (0.025M) of anhydrous disodium hydrogen phosphate, both previously dried at 110° to 130° for 2 hours, in sufficient water to produce 1000 ml.

Phosphate Buffer (pH 7.4): (a) dissolve 9.465 g of anhydrous disodium hydrogen phosphate in water and dilute to 1000 ml; (b) dissolve 9.073 g of potassium dihydrogen phosphate in water and dilute to 1000 ml. Mix 80 ml of (a) with 20 ml of (b) to obtain a solution of pH 7.4.

Phosphoric Acid: contains 84 to 90% w/w of H_3PO_4.

Potassium Cupri-tartrate Solution: Fehling's Solution: (a) dissolve 34.64 g of copper sulphate in a mixture of 0.5 ml of *sulphuric acid* and sufficient water to produce 500 ml; (b) dissolve 176 g of sodium potassium tartrate and 77 g of sodium hydroxide in sufficient water to produce 500 ml. Mix equal volumes of solutions (a) and (b) immediately before use.

Potassium Cyanide Solution: a 10% solution of potassium cyanide.

Potassium Permanganate Solution, Acidified: a 1% solution of potassium permanganate in 0.25M sulphuric acid.

Silver Nitrate Solution: a freshly-prepared 5% solution of silver nitrate.

Sodium Chloride–Potassium Chloride Solution: mix 140 ml of M sodium chloride with 50 ml of 0.1M potassium chloride, and dilute with water to 1000 ml.

Sodium Hydroxide Solution: a 20% solution of sodium hydroxide.

Sodium Hydroxide Solution, Dilute: a 5% solution of sodium hydroxide.

Sodium Hypobromite Solution: dissolve 5 ml of bromine in 50 ml of a 40% solution of sodium hydroxide, with agitation and cooling.

Starch-iodide Paper: impregnate unglazed white paper with *starch mucilage* diluted with an equal volume of a 0.4% solution of potassium iodide.

Starch Mucilage: triturate 0.5 g of starch with 5 ml of water and add this, with constant stirring, to sufficient water to produce about 100 ml. Boil for a few minutes, cool, and filter. It should be freshly prepared.

Sulphuric Acid: Concentrated: contains not less than 95% w/w of H_2SO_4.

Sulphuric Acid, Dilute: mix carefully 104 g of *sulphuric acid* with 896 g of water and cool. It contains about 10% w/w of H_2SO_4.

Sulphuric Acid, Fuming: Oleum: prepared by the addition of sulphur trioxide to *sulphuric acid* and is available containing about 30% of free SO_3.

Sulphuric Acid–Ethanol Reagent: add gradually 10 ml of *sulphuric acid* to 90 ml of ethanol.

Tetrabutylammonium Phosphate, 0.005M, pH 7.5: PIC Reagent A.
Marketed by Waters Associates Inc., Milford, MA 01757, USA; Waters Associates (Instruments) Ltd, Northwich, Cheshire, UK.

p-Toluenesulphonic Acid Solution: dissolve 4 g of *p*-toluenesulphonic acid in 20 ml of ethanol.

Trinder's Reagent: dissolve 40 mg of mercuric chloride in 850 ml of water, add 120 ml of M hydrochloric acid and 40 g of hydrated ferric nitrate, and dilute to 1000 ml with water.

Van Urk Reagent: dissolve 1 g of *p*-dimethylaminobenzaldehyde in 100 ml of ethanol and add 10 ml of *hydrochloric acid*.

Zwikker's Reagent: mix 40 ml of a 10% solution of copper sulphate with 10 ml of pyridine and add sufficient water to produce 100 ml.

Proprietary Test Materials

Amberlite XAD-2: polymeric adsorbent beads for adsorbing water-soluble organic substances.
Marketed by Rohm and Haas Company, Philadelphia, PA 19105, USA; Rohm and Haas (UK) Ltd, Croydon, Surrey, UK.

Anabolic Steroid Radioimmunoassay Kits: for nandrolone and for 17α-methyl substituted anabolic steroids.
Obtainable from Prof. R. V. Brooks, Dept of Chemical Pathology, St. Thomas' Hospital Medical School, London, UK.

Carbon Monoxide in Blood: Spectrophotometric Reference Standards.
Marketed by American Hospital Supply Corporation, Evanston, IL 60201, USA; American Hospital Supply (UK) Ltd, Ashford, Middlesex, UK.

Cholinesterase Activity Assay Kit: colorimetric method for plasma or serum.
Marketed by Sigma Chemical Co., St. Louis, MO 63178, USA; Sigma London Chemical Co. Ltd, Poole, Dorset, UK.

Co-oximeter, IL 282: for the determination of carbon monoxide in blood.
Marketed by Instrumentation Laboratory Inc., Lexington, MA 02173, USA; Instrumentation Lab. UK Ltd, Warrington, Cheshire, UK.

Dextrostix: reagent strips for the approximate estimation of glucose in blood.
Marketed by Ames, Division of Miles Laboratories Inc., Elkhart, IN 46515, USA; Ames Division of Miles Laboratories Ltd, Stoke Poges, Buckinghamshire, UK.

Ethanol Assay Kit: enzymatic method for the determination of ethanol in whole blood, plasma, or serum.
Marketed by Sigma Chemical Co., St Louis, MO 63178, USA; Sigma London Chemical Co. Ltd, Poole, Dorset, UK.

Extrelut: a column containing granules of diatomaceous earth with a large pore volume.
Marketed by E. Merck, D-6100 Darmstadt, W. Germany; BDH Chemicals Ltd, Poole, Dorset, UK.

High Performance Silica Gel TLC Plates: with fluorescent indicator and concentration zone.
Marketed by E. Merck, D-6100 Darmstadt, W. Germany; BDH Chemicals Ltd, Poole, Dorset, UK.

Labstix: reagent strips for urine testing to indicate pH, and the presence of protein, glucose, ketones, and blood.
Marketed by Ames, Division of Miles Laboratories Inc., Elkhart, IN 46515, USA; Ames Division of Miles Laboratories Ltd, Stoke Poges, Buckinghamshire, UK.

Paracetamol Assay Kit: enzymatic method for the determination of paracetamol in plasma.
Marketed by Cambridge Life Sciences, Cambridge, UK.

Sephadex LH-20: a bead-formed dextran gel with hydrophilic and lipophilic properties.
Marketed by Pharmacia (Great Britain) Ltd, Milton Keynes, Buckinghamshire, UK; Pharmacia Fine Chemicals, Division of Pharmacia Inc., Piscataway, NJ 08854, USA.

Sep-Pak C-18 Cartridge: a silica cartridge for column chromatography.
Marketed by Waters Associates Inc., Milford, MA 01757, USA; Waters Associates (Instruments) Ltd, Northwich, Cheshire, UK.

Serum-Iron Assay Kit
Marketed by Travenol Laboratories Inc., Deerfield, IL 60015, USA; Lorne Laboratories Ltd, Reading, Berkshire, UK.

Subtilisin A
Marketed by Novo Enzyme Products Ltd, Windsor, Berkshire, UK.

Tox Elut: a column containing granules of diatomaceous earth with a large pore volume.
Marketed by Analytichem International Inc., Lawndale, CA 90260, USA.

Urastrat: a complete quantitative system for the determination of urea nitrogen in serum.
Marketed by General Diagnostics, Warner-Lambert (UK) Ltd, Eastleigh, Hampshire, UK.

GENERAL INDEX

General Index

Aerolone, 689
Aerophylline, 561
Aeroseb-Dex, 518
Aerosol OT, 569
Aethacridinium lacticum, 591
Aethanolaminum, 594
Aethaphenum tartaricum, 836
Aethazolum, 985
Aethisteron, 598
Aethophyllinum, 607
Aethoxybenzamidum, 590
Aethylis biscoumacetas, 602
Aethylum hydroxybenzoicum, 603
Affel, 553
AFID, 183
Afko-Lube, 569
Afloben, 388
Afrazine, 842
African Tea, 437
Afrin, 842
Afrinol, 944
Aftate, 1032
Agarol, 885
Agedal, 828
17 AHPC, 672
Airbron, 318
Airet, 561
Ajan, 802
Ajmalandiol, 322
Ajmaline, 322
Ajmaline hydrochloride, 322
Ajmaline monoethanolate, 322
Akineton, 396
Akinophyl, 396
Akrotherm, 659
Alachlor, 81
Alba-Ce, 360
Albalon, 798
Alba-Temp, 849
Albego, 422
Albendazole, 323
Albiotic, 706
Albistat, 784
Albucid, 981
Albuterol, 963
Alcaine, 943
Alcanfor, 422
Alcaphor, 1054
Alclofenac, 323
Alcobon, 621
Alcohol, 593
    absolute, 593
    dehydrated, 593
    in postmortem samples, 115
    rubbing, 593
Alcohol isopropylicus, 691
Alcohol trichlorisobutylicus, 444
Alcohols, 18
    gas chromatography, 19
    test on blood, 6
    test on urine, 4
Alcojel, 691
Alcomicin, 637
Alcopar(a), 391
Alcuronium chloride, 324
Aldactide, 667, 973
Aldactone, 973
Aldecin, 374
Aldehyde, 311
Aldehydes,
    test on blood, 6
    test on urine, 4
Alderstan, 324

Aldicarb, 82
Aldoclor, 454, 764
Aldocorten, 324
Aldomet, 764, 766
Aldophosphamide, 504
Aldopur, 973
Aldoril, 663, 764
Aldosterone, 324
Aldrex, 324
Aldrin, 82, **324**
    mass spectrometry, 76
Alergicap, 557
Aletamine, 325
Aletamine hydrochloride, 325
Aleudrin(e), 689
Alexan, 506
Alfadolone, 329
AlfamesE, 605
Alfatesin(e), 329, 330
Alfathesin, 329, 330
Alfaxalone, 330
Alfentanil, 326
Alfentanil hydrochloride, 326
Alfetamine, 325
Algaphan, 522
Algipan, 762
Algodex, 522
Algopent, 860
Algoverine, 892
Alimemazine, 1046
Alisobumalum, 414
Alival, 818
Alkali flame ionisation detector, 183
Alkali halide disks, 244
Alkaloids, published infra-red spectra, 249
Alka-Seltzer, 361
Alkeran, 728
Alkron, 853
Allantoin, xvii
Allegron, 826
Allercur, 472
Aller-eze, 472
Allergefon, 433
Allergex, 457
Allerzine, 560
Allethrin, 77, 82
Allnortoxiferin chloride, 324
Allobarbital, 326
Allobarbitone, 326
Allocaine, 925
Allocor, 542
Alloferin, 324
Alloprin, 327
Allopur, 327
Allopurinol, 327
Allotropal, 769
Alloxanthine, 327
Allylbarbituric acid, 414
Allylbromoallylbarbituric acid, 398
Allyl-5-butylbarbituric acid, 1000
Allyl-5-sec-butylbarbituric acid, 678
Allylcarboxymethylpropylbarbi-turic acid, 952
Allylcyclohexenylthiobarbituric acid, 1014
Allylcyclopentenylbarbituric acid, 502
Allyldeoxydihydrohydroxyoxon-ormorphine, 797
Allyldihydrodibenzazepine, 366

Allylestrenol, 328
Allylguaiacol, 609
Allylhydroxymethylbutylbarbi-turic acid, 952
Allylhydroxypropylbarbituric acid, 398
Allylisobutylbarbituric acid, 414
Allylisopropylacetylurea, 359
Allylisopropylbarbituric acid, 358
Allylisopropylmalonylurea, 358
Allylisopropylmethylbarbituric acid, 582
Allylmethoxymethylenedioxyben-zene, 792
Allylmethoxyphenol, 609
Allylmethylbutylbarbituric acid, 951
Allylmethylmethylpentynylbarbi-turic acid, 753
Allylmethyloxobutylbarbituric acid, 952
Allylmorphinanol, 700
Allylneopentylbarbituric acid, 801
Allylnormorphine, 796
Allylnoroxymorphone, 797
Allyloestrenol, 328
Allyloxychlorophenylacetic acid, 323
Allyloxyphenoxyisopropylamino-propanol, 839
Allylphenethylamine, 325
Allylphenoxyisopropylaminopro-panol, 331
Allylprodine, xvii
Allypropymal, 358
Almazine, 711
Almond oil, artificial, 379
Almond seeds, 352
Alneobarbital, 801
Alnovin, 613
Aloes, 328
Aloin, 328
Alophen, 885
Alotano, 649
Aloxiprin, 328
Alpen, 351
Alpha Redisol, 669
Alpha tocopheryl acetate, 329
Alphadione, 329, 330
Alphadolone, 329
Alphadolone acetate, 329
Alpha-lobeline, 708
Alphameprodine, xvii
Alphamethadol, xvii
Alpha-methyldopa, 764
Alphanaphthol, 429
Alphaprodine, 329
Alphaprodine hydrochloride, 330
Alpha-Ruvite, 669
Alphaxalone, 330
Alprazolam, 331
Alprenolol, 331
Alprenolol hydrochloride, 332
AL-R, 457
Alrheumat, 697
Altex, 973
Althesin, 329, 330
Altilev, 826
Altocillin, 877
Aludrox SA, 335
Aluline, 327
Alumina, 160
Aluminium oxide, 328

Alunex, 457
Alupent, 833
Alupent Expectorant, 401
Alupram, 526
Alurate, 358
Aluzine, 634
Alverine, 332
Alverine citrate, 332
Alyrane, 584
Amal, 353
Amalic Acid Test, 129
Amanita, 407
Amantadine, 333
Amantadine hydrochloride, 333
Amantadine sulphate, 333
Amavil, 346
Ambaxin, 369
Ambazone, 334
Amben, 340
Ambenonium chloride, 334
Amberlite XAD-2, 1171
Ambestigmini chloridum, 334
Ambilhar, 814
Amblosin, 351
Ambodryl, 402
Ambroxol, 401
Ambucetamide, 334
Ambuphylline, 408
Ambutonium bromide, 335
Amcill, 351
Amen, 726
Americaine, 382
Amersol, 677
Amesec, 1011
Ametazole, 335
Ametazole hydrochloride, 335
Amethocaine, 335
Amethocaine hydrochloride, 335
Amethopterin, 756
Ametryn, 336
Ametryne, 82, 336
Amfepramone, 538
Amfetyline, 613
Amfipen, 351
Amicar, 341
Amicarbalide, 336
Amicarbalide isethionate, 336
Amidazofen, 337
Amidefrine, 337
Amidephrine, 337
Amidephrine mesylate, 337
Amidinodiaminochloropyrazine-carboxamide, 339
Amidinohydrazonocyclohexa-dienone thiosemicarbazone, 334
Amidinosulphanilamide, 986
Amidonal, 358
Amidone, 742
Amidopyrine, 337
Amidopyrine-Pyramidon, 337
Amid-Sal, 964
Amikacin, 338
    therapeutic drug monitoring, 107
Amikacin sulphate, 338
Amikin, 338
Amilco, 339, 663
Aminline, 346
Amiloride, 339
Amiloride hydrochloride, 339
Aminacrine, 339
Aminacrine hexylresorcinate, 340
Aminacrine hydrochloride, 340

Crematurm, 603, 659
Cresofin, 555
Cresol, 495
Cresol-ammonia test, on urine, 5
Cresoxydiol, 731
Cresylic acid, 495
Crilin, 860
Cristallovar, 831
Cromoglycate sodium, 970
Cromoglycic acid, 970
Cromolyn sodium, 970
Cromosil, 429
Cropropamide, 495
Cross-reactivity, 150
Crotalaria spectabilis, 788
Crotaline, 788
Crotamitex, 495
Crotamiton, 495
Crotetamide, 495
Crotethamide, 495
Croton-chloral hydrate, 420
Crozinal, 983
Crylène, 860
Cryofluorane, 532
Crystalline penicillin G, 390
Crystapen, 390
Crystapen G, 390
Crystapen V, 888
Crysticillin AS, 926
Crystodigin, 541
CSAG 144, 721
C-Tran, 446
Cuplex, 965
Cuprimine, 857
Curarin, 1057
Curling factor, 645
Curretab, 726
Cusum chart, 121
Cutisan, 1041
Cyanabin, 496
Cyanazine, 82
Cyanide,
    colour tests, 65, 145
    in postmortem samples, 116
    quantification in blood, 65
Cyanocobalamin, 496
Cyanodiphenylpropionic acid,
    395
Cyanodiphenylpropylpiperidino-
    piperidinecarboxamide, 910
Cyanoethyl silicone, 180
Cyanoethylamphetamine, 617
Cyanogen Bromide (test), 132
Cyanomethylmethylimidazolyl-
    methylthioethylguanidine, 467
Cyanopropyl phenylmethyl sili-
    cone, 180
Cyantin, 816
Cyclacur, 831
Cycladiene, 537
Cyclaine, 659
Cyclamic acid, xvii
Cyclandelate, 496
Cyclazocine, 496
Cyclimorph, 790
Cyclizine, 497, 561
Cyclizine hydrochloride, 497
Cyclizine lactate, 497
Cyclizinium chloride, 497
Cyclobarbital, 498
Cyclobarbitone, 498
Cyclobarbitone calcium, 498
Cyclobec, 535
Cyclobenzaprine, 499

Cyclobenzaprine hydrochloride,
    499
Cyclobral, 496
Cyclobutylmethyldihydrohydrox-
    ynormorphine, 794
Cyclobutylmethylmorphinandiol,
    417
Cyclodolum, 381
Cycloestrol, 657
Cyclofenil, 500
Cyclogest, 929
Cycloguanil, 500
    (metabolite), 931
Cycloguanil embonate, 500
Cycloguanil pamoate, 500
Cycloheptenylethylbarbituric
    acid, 651
Cyclohexadienylglycylamino-
    methylcephemcarboxylic acid,
    439
Cyclohexanedimethyl succinate,
    180
Cyclohexenyldimethylbarbituric
    acid, 656
Cyclohexenylethylbarbituric
    acid, 498
Cyclohexylacetoxime, 938
Cyclohexylaminomethylethyl
    benzoate, 659
Cyclohexyldimethylethylamine,
    938
Cyclohexylhydroxyphenylpropyl-
    methylpyrrolidinium chloride,
    1042
Cyclohexylhydroxyphenylpropyl-
    triethylammonium chloride,
    1043
Cyclohexylidenemethylenebis-
    phenyl acetate, 500
Cyclohexylmandeloyloxyethyl-
    diethylmethylammonium bro-
    mide, 846
Cyclohexylmethylpyrazinecar-
    boxamidoethylbenzenesul-
    phonylurea, 640
Cyclohexylphenylpiperidinopro-
    panol, 381
Cyclohexylphenylpyrrolidinylpro-
    panol, 928
Cyclomethycaine, 501
Cyclomethycaine sulphate, 501
Cyclopal, 502
Cyclopen, 503
Cyclopentadrin, 501
Cyclopentamine, 501
Cyclopentamine hydrochloride,
    502
Cyclopentaminium chloride, 502
Cyclopentenylallyl barbituric
    acid, 502
Cyclopenthiazide, 502
Cyclopentobarbital, 502
Cyclopentobarbitone, 502
Cyclopentolate, 503
Cyclopentolate hydrochloride,
    503
Cyclopentyldimethylethylamine,
    501
Cyclopentylmandeloyloxydimeth-
    ylpyrrolidinium bromide, 643
Cyclopentylphenylpiperidinopro-
    panol, 505

Cyclopentylthienylglycoloylox-
    yethyldiethylmethylammonium
    bromide, 862
Cyclophosphamide, 503
Cyclo-Progynova, 831
Cyclopropylmethylaminochloro-
    benzophenone, 197
Cyclopropylmethyldeoxydihydro-
    hydroxyoxonormorphine, 797
Cyclopropylmethyldihydro-
    hydroxymethylethylmethyl-
    ethanonormorphine, 561
Cyclopropylmethyldihydro-
    hydroxytrimethylpropylmethyl-
    ethanonormorphine, 411
Cyclopropylmethylhexahydrodi-
    methylmethanobenzazocinol,
    496
Cycloserine, 504
Cyclospasmol, 496
Cyclothiazide, 504
Cycobemin, 496
Cycogyl, 503
Cycrimine, 505
Cycrimine hydrochloride, 505
Cycriminium chloride, 505
Cylert, 856
Cynomel, 707
Cypermethrin, 77, 82
Cyprenorphine, xvii
Cyproheptadine, 505
Cyproheptadine hydrochloride,
    506
Cyren-A, 975
Cysteine-penicillamine disul-
    phide, 858
Cystospaz, 676
Cystospaz-M, 676
Cytacon, 496
Cytamen, 496
Cytarabine, 506
Cytarabine hydrochloride, 506
Cyteal, 447
Cytisine, 507
Cytisus scoparius, 972
Cytiton, 507
Cytolen, 1023
Cytomel, 707
Cytosar, 506
Cytosar-U, 506
Cytosine arabinoside, 506
Cytoxan, 503
Cyverm, 701

D

2,4-D, 83, 85, 531
Dactil, 907
DADPS, 509
Dagenan, 992
Dagga, 423
Dakryo Biciron, 401
Daktarin, 784
Dalacin, 473, 474
Dalacin C, 473, 474
Dalacine, 473
Dalapon, 82
Dalaron, 519
Dalmadorm, 630, 704
Dalmane, 630
Dalmate, 704
Dametine, 511
D-Amp, 351
Danabol, 744

Daneral-SA, 881
Danilone, 880
Dantamacrin, 508
Danthron, 507
Dantoin, 897
Dantrium, 508
Dantrolene, 508
Dantrolene sodium, 508
Dantron, 507
Daonil, 638
Dapotum, 629
Dapotum D, 629
Dapsone, 509
DAPT, 345
Daptazile, 345
Daptazole, 345
Daranide, 532
Daraphen, 522
Daraprim, 949
Darbid, 690
Daricon, 845
Darmol, 885
Dartal, 1018
Dartalan, 1018
Darvocet-N, 522
Darvon, 522
Darvon-N, 522
Datril, 849
Datura, 674
Davenol, 433, 898
Dazomet, 82
2,4-DB, 82, 85
DBD, 368
DBP, 530
DBPC, 420
DCPA, 532
DDA, 534
DDD, 534
DDE, 534
DDS, 509
DDT, 534
DEA, 491
Deacetyl-lanatoside C, 517
Dead-time, 189
Deanol chlorophenoxyacetate,
    723
Deapril-ST, 491
Debendox, 576, 949
Debrisoquine, 510
Debrisoquine sulphate, 510
Decaderm, 518
Decadron, 518, 519
Decadron-LA, 518
Decadron-TBA, 519
Deca-Durabolin, 798
Decalinium chloride, 514
Decalix, 518
Decamethonium bromide, 510
Decamethylenebisaminomethyl-
    quinolinium chloride, 514
Decamethylenebistrimethylam-
    monium dibromide, 510
Decaminum, 514
Decapryn, 576
Decaserpyl, 755
Decaserpyl Plus, 387
Decasone, 519
Decaspray, 518
Deccox, 511
Decentan, 866
Decicain, 335
Declinax, 510
Declomycin, 512
Declostatin, 512

Konakion, 901
Koppanyi-Zwikker Test, 135
Koro-Sulf, 986
Korum, 849
Krovar, 568
K-Strophanthin, 976
Kwell, 707
Kwellada, 707
Kwells, Quick, 674

L

LAAM, 702
Labetalol, 698
Labetalol hydrochloride, 699
LaBID, 1011
Labophylline, 1011
Labosept, 514
Labstix, 1171
Laburnine, 507
Laburnum anagyroides, 507
Lachesine chloride, 699
Laco, 397
Lactic acid, 603
Lactoacridine, 591
Lactoflavin, 959
Lactoxylidide, 1028
Ladropen, 621
Laevo-amphetamine, 701
Laevodopa, 702
Laevo-ecgonine, 579
Laevo-menthol, 729
Laevomycetinum, 443
LAM, 702
Lambert's Law, 222
Lamoryl, 645
Lampren(e), 476
Lanatoside C, 699
Lanatosides, 217
Lan-Dol, 733
Lanimerck, 699
Lanitop, 725
Lanocide, 699
Lanoxin(e), 542
Lanthanide shift reagents, 270
Lanvis, 1017
Lapudrine, 459
Laracor, 839
Laractone, 973
Laratrim, 988, 1049
Largactil, 460
Largon, 935
Larodopa, 702
Larotid, 348
Laroxyl, 346
Laryng-O-Jet, 705
Lasan, 567
Laser, 799
Lasikal, 634
Lasilactone, 634, 973
Lasilix, 634
Lasipressin, 634
Lasix, 634
Lasma, 1011
Laudamonium, 379
Laudexium methylsulphate, xvii
Lauryl gallate, 569
Laxatives,
    detection in urine, 33
    screening for abuse, 32
Laxbene, 397
Lead, 60
Lead acetate paper, 1170
Lead acetate solution, 1170

Ledercillin VK, 888
Ledercort, 1036
Ledercort diacetat, 1037
Lederfen, 611
Lederkyn, 990
Ledermycin, 511, 512
Ledermycine, 512
Lederspan, 1037
Ledertepa, 1020
Ledertrexate, 756
Lemiserp, 958
Lenacil, 84
Lénitral, 643
Lenoxin, 542
Lensen, 557
Lentizol, 346
Leodrine, 667
Leponex, 488
Leptanol, 617
Leptazol, 861
Lergoban, 560
Leritine, 355
Lethidrone, 796
Leucinocaine, xvii
Leukeran, 442
Leurocristine, 1063
Levacetylmethadol, 702
Levallorphan, 700
Levallorphan tartrate, 700
Levamisole, 701
Levamisole hydrochloride, 701
Levamphetamine, 701
Levant berries, 902
Levanxol, 1001
Levarterenol, 819
Levate, 346
Levo-BC-2627, 417
Levodopa, 702
Levo-Dromoran, 704
Levoid, 1023
Levomepromazine, 757
Levomethadyl acetate, 702
Levomethadyl acetate hydroch-
    loride, 703
Levomethorphan, xvii
Levomoramide, xvii
Levopa, 702
Levophed, 819
Levophenacylmorphan, xvii
Levoprome, 757
Levopropoxyphene, 704
Levopropoxyphene naphthalene-
    sulphonate, 704
Levopropoxyphene napsylate,
    704
Levorenin, 321
Levorphan, 704
Levorphanol, 704
Levorphanol bitartrate, 704
Levorphanol tartrate, 704
Levothroid, 1023
Levothyroxine, 1023
Levsin, 676
Levsinex, 676
Lexor, 663
Lexotan, 400
Lexotanil, 400
Liadren, 321
Libanil, 638
Librax, 446, 473
Libraxin, 446, 473
Libritabs, 446
Librium, 446
Librofem, 677

Lidemol, 625
Lidex, 625
Lidocaine, 705
Lidocaine hydrochloride, 705
Lidocaton, 705
Lidoflazine, 705
Lidone, 787
Liebermann's Test, 135
Lignocaine, 705
    therapeutic drug monitoring,
    108
Lignocaine hydrochloride, 705
Lignostab, 705
Likuden M, 645
Limbatril, 346, 446
Limbitrol, 346, 446
Limeciclina, 714
Limpidon, 422
Lincocin(e), 706
Lincomycin, 706
Lincomycin hydrochloride, 706
Linctifed, 944, 1053
Lindane, 84, **707**
Lingraine, 587
Linked scanning, 256
Linodil, 683
Linuron, 84
Linyl, 890
Lioresal, 369
Liothyronine, 707
    (metabolite), 1024
Liothyronine sodium, 707
Liotropina, 364
Lipavlon, 477
Lipo-Gantrisin, 986
Lipopill, 890
Liprin(al), 477
Liquamar, 889
Liquiprin, 849
Lisacort, 918
Liskantin, 922
Liskonum, 708
Listica, 672
Litalir, 673
Litarex, 708
Lithane, 708
Lithium,
    quantification in serum, 61
    therapeutic drug monitoring,
    109
Lithium carbonate, 708
Lithium citrate, 708
Lithizine, 708
Lithobid, 708
Lithonate, 708
Lithonate-S, 708
Lithotabs, 708
Liver, sampling of, 113
Lixaminol, 1011
Lobak, 449
Lobatox, 709
Lobelia inflata, 708
Lobeline, 708
Lobeline hydrochloride, 709
Lobeline sulphate, 709
Locacorten, 623
Local anaesthetics,
    gas chromatography, 197
    high pressure liquid chroma-
    tography, 218
    thin-layer chromatography,
    173
Locan, 335
Locapred, 518

Locorten, 623
Lofepramine, 709
Lofepramine hydrochloride, 709
Loftran, 695
Lomidine, 859
Lomotil, 558
Lomudal, 970
Lomusol, 970
Lonchocarpus urucu, 963
Lonchocarpus utilis, 963
Longatin, 827
Longifene, 405
Longum, 980
Loniten, 786
Lopemid, 709
Loperamide, 709
Loperamide hydrochloride, 709
Lophophora williamsii, 737
Lopirin, 426
Lopramine, 709
Loprazolam, 710
Loprazolam mesylate, 710
Lopresor, 779
Lopresoretic, 464, 779
Lopressor, 779
Lopurin, 327
Loqua, 663
Loramet, 712
Lorazepam, 711
    (metabolite), 713
Lorcainide, 711
Lorcainide hydrochloride, 712
Lorexane, 707
Lorfan, 700
Loridine, 438
Lorinon, 438
Lormetazepam, 712
Lorphen, 457
Lotrimin, 487
Loturine, 650
Lotusate, 1000
Lotussin, 520, 557
Low-dose preparations, 53
Loxapac, 713
Loxapine, 713
Loxapine succinate, 713
Loxitane, 713
Lozol, 681
LSD 25, 715
Lucanthone, xvii
Lucidril, 723
Ludiomil, 718
Ludobal, 955
Ludy Tenger reagent,
    1170
Lufyllin, 561
Lugacin, 637
Luminal, 883
Luminal Sodium, 883
Luminaletten, 883
Luminescence immunoassays,
    155
Lumirelax, 752
Lung, sampling of, 113
Lupanine, 99
Lupinidine, 972
Luteal hormone, 929
Luteine, 929
Luteodione, 726
Lutéran, 448
Lutogyl, 929
Lutométrodiol, 605
Luتوral, 726
Lycanol, 644

Lycine, 392
Lymecycline, 714
Lynenol, 714
Lynestrenol, 714
Lynoestrenol, 714
Lynoral, 596
Lyogen, 629
Lyogen-Depot, 629
Lyophrin, 321
Lysanxia, 915
Lyseptol, 495
Lysergamide, 714
Lysergic acid, 715
Lysergic acid amide, 714
Lysergic acid diethylamide, 715
Lysergide, 715
Lysivane, 599
Lysobex, 396
Lysoform, 633
Lysol, 495
Lyssipoll, 560
Lysthenon, 998
Lyteca, 849
Lytta vesicatoria, 425

M

M183, 316
M & B 693, 992
M & B Antiseptic Cream, 933
Macmiror, 812
Macocyn, 846
Maconha, 423
Macrodantin, 816
Madar, 821
Madopar, 378, 702
Madribon, 983
Maeva, 1001
Mafenide, 716
Mafenide acetate, 717
Mafenide hydrochloride, 717
Mafenide propionate, 717
Magnapen, 621
Magnesium silicate, 160
Magnetic sector mass spectrom-
   eter, 255
Majeptil, 1019
Malaoxon, 717
Malarivon, 453
Malatex, 384, 965
Malathion, 84, **717**
Malathion dicarboxylic acid, 717
Malathion monocarboxylic acid,
   717
Malgesic, 892
Malix, 638
Malogen, 1003
Malogen LA, 1003
Malogex, 1003
Malonal, 372
Malonylurea, 373
Maloprim, 509, 949
Mandaze, 654
Mandelamine, 654
Mandelic acid, 717
   (metabolite), 608, 856
Mandelin's reagent, 1170
Mandelin's Test, 137
Mandelonitrile, 352
Mandeloyloxymethyltropanium
   bromide, 661
Mandrax, 746
Manialith, 708
Manir, 845

Mannitol mustard, 718
Mannomustine, 718
Mannomustine hydrochloride,
   718
Mansonil, 805
Mantadix, 333
Manusept, 691, 1042
Maolate, 456
Maphenide, 717
Mappine, 407
Maprotiline, 718
Maprotiline hydrochloride, 718
Marboran, 751
Marcain(e), 411
Marcoumar, 889
Marcumar, 889
Mardon, 522
Marevan, 1064
Marezine, 497
Marihuana, 423
Marks Brushwood Killer, 1040
Marplan, 686
Marquis reagent, 1170
Marquis Test, 139
Marsilid, 685
Marsolone, 917
Marsone, 918
Marticarpine, 902
Marzine, 497
Masmoran, 673
Masopin, 661
Mass spectra,
   general notice, xvi
   interpretation of, 261
   reference collections, 260
Mass spectrometers,
   chromatography interfaces,
      252, 253
   double focussing, 256
   electrostatic analyser, 256
   instrumentation, 251-257
   ion detection, 257
   ion separation, 255
   magnetic sector, 255
   quadrupole filter, 255
   sample inlet system, 251
Mass spectrometry, 251-263
   chemical ionisation, 255
   electron impact ionisation,
      254
   gas chromatography and,
      185, 259
   high pressure liquid chroma-
      tography and, 260
   indexes, 1152-1165
   molecular weight determina-
      tion, 254, 256
   paper chromatography and,
      258
   pesticides, 74
   preparation of samples, 258
   presentation of results, 257
   quantification, 262
   thin-layer chromatography
      and, 258
Masterid, 577
Masteril, 577
Masteron, 577
Maté, 421
Matulane, 926
Maxeran, 776
Maxibolin, 605
Maxidex, 518
Maxifen, 911

Maximed, 942
Maxisporin, 439
Maxitrol, 518
Maxolon, 776
Mazanor, 719
Mazildene, 719
Mazindol, 719
M-Cillin B, 390
McNally's Test, 140
MCPA, 84, 86, **764**
MCPB, 84, 86
McReynolds Constant, 179
MDA, 766
Meadow saffron, 492
Meaverin, 732
Meballymal, 951
Meballymalnatrium, 951
Mebanazine, 720
Mebaral, 770
Mebendazole, 720
Mebeverine, 720
Mebeverine hydrochloride, 721
Mebezonium iodide, 721
Mebhydrolin, 721
Mebhydrolin napadisylate, 721
Mebhydrolin naphthalenedisul-
   phonate, 721
Mébubarbital, 863
Mebumal, 863
Mebumalnatrium, 863
Mebutamate, 722
Mebutina, 722
Mecamylamine, 722
Mecamylamine hydrochloride,
   722
Mechothane, 393
Meclastine, 472
Meclizine, 724
Meclizinium chloride, 724
Meclofenamate sodium, 723
Meclofenamic acid, 723
Meclofenoxane, 723
Meclofenoxate, 723
Meclofenoxate hydrochloride,
   723
Meclomen, 723
Mecloprodin, 472
Mecloqualone, 723
Meclozine, 724
Meclozine hydrochloride, 724
Mecoprop, 84
Medazepam, 724
Medigoxin, 725
Medihaler Epi, 321
Medihaler Iso, 689
Medihaler-duo, 689
Medilium, 446
Medimet-250, 764
Medised, 932
Meditran, 733
Medomet, 764
Medomin(e), 651
Medrol, 772
Medrone, 772
Medroxyprogesterone acetate,
   726
Mefenamic acid, 727
Mefrusal, 727
Mefruside, 727
Megace, 728
Megacef, 439
Megacillin, 390, 888, 926
Megaclor, 480
Megamin, 1014

Megascorb, 360
Megestrol acetate, 728
Megimide, 374
Meladinine, 758
Melfiat, 876
Melitase, 461
Melitoxin, 535
Mellaril, 1019
Mellaril-S, 1019
Melleretten, 1019
Melleril, 1019
Mellinese, 461
Mellitol, 1030
Melphalan, 728
Melting points, index to, 1085-
   1093
MEM, 898
Membrane separator, 253
Menadiol diacetate, 315
Menadione, 729
Menadione sodium bisulphite,
   729
Menaphthene, 729
Menaphthone, 729
Menolet, 773
Menospasm, 535
Menrium, 446
Mentha, 729
Menthanol, 729
Menthol, 729
Mentol, 729
Mepacrine, 729
Mepacrine hydrochloride, 729
Mepacrine mesylate, 730
Mepacrine methanesulphonate,
   730
Meparfynol, 769
Mepazine, 855
Mep-E, 733
Mepentamate, 769
Mepenzolate bromide, 730
Mepergan, 867, 932
Meperidine, 867
Mephenamine, 833
Mephenesin, 731
Mephenesin carbamate, 731
Mephenetoin, 754
Mephenon, 742
Mephenterdrine, 731
Mephentermine, 731
Mephentermine sulphate, 731
Mephenytoin, 754
Mephetedrine, 731
Mephobarbital, 770
Mephosfolan, 84
Mephyton, 901
Mepivacaine, 732
Mepivacaine hydrochloride, 732
Meprate, 733
Mepriam, 733
Meprobamate, 733
   (metabolite), 436, 1058
   test on stomach contents, 22
Mepron, 733
Meprospan, 733
Meprotanum, 733
Meprylcaine, 734
Meprylcaine hydrochloride, 734
Meptazinol, 734
Meptazinol hydrochloride, 734
Meptid, 734
Mepyramine, 734
Mepyramine maleate, 735
Mequin, 746